Drug Information Handbook *for* Dentistry

Oral Medicine for
Medically-Compromised Patients
& Specific Oral Conditions

8th Edition

lexi-comp
LEXI-COMP

Drug Information Handbook *for* Dentistry

Oral Medicine for Medically-Compromised Patients & Specific Oral Conditions

8th Edition

Richard L. Wynn, BSPharm, PhD
Professor of Pharmacology
Baltimore College of Dental Surgery
Dental School
University of Maryland at Baltimore
Baltimore, Maryland

Timothy F. Meiller, DDS, PhD
Professor
Diagnostic Sciences and Pathology
Baltimore College of Dental Surgery
Professor of Oncology
Greenebaum Cancer Center
University of Maryland at Baltimore
Baltimore, Maryland

Harold L. Crossley, DDS, PhD
Associate Professor of Pharmacology
Baltimore College of Dental Surgery
Dental School
University of Maryland at Baltimore
Baltimore, Maryland

LEXI-COMP, INC

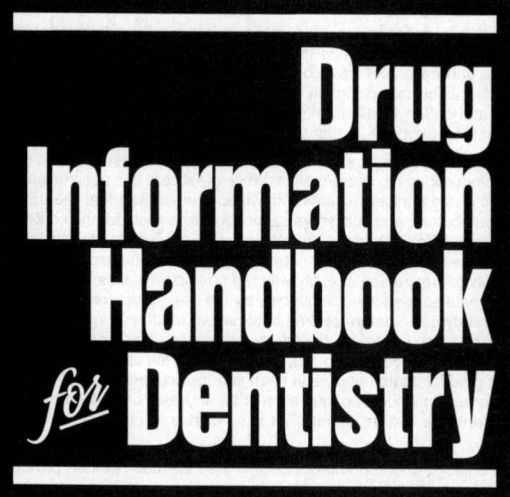

NOTICE

This handbook is intended to serve the user as a handy reference and not as a complete drug information resource. It does not include information on every therapeutic agent available. The publication covers a combination of commonly used drugs in dentistry and medicine and is specifically designed to present important aspects of drug data in a more concise format than is typically found in medical literature, exhaustive drug compendia, or product material supplied by manufacturers.

Drug information is constantly evolving because of ongoing research and clinical experience and is often subject to interpretation. While great care has been taken to ensure the accuracy of the information presented, the reader is advised that the authors, editors, reviewers, contributors, and publishers cannot be responsible for the continued currency of the information or for any errors, omissions, or the application of this information, or for any consequences arising therefrom. Therefore, the author(s) and/or the publisher shall have no liability to any person or entity with regard to claims, loss, or damage caused, or alleged to be caused, directly or indirectly, by the use of information contained herein. Because of the dynamic nature of drug information, readers are advised that decisions regarding drug therapy must be based on the independent judgment of the clinician, changing information about a drug (eg, as reflected in the literature and manufacturer's most current product information), and changing medical practices. The editors are not responsible for any inaccuracy of quotation or for any false or misleading implication that may arise due to the text or formulas as used or due to the quotation of revisions no longer official.

The editors, authors, and contributors have written this book in their private capacities. No official support or endorsement by any federal or state agency or pharmaceutical company is intended or inferred.

The publishers have made every effort to trace the copyright holders for borrowed material. If they have inadvertently overlooked any, they will be pleased to make the necessary arrangements at the first opportunity.

If you have any suggestions or questions regarding any information presented in this handbook, please contact our drug information pharmacist at

1-877-837-LEXI (5394)

This manual was produced using the FormuLex™ Program — a complete publishing service of Lexi-Comp, Inc.

lexi-comp

1100 Terex Road
Hudson, Ohio 44236
(330) 650-6506

LEXI-COMP, INC

ISBN 1-59195-024-4

TABLE OF CONTENTS

TABLE OF CONTENTS *(Continued)*

ABOUT THE AUTHORS

Richard L. Wynn, BSPharm, PhD

Richard L. Wynn, PhD, is Professor of Pharmacology at the Baltimore College of Dental Surgery, Dental School, University of Maryland at Baltimore. Dr Wynn has served as a dental educator, researcher, and teacher of dental pharmacology and dental hygiene pharmacology for his entire professional career. He holds a BS (pharmacy; registered pharmacist, Maryland), an MS (physiology) and a PhD (pharmacology) from the University of Maryland. Dr Wynn chaired the Department of Pharmacology at the University of Maryland Dental School from 1980 to 1995. Previously, he chaired the Department of Oral Biology at the University of Kentucky College of Dentistry.

Dr Wynn has to his credit over 250 publications including original research articles, textbooks, textbook chapters, monographs, and articles in continuing education journals. He has given over 400 continuing education seminars to dental professionals in the U.S., Canada, and Europe. Dr Wynn has been a consultant to the drug industry for 20 years and his research laboratories have contributed to the development of new analgesics and anesthetics. He is a consultant to the U.S. Pharmacopeia, Dental Drugs and Products section, the Academy of General Dentistry, the American Dental Association, and a former consultant to the Council on Dental Education, Commission on Accreditation. He is a featured columnist and his drug review articles, entitled *Pharmacology Today*, appear in each issue of General Dentistry, a journal published by the Academy. He is currently funded by drug industry and government agencies for research on the development of new drugs. One of his primary interests continues to be keeping dental professionals informed on all aspects of drug use in dental practice.

Timothy F. Meiller, DDS, PhD

Dr Meiller is Professor of Diagnostic Sciences and Pathology at the Baltimore College of Dental Surgery and Professor of Oncology in the Program of Oncology at the Greenebaum Cancer Center, University of Maryland at Baltimore.

Dr Meiller has held his position in Diagnostic Sciences at the Dental School for 25 years and serves as an attending faculty at the Greenebaum Cancer Center. He is a Diplomate of the American Board of Oral Medicine and a graduate of Johns Hopkins University and the University of Maryland Dental and Graduate Schools, holding a DDS and a PhD in Immunology/Virology. He has over 200 publications to his credit, maintains an active general dental practice, and is a consultant to the National Institutes of Health. He is currently engaged in ongoing investigations into cellular immune dysfunction in oral diseases associated with AIDS, in cancer patients, and in other medically compromised patients.

Harold L. Crossley, DDS, PhD

Dr Crossley is Associate Professor of Pharmacology at the Baltimore College of Dental Surgery, Dental School, University of Maryland at Baltimore. A native of Rhode Island, he received a Bachelor of Science degree in Pharmacy from the University of Rhode Island in 1964. He later was awarded the Master of Science (1970) and Doctorate degrees (1972) in the area of Pharmacology. The University of Maryland Dental School in Baltimore awarded Dr Crossley the DDS degree in 1980. He is the Director of Conjoint Sciences and Preclinical Studies at the School of Dentistry and maintains an intramural part-time private dental practice. Dr Crossley has co-authored a number of articles dealing with law enforcement on both a local and federal level. This liaison with law enforcement agencies keeps him well-acquainted with the "drug culture." He has been appointed to the Governor's Commission on Prescription Drug Abuse and the Maryland State Dental Association's Well-Being Committee.

Drawing on this unique background, Dr Crossley has become nationally and internationally recognized as an expert on street drugs and chemical dependency, as well as the clinical pharmacology of dental drugs.

EDITORIAL ADVISORY PANEL

Jeff Gonzales, PharmD
Critical Care Pharmacy Specialist
Cleveland Clinic Foundation
Cleveland, Ohio

Barbara L. Gracious, MD
Assistant Professor of Psychiatry and Pediatrics
Case Western Reserve University
Director of Child Psychiatry and Training & Education
University Hospitals of Cleveland
Cleveland, Ohio

Larry D. Gray, PhD
TriHealth
Clinical Microbiology Laboratory
Bethesda Oak Hospital
Cincinnati, Ohio

James L. Gutmann, DDS
Professor and Director of Graduate Endodontics
The Texas A & M University System
Baylor College of Dentistry
Dallas, Texas

Martin D. Higbee, PharmD, CGP
Associate Professor
Department of Pharmacy Practice and Science
The University of Arizona
Tucson, Arizona

Jane Hurlburt Hodding, PharmD
Director, Pharmacy
Miller Children's Hospital
Long Beach, California

Rebecca T. Horvat, PhD
Assistant Professor of Pathology and Laboratory Medicine
University of Kansas Medical Center
Kansas City, Kansas

Collin A. Hovinga, PharmD
Neuropharmacology Specialist
Cleveland Clinic Foundation
Cleveland, Ohio

Darrell T. Hulisz, PharmD
Department of Family Medicine
Case Western Reserve University
Cleveland, Ohio

Carlos M. Isada, MD
Department of Infectious Disease
Cleveland Clinic Foundation
Cleveland, Ohio

Sana Isa-Pratt, MD
Attending Physician
Department of Medicine
Overlake Hospital
Bellevue, Washington

David S. Jacobs, MD
President, Pathologists Chartered
Consultant in Pathology and Laboratory Medicine
Overland Park, Kansas

Bernard L. Kasten, Jr, MD, FCAP
Vice-President/Chief Medical Officer
Quest Diagnostics Inc
Teteroboro, New Jersey

Donna M. Kraus, PharmD, FAPhA
Associate Professor of Pharmacy Practice
Departments of Pharmacy Practice and Pediatrics
Pediatric Clinical Pharmacist
University of Illinois at Chicago
Chicago, Illinois

Charles Lacy, RPh, PharmD, FCSHP
Facilitative Officer, Clinical Programs
Nevada College of Pharmacy
Las Vegas, Nevada

Brenda R. Lance, RN, MSN
Nurse Coordinator
Ritzman Infusion Services
Akron, Ohio

Leonard L. Lance, RPh, BSPharm
Clinical Pharmacist
Lexi-Comp Inc
Hudson, Ohio

Jerrold B. Leikin, MD, FACP, FACEP, FACMT, FAACT
Director, Medical Toxicology
Evanston Northwestern Healthcare-OMEGA
Glenbrook Hospital
Glenview, Illinois
Associate Director
Toxikon Consortium at Cook County Hospital
Chicago, Illinois

Franklin A. Michota, Jr, MD
Head, Section of Hospital and Preoperative Medicine
Department of General Internal Medicine
Cleveland Clinic Foundation
Cleveland, Ohio

Michael A. Militello, PharmD, BCPS
Clinical Cardiology Specialist
Department of Pharmacy
Cleveland Clinic Foundation
Cleveland, Ohio

Suzanne Nesbit, PharmD
Clinical Pharmacy Specialist, Pain Management
Johns Hopkins Hospital
Baltimore, Maryland

Eugene S. Olsowka, MD, PhD
Pathologist
Institute of Pathology PC
Saginaw, Michigan

Dwight K. Oxley, MD
Medical Director of Pathology
Wesley Medical Center
Wichita, Kansas

EDITORIAL ADVISORY PANEL *(Continued)*

PREFACE TO THE EIGHTH EDITION

The authors of the *Drug Information Handbook for Dentistry* are gratified that the text has received many indicators of success over the years. We wish to thank the practitioners and students that have made each of the previous editions a success. In this new eighth edition, we have endeavored to respond to all of the comments and creative suggestions from our readership.

The philosophy of our book remains the same as in all previous editions. Complete cross-referencing of generic and brand names, medical and oral conditions, along with the therapeutic indication and example prescribing guidelines, have been the basis of the text and our indexing system has been the key to the success of this book. We are confident that dental practitioners and staff members can easily access needed information. Clinicians can cross-reference between an oral medicine problem, a suggested drug regimen, and the important pharmacologic information necessary to move ahead with a treatment selection. The alphabetical index now contains over 9,000 entries, including synonyms, as well as generic and name brands. By request, the natural products and Mexican brand names are now indexed, in addition to the generic drug names, synonyms, and U.S. and Canadian brand names. The therapeutic category index has been replaced with a new pharmacologic category index. The alphabetical listing of drug monographs contains 1474 drugs, including the most recent FDA-approved drugs as of July, 2002, in addition to 69 natural products. We've added more Canadian drugs and natural product monographs which now include a new "Effects on Bleeding" field.

This 8th edition includes easy-to-use algorithms to help the clinician make treatment decisions in evolving areas of patient care including preprocedural antibiotics related to endocarditis and joint prostheses. Many chapters include FAQs, or "Frequently Asked Questions", to help us focus on real-life scenarios. The sections on calcium channel blockers and gingival hyperplasia, cardiovascular disease, chemical dependency, dental office emergencies, diabetes, HIV infection and AIDS, odontogenic infections, oral bacterial infections, oral pain management, oral viral infections, pharmacology of drug metabolism and interactions, suggested readings, systemic viral diseases, and TMD have all been updated.

We know that our text remains an excellent companion to complete oral medicine and medical reference libraries that each clinician should have available. We hope that it compliments the sound foundation that each dental clinician has received during their education and by building on their knowledge of oral and systemic disease we have helped them with this text to focus on therapeutic considerations. Dental office management protocols, along with prescribing guidelines, should aid the busy practitioner. The active general practitioner, the specialist, the dental hygienist, and the advanced student of dentistry or dental hygiene will be better prepared for patient care with this new 8th edition.

Richard L. Wynn

Timothy F. Meiller

Harold L. Crossley

ACKNOWLEDGMENTS

This handbook exists in its present form as a result of the concerted efforts of many individuals, including Jack D. Bolinski, DDS, and Brad F. Bolinski, who recognized the need for a comprehensive dental and medical drug compendium; the publisher and president of Lexi-Comp, Inc, Robert D. Kerscher; Lynn D. Coppinger, managing editor; Barbara F. Kerscher, production manager; Mark F. Bonfiglio, BS, PharmD, RPh, Director of Pharmacotherapy Resources; Brad F. Bolinski, product manager; Sheila L. Digman, project manager; A. Nicole Springfield and Leeann F. Nemec, assistant project managers; and David C. Marcus, director of information systems.

Much of the material contained in this book was a result of contributions by pharmacists throughout the United States and Canada. Lexi-Comp has assisted many medical institutions in developing hospital-specific formulary manuals that contain clinical drug information, as well as dosing. Working with these clinical pharmacists, hospital pharmacy and therapeutics committees, and hospital drug information centers, Lexi-Comp has developed an evolutionary drug database that reflects the practice of pharmacy in these major institutions.

Special acknowledgment goes out to all Lexi-Comp staff members for their contributions to this handbook. In addition, the authors wish to thank their families, friends, and colleagues who supported them in their efforts to complete this handbook.

DESCRIPTION OF SECTIONS AND FIELDS USED IN THIS HANDBOOK

The *Drug Information Handbook for Dentistry, 8th Edition* is organized into six sections: Introductory text; drug monographs; natural products: herbal and dietary supplements; oral medicine topics; appendix; and the indexes, including a new pharmacologic category index and expanded alphabetical index containing synonyms, as well as U.S., Canadian, and Mexican brand names.

INTRODUCTORY TEXT

The first section is a compilation of information pertinent to the use of this handbook.

ALPHABETICAL LISTING OF DRUG MONOGRAPHS

The drug information section contains comprehensive monographs for drugs commonly prescribed in dentistry and concise monographs for other drugs which dental patients may be taking. Drug names and cross-references of U.S. brand names and synonyms are printed in red, in addition to the dental-specific fields. Monographs include all or most of the following fields:

Generic Name	U.S. adopted name
Pronunciation	Phonetic listing of generic name
Related Information	Cross-reference to other pertinent information found elsewhere in the book
U.S. Brand Names	Common trade names used in the United States
Canadian Brand Names	Trade names found in Canada if different from the U.S. brand name(s)
Mexican Brand Names	Trade names found in Mexico if different from the U.S. brand name(s)
Pharmacologic Category	Unique systematic classification of medications
Synonyms	Other names or accepted abbreviations of the generic drug
Use	Information pertaining to appropriate dental and medical indications of the drug; includes Orphan Drug status and Unlabeled/Investigational use which gives information pertaining to non-FDA approved and investigational indications of the drug
Local Anesthetic/Vasoconstrictor Precautions	Specific information to prevent potential drug interactions related to anesthesia
Effects on Dental Treatment	How drug therapy affects the dental treatment/diagnosis with suggested management approaches
Restrictions	DEA classification for federally scheduled controlled substances and their associated prescribing limits
Dosage	The amount of the drug to be typically given or taken during therapy
Mechanism of Action	How the drug works in the body to elicit a response
Other Adverse Effects	Side effects grouped by percentage of incidence and body systems
Contraindications	Information pertaining to inappropriate use of the drug
Warnings/Precautions	Cautions and hazardous conditions related to use of the drug
Drug Interactions	A list of agents that, when combined with the drug, may affect therapy
Dietary/Ethanol/Herb Considerations	Information regarding food, alcohol, herb/nutraceutical interactions with the drug and dietary/nutritional requirements resulting from use of the drug (given for dental-specific drugs only)
Drug Uptake	Information includes onset of action/effect, absorption and duration, time to peak concentration, and half-life.
Pregnancy Risk Factor	Five categories established by the FDA to indicate the potential of a systemically absorbed drug for causing birth defects
Breast-feeding Considerations	Information pertaining to drug administration while breast-feeding (given for dental-specific drugs only)
Dosage Forms	Information about the formulation(s), strength(s), and availability (given for dental-specific drugs only)
Generic Available	Indicated by a "yes" or "no"

Comments	Additional pertinent information
Selected Readings	Sources and literature where the user may find additional information

NATURAL PRODUCTS: HERBAL AND DIETARY SUPPLEMENTS

This section is divided into three parts. First, is a brief introduction to popular natural products, followed by an alphabetical listing of monographs. This second section has been expanded and contains concise monographs for products commonly purchased over-the-counter which dental patients may be taking. Names and synonyms are printed in red, in addition to the dental–specific fields. Monographs include all or most of the following fields:

Synonyms	Other names or accepted abbreviations of the product
Use	Information pertaining to appropriate medical indications for the product; some include recommendations from Commission E.
Effects on Bleeding	How the product affects bleeding during dental procedures
Local Anesthetic/Vasoconstrictor Precautions	Specific information to prevent potential interactions related to anesthesia
Dosage	The amount of the product to be typically given or taken during therapy
Mechanism of Action/Effect	How the product works in the body to elicit a response
Adverse Reactions	Side effects grouped by percentage of incidence and body systems
Contraindications	Information pertaining to inappropriate use of the product
Warnings	Cautions and hazardous conditions related to use of the product
Potential/Suspected Interactions	A list of drugs and other natural products that may affect therapy

Following the natural product monographs is a description of their known effects on the central nervous system, cardiovascular system, endocrine system, and gastrointestinal system.

ORAL MEDICINE TOPICS

This section is divided into two major parts and contains text on Oral Medicine topics. In each subsection, the systemic condition or the oral disease state is described briefly, followed by the pharmacologic considerations with which the dentist must be familiar. Selected readings have been listed for further inquiry.

Part I: **Dental Management and Therapeutic Considerations in Medically-Compromised Patients** focuses on common medical conditions and their associated drug therapies with which the dentist must be familiar. Patient profiles with commonly associated drug regimens are described.

Part II: **Dental Management and Therapeutic Considerations in Patients With Specific Oral Conditions** focus on therapies the dentist may choose to prescribe for patients suffering from oral disease or are in need of special care. Some overlap between these sections has resulted from systemic conditions that have oral manifestations and vice-versa. Cross-references to the descriptions and the monographs for individual drugs described elsewhere in this handbook allow for easy retrieval of information. Example prescriptions of selected drug therapies for each condition are presented so that the clinician can evaluate alternate approaches to treatment. Seldom is there a single drug of choice.

Those drug prescriptions listed represent prototype drugs and popular prescriptions and are examples only. The pharmacologic category index is available for cross-referencing if alternatives or additional drugs are sought.

Part III: **Other Oral Medicine Topics**

DESCRIPTION OF SECTIONS AND FIELDS USED IN THIS HANDBOOK *(Continued)*

APPENDIX

The appendix is broken down into various sections for easy use and offers a compilation of tables and guidelines which can often be helpful when considering patient care. It includes descriptions of most over-the-counter oral care products and dental drug interactions, in addition to, infectious disease information and the top 50 drugs prescribed in 2001.

INDEXES

This section includes a new pharmacologic index with an easy-to-use classification system in alphabetical order and an alphabetical index. The alphabetical index provides a quick reference for major topics within the sections, generic names, synonyms, U.S., Canadian, and Mexican brand names. From this index, the reader can cross-reference to the monographs, oral medicine topics, and appendix information.

FDA PREGNANCY CATEGORIES

Throughout this book there is a field labeled "Pregnancy Risk Factor" and the letter A, B, C, D, or X immediately following which signifies a category. The FDA has established these five categories to indicate the potential of a systemically absorbed drug for causing birth defects. The key differentiation among the categories rests upon the reliability of documentation and the risk:benefit ratio. Pregnancy category X is particularly notable, in that if any data exists that may implicate a drug as a teratogen and the risk:benefit ratio is clearly negative, the drug is contraindicated during pregnancy. These categories are summarized as follows:

A Controlled studies in pregnant women fail to demonstrate a risk to the fetus in the first trimester with no evidence of risk in later trimesters. The possibility of fetal harm appears remote.

B Either animal-reproductive studies have not demonstrated a fetal risk but there are no controlled studies in pregnant women, or animal-reproduction studies have shown an adverse effect (other than a decrease in fertility) that was not confirmed in controlled studies in women in the first trimester and there is no evidence of a risk in later trimesters.

C Either studies in animals have revealed adverse effects on the fetus (teratogenic or embryocidal effects or other) and there are no controlled studies in women, or studies in women and animals are not available. Drugs should be given only if the potential benefits justify the potential risk to the fetus.

D There is positive evidence of human fetal risk, but the benefits from use in pregnant women may be acceptable despite the risk (eg, if the drug is needed in a life-threatening situation or for a serious disease for which safer drugs cannot be used or are ineffective).

X Studies in animals or human beings have demonstrated fetal abnormalities or there is evidence of fetal risk based on human experience, or both, and the risk of the use of the drug in pregnant women clearly outweighs any possible benefit. The drug is contraindicated in women who are or may become pregnant.

FDA NAME DIFFERENTIATION PROJECT: THE USE OF TALL-MAN LETTERS

Confusion between similar drug names is an important cause of medication errors. For years, The Institute For Safe Medication Practices (ISMP), has urged generic manufacturers use a combination of large and small letters as well as bolding (ie, chlorpro**MAZINE** and chlorpro**PAMIDE**) to help distinguish drugs with look-alike names, especially when they share similar strengths. Recently the FDA's Division of Generic Drugs began to issue recommendation letters to manufacturers suggesting this novel way to label their products to help reduce this drug name confusion. Although this project has had marginal success, the method has successfully eliminated problems with products such as diphenhydr**AMINE** and dimenhy**DRINATE**. Hospitals should also follow suit by making similar changes in their own labels, preprinted order forms, computer screens and printouts, and drug storage location labels.

Lexi-Comp Medical Publishing, with this edition of the *Drug Information Handbook for Dentistry*, will begin using these "Tall-Man" letters for the drugs suggested by the FDA.

The following is a list of product names and recommended FDA revisions.

Drug Product	Recommended Revision
acetazolamide	aceta**ZOLAMIDE**
acetohexamide	aceto**HEXAMIDE**
bupropion	bu**PROP**ion
buspirone	bus**PIR**one
chlorpromazine	chlorpro**MAZINE**
chlorpropamide	chlorpro**PAMIDE**
clomiphene	clomi**PHENE**
clomipramine	clomi**PRAMINE**
cycloserine	cyclo**SERINE**
cyclosporine	cyclo**SPORINE**
daunorubicin	**DAUNO**rubicin
dimenhydrinate	dimenhy**DRINATE**
diphenhydramine	diphenhydr**AMINE**
dobutamine	**DOBUT**amine
dopamine	**DOP**amine
doxorubicin	**DOXO**rubicin
glipizide	glipi**ZIDE**
glyburide	gly**BURIDE**
hydralazine	hydr**ALAZINE**
hydroxyzine	hydr**OXY**zine
medroxyprogesterone	medroxy**PROGESTER**one
methylprednisolone	methyl**PREDNIS**olone
methyltestosterone	methyl**TESTOSTER**one
nicardipine	ni**CAR**dipine
nifedipine	**NIFE**dipine
prednisolone	predniso**LONE**
prednisone	predni**SONE**
sulfadiazine	sulfa**DIAZINE**
sulfisoxazole	sulfi**SOXAZOLE**
tolazamide	**TOLAZ**amide
tolbutamide	**TOLBUT**amide
vinblastine	vin**BLAS**tine
vincristine	vin**CRIS**tine

Institute for Safe Medication Practices. "New Tall-Man Lettering Will Reduce Mix-Ups Due to Generic Drug Name Confusion," *ISMP Medication Safety Alert*, September 19, 2001. Available at: http://www.ismp.org.

Institute for Safe Medication Practices. "Prescription Mapping, Can Improve Efficiency While Minimizing Errors With Look-Alike Products," *ISMP Medication Safety Alert*, October 6, 1999. Available at: http://www.ismp.org.

U.S. Pharmacopeia, "USP Quality Review: Use Caution-Avoid Confusion," March 2001, No. 76. Available at: http://www.usp.org.

CONTROLLED SUBSTANCES

Schedule I = C-I

The drugs and other substances in this schedule have no legal medical uses except research. They have a **high** potential for abuse. They include selected opiates such as heroin, opium derivatives, and hallucinogens.

Schedule II = C-II

The drugs and other substances in this schedule have legal medical uses and a **high** abuse potential which may lead to severe dependence. They include former "Class A" narcotics, amphetamines, barbiturates, and other drugs.

Schedule III = C-III

The drugs and other substances in this schedule have legal medical uses and a **lesser** degree of abuse potential which may lead to **moderate** dependence. They include former "Class B" narcotics and other drugs.

Schedule IV = C-IV

The drugs and other substances in this schedule have legal medial uses and **low** abuse potential which may lead to **moderate** dependence. They include barbiturates, benzodiazepines, propoxyphenes, and other drugs.

Schedule V = C-V

The drugs and other substances in this schedule have legal medical uses and **low** abuse potential which may lead to **moderate** dependence. They include narcotic cough preparations, diarrhea preparations, and other drugs.

Note: These are federal classifications. Your individual state may place a substance into a more restricted category. When this occurs, the more restricted category applies. Consult your state law.

PRESCRIPTION WRITING

Doctor's Name
Address
Phone Number

Patient's Name/Date

Patient's Address/Age

Rx	
	Drug Name/Dosage Size Disp: Number of tablets, capsules, ounces to be dispensed (roman numerals added as precaution for abused drugs) Sig: Direction on how drug is to be taken

Doctor's signature

State license number

DEA number (if required)

PRESCRIPTION REQUIREMENTS

1. Date
2. Full name and address of patient
3. Name and address of prescriber
4. Signature of prescriber

If Class II drug, Drug Enforcement Agency (DEA) number necessary.

If Class II and Class III narcotic, a triplicate prescription form (in the state of California) is necessary and it must be handwritten by the prescriber.

Please turn to appropriate oral medicine chapters for examples of prescriptions.

ABBREVIATIONS COMMONLY USED IN MEDICAL ORDERS

Abbreviation	From	Meaning
$\overline{aa}$, aa	ana	of each
ac	ante cibum	before meals or food
ad	ad	to, up to
a.d.	aurio dextra	right ear
ad lib	ad libitum	at pleasure
a.l.	aurio laeva	left ear
AM	ante meridiem	morning
amp		ampul
amt		amount
aq	aqua	water
aq. dest.	aqua destillata	distilled water
a.s.	aurio sinister	left ear
ASAP		as soon as possible
a.u.	aures utrae	each ear
bid	bis in die	twice daily
bm		bowel movement
bp		blood pressure
BSA		body surface area
c	cong	a gallon
$\bar{c}$	cum	with
cal		calorie
cap	capsula	capsule
cc		cubic centimeter
cm		centimeter
comp	compositus	compound
cont		continue
d	dies	day
d/c		discontinue
dil	dilue	dilute

PRESCRIPTION WRITING *(Continued)*

Abbreviation	From	Meaning
disp	dispensa	dispense
div	divide	divide
dtd	dentur tales doses	give of such a dose
elix, el	elixir	elixir
emp		as directed
et	et	and
ex aq		in water
f, ft	fac, fiat, fiant	make, let be made
FDA		Food and Drug Administration
g	gramma	gram
gr	granum	grain
gtt	gutta	a drop
h	hora	hour
hs	hora somni	at bedtime
I.M.		intramuscular
I.V.		intravenous
kcal		kilocalorie
kg		kilogram
L		liter
liq	liquor	a liquor, solution
mcg		microgram
mEq		milliequivalent
mg		milligram
mixt	mixtura	a mixture
mL		milliliter
mm		millimeter
M	misce	mix
m. dict	more dictor	as directed
NF		National Formulary
no.	numerus	number
noc	nocturnal	in the night
non rep	non repetatur	do not repeat, no refills
NPO		nothing by mouth
O, Oct	octarius	a pint
o.d.	oculus dexter	right eye
o.l.	oculus laevus	left eye
o.s.	oculus sinister	left eye
o.u.	oculo uterque	each eye
pc, post cib	post cibos	after meals
per		through or by
PM	post meridiem	afternoon or evening
P.O.	per os	by mouth
P.R.	per rectum	rectally
prn	pro re nata	as needed
pulv	pulvis	a powder
q		every
qad	quoque alternis die	every other day
qd		every day
qh	quiaque hora	every hour
qid	quater in die	four times a day
qod		every other day
qs	quantum sufficiat	a sufficient quantity
qs ad		a sufficient quantity to make
qty		quantity
qv	quam volueris	as much as you wish
Rx	recipe	take, a recipe
rep	repetatur	let it be repeated
$\bar{s}$	sine	without

Abbreviation	From	Meaning
sa	secundum artem	according to art
sat	sataratus	saturated
S.C.		subcutaneous
sig	signa	label, or let it be printed
sol	solutio	solution
solv		dissolve
$\overline{ss}$	semis	one-half
sos	si opus sit	if there is need
stat	statim	at once, immediately
supp	suppositorium	suppository
syr	syrupus	syrup
tab	tabella	tablet
tal		such
tid	ter in die	three times a day
tr, tinct	tincture	tincture
trit		triturate
tsp		teaspoonful
ung	unguentum	ointment
USAN		United States Adopted Names
USP		United States Pharmacopeia
u.d., ut dict	ut dictum	as directed
v.o.		verbal order
w.a.		while awake
x3		3 times
x4		4 times

SAFE WRITING PRACTICES

Health professionals and their support personnel frequently produce handwritten copies of information they see in print; therefore, such information is subjected to even greater possibilities for error or misinterpretation on the part of others. Thus, particular care must be given to how drug names and strengths are expressed when creating written health-care documents.

The following are a few examples of safe writing rules suggested by the Institute for Safe Medication Practices, Inc.*

1. There should be a space between a number and its units as it is easier to read. There should be no periods after the abbreviations mg or mL.

Correct	Incorrect
10 mg	10mg
100 mg	100mg

2. Never place a decimal and a zero after a whole number (2 mg is correct and 2.0 mg is **incorrect**). If the decimal point is not seen because it falls on a line or because individuals are working from copies where the decimal point is not seen, this causes a tenfold overdose.
3. Just the opposite is true for numbers less than one. Always place a zero before a naked decimal (0.5 mL is correct, .5 mL is **incorrect**).
4. Never abbreviate the word unit. The handwritten U or u, looks like a 0 (zero), and may cause a tenfold overdose error to be made.
5. IU is not a safe abbreviation for international units. The handwritten IU looks like IV. Write out international units or use int. units.
6. Q.D. is not a safe abbreviation for once daily, as when the Q is followed by a sloppy dot, it looks like QID which means four times daily.
7. O.D. is not a safe abbreviation for once daily, as it is properly interpreted as meaning "right eye" and has caused liquid medications such as saturated solution of potassium iodide and Lugol's solution to be administered incorrectly. There is no safe abbreviation for once daily. It must be written out in full.
8. Do not use chemical names such as 6-mercaptopurine or 6-thioguanine, as sixfold overdoses have been given when these were not recognized as chemical names. The proper names of these drugs are mercaptopurine or thioguanine.
9. Do not abbreviate drug names (5FC, 6MP, 5-ASA, MTX, HCTZ, CPZ, PBZ, etc) as they are misinterpreted and cause error.
10. Do not use the apothecary system or symbols.
11. Do not abbreviate microgram as µg; instead use mcg as there is less likelihood of misinterpretation.
12. When writing an outpatient prescription, write a complete prescription. A complete prescription can prevent the prescriber, the pharmacist, and/or the patient from making a mistake and can eliminate the need for further clarification. The legible prescriptions should contain:
    a. patient's full name
    b. for pediatric or geriatric patients: their age (or weight where applicable)
    c. drug name, dosage form and strength; if a drug is new or rarely prescribed, print this information
    d. number or amount to be dispensed
    e. complete instructions for the patient, including the purpose of the medication
    f. when there are recognized contraindications for a prescribed drug, indicate to the pharmacist that you are aware of this fact (ie, when prescribing a potassium salt for a patient receiving an ACE inhibitor, write "K serum leveling being monitored")

*From "Safe Writing" by Davis NM, PharmD and Cohen MR, MS, Lecturers and Consultants for Safe Medication Practices, 1143 Wright Drive, Huntington Valley, PA 19006. Phone: (215) 947-7566.

PHARMACOLOGY OF DRUG METABOLISM AND INTERACTIONS

Most drugs undergo metabolic transformation in the body prior to excretion. Drug metabolism is an enzyme-dependent process that developed as an adaptation to life on earth. Unlike fish, terrestrial vertebrates are unable to excrete lipid soluble compounds because kidney tubular reabsorption favors their retention. Excretion of these substances is accomplished in fish into the surrounding water. Although drug metabolism in humans results in the formation of compounds that are more polar in nature, it does not always result in the initial production of biologically inactive compounds. This means that a drug may stay active for some time during this metabolic process. Enzymatic modification of a parent drug can be distinguished by three basic patterns. First, an inactive parent drug may be transformed to an active compound. Second, an active parent drug may be converted to a second active compound which is subsequently converted to an inactive metabolite or byproduct. Third, an inactive compound may be formed directly from an active parent drug.

The most common reaction in drug metabolism is an oxidation reaction in which oxygen in the form of a hydroxyl group is attached to the drug molecule. With oxidation, the original drug molecule is changed just enough so that the drug metabolite will not attach to the receptor that is specific for the original molecule. This chemical change may render the drug inactive and is one mechanism of terminating drug activity. The overall process is called hydroxylation and is the direct incorporation of oxygen into the substrate drug molecule. Although the liver is the primary site for these hydroxylation enzyme reactions, these systems are also present in the kidney and gastrointestinal epithelium. This process is also called oxidative drug metabolism by an oxidative enzyme system.

This oxidative enzyme system relies on a particular cytochrome and numerous isoforms known as the cytochrome P450 system with designations CYP. Cytochrome P450 is a complex of protein and heme that contains an iron atom in its oxidized state. Through an energy transfer cascade, cytochrome P450 is reduced utilizing energy and reducing the iron to a ferrous form. This then binds with molecular oxygen and the cytochrome P450 eventually reverts to its oxidized form. The oxidized drug bound through this process to the cytochrome P450 is then released and the cytochrome is regenerated. The rate of drug biotransformation or metabolism appears to be directly related to the amounts of cytochrome P450 in the microsomal and enzyme cascade. In fact, there is a direct correlation between these systems.

There are five distinct groups of drug metabolizing enzymes which account for the majority of drug metabolism in humans. These enzyme "families", known as isoenzymes, are localized primarily in the liver. The nomenclature of this system has been standardized. Isoenzyme families are identified as a cytochrome (CYP prefix), followed by their numerical designation (eg, 1A2).

Enzymes may be inhibited (slowing metabolism through this pathway) or induced (increased in activity or number). Individual drugs metabolized by a specific enzyme are identified as substrates for the isoenzyme. Considerable effort has been expended in recent years to classify drugs metabolized by this system as either an inhibitor, inducer, or substrate of a specific isoenzyme. It should be noted that a drug may demonstrate complex activity within this scheme, acting as an inhibitor of one isoenzyme while serving as a substrate for another.

By recognizing that a substrate's metabolism may be dramatically altered by concurrent therapy with either an inducer or inhibitor, potential interactions may be identified and addressed. For example, a drug which inhibits CYP1A2 is likely to block metabolism of theophylline (a substrate for this isoenzyme). Because of this interaction, the dose of theophylline required to maintain a consistent level in the patient should be reduced when an inhibitor is added. Failure to make this adjustment may lead to supratherapeutic theophylline concentrations and potential toxicity.

This approach does have limitations. For example, the metabolism of specific drugs may have primary and secondary pathways. The contribution of secondary pathways to the overall metabolism may limit the impact of any given inhibitor. In addition, there may be up to a tenfold variation in the concentration of an isoenzyme across the broad population. In fact, a complete absence of an isoenzyme may occur in some genetic subgroups. Finally, the relative potency of inhibition, relative to the affinity of the enzyme for its substrate, demonstrates a high degree of variability. These issues make it difficult to anticipate whether a theoretical interaction will have a clinically relevant impact in a specific patient.

The details of this enzyme system continue to be investigated and information is expanding daily. However, to be complete, it should be noted that other enzyme systems also influence a drug's pharmacokinetic profile. For example, a key enzyme system regulating absorption of drugs is the p-glycoprotein system. Recent evidence suggests that some interaction originally attributed to the cytochrome system may, in fact, have been the result of inhibition of this enzyme.

The cytochrome P450 information provided in the "Drug Interactions" field of the drug monographs attempts to identify involvement of a particular isoenzyme in the drug's

PHARMACOLOGY OF DRUG METABOLISM AND INTERACTIONS *(Continued)*

metabolism. Within certain limits, it may be used to identify potential interactions, Many of the drugs used as antivirals, for instance, interfere with specific isoforms of the cytochrome P450 system and may, therefore, interact adversely with the metabolism of other drugs which the patient may be taking.

References

Baker GB, Urichuk CJ, and Coutts RT, "Drug Metabolism and Metabolic Drug-Drug Interactions in Psychiatry," *Child Adolescent Psychopharm News (Suppl).*

DeVane CL, "Pharmacogenetics and Drug Metabolism of Newer Antidepressant Agents," *J Clin Psychiatry*, 1994, 55(Suppl 12):38-45.

Drug Interactions Analysis and Management. Cytochrome (CYP) 450 Isozyme Drug Interactions, Vancouver, WA: Applied Therapeutics, Inc, 523-7.

Ereshefsky L, "Drug-Drug Interactions Involving Antidepressants: Focus on Venlafaxine," *J Clin Psychopharmacol*, 1996, 16(3 Suppl 2):375-535.

Ereshefsky L, *Psychiatr Annal*, 1996, 26:342-50.

Fleishaker JC and Hulst LK, "A Pharmacokinetic and Pharmacodynamic Evaluation of the Combined Administration of Alprazolam and Fluvoxamine," *Eur J Clin Pharmacol*, 1994, 46(1):35-9.

Flockhart DA, et al, *Clin Pharmacol Ther*, 1996, 59:189.

Ketter TA, Flockhart DA, Post RM, et al, "The Emerging Role of Cytochrome P450 3A in Psychopharmacology," *J Clin Psychopharmacol*, 1995, 15(6):387-98.

Michalets EL, "Update: Clinically Significant Cytochrome P450 Drug Interactions," *Pharmacotherapy*, 1998, 18(1):84-112.

Nemeroff CB, DeVane CL, and Pollock BG, "Newer Antidepressants and the Cytochrome P450 System," *Am J Psychiatry*, 1996, 153(3):311-20.

Pollock BG, "Recent Developments in Drug Metabolism of Relevance to Psychiatrists," *Harv Rev Psychiatry*, 1994, 2(4):204-13.

Richelson E, "Pharmacokinetic Drug Interactions of New Antidepressants: A Review of the Effects on the Metabolism of Other Drugs," *Mayo Clin Proc*, 1997, 72(9):835-47.

Riesenman C, "Antidepressant Drug Interactions and the Cytochrome P450 System: A Critical Appraisal," *Pharmacotherapy*, 1995, 15(6 Pt 2):84S-99S.

Schmider J, Greenblatt DJ, von Moltke LL, et al, "Relationship of *In Vitro* Data on Drug Metabolism to *In Vivo* Pharmacokinetics and Drug Interactions: Implications for Diazepam Disposition in Humans," *J Clin Psychopharmacol*, 1996, 16(4):267-72.

Slaughter RL, *Pharm Times*, 1996, 7:6-16.

Watkins PB, "Role of Cytochrome P450 in Drug Metabolism and Hepatotoxicity," *Semin Liver Dis*, 1990, 10(4):235-50.

CONJUGATION REACTIONS IN DRUG METABOLISM

Conjugation reactions involve coupling the drug or polar metabolite with an endogenous chemical compound present in cells such as glucuronic acid, sulfuric acid or acetic acid, or amino acids. The majority of conjugation reactions couple drugs to glucuronic acid. The product formed is called the glucuronide conjugate or glucuronide. The reaction is driven by a family of enzymes known as hepatic glucuronide transferases, found in the endoplasmic reticulum. Conjugation with glucuronic acid also occurs in the kidney and other tissues, but to a much lesser extent.

Conjugation of drugs results in polar, usually more water soluble, compounds that are most often therapeutically inactive. The drug conjugates formed are rapidly excreted in the urine and bile by transport systems favoring these types of water-soluble compounds. Thus, the parent drug is effectively rendered inactive and transported out of the body by this process.

SMOKING AND DRUG METABOLISM

Another area of intense interest involves smoking effects on drug metabolism, as well as, the effects of smoking cessation drugs. A review of the literature suggests that at least a dozen drugs interact with cigarette smoke in a clinically significant manner. Polycyclic aromatic hydrocarbons (PAHs) are largely responsible for enhancing drug metabolism. Cigarette smoke induces an increase in the concentration of CYP1A2, the isoenzyme responsible for metabolism of theophylline. Theophylline is, therefore, eliminated more quickly in smokers than in nonsmokers. As a result of hepatic induction of CYP1A2, serum concentrations of theophylline have been shown to be reduced in smokers. Cigarette smoking may substantially reduce tacrine plasma concentrations. The manufacturer states that mean plasma tacrine concentrations in smokers are about one-third of the concentration in nonsmokers (presumably after multiple doses of tacrine).

Patients with insulin-dependent diabetes who smoke heavily may require a higher dosage of insulin than nonsmokers. Cigarette smoking may also reduce serum concentrations of flecainide. Although the mechanism of this interaction is unknown, enhanced hepatic metabolism is possible. Propoxyphene, a pain reliever, has been found to be less effective in heavy smokers than in nonsmokers. The mechanism for the inefficacy of propoxyphene in smokers compared with nonsmokers may be enhanced biotransformation.

Frankl and Soloff reported in a study of five young, healthy, chronic smokers that propranolol, followed by smoking, significantly decreased cardiac output and significantly increased blood pressure and peripheral resistance compared with smoking alone. Steady-state concentrations of propranolol were found to be lower in smokers than in nonsmokers. Lastly, the incidence of drowsiness associated with the use of diazepam and chlordiazepoxide showed that drowsiness was less likely to occur in smokers than in nonsmokers. Smoking probably acts by producing arousal of the central nervous system rather than by accelerating metabolism and reducing concentrations of these drugs in the brain. Finally, the interaction between smoking and oral contraceptives is complex and may be deadly. Women >35 years of age who smoke >15 cigarettes daily may be at increased risk of myocardial infarction.

The norepinephrine and serotonin reuptake inhibitors, as a new class of smoking cessation drugs, have also received attention relative to metabolic interactions. *In vitro* studies indicate that bupropion is primarily metabolized to hydroxybupropion by the CYP2B6 isoenzyme. Therefore, the potential exists for a drug interaction between Zyban® and drugs that affect the CYP2B6 isoenzyme metabolism (eg, orphenadrine and cyclophosphamide). The hydroxybupropion metabolite of bupropion does not appear to be metabolized by the cytochrome P450 isoenzymes. No systemic data have been collected on the metabolism of Zyban® following concomitant administration with other drugs, or alternatively, the effect of concomitant administration of Zyban® on the metabolism of other drugs.

Animal data, however, indicated that bupropion may be an inducer of drug-metabolizing enzymes in humans. However, following chronic administration of bupropion, 100 mg 3 times/day, to 8 healthy male volunteers for 14 days, there was no evidence of induction of its own metabolism. Because bupropion is extensively metabolized, coadministration of other drugs may affect its clinical activity. Certain drugs may induce the metabolism of bupropion (eg, carbamazepine, phenobarbital, phenytoin), while other drugs may inhibit its metabolism (eg, cimetidine). Studies in animals demonstrated that the acute toxicity of bupropion is enhanced by the MAO inhibitor, phenelzine.

Limited clinical data suggest a higher incidence of adverse experiences in patients receiving concurrent administration of bupropion and levodopa. Administration of Zyban® to patients receiving levodopa concurrently should be undertaken with caution, using small initial doses and gradual dosage increases. Concurrent administration of Zyban® and agents that lower the seizure threshold should be undertaken only with extreme caution. Physiological changes resulting from smoking cessation itself, with or without treatment with Zyban®, may alter the pharmacokinetics of some concomitant medications, which may require dosage adjustment.

INTERACTIONS BETWEEN CIGARETTE SMOKE AND DRUGS

Drug	Mechanism	Effect on Cigarette Smokers
Theophylline	Induction of the CYP1A2 isoenzyme	May lead to reduced theophylline serum concentrations and decreased clinical effect; elimination of theophylline is considerably more rapid
Tacrine	Induction of the CYP1A2 isoenzyme	Effectiveness of tacrine may be decreased
Insulin	Decreased insulin absorption; may be related to peripheral vasoconstriction	Insulin-dependent diabetics who smoke heavily may require a 15% to 30% higher dose of insulin than nonsmokers
Flecainide	Unknown	May reduce flecainide serum concentrations
Propoxyphene	Unknown	May require higher dosage of propoxyphene to achieve analgesic effects
Propranolol	Increased release of catacholamines (eg, epinephrine) in smokers	May have increased blood pressure and heart rate relative to nonsmokers; consider effects on prevention of angina pectoris and stroke
Diazepam	Unclear as to whether pharmacokinetics are altered or end-organ responsiveness is decreased	May require larger doses of diazepam and chlordiazepoxide to achieve sedative effects

Adapted from Schein, JR, "Cigarette Smoking and Clinically Significant Drug Interactions," *Ann Pharmacother*, 1995, 29(11):1139-47.

SUMMARY

Once a drug has been metabolized in the liver, it is eliminated through several different mechanisms. One is directly through bile, into the intestine, and eventually excreted in feces. More commonly, the metabolites and the original drug pass back into the liver from the general circulation and are carried to other organs and tissues. Eventually, these metabolites are excreted through the kidney. In the kidney, the drug and its metabolites may be filtered by the glomerulus or secreted by the renal tubules into the urine. From the kidney, some of the drug may be reabsorbed and pass back into the

PHARMACOLOGY OF DRUG METABOLISM AND INTERACTIONS *(Continued)*

blood. The drug may also be carried to the lung. If the drug or its metabolite is volatile, it can pass from the blood into the alveolar air and be eliminated in the breath. To a minor extent, drugs and metabolites can be excreted by sweat and saliva. In nursing mothers, drugs are also excreted in mother's milk.

The clinical considerations of drug metabolism may affect which other drugs can and should be administered. Drug tolerance may be a consideration, in that larger doses of a drug may be necessary to obtain effect in patients in which the metabolism is extremely rapid. These interactions, via cytochrome P450 or its isoforms, can occasionally be used beneficially to increase/maintain blood levels of one drug by administering a second drug. Dental clinicians should attempt to stay current on this topic of drug interactions as knowledge evolves.

ALPHABETICAL LISTING OF DRUGS

A-200™ [OTC] *see* Pyrethrins *on page 1026*
A200® Lice [OTC] *see* Permethrin *on page 940*
A and D™ Ointment [OTC] *see* Vitamin A and Vitamin D *on page 1244*

Abacavir (a BAK a veer)

Related Information

HIV Infection and AIDS *on page 1334*

U.S. Brand Names Ziagen®

Canadian Brand Names Ziagen®

Pharmacologic Category Antiretroviral Agent, Reverse Transcriptase Inhibitor (Nucleoside)

Use Treatment of HIV infections in combination with other antiretroviral agents

Local Anesthetic/Vasoconstrictor Precautions No information available to require special precautions

Effects on Dental Treatment No effects or complications reported

Dosage Oral:

Children 3 months to 16 years: 8 mg/kg body weight twice daily (maximum: 300 mg twice daily) in combination with other antiretroviral agents

Adults: 300 mg twice daily in combination with other antiretroviral agents

Mechanism of Action Nucleoside reverse transcriptase inhibitor; abacavir is a guanosine analogue which is phosphorylated to carbovir triphosphate which interferes with HIV viral RNA dependent DNA polymerase resulting in inhibition of viral replication.

Other Adverse Effects Hypersensitivity reactions, which may be fatal, occur in ~5% of patients. Symptoms may include anaphylaxis, fever, rash, fatigue, diarrhea, abdominal pain, respiratory symptoms (eg, pharyngitis, dyspnea, or cough), headache, malaise, lethargy, myalgia, myolysis, arthralgia, edema, paresthesia, nausea and vomiting, mouth ulcerations, conjunctivitis, lymphadenopathy, hepatic failure, and renal failure.

Rates of adverse reactions were defined during combination therapy with lamivudine. Adverse reaction rates attributable to abacavir alone are not available.

Adults:

- Central nervous system: Insomnia (7%)
- Gastrointestinal: Nausea (47%), vomiting (16%), diarrhea (12%), anorexia (11%), pancreatitis
- Endocrine & metabolic: Hyperglycemia, hypertriglyceridemia (25%)
- Neuromuscular & skeletal: Weakness
- Miscellaneous: Elevated transaminases

Children:

- Central nervous system: Fever (19%), headache (16%)
- Dermatologic: Rash (11%)
- Gastrointestinal: Nausea (38%), vomiting (38%), diarrhea (16%), anorexia (9%)

Drug Interactions

Increased Effect/Toxicity: Increases the blood levels of amprenavir

Decreased Effect: May decrease the serum concentration of methadone in some patients

Drug Uptake

Half-life, elimination: 1.5 hours

Time to peak: 0.7-1.7 hours

Pregnancy Risk Factor C

Generic Available No

Abacavir, Lamivudine, and Zidovudine

(a BAK a veer, la MI vyoo deen, & zye DOE vyoo deen)

U.S. Brand Names Trizivir®

Pharmacologic Category Antiretroviral Agent, Reverse Transcriptase Inhibitor (Nucleoside)

Synonyms Azidothymidine, Abacavir, and Lamivudine; AZT, Abacavir, and Lamivudine; Compound S, Abacavir, and Lamivudine; Lamivudine, Abacavir, and Zidovudine; 3TC, Abacavir, and Zidovudine; ZDV, Abacavir, and Lamivudine; Zidovudine, Abacavir, and Lamivudine

Use Treatment of HIV infection (either alone or in combination with other antiretroviral agents) in patients whose regimen would otherwise contain the components of Trizivir® (based on analyses of surrogate markers in controlled studies with abacavir of up to 24 weeks; no clinical trials conducted with Trizivir®)

Local Anesthetic/Vasoconstrictor Precautions No information available to require special precautions

Effects on Dental Treatment No effects or complications reported

Dosage Oral:

Adolescents and Adults: 1 tablet twice daily; not recommended for patients <40 kg

Dosage adjustment in renal impairment: Because lamivudine and zidovudine require dosage adjustment in renal impairment, Trizivir® should not be used in patients with Cl_{cr} ≤50 mL/minute

Elderly: Use with caution

Mechanism of Action The combination of abacavir, lamivudine, and zidovudine is believed to act synergistically to inhibit reverse transcriptase via DNA chain termination after incorporation of the nucleoside analogue as well as to delay the emergence of mutations conferring resistance

Other Adverse Effects Fatal hypersensitivity reactions have occurred in patients taking abacavir (in Trizivir®). If Trizivir® is to be restarted following an interruption in therapy, first evaluate the patient for previously unsuspected symptoms of hypersensitivity. Do not restart if hypersensitivity is suspected or if hypersensitivity cannot be ruled out.

The following information is based on CNAAB3003 study data concerning effects noted in patients receiving abacavir, lamivudine, and zidovudine.

See Abacavir *on page 22*, Lamivudine *on page 683*, and Zidovudine *on page 1257* for additional information.

>10%:

Endocrine & metabolic: Increased triglycerides (25%)

Gastrointestinal: Nausea (47%), nausea and vomiting (16%), diarrhea (12%), loss of appetite/anorexia (11%)

1% to 10%:

Central nervous system: Insomnia (7%)

Miscellaneous: Hypersensitivity (5% based on abacavir component)

Other (frequency unknown): Pancreatitis, increased GGT

Drug Uptake See Abacavir *on page 22*, Lamivudine *on page 683* and Zidovudine *on page 1257*

Pregnancy Risk Factor C

Generic Available No

Abciximab (ab SIK si mab)

U.S. Brand Names ReoPro®

Canadian Brand Names ReoPro®

Pharmacologic Category Antiplatelet Agent, Glycoprotein IIb/IIIa Inhibitor

Synonyms C7E3; 7E3

Use Adjunct to percutaneous transluminal coronary angioplasty or atherectomy (PTCA) for the prevention of acute cardiac ischemic complications in patients at high risk for abrupt closure of the treated coronary vessel and patients at risk of restenosis; an adjunct with heparin to prevent cardiac ischemic complications in patients with unstable angina not responding to conventional therapy when a percutaneous coronary intervention is scheduled within 24 hours

Local Anesthetic/Vasoconstrictor Precautions No information available to require special precautions

Effects on Dental Treatment As with all anticoagulants, bleeding is a potential adverse effect of abciximab during dental surgery. Risk is dependent on multiple variables, including the intensity of anticoagulation and patient susceptibility. Medical consult is suggested. It is unlikely that ambulatory patients presenting for dental treatment will be taking intravenous anticoagulant therapy.

Dosage I.V.: 0.25 mg/kg bolus administered 10-60 minutes before the start of intervention followed by an infusion of 0.125 mcg/kg/minute (to a maximum of 10 mcg/minute) for 12 hours

Patients with unstable angina not responding to conventional medical therapy and who are planning to undergo percutaneous coronary intervention within 24 hours may be treated with abciximab 0.25 mg/kg I.V. bolus followed by an 18- to 24-hour I.V. infusion of 10 mcg/minute, concluding 1 hour after the percutaneous coronary intervention.

Mechanism of Action Fab antibody fragment of the chimeric human murine monoclonal antibody 7E3; abciximab binds to the glycoprotein GPIIb/IIIa receptor, a major receptor involved in the common pathway for platelet aggregation. Platelet aggregation is, therefore, inhibited.

Other Adverse Effects As with all drugs which may affect hemostasis, bleeding is associated with abciximab. Hemorrhage may occur at virtually any site. Risk is dependent on multiple variables, including the concurrent use of multiple agents which alter hemostasis and patient susceptibility.

>10%:

Cardiovascular: Hypotension (14.4%), chest pain (11.4%)

Gastrointestinal: Nausea (13.6%)

Hematologic: Minor bleeding (4.0% to 16.8%)

Neuromuscular & skeletal: Back pain (17.6%)

1% to 10%:

Cardiovascular: Bradycardia (4.5%), peripheral edema (1.6%)

Central nervous system: Headache (6.45)

Gastrointestinal: Vomiting (7.3%), abdominal pain (3.1%)

Hematologic: Major bleeding (1.1% to 14%), thrombocytopenia: <100,000 cells/mm^3 (2.5% to 5.6%); <50,000 cells/mm^3 (0.4% to 1.7%)

Local: Injection site pain (3.6%)

(Continued)

Abciximab *(Continued)*

Drug Interactions Increased Effect/Toxicity: The risk of bleeding is increased when given with heparin, other anticoagulants, thrombolytics, or antiplatelet drugs. However, aspirin and heparin were used concurrently in the majority of patients in the major clinical studies of abciximab. Allergic reactions may be increased in patients who have received diagnostic or therapeutic monoclonal antibodies due to the presence of HACA antibodies. Concomitant use of other glycoprotein IIb/IIIa antagonists is contraindicated.

Drug Uptake Half-life, elimination: ~30 minutes

Pregnancy Risk Factor C

Generic Available No

ABC Pack™ (Avelox®) *see* Moxifloxacin *on page 832*

Abelcet® *see* Amphotericin B Lipid Complex *on page 92*

Abreva™ [OTC] *see* Docosanol *on page 406*

Absorbine® Antifungal [OTC] *see* Tolnaftate *on page 1181*

Absorbine® Jock Itch [OTC] *see* Tolnaftate *on page 1181*

Absorbine Jr.® Antifungal [OTC] *see* Tolnaftate *on page 1181*

Acarbose (AY car bose)

Related Information

Endocrine Disorders and Pregnancy *on page 1331*

U.S. Brand Names Precose®

Canadian Brand Names Prandase®

Mexican Brand Names Glucobay®

Pharmacologic Category Antidiabetic Agent, Alpha-Glucosidase Inhibitor

Use

Monotherapy, as indicated as an adjunct to diet to lower blood glucose in patients with noninsulin-dependent diabetes mellitus (NIDDM) whose hyperglycemia cannot be managed on diet alone

Combined with a sulfonylurea, metformin, or insulin in patients with type 2 diabetes mellitus (noninsulin dependent, NIDDM) when diet plus acarbose does not result in adequate glycemic control. The effect of acarbose to enhance glycemic control is additive to that of other hypoglycemic agents when used in combination.

Local Anesthetic/Vasoconstrictor Precautions No information available to require special precautions

Effects on Dental Treatment No effects or complications reported

Dosage Oral:

Adults: Dosage must be individualized on the basis of effectiveness and tolerance while not exceeding the maximum recommended dose of 100 mg 3 times/day

Initial dose: 25 mg 3 times/day with the first bite of each main meal

Maintenance dose: Should be adjusted at 4- to 8-week intervals based on 1-hour postprandial glucose levels and tolerance. Dosage may be increased from 25 mg 3 times/day to 50 mg 3 times/day. Some patients may benefit from increasing the dose to 100 mg 3 times/day. Maintenance dose ranges: 50-100 mg 3 times/day.

Maximum dose:

≤60 kg: 50 mg 3 times/day

>60 kg: 100 mg 3 times/day

Patients receiving sulfonylureas: Acarbose given in combination with a sulfonylurea will cause a further lowering of blood glucose and may increase the hypoglycemic potential of the sulfonylurea. If hypoglycemia occurs, appropriate adjustments in the dosage of these agents should be made.

Elderly: Mean steady-state AUC and maximum concentrations of acarbose were 1.5 times higher in elderly compared to young volunteers; however, these differences were not statistically significant

Mechanism of Action Competitive inhibitor of pancreatic α-amylase and intestinal brush border α-glucosidases, resulting in delayed hydrolysis of ingested complex carbohydrates and disaccharides and absorption of glucose; dose-dependent reduction in postprandial serum insulin and glucose peaks; inhibits the metabolism of sucrose to glucose and fructose

Other Adverse Effects >10%:

Gastrointestinal: Abdominal pain (21%) and diarrhea (33%) tend to return to pretreatment levels over time, and the frequency and intensity of flatulence (77%) tend to abate with time

Hepatic: Elevated liver transaminases

Drug Interactions

Increased Effect/Toxicity: Acarbose may increase the risk of hypoglycemia when used with oral hypoglycemics.

Decreased Effect: The effect of acarbose is antagonized/decreased by thiazide and related diuretics, corticosteroids, phenothiazines, thyroid products, estrogens, oral contraceptives, phenytoin, nicotinic acid, sympathomimetics, calcium channel-blocking drugs, isoniazid, intestinal adsorbents (eg, charcoal) and digestive enzyme preparations (eg, amylase, pancreatin).

Drug Uptake Absorption: <2% absorbed as active drug

Pregnancy Risk Factor B

Generic Available No

A-Caro-25® *see* Beta-Carotene *on page 158*

Accolate® *see* Zafirlukast *on page 1253*

AccuNeb™ *see* Albuterol *on page 45*

Accupril® *see* Quinapril *on page 1031*

Accuretic™ *see* Quinapril and Hydrochlorothiazide *on page 1032*

Accutane® *see* Isotretinoin *on page 663*

Acebutolol (a se BYOO toe lole)

U.S. Brand Names Sectral®

Canadian Brand Names Apo®-Acebutolol; Gen-Acebutolol; Monitan®; Novo-Acebutolol; Nu-Acebutolol; Rhotral; Sectral®

Pharmacologic Category Antiarrhythmic Agent, Class II; Beta Blocker With Intrinsic Sympathomimetic Activity

Synonyms Acebutolol Hydrochloride

Use Treatment of hypertension, ventricular arrhythmias, angina

Local Anesthetic/Vasoconstrictor Precautions No information available to require special precautions

Effects on Dental Treatment Noncardioselective beta-blockers (ie, propranolol, nadolol) enhance the pressor response to epinephrine, resulting in hypertension and bradycardia. This has not been reported for acebutolol, a cardioselective beta-blocker. Therefore, local anesthetic with vasoconstrictor can be safely used in patients medicated with acebutolol. Many nonsteroidal anti-inflammatory drugs such as ibuprofen and indomethacin can reduce the hypotensive effect of beta-blockers after 3 or more weeks of therapy with the NSAID. Short-term NSAID use (ie, 3 days) requires no special precautions in patients taking beta-blockers.

Dosage Oral:

Adults:

- Hypertension: 400-800 mg/day (larger doses may be divided); maximum: 1200 mg/day
- Ventricular arrhythmias: Initial: 400 mg/day; maintenance: 600-1200 mg/day in divided doses

Elderly: Initial: 200-400 mg/day; dose reduction due to age related decrease in Cl_{cr} will be necessary; do not exceed 800 mg/day

Dosing adjustment in renal impairment:

- Cl_{cr} 25-49 mL/minute/1.73 m^2: Reduce dose by 50%.
- Cl_{cr} <25 mL/minute/1.73 m^2: Reduce dose by 75%.

Mechanism of Action Competitively blocks $beta_1$-adrenergic receptors with little or no effect on $beta_2$-receptors except at high doses; exhibits membrane stabilizing and intrinsic sympathomimetic activity

Other Adverse Effects

>10%: Central nervous system: Fatigue (11%)

1% to 10%:

- Cardiovascular: Chest pain (2%), edema (2%), bradycardia, hypotension, CHF
- Central nervous system: Headache (6%), dizziness (6%), insomnia (3%), depression (2%), abnormal dreams (2%), anxiety, hyperesthesia, hypoesthesia, impotence
- Dermatologic: Rash (2%), pruritus
- Gastrointestinal: Constipation (4%), diarrhea (4%), dyspepsia (4%), nausea (4%), flatulence (3%), vomiting, abdominal pain
- Genitourinary: Micturition frequency (3%), dysuria, nocturia, impotence (2%)
- Neuromuscular & skeletal: Arthralgia (2%), myalgia (2%), back pain, joint pain
- Ocular: Abnormal vision (2%), conjunctivitis, dry eyes, eye pain
- Respiratory: Dyspnea (4%), rhinitis (2%), cough (1%), pharyngitis, wheezing

Potential adverse effects (based on experience with other beta-blocking agents) include reversible mental depression, disorientation, catatonia, short-term memory loss, emotional lability, slightly clouded sensorium, laryngospasm, respiratory distress, allergic reactions, erythematous rash, agranulocytosis, purpura, thrombocytopenia, mesenteric artery thrombosis, ischemic colitis, alopecia, Peyronie's disease, claudication

Drug Interactions

Increased Effect/Toxicity: May increase the effects of other drugs which slow AV conduction (digoxin, verapamil, diltiazem), alpha-blockers (prazosin, terazosin), and alpha-adrenergic stimulants (epinephrine, phenylephrine); may mask the tachycardia from hypoglycemia caused by insulin and oral hypoglycemics. In patients receiving concurrent therapy, the risk of hypertensive crisis is increased when either clonidine or the beta-blocker is withdrawn. Reserpine has been shown to enhance the effect of acebutolol. Beta-blockers may increase the action or levels of disopyramide, nondepolarizing muscle relaxants, and theophylline although the effects are difficult to predict.

Decreased Effect: Decreased effect of acebutolol with aluminum salts, barbiturates, calcium salts, cholestyramine, colestipol, NSAIDs, penicillins (ampicillin),

(Continued)

Acebutolol *(Continued)*

rifampin, and salicylates due to decreased bioavailability and plasma concentrations. The effect of sulfonylureas may be decreased by beta-blockers; however, the decreased effect has not been shown with tolbutamide.

Drug Uptake

Onset of action: 1-2 hours
Duration: 12-24 hours
Absorption: Oral: 40%
Half-life, elimination: 6-7 hours
Time to peak: 2-4 hours

Pregnancy Risk Factor B (manufacturer); D (2nd and 3rd trimesters - expert analysis)

Generic Available Yes

Selected Readings

Foster CA and Aston SJ, "Propranolol-Epinephrine Interaction: A Potential Disaster," *Plast Reconstr Surg*, 1983, 72(1):74-8.
Wong DG, Spence JD, Lamki L, et al, "Effect of Nonsteroidal Anti-inflammatory Drugs on Control of Hypertension of Beta-Blockers and Diuretics," *Lancet*, 1986, 1(8488):997-1001.
Wynn RL, "Dental Nonsteroidal Anti-inflammatory Drugs and Prostaglandin-Based Drug Interactions, Part Two," *Gen Dent*, 1992, 40(2):104, 106, 108.
Wynn RL, "Epinephrine Interactions With Beta-Blockers," *Gen Dent*, 1994, 42(1):16, 18.

Aceon® *see* Perindopril Erbumine *on page 939*
Acephen® [OTC] *see* Acetaminophen *on page 26*

Acetaminophen (a seet a MIN oh fen)

Related Information

Acetaminophen and Pseudoephedrine *on page 30*
Acetaminophen, Dextromethorphan, and Pseudoephedrine *on page 34*
Butalbital, Acetaminophen, and Caffeine *on page 192*
Oral Pain *on page 1360*

U.S. Brand Names Acephen® [OTC]; Aspirin Free Anacin® Maximum Strength [OTC]; Cetafen® [OTC]; Cetafen Extra® [OTC]; Feverall® [OTC]; Genapap® [OTC]; Genapap® Children [OTC]; Genapap® Extra Strength [OTC]; Genapap® Infant [OTC]; Genebs® [OTC]; Genebs® Extra Strength [OTC]; Infantaire [OTC]; Liquiprin® for Children [OTC]; Mapap® [OTC]; Mapap® Children's [OTC]; Mapap® Extra Strength [OTC]; Mapap® Infants [OTC]; Redutemp® [OTC]; Silapap® Children's [OTC]; Silapap® Infants [OTC]; Tylenol® [OTC]; Tylenol® Arthritis Pain [OTC]; Tylenol® Children's [OTC]; Tylenol® Extra Strength [OTC]; Tylenol® Infants [OTC]; Tylenol® Junior Strength [OTC]; Tylenol® Sore Throat [OTC]; Valorin [OTC]; Valorin Extra [OTC]

Canadian Brand Names Abenol®; Apo®-Acetaminophen; Atasol®; Pediatrix; Tempra®; Tylenol®

Mexican Brand Names Algitrin®; Analphen; Andox®; Cilag®; Datril®; Febrin®; Magnidol®; Minofen®; Neodol; Neodolito®; Sedalito®; Sinedol; Sinedol 500; Temperal; Tempra®; Tylex®; Tylex 750; Winasorb

Pharmacologic Category Analgesic, Miscellaneous

Synonyms APAP; N-Acetyl-P-Aminophenol; Paracetamol

Use

Dental: Treatment of postoperative pain
Medical: Treatment of pain and fever; does not have anti-inflammatory effects

Local Anesthetic/Vasoconstrictor Precautions No information available to require special precautions

Effects on Dental Treatment No effects or complications reported

Dosage Oral, rectal (if fever not controlled with acetaminophen alone, administer with full doses of aspirin on an every 4- to 6-hour schedule, if aspirin is not otherwise contraindicated):

Children <12 years: 10-15 mg/kg/dose every 4-6 hours as needed; do **not** exceed 5 doses (2.6 g) in 24 hours; alternatively, the following age-based doses may be used (see table).

Acetaminophen Dosing

Age	Dosage (mg)	Age	Dosage (mg)
0-3 mo	40	4-5 y	240
4-11 mo	80	6-8 y	320
1-2 y	120	9-10 y	400
2-3 y	160	11 y	480

Adults: 325-650 mg every 4-6 hours or 1000 mg 3-4 times/day; do **not** exceed 4 g/day

Dosing interval in renal impairment:

Cl_{cr} 10-50 mL/minute: Administer every 6 hours
Cl_{cr} <10 mL/minute: Administer every 8 hours (metabolites accumulate)

Hemodialysis: Moderately dialyzable (20% to 50%)

Dosing adjustment/comments in hepatic impairment: Use with caution. Limited, low-dose therapy usually well tolerated in hepatic disease/cirrhosis. However, cases of hepatotoxicity at daily acetaminophen dosages <4 g/day have been reported. Avoid chronic use in hepatic impairment.

Mechanism of Action Inhibits the synthesis of prostaglandins in the CNS and peripherally blocks pain impulse generation; produces antipyresis by inhibition of hypothalamic heat-regulating center

Other Adverse Effects Frequency not defined:

Endocrine & metabolic: May increase chloride, uric acid, glucose; may decrease sodium, bicarbonate, calcium

Hepatic: May increase bilirubin, alkaline phosphatase

Renal: May increase ammonia

<1%: Rash, nausea, vomiting, blood dyscrasias (neutropenia, pancytopenia, leukopenia), anemia, analgesic nephropathy, nephrotoxicity with chronic overdose, hypersensitivity reactions (rare)

Contraindications Hypersensitivity to acetaminophen or any component of the formulation; G6PD deficiency

Warnings/Precautions May cause severe hepatic toxicity on overdose; use with caution in patients with alcoholic liver disease; chronic daily dosing in adults of 5-8 g of acetaminophen over several weeks or 3-4 g/day of acetaminophen for 1 year have resulted in liver damage

Drug Interactions

CYP1A2 enzyme substrate (minor), CYP2A6, CYP2C9, CYP2D6, CYP2E1 and 3A3/4 enzyme substrate

Increased Effect/Toxicity: Barbiturates, carbamazepine, hydantoins, isoniazid, rifampin, sulfinpyrazone may increase the hepatotoxic potential of acetaminophen; chronic ethanol abuse increases risk for acetaminophen toxicity; effect of warfarin may be enhanced

Decreased Effect: Barbiturates, carbamazepine, hydantoins, rifampin, sulfinpyrazone may decrease the analgesic effect of acetaminophen; cholestyramine may decrease acetaminophen absorption (separate dosing by at least 1 hour)

Dietary/Ethanol/Herb Considerations

Ethanol: Avoid or limit to <3 drinks/day; may cause hepatotoxicity.

Food: Administer oral form with food or milk; may decrease peak serum concentration and slightly delay absorption of extended-release form. Rate of absorption may be decreased with food high in carbohydrates.

Herb/Nutraceutical: Avoid St John's wort; may decrease serum concentration.

Drug Uptake

Onset of action: <1 hour

Duration: 4-6 hours

Half-life, elimination: Neonates: 2-5 hours; Adults: 1-3 hours

Time to peak: Oral: 10-60 minutes; may be delayed in acute overdoses

Pregnancy Risk Factor B

Breast-feeding Considerations May be taken while breast-feeding

Dosage Forms CAP: 500 mg. **CAPLET:** 500 mg. **CAPLET, extended release:** 650 mg. **ELIX:** 160 mg/5 mL (5 mL, 10 mL, 20 mL, 120 mL, 240 mL, 480 mL, 500 mL, 3780 mL). **GELCAP:** 500 mg. **GELTAB:** 500 mg. **LIQ, oral:** 160 mg/5 mL (120 mL, 240 mL, 480 mL, 3870 mL); 500 mg/15 mL (120 mL, 240 mL). **SOLN, oral drops:** 80 mg/0.8 mL (15 mL, 30 mL); 100 mg/mL (15 mL, 30 mL). **SUPP, rectal:** 80 mg, 120 mg, 325 mg, 650 mg. **SUSP, oral:** 160 mg/5 mL (120 mL, 240 mL). **SUSP, oral drops:** 80 mg/0.8 mL (15 mL, 30 mL); 100 mg/mL (15 mL, 30 mL). **SYR, oral:** 160 mg/5 mL (120 mL). **TAB:** 160 mg, 325 mg, 500 mg. **TAB, chewable:** 80 mg, 160 mg

Generic Available Yes

Comments Doses of acetaminophen >5 g/day for several weeks can produce severe, often fatal liver damage. Hepatotoxicity caused by acetaminophen is potentiated by chronic ethanol consumption. It has been reported that a combination of two quarts of whiskey a day with 8-10 acetaminophen tablets daily resulted in severe liver toxicity. People who consume ethanol at the same time that they use acetaminophen, even in therapeutic doses, are at risk of developing hepatotoxicity.

A study by Hylek, et al, suggested that the combination of acetaminophen with warfarin (Coumadin®) may cause enhanced anticoagulation. The following recommendations have been made by Hylek, et al, and supported by an editorial in *JAMA* by Bell.

Dose and duration of acetaminophen should be as low as possible, individualized and monitored.

The study by Hylek reported the following:

For patients who reported taking the equivalent of at least 4 regular strength (325 mg) tablets for longer than a week, the odds of having an INR >6.0 were increased 10-fold above those not taking acetaminophen. Risk decreased with lower intakes of acetaminophen reaching a background level of risk at a dose of 6 or fewer 325 mg tablets per week.

(Continued)

Acetaminophen *(Continued)*

Selected Readings

Ahmad N, Grad HA, Haas DA, et al, "The Efficacy of Nonopioid Analgesics for Postoperative Dental Pain: A Meta-Analysis," *Anesth Prog*, 1997, 44(4):119-26.

Bell WR, "Acetaminophen and Warfarin: Undesirable Synergy," *JAMA*, 1998, 279(9):702-3.

Botting RM, "Mechanism of Action of Acetaminophen: Is There a Cyclooxygenase 3?," *Clin Infect Dis*, 2000, Suppl 5:S202-10.

Dart RC, Kuffner EK, and Rumack BH, "Treatment of Pain or Fever with Paracetamol (Acetaminophen) in the Alcoholic Patient: A Systematic Review," *Am J Ther*, 2000, 7(2):123-34.

Dionne R, "Additive Analgesia Without Opioid Side Effects," *Compend Contin Educ Dent*, 2000, 21(7):572-4, 576-7.

Dionne RA and Berthold CW, "Therapeutic Uses of Nonsteroidal Anti-Inflammatory Drugs in Dentistry," *Crit Rev Oral Biol Med*, 2001, 12(4):315-30.

Dionne RA, Campbell RA, Cooper SA, et al, "Suppression of Postoperative Pain by Preoperative Administration of Ibuprofen in Comparison to Placebo, Acetaminophen, and Acetaminophen Plus Codeine," *J Clin Pharmacol*, 1983, 23(1):37-43.

Grant JA and Weiler JM, "A Report of a Rare Immediate Reaction After Ingestion of Acetaminophen," *Ann Allergy Asthma Immunol*, 2001, 87(3):227-9.

Hylek EM, Heiman H, Skates SJ, et al, "Acetaminophen and Other Risk Factors for Excessive Warfarin Anticoagulation," *JAMA*, 1998, 279(9):657-62.

Kwan D, Bartle WR, and Walker SE, "The Effects of Acetaminophen on Pharmacokinetics and Pharmacodynamics of Warfarin," *J Clin Pharmacol*, 1999, 39(1):68-75.

Lee WM, "Drug-Induced Hepatotoxicity," *N Engl J Med*, 1995, 333(17):1118-27.

Licht H, Seeff LB, and Zimmerman HJ, "Apparent Potentiation of Acetaminophen Hepatotoxicity by Alcohol," *Ann Intern Med*, 1980, 92(4):511.

McClain CJ, Price S, Barve S, et al, "Acetaminophen Hepatotoxicity: An Update," *Curr Gastroenterol Rep*, 1999, 1(1):42-9.

Murphy R, Swartz R, and Watkins PB, "Severe Acetaminophen Toxicity in a Patient Receiving Isoniazid," *Ann Intern Med*, 1990, 113(110):799-800.

Nguyen AM, Graham DY, Gage T, et al, "Nonsteroidal Anti-Inflammatory Drug Use in Dentistry: Gastrointestinal Implications," *Gen Dent*, 1999, 47(6):590-6.

Shek KL, Chan LN, and Nutescu E, "Warfarin-Acetaminophen Drug Interaction Revisited," *Pharmacotherapy*, 1999, 19(10):1153-8.

Tanaka E, Yamazaki K, and Misawa S, "Update: The Clinical Importance of Acetaminophen Hepatotoxicity in Nonalcoholic and Alcoholic Subjects," *J Clin Pharm Ther*, 2000, 25(5):325-32.

Acetaminophen and Codeine (a seet a MIN oh fen & KOE deen)

Related Information

Acetaminophen *on page 26*

U.S. Brand Names Capital® and Codeine; Phenaphen® With Codeine; Tylenol® With Codeine

Canadian Brand Names Empracet®-30; Empracet®-60; Emtec-30; Lenoltec; Triatec-8; Triatec-8 Strong; Triatec-30; Tylenol® with Codeine

Mexican Brand Names Tylex CD

Pharmacologic Category Analgesic, Narcotic

Synonyms Codeine and Acetaminophen

Use

Dental: Treatment of postoperative pain

Medical: Relief of mild to moderate pain

Local Anesthetic/Vasoconstrictor Precautions No information available to require special precautions

Effects on Dental Treatment <1%: Xerostomia

Restrictions C-III; C-V

Dosage Doses should be adjusted according to severity of pain and response of the patient. Adult doses ≥60 mg codeine fail to give commensurate relief of pain but merely prolong analgesia and are associated with an appreciably increased incidence of side effects.

Oral:

- Children: Analgesic:
  - Codeine: 0.5-1 mg codeine/kg/dose every 4-6 hours
  - Acetaminophen: 10-15 mg/kg/dose every 4 hours up to a maximum of 2.6 g/24 hours for children <12 years; **alternatively, the following can be used:**
    - 3-6 years: 5 mL 3-4 times/day as needed of elixir
    - 7-12 years: 10 mL 3-4 times/day as needed of elixir
    - >12 years: 15 mL every 4 hours as needed of elixir
- Adults:
  - Antitussive: Based on codeine (15-30 mg/dose) every 4-6 hours (maximum: 360 mg/24 hours based on codeine component)
  - Analgesic: Based on codeine (30-60 mg/dose) every 4-6 hours (maximum: 4000 mg/24 hours based on acetaminophen component)
- **Dosing adjustment in renal impairment:** See Acetaminophen *on page 26* and Codeine *on page 317*

Mechanism of Action Inhibits the synthesis of prostaglandins in the CNS and peripherally blocks pain impulse generation; produces antipyresis from inhibition of hypothalamic heat-regulating center; binds to opiate receptors in the CNS, causing inhibition of ascending pain pathways, altering the perception of and response to pain; causes cough supression by direct central action in the medulla; produces generalized CNS depression

Other Adverse Effects

>10%:

Central nervous system: Lightheadedness, dizziness, sedation
Gastrointestinal: Nausea, vomiting
Respiratory: Dyspnea

1% to 10%:

Central nervous system: Euphoria, dysphoria
Dermatologic: Pruritus
Gastrointestinal: Constipation, abdominal pain
Miscellaneous: Histamine release

<1%: Palpitations, hypotension, bradycardia, peripheral vasodilation, increased intracranial pressure, antidiuretic hormone release, biliary tract spasm, urinary retention, miosis, respiratory depression, physical and psychological dependence

Contraindications Hypersensitivity to acetaminophen, codeine phosphate, similar compounds, or any component of their formulation

Warnings/Precautions Use with caution in patients with hypersensitivity reactions to other phenanthrene derivative opioid agonists (morphine, hydrocodone, hydromorphone, levorphanol, oxycodone, oxymorphone); respiratory diseases including asthma, emphysema, COPD, or severe liver or renal insufficiency; some preparations contain sulfites which may cause allergic reactions; may be habit-forming

Enhanced analgesia has been seen in elderly patients on therapeutic doses of narcotics; duration of action may be increased in the elderly; the elderly may be particularly susceptible to the CNS depressant and constipating effects of narcotics

Drug Interactions Increased Effect/Toxicity: CNS depressants, phenothiazines, tricyclic antidepressants, guanabenz, MAO inhibitors (may also decrease BP); effect of warfarin may be enhanced

Dietary/Ethanol/Herb Considerations

Ethanol: Excessive intake may increase risk of acetaminophen-induced hepatotoxicity; avoid use or limit to <3 drinks/day.

Food: May be taken with food

Drug Uptake See Acetaminophen *on page 26* and Codeine *on page 317*

Pregnancy Risk Factor C

Breast-feeding Considerations Both acetaminophen and codeine may be taken while breast-feeding

Dosage Forms CAP [C-III]: #3: (Phenaphen® With Codeine): Acetaminophen 325 mg and codeine phosphate 30 mg. **ELIX, oral** [C-V]: Acetaminophen 120 mg and codeine phosphate 12 mg per 5 mL (5 mL, 10 mL, 12.5 mL, 15 mL, 120 mL, 480 mL, 3840 mL); (Tylenol® with Codeine): Acetaminophen 120 mg and codeine phosphate 12 mg per 5 mL (480 mL). **SUSP, oral** [C-V] (Capital® and Codeine): Acetaminophen 120 mg and codeine phosphate 12 mg per 5 mL (480 mL). **TAB** [C-III]: #2: Acetaminophen 300 mg and codeine phosphate 15 mg; #3 (Tylenol® with Codeine): Acetaminophen 300 mg and codeine phosphate 30 mg; #4 (Tylenol® with Codeine): Acetaminophen 300 mg and codeine phosphate 60 mg

Generic Available Yes

Comments Codeine products, as with other narcotic analgesics, are recommended only for acute dosing (ie, 3 days or less). The most common adverse effect you will see in your dental patients from codeine is nausea, followed by sedation and constipation. Codeine has narcotic addiction liability, especially when given long-term. Because of the acetaminophen component, this product should be used with caution in patients with alcoholic liver disease.

A study by Hylek, et al, suggested that the combination of acetaminophen with warfarin (Coumadin®) may cause enhanced anticoagulation. The following recommendations have been made by Hylek, et al, and supported by an editorial in *JAMA* by Bell.

Dose and duration of acetaminophen should be as low as possible, individualized and monitored.

The study by Hylek reported the following:

For patients who reported taking the equivalent of at least 4 regular strength (325 mg) tablets for longer than a week, the odds of having an INR >6.0 were increased 10-fold above those not taking acetaminophen. Risk decreased with lower intakes of acetaminophen reaching a background level of risk at a dose of 6 or fewer 325 mg tablets per week.

Selected Readings

Change DJ, Fricke JR, Bird SR, et al, "Rofecoxib Versus Codeine/Acetaminophen in Postoperative Dental Pain: A Double-Blind, Randomized, Placebo- and Active Comparator-Controlled Clinical Trial," *Clin Ther*, 2001, 23(9):1446-55.

Dionne RA, "New Approaches to Preventing and Treating Postoperative Pain," *J Am Dent Assoc*, 1992, 123(6):26-34.

Forbes JA, Butterworth GA, Burchfield WH, et al, "Evaluation of Ketorolac, Aspirin, and an Acetaminophen-Codeine Combination in Postoperative Oral Surgery Pain," *Pharmacotherapy*, 1990, 10(6 Pt 2):77S-93S.

Gobetti JP, "Controlling Dental Pain," *J Am Dent Assoc*, 1992, 123(6):47-52.

Mullican WS and Lacy JR, "Tramadol/Acetaminophen Combination Tablets and Codeine/Acetaminophen Combination Capsules for the Management of Chronic Pain: A Comparative Trial," *Clin Ther*, 2001, 23(9):1429-45.

(Continued)

Acetaminophen and Codeine *(Continued)*

Wynn RL, "Narcotic Analgesics for Dental Pain: Available Products, Strengths, and Formulations," *Gen Dent*, 2001, 49(2):126-8, 130, 132 passim.

Acetaminophen and Diphenhydramine

(a seet a MIN oh fen & dye fen HYE dra meen)

U.S. Brand Names Anacin PM Aspirin Free [OTC]; Excedrin® P.M. [OTC]; Goody's PM® Powder; Legatrin PM® [OTC]; Tylenol® PM Extra Strength [OTC]; Tylenol® Severe Allergy [OTC]

Pharmacologic Category Analgesic, Miscellaneous

Synonyms Diphenhydramine and Acetaminophen

Use Relief of mild to moderate pain, sinus headache; aid in the relief of insomnia

Local Anesthetic/Vasoconstrictor Precautions No information available to require special precautions

Effects on Dental Treatment 1% to 10%: Xerostomia

Dosage Adults: Oral: Take 2 caplets or 5 mL of liquid at bedtime or as directed by physician; do not exceed recommended dosage; not for use in children <12 years of age

Other Adverse Effects See Acetaminophen *on page 26* and diphenhydramine *on page 398*

Drug Uptake See Acetaminophen *on page 26* and Diphenhydramine *on page 398*

Generic Available Yes

Selected Readings

Barker JD Jr, de Carle DJ, and Anuras S, "Chronic Excessive Acetaminophen Use in Liver Damage," *Ann Intern Med*, 1977, 87(3):299-301.

Acetaminophen and Phenyltoloxamine

(a seet a MIN oh fen & fen il to LOKS a meen)

U.S. Brand Names Genesec® [OTC]; Percogesic® [OTC]; Phenylgesic® [OTC]

Pharmacologic Category Analgesic, Non-narcotic

Synonyms Phenyltoloxamine and Acetaminophen

Use Relief of mild to moderate pain

Local Anesthetic/Vasoconstrictor Precautions No information available to require special precautions

Effects on Dental Treatment No effects or complications reported

Dosage Oral:

Analgesic: Based on acetaminophen component:

Children: 10-15 mg/kg/dose every 4-6 hours as needed; do **not** exceed 5 doses/24 hours

Adults: 325-650 every 4-6 hours as needed; do **not** exceed 4 g/day

Product labeling:

Percogesic®:

Children 6-12 years: 1 tablet every 4 hours; do **not** exceed 4 tablets/24 hours

Adults: 1-2 tablets every 4 hours; do **not** exceed 8 tablets/24 hours

Pregnancy Risk Factor B

Generic Available Yes

Selected Readings

Botting RM, "Mechanism of Action of Acetaminophen: Is There a Cyclooxygenase 3?," *Clin Infect Dis*, 2000, Suppl 5:S202-10.

Dart RC, Kuffner EK, and Rumack BH, "Treatment of Pain or Fever with Paracetamol (Acetaminophen) in the Alcoholic Patient: A Systematic Review," *Am J Ther*, 2000, 7(2):123-34.

Dionne RA, Campbell RA, Cooper SA, et al, "Suppression of Postoperative Pain by Preoperative Administration of Ibuprofen in Comparison to Placebo, Acetaminophen, and Acetaminophen Plus Codeine," *J Clin Pharmacol*, 1983, 23(1):37-43.

Grant JA and Weiler JM, "A Report of a Rare Immediate Reaction After Ingestion of Acetaminophen," *Ann Allergy Asthma Immunol*, 2001, 87(3):227-9.

Kwan D, Bartle WR, and Walker SE, "The Effects of Acetaminophen on Pharmacokinetics and Pharmacodynamics of Warfarin," *J Clin Pharmacol*, 1999, 39(1):68-75.

Licht H, Seeff LB, and Zimmerman HJ, "Apparent Potentiation of Acetaminophen Hepatotoxicity by Alcohol," *Ann Intern Med*, 1980, 92(4):511.

McClain CJ, Price S, Barve S, et al, "Acetaminophen Hepatotoxicity: An Update," *Curr Gastroenterol Rep*, 1999, 1(1):42-9.

Shek KL, Chan LN, and Nutescu E, "Warfarin-Acetaminophen Drug Interaction Revisited," *Pharmacotherapy*, 1999, 19(10):1153-8.

Tanaka E, Yamazaki K, and Misawa S, "Update: The Clinical Importance of Acetaminophen Hepatotoxicity in Nonalcoholic and Alcoholic Subjects," *J Clin Pharm Ther*, 2000, 25(5):325-32.

Acetaminophen and Pseudoephedrine

(a seet a MIN oh fen & soo doe e FED rin)

U.S. Brand Names Alka-Seltzer Plus® Cold and Sinus [OTC]; Children's Tylenol® Sinus [OTC]; Infants Tylenol® Cold [OTC]; Medi-Synal [OTC]; Ornex® [OTC]; Ornex® Maximum Strength [OTC]; Sinus-Relief® [OTC]; Sinutab® Sinus Maximum Strength Without Drowsiness [OTC]; Sudafed® Cold and Sinus [OTC]; Sudafed® Sinus Headache [OTC]; Tylenol® Sinus Non-Drowsy [OTC]

Canadian Brand Names Dristan® N.D.; Dristan® N.D., Extra Strength; Sinutab® Non Drowsy; Sudafed® Head Cold and Sinus Extra Strength; Tylenol® Decongestant; Tylenol® Sinus

Pharmacologic Category Alpha/Beta Agonist; Analgesic, Miscellaneous
Synonyms Pseudoephedrine and Acetaminophen
Use Relief of mild to moderate pain, congestion
Local Anesthetic/Vasoconstrictor Precautions No information available to require special precautions
Effects on Dental Treatment No effects or complications reported
Dosage Oral:
Analgesic: Based on acetaminophen component:
Children: 10-15 mg/kg/dose every 4-6 hours as needed; do **not** exceed 5 doses in 24 hours
Adults: 325-650 mg every 4-6 hours as needed; do **not** exceed 4 g/day
Decongestant: Based on pseudoephedrine component:
Children:
2-6 years: 15 mg every 4 hours; do **not** exceed 90 mg/day
6-12 years: 30 mg every 4 hours; do **not** exceed 180 mg/day
Children >12 years and Adults: 60 mg every 4 hours; do **not** exceed 360 mg/day
Product labeling:
Alka-Seltzer Plus® Cold and Sinus:
Children 6-12 years: 1 dose with water every 4 hours (maximum: 4 doses/24 hours)
Adults: 2 doses with water every 4 hours (maximum: 4 doses/24 hours)
Children's Tylenol® Sinus: Children:
Liquid:
2-5 years (24-47 lbs): 1 teaspoonful every 4-6 hours (maximum: 4 doses/24 hours)
6-11 years (48-95 lbs): 2 teaspoonfuls every 4-6 hours (maximum: 4 doses/24 hours)
Tablet, chewable:
2-5 years (24-47 lbs): 2 tablets every 4-6 hours (maximum: 4 doses/24 hours)
6-11 years (48-95 lbs): 4 tablets every 4-6 hours (maximum: 4 doses/24 hours)
Sine-Aid® Maximum Strength, Tylenol® Sinus Maximum Strength: Children >12 years and Adults: 2 doses every 4-6 hours (maximum: 8 doses/24 hours)
Sinutab® Sinus Maximum Strength Without Drowsiness, Tavist® Sinus: Children >12 years and Adults: 2 doses every 6 hours; (maximum: 8 doses/24 hours)
Other Adverse Effects See Acetaminophen *on page 26* and Pseudoephedrine *on page 1022*
Drug Uptake See Acetaminophen *on page 26* and Pseudoephedrine *on page 1022*
Generic Available Yes

Acetaminophen and Tramadol (a seet a MIN oh fen & TRA ma dole)

U.S. Brand Names Ultracet™
Pharmacologic Category Analgesic, Non-narcotic; Analgesic, Miscellaneous
Synonyms APAP and Tramadol; Tramadol Hydrochloride and Acetaminophen
Use Short-term (≤5 days) management of acute pain
Local Anesthetic/Vasoconstrictor Precautions No information available to require special precautions
Effects on Dental Treatment No effects or complications reported
Dosage Oral: Adults: Acute pain: Two tablets every 4-6 hours as needed for pain relief (maximum: 8 tablets/day); treatment should not exceed 5 days
Dosage adjustment in renal impairment: Cl_{cr} <30 mL/minute: Maximum of 2 tablets every 12 hours; treatment should not exceed 5 days
Dosage adjustment in hepatic impairment: Use not recommended.
Mechanism of Action
Based on **acetaminophen** component: Inhibits the synthesis of prostaglandins in the CNS and peripherally blocks pain impulse generation; produces antipyresis from inhibition of hypothalamic heat-regulating center
Based on **tramadol** component: Binds to μ-opiate receptors in the CNS causing inhibition of ascending pain pathways, altering the perception of and response to pain; also inhibits the reuptake of norepinephrine and serotonin, which also modifies the ascending pain pathway
Other Adverse Effects
1% to 10%:
Central nervous system: Somnolence (6%), dizziness (3%), insomnia (2%), anxiety, confusion, euphoria, fatigue, headache, nervousness, somnolence, tremor
Dermatologic: Pruritus (2%), rash
Endocrine & metabolic: Hot flashes
Gastrointestinal: Constipation (6%), anorexia (3%), diarrhea (3%), nausea (3%), xerostomia (2%), abdominal pain, dyspepsia, flatulence, vomiting
Genitourinary: Prostatic disorder (2%)
Neuromuscular & skeletal: Weakness
Miscellaneous: Diaphoresis increased (4%)
<1%: Abnormal thinking, abnormal vision, albuminuria, amnesia, anemia, arrhythmia, ataxia, chest pain, convulsions, depersonalization, drug abuse,
(Continued)

Acetaminophen and Tramadol *(Continued)*

dysphagia, dyspnea, emotional lability, hallucination, hypertension, hypotension, hypertonia, impotence, liver function abnormalities, melena, micturition disorder, migraine, muscle contractions (involuntary), oliguria, palpitation, paresthesia, paroniria, rigors, stupor, syncope, tachycardia, tinnitus, tongue edema, urinary retention, weight loss, withdrawal syndrome, vertigo

Postmarketing and/or case reports: Agitation, allergic reactions, anaphylactoid reactions, anaphylaxis, cognitive dysfunction, coma, depression, diaphoresis, difficulty concentrating, fever, gastrointestinal bleeding, hepatitis, hyper-reflexia, mental status change, myocardial ischemia, orthostatic hypotension, liver failure, pulmonary edema, seizures, serotonin syndrome, shivering, Stevens-Johnson syndrome, suicidal tendency, toxic epidermal necrolysis, urticaria, vasodilation

Contraindications Hypersensitivity to acetaminophen, tramadol, opioids, or any component of their formulation; opioid-dependency; acute intoxication with ethanol, hypnotics, narcotics, centrally-acting analgesics, opioids, or psychotropic drugs; hepatic dysfunction

Warnings/Precautions Should be used only with extreme caution in patients receiving MAO inhibitors. Use with caution and reduce dosage when administering to patients receiving other CNS depressants. Seizures may occur when taken within the recommended dosage; risk is increased in patients receiving serotonin reuptake inhibitors (SSRIs or anorectics), tricyclic antidepressants, other cyclic compounds (including cyclobenzaprine, promethazine), neuroleptics, MAO inhibitors, or drugs which may lower seizure threshold. Patients with a history of seizures, or with a risk of seizures (head trauma, metabolic disorders, CNS infection, or malignancy, or during alcohol/drug withdrawal) are also at increased risk. Do not use with ethanol or other acetaminophen- or tramadol-containing products.

Elderly patients and patients with chronic respiratory disorders may be at greater risk of adverse events. Use with caution in patients with increased intracranial pressure or head injury. Use tramadol with caution and reduce dosage in patients with renal dysfunction and in patients with myxedema, hypothyroidism, or hypoadrenalism. Tolerance or drug dependence may result from extended use; abrupt discontinuation should be avoided. Safety and efficacy in pediatric patients have not been established.

Drug Interactions

Acetaminophen: CYP1A2, 2E1, and 3A3/4 enzyme substrate

Tramadol: CYP2D6 and 3A3/4 (minor) enzyme substrate

Amphetamines: May increase the risk of seizures with tramadol.

Anesthetic agents: May increase risk of CNS and respiratory depression; use together with caution and in reduced dosage.

Barbiturates: Barbiturates may increase the hepatotoxic effects of acetaminophen; in addition, acetaminophen levels may be lowered.

Carbamazepine: Carbamazepine decreases half-life of tramadol by 33% to 50%; also have increase risk of seizures; in addition, carbamazepine may increase the hepatotoxic effects and lower serum concentration of acetaminophen; concomitant use is not recommended.

CYP2D6 inhibitors: May increase tramadol serum concentration.

Digoxin: Rare reports of digoxin toxicity with concomitant tramadol use.

Hydantoin anticonvulsants: Phenytoin may increase the hepatotoxic effects of acetaminophen; in addition, acetaminophen levels may be lowered.

SSRIs: May increase the risk of seizures with tramadol by inhibiting CYP metabolism. Includes citalopram, fluoxetine, paroxetine, sertraline.

MAO inhibitors: May increases the risk of seizures.

Naloxone: May increase the risk of seizures (if administered in tramadol overdose).

Neuroleptic agents: May increase the risk of tramadol-associated seizures and may have additive CNS depressant effects.

Narcotics: May increase risk of CNS and respiratory depression; use together with caution and in reduced dosage.

Opioids: May increase the risk of seizures, and may have additive CNS depressant effects. Use together with caution and in reduced dosage.

Phenothiazines: May increase risk of CNS and respiratory depression; use together with caution and in reduced dosage.

Rifampin: Rifampin may increase the clearance of acetaminophen.

Quinidine: May increase the tramadol serum concentration by inhibiting CYP metabolism.

Sulfinpyrazone: Sulfinpyrazone may increase the hepatotoxic effects of acetaminophen; in addition, acetaminophen levels may be lowered.

Tricyclic antidepressants: May increase the risk of seizures.

Warfarin: Acetaminophen and tramadol may lead to an elevation of prothrombin times; monitor.

Dietary/Ethanol/Herb Considerations

Ethanol: Concomitant use increases liver toxicity.

Food may delay time to peak plasma concentrations; extent of absorption not affected.

Herb/Nutraceutical:

Based on **acetaminophen** component: Avoid St John's wort; may decrease acetaminophen levels.

Based on **tramadol** component: Avoid gotu kola, kava, SAMe, St John's wort, and valerian; may increase CNS depression.

Drug Uptake See Acetaminophen *on page 26* and Tramadol *on page 1187*

Pregnancy Risk Factor C

Breast-feeding Considerations Not recommended for postdelivery analgesia in nursing mothers.

Dosage Forms TAB: Acetaminophen 325 mg and tramadol 37.5 mg

Generic Available No

Selected Readings

Wynn RL, "NSAIDS and Cardiovascular Effects, Celecoxib for Dental Pain, and a New Analgesic - Tramadol with Acetaminophen," *Gen Dent*, 2002, 50(3):218-222.

Acetaminophen, Aspirin, and Caffeine

(a seet a MIN oh fen, AS pir in, & KAF een)

U.S. Brand Names Excedrin® Extra Strength [OTC]; Excedrin® Migraine [OTC]; Genaced [OTC]; Goody's® Extra Strength Headache Powder [OTC]; Vanquish® Extra Strength Pain Reliever [OTC]

Pharmacologic Category Analgesic, Miscellaneous

Synonyms Aspirin, Acetaminophen, and Caffeine; Aspirin, Caffeine and Acetaminophen; Caffeine, Acetaminophen, and Aspirin; Caffeine, Aspirin, and Acetaminophen

Use Relief of mild to moderate pain; pain associated with migraine headache

Local Anesthetic/Vasoconstrictor Precautions No information available to require special precautions

Effects on Dental Treatment No effects or complications reported

Dosage Oral: Adults:

Analgesic:

Based on **acetaminophen** component:

Mild to moderate pain: 325-650 mg every 4-6 hours as needed; do **not** exceed 4 g/day

Mild to moderate pain associated with migraine headache: 500 mg/dose (in combination with 500 mg aspirin and 130 mg caffeine) every 6 hours while symptoms persist; do not use for longer than 48 hours

Based on **aspirin** component:

Mild to moderate pain: 325-650 mg every 4-6 hours as needed; do **not** exceed 4 g/day

Mild to moderate pain associated with migraine headache: 500 mg/dose (in combination with 500 mg acetaminophen and 130 mg caffeine) every 6 hours; do not use for longer than 48 hours

Product labeling:

Excedrin® Extra Strength, Excedrin® Migraine: Children >12 years and Adults: 2 doses every 6 hours (maximum: 8 doses/24 hours)

Note: When used for migraine, do not use for longer than 48 hours

Goody's® Extra Strength Headache Powder: Children >12 years and Adults: 1 powder, placed on tongue or dissolved in water, every 4-6 hours (maximum: 4 powders/24 hours)

Goody's® Extra Strength Pain Relief Tablets: Children >12 years and Adults: 2 tablets every 4-6 hours (maximum: 8 tablets/24 hours)

Vanquish® Extra Strength Pain Reliever: Children >12 years and Adults: 2 tablets every 4 hours (maximum: 12 tablets/24 hours)

Other Adverse Effects See Acetaminophen *on page 26* and Aspirin *on page 119*

Drug Uptake See Acetaminophen *on page 26* and Aspirin *on page 119*

Pregnancy Risk Factor D

Generic Available Yes

Selected Readings

Desjardins PJ, Cooper SA, Gallegos TL, et al, "The Relative Analgesic Efficacy of Propiram Fumarate, Codeine Aspirin, and Placebo in Postimpaction Dental Pain," *J Clin Pharmacol*, 1984, 24(1):35-42.

Forbes JA, Butterworth GA, Burchfield WH, et al, "Evaluation of Ketorolac, Aspirin, and an Acetaminophen-Codeine Combination in Postoperative Oral Surgery Pain," *Pharmacotherapy*, 1990, 10(6 Pt 2):77S-93S.

Forbes JA, Keller CK, Smith JW, et al, "Analgesic Effect of Naproxen Sodium, Codeine, a Naproxen-Codeine Combination and Aspirin on the Postoperative Pain of Oral Surgery," *Pharmacotherapy*, 1986, 6(5):211-8.

Acetaminophen, Chlorpheniramine, and Pseudoephedrine

(a seet a MIN oh fen, klor fen IR a meen, & soo doe e FED rin)

U.S. Brand Names Alka-Seltzer® Plus Cold Liqui-Gels® [OTC]; Children's Tylenol® Cold [OTC]; Comtrex® Allergy-Sinus [OTC]; Sinutab® Sinus Allergy Maximum Strength [OTC]; Thera-Flu® Flu and Cold; Tylenol® Allergy Sinus [OTC]

Canadian Brand Names Sinutab® Sinus & Allergy; Tylenol® Allergy Sinus; Tylenol® Cold

Pharmacologic Category Analgesic, Miscellaneous; Antihistamine

(Continued)

Acetaminophen, Chlorpheniramine, and Pseudoephedrine *(Continued)*

Synonyms Acetaminophen, Pseudoephedrine, and Chlorpheniramine; Chlorpheniramine, Acetaminophen, and Pseudoephedrine; Chlorpheniramine, Pseudoephedrine, and Acetaminophen; Pseudoephedrine, Acetaminophen, and Chlorpheniramine; Pseudoephedrine, Chlorpheniramine, and Acetaminophen

Use Temporary relief of sinus symptoms

Local Anesthetic/Vasoconstrictor Precautions Use with caution since pseudoephedrine is a sympathomimetic amine which could interact with epinephrine to cause a pressor response

Effects on Dental Treatment

Chlorpheniramine: Prolonged use will cause significant xerostomia

Pseudoephedrine: Up to 10% of patients could experience tachycardia, palpitations, and xerostomia; use vasoconstrictor with caution

Dosage Oral:

Analgesic: Based on **acetaminophen** component:
- Children: 10-15 mg/kg/dose every 4-6 hours as needed; do **not** exceed 5 doses in 24 hours
- Adults: 325-650 mg every 4-6 hours as needed; do **not** exceed 4 g/day

Antihistamine: Based on chlorpheniramine maleate component:
- Children:
  - 2-6 years: 1 mg every 4-6 hours (maximum: 6 mg/24 hours)
  - 6-12 years: 2 mg every 4-6 hours (maximum: 12 mg/24 hours)
- Children >12 years and Adults: 4 mg every 4-6 hours (maximum: 24 mg/24 hours)

Decongestant: Based on **pseudoephedrine** component:
- Children:
  - 2-6 years: 15 mg every 4 hours (maximum: 90 mg/24 hours)
  - 6-12 years: 30 mg every 4 hours (maximum: 180 mg/24 hours)
- Children >12 years and Adults: 60 mg every 4 hours (maximum: 360 mg/24 hours)

Product labeling:

Alka-Seltzer Plus® Cold Medicine Liqui-Gels®:
- Children 6-12 years: 1 softgel every 4 hours with water (maximum: 4 doses/24 hours)
- Children >12 years and Adults: 2 softgels every 4 hours with water (maximum: 4 doses/24 hours)

Sinutab® Sinus Allergy Maximum Strength: Children >12 years and Adults: 2 tablets/caplets every 6 hours (maximum: 8 doses/24 hours)

Thera-Flu® Maximum Strength Flu and Cold Medicine for Sore Throat: Children >12 years and Adults: 1 packet dissolved in hot water every 6 hours (maximum: 4 packets/24 hours)

Other Adverse Effects See Acetaminophen *on page 26*, Chlorpheniramine *on page 268*, and Pseudoephedrine *on page 1022*

Drug Uptake See Acetaminophen *on page 26*, Chlorpheniramine *on page 268* and Pseudoephedrine *on page 1022*

Pregnancy Risk Factor B

Generic Available Yes

Selected Readings

Barker JD Jr, de Carle DJ, and Anuras S, "Chronic Excessive Acetaminophen Use in Liver Damage," *Ann Intern Med*, 1977, 87(3):299-301.

Acetaminophen, Dextromethorphan, and Pseudoephedrine

(a seet a MIN oh fen, deks troe meth OR fan, & soo doe e FED rin)

U.S. Brand Names Alka-Seltzer® Plus Flu Liqui-Gels® [OTC]; Comtrex® Non-Drowsy Cough and Cold [OTC]; Contac® Severe Cold and Flu/Non-Drowsy [OTC]; Infants' Tylenol® Cold Plus Cough Concentrated Drops [OTC]; Sudafed® Severe Cold [OTC]; Thera-Flu® Non-Drowsy Flu, Cold and Cough [OTC]; Triaminic® Sore Throat Formula [OTC]; Tylenol® Cold Non-Drowsy [OTC]; Tylenol® Flu Non-Drowsy Maximum Strength [OTC]; Vicks® DayQuil® Cold and Flu Non-Drowsy [OTC]

Canadian Brand Names Contac® Cough, Cold and Flu Day & Night™; Sudafed® Cold & Cough Extra Strength; Tylenol® Cold

Pharmacologic Category Antihistamine; Antitussive

Synonyms Dextromethorphan, Acetaminophen, and Pseudoephedrine; Pseudoephedrine, Acetaminophen, and Dextromethorphan; Pseudoephedrine, Dextromethorphan, and Acetaminophen

Use Treatment of mild to moderate pain and fever; symptomatic relief of cough and congestion

Local Anesthetic/Vasoconstrictor Precautions No information available to require special precautions

Effects on Dental Treatment No effects or complications reported

Dosage Oral:

Analgesic: Based on acetaminophen component:

Children: 10-15 mg/kg/dose every 4-6 hours as needed; do **not** exceed 5 doses/ 24 hours

Adults: 325-650 mg every 4-7 hours as needed; do **not** exceed 4 g/day

Cough suppressant: Based on dextromethorphan component:

Children 6-12 years: 15 mg every 6-8 hours; do **not** exceed 60 mg/24 hours

Children >12 years and Adults: 10-20 mg every 4-8 hours **or** 30 mg every 8 hours; do **not** exceed 120 mg/24 hours

Decongestant: Based on pseudoephedrine component:

Children:

2-6 years: 15 mg every 4 hours (maximum: 90 mg/24 hours)

6-12 years: 30 mg every 4 hours (maximum: 180 mg/24 hours)

Children >12 years and Adults: 60 mg every 4 hours (maximum: 360 mg/24 hours)

Product labeling:

Alka-Seltzer Plus® Cold and Flu Liqui-Gels®:

Children 6-12 years: 1 dose every 4 hours (maximum: 4 doses/24 hours)

Children >12 years and Adults: 2 dose every 4 hours (maximum: 4 doses/24 hours)

Infants' Tylenol® Cold Plus Cough Concentrated Drops: Children 2-3 years (24-55 lbs): 2 dropperfuls every 4-6 hours (maximum: 4 doses/24 hours)

Sudafed® Severe Cold, Thera-Flu® Non-Drowsy Maximum Strength (gelcap), Tylenol® Flu Non-Drowsy Maximum Strength: Children >12 years and Adults: 2 doses every 6 hours (maximum: 8 doses/24 hours)

Tylenol® Cold Non-Drowsy:

Children 6-11 years: 1 dose every 6 hours (maximum: 4 doses/24 hours)

Children ≥12 years and Adults: 2 doses every 6 hours (maximum: 8 doses/24 hours)

Thera-Flu® Non-Drowsy Maximum Strength: Children >12 years and Adults: 1 packet dissolved in hot water every 6 hours (maximum: 4 packets/24 hours)

Other Adverse Effects See Acetaminophen *on page 26*, Dextromethorphan *on page 372*, and Pseudoephedrine *on page 1022*

Warnings/Precautions Research on chicken embryos exposed to concentrations of dextromethorphan relative to those typically taken by humans has shown to cause birth defects and fetal death; more study is needed, but it is suggested that pregnant women should be advised not to use dextromethorphan-containing medications

Drug Uptake See Acetaminophen *on page 26*, Dextromethorphan *on page 372* and Pseudoephedrine *on page 1022*

Generic Available Yes

Acetaminophen, Isometheptene, and Dichloralphenazone

(a seet a MIN oh fen, eye soe me THEP teen, & dye KLOR al FEN a zone)

U.S. Brand Names Midrin®; Migratine®

Pharmacologic Category Analgesic, Miscellaneous

Synonyms Acetaminophen, Dichloralphenazone, and Isometheptene; Dichloralphenazone, Acetaminophen, and Isometheptene; Dichloralphenazone, Isometheptene, and Acetaminophen; Isometheptene, Acetaminophen, and Dichloralphenazone; Isometheptene, Dichloralphenazone, and Acetaminophen

Use Relief of migraine and tension headache

Local Anesthetic/Vasoconstrictor Precautions No information available to require special precautions

Effects on Dental Treatment No effects or complications reported

Restrictions C-IV

Dosage Adults: Oral:

Migraine headache: 2 capsules to start, followed by 1 capsule every hour until relief is obtained (maximum: 5 capsules/12 hours)

Tension headache: 1-2 capsules every 4 hours (maximum: 8 capsules/24 hours)

Other Adverse Effects Frequency not defined:

Central nervous system: Transient dizziness

Dermatological: Rash

Pregnancy Risk Factor B

Generic Available Yes

Comments Should not exceed 5 g in 12 hours; may cause drowsiness; avoid ethanol and other CNS depressants

Acetasol® HC *see* Acetic Acid, Propylene Glycol Diacetate, and Hydrocortisone *on page 37*

AcetaZOLAMIDE (a set a ZOLE a mide)

U.S. Brand Names Diamox®; Diamox Sequels®

Canadian Brand Names Apo®-Acetazolamide; Diamox®

Mexican Brand Names Acetadiazol®

(Continued)

AcetaZOLAMIDE *(Continued)*

Pharmacologic Category Anticonvulsant, Miscellaneous; Carbonic Anhydrase Inhibitor; Diuretic, Carbonic Anhydrase Inhibitor; Ophthalmic Agent, Antiglaucoma

Use Lowers intraocular pressure in the treatment of glaucoma, also as a diuretic, adjunct treatment of refractory seizures and acute altitude sickness; centrencephalic epilepsies (sustained release not recommended for anticonvulsant)

Local Anesthetic/Vasoconstrictor Precautions No information available to require special precautions

Effects on Dental Treatment >10%: Metallic taste; disappears upon drug withdrawal

Dosage Note: I.M. administration is not recommended because of pain secondary to the alkaline pH

Children:

Glaucoma:

Oral: 8-30 mg/kg/day or 300-900 mg/m^2/day divided every 8 hours

I.M., I.V.: 20-40 mg/kg/24 hours divided every 6 hours, not to exceed 1 g/day

Edema: Oral, I.M., I.V.: 5 mg/kg or 150 mg/m^2 once every day

Epilepsy: Oral: 8-30 mg/kg/day in 1-4 divided doses, not to exceed 1 g/day; sustained release capsule is not recommended for treatment of epilepsy

Adults:

Glaucoma:

Chronic simple (open-angle): Oral: 250 mg 1-4 times/day or 500 mg sustained release capsule twice daily

Secondary, acute (closed-angle): I.M., I.V.: 250-500 mg, may repeat in 2-4 hours to a maximum of 1 g/day

Edema: Oral, I.M., I.V.: 250-375 mg once daily

Epilepsy: Oral: 8-30 mg/kg/day in 1-4 divided doses, not to exceed 1 g/day; **sustained release capsule is not recommended for treatment of epilepsy**

Altitude sickness: Oral: 250 mg every 8-12 hours (or 500 mg extended release capsules every 12-24 hours). Therapy should begin 24-48 hours before and continue during ascent and for at least 48 hours after arrival at the high altitude.

Urine alkalinization: Oral: 5 mg/kg/dose repeated 2-3 times over 24 hours

Elderly: Oral: Initial: 250 mg twice daily; use lowest effective dose

Mechanism of Action Reversible inhibition of the enzyme carbonic anhydrase resulting in reduction of hydrogen ion secretion at renal tubule and an increased renal excretion of sodium, potassium, bicarbonate, and water to decrease production of aqueous humor; also inhibits carbonic anhydrase in CNS to retard abnormal and excessive discharge from CNS neurons

Other Adverse Effects

>10%:

Central nervous system: Malaise, unusual drowsiness or weakness

Gastrointestinal: Anorexia, weight loss, diarrhea, metallic taste, nausea, vomiting

Genitourinary: Polyuria

Neuromuscular & skeletal: Numbness, tingling, or burning in hands, fingers, feet, toes, mouth, tongue, lips, or anus

1% to 10%:

Central nervous system: Mental depression, drowsiness

Renal: Renal calculi

Warnings/Precautions Use in impaired hepatic function may result in coma. Use with caution in patients with respiratory acidosis and diabetes mellitus. Impairment of mental alertness and/or physical coordination may occur. Chemical similarities are present among sulfonamides, sulfonylureas, carbonic anhydrase inhibitors, thiazides, and loop diuretics (except ethacrynic acid). Use in patients with sulfonamide allergy is specifically contraindicated in product labeling, however a risk of cross-reaction exists in patients with allergy to any of these compounds; avoid use when previous reaction has been severe.

I.M. administration is painful because of the alkaline pH of the drug

Drug may cause substantial increase in blood glucose in some diabetic patients; malaise and complaints of tiredness and myalgia are signs of excessive dosing and acidosis in the elderly

Drug Interactions

Increased Effect/Toxicity: Concurrent use with diflunisal may increase the effect of acetazolamide causing a significant decrease in intraocular pressure. Cyclosporine concentrations may be increased by acetazolamide. Salicylate use may result in carbonic anhydrase inhibitor accumulation and toxicity. Acetazolamide-induced hypokalemia may increase the risk of toxicity with digoxin.

Decreased Effect: Use of acetazolamide may increase lithium excretion and alter excretion of other drugs by alkalinization of urine (eg, amphetamines, quinidine, procainamide, methenamine, phenobarbital, salicylates). Primidone serum concentration may be decreased.

Drug Uptake

Onset of action: Capsule, extended release: 2 hours; I.V.: 2 minutes

Peak effect: Capsule, extended release: 3-6 hours; I.V.: 15 minutes; Tablet: 1-4 hours

Duration: Capsule, extended release: 18-24 hours; I.V.: 4-5 hours; Tablet: 8-12 hours

Half-life, elimination: 2.4-5.8 hours

Pregnancy Risk Factor C

Generic Available Yes

Acetic Acid, Propylene Glycol Diacetate, and Hydrocortisone

(a SEE tik AS id, PRO pa leen GLY kole dye AS e tate, & hye droe KOR ti sone)

U.S. Brand Names Acetasol® HC; VōSol® HC

Canadian Brand Names VōSol® HC

Pharmacologic Category Otic Agent, Anti-infective

Synonyms Acetic Acid, Hydrocortisone, and Propylene Glycol Diacetate; Hydrocortisone, Acetic Acid, and Propylene Glycol Diacetate; Hydrocortisone, Propylene Glycol Diacetate, and Acetic Acid; Propylene Glycol Diacetate, Acetic Acid, and Hydrocortisone; Propylene Glycol Diacetate, Hydrocortisone, and Acetic Acid

Use Treatment of superficial infections of the external auditory canal caused by organisms susceptible to the action of the antimicrobial, complicated by swelling

Local Anesthetic/Vasoconstrictor Precautions No information available to require special precautions

Effects on Dental Treatment No effects or complications reported

Dosage Adults: Instill 4 drops in ear(s) 3-4 times/day

Other Adverse Effects Transient burning or stinging may be noticed occasionally when the solution is first instilled into the acutely inflamed ear.

Generic Available Yes

AcetoHEXAMIDE (a set oh HEKS a mide)

Related Information

Endocrine Disorders and Pregnancy *on page 1331*

Pharmacologic Category Antidiabetic Agent, Sulfonylurea

Synonyms Dymelor® [DSC]

Use Adjunct to diet for the management of mild to moderately severe, stable, noninsulin-dependent (type 2) diabetes mellitus

Local Anesthetic/Vasoconstrictor Precautions No information available to require special precautions

Effects on Dental Treatment Use salicylates with caution in patients taking acetohexamide due to potential increased hypoglycemia. NSAIDs such as ibuprofen, naproxen and others may be safely used. Acetohexamide-dependent diabetics (noninsulin-dependent, type 1) should be appointed for dental treatment in mornings to minimize chance of stress-induced hypoglycemia.

Dosage Adults: Oral (elderly patients may be more sensitive and should be started at a lower dosage initially):

Initial: 250 mg/day; increase in increments of 250-500 mg daily at intervals of 5-7 days up to 1.5 g/day. Patients on ≤1 g/day can be controlled with once daily administration. Patients receiving 1.5 g/day usually benefit from twice daily administration before the morning and evening meals. Doses >1.5 g daily are not recommended.

Mechanism of Action Believed to cause hypoglycemia by stimulating insulin release from the pancreatic beta cells; reduces glucose output from the liver (decreases gluconeogenesis); insulin sensitivity is increased at peripheral target sites (alters receptor sensitivity/receptor density); potentiates effects of ADH; may produce mild diuresis and significant uricosuric activity

Other Adverse Effects

>10%:

Central nervous system: Headache, dizziness

Gastrointestinal: Constipation, diarrhea, heartburn, anorexia, epigastric fullness

1% to 10%: Dermatologic: Rash, urticaria, photosensitivity

Warnings/Precautions Patients should be properly instructed in the early detection and treatment of hypoglycemia. Use caution in renal impairment. Chemical similarities are present among sulfonamides, sulfonylureas, carbonic anhydrase inhibitors, thiazides, and loop diuretics (except ethacrynic acid). Use in patients with sulfonylurea allergy is specifically contraindicated in product labeling, however a risk of cross-reaction exists in patients with allergy to any of these compounds; avoid use when previous reaction has been severe.

Product labeling states oral hypoglycemic drugs may be associated with an increased cardiovascular mortality as compared to treatment with diet alone or diet plus insulin. Data to support this association are limited, and several studies, including a large prospective trial (UKPDS) have not supported an association.

Drug Interactions

Increased Effect/Toxicity: Increases hypoglycemia when coadministered with salicylates or beta-adrenergic blockers; MAO inhibitors; oral anticoagulants, NSAIDs,

(Continued)

AcetoHEXAMIDE *(Continued)*

sulfonamides, phenylbutazone, insulin, clofibrate, fluconazole, gemfibrozil, H_2 antagonists, methyldopa, tricyclic antidepressants.

Decreased Effect: Decreases hypoglycemic effect when coadministered with cholestyramine, diazoxide, hydantoins, rifampin, thiazides, loop or thiazide diuretics, and phenylbutazone.

Drug Uptake

Onset of action: 1 hour; Peak effect: Hypoglycemic: 8-10 hours

Duration: 12-24 hours; prolonged with renal impairment

Half-life, elimination: Parent drug: 0.8-2.4 hours; Metabolite: 5-6 hours

Pregnancy Risk Factor D

Generic Available Yes

Acetohydroxamic Acid (a SEE toe hye droks am ik AS id)

U.S. Brand Names Lithostat®

Canadian Brand Names Lithostat®

Pharmacologic Category Urinary Tract Product

Synonyms AHA

Use Adjunctive therapy in chronic urea-splitting urinary infection

Local Anesthetic/Vasoconstrictor Precautions No information available to require special precautions

Effects on Dental Treatment No effects or complications reported

Dosage Oral:

Children: Initial: 10 mg/kg/day

Adults: 250 mg 3-4 times/day for a total daily dose of 10-15 mg/kg/day

Pregnancy Risk Factor X

Generic Available No

Acetylcholine (a se teel KOE leen)

U.S. Brand Names Miochol-E®

Canadian Brand Names Miochol®-E

Pharmacologic Category Cholinergic Agonist; Ophthalmic Agent, Miotic

Synonyms Acetylcholine Chloride

Use Produces complete miosis in cataract surgery, keratoplasty, iridectomy and other anterior segment surgery where rapid miosis is required

Local Anesthetic/Vasoconstrictor Precautions No information available to require special precautions

Effects on Dental Treatment Ophthalmic use of acetylcholine has no effect on dental treatment.

Dosage Adults: Intraocular: 0.5-2 mL of 1% injection (5-20 mg) instilled into anterior chamber before or after securing one or more sutures

Mechanism of Action Causes contraction of the sphincter muscles of the iris, resulting in miosis and contraction of the ciliary muscle, leading to accommodation spasm

Other Adverse Effects Frequency not defined:

Cardiovascular: Bradycardia, hypotension, flushing

Central nervous system: Headache

Ocular: Altered distance vision, decreased night vision, transient lenticular opacities

Respiratory: Dyspnea

Miscellaneous: Diaphoresis

Drug Interactions

Increased Effect/Toxicity: Effect may be prolonged or enhanced in patients receiving tacrine.

Decreased Effect: Effect may be decreased with flurbiprofen and suprofen, ophthalmic.

Drug Uptake

Onset of action: Rapid

Duration: ~10 minutes

Pregnancy Risk Factor C

Generic Available No

Acetylcysteine (a se teel SIS teen)

U.S. Brand Names Mucomyst®; Mucosil™

Canadian Brand Names Mucomyst®; Parvolex®

Pharmacologic Category Antidote; Mucolytic Agent

Synonyms Acetylcysteine Sodium; Mercapturic Acid; NAC; *N*-Acetylcysteine; *N*-Acetyl-L-cysteine

Use Adjunctive mucolytic therapy in patients with abnormal or viscid mucous secretions in acute and chronic bronchopulmonary diseases; pulmonary complications of surgery and cystic fibrosis; diagnostic bronchial studies; antidote for acute acetaminophen toxicity

Unlabeled/Investigational: Prevention of radiocontrast-induced renal dysfunction

Local Anesthetic/Vasoconstrictor Precautions No information available to require special precautions

Effects on Dental Treatment 1% to 10%: Stomatitis

Dosage

Acetaminophen poisoning: Children and Adults: Oral: 140 mg/kg; followed by 17 doses of 70 mg/kg every 4 hours; repeat dose if emesis occurs within 1 hour of administration; therapy should continue until all doses are administered even though the acetaminophen plasma concentration has dropped below the toxic range

Inhalation: Acetylcysteine 10% and 20% solution (Mucomyst®) (dilute 20% solution with sodium chloride or sterile water for inhalation); 10% solution may be used undiluted

Infants: 1-2 mL of 20% solution or 2-4 mL 10% solution until nebulized given 3-4 times/day

Children: 3-5 mL of 20% solution or 6-10 mL of 10% solution until nebulized given 3-4 times/day

Adolescents: 5-10 mL of 10% to 20% solution until nebulized given 3-4 times/day

Note: Patients should receive an aerosolized bronchodilator 10-15 minutes prior to acetylcysteine

Meconium ileus equivalent: Children and Adults: 100-300 mL of 4% to 10% solution by irrigation or orally

Prevention of radiocontrast-induced renal dysfunction (unlabeled use): Adults: Oral: 600 mg twice daily for 2 days (beginning the day before the procedure); may be given as powder in capsules, some centers use solution (diluted in cola beverage or juice). Hydrate patient with saline concurrently.

Mechanism of Action Exerts mucolytic action through its free sulfhydryl group which opens up the disulfide bonds in the mucoproteins thus lowering mucous viscosity. The exact mechanism of action in acetaminophen toxicity is unknown; thought to act by providing substrate for conjugation with the toxic metabolite.

Other Adverse Effects

Inhalation:

>10%:

Stickiness on face after nebulization
Miscellaneous: Unpleasant odor during administration

1% to 10%:

Central nervous system: Drowsiness, chills, fever
Gastrointestinal: Vomiting, nausea, stomatitis
Local: Irritation
Respiratory: Bronchospasm, rhinorrhea, hemoptysis
Miscellaneous: Clamminess

Systemic:

1% to 10%:

Central nervous system: Fever, drowsiness, dizziness (10%; prevention of radiocontrast-induced renal function)
Gastrointestinal: Nausea, stomatitis, vomiting

Drug Interactions Adsorbed by activated charcoal; clinical significance is minimal, though, once a pure acetaminophen ingestion requiring N-acetylcysteine is established; further charcoal dosing is unnecessary once the appropriate initial charcoal dose is achieved (5-10 g:g acetaminophen)

Drug Uptake

Onset of action: Inhalation: 5-10 minutes
Duration: Inhalation: >1 hour
Half-life, elimination: Reduced acetylcysteine: 2 hours; Total acetylcysteine: 5.5 hours
Time to peak, plasma: Oral: 1-2 hours

Pregnancy Risk Factor B

Generic Available Yes

Aciphex® *see* Rabeprazole *on page 1037*
Aclovate® *see* Alclometasone *on page 47*

Acrivastine and Pseudoephedrine

(AK ri vas teen & soo doe e FED rin)

U.S. Brand Names Semprex®-D

Pharmacologic Category Antihistamine

Synonyms Pseudoephedrine and Acrivastine

Use Temporary relief of nasal congestion, decongest sinus openings, running nose, itching of nose or throat, and itchy, watery eyes due to hay fever or other upper respiratory allergies

Local Anesthetic/Vasoconstrictor Precautions Use with caution since pseudoephedrine is a sympathomimetic amine which could interact with epinephrine to cause a pressor response

Effects on Dental Treatment ≤10%: Tachycardia, palpitations, xerostomia; use vasoconstrictor with caution

Dosage Adults: 1 capsule 3-4 times/day

(Continued)

Acrivastine and Pseudoephedrine *(Continued)*

Mechanism of Action Acrivastine is an analogue of triprolidine and it is considered to be relatively less sedating than traditional antihistamines; believed to involve competitive blockade of H_1-receptor sites resulting in the inability of histamine to combine with its receptor sites and exert its usual effects on target cells

Pseudoephedrine directly stimulates alpha-adrenergic receptors of respiratory mucosa causing vasoconstriction; directly stimulates beta-adrenergic receptors causing bronchial relaxation, increased heart rate and contractility

Other Adverse Effects

>10%: Central nervous system: Drowsiness, headache

1% to 10%:

- Cardiovascular: Tachycardia, palpitations
- Central nervous system: Nervousness, dizziness, insomnia, vertigo, lightheadedness, fatigue
- Gastrointestinal: Nausea, vomiting, xerostomia, diarrhea
- Genitourinary: Dysuria
- Neuromuscular & skeletal: Weakness
- Respiratory: Pharyngitis, cough increase
- Miscellaneous: Sweating

Drug Interactions

Increased Effect/Toxicity: Increased risk of hypertensive crisis when acrivastine and pseudoephedrine are given with MAO inhibitors or sympathomimetics; increased risk of severe CNS depression when given with CNS depressants

Decreased Effect: Decreases effect of guanethidine, reserpine, methyldopa, and beta-blockers when given in conjunction with acrivastine and pseudoephedrine

Drug Uptake See Pseudoephedrine *on page 1022*

Pregnancy Risk Factor B

Generic Available No

ACT® [OTC] *see* Fluoride *on page 514*

Act-A-Med® [OTC] *see* Triprolidine and Pseudoephedrine *on page 1213*

Actanol® [OTC] *see* Triprolidine and Pseudoephedrine *on page 1213*

Actedril® [OTC] *see* Triprolidine and Pseudoephedrine *on page 1213*

Acthar® *see* Corticotropin *on page 327*

ActHIB® *see Haemophilus* b Conjugate Vaccine *on page 575*

Acticin® *see* Permethrin *on page 940*

Actidose® [OTC] *see* Charcoal *on page 258*

Actidose-Aqua® [OTC] *see* Charcoal *on page 258*

Actifed® [OTC] *see* Triprolidine and Pseudoephedrine *on page 1213*

Actifed® Allergy (Night) [OTC] *see* Diphenhydramine and Pseudoephedrine *on page 400*

Actigall™ *see* Ursodiol *on page 1223*

Actimmune® *see* Interferon Gamma-1b *on page 649*

Actinex® *see* Masoprocol *on page 745*

Actiq® *see* Fentanyl *on page 493*

Actisite® *see* Tetracycline Periodontal Fibers *on page 1149*

Activase® *see* Alteplase *on page 59*

Activella™ *see* Estradiol and Norethindrone *on page 459*

Actonel® *see* Risedronate *on page 1056*

Actos® *see* Pioglitazone *on page 961*

ACU-dyne® [OTC] *see* Povidone-Iodine *on page 982*

Acular® *see* Ketorolac Tromethamine *on page 676*

Acular® PF *see* Ketorolac Tromethamine *on page 676*

Acyclovir (ay SYE kloe veer)

Related Information

Oral Viral Infections *on page 1380*

Systemic Viral Diseases *on page 1354*

U.S. Brand Names Zovirax®

Canadian Brand Names Apo®-Acyclovir; Avirax™; Nu-Acyclovir; Zovirax®

Mexican Brand Names Acifur; Cicloferon®; Isavir®; Laciken®; Opthavir®; Zovirax®; Zovirax I.V.®

Pharmacologic Category Antiviral Agent

Synonyms Aciclovir; ACV; Acycloguanosine

Use

Dental: Treatment of initial and prophylaxis of recurrent mucosal and cutaneous herpes simplex (HSV-1 and HSV-2) infections

Medical: Treatment of herpes simplex encephalitis, herpes zoster, genital herpes infection, varicella-zoster infections in healthy, nonpregnant persons >13 years of age, children <12 months of age who have a chronic skin or lung disorder or are receiving long-term aspirin therapy, and immunocompromised patients; for herpes zoster, acyclovir should be started within 72 hours of the appearance of the rash to be effective; acyclovir will not prevent postherpetic neuralgias

Local Anesthetic/Vasoconstrictor Precautions No information available to require special precautions

Effects on Dental Treatment No effects or complications reported

Dosage Dosing weight should be based on the smaller of lean body weight or total body weight.

Treatment of herpes simplex virus infections: Children >12 years and Adults:

I.V.:

Mucocutaneous HSV or severe initial herpes genitalis infection: 750 mg/m^2/day divided every 8 hours or 5 mg/kg/dose every 8 hours for 5-10 days

HSV encephalitis: 1500 mg/m^2/day divided every 8 hours or 10 mg/kg/dose for 10 days

Topical: Nonlife-threatening mucocutaneous HSV in immunocompromised patients: ½" ribbon of ointment for a 4" square surface area every 3 hours (6 times/day) for 7 days

Treatment of genital herpes simplex virus infections: Adults:

Oral: 200 mg every 4 hours while awake (5 times/day) for 10 days if initial episode; for 5 days if recurrence (begin at earliest signs of disease)

Topical: ½" ribbon of ointment for a 4" square surface area every 3 hours (6 times/day) for 7 days

Treatment of varicella-zoster virus (chickenpox) infections:

Oral:

Children: 10-20 mg/kg/dose (up to 800 mg) 4 times/day for 5 days; begin treatment within the first 24 hours of rash onset

Adults: 600-800 mg/dose every 4 hours while awake (5 times/day) for 7-10 days or 1000 mg every 6 hours for 5 days

I.V.: Children and Adults: 1500 mg/m^2/day divided every 8 hours or 10 mg/kg/dose every 8 hours for 7 days

Treatment of herpes zoster (shingles) infections:

Oral:

Children (immunocompromised): 250-600 mg/m^2/dose 4-5 times/day for 7-10 days

Adults (immunocompromised): 800 mg every 4 hours (5 times/day) for 7-10 days

I.V.:

Children and Adults (immunocompromised): 10 mg/kg/dose or 500 mg/m^2/dose every 8 hours

Older Adults (immunocompromised): 7.5 mg/kg/dose every 8 hours

If nephrotoxicity occurs: 5 mg/kg/dose every 8 hours

Prophylaxis in immunocompromised patients:

Varicella zoster or herpes zoster in HIV-positive patients: Adults: Oral: 400 mg every 4 hours (5 times/day) for 7-10 days

Bone marrow transplant recipients: Children and Adults: I.V.:

Allogeneic patients who are HSV seropositive: 150 mg/m^2/dose (5 mg/kg) every 12 hours; with clinical symptoms of herpes simplex: 150 mg/m^2/dose every 8 hours

Allogeneic patients who are CMV seropositive: 500 mg/m^2/dose (10 mg/kg) every 8 hours; for clinically symptomatic CMV infection, consider replacing acyclovir with ganciclovir

Chronic suppressive therapy for recurrent genital herpes simplex virus infections: Adults: 200 mg 3-4 times/day or 400 mg twice daily for up to 12 months, followed by re-evaluation

Dosing adjustment in renal impairment:

Oral: HSV/varicella-zoster:

Cl_{cr} 10-25 mL/minute: Administer dose every 8 hours

Cl_{cr} <10 mL/minute: Administer dose every 12 hours

I.V.:

Cl_{cr} 25-50 mL/minute: 5-10 mg/kg/dose: Administer every 12 hours

Cl_{cr} 10-25 mL/minute: 5-10 mg/kg/dose: Administer every 24 hours

Cl_{cr} <10 mL/minute: 2.5-5 mg/kg/dose: Administer every 24 hours

Hemodialysis: Dialyzable (50% to 100%); administer dose postdialysis

Peritoneal dialysis: Dose as for Cl_{cr} <10 mL/minute

Continuous arteriovenous or venovenous hemofiltration effects: Dose as for Cl_{cr} <10 mL/minute

Mechanism of Action Converted to acyclovir monophosphate by virus-specific thymidine kinase then further converted to acyclovir triphosphate by other cellular enzymes; acyclovir triphosphate inhibits DNA synthesis and viral replication by competing with deoxyguanosine triphosphate for viral DNA polymerase and being incorporated into viral DNA.

Other Adverse Effects

Systemic: Oral:

1% to 10%:

Central nervous system: Lightheadedness, headache

Gastrointestinal: Nausea, vomiting, abdominal pain

(Continued)

Acyclovir *(Continued)*

Systemic: Parenteral:

>10%:

Central nervous system: Lightheadedness

Gastrointestinal: Nausea, vomiting, anorexia

Local: Inflammation at injection site or phlebitis

1% to 10%: Renal: Acute renal failure

Topical:

>10%: Mild pain, burning, or stinging

1% to 10%: Itching

Contraindications Hypersensitivity to acyclovir, valacyclovir, or any component of their formulation

Warnings/Precautions Use with caution in patients with pre-existing renal disease or in those receiving other nephrotoxic drugs concurrently; maintain adequate urine output during the first 2 hours after I.V. infusion; use with caution in patients with underlying neurologic abnormalities, serious hepatic or electrolyte abnormalities, or substantial hypoxia. Use with caution in immunocompromised patients; thrombocytopenic purpura/hemolytic uremic syndrome (TTP/HUS) has been reported

Drug Interactions Increased CNS side effects with zidovudine and probenecid

Dietary/Ethanol/Herb Considerations Food: Administer oral forms with food to reduce GI upset; does not appear to affect absorption.

Drug Uptake

Absorption: Oral: 15% to 30%

Half-life, elimination: Terminal: Neonates: 4 hours; Children 1-12 years: 2-3 hours; Adults: 3 hours

Time to peak: Oral: ~1.5-2 hours; I.V.: ~1 hour

Pregnancy Risk Factor B

Breast-feeding Considerations May be taken while breast-feeding

Dosage Forms CAP: 200 mg. **INJ, powder for reconstitution:** 500 mg, 1000 mg. **INJ, solution** [preservative free]: 50 mg/mL (10 mL, 20 mL). **OINT, topical:** 5% (3 g, 15 g). **SUSP, oral:** 200 mg/5 mL (480 mL). **TAB:** 400 mg, 800 mg

Generic Available Yes

Adagen™ *see* Pegademase Bovine *on page 921*

Adalat® CC *see* NIFEdipine *on page 865*

Adapalene (a DAP a leen)

U.S. Brand Names Differin®

Canadian Brand Names Differin®

Mexican Brand Names Adaferin®

Pharmacologic Category Acne Products

Use Topical treatment of acne vulgaris

Local Anesthetic/Vasoconstrictor Precautions No information available to require special precautions

Effects on Dental Treatment No effects or complications reported

Dosage Children >12 years and Adults: Topical: Apply once daily before retiring; therapeutic results should be noticed after 8-12 weeks of treatment

Mechanism of Action Retinoid-like compound which is a modulator of cellular differentiation, keratinization and inflammatory processes, all of which represent important features in the pathology of acne vulgaris

Other Adverse Effects >10%: Dermatologic: Erythema, scaling, dryness, pruritus, burning, pruritus or burning immediately after application

Drug Uptake

Absorption: Topical: Minimal

Pregnancy Risk Factor C

Generic Available No

Adderall® *see* Dextroamphetamine and Amphetamine *on page 371*

Adderall XR™ *see* Dextroamphetamine and Amphetamine *on page 371*

Adenocard® *see* Adenosine *on page 42*

Adenoscan® *see* Adenosine *on page 42*

Adenosine (a DEN oh seen)

U.S. Brand Names Adenocard®; Adenoscan®

Canadian Brand Names Adenocard®

Pharmacologic Category Antiarrhythmic Agent, Class IV; Diagnostic Agent

Synonyms 9-Beta-D-ribofuranosyladenine

Use

Adenocard®: Treatment of paroxysmal supraventricular tachycardia (PSVT) including that associated with accessory bypass tracts (Wolff-Parkinson-White syndrome); when clinically advisable, appropriate vagal maneuvers should be attempted prior to adenosine administration; **not effective in atrial flutter, atrial fibrillation, or ventricular tachycardia**

Adenoscan®: Pharmacologic stress agent used in myocardial perfusion thallium-201 scintigraphy

Local Anesthetic/Vasoconstrictor Precautions No information available to require special precautions

Effects on Dental Treatment No effects or complications reported

Dosage

Adenocard®: **Rapid I.V. push (over 1-2 seconds) via peripheral line:**

Neonates: Initial dose: 0.05 mg/kg; if not effective within 2 minutes, increase dose by 0.05 mg/kg increments every 2 minutes to a maximum dose of 0.25 mg/kg or until termination of PSVT

Maximum single dose: 12 mg

Infants and Children: Pediatric advanced life support (PALS): Treatment of SVT: 0.1 mg/kg; if not effective, administer 0.2 mg/kg

Alternatively: Initial dose: 0.05 mg/kg; if not effective within 2 minutes, increase dose by 0.05 mg/kg increments every 2 minutes to a maximum dose of 0.25 mg/kg or until termination of PSVT; medium dose required: 0.15 mg/kg

Maximum single dose: 12 mg

Adults: 6 mg; if not effective within 1-2 minutes, 12 mg may be given; may repeat 12 mg bolus if needed

Maximum single dose: 12 mg

Follow each I.V. bolus of adenosine with normal saline flush

Note: Preliminary results in adults suggest adenosine may be administered via a central line at lower doses (ie, initial adult dose: 3 mg).

Adenoscan®: Continuous I.V. infusion via peripheral line: 140 mcg/kg/minute for 6 minutes using syringe or columetric infusion pump; total dose: 0.84 mg/kg. Thallium-201 is injected at midpoint (3 minutes) of infusion.

Hemodialysis: Significant drug removal is unlikely based on physiochemical characteristics.

Peritoneal dialysis: Significant drug removal is unlikely based on physiochemical characteristics.

Note: Patients who are receiving concomitant theophylline therapy may be less likely to respond to adenosine therapy.

Note: Higher doses may be needed for administration via peripheral versus central vein.

Mechanism of Action Slows conduction time through the A-V node, interrupting the re-entry pathways through the A-V node, restoring normal sinus rhythm

Other Adverse Effects

>10%:

Cardiovascular: Facial flushing (18%), palpitations, chest pain, hypotension

Central nervous system: Headache

Respiratory: Shortness of breath/dyspnea (12%)

Miscellaneous: Sweating

1% to 10%:

Central nervous system: Dizziness

Gastrointestinal: Nausea (3%)

Neuromuscular & skeletal: Paresthesia, numbness

Respiratory: Chest pressure (7%)

Drug Interactions

Increased Effect/Toxicity: Dipyridamole potentiates effects of adenosine. Use with carbamazepine may increase heart block.

Decreased Effect: Methylxanthines (eg, caffeine, theophylline) antagonize the effect of adenosine.

Drug Uptake

Onset of action: Rapid

Duration: Very brief

Half-life, elimination: <10 seconds

Pregnancy Risk Factor C

Generic Available No

Comments Short action an advantage; not effective in atrial flutter, atrial fibrillation, or ventricular tachycardia

Adipex-P® *see* Phentermine *on page 948*

Adoxa™ *see* Doxycycline *on page 418*

Adrenalin® *see* Epinephrine *on page 438*

Adrenalin® (Dental) *see* Epinephrine *on page 438*

Adriamycin PFS® *see* DOXOrubicin *on page 416*

Adriamycin RDF® *see* DOXOrubicin *on page 416*

Adrucil® *see* Fluorouracil *on page 516*

Adsorbonac® [DSC] *see* Sodium Chloride *on page 1094*

Advicor™ *see* Niacin and Lovastatin *on page 861*

Advil® [OTC] *see* Ibuprofen *on page 621*

Advil® Cold & Sinus Caplets [OTC] *see* Pseudoephedrine and Ibuprofen *on page 1024*

Advil® Migraine Liqui-Gels [OTC] *see* Ibuprofen *on page 621*

Aeroaid® [OTC] *see* Thimerosal *on page 1157*
AeroBid® *see* Flunisolide *on page 511*
AeroBid®-M *see* Flunisolide *on page 511*
Aerodine® [OTC] *see* Povidone-Iodine *on page 982*
Aerolate III® *see* Theophylline *on page 1152*
Aerolate JR® *see* Theophylline *on page 1152*
Aerolate SR® *see* Theophylline *on page 1152*
Afrin® Children's Nose Drops [OTC] *see* Oxymetazoline *on page 907*
Afrin® Sinus [OTC] *see* Oxymetazoline *on page 907*
Aftate® for Athlete's Foot [OTC] *see* Tolnaftate *on page 1181*
Aftate® for Jock Itch [OTC] *see* Tolnaftate *on page 1181*
Agenerase® *see* Amprenavir *on page 97*
Aggrastat® *see* Tirofiban *on page 1173*
Aggrenox™ *see* Aspirin and Dipyridamole *on page 123*
Agrylin® *see* Anagrelide *on page 99*
A-hydroCort® *see* Hydrocortisone *on page 608*
AKBeta® *see* Levobunolol *on page 696*
AK-Cide® *see* Sulfacetamide Sodium and Prednisolone *on page 1116*
AK-Con® *see* Naphazoline *on page 847*
AK-Dex® *see* Dexamethasone *on page 363*
AK-Dilate® Ophthalmic *see* Phenylephrine *on page 950*
Akineton® *see* Biperiden *on page 166*
AK-Nefrin® Ophthalmic *see* Phenylephrine *on page 950*
Akne-Mycin® *see* Erythromycin, Topical *on page 454*
AK-Neo-Dex® *see* Neomycin and Dexamethasone *on page 855*
AK-Pentolate® *see* Cyclopentolate *on page 334*
AK-Poly-Bac® *see* Bacitracin and Polymyxin B *on page 141*
AK-Pred® *see* PrednisoLONE *on page 988*
AKPro® *see* Dipivefrin *on page 401*
AK-Spore® H.C. *see* Bacitracin, Neomycin, Polymyxin B, and Hydrocortisone *on page 141*
AK-Spore® H.C. Otic *see* Neomycin, Polymyxin B, and Hydrocortisone *on page 857*
AK-Spore® Ophthalmic Solution *see* Neomycin, Polymyxin B, and Gramicidin *on page 856*
AK-Sulf® *see* Sulfacetamide Sodium *on page 1115*
AKTob® *see* Tobramycin *on page 1175*
AK-Tracin® *see* Bacitracin *on page 140*
AK-Trol® *see* Neomycin, Polymyxin B, and Dexamethasone *on page 856*
Akwa Tears® [OTC] *see* Artificial Tears *on page 117*
Ala-Cort® *see* Hydrocortisone *on page 608*
Alamast™ *see* Pemirolast *on page 924*
Ala-Scalp® *see* Hydrocortisone *on page 608*
Albalon® Liquifilm® *see* Naphazoline *on page 847*

Albendazole (al BEN da zole)

U.S. Brand Names Albenza®

Mexican Brand Names Bendapar®; Digezanol®; Endoplus®; Eskazole; Gascop®; Lurdex; Zentel®

Pharmacologic Category Anthelmintic

Use Treatment of parenchymal neurocysticercosis and cystic hydatid disease of the liver, lung, and peritoneum; albendazole may also be useful in the treatment of ascariasis, trichuriasis, enterobiasis, hookworm, strongyloidiasis, giardiasis, and microsporidiosis in AIDS

Local Anesthetic/Vasoconstrictor Precautions No information available to require special precautions

Effects on Dental Treatment No effects or complications reported

Dosage Oral:

Neurocysticercosis:

- <60 kg: 15 mg/kg/day in 2 divided doses (maximum: 800 mg/day) with meals for 8-30 days
- ≥60 kg: 400 mg twice daily for 8-30 days
- **Note:** Give concurrent anticonvulsant and steroid therapy during first week

Hydatid:

- <60 kg: 15 mg/kg/day in 2 divided doses with meals (maximum: 800 mg/day) for three 28-day cycles with 14-day drug-free interval in-between
- ≥60 kg: 400 mg twice daily for 3 cycles as above

Strongyloidiasis/tapeworm: Children >2 years and Adults: 400 mg/day for 3 days; may repeat in 3 weeks

Giardiasis: Adults: 400 mg/day for 3 days

Hookworm, pinworm, roundworm: Children >2 years and Adults: 400 mg as a single dose; may repeat in 3 weeks

Mechanism of Action Appears to cause selective degeneration of cytoplasmic microtubules in intestinal and tegmental cells of intestinal helminths, and larvae; glycogen is depleted, glucose uptake and cholinesterase secretion are impaired, and desecratory substances accumulate intracellularly. ATP production decreases causing energy depletion, immobilization, and worm death.

Other Adverse Effects 1% to 10%:

Central nervous system: Dizziness, headache, vertigo, fever

Dermatologic: Alopecia (reversible), rash, urticaria

Gastrointestinal: Abdominal pain, nausea, vomiting

Hepatic: Increased LFTs, jaundice

Drug Interactions CYP1A2 enzyme inhibitor (weak)

Dexamethasone: Increases plasma levels of albendazole metabolites; significance unknown

Enzyme inducers: May increase the metabolite formation of albendazole's active metabolite (primary activity is associated with this metabolite); limited information, no data concerning clinical effect; includes carbamazepine, rifampin, phenobarbital, and phenytoin

Praziquantel: May increase plasma concentrations of albendazole by 50%; significance unknown

Theophylline: Metabolism may be increased by albendazole; limited documentation suggests potential is low

Drug Uptake

Absorption: Oral absorption is poor (<5%); may increase ≥4.5 times with a fatty meal; albendazole itself is essentially undetectable in plasma; albendazole sulfoxide is probably the active agent

Half-life, elimination: 8-12 hours

Time to peak: 2-2.4 hours

Pregnancy Risk Factor C

Generic Available No

Albenza® *see* Albendazole *on page 44*

Albuterol (al BYOO ter ole)

Related Information

Dental Office Emergencies *on page 1418*

Ipratropium and Albuterol *on page 652*

Respiratory Diseases *on page 1328*

U.S. Brand Names AccuNeb™; Proventil®; Proventil® HFA; Proventil® Repetabs®; Ventolin®; Ventolin® HFA; Ventolin Rotacaps® [DSC]; Volmax®

Canadian Brand Names Alti-Salbutamol; Apo®-Salvent; Novo-Salmol

Mexican Brand Names Inspiryl®; Salbulin; Salbulin Autohaler®; Salbutalan; Ventolin®; Volmax®

Pharmacologic Category Beta$_2$ Agonist

Synonyms Salbutamol

Use Bronchodilator in reversible airway obstruction due to asthma or COPD; prevention of exercise-induced bronchospasm in patients ≥12 years of age

Local Anesthetic/Vasoconstrictor Precautions No information available to require special precautions

Effects on Dental Treatment No effects or complications reported

Dosage

Oral:

Children: Bronchospasm (treatment):

2-6 years: 0.1-0.2 mg/kg/dose 3 times/day; maximum dose not to exceed 12 mg/day (divided doses)

6-12 years: 2 mg/dose 3-4 times/day; maximum dose not to exceed 24 mg/day (divided doses)

Extended release: 4 mg every 12 hours; maximum dose not to exceed 24 mg/day (divided doses)

Children >12 years and Adults: Bronchospasm (treatment): 2-4 mg/dose 3-4 times/day; maximum dose not to exceed 32 mg/day (divided doses)

Extended release: 8 mg every 12 hours; maximum dose not to exceed 32 mg/day (divided doses). A 4 mg dose every 12 hours may be sufficient in some patients, such as adults of low body weight.

Elderly: Bronchospasm (treatment): 2 mg 3-4 times/day; maximum: 8 mg 4 times/day

Inhalation: Children ≥4 years and Adults:

Bronchospasm (treatment):

MDI: 90 mcg/spray: 1-2 inhalations every 4-6 hours; maximum: 12 inhalations/day

Capsule: 200-400 mcg every 4-6 hours

Exercise-induced bronchospasm (prophylaxis):

MDI-CFC aerosol: 2 inhalations 15 minutes before exercising

MDI-HFA aerosol: 2 inhalations 15-30 minutes before exercise

(Continued)

Albuterol *(Continued)*

Capsule: 200 mcg 15 minutes before exercise

Nebulization:

Children:

Bronchospasm (treatment): 0.01-0.05 mL/kg of 0.5% solution every 4-6 hours

2-12 years: AccuNeb™: 0.63 mg or 1.25 mg 3-4 times/day, as needed, delivered over 5-15 minutes

Children >40 kg, patients with more severe asthma, or children 11-12 years: May respond better with a 1.25 mg dose

Bronchospasm (acute): 0.01-0.05 mL/kg of 0.5% solution every 4-6 hours; intensive care patients may require more frequent administration; minimum dose: 0.1 mL; maximum dose: 1 mL diluted in 1-2 mL normal saline; continuous nebulized albuterol at 0.3 mg/kg/hour has been used safely in the treatment of severe status asthmaticus in children; continuous nebulized doses of 3 mg/kg/hour ± 2.2 mg/kg/hour in children whose mean age was 20.7 months resulted in no cardiac toxicity; the optimal dosage for continuous nebulization remains to be determined.

Adults:

Bronchospasm (treatment): 2.5 mg, diluted to a total of 3 mL, 3-4 times/day over 5-15 minutes

Bronchospasm (acute) in intensive care patients: 2.5-5 mg every 20 minutes for 3 doses, then 2.5-10 mg every 1-4 hours as needed, **or** 10-15 mg/hour continuously

Hemodialysis: Not removed

Peritoneal dialysis: Significant drug removal is unlikely based on physiochemical characteristics

Mechanism of Action Relaxes bronchial smooth muscle by action on beta$_2$-adrenergic receptors with little effect on heart rate

Other Adverse Effects Incidence of adverse effects is dependent upon age of patient, dose, and route of administration.

Frequency not defined:

Cardiovascular: Angina, atrial fibrillation, chest discomfort, extrasystoles, flushing, hypertension, palpitations, tachycardia

Central nervous system: CNS stimulation, dizziness, drowsiness, headache, insomnia, irritability, lightheadedness, migraine, nervousness, nightmares, restlessness, sleeplessness, tremor

Dermatologic: Angioedema, erythema multiforme, rash, Stevens-Johnson syndrome, urticaria

Endocrine & metabolic: Hypokalemia

Gastrointestinal: Diarrhea, xerostomia, gastroenteritis, nausea, unusual taste, vomiting, tooth discoloration

Genitourinary: Micturition difficulty

Neuromuscular & skeletal: Muscle cramps, weakness

Otic: Otitis media, vertigo

Respiratory: Asthma exacerbation, bronchospasm, cough, epistaxis, laryngitis, oropharyngeal drying/irritation, oropharyngeal edema

Miscellaneous: Allergic reaction, lymphadenopathy

Warnings/Precautions Use with caution in patients with hyperthyroidism, diabetes mellitus, or sensitivity to sympathomimetic amines; cardiovascular disorders including coronary insufficiency or hypertension; excessive use may result in tolerance. May cause paradoxical bronchospasm. Increased use may indicate a deterioration of condition and requires a re-evaluation of the patient. Excessive use of inhalers has been associated with fatalities.

Because of its minimal effect on beta$_1$-receptors and its relatively long duration of action, albuterol is a rational choice in the elderly when an inhaled beta agonist is indicated. Oral use should be avoided in the elderly due to adverse effects. All patients should utilize a spacer device when using a metered-dose inhaler; spacers and facemasks should be used in children <4 years. Patient response may vary between inhalers that contain chlorofluorocarbons and those which are chlorofluorocarbon-free.

Drug Interactions

Increased Effect/Toxicity: When used with inhaled ipratropium, an increased duration of bronchodilation may occur. Cardiovascular effects are potentiated in patients also receiving MAO inhibitors, tricyclic antidepressants, and sympathomimetic agents (eg, amphetamine, dopamine, dobutamine). Albuterol may increase the risk of malignant arrhythmias with inhaled anesthetics (eg, enflurane, halothane).

Decreased Effect: When used with nonselective beta-adrenergic blockers (eg, propranolol) the effect of albuterol is decreased.

Drug Uptake

Onset of action: Peak effect: Nebulization/oral inhalation: 0.5-2 hours; Oral: 2-3 hours

Duration: Nebulization/oral inhalation: 3-4 hours; Oral: 4-6 hours

Half-life elimination: Inhalation: 3.8 hours; Oral: 3.7-5 hours

Pregnancy Risk Factor C
Generic Available Yes

Alcaine® *see* Proparacaine *on page 1010*

Alclometasone (al kloe MET a sone)

U.S. Brand Names Aclovate®
Pharmacologic Category Corticosteroid, Topical
Synonyms Alclometasone Dipropionate
Use Treatment of inflammation of corticosteroid-responsive dermatosis (low potency topical corticosteroid)
Local Anesthetic/Vasoconstrictor Precautions No information available to require special precautions
Effects on Dental Treatment No effects or complications reported
Dosage Topical: Apply a thin film to the affected area 2-3 times/day
Therapy should be discontinued when control is achieved; if no improvement is seen, reassessment of diagnosis may be necessary.
Mechanism of Action Stimulates the synthesis of enzymes needed to decrease inflammation, suppress mitotic activity, and cause vasoconstriction
Other Adverse Effects 1% to 10%:
Dermatologic: Itching, erythema, dryness papular rashes
Local: Burning, irritation
Pregnancy Risk Factor C
Generic Available No

Alconefrin® Nasal [OTC] *see* Phenylephrine *on page 950*
Aldactazide® *see* Hydrochlorothiazide and Spironolactone *on page 596*
Aldactone® *see* Spironolactone *on page 1106*
Aldara™ *see* Imiquimod *on page 628*

Aldesleukin (al des LOO kin)

U.S. Brand Names Proleukin®
Canadian Brand Names Proleukin®
Mexican Brand Names Proleukin®
Pharmacologic Category Biological Response Modulator
Synonyms Epidermal Thymocyte Activating Factor; ETAF; IL-2; Interleukin-2; Lymphocyte Mitogenic Factor; NSC-373364; T-Cell Growth Factor; TCGF; Thymocyte Stimulating Factor
Use Treatment of metastatic renal cell cancer, melanoma
Unlabeled/Investigational: Multiple myeloma, HIV infection, and AIDS; may be used in conjunction with lymphokine-activated killer (LAK) cells, tumor-infiltrating lymphocyte (TIL) cells, interleukin-1, and interferons; colorectal cancer; non-Hodgkin's lymphoma
Local Anesthetic/Vasoconstrictor Precautions No information available to require special precautions
Effects on Dental Treatment >10%: Stomatitis
Mechanism of Action IL-2 promotes proliferation, differentiation, and recruitment of T and B cells, natural killer (NK) cells, and thymocytes; IL-2 also causes cytolytic activity in a subset of lymphocytes and subsequent interactions between the immune system and malignant cells; IL-2 can stimulate lymphokine-activated killer (LAK) cells and tumor-infiltrating lymphocytes (TIL) cells. LAK cells (which are derived from lymphocytes from a patient and incubated in IL-2) have the ability to lyse cells which are resistant to NK cells; TIL cells (which are derived from cancerous tissue from a patient and incubated in IL-2) have been shown to be 50% more effective than LAK cells.
Other Adverse Effects
>10%:
Cardiovascular: Sensory dysfunction, sinus tachycardia, arrhythmias, pulmonary congestion; hypotension (dose-limiting toxicity) which may require vasopressor support and hemodynamic changes resembling those seen in septic shock can be seen within 2 hours of administration; chest pain, acute myocardial infarction, SVT with hypotension has been reported, edema
Central nervous system: Dizziness, pain, fever, chills, cognitive changes, fatigue, malaise, disorientation, somnolence, paranoid delusion, and other behavioral changes; reversible and dose related; however, may continue to worsen for several days even after the infusion is stopped
Dermatologic: Pruritus, erythema, rash, dry skin, exfoliative dermatitis, macular erythema
Endocrine & metabolic: Fever, chills, low electrolyte levels (magnesium, calcium, phosphate, potassium, sodium)
Gastrointestinal: Nausea, vomiting, weight gain, diarrhea, stomatitis, anorexia, GI bleeding
Hematologic: Anemia, thrombocytopenia, leukopenia, eosinophilia, coagulation disorders
Hepatic: Elevated transaminase and alkaline phosphatase, jaundice
(Continued)

Aldesleukin *(Continued)*

Neuromuscular & skeletal: Weakness, rigors which can be decreased or ameliorated with acetaminophen or a nonsteroidal agent and meperidine

Renal: Oliguria, anuria, proteinuria; renal failure (dose-limiting toxicity) manifested as oliguria noted within 24-48 hours of initiation of therapy; marked fluid retention, azotemia, and increased serum creatinine seen, which may return to baseline within 7 days of discontinuation of therapy; hypophosphatemia

Respiratory: Dyspnea, pulmonary edema

Miscellaneous: Pain, infection (including sepsis and endocarditis) due to neutrophil impairment

1% to 10%:

Cardiovascular: Increase in vascular permeability: Capillary-leak syndrome manifested by severe peripheral edema, ascites, pulmonary infiltration, and pleural effusion; occurs in 2% to 4% of patients and is resolved after therapy ends.

Central nervous system: Seizures

Endocrine & metabolic: Hypo- and hyperglycemia; increased electrolyte levels (magnesium, calcium, phosphate, potassium, sodium), hypothyroidism

Hepatic: Ascites

Neuromuscular & skeletal: Arthralgia, myalgia

Renal: Hematuria, increased creatinine

Respiratory: Pleural effusions, edema

Drug Interactions

Aldesleukin may affect central nervous function; therefore, interactions could occur following concomitant administration of psychotropic drugs (eg, narcotics, analgesics, antiemetics, sedatives, tranquilizers).

Increased Effect/Toxicity: Concomitant administration of drugs possessing nephrotoxic (eg, aminoglycosides, indomethacin), myelotoxic (eg, cytotoxic chemotherapy), cardiotoxic (eg, doxorubicin), or hepatotoxic (eg, methotrexate, asparaginase) effects with aldesleukin may increase toxicity in these organ systems. The safety and efficacy of aldesleukin in combination with chemotherapies has not been established. Beta-blockers and other antihypertensives may potentiate the hypotension seen with aldesleukin.

Decreased Effect: Corticosteroids have been shown to decrease toxicity of IL-2, but have not been used since there is concern that they may reduce the efficacy of the lymphokine.

Drug Uptake

Absorption: Oral: Not absorbed

Half-life elimination: Initial: 6-13 minutes; Terminal: 80-120 minutes

Pregnancy Risk Factor C

Generic Available No

Comments 22 million units = 1.3 mg

1 Cetus Unit = 6 International Units

1.1 mg = 18 x 10^6 International Units (or 3 x 10^6 Cetus Units)

1 Roche Unit (Teceleukin) = 3 International Units

Aldoclor® *see* Chlorothiazide and Methyldopa *on page 267*

Aldomet® *see* Methyldopa *on page 793*

Aldoril® *see* Methyldopa and Hydrochlorothiazide *on page 794*

Alemtuzumab (ay lem TU zoo mab)

U.S. Brand Names Campath®

Pharmacologic Category Antineoplastic Agent, Monoclonal Antibody

Synonyms Campath-1H; DNA-derived Humanized Monoclonal Antibody; Humanized IgG1 Anti-CD52 Monoclonal Antibody

Use Treatment of B-cell chronic lymphocytic leukemia (B-CLL) in patients treated with alkylating agents and who have failed fludarabine therapy

Unlabeled/Investigational: Rheumatoid arthritis, graft versus host disease, multiple myeloma

Local Anesthetic/Vasoconstrictor Precautions No information available to require special precautions

Effects on Dental Treatment No effects or complications reported

Dosage Note: **Dose escalation is required;** usually accomplished in 3-7 days. Do not exceed single doses >30 mg or cumulative doses >90 mg/week. Premedicate with diphenhydramine and acetaminophen 30 minutes before initiation of infusion. Start anti-infective prophylaxis. Discontinue therapy during serious infection, serious hematologic or other serious toxicity until the event resolves. Permanently discontinue if evidence of autoimmune anemia or autoimmune thrombocytopenia occurs.

I.V. infusion: Adults: B-CLL:

Initial: 3 mg/day as a 2-hour infusion; when daily dose is tolerated (eg, infusion-related toxicities at or below Grade 2) increase to 10 mg/day and continue until tolerated; when 10 mg dose tolerated, increase to 30 mg/day

Maintenance: 30 mg/day 3 times/week on alternate days (ie, Monday, Wednesday, Friday) for up to 12 weeks

Dosage adjustment for hematologic toxicity (severe neutropenia or thrombocytopenia, not autoimmune):

First occurrence: ANC <250/µL and/or platelet count ≤25,000/µL: Hold therapy; resume at same dose when ANC ≥500/µL and platelet count ≥50,000/µL. If delay between dosing is ≥7 days, initiate at 3 mg/day and escalate dose as above according to patient tolerance

Second occurrence: ANC <250/µL and/or platelet count ≤25,000/µL: Hold therapy; resume at 10 mg/day when ANC ≥500/µL and platelet count ≥50,000/µL. If delay between dosing is ≥7 days, initiate at 3 mg/day and escalate dose to a maximum of 10 mg/day according to patient tolerance.

Third occurrence: ANC <250/µL and/or platelet count ≤25,000/µL: Permanently discontinue therapy

Patients with a baseline ANC ≤500/µL and/or a baseline platelet count ≤25,000/µL at initiation of therapy: If ANC and/or platelet counts decreased to ≤50% of the baseline value, hold therapy. When ANC and/or platelet count return to baseline, resume therapy. If delay between dosing is ≥7 days, initiate at 3 mg/day and escalate dose as above according to patient tolerance.

Mechanism of Action Recombinant monoclonal antibody binds to CD52, a nonmodulating antigen present on the surface of B and T lymphocytes, a majority of monocytes, macrophages, NK cells and a subpopulation of granulocytes. After binding to leukemic cells, an antibody-dependent lysis occurs.

Other Adverse Effects

>10%:

Cardiovascular: Hypotension (15% to 32%, infusion-related), peripheral edema (13%), hypertension (11%), tachycardia/SVT (11%)

Central nervous system: Drug-related fever (83%, infusion-related), fatigue (22% to 34%, infusion-related), headache (13% to 24%), dysthesias (15%), dizziness (12%), neutropenic fever (10%)

Dermatologic: Rash (30% to 40%, infusion-related), urticaria (22% to 30%, infusion-related), pruritus (14% to 24%, infusion-related)

Gastrointestinal: Nausea (47% to 54%), vomiting (33% to 41%), anorexia (20%), diarrhea (13% to 22%, infusion-related), stomatitis/mucositis (14%), abdominal pain (11%)

Hematologic: Lymphopenia, severe neutropenia (64% to 70%), severe anemia (38% to 47%), severe thrombocytopenia (50% to 52%)

Neuromuscular & skeletal: Rigors (89%, infusion-related), skeletal muscle pain (24%), weakness (13%), myalgia (11%)

Respiratory: Dyspnea (17% to 26%, infusion-related), cough (25%), bronchitis/pneumonitis (21%), pharyngitis (12%)

Miscellaneous: Infection (43% including sepsis, pneumonia, opportunistic infections; received PCP pneumonia and herpes prophylaxis); diaphoresis (19%)

1% to 10%:

Cardiovascular: Chest pain (10%)

Central nervous system: Insomnia (10%), malaise (9%), depression (7%), temperature change sensation (5%), somnolence (5%)

Dermatologic: Purpura (8%)

Gastrointestinal: Dyspepsia (10%), constipation (9%)

Hematologic: Pancytopenia/marrow hypoplasia (6%), positive Coombs' test without hemolysis (2%), autoimmune thrombocytopenia (2%), antibodies to alemtuzumab (2%), autoimmune hemolytic anemia (1%)

Neuromuscular & skeletal: Back pain (10%), tremor (7%)

Respiratory: Bronchospasm (9%), epistaxis (7%), rhinitis (7%)

Drug Uptake Serum half-life: 12 days

Pregnancy Risk Factor C

Generic Available No

Alendronate (a LEN droe nate)

U.S. Brand Names Fosamax®

Canadian Brand Names Fosamax®

Pharmacologic Category Bisphosphonate Derivative

Synonyms Alendronate Sodium

Use Treatment and prevention of osteoporosis in postmenopausal females; treatment of osteoporosis in males; Paget's disease of the bone in patients who are symptomatic, at risk for future complications, or with alkaline phosphatase ≥2 times the upper limit of normal; treatment of glucocorticoid-induced osteoporosis in males and females with low bone mineral density who are receiving a daily dosage ≥7.5 mg of prednisone (or equivalent)

Local Anesthetic/Vasoconstrictor Precautions No information available to require special precautions

Effects on Dental Treatment No effects or complications reported

Dosage Oral: Alendronate must be taken with a full glass (6-8 oz) of plain water first thing in the morning and ≥30 minutes before the first food, beverage, or other medication of the day. Patients should be instructed to stay upright (not to lie down) for at least 30 minutes **and** until after first food of the day (to reduce esophageal

(Continued)

Alendronate *(Continued)*

irritation). Patients should receive supplemental calcium and vitamin D if dietary intake is inadequate.

Adults:

Osteoporosis in postmenopausal females:

Prophylaxis: 5 mg once daily or 35 mg once weekly

Treatment: 10 mg once daily or 70 mg once weekly

Osteoporosis in males: 10 mg once daily

Paget's disease of bone: 40 mg once daily for 6 months

Retreatment: Relapses during the 12 months following therapy occurred in 9% of patients who responded to treatment. Specific retreatment data are not available. Retreatment with alendronate may be considered, following a 6-month post-treatment evaluation period, in patients who have relapsed based on increases in serum alkaline phosphatase, which should be measured periodically. Retreatment may also be considered in those who failed to normalize their serum alkaline phosphatase.

Glucocorticoid-induced osteoporosis: Treatment: 5 mg once daily; a dose of 10 mg once daily should be used in postmenopausal females who are not receiving estrogen. Patients treated with glucocorticoids should receive adequate amounts of calcium and vitamin D.

Dosage adjustment in renal impairment: Cl_{cr} <35 mL/minute: Use not recommended due to lack of experience

Mechanism of Action A bisphosphonate which inhibits bone resorption via actions on osteoclasts or on osteoclast precursors; decreases the rate of bone resorption direction, leading to an indirect decrease in bone formation

Other Adverse Effects Incidence of adverse effects increases significantly with Paget's disease at 40 mg/day (mostly GI adverse effects)

>10%: Endocrine & metabolic: Hypocalcemia (transient, mild, 18%); hypophosphatemia (transient, mild, 10%)

1% to 10%:

Central nervous system: Headache (0.2% to 3%)

Gastrointestinal: Abdominal pain (1% to 7%), acid reflux (1% to 5%), dyspepsia (1% to 4%), nausea (1% to 4%), flatulence (0.2% to 4%), diarrhea (0.6% to 3%), constipation (0.3% to 3%), esophageal ulcer (0.1% to 2%), abdominal distension (0.2% to 1%), gastritis (0.2% to 1%), vomiting (0.2% to 1%), dysphagia (0.1% to 1%), gastric ulcer (1%), melena (1%)

Neuromuscular & skeletal: Musculoskeletal pain (0.4% to 4%), muscle cramps (0.2% to 1%)

Warnings/Precautions Use caution in patients with renal impairment; hypocalcemia must be corrected before therapy initiation; ensure adequate calcium and vitamin D intake. May cause irritation to upper GI mucosa. Esophagitis, esophageal ulcers, esophageal erosions, and esophageal stricture (rare) have been reported; risk increases in patients unable to comply with dosing instructions. Use with caution in patients with dysphagia, esophageal disease, gastritis, duodenitis, or ulcers (may worsen underlying condition).

Drug Interactions

Increased Effect/Toxicity: I.V. ranitidine has been shown to double the bioavailability of alendronate. Estrogen replacement therapy, in combination with alendronate, may enhance the therapeutic effects of both agents on the maintenance of bone mineralization. An increased incidence of adverse GI effects has been noted when >10 mg alendronate is used in patients taking aspirin-containing products.

Decreased Effect: Oral medications (especially those containing multivalent cations, including calcium and antacids) may interfere with alendronate absorption; wait at least 30 minutes after taking alendronate before taking any oral medications.

Drug Uptake

Absorption: Oral: Male: 0.6% given in a fasting state; Female: 0.7%

Half-life, elimination: Terminal: Exceeds 10 years; >95% cleared in 6 hours

Pregnancy Risk Factor C

Generic Available No

Alesse® *see* Combination Hormonal Contraceptives *on page 323*

Aleve® [OTC] *see* Naproxen *on page 848*

Alfenta® *see* Alfentanil *on page 50*

Alfentanil (al FEN ta nil)

U.S. Brand Names Alfenta®

Canadian Brand Names Alfenta®

Mexican Brand Names Rapifen®

Pharmacologic Category Analgesic, Narcotic

Synonyms Alfentanil Hydrochloride

Use Analgesic adjunct given by continuous infusion or in incremental doses in maintenance of anesthesia with barbiturate or nitrous oxide (N_2O) or a primary anesthetic agent for the induction of anesthesia in patients undergoing general surgery in which endotracheal intubation and mechanical ventilation are required

Local Anesthetic/Vasoconstrictor Precautions No information available to require special precautions

Effects on Dental Treatment Erythromycin inhibits the liver metabolism of alfentanil resulting in increased sedation and prolonged respiratory depression.

Restrictions C-II

Dosage Doses should be titrated to appropriate effects; wide range of doses is dependent upon desired degree of analgesia/anesthesia

Children <12 years: Dose not established

Adults: Dose should be based on ideal body weight; see table.

Alfentanil

Indication	Approximate Duration of Anesthesia	Induction Period (Initial Dose)	Maintenance Period (Increments/ Infusion)	Total Dose	Effects
Incremental injection	≤30 minutes	8-20 mcg/kg	3-5 mcg/kg or 0.5-1 mcg/kg/ minute	8-40 mcg/kg	Spontaneously breathing or assisted ventilation when required
	30-60 minutes	20-50 mcg/kg	5-15 mcg/kg	Up to 75 mcg/kg	Assisted or controlled ventilation required; attenuation of response to laryngoscopy and intubation
Continuous infusion	>45 minutes	50-75 mcg/kg	0.5-3 mcg/kg/ minute; average infusion rate 1-1.5 mcg/kg/minute	Dependent on duration of procedure	Assisted or controlled ventilation required; some attenuation of response to intubation and incision, with intraoperative stability
Anesthetic induction	>45 minutes	130-245 mcg/kg	0.5-1.5 mcg/kg/ minute or general anesthetic	Dependent on duration of procedure	Assisted or controlled ventilation required; administer slowly (over 3 minutes); concentration of inhalation agents reduced by 30% to 50% for initial hour

Mechanism of Action Binds to opiate receptors (mu and kappa subtypes) in the CNS causing inhibition of ascending pain pathways, altering the perception of and response to pain; produces generalized CNS depression; is an ultra short-acting narcotic

Other Adverse Effects

>10%:

- Cardiovascular: Bradycardia, peripheral vasodilation
- Central nervous system: Drowsiness, sedation, increased intracranial pressure
- Endocrine & metabolic: Antidiuretic hormone release
- Gastrointestinal: Nausea, vomiting, constipation
- Ocular: Miosis

1% to 10%:

- Cardiovascular: Cardiac arrhythmias, orthostatic hypotension
- Central nervous system: Confusion, CNS depression
- Ocular: Blurred vision

Warnings/Precautions Use with caution in patients with drug dependence, head injury, acute asthma and respiratory conditions; hypotension has occurred in neonates with respiratory distress syndrome; use caution when administering to patients with bradyarrhythmias; rapid I.V. infusion may result in skeletal muscle and chest wall rigidity, impaired ventilation, or respiratory distress/arrest; inject slowly over 3-5 minutes. Alfentanil may produce more hypotension compared to fentanyl, therefore, be sure to administer slowly and ensure patient has adequate hydration.

Drug Interactions CYP3A3/4 enzyme substrate

Increased Effect/Toxicity: Dextroamphetamine may enhance the analgesic effect of morphine and other opiate agonists. CNS depressants (eg, benzodiazepines, barbiturates, phenothiazines, tricyclic antidepressants), erythromycin, reserpine, beta-blockers may increase the toxic effects of alfentanil.

Decreased Effect: Phenothiazines may antagonize the analgesic effect of opiate agonists.

Drug Uptake

Onset of action: Rapid

Duration: 30-60 minutes (dose dependent)

Half-life elimination: Newborns, premature: 5.33-8.75 hours; Children: 40-60 minutes; Adults: 83-97 minutes

Pregnancy Risk Factor C

Generic Available Yes

Selected Readings

Bartkowski RR, Goldberg ME, Larijani GE, et al, "Inhibition of Alfentanil Metabolism by Erythromycin," *Clin Pharmacol Ther*, 1989, 46(1):99-102.

(Continued)

Alfentanil *(Continued)*

Bartkowski RR and McDonnell TE, "Prolonged Alfentanil Effect Following Erythromycin Administration," *Anesthesiology*, 1990, 73(3):566-8.

Alferon® N *see* Interferon Alfa-n3 *on page 646*

Alglucerase (al GLOO ser ase)

U.S. Brand Names Ceredase®

Pharmacologic Category Enzyme

Synonyms Glucocerebrosidase

Use Treatment of anxiety disorder (GAD); panic disorder, with or without agoraphobia; anxiety associated with depression

Orphan drug: Replacement therapy for Gaucher's disease (type 1)

Local Anesthetic/Vasoconstrictor Precautions No information available to require special precautions

Effects on Dental Treatment No effects or complications reported

Dosage Usually administered as a 20-60 units/kg I.V. infusion given with a frequency ranging from 3 times/week to once every 2 weeks

Mechanism of Action Glucocerebrosidase is an enzyme prepared from human placental tissue. Gaucher's disease is an inherited metabolic disorder caused by the defective activity of beta-glucosidase and the resultant accumulation of glucosyl ceramide laden macrophages in the liver, bone, and spleen; acts by replacing the missing enzyme associated with Gaucher's disease.

Other Adverse Effects >10%: Local: Discomfort, burning, and edema at the site of injection

Drug Uptake Serum half-life, elimination: ~4-20 minutes

Pregnancy Risk Factor C

Generic Available No

Alitretinoin (a li TRET i noyn)

U.S. Brand Names Panretin®

Canadian Brand Names Panretin™

Pharmacologic Category Antineoplastic Agent, Miscellaneous

Use Orphan drug: Topical treatment of cutaneous lesions in AIDS-related Kaposi's sarcoma; not indicated when systemic therapy for Kaposi's sarcoma is indicated

Local Anesthetic/Vasoconstrictor Precautions No information available to require special precautions

Effects on Dental Treatment No effects or complications reported

Mechanism of Action Binds to retinoid receptors to inhibit growth of Kaposi's sarcoma.

Other Adverse Effects

>10%:

- Central nervous system: Pain (0% to 34%)
- Dermatologic: Rash (25% to 77%), pruritus (8% to 11%)
- Neuromuscular & skeletal: Paresthesia (3% to 22%)

1% to 10%:

- Cardiovascular: Edema (3% to 8%)
- Dermatologic: Exfoliative dermatitis (3% to 9%), skin disorder (0% to 8%)

Contraindications Hypersensitivity to alitretinoin, other retinoids, or any component of their formulation

Warnings/Precautions May cause fetal harm if absorbed by a woman who is pregnant. Patients with cutaneous T-cell lymphoma have a high incidence of treatment-limiting adverse reactions. May be photosensitizing (based on experience with other retinoids); minimize sun or other UV exposure of treated areas. Do not use concurrently with topical products containing DEET (increased toxicity may result). Safety in pediatric patients or geriatric patients has not been established. Occlusive dressing should not be used.

Drug Interactions Increased toxicity of DEET may occur if products containing this compound are used concurrently with alitretinoin. Due to limited absorption after topical application, interaction with systemic medications is unlikely.

Drug Uptake Absorption: Not extensive

Pregnancy Risk Factor D

Generic Available No

Alkaban-AQ® *see* VinBLAStine *on page 1240*

Alka-Mints® [OTC] *see* Calcium Carbonate *on page 201*

Alka-Seltzer Plus® Cold and Sinus [OTC] *see* Acetaminophen and Pseudoephedrine *on page 30*

Alka-Seltzer® Plus Cold Liqui-Gels® [OTC] *see* Acetaminophen, Chlorpheniramine, and Pseudoephedrine *on page 33*

Alka-Seltzer® Plus Flu Liqui-Gels® [OTC] *see* Acetaminophen, Dextromethorphan, and Pseudoephedrine *on page 34*

Alkeran® *see* Melphalan *on page 758*

Allbee® With C [OTC] *see* Vitamin B Complex With Vitamin C *on page 1244*

Allegra® *see* Fexofenadine *on page 500*
Allegra-D® *see* Fexofenadine and Pseudoephedrine *on page 501*
Aller-Chlor® [OTC] *see* Chlorpheniramine *on page 268*
Allerest® 12 Hour Nasal [OTC] *see* Oxymetazoline *on page 907*
Allerest® Maximum Strength [OTC] *see* Chlorpheniramine and Pseudoephedrine *on page 270*
Allerfed® [OTC] *see* Triprolidine and Pseudoephedrine *on page 1213*
Allerfrim® [OTC] *see* Triprolidine and Pseudoephedrine *on page 1213*
Allergen® *see* Antipyrine and Benzocaine *on page 107*
AllerMax® [OTC] *see* DiphenhydrAMINE *on page 398*
Allerphed® [OTC] *see* Triprolidine and Pseudoephedrine *on page 1213*
Allersol® *see* Naphazoline *on page 847*

Allopurinol (al oh PURE i nole)

U.S. Brand Names Aloprim™; Zyloprim®

Canadian Brand Names Apo®-Allopurinol; Zyloprim®

Mexican Brand Names Atisuril®; Unizuric 300; Zyloprim®

Pharmacologic Category Xanthine Oxidase Inhibitor

Synonyms Allopurinol Sodium Injection

Use Oral: Prevention of attack of gouty arthritis and nephropathy; treatment of secondary hyperuricemia which may occur during treatment of tumors or leukemia; prevention of recurrent calcium oxalate calculi

Orphan drug: I.V.: Management of patients with leukemia, lymphoma, and solid tumor malignancies who are receiving cancer chemotherapy which causes elevations of serum and urinary uric acid levels and who cannot tolerate oral therapy

Local Anesthetic/Vasoconstrictor Precautions No information available to require special precautions

Effects on Dental Treatment No effects or complications reported

Dosage

Oral:

Children ≤10 years: 10 mg/kg/day in 2-3 divided doses **or** 200-300 mg/m²/day in 2-4 divided doses, maximum: 800 mg/24 hours

Alternative: <6 years: 150 mg/day in 3 divided doses; 6-10 years: 300 mg/day in 2-3 divided doses

Children >10 years and Adults: Daily doses >300 mg should be administered in divided doses

Myeloproliferative neoplastic disorders: 600-800 mg/day in 2-3 divided doses for prevention of acute uric acid nephropathy for 2-3 days starting 1-2 days before chemotherapy

Gout: Mild: 200-300 mg/day; Severe: 400-600 mg/day

Elderly: Initial: 100 mg/day, increase until desired uric acid level is obtained

I.V.: Hyperuricemia secondary to chemotherapy: Intravenous daily dose can be given as a single infusion or in equally divided doses at 6-, 8-, or 12-hour intervals. A fluid intake sufficient to yield a daily urinary output of at least 2 L in adults and the maintenance of a neutral or, preferably, slightly alkaline urine are desirable.

Children: Starting dose: 200 mg/m²/day

Adults: 200-400 mg/m²/day (max: 600 mg/day)

Dosing adjustment in renal impairment: Must be adjusted due to accumulation of allopurinol and metabolites:

Oral: Removed by hemodialysis; adult maintenance doses of allopurinol* (mg) based on creatinine clearance (mL/minute): See table.

Adult Maintenance Doses of Allopurinol*

Creatinine Clearance (mL/min)	Maintenance Dose of Allopurinol (mg)
140	400 qd
120	350 qd
100	300 qd
80	250 qd
60	200 qd
40	150 qd
20	100 qd
10	100 q2d
0	100 q3d

*This table is based on a standard maintenance dose of 300 mg of allopurinol per day for a patient with a creatinine clearance of 100 mL/min.

Hemodialysis: Administer dose posthemodialysis or administer 50% supplemental dose

(Continued)

Allopurinol *(Continued)*

I.V.:

Cl_{cr} 10-20 mL/minute: 200 mg/day
Cl_{cr} 3-10 mL/minute: 100 mg/day
Cl_{cr} <3 mL/minute: 100 mg/day at extended intervals

Mechanism of Action Inhibits xanthine oxidase, the enzyme responsible for the conversion of hypoxanthine to xanthine to uric acid; allopurinol is metabolized to oxypurinol which is also an inhibitor of xanthine oxidase. Allopurinol acts on purine catabolism, reducing the production of uric acid without disrupting the biosynthesis of vital purines.

Other Adverse Effects The most common adverse reaction to allopurinol is a skin rash (usually maculopapular; however, more severe reactions, including Stevens-Johnson syndrome, have also been reported). While some studies cite an incidence of these reactions as high as >10% of cases (often in association with ampicillin or amoxicillin), the product labeling cites a much lower incidence, reflected below. Allopurinol should be discontinued at the first appearance of a rash or other sign of hypersensitivity.

>1%:

Dermatologic: Rash (1.5%)
Gastrointestinal: Nausea (1.3%), vomiting (1.2%)
Renal: Renal failure/impairment (1.2%)

Drug Interactions Hepatic enzyme inhibitor; isoenzyme profile not defined

Increased Effect/Toxicity: Allopurinol may increase the effects of azathioprine, chlorpropamide, mercaptopurine, theophylline, and oral anticoagulants. An increased risk of bone marrow suppression may occur when given with myelosuppressive agents (cyclophosphamide, possibly other alkylating agents). Amoxicillin/ampicillin, ACE inhibitors, and thiazide diuretics have been associated with hypersensitivity reactions when combined with allopurinol (rare), and the incidence of rash may be increased with penicillins (ampicillin, amoxicillin). Urinary acidification with large amounts of vitamin C may increase kidney stone formation.

Drug Uptake Allopurinol and oxypurinol are dialyzable

Onset of action: Peak effect: 1-2 weeks
Absorption: Oral: ~80%; Rectal: Poor and erratic
Half-life, elimination: Normal renal function: Parent drug: 1-3 hours; Oxypurinol: 18-30 hours; End-stage renal disease: Prolonged
Time to peak, plasma: Oral: 30-120 minutes

Pregnancy Risk Factor C

Generic Available Yes

Almotriptan (al moh TRIP tan)

U.S. Brand Names Axert™

Pharmacologic Category Serotonin $5\text{-}HT_{1D}$ Receptor Agonist

Use Acute treatment of migraine with or without aura

Local Anesthetic/Vasoconstrictor Precautions No information available to require special precautions

Effects on Dental Treatment No effects or complications reported

Dosage Oral: Adults: Migraine: Initial: 6.25-12.5 mg in a single dose; if the headache returns, repeat the dose after 2 hours; no more than 2 doses in 24-hour period

Note: If the first dose is ineffective, diagnosis needs to be re-evaluated. Safety of treating more than 4 migraines/month has not been established.

Dosage adjustment in renal impairment: Initial: 6.25 mg in a single dose; maximum daily dose: ≤12.5 mg

Dosage adjustment in hepatic impairment: Initial: 6.25 mg in a single dose; maximum daily dose: ≤12.5 mg

Mechanism of Action Selective agonist for serotonin ($5\text{-}HT_{1B}$, $5\text{-}HT_{1D}$, $5\text{-}HT_{1F}$ receptors) in cranial arteries; causes vasoconstriction and reduces sterile inflammation associated with antidromic neuronal transmission correlating with relief of migraine

Other Adverse Effects 1% to 10%:

Central nervous system: Headache (>1%), dizziness (>1%), somnolence (>1%)
Gastrointestinal: Nausea (1% to 2%), xerostomia (1%)
Neuromuscular & skeletal: Paresthesia (1%)

Drug Interactions CYP2D6 and 3A3/4 enzyme substrate

Increased Effect/Toxicity: Ergot-containing drugs prolong vasospastic reactions; ketoconazole and CYP3A4 inhibitors increase almotriptan serum concentration; select serotonin reuptake inhibitors may increase symptoms of hyper-reflexia, weakness, and incoordination; MAO inhibitors may increase toxicity

Drug Uptake

Absorption: Well absorbed
Half-life, elimination: 3-4 hours
Time to peak: 1-3 hours

Pregnancy Risk Factor C

Generic Available No

Alocril™ *see* Nedocromil Sodium *on page 851*

Aloe Vesta® 2-n-1 Antifungal [OTC] *see* Miconazole *on page 807*

Alomide® *see* Lodoxamide Tromethamine *on page 723*

Alophen® [OTC] *see* Bisacodyl *on page 166*

Aloprim™ *see* Allopurinol *on page 53*

Alora® *see* Estradiol *on page 457*

Alosetron (a LOE se tron)

U.S. Brand Names Lotronex®

Pharmacologic Category Selective 5-HT_3 Receptor Antagonist

Use Treatment of irritable bowel syndrome (IBS) in women with severe diarrhea-predominant IBS who have failed to respond to conventional therapy

Unlabeled/Investigational: Has demonstrated effectiveness as an antiemetic for a wide variety of causes of emesis

Local Anesthetic/Vasoconstrictor Precautions No information available to require special precautions

Effects on Dental Treatment No effects or complications reported

Restrictions Restricted distribution as of June 7, 2002; only physicians enrolled in GlaxoSmithKline's Prescribing Program may prescribe. Physicians must enroll in the plan prior to prescribing this medication. Program stickers must be affixed to all prescriptions; no phone, fax or computerized prescriptions are permitted. Patients are required to sign a "Patient-Physician Agreement" before receiving their initial prescription.

Dosage Discontinue immediately if constipation or signs/symptoms of ischemic colitis occur. Do not reinitiate in patients who develop ischemic colitis.

Adults: Female: Oral: 1 mg once daily for 4 weeks, with or without food; if tolerated, but response is inadequate, may be increased after 4 weeks to 1 mg twice daily. If response is inadequate after 4 weeks of twice daily dosing, discontinue treatment.

Dosage adjustment in renal/hepatic impairment: The need for dosage adjustment has not been defined (due to limited information on activity of metabolites).

Mechanism of Action Potent and selective antagonist of a subtype of the serotonin receptor, 5-HT_3 receptor, which is extensively distributed on enteric neurons in the human GI tract, as well as other peripheral and central locations; activation of these channels affects the regulation of visceral pain, colonic transit, and GI secretions. Improvement in pain, abdominal discomfort, urgency, and diarrhea may occur in patients with irritable bowel syndrome.

Other Adverse Effects

>10%: Gastrointestinal: Constipation (28%)

1% to 10%:

Cardiovascular: Hypertension (2%)

Central nervous system: Sleep disorders (3%), depression (2%)

Gastrointestinal: Nausea (7%), gastrointestinal discomfort and pain (5%), abdominal discomfort and pain (5%), gastrointestinal gaseous symptoms (3%), viral infections (2%), dyspepsia (3%), abdominal distention (2%), hemorrhoids (2%)

Otic: Bacterial ear infection (1%)

Respiratory: Allergic rhinitis (2%); throat and tonsil discomfort and pain (1%); bacterial nose and throat infection (1%)

Contraindications Do not start treatment in patients who are constipated. Hypersensitivity to alosetron or any component of the formulation; history of severe or chronic constipation; history of ischemic colitis, intestinal obstruction, stricture, toxic megacolon, GI perforation and/or adhesions; active diverticulitis, current or history of Crohn's disease or ulcerative colitis; history of impaired intestinal circulation, thrombophlebitis, or hypercoagulable state

Warnings/Precautions Lotronex® marketing is restricted due to serious and unpredictable GI adverse events, some leading to death. Discontinue immediately in patients with acute ischemic colitis, constipation, rectal bleeding, or sudden worsening of abdominal pain. Constipation is a frequent, dose-related side effect; serious complications have been infrequently reported (obstruction, perforation, impaction, toxic megacolon, secondary ischemia); risk may be increased in elderly, debilitated patients, or concurrent use of other medications which decrease GI motility. Use caution in hepatic or renal impairment. Safety and efficacy have not been established in pediatric or male patients.

Drug Interactions CYP2C9, CYP3A4, and CYP1A2 enzyme substrate; inhibits CYP1A2, 2E1 only at extremely high concentrations (no clinical significance)

Increased Effect/Toxicity: Inducers or inhibitors of these enzymes theoretically may change the clearance of alosetron, but this has not been evaluated. Alosetron inhibits N-acetyltransferase which may influence the metabolism of drugs such as isoniazid, procainamide, and hydralazine but there has not been any investigation of this. Drugs which decrease GI motility (opiates, anticholinergic agents, tricyclic antidepressants) may increase the risk of constipation and/or severe complications.

Drug Uptake

Half-life, elimination: 1.5 hours for alosetron

(Continued)

Alosetron *(Continued)*

Time to peak: 1 hour after oral administration

Pregnancy Risk Factor B

Generic Available No

Alpha$_1$-Proteinase Inhibitor (al fa won PRO tee in ase in HI bi tor)

U.S. Brand Names Prolastin®

Canadian Brand Names Prolastin®

Pharmacologic Category Antitrypsin Deficiency Agent

Synonyms Alpha$_1$-PI; Alpha$_1$-Proteinase Inhibitor, Human

Use Congenital alpha$_1$-antitrypsin deficiency

Local Anesthetic/Vasoconstrictor Precautions No information available to require special precautions

Effects on Dental Treatment No effects or complications reported

Dosage Adults: I.V.: 60 mg/kg once weekly (at a rate ≥0.08 mL/kg/minute)

Mechanism of Action Human alpha$_1$-proteinase inhibitor is prepared from the pooled human plasma of normal donors and is intended for use in the therapy of congenital alpha$_1$-antitrypsin deficiency. Alpha$_1$-antitrypsin (AAT) is the principal protease inhibitor in the serum and exists as a single polypeptide glycoprotein. Production of AAT occurs in the liver hepatocyte and secretion occurs at a rate to maintain serum concentration of 150-200 mg/dL. The major physiologic role of the antiprotease is that of combining with proteolytic enzymes to render them inactive. Several proteases can be inactivated by AAT including trypsin, chymotrypsin, coagulation factor XI, plasmin, thrombin, and neutrophil elastase.

Drug Uptake Serum half-life, elimination: Parent compound: 4.5-5.2 days

Pregnancy Risk Factor C

Generic Available No

Comments Sodium content of 1 L after reconstitution: 100-210 mEq

Alphagan® *see* Brimonidine *on page 177*
Alphagan® P *see* Brimonidine *on page 177*
Alphanate® *see* Antihemophilic Factor (Human) *on page 104*
AlphaNine® SD *see* Factor IX Complex (Human) *on page 484*
Alphatrex® *see* Betamethasone *on page 159*

Alprazolam (al PRAY zoe lam)

Related Information

Patients Requiring Sedation *on page 1400*
Temporomandibular Dysfunction (TMD) *on page 1397*

U.S. Brand Names Alprazolam Intensol®; Xanax®

Canadian Brand Names Alti-Alprazolam; Apo®-Alpraz; Gen-Alprazolam; Novo-Alprazol; Nu-Alprax; Xanax®; Xanax TS™

Mexican Brand Names Tafil

Pharmacologic Category Benzodiazepine

Use Treatment of anxiety disorder (GAD); panic disorder, with or without agoraphobia; anxiety associated with depression

Unlabeled/Investigational: Anxiety in children

Local Anesthetic/Vasoconstrictor Precautions No information available to require special precautions

Effects on Dental Treatment >10%: Significant xerostomia; normal salivary flow resumes with discontinuation

Restrictions C-IV

Dosage Oral:

Children: Anxiety (unlabeled use): Initial: 0.005 mg/kg or 0.125 mg/dose 3 times/day; increase in increments of 0.125-0.25 mg, up to a maximum of 0.02 mg/kg/dose or 0.06 mg/kg/day (0.375-3 mg/day)

Adults:

- Anxiety: Effective doses are 0.5-4 mg/day in divided doses; the manufacturer recommends starting at 0.25-0.5 mg 3 times/day; titrate dose upward; maximum: 4 mg/day
- Depression: Average dose required: 2.5-3 mg/day in divided doses
- Ethanol withdrawal: Usual dose: 2-2.5 mg/day in divided doses
- Panic disorder: Many patients obtain relief at 2 mg/day, as much as 10 mg/day may be required

Elderly: Elderly patients may be more sensitive to the effects of alprazolam including ataxia and oversedation. The elderly may also have impaired renal function leading to decreased clearance. The smallest effective dose should be used.

Dosing adjustment in hepatic impairment: Reduce dose by 50% to 60% or avoid in cirrhosis

Note: Treatment >4 months should be re-evaluated to determine the patient's need for the drug

Mechanism of Action Binds to stereospecific benzodiazepine receptors on the postsynaptic GABA neuron at several sites within the CNS, including the limbic system, reticular formation. Enhancement of the inhibitory effect of GABA on neuronal excitability results by increased neuronal membrane permeability to chloride ions. This shift in chloride ions results in hyperpolarization (a less excitable state) and stabilization.

Other Adverse Effects

>10%:

Central nervous system: Drowsiness, fatigue, ataxia, lightheadedness, memory impairment, dysarthria, irritability

Dermatologic: Rash

Endocrine & metabolic: Decreased libido, menstrual disorders

Gastrointestinal: Xerostomia, decreased salivation, increased or decreased appetite, weight gain or loss

Genitourinary: Micturition difficulties

1% to 10%:

Cardiovascular: Hypotension

Central nervous system: Confusion, dizziness, disinhibition, akathisia, increased libido

Dermatologic: Dermatitis, rash

Gastrointestinal: Increased salivation

Genitourinary: Sexual dysfunction, incontinence

Neuromuscular & skeletal: Rigidity, tremor, muscle cramps

Otic: Tinnitus

Respiratory: Nasal congestion

Warnings/Precautions Rebound or withdrawal symptoms, including seizures may occur 18 hours to 3 days following abrupt discontinuation or large decreases in dose (more common in patients receiving >4 mg/day or prolonged treatment). Dose reductions or tapering must be approached with extreme caution. Between dose, anxiety may also occur. Use with caution in patients receiving concurrent CYP3A4 inhibitors, particularly when these agents are added to therapy. Has weak uricosuric properties, use with caution in renal impairment or predisposition to urate nephropathy. Use with caution in elderly or debilitated patients, patients with hepatic disease (including alcoholics), renal impairment, or obese patients.

Causes CNS depression (dose-related) resulting in sedation, dizziness, confusion, or ataxia which may impair physical and mental capabilities. Patients must be cautioned about performing tasks which require mental alertness (ie, operating machinery or driving). Use with caution in patients receiving other CNS depressants or psychoactive agents. Effects with other sedative drugs or ethanol may be potentiated. Benzodiazepines have been associated with falls and traumatic injury and should be used with extreme caution in patients who are at risk of these events (especially the elderly). Use with caution in patients with respiratory disease or impaired gag reflex.

Use caution in patients with depression, particularly if suicidal risk may be present. Episodes of mania or hypomania have occurred in depressed patients treated with alprazolam. May cause physical or psychological dependence - use with caution in patients with a history of drug dependence. Acute withdrawal, including seizures, may be precipitated in patients after administration of flumazenil to patients receiving long-term benzodiazepine therapy.

Benzodiazepines have been associated with anterograde amnesia. Paradoxical reactions, including hyperactive or aggressive behavior, have been reported with benzodiazepines, particularly in adolescent/pediatric or psychiatric patients. Does not have analgesic, antidepressant, or antipsychotic properties.

Drug Interactions CYP3A3/4 enzyme substrate

Increased Effect/Toxicity: Alprazolam potentiates the CNS depressant effects of narcotic analgesics, barbiturates, phenothiazines, antihistamines, MAO inhibitors, sedative-hypnotics, and cyclic antidepressants. Serum levels and/or effects of alprazolam may be increased by inhibitors of CYP3A3/4, including amprenavir, cimetidine, ciprofloxacin, clarithromycin, clozapine, diltiazem, disulfiram, digoxin, erythromycin, ethanol, fluconazole, fluoxetine, fluvoxamine, isoniazid, itraconazole, ketoconazole, labetalol, levodopa, loxapine, metoprolol, metronidazole, miconazole, nefazodone, nelfinavir, omeprazole, phenytoin, rifabutin, rifampin, ritonavir, troleandomycin, valproic acid, and verapamil.

Decreased Effect: Carbamazepine, rifampin, rifabutin may enhance the metabolism of alprazolam and decrease its therapeutic effect.

Drug Uptake

Onset of action: Within 1 hour

Duration: 8-24 hours

Half-life, elimination: 12-15 hours

Time to peak: 1-2 hours

Pregnancy Risk Factor D

Generic Available Yes

Alprazolam Intensol® *see* Alprazolam *on page 56*

Alprostadil (al PROS ta dill)

U.S. Brand Names Caverject®; Edex®; Muse® Pellet; Prostin VR Pediatric®

Canadian Brand Names Caverject™; Prostin® VR

Mexican Brand Names Caverject®; Muse®

Pharmacologic Category Prostaglandin

Synonyms PGE_1; Prostaglandin E_1

Use Temporary maintenance of patency of ductus arteriosus in neonates with ductal-dependent congenital heart disease until surgery can be performed. These defects include cyanotic (eg, pulmonary atresia, pulmonary stenosis, tricuspid atresia, Fallot's tetralogy, transposition of the great vessels) and acyanotic (eg, interruption of aortic arch, coarctation of aorta, hypoplastic left ventricle) heart disease; diagnosis and treatment of erectile dysfunction of vasculogenic, psychogenic, or neurogenic etiology; adjunct in the diagnosis of erectile dysfunction

Unlabeled/Investigational: Treatment of pulmonary hypertension in infants and children with congenital heart defects with left-to-right shunts

Local Anesthetic/Vasoconstrictor Precautions No information available to require special precautions

Effects on Dental Treatment No effects or complications reported

Dosage

Patent ductus arteriosus (Prostin VR Pediatric®):

I.V. continuous infusion into a large vein, or alternatively through an umbilical artery catheter placed at the ductal opening: 0.05-0.1 mcg/kg/minute with therapeutic response, rate is reduced to lowest effective dosage; with unsatisfactory response, rate is increased gradually; maintenance: 0.01-0.4 mcg/kg/minute

PGE_1 is usually given at an infusion rate of 0.1 mcg/kg/minute, but it is often possible to reduce the dosage to 1/2 or even 1/10 without losing the therapeutic effect. The mixing schedule is shown in the table.

Add 1 Ampul (500 mcg) to:	Concentration (mcg/mL)	Infusion Rate mL/min/kg Needed to Infuse 0.1 mcg/kg/minute	Infusion Rate mL/kg/24 hours
250 mL	2	0.05	72
100 mL	5	0.02	28.8
50 mL	10	0.01	14.4
25 mL	20	0.005	7.2

Therapeutic response is indicated by increased pH in those with acidosis or by an increase in oxygenation (pO_2) usually evident within 30 minutes

Erectile dysfunction (Caverject®):

Vasculogenic, psychogenic, or mixed etiology: Individualize dose by careful titration; usual dose: 2.5-60 mcg (doses >60 mcg are not recommended); initiate dosage titration at 2.5 mcg, increasing by 2.5 mcg to a dose of 5 mcg and then in increments of 5-10 mcg depending on the erectile response until the dose produces an erection suitable for intercourse, not lasting >1 hour; if there is absolutely no response to initial 2.5 mcg dose, the second dose may increased to 7.5 mcg, followed by increments of 5-10 mcg

Neurogenic etiology (eg, spinal cord injury): Initiate dosage titration at 1.25 mcg, increasing to a doses of 2.5 mcg and then 5 mcg; increase further in increments 5 mcg until the dose is reached that produces an erection suitable for intercourse, not lasting >1 hour

Note: Patient must stay in the physician's office until complete detumescence occurs; if there is no response, then the next higher dose may be given within 1 hour; if there is still no response, a 1-day interval before giving the next dose is recommended; increasing the dose or concentration in the treatment of impotence results in increasing pain and discomfort

Muse® Pellet: Intraurethral: Administer as needed to achieve an erection; duration of action is about 30-60 minutes; use only two systems per 24-hour period

Elderly: Elderly patients may have a greater frequency of renal dysfunction; lowest effective dose should be used. In clinical studies with Edex®, higher minimally effective doses and a higher rate of lack of effect were noted.

Mechanism of Action Causes vasodilation by means of direct effect on vascular and ductus arteriosus smooth muscle; relaxes trabecular smooth muscle by dilation of cavernosal arteries when injected along the penile shaft, allowing blood flow to and entrapment in the lacunar spaces of the penis (ie, corporeal veno-occlusive mechanism)

Other Adverse Effects

>10%:

Cardiovascular: Flushing
Central nervous system: Fever
Genitourinary: Penile pain
Respiratory: Apnea

1% to 10%:

Cardiovascular: Bradycardia, hypotension, hypertension, tachycardia, cardiac arrest, edema

Central nervous system: Seizures, headache, dizziness

Endocrine & metabolic: Hypokalemia

Gastrointestinal: Diarrhea

Genitourinary: Priapism, penile fibrosis, penis disorder, penile rash, penile edema

Hematologic: Disseminated intravascular coagulation

Local: Injection site hematoma, injection site bruising

Neuromuscular & skeletal: Back pain

Respiratory: Upper respiratory infection, flu syndrome, sinusitis, nasal congestion, cough

Miscellaneous: Sepsis, localized pain in structures other than the injection site

Drug Interactions Increased Effect/Toxicity: Risk of hypotension and syncope may be increased with antihypertensives.

Drug Uptake

Onset of action: Rapid

Duration: <1 hour

Half-life elimination: 5-10 minutes

Pregnancy Risk Factor X

Generic Available Yes: Injection 5 mcg/mL

Alrex™ *see* Loteprednol *on page 733*

Altace® *see* Ramipril *on page 1040*

Altafed® [OTC] *see* Triprolidine and Pseudoephedrine *on page 1213*

Altamist [OTC] *see* Sodium Chloride *on page 1094*

Alteplase (AL te plase)

U.S. Brand Names Activase®; Cathflo™ Activase®

Canadian Brand Names Activase® rt-PA

Mexican Brand Names Actilyse®

Pharmacologic Category Thrombolytic Agent

Synonyms Alteplase, Recombinant; Alteplase, Tissue Plasminogen Activator, Recombinant; tPA

Use Management of acute myocardial infarction for the lysis of thrombi in coronary arteries; management of acute massive pulmonary embolism (PE) in adults

Acute myocardial infarction (AMI): Chest pain ≥20 minutes, ≤12-24 hours; S-T elevation ≥0.1 mV in at least two EKG leads

Acute pulmonary embolism (APE): Age ≤75 years: As soon as possible within 5 days of thrombotic event. Documented massive pulmonary embolism by pulmonary angiography or echocardiography or high probability lung scan with clinical shock.

Cathflo™ Activase®: Restoration of central venous catheter function

Unlabeled/Investigational: Peripheral arterial thrombotic obstruction

Local Anesthetic/Vasoconstrictor Precautions No information available to require special precautions

Effects on Dental Treatment No effects or complications reported

Dosage

I.V.:

Coronary artery thrombi: Front loading dose (weight-based):

Patients >67 kg: Total dose: 100 mg over 1.5 hours; infuse 15 mg (30 mL) over 1-2 minutes. Infuse 50 mg (100 mL) over 30 minutes. Concurrently, begin heparin 60 units/kg bolus (maximum: 4000 units) followed by continuous infusion of 12 units/kg/hour (maximum: 1000 units/hour) and adjust to aPTT target of 1.5-2 times the upper limit of control. Infuse remaining 35 mg (70 mL) of alteplase over the next hour.

Patients ≤67 kg: Total dose: 1.25 mg/kg; infuse 15 mg I.V. bolus over 1-2 minutes, then infuse 0.75 mg/kg (not to exceed 50 mg) over next 30 minutes, followed by 0.5 mg/kg over next 60 minutes (not to exceed 35 mg)

Acute pulmonary embolism: 100 mg over 2 hours.

Acute ischemic stroke: Doses should be given within the first 3 hours of the onset of symptoms. Load with 0.09 mg/kg as a bolus, followed by 0.81 mg/kg as a continuous infusion over 60 minutes. Maximum total dose should not exceed 90 mg. Heparin should not be started for at least 24 hours after starting alteplase for stroke.

Intracatheter: Central venous catheter clearance: Cathflo™ Activase®:

Patients ≥10 to <30 kg: 110% of the internal lumen volume of the catheter (≤2 mg [1 mg/mL]); retain in catheter for ≤2 hours; may instill a second dose if catheter remains occluded

Patients ≥30 kg: 2 mg (1 mg/mL); retain in catheter for ≤2 hours; may instill a second dose if catheter remains occluded

Intra-arterial: Peripheral arterial thrombotic obstruction (unlabeled use): 0.02-0.1 mg/kg/hour for 1-8 hours

Mechanism of Action Initiates local fibrinolysis by binding to fibrin in a thrombus (clot) and converts entrapped plasminogen to plasmin

(Continued)

Alteplase *(Continued)*

Other Adverse Effects As with all drugs which may affect hemostasis, bleeding is the major adverse effect associated with alteplase. Hemorrhage may occur at virtually any site. Risk is dependent on multiple variables, including the dosage administered, concurrent use of multiple agents which alter hemostasis, and patient predisposition. Rapid lysis of coronary artery thrombi by thrombolytic agents may be associated with reperfusion-related atrial and/or ventricular arrhythmias. **Note:** Lowest rate of bleeding complications expected with dose used to restore catheter function.

1% to 10%:

- Cardiovascular: Hypotension
- Central nervous system: Fever
- Dermatologic: Bruising (1%)
- Gastrointestinal: GI hemorrhage (5%), nausea, vomiting
- Genitourinary: GU hemorrhage (4%)
- Local: Bleeding at catheter puncture site (15.3%, accelerated administration)
- Hematologic: Bleeding (0.5% major, 7% minor: GUSTO trial)

Additional cardiovascular events associated **with use in myocardial infarction:** AV block, cardiogenic shock, heart failure, cardiac arrest, recurrent ischemia/infarction, myocardial rupture, electromechanical dissociation, pericardial effusion, pericarditis, mitral regurgitation, cardiac tamponade, thromboembolism, pulmonary edema, asystole, ventricular tachycardia, bradycardia, ruptured intracranial AV malformation, seizure, hemorrhagic bursitis, cholesterol crystal embolization

Additional events associated **with use in pulmonary embolism:** Pulmonary re-embolization, pulmonary edema, pleural effusion, thromboembolism

Additional events associated **with use in stroke:** Cerebral edema, cerebral herniation, seizure, new ischemic stroke

Drug Interactions

Increased Effect/Toxicity: The potential for hemorrhage with alteplase is increased by oral anticoagulants (warfarin), heparin, low molecular weight heparins, and drugs which affect platelet function (eg, NSAIDs, dipyridamole, ticlopidine, clopidogrel, IIb/IIIa antagonists). Concurrent use with aspirin and heparin may increase the risk of bleeding. However, aspirin and heparin were used concomitantly with alteplase in the majority of patients in clinical studies.

Decreased Effect: Aminocaproic acid (an antifibrinolytic agent) may decrease the effectiveness of thrombolytic therapy. Nitroglycerin may increase the hepatic clearance of alteplase, potentially reducing lytic activity (limited clinical information).

Drug Uptake Duration: >50% present in plasma cleared ~5 minutes after infusion terminated, ~80% cleared within 10 minutes

Pregnancy Risk Factor C

Generic Available No

ALternaGel® [OTC] *see* Aluminum Hydroxide *on page 61*

Altinac™ *see* Tretinoin, Topical *on page 1196*

Altocor™ *see* Lovastatin *on page 734*

Altretamine (al TRET a meen)

U.S. Brand Names Hexalen®

Canadian Brand Names Hexalen®

Pharmacologic Category Antineoplastic Agent, Miscellaneous

Synonyms Hexamethylmelamine; HEXM; HMM; HXM; NSC-13875

Use Palliative treatment of persistent or recurrent ovarian cancer following first-line therapy with a cisplatin- or alkylating agent-based combination

Local Anesthetic/Vasoconstrictor Precautions No information available to require special precautions

Effects on Dental Treatment No effects or complications reported

Mechanism of Action Although altretamine clinical antitumor spectrum resembles that of alkylating agents, the drug has demonstrated activity in alkylator-resistant patients; probably requires hepatic microsomal mixed-function oxidase enzyme activation to become cytotoxic. The drug selectively inhibits the incorporation of radioactive thymidine and uridine into DNA and RNA, inhibiting DNA and RNA synthesis; metabolized to reactive intermediates which covalently bind to microsomal proteins and DNA. These reactive intermediates can spontaneously degrade to demethylated melamines and formaldehyde which are also cytotoxic.

Other Adverse Effects

>10%:

- Central nervous system: Peripheral sensory neuropathy, neurotoxicity
- Gastrointestinal: Nausea, vomiting, anorexia, diarrhea
- Hematologic: Anemia, thrombocytopenia, leukopenia, neutropenia

1% to 10%:

- Central nervous system: Seizures
- Gastrointestinal: Anorexia, diarrhea, stomach cramps

Hepatic: Increased alkaline phosphatase

Drug Interactions

Increased Effect/Toxicity: Altretamine may cause severe orthostatic hypotension when administered with MAO inhibitors. Cimetidine may decrease metabolism of altretamine.

Decreased Effect: Phenobarbital may increase metabolism of altretamine which may decrease the effect.

Drug Uptake

Absorption: Well absorbed (75% to 89%)

Half-life, elimination: 13 hours

Time to peak, plasma: 0.5-3 hours

Pregnancy Risk Factor D

Generic Available No

Alu-Cap® [OTC] *see* Aluminum Hydroxide *on page 61*

Aluminum Acetate and Acetic Acid

(a LOO mi num AS e tate & a SEE tik AS id)

U.S. Brand Names Otic Domeboro®

Pharmacologic Category Antibiotic, Otic

Synonyms Acetic Acid and Aluminum Acetate Otic; Burow's Otic

Use Treatment of superficial infections of the external auditory canal

Local Anesthetic/Vasoconstrictor Precautions No information available to require special precautions

Effects on Dental Treatment No effects or complications reported

Dosage Instill 4-6 drops in ear(s) every 2-3 hours; insert saturated wick, keep moist for 24 hours

Other Adverse Effects 1% to 10%: Irritation

Generic Available Yes

Aluminum Chloride

(a LOO mi num KLOR ide)

U.S. Brand Names Gingi-Aid® Gingival Retraction Cord; Gingi-Aid® Solution; Hemodent® Gingival Retraction Cord

Pharmacologic Category Astringent

Use

Dental: Hemostatic; gingival retraction

Medical: Hemostatic

Local Anesthetic/Vasoconstrictor Precautions No information available to require special precautions

Effects on Dental Treatment No effects or complications reported

Mechanism of Action Precipitates tissue and blood proteins causing a mechanical obstruction to hemorrhage from injured blood vessels

Warnings/Precautions Since large amounts of astringents may cause tissue irritation and possible damage, only small amounts should be applied

Breast-feeding Considerations May be taken while breast-feeding

Dosage Forms RETRACTION CORD: [Impregnated with aqueous solution]: 1 mg/inch (72 inches); 2 mg/inch (72 inches); [Impregnated with aqueous 10% solution and dried]: 0.9 mg/inch (84 inches); 1.8 mg/inch (84 inches). **SOLN, aqueous:** 10 g/100 mL water (15 mL, 30 mL)

Generic Available Yes

Aluminum Hydroxide

(a LOO mi num hye DROKS ide)

U.S. Brand Names ALternaGel® [OTC]; Alu-Cap® [OTC]; Alu-Tab® [OTC]; Amphojel® [OTC]; Dialume® [OTC]

Canadian Brand Names Amphojel®; Basaljel®

Pharmacologic Category Antacid; Antidote

Use Treatment of hyperacidity; hyperphosphatemia

Local Anesthetic/Vasoconstrictor Precautions No information available to require special precautions

Effects on Dental Treatment Aluminum and magnesium ions prevent GI absorption of tetracycline by forming a large ionized chelated molecule with the aluminum ion and tetracyclines in the stomach. Aluminum hydroxide prevents GI absorption of ketoconazole and itraconazole by increasing the pH in the GI tract. Any of these drugs should be administered at least 1 hour before $Al(OH)_3$.

Dosage Oral:

Peptic ulcer disease (dosages empirical):

- Children: 5-15 mL/dose every 3-6 hours or 1 and 3 hours after meals and at bedtime
- Adults: 15-45 mL every 3-6 hours or 1 and 3 hours after meals and at bedtime

Prophylaxis against GI bleeding:

- Infants: 2-5 mL/dose every 1-2 hours
- Children: 5-15 mL/dose every 1-2 hours
- Adults: 30-60 mL/dose every hour

Titrate to maintain the gastric pH >5

(Continued)

Aluminum Hydroxide *(Continued)*

Hyperphosphatemia:

Children: 50-150 mg/kg/24 hours in divided doses every 4-6 hours, titrate dosage to maintain serum phosphorus within normal range

Adults: 500-1800 mg, 3-6 times/day, between meals and at bedtime; best taken with a meal or within 20 minutes of a meal

Antacid: Adults: 30 mL 1 and 3 hours postprandial and at bedtime

Amphojel®: 10 mL suspension or two 300 mg tablets 5-6 times/day between meals and at bedtime

Mechanism of Action Neutralizes hydrochloride in stomach to form Al $(Cl)_3$ salt + H_2O

Other Adverse Effects

>10%: Gastrointestinal: Constipation, chalky taste, stomach cramps, fecal impaction

1% to 10%: Gastrointestinal: Nausea, vomiting, discoloration of feces (white speckles)

Drug Interactions Aluminum hydroxide decreases the effect of tetracyclines, digoxin, indomethacin, iron salts, isoniazid, allopurinol, benzodiazepines, corticosteroids, penicillamine, phenothiazines, ranitidine, ketoconazole, and itraconazole.

Pregnancy Risk Factor C

Generic Available Yes

Aluminum Hydroxide and Magnesium Carbonate

(a LOO mi num hye DROKS ide & mag NEE zhum KAR bun nate)

U.S. Brand Names Gaviscon® Extra Strength [OTC]; Gaviscon® Liquid [OTC]

Pharmacologic Category Antacid

Synonyms Magnesium Carbonate and Aluminum Hydroxide

Use Temporary relief of symptoms associated with gastric acidity

Local Anesthetic/Vasoconstrictor Precautions No information available to require special precautions

Effects on Dental Treatment Aluminum and magnesium ions prevent GI absorption of tetracycline by forming a large ionized chelated molecule with the tetracyclines in the stomach. Aluminum hydroxide prevents GI absorption of ketoconazole and itraconazole by increasing the pH in the GI tract. Any of these drugs should be administered at least 1 hour before aluminum hydroxide.

Dosage Adults: Oral: 15-30 mL 4 times/day after meals and at bedtime

Other Adverse Effects 1% to 10%:

Endocrine & metabolic: Hypermagnesemia, aluminum intoxication (prolonged use and concomitant renal failure), hypophosphatemia

Gastrointestinal: Constipation, diarrhea

Neuromuscular & skeletal: Osteomalacia

Drug Interactions Decreased Effect: Tetracyclines, digoxin, indomethacin, or iron salts, isoniazid, allopurinol, benzodiazepines, corticosteroids, penicillamine, phenothiazines, ranitidine, ketoconazole, itraconazole

Generic Available Yes

Comments Sodium content per 5 mL (Gaviscon® liquid): 0.6 mEq

Aluminum Hydroxide and Magnesium Hydroxide

(a LOO mi num hye DROKS ide & mag NEE zhum hye DROK side)

U.S. Brand Names Maalox® [OTC]; Maalox® TC (Therapeutic Concentrate) [OTC]

Canadian Brand Names Diovol®; Diovol® Ex; Gelusil®; Gelusil® Extra Strength; Mylanta™; Univol®

Pharmacologic Category Antacid

Synonyms Magnesium Hydroxide and Aluminum Hydroxide

Use Antacid, hyperphosphatemia in renal failure

Local Anesthetic/Vasoconstrictor Precautions No information available to require special precautions

Effects on Dental Treatment Aluminum and magnesium ions prevent GI absorption of tetracycline by forming a large ionized chelated molecule with the tetracyclines in the stomach. Aluminum hydroxide prevents GI absorption of ketoconazole and itraconazole by increasing the pH in the GI tract. Any of these drugs should be administered at least 1 hour before aluminum hydroxide.

Dosage Oral: 5-10 mL or 1-2 tablets 4-6 times/day, between meals and at bedtime; may be used every hour for severe symptoms

Other Adverse Effects

>10%: Gastrointestinal: Constipation, chalky taste, stomach cramps, fecal impaction

1% to 10%: Gastrointestinal: Nausea, vomiting, discoloration of feces (white speckles)

Drug Interactions Decreased Effect: Tetracyclines, digoxin, indomethacin, or iron salts, isoniazid, allopurinol, benzodiazepines, corticosteroids, penicillamine, phenothiazines, ranitidine, ketoconazole, itraconazole

Pregnancy Risk Factor C

Generic Available Yes

Comments Sodium content of 5 mL (Maalox®): 1.3 mg (0.06 mEq)

Aluminum Hydroxide and Magnesium Trisilicate

(a LOO mi num hye DROKS ide & mag NEE zhum trye SIL i kate)

U.S. Brand Names Gaviscon® Tablet [OTC]

Pharmacologic Category Antacid

Synonyms Magnesium Trisilicate and Aluminum Hydroxide

Use Temporary relief of hyperacidity

Local Anesthetic/Vasoconstrictor Precautions No information available to require special precautions

Effects on Dental Treatment Aluminum and magnesium ions prevent GI absorption of tetracycline by forming a large ionized chelated molecule with the tetracyclines in the stomach. Aluminum hydroxide prevents GI absorption of ketoconazole and itraconazole by increasing the pH in the GI tract. Any of these drugs should be administered at least 1 hour before aluminum hydroxide.

Dosage Adults: Oral: Chew 2-4 tablets 4 times/day or as directed by physician

Drug Interactions Decreased Effect: Tetracyclines, digoxin, indomethacin, or iron salts, isoniazid, allopurinol, benzodiazepines, corticosteroids, penicillamine, phenothiazines, ranitidine, ketoconazole, itraconazole

Pregnancy Risk Factor C

Generic Available Yes

Comments Sodium content per tablet: (Gaviscon®): 0.8 mEq; (Gaviscon®-2): 1.6 mEq

Aluminum Hydroxide, Magnesium Hydroxide, and Simethicone

(a LOO mi num hye DROKS ide, mag NEE zhum hye DROKS ide, & sye METH i kone)

U.S. Brand Names Maalox® Fast Release Liquid [OTC]; Maalox® Max [OTC]; Mylanta® Extra Strength Liquid [OTC]; Mylanta® Liquid [OTC]

Canadian Brand Names Diovol Plus®; Mylanta™ Double Strength; Mylanta™ Extra Strength; Mylanta™ regular Strength

Pharmacologic Category Antacid; Antiflatulent

Synonyms Magnesium Hydroxide, Aluminum Hydroxide, and Simethicone; Simethicone, Aluminum Hydroxide, and Magnesium Hydroxide

Use Temporary relief of hyperacidity associated with gas; may also be used for indications associated with other antacids

Local Anesthetic/Vasoconstrictor Precautions No information available to require special precautions

Effects on Dental Treatment Aluminum and magnesium ions prevent GI absorption of tetracycline by forming a large ionized chelated molecule with the tetracyclines in the stomach. Aluminum hydroxide prevents GI absorption of ketoconazole and itraconazole by increasing the pH in the GI tract. Any of these drugs should be administered at least 1 hour before aluminum hydroxide.

Dosage Adults: 15-30 mL or 2-4 tablets 4-6 times/day between meals and at bedtime; may be used every hour for severe symptoms

Other Adverse Effects

>10%: Gastrointestinal: Chalky taste, stomach cramps, constipation, decreased bowel motility, fecal impaction, hemorrhoids

1% to 10%: Gastrointestinal: Nausea, vomiting, discoloration of feces (white speckles)

Drug Interactions Decreased Effect: Tetracyclines, digoxin, indomethacin, or iron salts, isoniazid, allopurinol, benzodiazepines, corticosteroids, penicillamine, phenothiazines, ranitidine, ketoconazole, itraconazole

Pregnancy Risk Factor C

Generic Available Yes

Comments Sodium content of 5 mL: (Maalox® Plus): 1.3 mg (0.06 mEq); (Mylanta®): 0.7 mg (0.03 mEq); (Mylanta®-II): 1.14 mg (0.05 mEq)

Aluminum Sulfate and Calcium Acetate

(a LOO mi num SUL fate & KAL see um AS e tate)

U.S. Brand Names Bluboro® [OTC]; Domeboro® [OTC]; Pedi-Boro® [OTC]

Pharmacologic Category Topical Skin Product

Synonyms Calcium Acetate and Aluminum Sulfate

Use Astringent wet dressing for relief of inflammatory conditions of the skin and to reduce weeping that may occur in dermatitis

Local Anesthetic/Vasoconstrictor Precautions No information available to require special precautions

Effects on Dental Treatment No effects or complications reported

(Continued)

Aluminum Sulfate and Calcium Acetate *(Continued)*

Dosage

Topical: Soak affected area in the solution 2-4 times/day for 15-30 minutes or apply wet dressing soaked in the solution 2-4 times/day for 30-minute treatment periods; rewet dressing with solution every few minutes to keep it moist

Domeboro®:

Wet dressing or compress: Saturate dressing and apply to affected area; saturate cloth every 15-30 minutes; repeat as needed

As a soak: Soak for 15-30 minutes 3 times/day

Generic Available Yes

Alupent® *see* Metaproterenol *on page 776*

Alu-Tab® [OTC] *see* Aluminum Hydroxide *on page 61*

Amantadine (a MAN ta deen)

Related Information

Respiratory Diseases *on page 1328*

Systemic Viral Diseases *on page 1354*

U.S. Brand Names Symmetrel®

Canadian Brand Names Endantadine®; PMS-Amantadine; Symmetrel®

Pharmacologic Category Anti-Parkinson's Agent, Dopamine Agonist; Antiviral Agent

Synonyms Adamantanamine Hydrochloride; Amantadine Hydrochloride

Use Symptomatic and adjunct treatment of parkinsonism; prophylaxis and treatment of influenza A viral infection; treatment of drug-induced extrapyramidal symptoms

Unlabeled/Investigational: Creutzfeldt-Jakob disease

Local Anesthetic/Vasoconstrictor Precautions No information available to require special precautions

Effects on Dental Treatment >10%: Xerostomia; prolonged use may cause significant xerostomia

Dosage Oral:

Children: Influenza A treatment:

1-9 years (<45 kg): 5-9 mg/kg/day in 1-2 divided doses to a maximum of 150 mg/day

10-12 years: 100-200 mg/day in 1-2 divided doses

Influenza prophylaxis: Administer for 10-21 days following exposure if the vaccine is concurrently given or for 90 days following exposure if the vaccine is unavailable or contraindicated and re-exposure is possible

Adults:

Drug-induced extrapyramidal reactions: 100 mg twice daily; may increase to 300-400 mg/day, if needed

Parkinson's disease or Creutzfeldt-Jakob disease (unlabeled use): 100 mg twice daily as sole therapy; may increase to 400 mg/day if needed with close monitoring; initial dose: 100 mg/day if with other serious illness or with high doses of other anti-Parkinson drugs

Influenza A viral infection: 200 mg/day in 1-2 divided doses; initiate within 24-48 hours after onset of symptoms; discontinue as soon as possible based on clinical response (generally within 3-5 days or within 24-48 hours after symptoms disappear)

Influenza prophylaxis: 200 mg/day in 1-2 doses; minimum 10-day course of therapy following exposure if the vaccine is concurrently given or for 90 days following exposure if the vaccine is unavailable or contraindicated and re-exposure is possible

Elderly patients should take the drug in 2 daily doses rather than a single dose to avoid adverse neurologic reactions

Dosing interval in renal impairment:

Cl_{cr} 50-60 mL/minute: Administer 200 mg alternating with 100 mg/day

Cl_{cr} 30-50 mL/minute: Administer 100 mg/day

Cl_{cr} 20-30 mL/minute: Administer 200 mg twice weekly

Cl_{cr} 10-20 mL/minute: Administer 100 mg 3 times/week

Cl_{cr} <10 mL/minute: Administer 200 mg alternating with 100 mg every 7 days

Hemodialysis: Slightly hemodialyzable (5% to 20%); no supplemental dose is needed

Peritoneal dialysis: No supplemental dose is needed

Continuous arterio-venous or venous-venous hemofiltration: No supplemental dose is needed

Mechanism of Action As an antiviral, blocks the uncoating of influenza A virus preventing penetration of virus into host; antiparkinsonian activity may be due to its blocking the reuptake of dopamine into presynaptic neurons and causing direct stimulation of postsynaptic receptors

Other Adverse Effects 1% to 10%:

Cardiovascular: Orthostatic hypotension, peripheral edema

Central nervous system: Insomnia, depression, anxiety, irritability, dizziness, hallucinations, ataxia, headache, somnolence, nervousness, dream abnormality, agitation, fatigue, confusion

Dermatologic: Livedo reticularis
Gastrointestinal: Nausea, anorexia, constipation, diarrhea, xerostomia
Respiratory: Dry nose

Drug Interactions Increased Effect/Toxicity: Anticholinergics (benztropine and trihexyphenidyl) may potentiate CNS side effects of amantadine. Hydrochlorothiazide, triamterene, and/or trimethoprim may increase toxicity of amantadine; monitor for altered response.

Drug Uptake
Onset of action: Antidyskinetic: Within 48 hours
Absorption: Well absorbed
Half-life, elimination: 10-28 hours; Impaired renal function: 7-10 days
Time to peak: 1-4 hours

Pregnancy Risk Factor C

Generic Available Yes

Amaryl® *see* Glimepiride *on page 557*

Ambenonium (am be NOE nee um)

U.S. Brand Names Mytelase®

Canadian Brand Names Mytelase®

Pharmacologic Category Cholinergic Agonist

Synonyms Ambenonium Chloride

Use Treatment of myasthenia gravis

Local Anesthetic/Vasoconstrictor Precautions No information available to require special precautions

Effects on Dental Treatment Increased salivation

Dosage Adults: Oral: 5-25 mg 3-4 times/day

Other Adverse Effects

>10%:
- Gastrointestinal: Diarrhea, increased salivation, nausea, stomach cramps, dysphagia
- Miscellaneous: Increased diaphoresis

1% to 10%:
- Genitourinary: Urge to urinate
- Ocular: Small pupils, lacrimation
- Respiratory: Increased bronchial secretions

Frequency not defined:
- Cardiovascular: Arrhythmias (especially bradycardia), hypotension, decreased carbon monoxide, tachycardia, AV block, nodal rhythm, nonspecific EKG changes, cardiac arrest, syncope, flushing
- Central nervous system: Convulsions, dysarthria, dysphonia, dizziness, loss of consciousness, drowsiness, headache
- Dermatologic: Skin rash, thrombophlebitis (I.V.), urticaria
- Gastrointestinal: Hyperperistalsis, nausea, vomiting, salivation, diarrhea, stomach cramps, dysphagia, flatulence
- Genitourinary: Urinary urgency
- Neuromuscular & skeletal: Weakness, fasciculations, muscle cramps, spasms, arthralgias
- Ocular: Small pupils, lacrimation
- Respiratory: Increased bronchial secretions, laryngospasm, bronchiolar constriction, respiratory muscle paralysis, dyspnea, respiratory depression, respiratory arrest, bronchospasm
- Miscellaneous: Diaphoresis (increased), anaphylaxis, allergic reactions

Drug Interactions
Increased Effect/Toxicity: Succinylcholine neuromuscular blockade may be prolonged.
Decreased Effect: Corticosteroids antagonize effects of anticholinesterases in myasthenia gravis. Procainamide or quinidine may reverse ambenonium cholinergic effects on muscle.

Pregnancy Risk Factor C

Generic Available No

Ambien® *see* Zolpidem *on page 1263*
Ambi® Skin Tone [OTC] *see* Hydroquinone *on page 611*
AmBisome® *see* Amphotericin B, Liposomal *on page 93*

Amcinonide (am SIN oh nide)

U.S. Brand Names Cyclocort®

Canadian Brand Names Cyclocort®

Pharmacologic Category Corticosteroid, Topical

Use Relief of the inflammatory and pruritic manifestations of corticosteroid-responsive dermatoses (high potency corticosteroid)

Local Anesthetic/Vasoconstrictor Precautions No information available to require special precautions

Effects on Dental Treatment No effects or complications reported

(Continued)

Amcinonide *(Continued)*

Dosage Adults: Topical: Apply in a thin film 2-3 times/day

Therapy should be discontinued when control is achieved; if no improvement is seen, reassessment of diagnosis may be necessary.

Mechanism of Action Stimulates the synthesis of enzymes needed to decrease inflammation, suppress mitotic activity, and cause vasoconstriction

Other Adverse Effects 1% to 10%: Topical: Itching, maceration of skin, skin atrophy, burning, erythema, dryness, irritation, papular rashes

Drug Uptake Absorption: Adequate through intact skin; increases with skin inflammation or occlusion

Pregnancy Risk Factor C

Generic Available No

Amcort® *see* Triamcinolone *on page 1197*

Amerge® *see* Naratriptan *on page 850*

Americaine® [OTC] *see* Benzocaine *on page 151*

Americaine® Anesthetic Lubricant *see* Benzocaine *on page 151*

A-methaPred® *see* MethylPREDNISolone *on page 797*

Amicar® *see* Aminocaproic Acid *on page 68*

Amidate® *see* Etomidate *on page 481*

Amifostine (am i FOS teen)

U.S. Brand Names Ethyol®

Canadian Brand Names Ethyol®

Mexican Brand Names Ethyol®

Pharmacologic Category Antidote

Synonyms Ethiofos; Gammaphos

Use Reduce the incidence of moderate to severe xerostomia in patients undergoing postoperative radiation treatment for head and neck cancer, where the radiation port includes a substantial portion of the parotid glands. Reduce the cumulative renal toxicity associated with repeated administration of cisplatin in patients with advanced ovarian cancer or nonsmall cell lung cancer. In these settings, the clinical data does not suggest that the effectiveness of cisplatin-based chemotherapy regimens is altered by amifostine.

Local Anesthetic/Vasoconstrictor Precautions No information available to require special precautions

Effects on Dental Treatment Nausea/vomiting (may be severe)

Dosage Adults: I.V. (refer to individual protocols): 910 mg/m^2 administered once daily as a 15-minute I.V. infusion, starting 30 minutes prior to chemotherapy

Reduction of xerostomia from head and neck radiation: 200 mg/m^2 I.V. (as a 3-minute infusion) once daily, starting 15-30 minutes before standard fraction radiation therapy

Note: 15-minute infusion is better tolerated than more extended infusions. Further reductions in infusion times have not been systematically investigated. The infusion of amifostine should be interrupted if the systolic BP (mm Hg) decreases significantly from the following baseline values:

Decrease of 20 if baseline systolic BP <100
Decrease of 25 if baseline systolic BP 100-119
Decrease of 30 if baseline systolic BP 120-139
Decrease of 40 if baseline systolic BP 140-179
Decrease of 50 if baseline systolic BP ≥180

Mean onset of hypotension is 14 minutes into the 15-minute infusion and the mean duration was 6 minutes. Hypotension should be treated with fluid infusion and postural management of the patient (supine or Trendelenburg position). If the BP returns to normal within 5 minutes and the patient is asymptomatic, the infusion may be restarted so that the full dose of amifostine may be administered. If the full dose of amifostine cannot be administered, the dose of amifostine for subsequent cycles should be 740 mg/m^2.

Mechanism of Action Prodrug that is dephosphorylated by alkaline phosphatase in tissues to a pharmacologically active free thiol metabolite that can reduce the toxic effects of cisplatin, and reduce toxicity of radiation. The free thiol is available to bind to, and detoxify, reactive metabolites of cisplatin; and can also act as a scavenger of free radicals that may be generated in tissues exposed to cisplatin or radiation.

Other Adverse Effects >10%:

Cardiovascular: Flushing; hypotension (62%)
Central nervous system: Chills, dizziness, somnolence
Gastrointestinal: Nausea/vomiting (may be severe)
Respiratory: Sneezing
Miscellaneous: Feeling of warmth/coldness, hiccups

Drug Interactions Special consideration should be given to patients receiving antihypertensive medications or other drugs that could potentiate hypotension.

Drug Uptake

Absorption: Oral: Poor

Serum half-life: 9 minutes

Pregnancy Risk Factor C

Generic Available No

Amigesic® *see* Salsalate *on page 1074*

Amikacin (am i KAY sin)

U.S. Brand Names Amikin®

Canadian Brand Names Amikin®

Mexican Brand Names Akacin®; Amikafur®; Amikalem®; Amikayect; Amikin®; A.M.K.®; Biclin; Gamikal®; Oprad®; Yectamid

Pharmacologic Category Antibiotic, Aminoglycoside

Synonyms Amikacin Sulfate

Use Treatment of documented gram-negative enteric infection resistant to gentamicin and tobramycin (bone infections, respiratory tract infections, endocarditis, and septicemia); documented infection of mycobacterial organisms susceptible to amikacin including *Pseudomonas, Proteus, Serratia*, and gram-positive *Staphylococcus*

Local Anesthetic/Vasoconstrictor Precautions No information available to require special precautions

Effects on Dental Treatment No effects or complications reported

Dosage Individualization is critical because of the low therapeutic index

Use of ideal body weight (IBW) for determining the mg/kg/dose appears to be more accurate than dosing on the basis of total body weight (TBW)

In morbid obesity, dosage requirement may best be estimated using a dosing weight of IBW + 0.4 (TBW - IBW)

Initial and periodic peak and trough plasma drug levels should be determined, particularly in critically ill patients with serious infections or in disease states known to significantly alter aminoglycoside pharmacokinetics (eg, cystic fibrosis, burns, or major surgery)

Once daily dosing: Higher peak serum drug concentration to MIC ratios, demonstrated aminoglycoside postantibiotic effect, decreased renal cortex drug uptake, and improved cost-time efficiency are supportive reasons for the use of once daily dosing regimens for aminoglycosides. Current research indicates these regimens to be as effective for nonlife-threatening infections, with no higher incidence of nephrotoxicity, than those requiring multiple daily doses. Doses are determined by calculating the entire day's dose via usual multiple dose calculation techniques and administering this quantity as a single dose. Doses are then adjusted to maintain mean serum concentration above the MIC(s) of the causative organism(s). (Example: 14-35 mg/kg as a single dose/24 hours; peak (maximum) serum concentration may approximate 40-55 μg/mL and trough (minimum) serum concentration <3 μg/L). Further research is needed for universal recommendation in all patient populations and gram-negative disease; exceptions may include those with known high clearance (eg, children, patients with cystic fibrosis or burns who may require shorter dosage intervals) and patients with renal function impairment for whom longer than conventional dosage intervals are usually required.

Children and Adults: I.M., I.V.: 5-7.5 mg/kg/dose every 8 hours

Mechanism of Action Inhibits protein synthesis in susceptible bacteria by binding to ribosomal subunits

Other Adverse Effects 1% to 10%:

Central nervous system: Neurotoxicity

Otic: Ototoxicity (auditory), ototoxicity (vestibular)

Renal: Nephrotoxicity

Drug Interactions Increased Effect/Toxicity: Amikacin may increase or prolong the effect of neuromuscular blocking agents. Concurrent use of amphotericin (or other nephrotoxic drugs) may increase the risk of amikacin-induced nephrotoxicity. The risk of ototoxicity from amikacin may be increased with other ototoxic drugs.

Drug Uptake

Absorption: I.M.: May be delayed in bedridden patients

Half-life, elimination (dependent on renal function and age):

Infants: Low birthweight (1-3 days): 7-9 hours; Full-term >7 days: 4-5 hours

Children: 1.6-2.5 hours

Adults: Normal renal function: 1.4-2.3 hours; Anuria/end-stage renal disease: 28-86 hours

Time to peak: I.M.: 45-120 minutes; I.V.: ≤30 minutes following 30-minute infusion

Pregnancy Risk Factor C

Generic Available Yes

Amikin® *see* Amikacin *on page 67*

Amiloride (a MIL oh ride)

U.S. Brand Names Midamor®

Canadian Brand Names Midamor®

Pharmacologic Category Diuretic, Potassium Sparing

Synonyms Amiloride Hydrochloride

(Continued)

Amiloride *(Continued)*

Use Counteracts potassium loss induced by other diuretics in the treatment of hypertension or edematous conditions including CHF, hepatic cirrhosis, and hypoaldosteronism; usually used in conjunction with more potent diuretics such as thiazides or loop diuretics

Unlabeled/Investigational: Cystic fibrosis; reduction of lithium-induced polyuria

Local Anesthetic/Vasoconstrictor Precautions No information available to require special precautions

Effects on Dental Treatment No effects or complications reported

Dosage Oral:

Children: Although safety and efficacy have not been established by the FDA in children, a dosage of 0.625 mg/kg/day has been used in children weighing 6-20 kg

Adults: 5-10 mg/day (up to 20 mg)

Elderly: Initial: 5 mg once daily or every other day

Mechanism of Action Interferes with potassium/sodium exchange (active transport) in the distal tubule, cortical collecting tubule and collecting duct by inhibiting sodium, potassium-ATPase; decreases calcium excretion; increases magnesium loss

Other Adverse Effects 1% to 10%:

Central nervous system: Headache, fatigue, dizziness

Endocrine & metabolic: Hyperkalemia, hyperchloremic metabolic acidosis, dehydration, hyponatremia, gynecomastia

Gastrointestinal: Nausea, diarrhea, vomiting, abdominal pain, gas pain, appetite changes, constipation

Genitourinary: Impotence

Neuromuscular & skeletal: Muscle cramps, weakness

Respiratory: Cough, dyspnea

Drug Interactions

Increased Effect/Toxicity: Increased risk of amiloride-associated hyperkalemia with triamterene, spironolactone, angiotensin-converting enzyme (ACE) inhibitors, potassium preparations, cyclosporine, tacrolimus, and indomethacin. Amiloride may increase the toxicity of amantadine and lithium by reduction of renal excretion. Quinidine and amiloride together may increase risk of malignant arrhythmias.

Decreased Effect: Effect of amiloride decreased with use of nonsteroidal anti-inflammatory agents. Amoxicillin's absorption may be reduced with concurrent use.

Drug Uptake

Onset of action: 2 hours

Absorption: Oral: ~15% to 25%

Duration: 24 hours

Half-life, elimination: 6-9 hours; End-stage renal disease: 8-144 hours

Time to peak: 6-10 hours

Pregnancy Risk Factor B

Generic Available Yes

Amiloride and Hydrochlorothiazide

(a MIL oh ride & hye droe klor oh THYE a zide)

U.S. Brand Names Moduretic®

Canadian Brand Names Alti-Amiloride HCTZ; Apo®-Amilzide; Moduret®; Moduretic®; Novamilor; Nu-Amilzide

Pharmacologic Category Diuretic, Combination

Synonyms Hydrochlorothiazide and Amiloride

Use Antikaliuretic diuretic, antihypertensive

Local Anesthetic/Vasoconstrictor Precautions No information available to require special precautions

Effects on Dental Treatment No effects or complications reported

Dosage Adults: Oral: Start with 1 tablet/day, then may be increased to 2 tablets/day if needed; usually given in a single dose

Other Adverse Effects See Amiloride *on page 67* and Hydrochlorothiazide *on page 595*

Drug Interactions See Amiloride *on page 67* and Hydrochlorothiazide *on page 68*

Drug Uptake See Amiloride *on page 67* and Hydrochlorothiazide *on page 595*

Pregnancy Risk Factor B

Generic Available Yes

Aminocaproic Acid (a mee noe ka PROE ik AS id)

U.S. Brand Names Amicar®

Canadian Brand Names Amicar®

Pharmacologic Category Hemostatic Agent

Use Treatment of excessive bleeding from fibrinolysis

Local Anesthetic/Vasoconstrictor Precautions No information available to require special precautions

Effects on Dental Treatment No effects or complications reported

Dosage In the management of acute bleeding syndromes, oral dosage regimens are the same as the I.V. dosage regimens in adults and children

Chronic bleeding: Oral, I.V.: 5-30 g/day in divided doses at 3- to 6-hour intervals
Acute bleeding syndrome:
- Children: Oral, I.V.: 100 mg/kg or 3 g/m^2 during the first hour, followed by continuous infusion at the rate of 33.3 mg/kg/hour or 1 g/m^2/hour; total dosage should not exceed 18 g/m^2/24 hours
  - Traumatic hyphema: Oral: 100 mg/kg/dose every 6-8 hours
- Adults:
  - Oral: For elevated fibrinolytic activity, give 5 g during first hour, followed by 1-1.25 g/hour for ~ 8 hours or until bleeding stops
  - I.V.: Administer 4-5 g in 250 mL of diluent during first hour followed by continuous infusion at the rate of 1-1.25 g/hour in 50 mL of diluent, continue for 8 hours or until bleeding stops
  - Maximum daily dose: Oral, I.V.: 30 g

Mechanism of Action Competitively inhibits activation of plasminogen to plasmin, also, a lesser antiplasmin effect

Other Adverse Effects

>10%: Gastrointestinal: Anorexia, nausea

1% to 10%:
- Cardiovascular: Hypotension, bradycardia, arrhythmia
- Central nervous system: Dizziness, headache, malaise, fatigue
- Dermatologic: Rash (measles-like skin rash or itching on face and/or palms of hands); masculinization and hirsutism in females
- Endocrine & metabolic: Adrenocortical insufficiency
- Gastrointestinal: GI irritation, vomiting, cramps, diarrhea
- Hematologic: Decreased platelet function, elevated serum enzymes, leukopenia, agranulocytosis, thrombocytopenia
- Neuromuscular & skeletal: Myopathy, weakness
- Otic: Tinnitus
- Respiratory: Nasal congestion

Drug Interactions Increased Effect/Toxicity: Increased risk of hypercoagulability with oral contraceptives, estrogens. Should not be administered with factor IX complex concentrated or anti-inhibitor complex concentrates due to an increased risk of thrombosis.

Drug Uptake

Onset of action: ~1-72 hours
Half-life, elimination: 1-2 hours
Time to peak: Oral: ~2 hours

Pregnancy Risk Factor C

Generic Available Yes: Injection, syrup

Comments Antifibrinolytic drugs are useful to control bleeding after dental extractions in patients with hemophilia. A clinical trial reported that aminocaproic acid or tranexamic acid reduces both recurrent bleeding and the amount of clotting factor replacement therapy required. In adults, the oral dose was 50-60 mg aminocaproic acid per kg every 4 hours until dental sockets were completely healed.

Amino-Cerv™ Vaginal Cream *see* Urea *on page 1221*

Aminoglutethimide (a mee noe gloo TETH i mide)

U.S. Brand Names Cytadren®

Pharmacologic Category Antineoplastic Agent, Miscellaneous

Use Suppression of adrenal function in selected patients with Cushing's syndrome; also used successfully in postmenopausal patients with advanced breast carcinoma and in patients with metastatic prostate carcinoma as salvage (third-line hormonal agent)

Local Anesthetic/Vasoconstrictor Precautions No information available to require special precautions

Effects on Dental Treatment >10%: Nausea; ~10%: Orthostatic hypotension

Mechanism of Action Blocks the enzymatic conversion of cholesterol to delta-5-pregnenolone, thereby reducing the synthesis of adrenal glucocorticoids, mineralocorticoids, estrogens, aldosterone, and androgens

Other Adverse Effects Most will diminish in incidence and severity after 2-6 weeks

>10%:
- Central nervous system: Headache, dizziness, drowsiness, and lethargy are frequent at the start of therapy, clumsiness
- Dermatologic: Skin rash
- Gastrointestinal: Nausea, vomiting, anorexia
- Hepatic: Cholestatic jaundice
- Neuromuscular & skeletal: Myalgia
- Renal: Nephrotoxicity
- Respiratory: Pulmonary alveolar damage

(Continued)

Aminoglutethimide *(Continued)*

Miscellaneous: Systemic lupus erythematosus

1% to 10%:

Cardiovascular: Hypotension and tachycardia, orthostatic hypotension

Central nervous system: Headache

Dermatologic: Hirsutism in females, pruritus

Endocrine & metabolic: Adrenocortical insufficiency

Hematologic: Rare cases of neutropenia, leukopenia, thrombocytopenia, pancytopenia, and agranulocytosis have been reported

Neuromuscular & skeletal: Myalgia

Drug Interactions Cytochrome P450 hepatic microsomal enzyme inducer; isoenzymes undefined

Decreased Effect: May decrease therapeutic effect of dexamethasone, digitoxin (after 3-8 weeks), theophylline, warfarin, and medroxyprogesterone

Drug Uptake

Onset of action: Adrenal suppression: 3-5 days

Absorption: 90%

Half-life elimination: 7-15 hours; shorter following multiple doses.

Pregnancy Risk Factor D

Generic Available No

Aminolevulinic Acid (a MEE noh lev yoo lin ik AS id)

U.S. Brand Names Levulan® Kerastick™

Canadian Brand Names Levulan®

Pharmacologic Category Photosensitizing Agent, Topical; Topical Skin Product

Synonyms Aminolevulinic Acid Hydrochloride

Use Treatment of nonhyperkeratotic actinic keratoses of the face or scalp; to be used in conjunction with blue light illumination

Local Anesthetic/Vasoconstrictor Precautions No information available to require special precautions

Effects on Dental Treatment No effects or complications reported

Dosage Adults: Topical: Apply to actinic keratoses (**not** perilesional skin) followed 14-18 hours later by blue light illumination. Application/treatment may be repeated at a treatment site after 8 weeks.

Mechanism of Action A metabolic precursor of protoporphyrin IX (PpIX), which is a photosensitizer; photosensitization following application of aminolevulinic acid topical solution occurs through the metabolic conversion to PpIX. When exposed to light of appropriate wavelength and energy, accumulated PpIX produces a photodynamic reaction.

Other Adverse Effects

>10%: Dermatologic: Severe stinging or burning (50%), scaling of the skin/crusted skin (64% to 71%), hyperpigmentation/hypopigmentation (22% to 36%), itching (14% to 25%), erosion (2% to 14%)

Symptoms subside between 1 minute and 24 hours after turning off the blue light illuminator. Severe stinging or burning was reported in at least 50% of patients from at least 1 lesional site treatment.

1% to 10%:

Central nervous system: Dysesthesia (0% to 2%)

Dermatologic: Skin ulceration (2% to 4%), vesiculation (4% to 5%), pustular drug eruption (0% to 4%), skin disorder (5% to 12%)

Hematologic: Bleeding/hemorrhage (2% to 4%)

Local: Wheal/flare (2% to 7%), local pain (1%), tenderness (1%), edema (1%), scabbing (0% to 2%)

Warnings/Precautions For external use only. Do not apply to eyes or mucous membranes. Treatment site will become photosensitive following application. Patients should be instructed to avoid exposure to sunlight, bright indoor lights, or tanning beds during the period prior to blue light treatment. Should be applied by a qualified health professional to avoid application to perilesional skin. Has not been tested in individuals with coagulation defects (acquired or inherited).

Drug Interactions Increased Effect/Toxicity: Photosensitizing agents such as griseofulvin, thiazide diuretics, sulfonamides, sulfonylureas, phenothiazines, and tetracyclines theoretically may increase the photosensitizing potential of aminolevulinic acid.

Drug Uptake

Aminolevulinic acid:

Serum half-life, mean: 0.7 ± 0.18 hours after oral

PpIX:

Serum half-life, mean clearance for lesions: 30 ± 10 hours

Time to peak fluorescence intensity: 11 ± 1 hour

Pregnancy Risk Factor C

Generic Available No

Amino-Opti-E® [OTC] *see* Vitamin E *on page 1245*

Aminophylline (am in OFF i lin)

Related Information

Dental Drug Interactions: Update on Drug Combinations Requiring Special Considerations *on page 1434*

Respiratory Diseases *on page 1328*

Theophylline *on page 1152*

U.S. Brand Names Truphylline®

Canadian Brand Names Phyllocontin®; Phyllocontin®-350

Mexican Brand Names Drafilyn®

Pharmacologic Category Theophylline Derivative

Synonyms Theophylline Ethylenediamine

Use Bronchodilator in reversible airway obstruction due to asthma or COPD; increase diaphragmatic contractility; neonatal idiopathic apnea of prematurity

Local Anesthetic/Vasoconstrictor Precautions No information available to require special precautions

Effects on Dental Treatment Prescribe erythromycin with caution to patients taking theophylline products. Erythromycin will delay the normal metabolic inactivation of theophyllines leading to increased blood levels; this has resulted in nausea, vomiting and CNS restlessness

Dosage

Neonates: Apnea of prematurity:

Loading dose: 5 mg/kg for one dose

Maintenance: I.V.:

0-24 days: Begin at 2 mg/kg/day divided every 12 hours and titrate to desired levels and effects

>24 days: 3 mg/kg/day divided every 12 hours; increased dosages may be indicated as liver metabolism matures (usually >30 days of life); monitor serum concentration to determine appropriate dosages

Theophylline levels should be initially drawn after 3 days of therapy; repeat levels are indicated 3 days after each increase in dosage or weekly if on a stabilized dosage

Treatment of acute bronchospasm:

Loading dose (in patients not currently receiving aminophylline or theophylline): 6 mg/kg (based on aminophylline) administered I.V. over 20-30 minutes; administration rate should not exceed 25 mg/minute (aminophylline)

Approximate I.V. maintenance dosages are based upon **continuous infusions**; bolus dosing (often used in children <6 months of age) may be determined by multiplying the hourly infusion rate by 24 hours and dividing by the desired number of doses/day

6 weeks to 6 months: 0.5 mg/kg/hour

6 months to 1 year: 0.6-0.7 mg/kg/hour

1-9 years: 1-1.2 mg/kg/hour

9-12 years and young adult smokers: 0.9 mg/kg/hour

12-16 years: 0.7 mg/kg/hour

Adults (healthy, nonsmoking): 0.7 mg/kg/hour

Older patients and patients with cor pulmonale, patients with CHF or liver failure: 0.25 mg/kg/hour

Dosage should be adjusted according to serum concentration measurements during the first 12- to 24-hour period; avoid using suppositories due to erratic, unreliable absorption.

Rectal: Adults: 500 mg 3 times/day

Mechanism of Action Causes bronchodilatation, diuresis, CNS and cardiac stimulation, and gastric acid secretion by blocking phosphodiesterase which increases tissue concentrations of cyclic adenine monophosphate (cAMP) which in turn promotes catecholamine stimulation of lipolysis, glycogenolysis, and gluconeogenesis and induces release of epinephrine from adrenal medulla cells

Other Adverse Effects

Uncommon at serum theophylline concentrations ≤20 mcg/mL

1% to 10%:

Cardiovascular: Tachycardia

Central nervous system: Nervousness, restlessness

Gastrointestinal: Nausea, vomiting

Drug Interactions

Increased Effect/Toxicity:

Increased theophylline level

Allopurinol (>600 mg/day), beta-blockers, calcium channel blockers, carbamazepine, CHF, cimetidine, ciprofloxacin, cor pulmonale, corticosteroids, disulfiram, ephedrine, erythromycin, fever/viral illness, hepatic cirrhosis, influenza virus vaccine, interferon, isoniazid, loop diuretics, macrolides, mexiletine, oral contraceptives, propranolol, quinolones, thiabendazole, thyroid hormones, troleandomycin

(Continued)

Aminophylline *(Continued)*

Decreased Effect/Increased Toxicity: Changes in diet may affect the elimination of theophylline; charcoal-broiled foods may increase elimination, reducing half-life by 50%; other factors reported to affect serum theophylline levels:

Decreased theophylline level

Aminoglutethimide, barbiturates, carbamazepine, charcoal, high protein/low carbohydrate diet, hydantoins, isoniazid, I.V. isoproterenol, ketoconazole, loop diuretics, phenobarbital, phenytoin, rifampin, smoking (cigarettes, marijuana), sulfinpyrazone, sympathomimetics

Drug Uptake

Theophylline:

Absorption: Oral: Depends upon dosage form

Half-life, elimination: Highly variable; dependent on liver and cardiac function, age, lung disease and smoking history

Time to peak: Oral: 1 hour; Uncoated tablet: 2 hours; Chewable tablet: 1-1.5 hours; Enteric-coated tablet: 5 hours; I.V.: ≤30 minutes

Pregnancy Risk Factor C

Generic Available Yes

Selected Readings

Delaforge M and Sartori E, "*In Vivo* Effects of Erythromycin, Oleandomycin, and Erythralosamine Derivatives on Hepatic Cytochrome P450," *Biochem Pharmacol*, 1990, 40(2):223-8.

Ludden TM, "Pharmacokinetic Interactions of the Macrolide Antibiotics," *Clin Pharmacokinet*, 1985, 10(1):63-79.

Aminosalicylate Sodium (a MEE noe sa LIS i late SOW dee um)

Related Information

Rheumatoid Arthritis and Osteoarthritis *on page 1340*

Temporomandibular Dysfunction (TMD) *on page 1397*

Canadian Brand Names Nemasol® Sodium

Mexican Brand Names Salofalk

Pharmacologic Category Salicylate

Synonyms Para-Aminosalicylate Sodium; PAS

Use Treatment of tuberculosis with combination drugs; has also been used in Crohn's disease

Local Anesthetic/Vasoconstrictor Precautions No information available to require special precautions

Effects on Dental Treatment NSAID formulations are known to reversibly decrease platelet aggregation via mechanisms different than observed with aspirin. The dentist should be aware of the potential of abnormal coagulation. Caution should also be exercised in the use of NSAIDs in patients already on anticoagulant therapy with drugs such as warfarin (Coumadin®).

Dosage Oral:

Children: 150-300 mg/kg/day in 3-4 equally divided doses

Adults: 150 mg/kg/day in 2-3 equally divided doses (usually 12-14 g/day)

Mechanism of Action Aminosalicylic acid (PAS) is a highly specific bacteriostatic agent active against *M. tuberculosis.* Most strains of *M. tuberculosis* are sensitive to a concentration of 1 µg/mL; structurally related to para-aminobenzoic acid (PABA) and its mechanism of action is thought to be similar to the sulfonamides, a competitive antagonism with PABA; disrupts plate biosynthesis in sensitive organisms

Other Adverse Effects 1% to 10%: Gastrointestinal: Nausea, vomiting, diarrhea, abdominal pain

Warnings/Precautions Use with caution in patients with CHF, dehydration, hypertension, decreased renal or hepatic function, history of GI disease, active GI ulceration or bleeding, or those receiving anticoagulants; patients who are sodium restricted. Withhold for at least 4-6 half-lives prior to surgical or dental procedures.

Drug Interactions Decreased Effect: May decrease serum concentration of digoxin and vitamin B_{12}

Drug Uptake

Absorption: Readily, >90%

Half-life elimination: Reduced with renal dysfunction

Pregnancy Risk Factor C

Generic Available Yes

Aminoxin® [OTC] *see* Pyridoxine *on page 1027*

Amiodarone (a MEE oh da rone)

Related Information

Cardiovascular Diseases *on page 1308*

U.S. Brand Names Cordarone®; Pacerone®

Canadian Brand Names Alti-Amiodarone; Cordarone®; Gen-Amiodarone; Novo-Amiodarone

Mexican Brand Names Braxan; Cardiorona; Cordarone®

Pharmacologic Category Antiarrhythmic Agent, Class III

Synonyms Amiodarone Hydrochloride

Use

Oral: Management of life-threatening recurrent ventricular fibrillation (VF) or hemodynamically unstable ventricular tachycardia (VT)

I.V.: Initiation of treatment and prophylaxis of frequency recurring VF and unstable VT in patients refractory to other therapy. Also, used for patients when oral amiodarone is indicated, but who are unable to take oral medication.

Unlabeled/Investigational:

Conversion of atrial fibrillation to normal sinus rhythm; maintenance of normal sinus rhythm

Prevention of postoperative atrial fibrillation during cardiothoracic surgery

Paroxysmal supraventricular tachycardia (SVT)

Control of rapid ventricular rate due to accessory pathway conduction in pre-excited atrial arrhythmias [ACLS guidelines]

After defibrillation and epinephrine in cardiac arrest with persistent ventricular tachycardia (VT) or ventricular fibrillation (VF) [ACLS guidelines]

Control of hemodynamically stable VT, polymorphic VT, or wide-complex tachycardia of uncertain origin [ACLS guidelines]

Local Anesthetic/Vasoconstrictor Precautions No information available to require special precautions

Effects on Dental Treatment No effects or complications reported

Dosage

Oral:

Children (calculate doses for children <1 year on body surface area): Loading dose: 10-15 mg/kg/day or 600-800 mg/1.73 m^2/day for 4-14 days or until adequate control of arrhythmia or prominent adverse effects occur (this loading dose may be given in 1-2 divided doses/day). Dosage should then be reduced to 5 mg/kg/day or 200-400 mg/1.73 m^2/day given once daily for several weeks. If arrhythmia does not recur, reduce to lowest effective dosage possible. Usual daily minimal dose: 2.5 mg/kg/day; maintenance doses may be given for 5 of 7 days/week.

Adults: Ventricular arrhythmias: 800-1600 mg/day in 1-2 doses for 1-3 weeks, then when adequate arrhythmia control is achieved, decrease to 600-800 mg/day in 1-2 doses for 1 month; maintenance: 400 mg/day. Lower doses are recommended for supraventricular arrhythmias.

I.V.:

Children: Ventricular arrhythmias: A multicenter study (Perry, 1996; n=40; mean age 5.4 years with 24 of 40 children <2 years of age) used an I.V. loading dose of 5 mg/kg that was divided into five 1 mg/kg aliquots, with each aliquot given over 5-10 minutes. Additional 1-5 mg/kg doses could be administered 30 minutes later in a similar fashion if needed. The mean loading dose was 6.3 mg/kg. A maintenance dose (continuous infusion of 10-15 mg/kg/day) was administered to 21 of the 40 patients. Further studies are needed.

Note: I.V. administration at low flow rates (potentially associated with use in pediatrics) may result in leaching of plasticizers (DEHP) from I.V. tubing. DEHP may adversely affect male reproductive tract development. Alternative means of dosing and administration (1 mg/kg aliquots) may need to be considered.

Adults:

Stable VT or SVT (unlabeled uses): First 24 hours: 1000 mg according to following regimen

Step 1: 150 mg (100 mL) over first 10 minutes (mix 3 mL in 100 mL D_5W)

Step 2: 360 mg (200 mL) over next 6 hours (mix 18 mL in 500 mL D_5W): 1 mg/minute

Step 3: 540 mg (300 mL) over next 18 hours: 0.5 mg/minute

Note: After the first 24 hours: 0.5 mg/minute utilizing concentration of 1-6 mg/mL

Breakthrough VF or VT: 150 mg supplemental doses in 100 mL D_5W over 10 minutes

Pulseless VF or VT: I.V. push: Initial: 300 mg in 20-30 mL NS or D_5W; if VF or VT recurs, supplemental dose of 150 mg followed by infusion of 1 mg/minute for 6 hours, then 0.5 mg/minute (maximum daily dose: 2.2 g)

Note: When switching from I.V. to oral therapy, use the following as a guide:

<1-week I.V. infusion: 800-1600 mg/day

1- to 3-week I.V. infusion: 600-800 mg/day

>3-week I.V. infusion: 400 mg/day

Recommendations for conversion to I.V. amiodarone after oral administration: During long-term amiodarone therapy (ie, ≥4 months), the mean plasma-elimination half-life of the active metabolite of amiodarone is 61 days. Replacement therapy may not be necessary in such patients if oral therapy is discontinued for a period <2 weeks, since any changes in serum amiodarone concentrations during this period may **not** be clinically significant.

Dosing adjustment in hepatic impairment: Probably necessary in substantial hepatic impairment.

Hemodialysis: Not dialyzable (0% to 5%); supplemental dose is not necessary.

Peritoneal dialysis effects: Not dialyzable (0% to 5%); supplemental dose is not necessary.

(Continued)

Amiodarone *(Continued)*

Mechanism of Action Class III antiarrhythmic agent which inhibits adrenergic stimulation, prolongs the action potential and refractory period in myocardial tissue; decreases A-V conduction and sinus node function

Other Adverse Effects With large dosages (>400 mg/day), adverse reactions occur in ~75% of patients and require discontinuance in 5% to 20%.

>10%:

Cardiovascular: Hypotension (I.V. 16%)

Central nervous system: Between 20% and 40% of patients experience some form of neurologic adverse events (see central nervous system and neuromuscular effects: 1% to 10% frequencies).

Gastrointestinal: Nausea, vomiting

1% to 10%:

Cardiovascular: Congestive heart failure, arrhythmias (including atropine-resistant bradycardia, heart block, sinus arrest, ventricular tachycardia), myocardial depression, flushing, edema. Additional effects associated with I.V. administration include asystole, cardiac arrest, electromechanical dissociation, ventricular tachycardia and cardiogenic shock.

Central nervous system: Fever, fatigue, involuntary movements, incoordination, malaise, sleep disturbances, ataxia, dizziness, headache

Dermatologic: Photosensitivity (10%)

Endocrine & metabolic: Hypothyroidism or hyperthyroidism (less common), decreased libido

Gastrointestinal: Constipation, anorexia, abdominal pain, abnormal salivation, abnormal taste (oral form)

Genitourinary: Noninfectious epididymitis (3% to 11%)

Hematologic: Coagulation abnormalities

Hepatic: Abnormal LFTs

Local: Phlebitis (I.V., with concentrations >3 mg/mL)

Neuromuscular & skeletal: Paresthesia, tremor, muscular weakness, peripheral neuropathy

Ocular: Visual disturbances, corneal microdeposits (occur in a majority of patients, and lead to visual disturbance in ~10%)

Respiratory: Pulmonary toxicity has been estimated to occur at a frequency between 2% and 7% of patients (some reports indicate a frequency as high as 17%). Toxicity may present as hypersensitivity pneumonitis, pulmonary fibrosis (cough, fever, malaise), pulmonary inflammation, interstitial pneumonitis, or alveolar pneumonitis

Miscellaneous: Abnormal smell (oral form)

Drug Interactions CYP3A3/4 enzyme substrate; CYP2C9, 2D6, and 3A3/4 enzyme inhibitor

Due to the long half-life of amiodarone, drug interactions may take 1 or more weeks to develop.

Increased Effect/Toxicity: Cisapride, gatifloxacin, moxifloxacin, and sparfloxacin are contraindicated. Use of amiodarone with diltiazem, verapamil, digoxin, beta-blockers, and other drugs which delay AV conduction may cause excessive AV block (amiodarone may also decrease the metabolism of some of these agents - see below). Amprenavir, cimetidine, nelfinavir, and ritonavir increase amiodarone levels. Amiodarone may increase the levels of digoxin (reduce dose by 50% on initiation), clonazepam, cyclosporine, flecainide (decrease dose up to 33%), metoprolol, phenothiazines, phenytoin, procainamide (reduce dose), propranolol, quinidine, tricyclic antidepressants, and warfarin. Concurrent use of fentanyl may lead to bradycardia, sinus arrest, and hypotension. The effect of drugs which prolong the QT interval, including amitriptyline, astemizole, bepridil, cisapride, disopyramide, erythromycin, gatifloxacin, haloperidol, imipramine, moxifloxacin, quinidine, pimozide, procainamide, sotalol, sparfloxacin, theophylline, and thioridazine may be increased. Amiodarone may alter thyroid function and response to thyroid supplements. Amiodarone enhances the myocardial depressant and conduction defects of inhalation anesthetics (monitor).

Decreased Effect: Amiodarone blood levels may be decreased by phenytoin and rifampin. Amiodarone may alter thyroid function and response to thyroid supplements; monitor closely.

Drug Uptake

Onset of action: Oral: 3 days to 3 weeks; I.V.: May be more rapid

Peak effect: 1 week to 5 months

Duration after discontinuation: 7-50 days

Note: Mean onset of effect and duration after discontinuation may be shorter in children than adults

Serum half-life, elimination: 40-55 days (range: 26-107 days); shorter in children than adults

Pregnancy Risk Factor D

Generic Available Yes: Tablet

Amipaque® *see* Radiological/Contrast Media (Nonionic) *on page 1039*

Amitone® [OTC] *see* Calcium Carbonate *on page 201*

Amitriptyline (a mee TRIP ti leen)

Related Information

Temporomandibular Dysfunction (TMD) *on page 1397*

U.S. Brand Names Elavil®; Vanatrip®

Canadian Brand Names Apo®-Amitriptyline; Elavil®

Mexican Brand Names Anapsique; Tryptanol®

Pharmacologic Category Antidepressant, Tricyclic (Tertiary Amine)

Synonyms Amitriptyline Hydrochloride

Use Relief of symptoms of depression

Unlabeled/Investigational: Analgesic for certain chronic and neuropathic pain; prophylaxis against migraine headaches; treatment of depressive disorders in children

Local Anesthetic/Vasoconstrictor Precautions Use with caution; epinephrine, norepinephrine and levonordefrin have been shown to have an increased pressor response in combination with TCAs

Effects on Dental Treatment

>10%: Xerostomia

Amitriptyline is the most anticholinergic and sedating of the antidepressants; pronounced effects on the cardiovascular system; long-term treatment with TCAs such as amitriptyline increases the risk of caries by reducing salivation and salivary buffer capacity. In a study by Rundergren, et al, pathological alterations were observed in the oral mucosa of 72% of 58 patients; 55% had new carious lesions after taking TCAs for a median of 5$^1/_2$ years. Current research is investigating the use of the salivary stimulant pilocarpine (Salagen®) to overcome the xerostomia from amitriptyline.

Dosage

Children:

Chronic pain management (unlabeled use): Oral: Initial: 0.1 mg/kg at bedtime, may advance as tolerated over 2-3 weeks to 0.5-2 mg/kg at bedtime

Depressive disorders (unlabeled use): Oral: Initial doses of 1 mg/kg/day given in 3 divided doses with increases to 1.5 mg/kg/day have been reported in a small number of children (n=9) 9-12 years of age; clinically, doses up to 3 mg/kg/day (5 mg/kg/day if monitored closely) have been proposed

Adolescents: Depressive disorders: Oral: Initial: 25-50 mg/day; may administer in divided doses; increase gradually to 100 mg/day in divided doses

Adults:

Depression:

Oral: 50-150 mg/day single dose at bedtime or in divided doses; dose may be gradually increased up to 300 mg/day

I.M.: 20-30 mg 4 times/day

Pain management (unlabeled use): Oral: Initial: 25 mg at bedtime; may increase as tolerated to 100 mg/day

Dosing interval in hepatic impairment: Use with caution and monitor plasma concentrations and patient response

Hemodialysis: Nondialyzable

Mechanism of Action Increases the synaptic concentration of serotonin and/or norepinephrine in the CNS by inhibition of their reuptake at the presynaptic neuronal membrane

Other Adverse Effects Anticholinergic effects may be pronounced; moderate to marked sedation can occur (tolerance to these effects usually occurs)

Cardiovascular: Orthostatic hypotension, tachycardia, nonspecific EKG changes, changes in A-V conduction

Central nervous system: Restlessness, dizziness, insomnia, sedation, fatigue, anxiety, impaired cognitive function, seizures, extrapyramidal symptoms

Dermatologic: Allergic rash, urticaria, photosensitivity

Gastrointestinal: Weight gain, xerostomia, constipation

Genitourinary: Urinary retention

Ocular: Blurred vision, mydriasis

Miscellaneous: Diaphoresis

Contraindications Hypersensitivity to amitriptyline or any component of the formulation (cross-sensitivity with other tricyclics may occur); use with MAO inhibitors or within past 14 days; recovery from acute myocardial infarction; concurrent use of cisapride; pregnancy

Drug Interactions CYP1A2, 2C9, 2C19, 2D6, and 3A3/4 enzyme substrate

Increased Effect/Toxicity: Amitriptyline increases the effects of amphetamines, anticholinergics, other CNS depressants (sedatives, hypnotics) carbamazepine, tolazamide, chlorpropamide, and warfarin. When used with MAO inhibitors, hyperpyrexia, hypertension, tachycardia, confusion, seizures, and **deaths have been reported** (serotonin syndrome). The SSRIs (to varying degrees), cimetidine, fenfluramine, indinavir, methylphenidate, ritonavir, quinidine, diltiazem, valproate, and verapamil inhibit the metabolism of TCAs and clinical toxicity may result. Use of lithium with a TCA may increase the risk for neurotoxicity. Phenothiazines may increase concentration of some TCAs and TCAs may increase the

(Continued)

Amitriptyline *(Continued)*

concentration of phenothiazines. Pressor response to I.V. epinephrine, norepinephrine, and phenylephrine may be enhanced in patients receiving TCAs (**Note:** Effect is unlikely with epinephrine or levonordefrin dosages typically administered as infiltration in combination with local anesthetics). Combined use of beta-agonists or drugs which prolong QT_c (including quinidine, procainamide, disopyramide, cisapride, sparfloxacin, gatifloxacin, moxifloxacin) with TCAs may predispose patients to cardiac arrhythmias.

Decreased Effect: Carbamazepine, phenobarbital, and rifampin may increase the metabolism of amitriptyline resulting in a decreased effect of amitriptyline. Amitriptyline inhibits the antihypertensive response to bethanidine, clonidine, debrisoquin, guanadrel, guanethidine, guanabenz, or guanfacine. Cholestyramine and colestipol may bind TCAs and reduce their absorption.

Drug Uptake

Onset of action: Migraine prophylaxis: 6 weeks, higher dosage may be required in heavy smokers because of increased metabolism; Depression: 3-4 weeks, reduce dosage to lowest effective level

Half-life, elimination: Adults: 9-25 hours (15-hour average)

Time to peak: ~4 hours

Pregnancy Risk Factor D

Generic Available Yes

Selected Readings

Boakes AJ, Laurence DR, Teoh PC, et al, "Interactions Between Sympathomimetic Amines and Antidepressant Agents in Man," *Br Med J*, 1973, 1(849):311-5.

Friedlander AH, Mahler ME, "Major Depressive Disorder. Psychopathology, Medical Management, and Dental Implications," *J Am Dent Assoc*, 201, 132(5):629-38.

Ganzberg S, "Psychoactive Drugs," *ADA Guide to Dental Therapeutics*, 2nd ed, Chicago, IL: ADA Publishing, a Division of ADA Business Enterprises, Inc, 2000, 376-405.

Jastak JT and Yagiela JA, "Vasoconstrictors and Local Anesthesia: A Review and Rationale for Use," *J Am Dent Assoc*, 1983, 107(4):623-30.

Rundegren J, van Dijken J, Mörnstad H, et al, "Oral Conditions in Patients Receiving Long-Term Treatment With Cyclic Antidepressant Drugs," *Swed Dent J*, 1985, 9(2):55-64.

Yagiela JA, "Adverse Drug Interactions in Dental Practice: Interactions Associated With Vasoconstrictors. Part V of a Series," *J Am Dent Assoc*, 1999, 130(5):701-9.

Amitriptyline and Chlordiazepoxide

(a mee TRIP ti leen & klor dye az e POKS ide)

U.S. Brand Names Limbitrol®; Limbitrol® DS

Canadian Brand Names Limbitrol®

Pharmacologic Category Antidepressant, Tricyclic (Tertiary Amine); Benzodiazepine

Synonyms Chlordiazepoxide and Amitriptyline

Use Treatment of moderate to severe anxiety and/or agitation and depression

Local Anesthetic/Vasoconstrictor Precautions Use with caution; epinephrine, norepinephrine and levonordefrin have been shown to have an increased pressor response in combination with TCAs

Effects on Dental Treatment

Amitriptyline: The most anticholinergic and sedating of the antidepressants; pronounced effects on the cardiovascular system; long-term treatment with TCAs such as amitriptyline increases the risk of caries by reducing salivation and salivary buffer capacity. In a study by Rundergren, et al, pathological alterations were observed in the oral mucosa of 72% of 58 patients; 55% had new carious lesions after taking TCAs for a median of 5½ years. Current research is investigating the use of the salivary stimulant pilocarpine (Salagen®) to overcome the xerostomia from amitriptyline.

Chlordiazepoxide: Over 10% of patients will experience xerostomia which disappears with cessation of drug therapy

Restrictions C-IV

Dosage Initial: 3-4 tablets in divided doses; this may be increased to 6 tablets/day as required; some patients respond to smaller doses and can be maintained on 2 tablets

Other Adverse Effects See Amitriptyline *on page 75* and Chlordiazepoxide *on page 262*

Warnings/Precautions

Based on **amitriptyline** component:

Often causes drowsiness/sedation, resulting in impaired performance of tasks requiring alertness (ie, operating machinery or driving). Sedative effects may be additive with other CNS depressants and/or ethanol. The degree of sedation is very high relative to other antidepressants. May worsen psychosis in some patients or precipitate a shift to mania or hypomania in patients with bipolar disease. May cause hyponatremia/SIADH. May increase the risks associated with electroconvulsive therapy. This agent should be discontinued, when possible, prior to elective surgery. Therapy should not be abruptly discontinued in patients receiving high doses for prolonged periods.

May cause orthostatic hypotension; the risk of this problem is very high relative to other antidepressants. Use with caution in patients at risk of hypotension or in patients where transient hypotensive episodes would be poorly tolerated (cardiovascular disease or cerebrovascular disease). The degree of anticholinergic blockade produced by this agent is very high relative to other cyclic antidepressants; use with caution in patients with urinary retention, benign prostatic hyperplasia, narrow-angle glaucoma, xerostomia, visual problems, constipation, or a history of bowel obstruction. May alter glucose control - use with caution in patients with diabetes.

Use caution in patients with depression, particularly if suicidal risk may be present. Use with caution in patients with a history of cardiovascular disease (including previous MI, stroke, tachycardia, or conduction abnormalities). The risk of conduction abnormalities with this agent is high relative to other antidepressants. May lower seizure threshold - use caution in patients with a previous seizure disorder or condition predisposing to seizures such as brain damage, alcoholism, or concurrent therapy with other drugs which lower the seizure threshold. Use with caution in hyperthyroid patients or those receiving thyroid supplementation. Use with caution in patients with hepatic or renal dysfunction and in elderly patients. Not recommended for use in patients <12 years of age.

Based on **chlordiazepoxide** component:

Active metabolites with extended half-lives may lead to delayed accumulation and adverse effects. Use with caution in elderly or debilitated patients, pediatric patients, patients with hepatic disease (including alcoholics) or renal impairment. Use with caution in patients with respiratory disease or impaired gag reflex. Use with caution in patients with porphyria.

Parenteral administration should be avoided in comatose patients or shock. Adequate resuscitative equipment/personnel should be available, and appropriate monitoring should be conducted at the time of injection and for several hours following administration. The parenteral formulation should be diluted for I.M. administration with the supplied diluent only. This diluent should not be used when preparing the drug for I.V. administration.

Causes CNS depression (dose-related) resulting in sedation, dizziness, confusion, or ataxia which may impair physical and mental capabilities. Patients must be cautioned about performing tasks which require mental alertness (ie, operating machinery or driving). Use with caution in patients receiving other CNS depressants or psychoactive agents (lithium, phenothiazines). Effects with other sedative drugs or ethanol may be potentiated. Benzodiazepines have been associated with falls and traumatic injury and should be used with extreme caution in patients who are at risk of these events (especially the elderly).

Use caution in patients with depression, particularly if suicidal risk may be present. Use with caution in patients with a history of drug dependence. Benzodiazepines have been associated with dependence and acute withdrawal symptoms on discontinuation or reduction in dose. Acute withdrawal, including seizures, may be precipitated in patients after administration of flumazenil to patients receiving long-term benzodiazepine therapy.

Benzodiazepines have been associated with anterograde amnesia. Paradoxical reactions, including hyperactive or aggressive behavior have been reported with benzodiazepines, particularly in adolescent/pediatric or psychiatric patients. Does not have analgesic, antidepressant, or antipsychotic properties.

Drug Interactions

See Amitriptyline *on page 75* and Chlordiazepoxide *on page 262*

Amitriptyline: CYP1A2, 2C9, 2C19, 2D6, and 3A3/4 enzyme substrate

Chlordiazepoxide: CYP3A3/4 enzyme substrate

Drug Uptake See Amitriptyline *on page 75* and Chlordiazepoxide *on page 262*

Pregnancy Risk Factor D

Generic Available Yes

Selected Readings

Boakes AJ, Laurence DR, Teoh PC, et al, "Interactions Between Sympathomimetic Amines and Antidepressant Agents in Man," *Br Med J*, 1973, 1(849):311-5.

Jastak JT and Yagiela JA, "Vasoconstrictors and Local Anesthesia: A Review and Rationale for Use," *J Am Dent Assoc*, 1983, 107(4):623-30.

Mitchell JR, "Guanethidine and Related Agents. III Antagonism by Drugs Which Inhibit the Norepinephrine Pump in Man," *J Clin Invest*, 1970, 49(8):1596-604.

Rundegren J, van Dijken J, Mörnstad H, et al, "Oral Conditions in Patients Receiving Long-Term Treatment With Cyclic Antidepressant Drugs," *Swed Dent J*, 1985, 9(2):55-64.

Amitriptyline and Perphenazine

(a mee TRIP ti leen & per FEN a zeen)

U.S. Brand Names Etrafon®; Triavil®

Canadian Brand Names Etrafon®; Triavil®

Pharmacologic Category Antidepressant, Tricyclic (Tertiary Amine); Antipsychotic Agent, Phenothiazine, Piperazine

Synonyms Perphenazine and Amitriptyline

Use Treatment of patients with moderate to severe anxiety and depression

Local Anesthetic/Vasoconstrictor Precautions

Amitriptyline: Use with caution; epinephrine, norepinephrine and levonordefrin have been shown to have an increased pressor response in combination with TCAs

(Continued)

Amitriptyline and Perphenazine *(Continued)*

Perphenazine: No information available to require special precautions

Effects on Dental Treatment

>10%: Xerostomia

Amitriptyline: The most anticholinergic and sedating of the antidepressants; pronounced effects on the cardiovascular system; long-term treatment with TCAs such as amitriptyline increases the risk of caries by reducing salivation and salivary buffer capacity. In a study by Rundergren, et al, pathological alterations were observed in the oral mucosa of 72% of 58 patients; 55% had new carious lesions after taking TCAs for a median of 5½ years. Current research is investigating the use of the salivary stimulant pilocarpine (Salagen®) to overcome the xerostomia from amitriptyline.

Perphenazine: Significant hypotension may occur, especially when the drug is administered parenterally; orthostatic hypotension is due to alpha-receptor blockade, the elderly are at greater risk for orthostatic hypotension.

Tardive dyskinesia: Prevalence rate may be 40% in elderly; development of the syndrome and the irreversible nature are proportional to duration and total cumulative dose over time. Extrapyramidal reactions are more common in elderly with up to 50% developing these reactions after 60 years of age; drug-induced **Parkinson's syndrome** occurs often; **Akathisia** is the most common extrapyramidal reaction in elderly.

Increased confusion, memory loss, psychotic behavior, and agitation frequently occur as a consequence of anticholinergic effects. Antipsychotic associated sedation in nonpsychotic patients is extremely unpleasant due to feelings of depersonalization, derealization, and dysphoria.

Dosage Oral: 1 tablet 2-4 times/day

Other Adverse Effects

Based on **amitriptyline** component: Anticholinergic effects may be pronounced; moderate to marked sedation can occur (tolerance to these effects usually occurs).

Frequency not defined:

- Cardiovascular: Orthostatic hypotension, tachycardia, nonspecific EKG changes, changes in AV conduction
- Central nervous system: Restlessness, dizziness, insomnia, sedation, fatigue, anxiety, impaired cognitive function, seizures, extrapyramidal symptoms
- Dermatologic: Allergic rash, urticaria, photosensitivity
- Gastrointestinal: Weight gain, xerostomia, constipation
- Genitourinary: Urinary retention

Based on **perphenazine** component:

- Cardiovascular: Hypotension, orthostatic hypotension, hypertension, tachycardia, bradycardia, dizziness, cardiac arrest
- Central nervous system: Extrapyramidal symptoms (pseudoparkinsonism, akathisia, dystonias, tardive dyskinesia), dizziness, cerebral edema, seizures, headache, drowsiness, paradoxical excitement, restlessness, hyperactivity, insomnia, neuroleptic malignant syndrome (NMS), impairment of temperature regulation
- Dermatologic: Increased sensitivity to sun, rash, discoloration of skin (blue-gray)
- Endocrine & metabolic: Hypoglycemia, hyperglycemia, galactorrhea, lactation, breast enlargement, gynecomastia, menstrual irregularity, amenorrhea, SIADH, changes in libido
- Gastrointestinal: Constipation, weight gain,. vomiting, stomach pain, nausea, xerostomia, salivation, diarrhea, anorexia, ileus
- Genitourinary: Difficulty in urination, ejaculatory disturbances, incontinence, polyuria, ejaculating dysfunction, priapism
- Hematologic: Agranulocytosis, leukopenia, eosinophilia, hemolytic anemia, thrombocytopenic purpura, pancytopenia
- Hepatic: Cholestatic jaundice, hepatotoxicity
- Neuromuscular & skeletal: Tremor
- Ocular: Pigmentary retinopathy, blurred vision, cornea and lens changes
- Respiratory: Nasal congestion
- Miscellaneous: Diaphoresis

Warnings/Precautions Safe use of tricyclic antidepressants in children <12 years of age has not been established; amitriptyline should not be abruptly discontinued in patients receiving high doses for prolonged periods; do not drink alcoholic beverages

Drug Interactions

Based on **amitriptyline** component: CYP1A2, 2C9, 2C19, 2D6, and 3A3/4 enzyme substrate

- Altretamine: Concurrent use may cause orthostatic hypertension
- Amphetamines: TCAs may enhance the effect of amphetamines; monitor for adverse CV effects
- Anticholinergics: Combined use with TCAs may produce additive anticholinergic effects

Antihypertensives: Amitriptyline inhibits the antihypertensive response to bethanidine, clonidine, debrisoquin, guanadrel, guanethidine, guanabenz, guanfacine; monitor BP; consider alternate antihypertensive agent

Beta-agonists: When combined with TCAs may predispose patients to cardiac arrhythmias

Bupropion: May increase the levels of tricyclic antidepressants. Based on limited information; monitor response

Carbamazepine: Tricyclic antidepressants may increase carbamazepine levels; monitor

Cholestyramine and colestipol: May bind TCAs and reduce their absorption; monitor for altered response

Clonidine: Abrupt discontinuation of clonidine may cause hypertensive crisis, amitriptyline may enhance the response (also see note on antihypertensives)

CNS depressants: Sedative effects may be additive with TCAs; monitor for increased effect; includes benzodiazepines, barbiturates, antipsychotics, ethanol, and other sedative medications.

CYP1A2 inhibitors: Metabolism of amitriptyline may be decreased; increasing clinical effect or toxicity; inhibitors include cimetidine, ciprofloxacin, fluvoxamine, isoniazid, ritonavir, and zileuton

CYP2C8/9 inhibitors: Serum levels and/or toxicity of some tricyclic antidepressants may be increased; inhibitors include amiodarone, cimetidine, fluvoxamine, some NSAIDs, metronidazole, ritonavir, sulfonamides, troglitazone, valproic acid, and zafirlukast; monitor for increased effect/toxicity

CYP2C19 inhibitors: Serum levels of amitriptyline may be increased; inhibitors include cimetidine, felbamate, fluconazole, fluoxetine, fluvoxamine, omeprazole, teniposide, tolbutamide, and troglitazone

CYP2D6 inhibitors: Serum levels and/or toxicity of some tricyclic antidepressants may be increased; inhibitors include amiodarone, cimetidine, delavirdine, fluoxetine, paroxetine, propafenone, quinidine, and ritonavir; monitor for increased effect/toxicity

CYP3A3/4 inhibitors: Serum level and/or toxicity of some tricyclic antidepressants may be increased. Inhibitors include amiodarone, cimetidine, clarithromycin, erythromycin, delavirdine, diltiazem, dirithromycin, disulfiram, fluoxetine, fluvoxamine, grapefruit juice, indinavir, itraconazole, ketoconazole, nefazodone, nevirapine, propoxyphene, quinupristin-dalfopristin, ritonavir, saquinavir, verapamil, zafirlukast, zileuton. Monitor for altered effects; a decrease in TCA dosage may be required

Enzyme inducers: May increase the metabolism of amitriptyline resulting in decreased effect; includes carbamazepine, phenobarbital, phenytoin, and rifampin; monitor for decreased response

Epinephrine (and other direct alpha-agonists): Pressor response to I.V. epinephrine, norepinephrine, and phenylephrine may be enhanced in patients receiving TCAs (**Note:** Effect is unlikely with epinephrine or levonordefrin dosages typically administered as infiltration in combination with local anesthetics)

Fenfluramine: May increase tricyclic antidepressant levels/effects

Hypoglycemic agents (including insulin): TCAs may enhance the hypoglycemic effects of tolazamide, chlorpropamide, or insulin; monitor for changes in blood glucose levels; reported with chlorpropamide, tolazamide, and insulin

Levodopa: Tricyclic antidepressants may decrease the absorption (bioavailability) of levodopa; rare hypertensive episodes have also been attributed to this combination

Linezolid: Hyperpyrexia, hypertension, tachycardia, confusion, seizures, and **deaths have been reported** with agents which inhibit MAO (serotonin syndrome); this combination should be avoided

Lithium: Concurrent use with a TCA may increase the risk for neurotoxicity

MAO inhibitors: Hyperpyrexia, hypertension, tachycardia, confusion, seizures, and **deaths have been reported** (serotonin syndrome); this combination should be avoided

Methylphenidate: Metabolism of amitriptyline may be decreased

Phenothiazines: Serum concentrations of some TCAs may be increased; in addition, TCAs may increase concentration of phenothiazines; monitor for altered clinical response

QT_c-prolonging agents: Concurrent use of tricyclic agents with other drugs which may prolong QT_c interval may increase the risk of potentially fatal arrhythmias; includes type Ia and type III antiarrhythmics agents, selected quinolones (sparfloxacin, gatifloxacin, moxifloxacin, grepafloxacin), cisapride, and other agents

Ritonavir: Combined use of high-dose tricyclic antidepressants with ritonavir may cause serotonin syndrome in HIV-positive patients; monitor

Sucralfate: Absorption of tricyclic antidepressants may be reduced with coadministration

Sympathomimetics, indirect-acting: Tricyclic antidepressants may result in a decreased sensitivity to indirect-acting sympathomimetics; includes dopamine and ephedrine; also see interaction with epinephrine (and direct-acting sympathomimetics)

Tramadol: Tramadol's risk of seizures may be increased with TCAs

(Continued)

Amitriptyline and Perphenazine *(Continued)*

Valproic acid: May increase serum concentrations/adverse effects of some tricyclic antidepressants

Warfarin (and other oral anticoagulants): Amitriptyline may increase the anticoagulant effect in patients stabilized on warfarin; monitor INR

Based on **perphenazine** component: CYP2D6 enzyme substrate; CYP2D6 enzyme inhibitor

Aluminum salts: May decrease the absorption of phenothiazines; monitor

Amphetamines: Efficacy may be diminished by antipsychotics; in addition, amphetamines may increase psychotic symptoms; avoid concurrent use

Anticholinergics: May inhibit the therapeutic response to phenothiazines and excess anticholinergic effects may occur; includes benztropine, trihexyphenidyl, biperiden, and drugs with significant anticholinergic activity (TCAs, antihistamines, disopyramide)

Antihypertensives: Concurrent use of phenothiazines with an antihypertensive may produce additive hypotensive effects (particularly orthostasis)

Bromocriptine: Phenothiazines inhibit the ability of bromocriptine to lower serum prolactin concentrations

CNS depressants: Sedative effects may be additive with phenothiazines; monitor for increased effect; includes barbiturates, benzodiazepines, narcotic analgesics, ethanol, and other sedative agents

CYP2D6 inhibitors: Metabolism of phenothiazines may be decreased; increasing clinical effect or toxicity; inhibitors include amiodarone, cimetidine, delavirdine, fluoxetine, paroxetine, propafenone, quinidine, and ritonavir; monitor for increased effect/toxicity

Enzyme inducers: May enhance the hepatic metabolism of phenothiazines; larger doses may be required; includes rifampin, rifabutin, barbiturates, phenytoin, and cigarette smoking

Epinephrine: Chlorpromazine (and possibly other low potency antipsychotics) may diminish the pressor effects of epinephrine

Guanethidine and guanadrel: Antihypertensive effects may be inhibited by phenothiazines

Levodopa: Phenothiazines may inhibit the antiparkinsonian effect of levodopa; avoid this combination

Lithium: Phenothiazines may produce neurotoxicity with lithium; this is a rare effect

Metoclopramide: May increase extrapyramidal symptoms (EPS) or risk.

Phenytoin: May reduce serum levels of phenothiazines; phenothiazines may increase phenytoin serum levels

Propranolol: Serum concentrations of phenothiazines may be increased; propranolol also increases phenothiazine concentrations

Polypeptide antibiotics: Rare cases of respiratory paralysis have been reported with concurrent use of phenothiazines

QT_c prolonging agents: Effects on QT_c interval may be additive with phenothiazines, increasing the risk of malignant arrhythmias; includes type Ia antiarrhythmics, TCAs, and some quinolone antibiotics (sparfloxacin, moxifloxacin, and gatifloxacin)

Sulfadoxine-pyrimethamine: May increase phenothiazine concentrations

Tricyclic antidepressants: Concurrent use may produce increased toxicity or altered therapeutic response

Trazodone: Phenothiazines and trazodone may produce additive hypotensive effects

Valproic acid: Serum levels may be increased by phenothiazines

Drug Uptake See Amitriptyline *on page 75* and Perphenazine *on page 941*

Pregnancy Risk Factor D

Generic Available Yes

Selected Readings

Boakes AJ, Laurence DR, Teoh PC, et al, "Interactions Between Sympathomimetic Amines and Antidepressant Agents in Man," *Br Med J*, 1973, 1(849):311-5.

Jastak JT and Yagiela JA, "Vasoconstrictors and Local Anesthesia: A Review and Rationale for Use," *J Am Dent Assoc*, 1983, 107(4):623-30.

Mitchell JR, "Guanethidine and Related Agents. III Antagonism by Drugs Which Inhibit the Norepinephrine Pump in Man," *J Clin Invest*, 1970, 49(8):1596-604.

Rundegren J, van Dijken J, Mörnstad H, et al, "Oral Conditions in Patients Receiving Long-Term Treatment With Cyclic Antidepressant Drugs," *Swed Dent J*, 1985, 9(2):55-64.

Amlexanox (am LEKS an oks)

Related Information

Oral Nonviral Soft Tissue Ulcerations or Erosions *on page 1384*

U.S. Brand Names Aphthasol™

Pharmacologic Category Anti-inflammatory, Locally Applied

Use Treatment of aphthous ulcers (ie, canker sores); has been investigated in many allergic disorders

Local Anesthetic/Vasoconstrictor Precautions No information available to require special precautions

Effects on Dental Treatment Discontinue therapy if rash or contact mucositis develops.

Dosage Administer (0.5 cm - 1/4") directly on ulcers 4 times/day following oral hygiene, after meals, and at bedtime.

Mechanism of Action As a benzopyrano-bipyridine carboxylic acid derivative, amlexanox has anti-inflammatory and antiallergic properties; it inhibits chemical mediatory release of the slow-reacting substance of anaphylaxis (SRS-A) and may have antagonistic effects on interleukin-3

Other Adverse Effects 1% to 2%:

Dermatologic: Allergic contact dermatitis

Gastrointestinal: Oral irritation

Contraindications Hypersensitivity to amlexanox or any component of the formulation

Drug Uptake

Absorption: Some from swallowed paste

Half-life, elimination: 3.5 hours

Time to peak: 2 hours

Pregnancy Risk Factor B

Generic Available No

Comments Treatment of canker sores with amlexanox showed a 76% median reduction in ulcer size compared to a 40% reduction with placebo. Greer, et al, reported an overall mean reduction in ulcer size of 1.82 mm^2 for patients treated with 5% amlexanox versus an average reduction of 0.52 mm^2 for the control group. Recent studies in over thousands of patients have confirmed that amlexanox accelerates the resolution of pain and healing of aphthous ulcers more significantly than vehicle and no treatment.

Selected Readings

Binnie WH, Curro FA, Khandwala A, et al, "Amlexanox Oral Paste: A Novel Treatment That Accelerates the Healing of Aphthous Ulcers," *Compend Contin Educ Dent*, 1997, 18(11):1116-8, 1120-2, 1124.

Greer RO Jr, Lindenmuth JE, Juarez T, et al, "A Double-Blind Study of Topically Applied 5% Amlexanox in the Treatment of Aphthous Ulcers," *J Oral Maxillofac Surg*, 1993, 51(3):243-8.

Khandwala A, Van Inwegen RG, and Alfano MC, "5% Amlexanox Oral Paste, A New Treatment for Recurrent Minor Aphthous Ulcers: I. Clinical Demonstration of Acceleration of Healing and Resolution of Pain," *Oral Surg Oral Med Oral Pathol Oral Radiol Endod*, 1997, 83(2):222-30.

Khandwala A, Van Inwegen RG, Charney MR, et al, "5% Amlexanox Oral Paste, A New Treatment for Recurrent Minor Aphthous Ulcers: II. Pharmacokinetics and Demonstration of Clinical Safety," *Oral Surg Oral Med Oral Pathol Oral Radiol Endod*, 1997, 83(2):231-8.

Amlodipine (am LOE di peen)

Related Information

Calcium Channel Blockers and Gingival Hyperplasia *on page 1432*

Cardiovascular Diseases *on page 1308*

U.S. Brand Names Norvasc®

Canadian Brand Names Norvasc®

Mexican Brand Names Norvas

Pharmacologic Category Calcium Channel Blocker

Use Treatment of hypertension and angina

Local Anesthetic/Vasoconstrictor Precautions No information available to require special precautions

Effects on Dental Treatment ~1%: Gingival hyperplasia (fewer reports with amlodipine than with other CCBs); usually disappears with discontinuation (consultation with physician is suggested)

Dosage Adults: Oral:

Hypertension: Initial dose: 2.5-5 mg once daily; usual dose: 5 mg once daily; maximum dose: 10 mg once daily. In general, titrate in 2.5 mg increments over 7-14 days.

Angina: Usual dose: 5-10 mg; use lower doses for elderly or those with hepatic insufficiency (eg, 2.5-5 mg).

Dialysis: Hemodialysis and peritoneal dialysis does not enhance elimination. Supplemental dose is not necessary.

Dosage adjustment in hepatic impairment: Administer 2.5 mg once daily.

Elderly: Dosing should start at the lower end of dosing range due to possible increased incidence of hepatic, renal, or cardiac impairment. Elderly patients also show decreased clearance of amlodipine.

Mechanism of Action Inhibits calcium ion from entering the "slow channels" or select voltage-sensitive areas of vascular smooth muscle and myocardium during depolarization, producing a relaxation of coronary vascular smooth muscle and coronary vasodilation; increases myocardial oxygen delivery in patients with vasospastic angina

Other Adverse Effects

>10%: Cardiovascular: Peripheral edema (1.8% to 14.6% dose-related)

1% to 10%:

- Central nervous system: Headache (7.3%; similar to placebo)
- Cardiovascular: Flushing (0.7% to 2.6%), palpitations (0.7% to 4.5%)
- Dermatologic: Rash (1% to 2%), pruritus (1% to 2%)
- Endocrine & metabolic: Male sexual dysfunction (1% to 2%)

(Continued)

Amlodipine *(Continued)*

Gastrointestinal: Nausea (2.9%), abdominal pain (1% to 2%), dyspepsia (1% to 2%), gingival hyperplasia

Neuromuscular & skeletal: Muscle cramps (1% to 2%), weakness (1% to 2%)

Respiratory: Shortness of breath (1% to 2%), pulmonary edema (15% from PRAISE trial, CHF population)

Drug Interactions CYP3A3/4 enzyme substrate

Increased Effect/Toxicity: Azole antifungals (itraconazole, ketoconazole, fluconazole), erythromycin, and other inhibitors of cytochrome P450 isoenzyme 3A4 may inhibit amlodipine's metabolism. Cyclosporine levels may be increased by amlodipine. Blood pressure-lowering effects of sildenafil are additive with amlodipine. Grapefruit juice may modestly increase amlodipine levels.

Decreased Effect: Rifampin (and potentially other enzyme inducers) increase the metabolism of amlodipine. Calcium may reduce the calcium channel blocker's hypotensive effects.

Drug Uptake

Onset of action: 30-50 minutes

Peak effect: 6-12 hours

Duration: 24 hours

Absorption: Oral: Well absorbed

Half-life elimination: 30-50 hours

Pregnancy Risk Factor C

Generic Available No

Selected Readings

Jorgensen MG, "Prevalence of Amlodipine-Related Gingival Hyperplasia," *J Periodontol*, 1997, 68(7):676-8.

Wynn RL, "An Update on Calcium Channel Blocker-Induced Gingival Hyperplasia," *Gen Dent*, 1995, 43(3):218-22.

Wynn RL, "Calcium Channel Blockers and Gingival Hyperplasia," *Gen Dent*, 1991, 39(4):240-3.

Amlodipine and Benazepril (am LOE di peen & ben AY ze pril)

U.S. Brand Names Lotrel®

Canadian Brand Names Lotrel®

Pharmacologic Category Antihypertensive Agent Combination

Synonyms Benazepril and Amlodipine

Use Treatment of hypertension

Local Anesthetic/Vasoconstrictor Precautions No information available to require special precautions

Effects on Dental Treatment ~1%: Gingival hyperplasia (fewer reports with amlodipine than with other CCBs); usually disappears with discontinuation (consultation with physician is suggested)

Dosage Adults: Oral: 1 capsule daily

Mechanism of Action The mechanism through which benazepril lowers BP is believed to be primarily suppression of the renin-angiotensin-aldosterone system, benazepril has an antihypertensive effect even in patients with low-renin hypertension; amlodipine is a dihydropyridine calcium antagonist that inhibits the transmembrane influx of calcium ions into vascular smooth muscle and cardiac muscle; amlodipine is a peripheral arterial vasodilator that acts directly on vascular smooth muscle to cause a reduction in peripheral vascular resistance and reduction in BP

Drug Uptake

See Benazepril *on page 149* and Amlodipine *on page 81*

Absorption: Not influenced by the presence of food in the GI tract; food effects on absorption have not been studied

Amlodipine: 64% to 90%

Benazepril: 37%

Time to peak:

Amlodipine: 6-12 hours

Benazepril: 0.5-2 hours

Pregnancy Risk Factor C/D (2nd and 3rd trimesters)

Generic Available No

Selected Readings

Wynn RL, "An Update on Calcium Channel Blocker-Induced Gingival Hyperplasia," *Gen Dent*, 1995, 43(3):218-22.

Wynn RL, "Calcium Channel Blockers and Gingival Hyperplasia," *Gen Dent*, 1991, 39(4):240-3.

Ammens® Medicated Deodorant [OTC] *see* Zinc Oxide *on page 1260*

Ammonia Spirit, Aromatic (a MOE nee ah SPEAR it, air oh MAT ik)

Related Information

Dental Office Emergencies *on page 1418*

U.S. Brand Names Aromatic Ammonia Aspirols®

Pharmacologic Category Respiratory Stimulant

Synonyms Smelling Salts

Use Respiratory and circulatory stimulant, treatment of fainting

Local Anesthetic/Vasoconstrictor Precautions No information available to require special precautions

Effects on Dental Treatment No effects or complications reported

Dosage Used as "smelling salts" as treatment or prevention of fainting

Other Adverse Effects 1% to 10%:

Gastrointestinal: Nausea, vomiting

Respiratory: Irritation to nasal mucosa, coughing

Contraindications Hypersensitivity to ammonia or any component of the formulation

Pregnancy Risk Factor C

Dosage Forms SOLN: 60 mL, 480 mL. **VAPOR, inhalation** [ampul]: 0.33 mL

Generic Available Yes

Ammonium Chloride (a MOE nee um KLOR ide)

Pharmacologic Category Electrolyte Supplement, Parenteral; Urinary Acidifying Agent

Use Diuretic or systemic and urinary acidifying agent; treatment of hypochloremic states

Local Anesthetic/Vasoconstrictor Precautions No information available to require special precautions

Effects on Dental Treatment No effects or complications reported

Dosage Metabolic alkalosis: The following equations represent different methods of correction utilizing either the serum HCO_3^-, the serum chloride, or the base excess

Dosing of mEq NH_4Cl via the chloride-deficit method (hypochloremia):

Dose of mEq NH_4Cl = [0.2 L/kg x body weight (kg)] x [103 - observed serum chloride]; administer 100% of dose over 12 hours, then re-evaluate

Note: 0.2 L/kg is the estimated chloride space and 103 is the average normal serum chloride concentration

Dosing of mEq NH_4Cl via the bicarbonate-excess method (refractory hypochloremic metabolic alkalosis):

Dose of NH_4Cl = [0.5 L/kg x body weight (kg)] x (observed serum HCO_3^- - 24); administer 50% of dose over 12 hours, then re-evaluate

Note: 0.5 L/kg is the estimated bicarbonate space and 24 is the average normal serum bicarbonate concentration

Dosing of mEq NH_4Cl via the base-excess method:

Dose of NH_4Cl = [0.3 L/kg x body weight (kg)] x measured base excess (mEq/L); administer 50% of dose over 12 hours, then re-evaluate

Note: 0.3 L/kg is the estimated extracellular bicarbonate and base excess is measured by the chemistry lab and reported with arterial blood gases

These equations will yield different requirements of ammonium chloride

Equation #1 is inappropriate to use if the patient has severe metabolic alkalosis without hypochloremia or if the patient has uremia

Equation #3 is the most useful for the first estimation of ammonium chloride dosage

Children: Urinary acidifying agents: Oral, I.V.: 75 mg/kg/day in 4 divided doses; maximum daily dose: 6 g

Adults: Urinary acidifying agent/diuretic:

Oral: 1-2 g every 4-6 hours

I.V.: 1.5 g/dose every 6 hours

Mechanism of Action Increases acidity by increasing free hydrogen ion concentration

Other Adverse Effects Frequency not defined:

Cardiovascular: Bradycardia

Central nervous system: Headache (with large doses), coma, mental confusion

Dermatologic: Rash

Endocrine & metabolic: Hypokalemia (with large doses), metabolic acidosis, potassium and sodium may be decreased, hyperchloremia

Gastrointestinal: Vomiting, gastric irritation, nausea

Hepatic: Ammonia may be increased

Local: Pain at site of injection

Respiratory: Hyperventilation (with large doses)

Drug Uptake Absorption: Rapid from GI tract, complete within 3-6 hours

Pregnancy Risk Factor C

Generic Available Yes

Amobarbital (am oh BAR bi tal)

U.S. Brand Names Amytal®

Canadian Brand Names Amytal®

Pharmacologic Category Barbiturate

Synonyms Amylobarbitone

Use

Oral: Hypnotic in short-term treatment of insomnia, to reduce anxiety and provide sedation preoperatively

I.M., I.V.: Control status epilepticus or acute seizure episodes. Also used in catatonic, negativistic, or manic reactions and in "Amytal® Interviewing" for narcoanalysis

(Continued)

Amobarbital *(Continued)*

Local Anesthetic/Vasoconstrictor Precautions No information available to require special precautions

Effects on Dental Treatment No effects or complications reported

Restrictions C-II

Dosage

Children: Oral:
- Sedation: 6 mg/kg/day divided every 6-8 hours
- Insomnia: 2 mg/kg or 70 mg/m²/day in 4 equally divided doses
- Hypnotic: 2-3 mg/kg

Adults:
- Insomnia: Oral: 65-200 mg at bedtime
- Sedation: Oral: 30-50 mg 2-3 times/day
- Preanesthetic: Oral: 200 mg 1-2 hours before surgery
- Hypnotic:
  - Oral: 65-200 mg at bedtime
  - I.M., I.V.: 65-500 mg, should not exceed 500 mg I.M. or 1000 mg I.V.
- Acute episode of agitated behavior:
  - Oral: 30-50 mg 2-3 times/day
  - I.M., I.V.: 65-500 mg, should not exceed 500 mg I.M. or 1000 mg I.V.
- Status epilepticus/acute seizure episode: I.M., I.V.: 65-500 mg, should not exceed 500 mg I.M. or 1000 mg I.V.
- Amobarbital (Amytal®) interview: I.V.: 50 mg/minute for total dose up to 300 mg

Mechanism of Action Interferes with transmission of impulses from the thalamus to the cortex of the brain resulting in an imbalance in central inhibitory and facilitatory mechanisms

Other Adverse Effects

>10%:
- Central nervous system: Dizziness, lightheadedness, "hangover" effect, drowsiness, CNS depression, fever
- Local: Pain at injection site

1% to 10%:
- Central nervous system: Confusion, mental depression, unusual excitement, nervousness, faint feeling, headache, insomnia, nightmares
- Gastrointestinal: Nausea, vomiting, constipation

Drug Interactions CYP1A2, 2B6, 2C, 2C8, 2C9, 2C18, 2C19, 3A3/4, and 3A5-7 enzyme inducer

Barbiturates are cytochrome P450 enzyme inducers; patients should be monitored when these drugs are started or stopped for a decreased or increased therapeutic effect respectively.

Increased Effect/Toxicity: When combined with other CNS depressants, narcotic analgesics, antidepressants, or benzodiazepines, additive respiratory and CNS depression may occur. Barbiturates may enhance the hepatotoxic potential of acetaminophen overdoses. Chloramphenicol, MAO inhibitors, valproic acid, and felbamate may inhibit barbiturate metabolism. Barbiturates may impair the absorption of griseofulvin, and may enhance the nephrotoxic effects of methoxyflurane. Concurrent use of meperidine may result in increased CNS depression.

Decreased Effect: Barbiturates are hepatic enzyme inducers, and may increase the metabolism of antipsychotics, some beta-blockers (unlikely with atenolol and nadolol), calcium channel blockers, chloramphenicol, cimetidine, corticosteroids, cyclosporine, disopyramide, doxycycline, ethosuximide, felbamate, furosemide, griseofulvin, lamotrigine, phenytoin, propafenone, quinidine, tacrolimus, TCAs, and theophylline. Barbiturates may increase the metabolism of estrogens and reduce the efficacy of oral contraceptives; an alternative method of contraception should be considered. Barbiturates inhibit the hypoprothrombinemic effects of oral anticoagulants via increased metabolism. Barbiturates may enhance the metabolism of methadone resulting in methadone withdrawal.

Drug Uptake

Onset of action: Oral: Within 1 hour; I.V.: Within 5 minutes

Half-life elimination: Biphasic: Initial: 40 minutes; Terminal: 20 hours

Pregnancy Risk Factor D

Generic Available Yes: Capsule

Amobarbital and Secobarbital

(am oh BAR bi tal & see koe BAR bi tal)

U.S. Brand Names Tuinal®

Pharmacologic Category Barbiturate

Synonyms Secobarbital and Amobarbital

Use Short-term treatment of insomnia

Local Anesthetic/Vasoconstrictor Precautions No information available to require special precautions

Effects on Dental Treatment No effects or complications reported

Restrictions C-II

Dosage Adults: Oral: 1-2 capsules at bedtime

Other Adverse Effects
>10%:
Central nervous system: Dizziness, lightheadedness, drowsiness, "hangover" effect
Local: Pain at injection site
1% to 10%:
Central nervous system: Confusion, mental depression, unusual excitement, nervousness, faint feeling, headache, insomnia, nightmares
Gastrointestinal: Constipation, nausea, vomiting

Drug Interactions Amobarbital: CYP1A2, 2B6, 2C, 2C8, 2C9, 2C18, 2C19, 3A3/4, and 3A5-7 enzyme inducer; barbiturates are cytochrome P450 enzyme inducers; patients should be monitored when these drugs are started or stopped for a decreased or increased therapeutic effect respectively.

Drug Uptake See Amobarbital *on page 83* and Secobarbital *on page 1078*

Pregnancy Risk Factor D

Generic Available No

AMO Vitrax® *see* Sodium Hyaluronate *on page 1097*

Amoxapine (a MOKS a peen)

Canadian Brand Names Asendin®

Mexican Brand Names Demolox

Pharmacologic Category Antidepressant, Tricyclic (Secondary Amine)

Synonyms Asendin® [DSC]

Use Treatment of depression, psychotic depression, depression accompanied by anxiety or agitation

Local Anesthetic/Vasoconstrictor Precautions Use with caution; epinephrine, norepinephrine and levonordefrin have been shown to have an increased pressor response in combination with TCAs

Effects on Dental Treatment
>10%: Xerostomia
Long-term treatment with TCAs such as amoxapine increases the risk of caries by reducing salivation and salivary buffer capacity.

Dosage Once symptoms are controlled, decrease gradually to lowest effective dose. Maintenance dose is usually given at bedtime to reduce daytime sedation. Oral:
Children: Not established in children <16 years of age
Adolescents: Initial: 25-50 mg/day; increase gradually to 100 mg/day; may give as divided doses or as a single dose at bedtime
Adults: Initial: 25 mg 2-3 times/day, if tolerated, dosage may be increased to 100 mg 2-3 times/day; may be given in a single bedtime dose when dosage <300 mg/day
Elderly: Initial: 25 mg at bedtime increased by 25 mg weekly for outpatients and every 3 days for inpatients if tolerated; usual dose: 50-150 mg/day, but doses up to 300 mg may be necessary
Maximum daily dose:
Inpatient: 600 mg
Outpatient: 400 mg

Mechanism of Action Reduces the reuptake of serotonin and norepinephrine. The metabolite, 7-OH-amoxapine has significant dopamine receptor blocking activity similar to haloperidol.

Other Adverse Effects
>10%:
Central nervous system: Drowsiness
Gastrointestinal: Xerostomia, constipation
1% to 10%:
Central nervous system: Dizziness, headache, confusion, nervousness, restlessness, insomnia, ataxia, excitement, anxiety
Dermatologic: Edema, skin rash
Endocrine: Elevated prolactin levels
Gastrointestinal: Nausea
Neuromuscular & skeletal: Tremor, weakness
Ocular: Blurred vision
Miscellaneous: Diaphoresis

Drug Interactions CYP1A2, 2C9, 2C19, 2D6, and 3A3/4 enzyme substrate
Increased Effect/Toxicity: Amoxapine increases the effects of amphetamines, anticholinergics, other CNS depressants (sedatives, hypnotics), chlorpropamide, tolazamide, and warfarin. When used with MAO inhibitors, hyperpyrexia, hypertension, tachycardia, confusion, seizures, and **deaths have been reported** (serotonin syndrome). The SSRIs (to varying degrees), cimetidine, indinavir, methylphenidate, ritonavir, quinidine, diltiazem, and verapamil inhibit the metabolism of TCAs and clinical toxicity may result. Use of lithium with a TCA may increase the risk for neurotoxicity. Phenothiazines may increase concentration of some TCAs and TCAs may increase the concentration of phenothiazines. Pressor response to I.V. epinephrine, norepinephrine, and phenylephrine may be enhanced in patients receiving TCAs (**Note:** Effect is unlikely with epinephrine or

(Continued)

Amoxapine *(Continued)*

levonordefrin dosages typically administered as infiltration in combination with local anesthetics). Combined use of beta-agonists or drugs which prolong QT_c (including quinidine, procainamide, disopyramide, cisapride, sparfloxacin, gatifloxacin, moxifloxacin) with TCAs may predispose patients to cardiac arrhythmias.

Decreased Effect: Carbamazepine, phenobarbital, and rifampin may increase the metabolism of amoxapine resulting in decreased effect of amoxapine. Amoxapine inhibits the antihypertensive effects of bethanidine, clonidine, debrisoquin, guanadrel, guanethidine, guanabenz, or guanfacine. Cholestyramine and colestipol may bind TCAs and reduce their absorption.

Drug Uptake

Onset of action: Therapeutic: Usually 1-2 weeks

Absorption: Oral: Rapid; well absorbed

Half-life, elimination: Parent drug: 11-16 hours; Active metabolite (8-hydroxy): Adults: 30 hours

Time to peak: 1-2 hours

Pregnancy Risk Factor C

Generic Available Yes

Selected Readings

Friedlander AH and Mahler ME, "Major Depressive Disorder. Psychopathology, Medical Management, and Dental Implications," *J Am Dent Assoc*, 2001, 132(5):629-38.

Ganzberg S, "Psychoactive Drugs," *ADA Guide to Dental Therapeutics*, 2nd ed, Chicago, IL: ADA Publishing, a Division of ADA Business Enterprises, Inc, 2000, 376-405.

Jastak JT and Yagiela JA, "Vasoconstrictors and Local Anesthesia: A Review and Rationale for Use," *J Am Dent Assoc*, 1983, 107(4):623-30.

Mitchell JR, "Guanethidine and Related Agents. III Antagonism by Drugs Which Inhibit the Norepinephrine Pump in Man," *J Clin Invest*, 1970, 49(8):1596-604.

Rundegren J, van Dijken J, Mörnstad H, et al, "Oral Conditions in Patients Receiving Long-Term Treatment With Cyclic Antidepressant Drugs," *Swed Dent J*, 1985, 9(2):55-64.

Yagiela JA, "Adverse Drug Interactions in Dental Practice: Interactions Associated With Vasoconstrictors. Part V of a Series," *J Am Dent Assoc*, 1999, 130(5):701-9.

Amoxicillin (a moks i SIL in)

Related Information

Animal and Human Bites Guidelines *on page 1416*

Antibiotic Prophylaxis, Preprocedural Guidelines for Dental Patients *on page 1344*

Cardiovascular Diseases *on page 1308*

Gastrointestinal Disorders *on page 1326*

Oral Bacterial Infections *on page 1367*

Periodontal Diseases *on page 1375*

U.S. Brand Names Amoxicot®; Amoxil®; Moxilin®; Trimox®; Wymox®

Canadian Brand Names Amoxil®; Apo®-Amoxi; Gen-Amoxicillin; Lin-Amox; Novamoxin®; Nu-Amoxi; Scheinpharm™ Amoxicillin

Mexican Brand Names Acimox; Aclimafel®; Acroxil®; Amoxifur; Amoxil®; Amoxinovag®; Amoxisol; Amoxivet; Ampliron®; Ardine®; Eumetinex®; Flemoxon; Gimalxina; Grunicina; Hidramox®; Moxlin®; Penamox®; Polymox®; Servamox®; Solciclina®; Xalyn-Or®

Pharmacologic Category Antibiotic, Penicillin

Synonyms Amoxicillin Trihydrate; Amoxycillin; *p*-Hydroxyampicillin

Use Treatment of otitis media, sinusitis, and infections caused by susceptible organisms involving the respiratory tract, skin, and urinary tract; prophylaxis of bacterial endocarditis in patients undergoing surgical or dental procedures; as part of a multidrug regimen for *H. pylori* eradication; treatment of oral-facial infections

Unlabeled/Investigational: Postexposure prophylaxis for anthrax exposure with documented susceptible organisms

Local Anesthetic/Vasoconstrictor Precautions No information available to require special precautions

Effects on Dental Treatment Prolonged use of penicillins may lead to development of oral candidiasis.

Dosage Oral:

Children: 20-50 mg/kg/day in divided doses every 8 hours

Acute otitis media due to highly-resistant strains of *S. pneumoniae*: Doses as high as 80-90 mg/kg/day divided every 12 hours have been used

Subacute bacterial endocarditis prophylaxis (standard regimen): 50 mg/kg 1 hour before dental procedure with no follow-up dose needed; total children's dose should not exceed adult dose.

Anthrax exposure (unlabeled use): **Note:** Postexposure prophylaxis only with documented susceptible organisms:

<40 kg: 15 mg/kg every 8 hours

≥40 kg: 500 mg every 8 hours

Adults: 250-500 mg every 8 hours or 500-875 mg twice daily; maximum dose: 2-3 g/day

Endocarditis prophylaxis (standard regimen): 2 g 1 hour before dental procedure with no follow-up dose.

Joint replacement prophylaxis: 2 g 1 hour before dental procedure with no follow-up dose.

Helicobacter pylori eradication: 1000 mg twice daily; requires combination therapy with at least one other antibiotic and an acid-suppressing agent (proton pump inhibitor or H_2 blocker)

Anthrax exposure (unlabeled use): **Note:** Postexposure prophylaxis only with documented susceptible organisms: 500 mg every 8 hours

Dosing interval in renal impairment:

Cl_{cr} 10-50 mL/minute: Administer every 12 hours

Cl_{cr} <10 mL/minute: Administer every 24 hours

Dialysis: Moderately dialyzable (20% to 50%) by hemo- or peritoneal dialysis; ~ 50 mg of amoxicillin per liter of filtrate is removed by continuous arteriovenous or venovenous hemofiltration; dose as per Cl_{cr} <10 mL/minute guidelines

Mechanism of Action Inhibits bacterial cell wall synthesis by binding to one or more of the penicillin binding proteins (PBPs); which in turn inhibits the final transpeptidation step of peptidoglycan synthesis in bacterial cell walls, thus inhibiting cell wall biosynthesis. Bacteria eventually lyse due to ongoing activity of cell wall autolytic enzymes (autolysins and murein hydrolases) while cell wall assembly is arrested.

Other Adverse Effects Frequency not defined:

Central nervous system: Hyperactivity, agitation, anxiety, insomnia, confusion, convulsions, behavioral changes, dizziness

Dermatologic: Erythematous maculopapular rashes, erythema multiforme, Stevens-Johnson syndrome, exfoliative dermatitis, toxic epidermal necrolysis, hypersensitivity vasculitis, urticaria

Gastrointestinal: Nausea, vomiting, diarrhea, hemorrhagic colitis, pseudomembranous colitis

Hematologic: Anemia, hemolytic anemia, thrombocytopenia, thrombocytopenia purpura, eosinophilia, leukopenia, agranulocytosis

Hepatic: Elevated AST (SGOT) and ALT (SGPT), cholestatic jaundice, hepatic cholestasis, acute cytolytic hepatitis

Contraindications Hypersensitivity to amoxicillin, penicillin, or any component of their formulation

Warnings/Precautions In patients with renal impairment, doses and/or frequency of administration should be modified in response to the degree of renal impairment; a high percentage of patients with infectious mononucleosis have developed rash during therapy with amoxicillin; a low incidence of cross-allergy with other beta-lactams and cephalosporins exists

Drug Interactions

Allopurinol theoretically has an additive potential for amoxicillin rash.

Aminoglycosides may be synergistic against selected organisms.

Oral contraceptive efficacy may be reduced.

Probenecid, disulfiram may increase levels of penicillins (amoxicillin).

Warfarin's effects may be increased.

Dietary/Ethanol/Herb Considerations Food: Administer with food, milk, or juice; does not interfere with absorption. Yogurt, boiled milk, or buttermilk may reduce diarrhea. Fruit, fluids, and fiber may reduce constipation.

Drug Uptake

Absorption: Oral: Rapid and nearly complete; food does not interfere

Half-life, elimination:

Neonates, full term: 3.7 hours

Infants and Children: 1-2 hours

Adults: Normal renal function: 0.7-1.4 hours

Cl_{cr} <10 mL/minute: 7-21 hours

Time to peak: Capsule: 2 hours; Suspension: 1 hour

Pregnancy Risk Factor B

Breast-feeding Considerations May be taken while breast-feeding

Dosage Forms CAP: 250 mg, 500 mg; (Amoxicot®, Amoxil®, Moxilin®, Trimox®): 250 mg, 500 mg; (Wymox®): 250 mg. **POWDER, oral suspension:** 125 mg/5 mL (5 mL, 80 mL, 100 mL, 150 mL), 250 mg/5 mL (5 mL, 80 mL, 100 mL, 150 mL); (Amoxicot®): 125 mg/5 mL (100 mL, 150 mL), 250 mg/5 mL (100 mL, 150 mL). **POWDER, oral suspension** [drops] (Amoxil®): 50 mg/mL (15 mL, 30 mL). **TAB, chewable:** 125 mg, 200 mg, 250 mg, 400 mg; (Amoxil®): 200 mg, 400 mg. **TAB, film coated** (Amoxil®): 500 mg, 875 mg

Generic Available Yes

Selected Readings

Dajani AS, Taubert KA, Wilson W, et al, "Prevention of Bacterial Endocarditis. Recommendations by the American Heart Association," *JAMA* 1997, 277(22):1794-801.

Dajani AS, Taubert KA, Wilson W, et al, "Prevention of Bacterial Endocarditis: Recommendations by the American Heart Association," *J Am Dent Assoc* 1997, 128(8):1142-51.

Wynn RL, Bergman SA, Meiller TF, et al, "Antibiotics in Treating Oral-Facial Infections of Odontogenic Origin: An Update", *Gen Dent*, 2001, 49(3):238-40, 242, 244 passim.

Amoxicillin and Clavulanate Potassium

(a moks i SIL in & klav yoo LAN ate poe TASS ee um)

Related Information

Animal and Human Bites Guidelines *on page 1416*

Oral Bacterial Infections *on page 1367*

U.S. Brand Names Augmentin®; Augmentin ES-600™

Canadian Brand Names Augmentin®; Clavulin®

Mexican Brand Names Amoxiclav®; Augmentin®; Clavulin®; Servamox Clv®

Pharmacologic Category Antibiotic, Penicillin

Synonyms Amoxicillin and Clavulanic Acid

Use

Dental: Treatment of orofacial infections when beta-lactamase-producing staphylococci and beta-lactamase-producing *Bacteroides* are present

Medical: Treatment of otitis media, sinusitis, and infections caused by susceptible organisms involving the lower respiratory tract, skin and skin structure, and urinary tract; spectrum same as amoxicillin with additional coverage of beta-lactamase producing *B. catarrhalis*, *H. influenzae*, *N. gonorrhoeae*, and *S. aureus* (not MRSA). The expanded coverage of this combination makes it a useful alternative when penicillinase-producing bacteria are present and patients cannot tolerate alternative treatments.

Local Anesthetic/Vasoconstrictor Precautions No information available to require special precautions

Effects on Dental Treatment Prolonged use of penicillins may lead to development of oral candidiasis.

Dosage Dose is based on the amoxicillin component (see table).

Infants <3 months: 30 mg/kg/day divided every 12 hours using the 125 mg/5 mL suspension

Children ≥3 months and <40 kg:

- Otitis media: 90 mg/kg/day divided every 12 hours for 10 days
- Lower respiratory tract infections, severe infections, sinusitis: 45 mg/kg/day divided every 12 hours **or** 40 mg/kg/day divided every 8 hours
- Less severe infections: 25 mg/kg/day divided every 12 hours or 20 mg/kg/day divided every 8 hours

Children >40 kg and Adults: 250-500 mg every 8 hours or 875 mg every 12 hours

Dosing interval in renal impairment:

- Cl_{cr} <30 mL/minute: Do not use 875 mg tablet
- Cl_{cr} 10-30 mL/minute: 250-500 mg every 12 hours
- Cl_{cr} <10 mL/minute: 250-500 every 24 hours

Hemodialysis: Moderately dialyzable (20% to 50%)

250-500 mg every 24 hours; administer dose during and after dialysis

Peritoneal dialysis: Moderately dialyzable (20% to 50%)

Amoxicillin: Administer 250 mg every 12 hours

Clavulanic acid: Dose for Cl_{cr} <10 mL/minute

Augmentin® Product-Specific Considerations

Strength	Form	Consideration
125 mg	CT, S	Dosing every 8 hours
	S	For adults having difficulty swallowing tablets, 125 mg/5 mL suspension may be substituted for 500 mg tablet.
200 mg	CT, S	Dosing every 12 hours
	CT	Contains phenylalanine
	S	For adults having difficulty swallowing tablets, 200 mg/5 mL suspension may be substituted for 875 mg tablet.
250 mg	CT, S, T	Dosing every 8 hours
	CT	Contains phenylalanine
	T	Not for use in patients <40 kg
	CT, T	Tablet and chewable tablet are not interchangeable due to differences in clavulanic acid.
	S	For adults having difficulty swallowing tablets, 250 mg/5 mL suspension may be substituted for 500 mg tablet.
400 mg	CT, S	Dosing every 12 hours
	CT	Contains phenylalanine
	S	For adults having difficulty swallowing tablets, 400 mg/5 mL suspension may be substituted for 875 mg tablet.
500 mg	T	Dosing every 8 hours or every 12 hours
600 mg	S	Dosing every 12 hours
		Contains phenylalanine
		Not for use in adults or children ≥40 kg
		600 mg/5 mL suspension is not equivalent to or interchangeable with 200 mg/5 mL or 400 mg/5 mL due to differences in clavulanic acid.
875 mg	T	Not for use in Cl_{cr}<30 mL/minute

Legend: CT = chewable tablet, S = suspension, T = tablet

Continuous arteriovenous or venovenous hemofiltration effects:
Amoxicillin: ~50 mg of amoxicillin/L of filtrate is removed
Clavulanic acid: Dose for Cl_{cr} <10 mL/minute
See table on previous page.

Mechanism of Action Clavulanic acid binds and inhibits beta-lactamases that inactivate amoxicillin resulting in amoxicillin having an expanded spectrum of activity. Amoxicillin inhibits bacterial cell wall synthesis by binding to one or more of the penicillin binding proteins (PBPs); which in turn inhibits the final transpeptidation step of peptidoglycan synthesis in bacterial cell walls, thus inhibiting cell wall biosynthesis. Bacteria eventually lyse due to ongoing activity of cell wall autolytic enzymes (autolysins and murein hydrolases) while cell wall assembly is arrested.

Other Adverse Effects

>10%: Gastrointestinal: Diarrhea (3% to 34% incidence varies upon dose and regimen used)

1% to 10%:
Dermatologic: Diaper rash, skin rash, urticaria
Gastrointestinal: Loose stools, nausea, vomiting
Genitourinary: Vaginitis
Miscellaneous: Moniliasis

Additional adverse reactions seen with **ampicillin-class antibiotics:** Agitation, agranulocytosis, ALT elevated, anaphylaxis, anemia, angioedema, anxiety, AST elevated, behavioral changes, black "hairy" tongue, confusion, convulsions, dizziness, enterocolitis, eosinophilia, erythema multiforme, exanthematous pustulosis, exfoliative dermatitis, gastritis, glossitis, hematuria, hemolytic anemia, hemorrhagic colitis, indigestion, insomnia, hyperactivity, interstitial nephritis, leukopenia, mucocutaneous candidiasis, pruritus, pseudomembranous colitis, serum sickness-like reaction, Stevens-Johnson syndrome, stomatitis, thrombocytopenia, thrombocytopenic purpura, tooth discoloration, toxic epidermal necrolysis

Contraindications Hypersensitivity to amoxicillin, clavulanic acid, penicillin, or any component of their formulation; concomitant use of disulfiram; history of cholestatic jaundice or hepatic dysfunction with amoxicillin/clavulanate potassium therapy

Warnings/Precautions Prolonged use may result in superinfection; in patients with renal impairment, doses and/or frequency of administration should be modified in response to the degree of renal impairment; high percentage of patients with infectious mononucleosis have developed rash during therapy; a low incidence of cross-allergy with cephalosporins exists; incidence of diarrhea is higher than with amoxicillin alone. Use caution in patients with hepatic dysfunction. Hepatic dysfunction, although rare, is more common in elderly and/or males, and occurs more frequently with prolonged treatment, and may occur after therapy is complete. Due to differing content of clavulanic acid, not all formulations are interchangeable. Some products contain phenylalanine.

Drug Interactions

Allopurinol: Additive potential for amoxicillin rash
Aminoglycosides may be synergistic against selected organisms.
Oral contraceptives: Pregnancy has been reported following concomitant use with antibiotics, however pharmacokinetic studies have not shown consistent effects on plasma concentrations of synthetic steroids. Use of a nonhormonal contraceptive product is recommended.
Probenecid may increase levels of penicillins (amoxicillin).
Warfarin's effects may be increased.

Dietary/Ethanol/Herb Considerations Food has no affect on amoxicillin absorption but increases clavulanic acid absorption. Administer with meals to increase absorption and reduce GI upset; may mix with milk, formula, or juice. All dosage forms contain potassium.

Drug Uptake Amoxicillin pharmacokinetics are not affected by clavulanic acid. See Amoxicillin *on page 86*

Pregnancy Risk Factor B

Breast-feeding Considerations

Amoxicillin: May be taken while breast-feeding
Clavulanic acid: No data reported

Dosage Forms POWDER, oral suspension: 125: Amoxicillin 125 mg and clavulanate potassium 31.25 mg per 5 mL (75 mL, 100 mL, 150 mL); 200: Amoxicillin 200 mg and clavulanate potassium 28.5 mg per 5 mL (50 mL, 75 mL, 100 mL); 250: Amoxicillin 250 mg and clavulanate potassium 62.5 mg per 5 mL (75 mL, 100 mL, 150 mL); 400: Amoxicillin 400 mg and clavulanate potassium 57 mg per 5 mL (50 mL, 75 mL, 100 mL); 600 (ES-600™): Amoxicillin 600 mg and clavulanic potassium 42.9 mg per 5 mL (50 mL, 75 mL, 100 mL, 150 mL). **TAB:** 250: Amoxicillin 250 mg and clavulanate potassium 125 mg; 500: Amoxicillin 500 mg and clavulanate potassium 125 mg; 875: Amoxicillin 875 mg and clavulanate potassium 125 mg. **TAB, chewable:** 125: Amoxicillin 125 mg and clavulanate potassium 31.25 mg; 200: Amoxicillin 200 mg and clavulanate potassium 28.5 mg; 250: Amoxicillin 250 mg and clavulanate potassium 62.5 mg; 400: Amoxicillin 400 mg and clavulanate potassium 57 mg

Generic Available No

(Continued)

Amoxicillin and Clavulanate Potassium *(Continued)*

Comments In maxillary sinus, anterior nasal cavity, and deep neck infections, beta-lactamase-producing staphylococci and beta-lactamase-producing *Bacteroides* usually are present. In these situations, antibiotics that resist the beta-lactamase enzyme are indicated. Amoxicillin and clavulanic acid is administered orally for moderate infections. Ampicillin sodium and sulbactam sodium (Unasyn®) is administered parenterally for more severe infections.

Selected Readings

Wynn RL and Bergman SA, "Antibiotics and Their Use in the Treatment of Orofacial Infections, Part I," *Gen Dent*, 1994, 42(5):398, 400, 402.

Wynn RL and Bergman SA, "Antibiotics and Their Use in the Treatment of Orofacial Infections, Part II," *Gen Dent*, 1994, 42(6):498-502.

Amoxicot® *see* Amoxicillin *on page 86*

Amoxil® *see* Amoxicillin *on page 86*

Amphocin® *see* Amphotericin B (Conventional) *on page 91*

Amphojel® [OTC] *see* Aluminum Hydroxide *on page 61*

Amphotec® *see* Amphotericin B Cholesteryl Sulfate Complex *on page 90*

Amphotericin B Cholesteryl Sulfate Complex

(am foe TER i sin bee kole LES te ril SUL fate KOM plecks)

U.S. Brand Names Amphotec®

Pharmacologic Category Antifungal Agent, Parenteral

Synonyms ABCD; Amphotericin B Colloidal Dispersion

Use Treatment of invasive aspergillosis in patients who have failed amphotericin B deoxycholate treatment, or who have renal impairment or experience unacceptable toxicity which precludes treatment with amphotericin B deoxycholate in effective does.

Local Anesthetic/Vasoconstrictor Precautions No information available to require special precautions

Effects on Dental Treatment No effects or complications reported

Dosage Children and Adults: I.V.:

Premedication: For patients who experience chills, fever, hypotension, nausea, or other nonanaphylactic infusion-related immediate reactions, premedicate with the following drugs, 30-60 minutes prior to drug administration: a nonsteroidal (eg, ibuprofen, choline magnesium trisalicylate, etc) with or without diphenhydramine; or acetaminophen with diphenhydramine; or hydrocortisone 50-100 mg. If the patient experiences rigors during the infusion, meperidine may be administered.

Range: 3-4 mg/kg/day (infusion of 1 mg/kg/hour); maximum: 7.5 mg/kg/day

Mechanism of Action Binds to ergosterol altering cll membrane permeability in susceptible fungi and causing leakage of cell components with subsequent cell death

Other Adverse Effects 1% to 10%:

Cardiovascular: Hypotension, tachycardia

Central nervous system: Headache, chills, fever

Dermatologic: Rash

Endocrine & metabolic: Hypokalemia, hypomagnesemia

Gastrointestinal: Nausea, diarrhea, abdominal pain

Hematologic: Thrombocytopenia

Hepatic: Abnormal LFTs

Neuromuscular & skeletal: Rigors

Renal: Elevated creatinine

Respiratory: Dyspnea

Note: Amphotericin B colloidal dispersion has an improved therapeutic index compared to conventional amphotericin B, and has been used safely in patients with amphotericin B-related nephrotoxicity; however, continued decline of renal function has occurred in some patients.

Warnings/Precautions Anaphylaxis has been reported; facilities for cardiopulmonary resuscitation should be available; infusion reactions, sometimes, severe, usually subside with continued therapy

Drug Interactions

Increased Effect/Toxicity: Toxic effect with other nephrotoxic drugs (eg, cyclosporine and aminoglycosides) may be additive. Corticosteroids may increase potassium depletion caused by amphotericin. Amphotericin B may predispose patients receiving digitalis glycosides or neuromuscular blocking agents to toxicity secondary to hypokalemia.

Decreased Effect: Pharmacologic antagonism may occur with azole antifungals (ketoconazole, miconazole, etc).

Drug Uptake Serum, half-life: 28-29 hours (increases with higher doses)

Pregnancy Risk Factor B

Generic Available No

Amphotericin B (Conventional)

(am foe TER i sin bee con VEN sha nal)

Related Information

Oral Fungal Infections *on page 1377*

U.S. Brand Names Amphocin®; Fungizone®

Canadian Brand Names Fungizone®

Pharmacologic Category Antifungal Agent, Parenteral; Antifungal Agent, Topical

Synonyms Amphotericin B Desoxycholate

Use Treatment of severe systemic and CNS infections caused by susceptible fungi such as *Candida* species, *Histoplasma capsulatum*, *Cryptococcus neoformans*, *Aspergillus* species, *Blastomyces dermatitidis*, *Torulopsis glabrata*, and *Coccidioides immitis*; fungal peritonitis; irrigant for bladder fungal infections; and topically for cutaneous and mucocutaneous candidal infections; used in fungal infection in patients with bone marrow transplantation, amebic meningoencephalitis, ocular aspergillosis (intraocular injection), candidal cystitis (bladder irrigation), chemoprophylaxis (low-dose I.V.), immunocompromised patients at risk of aspergillosis (intranasal/nebulized), refractory meningitis (intrathecal), coccidioidal arthritis (intra-articular/I.M.).

Low-dose amphotericin B 0.1-0.25 mg/kg/day has been administered after bone marrow transplantation to reduce the risk of invasive fungal disease. Alternative routes of administration and extemporaneous preparations have been used when standard antifungal therapy is not available (eg, inhalation, intraocular injection, subconjunctival application, intracavitary administration into various joints and the pleural space).

Local Anesthetic/Vasoconstrictor Precautions No information available to require special precautions

Effects on Dental Treatment No effects or complications reported

Dosage

I.V.:

- Children:
  - Test dose (not required): I.V.: 0.1 mg/kg/dose to a maximum of 1 mg; infuse over 30-60 minutes
  - Initial therapeutic dose: 0.25 mg/kg gradually increased, usually in 0.25 mg/kg increments on each subsequent day, until the desired daily dose is reached
  - Maintenance dose: 0.25-1 mg/kg/day given once daily; infuse over 2-6 hours. Once therapy has been established, amphotericin B can be administered on an every other day basis at 1-1.5 mg/kg/dose; cumulative dose: 1.5-2 g over 6-10 weeks
- Adults:
  - Test dose (not required).: 1 mg infused over 20-30 minutes
  - Initial dose: 0.25 mg/kg administered over 2-6 hours, gradually increased on subsequent days to the desired level by 0.25 mg/kg increments per day; in critically ill patients, may initiate with 1-1.5 mg/kg/day with close observation
  - Maintenance dose: 0.25-1 mg/kg/day or 1.5 mg/kg over 4-6 hours every other day; do not exceed 1.5 mg/kg/day; cumulative dose: 1-4 g over 4-10 weeks
  - Duration of therapy varies with nature of infection: Histoplasmosis, *Cryptococcus*, or blastomycosis may be treated with total dose of 2-4 g

I.T.:

- Children.: 25-100 mcg every 48-72 hours; increase to 500 mcg as tolerated
- Adults: 25-300 mcg every 48-72 hours; increase to 500 mcg to 1 mg as tolerated

Oral: 1 mL (100 mg) 4 times/day

Topical: Apply to affected areas 2-4 times/day for 1-4 weeks of therapy depending on nature and severity of infection

Mechanism of Action Binds to ergosterol altering cell membrane permeability in susceptible fungi and causing leakage of cell components with subsequent cell death

Other Adverse Effects

>10%:

- Cardiovascular: Hypotension, tachypnea
- Central nervous system: Fever, chills, headache (less frequent with I.T.), malaise, generalized pain
- Endocrine & metabolic: Hypokalemia, hypomagnesemia
- Gastrointestinal: Anorexia, nausea (less frequent with I.T.), vomiting (less frequent with I.T.), diarrhea, heartburn, cramping epigastric pain
- Hematologic: Normochromic-normocytic anemia
- Local: Pain at injection site with or without phlebitis or thrombophlebitis (incidence may increase with peripheral infusion of admixtures >0.1 mg/mL)
- Neuromuscular & skeletal: Generalized pain, including muscle and joint pains (less frequent with I.T.)
- Renal: Decreased renal function and renal function abnormalities including: azotemia, renal tubular acidosis, nephrocalcinosis

1% to 10%:

- Cardiovascular: Hypertension, hypotension, flushing

(Continued)

Amphotericin B (Conventional) *(Continued)*

Central nervous system: Delirium, arachnoiditis, pain along lumbar nerves (especially I.T. therapy)
Gastrointestinal: Nausea, vomiting
Genitourinary: Urinary retention
Hematologic: Leukocytosis
Local: Thrombophlebitis
Neuromuscular & skeletal: Paresthesia (especially with I.T. therapy)
Renal: Renal tubular acidosis, renal failure

Drug Interactions
Increased Effect/Toxicity: Use of amphotericin with other nephrotoxic drugs (eg, cyclosporine and aminoglycosides) may result in additive toxicity. Amphotericin may increase the toxicity of flucytosine. Antineoplastic agents may increase the risk of amphotericin-induced nephrotoxicity, bronchospasms, and hypotension. Corticosteroids may increase potassium depletion caused by amphotericin. Amphotericin B may predispose patients receiving digitalis glycosides or neuromuscular-blocking agents to toxicity secondary to hypokalemia.
Decreased Effect: Pharmacologic antagonism may occur with azole antifungal agents (ketoconazole, miconazole).

Drug Uptake
Half-life, elimination: Biphasic: Initial: 15-48 hours; Terminal: 15 days
Time to peak: ≤1 hour (4- to 6-hour dose)

Pregnancy Risk Factor B

Generic Available Yes: Powder for reconstitution

Amphotericin B Lipid Complex

(am foe TER i sin bee LIP id KOM pleks)

U.S. Brand Names Abelcet®

Canadian Brand Names Abelcet®

Pharmacologic Category Antifungal Agent, Parenteral

Synonyms ABLC

Use Treatment of aspergillosis or any type of progressive fungal infection in patients who are refractory to or intolerant of conventional amphotericin B therapy
Orphan drug: Cryptococcal meningitis

Local Anesthetic/Vasoconstrictor Precautions No information available to require special precautions

Effects on Dental Treatment No effects or complications reported

Dosage Children and Adults: I.V.:
Premedication: For patients who experience chills, fever, hypotension, nausea, or other nonanaphylactic infusion-related immediate reactions, premedicate with the following drugs, 30-60 minutes prior to drug administration: a nonsteroidal (eg, ibuprofen, choline magnesium trisalicylate, etc) with or without diphenhydramine; or acetaminophen with diphenhydramine; or hydrocortisone 50-100 mg. If the patient experiences rigors during the infusion, meperidine may be administered.
Range: 2.5-5 mg/kg/day as a single infusion
Hemodialysis/peritoneal dialysis: No supplemental dosage necessary
Continuous arteriovenous or venovenous hemofiltration: No supplemental dosage necessary

Mechanism of Action Binds to ergosterol altering cell membrane permeability in susceptible fungi and causing leakage of cell components with subsequent cell death

Other Adverse Effects Nephrotoxicity and infusion-related hyperpyrexia, rigor, and chilling are reduced relative to amphotericin deoxycholate.
>10%:
Central nervous system: Chills, fever
Renal: Increased serum creatinine
Miscellaneous: Multiple organ failure
1% to 10%:
Cardiovascular: Hypotension, cardiac arrest
Central nervous system: Headache, pain
Dermatologic: Rash
Endocrine & metabolic: Bilirubinemia, hypokalemia, acidosis
Gastrointestinal: Nausea, vomiting, diarrhea, gastrointestinal hemorrhage, abdominal pain
Renal: Renal failure
Respiratory: Respiratory failure, dyspnea, pneumonia

Warnings/Precautions Anaphylaxis has been reported with amphotericin B desoxycholate and other amphotericin B-containing drugs. Facilities for cardiopulmonary resuscitation should be available during administration due to the possibility of anaphylactic reaction. If severe respiratory distress occurs, the infusion should be immediately discontinued and the patient should not receive further infusions. During the initial dosing, the drug should be administered I.V. and under close clinical observation by medically trained personnel. Acute reactions (including fever and chills) may occur 1-2 hours after starting an I.V. infusion. These reactions are usually more common with the first few doses and generally diminish with subsequent doses.

Drug Interactions

Increased Effect/Toxicity: See Amphotericin B (Conventional) *on page 91*

Decreased Effect: Pharmacologic antagonism may occur with azole antifungal agents (ketoconazole, miconazole).

Drug Uptake Serum half-life: ~24 hours

Pregnancy Risk Factor B

Generic Available No

Amphotericin B, Liposomal (am foe TER i sin bee lye po SO mal)

U.S. Brand Names AmBisome®

Canadian Brand Names AmBisôme®

Pharmacologic Category Antifungal Agent, Parenteral

Synonyms L-AmB

Use Empirical therapy for presumed fungal infection in febrile, neutropenic patients. Treatment of patients with *Aspergillus* species, *Candida* species and/or *Cryptococcus* species infections refractory to amphotericin B desoxycholate, or in patients where renal impairment or unacceptable toxicity precludes the use of amphotericin B desoxycholate. Treatment of visceral leishmaniasis. In immunocompromised patients with visceral leishmaniasis treated with amphotericin B (liposomal), relapse rates were high following initial clearance of parasites. Treatment of cryptococcal meningitis in HIV-infected patients.

Local Anesthetic/Vasoconstrictor Precautions No information available to require special precautions

Effects on Dental Treatment No effects or complications reported

Dosage Children and Adults: I.V.:

Premedication: For patients who experience chills, fever, hypotension, nausea, or other nonanaphylactic infusion-related immediate reactions, premedicate with the following drugs, 30-60 minutes prior to drug administration: a nonsteroidal (eg, ibuprofen, choline magnesium trisalicylate, etc) with or without diphenhydramine; or acetaminophen with diphenhydramine; or hydrocortisone 50-100 mg. If the patient experiences rigors during the infusion, meperidine may be administered.

Empiric therapy: Recommended initial dose: 3 mg/kg/day

Systemic fungal infections (*Aspergillus, Candida, Cryptococcus*): Recommended initial dose of 3-5 mg/kg/day

Cryptococcal meningitis in HIV-infected patients: 6 mg/kg/day

Treatment of visceral leishmaniasis:

- Immunocompetent patients: 3 mg/kg/day on days 1-5, and 3 mg/kg/day on days 14 and 21; a repeat course may be given in patients who do not achieve parasitic clearance
- Immunocompromised patients: 4 mg/kg/day on days 1-5, and 4 mg/kg/day on days 10, 17, 24, 31, and 38

Mechanism of Action Binds to ergosterol altering cell membrane permeability in susceptible fungi and causing leakage of cell components with subsequent cell death

Other Adverse Effects Percentage is dependent upon population studied and may vary with respect to premedications and underlying illness.

>10%:

- Cardiovascular: Peripheral edema (15%), edema (12% to 14%), tachycardia (9% to 18%), hypotension (7% to 14%), hypertension (8% to 20%), chest pain (8% to 12%), hypervolemia (8% to 12%)
- Central nervous system: Chills (29% to 48%), insomnia (17% to 22%), headache (9% to 20%), anxiety (7% to 14%), pain (14%), confusion (9% to 13%)
- Dermatologic: Rash (5% to 25%), pruritus (11%)
- Endocrine & metabolic: Hypokalemia (31% to 51%), hypomagnesemia (15% to 50%), hyperglycemia (8% to 23%), hypocalcemia (5% to 18%), hyponatremia (8% to 12%)
- Gastrointestinal: Nausea (16% to 40%), vomiting (10% to 32%), diarrhea (11% to 30%), abdominal pain (7% to 20%), constipation (15%), anorexia (10% to 14%),
- Hematologic: Anemia (27% to 48%), blood transfusion reaction (9% to 18%), leukopenia (15% to 17%), thrombocytopenia (6% to 13%)
- Hepatic: Increased alkaline phosphatase (7% to 22%), increased BUN (7% to 21%), bilirubinemia (9% to 18%), increased ALT (15%), increased AST (13%), abnormal LFTs (not specified) (4% to 13%)
- Local: Phlebitis (9% to 11%)
- Neuromuscular & skeletal: Weakness (6% to 13%), back pain (12%)
- Renal: Increased creatinine (18% to 40%), hematuria (14%)
- Respiratory: Dyspnea (18% to 23%), lung disorder (14% to 18%), increased cough (2% to 18%), epistaxis (8% to 15%), pleural effusion (12%), rhinitis (11%)
- Miscellaneous: Sepsis (7% to 14%), infection (11% to 12%)

(Continued)

Amphotericin B, Liposomal *(Continued)*

2% to 10%:

Cardiovascular: Arrhythmia, atrial fibrillation, bradycardia, cardiac arrest, cardiomegaly, facial swelling, flushing, postural hypotension, valvular heart disease, vascular disorder

Central nervous system: Agitation, abnormal thinking, coma, convulsion, depression, dysesthesia, dizziness (7% to 8%), hallucinations, malaise, nervousness, somnolence

Dermatologic: Alopecia, bruising, cellulitis, dry skin, maculopapular rash, petechia, purpura, skin discoloration, skin disorder, skin ulcer, urticaria, vesiculobullous rash

Endocrine & metabolic: Acidosis, increased amylase, fluid overload, hypernatremia (4%), hyperchloremia, hyperkalemia, hypermagnesemia, hyperphosphatemia, hypophosphatemia, hypoproteinemia, increased lactate dehydrogenase, increased nonprotein nitrogen

Gastrointestinal: Constipation, xerostomia, dyspepsia, enlarged abdomen, eructation, fecal incontinence, flatulence, gastrointestinal hemorrhage (10%), hematemesis, hemorrhoids, gum/oral hemorrhage, ileus, mucositis, rectal disorder, stomatitis, ulcerative stomatitis

Genitourinary: Vaginal hemorrhage

Hematologic: Coagulation disorder, hemorrhage, decreased prothrombin, thrombocytopenia

Hepatic: Hepatocellular damage, hepatomegaly, veno-occlusive liver disease

Local: Injection site inflammation

Neuromuscular & skeletal: Arthralgia, bone pain, dystonia, myalgia, neck pain, paresthesia, rigors, tremor

Ocular: Conjunctivitis, dry eyes, eye hemorrhage

Renal: Abnormal renal function, acute kidney failure, dysuria, kidney failure, toxic nephropathy, urinary incontinence

Respiratory: Asthma, atelectasis, cough, dry nose, hemoptysis, hyperventilation, lung edema, pharyngitis, pneumonia, respiratory alkalosis, respiratory insufficiency, respiratory failure, sinusitis, hypoxia (6% to 8%)

Miscellaneous: Allergic reaction, cell-mediated immunological reaction, flu-like syndrome, graft versus host disease, herpes simplex, hiccup, procedural complication (8% to 10%), sweating (7%)

Contraindications Hypersensitivity to amphotericin B or any components of the formulation, unless, in the opinion of the treating physician, the benefit of therapy outweighs the risk

Warnings/Precautions Anaphylaxis has been reported with amphotericin B desoxycholate and other amphotericin B-containing drugs. Facilities for cardiopulmonary resuscitation should be available during administration due to the possibility of anaphylactic reaction. As with any amphotericin B-containing product the drug should be administered by medically trained personnel. During the initial dosing period, patients should be under close clinical observation. Amphotericin B, liposomal has been shown to be significantly less toxic than amphotericin B desoxycholate; however, adverse events may still occur. If severe respiratory distress occurs, the infusion should be immediately discontinued and the patient should not receive further infusions. Acute reactions (including fever and chills) may occur 1-2 hours after starting an I.V. infusion. These reactions are usually more common with the first few doses and generally diminish with subsequent doses.

Drug Interactions Increased Effect/Toxicity: Drug interactions have not been studied in a controlled manner; however, drugs that interact with conventional amphotericin B may also interact with amphotericin B liposome for injection. The following drug interactions have been described for conventional amphotericin B. See Drug Interactions - Increased Effect/Toxicity in Amphotericin B monograph.

Drug Uptake Serum, half-life: Terminal: 174 hours

Pregnancy Risk Factor B

Generic Available No

Comments Amphotericin B, liposomal is a true single bilayer liposomal drug delivery system. Liposomes are closed, spherical vesicles created by mixing specific proportions of amphophilic substances such as phospholipids and cholesterol so that they arrange themselves into multiple concentric bilayer membranes when hydrated in aqueous solutions. Single bilayer liposomes are then formed by microemulsification of multilamellar vesicles using a homogenizer. Amphotericin B, liposomal consists of these unilamellar bilayer liposomes with amphotericin B intercalated within the membrane. Due to the nature and quantity of amphophilic substances used, and the lipophilic moiety in the amphotericin B molecule, the drug is an integral part of the overall structure of the amphotericin B liposomes. Amphotericin B, liposomal contains true liposomes that are <100 nm in diameter.

Ampicillin (am pi SIL in)

Related Information

Antibiotic Prophylaxis, Preprocedural Guidelines for Dental Patients *on page 1344*

Cardiovascular Diseases *on page 1308*

Dental Drug Interactions: Update on Drug Combinations Requiring Special Considerations *on page 1434*

U.S. Brand Names Marcillin®; Principen®

Canadian Brand Names Apo®-Ampi; Novo-Ampicillin; Nu-Ampi

Mexican Brand Names Anglopen; Binotal; Dibacilina; Flamicina®; Lampicin; Marovilina®; Omnipen®; Pentrexyl; Sinaplin®

Pharmacologic Category Antibiotic, Penicillin

Synonyms Aminobenzylpenicillin; Ampicillin Sodium; Ampicillin Trihydrate

Use

Dental: Alternate antibiotic for the prevention of bacterial endocarditis in patients undergoing dental procedures; used in patients unable to take oral medications

Medical: Treatment of susceptible bacterial infections (nonbeta-lactamase-producing organisms); susceptible bacterial infections caused by streptococci, pneumococci, nonpenicillinase-producing staphylococci, *Listeria*, meningococci; some strains of *H. influenzae*, *Salmonella*, *Shigella*, *E. coli*, *Enterobacter*, and *Klebsiella*

Local Anesthetic/Vasoconstrictor Precautions No information available to require special precautions

Effects on Dental Treatment Prolonged use of penicillins may lead to development of oral candidiasis.

Dosage

Neonates: I.M., I.V.:

Postnatal age ≤7 days:

≤2000 g: Meningitis: 50 mg/kg/dose every 12 hours; other infections: 25 mg/kg/dose every 12 hours

>2000 g: Meningitis: 50 mg/kg/dose every 8 hours; other infections: 25 mg/kg/dose every 8 hours

Postnatal age >7 days:

<1200 g: Meningitis: 50 mg/kg/dose every 12 hours; other infections: 25 mg/kg/dose every 12 hours

1200-2000 g: Meningitis: 50 mg/kg/dose every 8 hours; other infections: 25 mg/kg/dose every 8 hours

>2000 g: Meningitis: 50 mg/kg/dose every 6 hours; other infections: 25 mg/kg/dose every 6 hours

Infants and Children: I.M., I.V.: 100-400 mg/kg/day in doses divided every 4-6 hours

Meningitis: 200 mg/kg/day in doses divided every 4-6 hours; maximum dose: 12 g/day

Children: Oral: 50-100 mg/kg/day in doses divided every 6 hours; maximum dose: 2-3 g/day

Adults:

Oral: 250-500 mg every 6 hours

I.M.: 500 mg to 1.5 g every 4-6 hours

I.V.: 500 mg to 3 g every 4-6 hours; maximum dose: 12 g/day

Sepsis/meningitis: 150-250 mg/kg/24 hours divided every 3-4 hours

Dosing interval in renal impairment:

Cl_{cr} 30-50 mL/minute: Administer every 6-8 hours

Cl_{cr} 10-30 mL/minute: Administer every 8-12 hours

Cl_{cr} <10 mL/minute: Administer every 12 hours

Hemodialysis: Moderately dialyzable (20% to 50%); administer dose after dialysis

Peritoneal dialysis: Moderately dialyzable (20% to 50%)

Administer 250 mg every 12 hours

Continuous arteriovenous or venovenous hemofiltration effects: Dose as for Cl_{cr} 10-50 mL/minute; ~50 mg of ampicillin per liter of filtrate is removed

Mechanism of Action Inhibits bacterial cell wall synthesis by binding to one or more of the penicillin binding proteins (PBPs); which in turn inhibits the final transpeptidation step of peptidoglycan synthesis in bacterial cell walls, thus inhibiting cell wall biosynthesis. Bacteria eventually lyse due to ongoing activity of cell wall autolytic enzymes (autolysins and murein hydrolases) while cell wall assembly is arrested.

Other Adverse Effects

>10%: Local: Pain at injection site

1% to 10%:

Dermatologic: Rash (appearance of a rash should be carefully evaluated to differentiate, if possible; nonallergic ampicillin rash from hypersensitivity reaction; incidence is higher in patients with viral infections, *Salmonella* infections, lymphocytic leukemia, or patients that have hyperuricemia)

Gastrointestinal: Diarrhea, vomiting, oral candidiasis, abdominal cramps

Miscellaneous: Allergic reaction (includes serum sickness, urticaria, angioedema, bronchospasm, hypotension, etc)

<1%: Penicillin encephalopathy, seizures (with large I.V. doses or patients with renal dysfunction), anemia, hemolytic anemia, thrombocytopenia, thrombocytopenic purpura, eosinophilia, leukopenia, granulocytopenia, decreased lymphocytes, interstitial nephritis (rare)

Contraindications Hypersensitivity to ampicillin, other penicillins, or any component of their formulation

(Continued)

Ampicillin *(Continued)*

Warnings/Precautions Dosage adjustment may be necessary in patients with renal impairment; a low incidence of cross-allergy with other beta-lactams exists; high percentage of patients with infectious mononucleosis have developed rash during therapy with ampicillin. Appearance of a rash should be carefully evaluated to differentiate a nonallergic ampicillin rash from a hypersensitivity reaction. Ampicillin rash occurs in 5% to 10% of children receiving ampicillin and is a generalized dull red, maculopapular rash, generally appearing 3-14 days after the start of therapy. It normally begins on the trunk and spreads over most of the body. It may be most intense at pressure areas, elbows, and knees.

Drug Interactions

Allopurinol theoretically has an additive potential for ampicillin/amoxicillin rash.
Aminoglycosides may be synergistic against selected organisms.
Oral contraceptive efficacy may be reduced.
Probenecid, disulfiram may increase levels of penicillins (ampicillin).
Warfarin's effects may be increased.

Dietary/Ethanol/Herb Considerations Food decreases absorption rate and may decrease serum concentration; administer on an empty stomach.

Drug Uptake

Absorption: Oral: 50%
Half-life, elimination: Adults and Children: 1-1.8 hours
Time to peak: Oral: ~1-2 hours

Pregnancy Risk Factor B

Breast-feeding Considerations Excreted into breast milk in small amounts like amoxicillin which is compatible with breast-feeding

Dosage Forms CAP: 250 mg, 500 mg; (Marcillin®): 500 mg; (Principen®): 250 mg, 500 mg. **INJ, powder for reconstitution:** 125 mg, 250 mg, 500 mg, 1 g, 2 g, 10 g. **POWDER, oral suspension** (Principen®): 125 mg/5 mL (100 mL, 200 mL); 250 mg/5 mL (100 mL, 200 mL)

Generic Available Yes

Selected Readings

Dajani AS, Taubert KA, Wilson W, et al, "Prevention of Bacterial Endocarditis. Recommendations by the American Heart Association," *JAMA* 1997, 277(22):1794-801.
Dajani AS, Taubert KA, Wilson W, et al, "Prevention of Bacterial Endocarditis: Recommendations by the American Heart Association," *J Am Dent Assoc* 1997, 128(8):1142-51.
Wynn RL, Bergman SA, Meiller TF, et al, "Antibiotics in Treating Oral-Facial Infections of Odontogenic Origin: An Update", *Gen Dent*, 2001, 49(3):238-40, 242, 244 passim.

Ampicillin and Sulbactam (am pi SIL in & SUL bak tam)

Related Information

Dental Drug Interactions: Update on Drug Combinations Requiring Special Considerations *on page 1434*

U.S. Brand Names Unasyn®

Canadian Brand Names Unasyn®

Mexican Brand Names Unasyna

Pharmacologic Category Antibiotic, Penicillin

Synonyms Sulbactam and Ampicillin

Use

Dental: Parenteral beta-lactamase-resistant antibiotic combination in treatment of more severe orofacial infections where beta-lactamase-producing staphylococci and beta-lactamase-producing *Bacteroides* are present

Medical: Treatment of susceptible bacterial infections involved with skin and skin structure, intra-abdominal infections, gynecological infections; spectrum is that of ampicillin plus organisms producing beta-lactamases such as *S. aureus*, *H. influenzae*, *E. coli*, *Klebsiella*, *Acinetobacter*, *Enterobacter*, and anaerobes

Local Anesthetic/Vasoconstrictor Precautions No information available to require special precautions

Effects on Dental Treatment Prolonged use of penicillins may lead to development of oral candidiasis. Some patients may experience hairy tongue.

Dosage Unasyn® (ampicillin/sulbactam) is a combination product. Each 3 g vial contains 2 g of ampicillin and 1 g of sulbactam. Sulbactam has very little antibacterial activity by itself, but effectively extends the spectrum of ampicillin to include beta-lactamase producing strains that are resistant to ampicillin alone. Therefore, dosage recommendations for Unasyn® are based on the ampicillin component.

I.M., I.V.:

Children: 100-200 mg ampicillin/kg/day divided every 6 hours; maximum dose: 8 g ampicillin/day

Adults: 1-2 g ampicillin every 6-8 hours; maximum dose: 8 g ampicillin/day

Mechanism of Action The addition of sulbactam, a beta-lactamase inhibitor, to ampicillin extends the spectrum of ampicillin to include some beta-lactamase producing organisms; inhibits bacterial cell wall synthesis by binding to one or more of the penicillin binding proteins (PBPs); which in turn inhibits the final transpeptidation step of peptidoglycan synthesis in bacterial cell walls, thus inhibiting cell wall biosynthesis. Bacteria eventually lyse due to ongoing activity of cell wall autolytic enzymes (autolysins and murein hydrolases) while cell wall assembly is arrested.

Other Adverse Effects

>10%: Local: Pain at injection site (I.M.)

1% to 10%:

Dermatologic: Rash

Gastrointestinal: Diarrhea

Local: Pain at injection site (I.V.)

Miscellaneous: Allergic reaction (may include serum sickness, urticaria, bronchospasm, hypotension, etc)

<1%: Chest pain, fatigue, malaise, headache, chills, penicillin encephalopathy, seizures (with large I.V. doses or patients with renal dysfunction), itching, nausea, vomiting, enterocolitis, pseudomembranous colitis, hairy tongue, dysuria, vaginitis, leukopenia, neutropenia, thrombocytopenia, decreased hemoglobin and hematocrit, increased liver enzymes, thrombophlebitis, increased BUN/creatinine, interstitial nephritis (rare)

Contraindications Hypersensitivity to ampicillin, sulbactam, penicillins, or any component of their formulation

Warnings/Precautions Dosage adjustment may be necessary in patients with renal impairment; a low incidence of cross-allergy with other beta-lactams exists; high percentage of patients with infectious mononucleosis have developed rash during therapy with ampicillin. Appearance of a rash should be carefully evaluated to differentiate a nonallergic ampicillin rash from a hypersensitivity reaction. Ampicillin rash occurs in 5% to 10% of children receiving ampicillin and is a generalized dull red, maculopapular rash, generally appearing 3-14 days after the start of therapy. It normally begins on the trunk and spreads over most of the body. It may be most intense at pressure areas, elbows, and knees.

Drug Interactions

Allopurinol theoretically has an additive potential for ampicillin/amoxicillin rash.

Aminoglycosides may be synergistic against selected organisms.

Oral contraceptive efficacy may be reduced.

Probenecid, disulfiram may increase levels of penicillins (ampicillin).

Warfarin's effects may be increased.

Drug Uptake

Absorption: Oral: 50%

Duration: Ampicillin: 6 hours

Half-life, elimination: Ampicillin: 1-1.8 hours; Sulbactam: 1-1.3 hours

Time to peak: Ampicillin: 1-2 hours

Pregnancy Risk Factor B

Breast-feeding Considerations

Ampicillin: Excreted into breast milk in small amounts like amoxicillin which is compatible with breast-feeding

Sulbactam sodium: No data reported

Dosage Forms INJ, powder for reconstitution: 1.5 g [ampicillin sodium 1 g and sulbactam sodium 0.5 g]; 3 g [ampicillin sodium 2 g and sulbactam sodium 1 g]; 15 g [ampicillin sodium 10 g and sulbactam sodium 5 g] [bulk package]

Generic Available No

Comments In maxillary sinus, anterior nasal cavity, and deep neck infections, beta-lactamase-producing staphylococci and beta-lactamase-producing *Bacteroides* usually are present. In these situations, antibiotics that resist the beta-lactamase enzyme should be administered. Amoxicillin and clavulanic acid is administered orally for moderate infections. Ampicillin sodium and sulbactam sodium (Unasyn®) is administered parenterally for more severe infections.

Selected Readings

Wynn RL and Bergman SA, "Antibiotics and Their Use in the Treatment of Orofacial Infections, Part I," *Gen Dent*, 1994, 42(5):398, 400, 402.

Wynn RL and Bergman SA, "Antibiotics and Their Use in the Treatment of Orofacial Infections, Part II," *Gen Dent*, 1994, 42(6):498-502.

Amprenavir (am PRE na veer)

Related Information

HIV Infection and AIDS *on page 1334*

U.S. Brand Names Agenerase®

Canadian Brand Names Agenerase®

Pharmacologic Category Antiretroviral Agent, Protease Inhibitor

Use Treatment of HIV infections in combination with at least two other antiretroviral agents

Note: Oral solution should be used only when capsules or other protease inhibitors are not therapeutic options.

Local Anesthetic/Vasoconstrictor Precautions No information available to require special precautions

Effects on Dental Treatment ≤10%: Perioral tingling/numbness, taste disorders

Dosage Oral: **Note:** Capsule and oral solution are **not** interchangeable on a mg-per-mg basis.

(Continued)

Amprenavir *(Continued)*

Capsule:

Children 4-12 years and older (<50 kg): 20 mg/kg twice daily or 15 mg/kg 3 times daily; maximum: 2400 mg/day

Children >13 years (>50 kg) and Adults: 1200 mg twice daily

Note: Dosage adjustments for amprenavir when administered in combination therapy:

Efavirenz: Adjustments necessary for both agents:

Amprenavir 1200 mg 3 times/day (single protease inhibitor) **or**

Amprenavir 1200 mg twice daily plus ritonavir 200 mg twice daily

Ritonavir: Adjustments necessary for both agents:

Amprenavir 1200 mg plus ritonavir 200 mg once daily **or**

Amprenavir 600 mg plus ritonavir 100 mg twice daily

Solution:

Children 4-12 years or older (up to 16 years weighing <50 kg): 22.5 mg/kg twice daily or 17 mg/kg 3 times daily; maximum: 2800 mg/day

Children 13-16 years (weighing at least 50 kg) or >16 years and Adults: 1400 mg twice daily

Dosage adjustment in renal impairment: Oral solution is contraindicated in renal failure.

Dosage adjustment in hepatic impairment:

Child-Pugh score between 5-8:

Capsule: 450 mg twice daily

Solution: 513 mg twice daily; contraindicated in hepatic failure

Child-Pugh score between 9-12:

Capsule: 300 mg twice daily

Solution: 342 mg twice daily; contraindicated in hepatic failure

Mechanism of Action Binds to the protease activity site and inhibits the activity of the enzyme. HIV protease is required for the cleavage of viral polyprotein precursors into individual functional proteins found in infectious HIV. Inhibition prevents cleavage of these polyproteins, resulting in the formation of immature, noninfectious viral particles.

Other Adverse Effects Protease inhibitors cause dyslipidemia which includes elevated cholesterol and triglycerides and a redistribution of body fat centrally to cause "protease paunch," buffalo hump, facial atrophy, and breast enlargement. These agents also cause hyperglycemia.

>10%:

Dermatologic: Rash (28%)

Endocrine & metabolic: Hyperglycemia (37% to 41%), hypertriglyceridemia (38% to 27%)

Gastrointestinal: Nausea (38% to 73%), vomiting (20% to 29%), diarrhea (33% to 56%)

Miscellaneous: Perioral tingling/numbness

1% to 10%:

Central nervous system: Depression (4% to 15%), headache, paresthesia, fatigue

Dermatologic: Stevens-Johnson syndrome (1% of total, 4% of patients who develop a rash)

Endocrine and metabolic: Hypercholesterolemia (4% to 9%)

Gastrointestinal: Taste disorders (1% to 10%)

Contraindications Hypersensitivity to amprenavir or any component of the formulation; concurrent therapy with rifampin, astemizole, bepridil, cisapride, dihydroergotamine, ergotamine, midazolam, and triazolam; severe previous allergic reaction to sulfonamides; oral solution in infants and children <4 years of age, pregnant women, renal or hepatic failure, and use of metronidazole or disulfiram

Warnings/Precautions Because of hepatic metabolism and effect on cytochrome P450 enzymes, amprenavir should be used with caution in combination with other agents metabolized by this system (see Contraindications and Drug Interactions). Use with caution in patients with diabetes mellitus, sulfonamide allergy, hepatic impairment, or hemophilia. Redistribution of fat may occur (eg, buffalo hump, peripheral wasting, cushingoid appearance). Additional vitamin E supplements should be avoided. Concurrent use of sildenafil should be avoided.

Certain ethnic populations (Asians, Eskimos, Native Americans) may be at increased risk of propylene glycol-associated adverse events, and the oral solution of amprenavir should be avoided.

Drug Interactions CYP3A3/4 enzyme substrate and inhibitor

Increased Effect/Toxicity: Concurrent use of cisapride, pimozide, quinidine, and rifampin is contraindicated. Serum concentrations/effect of many benzodiazepines may be increased; concurrent use of midazolam or triazolam is contraindicated. Concurrent use of ergot alkaloids (dihydroergotamine, ergotamine, ergonovine, methylergonovine) with amprenavir is also contraindicated (may cause vasospasm and peripheral ischemia).

Concurrent use of oral solution with disulfiram or metronidazole is contraindicated (risk of propylene glycol toxicity). Serum concentrations of amiodarone, lidocaine, quinidine and other antiarrhythmics may be increased, potentially leading to toxicity. HMG-CoA reductase inhibitors serum concentration may be increased by amprenavir, increasing the risk of myopathy/rhabdomyolysis; lovastatin and simvastatin are contraindicated; fluvastatin and pravastatin may be safer alternatives. Serum concentrations/effect of benzodiazepines, calcium channel blockers, cyclosporine, itraconazole, ketoconazole, rifabutin, tacrolimus, tricyclic antidepressants may be increased. May increase warfarin's effects, monitor INR.

Sildenafil serum concentration may be increased by amprenavir; when used concurrently, do not exceed a maximum sildenafil dose of 25 mg in a 48-hour period. Concurrent therapy with ritonavir may result in increased serum concentration: dosage adjustment is recommended. Clarithromycin, indinavir, nelfinavir may increase serum concentration of amprenavir.

Decreased Effect: Enzyme-inducing agents (rifampin, phenobarbital, phenytoin) may decrease serum concentration/effect of amprenavir; rifampin is contraindicated. The administration of didanosine (buffered formulation) should be separated from amprenavir by 1 hour to limit interaction between formulations. Serum concentrations of estrogen may be decreased, use alternative (nonhormonal) forms of contraception. Dexamethasone may decrease the therapeutic effect of amprenavir. Efavirenz and nevirapine may decrease serum concentration of amprenavir (dosing for combinations not established). Avoid St John's wort (may lead to subtherapeutic concentrations of amprenavir).

Drug Uptake

Absorption: 63%

Half-life, elimination: 7.1-10.6 hours

Time to peak: 1-2 hours

Pregnancy Risk Factor C

Generic Available No

Comments Propylene glycol is included in the oral solution; a dose of 22.5 mg/kg twice daily corresponds to an intake of 1650 mg/kg of propylene glycol.

Selected Readings Kaul DR, Cinti SK, Carver PL, et al, "HIV Protease Inhibitors: Advances in Therapy and Adverse Reactions, Including Metabolic Complications," *Pharmacotherapy*, 1999, 19(3):281-98.

Amvisc® *see* Sodium Hyaluronate *on page 1097*

Amvisc® Plus *see* Sodium Hyaluronate *on page 1097*

Amyl Nitrite (AM il NYE trite)

Pharmacologic Category Antidote; Vasodilator

Synonyms Isoamyl Nitrite

Use Coronary vasodilator in angina pectoris; adjunct in treatment of cyanide poisoning; used to produce changes in the intensity of heart murmurs

Local Anesthetic/Vasoconstrictor Precautions No information available to require special precautions

Effects on Dental Treatment No effects or complications reported

Dosage Nasal inhalation:

Cyanide poisoning: Children and Adults: Inhale the vapor from a 0.3 mL crushed ampul every minute for 15-30 seconds until I.V. sodium nitrite infusion is available

Angina: Adults: 1-6 inhalations from 1 crushed ampul; may repeat in 3-5 minutes

Other Adverse Effects 1% to 10%:

Cardiovascular: Postural hypotension, cutaneous flushing of head, neck, and clavicular area, tachycardia

Central nervous system: Headache, restlessness

Gastrointestinal: Nausea, vomiting

Drug Interactions Avoid concurrent use of sildenafil; severe reactions may result.

Drug Uptake

Onset of action: Angina: Within 30 seconds

Duration: 3-15 minutes

Pregnancy Risk Factor X

Generic Available Yes

Amytal® *see* Amobarbital *on page 83*

Anacin PM Aspirin Free [OTC] *see* Acetaminophen and Diphenhydramine *on page 30*

Anadrol® *see* Oxymetholone *on page 907*

Anafranil® *see* ClomiPRAMINE *on page 306*

Anagrelide (an AG gre lide)

U.S. Brand Names Agrylin®

Canadian Brand Names Agrylin®

Pharmacologic Category Phospholipase A_2 Inhibitor

Synonyms Anagrelide Hydrochloride

Use Treatment of thrombocythemia (ET), secondary to myeloproliferative disorders, to reduce the elevated platelet count and the risk of thrombosis, and to ameliorate associated symptoms (including thrombohemorrhagic events)

(Continued)

Anagrelide *(Continued)*

Local Anesthetic/Vasoconstrictor Precautions No information available to require special precautions

Effects on Dental Treatment No effects or complications reported

Dosage Adults: Oral: 0.5 mg 4 times/day or 1 mg twice daily; maintain for ≥1 week, then adjust to the lowest effective dose to reduce and maintain platelet count <600,000/µL ideally to the normal range; the dose must not be increased by >0.5 mg/day in any 1 week; maximum dose: 10 mg/day or 2.5 mg/dose

Mechanism of Action Appears to inhibit cyclic nucleotide phosphodiesterase and the release of arachidonic acid from phospholipase, possibly by inhibiting phospholipase A2; causes a dose-related reduction in platelet production, which results from decreased megakaryocyte hypermaturation; disrupts the postmitotic phase of maturation

Other Adverse Effects Frequency not defined:

- Cardiovascular: Palpitations (27%), chest pain (8%), tachycardia (7%), orthostatic hypotension, CHF, cardiomyopathy, myocardial infarction (rare), complete heart block, angina, and atrial fibrillation, hypertension, pericardial perfusion (rare)
- Central nervous system: Headache (44%), dizziness (15%), bad dreams, impaired concentration ability
- Hematologic: Anemia, thrombocytopenia, ecchymosis and lymphadenoma have been reported rarely
- Respiratory: Pleural effusion

Drug Interactions There is a single case report that suggests sucralfate may interfere with anagrelide absorption.

Drug Uptake

- Duration: 6-24 hours
- Half-life elimination, plasma: 1.3 hours
- Time to peak, serum: 1 hour

Pregnancy Risk Factor C

Generic Available No

Anakinra (an a KIN ra)

U.S. Brand Names Kineret™

Pharmacologic Category Antirheumatic, Disease Modifying; Interleukin-1 Receptor Antagonist

Synonyms IL-1Ra; Interleukin-1 Receptor antagonist

Use Reduction of signs and symptoms of moderately- to severely-active rheumatoid arthritis in adult patients who have failed one or more disease-modifying antirheumatic drugs (DMARDs); may be used alone or in combination with DMARDs (other than tumor necrosis factor-blocking agents)

Local Anesthetic/Vasoconstrictor Precautions No information available to require special precautions

Effects on Dental Treatment No effects or complications reported

Dosage

Adults: S.C.: Rheumatoid arthritis: 100 mg once daily (administer at ~ the same time each day)

Dosage adjustment in renal impairment: No specific guidelines for adjustment (clearance decreased by 70% to 75% in patients with Cl_{cr} <30 mL/minute)

Mechanism of Action Binds to the interleukin-1 (IL-1) receptor which is induced by inflammatory stimuli and mediates a variety of immunological responses, including degradation of cartilage (loss of proteoglycans) and stimulation of bone resorption

Other Adverse Effects

>10%

- Central nervous system: Headache (12%)
- Local: Injection site reaction (majority mild, typically lasting 14-28 days, characterized by erythema, ecchymosis, inflammation and pain; up to 71%)
- Miscellaneous: Infection (40% versus 35% in placebo; serious infections in 2% to 7%)

1% to 10%

- Gastrointestinal: Nausea (8%), diarrhea (7%), abdominal pain (5%)
- Hematologic: Decreased WBCs (8%)
- Respiratory: Sinusitis (7%)
- Miscellaneous: Flu-like symptoms (6%)

Drug Interactions Etanercept may increase risk of serious infection. Use caution with other drugs known to block or decrease the activity of TNF - tumor necrosis factor (eg, infliximab and thalidomide).

Drug Uptake

- Half-life, elimination: Terminal: 4-6 hours
- Time to peak: S.C.: 3-7 hours

Pregnancy Risk Factor B

Generic Available No

Ana-Kit® *see* Insect Sting Kit *on page 638*

Analpram-HC® *see* Pramoxine and Hydrocortisone *on page 984*

Anamine® [OTC] *see* Chlorpheniramine and Pseudoephedrine *on page 270*
Anaplex® [OTC] *see* Chlorpheniramine and Pseudoephedrine *on page 270*
Anaprox® *see* Naproxen *on page 848*
Anaspaz® *see* Hyoscyamine *on page 617*

Anastrozole (an AS troe zole)

U.S. Brand Names Arimidex®
Canadian Brand Names Arimidex®
Mexican Brand Names Arimidex®
Pharmacologic Category Antineoplastic Agent, Miscellaneous
Use Treatment of locally-advanced or metastatic breast cancer (ER-positive or hormone receptor unknown) in postmenopausal women; treatment of advanced breast cancer in postmenopausal women with disease progression following tamoxifen therapy. Patients with ER-negative disease and patients who did not respond to tamoxifen therapy rarely responded to anastrozole.
Local Anesthetic/Vasoconstrictor Precautions No information available to require special precautions
Effects on Dental Treatment No effects or complications reported
Mechanism of Action Potent and selective nonsteroidal aromatase inhibitor. It significantly lowers serum estradiol concentrations and has not detectable effect on formation of adrenal corticosteroids or aldosterone. In postmenopausal women, the principal source of circulating estrogen is conversion of adrenally generated androstenedione to estrone by aromatase in peripheral tissues.
Other Adverse Effects
>5%:
Central nervous system: Headache, dizziness, depression
Cardiovascular: Flushing, peripheral edema, chest pain
Dermatologic: Rash
Gastrointestinal: Little to mild nausea (10%), vomiting, diarrhea, abdominal pain, anorexia, xerostomia
Genitourinary: Pelvic pain
Neuromuscular & skeletal: Increased bone and tumor pain, muscle weakness, paresthesia
Respiratory: Dyspnea, cough, pharyngitis
2% to 5%:
Cardiovascular: Hypertension
Central nervous system: Somnolence, confusion, insomnia, anxiety, nervousness, fever, malaise, accidental injury
Dermatologic: Hair thinning, pruritus
Endocrine & metabolic: Breast pain
Gastrointestinal: Weight loss
Genitourinary: Urinary tract infection
Hematologic: Anemia, leukopenia
Local: Thrombophlebitis
Neuromuscular & skeletal: Myalgia, arthralgia, pathological fracture, neck pain
Respiratory: Sinusitis, bronchitis, rhinitis
Miscellaneous: Flu-like syndrome, infection
Drug Interactions CYP3A3/4 enzyme substrate; CYP1A2, 2C8, 2C9, and 3A3/4 enzyme inhibitor (only at high concentrations)
Increased Effect/Toxicity: At therapeutic concentrations, it is unlikely that coadministration of anastrozole with other drugs will result in clinically significant inhibition of cytochrome P450-mediated drug metabolism. Inhibitors of CYP3A4 may increase anastrozole concentrations.
Drug Uptake
Absorption: Well absorbed from GI tract; food does not affect absorption
Half-life, elimination: 50 hours
Pregnancy Risk Factor D
Generic Available No

Anatuss® DM [OTC] *see* Guaifenesin, Pseudoephedrine, and Dextromethorphan *on page 571*
Anbesol® [OTC] *see* Benzocaine *on page 151*
Anbesol® Baby [OTC] *see* Benzocaine *on page 151*
Anbesol® Maximum Strength [OTC] *see* Benzocaine *on page 151*
Ancef® *see* Cefazolin *on page 234*
Ancobon® *see* Flucytosine *on page 508*
Andehist DM NR Drops *see* Carbinoxamine, Pseudoephedrine, and Dextromethorphan *on page 221*
Andehist NR Drops *see* Carbinoxamine and Pseudoephedrine *on page 221*
Andehist NR Syrup *see* Brompheniramine and Pseudoephedrine *on page 180*
Androderm® *see* Testosterone *on page 1143*
AndroGel® *see* Testosterone *on page 1143*
Android® *see* MethylTESTOSTERone *on page 799*
Anergan® *see* Promethazine *on page 1006*

Anestacon® *see* Lidocaine *on page 706*
Anexsia® *see* Hydrocodone and Acetaminophen *on page 598*

Anisindione (an is in DY one)

U.S. Brand Names Miradon®

Pharmacologic Category Anticoagulant, Indanedione

Use Prophylaxis and treatment of venous thrombosis, pulmonary embolism, and thromboembolic disorders; atrial fibrillation with risk of embolism; adjunct in the prophylaxis of systemic embolism following myocardial infarction

Local Anesthetic/Vasoconstrictor Precautions No information available to require special precautions

Effects on Dental Treatment Signs of anisindione overdose may first appear as bleeding from gingival tissue; consultation with prescribing physician is advisable prior to surgery to determine temporary dose reduction or withdrawal of medication.

Dosage When discontinuing therapy, the manufacturer recommends tapering the dose over 3-4 weeks.

Oral: Adults:

Initial: 300 mg on first day, 200 mg on second day, 100 mg on third day

Maintenance: Established by daily PT/INR determinations; range: 25-250 mg/day

Mechanism of Action Interferes with hepatic synthesis of vitamin K-dependent coagulation factors (II, VII, IX, X).

Other Adverse Effects As with all anticoagulants, bleeding is the major adverse effect of warfarin. Hemorrhage may occur at virtually any site. Risk is dependent on multiple variables, including the intensity of anticoagulation and patient susceptibility. Additional adverse effects are often related to idiosyncratic reactions, and the frequency cannot be accurately estimated.

Cardiovascular: Vasculitis, edema, hemorrhagic shock
Central nervous system: Fever, headache,
Dermatologic: Rash, dermatitis, exfoliative dermatitis, urticaria, alopecia
Gastrointestinal: Nausea, diarrhea, gastrointestinal bleeding, steatorrhea
Genitourinary: Hematuria
Hematologic: Hemorrhage, leukopenia, unrecognized bleeding sites (eg, colon cancer) may be uncovered by anticoagulation, retroperitoneal hematoma, agranulocytosis (higher incidence vs warfarin), red cell aplasia, anemia, thrombocytopenia, eosinophilia
Hepatic: Hepatitis, jaundice
Ocular: Paralysis of accommodation
Renal: Renal tubular necrosis, albuminuria, anuria, urine discoloration (red-orange)
Respiratory: Hemoptysis, epistaxis, pulmonary hemorrhage, pharyngitis
Miscellaneous: Hypersensitivity/allergic reactions

Skin necrosis/gangrene, due to paradoxical local thrombosis, is a known but rare risk of oral anticoagulant therapy. Its onset is usually within the first few days of therapy and is frequently localized to the limbs, breast, or penis. The risk of this effect is increased in patients with protein C or S deficiency. Additional adverse reactions associated with warfarin, but likely to also occur with indanediones, include priapism and skin necrosis ("purple toes" syndrome or cutaneous gangrene).

Drug Interactions Potential drug interactions are generally inferred from documented interactions with warfarin. Since anisindione has not been specifically characterized, it is difficult to extrapolate CYP-mediated interactions to this agent, and interactions based on this mechanism are speculative. See Warfarin *on page 1250*

Drug Uptake

Onset of action: Anticoagulation: 36-72 hours

Peak effect: Full therapeutic effect: 5-7 days; INR may increase in 36-72 hours

Duration: 1-3 days

Pregnancy Risk Factor X

Generic Available No

Anodynos-DHC® *see* Hydrocodone and Acetaminophen *on page 598*
Ansaid® Oral *see* Flurbiprofen *on page 522*
Antabuse® *see* Disulfiram *on page 404*
Antagon® *see* Ganirelix *on page 548*
Anthra-Derm® *see* Anthralin *on page 102*

Anthralin (AN thra lin)

U.S. Brand Names Anthra-Derm®; Drithocreme®; Drithocreme® HP 1%; Dritho-Scalp®; Micanol®

Canadian Brand Names Anthraforte®; Anthranol®; Anthrascalp®; Micanol®

Mexican Brand Names Anthranol®

Pharmacologic Category Antipsoriatic Agent; Keratolytic Agent

Synonyms Dithranol

Use Treatment of psoriasis (quiescent or chronic psoriasis)

Local Anesthetic/Vasoconstrictor Precautions No information available to require special precautions

Effects on Dental Treatment No effects or complications reported

Dosage Adults: Topical: Generally, apply once a day or as directed. The irritant potential of anthralin is directly related to the strength being used and each patient's individual tolerance. Always commence treatment for at least 1 week using the lowest strength possible.

Skin application: Apply sparingly only to psoriatic lesions and rub gently and carefully into the skin until absorbed. Avoid applying an excessive quantity which may cause unnecessary soiling and staining of the clothing or bed linen.

Scalp application: Comb hair to remove scalar debris and, after suitably parting, rub cream well into the lesions, taking care to prevent the cream from spreading onto the forehead

Remove by washing or showering; optimal period of contact will vary according to the strength used and the patient's response to treatment. Continue treatment until the skin is entirely clear (ie, when there is nothing to feel with the fingers and the texture is normal)

Mechanism of Action Reduction of the mitotic rate and proliferation of epidermal cells in psoriasis by inhibiting synthesis of nucleic protein from inhibition of DNA synthesis to affected areas

Other Adverse Effects 1% to 10%: Dermatologic: Transient primary irritation of uninvolved skin; temporary discoloration of hair and fingernails, may stain skin, hair, or fabrics

Drug Interactions Long-term use of topical corticosteroids may destabilize psoriasis and withdrawal may also give rise to a "rebound" phenomenon. Allow an interval of at least 1 week between the discontinuance of topical corticosteroids and the commencement of therapy.

Pregnancy Risk Factor C

Generic Available No

Anthrax Vaccine Adsorbed (AN thraks vak SEEN ad SORBED)

U.S. Brand Names BioThrax™

Pharmacologic Category Vaccine

Synonyms AVA

Use Recommended for individuals who may come in contact with animal products which come from anthrax endemic areas and may be contaminated with *Bacillus anthracis* spores; recommended for high-risk persons such as veterinarians and other handling potentially infected animals. The Department of Defense is implementing an anthrax vaccination program against the biological warfare agent anthrax, which will be administered to all active duty and reserve personnel. Routine immunization for the general population is not recommended.

Unlabeled/Investigational: Postexposure prophylaxis in combination with antibiotics

Local Anesthetic/Vasoconstrictor Precautions No information available to require special precautions

Effects on Dental Treatment No effects or complications reported

Restrictions Not available commercially; presently, all anthrax vaccine lots are owned by the U.S. Department of Defense. The Centers for Disease Control (CDC) does not currently recommend routine vaccination of the general public.

Dosage S.C.:

Children <18 years: Safety and efficacy have not been established

Children ≥18 years and Adults:

Primary immunization: Three injections of 0.5 mL each given 2 weeks apart, followed by three additional injections given at 6-, 12-, and 18 months; it is not necessary to restart the series if a dose is not given on time; resume as soon as practical

Subsequent booster injections: 0.5 mL at 1-year intervals are recommended for immunity to be maintained

Patients receiving long-term corticosteroids or other immunosuppressants should be given an additional dose ≥1 month after discontinuation of immunosuppressant

Elderly: Safety and efficacy have not been established for patients >65 years of age

Mechanism of Action Active immunization against *Bacillus anthracis.* The vaccine is prepared from a cell-free filtrate of *B. anthracis*, but no dead or live bacteria.

Other Adverse Effects Includes pre- and post-licensure data; systemic reactions reported more often in women than in men

>10%:

Central nervous system: Malaise (4% to 11%)

Local: Tenderness (58% to 71%), erythema (12% to 43%), subcutaneous nodule (4% to 39%), induration (8% to 21%), warmth (11% to 19%), local pruritus (7% to 19%)

Neuromuscular & skeletal: Arm motion limitation (7% to 12%)

1% to 10%:

Central nervous system: Headache (4% to 7%), fever (<1% to 7%)

Gastrointestinal: Anorexia (4%), vomiting (4%), nausea (<1% to 4%)

(Continued)

Anthrax Vaccine Adsorbed *(Continued)*

Local: Mild local reactions (>5 cm) (edema/induration <30mm) (9%), with inflammation and pruritus, subcutaneous nodules (4%); all local reactions have been reversible

Neuromuscular & skeletal: Myalgia (4% to 7%)

Respiratory: Respiratory difficulty (4%)

Contraindications Hypersensitivity to anthrax vaccine or any component of the formulation; severe anaphylactic reaction to a previous dose of anthrax vaccine; history of anthrax

Warnings/Precautions Injection may be deferred in patients with any acute respiratory disease or other active infection. Persons receiving immunosuppressive agents may not have adequate response to immunization. If immunosuppressive therapy is short-term, immunization should be delayed. If immunosuppressive therapy is long-term, an extra dose of vaccine should be given a month or more after immunosuppressive therapy is discontinued.

Drug Uptake Duration: Unknown; may be 1-2 years following 2 inoculations, based on animal data

Pregnancy Risk Factor D

Generic Available No

Selected Readings "Anthrax Vaccine," *Med Lett Drugs Ther*, 1998, May 8;40(1026):52-3.

AntibiOtic® **Otic** *see* Neomycin, Polymyxin B, and Hydrocortisone *on page 857*

Antihemophilic Factor (Human)

(an tee hee moe FIL ik FAK tor HYU man)

U.S. Brand Names Alphanate®; Hemofil® M; Humate-P®; Koāte®-DVI; Monarc® M; Monoclate-P®

Canadian Brand Names Hemofil® M; Humate-P®

Pharmacologic Category Antihemophilic Agent; Blood Product Derivative

Synonyms AHF (Human); Factor VIII (Human)

Use Management of hemophilia A in patients whom a deficiency in factor VIII has been demonstrated

Humate-P®: Also indicated as treatment of spontaneous bleeding in patients with severe von Willebrand disease and in mild and moderate von Willebrand disease where desmopressin is known or suspected to be inadequate

Orphan drug: Alphanate®: Management of von Willebrand disease

Local Anesthetic/Vasoconstrictor Precautions No information available to require special precautions

Effects on Dental Treatment No effects or complications reported

Dosage Children and Adults: I.V.: Individualize dosage based on coagulation studies performed prior to treatment and at regular intervals during treatment; 1 AHF unit is the activity present in 1 mL of normal pooled human plasma; dosage should be adjusted to actual vial size currently stocked in the pharmacy. (General guidelines presented; consult individual product labeling for specific dosing recommendations.)

Dosage based on desired factor VIII increase (%):

To calculate dosage needed based on desired factor VIII increase (%):

Body weight (kg) X 0.5 int. units/kg X desired factor VIII increase (%) = int. units factor VIII required

For example:

50 kg X 0.5 int. units/kg X 30 (% increase) = 750 int. units factor VIII

Dosage based on expected factor VIII increase (%):

It is also possible to calculate the **expected** % factor VIII increase:

(# int. units administered X 2%/int. units/kg) divided by body weight (kg) = expected % factor VIII increase

For example:

(1400 int. units X 2%/int. units/kg) divided by 70 kg = 40%

General guidelines:

Minor Hemorrhage: Required peak postinfusion AHF level: 20% to 40% (10-20 int. units/kg), repeat dose every 12-24 hours for 1-3 days until bleeding is resolved or healing achieved; mild superficial or early hemorrhages may respond to a single dose

Moderate hemorrhage: Required peak postinfusion AHF level: 30% to 60% (15-30 int. units/kg): Infuse every 12-24 hours for ≥ 3 days until pain and disability are resolved

Alternatively, a loading dose to achieve 50% (25 int. units/kg) may be given, followed by 10-15 int. units/kg dose given every 8-12 hours; may be needed for >7 days

Severe/life-threatening hemorrhage: Required peak postinfusion AHF level: 60% to 100% (30-50 int. units/kg): Infuse every 8-24 hours until threat is resolved

Alternatively, a loading dose to achieve 80% to 100% (40-50 int. units/kg) may be given, followed by 20-25 int. units/kg dose given every 8-12 hours for ≥14 days

Minor surgery: Required peak postinfusion AHF level: 30% to 80% (15-40 int. units/kg): Highly dependent upon procedure and specific product recommendations; for some procedures, may be administered as a single infusion plus oral antifibrinolytic therapy within 1 hour; in other procedures, may repeat dose every 12-24 hours as needed

Major surgery: Required peak pre- and postsurgery AHF level: 80% to 100% (40-50 int. units/kg): Administer every 6-24 hours until healing is complete (10-14 days)

Prophylaxis: May also be given on a regular schedule to prevent bleeding

If bleeding is not controlled with adequate dose, test for presence of inhibitor. It may not be possible or practical to control bleeding if inhibitor titers >10 Bethesda units/mL; antihemophilic factor (porcine) may be considered as an alternative

von Willebrand disease:

Treatment of hemorrhage in von Willebrand disease (Humate-P®): 1 int. units of factor VIII per kg of body weight would be expected to raise circulating vWR:RCof ~ 3.5-4 int. units/dL

Type 1, mild (if desmopressin is not appropriate): Major hemorrhage:
- Loading dose: 40-60 int. units/kg
- Maintenance dose: 40-50 int. units/kg every 8-12 hours for 3 days, keeping vWF:RCof nadir >50%; follow with 40-50 int. units/kg daily for up to 7 days

Type 1, moderate or severe:
- Minor hemorrhage: 40-50 int. units/kg for 1-2 doses
- Major hemorrhage:
  - Loading dose: 50-75 int. units/kg
  - Maintenance dose: 40-60 int. units/kg daily for up to 7 days

Types 2 and 3:
- Minor hemorrhage: 40-50 int. units/kg for 1-2 doses
- Major hemorrhage:
  - Loading dose: 60-80 int. units/kg
  - Maintenance dose: 40-60 int. units/kg every 8-12 hours for 3 days, keeping vWF:RCof nadir >50%; follow with 40-60 int. units/kg daily for up to 7 days

Elderly: Response in the elderly is not expected to differ from that of younger patients; dosage should be individualized

Mechanism of Action Protein (factor VIII) in normal plasma which is necessary for clot formation and maintenance of hemostasis; activates factor X in conjunction with activated factor IX; activated factor X converts prothrombin to thrombin, which converts fibrinogen to fibrin and with factor XIII forms a stable clot

Drug Uptake Half-life, elimination: Mean $t_{1/2}$: 12-17 hours in patients with hemophilia A; consult specific product labeling

Pregnancy Risk Factor C

Generic Available Yes

Antihemophilic Factor (Porcine)

(an tee hee moe FIL ik FAK ter POR seen)

U.S. Brand Names Hyate:C®

Pharmacologic Category Antihemophilic Agent

Synonyms AHF (Porcine); Factor VIII (Porcine)

Use Management of hemophilia A in patients with antibodies to human factor VIII (consider use of human factor VIII in patients with antibody titer of <5 Bethesda units/mL); management of previously nonhemophilic patients with spontaneously-acquired inhibitors to human factor VIII, regardless of initial antihuman inhibitor titer

Local Anesthetic/Vasoconstrictor Precautions No information available to require special precautions

Effects on Dental Treatment No effects or complications reported

Dosage Clinical response should be used to assess efficacy.

Initial dose:

Antibody level to human factor VIII <50 Bethesda units/mL: 100-150 porcine units/kg (body weight) is recommended

Antibody level to human factor VIII >50 Bethesda units/mL: Activity of the antibody to antihemophilic (porcine) should be determined; **an antiporcine antibody level** >20 Bethesda units/mL indicates that the patient is unlikely to benefit from treatment; for lower titers, a dose of 100-150 porcine units/kg is recommended

The initial dose may also be calculated using the following method:

1. Determine patient's antibody titer against porcine factor VIII
2. Calculate average plasma volume:
   (Body weight kg)(average blood volume)(1 - hematocrit) = Plasma volume
   (Body weight kg)(80 mL/kg)(1 - hematocrit) = Plasma volume
   Note: A hematocrit of 50% = 0.5 for the equation
3. Neutralizing dose:
   (Plasma volume mL)(antibody titer Bethesda units/mL) = Neutralizing Dose Units

(Continued)

Antihemophilic Factor (Porcine) *(Continued)*

This is the predicted dose required to neutralize the circulating antibodies. An incremental dose must be added to the neutralizing dose in order to increase the plasma factor VIII to the desired level.

4. Incremental dose:
   (Desired plasma factor VIII level)(Body weight) divided by 1.5 = Incremental Dose Units
5. Total Dose: Neutralizing dose + Incremental Dose = Total Dose Units

If a patient has previously been treated with Hyate:C®, this may provide a guide to his likely response and, therefore, assist in estimation of the preliminary dose

Subsequent doses: Following administration of the initial dose, if the recovery of factor VIII in the patient's plasma is not sufficient, another larger dose should be administered; if recovery after the second dose is still insufficient, a third and larger dose may prove effective. Once appropriate factor VIII levels are achieved, dosing can be repeated every 6-8 hours.

Mechanism of Action Factor VIII is the coagulation portion of the factor VIII complex in plasma. Factor VIII acts as a cofactor for factor IX to activate factor X in the intrinsic pathway of blood coagulation.

Other Adverse Effects Reactions tend to lessen in frequency and severity as further infusions are given; hydrocortisone and/or antihistamines may help to prevent or alleviate side effects and may be prescribed as precautionary measures.

1% to 10%:

Central nervous system: Fever, headache, chills
Dermatologic: Rashes
Gastrointestinal: Nausea, vomiting

Drug Uptake Half-life, elimination: 10-11 hours (patients without detectable inhibitors)

Pregnancy Risk Factor C

Generic Available No

Antihemophilic Factor (Recombinant)

(an tee hee moe FIL ik FAK tor ree KOM be nant)

U.S. Brand Names Helixate® FS; Kogenate® FS; Recombinate™; ReFacto®

Canadian Brand Names Kogenate®; Recombinate™

Pharmacologic Category Antihemophilic Agent

Synonyms AHF (Recombinant); Factor VIII (Recombinant); rAHF

Use Management of hemophilia A for patients in whom a deficiency in factor VIII has been demonstrated; can be of significant therapeutic value in patients with acquired factor VIII inhibitors not exceeding 10 Bethesda units/mL

Orphan drug:

Kogenate®: Prophylaxis and treatment of bleeding with hemophilia A; prophylaxis for hemophilia A surgery

ReFacto®: Control and prevention of hemorrhagic episodes; surgical prophylaxis for hemophilia A (congenital factor VIII deficiency or classic hemophilia)

Local Anesthetic/Vasoconstrictor Precautions No information available to require special precautions

Effects on Dental Treatment No effects or complications reported

Dosage I.V.: Individualize dosage based on coagulation studies performed prior to and during treatment at regular intervals. One AHF unit is the activity present in 1 mL of normal pooled human plasma; dosage should be adjusted to actual vial size currently stocked in the pharmacy.

Hospitalized patients: 20-50 units/kg/dose; may be higher for special circumstances; dose can be given every 12-24 hours and more frequently in special circumstances

Formula to approximate percentage increase in plasma antihemophilic factor:

Units required = desired level increase (desired level - actual level) x plasma volume (mL)

Total blood volume (mL blood/kg) = 70 mL/kg (adults); 80 mL/kg (children).

Plasma volume = total blood volume (mL) x [1 - Hct (in decimals)]

ie, for a 70 kg adult with a Hct = 40% : plasma volume = [70 kg x 70 mL/kg] x [1 - 0.4] = 2940 mL

To calculate number of units of factor VIII needed to increase level to desired range (highly individualized and dependent on patient's condition):

Number of units = desired level increase [desired level - actual level] x plasma volume (in mL)

ie, for a 100% level in the above patient who has an actual level of 20% the number of units needed = [1 (for a 100% level) - 0.2] x 2940 mL = 2352 units

Mechanism of Action Protein (factor VIII) in normal plasma which is necessary for clot formation and maintenance of hemostasis; activates factor X in conjunction with activated factor IX; activated factor X converts prothrombin to thrombin, which converts fibrinogen to fibrin, and with factor XIII forms a stable clot

Drug Uptake Half-life, elimination: Mean $t^1/_2$: 14-16 hours

Pregnancy Risk Factor C

Generic Available No

Antihist-1® [OTC] *see* Clemastine *on page 299*

Anti-inhibitor Coagulant Complex

(an tee-in HI bi tor coe AG yoo lant KOM pleks)

U.S. Brand Names Autoplex® T; Feiba VH Immuno®

Canadian Brand Names Feiba® VH Immuno

Pharmacologic Category Antihemophilic Agent; Blood Product Derivative

Synonyms Coagulant Complex Inhibitor

Use Patients with factor VIII inhibitors who are to undergo surgery or those who are bleeding

Local Anesthetic/Vasoconstrictor Precautions No information available to require special precautions

Effects on Dental Treatment No effects or complications reported

Dosage Dosage range: 25-100 factor VIII correctional units per kg depending on the severity of hemorrhage

Pregnancy Risk Factor C

Generic Available No

Antilirium® *see* Physostigmine *on page 953*

Antiminth® [OTC] *see* Pyrantel Pamoate *on page 1025*

Antipyrine and Benzocaine (an tee PYE reen & BEN zoe kane)

U.S. Brand Names Allergen®; Auralgan®; Auroto®

Canadian Brand Names Auralgan®

Pharmacologic Category Otic Agent, Analgesic; Otic Agent, Cerumenolytic

Synonyms Benzocaine and Antipyrine

Use Temporary relief of pain and reduction of swelling associated with acute congestive and serous otitis media, swimmer's ear, otitis externa; facilitates ear wax removal

Local Anesthetic/Vasoconstrictor Precautions Information available to require special precautions

Effects on Dental Treatment No effects or complications reported

Dosage Otic: Fill ear canal; moisten cotton pledget, place in external ear, repeat every 1-2 hours until pain and congestion is relieved; for ear wax removal instill drops 3-4 times/day for 2-3 days

Pregnancy Risk Factor C

Generic Available Yes

Antispas® *see* Dicyclomine *on page 382*

Antithrombin III (an tee THROM bin three)

U.S. Brand Names Thrombate III™

Canadian Brand Names Thrombate III®

Pharmacologic Category Anticoagulant; Blood Product Derivative

Synonyms AT III; Heparin Cofactor I

Use Agent for hereditary antithrombin III deficiency; has been used effectively for acquired antithrombin III deficiencies related to disseminated intravascular coagulation (DIC); may be useful during acute management of hepatic veno-occlusive disease

Orphan drug:

ATnativ®: Treatment of hereditary antithrombin III deficiency in connection with surgical or obstetrical procedures; treatment of thromboembolism

Thrombate III™: Replacement therapy in congenital deficiency of antithrombin III for prevention and treatment of thrombosis and pulmonary emboli

Local Anesthetic/Vasoconstrictor Precautions No information available to require special precautions

Effects on Dental Treatment No effects or complications reported

Dosage After first dose of antithrombin III, level should increase to 120% of normal; thereafter maintain at levels >80%. Generally, achieved by administration of maintenance doses once every 24 hours; initially and until patient is stabilized, measure antithrombin III level at least twice daily, thereafter once daily and always immediately before next infusion. 1 unit = quantity of antithrombin III in 1 mL of normal pooled human plasma; administration of 1 unit/1 kg raises AT-III level by 1% to 2%; assume plasma volume of 40 mL/kg

Initial dosage (units) = [desired AT-III level % - baseline AT-III level %] x body weight (kg) divided by 1%/units/kg, eg, if a 70 kg adult patient had a baseline AT-III level of 57%, the initial dose would be (120% - 57%) x 70/1%/units/kg = 4,410 units

Measure antithrombin III preceding and 30 minutes after dose to calculate *in vivo* recovery rate; maintain level within normal range for 2-8 days depending on type of surgery or procedure

(Continued)

Antithrombin III *(Continued)*

Mechanism of Action The primary physiologic inhibitor of *in vivo* coagulation; it is an alpha$_2$-globulin. Its principal actions are the inactivation of thrombin, plasmin, and other active serine proteases of coagulation, including factors IXa, Xa, XIa, XIIa, and VIIa. The inactivation of proteases is a major step in the normal clotting process. The strong activation of clotting enzymes at the site of every bleeding injury facilitates fibrin formation and maintains normal hemostasis. Thrombosis in the circulation would be caused by active serine proteases if they were not inhibited by antithrombin III after the localized clotting process. Patients with congenital deficiency are in a prethrombotic state, even if asymptomatic, as evidenced by elevated plasma concentrations of prothrombin activation fragment, which are normalized following infusions of antithrombin III concentrate.

Other Adverse Effects 1% to 10%: Central nervous system: Dizziness (2%)

Drug Interactions Increased Effect/Toxicity: Heparin's anticoagulant effects are potentiated by antithrombin III. Risk of hemorrhage with antithrombin III may be increased by thrombolytic agents, oral anticoagulants (warfarin), and drugs which affect platelet function (eg, aspirin, NSAIDs, dipyridamole, ticlopidine, clopidogrel, and IIb/IIIa antagonists).

Pregnancy Risk Factor C

Generic Available No

Anti-Tuss® Expectorant [OTC] *see* Guaifenesin *on page 568*

Antivert® *see* Meclizine *on page 750*

Antizol® *see* Fomepizole *on page 533*

Antrizine® *see* Meclizine *on page 750*

Anturane® *see* Sulfinpyrazone *on page 1123*

Anucort-HC® Suppository *see* Hydrocortisone *on page 608*

Anusol® [OTC] *see* Pramoxine *on page 984*

Anusol® HC 1 [OTC] *see* Hydrocortisone *on page 608*

Anusol® HC 2.5% [OTC] *see* Hydrocortisone *on page 608*

Anusol-HC® Suppository *see* Hydrocortisone *on page 608*

ANX® *see* HydrOXYzine *on page 616*

Anzemet® *see* Dolasetron *on page 409*

Apatate® [OTC] *see* Vitamin B Complex *on page 1244*

Aphedrid™ [OTC] *see* Triprolidine and Pseudoephedrine *on page 1213*

Aphrodyne® *see* Yohimbine *on page 1253*

Aphthasol™ *see* Amlexanox *on page 80*

Aplisol® *see* Tuberculin Purified Protein Derivative *on page 1218*

Apraclonidine (a pra KLOE ni deen)

U.S. Brand Names Iopidine®

Canadian Brand Names Iopidine®

Pharmacologic Category Alpha$_2$ Agonist, Ophthalmic

Synonyms Aplonidine; Apraclonidine Hydrochloride; p-Aminoclonidine

Use Prevention and treatment of postsurgical intraocular pressure elevation

Local Anesthetic/Vasoconstrictor Precautions No information available to require special precautions

Effects on Dental Treatment No effects or complications reported

Dosage Adults: Ophthalmic:

0.5%: Instill 1-2 drops in the affected eye(s) 3 times/day; since apraclonidine 0.5% will be used with other ocular glaucoma therapies, use an approximate 5-minute interval between instillation of each medication to prevent washout of the previous dose

1%: Instill 1 drop in operative eye 1 hour prior to anterior segment laser surgery, second drop in eye immediately upon completion of procedure

Dosing adjustment in renal impairment: Although the topical use of apraclonidine has not been studied in renal failure patients, structurally related clonidine undergoes a significant increase in half-life in patients with severe renal impairment; close monitoring of cardiovascular parameters in patients with impaired renal function is advised if they are candidates for topical apraclonidine therapy

Dosing adjustment in hepatic impairment: Close monitoring of cardiovascular parameters in patients with impaired liver function is advised because the systemic dosage form of clonidine is partially metabolized in the liver

Mechanism of Action A potent alpha-adrenergic agent similar to clonidine; relatively selective for alpha$_2$-receptors but does retain some binding to alpha$_1$-receptors; appears to result in reduction of aqueous humor formation; its penetration through the blood-brain barrier is more polar than clonidine which reduces its penetration through the blood-brain barrier and suggests that its pharmacological profile is characterized by peripheral rather than central effects.

Other Adverse Effects

1% to 10%:

Cardiovascular: Arrhythmia, chest pain, facial edema, peripheral edema

Central nervous system: Depression, dizziness, headache, insomnia, lethargy, malaise, nervousness, somnolence
Dermatologic: Contact dermatitis, dermatitis
Gastrointestinal: Constipation, xerostomia, nausea, taste perversion
Neuromuscular & skeletal: Abnormal coordination, myalgia, paresthesia, weakness
Ocular: Upper lid elevation, conjunctival blanching, mydriasis, burning and itching eyes, discomfort, conjunctival microhemorrhage, blurred vision
Respiratory: Asthma, dry nose, parosmia, pharyngitis, rhinitis

Drug Interactions Topical beta-blockers or pilocarpine may have an additive effect on intraocular pressure.

Drug Uptake
Onset of action: 1 hour; Peak effect: Intraocular pressure: 3-5 hours

Pregnancy Risk Factor C

Generic Available No

Apresoline® *see* HydrALAZINE *on page 593*
Apri® *see* Combination Hormonal Contraceptives *on page 323*
Aprodine® [OTC] *see* Triprolidine and Pseudoephedrine *on page 1213*
Aprodine® w/C *see* Triprolidine, Pseudoephedrine, and Codeine *on page 1214*

Aprotinin (a proe TYE nin)

U.S. Brand Names Trasylol®

Canadian Brand Names Trasylol®

Mexican Brand Names Trasylol®

Pharmacologic Category Blood Product Derivative; Hemostatic Agent

Use Reduction or prevention of blood loss in patients undergoing coronary artery bypass surgery when a high index of suspicion of excessive bleeding potential exists; this includes open heart reoperation, pre-existing coagulopathy, operations on the great vessels, and patients whose religious beliefs prohibit blood transfusions

Local Anesthetic/Vasoconstrictor Precautions No information available to require special precautions

Effects on Dental Treatment No effects or complications reported

Dosage
Test dose: **All** patients should receive a 1 mL I.V. test dose at least 10 minutes prior to the loading dose to assess the potential for allergic reactions. **Note:** To avoid physical incompatibility with heparin when adding to pump-prime solution, each agent should be added during recirculation to assure adequate dilution.
Regimen A (standard dose):
2 million units (280 mg) loading dose I.V. over 20-30 minutes
2 million units (280 mg) into pump prime volume
500,000 units/hour (70 mg/hour) I.V. during operation
Regimen B (low dose):
1 million units (140 mg) loading dose I.V. over 20-30 minutes
1 million units (140 mg) into pump prime volume
250,000 units/hour (35 mg/hour) I.V. during operation

Mechanism of Action Serine protease inhibitor; inhibits plasmin, kallikrein, and platelet activation producing antifibrinolytic effects; a weak inhibitor of plasma pseudocholinesterase. It also inhibits the contact phase activation of coagulation and preserves adhesive platelet glycoproteins making them resistant to damage from increased circulating plasmin or mechanical injury occurring during bypass

Other Adverse Effects 1% to 10%
Cardiovascular: Atrial fibrillation, myocardial infarction, heart failure, atrial flutter, ventricular tachycardia, hypotension, supraventricular tachycardia
Central nervous system: Fever, mental confusion
Local: Phlebitis
Renal: Increased potential for postoperative renal dysfunction
Respiratory: Dyspnea, bronchoconstriction

Drug Interactions
Increased Effect/Toxicity: Heparin and aprotinin prolong ACT; the ACT becomes a poor measure of adequate anticoagulation with the concurrent use of these drugs. Use with succinylcholine or tubocurarine may produce prolonged or recurring apnea.
Decreased Effect: Aprotinin blocks the fibrinolytic activity of thrombolytic agents (alteplase, streptokinase). The antihypertensive effects of captopril (and other ACE inhibitors) may be blocked; avoid concurrent use.

Drug Uptake Half-life, elimination: 2.5 hours

Pregnancy Risk Factor B

Generic Available No

Aquacare® [OTC] *see* Urea *on page 1221*
Aquachloral® Supprettes® *see* Chloral Hydrate *on page 259*
AquaMEPHYTON® *see* Phytonadione *on page 954*
AquaSite® [OTC] *see* Artificial Tears *on page 117*

Aquasol A® *see* Vitamin A *on page 1243*
Aquasol E® [OTC] *see* Vitamin E *on page 1245*
Aquatensen® *see* Methyclothiazide *on page 792*
Aquazide® *see* Hydrochlorothiazide *on page 595*
Aralen® Phosphate *see* Chloroquine Phosphate *on page 266*
Aranesp™ *see* Darbepoetin Alfa *on page 351*
Arava™ *see* Leflunomide *on page 687*
Aredia® *see* Pamidronate *on page 912*
Arestin™ *see* Minocycline Hydrochloride Periodontal Microspheres *on page 817*

Argatroban (*Marketed Without Brand Name*) (ar GA troh ban)

Pharmacologic Category Anticoagulant, Thrombin Inhibitor

Use Prophylaxis or treatment of thrombosis in adults with heparin-induced thrombocytopenia; adjunct to percutaneous coronary intervention (PCI) in patients who have or are at risk of thrombosis associated with heparin-induced thrombocytopenia

Local Anesthetic/Vasoconstrictor Precautions No information available to require special precautions

Effects on Dental Treatment As with all anticoagulants, bleeding is a potential adverse effect of argatroban during dental surgery. Risk is dependent on multiple variables, including the intensity of anticoagulation and patient susceptibility. Medical consult is suggested. It is unlikely that ambulatory patients presenting for dental treatment will be taking intravenous anticoagulant therapy.

Dosage I.V.: Adults:

Heparin-induced thrombocytopenia:

Initial dose: 2 mcg/kg/minute

Maintenance dose: Measure aPTT after 2 hours, adjust dose until the steady-state aPTT is 1.5-3.0 times the initial baseline value, not exceeding 100 seconds; dosage should not exceed 10 mcg/kg/minute

Conversion to oral anticoagulant: Because there may be a combined effect on the INR when argatroban is combined with warfarin, loading doses of warfarin should not be used. Warfarin therapy should be started at the expected daily dose.

Patients receiving ≤2 mcg/kg/minute of argatroban: Argatroban therapy can be stopped when the combined INR on warfarin and argatroban is >4; repeat INR measurement in 4-6 hours; if INR is below therapeutic level, argatroban therapy may be restarted. Repeat procedure daily until desired INR on warfarin alone is obtained.

Patients receiving >2 mcg/kg/minute of argatroban: Reduce dose of argatroban to 2 mcg/kg/minute; measure INR for argatroban and warfarin 4-6 hours after dose reduction; argatroban therapy can be stopped when the combined INR on warfarin and argatroban is >4. Repeat INR measurement in 4-6 hours; if INR is below therapeutic level, argatroban therapy may be restarted. Repeat procedure daily until desired INR on warfarin alone is obtained.

Percutaneous coronary intervention (PCI):

Initial: Begin infusion of 25 mcg/kg/minute and administer bolus dose of 350 mcg/kg (over 3-5 minutes). ACT should be checked 5-10 minutes after bolus infusion; proceed with procedure if ACT >300 seconds. Following initial bolus:

ACT <300 seconds: Give an additional 150 mcg/kg bolus, and increase infusion rate to 30 mcg/kg/minute (recheck ACT in 5-10 minutes)

ACT >450 seconds: Decrease infusion rate to 15 mcg/kg/minute (recheck ACT in 5-10 minutes)

Once a therapeutic ACT (300-450 seconds) is achieved, infusion should be continued at this dose for the duration of the procedure.

Impending abrupt closure, thrombus formation during PCI, or inability to achieve ACT >300 sec: An additional bolus of 150 mcg/kg, followed by an increase in infusion rate to 40 mcg/kg/minute may be administered.

Dosage adjustment in hepatic impairment: Decreased clearance and increased elimination half-life are seen with hepatic impairment; dose should be reduced. Initial dose for moderate hepatic impairment is 0.5 mcg/kg/minute. **Note:** During PCI, avoid use in patients with elevations of ALT/AST (>3 x ULN); the use of argatroban in these patients has not been evaluated.

Elderly: No adjustment is necessary for patients with normal liver function

Mechanism of Action A direct, highly selective thrombin inhibitor. Reversibly binds to the active thrombin site of free and clot-associated thrombin. Inhibits fibrin formation; activation of coagulation factors V, VIII, and XIII; protein C; and platelet aggregation.

Other Adverse Effects As with all anticoagulants, bleeding is the major adverse effect of argatroban. Hemorrhage may occur at virtually any site. Risk is dependent on multiple variables, including the intensity of anticoagulation and patient susceptibility.

>10%:

Gastrointestinal: Gastrointestinal bleed (minor, 14%)

Genitourinary: Genitourinary bleed and hematuria (minor, 12%)

1% to 10%:

Cardiovascular: Hypotension (7%), cardiac arrest (6%), ventricular tachycardia (5%), atrial fibrillation (3%), cerebrovascular disorder (2%)

Central nervous system: Fever (7%), pain (5%), intracranial bleeding (1%, only observed in patients also receiving streptokinase or tissue plasminogen activator)

Gastrointestinal: Diarrhea (6%), nausea (5%), vomiting (4%), abdominal pain (3%), bleeding (major, 2%)

Genitourinary: Urinary tract infection (5%)

Hematologic: Decreased hemoglobin <2 g/dL and hematocrit (minor, 10%)

Local: Bleeding at the injection site (minor, 2% to 5%)

Renal: Abnormal renal function (3%)

Respiratory: Dyspnea (8%), coughing (3%), hemoptysis (minor, 3%), pneumonia (3%)

Miscellaneous: Sepsis (6%), infection (4%)

Drug Interactions CYP3A4/5 enzyme substrate (minor pathway)

Drugs which affect platelet function (eg, aspirin, NSAIDs, dipyridamole, ticlopidine, clopidogrel): May potentiate the risk of hemorrhage.

Erythromycin: Concurrent therapy failed to demonstrate a significant effect on argatroban pharmacokinetics, indicating CYP3A4/5 is not a major route of argatroban metabolism.

Glycoprotein IIb/IIIa antagonists: Concurrent therapy has not been evaluated. An increased risk of bleeding would be expected.

Heparin: Sufficient time must pass after heparin therapy is discontinued; allow heparin's effect on the aPTT to decrease

Thrombolytics: Safety and efficacy for concomitant use have not been established. May increase risk of bleeding. Intracranial bleeding has been reported.

Warfarin: Concomitant use with argatroban increases PT and INR greater than that of warfarin alone. Argatroban is commonly continued during the initiation of warfarin therapy to assure anticoagulation and to protect against possible transient hypercoagulability.

Drug Uptake

Onset of action: Immediate

Half-life, elimination (dependent on hepatic function): 39-51; Hepatic dysfunction: 181 minutes

Time to peak: Steady-state: 1-3 hours

Pregnancy Risk Factor B

Generic Available No

Argesic®-SA *see* Salsalate *on page 1074*

Arginine (AR ji neen)

U.S. Brand Names R-Gene®

Pharmacologic Category Amino Acid; Diagnostic Agent

Synonyms Arginine Hydrochloride; L-Arginine

Use Pituitary function test (growth hormone)

Unlabeled/Investigational: Treatment and management of severe, uncompensated, metabolic alkalosis (pH ≥7.55) **after** optimizing therapy with sodium, potassium, or ammonium chloride supplements hypercholesterolemia, inflammatory bowel disease, male infertility, poor circulation, urea cycle disorders; wound-healing agent, enhances libido, increases lean body mass, immunosupportive

Local Anesthetic/Vasoconstrictor Precautions No information available to require special precautions

Effects on Dental Treatment No effects or complications reported

Dosage Do not use as an alternative to chloride supplementation; may be used in patients unresponsive to sodium chloride or potassium chloride supplementation.

I.V.

Acidifying agent: 10 g infused over 30 minutes

Ammonia intoxication in cirrhotics: 37.5-100 g (4 doses in 10 days) followed by 50 g/day for 5 days

Growth hormone/pituitary function test (administered over 30 minutes): Children: 0.5 g/kg; Adults: 30 g (300 mL of a 10% solution)

Hypochloremia: Infants, Children, and Adults: Dose (mL) = 0.4 x weight (kg) x ($103-Cl^-$) where Cl^- = the patient's serum chloride concentration in mEq/L; give 1/2 to 1/3 dose calculated then re-evaluate

Inborn errors of urea synthesis: Initial: 0.8 g/kg, then 0.2-0.8 g/kg/day as a continuous infusion

Intermittent hyperammonemic crisis in patients with urea cycle disorders: Neonates, Infants, Children, and Adults:

ASL or ASS: 0.6 g/kg or 12 g/m2 loading dose, followed by 0.6 g/kg/day or 12 g/m2/day continuous infusion

CPS or OTC: 0.2 g/kg or 4 g/m2 loading dose, followed by 0.2 g/kg/day or 4 g/m2/day continuous infusion

(Continued)

Arginine *(Continued)*

Metabolic alkalosis (**Fourth-line treatment** for uncompensated metabolic alkalosis after sodium chloride, potassium chloride, and ammonium chloride supplementation has been optimized): Neonates, Infants, Children, and Adults: dose (G) = weight (kg) x 0.1 x (HCO_3^- - 24) where HCO_3^- = the patient's serum bicarbonate concentration in mEq/L; give ½ to ⅓ dose calculated then re-evaluate

Urea cycle disorders: Neonates, Infants, Children, and Adults:

Argininosuccinic acid lyase (ASL) or argininosuccinic acid synthetase (ASS) disorders or pending definitive diagnosis: 600 mg/kg as a loading dose, followed by 600 mg/kg/day as a continuous infusion

Carbamyl phosphate synthetase (CPS) or ornithine transcarbamylase (OTC) disorder: 200 mg/kg as a loading dose followed by 200 mg/kg/day as a continuous infusion

Oral:

3-6 g/day

Oligospermia: 2-4 g/day

Mechanism of Action Precursor to nitric oxide, the neurotransmitter that relaxes blood vessels and improves circulation; stimulates pituitary release of growth hormone and prolactin, as well as, pancreatic release of glucagon and insulin. Patients with impaired pituitary function have lower or no increase in plasma concentrations of growth hormone after administration of arginine. Arginine is metabolized by the liver to produce hydrogen ions; has acidifying properties and may be used in patients with relative hepatic insufficiency because it combines with ammonia in the body to produce urea. It is an integral part of the urea cycle, which is the biochemical pathway that metabolizes protein and other nitrogen-containing compounds; used in urea cycle disorders to increase arginine serum concentration and prevent breakdown of endogenous protein. Arginine hydrochloride has been used investigationally in treatment of metabolic alkalosis due to its high chloride content; contains 475 mEq of hydrogen ions and 475 mEq of chloride ions/L.

Other Adverse Effects

1% to 10%:

Cardiovascular: Flushing (after rapid I.V. administration)

Central nervous system: Headache (after rapid I.V. administration)

Gastrointestinal: Nausea, vomiting

Neuromuscular & skeletal: Numbness

Local: Venous irritation

Frequency not defined:

Cardiovascular: Hypotension (due to vasodilation)

Central nervous system: Increased intracranial pressure

Endocrine & metabolic: Hyperglycemia, hyperkalemia, hyponatremia, metabolic acidosis (secondary to hyperchloremia)

Gastrointestinal: Abdominal pain, bloating

Local: Severe tissue necrosis with extravasation

Neuromuscular & skeletal: Numbness

Miscellaneous: Increased serum gastrin concentration

Contraindications Hypersensitivity to arginine or any component of the formulation, hepatic or renal failure

Warnings/Precautions Accumulation of excess arginine may result in overproduction of nitric oxide, leading to vasodilation and hypotension. Use with caution in individuals with herpes simplex; may stimulate growth of the virus, especially in those with low lysine levels. Hyperkalemia may occur in patients with renal or hepatic failure.

Drug Interactions Increased Effect/Toxicity: Estrogen-progesterone combinations (increases growth hormone response and decreases glucagon and insulin effects), nitroglycerin, sildenafil, spironolactone (potentially fatal hyperkalemia reported in individuals with hepatic disease)

Drug Uptake

Absorption: Oral: Well absorbed

Time to peak: ~2 hours

Pregnancy Risk Factor C

Generic Available No

Argyrol® S.S. 20% *see* Silver Protein, Mild *on page 1087*
Aricept® *see* Donepezil *on page 410*
Arimidex® *see* Anastrozole *on page 101*
Aristocort® *see* Triamcinolone *on page 1197*
Aristocort® A *see* Triamcinolone *on page 1197*
Aristocort® Forte *see* Triamcinolone *on page 1197*
Aristocort® Intralesional *see* Triamcinolone *on page 1197*
Aristospan® Intra-Articular *see* Triamcinolone *on page 1197*
Aristospan® Intralesional *see* Triamcinolone *on page 1197*
Arixtra® *see* Fondaparinux *on page 535*
Arlex® *see* Sorbitol *on page 1101*

Arlidin® *see* Nylidrin *on page 880*
Arm-a-Med® Isoetharine *see* Isoetharine *on page 658*
Armour® Thyroid *see* Thyroid *on page 1164*
Aromasin® *see* Exemestane *on page 483*
Aromatic Ammonia Aspirols® *see* Ammonia Spirit, Aromatic *on page 82*
Artane® *see* Trihexyphenidyl *on page 1208*
Arthropan® [OTC] *see* Choline Salicylate *on page 280*
Arthrotec® *see* Diclofenac and Misoprostol *on page 380*

Articaine Hydrochloride and Epinephrine *Canada*

(AR ti kane hye droe KLOR ide & ep i NEF rin)

Related Information
Oral Pain *on page 1360*

Canadian Brand Names Astracaine®; Astracaine® Forte; Septocaine®

Pharmacologic Category Local Anesthetic

Synonyms Articaine Hydrochloride and Epinephrine [Dental]

Use Dental: Anesthesia for infiltration and nerve block anesthesia in clinical dentistry

Local Anesthetic/Vasoconstrictor Precautions No information available to require special precautions

Effects on Dental Treatment No effects or complications reported

Dosage Adults:
Ultracaine DS® Forte:
Infiltration: Volume: 0.5-2.5 mL; Total dose: 20-100 mg;
Nerve block: Volume: 0.5-3.4 mL; Total dose: 20-136 mg
Oral surgery: Volume: 1-5.1 mL; Total dose: 40-204 mg
Ultracaine DS®:
Infiltration: Volume: 0.5-2.5 mL; Total dose: 20-100 mg
Nerve block: Volume: 0.5-3.4 mL; Total dose: 20-136 mg
Oral surgery: Volume: 1-5.1 mL; Total dose: 40-204 mg
Maximum dose: 7 mg/kg
To date, Ultracaine® has not been administered to children <4 years of age, nor in doses >5 mg/kg in children between the ages of 4 and 12

Mechanism of Action Blocks nerve conduction by interfering with the permeability of the nerve axonal membrane to sodium ions; this results in the loss of the generation of the nerve axon potential. Local anesthetics reversibly prevent generation and conduction of electrical impulses in neurons by decreasing the transient increase in permeability to sodium. The differential sensitivity generally depends on the size of the fiber; small fibers are more sensitive than larger fibers and require a longer period for recovery. Sensory pain fibers are usually blocked first, followed by fibers that transmit sensations of temperature, touch, and deep pressure. High concentrations block sympathetic somatic sensory and somatic motor fibers. The spread of anesthesia depends upon the distribution of the solution. This is primarily dependent on the site of administration and volume of drug injected.

Other Adverse Effects Frequency not defined:
Cardiovascular: Myocardial depression, arrhythmias, tachycardia, bradycardia, BP changes, edema
Central nervous system: Excitation, depression, nervousness, dizziness, headache, somnolence, unconsciousness, convulsions, chills
Dermatologic: Allergic reactions include cutaneous lesions, urticaria, itching, reddening of skin
Gastrointestinal: Vomiting, allergic reactions include nausea and diarrhea
Local: Reactions at the site of injection, swelling, burning, ischemia, tissue necrosis
Neuromuscular & skeletal: Tremors
Ocular: Visual disturbances, blurred vision, blindness, diplopia, pupillary constriction
Otic: Tinnitus
Respiratory: Allergic reactions include wheezing, acute asthmatic attacks

Contraindications Hypersensitivity to articaine hydrochloride, epinephrine, local anesthetics of the amide group, or any component of their formulation; inflammation and/or sepsis near the injection site; severe shock; any degree of heart block, paroxysmal tachycardia, or known arrhythmia with rapid heart rate; narrow-angle glaucoma; cholinesterase deficiency; existing neurologic disease; severe hypertension; caution required of any vasopressor drug should be followed

Warnings/Precautions Articaine should be used cautiously in persons with known drug allergies or sensitivities, or suspected sensitivity to the amide-type local anesthetics. Avoid excessive premedications with sedatives, tranquilizers, and antiemetic agents. Inject slowly with frequent aspirations and if blood is aspirated, relocate needle. Articaine should be used with extreme caution in patients having a history of thyrotoxicosis or diabetes. Due to the sulfite component of the articaine preparation, hypersensitivity reactions may occur occasionally in patients with bronchial asthma.

Drug Interactions
MAO inhibitors: Administration of local anesthetic solutions containing epinephrine may produce severe, prolonged hypertension
(Continued)

Articaine Hydrochloride and Epinephrine *Canada* *(Continued)*

Tricyclic antidepressants: Pressor response to I.V. epinephrine, norepinephrine, and phenylephrine may be enhanced in patients receiving TCAs (**Note:** Effect is unlikely with epinephrine or levonordefrin dosages typically administered as infiltration in combination with local anesthetics)

Breast-feeding Considerations Articaine is unlikely to be transferred to mother's milk since it is rapidly metabolized and eliminated

Dosage Forms INJ: (Ultracaine DS®): Articaine hydrochloride with epinephrine [1:200,000] and sodium metabisulfite [0.5 mg/mL] and an antioxidant and water for injection (1.7 mL) [50s]; (Ultracaine DS Forte®): Articaine hydrochloride 4% with epinephrine [1:100,000] and sodium metabisulfite [0.5 mg/mL] and an antioxidant and water for injection (1.7 mL) [50s]

Selected Readings

Weaver JM, "Articaine, A New Local Anesthetic for American Dentists: Will It Supersede Lidocaine?" *Anesth Prog*, 1999, 46(4):111-2.

Articaine Hydrochloride and Epinephrine *U.S.*

(AR ti kane hye droe KLOR ide & ep i NEF rin)

Related Information

Oral Pain *on page 1360*

U.S. Brand Names Septocaine™

Pharmacologic Category Local Anesthetic

Synonyms Articaine Hydrochloride and Epinephrine [Dental]

Use Dental: Anesthesia agent for infiltration and nerve block anesthesia in clinical dentistry; Septocaine™ is indicated for local, infiltrative, or conductive anesthesia in both simple and complex dental and periodontal procedures

Local Anesthetic/Vasoconstrictor Precautions No information available to require special precautions

Effects on Dental Treatment No effects or complications reported

Dosage Summary of recommended volumes and concentrations for various types of anesthetic procedures; dosages (administered by submucosal injection and/or nerve block) apply to normal healthy adults.

Recommended Septocaine™ Dosages Based on Anesthetic Procedure

Procedure	Injection (4% Solution) Volume (mL)	Total Dose of Articaine HCl (mg)
Infiltration	0.5-2.5	20-100
Nerve Block	0.5-3.4	20-136
Oral Surgery	1.0-5.1	40-204

This table provides dosage guides only. Other dosages may be used; however, do not exceed maximum recommended dose.

The clinician is reminded that these doses serve only as a guide to the amount of anesthetic required for most routine procedures. The actual volumes to be used depend upon a number of factors, such as type and extent of surgical procedure, depth of anesthesia, degree of muscular relaxation, and condition of the patient. In all cases, the smallest dose that will produce the desired result should be given. Dosages should be reduced for pediatric patients, elderly patients, and patients with cardiac and/or liver disease.

Children <4 years: Safety and efficacy have not been established

Children 4-16 years (dosages in a clinical trial of 61 patients):

- Simple procedures: 0.76-5.65 mg/kg (0.9-5.1 mL) was administered safely to 51 patients
- Complex procedures: 0.37-7.48 mg/kg (0.7-3.9 mL) was administered safely to 10 patients
- **Note:** Approximately 13% of the pediatric patients required additional injections for complete anesthesia

Geriatric patients (dosages in a clinical trial):

- 65-75 years
  - Simple procedures: 0.43-4.76 mg/kg (0.9-11.9 mL) was administered safely to 35 patients
  - Complex procedures: 1.05-4.27 mg/kg (1.3-6.8 mL) was administered safely to 19 patients
- ≥75 years:
  - Simple procedures: 0.78-4.76 mg/kg (1.3-11.9 mL) was administered safely to 7 patients
  - Complex procedures: 1.12-2.17 mg/kg (1.3-5.1 mL) was administered safely to 4 patients
- **Note:** Approximately 6% of the patients 65-75 years of age (none of the patients ≥75 years of age) required additional injections for complete anesthesia,

compared to 11% of the patients 17-65 years of age who required additional injections.

Maximum recommended dosages:

Children (use in pediatric patients <4 years is not recommended): Not to exceed 7 mg/kg (0.175 mL/kg) **or** 3.2 mg/lb (0.0795 mL/lb) of body weight

Adults (normal, healthy): Submucosal infiltration and/or nerve block: Not to exceed 7 mg/kg (0.175 mL/kg) **or** 3.2 mg/lb (0.0795 mL/lb) of body weight

The following numbers of dental cartridges (1.7 mL) provide the indicated amounts of articaine hydrochloride 4% and epinephrine 1:100,000.

# of Cartridges (1.7 mL)	Articaine HCl (4%) (mg)	Epinephrine 1:100,000 (mg)
1	68	0.017
2	136	0.034
3	204	0.051
4	272	0.068
5	340	0.085
6	408	0.102
7	476	0.119
8	544	0.136

Mechanism of Action Local anesthetics block the generation and conduction of nerve impulses, presumably by increasing the threshold for electrical excitation in the nerve, by slowing the propagation of the nerve impulse, and by reducing the rate of rise of the action potential. In general, the progression of anesthesia is related to the diameter, myelination, and conduction velocity of the affected nerve fibers. Clinically, the order of loss of nerve function is as follows: 1) pain, 2) temperature, 3) touch, 4) proprioception, and 5) skeletal muscle tone.

Other Adverse Effects Adverse reactions to Septocaine™ are characteristic of those associated with other amide-type local anesthetics; adverse reactions to this group of drugs may also result from excessive plasma levels which may be due to overdosage, unintentional intravascular injection, or slow metabolic degradation.

≥1% (in controlled trial of 882 patients):

Central nervous system: Headache (4%), paresthesia (1%)

Gastrointestinal: Gingivitis (1%)

Miscellaneous: Pain (body as a whole 13%), facial edema (1%)

<1% (adverse and intercurrent events recorded in 1 or more patients in controlled trials, occurring at an overall rate of <1%, and considered clinically significant): Abdominal pain, accidental injury, arthralgia, asthenia, back pain, constipation, diarrhea, dizziness, dysmenorrhea, dyspepsia, ear pain, ecchymosis, edema, facial paralysis, glossitis, gum hemorrhage, hemorrhage, hyperesthesia, increased salivation, injection site pain, lymphadenopathy, malaise, migraine, mouth ulceration, myalgia, nausea, neck pain, nervousness, neuropathy, osteomyelitis, paresthesia, pharyngitis, pruritus, rhinitis, skin disorder, somnolence, stomatitis, syncope, tachycardia, taste perversion, thirst, tongue edema, tooth disorder, vomiting, xerostomia

Contraindications Hypersensitivity to local anesthetics of the amide type, sodium metabisulfite, or any component of their formulation

Warnings/Precautions Intravascular injections should be avoided; aspiration should be performed prior to administration of Septocaine™; the needle must be repositioned until no return of blood can be elicited by aspiration; however, absence of blood in the syringe does not guarantee that intravascular injection has been avoided. **Accidental intravascular injection may be associated with convulsions, followed by CNS or cardiorespiratory depression and coma, ultimately progressing to respiratory arrest.** Dental practitioners and/or clinicians using local anesthetic agents should be well trained in diagnosis and management of emergencies that may arise from the use of these agents. Resuscitative equipment, oxygen, and other resuscitative drugs should be available for immediate use.

Because Septocaine™ contains epinephrine, which can cause local tissue necrosis or systemic toxicity, usual precautions for epinephrine administration should be observed. It also contains sodium metabisulfite, which may cause allergic-type reactions (including anaphylactic symptoms, and life-threatening or less severe asthmatic episodes) in certain susceptible patients. The overall prevalence of the sulfite sensitivity in the general population is unknown, and is seen more frequently in asthmatic than in nonasthmatic persons.

To avoid serious adverse effects and high plasma concentrations, the lowest dosage resulting in effective anesthesia should be administered. Repeated doses may cause significant increases in blood levels with each repeated dose due to the possibility of accumulation of the drug or its metabolites. Tolerance to elevated blood levels varies with patient status. Reduced dosages, commensurate with age and physical condition, should be given to debilitated patients, elderly patients,
(Continued)

Articaine Hydrochloride and Epinephrine *U.S.* *(Continued)*

acutely-ill patients, and pediatric patients. Septocaine™ should also be used with caution in patients with heart block.

Local anesthetic solutions containing a vasoconstrictor (such as Septocaine™) should be used cautiously. Patients with peripheral vascular disease or hypertensive vascular disease may exhibit exaggerated vasoconstrictor response, possibly resulting in ischemic injury or necrosis. It should also be used cautiously in patients during or following the administration of a potent general anesthetic agent, since cardiac arrhythmias may occur under these conditions.

Systemic absorption of local anesthetics may produce CNS and cardiovascular effects. Changes in cardiac conduction, excitability, refractoriness, contractility, and peripheral vascular resistance are minimal at blood concentrations produced by therapeutic doses. However, toxic blood concentrations depress cardiac conduction and excitability, which may lead to A-V block, ventricular arrhythmias, and cardiac arrest (sometimes resulting in death). In addition, myocardial contractility is depressed and peripheral vasodilation occurs, leading to decreased cardiac output and arterial BP.

Careful and constant monitoring of cardiovascular and respiratory (adequacy of ventilation) vital signs and the patient's state of consciousness should be done following each local anesthetic injection; at such times, restlessness, anxiety, tinnitus, dizziness, blurred vision, tremors, depression, or drowsiness may be early warning signs of CNS toxicity.

In vitro studies show that ~5% to 10% of articaine is metabolized by the human liver microsomal P450 isoenzyme system; however, no studies have been performed in patient with liver dysfunction, and caution should be used in patients with severe hepatic disease. Use with caution in patients with impaired cardiovascular function, since they may be less able to compensate for function changes associated with prolonged A-V conduction produced by these drugs.

Small doses of local anesthetics injected into dental blocks may produce adverse reactions similar to systemic toxicity seen in unintentional intravascular injections at larger doses. Confusion, convulsions, respiratory depression and/or respiratory arrest, and cardiovascular stimulation or depression have been reported. These reactions may be due to intra-arterial injection of the local anesthetic with retrograde flow to the cerebral circulation. Patients receiving such blocks should be observed constantly with resuscitative equipment and personnel trained in treatment of adverse reactions immediately available. Dosage recommendations should not be exceeded; see Dosage

Drug Interactions

MAO inhibitors: Administration of local anesthetic solutions containing epinephrine may produce severe, prolonged hypertension

Phenothiazines, butyrophenones may reduce or reverse the pressor effects of epinephrine; concurrent use of these agents should be avoided; in situations when concurrent therapy is necessary, careful patient monitoring is essential.

Tricyclic antidepressants: Pressor response to I.V. epinephrine, norepinephrine, and phenylephrine may be enhanced in patients receiving TCAs (**Note:** Effect is unlikely with epinephrine or levonordefrin dosages typically administered as infiltration in combination with local anesthetics)

Drug Uptake Administration of articaine HCl with epinephrine results in a 3- to 5-fold increase in plasma epinephrine concentrations compared to baseline; however, in healthy adults, it does not appear to be associated with marked increases in BP or HR, except in the case of accidental intravascular, injection.

Onset of action: 1-6 minutes

Duration: Complete anesthesia: ~1 hour

Pregnancy Risk Factor C

Breast-feeding Considerations It is not known whether articaine is excreted in human milk. Because many drugs are excreted in human milk, caution should be exercised when Septocaine™ is administered to a nursing woman.

Dosage Forms INJ: (Septocaine™): Articaine hydrochloride 4% with epinephrine (as bitartrate) 1:100,000, sodium chloride 1.6 mg/mL, sodium bisulfite 0.5 mg/mL, and sodium hydroxide (to adjust pH to 5.0) (1.7 mL) [cartridge, 50/box]

Generic Available No

Comments Septocaine™ (articaine hydrochloride 4% and epinephrine 1:100,000) is the first FDA approval in 30 years of a new local dental anesthetic providing complete pulpal anesthesia for approximately 1 hour. Chemically, articaine contains both an amide linkage and an ester linkage, making it chemically unique in the class of local anesthetics. Since it contains the ester linkage, articaine HCl is rapidly metabolized by plasma carboxyesterase to its primary metabolite, articainic acid, which is an inactive product of this metabolism. According to the manufacturer, *in vitro* studies show that the human liver microsomal P450 isoenzyme system metabolizes approximately 5% to 10% of available articaine with nearly quantitative conversion to articainic acid. The elimination half-life of articaine is about 1.8 hours, and that of articainic acid is about 1.5 hours. Articaine is excreted primarily through urine with 53% to 57% of the administered dose eliminated in the first 24 hours following submucosal administration. Articainic acid is the primary metabolite in urine. A minor metabolite, articainic acid glucuronide, is also excreted in the urine. Articaine constitutes only 2% of the total dose excreted in urine.

Selected Readings

Malamed SF, Gagnon S, Leblanc D, "A Comparison Between Articaine HCl and Lidocaine HCl in Pediatric Dental Patients," *Pediatr Dent*, 2000, 22(4):307-11.

Malamed SF, Gagnon S, Leblanc D, "Articaine Hydrochloride: A Study of the Safety of a New Amide Local Anesthetic," *J Am Dent Assoc*, 2001, 132(2):177-85.

Malamed SF, Gagnon S, Leblanc D, "Efficacy of Articaine: A New Amide Local Anesthetic," *J Am Dent Assoc*, 2000, 131(5):635-42.

Schertzer ER Jr, "Articaine vs lidocaine," *J Am Dent Assoc*, 2000, 131(9):1248, 1250.

Weaver JM, "Articaine, A New Local Anesthetic for American Dentists: Will It Supersede Lidocaine?" *Anesth Prog*, 1999, 46(4):111-2.

Artificial Tears (ar ti FISH il tears)

U.S. Brand Names Akwa Tears® [OTC]; AquaSite® [OTC]; Bion® Tears [OTC]; HypoTears [OTC]; HypoTears PF [OTC]; Isopto® Tears [OTC]; Liquifilm® Tears [OTC]; Moisture® Eyes [OTC]; Moisture® Eyes PM [OTC]; Murine® Tears [OTC]; Murocel® [OTC]; Nature's Tears® [OTC]; Nu-Tears® [OTC]; Nu-Tears® II [OTC]; OcuCoat® [OTC]; OcuCoat® PF [OTC]; Puralube® Tears [OTC]; Refresh® [OTC]; Refresh® Plus [OTC]; Refresh® Tears [OTC]; Teargen® [OTC]; Teargen® II [OTC]; Tearisol® [OTC]; Tears Again® [OTC]; Tears Naturale® [OTC]; Tears Naturale® Free [OTC]; Tears Naturale® II [OTC]; Tears Plus® [OTC]; Tears Renewed® [OTC]; Ultra Tears® [OTC]; Viva-Drops® [OTC]

Canadian Brand Names Teardrops®

Pharmacologic Category Ophthalmic Agent, Miscellaneous

Synonyms Hydroxyethylcellulose; Polyvinyl Alcohol

Use Ophthalmic lubricant; for relief of dry eyes and eye irritation

Local Anesthetic/Vasoconstrictor Precautions No information available to require special precautions

Effects on Dental Treatment No effects or complications reported

Dosage Use as needed to relieve symptoms, 1-2 drops into eye(s) 3-4 times/day

Other Adverse Effects 1% to 10%: Ocular: May cause mild stinging or temporary blurred vision

Pregnancy Risk Factor C

Generic Available Yes

Asacol® *see* Mesalamine *on page 772*

Ascorbic Acid (a SKOR bik AS id)

U.S. Brand Names C-500-GR™ [OTC]; Cecon® [OTC]; Cevi-Bid® [OTC]; C-Gram [OTC]; Dull-C® [OTC]; Vita-C® [OTC]

Canadian Brand Names Apo®-C; Proflavanol C™; Revitalose C-1000®

Mexican Brand Names Cevalin®; Ce-Vi-Sol®; Redoxon®; Redoxon® Forte

Pharmacologic Category Vitamin, Water Soluble

Synonyms Vitamin C

Use Prevention and treatment of scurvy and to acidify the urine

Unlabeled/Investigational: In large doses to decrease the severity of "colds"; dietary supplementation; a 20-year study was recently completed involving 730 individuals which indicates a possible decreased risk of death by stroke when ascorbic acid at doses ≥45 mg/day was administered

Local Anesthetic/Vasoconstrictor Precautions No information available to require special precautions

Effects on Dental Treatment No effects or complications reported

Dosage Oral, I.M., I.V., S.C.:

Recommended daily allowance (RDA):
- <6 months: 30 mg
- 6 months to 1 year: 35 mg
- 1-3 years: 15 mg; upper limit of intake should not exceed 400 mg/day
- 4-8 years: 25 mg; upper limit of intake should not exceed 650 mg/day
- 9-13 years: 45 mg; upper limit of intake should not exceed 1200 mg/day
- 14-18 years: Upper limit of intake should not exceed 1800 mg/day
  - Male: 75 mg
  - Female: 65 mg
- Adults: Upper limit of intake should not exceed 2000 mg/day
  - Male: 90 mg
  - Female: 75 mg;
- Pregnant female:
  - ≤18 years: 80 mg; upper limit of intake should not exceed 1800 mg/day
  - 19-50 years: 85 mg; upper limit of intake should not exceed 2000 mg/day
- Lactating female:
  - ≤18 years: 15 mg; upper limit of intake should not exceed 1800 mg/day
  - 19-50 years: 20 mg; upper limit of intake should not exceed 2000 mg/day
- Adult smoker: Add an additional 35 mg/day

(Continued)

Ascorbic Acid *(Continued)*

Children:
- Scurvy: 100-300 mg/day in divided doses for at least 2 weeks
- Urinary acidification: 500 mg every 6-8 hours
- Dietary supplement: 35-100 mg/day

Adults:
- Scurvy: 100-250 mg 1-2 times/day for at least 2 weeks
- Urinary acidification: 4-12 g/day in 3-4 divided doses
- Prevention and treatment of colds: 1-3 g/day
- Dietary supplement: 50-200 mg/day

Mechanism of Action Not fully understood; necessary for collagen formation and tissue repair; involved in some oxidation-reduction reactions as well as other metabolic pathways, such as synthesis of carnitine, steroids, and catecholamines and conversion of folic acid to folinic acid

Other Adverse Effects 1% to 10%: Renal: Hyperoxaluria (incidence dose-related)

Contraindications Large doses during pregnancy

Warnings/Precautions Diabetics and patients prone to recurrent renal calculi (eg, dialysis patients) should not take excessive doses for extended periods of time

Drug Interactions

Increased Effect/Toxicity: Ascorbic acid enhances iron absorption from the GI tract. Concomitant ascorbic acid taken with oral contraceptives may increase contraceptive effect.

Decreased Effect:Ascorbic acid and fluphenazine may decrease fluphenazine levels. Ascorbic acid and warfarin may decrease anticoagulant effect. Changes in dose of ascorbic acid when taken with oral contraceptives may reduce the contraceptive effect.

Drug Uptake Absorption: Oral: Readily absorbed; an active process and is thought to be dose-dependent

Pregnancy Risk Factor A/C (dose exceeding RDA recommendation)

Generic Available Yes

Ascriptin® [OTC] *see* Aspirin *on page 119*
Ascriptin® Arthritis Pain [OTC] *see* Aspirin *on page 119*
Ascriptin® Enteric [OTC] *see* Aspirin *on page 119*
Ascriptin® Extra Strength [OTC] *see* Aspirin *on page 119*

Asparaginase (a SPIR a ji nase)

U.S. Brand Names Elspar®

Canadian Brand Names Elspar®; Kidrolase®

Mexican Brand Names Leunase

Pharmacologic Category Antineoplastic Agent, Miscellaneous

Synonyms *E. coli* Asparaginase; *Erwinia* Asparaginase; L-asparaginase; NSC-106977 (*Erwinia*); NSC-109229 (*E. coli*)

Use Treatment of acute lymphocytic leukemia, lymphoma; used for induction therapy

Local Anesthetic/Vasoconstrictor Precautions No information available to require special precautions

Effects on Dental Treatment No effects or complications reported

Mechanism of Action Some malignant cells (ie, lymphoblastic leukemia cells and those of lymphocyte derivation) must acquire the amino acid asparagine from surrounding fluid such as blood, whereas normal cells can synthesize their own asparagine. Asparaginase is an enzyme that deaminates asparagine to aspartic acid and ammonia in the plasma and extracellular fluid and therefore deprives tumor cells of the amino acid for protein synthesis.

There are two purified preparations of the enzyme, one from *Escherichia coli* and one from *Erwinia carotovora.* These two preparations vary slightly in the gene sequencing and have slight differences in enzyme characteristics. Both are highly specific for asparagine and have <10% activity for the D-isomer. The preparation from *E. coli* has had the most use in clinical and research practice.

Other Adverse Effects

>10%:

Central nervous system: Fatigue, somnolence, depression, hallucinations, agitation, disorientation or convulsions (10% to 60%), stupor, confusion, coma (25%)

Endocrine & metabolic: Fever, chills (50% to 60%), hyperglycemia (10%)

Gastrointestinal: Nausea, vomiting (50% to 60%), anorexia, abdominal cramps (70%), acute pancreatitis (15%, may be severe in some patients)

Hematologic: Hypofibrinogenemia and depression of clotting factors V and VIII, variable decreased in factors VII and IX, severe protein C deficiency and decrease in antithrombin III (may be dose-limiting or fatal)

Hepatic: Transient elevations of transaminases, bilirubin, and alkaline phosphatase

Hypersensitivity: Acute allergic reactions (fever, rash, urticaria, arthralgia, hypotension, angioedema, bronchospasm, anaphylaxis (15% to 35%); may be dose-limiting in some patients, may be fatal)

Renal: Azotemia (66%)

1% to 10%:

Endocrine & metabolic: Hyperuricemia

Gastrointestinal: Stomatitis

Drug Interactions

Increased Effect/Toxicity: Increased toxicity has been noticed when asparaginase is administered with vincristine (neuropathy) and prednisone (hyperglycemia). Increased hepatotoxicity when used with mercaptopurine.

Decreased Effect: Asparaginase terminates methotrexate action. Asparaginase metabolism is decreased when used with cyclophosphamide.

Drug Uptake

Absorption: Not absorbed from GI tract, therefore, requires parenteral administration; I.M. administration produces peak blood concentration 50% lower than those from I.V. administration (I.M. may be less immunogenic).

Half-life, elimination: 8-30 hours

Pregnancy Risk Factor C

Generic Available No

A-Spas® S/L *see* Hyoscyamine *on page 617*

Aspercin [OTC] *see* Aspirin *on page 119*

Aspercin Extra [OTC] *see* Aspirin *on page 119*

Aspergum® [OTC] *see* Aspirin *on page 119*

Aspirin (AS pir in)

Related Information

Butalbital, Aspirin, and Caffeine *on page 194*

Cardiovascular Diseases *on page 1308*

Carisoprodol and Aspirin *on page 224*

Dental Drug Interactions: Update on Drug Combinations Requiring Special Considerations *on page 1434*

Oral Pain *on page 1360*

Rheumatoid Arthritis and Osteoarthritis *on page 1340*

U.S. Brand Names Ascriptin® [OTC]; Ascriptin® Arthritis Pain [OTC]; Ascriptin® Enteric [OTC]; Ascriptin® Extra Strength [OTC]; Aspercin [OTC]; Aspercin Extra [OTC]; Aspergum® [OTC]; Bayer® Aspirin [OTC]; Bayer® Aspirin Extra Strength [OTC]; Bayer® Aspirin Regimen Adult Low Strength [OTC]; Bayer® Aspirin Regimen Adult Low Strength with Calcium [OTC]; Bayer® Aspirin Regimen Children's [OTC]; Bayer® Aspirin Regimen Regular Strength [OTC]; Bayer® Plus Extra Strength [OTC]; Bufferin® [OTC]; Bufferin® Arthritis Strength [OTC]; Bufferin® Extra Strength [OTC]; Easprin®; Ecotrin® [OTC]; Ecotrin® Low Adult Strength [OTC]; Ecotrin® Maximum Strength [OTC]; Halfprin® [OTC]; St. Joseph® Pain Reliever [OTC]; Sureprin 81™ [OTC]; ZORprin®

Canadian Brand Names Apo®-ASA; Asaphen; Asaphen E.C.; Entrophen®; Novasen

Mexican Brand Names ASA 500®; Aspirina Protect®; Ecotrin®

Pharmacologic Category Salicylate

Synonyms Acetylsalicylic Acid; ASA

Use

Dental: Treatment of postoperative pain

Medical: Treatment of mild to moderate pain, inflammation, and fever; may be used as prophylaxis of myocardial infarction; prophylaxis of stroke and/or transient ischemic episodes; management of rheumatoid arthritis, rheumatic fever, osteoarthritis, and gout (high dose); adjunctive therapy in revascularization procedures (coronary artery bypass graft [CABG], percutaneous transluminal coronary angioplasty [PTCA], carotid endarterectomy)

Unlabeled/Investigational: Low doses have been used in the prevention of pre-eclampsia, recurrent spontaneous abortions, prematurity, fetal growth retardation (including complications associated with autoimmune disorders such as lupus or antiphospholipid syndrome)

Local Anesthetic/Vasoconstrictor Precautions No information available to require special precautions

Effects on Dental Treatment Avoid aspirin, if possible, for 1 week prior to surgery due to possibility of postoperative bleeding.

Dosage

Children:

Analgesic and antipyretic: Oral, rectal: 10-15 mg/kg/dose every 4-6 hours, up to a total of 4 g/day

Anti-inflammatory: Oral: Initial: 60-90 mg/kg/day in divided doses; usual maintenance: 80-100 mg/kg/day divided every 6-8 hours; monitor serum concentration

Antiplatelet effects: Adequate pediatric studies have not been performed; pediatric dosage is derived from adult studies and clinical experience and is not well established; suggested doses have ranged from 3-5 mg/kg/day to 5-10 mg/kg/day given as a single daily dose. Doses are rounded to a convenient amount (eg, 1/2 of 80 mg tablet).

(Continued)

Aspirin *(Continued)*

Mechanical prosthetic heart valves: 6-20 mg/kg/day given as a single daily dose (used in combination with an oral anticoagulant in children who have systemic embolism despite adequate oral anticoagulation therapy (INR 2.5-3.5) and used in combination with low-dose anticoagulation (INR 2-3) and dipyridamole when full-dose oral anticoagulation is contraindicated)

Blalock-Taussig shunts: 3-5 mg/kg/day given as a single daily dose

Kawasaki disease: Oral: 80-100 mg/kg/day divided every 6 hours; monitor serum concentration; after fever resolves: 3-5 mg/kg/day once daily; in patients without coronary artery abnormalities, give lower dose for at least 6-8 weeks or until ESR and platelet count are normal; in patients with coronary artery abnormalities, low-dose aspirin should be continued indefinitely

Antirheumatic: Oral: 60-100 mg/kg/day in divided doses every 4 hours

Adults:

Analgesic and antipyretic: Oral, rectal: 325-650 mg every 4-6 hours up to 4 g/day

Anti-inflammatory: Oral: Initial: 2.4-3.6 g/day in divided doses; usual maintenance: 3.6-5.4 g/day; monitor serum concentration

Myocardial infarction prophylaxis: 75-325 mg/day; use of a lower aspirin dosage has been recommended in patients receiving ACE inhibitors

Acute myocardial infarction: 160-325 mg/day

CABG: 325 mg/day starting 6 hours following procedure

PTCA: Initial: 80-325 mg/day starting 2 hours before procedure; longer pretreatment durations (up to 24 hours) should be considered if lower dosages (80-100 mg) are used

Carotid endarterectomy: 81-325 mg/day preoperatively and daily thereafter

Acute stroke : 160-325 mg/day, initiated within 48 hours (in patients who are not candidates for thrombolytics and are not receiving systemic anticoagulation)

Stroke prevention/TIA: 30-325 mg/day (dosages up to 1300 mg/day in 2-4 divided doses have been used in clinical trials)

Pre-eclampsia prevention (unlabeled use): 60-80 mg/day during gestational weeks 13-26 (patient selection criteria not established)

Dosing adjustment in renal impairment: Cl_{cr} <10 mL/minute: Avoid use.

Hemodialysis: Dialyzable (50% to 100%)

Dosing adjustment in hepatic disease: Avoid use in severe liver disease.

Mechanism of Action Inhibits prostaglandin synthesis by decreasing the activity of the enzyme, cyclooxygenase, which results in decreased formation of prostaglandin precursors; acts on the hypothalamic heat-regulating center to reduce fever; blocks thromboxane synthetase action which prevents formation of the platelet-aggregating substance thromboxane A_2

Other Adverse Effects As with all drugs which may affect hemostasis, bleeding is associated with aspirin. Hemorrhage may occur at virtually any site. Risk is dependent on multiple variables including dosage, concurrent use of multiple agents which alter hemostasis, and patient susceptibility. Many adverse effects of aspirin are dose-related, and are rare at low dosages. Other serious reactions are idiosyncratic, related to allergy or individual sensitivity. Accurate estimation of frequencies is not possible.

Cardiovascular: Hypotension, tachycardia, dysrhythmias, edema

Central nervous system: Fatigue, insomnia, nervousness, agitation, confusion, dizziness, headache, lethargy, cerebral edema, hyperthermia, coma

Dermatologic: Rash, angioedema, urticaria

Endocrine and metabolic: Acidosis, hyperkalemia, dehydration, hypoglycemia (children), hyperglycemia, hypernatremia (buffered forms)

Gastrointestinal: Nausea, vomiting, dyspepsia, epigastric discomfort, heartburn, stomach pains, gastrointestinal ulceration (6% to 31%), gastric erosions, gastric erythema, duodenal ulcers

Hematologic: Anemia, disseminated intravascular coagulation, prolongation of prothrombin times, coagulopathy, thrombocytopenia, hemolytic anemia, bleeding, iron-deficiency anemia

Hepatic: Hepatotoxicity, increased transaminases, hepatitis (reversible)

Neuromuscular and skeletal: Rhabdomyolysis, weakness, acetabular bone destruction (OA)

Otic: Hearing loss, tinnitus

Renal: Interstitial nephritis, papillary necrosis, proteinuria, renal impairment, renal failure (including cases caused by rhabdomyolysis), increased BUN, increased serum creatinine

Respiratory: Asthma, bronchospasm, dyspnea, laryngeal edema, hyperpnea, tachypnea, respiratory alkalosis, noncardiogenic pulmonary edema

Miscellaneous: Anaphylaxis, prolonged pregnancy and labor, stillbirths, low birth weight, peripartum bleeding, Reye's syndrome

Case reports: Colonic ulceration, esophageal stricture, esophagitis with esophageal ulcer, esophageal hematoma, oral mucosal ulcers (aspirin-containing chewing gum), coronary artery spasm, conduction defect and atrial fibrillation (toxicity), delirium, ischemic brain infarction, colitis, rectal stenosis (suppository), cholestatic jaundice, periorbital edema, rhinosinusitis

Contraindications Hypersensitivity to salicylates, other NSAIDs, or any component of their formulation; asthma; rhinitis; nasal polyps; inherited or acquired bleeding disorders (including factor VII and factor IX deficiency); children (<16 years of age) for viral infections (chickenpox or flu symptoms), with or without fever (due to a potential association with Reye's syndrome); pregnancy (3rd trimester especially)

Warnings/Precautions Use with caution in patients with platelet and bleeding disorders, renal dysfunction, dehydration, erosive gastritis, or peptic ulcer disease. Heavy ethanol use (>3 drinks/day) can increase bleeding risks. Avoid use in severe renal failure or in severe hepatic failure. Discontinue use if tinnitus or impaired hearing occurs. Caution in mild-moderate renal failure (only at high dosages). Patients with sensitivity to tartrazine dyes, nasal polyps and asthma may have an increased risk of salicylate sensitivity. Surgical patients should avoid ASA if possible, for 1-2 weeks prior to surgery, to reduce the risk of excessive bleeding.

Drug Interactions

ACE inhibitors: The effects of ACE inhibitors may be blunted by aspirin administration, particularly at higher dosages.

Buspirone increases aspirin's free % *in vitro*.

Carbonic anhydrase inhibitors and corticosteroids have been associated with alteration in salicylate serum concentration.

Heparin and low molecular weight heparins: Concurrent use may increase the risk of bleeding.

Methotrexate serum concentration may be increased; consider discontinuing aspirin 2-3 days before high-dose methotrexate treatment or avoid concurrent use.

NSAIDs may increase the risk of GI adverse effects and bleeding. Serum concentrations of some NSAIDs may be decreased by aspirin.

Platelet inhibitors (IIb/IIIa antagonists): Risk of bleeding may be increased.

Probenecid effects may be antagonized by aspirin.

Sulfonylureas: The effects of older sulfonylurea agents (tolazamide, tolbutamide) may be potentiated due to displacement from plasma proteins. This effect does not appear to be clinically significant for newer sulfonylurea agents (glyburide, glipizide, glimepiride).

Valproic acid may be displaced from its binding sites which can result in toxicity.

Verapamil may potentiate the prolongation of bleeding time associated with aspirin.

Warfarin and oral anticoagulants may increase the risk of bleeding.

Dietary/Ethanol/Herb Considerations

Ethanol: Avoid use; may enhance gastric mucosal irritation.

Food may decrease the rate but not extent of oral absorption. Administer with food or milk to reduce GI upset. Fresh fruits containing vitamin C displace drug from binding sites, resulting in increased urinary excretion of aspirin. Limit Benedictine liqueur, curry powder, gherkins, licorice, paprika, prunes, raisins, and tea due to potential salicylate accumulation. Diet may require folic acid and/or iron supplementation; doses of 3-4 g/day may cause iron-deficiency and folic acid deficiency leading to macrocytic anemia. Avoid garlic, ginger, and green tea.

Herb/Nutraceutical: Avoid cat's claw, dong quai, evening primrose, feverfew, garlic, ginger, ginkgo biloba, ginseng, green tea, horse chestnut, and red clover due to additional antiplatelet activity. Limit licorice due to salicylate content.

Drug Uptake

Absorption: Rapid

Duration: 4-6 hours

Half-life, elimination: Parent drug: 15-20 minutes; Salicylates (dose dependent): 3 hours at lower doses (300-600 mg), 5-6 hours (after 1 g), 10 hours with higher doses

Time to peak: ~1-2 hours

Pregnancy Risk Factor C/D (full-dose aspirin in 3rd trimester - expert analysis)

Breast-feeding Considerations Use cautiously due to potential adverse effects in nursing infants

Dosage Forms CAPLET, buffered: 325 mg, 500 mg. **GELCAP:** 325 mg, 500 mg. **GUM:** 227 mg. **SUPP, rectal:** 60 mg, 120 mg, 125 mg, 200 mg, 300 mg, 325 mg, 600 mg, 650 mg. **TAB:** 325 mg, 500 mg; film coated: 325 mg. **TAB, buffered:** 325 mg, 500 mg. **TAB, chewable:** 81 mg. **TAB, controlled release** (ZORprin®): 800 mg. **TAB, enteric coated:** 81 mg, 162 mg, 325 mg, 500 mg, 650 mg, 975 mg; (Easprin®): 975 mg

Generic Available Yes

Comments Anti-inflammatory actions of aspirin are not seen clinically at doses <3500 mg/day. Patients taking one aspirin tablet daily as an antithrombotic and who require dental surgery should be given special consideration in consultation with the physician before removal of the aspirin relative to prevention of postoperative bleeding.

Selected Readings

Desjardins PJ, Cooper SA, Gallegos TL, et al, "The Relative Analgesic Efficacy of Propiram Fumarate, Codeine Aspirin, and Placebo in Post-Impaction Dental Pain," *J Clin Pharmacol*, 1984, 24(1):35-42.

Forbes JA, Butterworth GA, Burchfield WH, et al, "Evaluation of Ketorolac, Aspirin, and an Acetaminophen-Codeine Combination in Postoperative Oral Surgery Pain," *Pharmacotherapy*, 1990, 10(6 Pt 2):77S-93S.

(Continued)

Aspirin *(Continued)*

Hurlen M, Erikssen J, Smith P, et al, "Comparison of Bleeding Complications of Warfarin and Warfarin Plus Acetylsalicylic Acid: A Study in 3166 Outpatients," *J Intern Med*, 1994, 236(3):299-304.

Aspirin and Codeine (AS pir in & KOE deen)

Related Information

Dental Drug Interactions: Update on Drug Combinations Requiring Special Considerations *on page 1434*

Oral Pain *on page 1360*

U.S. Brand Names Empirin® With Codeine

Canadian Brand Names Coryphen® Codeine

Pharmacologic Category Analgesic, Narcotic

Synonyms Codeine and Aspirin

Use

Dental: Treatment of postoperative pain

Medical: Relief of pain

Local Anesthetic/Vasoconstrictor Precautions No information available to require special precautions

Effects on Dental Treatment

<1%: Xerostomia

Use with caution in impaired hepatic function; use with caution in patients with platelet and bleeding disorders, renal dysfunction, erosive gastritis, or peptic ulcer disease, previous nonreaction does not guarantee future safe taking of medication; do not use aspirin in children <16 years of age for chickenpox or flu symptoms due to the association with Reye's syndrome

Avoid aspirin, if possible, for 1 week prior to surgery due to possibility of postoperative bleeding

Elderly are a high-risk population for adverse effects from nonsteroidal anti-inflammatory agents. As much as 60% of elderly with GI complications to NSAIDs can develop peptic ulceration and/or hemorrhage asymptomatically. Also, concomitant disease and drug use contribute to the risk for GI adverse effects. Use lowest effective dose for shortest period possible. Consider renal function decline with age. Use with caution in patients with history of asthma.

Restrictions C-III

Dosage Oral:

Children:

- Aspirin: 10 mg/kg/dose every 4 hours
- Codeine: 0.5-1 mg/kg/dose every 4 hours

Adults: 1-2 tablets every 4-6 hours as needed for pain

Dosing adjustment in renal impairment:

- Cl_{cr} 10-50 mL/minute: Administer 75% of dose
- Cl_{cr} <10 mL/minute: Avoid use

Dosing interval in hepatic disease: Avoid use in severe liver disease

Mechanism of Action Aspirin inhibits prostaglandin synthesis, acts on the hypothalamus heat-regulating center to reduce fever, blocks prostaglandin synthetase action which prevents formation of the platelet-aggregating substance thromboxane A_2; codeine binds to opiate receptors (mu and kappa subtypes) in the CNS causing inhibition of ascending pain pathways, altering the perception of and response to pain

Other Adverse Effects

>10%:

- Central nervous system: Lightheadedness, dizziness, sedation
- Gastrointestinal: Nausea, heartburn, stomach pains, dyspepsia, epigastric discomfort, vomiting
- Respiratory: Dyspnea

1% to 10%:

- Central nervous system: Fatigue, euphoria, dysphoria
- Dermatologic: Rash, pruritus
- Gastrointestinal: Gastrointestinal ulceration, constipation
- Hematologic: Hemolytic anemia
- Neuromuscular & skeletal: Weakness
- Respiratory: Dyspnea
- Miscellaneous: Anaphylactic shock

Contraindications Hypersensitivity to aspirin, codeine, or any component of their formulation; premature infants or during labor for delivery of a premature infant; pregnancy

Warnings/Precautions

Use with caution in patients with impaired renal function, erosive gastritis, or peptic ulcer disease

Enhanced analgesia has been seen in elderly patients on therapeutic doses of narcotics; duration of action may be increased in the elderly; the elderly may be particularly susceptible to the CNS depressant and constipating effects of narcotics

Drug Interactions See Aspirin *on page 119* and Codeine *on page 317*

Dietary/Ethanol/Herb Considerations

Ethanol: Avoid use; may enhance gastric mucosal irritation and increase CNS depression.

Food: Administer with food or milk to reduce GI upset; food decreases the rate but not extent of oral absorption.

Herb/Nutraceutical: Avoid gotu kola, kava, SAMe, St John's wort, and valerian; may increase CNS depression.

Drug Uptake

Aspirin:

Absorption: Rapid

Half-life, elimination: Parent drug: 15-20 minutes; Salicylates (dose-dependent): From 3 hours at lower doses (300-600 mg), to 5-6 hours (after 1 g) to 10 hours with higher doses

Time to peak: ~1-2 hours

Codeine:

Onset of action: 0.5-1 hour

Duration: 4-6 hours

Half-life, elimination: 2.5-3.5 hours

Time to peak: 1-1.5 hours

Pregnancy Risk Factor D

Breast-feeding Considerations

Aspirin: Cautious use due to potential adverse effects in nursing infants

Codeine: Codeine not contraindicated with breast-feeding

Dosage Forms TAB: #3: Aspirin 325 mg and codeine 30 mg; #4: Aspirin 325 mg and codeine 60 mg

Generic Available Yes

Comments Codeine products, as with other narcotic analgesics, are recommended only for limited acute dosing (ie, 3 days or less). The most common adverse effect you will see in your dental patients from codeine is nausea, followed by sedation and constipation. Codeine has narcotic addiction liability, especially when given long-term. The aspirin component has anticoagulant effects and can affect bleeding times.

Selected Readings

Dionne RA, "New Approaches to Preventing and Treating Postoperative Pain," *J Am Dent Assoc*, 1992, 123(6):26-34.

Gobetti JP, "Controlling Dental Pain," *J Am Dent Assoc*, 1992, 123(6):47-52.

Aspirin and Dipyridamole

(AS pir in & ek STEN did ri LEES dye peer ID a mole)

U.S. Brand Names Aggrenox™

Canadian Brand Names Aggrenox®

Pharmacologic Category Antiplatelet Agent

Synonyms Dipyridamole and Aspirin

Use Reduction in the risk of stroke in patients who have had transient ischemia of the brain or completed ischemic stroke due to thrombosis

Local Anesthetic/Vasoconstrictor Precautions No information available to require special precautions

Effects on Dental Treatment No effects or complications reported

Dosage Oral:

Adults: 1 capsule (dipyridamole 200 mg, aspirin 25 mg) twice daily.

Dosage adjustment in renal impairment: Avoid use in patients with severe renal dysfunction (Cl_{cr} <10 mL/minute). Studies have not been done in patients with renal impairment.

Dosage adjustment in hepatic impairment: Avoid use in patients with severe hepatic impairment; studies have not been done in patients with varying degrees of hepatic impairment

Elderly: Plasma concentrations were 40% higher, but specific dosage adjustments have not been recommended

Mechanism of Action The antithrombotic action results from additive antiplatelet effects. Dipyridamole inhibits the uptake of adenosine into platelets, endothelial cells, and erythrocytes. Aspirin inhibits platelet aggregation by irreversible inhibition of platelet cyclo-oxygenase and thus inhibits the generation of thromboxane A2.

Other Adverse Effects

>10%:

Central nervous system: Headache (38%)

Gastrointestinal: Dyspepsia, abdominal pain (18%), nausea (16%), diarrhea (13%)

1% to 10%:

Cardiovascular: Cardiac failure (2%)

Central nervous system: Pain (6%), seizures (2%), fatigue (6%), malaise (2%), syncope (1%), amnesia (2%), confusion (1%), somnolence (1%)

Dermatologic: Purpura (1%)

Gastrointestinal: Vomiting (8%), bleeding (4%), rectal bleeding (2%), hemorrhoids (1%), hemorrhage (1%), anorexia (1%)

Hematologic: Anemia (2%)

(Continued)

Aspirin and Dipyridamole *(Continued)*

Neuromuscular & skeletal: Back pain (5%), weakness (2%), arthralgia (6%), arthritis (2%), arthrosis (1%), myalgia (1%)

Respiratory: Cough (2%), upper respiratory tract infections (1%), epistaxis (2%)

Contraindications Hypersensitivity to dipyridamole, aspirin, or any component of their formulation; allergy to NSAIDs; asthma, rhinitis, and nasal polyps; bleeding disorders (factor VII or IX deficiencies); children <16 years of age with viral infections; pregnancy (especially third trimester)

Warnings/Precautions Patients who consume ≥3 alcoholic drinks per day are at risk of bleeding. Cautious use in patients with inherited or acquired bleeding disorders including those of liver disease or vitamin K deficiency. Watch for signs and symptoms of GI ulcers and bleeding. Avoid use in patients with active peptic ulcer disease. Discontinue use if dizziness, tinnitus, or impaired hearing occurs. Stop 1-2 weeks before elective surgical procedures to avoid bleeding. Use caution in the elderly who are at high risk for adverse events. Cautious use in patients with hypotension, patients with unstable angina, recent MI, and hepatic dysfunction. Avoid in patients with severe renal failure. Safety and efficacy in children have not been established.

Drug Interactions See Aspirin *on page 119* and Dipyridamole *on page 401*

Drug Uptake

Aggrenox™:

Half-life, elimination: Salicylic acid: 1.71 hours

Time to peak: 0.63 hours

Aspirin: See Aspirin *on page 119*

Dipyridamole:

Half-life, elimination: 13.6 hours

Time to peak: 2 hours

Pregnancy Risk Factor B (dipyridamole); D (aspirin)

Generic Available No

Aspirin and Meprobamate (AS pir in & me proe BA mate)

U.S. Brand Names Equagesic®

Canadian Brand Names 292 MEP®

Pharmacologic Category Antianxiety Agent, Miscellaneous

Synonyms Meprobamate and Aspirin

Use Adjunct to treatment of skeletal muscular disease in patients exhibiting tension and/or anxiety

Local Anesthetic/Vasoconstrictor Precautions No information available to require special precautions

Effects on Dental Treatment Use with caution in impaired hepatic function; use with caution in patients with platelet and bleeding disorders, renal dysfunction, erosive gastritis, or peptic ulcer disease, previous nonreaction does not guarantee future safe taking of medication; do not use aspirin in children <16 years of age for chickenpox or flu symptoms due to the association with Reye's syndrome. Avoid aspirin, if possible, for 1 week prior to surgery due to possibility of postoperative bleeding

Elderly are a high-risk population for adverse effects from nonsteroidal anti-inflammatory agents. As much as 60% of elderly with GI complications to NSAIDs can develop peptic ulceration and/or hemorrhage asymptomatically. Also, concomitant disease and drug use contribute to the risk for GI adverse effects. Use lowest effective dose for shortest period possible. Consider renal function decline with age. Use with caution in patients with history of asthma

Restrictions C-IV

Dosage Oral: 1 tablet 3-4 times/day

Other Adverse Effects See Aspirin *on page 119* and Meprobamate *on page 768*

Drug Interactions See Aspirin *on page 119* and Meprobamate *on page 768*

Drug Uptake See Aspirin *on page 119* and Meprobamate *on page 768*

Pregnancy Risk Factor D

Generic Available Yes

Comments Abrupt discontinuation after sustained use (generally >10 days) may cause withdrawal symptoms

Selected Readings

Desjardins PJ, Cooper SA, Gallegos TL, et al, "The Relative Analgesic Efficacy of Propiram Fumarate, Codeine Aspirin, and Placebo in Postimpaction Dental Pain," *J Clin Pharmacol*, 1984, 24(1):35-42.

Forbes JA, Butterworth GA, Burchfield WH, et al, "Evaluation of Ketorolac, Aspirin, and an Acetaminophen-Codeine Combination in Postoperative Oral Surgery Pain," *Pharmacotherapy*, 1990, 10(6 Pt 2):77S-93S.

Forbes JA, Keller CK, Smith JW, et al, "Analgesic Effect of Naproxen Sodium, Codeine, a Naproxen-Codeine Combination and Aspirin on the Postoperative Pain of Oral Surgery," *Pharmacotherapy*, 1986, 6(5):211-8.

Aspirin Free Anacin® Maximum Strength [OTC] *see* Acetaminophen *on page 26*

Astelin® *see* Azelastine *on page 136*

AsthmaHaler® *see* Epinephrine *on page 438*

AsthmaNefrin® *see* Epinephrine, Racemic *on page 440*
Astramorph™ PF *see* Morphine Sulfate *on page 829*
Atacand® *see* Candesartan *on page 208*
Atacand HCT™ *see* Candesartan and Hydrochlorothiazide *on page 209*
Atapryl® *see* Selegiline *on page 1079*
Atarax® *see* HydrOXYzine *on page 616*

Atenolol (a TEN oh lole)

Related Information

Cardiovascular Diseases *on page 1308*

U.S. Brand Names Tenormin®

Canadian Brand Names Apo®-Atenol; Gen-Atenolol; Novo-Atenol; Nu-Atenol; PMS-Atenolol; Rhoxal-atenolol; Scheinpharm Atenolol; Tenolin; Tenormin®

Mexican Brand Names Blokium®; Tenormin®

Pharmacologic Category Beta Blocker, $Beta_1$ Selective

Use Treatment of hypertension, alone or in combination with other agents; management of angina pectoris, postmyocardial infarction patients

Unlabeled/Investigational: Acute alcohol withdrawal, supraventricular and ventricular arrhythmias, and migraine headache prophylaxis

Local Anesthetic/Vasoconstrictor Precautions No information available to require special precautions

Effects on Dental Treatment Noncardioselective beta-blockers (ie, propranolol, nadolol) enhance the pressor response to epinephrine, resulting in hypertension and bradycardia. This has not been reported for atenolol, a cardioselective beta-blocker. Therefore, local anesthetic with vasoconstrictor can be safely used in patients medicated with atenolol. Many nonsteroidal anti-inflammatory drugs such as ibuprofen and indomethacin can reduce the hypotensive effect of beta-blockers after 3 or more weeks of therapy with the NSAID. Short-term NSAID use (ie, 3 days) requires no special precautions in patients taking beta-blockers.

Dosage

Oral:

Children: 0.8-1 mg/kg/dose given daily; range of 0.8-1.5 mg/kg/day; maximum dose: 2 mg/kg/day

Adults:

Hypertension: 50 mg once daily, may increase to 100 mg/day. Doses >100 mg are unlikely to produce any further benefit.

Angina pectoris: 50 mg once daily, may increase to 100 mg/day. Some patients may require 200 mg/day.

Postmyocardial infarction: Follow I.V. dose with 100 mg/day or 50 mg twice daily for 6-9 days postmyocardial infarction.

I.V.:

Hypertension: Dosages of 1.25-5 mg every 6-12 hours have been used in short-term management of patients unable to take oral enteral beta-blockers

Postmyocardial infarction: Early treatment: 5 mg slow I.V. over 5 minutes; may repeat in 10 minutes. If both doses are tolerated, may start oral atenolol 50 mg every 12 hours or 100 mg/day for 6-9 days postmyocardial infarction.

Dosing interval for oral atenolol in renal impairment:

Cl_{cr} 15-35 mL/minute: Administer 50 mg/day maximum.

Cl_{cr} <15 mL/minute: Administer 50 mg every other day maximum.

Hemodialysis: Moderately dialyzable (20% to 50%) via hemodialysis; administer dose postdialysis or administer 25-50 mg supplemental dose.

Peritoneal dialysis: Elimination is not enhanced; supplemental dose is not necessary.

Mechanism of Action Competitively blocks response to beta-adrenergic stimulation, selectively blocks $beta_1$-receptors with little or no effect on $beta_2$-receptors except at high doses

Other Adverse Effects 1% to 10%:

Cardiovascular: Persistent bradycardia, hypotension, chest pain, edema, heart failure, second- or third-degree AV block, Raynaud's phenomenon

Central nervous system: Dizziness, fatigue, insomnia, lethargy, confusion, mental impairment, depression, headache, nightmares

Gastrointestinal: Constipation, diarrhea, nausea

Genitourinary: Impotence

Miscellaneous: Cold extremities

Drug Interactions

Increased Effect/Toxicity: Atenolol may increase the effects of other drugs which slow AV conduction (digoxin, verapamil, diltiazem), alpha-blockers (prazosin, terazosin), and alpha-adrenergic stimulants (epinephrine, phenylephrine). Atenolol may mask the tachycardia from hypoglycemia caused by insulin and oral hypoglycemics. In patients receiving concurrent therapy, the risk of hypertensive crisis is increased when either clonidine or the beta-blocker is withdrawn. Reserpine has been shown to enhance the effect of atenolol. Beta-blockers may increase the action or levels of disopyramide, nondepolarizing muscle relaxants, and theophylline although the effects are difficult to predict.

(Continued)

Atenolol *(Continued)*

Decreased Effect: Decreased effect of atenolol with aluminum salts, barbiturates, calcium salts, cholestyramine, colestipol, NSAIDs, penicillins (ampicillin), rifampin, salicylates, and sulfinpyrazone due to decreased bioavailability and plasma concentrations. Beta-blockers may decrease the effect of sulfonylureas.

Drug Uptake

Onset of action: Peak effect: Oral: 2-4 hours

Duration: Normal renal function: 12-24 hours

Absorption: Incomplete

Half-life, elimination: Beta:

Neonates: ≤35 hours; Mean: 16 hours

Children: 4.6 hours; children >10 years may have longer half-life (>5 hours) compared to children 5-10 years (<5 hours)

Adults: Normal renal function: 6-9 hours, longer with renal impairment; End-stage renal disease: 15-35 hours

Pregnancy Risk Factor D

Generic Available Yes: Tablet

Selected Readings

Foster CA and Aston SJ, "Propranolol-Epinephrine Interaction: A Potential Disaster," *Plast Reconstr Surg*, 1983, 72(1):74-8.

Wong DG, Spence JD, Lamki L, et al, "Effect of Nonsteroidal Anti-inflammatory Drugs on Control of Hypertension of Beta-Blockers and Diuretics," *Lancet*, 1986, 1(8488):997-1001.

Wynn RL, "Dental Nonsteroidal Anti-inflammatory Drugs and Prostaglandin-Based Drug Interactions-Part Two," *Gen Dent*, 1992, 40(2):104, 106, 108.

Wynn RL, "Epinephrine Interactions With Beta-Blockers," *Gen Dent*, 1994, 42(1):16, 18.

Atenolol and Chlorthalidone (a TEN oh lole & klor THAL i done)

U.S. Brand Names Tenoretic®

Canadian Brand Names Tenoretic®

Pharmacologic Category Antihypertensive Agent Combination

Synonyms Chlorthalidone and Atenolol

Use Treatment of hypertension with a cardioselective beta-blocker and a diuretic

Local Anesthetic/Vasoconstrictor Precautions No information available to require special precautions

Effects on Dental Treatment Noncardioselective beta-blockers (ie, propranolol, nadolol) enhance the pressor response to epinephrine, resulting in hypertension and bradycardia. This has not been reported for atenolol, a cardioselective beta-blocker. Therefore local anesthetic with vasoconstrictor can be safely used in patients medicated with atenolol. Many nonsteroidal anti-inflammatory drugs such as ibuprofen and indomethacin can reduce the hypotensive effect of beta-blockers after 3 or more weeks of therapy with the NSAID. Short-term NSAID use (ie, 3 days) requires no special precautions in patients taking beta-blockers.

Dosage Adults: Oral: Initial: One (50) tablet once daily, then individualize dose until optimal dose is achieved

Other Adverse Effects See Atenolol *on page 125* and Chlorthalidone *on page 277*

Drug Uptake See Atenolol *on page 125* and Chlorthalidone *on page 277*

Pregnancy Risk Factor D

Generic Available Yes

Comments May contain povidone as inactive ingredient

Selected Readings

Foster CA and Aston SJ, "Propranolol-Epinephrine Interaction: A Potential Disaster," *Plast Reconstr Surg*, 1983, 72(1):74-8.

Wong DG, Spence JD, Lamki L, et al, "Effect of Nonsteroidal Anti-inflammatory Drugs on Control of Hypertension of Beta-Blockers and Diuretics," *Lancet*, 1986, 1(8488):997-1001.

Wynn RL, "Dental Nonsteroidal Anti-inflammatory Drugs and Prostaglandin-Based Drug Interactions - Part Two," *Gen Dent*, 1992, 40(2):104, 106, 108.

Wynn RL, "Epinephrine Interactions With Beta-Blockers," *Gen Dent*, 1994, 42(1):16, 18.

Atgam® *see* Lymphocyte Immune Globulin *on page 737*

Ativan® *see* Lorazepam *on page 729*

Atolone® *see* Triamcinolone *on page 1197*

Atorvastatin (a TORE va sta tin)

U.S. Brand Names Lipitor®

Canadian Brand Names Lipitor®

Mexican Brand Names Lipitor®

Pharmacologic Category Antilipemic Agent, HMG-CoA Reductase Inhibitor

Use Adjunct to diet for the reduction of elevated total and LDL cholesterol, apolipoprotein B, and triglyceride levels in patients with hypercholesterolemia (types IIA, IIB, and IIC); adjunctive therapy to diet for treatment of elevated serum triglyceride levels (type IV); treatment of primary dysbetalipoproteinemia (type III) in patients who do not respond adequately to diet; to increase HDL cholesterol in patients with primary hypercholesterolemia (heterozygous familial and nonfamilial) and mixed dyslipidemia (Fredrickson types IIa and IIb). Also may be used in hypercholesterolemic patients without clinically evident heart disease to reduce the risk of myocardial infarction, to reduce the risk for revascularization, and reduce the risk of death due to cardiovascular causes

Local Anesthetic/Vasoconstrictor Precautions No information available to require special precautions

Effects on Dental Treatment No effects or complications reported

Dosage Adults: Oral: Initial: 10-20 mg once daily; patients requiring >45% reduction in LDL-C may be started at 40 mg once daily; titrate initial dose to achieve goal (maximum dose: 80 mg once daily)

Dosing adjustment in hepatic impairment: Do not use in active liver disease. Adults: Oral: Initial: 10 mg once daily, titrate up to 80 mg/day if needed

Mechanism of Action Inhibitor of 3-hydroxy-3-methylglutaryl coenzyme A (HMG-CoA) reductase, the rate limiting enzyme in cholesterol synthesis (reduces the production of mevalonic acid from HMG-CoA); this then results in a compensatory increase in the expression of LDL receptors on hepatocyte membranes and a stimulation of LDL catabolism

Other Adverse Effects

>10%: Central nervous system: Headache (3% to 17%)

2% to 10%:

Cardiovascular: Chest pain, peripheral edema

Central nervous system: Weakness (0% to 4%), insomnia, dizziness

Dermatologic: Rash (1% to 4%)

Gastrointestinal: Abdominal pain (0% to 4%), constipation (0% to 3%), diarrhea (0% to 4%), dyspepsia (1% to 3%), flatulence (1% to 3%), nausea

Genitourinary: Urinary tract infection

Neuromuscular & skeletal: Arthralgia (0% to 5%), myalgia (0% to 6%), back pain (0% to 4%), arthritis

Respiratory: Sinusitis (0% to 6%), pharyngitis (0% to 3%), bronchitis, rhinitis

Miscellaneous: Infection (2% to 10%), flu-like syndrome (0% to 3%), allergic reaction (0% to 3%)

<2% (Limited to important or life-threatening): Pneumonia, dyspnea, epistaxis, face edema, fever, photosensitivity, malaise, edema, gastroenteritis, elevated transaminases, colitis, vomiting, gastritis, xerostomia, rectal hemorrhage, esophagitis, eructation, glossitis, stomatitis, anorexia, increased appetite, biliary pain, cheilitis, duodenal ulcer, dysphagia, enteritis, melena, gingival hemorrhage, tenesmus, hepatitis, pancreatitis, cholestatic jaundice, paresthesia, somnolence, abnormal dreams, decreased libido, emotional lability, incoordination, peripheral neuropathy, torticollis, facial paralysis, hyperkinesia, depression, hypesthesia, hypertonia, leg cramps, bursitis, myasthenia, myositis, tendinous contracture, pruritus, alopecia, dry skin, urticaria, acne, eczema, seborrhea, skin ulcer, cystitis, hematuria, impotence, dysuria, nocturia, epididymitis, fibrocystic breast disease, vaginal hemorrhage, nephritis, abnormal urination, amblyopia, tinnitus, deafness, glaucoma, taste loss, taste perversion, palpitation, vasodilation, syncope, migraine, postural hypotension, phlebitis, arrhythmia, angina, hypertension, hyperglycemia, gout, weight gain, hypoglycemia, ecchymosis, anemia, lymphadenopathy, thrombocytopenia, petechiae, pharyngitis, rhinitis, myopathy

Additional class-related events or case reports (not necessarily reported with atorvastatin therapy): Myopathy, increased CPK (>10x normal), rhabdomyolysis, renal failure (secondary to rhabdomyolysis), alteration in taste, impaired extraocular muscle movement, facial paresis, tremor, memory loss, vertigo, paresthesia, peripheral neuropathy, peripheral nerve palsy, anxiety, depression, psychic disturbance, hypersensitivity reaction, angioedema, anaphylaxis, systemic lupus erythematosus-like syndrome, polymyalgia rheumatica, dermatomyositis, vasculitis, purpura, thrombocytopenia, leukopenia, hemolytic anemia, positive ANA, increased ESR, eosinophilia, arthritis, urticaria, photosensitivity, fever, chills, flushing, malaise, dyspnea, rash, toxic epidermal necrolysis, erythema multiforme, Stevens-Johnson syndrome, pancreatitis, hepatitis, cholestatic jaundice, fatty liver, cirrhosis, fulminant hepatic necrosis, hepatoma, anorexia, vomiting, alopecia, nodules, skin discoloration, dryness of skin/mucous membranes, nail changes, gynecomastia, decreased libido, erectile dysfunction, impotence, cataracts, ophthalmoplegia, elevated transaminases, increased alkaline phosphatase, increased GGT, hyperbilirubinemia, thyroid dysfunction

Warnings/Precautions Liver function must be monitored by periodic laboratory assessment. Rhabdomyolysis with acute renal failure has occurred. Risk is dose-related and is increased with concurrent use of lipid-lowering agents which may cause rhabdomyolysis (gemfibrozil, fibric acid derivatives, or niacin at doses ≥1 g/day) or during concurrent use with potent CYP3A3/4 inhibitors (including amiodarone, clarithromycin, cyclosporine, erythromycin, itraconazole, ketoconazole, nefazodone, grapefruit juice in large quantities, verapamil, or protease inhibitors such as indinavir, nelfinavir, or ritonavir). Weigh the risk versus benefit when combining any of these drugs with atorvastatin. Discontinue in any patient experiencing an acute or serious condition predisposing to renal failure secondary to rhabdomyolysis.

Drug Interactions CYP3A3/4 enzyme substrate

(Continued)

Atorvastatin *(Continued)*

Increased Effect/Toxicity: Inhibitors of CYP3A3/4 (amiodarone, amprenavir, clarithromycin, cyclosporine, diltiazem, fluvoxamine, erythromycin, fluconazole, indinavir, itraconazole, ketoconazole, miconazole, nefazodone, nelfinavir, ritonavir, troleandomycin, and verapamil) may increase atorvastatin blood levels and may increase the risk of atorvastatin-induced myopathy and rhabdomyolysis. The risk of myopathy and rhabdomyolysis due to concurrent use of a CYP3A3/4 inhibitor with atorvastatin is probably less than lovastatin or simvastatin. Cyclosporine, clofibrate, fenofibrate, gemfibrozil, and niacin also may increase the risk of myopathy and rhabdomyolysis. The effect/toxicity of levothyroxine may be increased by atorvastatin. Levels of digoxin and ethinyl estradiol may be increased by atorvastatin.

Decreased Effect: Colestipol, antacids decreased plasma concentrations but effect on LDL cholesterol was not altered. Cholestyramine may decrease absorption of atorvastatin when administered concurrently.

Drug Uptake

Onset of action: Initial changes: 3-5 days; Maximal reduction in plasma cholesterol and triglycerides: 2 weeks

Absorption: Rapid

Half-life, elimination: Parent drug: 14 hours

Time to peak: 1-2 hours

Pregnancy Risk Factor X

Generic Available No

Selected Readings Siedlik PH, Olson, SC, Yang BB, et al, "Erythromycin Coadministration Increases Plasma Atorvastatin Concentrations," *J Clin Pharmacol*, 1999, 39(5):501-4.

Atovaquone (a TOE va kwone)

Related Information

Systemic Viral Diseases *on page 1354*

U.S. Brand Names Mepron™

Canadian Brand Names Mepron®

Pharmacologic Category Antiprotozoal

Use Acute oral treatment of mild to moderate *Pneumocystis carinii* pneumonia (PCP) in patients who are intolerant to co-trimoxazole; treatment/suppression of *Toxoplasma gondii* encephalitis, primary prophylaxis of HIV-infected persons at high risk for developing *Toxoplasma gondii* encephalitis

Local Anesthetic/Vasoconstrictor Precautions No information available to require special precautions

Effects on Dental Treatment No effects or complications reported

Dosage Adults: Oral: 750 mg 2 times/day with food for 21 days

Mechanism of Action Mechanism has not been fully elucidated; may inhibit electron transport in mitochondria inhibiting metabolic enzymes

Other Adverse Effects

>10%:

- Central nervous system: Headache, fever, insomnia, anxiety
- Dermatologic: Rash
- Gastrointestinal: Nausea, diarrhea, vomiting
- Respiratory: Cough

1% to 10%:

- Central nervous system: Dizziness
- Dermatologic: Pruritus
- Endocrine & metabolic: Hypoglycemia, hyponatremia
- Gastrointestinal: Abdominal pain, constipation, anorexia, heartburn
- Hematologic: Anemia, neutropenia, leukopenia
- Hepatic: Elevated amylase and liver enzymes
- Neuromuscular & skeletal: Weakness
- Renal: Elevated BUN/creatinine
- Respiratory: Cough
- Miscellaneous: Oral *Monilia* **Note:** Adverse reaction statistics have been compiled from studies including patients with advanced HIV disease; consequently, it is difficult to distinguish reactions attributed to atovaquone from those caused by the underlying disease or a combination, thereof.

Drug Interactions

Increased Effect/Toxicity: Possible increased toxicity with other highly protein-bound drugs.

Decreased Effect: Rifamycins (rifampin) used concurrently decrease the steady-state plasma concentrations of atovaquone.

Drug Uptake

Absorption: Significantly increased with a high-fat meal

Half-life, elimination: 2-3 days

Pregnancy Risk Factor C

Generic Available No

Atovaquone and Proguanil (a TOE va kwone & pro GWA nil)

U.S. Brand Names Malarone™

Canadian Brand Names Malarone™

Pharmacologic Category Antimalarial Agent

Synonyms Proguanil and Atovaquone

Use Prevention or treatment of acute, uncomplicated *P. falciparum* malaria

Local Anesthetic/Vasoconstrictor Precautions No information available to require special precautions

Effects on Dental Treatment No effects or complications reported

Dosage Oral (doses given in mg of atovaquone and proguanil):

Children (dosage based on body weight):

Prevention of malaria: Start 1-2 days prior to entering a malaria-endemic area, continue throughout the stay and for 7 days after returning. Take as a single dose, once daily.

11-20 kg: Atovaquone/proguanil 62.5 mg/25 mg
21-30 kg: Atovaquone/proguanil 125 mg/50 mg
31-40 kg: Atovaquone/proguanil 187.5 mg/75 mg
>40 kg: Atovaquone/proguanil 250 mg/100 mg

Treatment of acute malaria: Take as a single dose, once daily for 3 consecutive days.

11-20 kg: Atovaquone/proguanil 250 mg/100 mg
21-30 kg: Atovaquone/proguanil 500 mg/200 mg
31-40 kg: Atovaquone/proguanil 750 mg/300 mg
>40 kg: Atovaquone/proguanil 1 g/400 mg

Adults:

Prevention of malaria: Atovaquone/proguanil 250 mg/100 mg once daily; start 1-2 days prior to entering a malaria-endemic area, continue throughout the stay and for 7 days after returning

Treatment of acute malaria: Atovaquone/proguanil 1 g/400 mg as a single dose, once daily for 3 consecutive days

Dosage adjustment in renal/hepatic impairment: No information available, use with caution.

Elderly: Use with caution due to possible decrease in renal and hepatic function, as well as possible decreases in cardiac function, concomitant diseases, or other drug therapy.

Mechanism of Action

Atovaquone: Selectively inhibits parasite mitochondrial electron transport.

Proguanil: The metabolite cycloguanil inhibits dihydrofolate reductase, disrupting deoxythymidylate synthesis. Together, atovaquone/cycloguanil affect the erythrocytic and exoerythrocytic stages of development.

Other Adverse Effects

>10%: Gastrointestinal: Abdominal pain (17%), nausea (12%), vomiting (12% adults, 10% to 13% children)

1% to 10%:

Central nervous system: Headache (10%), dizziness (5%)
Dermatologic: Pruritus (6% children)
Gastrointestinal: Diarrhea (8%), anorexia (5%)
Neuromuscular & skeletal: Weakness (8%)

Adverse reactions reported in placebo-controlled clinical trials when used for prophylaxis. In general, reactions were similar to those seen with placebo:

>10%:

Central nervous system: Headache (22% adults, 19% children)
Gastrointestinal: Abdominal pain (33% children)
Neuromuscular & skeletal: Myalgia (12% adults)

1% to 10%:

Central nervous system: Fever (5% adults, 6% children)
Gastrointestinal: Abdominal pain (9% adults), diarrhea (6% adults, 2% children), dyspepsia (3% adults), gastritis (3% adults), vomiting (1% adults, 7% children)
Neuromuscular & skeletal: Back pain (8% adults)
Respiratory: Upper respiratory tract infection (8% adults), cough (6% adults, 9% children)
Miscellaneous: Flu-like syndrome (2% adults, 9% children)

In addition, 54% of adults in the placebo-controlled trials reported any adverse event (65% for placebo) and 60% of children reported adverse events (62% for placebo).

Drug Interactions Proguanil: CYP2C19 enzyme substrate

Decreased Effect: Metoclopramide decreases bioavailability of atovaquone. Rifampin decreases atovaquone levels by 50%. Tetracycline decreases plasma concentrations of atovaquone by 40%.

Drug Uptake

Absorption: Atovaquone has low aqueous solubility, when taken with food the bioavailability is 23%; proguanil is extensively absorbed

Half-life, elimination: Atovaquone 2-3 days in adults, 1-2 days in children; proguanil 12-21 hours

(Continued)

Atovaquone and Proguanil *(Continued)*

Pregnancy Risk Factor C

Generic Available No

Atridox™ *see* Doxycycline Hyclate Periodontal Extended-Release Liquid *on page 421*

Atromid-S® *see* Clofibrate *on page 305*

Atropine (A troe peen)

Related Information

Cardiovascular Diseases *on page 1308*

U.S. Brand Names Atropine-Care®; Atropisol®; Isopto® Atropine; Sal-Tropine™

Canadian Brand Names Atropisol®; Isopto® Atropine

Mexican Brand Names Lomotil®; Tropyn Z

Pharmacologic Category Anticholinergic Agent; Anticholinergic Agent, Ophthalmic; Antidote; Antispasmodic Agent, Gastrointestinal; Ophthalmic Agent, Mydriatic

Synonyms Atropine Sulfate

Use Preoperative medication to inhibit salivation and secretions; treatment of symptomatic sinus bradycardia; antidote for organophosphate pesticide poisoning; to produce mydriasis and cycloplegia for examination of the retina and optic disc and accurate measurement of refractive errors; uveitis; AV block (nodal level); ventricular asystole; treatment of GI disorders (eg, peptic ulcer disease, irritable bowel syndrome, hypermotility of colon)

Local Anesthetic/Vasoconstrictor Precautions No information available to require special precautions

Effects on Dental Treatment >10%: Xerostomia

Dosage

Neonates, Infants, and Children: Doses <0.1 mg have been associated with paradoxical bradycardia.

Preanesthetic: Oral, I.M., I.V., S.C.:

<5 kg: 0.02 mg/kg/dose 30-60 minutes preop then every 4-6 hours as needed. Use of a minimum dosage of 0.1 mg in neonates <5 kg will result in dosages >0.02 mg/kg. There is no documented minimum dosage in this age group.

>5 kg: 0.01-0.02 mg/kg/dose to a maximum 0.4 mg/dose 30-60 minutes preop; minimum dose: 0.1 mg

Bradycardia: I.V., intratracheal: 0.02 mg/kg, minimum dose 0.1 mg, maximum single dose: 0.5 mg in children and 1 mg in adolescents; may repeat in 5-minute intervals to a maximum total dose of 1 mg in children or 2 mg in adolescents. (**Note:** For intratracheal administration, the dosage must be diluted with normal saline to a total volume of 1-2 mL). When treating bradycardia in neonates, reserve use for those patients unresponsive to improved oxygenation and epinephrine.

Children:

Mydriasis, cycloplegia (preprocedure): Ophthalmic: 0.5% solution: Instill 1-2 drops twice daily for 1-3 days before the procedure

Uveitis: Ophthalmic: 0.5% solution: Instill 1-2 drops up to 3 times/day

Adults (doses <0.5 mg have been associated with paradoxical bradycardia):

Asystole or pulseless electrical activity: I.V.: 1 mg; repeat in 3-5 minutes if asystole persists; total dose of 0.04 mg/kg; may give intratracheally in 10 mL NS (intratracheal dose should be 2-2.5 times the I.V. dose)

Preanesthetic: I.M., I.V., S.C.: 0.4-0.6 mg 30-60 minutes preop and repeat every 4-6 hours as needed

Bradycardia: I.V.: 0.5-1 mg every 5 minutes, not to exceed a total of 3 mg or 0.04 mg/kg; may give intratracheally in 10 mL NS (intratracheal dose should be 2-2.5 times the I.V. dose)

Neuromuscular blockade reversal: I.V.: 25-30 mcg/kg 60 seconds before neostigmine or 7-10 mcg/kg in combination with edrophonium

Organophosphate or carbamate poisoning: I.V.: 1-2 mg/dose every 10-20 minutes until atropine effect (dry flushed skin, tachycardia, mydriasis, fever) is observed, then every 1-4 hours for at least 24 hours; up to 50 mg in first 24 hours and 2 g over several days may be given in cases of severe intoxication

GI disorders: Oral: 0.4-0.6 mg every 4-6 hours

Ophthalmic:

Solution: 1%:

Mydriasis, cycloplegia (preprocedure): Instill 1-2 drops 1 hour before the procedure.

Uveitis: Instill 1-2 drops 4 times/day.

Ointment: Uveitis: Apply a small amount in the conjunctival sac up to 3 times/day. Compress the lacrimal sac by digital pressure for 1-3 minutes after instillation.

Mechanism of Action Blocks the action of acetylcholine at parasympathetic sites in smooth muscle, secretory glands, and the CNS; increases cardiac output, dries secretions, antagonizes histamine and serotonin

Other Adverse Effects

>10%:

Dermatologic: Dry, hot skin
Gastrointestinal: Impaired GI motility, constipation, xerostomia and throat
Local: Irritation at injection site
Respiratory: Dry nose
Miscellaneous: Diaphoresis (decreased)

1% to 10%:

Dermatologic: Increased sensitivity to light
Endocrine & metabolic: Decreased flow of breast milk
Gastrointestinal: Dysphagia

Contraindications Hypersensitivity to atropine sulfate or any component of the formulation; angle-closure glaucoma; tachycardia; thyrotoxicosis; obstructive disease of the GI tract; obstructive uropathy; clarithromycin, erythromycin, ketoconazole, fluconazole, and itraconazole

Warnings/Precautions Use with caution in children with spastic paralysis; use with caution in elderly patients. Low doses cause a paradoxical decrease in heart rates. Some commercial products contain sodium metabisulfite, which can cause allergic-type reactions. May accumulate with multiple inhalational administration, particularly in the elderly. Heat prostration may occur in hot weather. Use with caution in patients with autonomic neuropathy, prostatic hypertrophy, hyperthyroidism, CHF, cardiac arrhythmias, chronic lung disease, biliary tract disease.

Drug Interactions

Increased Effect/Toxicity: Amantadine, antihistamines, phenothiazines, and TCAs may increase anticholinergic effects of atropine when used concurrently. Sympathomimetic amines may cause tachyarrhythmias; avoid concurrent use.

Decreased Effect: Effect of some phenothiazines may be antagonized. Levodopa effects may be decreased (limited clinical validation). Drugs with cholinergic mechanisms (metoclopramide, cisapride, bethanechol) decrease anticholinergic effects of atropine.

Drug Uptake

Onset of action: I.V.: Rapid
Absorption: Complete and well from all dosage forms
Half-life, elimination: 2-3 hours

Pregnancy Risk Factor C

Generic Available Yes

Atropine-Care® *see* Atropine *on page 130*

Atropine Sulfate Dental Tablets

(A troe peen SUL fate DEN tal TAB lets)

Related Information

Atropine *on page 130*

U.S. Brand Names Sal-Tropine™

Pharmacologic Category Anticholinergic Agent

Use Reduce salivation and bronchial secretions

Local Anesthetic/Vasoconstrictor Precautions No information available to require special precautions

Effects on Dental Treatment When used in therapeutic doses, causes significant xerostomia

Dosage Oral:

Children:

7-16 lbs: 0.1 mg
17-24 lbs: 0.15 mg
24-40 lbs: 0.2 mg
40-65 lbs: 0.3 mg
65-90 lbs: 0.4 mg
>90 lbs: 0.4 mg

Adults: 0.4 mg

Mechanism of Action Blocks the action of acetylcholine at parasympathetic sites in smooth muscle, secretory glands, and the CNS; increases cardiac output, dries secretions, antagonizes histamine and serotonin

Other Adverse Effects Frequency not defined (dose-related):

0.5 mg: Slight dryness of nose and mouth; bradycardia

1 mg: Increased dryness of nose and mouth; thirst; slowing then acceleration of heart rate; mydriasis

2 mg: Significant xerostomia; tachycardia with palpitations; mydriasis; slight blurring of vision; flushed, dry skin

5 mg: Increase in above symptoms plus disturbance of speech; difficulty swallowing; headache; hot, dry skin; restlessness with asthenia

10 mg: Above symptoms to extreme degree plus ataxia, excitement, disorientation, hallucinations, delirium, coma

In addition to the above, atropine may produce fever, particularly in children by inhibiting heat loss loss by evaporation; a scarlitiniform rash may occur

(Continued)

Atropine Sulfate Dental Tablets *(Continued)*

Contraindications Glaucoma; adhesions (synechiae) between the iris and lens of the eye; asthma

Warnings/Precautions Doses of 0.5-1 mg of atropine are mildly stimulating to the CNS. Larger doses may produce mental disturbances; still larger doses are CNS-depressant. Death from atropine poisoning, though rare, is usually due to paralysis of the medullary centers. Signs and symptoms of atropine overdose include mydriasis, tachycardia, decreased salivation, decreased sweating, diminished bowel sounds, urinary retention, hypertension, and vasodilation. CNS symptoms include anxiety, disorientation, hallucinations, hyperactivity, and convulsions or coma. Hyperthermia may occur.

Drug Interactions

Increased Effect: Atropine-induced mouth dryness may be increased if it is given with other drugs that have anticholinergic actions such as tricyclic antidepressants, antipsychotics, some antihistamines, and antiparkinsonism drugs

Decreased Effect: May interfere with absorption of other medications due to its actions on slowing GI motility and gastric emptying

Dosage Forms TAB, as sulfate: 0.4 mg

Atropisol® *see* Atropine *on page 130*

Atrovent® *see* Ipratropium *on page 651*

A/T/S® *see* Erythromycin, Topical *on page 454*

Attapulgite (at a PULL gite)

Related Information

Oral Nonviral Soft Tissue Ulcerations or Erosions *on page 1384*

U.S. Brand Names Children's Kaopectate® [OTC]; Diasorb® [OTC]; Kaopectate® Advanced Formula [OTC]; Kaopectate® Maximum Strength Caplets [OTC]; K-Pek® [OTC]

Canadian Brand Names Kaopectate®

Pharmacologic Category Antidiarrheal

Use Symptomatic treatment of diarrhea

Local Anesthetic/Vasoconstrictor Precautions No information available to require special precautions

Effects on Dental Treatment Do not give oral drugs concomitantly with Kaopectate® due to decreased GI absorption.

Dosage Adequate controlled clinical studies documenting the efficacy of attapulgite are lacking; its usage and dosage has been primarily empiric; the following are manufacturer's recommended dosages

Oral: Give after each bowel movement

Children:

- 3-6 years: 300-750 mg/dose; maximum dose: 7 doses/day or 2250 mg/day
- 6-12 years: 600-1500 mg/dose; maximum dose: 7 doses/day or 4500 mg/day

Children >12 years and Adults: 1200-3000 mg/dose; maximum dose: 8 doses/day or 9000 mg/day

Mechanism of Action Controls diarrhea because of its absorbent action

Other Adverse Effects The powder, if chronically inhaled, can cause pneumoconiosis, since it contains large amounts of silica

1% to 10%: Constipation (dose related)

Drug Interactions May decrease GI absorption of orally administered clindamycin, tetracyclines, penicillamine, digoxin

Drug Uptake Absorption: Not absorbed

Pregnancy Risk Factor B

Generic Available Yes

Attenuvax® *see* Measles Virus Vaccine, Live *on page 748*

Augmentin® *see* Amoxicillin and Clavulanate Potassium *on page 88*

Augmentin ES-600™ *see* Amoxicillin and Clavulanate Potassium *on page 88*

Auralgan® *see* Antipyrine and Benzocaine *on page 107*

Auranofin (au RANE oh fin)

Related Information

Rheumatoid Arthritis and Osteoarthritis *on page 1340*

U.S. Brand Names Ridaura®

Canadian Brand Names Ridaura®

Pharmacologic Category Gold Compound

Use Management of active stage of classic or definite rheumatoid arthritis in patients that do not respond to or tolerate other agents; psoriatic arthritis; adjunctive or alternative therapy for pemphigus

Local Anesthetic/Vasoconstrictor Precautions No information available to require special precautions

Effects on Dental Treatment No effects or complications reported

Dosage Oral:

Children: Initial: 0.1 mg/kg/day divided daily; usual maintenance: 0.15 mg/kg/day in 1-2 divided doses; maximum: 0.2 mg/kg/day in 1-2 divided doses

Adults: 6 mg/day in 1-2 divided doses; after 3 months may be increased to 9 mg/day in 3 divided doses; if still no response after 3 months at 9 mg/day, discontinue drug

Dosing adjustment in renal impairment:

Cl_{cr} 50-80 mL/minute: Reduce dose to 50%

Cl_{cr} <50 mL/minute: Avoid use

Mechanism of Action Exact mechanism unknown; gold is taken up by macrophages which results in inhibition of phagocytosis and lysosomal membrane stabilization. Other actions observed are decreased serum rheumatoid factor and alterations in immunoglobulins. Additionally, complement activation is decreased, prostaglandin synthesis is inhibited, and lysosomal enzyme activity is decreased.

Other Adverse Effects

>10%:

Dermatologic: Itching, rash
Gastrointestinal: Stomatitis
Ocular: Conjunctivitis
Renal: Proteinuria

1% to 10%:

Dermatologic: Urticaria, alopecia
Gastrointestinal: Glossitis
Hematologic: Eosinophilia, leukopenia, thrombocytopenia
Renal: Hematuria

Drug Interactions Toxicity of penicillamine, antimalarials, hydroxychloroquine, cytotoxic agents, and immunosuppressants may be increased.

Drug Uptake

Onset of action: Delayed; therapeutic response may require 3-4 months
Absorption: Oral: ~20% gold in dose is absorbed
Duration: Prolonged
Half-life, elimination: 21-31 days (dose-dependent)
Time to peak: ~2 hours

Pregnancy Risk Factor C

Generic Available No

Auro® Ear Drops [OTC] *see* Carbamide Peroxide *on page 218*

Aurolate® *see* Gold Sodium Thiomalate *on page 564*

Aurothioglucose (aur oh thye oh GLOO kose)

Related Information

Rheumatoid Arthritis and Osteoarthritis *on page 1340*

U.S. Brand Names Solganal®

Canadian Brand Names Solganal®

Pharmacologic Category Gold Compound

Use Adjunctive treatment in adult and juvenile active rheumatoid arthritis; alternative or adjunct in treatment of pemphigus; psoriatic patients who do not respond to NSAIDs

Local Anesthetic/Vasoconstrictor Precautions No information available to require special precautions

Effects on Dental Treatment No effects or complications reported

Dosage I.M.: Doses should initially be given at weekly intervals

Children 6-12 years: Initial: 0.25 mg/kg/dose first week; increment at 0.25 mg/kg/dose increasing with each weekly dose; maintenance: 0.75-1 mg/kg/dose weekly not to exceed 25 mg/dose to a total of 20 doses, then every 2-4 weeks

Adults: 10 mg first week; 25 mg second and third week; then 50 mg/week until 800 mg to 1 g cumulative dose has been given; if improvement occurs without adverse reactions, give 25-50 mg every 2-3 weeks, then every 3-4 weeks

Mechanism of Action Unknown, may decrease prostaglandin synthesis or may alter cellular mechanisms by inhibiting sulfhydryl systems

Other Adverse Effects

>10%:

Dermatologic: Itching, rash, exfoliative dermatitis, reddened skin
Gastrointestinal: Gingivitis, glossitis, metallic taste, stomatitis

1% to 10%: Renal: Proteinuria

Drug Interactions Toxicity of penicillamine, antimalarials, hydroxychloroquine, cytotoxic agents, and immunosuppressants may be increased.

Drug Uptake

Absorption: I.M.: Erratic and slow
Half-life, elimination: 3-27 days (dose-dependent)
Time to peak: 4-6 hours

Pregnancy Risk Factor C

Generic Available No

Auroto® *see* Antipyrine and Benzocaine *on page 107*

Autoplex® T *see* Anti-inhibitor Coagulant Complex *on page 107*
Avagard™ [OTC] *see* Chlorhexidine Gluconate *on page 263*
Avalide® *see* Irbesartan and Hydrochlorothiazide *on page 653*
Avandia® *see* Rosiglitazone *on page 1069*
Avapro® *see* Irbesartan *on page 653*
AVC™ *see* Sulfanilamide *on page 1121*
Avelox® *see* Moxifloxacin *on page 832*
Aventyl® *see* Nortriptyline *on page 878*
Aviane™ *see* Combination Hormonal Contraceptives *on page 323*
Avinza™ *see* Morphine Sulfate *on page 829*
Avita® *see* Tretinoin, Topical *on page 1196*
Avitene® *see* Microfibrillar Collagen Hemostat *on page 808*
Avonex® *see* Interferon Beta-1a *on page 647*
Axert™ *see* Almotriptan *on page 54*
Axid® *see* Nizatidine *on page 874*
Axid® AR [OTC] *see* Nizatidine *on page 874*
Aygestin® *see* Norethindrone *on page 876*
Ayr® Baby Saline [OTC] *see* Sodium Chloride *on page 1094*
Ayr® Saline [OTC] *see* Sodium Chloride *on page 1094*

Azacitidine (ay za SYE ti deen)

Pharmacologic Category Antineoplastic Agent, Miscellaneous

Synonyms AZA-CR; 5-Azacytidine; 5-AZC; Ladakamycin; NSC-102816

Use Refractory acute lymphocytic and myelogenous leukemia; myelodysplastic syndrome

Local Anesthetic/Vasoconstrictor Precautions No information available to require special precautions

Effects on Dental Treatment No effects or complications reported

Restrictions Available through NCI (Group C) at 301-496-5725.

Other Adverse Effects

>10%:

Central nervous system: Coma (at doses of 300-750 mg/m^2)
Gastrointestinal: Nausea, vomiting, diarrhea, mucositis
Hematologic: Leukopenia, thrombocytopenia,

1% to 10%:

Cardiovascular: Hypotension,
Central nervous system: Coma
Dermatologic: Rash
Hepatic: Hepatic abnormalities (increased enzyme levels up to coma)
Renal: Renal toxicity (azotemia, hypophosphatemia, tubular acidosis)

Drug Uptake

Absorption: S.C.: Rapid and complete
Half-life, elimination: ~4 hours

Pregnancy Risk Factor C

Generic Available No

Azactam® *see* Aztreonam *on page 139*

Azatadine (a ZA ta deen)

U.S. Brand Names Optimine®

Canadian Brand Names Optimine®

Mexican Brand Names Idulamine®

Pharmacologic Category Antihistamine

Synonyms Azatadine Maleate

Use Treatment of perennial and seasonal allergic rhinitis and chronic urticaria

Local Anesthetic/Vasoconstrictor Precautions No information available to require special precautions

Effects on Dental Treatment This drug has atropine-like effects and the patient may experience drowsiness; dry mouth, nose, and throat.

Dosage Children >12 years and Adults: Oral: 1-2 mg twice daily

Mechanism of Action Piperidine-derivative antihistamine with both anticholinergic and antiserotonin activity; demonstrated to inhibit mediator release from human mast cells *in vitro*; mechanism of this action is suggested to prevent calcium entry into the mast cell through voltage-dependent calcium channels

Other Adverse Effects

>10%:

Central nervous system: Slight to moderate drowsiness
Respiratory: Thickening of bronchial secretions

1% to 10%:

Central nervous system: Headache, fatigue, nervousness, dizziness
Gastrointestinal: Appetite increase, weight gain, nausea, diarrhea, abdominal pain, xerostomia
Neuromuscular & skeletal: Arthralgia

Respiratory: Pharyngitis

Drug Interactions Increased Effect/Toxicity: Procarbazine, CNS depressants, tricyclic antidepressants, ethanol

Drug Uptake

Onset of action: 1-2 hours

Absorption: Rapid and extensive

Half-life, elimination: ~8.7 hours

Time to peak: 4 hours

Pregnancy Risk Factor B

Generic Available No

Azatadine and Pseudoephedrine

(a ZA ta deen & soo doe e FED rin)

U.S. Brand Names Rynatan® Tablet; Trinalin®

Canadian Brand Names Trinalin®

Pharmacologic Category Antihistamine/Decongestant Combination

Synonyms Pseudoephedrine and Azatadine

Use Perennial and seasonal allergic rhinitis and other allergic symptoms including urticaria

Local Anesthetic/Vasoconstrictor Precautions

Azatadine: No information available to require special precautions

Pseudoephedrine: Use with caution since pseudoephedrine is a sympathomimetic amine which could interact with epinephrine to cause a pressor response

Effects on Dental Treatment

Azatadine: This drug has atropine-like effects and the patient may experience drowsiness, and dry mouth, nose, and throat

Pseudoephedrine: Up to 10% of patients could experience tachycardia, palpitations, and xerostomia; use vasoconstrictor with caution

Dosage Adults: 1-2 mg twice daily

Other Adverse Effects See Azatadine *on page 134* and Pseudoephedrine *on page 1022*

Drug Uptake See Azatadine *on page 134* and Pseudoephedrine *on page 1022*

Pregnancy Risk Factor C

Generic Available No

Azathioprine (ay za THYE oh preen)

U.S. Brand Names Imuran®

Canadian Brand Names Alti-Azathioprine; Gen-Azathioprine; Imuran®

Mexican Brand Names Azatrilem; Imuran®

Pharmacologic Category Immunosuppressant Agent

Synonyms Azathioprine Sodium

Use Adjunct with other agents in prevention of rejection of solid organ transplants; also used in severe active rheumatoid arthritis unresponsive to other agents; other autoimmune diseases (ITP, SLE, MS, Crohn's disease); **azathioprine is an imidazolyl derivative of 6-mercaptopurine**

Local Anesthetic/Vasoconstrictor Precautions No information available to require special precautions

Effects on Dental Treatment No effects or complications reported

Dosage I.V. dose is equivalent to oral dose

Children and Adults: Renal transplantation: Oral, I.V.: 2-5 mg/kg/day to start, then 1-3 mg/kg/day maintenance

Adults: Rheumatoid arthritis: Oral: 1 mg/kg/day for 6-8 weeks; increase by 0.5 mg/kg every 4 weeks until response or up to 2.5 mg/kg/day

Mechanism of Action Antagonizes purine metabolism and may inhibit synthesis of DNA, RNA, and proteins; may also interfere with cellular metabolism and inhibit mitosis

Other Adverse Effects Dose reduction or temporary withdrawal allows reversal.

>10%:

- Central nervous system: Fever, chills
- Gastrointestinal: Nausea, vomiting, anorexia, diarrhea
- Hematologic: Thrombocytopenia, leukopenia, anemia
- Miscellaneous: Secondary infection

1% to 10%:

- Dermatologic: Rash
- Hematologic: Pancytopenia
- Hepatic: Hepatotoxicity

Drug Interactions

Increased Effect/Toxicity: Allopurinol may increase serum concentration of azathioprine's active metabolite (6-MP). Decrease azathioprine dose to $1/3$ to $1/4$ of normal dose. Azathioprine and ACE inhibitors may induce severe leukopenia. Azathioprine and methotrexate may result in elevated levels of the metabolite 6-MP.

Decreased Effect: Azathioprine and cyclosporine may result in a decrease in cyclosporine levels. Azathioprine and nondepolarizing neuromuscular blockers may cause the action of the neuromuscular blocker to be decreased or reversed.

(Continued)

Azathioprine *(Continued)*

Azathioprine and anticoagulants may result in decreased action of the anticoagulant.

Drug Uptake Half-life, elimination: Parent drug: 12 minutes; 6-mercaptopurine: 0.7-3 hours; End-stage renal disease: Slightly prolonged

Pregnancy Risk Factor D

Generic Available Yes

Azelaic Acid (a zeh LAY ik AS id)

U.S. Brand Names Azelex®; Finevin™

Mexican Brand Names Cutacelan®

Pharmacologic Category Topical Skin Product, Acne

Use *Acne vulgaris*: Topical treatment of mild to moderate inflammatory acne vulgaris

Local Anesthetic/Vasoconstrictor Precautions No information available to require special precautions

Effects on Dental Treatment No effects or complications reported

Dosage Topical: Adolescents >12 years and Adults: Acne vulgaris: After skin is thoroughly washed and patted dry, gently but thoroughly massage a thin film of azelaic acid cream into the affected areas twice daily, in the morning and evening. The duration of use can vary and depends on the severity of the acne. In the majority of patients with inflammatory lesions, improvement of the condition occurs within 4 weeks.

Mechanism of Action A dietary constituent normally found in whole grain cereals; can be formed endogenously; exact mechanism is not known; *in vitro*, azelaic acid possesses antimicrobial activity against *Propionibacterium acnes* and *Staphylococcus epidermidis*; may decrease microcomedo formation

Other Adverse Effects 1% to 10%:

Dermatologic: Pruritus, stinging

Local: Burning

Neuromuscular & skeletal: Paresthesia

Drug Uptake

Absorption: ~3% to 5% penetrates the stratum corneum; up to 10% is found in the epidermis and dermis; 4% is systemically absorbed

Half-life, elimination: 12 hours after topical dosing

Pregnancy Risk Factor B

Generic Available No

Azelastine (a ZEL as teen)

U.S. Brand Names Astelin®; Optivar™

Canadian Brand Names Astelin®

Mexican Brand Names Astelin®

Pharmacologic Category Antihistamine

Synonyms Azelastine Hydrochloride

Use

Nasal spray: Treatment of the symptoms of seasonal allergic rhinitis such as rhinorrhea, sneezing, and nasal pruritus in adults and children ≥5 years of age

Ophthalmic: Treatment of itching of the eye associated with seasonal allergic conjunctivitis

Local Anesthetic/Vasoconstrictor Precautions No information available to require special precautions

Effects on Dental Treatment

2% to 10%: Xerostomia

Chronic use of antihistamines will inhibit salivary flows particularly in elderly patients; may contribute to periodontal disease and oral discomfort.

Dosage

Nasal spray: Children ≥5 years and Adults: 2 sprays (137 mcg/spray) each nostril twice daily. Before initial use, the delivery system should be primed with 4 sprays or until a fine mist appears. If 3 or more days have elapsed since last use, the delivery system should be reprimed.

Ophthalmic: Instill 1 drop into affected eye(s) twice daily

Mechanism of Action Competes with histamine for histamine$_1$-receptor sites on effector cells in the GI tract, blood vessels, and respiratory tract which inhibits the symptoms associated with seasonal allergic rhinitis (ie, sneezing, pruritus, increased mucus production); when used intranasally, reduces hyper-reactivity of the airways; increases the motility of bronchial epithelial cilia, improving mucociliary transport

Other Adverse Effects

Nasal spray:

>10%:

Central nervous system: Headache (15%), somnolence (12%)

Gastrointestinal: Bitter taste (20%)

2% to 10%:

Central nervous system: Dizziness (2%), fatigue (2%)

Gastrointestinal: Nausea (3%), weight gain (2%), xerostomia (3%)
Respiratory: Nasal burning (4%), pharyngitis (4%), paroxysmal sneezing (3%), rhinitis (2%), epistaxis (2%)

<2%:

Cardiovascular: Flushing, hypertension, tachycardia
Central nervous system: Drowsiness, fatigue, vertigo, depression, nervousness, hypoesthesia, anxiety, depersonalization, sleep disorder, abnormal thinking, malaise
Dermatologic: Contact dermatitis, eczema, hair and follicle infection, furunculosis
Gastrointestinal: Constipation, gastroenteritis, glossitis, increased appetite, ulcerative stomatitis, vomiting, increased ALT, aphthous stomatitis, abdominal pain
Genitourinary: Urinary frequency, hematuria, albuminuria, amenorrhea
Neuromuscular & skeletal: Myalgia, vertigo, temporomandibular dislocation, hypoesthesia, hyperkinesia, back pain, extremity pain
Ocular: Conjunctivitis, watery eyes, eye pain
Respiratory: Bronchospasm, coughing, throat burning, laryngitis
Miscellaneous: Allergic reactions, viral infections

Ophthalmic:

>10%:

Central nervous system: Headache (15%)
Ocular: Transient burning/stinging (30%)

1% to 10%:

Central nervous system: Fatigue
Genitourinary: Bitter taste (10%)
Ocular: Conjunctivitis, eye pain, blurred vision (temporary)
Respiratory: Asthma, dyspnea, pharyngitis
Miscellaneous: Flu-like syndrome

Contraindications Hypersensitivity to azelastine or any component of the formulation

Warnings/Precautions Azelastine causes somnolence. Caution should be exercised when performing activities that require mental alertness. Concurrent use of ethanol or other CNS depressants with azelastine should be avoided. Avoid use of azelastine with other antihistamines unless advised by a physician.

Drug Interactions Increased Effect/Toxicity: May cause additive sedation when concomitantly administered with other CNS depressant medications; cimetidine can increase the AUC and C_{max} of azelastine by as much as 65%.

Drug Uptake

Onset of action: Peak effect: Nasal spray: 3 hours; Ophthalmic solution: 3 minutes
Duration: Nasal spray: 12 hours; Ophthalmic solution: 8 hours
Half-life, elimination: Azelastine 22 hours; desmethylazelastine 54 hours
Time to peak: 2-3 hours

Pregnancy Risk Factor C

Generic Available No

Comments Azelastine is absorbed systemically will cause sedation in some patients. Although this agent is clinically effective, the side effects of sedation, bitter taste, and high cost will limits its use in many patients.

Azelex® *see* Azelaic Acid *on page 136*

Azithromycin (az ith roe MYE sin)

Related Information

Antibiotic Prophylaxis, Preprocedural Guidelines for Dental Patients *on page 1344*

U.S. Brand Names Zithromax®; Zithromax® Z-PAK®

Canadian Brand Names Zithromax®; Zithromax® Z-PAK®

Mexican Brand Names Azitrocin®

Pharmacologic Category Antibiotic, Macrolide

Synonyms Azithromycin Dihydrate

Use

Dental: Alternate antibiotic in the treatment of common orofacial infections caused by aerobic gram-positive cocci and susceptible anaerobes; alternate antibiotic for the prevention of bacterial endocarditis in patients undergoing dental procedures

Medical:

Children: Treatment of acute otitis media due to *H. influenzae*, *M. catarrhalis*, or *S. pneumoniae*; pharyngitis/tonsillitis due to *S. pyogenes*

Adults:

Treatment of bacterial exacerbations of Chronic Obstructive Pulmonary Disease (COPD) due to *Hemophilus influenzae*, *Moraxella catarrhalis*, or *Streptococcus pneumoniae*

Treatment of mild to moderate upper and lower respiratory tract infections, infections of the skin and skin structure, and sexually transmitted diseases due to susceptible strains of *C. trachomatis*, *M. catarrhalis*, *H. influenzae*, *S. aureus*, *S. pneumoniae*, *Mycoplasma pneumoniae*, and *C. psittaci*; community-acquired pneumonia, pelvic inflammatory disease (PID)

(Continued)

Azithromycin *(Continued)*

Prevention (or to delay onset) of infection with *Mycobacterium avium* complex (MAC)

Prevention (or to delay onset) or treatment of MAC in patients with advanced HIV infection

Prophylaxis of bacterial endocarditis in patients who are allergic to penicillin and undergoing surgical procedures

Unlabeled/Investigational: Uncomplicated gonococcal pharyngitis of the cervix, urethra, and rectum caused by *N. gonorrhoeae*; gonococcal pharyngitis due to *N. gonorrhoeae*; chlamydial infections due to *C. trachomatis*

Local Anesthetic/Vasoconstrictor Precautions No information available to require special precautions

Effects on Dental Treatment No effects or complications reported

Dosage

Oral:

Children ≥6 months:

Community-acquired pneumonia: 10 mg/kg on day 1 (maximum: 500 mg/day) followed by 5 mg/kg/day once daily on days 2-5 (maximum: 250 mg/day)

Otitis media:

1-day regimen: 30 mg/kg as a single dose

3-day regimen: 10 mg/kg once daily for 3 days

5-day regimen: 10 mg/kg on day 1 (maximum: 250 mg/day) followed by 5 mg/kg/day once daily on days 2-5 (maximum: 250 mg/day)

Children ≥2 years: Pharyngitis, tonsillitis: 12 mg/kg/day once daily for 5 days (maximum: 500 mg/day)

Children:

M. avium-infected patients with acquired immunodeficiency syndrome: Not currently FDA approved for use; 10-20 mg/kg/day once daily (maximum: 40 mg/kg/day) has been used in clinical trials; prophylaxis for first episode of MAC: 5-12 mg/kg/day once daily (maximum: 500 mg/day)

Prophylaxis for bacterial endocarditis: 15 mg/kg 1 hour before procedure

Adolescents ≥16 years and Adults:

Treatment of bacterial exacerbations of Chronic Obstructive Pulmonary Disease (COPD) due to *Haemophilus influenzae*, *Moraxella catarrhalis*, or *Streptococcus pneumoniae*: 500 mg/day for 3 days

Respiratory tract, skin and soft tissue infections: 500 mg on day 1 followed by 250 mg/day on days 2-5 (maximum: 500 mg/day)

Nongonococcal urethritis/cervicitis (due to *C. trachomatis*): 1 g as a single dose

Prophylaxis of disseminated *M. avium* complex disease in patient with advanced HIV infection: 1200 mg once weekly (may be combined with rifabutin)

Treatment of disseminated *M. avium* complex disease in patient with advanced HIV infection: 600 mg daily (in combination with ethambutol 15 mg/kg)

Prophylaxis for bacterial endocarditis: 500 mg 1 hour prior to the procedure

I.V.: Adults:

Community-acquired pneumonia: 500 mg as a single dose for at least 2 days, follow I.V. therapy by the oral route with a single daily dose of 500 mg to complete a 7-10 day course of therapy

Pelvic inflammatory disease (PID): 500 mg as a single dose for 1-2 days, follow I.V. therapy by the oral route with a single daily dose of 250 mg to complete a 7-day course of therapy

Mechanism of Action Inhibits RNA-dependent protein synthesis at the chain elongation step; binds to the 50S ribosomal subunit resulting in blockage of transpeptidation

Other Adverse Effects

1% to 10%: Gastrointestinal: Diarrhea, nausea, abdominal pain, cramping, vomiting (especially with high single-dose regimens)

<1%: Ventricular arrhythmias, fever, headache, dizziness, rash, angioedema, hypertrophic pyloric stenosis, vaginitis, eosinophilia, elevated LFTs, cholestatic jaundice, thrombophlebitis, ototoxicity, nephritis, allergic reactions

Contraindications Hypersensitivity to azithromycin, other macrolide antibiotics, or any component of their formulation; hepatic impairment; use with pimozide

Warnings/Precautions Use with caution in patients with hepatic dysfunction; hepatic impairment with or without jaundice has occurred chiefly in older children and adults; it may be accompanied by malaise, nausea, vomiting, abdominal colic, and fever; discontinue use if these occur; may mask or delay symptoms of incubating gonorrhea or syphilis, so appropriate culture and susceptibility tests should be performed prior to initiating azithromycin; pseudomembranous colitis has been reported with use of macrolide antibiotics; safety and efficacy have not been established in children <6 months of age with acute otitis media and in children <2 years of age with pharyngitis/tonsillitis

Drug Interactions

Increased Effect/Toxicity: May increase levels of tacrolimus, phenytoin, ergot alkaloids, alfentanil, astemizole, terfenadine, bromocriptine, carbamazepine, cyclosporine, digoxin, disopyramide, and triazolam; azithromycin did not affect the response to warfarin or theophylline although caution is advised when administered together; avoid use with pimozide due to significant risk of cardiotoxicity

Decreased peak serum concentration: Aluminum- and magnesium-containing antacids by 24% but not total absorption

Dietary/Ethanol/Herb Considerations Food may alter rate and extent of GI absorption depending upon the formulation. Administer suspension and capsules 1 hour before or 2 hours following meals. Oral suspension may be administered with food but absorption is significantly increased (46%). Administer tablet with food to reduce GI upset.

Drug Uptake

Absorption: Rapid

Half-life, elimination: Terminal: 68 hours

Time to peak: 2.3-4 hours

Pregnancy Risk Factor B

Dosage Forms INJ, powder for reconstitution: 500 mg. **POWDER, oral suspension:** 100 mg/5 mL (15 mL); 200 mg/5 mL (15 mL, 22.5 mL, 30 mL); 1 g. **TAB:** 250 mg, 600 mg; (Zithromax® Z-PAK®): 250 mg (6s)

Generic Available No

Comments Although the erythromycins inhibit the hepatic metabolism of theophylline and carbamazepine to enhance their effects, azithromycin has not been shown to inhibit the hepatic metabolism of these drugs. Clauzel, et al, reported that azithromycin did not inhibit the metabolism of theophylline after a standard 5-day regimen (500 mg on day one followed by 250 mg daily). Rapeport, et al, reported that azithromycin did not affect the blood levels of carbamazepine.

Selected Readings

Dajani AS, Taubert KA, Wilson W, et al, "Prevention of Bacterial Endocarditis. Recommendations by the American Heart Association," *JAMA*, 1997, 277(22):1794-801.

Dajani AS, Taubert KA, Wilson W, et al, "Prevention of Bacterial Endocarditis: Recommendations by the American Heart Association," *J Am Dent Assoc*, 1997, 128(8):1142-51.

Wynn RL, "New Erythromycins," *Gen Dent*, 1996, 44(4):304-7.

Wynn RL, Bergman SA, Meiller TF, et al, "Antibiotics in Treating Oral-Facial Infections of Odontogenic Origin: An Update", *Gen Dent*, 2001, 49(3):238-40, 242, 244 passim.

Azmacort® *see* Triamcinolone *on page 1197*

Azo-Dine® [OTC] *see* Phenazopyridine *on page 943*

Azo-Gesic® [OTC] *see* Phenazopyridine *on page 943*

Azopt® *see* Brinzolamide *on page 178*

Azo-Standard® *see* Phenazopyridine *on page 943*

Aztreonam (AZ tree oh nam)

U.S. Brand Names Azactam®

Canadian Brand Names Azactam®

Pharmacologic Category Antibiotic, Miscellaneous

Synonyms Azthreonam

Use Treatment of patients with documented aerobic gram-negative bacillary infection in which beta-lactam therapy is contraindicated (eg, penicillin or cephalosporin allergy); used for urinary tract infections, lower respiratory tract infections, septicemia, skin/skin structure infections, intra-abdominal infections, and gynecological infections; as part of a multiple-drug regimen for the empirical treatment of neutropenic fever in persons with a history of beta-lactam allergy or with known multidrug-resistant organisms

Local Anesthetic/Vasoconstrictor Precautions No information available to require special precautions

Effects on Dental Treatment No effects or complications reported

Dosage

Neonates: I.M., I.V.:

Postnatal age ≤7 days:

<2000 g: 30 mg/kg/dose every 12 hours

>2000 g: 30 mg/kg/dose every 8 hours

Postnatal age >7 days:

<1200 g: 30 mg/kg/dose every 12 hours

1200-2000 g: 30 mg/kg/dose every 8 hours

>2000 g: 30 mg/kg/dose every 6 hours

Children >1 month: I.M., I.V.: 90-120 mg/kg/day divided every 6-8 hours

Cystic fibrosis: 50 mg/kg/dose every 6-8 hours (ie, up to 200 mg/kg/day); maximum: 6-8 g/day

Adults:

Urinary tract infection: I.M., I.V.: 500 mg to 1 g every 8-12 hours

Moderately severe systemic infections: 1 g I.V. or I.M. or 2 g I.V. every 8-12 hours

Severe systemic or life-threatening infections (especially caused by *Pseudomonas aeruginosa*): I.V.: 2 g every 6-8 hours; maximum: 8 g/day

Dosing adjustment in renal impairment: Adults:

Cl_{cr} >50 mL/minute: 500 mg to 1 g every 6-8 hours

Cl_{cr} 10-50 mL/minute: 50% to 75% of usual dose given at the usual interval

Cl_{cr} <10 mL/minute: 25% of usual dosage given at the usual interval

(Continued)

Aztreonam *(Continued)*

Hemodialysis: Moderately dialyzable (20% to 50%); administer dose postdialysis or supplemental dose of 500 mg after dialysis

Peritoneal dialysis: Administer as for Cl_{cr} <10 mL/minute

Continuous arteriovenous or venovenous hemofiltration: Dose as for Cl_{cr} 10-50 mL/minute

Mechanism of Action Inhibits bacterial cell wall synthesis by binding to one or more of the penicillin binding proteins (PBPs); which in turn inhibits the final transpeptidation step of peptidoglycan synthesis in bacterial cell walls, thus inhibiting cell wall biosynthesis. Bacteria eventually lyse due to ongoing activity of cell wall autolytic enzymes (autolysins and murein hydrolases) while cell wall assembly is arrested. Monobactam structure makes cross-allergenicity with beta-lactams unlikely.

Other Adverse Effects 1% to 10%:

Dermatologic: Rash

Gastrointestinal: Diarrhea, nausea, vomiting

Local: Thrombophlebitis, pain at injection site

Drug Interactions Avoid antibiotics that induce beta-lactamase production (cefoxitin, imipenem).

Drug Uptake

Absorption: I.M.: Well absorbed; I.M. and I.V. doses produce comparable serum concentrations

Half-life, elimination:

Neonates: <7 days, ≤2.5 kg: 5.5-9.9 hours; <7 days, >2.5 kg: 2.6 hours; 1 week to 1 month: 2.4 hours

Children 2 months to 12 years: 1.7 hours

Adults: Normal renal function: 1.7-2.9 hours

End-stage renal disease: 6-8 hours

Time to peak: I.M., I.V. push: ~60 minutes; I.V. infusion: 1.5 hours

Pregnancy Risk Factor B

Generic Available No

Azulfidine® *see* Sulfasalazine *on page 1121*

Azulfidine® EN-tabs® *see* Sulfasalazine *on page 1121*

Babee® Teething® [OTC] *see* Benzocaine *on page 151*

Bacid® [OTC] *see Lactobacillus acidophilus* and *Lactobacillus bulgaricus on page 682*

Baciguent® [OTC] *see* Bacitracin *on page 140*

Baci-IM® *see* Bacitracin *on page 140*

Bacitracin (bas i TRAY sin)

U.S. Brand Names AK-Tracin®; Baciguent® [OTC]; Baci-IM®

Canadian Brand Names Baciguent®

Pharmacologic Category Antibiotic, Ophthalmic; Antibiotic, Topical; Antibiotic, Miscellaneous

Use Treatment of susceptible bacterial infections (staphylococcal pneumonia and empyema); due to toxicity risks, systemic and irrigant uses of bacitracin should be limited to situations where less toxic alternatives would not be effective; oral administration has been successful in antibiotic-associated colitis and has been used for enteric eradication of vancomycin-resistant enterococci (VRE)

Local Anesthetic/Vasoconstrictor Precautions No information available to require special precautions

Effects on Dental Treatment No effects or complications reported

Dosage Do not administer I.V.:

Children: I.M.: 800-1200 units/kg/day divided every 8 hours

Adults: Antibiotic-associated colitis: Oral: 25,000 units 4 times/day for 7-10 days

Topical: Apply 1-5 times/day

Ophthalmic, ointment: Instill 1/4" to 1/2" ribbon every 3-4 hours into conjunctival sac for acute infections, or 2-3 times/day for mild to moderate infections for 7-10 days

Irrigation, solution: 50-100 units/mL in normal saline, lactated Ringer's, or sterile water for irrigation; soak sponges in solution for topical compresses 1-5 times/day or as needed during surgical procedures

Mechanism of Action Inhibits bacterial cell wall synthesis by preventing transfer of mucopeptides into the growing cell wall

Other Adverse Effects 1% to 10%:

Cardiovascular: Hypotension, edema of the face/lips, tightness of chest

Central nervous system: Pain

Dermatologic: Rash, itching

Gastrointestinal: Anorexia, nausea, vomiting, diarrhea, rectal itching

Hematologic: Blood dyscrasias

Miscellaneous: Sweating

Drug Interactions Increased neuromuscular blockade: Nephrotoxic drugs, neuromuscular blocking agents, and anesthetics

Drug Uptake
Absorption: Poor from mucous membranes and intact or denuded skin; rapidly absorbed following I.M. administration; not absorbed by bladder irrigation, but absorption can occur from peritoneal or mediastinal lavage
Duration: 6-8 hours
Time to peak: I.M.: 1-2 hours
Pregnancy Risk Factor C
Generic Available Yes

Bacitracin and Polymyxin B (bas i TRAY sin & pol i MIKS in bee)

U.S. Brand Names AK-Poly-Bac®; Betadine® First Aid Antibiotics + Moisturizer [OTC]; Polysporin® Ophthalmic; Polysporin® Topical [OTC]
Canadian Brand Names LID-Pack®; Optimyxin®; Optimyxin Plus®; Polycidin® Ophthalmic Ointment
Pharmacologic Category Antibiotic, Ophthalmic; Antibiotic, Topical
Synonyms Polymyxin B and Bacitracin
Use Treatment of superficial infections caused by susceptible organisms
Local Anesthetic/Vasoconstrictor Precautions No information available to require special precautions
Effects on Dental Treatment No effects or complications reported
Dosage Children and Adults:
Ophthalmic ointment: Instill 1/2" ribbon in the affected eye(s) every 3-4 hours for acute infections or 2-3 times/day for mild to moderate infections for 7-10 days
Topical ointment/powder: Apply to affected area 1-4 times/day; may cover with sterile bandage if needed
Mechanism of Action See Bacitracin *on page 140* and Polymyxin B *on page 971*
Other Adverse Effects 1% to 10%: Local: Rash, itching, burning, anaphylactoid reactions, swelling, conjunctival erythema
Drug Uptake See Bacitracin *on page 140* and Polymyxin B *on page 971*
Pregnancy Risk Factor C
Generic Available Yes

Bacitracin, Neomycin, and Polymyxin B
(bas i TRAY sin, nee oh MYE sin & pol i MIKS in bee)

U.S. Brand Names Mycitracin® [OTC]; Neosporin® Ophthalmic Ointment; Neosporin® Topical [OTC]; Triple Antibiotic®
Canadian Brand Names Neosporin® Ophthalmic Ointment; Neotopic®
Pharmacologic Category Antibiotic, Ophthalmic; Antibiotic, Topical
Synonyms Neomycin, Bacitracin, and Polymyxin B; Polymyxin B, Bacitracin, and Neomycin
Use Aids in the prevention of infection in minor abrasions, burns, and cuts; short-term treatment of superficial external ocular infections caused by susceptible organisms
Local Anesthetic/Vasoconstrictor Precautions No information available to require special precautions
Effects on Dental Treatment No effects or complications reported
Dosage Children and Adults:
Ophthalmic ointment: Instill 1/2" ribbon into the conjunctival sac every 3-4 hours for acute infections or 2-3 times/day for mild to moderate infections for 7-10 days
Topical: Apply 1-4 times/day to affected areas and cover with sterile bandage if necessary
Mechanism of Action See Bacitracin *on page 140*, Neomycin *on page 854*, and Polymyxin B *on page 971*
Other Adverse Effects 1% to 10%:
Cardiovascular: Edema
Dermatologic: Reddening, allergic contact dermatitis
Local: Itching, failure to heal
Drug Uptake See Bacitracin *on page 140*, Neomycin *on page 854* and Polymyxin B *on page 971*
Pregnancy Risk Factor C
Generic Available Yes

Bacitracin, Neomycin, Polymyxin B, and Hydrocortisone
(bas i TRAY sin, nee oh MYE sin, pol i MIKS in bee & hye droe KOR ti sone)

U.S. Brand Names AK-Spore® H.C.; Cortisporin® Ointment
Canadian Brand Names Cortisporin®
Pharmacologic Category Antibiotic, Ophthalmic; Antibiotic, Otic; Antibiotic, Topical; Corticosteroid, Ophthalmic; Corticosteroid, Otic; Corticosteroid, Topical
Synonyms Hydrocortisone, Bacitracin, Neomycin, and Polymyxin B; Neomycin, Bacitracin, Polymyxin B, and Hydrocortisone; Polymyxin B, Bacitracin, Neomycin, and Hydrocortisone
Use Prevention and treatment of susceptible superficial topical infections
Local Anesthetic/Vasoconstrictor Precautions No information available to require special precautions
(Continued)

Bacitracin, Neomycin, Polymyxin B, and Hydrocortisone *(Continued)*

Effects on Dental Treatment No effects or complications reported

Dosage Discontinue when control is achieved; if no improvement is seen, reassessment of diagnosis may be necessary.

Children and Adults:

Ophthalmic ointment: Instill ½" ribbon to inside of lower lid every 3-4 hours until improvement occurs

Topical: Apply sparingly 2-4 times/day

Mechanism of Action See Bacitracin *on page 140*, Neomycin *on page 854*, Polymyxin B *on page 971*, and Hydrocortisone *on page 608*

Other Adverse Effects 1% to 10%:

Dermatologic: Rash, generalized itching

Respiratory: Apnea

Drug Uptake See Bacitracin *on page 140*, Neomycin *on page 854*, Polymyxin B *on page 971* and Hydrocortisone *on page 608*

Pregnancy Risk Factor C

Generic Available Yes

Bacitracin, Neomycin, Polymyxin B, and Lidocaine

(bas i TRAY sin, nee oh MYE sin, pol i MIKS in bee & LYE doe kane)

U.S. Brand Names Spectrocin Plus® [OTC]

Pharmacologic Category Antibiotic, Topical

Use Prevention and treatment of susceptible superficial topical infections

Local Anesthetic/Vasoconstrictor Precautions No information available to require special precautions

Effects on Dental Treatment No effects or complications reported

Dosage Adults: Topical: Apply 1-4 times/day to infected areas; cover with sterile bandage if needed

Drug Uptake See Bacitracin *on page 140*, Neomycin *on page 854* and Polymyxin B *on page 971* Lidocaine *on page 706*

Generic Available Yes

Backache Pain Relief Extra Strength *see* Magnesium Salicylate *on page 742*

Baclofen (BAK loe fen)

U.S. Brand Names Lioresal®

Canadian Brand Names Apo®-Baclofen; Gen-Baclofen; Lioresal®; Liotec; Novo-Baclofen; Nu-Baclo; PMS-Baclofen

Pharmacologic Category Skeletal Muscle Relaxant

Use

Orphan drug: Intrathecal: Treatment of intractable spasticity caused by spinal cord injury, multiple sclerosis, and other spinal disease (spinal ischemia or tumor, transverse myelitis, cervical spondylosis, degenerative myelopathy)

Unlabeled/Investigational: Intractable hiccups, intractable pain relief, bladder spasticity, trigeminal neuralgia, cerebral palsy, Huntington's chorea

Local Anesthetic/Vasoconstrictor Precautions No information available to require special precautions

Effects on Dental Treatment No effects or complications reported

Dosage

Oral:

Children:

2-7 years: Initial: 10-15 mg/24 hours divided every 8 hours; titrate dose every 3 days in increments of 5-15 mg/day to a maximum of 40 mg/day

≥8 years: Maximum: 60 mg/day in 3 divided doses

Adults: 5 mg 3 times/day, may increase 5 mg/dose every 3 days to a maximum of 80 mg/day

Intrathecal:

Test dose: 50-100 mcg, doses >50 mcg should be given in 25 mcg increments, separated by 24 hours

Maintenance: After positive response to test dose, a maintenance intrathecal infusion can be administered via an implanted intrathecal pump. Initial dose via pump: Infusion at a 24-hourly rate dosed at twice the test dose.

Mechanism of Action Inhibits the transmission of both monosynaptic and polysynaptic reflexes at the spinal cord level, possibly by hyperpolarization of primary afferent fiber terminals, with resultant relief of muscle spasticity

Other Adverse Effects Withdrawal reactions have occurred with abrupt discontinuation (particularly severe with intrathecal use).

>10%:

Central nervous system: Drowsiness, vertigo, psychiatric disturbances, insomnia, slurred speech, ataxia, hypotonia

Neuromuscular & skeletal: Weakness

1% to 10%:

Cardiovascular: Hypotension

Central nervous system: Fatigue, confusion, headache
Dermatologic: Rash
Gastrointestinal: Nausea, constipation
Genitourinary: Polyuria

Warnings/Precautions Use with caution in patients with seizure disorder or impaired renal function. Avoid abrupt withdrawal; abrupt withdrawal of intrathecal baclofen has resulted in altered mental status and severe sequelae (hyperpyrexia, obtundation, rebound/exaggerated spasticity, muscle rigidity, and rhabdomyolysis), leading to organ failure and some fatalities. Risk may be higher in patients with injuries at T-6 or above, history of baclofen withdrawal, or limited ability to communicate. Elderly are more sensitive to the effects of baclofen and are more likely to experience adverse CNS effects at higher doses. Patients and caregivers are advised to keep refill appointments and to be alert to early symptoms of withdrawal.

Drug Interactions Increased Effect/Toxicity: May decrease the clearance of ibuprofen or other NSAIDs and increase the potential for renal toxicity; effects may be additive with CNS depressants.

Drug Uptake
Onset of action: 3-4 days; Peak effect: 5-10 days
Absorption: Oral: Rapid; dose-dependent
Half-life, elimination: 3.5 hours
Time to peak: Oral: ~2-3 hours

Pregnancy Risk Factor C

Generic Available Yes: Tablets only

Bactocill® *see* Oxacillin *on page 893*
BactoShield® [OTC] *see* Chlorhexidine Gluconate *on page 263*
Bactrim™ *see* Sulfamethoxazole and Trimethoprim *on page 1120*
Bactrim™ DS *see* Sulfamethoxazole and Trimethoprim *on page 1120*
Bactroban® *see* Mupirocin *on page 834*
Bactroban® Nasal *see* Mupirocin *on page 834*
Baker's P & S [OTC] *see* Phenol *on page 946*

Balanced Salt Solution (BAL anced salt soe LOO shun)

U.S. Brand Names BSS®

Canadian Brand Names BSS®; BSS® Plus; Eye-Stream®

Pharmacologic Category Ophthalmic Agent, Miscellaneous

Use Intraocular irrigating solution; also used to soothe and cleanse the eye in conjunction with hard contact lenses

Local Anesthetic/Vasoconstrictor Precautions No information available to require special precautions

Effects on Dental Treatment No effects or complications reported

Dosage Use as needed for foreign body removal, gonioscopy and other general ophthalmic office procedures

Generic Available Yes

Baldex® *see* Dexamethasone *on page 363*
BAL in Oil® *see* Dimercaprol *on page 397*
Balmex® [OTC] *see* Zinc Oxide *on page 1260*
Balnetar® [OTC] *see* Coal Tar, Lanolin, and Mineral Oil *on page 315*
Bancap HC® *see* Hydrocodone and Acetaminophen *on page 598*
Banophen® [OTC] *see* DiphenhydrAMINE *on page 398*
Banophen® Decongestant [OTC] *see* Diphenhydramine and Pseudoephedrine *on page 400*
Banthine® *see* Methantheline *on page 780*
Barbidonna® *see* Hyoscyamine, Atropine, Scopolamine, and Phenobarbital *on page 618*
Baridium® *see* Phenazopyridine *on page 943*

Basiliximab (ba si LIKS i mab)

U.S. Brand Names Simulect®

Canadian Brand Names Simulect®

Mexican Brand Names Simulect®

Pharmacologic Category Monoclonal Antibody

Use Prophylaxis of acute organ rejection in renal transplantation

Local Anesthetic/Vasoconstrictor Precautions No information available to require special precautions

Effects on Dental Treatment Causes gingival hypertrophy (GH) similar to that caused by cyclosporine; early reports indicate that frequency/incidence of basiliximab-induced GH not as high as cyclosporine-induced GH

Dosage **Note:** Patients previously administered basiliximab should only be re-exposed to a subsequent course of therapy with extreme caution.
I.V.:
Children 2-15 years of age: 12 mg/m^2 (maximum: 20 mg) within 2 hours prior to transplant surgery, followed by a second dose of 12 mg/m^2 (maximum: 20 mg/

(Continued)

Basiliximab *(Continued)*

dose) 4 days after transplantation; the second dose should be withheld if complications occur (including severe hypersensitivity reactions or graft loss)

Adults: 20 mg within 2 hours prior to transplant surgery, followed by a second 20 mg dose 4 days after transplantation; the second dose should be withheld if complications occur (including severe hypersensitivity reactions or graft loss)

Dosing adjustment/comments in renal or hepatic impairment: No specific dosing adjustment recommended

Mechanism of Action Chimeric (murine/human) monoclonal antibody which blocks the alpha-chain of the interleukin-2 (IL-2) receptor complex; this receptor is expressed on activated T lymphocytes and is a critical pathway for activating cell-mediated allograft rejection

Other Adverse Effects Reported in 96% of placebo and basiliximab groups:

>10%:
- Cardiovascular: Peripheral edema, hypertension, atrial fibrillation
- Central nervous system: Fever, headache, insomnia, pain
- Dermatologic: Wound complications, acne
- Endocrine & metabolic: Hypokalemia, hyperkalemia, hyperglycemia, hyperuricemia, hypophosphatemia, hypercholesterolemia
- Gastrointestinal: Constipation, nausea, diarrhea, abdominal pain, vomiting, dyspepsia
- Genitourinary: Urinary tract infection
- Hematologic: Anemia
- Neuromuscular & skeletal: Tremor
- Respiratory: Dyspnea, infection (upper respiratory)
- Miscellaneous: Viral infection

3% to 10%:
- Cardiovascular: Chest pain, cardiac failure, hypotension, arrhythmia, tachycardia, generalized edema, abnormal heart sounds, angina pectoris
- Central nervous system: Hypoesthesia, neuropathy, agitation, anxiety, depression, malaise, fatigue, rigors, dizziness
- Dermatologic: Cyst, hypertrichosis, pruritus, rash, skin disorder, skin ulceration
- Endocrine & metabolic: Dehydration, diabetes mellitus, fluid overload, hypercalcemia, hyperlipidemia, hypoglycemia, hypomagnesemia, acidosis, hypertriglyceridemia, hypocalcemia, hyponatremia
- Gastrointestinal: Flatulence, gastroenteritis, GI hemorrhage, gingival hyperplasia, melena, esophagitis, stomatitis, enlarged abdomen, moniliasis, ulcerative stomatitis, weight gain
- Genitourinary: Impotence, genital edema, albuminuria, bladder disorder, hematuria, urinary frequency, oliguria, abnormal renal function, renal tubular necrosis, ureteral disorder, urinary retention, dysuria
- Hematologic: Hematoma, hemorrhage, purpura, thrombocytopenia, thrombosis, polycythemia, leukopenia
- Neuromuscular & skeletal: Arthralgia, arthropathy, cramps, fracture, hernia, myalgia, paresthesia, weakness, back pain, leg pain
- Ocular: Cataract, conjunctivitis, abnormal vision
- Respiratory: Bronchitis, bronchospasm, pneumonia, pulmonary edema, sinusitis, rhinitis, coughing, pharyngitis
- Miscellaneous: Accidental trauma, facial edema, sepsis, infection, increased glucocorticoids, herpes infection

Drug Interactions Basiliximab is an immunoglobulin; specific drug interactions have not been evaluated, but are not anticipated. It is not known if the immune response to vaccines will be impaired during or following basiliximab therapy.

Drug Uptake

Duration, mean: 36 days (determined by IL-2R alpha saturation); duration increased with concomitant use of cyclosporine, corticosteroids, and azathioprine

Half-life, elimination, mean: Children: 1-11 years: 9.5 ± 4.5 days; 12-16 years: 9.1 ± 3.9 days; Adults: 7.2 days ± 3.2 days

Pregnancy Risk Factor B (manufacturer)

Generic Available No

Bayer® Aspirin [OTC] *see* Aspirin *on page 119*

Bayer® Aspirin Extra Strength [OTC] *see* Aspirin *on page 119*

Bayer® Aspirin Regimen Adult Low Strength [OTC] *see* Aspirin *on page 119*

Bayer® Aspirin Regimen Adult Low Strength with Calcium [OTC] *see* Aspirin *on page 119*

Bayer® Aspirin Regimen Children's [OTC] *see* Aspirin *on page 119*

Bayer® Aspirin Regimen Regular Strength [OTC] *see* Aspirin *on page 119*

Bayer® Plus Extra Strength [OTC] *see* Aspirin *on page 119*

BayGam® *see* Immune Globulin, Intramuscular *on page 629*

BayHep B™ *see* Hepatitis B Immune Globulin *on page 584*

BayRab® *see* Rabies Immune Globulin (Human) *on page 1038*

BayRho-D® *see* Rh_o(D) Immune Globulin *on page 1048*

BayRho-D® Mini-Dose *see* Rh_o(D) Immune Globulin *on page 1048*

BayTet™ *see* Tetanus Immune Globulin (Human) *on page 1145*
Baza® Antifungal [OTC] *see* Miconazole *on page 807*
B-Caro-T™ *see* Beta-Carotene *on page 158*

BCG Vaccine (bee see jee vak SEEN)

U.S. Brand Names TheraCys®; TICE® BCG

Canadian Brand Names ImmuCyst®; Oncotice™; Pacis™

Pharmacologic Category Biological Response Modulator; Vaccine

Synonyms Bacillus Calmette-Guérin (BCG) Live; BCG, Live

Use Immunization against tuberculosis and immunotherapy for cancer; treatment of bladder cancer; not routinely recommended for use in the U.S. for prevention of tuberculosis

Strongly recommended for infants and children with negative tuberculin skin tests who:

- Are at high risk of intimate and prolonged exposure to persistently untreated or ineffectively treated patients with infectious pulmonary tuberculosis, and
  - Cannot be removed from the source of exposure, and
  - Cannot be placed on long-term preventive therapy
  - Are continuously exposed with tuberculosis who have bacilli resistant to isoniazid and rifampin
- BCG is also recommended for tuberculin-negative infants and children in groups in which the rate of new infections exceeds 1% per year and for whom the usual surveillance and treatment programs have been attempted but are not operationally feasible

BCG should be administered with caution to persons in groups at high risk for HIV infection or persons known to be severely immunocompromised. Although limited data suggest that the vaccine may be safe for use in asymptomatic children infected with HIV, BCG vaccination is not recommended for HIV infected adults or for persons with symptomatic disease. Until further research can clearly define the risks and benefits of BCG vaccination for this population, vaccination should be restricted to persons at exceptionally high risk for tuberculosis infection. HIV infected persons thought to be infected with *Mycobacterium tuberculosis* should be strongly recommended for tuberculosis preventive therapy.

Local Anesthetic/Vasoconstrictor Precautions No information available to require special precautions

Effects on Dental Treatment No effects or complications reported

Dosage Children >1 month and Adults:

Immunization against tuberculosis (TICE® BCG): 0.2-0.3 mL percutaneous; initial lesion usually appears after 10-14 days consisting of small red papule at injection site and reaches maximum diameter of 3 mm in 4-6 weeks; conduct postvaccinal tuberculin test (ie, 5 TU of PPD) in 2-3 months; if test is negative, repeat vaccination

Immunotherapy for bladder cancer:

- Intravesical treatment: Instill into bladder for 2 hours
- TheraCys®: One dose diluted in 50 mL NS (preservative free) instilled into bladder once weekly for 6 weeks followed by one treatment at 3, 6, 12, 18, and 24 months after initial treatment
- TICE® BCG: One dose diluted in 50 mL NS (preservative free) instilled into the bladder once weekly for 6 weeks followed by once monthly for 6-12 months

Mechanism of Action BCG live is an attenuated strain of Bacillus Calmette-Guérin used as a biological response modifier; BCG live, when used intravesicular for treatment of bladder carcinoma *in situ*, is thought to cause a local, chronic inflammatory response involving macrophage and leukocyte infiltration of the bladder. By a mechanism not fully understood, this local inflammatory response leads to destruction of superficial tumor cells of the urothelium. Evidence of systemic immune response is also commonly seen, manifested by a positive PPD tuberculin skin test reaction, however, its relationship to clinical efficacy is not well-established. BCG is active immunotherapy which stimulates the host's immune mechanism to reject the tumor.

Other Adverse Effects All serious adverse reactions must be reported to the U.S. Department of Health and Human Services (DHHS) Vaccine Adverse Event Reporting System (VAERS) 1-800-822-7967.

1% to 10%:

- Genitourinary: Bladder infection, dysuria, polyuria, prostatitis
- Miscellaneous: Flu-like syndrome

Drug Interactions Antimicrobial or immunosuppressive drugs may impair response to BCG or increase risk of infection; antituberculosis drugs

Pregnancy Risk Factor C

Generic Available No

Comments Live, attenuated vaccine; live culture preparation of bacillus Calmette-Guérin (BCG) strain of *Mycobacterium bovis* and is a substrain of Pasteur Institute strain designed for use as active immunizing agent against tuberculosis

B-D Glucose® [OTC] *see* Glucose *on page 559*

Becaplermin (be KAP ler min)

U.S. Brand Names Regranex®

Canadian Brand Names Regranex®

Pharmacologic Category Growth Factor, Platelet-derived; Topical Skin Product

Synonyms Recombinant Human Platelet-Derived Growth Factor B; rPDGF-BB

Use Treatment of diabetic ulcers that occur on the lower limbs and feet

Local Anesthetic/Vasoconstrictor Precautions No information available to require special precautions

Effects on Dental Treatment No effects or complications reported

Dosage Adults: Topical: Apply once daily; applied with a cotton swab or similar tool, as a coating over the ulcer

Mechanism of Action A genetically engineered form of platelet-derived growth factor, a naturally occurring protein in the body that stimulates wound healing.

Drug Uptake

Onset of action (complete healing): 15% of patients within 8 weeks, 25% at 10 weeks

Absorption: Minimal

Pregnancy Risk Factor C

Generic Available No

Because® [OTC] *see* Nonoxynol 9 *on page 874*

Beclomethasone (be kloe METH a sone)

Related Information

Respiratory Diseases *on page 1328*

U.S. Brand Names Beconase®; Beconase® AQ; QVAR™; Vancenase® AQ 84 mcg; Vancenase® Pockethaler®; Vanceril®

Canadian Brand Names Alti-Beclomethasone; Apo®-Beclomethasone; Gen-Beclo; Nu-Beclomethasone; Propaderm®; QVAR™; Rivanase AQ; Vancenase®; Vanceril®

Mexican Brand Names Aerobec; Beconase Aqua; Becotide

Pharmacologic Category Corticosteroid, Inhalant (Oral); Corticosteroid, Nasal

Synonyms Beclomethasone Dipropionate; Beclovent® [DSC]

Use

Oral inhalation: Maintenance and prophylactic treatment of asthma; includes those who require corticosteroids and those who may benefit from a dose reduction/elimination of systemically administered corticosteroids. Not for relief of acute bronchospasm

Nasal aerosol: Symptomatic treatment of seasonal or perennial rhinitis and to prevent recurrence of nasal polyps following surgery

Local Anesthetic/Vasoconstrictor Precautions No information available to require special precautions

Effects on Dental Treatment Localized infections with *Candida albicans* or *Aspergillus niger* have occurred frequently in the mouth and pharynx with repetitive use of oral inhaler of beclomethasone. Positive cultures for oral *Candida* may be present in up to 75% of patients. These infections may require treatment with appropriate antifungal therapy or discontinuance of treatment with beclomethasone inhaler.

Dosage Nasal inhalation and oral inhalation dosage forms are not to be used interchangeably.

Aqueous inhalation, nasal:

- Vancenase® AQ, Beconase® AQ: Children ≥6 years and Adults: 1-2 inhalations each nostril twice daily; total dose 168-336 mcg/day
- Vancenase® AQ 84 mcg: Children ≥6 years and Adults: 1-2 inhalations in each nostril once daily; total dose 168-336 mcg/day

Intranasal (Vancenase®, Beconase®):

- Children 6-12 years: 1 inhalation in each nostril 3 times/day; total dose 252 mcg/day
- Children ≥12 years and Adults: 1 inhalation in each nostril 2-4 times/day or 2 inhalations each nostril twice daily (total dose 168-336 mcg/day); usual maximum maintenance: 1 inhalation in each nostril 3 times/day (252 mcg/day)

Oral inhalation (doses should be titrated to the lowest effective dose once asthma is controlled):

- Beclovent®, Vanceril®:
  - Children 6-12 years: 1-2 inhalations 3-4 times/day (alternatively: 2-4 inhalations twice daily); maximum dose: 10 inhalations/day (420 mcg)
  - Children ≥12 years and Adults: 2 inhalations 3-4 times/day (alternatively: 4 inhalations twice daily); maximum dose: 20 inhalations/day (840 mcg/day); patients with severe asthma: Initial: 12-16 inhalations/day (divided 3-4 times/day); dose should be adjusted downward according to patient's response
- Vanceril® 84 mcg double strength:
  - Children 6-12 years: 2 inhalations twice daily; maximum dose: 5 inhalations/day (420 mcg)
  - Children ≥12 years and Adults: 2 inhalations twice daily; maximum dose: 10 inhalations/day (840 mcg); patients with severe asthma: Initial: 6-8 inhalations/day (divided twice daily); dose should be adjusted downward according to patient's response

QVAR™:
Children ≥ 12 years and Adults:
Patients previously on bronchodilators only: Initial dose 40-80 mcg twice daily; maximum dose 320 mcg twice day
Patients previously on inhaled corticosteroids: Initial dose 40-160 mcg twice daily; maximum dose 320 mcg twice daily
NIH Guidelines (NIH, 1997) (give in divided doses):
Children:
"Low" dose: 84-336 mcg/day (42 mcg/puff: 2-8 puffs/day or 84 mcg/puff: 1-4 puffs/day)
"Medium" dose: 336-672 mcg/day (42 mcg/puff: 8-16 puffs/day or 84 mcg/puff: 4-8 puffs/day)
"High" dose: >672 mcg/day (42 mcg/puff: >16 puffs/day or 84 mcg/puff >8 puffs/day)
Adults:
"Low" dose: 168-504 mcg/day (42 mcg/puff: 4-12 puffs/day or 84 mcg/puff: 2-6 puffs/day)
"Medium" dose: 504-840 mcg/day (42 mcg/puff: 12-20 puffs/day or 84 mcg/puff: 6-10 puffs/day)
"High" dose: >840 mcg/day (42 mcg/puff: >20 puffs/day or 84 mcg/puff: >10 puffs/day)

Mechanism of Action Controls the rate of protein synthesis, depresses the migration of polymorphonuclear leukocytes, fibroblasts, reverses capillary permeability, and lysosomal stabilization at the cellular level to prevent or control inflammation

Other Adverse Effects Frequency not defined:
Central nervous system: Agitation, depression, dizziness, dysphonia, headache, lightheadedness, mental disturbances
Dermatologic: Acneiform lesions, angioedema, atrophy, bruising, pruritus, purpura, striae, rash, urticaria
Endocrine & metabolic: Cushingoid features, growth velocity reduction in children and adolescents, HPA function suppression, weight gain
Gastrointestinal: Dry/irritated nose, throat and mouth, hoarseness, localized *Candida* or *Aspergillus* infections, loss of smell, loss of taste, nausea, unpleasant smell, unpleasant taste, vomiting
Local: Nasal spray: Burning, epistaxis, localized *Candida* infections, nasal septum perforation (rare), nasal stuffiness, nosebleeds, rhinorrhea, sneezing, transient irritation, ulceration of nasal mucosa (rare)
Ocular: Cataracts, glaucoma, increased intraocular pressure
Respiratory: Cough, paradoxical bronchospasm, pharyngitis, sinusitis, wheezing
Miscellaneous: Anaphylactic/anaphylactoid reactions, death (due to adrenal insufficiency, reported during and after transfer from systemic corticosteroids to aerosol in asthmatic patients), immediate and delayed hypersensitivity reactions

Drug Interactions The addition of salmeterol has been demonstrated to improve response to inhaled corticosteroids (as compared to increasing steroid dosage).

Drug Uptake
Onset of action: Therapeutic effect: 1-4 weeks
Absorption: Inhalation: Readily absorbed; quickly hydrolyzed by pulmonary esterases prior to absorption
Half-life, elimination: Inhalation: Initial: 3 hours; Terminal: 15 hours

Pregnancy Risk Factor C

Generic Available No

Beconase® *see* Beclomethasone *on page 146*
Beconase® AQ *see* Beclomethasone *on page 146*
Becotin® Pulvules® *see* Vitamins, Multiple *on page 1246*

Belladonna and Opium (bel a DON a & OH pee um)

U.S. Brand Names B&O Supprettes®

Pharmacologic Category Analgesic Combination (Narcotic); Antispasmodic Agent, Urinary

Synonyms Opium and Belladonna

Use Relief of moderate to severe pain associated with rectal or bladder tenesmus that may occur in postoperative states and neoplastic situations; pain associated with ureteral spasms not responsive to non-narcotic analgesics and to space intervals between injections of opiates

Local Anesthetic/Vasoconstrictor Precautions No information available to require special precautions

Effects on Dental Treatment This drug has atropine-like effects and the patient may experience drowsiness, and dry mouth, nose, and throat.

Restrictions C-II

Dosage Adults: Rectal: 1 suppository 1-2 times/day, up to 4 doses/day

Mechanism of Action Anticholinergic alkaloids act primarily by competitive inhibition of the muscarinic actions of acetylcholine on structures innervated by postganglionic cholinergic neurons and on smooth muscle; resulting effects include antisecretory activity on exocrine glands and intestinal mucosa and smooth muscle
(Continued)

Belladonna and Opium *(Continued)*

relaxation. The opium component contains many narcotic alkaloids including morphine; its mechanism for gastric motility inhibition is primarily due to this morphine content; it results in a decrease in digestive secretions, an increase in GI muscle tone, and therefore a reduction in GI propulsion.

Other Adverse Effects

>10%:
- Dermatologic: Dry skin
- Gastrointestinal: Constipation, xerostomia and throat
- Respiratory: Dry nose
- Miscellaneous: Diaphoresis (decreased)

1% to 10%:
- Dermatologic: Increased sensitivity to light
- Endocrine & metabolic: Decreased flow of breast milk
- Gastrointestinal: Dysphagia

Drug Interactions

Increased Effect/Toxicity: Additive effects with CNS depressants. May increase effects of digoxin and atenolol. Coadministration with other anticholinergic agents (phenothiazines, tricyclic antidepressants, amantadine, and antihistamines) may increase effects such as xerostomia, constipation, and urinary retention.

Decreased Effect: May decrease effects of drugs with cholinergic mechanisms; antipsychotic efficacy of phenothiazines may be decreased.

Drug Uptake Onset of action: Belladonna: 1-2 hours; Opium: ≤30 minutes

Pregnancy Risk Factor C

Generic Available Yes

Belladonna, Phenobarbital, and Ergotamine Tartrate

(bel a DON a, fee noe BAR bi tal, & er GOT a meen TAR trate)

U.S. Brand Names Bellamine S; Bel-Phen-Ergot S®; Bel-Tabs

Canadian Brand Names Bellergal® Spacetabs®

Pharmacologic Category Ergot Derivative

Synonyms Ergotamine Tartrate, Belladonna, and Phenobarbital; Phenobarbital, Belladonna, and Ergotamine Tartrate

Use Management and treatment of menopausal disorders, GI disorders and recurrent throbbing headache

Local Anesthetic/Vasoconstrictor Precautions No information available to require special precautions

Effects on Dental Treatment >10%: Xerostomia

Dosage Oral: 1 tablet each morning and evening

Other Adverse Effects

>10%:
- Cardiovascular: Peripheral vascular effects (numbness and tingling of fingers and toes)
- Central nervous system: Drowsiness, dizziness,
- Dermatologic: Dry skin
- Gastrointestinal: Constipation, xerostomia and throat, diarrhea, nausea, vomiting
- Respiratory: Dry nose
- Miscellaneous: Decreased diaphoresis

1% to 10%:
- Cardiovascular: Precordial distress and pain, transient tachycardia or bradycardia
- Dermatologic: Photosensitivity
- Endocrine & metabolic: Decreased flow of breast milk
- Gastrointestinal: Difficulty in swallowing
- Neuromuscular & skeletal: Muscle pains in the extremities, weakness in the legs

Drug Interactions

Increased Effect/Toxicity: Combined administration of phenobarbital and CNS depressants such as alcohol, tricyclic depressants, phenothiazines, and narcotic analgesics may result in potentiation of depressant actions. **Phenobarbital taken with warfarin induces liver enzymes that enhance clearance of warfarin. A reduction in phenobarbital dose in patients receiving warfarin has resulted in fatal bleeding episodes**. Griseofulvin, quinidine, doxycycline, and estrogen have been shown to be metabolized at an increased rate. Belladonna and concomitant administration of tricyclic antidepressants may result in additive anticholinergic effects. Valproic acid appears to decrease barbiturate metabolism (increased barbiturate levels). A similar reaction is possible with phenytoin.

Decreased Effect: Phenobarbital may lower plasma concentrations of dicumarol due to decreased absorption. Possible interaction between ergot alkaloids and beta-blockers.

Drug Uptake See Ergotamine *on page 448*, Phenobarbital *on page 945*

Pregnancy Risk Factor X

Generic Available Yes

Bellamine S *see* Belladonna, Phenobarbital, and Ergotamine Tartrate *on page 148*
Bellatal® *see* Hyoscyamine, Atropine, Scopolamine, and Phenobarbital *on page 618*

Bel-Phen-Ergot S® *see* Belladonna, Phenobarbital, and Ergotamine Tartrate *on page 148*

Bel-Tabs *see* Belladonna, Phenobarbital, and Ergotamine Tartrate *on page 148*

Benadryl® [OTC] *see* DiphenhydrAMINE *on page 398*

Benadryl® Decongestant Allergy [OTC] *see* Diphenhydramine and Pseudoephedrine *on page 400*

Benazepril (ben AY ze pril)

Related Information

Cardiovascular Diseases *on page 1308*

U.S. Brand Names Lotensin®

Canadian Brand Names Lotensin®

Mexican Brand Names Lotensin®

Pharmacologic Category Angiotensin-Converting Enzyme (ACE) Inhibitor

Synonyms Benazepril Hydrochloride

Use Treatment of hypertension, either alone or in combination with other antihypertensive agents; treatment of left ventricular dysfunction after myocardial infarction

Local Anesthetic/Vasoconstrictor Precautions No information available to require special precautions

Effects on Dental Treatment No effects or complications reported

Dosage Adults: Oral: 20-40 mg/day as a single dose or 2 divided doses; maximum daily dose: 80 mg

Mechanism of Action Competitive inhibition of angiotensin I being converted to angiotensin II, a potent vasoconstrictor, through the angiotensin I-converting enzyme (ACE) activity, with resultant lower levels of angiotensin II which causes an increase in plasma renin activity and a reduction in aldosterone secretion

Other Adverse Effects 1% to 10%:

Cardiovascular: Postural dizziness (1.5%)

Central nervous system: Headache (6.2%), dizziness (3.6%), fatigue (2.4%), somnolence (1.6%)

Endocrine & metabolic: Hyperkalemia (1%), increased uric acid

Gastrointestinal: Nausea (1.3%)

Renal: Increased serum creatinine (2%), worsening of renal function may occur in patients with bilateral renal artery stenosis or hypovolemia

Respiratory: Cough (1.2% to 10%)

Eosinophilic pneumonitis, neutropenia, anaphylaxis, renal insufficiency and renal failure have been reported with other ACE inhibitors. In addition, a syndrome including fever, myalgia, arthralgia, interstitial nephritis, vasculitis, rash, eosinophilia, and elevated ESR has been reported to be associated with ACE inhibitors.

Drug Interactions

Increased Effect/Toxicity: Potassium supplements, co-trimoxazole (high dose), angiotensin II receptor antagonists (candesartan, losartan, irbesartan, etc), or potassium-sparing diuretics (amiloride, spironolactone, triamterene) may result in elevated serum potassium levels when combined with benazepril. ACE inhibitor effects may be increased by phenothiazines or probenecid (increases levels of captopril). ACE inhibitors may increase serum concentration/effects of digoxin, lithium, and sulfonlyureas. Diuretics have additive hypotensive effects with ACE inhibitors, and hypovolemia increases the potential for adverse renal effects of ACE inhibitors. In patients with compromised renal function, coadministration with nonsteroidal anti-inflammatory drugs may result in further deterioration of renal function. Allopurinol and ACE inhibitors may cause a higher risk of hypersensitivity reaction when taken concurrently.

Decreased Effect: Aspirin (high dose) may reduce the therapeutic effects of ACE inhibitors; at low dosages this does not appear to be significant. Rifampin may decrease the effect of ACE inhibitors. Antacids may decrease the bioavailability of ACE inhibitors (may be more likely to occur with captopril); separate administration times by 1-2 hours. NSAIDs, specifically indomethacin, may reduce the hypotensive effects of ACE inhibitors.

Drug Uptake

Reduction in plasma angiotensin-converting enzyme activity:

Peak effect: 1-2 hours after 2-20 mg dose

Duration: >90% inhibition for 24 hours after 5-20 mg dose

Reduction in blood pressure:

Peak effect: 2-4 hours after single dose; 2 weeks with continuous therapy

Absorption: Rapid (37%); food does not alter significantly; metabolite (benazeprilat) itself unsuitable for oral administration due to poor absorption

Half-life, elimination: Effective: 10-11 hours; Benazeprilat: Terminal: 22 hours

Time to peak: Parent drug: 1-1.5 hours

Dialysis: ~6% of metabolite removed in 4 hours of dialysis following 10 mg of benazepril administered 2 hours prior to procedure; parent compound was not found in the dialysate

Pregnancy Risk Factor C/D (2nd and 3rd trimesters)

Generic Available No

Benazepril and Hydrochlorothiazide

(ben AY ze pril & hye droe klor oh THYE a zide)

U.S. Brand Names Lotensin® HCT

Canadian Brand Names Lotrel®

Pharmacologic Category Antihypertensive Agent Combination

Synonyms Hydrochlorothiazide and Benazepril

Use Treatment of hypertension

Local Anesthetic/Vasoconstrictor Precautions No information available to require special precautions

Effects on Dental Treatment No effects or complications reported

Dosage Dose is individualized

Drug Uptake See Benazepril *on page 149* and Hydrochlorothiazide *on page 595*

Pregnancy Risk Factor C/D (2nd and 3rd trimesters)

Generic Available No

Bendroflumethiazide (ben droe floo meth EYE a zide)

Related Information

Cardiovascular Diseases *on page 1308*

U.S. Brand Names Naturetin®

Pharmacologic Category Diuretic, Thiazide

Use Management of mild to moderate hypertension; treatment of edema associated with CHF, pregnancy, or nephrotic syndrome; reportedly does not alter serum electrolyte concentrations appreciably at recommended doses

Local Anesthetic/Vasoconstrictor Precautions No information available to require special precautions

Effects on Dental Treatment No effects or complications reported

Dosage Oral:

Children: Initial: 0.1-0.4 mg/kg/day in 1-2 doses; maintenance dose: 0.05-0.1 mg/kg/day in 1-2 doses

Adults: 2.5-20 mg/day or twice daily in divided doses

Mechanism of Action Like other thiazide diuretics, it inhibits sodium, chloride, and water reabsorption in the renal distal tubules, thereby producing diuresis with a resultant reduction in plasma volume; hypothetically may reduce peripheral resistance through increased prostacyclin synthesis

Other Adverse Effects 1% to 10%:

Cardiovascular: Orthostatic hypotension

Endocrine & metabolic: Hyponatremia, hypokalemia

Gastrointestinal: Anorexia, gastritis, diarrhea

Warnings/Precautions Use with caution in severe renal disease. Electrolyte disturbances (hypokalemia, hypochloremic alkalosis, hyponatremia) can occur. Use with caution in severe hepatic dysfunction; hepatic encephalopathy can be caused by electrolyte disturbances. Gout can be precipitated in certain patients with a history of gout, a familial predisposition to gout, or chronic renal failure. Cautious use in diabetics; may see a change in glucose control. Hypersensitivity reactions can occur. Can cause SLE exacerbation or activation. Use with caution in patients with moderate or high cholesterol concentrations. Photosensitization may occur.

Chemical similarities are present among sulfonamides, sulfonylureas, carbonic anhydrase inhibitors, thiazides, and loop diuretics (except ethacrynic acid). Use in patients with thiazide or sulfonamide allergy is specifically contraindicated in product labeling, however a risk of cross-reaction exists in patients with allergy to any of these compounds; avoid use when previous reaction has been severe.

Drug Interactions

Increased Effect/Toxicity: Increased effect of thiazides with furosemide and other loop diuretics. Increased hypotension and/or renal adverse effects of ACE inhibitors may result in aggressively diuresed patients. Beta-blockers increase hyperglycemic effects of thiazides in type 2 diabetes mellitus. Cyclosporine and thiazides can increase the risk of gout or renal toxicity. Digoxin toxicity can be exacerbated if a thiazide induces hypokalemia or hypomagnesemia. Lithium toxicity can occur with thiazides due to reduced renal excretion of lithium. Thiazides may prolong the duration of action with neuromuscular blocking agents.

Decreased Effect: Effects of oral hypoglycemics may be decreased. Decreased absorption of hydrochlorothiazide with cholestyramine and colestipol. NSAIDs can decrease the efficacy of thiazides, reducing the diuretic and antihypertensive effects.

Pregnancy Risk Factor D

Generic Available No

BeneFix™ *see* Factor IX Complex (Human) *on page 484*

Benicar™ *see* Olmesartan *on page 885*

Benoquin® *see* Monobenzone *on page 827*

Bentoquatam (ben to KWA tam)

U.S. Brand Names IvyBlock® [OTC]

Pharmacologic Category Topical Skin Product

Synonyms Quaternium-18 Bentonite

Use To protect the skin from rash due to exposure to poison sumac, poison ivy or poison oak

Local Anesthetic/Vasoconstrictor Precautions No information available to require special precautions

Effects on Dental Treatment No effects or complications reported

Dosage Topical: Apply to exposed skin at least 15 minutes before potential contact and reapply every 4 hours

Mechanism of Action An organoclay substance which is capable of absorbing or binding to urushiol, the active principle in poison oak, ivy, and sumac. Bentoquatam serves as a barrier, blocking urushiol skin contact/absorption.

Drug Uptake Absorption: Has not been studied

Generic Available No

Bentyl® *see* Dicyclomine *on page 382*

Benylin DM® [OTC] *see* Dextromethorphan *on page 372*

Benylin® Expectorant [OTC] *see* Guaifenesin and Dextromethorphan *on page 569*

Benylin® Pediatric [OTC] *see* Dextromethorphan *on page 372*

Benza® [OTC] *see* Benzalkonium Chloride *on page 151*

Benzac® *see* Benzoyl Peroxide *on page 153*

Benzac® AC *see* Benzoyl Peroxide *on page 153*

Benzac® AC Wash *see* Benzoyl Peroxide *on page 153*

BenzaClin™ *see* Clindamycin and Benzoyl Peroxide *on page 301*

Benzacot® *see* Trimethobenzamide *on page 1209*

Benzac® W *see* Benzoyl Peroxide *on page 153*

Benzac® W Wash *see* Benzoyl Peroxide *on page 153*

Benzagel® *see* Benzoyl Peroxide *on page 153*

Benzagel® Wash *see* Benzoyl Peroxide *on page 153*

Benzalkonium Chloride (benz al KOE nee um KLOR ide)

Related Information

Periodontal Diseases *on page 1375*

U.S. Brand Names Benza® [OTC]; 3M™ Cavilon™ Skin Cleanser [OTC]; Ony-Clear [OTC]; Zephiran® [OTC]

Pharmacologic Category Antibiotic, Topical

Synonyms BAC

Use Surface antiseptic and germicidal preservative

Local Anesthetic/Vasoconstrictor Precautions No information available to require special precautions

Effects on Dental Treatment No effects or complications reported

Dosage Thoroughly rinse anionic detergents and soaps from the skin or other areas prior to use of solutions because they reduce the antibacterial activity of BAC. To protect metal instruments stored in BAC solution, add crushed Anti-Rust Tablets, 4 tablets/quart, to antiseptic solution, change solution at least once weekly. Not to be used for storage of aluminum or zinc instruments, instruments with lenses fastened by cement, lacquered catheters, or some synthetic rubber goods.

Other Adverse Effects 1% to 10%: Hypersensitivity

Pregnancy Risk Factor C

Generic Available Yes

Benzamycin® *see* Erythromycin and Benzoyl Peroxide *on page 453*

Benzashave® *see* Benzoyl Peroxide *on page 153*

Benzedrex® [OTC] *see* Propylhexedrine *on page 1019*

Benzocaine (BEN zoe kane)

Related Information

Mouth Pain, Cold Sore, and Canker Sore Products *on page 1458*
Oral Pain *on page 1360*

U.S. Brand Names Americaine® [OTC]; Americaine® Anesthetic Lubricant; Anbesol® [OTC]; Anbesol® Baby [OTC]; Anbesol® Maximum Strength [OTC]; Babee® Teething® [OTC]; Benzodent® [OTC]; Chiggerex® [OTC]; Chiggertox® [OTC]; Cylex® [OTC]; Detane® [OTC]; Foille® [OTC]; Foille® Medicated First Aid [OTC]; Foille® Plus [OTC]; HDA® Toothache [OTC]; Hurricaine®; Lanacane® [OTC]; Mycinettes® [OTC]; Orabase®-B [OTC]; Orajel® [OTC]; Orajel® Baby [OTC]; Orajel® Baby Nighttime [OTC]; Orajel® Maximum Strength [OTC]; Orasol® [OTC]; Solarcaine® [OTC]; Trocaine® [OTC]; Zilactin®-B [OTC]; Zilactin® Baby [OTC]

Canadian Brand Names Anbesol® Baby; Zilactin-B®; Zilactin Baby®

Mexican Brand Names Graneodin-B

Pharmacologic Category Local Anesthetic

Synonyms Ethyl Aminobenzoate

Use

Dental: Ester-type topical local anesthetic for temporary relief of pain associated with toothache, minor sore throat pain and canker sore

(Continued)

Benzocaine *(Continued)*

Medical: Local anesthetic (ester derivative); temporary relief of pain associated with pruritic dermatosis, pruritus, minor burns, acute congestive and serious otitis media, swimmer's ear, otitis externa, hemorrhoids, rectal fissures, anesthetic lubricant for passage of catheters and endoscopic tubes; nonprescription diet aid

Local Anesthetic/Vasoconstrictor Precautions No information available to require special precautions

Effects on Dental Treatment No effects or complications reported

Dosage Children and Adults:

Mucous membranes: Dosage varies depending on area to be anesthetized and vascularity of tissues

Oral mouth/throat preparations: Do not administer for >2 days or in children <2 years of age, unless directed by a physician; refer to specific package labeling

Topical: Apply to affected area as needed

Mechanism of Action Local anesthetics bind selectively to the intracellular surface of sodium channels to block influx of sodium into the axon. As a result, depolarization necessary for action potential propagation and subsequent nerve function is prevented. The block at the sodium channel is reversible. When drug diffuses away from the axon, sodium channel function is restored and nerve propagation returns.

Other Adverse Effects Dose-related and may result in high plasma levels

1% to 10%:

Dermatologic: Angioedema, contact dermatitis

Local: Burning, stinging

<1%: Edema, urticaria, urethritis, methemoglobinemia (risk may be increased in infants), tenderness

Contraindications Hypersensitivity to benzocaine, other ester-type local anesthetics, or any component of their formulation; secondary bacterial infection of area; ophthalmic use; see package labeling for specific contraindications

Warnings/Precautions Not intended for use when infections are present

Drug Interactions May antagonize actions of sulfonamides

Drug Uptake

Onset of action: ~1 minute

Absorption: Topical: Poorly absorbed after administration to intact skin, but well absorbed from mucous membranes and traumatized skin

Duration: 15-20 minutes

Pregnancy Risk Factor C

Dosage Forms AERO, oral spray: 20% (60 mL). **AERO, topical spray:** 5% (97.5 mL, 105 mL); 20% (20 mL, 90 mL, 120 mL, 135 mL). **CRM, topical:** 5% (30 g, 454 g); 20% (30 g). **GEL, oral:** 6.3% (7.5 g); 6.5% (15 mL); 7.5% (7.5 g, 10 g, 15 g); 10% (6 g, 7.5 g, 10 g); 20% (6 g, 7 g, 7.5 g, 10 g); (Hurricaine®): 20% (5 g, 30 g). **GEL, topical:** 20% (2.5 g, 28 g). **LIQ, oral:** 6.3% (9 mL, 15 mL, 30 mL); 7.5% (13 mL); 10% (13 mL); 20% (9 mL, 14 mL, 30 mL). **LIQ, topical:** 2% (30 mL). **LOT, oral:** 2.5% (15 mL). **LOZ:** 10 mg, 15 mg. **OINT, oral:** 20% (30 g). **OINT, topical:** 2% (52 g); 5% (3.5 g, 28 g). **PASTE, oral:** 20% (7 g)

Generic Available Yes

Benzocaine, Butyl Aminobenzoate, Tetracaine, and Benzalkonium Chloride

(BEN zoe kane, BYOO til a meen oh BENZ oh ate, TET ra kane, & benz al KOE nee um KLOR ide)

U.S. Brand Names Cetacaine®

Pharmacologic Category Local Anesthetic

Synonyms Tetracaine Hydrochloride, Benzocaine Butyl Aminobenzoate, and Benzalkonium Chloride

Use Dental: Topical anesthetic to control pain or gagging

Local Anesthetic/Vasoconstrictor Precautions No information available to require special precautions

Effects on Dental Treatment No effects or complications reported

Dosage Apply to affected area for ~ 1 second or less

Other Adverse Effects Dose related and may result from high plasma levels

1% to 10%:

Dermatologic: Contact dermatitis, angioedema

Local: Burning, stinging

<1%: Edema, urticaria, urethritis, methemoglobinemia (risk may be increased in infants), tenderness

Pregnancy Risk Factor C

Dosage Forms AERO, topical: Benzocaine 14%, butyl aminobenzoate 2%, tetracaine 2%, and benzalkonium 0.5% (56 g). **GEL, topical:** Benzocaine 14%, butyl aminobenzoate 2%, tetracaine 2%, and benzalkonium 0.5% (29 g). **LIQ, topical:** Benzocaine 14%, butyl aminobenzoate 2%, tetracaine 2%, and benzalkonium 0.5% (56 mL)

Generic Available No

Benzocaine, Gelatin, Pectin, and Sodium Carboxymethylcellulose

(BEN zoe kane, JEL a tin, PEK tin, & SOW dee um kar box ee meth il SEL yoo lose)

U.S. Brand Names Orabase® With Benzocaine [OTC]

Pharmacologic Category Local Anesthetic

Use Dental: Topical anesthetic and emollient for oral lesions

Local Anesthetic/Vasoconstrictor Precautions No information available to require special precautions

Effects on Dental Treatment No effects or complications reported

Dosage Apply 2-4 times/day

Other Adverse Effects Dose related and may result from high plasma levels

1% to 10%:

Dermatologic: Contact dermatitis, angioedema

Local: Burning, stinging

<1%: Edema, urticaria, urethritis, methemoglobinemia (risk may be increased in infants), tenderness

Pregnancy Risk Factor C

Dosage Forms PASTE: Benzocaine 20%, gelatin, pectin, and sodium carboxymethylcellulose (5 g, 15 g)

Generic Available No

Benzodent® [OTC] *see* Benzocaine *on page 151*

Benzoin (BEN zoyn)

U.S. Brand Names TinBen® [OTC]

Pharmacologic Category Antibiotic, Topical; Topical Skin Product

Synonyms Gum Benjamin

Use Protective application for irritations of the skin; sometimes used in boiling water as steam inhalants for their expectorant and soothing action

Local Anesthetic/Vasoconstrictor Precautions No information available to require special precautions

Effects on Dental Treatment No effects or complications reported

Dosage Apply 1-2 times/day

Generic Available Yes

Benzonatate (ben ZOE na tate)

Related Information

Management of Patients Undergoing Cancer Therapy *on page 1402*

U.S. Brand Names Tessalon®

Canadian Brand Names Tessalon®

Mexican Brand Names Beknol; Pebegal; Tesalon; Tusical®; Tusitato®

Pharmacologic Category Antitussive

Use Symptomatic relief of nonproductive cough

Local Anesthetic/Vasoconstrictor Precautions No information available to require special precautions

Effects on Dental Treatment No effects or complications reported

Dosage Children >10 years and Adults: Oral: 100 mg 3 times/day or every 4 hours up to 600 mg/day

Mechanism of Action Tetracaine congener with antitussive properties; suppresses cough by topical anesthetic action on the respiratory stretch receptors

Other Adverse Effects 1% to 10%:

Central nervous system: Sedation, headache, dizziness

Dermatologic: Rash

Gastrointestinal: GI upset

Neuromuscular & skeletal: Numbness in chest

Ocular: Burning sensation in eyes

Respiratory: Nasal congestion

Drug Uptake

Onset of action: 15-20 minutes

Duration: 3-8 hours

Pregnancy Risk Factor C

Generic Available Yes

Benzoyl Peroxide (BEN zoe il peer OKS ide)

U.S. Brand Names Benzac®; Benzac® AC; Benzac® AC Wash; Benzac® W; Benzac® W Wash; Benzagel®; Benzagel® Wash; Benzashave®; Brevoxyl®; Brevoxyl® Cleansing; Brevoxyl® Wash; Clinac™ BPO; Del Aqua®; Desquam-E™; Desquam-X®; Exact® Acne Medication [OTC]; Fostex® 10% BPO [OTC]; Loroxide® [OTC]; Neutrogena® Acne Mask [OTC]; Neutrogena® On The Spot® Acne Treatment [OTC]; Oxy 10® Balanced Medicated Face Wash [OTC]; Palmer's® Skin Success Acne [OTC]; PanOxyl®; PanOxyl®-AQ; PanOxyl® Bar [OTC]; Seba-Gel™; Triaz®; Triaz® Cleanser; Zapzyt® [OTC]

(Continued)

Benzoyl Peroxide *(Continued)*

Canadian Brand Names Acetoxyl®; Benoxyl®; Benzac AC®; Benzac W® Gel; Benzac W® Wash; Desquam-X®; Oxyderm™; PanOxyl®; PanOxyl®-AQ; Solugel®

Mexican Brand Names Benoxyl®; Benzac®; Benzaderm®; Solugel®

Pharmacologic Category Topical Skin Product; Topical Skin Product, Acne

Use Adjunctive treatment of mild to moderate acne vulgaris and acne rosacea

Local Anesthetic/Vasoconstrictor Precautions No information available to require special precautions

Effects on Dental Treatment No effects or complications reported

Dosage Children and Adults:

Cleansers: Wash once or twice daily; control amount of drying or peeling by modifying dose frequency or concentration

Topical: Apply sparingly once daily; gradually increase to 2-3 times/day if needed. If excessive dryness or peeling occurs, reduce dose frequency or concentration; if excessive stinging or burning occurs, remove with mild soap and water; resume use the next day.

Mechanism of Action Releases free-radical oxygen which oxidizes bacterial proteins in the sebaceous follicles decreasing the number of anaerobic bacteria and decreasing irritating-type free fatty acids

Other Adverse Effects 1% to 10%: Dermatologic: Irritation, contact dermatitis, dryness, erythema, peeling, stinging

Drug Interactions Increased Toxicity: Benzoyl peroxide potentiates adverse reactions seen with tretinoin

Drug Uptake Absorption: ~5% through the skin; gels are more penetrating than creams

Pregnancy Risk Factor C

Generic Available Yes

Benzoyl Peroxide and Hydrocortisone

(BEN zoe il peer OKS ide & hye droe KOR ti sone)

U.S. Brand Names Vanoxide-HC®

Canadian Brand Names Vanoxide-HC

Pharmacologic Category Topical Skin Product; Topical Skin Product, Acne

Synonyms Hydrocortisone and Benzoyl Peroxide

Use Treatment of acne vulgaris and oily skin

Local Anesthetic/Vasoconstrictor Precautions No information available to require special precautions

Effects on Dental Treatment No effects or complications reported

Dosage Shake well; apply thin film 1-3 times/day, gently massage into skin

Therapy should be discontinued when control is achieved; if no improvement is seen, reassessment of diagnosis may be necessary.

Other Adverse Effects See Benzoyl Peroxide *on page 153* and Hydrocortisone *on page 608*

Drug Uptake See Hydrocortisone *on page 608* and Benzoyl Peroxide *on page 153*

Pregnancy Risk Factor C

Generic Available No

Benzphetamine (benz FET a meen)

U.S. Brand Names Didrex®

Canadian Brand Names Didrex®

Pharmacologic Category Anorexiant

Synonyms Benzphetamine Hydrochloride

Use Short-term adjunct in exogenous obesity

Local Anesthetic/Vasoconstrictor Precautions Use with caution since amphetamines have actions similar to epinephrine and norepinephrine

Effects on Dental Treatment No effects or complications reported

Restrictions C-III

Dosage Adults: Oral: 25-50 mg 2-3 times/day, preferably twice daily, midmorning and midafternoon; maximum dose: 50 mg 3 times/day

Mechanism of Action Noncatechol sympathomimetic amines with pharmacologic actions similar to ephedrine; require breakdown by monoamine oxidase for inactivation; produce CNS and respiratory stimulation, a pressor response, mydriasis, bronchodilation, and contraction of the urinary sphincter; thought to have a direct effect on both alpha- and beta-receptor sites in the peripheral system, as well as release stores of norepinephrine in adrenergic nerve terminals; CNS action is thought to occur in the cerebral cortex and reticular-activating system; anorexigenic effect is probably secondary to the CNS-stimulating effect; the site of action is probably the hypothalamic feeding center

Other Adverse Effects Frequency not defined:

Cardiovascular: Hypertension, palpitations, tachycardia, chest pain, T-wave changes, arrhythmias, pulmonary hypertension, valvulopathy

Central nervous system: Euphoria, nervousness, insomnia, restlessness, dizziness, anxiety, headache, agitation, confusion, mental depression, psychosis, CVA, seizure

Dermatologic: Alopecia, urticaria, skin rash, ecchymosis, erythema

Endocrine & metabolic: Changes in libido, gynecomastia, menstrual irregularities, porphyria

Gastrointestinal: Nausea, vomiting, abdominal cramps, constipation, xerostomia, metallic taste

Genitourinary: Impotence

Hematologic: Bone marrow depression, agranulocytosis, leukopenia

Neuromuscular & skeletal: Tremor

Ocular: Blurred vision, mydriasis

Drug Interactions CYP3A3/4 enzyme substrate

Increased Effect/Toxicity: Amphetamines may precipitate hypertensive crisis or serotonin syndrome in patients receiving MAO inhibitors (selegiline >10 mg/day, isocarboxazid, phenelzine, tranylcypromine, furazolidone). Serotonin syndrome has also been associated with combinations of amphetamines and SSRIs; these combinations should be avoided. TCAs may enhance the effects of amphetamines, potentially leading to hypertensive crisis. Large doses of antacids or urinary alkalinizers increase the half-life and duration of action of amphetamines. May precipitate arrhythmias in patients receiving general anesthetics. Inhibitors of CYP2D6 may increase the effects of amphetamines (includes amiodarone, cimetidine, delavirdine, fluoxetine, paroxetine, propafenone, quinidine, and ritonavir).

Decreased Effect: Amphetamines inhibit the antihypertensive response to guanethidine and guanadrel. Urinary acidifiers decrease the half-life and duration of action of amphetamines. Enzyme inducers (barbiturates, carbamazepine, phenytoin, and rifampin) may decrease serum concentration of amphetamines.

Pregnancy Risk Factor X

Generic Available No

Benztropine (BENZ troe peen)

U.S. Brand Names Cogentin®

Canadian Brand Names Apo®-Benztropine; Cogentin®

Pharmacologic Category Anticholinergic Agent; Anti-Parkinson's Agent, Anticholinergic

Synonyms Benztropine Mesylate

Use Adjunctive treatment of Parkinson's disease; also used in treatment of drug-induced extrapyramidal effects (except tardive dyskinesia) and acute dystonic reactions

Local Anesthetic/Vasoconstrictor Precautions No information available to require special precautions

Effects on Dental Treatment Dry mouth, nose, and throat very prevalent

Dosage Use in children <3 years of age should be reserved for life-threatening emergencies

Drug-induced extrapyramidal reaction: Oral, I.M., I.V.:

Children >3 years: 0.02-0.05 mg/kg/dose 1-2 times/day

Adults: 1-4 mg/dose 1-2 times/day

Acute dystonia: Adults: I.M., I.V.: 1-2 mg

Parkinsonism: Oral:

Adults: 0.5-6 mg/day in 1-2 divided doses; if one dose is greater, give at bedtime; titrate dose in 0.5 mg increments at 5- to 6-day intervals

Elderly: Initial: 0.5 mg once or twice daily; increase by 0.5 mg as needed at 5-6 days; maximum: 6 mg/day

Mechanism of Action Thought to partially block striatal cholinergic receptors to help balance cholinergic and dopaminergic activity. Possesses both anticholinergic and antihistaminic effects. *In vitro* anticholinergic activity approximates that of atropine; *in vivo* it is only about half as active as atropine. Animal data suggest its antihistaminic activity and duration of action approach that of pyrilamine maleate. May also inhibit the reuptake and storage of dopamine and thereby, prolong the action of dopamine.

Other Adverse Effects Frequency not defined:

Cardiovascular: Tachycardia

Central nervous system: Confusion, disorientation, memory impairment, toxic psychosis, visual hallucinations

Dermatologic: Rash

Endocrine & metabolic: Heat stroke, hyperthermia

Gastrointestinal: Xerostomia, nausea, vomiting, constipation, ileus

Genitourinary: Urinary retention, dysuria

Ocular: Blurred vision, mydriasis

Miscellaneous: Fever

Drug Interactions

Increased Effect/Toxicity: Central and/or peripheral anticholinergic syndrome can occur when benztropine is administered with amantadine, rimantadine, narcotic

(Continued)

Benztropine *(Continued)*

analgesics, phenothiazines and other antipsychotics (especially with high anticholinergic activity), tricyclic antidepressants, quinidine and some other antiarrhythmics, and antihistamines. Benztropine may increase the absorption of digoxin.

Decreased Effect: May increase gastric degradation of levodopa and decrease the amount of levodopa absorbed by delaying gastric emptying; therapeutic effects of cholinergic agents (tacrine, donepezil) and neuroleptics may be antagonized.

Drug Uptake

Onset of action: Oral: ≤1 hour; Parenteral: ≤15 minutes

Duration: 6-48 hours

Pregnancy Risk Factor C

Generic Available Yes: Tablet

Benzylpenicilloyl-polylysine (BEN zil pen i SIL oyl pol i LIE seen)

U.S. Brand Names Pre-Pen®

Pharmacologic Category Diagnostic Agent

Synonyms Penicilloyl-polylysine; PPL

Use Adjunct in assessing the risk of administering penicillin (penicillin or benzylpenicillin) in adults with a history of clinical penicillin hypersensitivity

Local Anesthetic/Vasoconstrictor Precautions No information available to require special precautions

Effects on Dental Treatment No effects or complications reported

Dosage PPL is administered by a scratch technique or by intradermal injection. For initial testing, PPL should always be applied via the scratch technique. **Do not give intradermally to patients who have positive reactions to a scratch test.** PPL test alone does not identify those patients who react to a minor antigenic determinant and does not appear to predict reliably the occurrence of late reactions.

Scratch test: Use scratch technique with a 20-gauge needle to make 3-5 mm nonbleeding scratch on epidermis, apply a small drop of solution to scratch, rub in gently with applicator or toothpick. A positive reaction consists of a pale wheal surrounding the scratch site which develops within 10 minutes and ranges from 5-15 mm or more in diameter.

Intradermal test: Use intradermal test with a tuberculin syringe with a 26- to 30-gauge short bevel needle; a dose of 0.01-0.02 mL is injected intradermally. A control of 0.9% sodium chloride should be injected at least 1.5" from the PPL test site. Most skin responses to the intradermal test will develop within 5-15 minutes.

Interpretation:

(-) Negative: No reaction

(±) Ambiguous: Wheal only slightly larger than original bleb with or without erythematous flare and larger than control site

(+) Positive: Itching and marked increase in size of original bleb

Control site should be reactionless

Mechanism of Action Elicits IgE antibodies which produce type I accelerate urticarial reactions to penicillins

Other Adverse Effects 1% to 10%: Local: Intense local inflammatory response at skin test site

Frequency not defined:

Cardiovascular: Hypotension

Dermatologic: Angioneurotic edema, pruritus, erythema, urticaria

Local: Intense local inflammatory response at skin test site, wheal (locally)

Respiratory: Dyspnea

Miscellaneous: Systemic allergic reactions occur rarely

Drug Interactions Corticosteroids and other immunosuppressive agents may inhibit the immune response to the skin test.

Pregnancy Risk Factor C

Generic Available No

Bepridil (BE pri dil)

Related Information

Calcium Channel Blockers and Gingival Hyperplasia *on page 1432*

Cardiovascular Diseases *on page 1308*

U.S. Brand Names Vascor®

Canadian Brand Names Vascor®

Pharmacologic Category Calcium Channel Blocker

Synonyms Bepridil Hydrochloride

Use Treatment of chronic stable angina; due to side effect profile, reserve for patients who have been intolerant of other antianginal therapy; bepridil may be used alone or in combination with nitrates or beta-blockers

Local Anesthetic/Vasoconstrictor Precautions No information available to require special precautions

Effects on Dental Treatment Other drugs of this class can cause gingival hyperplasia (ie, nifedipine) but there have been no reports for bepridil.

Dosage Adults: Oral: Initial: 200 mg/day, then adjust dose at 10-day intervals until optimal response is achieved; maximum daily dose: 400 mg

Mechanism of Action A type 4 calcium antagonist which possesses characteristics of the traditional calcium antagonist, inhibiting calcium ion from entering the "slow channels" or select voltage-sensitive areas of vascular smooth muscle and myocardium during depolarization and producing a relaxation of coronary vascular smooth muscle and coronary vasodilation; may also inhibit fast sodium channels (inward) which may account for some of its side effects (eg, arrhythmias); a direct bradycardia effect of bepridil has been postulated via direct action on the S-A node.

Other Adverse Effects

>10%:

- Central nervous system: Dizziness
- Gastrointestinal: Nausea, dyspepsia

1% to 10%:

- Cardiovascular: Bradycardia, edema, palpitations, QT prolongation (dose-related; up to 5% with prolongation of ≥25%), CHF (1%)
- Central nervous system: Nervousness, headache (7% to 13%), drowsiness, psychiatric disturbances (<2%), insomnia (2% to 3%)
- Dermatologic: Rash (≤2%)
- Endocrine & metabolic: Sexual dysfunction
- Gastrointestinal: Diarrhea, anorexia, xerostomia, constipation, abdominal pain, dyspepsia, flatulence
- Neuromuscular & skeletal: Weakness (7% to 14%), tremor (<9%), paresthesia (3%)
- Ocular: Blurred vision
- Otic: Tinnitus
- Respiratory: Rhinitis, dyspnea (≤9%), cough (≤2%)
- Miscellaneous (≤2%): Flu syndrome, diaphoresis

Drug Interactions CYP3A3/4 enzyme substrate

Increased Effect/Toxicity: Use with H_2 blockers may increase bioavailability and cardiac depressant effects on AV conduction. Bepridil may increase serum concentration/effects of carbamazepine, cyclosporine, digitalis, quinidine, and theophylline. Concurrent use of fentanyl with bepridil may increase hypotension. Use with amprenavir, ritonavir, sparfloxacin (possibly also gatifloxacin and moxifloxacin) may increase risk of bepridil toxicity, especially its cardiotoxicity. Use with cisapride may increase the risk of malignant arrhythmias, concurrent use is contraindicated.

Drug Uptake

Onset of action: 1 hour
Absorption: Oral: 100%
Half-life, elimination: 24 hours
Time to peak: 2-3 hours

Pregnancy Risk Factor C

Generic Available No

Beractant (ber AKT ant)

U.S. Brand Names Survanta®

Canadian Brand Names Survanta®

Mexican Brand Names Survanta®

Pharmacologic Category Lung Surfactant

Synonyms Bovine Lung Surfactant; Natural Lung Surfactant

Use Prevention and treatment of respiratory distress syndrome (RDS) in premature infants

Prophylactic therapy: Body weight <1250 g in infants at risk for developing or with evidence of surfactant deficiency

Rescue therapy: Treatment of infants with RDS confirmed by x-ray and requiring mechanical ventilation (administer as soon as possible - within 8 hours of age)

Local Anesthetic/Vasoconstrictor Precautions No information available to require special precautions

Effects on Dental Treatment No effects or complications reported

Dosage

Prophylactic treatment: Give 100 mg phospholipids (4 mL/kg) intratracheally as soon as possible; as many as 4 doses may be administered during the first 48 hours of life, no more frequently than 6 hours apart. The need for additional doses is determined by evidence of continuing respiratory distress; if the infant is still intubated and requiring at least 30% inspired oxygen to maintain a PAO_2 ≤80 torr.

Rescue treatment: Administer 100 mg phospholipids (4 mL/kg) as soon as the diagnosis of RDS is made

Mechanism of Action Replaces deficient or ineffective endogenous lung surfactant in neonates with respiratory distress syndrome (RDS) or in neonates at risk of developing RDS. Surfactant prevents the alveoli from collapsing during expiration by lowering surface tension between air and alveolar surfaces.

(Continued)

Beractant *(Continued)*

Other Adverse Effects During the dosing procedure:

>10%: Cardiovascular: Transient bradycardia

1% to 10%: Respiratory: Oxygen desaturation

Generic Available No

Berocca® *see* Vitamin B Complex With Vitamin C and Folic Acid *on page 1244*

Beta-2® *see* Isoetharine *on page 658*

Beta-Carotene (BAY tah KARE oh teen)

U.S. Brand Names A-Caro-25®; B-Caro-T™; Lumitene™

Pharmacologic Category Vitamin, Fat Soluble

Use Prophylaxis and treatment of polymorphous light eruption; prophylaxis against photosensitivity reactions in patients with erythropoietic protoporphyria (EPP)

Local Anesthetic/Vasoconstrictor Precautions No information available to require special precautions

Effects on Dental Treatment No effects or complications reported

Dosage Topical administration is considerably less effective than systemic therapy.

Oral:

Children <14 years: 30-150 mg/day

Adults: 30-300 mg/day; 10,000-30,000 int. units/day (no RDI established)

Prophylaxis/treatment of polymorphous light eruption or prophylaxis against photosensitivity reactions in erythropoietic protoporphyria: 30-300 mg/day

Mechanism of Action One of more than 400 carotenoids found in fruits and the chloroplasts and chlorophyll of green, leafy vegetables; as a general rule, the deeper the color, the higher the concentration of beta-carotene. Carotenoids in green vegetables are absorbed two to three times better than those in red or yellow vegetables. Beta-carotene is a precursor to vitamin A and is converted in the GI tract. Conversion is affected by the age and overall health of the individual and requires adequate levels of protein, thyroid hormones, bile, zinc and vitamin C. Natural form is an efficient free radical scavenger of singlet oxygen; synthetic form ("trans" form) has recently been found to be pro-oxidant. It is capable of blocking chain-reaction lipid peroxidation and is critical in both cell-mediated and humoral immunity. Retinoids interact with nuclear receptors, influencing apoptosis (cell death) and gene expression. The exact mechanism in erythropoietic protoporphyria has not been elucidated; although patient must become carotenemic before effects are observed, there appears to be more than a simple internal light screen responsible for the action.

Other Adverse Effects >10%: Dermatologic: Carotenodermia (yellowing of palms, hands, or soles of feet, and to a lesser extent the face)

Drug Interactions

Increased Toxicity: Additional vitamin A supplementation

Decreased Effect: Orlistat and drugs which can cause depletion of beta-carotene and/or vitamin A: Cholestyramine, colchicine, colestipol, mineral oil, and neomycin

Pregnancy Risk Factor C

Generic Available Yes

Betadine® [OTC] *see* Povidone-Iodine *on page 982*

Betadine® 5% Sterile Ophthalmic Prep Solution *see* Povidone-Iodine *on page 982*

Betadine® First Aid Antibiotics + Moisturizer [OTC] *see* Bacitracin and Polymyxin B *on page 141*

Betagan® [OTC] *see* Povidone-Iodine *on page 982*

Betagan® Liquifilm® *see* Levobunolol *on page 696*

Betaine Anhydrous (BAY tayne an HY drus)

U.S. Brand Names Cystadane®

Canadian Brand Names Cystadane™

Pharmacologic Category Homocystinuria, Treatment Agent

Use Orphan drug: Treatment of homocystinuria to decrease elevated homocysteine blood levels; included within the category of homocystinuria are deficiencies or defects in cystathionine beta-synthase (CBS), 5,10-methylenetetrahydrofolate reductase (MTHFR), and cobalamin cofactor metabolism (CBL).

Local Anesthetic/Vasoconstrictor Precautions No information available to require special precautions

Effects on Dental Treatment No effects or complications reported

Dosage Oral: 6 g/day, usually give in two 3 g doses

Other Adverse Effects Minimal; have included nausea, GI distress, and diarrhea

Pregnancy Risk Factor C

Generic Available No

Betamethasone (bay ta METH a sone)

Related Information

Respiratory Diseases *on page 1328*

U.S. Brand Names Alphatrex®; Betatrex®; Beta-Val®; Celestone®; Celestone® Phosphate; Celestone® Soluspan®; Diprolene®; Diprolene® AF; Diprosone®; Luxiq™; Maxivate®; Valisone® [DSC]

Canadian Brand Names Betaderm; Betaject™; Betnesol®; Betnovate®; Celestoderm®-EV/2; Celestoderm®-V; Celestone® Soluspan®; Diprolene® Glycol; Diprosone®; Ectosone; Prevex® B; Taro-Sone®; Topilene®; Topisone®; Valisone® Scalp Lotion

Mexican Brand Names Celestone®

Pharmacologic Category Corticosteroid, Systemic; Corticosteroid, Topical

Synonyms Betamethasone Dipropionate; Betamethasone Dipropionate, Augmented; Betamethasone Sodium Phosphate; Betamethasone Valerate; Flubenisolone

Use

Dental: Treatment of a variety of oral diseases of allergic, inflammatory or autoimmune origin

Medical: Inflammatory dermatoses such as seborrheic or atopic dermatitis, neurodermatitis, anogenital pruritus, psoriasis, inflammatory phase of xerosis

Local Anesthetic/Vasoconstrictor Precautions No information available to require special precautions

Effects on Dental Treatment No effects or complications reported

Dosage Base dosage on severity of disease and patient response.

Children: Use lowest dose listed as initial dose for adrenocortical insufficiency (physiologic replacement)

I.M.: 0.0175-0.125 mg base/kg/day divided every 6-12 hours **or** 0.5-7.5 mg base/m²/day divided every 6-12 hours

Oral: 0.0175-0.25 mg/kg/day divided every 6-8 hours **or** 0.5-7.5 mg/m²/day divided every 6-8 hours

Topical:

≤12 years: Use is not recommended.

>12 years: Apply a thin film twice daily; use minimal amount for shortest period of time to avoid HPA axis suppression

Adolescents and Adults:

Oral: 2.4-4.8 mg/day in 2-4 doses; range: 0.6-7.2 mg/day

I.M.: Betamethasone sodium phosphate and betamethasone acetate: 0.6-9 mg/day (generally, 1/3 to 1/2 of oral dose) divided every 12-24 hours

Foam: Apply twice daily, once in the morning and once at night to scalp

Dosing adjustment in hepatic impairment: Adjustments may be necessary in patients with liver failure because betamethasone is extensively metabolized in the liver

Adults:

Intrabursal, intra-articular, intradermal: 0.25-2 mL

Intralesional: Rheumatoid arthritis/osteoarthritis:

Very large joints: 1-2 mL

Large joints: 1 mL

Medium joints: 0.5-1 mL

Small joints: 0.25-0.5 mL

Topical: Apply thin film 2-4 times/day. Therapy should be discontinued when control is achieved; if no improvement is seen, reassessment of diagnosis may be necessary.

Mechanism of Action Controls the rate of protein synthesis, depresses the migration of polymorphonuclear leukocytes, fibroblasts, reverses capillary permeability, and lysosomal stabilization at the cellular level to prevent or control inflammation

Other Adverse Effects

Systemic:

>10%:

Central nervous system: Insomnia, nervousness

Gastrointestinal: Increased appetite, indigestion

1% to 10%:

Central nervous system: Dizziness or lightheadedness, headache

Dermatologic: Hirsutism, hypopigmentation

Endocrine & metabolic: Diabetes mellitus

Neuromuscular & skeletal: Arthralgia

Ocular: Cataracts, glaucoma

Respiratory: Epistaxis

Miscellaneous: Diaphoresis

<1% (Limited to important or life-threatening): Vertigo, seizures, psychoses, pseudotumor cerebri, mood swings, delirium, hallucinations, euphoria, Cushing's syndrome, pituitary-adrenal axis suppression, growth suppression, glucose intolerance, hypokalemia, alkalosis, amenorrhea, sodium and water retention, hyperglycemia

(Continued)

Betamethasone *(Continued)*

Topical:

1% to 10%:

Dermatologic: Itching, allergic contact dermatitis, erythema, dryness papular rashes, folliculitis, furunculosis, pustules, pyoderma, vesiculation, hyperesthesia, skin infection (secondary)

Local: Burning, irritation

<1% (Limited to important or life-threatening): Cushing's syndrome, hypokalemic syndrome, glaucoma, cataracts (posterior subcapsular)

Contraindications Hypersensitivity to betamethasone or any component of the formulation; systemic fungal infections

Warnings/Precautions Fatalities have occurred due to adrenal insufficiency in asthmatic patients during and after transfer from systemic corticosteroids to aerosol steroids. Several months may be required for recovery of this syndrome; during this period, aerosol steroids do **not** provide the systemic steroid needed to treat patients having trauma, surgery, or infections. Use with caution in patients with hypothyroidism, cirrhosis, ulcerative colitis. Do not use occlusive dressings on weeping or exudative lesions and general caution with occlusive dressings should be observed. Discontinue if skin irritation or contact dermatitis should occur; do not use in patients with decreased skin circulation. Topical use in patients ≤ 12 years of age is not recommended.

Drug Interactions CYP3A3/4 enzyme substrate

Insulin or oral hypoglycemics: Betamethasone may increase blood glucose.

Phenytoin, phenobarbital, rifampin increase clearance of betamethasone.

Potassium-depleting diuretics increase potassium loss.

Skin test antigens, immunizations: Betamethasone may decrease response and increase potential infections.

Dietary/Ethanol/Herb Considerations

Ethanol: Avoid use; may enhance gastric mucosal irritation.

Food: Administer with food to reduce GI upset. Betamethasone interferes with calcium absorption. Limit caffeine.

Herb/Nutraceutical: Avoid cat's claw and echinacea due to immunostimulant properties.

Drug Uptake

Half-life, elimination: Oral: 6.5 hours

Time to peak: I.V.: 10-36 minutes

Pregnancy Risk Factor C

Dosage Forms CRM, topical, as dipropionate: 0.05% (15 g, 45 g, 60 g); (Alphatrex®, Diprosone®): 0.05% (15 g, 45 g); (Maxivate®): 0.05% (45 g). **CRM, topical, as dipropionate augmented** (Diprolene® AF): 0.05% (15 g, 50 g). **CRM, topical, as valerate:** 0.1% (15 g, 45 g); (Betatrex®, Valisone® [DSC]): 0.1% (15 g, 45 g); (Beta-Val®): 0.1% (15 g, 45 g). **FOAM, topical, as valerate** (Luxiq™): 0.12% (50 g, 100 g). **GEL, topical, as dipropionate augmented** (Diprolene®): 0.05% (15 g, 50 g). **INJ, solution, as sodium phosphate** (Celestone® Phosphate): 4 mg/mL (5 mL). **INJ, suspension** (Celestone® Soluspan®): Betamethasone sodium phosphate 3 mg/mL and betamethasone acetate 3 mg/mL [6 mg/mL] (5 mL) **LOT, topical, as dipropionate**: 0.05% (20 mL, 60 mL); (Alphatrex®, Maxivate®): 0.05% (60 mL); (Diprosone®): 0.05% (20 mL, 60 mL). **LOT, topical, as dipropionate augmented** (Diprolene®): 0.05% (30 mL, 60 mL). **LOT, topical, as valerate** (Beta-Val®, Betatrex®, Valisone® [DSC]): 0.1% (60 mL). **OINT, topical, as dipropionate**: 0.05% (15 g, 45 g); (Alphatrex®, Maxivate®): 0.05% (45 g); (Diprosone®): 0.05% (15 g, 45 g). **OINT, topical, as dipropionate augmented**: 0.05% (15 g, 45 g, 50 g); (Diprolene®): 0.05% (15 g, 50 g). **OINT, topical, as valerate** (Betatrex®, Valisone® [DSC]): 0.1% (15 g, 45 g). **SYR, as base** (Celestone®): 0.6 mg/5 mL (118 mL). **TAB, as base** (Celestone®): 0.6 mg

Generic Available Yes

Betamethasone and Clotrimazole

(bay ta METH a sone & kloe TRIM a zole)

U.S. Brand Names Lotrisone®

Canadian Brand Names Lotriderm®

Pharmacologic Category Antifungal Agent, Topical; Corticosteroid, Topical

Synonyms Clotrimazole and Betamethasone

Use Topical treatment of various dermal fungal infections (including tinea pedis, cruris, and corpora in patients ≥17 years of age)

Local Anesthetic/Vasoconstrictor Precautions No information available to require special precautions

Effects on Dental Treatment No effects or complications reported

Dosage

Children <17 years: Do not use

Children ≥17 years and Adults:

Tinea corporis, tinea cruris: Topical: Massage into affected area twice daily, morning and evening; do not use for longer than 2 weeks; re-evaluate after 1 week if no clinical improvement; do not exceed 45 g cream/week or 45 mL lotion/week

Tinea pedis: Topical: Massage into affected area twice daily, morning and evening; do not use for longer than 4 weeks; re-evaluate after 2 weeks if no clinical improvement; do not exceed 45 g cream/week or 45 mL lotion/week

Elderly: Use with caution; skin atrophy and skin ulceration (rare) have been reported in patients with thinning skin; do not use for diaper dermatitis or under occlusive dressings

Mechanism of Action Betamethasone dipropionate is a corticosteroid. Clotrimazole is an antifungal agent.

Other Adverse Effects 1% to 10%:

Dermatologic: Dry skin (2%)

Local: Burning (2%)

Neuromuscular & skeletal: Paresthesia (2%)

See Betamethasone *on page 159* and Clotrimazole *on page 312*

Contraindications Hypersensitivity to betamethasone dipropionate, clotrimazole, other corticosteroids or imidazoles, or any component of their formulation

Warnings/Precautions Systemic absorption of topical corticosteroids may cause hypothalamic-pituitary-adrenal (HPA) axis suppression (reversible); may lead to manifestations of Cushing's syndrome, hyperglycemia, and glucosuria; risk is increased when used over large surface areas, for prolonged periods of time, or with occlusive dressings; not for use in patients <17 years of age (striae and growth retardation have been reported with use in infants and children); do not use for diaper dermatitis.

Drug Uptake See Clotrimazole *on page 312* and Betamethasone *on page 159*

Pregnancy Risk Factor C

Generic Available Yes: Cream

Betapace® *see* Sotalol *on page 1102*

Betapace AF™ *see* Sotalol *on page 1102*

Betasept® [OTC] *see* Chlorhexidine Gluconate *on page 263*

Betaseron® *see* Interferon Beta-1b *on page 648*

Betatrex® *see* Betamethasone *on page 159*

Beta-Val® *see* Betamethasone *on page 159*

Betaxolol (be TAKS oh lol)

Related Information

Cardiovascular Diseases *on page 1308*

U.S. Brand Names Betoptic® S; Kerlone®

Canadian Brand Names Betoptic® S

Pharmacologic Category Beta Blocker, $Beta_1$ Selective

Synonyms Betaxolol Hydrochloride

Use Treatment of chronic open-angle glaucoma and ocular hypertension; management of hypertension

Local Anesthetic/Vasoconstrictor Precautions No information available to require special precautions

Effects on Dental Treatment Noncardioselective beta-blockers (ie, propranolol, nadolol) enhance the pressor response to epinephrine, resulting in hypertension and bradycardia. This has not been reported for betaxolol, a cardioselective beta-blocker. Therefore local anesthetic with vasoconstrictor can be safely used in patients medicated with betaxolol. Many nonsteroidal anti-inflammatory drugs such as ibuprofen and indomethacin can reduce the hypotensive effect of beta-blockers after 3 or more weeks of therapy with the NSAID. Short-term NSAID use (ie, 3 days) requires no special precautions in patients taking beta-blockers.

Dosage Adults:

Ophthalmic: Instill 1 drop twice daily

Oral: 10 mg/day; may increase dose to 20 mg/day after 7-14 days if desired response is not achieved; initial dose in elderly patients: 5 mg/day

Mechanism of Action Competitively blocks $beta_1$-receptors, with little or no effect on $beta_2$-receptors; ophthalmic reduces intraocular pressure by reducing the production of aqueous humor

Other Adverse Effects

Ophthalmic:

>10%: Ocular: Conjunctival hyperemia

1% to 10%:

Ocular: Anisocoria, corneal punctate keratitis, keratitis, corneal staining, decreased corneal sensitivity, eye pain, vision disturbances

Systemic:

>10%:

Central nervous system: Drowsiness, insomnia

Endocrine & metabolic: Decreased sexual ability

1% to 10%:

Cardiovascular: Bradycardia, palpitations, edema, CHF, reduced peripheral circulation

Central nervous system: Mental depression

(Continued)

Betaxolol *(Continued)*

Gastrointestinal: Diarrhea or constipation, nausea, vomiting, stomach discomfort
Respiratory: Bronchospasm
Miscellaneous: Cold extremities

Drug Interactions CYP1A2 and 2D6 enzyme substrate

Increased Effect/Toxicity: The heart rate lowering effects of betaxolol are additive with other drugs which slow AV conduction (digoxin, verapamil, diltiazem). Reserpine increases the effects of betaxolol. Concurrent use of betaxolol may increase the effects of alpha-blockers (prazosin, terazosin), alpha-adrenergic stimulants (epinephrine, phenylephrine), and the vasoconstrictive effects of ergot alkaloids. Betaxolol may mask the tachycardia from hypoglycemia caused by insulin and oral hypoglycemics. In patients receiving concurrent therapy, the risk of hypertensive crisis is increased when either clonidine or the beta-blocker is withdrawn. Beta-blockers may increase the action or levels of disopyramide, nondepolarizing muscle relaxants, and theophylline although the effects are difficult to predict.

Decreased Effect: Decreased effect of betaxolol with aluminum salts, barbiturates, calcium salts, cholestyramine, colestipol, NSAIDs, penicillins (ampicillin), rifampin, salicylates, and sulfinpyrazone due to decreased bioavailability and plasma concentrations. Beta-blockers may decrease the effect of sulfonylureas.

Drug Uptake

Onset of action: Ophthalmic: 30 minutes; Oral: 1-1.5 hours
Absorption: Ophthalmic: Some systemic; Oral: ~100%
Duration: Ophthalmic: ≥12 hours
Half-life, elimination: Oral: 12-22 hours
Time to peak: Ophthalmic: ~2 hours; Oral: 1.5-6 hours

Pregnancy Risk Factor C (manufacturer); D (2nd and 3rd trimesters - expert analysis)

Generic Available Yes: Solution

Selected Readings

Foster CA and Aston SJ, "Propranolol-Epinephrine Interaction: A Potential Disaster," *Plast Reconstr Surg*, 1983, 72(1):74-8.
Wong DG, Spence JD, Lamki L, et al, "Effect of Nonsteroidal Anti-inflammatory Drugs on Control of Hypertension of Beta-Blockers and Diuretics," *Lancet*, 1986, 1(8488):997-1001.
Wynn RL, "Dental Nonsteroidal Anti-inflammatory Drugs and Prostaglandin-Based Drug Interactions, Part Two," *Gen Dent*, 1992, 40(2):104, 106, 108.
Wynn RL, "Epinephrine Interactions With Beta-Blockers," *Gen Dent*, 1994, 42(1):16, 18.

Betaxon® *see* Levobetaxolol *on page 695*

Bethanechol (be THAN e kole)

U.S. Brand Names Urecholine®

Canadian Brand Names Duvoid®; Myotonachol®; Urecholine®

Pharmacologic Category Cholinergic Agonist

Synonyms Bethanechol Chloride

Use Nonobstructive urinary retention and retention due to neurogenic bladder; treatment and prevention of bladder dysfunction caused by phenothiazines; diagnosis of flaccid or atonic neurogenic bladder; gastroesophageal reflux

Local Anesthetic/Vasoconstrictor Precautions No information available to require special precautions

Effects on Dental Treatment This is a cholinergic agent similar to pilocarpine and expect to see salivation and sweating in patients.

Dosage

Children:
Oral:
Abdominal distention or urinary retention: 0.6 mg/kg/day divided 3-4 times/day
Gastroesophageal reflux: 0.1-0.2 mg/kg/dose given 30 minutes to 1 hour before each meal to a maximum of 4 times/day
S.C.: 0.15-0.2 mg/kg/day divided 3-4 times/day

Adults:
Oral: 10-50 mg 2-4 times/day
S.C.: 2.5-5 mg 3-4 times/day, up to 7.5-10 mg every 4 hours for neurogenic bladder

Mechanism of Action Stimulates cholinergic receptors in the smooth muscle of the urinary bladder and GI tract resulting in increased peristalsis, increased GI and pancreatic secretions, bladder muscle contraction, and increased ureteral peristaltic waves

Other Adverse Effects More common with S.C. administration. Frequency not defined:

Cardiovascular: Hypotension, tachycardia, flushed skin
Central nervous system: Headache, malaise
Gastrointestinal: Abdominal cramps, diarrhea, nausea, vomiting, salivation, eructation
Genitourinary: Urinary urgency
Ocular: Lacrimation, miosis
Respiratory: Asthmatic attacks

Miscellaneous: Diaphoresis

Drug Interactions

Increased Effect/Toxicity: Bethanechol and ganglionic blockers may cause a critical fall in BP. Cholinergic drugs or anticholinesterase agents may have additive effects with bethanechol.

Decreased Effect: Procainamide, quinidine may decrease the effects of bethanechol. Anticholinergic agents (atropine, antihistamines, TCAs, phenothiazines) may decrease effects.

Drug Uptake

Onset of action: Oral: 30-90 minutes; S.C.: 5-15 minutes

Absorption: Oral: Variable

Duration: Oral: ≤6 hours; S.C.: 2 hours

Pregnancy Risk Factor C

Generic Available Yes

Betimol® *see* Timolol *on page 1170*

Betoptic® S *see* Betaxolol *on page 161*

Bexarotene (beks AIR oh teen)

U.S. Brand Names Targretin®

Canadian Brand Names Targretin®

Pharmacologic Category Antineoplastic Agent, Miscellaneous

Use

Oral: Treatment of cutaneous manifestations of cutaneous T-cell lymphoma in patients who are refractory to at least one prior systemic therapy

Topical: Treatment of cutaneous lesions in patients with cutaneous T-cell lymphoma (stage 1A and 1B) who have refractory or persistent disease after other therapies or who have not tolerated other therapies

Local Anesthetic/Vasoconstrictor Precautions No information available to require special precautions

Effects on Dental Treatment No effects or complications reported

Dosage

Adults:

Oral: 300 mg/m²/day taken as a single daily dose. If there is no tumor response after 8 weeks and the initial dose was well tolerated, then an increase to 400 mg/m²/day can be made with careful monitoring. Maintain as long as the patient is deriving benefit.

If the initial dose is not tolerated, then it may be adjusted to 200 mg/m²/day, then to 100 mg/m²/day or temporarily suspended if necessary to manage toxicity

Gel: Apply once every other day for first week, then increase on a weekly basis to once daily, 2 times/day, 3 times/day, and finally 4 times/day, according to tolerance

Mechanism of Action The exact mechanism in the treatment of cutaneous T-cell lymphoma is unknown. Binds and activates retinoid X receptor subtypes. Retinoid receptor subtypes can form heterodimers with various receptor partners such as retinoic acid receptors, vitamin D receptor, thyroid receptor and peroxisome proliferator activator receptors. Once activated, these receptors function as transcription factors that regulate the expression of genes which control cellular differentiation and proliferation. Bexarotene inhibits the growth *in vitro* of some tumor cell lines of hematopoietic and squamous cell origin.

Other Adverse Effects The first percentage is at a dose of 300 mg/m²/day; the second percentage is at a dose >300 mg/m²/day. Grade 3 and grade 4 events that occurred more frequently in patients at both doses were hyperlipidemia, hypertriglyceridemia, pruritus, headache, peripheral edema, leukopenia, rash, and hypercholesterolemia. Frequency of events was dose-related.

Oral:

>10%:

Cardiovascular: Peripheral edema (13% to 11%)

Central nervous system: Headache (30% to 42%), chills (10% to 13%)

Dermatologic: Rash (17% to 23%), exfoliative dermatitis (10% to 28%)

Endocrine & metabolic: Hyperlipidemia (about 79% in both dosing ranges), hypercholesteremia (32% to 62%), hypothyroidism (29% to 53%)

Hematologic: Leukopenia (17% to 47%)

Neuromuscular & skeletal: Weakness (20% to 45%)

Miscellaneous: Infection (13% to 23%)

<10%:

Cardiovascular: Hemorrhage, hypertension, angina pectoris, right heart failure, tachycardia, cerebrovascular accident

Central nervous system: Fever (5% to 17%), insomnia (5% to 11%), subdural hematoma, syncope, depression, agitation, ataxia, confusion, dizziness, hyperesthesia

Dermatologic: Dry skin (about 10% for both dosing ranges), alopecia (4% to 11%), skin ulceration, acne, skin nodule, maculopapular rash, serous drainage, vesicular bullous rash, cheilitis

(Continued)

Bexarotene *(Continued)*

Endocrine & metabolic: Hypoproteinemia, hyperglycemia, weight loss/gain, serum amylase (elevated), breast pain
Gastrointestinal: Abdominal pain (11% to 4%), nausea (16% to 8%), diarrhea (7% to 42%), vomiting (4% to 13%), anorexia (2% to 23%), constipation, xerostomia, flatulence, colitis, dyspepsia, gastroenteritis, gingivitis, melena, pancreatitis,
Genitourinary: Albuminuria, hematuria, urinary incontinence, urinary tract infection, urinary urgency, dysuria, kidney function abnormality
Hematologic: Hypochromic anemia (4% to 13%), anemia (6% to 25%), eosinophilia, thrombocythemia, coagulation time increased, lymphocytosis, thrombocytopenia
Hepatic: LDH increase (7% to 13%), hepatic failure
Neuromuscular & skeletal: Back pain (2% to 11%), arthralgia, myalgia, bone pain, myasthenia, arthrosis, neuropathy
Ocular: Dry eyes, conjunctivitis, blepharitis, corneal lesion, visual field defects, keratitis
Otic: Ear pain, otitis externa
Renal: Creatinine (elevated)
Respiratory: Pharyngitis, rhinitis, dyspnea, pleural effusion, bronchitis, increased cough, lung edema, hemoptysis, hypoxia
Miscellaneous: Flu-like syndrome (4% to 13%), bacterial infection (1% to 13%)

Topical:
Cardiovascular: Edema (10%)
Central nervous system: Headache (14%), weakness (6%), pain (30%)
Dermatologic: Rash (14% to 72%), pruritus (6% to 40%), contact dermatitis (14%), exfoliative dermatitis (6%)
Hematologic: Leukopenia (6%), lymphadenopathy (6%)
Neuromuscular & skeletal: Paresthesia (6%)
Respiratory: Cough (6%), pharyngitis (6%)
Miscellaneous: Diaphoresis (6%), infection (18%)

Drug Interactions CYP3A3/4 enzyme substrate
Increased Effect/Toxicity: Bexarotene plasma concentrations may be increased by azole antifungals, clarithromycin, erythromycin, fluvoxamine, nefazodone, quinine, ritonavir, or gemfibrozil.
Decreased Effect: Bexarotene plasma concentrations may be decreased by rifampin, phenytoin, phenobarbital, or nafcillin.

Drug Uptake
Absorption: Significantly improved by a fat-containing meal
Half-life, elimination: 7 hours
Time to peak: 2 hours

Pregnancy Risk Factor X
Generic Available No

Bextra® *see* Valdecoxib *on page 1225*
Biaxin® *see* Clarithromycin *on page 296*
Biaxin® XL *see* Clarithromycin *on page 296*

Bicalutamide (bye ka LOO ta mide)

U.S. Brand Names Casodex®
Canadian Brand Names Casodex®
Mexican Brand Names Casodex®
Pharmacologic Category Antiandrogen
Use Combination therapy with a luteinizing hormone-releasing hormone (LHRH) analog for the treatment of advanced prostate cancer
Local Anesthetic/Vasoconstrictor Precautions No information available to require special precautions
Effects on Dental Treatment No effects or complications reported
Mechanism of Action Pure nonsteroidal antiandrogen that binds to androgen receptors; specifically a competitive inhibitor for the binding of dihydrotestosterone and testosterone; prevents testosterone stimulation of cell growth in prostate cancer

Other Adverse Effects
>10%: Endocrine & metabolic: Hot flashes (49%)
≥2% to <5%:
Cardiovascular: Angina pectoris, CHF, edema
Central nervous system: Anxiety, depression, confusion, somnolence, nervousness, fever, chills
Dermatologic: Dry skin, pruritus, alopecia
Endocrine & metabolic: Breast pain, diabetes mellitus, decreased libido, dehydration, gout
Gastrointestinal: Anorexia, dyspepsia, rectal hemorrhage, xerostomia, melena, weight gain
Genitourinary: Polyuria, urinary impairment, dysuria, urinary retention, urinary urgency

Hepatic: Alkaline phosphatase increased

Neuromuscular & skeletal: Myasthenia, arthritis, myalgia, leg cramps, pathological fracture, neck pain, hypertonia, neuropathy

Renal: Creatinine increased

Respiratory: Cough increased, pharyngitis, bronchitis, pneumonia, rhinitis, lung disorder

Miscellaneous: Sepsis, neoplasma

Drug Interactions Bicalutamide may displace warfarin from protein binding sites which may result in an increased anticoagulant effect, especially when bicalutamide therapy is started after the patient is already on warfarin.

Drug Uptake

Absorption: Rapid and complete

Half-life, elimination: ≤10 days; Active enantiomer is 5.8 days

Pregnancy Risk Factor X

Generic Available No

Bicillin® C-R *see* Penicillin G Benzathine and Procaine Combined *on page 929*

Bicillin® C-R 900/300 *see* Penicillin G Benzathine and Procaine Combined *on page 929*

Bicillin® L-A *see* Penicillin G Benzathine *on page 928*

Bicitra® *see* Sodium Citrate and Citric Acid *on page 1096*

BiCNU® *see* Carmustine *on page 225*

Biltricide® *see* Praziquantel *on page 986*

Bimatoprost (bi MAT oh prost)

U.S. Brand Names Lumigan™

Pharmacologic Category Ophthalmic Agent, Miscellaneous

Use Reduction of intraocular pressure (IOP) in patients with open-angle glaucoma or ocular hypertension; should be used in patients who are intolerant of other IOP-lowering medications or failed treatment with another IOP-lowering medication

Local Anesthetic/Vasoconstrictor Precautions No information available to require special precautions

Effects on Dental Treatment No effects or complications reported

Dosage Ophthalmic: Adult: Open-angle glaucoma or ocular hypertension: Instill 1 drop into affected eye(s) once daily in the evening; do not exceed once-daily dosing (may decrease IOP-lowering effect). If used with other topical ophthalmic agents, separate administration by at least 5 minutes.

Mechanism of Action As a synthetic analog of prostaglandin with ocular hypotensive activity, bimatoprost decreases intraocular pressure by increasing the outflow of aqueous humor.

Other Adverse Effects

>10%: Ocular (15% to 45%): Conjunctival hyperemia, growth of eyelashes, ocular pruritus

1% to 10%:

Central nervous system: Headache (1% to 5%)

Dermatologic: Hirsutism (1% to 5%)

Hepatic: Abnormal LFTs (1% to 5%)

Neuromuscular & skeletal: Weakness (1% to 5%)

Ocular:

3% to 10%: Blepharitis, burning, cataract, dryness, eyelid redness, eyelash darkening, foreign body sensation, irritation, pain, pigmentation of periocular skin, superficial punctate keratitis, visual disturbance

1% to 3%: Allergic conjunctivitis, asthenopia, conjunctival edema, discharge, increased iris pigmentation, photophobia, tearing

Respiratory: Upper respiratory tract infection (10%)

Contraindications Hypersensitivity to bimatoprost or any component of the formulation

Drug Interactions Specific drug interactions have not been reported. When using more than one ophthalmic product, wait at least 5 minutes between application of each medication.

Drug Uptake

Onset of IOP reducing effect: ~4 hours; Peak effect: Maximum reduction of IOP: ~8-12 hours

Half-life, elimination: I.V.: 45 minutes in systemic circulation

Time to peak, plasma: 10 minutes

Pregnancy Risk Factor C

Generic Available No

Biocef *see* Cephalexin *on page 251*

Biodine [OTC] *see* Povidone-Iodine *on page 982*

Biofed-PE® [OTC] *see* Triprolidine and Pseudoephedrine *on page 1213*

Bion® Tears [OTC] *see* Artificial Tears *on page 117*

Biopatch® [OTC] *see* Chlorhexidine Gluconate *on page 263*

Bio-Statin® *see* Nystatin *on page 880*

BioThrax™ *see* Anthrax Vaccine Adsorbed *on page 103*

Biperiden (bye PER i den)

U.S. Brand Names Akineton®

Canadian Brand Names Akineton®

Mexican Brand Names Akineton®

Pharmacologic Category Anticholinergic Agent; Anti-Parkinson's Agent, Anticholinergic

Synonyms Biperiden Hydrochloride; Biperiden Lactate

Use Adjunct in the therapy of all forms of Parkinsonism; control of extrapyramidal symptoms secondary to antipsychotics

Local Anesthetic/Vasoconstrictor Precautions No information available to require special precautions

Effects on Dental Treatment Dry mouth, nose, and throat very prevalent

Dosage Oral: Adults:

Parkinsonism: 2 mg 3-4 times/day

Extrapyramidal: 2 mg 1-3 times/day

Mechanism of Action A weak anticholinergic agent; beneficial effects in Parkinson's disease and neuroleptic-induced extrapyramidal reactions are believed to be due to the inhibition of striatal cholinergic receptors.

Other Adverse Effects Frequency not defined:

Cardiovascular: Orthostatic hypotension, bradycardia

Central nervous system: Drowsiness, euphoria, disorientation, agitation, sleep disorder (decreased REM sleep and increased REM latency)

Gastrointestinal: Constipation, xerostomia

Genitourinary: Urinary retention

Neuromuscular & skeletal: Choreic movements

Ocular: Blurred vision

Drug Interactions

Increased Effect/Toxicity: Central and/or peripheral anticholinergic syndrome can occur when administered with amantadine (or rimantadine), narcotic analgesics, phenothiazines and other antipsychotics (especially with high anticholinergic activity), tricyclic antidepressants, quinidine and some other antiarrhythmics, and antihistamines. Anticholinergics may increase the bioavailability of atenolol (and possibly other beta-blockers). Anticholinergics may decrease gastric degradation and increase the amount of digoxin or levodopa absorbed by delaying gastric emptying.

Decreased Effect: Anticholinergics may antagonize the therapeutic effect of neuroleptics and cholinergic agents (includes tacrine and donepezil).

Drug Uptake

Half-life, elimination: 18.4-24.3 hours

Time to peak: 1-1.5 hours

Pregnancy Risk Factor C

Generic Available No

Bisac-Evac™ [OTC] *see* Bisacodyl *on page 166*

Bisacodyl (bis a KOE dil)

U.S. Brand Names Alophen® [OTC]; Bisac-Evac™ [OTC]; Bisacodyl Uniserts® [OTC]; Dulcolax® [OTC]; Feen-A-Mint® [OTC]; Femilax™ [OTC]; Fleet® Bisacodyl Enema [OTC]; Fleet® Stimulant Laxative [OTC]; Modane Tablets® [OTC]

Canadian Brand Names Apo®-Bisacodyl; Dulcolax®

Mexican Brand Names Dulcolan®

Pharmacologic Category Laxative, Stimulant

Use Treatment of constipation; colonic evacuation prior to procedures or examination

Local Anesthetic/Vasoconstrictor Precautions No information available to require special precautions

Effects on Dental Treatment No effects or complications reported

Dosage

Children:

Oral: >6 years: 5-10 mg (0.3 mg/kg) at bedtime or before breakfast

Rectal suppository:

<2 years: 5 mg as a single dose

>2 years: 10 mg

Adults:

Oral: 5-15 mg as single dose (up to 30 mg when complete evacuation of bowel is required)

Rectal suppository: 10 mg as single dose

Mechanism of Action Stimulates peristalsis by directly irritating the smooth muscle of the intestine, possibly the colonic intramural plexus; alters water and electrolyte secretion producing net intestinal fluid accumulation and laxation

Other Adverse Effects Frequency not defined:

Central nervous system: Vertigo

Endocrine & metabolic: Electrolyte and fluid imbalance (metabolic acidosis or alkalosis, hypocalcemia)

Gastrointestinal: Mild abdominal cramps, nausea, vomiting, rectal burning

Drug Interactions Decreased Effect: Antacids may decrease the effect of bisacodyl. Bisacodyl may decrease the effect of warfarin.

Drug Uptake

Onset of action: Oral: 6-10 hours; Rectal: 0.25-1 hour

Absorption: Oral, rectal: <5% absorbed systemically

Pregnancy Risk Factor C

Generic Available Yes

Bisacodyl Uniserts® [OTC] *see* Bisacodyl *on page 166*

Bismatrol® [OTC] *see* Bismuth *on page 167*

Bismuth (BIZ muth)

Related Information

Gastrointestinal Disorders *on page 1326*

Ranitidine Bismuth Citrate *on page 1041*

U.S. Brand Names Bismatrol® [OTC]; Colo-Fresh™ [OTC]; Diotame® [OTC]; Pepto-Bismol® [OTC]; Pepto-Bismol® Maximum Strength [OTC]

Pharmacologic Category Antidiarrheal

Synonyms Bismuth Subgallate; Bismuth Subsalicylate; Pink Bismuth

Use Symptomatic treatment of mild, nonspecific diarrhea; indigestion, nausea, control of traveler's diarrhea (enterotoxigenic *Escherichia coli*); as part of a multidrug regimen for *H. pylori* eradication to reduce the risk of duodenal ulcer recurrence; subgallate formulation to control fecal odors in colostomy, ileostomy, or fecal incontinence

Local Anesthetic/Vasoconstrictor Precautions No information available to require special precautions

Effects on Dental Treatment No effects or complications reported

Dosage Oral:

Nonspecific diarrhea: Subsalicylate:

- Children: Up to 8 doses/24 hours:
  - 3-6 years: 1/3 tablet or 5 mL (regular strength) every 30 minutes to 1 hour as needed
  - 6-9 years: 2/3 tablet or 10 mL (regular strength) every 30 minutes to 1 hour as needed
  - 9-12 years: 1 tablet or 15 mL (regular strength) every 30 minutes to 1 hour as needed
- Adults: 2 tablets or 30 mL every 30 minutes to 1 hour as needed up to 8 doses/24 hours

Prevention of traveler's diarrhea: 2.1 g/day or 2 tablets 4 times/day before meals and at bedtime

Helicobacter pylori eradication: 524 mg 4 times/day with meals and at bedtime; requires combination therapy

Control of fecal odor in ileostomy or colostomy: Subgallate: 1-2 tablets 3 times/day with meals (maximum: 5 tablets/day)

Dosing adjustment in renal impairment: Should probably be avoided in patients with renal failure

Mechanism of Action Exhibits both antisecretory and antimicrobial action; may provide some antacid and anti-inflammatory action. The salicylate moiety provides antisecretory effect and the bismuth exhibits antimicrobial directly against bacterial and viral GI pathogens.

Other Adverse Effects >10%: Gastrointestinal: Discoloration of the tongue (darkening), grayish black stools

Drug Interactions

Increased Toxicity: Aspirin, warfarin, hypoglycemics

Decreased Effect: Tetracyclines and uricosurics

Drug Uptake

Absorption: Minimal (<1%) across GI tract, salt (eg, salicylate) may be readily absorbed (80%); bismuth subsalicylate is rapidly cleaved to bismuth and salicylic acid in the stomach

Half-life elimination: Terminal: Bismuth: 21-72 days; Salicylate: 2-5 hours

Pregnancy Risk Factor C/D (3rd trimester)

Generic Available Yes

Bismuth, Metronidazole, and Tetracycline

(BIZ muth sub sa LIS i late, me troe NI da zole, & tet ra SYE kleen)

U.S. Brand Names Helidac®

Pharmacologic Category Antibiotic, Tetracycline Derivative; Antidiarrheal

Synonyms Bismuth Subsalicylate, Tetracycline, and Metronidazole; Metronidazole, Bismuth Subsalicylate, and Tetracycline; Metronidazole, Tetracycline, and Bismuth Subsalicylate; Tetracycline, Bismuth Subsalicylate, and Metronidazole; Tetracycline, Metronidazole, and Bismuth Subsalicylate

Use Combination therapy with an H_2 antagonist, used in treatment of and to decrease rate of recurrence of active duodenal ulcer associated with *H. pylori* infection

(Continued)

Bismuth, Metronidazole, and Tetracycline *(Continued)*

Local Anesthetic/Vasoconstrictor Precautions No information available to require special precautions

Effects on Dental Treatment Tetracyclines are not recommended for use during pregnancy since they can cause enamel hypoplasia and permanent teeth discoloration; long-term use associated with oral candidiasis.

Dosage Adults: Chew 2 bismuth subsalicylate 262.4 mg tablets, swallow 1 metronidazole 250 mg tablet, and swallow 1 tetracycline 500 mg capsule plus an H_2 antagonist 4 times/day at meals and bedtime for 14 days; follow with 8 oz of water

Mechanism of Action Bismuth subsalicylate, metronidazole, and tetracycline individually have demonstrated *in vitro* activity against most susceptible strains of *H. pylori* isolated from patients with duodenal ulcers. Resistance to metronidazole is increasing in the U.S.; an alternative regimen, not containing metronidazole, if *H. pylori* is not eradicated follow therapy.

Other Adverse Effects See Bismuth *on page 167*, Metronidazole *on page 804*, and Tetracycline *on page 1147*

Contraindications Hypersensitivity to salicylates, bismuth, metronidazole, tetracycline, or any component of their formulation; pregnancy or lactation; children; significant renal/hepatic impairment

Warnings/Precautions See Bismuth *on page 167*, Metronidazole *on page 804*, and Tetracycline *on page 1147*

Drug Interactions See Metronidazole *on page 804* and Tetracycline *on page 1147*

Drug Uptake No data on combination; see Bismuth *on page 167*, Metronidazole *on page 804*, and Tetracycline *on page 1147*

Pregnancy Risk Factor D (tetracycline); B (metronidazole)

Generic Available No

Bisoprolol (bis OH proe lol)

Related Information

Cardiovascular Diseases *on page 1308*

U.S. Brand Names Zebeta®

Canadian Brand Names Monocor®; Zebeta®

Pharmacologic Category Beta Blocker, $Beta_1$ Selective

Synonyms Bisoprolol Fumarate

Use Treatment of hypertension, alone or in combination with other agents

Unlabeled/Investigational: Angina pectoris, supraventricular arrhythmias, PVCs

Local Anesthetic/Vasoconstrictor Precautions No information available to require special precautions

Effects on Dental Treatment Noncardioselective beta-blockers (ie, propranolol, nadolol) enhance the pressor response to epinephrine, resulting in hypertension and bradycardia. This has not been reported for bisoprolol, a cardioselective beta-blocker. Therefore local anesthetic with vasoconstrictor can be safely used in patients medicated with bisoprolol. Many nonsteroidal anti-inflammatory drugs such as ibuprofen and indomethacin can reduce the hypotensive effect of beta-blockers after 3 or more weeks of therapy with the NSAID. Short-term NSAID use (ie, 3 days) requires no special precautions in patients taking beta-blockers.

Dosage Oral:

Adults: 5 mg once daily, may be increased to 10 mg, and then up to 20 mg once daily, if necessary

Elderly: Initial dose: 2.5 mg/day; may be increased by 2.5-5 mg/day; maximum recommended dose: 20 mg/day

Mechanism of Action Selective inhibitor of $beta_1$-adrenergic receptors; competitively blocks $beta_1$-receptors, with little or no effect on $beta_2$-receptors at doses <10 mg

Other Adverse Effects

>10%

- Central nervous system: Drowsiness, insomnia
- Endocrine & metabolic: Decreased sexual ability

1% to 10%:

- Cardiovascular: Bradycardia, palpitations, edema, CHF, reduced peripheral circulation
- Central nervous system: Mental depression
- Gastrointestinal: Diarrhea or constipation, nausea, vomiting, stomach discomfort
- Ocular: Mild ocular stinging and discomfort, tearing, photophobia, decreased corneal sensitivity, keratitis
- Respiratory: Bronchospasm
- Miscellaneous: Cold extremities

Drug Interactions CYP2D6 enzyme substrate

Increased Effect/Toxicity: Bisoprolol may increase the effects of other drugs which slow AV conduction (digoxin, verapamil, diltiazem), alpha-blockers (prazosin, terazosin), and alpha-adrenergic stimulants (epinephrine, phenylephrine). Bisoprolol may mask the tachycardia from hypoglycemia caused by insulin and oral hypoglycemics. In patients receiving concurrent therapy, the risk of hypertensive crisis is increased when either clonidine or the beta-blocker is withdrawn. Reserpine has been shown to enhance the effect of beta-blockers. Beta-blockers may increase the action or levels of disopyramide, nondepolarizing muscle relaxants, and theophylline although the effects are difficult to predict.

Decreased Effect: Decreased effect of bisoprolol with aluminum salts, barbiturates, calcium salts, cholestyramine, colestipol, NSAIDs, penicillins (ampicillin), rifampin, and salicylates due to decreased bioavailability and plasma concentrations. The effect of sulfonylureas may be decreased by beta-blockers.

Drug Uptake

Onset of action: 1-2 hours

Absorption: Rapid and almost complete from GI tract

Half-life, elimination: 9-12 hours

Time to peak: 1.7-3 hours

Pregnancy Risk Factor C (manufacturer); D (2nd and 3rd trimesters - expert analysis)

Generic Available Yes

Selected Readings

Foster CA and Aston SJ, "Propranolol-Epinephrine Interaction: A Potential Disaster," *Plast Reconstr Surg*, 1983, 72(1):74-8.

Wong DG, Spence JD, Lamki L, et al, "Effect of Nonsteroidal Anti-inflammatory Drugs on Control of Hypertension of Beta-Blockers and Diuretics," *Lancet*, 1986, 1(8488):997-1001.

Wynn RL, "Dental Nonsteroidal Anti-inflammatory Drugs and Prostaglandin-Based Drug Interactions, Part Two," *Gen Dent*, 1992, 40(2):104, 106, 108.

Wynn RL, "Epinephrine Interactions With Beta-Blockers," *Gen Dent*, 1994, 42(1):16, 18.

Bisoprolol and Hydrochlorothiazide

(bis OH proe lol & hye droe klor oh THYE a zide)

U.S. Brand Names Ziac®

Canadian Brand Names Ziac™

Pharmacologic Category Antihypertensive Agent Combination

Synonyms Hydrochlorothiazide and Bisoprolol

Use Treatment of hypertension

Local Anesthetic/Vasoconstrictor Precautions No information available to require special precautions

Effects on Dental Treatment Noncardioselective beta-blockers (ie, propranolol, nadolol) enhance the pressor response to epinephrine, resulting in hypertension and bradycardia. This has not been reported for bisoprolol, a cardioselective beta-blocker. Therefore local anesthetic with vasoconstrictor can be safely used in patients medicated with bisoprolol. Many nonsteroidal anti-inflammatory drugs such as ibuprofen and indomethacin can reduce the hypotensive effect of beta-blockers after 3 or more weeks of therapy with the NSAID. Short-term NSAID use (ie, 3 days) requires no special precautions in patients taking beta-blockers.

Dosage Adults: Oral: Dose is individualized, given once daily

Other Adverse Effects

>10%: Central nervous system: Fatigue

1% to 10%:

- Cardiovascular: Chest pain, edema, bradycardia, hypotension
- Central nervous system: Headache, dizziness, depression, abnormal dreams
- Dermatologic: Rash, photosensitivity
- Endocrine & metabolic: Hypokalemia, fluid and electrolyte imbalances (hypocalcemia, hypomagnesemia, hyponatremia), hyperglycemia
- Gastrointestinal: Constipation, diarrhea, dyspepsia, nausea, insomnia, flatulence
- Genitourinary: Micturition (frequency)
- Hematologic: Rarely blood dyscrasias
- Neuromuscular & skeletal: Arthralgia, myalgia
- Ocular: Abnormal vision
- Renal: Prerenal azotemia
- Respiratory: Rhinitis, cough, dyspnea

Drug Interactions

Based on **bisoprolol** component: CYP2D6 enzyme substrate

- Alpha-blockers (prazosin, terazosin): Concurrent use of beta-blockers may increase risk of orthostasis.
- Clonidine: Hypertensive crisis after or during withdrawal of either agent.
- Drugs which slow AV conduction (digoxin): Effects may be additive with beta-blockers.
- Glucagon: Bisoprolol may blunt the hyperglycemic action of glucagon.
- Insulin: Bisoprolol may mask tachycardia from hypoglycemia.
- NSAIDs (ibuprofen, indomethacin, naproxen, piroxicam) may reduce the antihypertensive effects of beta-blockers.
- Salicylates may reduce the antihypertensive effects of beta-blockers.
- Sulfonylureas: Beta-blockers may alter response to hypoglycemic agents.

Based on **hydrochlorothiazide** component:

- ACE inhibitors: Increased hypotension if aggressively diuresed with a thiazide diuretic.

(Continued)

Bisoprolol and Hydrochlorothiazide *(Continued)*

Beta-blockers increase hyperglycemic effects in type 2 diabetes mellitus (noninsulin dependent, NIDDM)

Cyclosporine and thiazides can increase the risk of gout or renal toxicity; avoid concurrent use.

Digoxin toxicity can be exacerbated if a thiazide induces hypokalemia or hypomagnesemia.

Lithium toxicity can occur by reducing renal excretion of lithium; monitor lithium concentration and adjust as needed.

Neuromuscular blocking agents can prolong blockade; monitor serum potassium and neuromuscular status.

NSAIDs can decrease the efficacy of thiazides reducing the diuretic and antihypertensive effects.

Drug Uptake See Bisoprolol *on page 168* and Hydrochlorothiazide *on page 595*

Pregnancy Risk Factor C/D (2nd and 3rd trimesters)

Generic Available Yes

Bitolterol (bye TOLE ter ole)

Related Information

Respiratory Diseases *on page 1328*

U.S. Brand Names Tornalate®

Canadian Brand Names Tornalate®

Pharmacologic Category $Beta_2$ Agonist

Synonyms Bitolterol Mesylate; Tornalate® [DSC]

Use Prevention and treatment of bronchial asthma and bronchospasm

Local Anesthetic/Vasoconstrictor Precautions No information available to require special precautions

Effects on Dental Treatment No effects or complications reported

Dosage Children >12 years and Adults:

Bronchospasm: 2 inhalations at an interval of at least 1-3 minutes, followed by a third inhalation if needed

Prevention of bronchospasm: 2 inhalations every 8 hours; do not exceed 3 inhalations every 6 hours or 2 inhalations every 4 hours

Mechanism of Action Selectively stimulates $beta_2$-adrenergic receptors in the lungs producing bronchial smooth muscle relaxation; minor $beta_1$ activity

Other Adverse Effects

>10%: Neuromuscular & skeletal: Tremors (14%)

1% to 10%:

- Cardiovascular: Palpitations (3%), chest tightness (1%)
- Central nervous system: Nervousness (5%), headache (4%), dizziness (3%), lightheadedness (3%)
- Gastrointestinal: Xerostomia, nausea (3%), unpleasant taste
- Respiratory: Bronchial irritation (5%), coughing (4%)

Drug Interactions

Increased Effect/Toxicity: Increased toxicity with MAO inhibitors, tricyclic antidepressants, sympathomimetic agents (eg, amphetamine, dopamine, dobutamine), inhaled anesthetics (eg, enflurane). Increased toxicity (cardiotoxicity) with aminophylline, theophylline, or oxtriphylline.

Decreased Effect: Decreased effect with beta-adrenergic blockers (eg, propranolol).

Drug Uptake

Onset of action: Rapid

Duration: 4-8 hours

Half-life, elimination: 3 hours

Time to peak (colterol): Inhalation: ≤1 hour

Pregnancy Risk Factor C

Generic Available No

Black Draught® [OTC] *see* Senna *on page 1081*

Blenoxane® *see* Bleomycin *on page 170*

Bleomycin (blee oh MYE sin)

U.S. Brand Names Blenoxane®

Canadian Brand Names Blenoxane®

Mexican Brand Names Blanoxan®; Bleolem

Pharmacologic Category Antineoplastic Agent, Antibiotic

Synonyms Bleo; Bleomycin Sulfate; BLM; NSC-125066

Use Treatment of squamous cell carcinomas, melanomas, sarcomas, testicular carcinoma, Hodgkin's lymphoma, and non-Hodgkin's lymphoma

Orphan drug: Sclerosing agent for malignant pleural effusion

Local Anesthetic/Vasoconstrictor Precautions No information available to require special precautions

Effects on Dental Treatment No effects or complications reported

Mechanism of Action Inhibits synthesis of DNA; binds to DNA leading to single- and double-strand breaks; isolated from *Streptomyces verticillus*

Other Adverse Effects

>10%:

Cardiovascular: Raynaud's phenomenon

Central nervous system: Mild febrile reaction, fever, chills, patients may become febrile after intracavitary administration

Dermatologic: Pruritic erythema

Integument: ~50% of patients will develop erythema, induration, and hyperkeratosis and peeling of the skin; hyperpigmentation, alopecia, nailbed changes may occur; this appears to be dose-related and is reversible after cessation of therapy

Irritant chemotherapy

Gastrointestinal: Mucocutaneous toxicity, stomatitis, nausea, vomiting, anorexia

Emetic potential: Moderately low (10% to 30%)

Local: Phlebitis, pain at tumor site

1% to 10%:

Dermatologic: Alopecia

Gastrointestinal: Weight loss

Respiratory: Toxicities (usually pneumonitis) occur in 10% of treated patients; 1% of patients progress to pulmonary fibrosis and death

Miscellaneous: Idiosyncratic: Similar to anaphylaxis and occurs in 1% of lymphoma patients; may include hypotension, confusion, fever, chills, and wheezing. May be immediate or delayed for several hours; symptomatic treatment includes volume expansion, pressor agents, antihistamines, and steroids

Drug Interactions

Increased Effect/Toxicity: Bleomycin with digoxin may result in elevated serum digoxin levels due to decreased renal clearance. CCNU (lomustine) increases severity of leukopenia. Results in delayed bleomycin elimination due to a decrease in creatinine clearance secondary to cisplatin.

Decreased Effect: Bleomycin and digitalis glycosides may decrease plasma concentrations of digoxin. Concomitant therapy with phenytoin results in decreased phenytoin levels, possibly due to decreased oral absorption.

Drug Uptake

Absorption: I.M. and intrapleural administration produces serum concentration of 30% of I.V. administration; intraperitoneal and S.C. routes produce serum concentration equal to those of I.V.

Half-life, elimination (dependent upon renal function): Biphasic:

Initial: 1.3 hours; Terminal: 9 hours

End-stage renal disease: Initial: 2 hours; Terminal: 30 hours

Time to peak: I.M.: ≤30 minutes

Pregnancy Risk Factor D

Generic Available Yes

Bleph®-10 *see* Sulfacetamide Sodium *on page 1115*

Blephamide® *see* Sulfacetamide Sodium and Prednisolone *on page 1116*

Blis-To-Sol® [OTC] *see* Tolnaftate *on page 1181*

Blocadren® *see* Timolol *on page 1170*

Bluboro® [OTC] *see* Aluminum Sulfate and Calcium Acetate *on page 63*

Bonine® [OTC] *see* Meclizine *on page 750*

Bontril PDM® *see* Phendimetrazine *on page 943*

Bontril® Slow-Release *see* Phendimetrazine *on page 943*

Boric Acid (BOR ik AS id)

U.S. Brand Names Borofax® [OTC]; Dri-Ear® Otic [OTC]; Swim-Ear® Otic [OTC]

Pharmacologic Category Pharmaceutical Aid; Topical Skin Product

Use

Ophthalmic: Mild antiseptic used for inflamed eyelids

Otic: Prophylaxis of swimmer's ear

Topical ointment: Temporary relief of chapped/chafed/dry skin or diaper rash; minor abrasions, burns, insect bites and other skin irritations

Local Anesthetic/Vasoconstrictor Precautions No information available to require special precautions

Effects on Dental Treatment No effects or complications reported

Dosage Apply to lower eyelid 1-2 times/day

Generic Available Yes

Comments Not a corrosive substance

Borofax® [OTC] *see* Boric Acid *on page 171*

Bosentan (boe SEN tan)

U.S. Brand Names Tracleer™

Pharmacologic Category Endothelin Antagonist

(Continued)

Bosentan *(Continued)*

Use Treatment of pulmonary artery hypertension (PAH) in patients with World Health Organization (WHO) Class III or IV symptoms to improve exercise capacity and decrease the rate of clinical deterioration

Unlabeled/Investigational: Congestive heart failure

Local Anesthetic/Vasoconstrictor Precautions No information available to require special precautions

Effects on Dental Treatment No effects or complications reported

Restrictions Not available through wholesalers or individual pharmacies; available only through a limited distribution program directly from the manufacturer (Actelion Pharmaceuticals 1-866-228-3546)

Dosage Oral: Adults: Initial: 62.5 mg twice daily for 4 weeks; increase to maintenance dose of 125 mg twice daily; adults <40 kg should be maintained at 62.5 mg twice daily

Note: When discontinuing treatment, consider a reduction in dosage to 62.5 mg twice daily for 3-7 days (to avoid clinical deterioration).

Dosage adjustment in hepatic impairment: Avoid use in patients with **pretreatment** moderate to severe hepatic insufficiency.

Modification based on transaminase elevation:

If any elevation, regardless of degree, is accompanied by clinical symptoms of hepatic injury (unusual fatigue, nausea, vomiting, abdominal pain, fever, or jaundice) or a serum bilirubin ≥2 times the upper limit of normal, treatment should be stopped.

AST/ALT >3 times but ≤5 times upper limit of normal: Confirm with additional test; if confirmed, reduce dose or interrupt treatment. Monitor transaminase levels at least every 2 weeks. May continue or reintroduce treatment, as appropriate, following return to pretreatment values. Begin with initial dose (above) and recheck transaminases within 3 days

AST/ALT >5 times but ≤8 times upper limit of normal: Confirm with additional test; if confirmed, stop treatment. Monitor transaminase levels at least every 2 weeks. May reintroduce treatment, as appropriate, following return to pretreatment values.

AST/ALT >8 times upper limit of normal: Stop treatment.

Mechanism of Action Blocks endothelin receptors on vascular endothelium and smooth muscle. Stimulation of these receptors is associated with vasoconstriction. Although bosentan blocks both ET_A and ET_B receptors, the affinity is higher for the A subtype. Improvement in symptoms of primary pulmonary hypertension and a decrease in the rate of clinical deterioration have been demonstrated in clinical trials.

Other Adverse Effects

>10% :

Central nervous system: Headache (16% to 22%)

Gastrointestinal: Dyspepsia (4%)

Hematologic: Decreased hemoglobin (≥1 g/dL in up to 57%; typically in first 6 weeks of therapy)

Hepatic: Increased serum transaminases (>3 times upper limit of normal; up to 11%)

Respiratory: Nasopharyngitis (11%)

1% to 10%:

Cardiovascular: Flushing (7% to 9%), edema (lower limb, 8%; generalized 4%), hypotension (7%), palpitations (5%)

Central nervous system: Fatigue (4%)

Dermatologic: Pruritus (4%)

Hematologic: Anemia (3%)

Hepatic: Abnormal hepatic function (6% to 8%)

Drug Interactions CYP2C9 and CYP3A3/4 enzyme substrate; CYP2C9 and CYP3A3/4 enzyme inducer

Cyclosporine: Bosentan may enhance the metabolism of cyclosporine, decreasing its serum concentrations by ~50%; effect on sirolimus and/or tacrolimus has not been specifically evaluated, but may be similar. Cyclosporine increases serum concentrations of bosentan (approximately 3-4 times baseline). Concurrent use of cyclosporine is contraindicated.

Glyburide: An increased risk of serum transaminase elevations was observed during concurrent therapy with bosentan. Concurrent use is contraindicated.

HMG-CoA reductase inhibitors: Agents metabolized via CYP3A3/4 may be decreased by bosentan; includes atorvastatin, lovastatin, and simvastatin.

Ketoconazole: May increase the serum concentrations of bosentan; concentrations are increased approximately two-fold; monitor for increased effects.

Many interactions have not been specifically evaluated, but may be extrapolated from similar interactions with inducers/inhibitors of CYP3A3/4 and CYP2C9 isoenzymes. Key potential interactions are summarized as follows:

Anticonvulsants: Bosentan may increase the metabolism of selected anticonvulsants; includes ethosuximide, phenytoin, tiagabine, and zonisamide. The effect of concurrent therapy with enzyme-inducing anticonvulsants on bosentan concentrations has not been established.

Antipsychotics: Bosentan may enhance the metabolism (decrease the efficacy) of antipsychotics; monitor for altered response; dosage adjustment may be needed

Calcium channel blockers: Bosentan may enhance the metabolism of calcium channel blockers, decreasing their clinical effect.

Corticosteroids: Bosentan may enhance the metabolism of corticosteroids, decreasing their clinical effect.

CYP2C9 inhibitors: May increase the serum concentrations of bosentan; includes amiodarone, fluoxetine, sulfonamides, ritonavir, zafirlukast.

CYP3A3/4 inhibitors: May increase the serum concentrations of bosentan; includes amiodarone, cimetidine, clarithromycin, erythromycin, delavirdine, diltiazem, dirithromycin, disulfiram, fluoxetine, fluvoxamine, grapefruit juice, indinavir, itraconazole, ketoconazole, nefazodone, nevirapine, propoxyphene, quinupristin-dalfopristin, ritonavir, saquinavir, verapamil, zafirlukast, zileuton

Doxycycline: Bosentan may enhance the metabolism of doxycycline, decreasing its clinical effect; higher dosages may be required

Estrogens: Bosentan may increase the metabolism of estrogens and reduce their efficacy

Hormonal contraceptives: Bosentan may enhance the metabolism of hormonal contraceptives, decreasing their clinical effect; an alternative method of contraception should be considered

Methadone: Bosentan may enhance the metabolism of methadone resulting in methadone withdrawal

Protease inhibitors: Serum concentrations may be decreased by bosentan. Avoid concurrent use of agents metabolized by CYP3A3/4 or CYP2C9.

Warfarin: Bosentan may increase the metabolism of oral anticoagulants; monitor for changes in INR. Significant changes in INR not observed in clinical trials.

Drug Uptake Half-life, elimination: 5 hours (increases in heart failure, possibly in PAH)

Pregnancy Risk Factor X

Generic Available No

B&O Supprettes® *see* Belladonna and Opium *on page 147*

Botox® *see* Botulinum Toxin Type A *on page 173*

Botox® Cosmetic *see* Botulinum Toxin Type A *on page 173*

Botulinum Toxin Type A (BOT yoo lin num TOKS in type aye)

U.S. Brand Names Botox®; Botox® Cosmetic

Canadian Brand Names Botox®

Pharmacologic Category Neuromuscular Blocker Agent, Toxin; Ophthalmic Agent, Toxin

Use Treatment of strabismus and blepharospasm associated with dystonia (including benign essential blepharospasm or VII nerve disorders in patients ≥12 years of age); cervical dystonia (spasmodic torticollis) in patients ≥16 years of age; temporary improvement in the appearance of lines/wrinkles of the face (moderate to severe glabellar lines associated with corrugator and/or procerus muscle activity) in adult patient ≤65 years of age

Orphan drug: Treatment of dynamic muscle contracture in pediatric cerebral palsy patients

Unlabeled/Investigational: Treatment of oromandibular dystonia, spasmodic dysphonia (laryngeal dystonia) and other dystonias (ie, writer's cramp, focal task-specific dystonias); migraine treatment and prophylaxis; cosmetic use to decrease lines and wrinkles of the face and neck; chronic anal fissure

Local Anesthetic/Vasoconstrictor Precautions No information available to require special precautions

Effects on Dental Treatment No effects or complications reported

Dosage I.M.:

Children ≥16 years and Adults: Cervical dystonia: For dosing guidance, the mean dose is 236 units (25th to 75th percentile range 198-300 units) divided among the affected muscles in patients previously treated with botulinum toxin. Initial dose in previously untreated patients should be lower. Sequential dosing should be based on the patient's head and neck position, localization of pain, muscle hypertrophy, patient response, and previous adverse reactions. The total dose injected into the sternocleidomastoid muscles should be ≤100 units to decrease the occurrence of dysphagia.

Children ≥12 years and Adults:

Blepharospasm: Initial dose: 1.25-2.5 units injected into the medial and lateral pretarsal orbicularis oculi of the upper and lower lid; dose may be increased up to twice the previous dose if the response from the initial dose lasted ≤2 months; maximum dose per site: 5 units; cumulative dose in a 30-day period: ≤200 units. Tolerance may occur if treatments are given more often than every 3 months, but the effect is not usually permanent.

(Continued)

Botulinum Toxin Type A *(Continued)*

Strabismus:
Initial dose:
Vertical muscles and for horizontal strabismus <20 prism diopters: 1.25-2.5 units in any one muscle
Horizontal strabismus of 20-50 prism diopters: 2.5-5 units in any one muscle
Persistent VI nerve palsy >1 month: 1.5-2.5 units in the medial rectus muscle
Re-examine patients 7-14 days after each injection to assess the effect of that dose. Subsequent doses for patients experiencing incomplete paralysis of the target may be increased up to twice the previous administered dose. The maximum recommended dose as a single injection for any one muscle is 25 units. Do not administer subsequent injections until the effects of the previous dose are gone.

Adults ≤65 years: Reduction of glabellar lines: An effective dose is determined by gross observation of the patient's ability to activate the superficial muscles injected. The location, size and use of muscles may vary markedly among individuals. Inject 0.1 mL dose into each of five sites, two in each corrugator muscle and one in the procerus muscle (total dose 0.5 mL).

Mechanism of Action A neurotoxin produced by *Clostridium botulinum*, spore-forming anaerobic bacillus, which appears to affect only the presynaptic membrane of the neuromuscular junction in humans; prevents calcium-dependent release of acetylcholine and produces a state of denervation; muscle inactivation persists until new fibrils grow from the nerve and form junction plates on new areas of the muscle-cell walls. The antagonist muscle shortens simultaneously ("contracture"), taking up the slack created by agonist paralysis; following several weeks of paralysis, alignment of the eye is measurably changed, despite return of innervation to the injected muscle.

Other Adverse Effects Adverse effects usually occur in 1 week and may last up to several months

>10% :
Central nervous system: Headache (cervical dystonia up to 11%, reduction of glabellar lines up to 13%; can occur with other uses)
Gastrointestinal: Dysphagia (cervical dystonia 19%)
Neuromuscular & skeletal: Neck pain (cervical dystonia 11%)
Ocular: Ptosis (blepharospasm 10% to 40%, strabismus 1% to 38%, reduction of glabellar lines 1% to 5%); vertical deviation (strabismus 17%)
Respiratory: Upper respiratory infection (cervical dystonia 12%),

2% to 10%:
Central nervous system: Dizziness (cervical dystonia, reduction of glabellar lines); speech disorder (cervical dystonia), fever (cervical dystonia), drowsiness (cervical dystonia)
Gastrointestinal: Xerostomia (cervical dystonia), nausea (cervical dystonia, reduction of glabellar lines)
Local: Injection site reaction
Neuromuscular & skeletal: Back pain (cervical dystonia); hypertonia (cervical dystonia); weakness (cervical dystonia, reduction of glabellar lines); facial pain (reduction of glabellar lines)
Ocular: Dry eyes (blepharospasm 6%), superficial punctate keratitis (blepharospasm 6%)
Respiratory: Cough (cervical dystonia), rhinitis (cervical dystonia), infection (reduction of glabellar lines)
Miscellaneous: Flu syndrome (cervical dystonia, reduction of glabellar lines)

<2%: Stiffness, diplopia (cervical dystonia, blepharospasm), ptosis (cervical dystonia), dyspnea (cervical dystonia), numbness (cervical dystonia), ectropion (blepharospasm), lagophthalmos (blepharospasm), facial weakness (blepharospasm), ecchymoses (blepharospasm), eyelid edema (blepharospasm), tearing (blepharospasm), photophobia (blepharospasm), entropion (blepharospasm)

Drug Interactions
Aminoglycosides: May increase neuromuscular blockade
Neuromuscular-blocking agents: May increase neuromuscular blockade
Other agents which may have neuromuscular-blocking activity: Calcium channel blockers, catecholamines, chloroquine, clindamycin, colistin, corticosteroids, digitalis glycosides, diuretics, inhalation anesthetics, lidocaine, lincomycin, magnesium salts, opioids, phenytoin, phenelzine, polymixin B, procainamide, propranolol, quinidine, tetracyclines

Drug Uptake
Onset of action (improvement):
Blepharospasm: ~3 days
Cervical dystonia: ~2 weeks
Strabismus: ~1-2 days
Reduction of glabellar lines (Botox® Cosmetic): 1-2 days, increasing in intensity during first week
Duration:
Blepharospasm: ~3 months
Cervical dystonia: <3 months

Strabismus: ~2-6 weeks
Reduction of glabellar lines (Botox® Cosmetic): ≤3 months
Absorption: Not expected to be present in peripheral blood at recommended doses
Time to peak:
Blepharospasm: 1-2 weeks
Cervical dystonia: ~6 weeks
Strabismus: Within first week

Pregnancy Risk Factor C (manufacturer)

Generic Available No

Botulinum Toxin Type B (BOT yoo lin num TOKS in type bee)

U.S. Brand Names Myobloc®

Pharmacologic Category Neuromuscular Blocker Agent, Toxin

Use Treatment of cervical dystonia (spasmodic torticollis)

Unlabeled/Investigational: Treatment of cervical dystonia in patients who have developed resistance to botulinum toxin type A

Local Anesthetic/Vasoconstrictor Precautions No information available to require special precautions

Effects on Dental Treatment No effects or complications reported

Dosage

Children: Not established in pediatric patients

Adults: Cervical dystonia: I.M.: Initial: 2500-5000 units divided among the affected muscles in patients **previously treated** with botulinum toxin; initial dose in **previously untreated** patients should be lower. Subsequent dosing should be optimized according to patient's response.

Elderly: No dosage adjustments required, but limited experience in patients ≥75 years old

Mechanism of Action A neurotoxin produced by *Clostridium botulinum,* spore-forming anaerobic bacillus; cleaves synaptic Vesicle Association Membrane Protein (VAMP; synaptobrevin) which is a component of the protein complex responsible for docking and fusion of the synaptic vesicle to the presynaptic membrane; paralyzes the muscle by blocking neurotransmitter release

Other Adverse Effects

>10%:

Central nervous system: Headache (10% to 16%), pain (6% to 13%; placebo 10%)
Gastrointestinal: Dysphagia (10% to 25%), xerostomia (3% to 34%)
Local: Injection site pain (12% to 16%)
Neuromuscular & skeletal: Neck pain (up to 17%; placebo: 16%)
Miscellaneous: Infection (13% to 19%; placebo: 15%)

1% to 10%:

Cardiovascular: Chest pain, vasodilation, peripheral edema
Central nervous system: Dizziness (3% to 6%), fever, malaise, migraine, anxiety, tremor, hyperesthesia, somnolence, confusion, vertigo
Dermatologic: Pruritus, bruising
Gastrointestinal: Nausea (3% to 10%; placebo: 5%), dyspepsia (up to 10%; placebo: 5%), vomiting, stomatitis, taste perversion
Genitourinary: Urinary tract infection, cystitis, vaginal moniliasis
Hematologic: Serum neutralizing activity
Neuromuscular & skeletal: Torticollis (up to 8%; placebo: 7%), arthralgia (up to 7%; placebo: 5%), back pain (3% to 7%; placebo: 3%), myasthenia (3% to 6%; placebo: 3%), weakness (up to 6%; placebo: 4%), arthritis
Ocular: Amblyopia, abnormal vision
Otic: Otitis media, tinnitus
Respiratory: Cough (3% to 7%; placebo: 3%), rhinitis (1% to 5%; placebo: 6%), dyspnea, pneumonia
Miscellaneous: Flu-syndrome (6% to 9%), allergic reaction, viral infection, abscess, cyst

Contraindications Hypersensitivity to albumin, botulinum toxin, or any component of their formulation; infection at the injection site(s); pregnancy; coadministration of agents known to potentiate neuromuscular blockade; relative contraindications include diseases of neuromuscular transmission; coagulopathy, including therapeutic anticoagulation; inability of patient to cooperate

Drug Interactions

Aminoglycosides: May increase neuromuscular blockade
Neuromuscular-blocking agents: May increase neuromuscular blockade
Botulinum toxin type A: Potentiation of paralysis with concurrent or overlapping use; separate by ≥4 months
Other agents which may have neuromuscular-blocking activity: Inhalation anesthetics, calcium channel blockers, catecholamines, chloroquine, clarithromycin, clindamycin, colistin, corticosteroids, digitalis glycosides, diuretics, erythromycin, inhalation anesthetics, lidocaine, lincomycin, magnesium salts, opioids, phenytoin, phenelzine, polymixin B, procainamide, propranolol, quinidine, tetracyclines, vancomycin

(Continued)

Botulinum Toxin Type B *(Continued)*

Drug Uptake

Absorption: Not expected to be present in the peripheral blood at measurable levels following I.M. injection at the recommended doses

Duration: 12-16 weeks

Pregnancy Risk Factor C (manufacturer)

Generic Available No

Boudreaux's® Butt Paste [OTC] *see* Zinc Oxide *on page 1260*
Bravelle™ *see* Follitropins *on page 531*
Breathe Free® [OTC] *see* Sodium Chloride *on page 1094*
Breathe Right® Saline [OTC] *see* Sodium Chloride *on page 1094*
Breonesin® [OTC] *see* Guaifenesin *on page 568*
Brethine® *see* Terbutaline *on page 1141*

Bretylium (bre TIL ee um)

Related Information

Cardiovascular Diseases *on page 1308*

Pharmacologic Category Antiarrhythmic Agent, Class III

Synonyms Bretylium Tosylate

Use Treatment of ventricular tachycardia and fibrillation; used in the treatment of other serious ventricular arrhythmias resistant to lidocaine

Local Anesthetic/Vasoconstrictor Precautions No information available to require special precautions

Effects on Dental Treatment No effects or complications reported

Dosage (Note: Patients should undergo defibrillation/cardioversion before and after bretylium doses as necessary)

Children:

I.M.: 2-5 mg/kg as a single dose

I.V.: Initial: 5 mg/kg, then attempt electrical defibrillation; repeat with 10 mg/kg if ventricular fibrillation persists at 15-minute intervals to maximum total of 30 mg/kg

Maintenance dose: I.M., I.V.: 5 mg/kg every 6-8 hours

Adults:

Immediate life-threatening ventricular arrhythmias, ventricular fibrillation, unstable ventricular tachycardia: Initial dose: I.V.: 5 mg/kg (undiluted) over 1 minute; if arrhythmia persists, give 10 mg/kg (undiluted) over 1 minute and repeat as necessary (usually at 15- to 30-minute intervals) up to a total dose of 30-35 mg/kg

Other life-threatening ventricular arrhythmias:

Initial dose: I.M., I.V.: 5-10 mg/kg, may repeat every 1-2 hours if arrhythmia persist; give I.V. dose (diluted) over 8-10 minutes

Maintenance dose: I.M.: 5-10 mg/kg every 6-8 hours; I.V. (diluted): 5-10 mg/kg every 6 hours; I.V. infusion (diluted): 1-2 mg/minute (little experience with doses >40 mg/kg/day)

2 g/250 mL D_5W (infusion pump should be used for I.V. infusion administration)

Rate of I.V. infusion: 1-4 mg/minute

1 mg/minute = 7 mL/hour
2 mg/minute = 15 mL/hour
3 mg/minute = 22 mL/hour
4 mg/minute = 30 mL/hour

Mechanism of Action Class II antiarrhythmic; after an initial release of norepinephrine at the peripheral adrenergic nerve terminals, inhibits further release by postganglionic nerve endings in response to sympathetic nerve stimulation

Other Adverse Effects

>10%: Cardiovascular: Hypotension (both postural and supine)

1% to 10%: Gastrointestinal: Nausea, vomiting

Drug Interactions Increased Effect/Toxicity: Other antiarrhythmic agents may potentiate or antagonize cardiac effects of bretylium. Toxic effects may be additive. The vasopressor effects of catecholamines may be enhanced by bretylium. Toxicity of agents which may prolong QT interval (including cisapride, tricyclic antidepressants, antipsychotics, erythromycin, Class Ia and Class III antiarrhythmics) and specific quinolones (sparfloxacin, gatifloxacin, moxifloxacin) may be increased. Digoxin toxicity may be aggravated by bretylium.

Drug Uptake

Onset of antiarrhythmic effect: I.M.: ≤2 hours; I.V.: 6-20 minutes

Peak effect: 6-9 hours

Duration: 6-24 hours

Half-life, elimination: 7-11 hours; Average: 4-17 hours; End-stage renal disease: 16-32 hours

Pregnancy Risk Factor C

Generic Available Yes

Brevibloc® *see* Esmolol *on page 454*
Brevicon® *see* Combination Hormonal Contraceptives *on page 323*

Brevital® Sodium *see* Methohexital *on page 786*
Brevoxyl® *see* Benzoyl Peroxide *on page 153*
Brevoxyl® Cleansing *see* Benzoyl Peroxide *on page 153*
Brevoxyl® Wash *see* Benzoyl Peroxide *on page 153*

Brimonidine (bri MOE ni deen)

U.S. Brand Names Alphagan®; Alphagan® P

Canadian Brand Names Alphagan™

Mexican Brand Names Alphagan®

Pharmacologic Category $Alpha_2$ Agonist, Ophthalmic; Ophthalmic Agent, Antiglaucoma

Synonyms Brimonidine Tartrate

Use Lowering of intraocular pressure in patients with open-angle glaucoma or ocular hypertension

Local Anesthetic/Vasoconstrictor Precautions No information available to require special precautions

Effects on Dental Treatment No effects or complications reported

Dosage Ophthalmic: Children ≥2 years of age and Adults: Glaucoma (Alphagan®, Alphagan® P): Instill 1 drop in affected eye(s) 3 times/day (~ every 8 hours)

Mechanism of Action Selective for $alpha_2$-receptors; appears to result in reduction of aqueous humor formation and increase uveoscleral outflow

Other Adverse Effects

Alphagan®:

>10%:

Central nervous system: Drowsiness, fatigue, headache

Gastrointestinal: Xerostomia

Ocular: Allergic reactions, blurring, burning, follicular conjunctivitis, foreign body sensation, hyperemia, pruritus, stinging

1% to 10% (unless otherwise noted 3% to 9%):

Cardiovascular: Arrhythmias (<3%), hypertension (<3%), palpitations (<3%), syncope (<3%)

Central nervous system: Dizziness, anxiety (<3%), depression (<3%), insomnia (<3%)

Gastrointestinal: Abnormal taste, nasal dryness (<3%)

Neuromuscular & skeletal: Muscular pain, weakness

Ocular: Corneal staining, corneal erosion, photophobia, eyelid erythema, ocular ache/pain, ocular dryness, tearing, eyelid edema, conjunctival edema, blepharitis, ocular irritation, conjunctival blanching, abnormal vision, lid crusting, conjunctival hemorrhage, conjunctival discharge

Respiratory: Upper respiratory symptoms

Pediatric use: Somnolence and lethargy were reported in up to 83% of patients 2-6 years of age. Children ≥7 years of age experienced somnolence less frequently (25%).

Alphagan® P:

>10%: Ocular: Allergic conjunctivitis, conjunctival hyperemia, eye pruritus

1% to 10% (unless otherwise noted 1% to 4%):

Cardiovascular: Hypertension (5& to 9%)

Central nervous system: Dizziness, headache

Dermatologic: Rash

Gastrointestinal: Xerostomia (5% to 9%), dyspepsia

Ocular: Burning sensation (5% to 9%), conjunctival folliculosis (5% to 9%), visual disturbance (5% to 9%), blepharitis, conjunctival edema, conjunctival hemorrhage, conjunctivitis, eye discharge, irritation, eyelid edema, eyelid erythema, follicular conjunctivitis, foreign body sensation, pain, photophobia, stinging, superficial punctate keratopathy, visual field defect, vitreous floaters, watery eyes, worsened visual acuity

Respiratory: Bronchitis, cough, dyspnea, pharyngitis, rhinitis, sinus infection

Miscellaneous: Allergic reaction, flu-like syndrome

Drug Interactions

Increased Effect/Toxicity: CNS depressants (eg, alcohol, barbiturates, opiates, sedatives, anesthetics) may have additive or potentiating effect; topical beta-blockers, pilocarpine may have additive decreased intraocular pressure; antihypertensives, cardiac glycosides may increase effects.

Decreased Effect: Tricyclic antidepressants can affect the metabolism and uptake of circulating amines.

Drug Uptake

Onset of action: Peak effect: 2 hours

Half-life, elimination: 2-3 hours

Time to peak, plasma: Alphagan®: 1-4 hours; Alphagan® P: 0.5-2.5 hours

Pregnancy Risk Factor B

Generic Available No

Comments The use of Purite® as a preservative in Alphagan® P has lead to a reduced incidence of certain adverse effects associated with Alphagan®, which uses benzalkonium chloride as a preservative.

Brinzolamide (brin ZOH la mide)

U.S. Brand Names Azopt®

Canadian Brand Names Azopt™

Pharmacologic Category Carbonic Anhydrase Inhibitor; Ophthalmic Agent, Antiglaucoma

Use Lowers intraocular pressure in the treatment of glaucoma in patients with ocular hypertension or open-angle glaucoma

Local Anesthetic/Vasoconstrictor Precautions No information available to require special precautions

Effects on Dental Treatment 5% to 10%: Taste disturbances

Dosage Adults: Ophthalmic: Instill 1 drop in eye(s) 3 times/day

Mechanism of Action Inhibition of carbonic anhydrase decreases aqueous humor secretion. This results in a reduction of intraocular pressure.

Other Adverse Effects 1% to 10%:

Dermatologic: Dermatitis (1% to 5%)

Gastrointestinal: Taste disturbances (5% to 10%)

Ocular: Blurred vision (5% to 10%), blepharitis (1% to 5%), dry eye (1% to 5%), foreign body sensation (1% to 5%), eye discharge (1% to 5%), eye pain (1% to 5%), itching of eye (1% to 5%)

Respiratory: Rhinitis

Warnings/Precautions Effects of prolonged use on corneal epithelial cells have not been evaluated; has not been studied in acute angle-closure glaucoma; renal impairment (parent and metabolite may accumulate). Patients with allergy to sulfonamides (brinzolamide is a sulfonamide); systemic absorption may cause serious hypersensitivity reactions to recur. Chemical similarities are present among sulfonamides, sulfonylureas, carbonic anhydrase inhibitors, thiazides, and loop diuretics (except ethacrynic acid). In patients with allergy to one of these compounds, a risk of cross-reaction exists; avoid use when previous reaction has been severe.

Drug Interactions Increased Effect/Toxicity: Concurrent use of oral carbonic anhydrase inhibitors (CAIs) may lead to additive effects and toxicity. High-dose salicylates may result in toxicity from CAIs.

Drug Uptake

Onset of action: Peak effect: 2 hours

Absorption: Topical: Into the systemic circulation

Duration: 8-12 hours

Pregnancy Risk Factor C

Generic Available No

Brodspec® *see* Tetracycline *on page 1147*

Brofed® *see* Brompheniramine and Pseudoephedrine *on page 180*

Bromanate® [OTC] *see* Brompheniramine and Pseudoephedrine *on page 180*

Bromazepam *Not Available in U.S.* (broe MA ze pam)

Canadian Brand Names Alti-Bromazepam; Apo®-Bromazepam; Gen-Bromazepam; Lectopam®; Novo-Bromazepam; Nu-Bromazepam

Pharmacologic Category Benzodiazepine

Use Short-term, symptomatic treatment of anxiety

Local Anesthetic/Vasoconstrictor Precautions No information available to require special precautions

Effects on Dental Treatment No effects or complications reported

Restrictions CDSA IV

Dosage Oral:

Adults: Initial: 6-18 mg/day in equally divided doses; initial course of treatment should not last longer than 1 week; optimal dosage range: 6-30 mg/day

Elderly/debilitated: Initial dose: 3 mg/day in divided doses

Mechanism of Action Binds to stereospecific benzodiazepine receptors on the postsynaptic GABA neuron at several sites within the CNS, including the limbic system, reticular formation. Enhancement of the inhibitory effect of GABA on neuronal excitability results by increased neuronal membrane permeability to chloride ions. This shift in chloride ions results in hyperpolarization (a less excitable state) and stabilization.

Other Adverse Effects Frequency not defined:

Cardiovascular: Hypotension, palpitations, tachycardia

Central nervous system: Drowsiness, ataxia, dizziness, confusion, depression, euphoria, lethargy, slurred speech, stupor, headache, seizures, anterograde amnesia. In addition, paradoxical reactions (including excitation, agitation, hallucinations, and psychosis) are known to occur with benzodiazepines.

Dermatologic: Rash, pruritus

Endocrine & metabolic: Hyperglycemia, hypoglycemia

Gastrointestinal: Xerostomia, nausea, vomiting

Genitourinary: Incontinence, libido decreased

Hematologic: Hemoglobin decreased, hematocrit decreased, WBCs increased/decreased

Hepatic: Transaminases increased, alkaline phosphatase increased, bilirubin increased
Neuromuscular & skeletal: Weakness, muscle spasm
Ocular: Blurred vision, depth perception decreased

Drug Interactions Possible CYP3A3/4 enzyme substrate (not established)
Increased Effect/Toxicity: Benzodiazepines potentiate the CNS depressant effects of narcotic analgesics, barbiturates, phenothiazines, ethanol, antihistamines, MAO inhibitors, sedative-hypnotics, and cyclic antidepressants. Serum levels and/or effects of benzodiazepines may be increased by inhibitors of CYP3A3/4 including amiodarone, amprenavir, cimetidine, clarithromycin, erythromycin, delavirdine, diltiazem, dirithromycin, disulfiram, fluoxetine, fluvoxamine, grapefruit juice, indinavir, itraconazole, ketoconazole, nefazodone, nevirapine, propoxyphene, quinupristin-dalfopristin, ritonavir, saquinavir, verapamil, zafirlukast, zileuton.
Decreased Effect: Carbamazepine, rifampin, rifabutin may enhance the metabolism of benzodiazepines and decrease therapeutic effect.

Drug Uptake Half-life, elimination: 20 hours
Pregnancy Risk Factor D (based on other benzodiazepines)
Generic Available Yes

Bromfed® [OTC] *see* Brompheniramine and Pseudoephedrine *on page 180*
Bromfed-PD® [OTC] *see* Brompheniramine and Pseudoephedrine *on page 180*
Bromfenex® *see* Brompheniramine and Pseudoephedrine *on page 180*
Bromfenex® PD *see* Brompheniramine and Pseudoephedrine *on page 180*

Bromocriptine (broe moe KRIP teen)

U.S. Brand Names Parlodel®
Canadian Brand Names Apo® Bromocriptine; Parlodel®; PMS-Bromocriptine
Mexican Brand Names Cryocriptina; Parlodel®; Serocryptin®
Pharmacologic Category Anti-Parkinson's Agent, Dopamine Agonist; Ergot Derivative
Synonyms Bromocriptine Mesylate
Use
Usually used with levodopa or levodopa/carbidopa in treatment of Parkinson's disease - treatment of parkinsonism in patients unresponsive or allergic to levodopa
Prolactin-secreting pituitary adenomas, acromegaly, amenorrhea/galactorrhea secondary to hyperprolactinemia in the absence of primary tumor
The indication for prevention of postpartum lactation has been withdrawn voluntarily by Sandoz Pharmaceuticals Corporation
Neuroleptic malignant syndrome

Local Anesthetic/Vasoconstrictor Precautions No information available to require special precautions
Effects on Dental Treatment No effects or complications reported
Dosage Adults: Oral:
Parkinsonism: 1.25 mg 2 times/day, increased by 2.5 mg/day in 2- to 4-week intervals (usual dose range is 30-90 mg/day in 3 divided doses), though elderly patients can usually be managed on lower doses
Hyperprolactinemia: 2.5 mg 2-3 times/day
Acromegaly: Initial: 1.25-2.5 mg increasing as necessary every 3-7 days; usual dose: 20-30 mg/day

Mechanism of Action Semisynthetic ergot alkaloid derivative with dopaminergic properties; inhibits prolactin secretion and can improve symptoms of Parkinson's disease by directly stimulating dopamine receptors in the corpus stratum
Other Adverse Effects
>10%:
Central nervous system: Headache, dizziness
Gastrointestinal: Nausea
1% to 10%:
Cardiovascular: Orthostatic hypotension
Central nervous system: Fatigue, lightheadedness, drowsiness
Gastrointestinal: Anorexia, vomiting, abdominal cramps, constipation
Respiratory: Nasal congestion

Drug Interactions CYP3A3/4 enzyme substrate
Increased Effect/Toxicity: Isometheptene and phenylpropanolamine (and other sympathomimetics) should be avoided in patients receiving bromocriptine - may increase risk of hypertension and seizure. Erythromycin, fluvoxamine, and nefazodone may increase bromocriptine concentrations.
Decreased Effect: Antipsychotics may inhibit bromocriptine's ability to lower prolactin.

Drug Uptake
Half-life, elimination: Biphasic: Initial: 6-8 hours; Terminal: 50 hours
Time to peak: Oral: 1-2 hours
Pregnancy Risk Factor B
Generic Available No

Bromodiphenhydramine and Codeine

(brome oh dye fen HYE dra meen & KOE deen)

Pharmacologic Category Antihistamine/Antitussive

Synonyms Codeine and Bromodiphenhydramine

Use Relief of upper respiratory symptoms and cough associated with allergies or common cold

Local Anesthetic/Vasoconstrictor Precautions No information available to require special precautions

Effects on Dental Treatment

Bromodiphenhydramine: 1% to 10%: Xerostomia

Codeine: <1%: Xerostomia

Restrictions C-V

Dosage Adults: Oral: 5-10 mL every 4-6 hours

Pregnancy Risk Factor C

Generic Available Yes

Brompheniramine and Pseudoephedrine

(brome fen IR a meen & soo doe e FED rin)

U.S. Brand Names Andehist NR Syrup; Brofed®; Bromanate® [OTC]; Bromfed® [OTC]; Bromfed-PD® [OTC]; Bromfenex®; Bromfenex® PD; Children's Dimetapp® Elixir Cold & Allergy [OTC]; Rondec® Syrup; Touro™ Allergy

Pharmacologic Category Antihistamine/Decongestant Combination

Synonyms Pseudoephedrine and Brompheniramine

Use Temporary relief of symptoms of seasonal and perennial allergic rhinitis, and vasomotor rhinitis, including nasal obstruction

Local Anesthetic/Vasoconstrictor Precautions Use with caution since pseudoephedrine is a sympathomimetic amine which could interact with epinephrine to cause a pressor response

Effects on Dental Treatment

Brompheniramine: Prolonged use may decrease salivary flow

Pseudoephedrine: Up to 10% of patients could experience tachycardia, palpitations, and xerostomia; use vasoconstrictor with caution

Dosage Children >12 years and Adults: Oral: 10 mL every 4-6 hours, up to 40 mL/day

Mechanism of Action Brompheniramine maleate is an antihistamine with H_1-receptor activity; pseudoephedrine, a sympathomimetic amine and isomer of ephedrine, acts as a decongestant in respiratory tract mucous membranes with less vasoconstrictor action than ephedrine in normotensive individuals.

Other Adverse Effects

>10%:
- Cardiovascular: Tachycardia
- Central nervous system: Slight to moderate drowsiness, nervousness, transient stimulation, insomnia
- Respiratory: Thickening of bronchial secretions

1% to 10%:
- Central nervous system: Headache, fatigue, dizziness
- Gastrointestinal: Appetite increase, weight gain, nausea, diarrhea, abdominal pain, xerostomia
- Genitourinary: Dysuria
- Neuromuscular & skeletal: Arthralgia, weakness
- Respiratory: Pharyngitis
- Miscellaneous: Diaphoresis

Drug Interactions CNS depressants, MAO inhibitors, sympathomimetics, Rauwolfia alkaloids, tricyclic antidepressants, ganglionic blocking agents, propranolol

Drug Uptake See Pseudoephedrine *on page 1022*

Pregnancy Risk Factor C

Generic Available Yes

Brompheril® [OTC] *see* Dexbrompheniramine and Pseudoephedrine *on page 365*

Bronchial® *see* Theophylline and Guaifenesin *on page 1155*

Broncho Saline® *see* Sodium Chloride *on page 1094*

Bronitin® *see* Epinephrine *on page 438*

Bronkometer® *see* Isoetharine *on page 658*

Bronkosol® *see* Isoetharine *on page 658*

Brontex® Liquid *see* Guaifenesin and Codeine *on page 568*

Brontex® Tablet *see* Guaifenesin and Codeine *on page 568*

BSS® *see* Balanced Salt Solution *on page 143*

Budesonide (byoo DES oh nide)

U.S. Brand Names Entocort™ EC; Pulmicort Respules™; Pulmicort Turbuhaler®; Rhinocort®; Rhinocort® Aqua™

Canadian Brand Names Entocort®; Gen-Budesonide AQ; Pulmicort®; Rhinocort® Turbuhaler®

Mexican Brand Names Pulmicort®; Rhinocort®

Pharmacologic Category Corticosteroid, Inhalant (Oral); Corticosteroid, Nasal; Corticosteroid, Systemic

Use

Intranasal: Children ≥6 years of age and Adults: Management of symptoms of seasonal or perennial rhinitis

Nebulization: Children 12 months to 8 years: Maintenance and prophylactic treatment of asthma

Oral capsule: Treatment of active Crohn's disease (mild to moderate) involving the ileum and/or ascending colon

Oral inhalation: Maintenance and prophylactic treatment of asthma; includes patients who require corticosteroids and those who may benefit from systemic dose reduction/elimination

Local Anesthetic/Vasoconstrictor Precautions No information available to require special precautions

Effects on Dental Treatment Localized infections with *Candida albicans* or *Aspergillus niger* have occurred frequently in the mouth and pharynx with repetitive use of oral inhaler of corticosteroids. These infections may require treatment with appropriate antifungal therapy or discontinuance of treatment with corticosteroid inhaler.

Dosage

Nasal inhalation: Children ≥6 years and Adults:

Rhinocort®: Initial: 8 sprays (4 sprays/nostril) per day (256 mcg/day), given as either 2 sprays in each nostril in the morning and evening or as 4 sprays in each nostril in the morning; after symptoms decrease (usually by 3-7 days), reduce dose slowly every 2-4 weeks to the smallest amount needed to control symptoms

Rhinocort® Aqua™: 64 mcg/day as a single 32 mcg spray in each nostril. Some patients who do not achieve adequate control may benefit from increased dosage. A reduced dosage may be effective after initial control is achieved.

Maximum dose: Children <12 years: 128 mcg/day; Adults: 256 mcg/day

Nebulization: Children 12 months to 8 years: Pulmicort Respules™: Titrate to lowest effective dose once patient is stable; start at 0.25 mg/day or use as follows:

Previous therapy of bronchodilators alone: 0.5 mg/day administered as a single dose or divided twice daily (maximum daily dose: 0.5 mg)

Previous therapy of inhaled corticosteroids: 0.5 mg/day administered as a single dose or divided twice daily (maximum daily dose: 1 mg)

Previous therapy of oral corticosteroids: 1 mg/day administered as a single dose or divided twice daily (maximum daily dose: 1 mg)

Oral inhalation:

Children ≥6 years:

Previous therapy of bronchodilators alone: 200 mcg twice initially which may be increased up to 400 mcg twice daily

Previous therapy of inhaled corticosteroids: 200 mcg twice initially which may be increased up to 400 mcg twice daily

Previous therapy of oral corticosteroids: The highest recommended dose in children is 400 mcg twice daily

Adults:

Previous therapy of bronchodilators alone: 200-400 mcg twice initially which may be increased up to 400 mcg twice daily

Previous therapy of inhaled corticosteroids: 200-400 mcg twice initially which may be increased up to 800 mcg twice daily

Previous therapy of oral corticosteroids: 400-800 mcg twice daily which may be increased up to 800 mcg twice daily

NIH Guidelines (NIH, 1997) (give in divided doses twice daily):

Children:

"Low" dose: 100-200 mcg/day

"Medium" dose: 200-400 mcg/day (1-2 inhalations/day)

"High" dose: >400 mcg/day (>2 inhalation/day)

Adults:

"Low" dose: 200-400 mcg/day (1-2 inhalations/day)

"Medium" dose: 400-600 mcg/day (2-3 inhalations/day)

"High" dose: >600 mcg/day (>3 inhalation/day)

Oral: Adults: Crohn's disease: 9 mg once daily in the morning; safety and efficacy have not been established for therapy duration >8 weeks; recurring episodes may be treated with a repeat 8-week course of treatment

Note: Treatment may be tapered to 6 mg once daily for 2 weeks prior to complete cessation. Patients receiving CYP3A3/4 inhibitors should be monitored closely for signs and symptoms of hypercorticism; dosage reduction may be required.

Dosage adjustment in hepatic impairment: Monitor closely for signs and symptoms of hypercorticism; dosage reduction may be required.

Mechanism of Action Controls the rate of protein synthesis, depresses the migration of polymorphonuclear leukocytes, fibroblasts, reverses capillary permeability, and lysosomal stabilization at the cellular level to prevent or control inflammation

(Continued)

Budesonide *(Continued)*

Other Adverse Effects Reaction severity varies by dose and duration; not all adverse reactions have been reported with each dosage form.

>10%:

Central nervous system: Oral capsule: Headache (up to 21%)

Gastrointestinal: Oral capsule: Nausea (up to 11%)

Respiratory: Respiratory infection, rhinitis

Miscellaneous: Symptoms of HPA axis suppression and/or hypercorticism (acne, easy bruising, fat redistribution, striae, edema) may occur in >10% of patients following administration of dosage forms which result in higher systemic exposure (ie, oral capsule), but may be less frequent than rates observed with comparator drugs (prednisolone). These symptoms may be rare (<1%) following administration via methods which result in lower exposures (topical).

1% to 10%:

Cardiovascular: Syncope, edema, hypertension

Central nervous system: Chest pain, dysphonia, emotional lability, fatigue, fever, insomnia, migraine, nervousness, pain, dizziness, vertigo

Dermatologic: Bruising, contact dermatitis, eczema, pruritus, pustular rash, rash

Endocrine & metabolic: Hypokalemia, adrenal insufficiency

Gastrointestinal: Abdominal pain, anorexia, diarrhea, xerostomia, dyspepsia, gastroenteritis, oral candidiasis, taste perversion, vomiting, weight gain, flatulence

Hematologic: Cervical lymphadenopathy, purpura, leukocytosis

Neuromuscular & skeletal: Arthralgia, fracture, hyperkinesis, hypertonia, myalgia, neck pain, weakness, paresthesia, back pain

Ocular: Conjunctivitis, eye infection

Otic: Earache, ear infection, external ear infection

Respiratory: Bronchitis, bronchospasm, cough, epistaxis, nasal irritation, pharyngitis, sinusitis, stridor

Miscellaneous: Allergic reaction, flu-like syndrome, herpes simplex, infection, moniliasis, viral infection, voice alteration

Contraindications

Hypersensitivity to budesonide or any component of the formulation.

Inhalation: Contraindicated in primary treatment of status asthmaticus, acute episodes of asthma; not for relief of acute bronchospasm

Warnings/Precautions May cause hypercorticism and/or suppression of hypothalamic-pituitary-adrenal (HPA) axis, particularly in younger children or in patients receiving high doses for prolonged periods. Particular care is required when patients are transferred from systemic corticosteroids to products with lower systemic bioavailability (ie, inhalation). May lead to possible adrenal insufficiency or withdrawal from steroids, including an increase in allergic symptoms. Patients receiving prolonged therapy of ≥20 mg per day of prednisone (or equivalent) may be most susceptible. Aerosol steroids do **not** provide the systemic steroid needed to treat patients having trauma, surgery, or infections.

Controlled clinical studies have shown that orally-inhaled and intranasal corticosteroids may cause a reduction in growth velocity in pediatric patients. (In studies of orally-inhaled corticosteroids, the mean reduction in growth velocity was approximately 1 centimeter per year [range 0.3-1.8 cm per year] and appears to be related to dose and duration of exposure.) To minimize the systemic effects of orally-inhaled and intranasal corticosteroids, each patient should be titrated to the lowest effective dose. Growth should be routinely monitored in pediatric patients.

May suppress the immune system, patients may be more susceptible to infection. Use with caution in patients with systemic infections or ocular herpes simplex. Avoid exposure to chickenpox and measles. Corticosteroids should be used with caution in patients with diabetes, hypertension, osteoporosis, peptic ulcer, glaucoma, cataracts, or tuberculosis. Use caution in hepatic impairment. Enteric-coated capsules should not be crushed or chewed.

Drug Interactions CYP3A3/4 enzyme substrate

Increased Effect/Toxicity: Cimetidine may decrease the clearance and increase the bioavailability of budesonide, increasing its serum concentration. In addition, CYP3A3/4 inhibitors may increase the serum concentration and/or toxicity of budesonide; effect was shown with ketoconazole but not erythromycin. Other potential inhibitors include amiodarone, cimetidine, clarithromycin, delavirdine, diltiazem, dirithromycin, disulfiram, fluoxetine, fluvoxamine, indinavir, itraconazole, ketoconazole, nefazodone, nevirapine, propoxyphene, quinupristin-dalfopristin, ritonavir, saquinavir, verapamil, zafirlukast, zileuton. The addition of salmeterol has been demonstrated to improve response to inhaled corticosteroids (as compared to increasing steroid dosage).

Decreased Effect: CYP3A3/4 inducers (including carbamazepine, phenytoin, phenobarbital, rifampin) may decrease budesonide levels and/or effects. Theoretically, proton pump inhibitors (omeprazole, pantoprazole) alter gastric pH may affect the rate of dissolution of enteric-coated capsules. Administration with omeprazole did not alter kinetics of budesonide capsules.

Drug Uptake

Onset of action: Respules™: 2-8 days; Rhinocort® Aqua™: ~10 hours; Turbuhaler®: 24 hours

Peak effect: Respules™: 4-6 weeks; Rhinocort® Aqua™: ~2 weeks; Turbuhaler®: 1-2 weeks

Absorption: Capsule: Rapid and complete

Half-life, elimination: 2-3.6 hours

Time to peak: Capsule: 30-600 minutes (variable in Crohn's disease); Respules™: 10-30 minutes; Turbuhaler®: 1-2 hours; Nasal: 1 hour

Pregnancy Risk Factor C/B (Pulmicort Turbuhaler®)

Generic Available No

Bufferin® [OTC] *see* Aspirin *on page 119*

Bufferin® Arthritis Strength [OTC] *see* Aspirin *on page 119*

Bufferin® Extra Strength [OTC] *see* Aspirin *on page 119*

Bumetanide (byoo MET a nide)

Related Information

Cardiovascular Diseases *on page 1308*

U.S. Brand Names Bumex®

Canadian Brand Names Bumex®; Burinex®

Mexican Brand Names Bumedyl®; Drenural®; Miccil®

Pharmacologic Category Diuretic, Loop

Use Management of edema secondary to CHF or hepatic or renal disease including nephrotic syndrome; may be used alone or in combination with antihypertensives in the treatment of hypertension; can be used in furosemide-allergic patients; (1 mg = 40 mg furosemide)

Local Anesthetic/Vasoconstrictor Precautions No information available to require special precautions

Effects on Dental Treatment No effects or complications reported

Dosage

Children:

<6 months: Dose not established

>6 months:

Oral: Initial: 0.015 mg/kg/dose once daily or every other day; maximum dose: 0.1 mg/kg/day

I.M., I.V.: Dose not established

Adults:

Oral: 0.5-2 mg/dose 1-2 times/day; maximum: 10 mg/day

I.M., I.V.: 0.5-1 mg/dose; maximum: 10 mg/day

Continuous I.V. infusions of 0.9-1 mg/hour may be more effective than bolus dosing

Mechanism of Action Inhibits reabsorption of sodium and chloride in the ascending loop of Henle and proximal renal tubule, interfering with the chloride-binding cotransport system, thus causing increased excretion of water, sodium, chloride, magnesium, phosphate and calcium; it does not appear to act on the distal tubule

Other Adverse Effects

>10%:

Endocrine & metabolic: Hyperuricemia (18%), hypochloremia (14.9%), hypokalemia (14.7%)

Renal: Azotemia (10.6%)

1% to 10%:

Neuromuscular & skeletal: Muscle cramps (1.1%)

Central nervous system: Dizziness (1.1%)

Endocrine & metabolic: Hyponatremia (9.2%), hyperglycemia (6.6%), variations in phosphorus (4.5%), CO_2 content (4.3%), bicarbonate (3.1%), and calcium (2.4%)

Renal: Increased serum creatinine (7.4%)

Otic: Ototoxicity (1.1%)

Warnings/Precautions Adjust dose to avoid dehydration. In cirrhosis, avoid electrolyte and acid/base imbalances that might lead to hepatic encephalopathy. Ototoxicity is associated with I.V. rapid administration, renal impairment, excessive doses, and concurrent use of other ototoxins. Hypersensitivity reactions can rarely occur. Monitor fluid status and renal function in an attempt to prevent oliguria, azotemia, and reversible increases in BUN and creatinine. Close medical supervision of aggressive diuresis required. Watch for and correct electrolyte disturbances. Coadministration of antihypertensives may increase the risk of hypotension.

Chemical similarities are present among sulfonamides, sulfonylureas, carbonic anhydrase inhibitors, thiazides, and loop diuretics (except ethacrynic acid). Use in patients with sulfonylurea allergy is specifically contraindicated in product labeling, however a risk of cross-reaction exists in patients with allergy to any of these compounds; avoid use when previous reaction has been severe.

(Continued)

Bumetanide *(Continued)*

Loop diuretics are potent diuretics; excess amounts can lead to profound diuresis with fluid and electrolyte loss; close medical supervision and dose evaluation is required; *in vitro* studies using pooled sera from critically ill neonates have shown bumetanide to be a potent displacer of bilirubin; avoid use in neonates at risk for kernicterus.

Drug Interactions

Increased Effect/Toxicity: Bumetanide-induced hypokalemia may predispose to digoxin toxicity and may increase the risk of arrhythmia with drugs which may prolong QT interval, including type Ia and type III antiarrhythmic agents, cisapride, terfenadine, and some quinolones (sparfloxacin, gatifloxacin, and moxifloxacin). The risk of toxicity from lithium and salicylates (high dose) may be increased by loop diuretics. Hypotensive effects and/or adverse renal effects of ACE inhibitors and NSAIDs are potentiated by bumetanide-induced hypovolemia. The effects of peripheral adrenergic-blocking drugs or ganglionic blockers may be increased by bumetanide. Bumetanide may increase the risk of ototoxicity with other ototoxic agents (aminoglycosides, cis-platinum), especially in patients with renal dysfunction. Synergistic diuretic effects occur with thiazide-type diuretics. Diuretics tend to be synergistic with other antihypertensive agents, and hypotension may occur.

Decreased Effect: Glucose tolerance may be decreased by loop diuretics, requiring adjustment of hypoglycemic agents. Cholestyramine or colestipol may reduce bioavailability of bumetanide. Indomethacin (and other NSAIDs) may reduce natriuretic and hypotensive effects of diuretics. Hypokalemia may reduce the efficacy of some antiarrhythmics.

Drug Uptake

Onset of action: Oral, I.M.: 0.5-1 hour; I.V.: 2-3 minutes

Duration: 6 hours

Half-life, elimination: Infants <6 months: Possibly 2.5 hours; Children and Adults: 1-1.5 hours

Pregnancy Risk Factor C (manufacturer); D (expert analysis)

Generic Available Yes

Bumex® *see* Bumetanide *on page 183*

Buphenyl® *see* Sodium Phenylbutyrate *on page 1097*

Bupivacaine (byoo PIV a kane)

Related Information

Oral Pain *on page 1360*

U.S. Brand Names Marcaine®; Marcaine® Spinal; Sensorcaine®; Sensorcaine®-MPF

Canadian Brand Names Marcaine®; Sensorcaine®

Mexican Brand Names Buvacaina

Pharmacologic Category Local Anesthetic

Synonyms Bupivacaine Hydrochloride

Use

Dental: Local anesthetic (injectable) for infiltration

Medical: Local anesthetic (injectable) for peripheral nerve block, infiltration, sympathetic block, caudal or epidural block, retrobulbar block

Local Anesthetic/Vasoconstrictor Precautions No information available to require special precautions

Effects on Dental Treatment No effects or complications reported

Dosage Dose varies with procedure, depth of anesthesia, vascularity of tissues, duration of anesthesia and condition of patient. Some formulations contain metabisulfites (in epinephrine-containing injection); do not use solutions containing preservatives for caudal or epidural block.

Local anesthesia: Infiltration: 0.25% infiltrated locally; maximum: 175 mg

Caudal block (with or without epinephrine, preservative free):
- Children: 1-3.7 mg/kg
- Adults: 15-30 mL of 0.25% or 0.5%

Epidural block (other than caudal block - with or without epinephrine, preservative free):
- Administer in 3-5 mL increments, allowing sufficient time to detect toxic manifestations of inadvertent I.V. or I.T. administration:
  - Children: 1.25 mg/kg/dose
  - Adults: 10-20 mL of 0.25% or 0.5%
  - Surgical procedures requiring a high degree of muscle relaxation and prolonged effects **only**: 10-20 mL of 0.75% (**Note:** Not to be used in obstetrical cases)

Maxillary and mandibular infiltration and nerve block: 9 mg (1.8 mL) of 0.5% (with epinephrine) per injection site; a second dose may be administered if necessary to produce adequate anesthesia after allowing up to 10 minutes for onset, up to a maximum of 90 mg per dental appointment

Obstetrical anesthesia: Incremental dose: 3-5 mL of 0.5% (not exceeding 50-100 mg in any dosing interval); allow sufficient time to detect toxic manifestations or inadvertent I.V. or I.T. injection

Peripheral nerve block: 5 mL of 0.25 or 0.5%; maximum: 400 mg/day

Sympathetic nerve block: 20-50 mL of 0.25%

Retrobulbar anesthesia: 2-4 mL of 0.75%

Spinal anesthesia: Solution of 0.75% bupivacaine in 8.25% dextrose is used:
- Lower extremity and perineal procedures: 1 mL
- Lower abdominal procedures: 1.6 mL
- Obstetrical:
  - Normal vaginal delivery: 0.8 mL (higher doses may be required in some patients)
  - Cesarean section: 1-1.4 mL

Mechanism of Action Blocks both the initiation and conduction of nerve impulses by decreasing the neuronal membrane's permeability to sodium ions, which results in inhibition of depolarization with resultant blockade of conduction. Local anesthetics reversibly prevent generation and conduction of electrical impulses in neurons by decreasing the transient increase in permeability to sodium. The differential sensitivity generally depends on the size of the fiber; small fibers are more sensitive than larger fibers and require a longer period for recovery. Sensory pain fibers are usually blocked first, followed by fibers that transmit sensations of temperature, touch, and deep pressure. High concentrations block sympathetic somatic sensory and somatic motor fibers. The spread of anesthesia depends upon the distribution of the solution. This is primarily dependent on the site of administration and volume of drug injected.

Other Adverse Effects Most effects are dose-related, and are often due to accelerated absorption from the injection site, unintentional intravascular injection, or slow metabolic degradation. The development of any central nervous system symptoms may be an early indication of more significant toxicity (seizures). Frequency not defined:

Cardiovascular: Hypotension, bradycardia, palpitations, heart block, ventricular arrhythmias, cardiac arrest

Central nervous system: Restlessness, anxiety, dizziness, seizures (0.1%); rare symptoms (usually associated with unintentional subarachnoid injection during high spinal anesthesia) include persistent anesthesia, paresthesia, paralysis, headache, septic meningitis, and cranial nerve palsies

Gastrointestinal: Nausea, vomiting; rare symptoms (usually associated with unintentional subarachnoid injection during high spinal anesthesia) include fecal incontinence and loss of sphincter control

Genitourinary: Rare symptoms (usually associated with unintentional subarachnoid injection during high spinal anesthesia) include urinary incontinence, loss of perineal sensation, and loss of sexual function

Neuromuscular & skeletal: Weakness

Ocular: Blurred vision, pupillary constriction

Otic: Tinnitus

Respiratory: Apnea, hypoventilation (usually associated with unintentional subarachnoid injection during high spinal anesthesia)

Miscellaneous; Allergic reactions (urticaria, pruritus, angioedema), anaphylactoid reactions

Contraindications Hypersensitivity to bupivacaine hydrochloride, amide-type local anesthetics (etidocaine, lidocaine, mepivacaine, prilocaine, ropivacaine), or any component of their formulation (para-aminobenzoic acid or parabens in specific formulations); obstetrical paracervical block anesthesia

Warnings/Precautions Use with caution in patients with hepatic impairment. Some commercially available formulations contain sodium metabisulfite, which may cause allergic-type reactions; not recommended for use in children <12 years of age. The solution for spinal anesthesia should not be used in children <18 years of age. **Do not use solutions containing preservatives for caudal or epidural block**. Local anesthetics have been associated with rare occurrences of sudden respiratory arrest; convulsions due to systemic toxicity leading to cardiac arrest have also been reported, presumably following unintentional intravascular injection. The 0.75% is **not** recommended for obstetrical anesthesia. A test dose is recommended prior to epidural administration (prior to initial dose) and all reinforcing doses with continuous catheter technique.

Drug Interactions

Increased Effect: Hyaluronidase

Increased Toxicity: Beta-blockers, ergot-type oxytocics, MAO inhibitors, TCAs, phenothiazines, vasopressors

Drug Uptake

Onset of action: Anesthesia (route-dependent): 4-10 minutes

Duration: 1.5-8.5 hours

Half-life, elimination (age-dependent): Neonates: 8.1 hours; Adults: 1.5-5.5 hours

Pregnancy Risk Factor C

Dosage Forms INJ, solution [preservative free]: 0.25% [2.5 mg/mL] (20 mL, 30 mL, 50 mL), 0.5% [5 mg/mL] (20 mL, 30 mL), 0.75% [7.5 mg/mL] (20 mL, 30 mL); (Continued)

Bupivacaine *(Continued)*

(Marcaine®): 0.25% [2.5 mg/mL] (10 mL, 30 mL, 50 mL), 0.5% [5 mg/mL] (10 mL, 30 mL), 0.75% [7.5 mg/mL] (10 mL, 30 mL); (Marcaine® Spinal): 0.75% [7.5 mg/mL] (2 mL); (Sensorcaine®-MPF): 0.25% [2.5 mg/mL] (10 mL, 30 mL), 0.5% [5 mg/mL] (10 mL, 30 mL), 0.75% [7.5 mg/mL] (10 mL, 30 mL). **INJ, solution:** 0.25% [2.5 mg/mL] (10 mL, 30 mL, 50 mL), 0.5% [5 mg/mL] (10 mL, 30 mL, 50 mL), 0.75% [7.5 mg/mL] (10 mL, 30 mL); (Marcaine®, Sensorcaine®): 0.25% [2.5 mg/mL] (50 mL), 0.5% [5 mg/mL] (50 mL). **INJ, solution, with epinephrine 1:200,000** [preservative free]: (Marcaine®): 0.25% [2.5 mg/mL] (10 mL, 30 mL, 50 mL), 0.5% [5 mg/mL] (3 mL, 10 mL, 30 mL), 0.75% [7.5 mg/mL] (30 mL); (Sensorcaine®-MPF): 0.25% [2.5 mg/mL] (10 mL, 30 mL), 0.5% [5 mg/mL] (5 mL, 10 mL, 30 mL). **INJ, solution, with epinephrine 1:200,000** (Marcaine®, Sensorcaine®): 0.25% [2.5 mg/mL] (50 mL); 0.5% [5 mg/mL] (50 mL)

Generic Available Yes

Bupivacaine and Epinephrine (byoo PIV a kane & ep i NEF rin)

Related Information

Oral Pain *on page 1360*

U.S. Brand Names Marcaine® with Epinephrine

Canadian Brand Names Sensorcaine® With Epinephrine

Pharmacologic Category Local Anesthetic

Use Local anesthesia

Local Anesthetic/Vasoconstrictor Precautions No information available to require special precautions

Effects on Dental Treatment No effects or complications reported

Dosage

Children <10 years: Dosage has not been established.

Children >10 years and Adults: Infiltration and nerve block in maxillary and mandibular area: 9 mg (1.8 mL) of bupivacaine as a 0.5% solution with epinephrine 1:200,000 per injection site. A second dose may be administered if necessary to produce adequate anesthesia after allowing up to 10 minutes for onset. Up to a maximum of 90 mg of bupivacaine hydrochloride per dental appointment. The effective anesthetic dose varies with procedure, intensity of anesthesia needed, duration of anesthesia required, and physical condition of the patient; always use the lowest effective dose along with careful aspiration.

The following numbers of dental carpules (1.8 mL) provide the indicated amounts of bupivacaine hydrochloride 0.5% and epinephrine 1:200,000. See table.

# of Cartridges (1.8 mL)	Bupivacaine HCl (0.5%) (mg)	Epinephrine 1:200,000 (mg)
1	9	0.009
2	18	0.018
3	27	0.027
4	36	0.036
5	45	0.045
6	54	0.054
7	63	0.063
8	72	0.072
9	81	0.081
10	90	0.090

Note: Doses of bupivacaine hydrochloride with epinephrine cited from USP Dispensing Information (USP DI), 17th ed, The United States Pharmacopeial Convention, Inc, Rockville, MD, 1997, 134.

Mechanism of Action Local anesthetics bind selectively to the intracellular surface of sodium channels to block influx of sodium into the axon. As a result, depolarization necessary for action potential propagation and subsequent nerve function is prevented. Local anesthetics reversibly prevent generation and conduction of electrical impulses in neurons by decreasing the transient increase in permeability to sodium. The differential sensitivity generally depends on the size of the fiber; small fibers are more sensitive than larger fibers and require a longer period for recovery. Sensory pain fibers are usually blocked first, followed by fibers that transmit sensations of temperature, touch, and deep pressure. High concentrations block sympathetic somatic sensory and somatic motor fibers. The spread of anesthesia depends upon the distribution of the solution. This is primarily dependent on the site of administration and volume of drug injected. The block at the sodium channel is reversible. When drug diffuses away from the axon, sodium channel function is restored and nerve propagation returns.

Epinephrine prolongs the duration of the anesthetic actions of bupivacaine by causing vasoconstriction (alpha adrenergic receptor agonist) of the vasculature surrounding the nerve axons. This prevents the diffusion of bupivacaine away from the nerves resulting in a longer retention in the axon

Other Adverse Effects The degree of adverse effects in the central nervous system and cardiovascular system is directly related to the blood levels of bupivacaine. Frequency not defined:

Cardiovascular: Myocardial effects include a decrease in contraction force as well as a decrease in electrical excitability and myocardial conduction rate resulting in bradycardia and reduction in cardiac output.

Central nervous system: High blood levels result in anxiety, restlessness, disorientation, confusion, dizziness, tremors and seizures. This is followed by depression of CNS resulting in somnolence, unconsciousness and possible respiratory arrest. Nausea and vomiting may also occur. In some cases, symptoms of CNS stimulation may be absent and the primary CNS effects are somnolence and unconsciousness.

Hypersensitivity reactions: Extremely rare, but may be manifest as dermatologic reactions and edema at injection site. Asthmatic syndromes have occurred. Patients may exhibit hypersensitivity to bisulfites contained in local anesthetic solution to prevent oxidation of epinephrine. In general, patients reacting to bisulfites have a history of asthma and their airways are hyper-reactive to asthmatic syndrome.

Psychogenic reactions: It is common to misinterpret psychogenic responses to local anesthetic injection as an allergic reaction. Intraoral injections are perceived by many patients as a stressful procedure in dentistry. Common symptoms to this stress are diaphoresis, palpitations, hyperventilation, generalized pallor and a fainting feeling.

Contraindications Hypersensitivity to bupivacaine or any component of the formulation

Warnings/Precautions Should be avoided in patients with uncontrolled hyperthyroidism

Drug Interactions

Due to bupivacaine component:

Increased Effect: Hyaluronidase

Increased Toxicity: Beta-blockers, ergot-type oxytocics, MAO inhibitors, TCAs, phenothiazines, vasopressors

Due to epinephrine component:

With MAO inhibitors: May result in increased pressor response

With tricyclic antidepressants: Pressor response to I.V. epinephrine, norepinephrine, and phenylephrine may be enhanced in patients receiving TCAs (**Note:** Effect is unlikely with epinephrine or levonordefrin dosages typically administered as infiltration in combination with local anesthetics)

With nonselective beta-blockers (ie, propranolol): May result in serious hypertension and reflex bradycardia

Drug Uptake

Onset of action: Infiltration and nerve block: 2-20 minutes

Duration: Infiltration: 1 hour; Nerve block: 5-7 hours

Half-life, elimination, serum: Adults: 1.5-5.5 hours

Pregnancy Risk Factor C

Breast-feeding Considerations Usual infiltration doses of bupivacaine with epinephrine given to nursing mothers has not been shown to affect the health of the nursing infant

Dosage Forms INJ: Bupivacaine hydrochloride 0.5% with epinephrine 1:200,000 (1.8 mL) [cartridge, 50/box]

Generic Available Yes

Selected Readings

Ayoub ST and Coleman AE, "A Review of Local Anesthetics," *Gen Dent*, 1992, 40(4):285-7, 289-90.

Jastak JT and Yagiela JA, "Vasoconstrictors and Local Anesthesia: A Review and Rationale for Use," *J Am Dent Assoc*, 1983, 107(4):623-30.

MacKenzie TA and Young ER, "Local Anesthetic Update," *Anesth Prog*, 1993, 40(2):29-34.

Wynn RL, "Epinephrine Interactions With Beta-Blockers," *Gen Dent*, 1994, 42(1):16, 18.

Yagiela JA, "Local Anesthetics," *Anesth Prog*, 1991, 38(4-5):128-41.

Buprenex® *see* Buprenorphine *on page 187*

Buprenorphine (byoo pre NOR feen)

U.S. Brand Names Buprenex®

Canadian Brand Names Buprenex®

Mexican Brand Names Temgesic®

Pharmacologic Category Analgesic, Narcotic

Synonyms Buprenorphine Hydrochloride

Use Management of moderate to severe pain

Unlabeled/Investigational: Heroin and opioid withdrawal

Local Anesthetic/Vasoconstrictor Precautions No information available to require special precautions

Effects on Dental Treatment No effects or complications reported

Restrictions C-V

Dosage Long-term use is not recommended.

(Continued)

Buprenorphine *(Continued)*

I.M., slow I.V.:
Children ≥13 years and Adults:
Moderate to severe pain: 0.3-0.6 mg every 6 hours as needed
Heroin or opiate withdrawal (unlabeled use): Variable; 0.1-0.4 mg every 6 hours
Elderly: Moderate to severe pain: 0.15 mg every 6 hours; elderly patients are more likely to suffer from confusion and drowsiness compared to younger patients

Mechanism of Action Opiate agonist/antagonist that produces analgesia by binding to mu and kappa opiate receptors in the CNS

Other Adverse Effects
>10%: Central nervous system: Sedation
1% to 10%:
Cardiovascular: Hypotension
Central nervous system: Respiratory depression, dizziness, headache
Gastrointestinal: Vomiting, nausea
Ocular: Miosis
Miscellaneous: Diaphoresis

Drug Interactions CYP3A3/4 enzyme substrate
Cimetidine: May increase sedation from narcotic analgesics; however, histamine blockers may attenuate the cardiovascular response from histamine release associated with narcotic analgesics
CNS depressants: May produce additive respiratory and CNS depression; includes benzodiazepines, barbiturates, ethanol, and other sedatives. Respiratory and CV collapse was reported in a patient who received diazepam and buprenorphine.
CYP3A3/4 inhibitors: Serum level and/or toxicity of buprenorphine may be increased; inhibitors include amiodarone, cimetidine, clarithromycin, erythromycin, delavirdine, diltiazem, dirithromycin, disulfiram, fluoxetine, fluvoxamine, grapefruit juice, indinavir, itraconazole, ketoconazole, nefazodone, nevirapine, propoxyphene, quinupristin-dalfopristin, ritonavir, saquinavir, verapamil, zafirlukast, and zileuton. Monitor for altered effects; a decrease in buprenorphine dosage may be required.
Enzyme inducers: May reduce serum concentrations of buprenorphine, resulting in loss of efficacy; includes barbiturates, carbamazepine, phenytoin, rifabutin, and rifampin.
Naltrexone: May antagonize the effect of narcotic analgesics; concurrent use or use within 7-10 days is contraindicated

Drug Uptake
Onset of analgesic effect: 10-30 minutes
Absorption: I.M., S.C.: 30% to 40%
Duration: 6-8 hours
Half-life, elimination: 2.2-3 hours

Pregnancy Risk Factor C

Generic Available Yes

BuPROPion (byoo PROE pee on)

Related Information
Chemical Dependency and Smoking Cessation *on page 1410*

U.S. Brand Names Wellbutrin®; Wellbutrin SR®; Zyban®

Canadian Brand Names Wellbutrin®; Zyban™

Mexican Brand Names Wellbutrin®

Pharmacologic Category Antidepressant, Dopamine-Reuptake Inhibitor; Smoking Cessation Aid

Use Treatment of depression; adjunct in smoking cessation
Unlabeled/Investigational: Attention-deficit/hyperactivity disorder (ADHD)

Local Anesthetic/Vasoconstrictor Precautions Although this is not a tricyclic antidepressant, it can cause hypertensive episodes and should be used with caution in the presence of a vasoconstrictor.

Effects on Dental Treatment >10%: Significant xerostomia; normal salivary flow resumes with discontinuation

Dosage Oral:
Children and Adolescents: ADHD (unlabeled use): 1.4-6 mg/kg/day
Adults:
Depression:
Immediate release: 100 mg 3 times/day; begin at 100 mg twice daily; may increase to a maximum dose of 450 mg/day
Sustained release: Initial: 150 mg/day in the morning; may increase to 150 mg twice daily by day 4 if tolerated; target dose: 300 mg/day given as 150 mg twice daily; maximum dose: 400 mg/day given as 200 mg twice daily
Smoking cessation: Initiate with 150 mg once daily for 3 days; increase to 150 mg twice daily; treatment should continue for 7-12 weeks
Elderly: Depression: 50-100 mg/day, increase by 50-100 mg every 3-4 days as tolerated; there is evidence that the elderly respond at 150 mg/day in divided doses, but some may require a higher dose

Dosing adjustment/comments in renal or hepatic impairment: Patients with renal or hepatic failure should receive a reduced dosage initially and be closely monitored

Mechanism of Action Antidepressant structurally different from all other previously marketed antidepressants; like other antidepressants the mechanism of bupropion's activity is not fully understood; weak blocker of serotonin and norepinephrine re-uptake, inhibits neuronal dopamine re-uptake and is **not** a monoamine oxidase A or B inhibitor

Other Adverse Effects

>10%:

Cardiovascular: Tachycardia

Central nervous system: Agitation, insomnia, headache, dizziness, sedation

Gastrointestinal: Nausea, vomiting, xerostomia, constipation

Neuromuscular & skeletal: Tremor

Ocular: Blurred vision

Respiratory: Rhinitis

Miscellaneous: Diaphoresis

1% to 10%:

Cardiovascular: Hypertension (2.5% alone, up to 6.1% in combination with nicotine patch), palpitations

Central nervous system: Anxiety, nervousness, confusion, hostility, abnormal dreams

Dermatologic: Rash, acne, dry skin

Endocrine & metabolic: Hyper- or hypoglycemia

Gastrointestinal: Anorexia, diarrhea, dyspepsia

Neuromuscular & skeletal: Arthralgia, myalgia

Otic: Tinnitus

Postintroduction adverse reactions: Arthralgia, myalgia, and fever with rash and other symptoms suggestive of delayed hypersensitivity resembling serum sickness reported

Hypertension (in some cases severe) requiring acute treatment has been reported in patients receiving bupropion alone and in combination with nicotine replacement therapy, orthostatic hypotension, third degree heart block, extrasystoles, myocardial infarction, phlebitis, pulmonary embolism

Contraindications Hypersensitivity to bupropion or any component of formulation; seizure disorder; current profile of bulimia or anorexia nervosa; concurrent administration of an MAO inhibitor

Warnings/Precautions Use of bupropion is associated with dose-dependent risk of seizures; therefore, doses of >300 mg/day should not be prescribed

Use caution in patients with cardiovascular disease, history of hypertension, or coronary artery disease; treatment-emergent hypertension (including some severe cases) has been reported, both with bupropion alone and in combination with nicotine transdermal systems.

Drug Interactions CYP2B6 enzyme substrate; CYP3A3/4 enzyme substrate (minor)

Increased Effect/Toxicity: Treatment-emergent hypertension may occur in patients treated with bupropion and nicotine patch. Cimetidine may inhibit the metabolism (increase clinical/adverse effects) of bupropion. Toxicity of bupropion is enhanced by levodopa and phenelzine (MAO inhibitors). Risk of seizures may be increased with agents that may lower seizure threshold (antipsychotics, antidepressants, theophylline, abrupt discontinuation of benzodiazepines, systemic steroids).

Decreased Effect: Carbamazepine, phenobarbital, and phenytoin may increase the metabolism (decrease clinical effect) of bupropion.

Drug Uptake

Onset of therapeutic effect: >2 weeks

Absorption: Rapidly absorbed from GI tract

Half-life, elimination: 14 hours

Time to peak: ~3 hours

Pregnancy Risk Factor B

Generic Available Yes: Wellbutrin® strength only

BuSpar® *see* BusPIRone *on page 189*

BusPIRone (byoo SPYE rone)

Related Information

Patients Requiring Sedation *on page 1400*

U.S. Brand Names BuSpar®

Canadian Brand Names Apo®-Buspirone; BuSpar®; Buspirex; Bustab®; Gen-Buspirone; Lin-Buspirone; Novo-Buspirone; Nu-Buspirone; PMS-Buspirone

Mexican Brand Names Neurosine

Pharmacologic Category Antianxiety Agent, Miscellaneous

Synonyms Buspirone Hydrochloride

Use Management of anxiety; has shown little potential for abuse

(Continued)

BusPIRone *(Continued)*

Unlabeled/Investigational: Panic attacks; management of aggression in mental retardation and secondary mental disorders; major depression; potential augmenting agent for antidepressants; premenstrual syndrome

Local Anesthetic/Vasoconstrictor Precautions No information available to require special precautions

Effects on Dental Treatment No effects or complications reported

Dosage Oral:

Generalized anxiety disorder:

Children and Adolescents: Initial: 5 mg daily; increase in increments of 5 mg/day at weekly intervals as needed, to a maximum dose of 60 mg/day divided into 2-3 doses

Adults: Oral: 15 mg/day (7.5 mg twice daily); may increase in increments of 5 mg/day every 2-4 days to a maximum of 60 mg/day; target dose for most people is 30 mg/day (15 mg twice daily)

Dosing adjustment in renal or hepatic impairment: Buspirone is metabolized by the liver and excreted by the kidneys. Patients with impaired hepatic or renal function demonstrated increased plasma concentrations and a prolonged half-life of buspirone. Therefore, use in patients with severe hepatic or renal impairment cannot be recommended.

Mechanism of Action Selectively antagonizes CNS serotonin 5-HT_1A receptors without affecting benzodiazepine-GABA receptors; may down-regulate postsynaptic 5-HT_2 receptors as do antidepressants

Other Adverse Effects

>10%: Central nervous system: Dizziness

1% to 10%:

Central nervous system: Drowsiness, EPS, serotonin syndrome, confusion, nervousness, lightheadedness, excitement, anger, hostility, headache

Dermatologic: Rash

Gastrointestinal: Diarrhea, nausea

Neuromuscular & skeletal: Muscle weakness, numbness, paresthesia, incoordination, tremor

Ocular: Blurred vision, tunnel vision

Miscellaneous: Diaphoresis, allergic reactions

Drug Interactions CYP3A3/4 enzyme substrate

Increased Effect/Toxicity: Concurrent use of buspirone with SSRIs or trazodone may cause serotonin syndrome. Erythromycin, clarithromycin, diltiazem, itraconazole, ketoconazole, or verapamil may result in increases in buspirone concentrations. Buspirone should not be used concurrently with an MAO inhibitor due to reports of increased BP; theoretically, a selective MAO type B inhibitors (selegiline) has a lower risk of this reaction.

Decreased Effect: Enzyme inducers (phenobarbital, carbamazepine, phenytoin, rifampin) may reduce serum concentration of buspirone resulting in loss of efficacy.

Drug Uptake

Half-life, elimination: 2-3 hours

Time to peak: Oral: 40-60 minutes

Pregnancy Risk Factor B

Generic Available Yes

Busulfan (byoo SUL fan)

U.S. Brand Names Busulfex®; Myleran®

Canadian Brand Names Busulfex®; Myleran®

Mexican Brand Names Myleran®

Pharmacologic Category Antineoplastic Agent, Alkylating Agent

Use

Oral: Chronic myelogenous leukemia and bone marrow disorders, such as polycythemia vera and myeloid metaplasia, conditioning regimens for bone marrow transplantation

I.V.: Combination therapy with cyclophosphamide as a conditioning regimen prior to allogeneic hematopoietic progenitor cell transplantation for chronic myelogenous leukemia

Local Anesthetic/Vasoconstrictor Precautions No information available to require special precautions

Effects on Dental Treatment No effects or complications reported

Mechanism of Action Reacts with N-7 position of guanosine and interferes with DNA replication and transcription of RNA. Busulfan has a more marked effect on myeloid cells (and is, therefore, useful in the treatment of CML) than on lymphoid cells. The drug is also very toxic to hematopoietic stem cells (thus its usefulness in high doses in BMT preparative regimens). Busulfan exhibits little immunosuppressive activity. Interferes with the normal function of DNA by alkylation and cross-linking the strands of DNA.

Other Adverse Effects

>10%:

Hematologic: Severe pancytopenia, leukopenia, thrombocytopenia, anemia, and bone marrow suppression are common and patients should be monitored closely while on therapy. Since this is a delayed effect (busulfan affects the stem cells), the drug should be discontinued temporarily at the first sign of a large or rapid fall in any blood element. Some patients may develop bone marrow fibrosis or chronic aplasia which is probably due to the busulfan toxicity. In large doses, busulfan is myeloablative and is used for this reason in BMT.

Myelosuppressive:
- WBC: Moderate
- Platelets: Moderate
- Onset: 7-10 days
- Nadir: 14-21 days
- Recovery 28 days

1% to 10%:

Dermatologic: Hyperpigmentation skin (busulfan tan), urticaria, erythema, alopecia

Endocrine & metabolic: Amenorrhea

Gastrointestinal: Nausea, vomiting, diarrhea; drug has little effect on the GI mucosal lining

Neuromuscular & skeletal: Weakness

Frequency not defined: Fertility/carcinogenesis: Sterility, ovarian suppression, amenorrhea, azoospermia, and testicular atrophy; malignant tumors have been reported in patients on busulfan therapy.

Drug Interactions CYP3A3/4 enzyme substrate. Itraconazole or other cytotoxic agents may increase risk of pulmonary toxicity.

Drug Uptake

Absorption: Rapid and complete from the GI tract
Duration: 28 days
Half-life, elimination: After first dose: 3.4 hours; After last dose: 2.3 hours
Time to peak: Oral: ≤4 hours; I.V.: ≤5 minutes

Pregnancy Risk Factor D

Generic Available No

Busulfex® *see* Busulfan *on page 190*

Butabarbital Sodium (byoo ta BAR bi tal)

U.S. Brand Names Butisol Sodium®

Pharmacologic Category Barbiturate

Use Sedative, hypnotic

Local Anesthetic/Vasoconstrictor Precautions No information available to require special precautions

Effects on Dental Treatment No effects or complications reported

Restrictions C-III

Dosage Oral:

Children: Preop: 2-6 mg/kg/dose; maximum: 100 mg

Adults:
- Sedative: 15-30 mg 3-4 times/day
- Hypnotic: 50-100 mg
- Preop: 50-100 mg 1-1½ hours before surgery

Mechanism of Action Interferes with transmission of impulses from the thalamus to the cortex of the brain resulting in an imbalance in central inhibitory and facilitatory mechanisms

Other Adverse Effects

>10%: Central nervous system: Dizziness, lightheadedness, drowsiness, "hang-over" effect

1% to 10%:

Central nervous system: Confusion, mental depression, unusual excitement, nervousness, faint feeling, headache, insomnia, nightmares

Gastrointestinal: Constipation, nausea, vomiting

Drug Interactions Barbiturates are cytochrome P450 enzyme inducers. Patients should be monitored when these drugs are started or stopped for a decreased or increased therapeutic effect respectively.

Increased Effect/Toxicity: When butabarbital is combined with other CNS depressants, narcotic analgesics, antidepressants, or benzodiazepines, additive respiratory and CNS depression may occur. Barbiturates may enhance the hepatotoxic potential of acetaminophen overdoses. Chloramphenicol, MAO inhibitors, valproic acid, and felbamate may inhibit barbiturate metabolism. Barbiturates may impair the absorption of griseofulvin, and may enhance the nephrotoxic effects of methoxyflurane.

Decreased Effect: Barbiturates such as butabarbital are hepatic enzyme inducers, and may increase the metabolism of antipsychotics, some beta-blockers (unlikely with atenolol and nadolol), calcium channel blockers, chloramphenicol, cimetidine, corticosteroids, cyclosporine, disopyramide, doxycycline, ethosuximide,

(Continued)

Butabarbital Sodium *(Continued)*

felbamate, furosemide, griseofulvin, lamotrigine, phenytoin, propafenone, quinidine, tacrolimus, TCAs, and theophylline. Barbiturates may increase the metabolism of estrogens and reduce the efficacy of oral contraceptives; an alternative method of contraception should be considered. Barbiturates inhibit the hypoprothrombinemic effects of oral anticoagulants via increased metabolism. Barbiturates may enhance the metabolism of methadone resulting in methadone withdrawal.

Drug Uptake

Half-life, elimination: 40-140 hours

Time to peak: Oral: 40-60 minutes

Pregnancy Risk Factor D

Generic Available Yes

Butalbital, Acetaminophen, and Caffeine

(byoo TAL bi tal, a seet a MIN oh fen, & KAF een)

U.S. Brand Names Esgic®; Esgic-Plus™; Fioricet®; Repan®

Pharmacologic Category Barbiturate

Synonyms Acetaminophen, Butalbital, and Caffeine

Use Relief of the symptomatic complex of tension or muscle contraction headache

Local Anesthetic/Vasoconstrictor Precautions No information available to require special precautions

Effects on Dental Treatment No effects or complications reported

Dosage Adults: Oral: 1-2 tablets or capsules every 4 hours; not to exceed 6/day

Other Adverse Effects

>10%:

- Central nervous system: Dizziness, lightheadedness, drowsiness
- Gastrointestinal: Nausea, heartburn, stomach pains, dyspepsia, epigastric discomfort

1% to 10%:

- Central nervous system: Confusion, mental depression, unusual excitement, nervousness, faint feeling, insomnia, nightmares, intoxicated feeling
- Dermatologic: Rash
- Gastrointestinal: Constipation, GI ulceration
- Hematologic: Hemolytic anemia
- Neuromuscular & skeletal: Weakness
- Respiratory: Troubled breathing
- Miscellaneous: Anaphylactic shock

Drug Interactions Also see Acetaminophen *on page 26*

Barbiturates are enzyme inducers. Patients should be monitored when these drugs are started or stopped for a decreased or increased therapeutic effect respectively.

Decreased effect: Butalbital compound may reduce the efficacy of beta-blockers, chloramphenicol, cimetidine, clozapine, corticosteroids, cyclosporine, disopyramide, doxycycline, ethosuximide, furosemide, griseofulvin, haloperidol, lamotrigine, methadone, nifedipine, oral contraceptives, phenothiazine, phenytoin, propafenone, quinidine, tacrolimus, TCAs, theophylline, warfarin, and verapamil

Increased toxicity when combined with other CNS depressants, benzodiazepine, valproic acid, chloramphenicol, or antidepressants; respiratory and CNS depression may be additive. MAO inhibitors may prolong the effect of butalbital compound

Pregnancy Risk Factor D

Generic Available Yes

Selected Readings

Botting RM, "Mechanism of Action of Acetaminophen: Is There a Cyclooxygenase 3?," *Clin Infect Dis*, 2000, Suppl 5:S202-10.

Dart RC, Kuffner EK, and Rumack BH, "Treatment of Pain or Fever with Paracetamol (Acetaminophen) in the Alcoholic Patient: A Systematic Review," *Am J Ther*, 2000, 7(2):123-34.

Grant JA and Weiler JM, "A Report of a Rare Immediate Reaction After Ingestion of Acetaminophen," *Ann Allergy Asthma Immunol*, 2001, 87(3):227-9.

Kwan D, Bartle WR, and Walker SE, "The Effects of Acetaminophen on Pharmacokinetics and Pharmacodynamics of Warfarin," *J Clin Pharmacol*, 1999, 39(1):68-75.

McClain CJ, Price S, Barve S, et al, "Acetaminophen Hepatotoxicity: An Update," *Curr Gastroenterol Rep*, 1999, 1(1):42-9.

Shek KL, Chan LN, and Nutescu E, "Warfarin-Acetaminophen Drug Interaction Revisited," *Pharmacotherapy*, 1999, 19(10):1153-8.

Tanaka E, Yamazaki K, and Misawa S, "Update: The Clinical Importance of Acetaminophen Hepatotoxicity in Nonalcoholic and Alcoholic Subjects," *J Clin Pharm Ther*, 2000, 25(5):325-32.

Butalbital, Acetaminophen, Caffeine, and Codeine

(byoo TAL bi tal, a seet a MIN oh fen, KAF een, & KOE deen)

U.S. Brand Names Fioricet® with Codeine

Pharmacologic Category Analgesic Combination (Narcotic); Barbiturate

Synonyms Acetaminophen, Caffeine, Codeine, and Butalbital; Caffeine, Acetaminophen, Butalbital, and Codeine; Codeine, Acetaminophen, Butalbital, and Caffeine

Use Relief of symptoms of complex tension (muscle contraction) headache

Local Anesthetic/Vasoconstrictor Precautions No information available to require special precautions

Effects on Dental Treatment No effects or complications reported

Restrictions C-III

Dosage Oral:

Adults: 1-2 capsules every 4 hours. Total daily dosage should not exceed 6 capsules.

Dosing adjustment/comments in hepatic impairment: Use with caution. Limited, low-dose therapy usually well tolerated in hepatic disease/cirrhosis. However, cases of hepatotoxicity at daily acetaminophen dosages <4 g/day have been reported. Avoid chronic use in hepatic impairment.

Mechanism of Action Combination product for the treatment of tension headache. Contains codeine (narcotic analgesic), butalbital (barbiturate), caffeine (CNS stimulant), and acetaminophen (nonopiate, nonsalicylate analgesic).

Other Adverse Effects Frequency not defined:

Cardiovascular: Tachycardia, palpitation, hypotension, edema, syncope

Central nervous system: Drowsiness, fatigue, mental confusion, disorientation, nervousness, hallucination, euphoria, depression, seizure, headache, agitation, fainting, excitement, fever

Dermatologic: Rash, erythema, pruritus, urticaria, erythema multiforme, exfoliative dermatitis, toxic epidermal necrolysis

Gastrointestinal: Nausea, xerostomia, constipation, gastrointestinal spasm, heartburn, flatulence

Genitourinary: Urinary retention, diuresis

Neuromuscular & skeletal: Leg pain, weakness, numbness

Otic: Tinnitus

Miscellaneous: Allergic reaction, anaphylaxis

Note: Potential reactions associated with components of Fioricet® with Codeine include agranulocytosis, irritability, nausea, thrombocytopenia, tremor, vomiting

Contraindications Hypersensitivity to butalbital, codeine, caffeine, acetaminophen, or any component of the formulation; porphyria; known G6PD deficiency; pregnancy (prolonged use or high doses at term)

Warnings/Precautions May cause severe hepatic toxicity on overdose; use with caution in patients with alcoholic liver disease; chronic daily dosing in adults of 5-8 g of acetaminophen over several weeks or 3-4 g/day of acetaminophen for 1 year have resulted in liver damage. Use with caution in patients with hypersensitivity reactions to other phenanthrene derivative opioid agonists (eg, morphine, hydrocodone, oxycodone). Use caution with Addison's disease, severe renal or hepatic impairment. Use caution in patients with head injury or other intracranial lesions, acute abdominal conditions, urethral stricture of BPH, or in patients with respiratory diseases. Elderly and/or debilitated patients may be more susceptible to CNS depressants, as well as constipating effects of narcotics. Tolerance or drug dependence may result from extended use. Safety and efficacy in pediatric patients have not been established.

Drug Interactions

Acetaminophen: CYP1A2 enzyme substrate (minor); CYP2E1 and 3A3/4 enzyme substrate

Codeine: CYP2D6 and 3A3/4 substrate; CYP2D6 enzyme inhibitor

See Butalbital Compound and Codeine *on page 194*

Dietary/Ethanol/Herb Considerations

Ethanol: Avoid use; may increase CNS depression.

Herb/Nutraceutical: Avoid gotu kola, kava, SAMe, St John's wort, and valerian; may increase CNS depression.

Pregnancy Risk Factor C (per manufacturer)/D (prolonged use or high doses at term)

Breast-feeding Considerations Codeine, caffeine, barbiturates, and acetaminophen are excreted in breast milk in small amounts. Discontinuation of breast-feeding or discontinuation of the drug should be considered.

Dosage Forms CAP: Butalbital 50 mg, caffeine 40 mg, acetaminophen 325 mg, and codeine phosphate 30 mg

Generic Available Yes

Selected Readings

Botting RM, "Mechanism of Action of Acetaminophen: Is There a Cyclooxygenase 3?," *Clin Infect Dis*, 2000, Suppl 5:S202-10.

Dart RC, Kuffner EK, and Rumack BH, "Treatment of Pain or Fever with Paracetamol (Acetaminophen) in the Alcoholic Patient: A Systematic Review," *Am J Ther*, 2000, 7(2):123-34.

Grant JA and Weiler JM, "A Report of a Rare Immediate Reaction After Ingestion of Acetaminophen," *Ann Allergy Asthma Immunol*, 2001, 87(3):227-9.

Kwan D, Bartle WR, and Walker SE, "The Effects of Acetaminophen on Pharmacokinetics and Pharmacodynamics of Warfarin," *J Clin Pharmacol*, 1999, 39(1):68-75.

McClain CJ, Price S, Barve S, et al, "Acetaminophen Hepatotoxicity: An Update," *Curr Gastroenterol Rep*, 1999, 1(1):42-9.

Shek KL, Chan LN, and Nutescu E, "Warfarin-Acetaminophen Drug Interaction Revisited," *Pharmacotherapy*, 1999, 19(10):1153-8.

Tanaka E, Yamazaki K, and Misawa S, "Update: The Clinical Importance of Acetaminophen Hepatotoxicity in Nonalcoholic and Alcoholic Subjects," *J Clin Pharm Ther*, 2000, 25(5):325-32.

Butalbital, Aspirin, and Caffeine

(byoo TAL bi tal, AS pir in, & KAF een)

U.S. Brand Names Fiorinal®

Pharmacologic Category Barbiturate

Synonyms Aspirin, Caffeine, and Butalbital; Butalbital Compound

Use Relief of the symptomatic complex of tension or muscle contraction headache

Local Anesthetic/Vasoconstrictor Precautions No information available to require special precautions

Effects on Dental Treatment Avoid aspirin products, if possible, for 1 week prior to surgery due to possibility of postoperative bleeding.

Restrictions C-III

Dosage Adults: Oral: 1-2 tablets or capsules every 4 hours; not to exceed 6/day

Other Adverse Effects

>10%:

Central nervous system: Dizziness, lightheadedness, drowsiness, "hangover" effect

Gastrointestinal: Heartburn, stomach pains, dyspepsia, epigastric discomfort, nausea

1% to 10%:

Central nervous system: Confusion, mental depression, unusual excitement, nervousness, faint feeling, headache, insomnia, nightmares, fatigue

Dermatologic: Skin rash

Gastrointestinal: Constipation, vomiting, gastrointestinal ulceration

Hematologic: Hemolytic anemia

Neuromuscular & skeletal: Weakness

Respiratory: Troubled breathing

Miscellaneous: Anaphylactic shock

Drug Interactions

Barbiturates are enzyme inducers. Patients should be monitored when these drugs are started or stopped for a decreased or increased therapeutic effect respectively.

Decreased effect: Butalbital compound may reduce the efficacy of beta-blockers, chloramphenicol, cimetidine, clozapine, corticosteroids, cyclosporine, disopyramide, doxycycline, ethosuximide, furosemide, griseofulvin, haloperidol, lamotrigine, methadone, nifedipine, oral contraceptives, phenothiazine, phenytoin, propafenone, quinidine, tacrolimus, TCAs, theophylline, warfarin, and verapamil

Increased toxicity when combined with other CNS depressants, benzodiazepine, valproic acid, chloramphenicol, or antidepressants; respiratory and CNS depression may be additive. MAO inhibitors may prolong the effect of butalbital compound

Pregnancy Risk Factor C/D (prolonged use or high doses at term)

Generic Available Yes

Butalbital, Aspirin, Caffeine, and Codeine

(byoo TAL bi tal, AS pir in, KAF een, & KOE deen)

U.S. Brand Names Fiorinal® With Codeine

Canadian Brand Names Fiorinal®-C 1/2; Fiorinal®-C 1/4; Tecnal C 1/2; Tecnal C 1/4

Pharmacologic Category Analgesic Combination (Narcotic); Barbiturate

Synonyms Codeine and Butalbital Compound; Codeine, Butalbital, Aspirin, and Caffeine

Use Mild to moderate pain when sedation is needed

Local Anesthetic/Vasoconstrictor Precautions No information available to require special precautions

Effects on Dental Treatment <1%: Xerostomia

Restrictions C-III

Dosage Adults: Oral: 1-2 capsules every 4 hours as needed for pain; up to 6/day

Other Adverse Effects

>10%:

Central nervous system: Dizziness, lightheadedness, drowsiness

Gastrointestinal: Nausea, heartburn, stomach pains, dyspepsia, epigastric discomfort

1% to 10%:

Central nervous system: Confusion, mental depression, unusual excitement, nervousness, faint feeling, insomnia, nightmares, intoxicated feeling

Dermatologic: Rash

Gastrointestinal: Constipation, GI ulceration

Warnings/Precautions Children and teenagers should not use for chickenpox or flu symptoms before a physician is consulted about Reye's syndrome

Drug Interactions

Increased Effect/Toxicity: MAO inhibitors may enhance the CNS effects of butalbital. In patients receiving concomitant corticosteroids during the chronic use of ASA, withdrawal of corticosteroids may result in salicylism. Butalbital compound and codeine may enhance effects of oral anticoagulants. Increased effect with oral antidiabetic agents and insulin, 6-mercaptopurine and methotrexate, NSAIDs, other narcotic analgesics, alcohol, general anesthetics, tranquilizers such as chlordiazepoxide, sedative hypnotics, or other CNS depressants.

Decreased Effect: Aspirin, butalbital, caffeine, and codeine may diminish effects of uricosuric agents such as probenecid and sulfinpyrazone.

Pregnancy Risk Factor C/D (prolonged use or high doses at term)

Generic Available Yes

Comments Abrupt discontinuation after sustained use (generally >10 days) may cause withdrawal symptoms

Butenafine (byoo TEN a fine)

U.S. Brand Names Lotrimin® Ultra™ [OTC]; Mentax®

Pharmacologic Category Antifungal Agent, Topical

Synonyms Butenafine Hydrochloride

Use Topical treatment of tinea pedis (athlete's foot), tinea cruris (jock itch), tinea corporis (ringworm), and tinea versicolor

Local Anesthetic/Vasoconstrictor Precautions No information available to require special precautions

Effects on Dental Treatment No effects or complications reported

Dosage Children >12 years and Adults: Topical:

Tinea corporis, tinea cruris, or tinea versicolor: Apply once daily for 2 weeks to affected area and surrounding skin

Tinea pedis: Apply once daily for 4 weeks or twice daily for 7 days to affected area and surrounding skin (7-day regimen may have lower efficacy)

Mechanism of Action Exerts antifungal activity by blocking squalene epoxidation, resulting in inhibition of ergosterol synthesis (antidermatophyte and *Sporothrix schenckii* activity); in higher concentrations, the drug disrupts fungal cell membranes (anticandidal activity)

Other Adverse Effects >1%: Dermatologic: Burning, stinging, irritation, erythema, pruritus (2%)

Drug Uptake

Absorption: Minimal systemic absorption when topically applied

Half-life, elimination: 35 hours

Time to peak: 6 hours (10 ng/mL)

Pregnancy Risk Factor B

Generic Available No

Butisol Sodium® *see* Butabarbital Sodium *on page 191*

Butoconazole (byoo toe KOE na zole)

U.S. Brand Names Gynazole-1™; Mycelex®-3 [OTC]

Canadian Brand Names Femstat® One

Mexican Brand Names Femstal®

Pharmacologic Category Antifungal Agent, Vaginal

Synonyms Butoconazole Nitrate

Use Local treatment of vulvovaginal candidiasis

Local Anesthetic/Vasoconstrictor Precautions No information available to require special precautions

Effects on Dental Treatment No effects or complications reported

Dosage Adults:

Femstat®-3 [OTC]: Insert 1 applicatorful (~5 g) intravaginally at bedtime for 3 consecutive days

Gynazole-1™: Insert 1 applicatorful (~5 g) intravaginally as a single dose; treatment may need to be extended for up to 6 days in pregnant women (use in pregnancy during 2nd or 3rd trimester only)

Mechanism of Action Increases cell membrane permeability in susceptible fungi (*Candida*)

Other Adverse Effects Frequency not defined:

Gastrointestinal: Abdominal pain or cramping

Genitourinary: Pelvic pain; vulvar/vaginal burning, itching, soreness, and swelling

Drug Uptake

Absorption: 2%

Time to peak: 12-24 hours

Pregnancy Risk Factor C (use only in 2nd or 3rd trimester)

Generic Available No

Butorphanol (byoo TOR fa nole)

U.S. Brand Names Stadol®; Stadol® NS

Canadian Brand Names Stadol NS™

Pharmacologic Category Analgesic, Narcotic

Synonyms Butorphanol Tartrate

Use

Nasal spray: Management of moderate to severe pain, including migraine headache pain

(Continued)

Butorphanol *(Continued)*

Parenteral: Management of moderate to severe pain; preoperative medication; supplement to balanced anesthesia; management of pain during labor

Local Anesthetic/Vasoconstrictor Precautions No information available to require special precautions

Effects on Dental Treatment No effects or complications reported

Restrictions C-IV

Dosage Adults:

Nasal spray:

Moderate to severe pain (including migraine headache pain): Initial: 1 spray (~1 mg per spray) in 1 nostril; if adequate pain relief is not achieved within 60-90 minutes, an additional 1 spray in 1 nostril may be given; may repeat initial dose sequence in 3-4 hours after the last dose as needed

Alternatively, an initial dose of 2 mg (1 spray in each nostril) may be used in patients who will be able to remain recumbent (in the event drowsiness or dizziness occurs); additional 2 mg doses should not be given for 3-4 hours

Note: In some clinical trials, an initial dose of 2 mg (as 2 doses 1 hour apart or 2 mg initially - 1 spray in each nostril) has been used, followed by 1 mg in 1 hour; side effects were greater at these dosages

Parenteral:

Moderate to severe pain:

I.M. Initial: 2 mg, may repeat every 3-4 hours as needed

I.V.: Initial: 1 mg, may repeat every 3-4 hours as needed

Preoperative medication: I.M.: 2 mg 60-90 minutes before surgery

Supplement to balanced anesthesia: I.V.: 2 mg shortly before induction and/or an incremental dose of 0.5-1 mg (up to 0.06 mg/kg), depending on previously administered sedative, analgesic, and hypnotic medications

Pain during labor (fetus >37 weeks gestation and no signs of fetal distress):

I.M., I.V.: 1-2 mg; may repeat in 4 hours

Note: Alternative analgesia should be used for pain associated with delivery or if delivery is anticipated within 4 hours

Dosage adjustment in renal impairment:

I.M., I.V.: Initial dosage should generally be $1/2$ of the recommended dose; repeated dosing must be based on initial response rather than fixed intervals, but generally should be at least 6 hours apart

Nasal spray: Initial dose should not exceed 1 mg; a second dose may be given after 90-120 minutes

Dosage adjustment in hepatic impairment:

I.M., I.V.: Initial dosage should generally be $1/2$ of the recommended dose; repeated dosing must be based on initial response rather than fixed intervals, but generally should be at least 6 hours apart

Nasal spray: Initial dose should not exceed 1 mg; a second dose may be given after 90-120 minutes

Elderly:

I.M., I.V.: Initial dosage should generally be $1/2$ of the recommended dose; repeated dosing must be based on initial response rather than fixed intervals, but generally should be at least 6 hours apart

Nasal Spray: Initial dose should not exceed 1 mg; a second dose may be given after 90-120 minutes

Mechanism of Action Mixed narcotic agonist-antagonist with central analgesic actions; binds to opiate receptors in the CNS, causing inhibition of ascending pain pathways, altering the perception of and response to pain; produces generalized CNS depression

Other Adverse Effects

>10%:

Central nervous system: Drowsiness (43%), dizziness (19%), insomnia (Stadol® NS)

Gastrointestinal: Nausea/vomiting (13%)

Respiratory: Nasal congestion (Stadol® NS)

1% to 10%:

Cardiovascular: Vasodilation, palpitations

Central nervous system: Lightheadedness, headache, lethargy, anxiety, confusion, euphoria, somnolence

Dermatologic: Pruritus

Gastrointestinal: Anorexia, constipation, xerostomia, stomach pain, unpleasant aftertaste

Neuromuscular & skeletal: Tremor, paresthesia, weakness

Ocular: Blurred vision

Otic: Ear pain, tinnitus

Respiratory: Bronchitis, cough, dyspnea, epistaxis, nasal irritation, pharyngitis, rhinitis, sinus congestion, sinusitis, upper respiratory infection

Miscellaneous: Diaphoresis (increased)

Drug Interactions Increased toxicity with CNS depressants, phenothiazines, barbiturates, skeletal muscle relaxants, alfentanil, guanabenz, and MAO inhibitors

Drug Uptake

Onset of action: I.M.: 5-10 minutes; I.V.: <10 minutes; Nasal: ~15 minutes

Peak Effect: I.M.: 0.5-1 hour; I.V.: 4-5 minutes

Absorption: Rapid and well

Duration: I.M., I.V.: 3-4 hours; Nasal: 4-5 hours

Half-life, elimination: 2.5-4 hours

Pregnancy Risk Factor C/D (prolonged use or high doses at term)

Generic Available Yes: Injection

Byclomine® *see* Dicyclomine *on page 382*

Bydramine® Cough Syrup [OTC] *see* DiphenhydrAMINE *on page 398*

C-500-GR™ [OTC] *see* Ascorbic Acid *on page 117*

Cabergoline (ca BER go leen)

U.S. Brand Names Dostinex®

Pharmacologic Category Ergot Derivative

Use Treatment of hyperprolactinemia

Adjunct for the treatment of Parkinson's disease

Local Anesthetic/Vasoconstrictor Precautions No information available to require special precautions

Effects on Dental Treatment No effects or complications reported

Dosage Adults: Oral: 0.25 mg twice a week; dosage may be increased by 0.25 mg twice weekly to a dose of up to 1 mg twice a week (according to the patient's prolactin level)

Mechanism of Action A long-acting dopamine receptor agonist with a high affinity for D_2 receptors; prolactin secretion by the anterior pituitary is predominantly under hypothalamic inhibitory control exerted through the release of dopamine

Other Adverse Effects

>10%:

Central nervous system: Headache (26%), dizziness (17%)

Gastrointestinal: Nausea (29%)

1% to 10%:

Body as whole: Asthenia (6%), fatigue (5%), syncope (1%), influenza-like symptoms (1%), malaise (1%), periorbital edema (1%), peripheral edema (1%)

Cardiovascular: Hot flashes (3%), hypotension (1%), dependent edema (1%), palpitations (1%)

Central nervous system: Vertigo (4%), depression (3%), somnolence (2%), anxiety (1%), insomnia (1%), impaired concentration (1%), nervousness (1%)

Dermatologic: Acne (1%), pruritus (1%)

Endocrine: Breast pain (2%), dysmenorrhea (1%)

Gastrointestinal: Constipation (7%), abdominal pain (5%), dyspepsia (5%), vomiting (4%), xerostomia (2%), diarrhea (2%), flatulence (2%), throat irritation (1%), toothache (1%), anorexia (1%)

Neuromuscular & skeletal: Pain (2%), arthralgia (1%), paresthesias (2%)

Ocular: Abnormal vision (1%)

Respiratory: Rhinitis (1%)

Drug Interactions

Increased Effect/Toxicity: Additive hypotensive effects may occur when cabergoline is administered with antihypertensive medications; dosage adjustment of the antihypertensive medication may be required.

Decreased Effect: Dopamine antagonists (eg, phenothiazines, butyrophenones, thioxanthenes, or metoclopramide) may reduce the therapeutic effects of cabergoline and should not be used concomitantly.

Drug Uptake

Half-life, elimination: 63-69 hours

Time to peak: 2-3 hours

Pregnancy Risk Factor B

Generic Available No

Cafergot® *see* Ergotamine *on page 448*

Caffeine and Sodium Benzoate

(KAF een & SOW dee um BEN zoe ate)

Pharmacologic Category Diuretic, Miscellaneous

Synonyms Sodium Benzoate and Caffeine

Use Emergency stimulant in acute circulatory failure; as a diuretic; and to relieve spinal puncture headache

Local Anesthetic/Vasoconstrictor Precautions No information available to require special precautions

Effects on Dental Treatment No effects or complications reported

Dosage

Adults:

Stimulant/diuretic: I.M., I.V.: 500 mg, maximum single dose: 1 g

(Continued)

Caffeine and Sodium Benzoate *(Continued)*

Spinal puncture headaches:

I.V.: 500 mg in 1000 mL NS infused over 1 hour, followed by 1000 mL NS infused over 1 hour; a second course of caffeine can be given for unrelieved headache pain in 4 hours.

Oral: 300 mg

Children: Stimulant: I.M., I.V., S.C.: 8 mg/kg every 4 hours as needed

Other Adverse Effects 1% to 10%:

Cardiovascular: Tachycardia, extrasystoles, palpitations

Central nervous system: Insomnia, restlessness, nervousness, mild delirium, headache, anxiety

Gastrointestinal: Nausea, vomiting, gastric irritation

Neuromuscular & skeletal: Muscle tension following abrupt cessation of drug after regular consumption of 500-600 mg/day

Renal: Diuresis

Pregnancy Risk Factor C

Generic Available Yes

Calan® *see* Verapamil *on page 1236*

Calan® SR *see* Verapamil *on page 1236*

Calbon® *see* Calcium Lactate *on page 206*

Cal Carb-HD® [OTC] *see* Calcium Carbonate *on page 201*

Calcibind® *see* Cellulose Sodium Phosphate *on page 250*

Calci-Chew™ [OTC] *see* Calcium Carbonate *on page 201*

Calciday-667® [OTC] *see* Calcium Carbonate *on page 201*

Calcifediol (kal si fe DYE ole)

U.S. Brand Names Calderol®

Canadian Brand Names Calderol®

Pharmacologic Category Vitamin D Analog

Synonyms 25-HCC; 25-Hydroxycholecalciferol; 25-Hydroxyvitamin D_3

Use Treatment and management of metabolic bone disease associated with chronic renal failure or hypocalcemia in patients on chronic renal dialysis

Local Anesthetic/Vasoconstrictor Precautions No information available to require special precautions

Effects on Dental Treatment No effects or complications reported

Dosage Children and Adults: Hepatic osteodystrophy: Oral: 20-100 mcg/day or every other day; titrate to obtain normal serum calcium/phosphate levels; increase dose at 4-week intervals

Mechanism of Action Vitamin D analog that (along with calcitonin and parathyroid hormone) regulates serum calcium homeostasis by promoting absorption of calcium and phosphorus in the small intestine; promotes renal tubule resorption of phosphate; increases rate of accretion and resorption in bone minerals

Other Adverse Effects Frequency not defined:

Cardiovascular: Hypotension, cardiac arrhythmias, hypertension

Central nervous system: Irritability, headache, somnolence, seizures (rare)

Dermatologic: Pruritus,

Endocrine & metabolic: Hypercalcemia, polydipsia, hypermagnesemia

Gastrointestinal: Nausea, vomiting, constipation, anorexia, pancreatitis, metallic taste, xerostomia

Hepatic: Elevated LFTs

Neuromuscular & skeletal: Myalgia, bone pain,

Ocular: Conjunctivitis, photophobia

Renal: Polyuria

Drug Interactions

Increased Effect/Toxicity: The effect of calcifediol is increased with thiazide diuretics. Additive effect with antacids (magnesium).

Decreased Effect: The effect of calcifediol is decreased when taken with cholestyramine or colestipol.

Drug Uptake

Absorption: Rapid from the small intestines

Half-life, elimination: 12-22 days

Time to peak: Oral: ≤4 hours

Pregnancy Risk Factor C (manufacturer); A/D (dose exceeding RDA recommendation) (expert analysis)

Generic Available No

Calciferol™ *see* Ergocalciferol *on page 446*

Calcijex™ *see* Calcitriol *on page 199*

Calcimar® *see* Calcitonin *on page 199*

Calci-Mix™ [OTC] *see* Calcium Carbonate *on page 201*

Calcipotriene (kal si POE try een)

U.S. Brand Names Dovonex®

Pharmacologic Category Topical Skin Product; Vitamin D Analog

Use Treatment of moderate plaque psoriasis

Local Anesthetic/Vasoconstrictor Precautions No information available to require special precautions

Effects on Dental Treatment No effects or complications reported

Dosage Adults: Topical: Apply in a thin film to the affected skin twice daily and rub in gently and completely

Mechanism of Action Synthetic vitamin D_3 analog which regulates skin cell production and proliferation

Other Adverse Effects

>10%: Dermatologic: Burning, itching, skin irritation, erythema, dry skin, peeling, rash, worsening of psoriasis

1% to 10%: Dermatologic: Dermatitis

Pregnancy Risk Factor C

Generic Available No

Calcitonin (kal si TOE nin)

U.S. Brand Names Calcimar®; Miacalcin®

Canadian Brand Names Calcimar®; Caltine®; Miacalcin® NS

Mexican Brand Names Miacalcic®; Oseum®; Tonocalcin®

Pharmacologic Category Antidote

Synonyms Calcitonin (Salmon)

Use

Calcitonin (human): Treatment of Paget's disease of bone

Calcitonin (salmon): Treatment of Paget's disease of bone and as adjunctive therapy for hypercalcemia; also used in postmenopausal osteoporosis

Local Anesthetic/Vasoconstrictor Precautions No information available to require special precautions

Effects on Dental Treatment No effects or complications reported

Dosage

Children: Dosage not established

Adults:

Paget's disease:

Salmon calcitonin: I.M., S.C.: 100 units/day to start, 50 units/day or 50-100 units every 1-3 days maintenance dose; Intranasal: 200-400 units (1-2 sprays)/day

Human calcitonin: S.C.: Initial: 0.5 mg/day (maximum: 0.5 mg twice daily); maintenance: 0.5 mg 2-3 times/week or 0.25 mg/day

Hypercalcemia: Initial: Salmon calcitonin: I.M., S.C.: 4 units/kg every 12 hours; may increase up to 8 units/kg every 12 hours to a maximum of every 6 hours

Osteogenesis imperfecta: Salmon calcitonin: I.M., S.C.: 2 units/kg 3 times/week

Postmenopausal osteoporosis: Salmon calcitonin:

I.M., S.C.: 100 units/day

Intranasal: 200 units (1 spray)/day

Mechanism of Action Structurally similar to human calcitonin; it directly inhibits osteoclastic bone resorption; promotes the renal excretion of calcium, phosphate, sodium, magnesium and potassium by decreasing tubular reabsorption; increases the jejunal secretion of water, sodium, potassium, and chloride

Other Adverse Effects

>10%:

Cardiovascular: Facial flushing

Gastrointestinal: Nausea, diarrhea, anorexia

Local: Edema at injection site

1% to 10%:

Genitourinary: Polyuria

Neuromuscular & skeletal: Back/joint pain

Respiratory: Nasal bleeding/crusting (following intranasal administration)

Drug Interactions Plicamycin may enhance hypocalcemic effect.

Drug Uptake

Hypercalcemia:

Onset of action: ~2 hours

Duration: 6-8 hours

Half-life, elimination: S.C.: 1.2 hours

Pregnancy Risk Factor C

Generic Available No

Cal-Citrate® 250 [OTC] *see* Calcium Citrate *on page 203*

Calcitriol (kal si TRYE ole)

U.S. Brand Names Calcijex™; Rocaltrol®

Canadian Brand Names Rocaltrol®

Mexican Brand Names Rocaltrol®; Tirocal®

(Continued)

Calcitriol *(Continued)*

Pharmacologic Category Vitamin D Analog

Synonyms 1,25 Dihydroxycholecalciferol

Use Management of hypocalcemia in patients on chronic renal dialysis; reduce elevated parathyroid hormone levels; decrease severity of psoriatic lesions in psoriatic vulgaris; oral solution is indicated for the management of secondary hyperparathyroidism and resultant metabolic bone disease in predialysis (moderate to severe chronic renal failure) patients (adults, neonates, and older infants).

Unlabeled/Investigational: Vitamin D resistant rickets

Local Anesthetic/Vasoconstrictor Precautions No information available to require special precautions

Effects on Dental Treatment No effects or complications reported

Dosage Individualize dosage to maintain calcium levels of 9-10 mg/dL

Renal failure:

Oral:

Children: Initial: 15 ng/kg/day; maintenance: 5-40 ng/kg/day

Adults: 0.25 mcg/day or every other day (may require 0.5-1 mcg/day)

I.V.: Adults: 0.5 mcg (0.01 mcg/kg) 3 times/week; most doses in the range of 0.5-3 mcg (0.01-0.05 mcg/kg) 3 times/week

Hypoparathyroidism/pseudohypoparathyroidism: Oral:

Children:

<1 year: 0.04-0.08 mcg/kg/day

1-6 years: Initial: 0.25 mcg/day, increase at 2- to 4-week intervals

Children >6 years and Adults: 0.5-2 mcg/day

Vitamin D-resistant rickets (familial hypophosphatemia): Oral: 2 mcg/day; initial: 15-20 ng/kg/day; maintenance: 30-60 ng/kg/day

Mechanism of Action Promotes absorption of calcium in the intestines and retention at the kidneys thereby increasing calcium levels in the serum; decreases excessive serum phosphatase levels, parathyroid hormone levels, and decreases bone resorption; increases renal tubule phosphate resorption

Other Adverse Effects

>10%: Endocrine & metabolic: Hypercalcemia (33%)

Frequency not defined:

Cardiovascular: Cardiac arrhythmias, hypertension, hypotension

Central nervous system: Headache, irritability, seizures (rare), somnolence

Dermatologic: Pruritus

Endocrine & metabolic: Hypermagnesemia, polydipsia

Gastrointestinal: Anorexia, constipation, metallic taste, nausea, pancreatitis, vomiting, xerostomia

Hepatic: Elevated LFTs

Neuromuscular & skeletal: Bone pain, myalgia

Ocular: Conjunctivitis, photophobia

Renal: Polyuria

Drug Interactions

Increased Effect/Toxicity: Risk of hypercalcemia with thiazide diuretics. Risk of hypermagnesemia with magnesium-containing antacids.

Decreased Effect: Cholestyramine and colestipol decrease absorption/effect of calcitriol.

Drug Uptake

Onset of action: ~2-6 hours

Absorption: Oral: Rapid

Duration: 3-5 days

Half-life, elimination: 3-8 hours

Pregnancy Risk Factor C (manufacturer); A/D (dose exceeding RDA recommendation) (expert analysis)

Generic Available Yes

Calcium Acetate (KAL see um AS e tate)

U.S. Brand Names PhosLo®

Pharmacologic Category Antidote; Calcium Salt; Electrolyte Supplement, Parenteral

Use Calcium acetate binds phosphorus in the GI tract better than other calcium salts due to its lower solubility and subsequent reduced absorption and increased formation of calcium phosphate; calcium acetate does not promote aluminum absorption

Oral: Control of hyperphosphatemia in end-stage renal failure; does not promote aluminum absorption

I.V.: Calcium supplementation in parenteral nutrition therapy

Local Anesthetic/Vasoconstrictor Precautions No information available to require special precautions

Effects on Dental Treatment No effects or complications reported

Dosage Adults: Oral: 2 tablets with each meal; dosage may be increased to bring serum phosphate value to <6 mg/dL; most patients require 3-4 tablets with each meal

Mechanism of Action Moderates nerve and muscle performance via action potential excitation threshold regulation; combines with dietary phosphate to form insoluble calcium phosphate which is excreted in feces

Other Adverse Effects Frequency not defined:

Mild hypercalcemia (calcium: >10.5 mg/dL to ≤12 mg/dL) may be asymptomatic or manifest itself as constipation, anorexia, nausea, and vomiting

More severe hypercalcemia (calcium: >12 mg/dL) is associated with confusion, delirium, stupor, and coma

Drug Interactions

Increased Effect/Toxicity: High doses of calcium with thiazide diuretics may result in milk-alkali syndrome and hypercalcemia; monitor response. Calcium salts may decrease T_4 absorption; separate dose from levothyroxine by at least 4 hours. Calcium acetate may potentiate digoxin toxicity.

Decreased Effect: Absorption of tetracycline, atenolol (and potentially other beta-blockers), iron, quinolone antibiotics, alendronate, sodium fluoride, and zinc absorption may be significantly decreased; space administration times. Effects of calcium channel blockers (eg, verapamil) effects may be diminished. Polystyrene sulfonate's potassium-binding ability may be reduced; avoid concurrent administration.

Drug Uptake Absorption: Requires vitamin D; minimal unless chronic, high doses are given; calcium is absorbed in soluble, ionized form; solubility of calcium is increased in an acid environment

Pregnancy Risk Factor C

Generic Available No

Calcium Carbonate (KAL see um KAR bun ate)

Related Information

Calcium Carbonate and Magnesium Carbonate *on page 202*

U.S. Brand Names Alka-Mints® [OTC]; Amitone® [OTC]; Cal Carb-HD® [OTC]; Calci-Chew™ [OTC]; Calciday-667® [OTC]; Calci-Mix™ [OTC]; Cal-Plus® [OTC]; Caltrate® 600 [OTC]; Caltrate, Jr.® [OTC]; Chooz® [OTC]; Dicarbosil® [OTC]; Equilet® [OTC]; Florical® [OTC]; Gencalc® 600 [OTC]; Mallamint® [OTC]; Nephro-Calci® [OTC]; Os-Cal® 500 [OTC]; Oyst-Cal 500 [OTC]; Oystercal® 500; Rolaids® Calcium Rich [OTC]; Tums® [OTC]; Tums® E-X Extra Strength Tablet [OTC]; Tums® Ultra [OTC]

Canadian Brand Names Apo®-Cal; Calcite-500; Caltrate®; Os-Cal®

Mexican Brand Names Calsan®; Caltrate®; Osteomin®

Pharmacologic Category Antacid; Antidote; Calcium Salt; Electrolyte Supplement, Oral

Use Adjunct in prevention of postmenopausal osteoporosis, antacid, treatment and prevention of calcium depletion (osteoporosis, osteomalacia, etc); control of hyperphosphatemia in end-stage renal disease; has been known to bind phosphate

Local Anesthetic/Vasoconstrictor Precautions No information available to require special precautions

Effects on Dental Treatment No effects or complications reported

Dosage Oral (dosage is in terms of elemental calcium):

Dietary Reference Intake:

- 0-6 months: 210 mg/day
- 7-12 months: 270 mg/day
- 1-3 years: 500 mg/day
- 4-8 years: 800 mg/day
- Adults, Male/Female:
  - 9-18 years: 1300 mg/day
  - 19-50 years: 1000 mg/day
  - ≥51 years: 1200 mg/day
- Female: Pregnancy: Same as for Adults, Male/Female
- Female: Lactating: Same as for Adults, Male/Female

Hypocalcemia (dose depends on clinical condition and serum calcium level): Dose expressed in mg of **elemental calcium**

- Neonates: 50-150 mg/kg/day in 4-6 divided doses; not to exceed 1 g/day
- Children: 45-65 mg/kg/day in 4 divided doses
- Adults: 1-2 g or more/day in 3-4 divided doses

Adults:

- Dietary supplementation: 500 mg to 2 g divided 2-4 times/day
- Antacid: Dosage based on acid-neutralizing capacity of specific product; generally, 1-2 tablets or 5-10 mL every 2 hours; maximum: 7000 mg calcium carbonate per 24 hours; specific product labeling should be consulted

Adults >51 years of age: Osteoporosis: 1200 mg/day

Dosing adjustment in renal impairment: Cl_{cr} <25 mL/minute: Dosage adjustments may be necessary depending on the serum calcium levels

Mechanism of Action As dietary supplement, used to prevent or treat negative calcium balance; in osteoporosis, it helps to prevent or decrease the rate of bone loss. The calcium in calcium salts moderates nerve and muscle performance and allows normal cardiac function. Also used to treat hyperphosphatemia in patients with advanced renal insufficiency by combining with dietary phosphate to form

(Continued)

Calcium Carbonate *(Continued)*

insoluble calcium phosphate, which is excreted in feces. Calcium salts as antacids neutralize gastric acidity resulting in increased gastric an duodenal bulb pH; they additionally inhibit proteolytic activity of peptic if the pH is increased >4 and increase lower esophageal sphincter tone.

Other Adverse Effects Well tolerated; 1% to 10%:

Central nervous system: Headache

Endocrine & metabolic: Hypophosphatemia, hypercalcemia

Gastrointestinal: Constipation, laxative effect, acid rebound, nausea, vomiting, anorexia, abdominal pain, xerostomia, flatulence

Miscellaneous: Milk alkali syndrome with very high, chronic dosing and/or renal failure (headache, nausea, irritability, and weakness or alkalosis, hypercalcemia, renal impairment)

Drug Interactions

Increased Effect/Toxicity: High doses of calcium with thiazide diuretics may result in milk-alkali syndrome and hypercalcemia; monitor response. Calcium salts may decrease T_4 absorption; separate dose from levothyroxine by at least 4 hours. Calcium acetate may potentiate digoxin toxicity.

Decreased Effect: Absorption of tetracycline, atenolol (and potentially other beta-blockers), iron, quinolone antibiotics, alendronate, sodium fluoride, and zinc absorption may be significantly decreased; space administration times. Effects of calcium channel blockers (eg, verapamil) effects may be diminished. Polystyrene sulfonate's potassium-binding ability may be reduced; avoid concurrent administration.

Drug Uptake Absorption: Requires vitamin D; minimal unless chronic, high doses are given; calcium is absorbed in soluble, ionized form; solubility of calcium is increased in an acid environment

Pregnancy Risk Factor C

Generic Available Yes

Calcium Carbonate and Magnesium Carbonate

(KAL see um KAR bun ate & mag NEE zhum KAR bun ate)

Pharmacologic Category Antacid

Use Hyperacidity

Local Anesthetic/Vasoconstrictor Precautions No information available to require special precautions

Effects on Dental Treatment Do not give tetracyclines concomitantly.

Calcium Carbonate and Simethicone

(KAL see um KAR bun ate & sye METH i kone)

U.S. Brand Names Titralac® Plus Liquid [OTC]

Pharmacologic Category Antacid; Antiflatulent

Synonyms Simethicone and Calcium Carbonate

Use Relief of acid indigestion, heartburn, peptic esophagitis, hiatal hernia, and gas

Local Anesthetic/Vasoconstrictor Precautions No information available to require special precautions

Effects on Dental Treatment Do not give tetracyclines concomitantly.

Dosage Oral: 0.5-2 g 4-6 times/day

Drug Uptake See Calcium Carbonate *on page 201* and Simethicone *on page 1088*

Pregnancy Risk Factor C

Generic Available Yes

Calcium Chloride (KAL see um KLOR ide)

Pharmacologic Category Calcium Salt; Electrolyte Supplement, Parenteral

Use Cardiac resuscitation when epinephrine fails to improve myocardial contractions, cardiac disturbances of hyperkalemia, hypocalcemia, or calcium channel blocking agent toxicity; emergent treatment of hypocalcemic tetany, treatment of hypermagnesemia

Local Anesthetic/Vasoconstrictor Precautions No information available to require special precautions

Effects on Dental Treatment No effects or complications reported

Dosage Note: Calcium chloride is 3 times as potent as calcium gluconate

Cardiac arrest in the presence of hyperkalemia or hypocalcemia, magnesium toxicity, or calcium antagonist toxicity: I.V.:

- Infants and Children: 20 mg/kg; may repeat in 10 minutes if necessary
- Adults: 2-4 mg/kg (10% solution), repeated every 10 minutes if necessary

Hypocalcemia: I.V.:

- Children (manufacturer's recommendation): 2.7-5 mg/kg/dose every 4-6 hours
- Alternative pediatric dosing: Infants and Children: 10-20 mg/kg/dose (infants <1 mEq; children 1-7 mEq), repeat every 4-6 hours if needed
- Adults: 500 mg to 1 g (7-14 mEq)/dose repeated every 4-6 hours if needed

Hypocalcemic tetany: I.V.:

Infants and Children: 10 mg/kg (0.5-0.7 mEq/kg) over 5-10 minutes; may repeat after 6-8 hours or follow with an infusion with a maximum dose of 200 mg/kg/day

Adults: 1 g over 10-30 minutes; may repeat after 6 hours

Hypocalcemia secondary to citrated blood transfusion: I.V.:

Neonates, Infants, and Children: Give 0.45 mEq **elemental** calcium for each 100 mL citrated blood infused

Adults: 1.35 mEq calcium with each 100 mL of citrated blood infused

Dosing adjustment in renal impairment: Cl_{cr} <25 mL/minute: Dosage adjustments may be necessary depending on the serum calcium levels

Mechanism of Action Moderates nerve and muscle performance via action potential excitation threshold regulation

Drug Interactions

Increased Effect/Toxicity: High doses of calcium with thiazide diuretics may result in milk-alkali syndrome and hypercalcemia; monitor response. Calcium may potentiate digoxin toxicity.

Decreased Effect: Effects of calcium channel blockers (eg, verapamil) effects may be diminished.

Drug Uptake Absorption: I.V. calcium salts are absorbed directly into the bloodstream

Pregnancy Risk Factor C

Generic Available Yes

Calcium Citrate (KAL see um SIT rate)

U.S. Brand Names Cal-Citrate® 250 [OTC]; Citracal® [OTC]

Pharmacologic Category Calcium Salt

Use Adjunct in prevention of postmenopausal osteoporosis; treatment and prevention of calcium depletion

Local Anesthetic/Vasoconstrictor Precautions No information available to require special precautions

Effects on Dental Treatment No effects or complications reported

Dosage Oral: Dosage is in terms of elemental calcium

Dietary Reference Intake:

0-6 months: 210 mg/day
7-12 months: 270 mg/day
1-3 years: 500 mg/day
4-8 years: 800 mg/day
Adults, Male/Female:
9-18 years: 1300 mg/day
19-50 years: 1000 mg/day
≥51 years: 1200 mg/day
Female: Pregnancy: Same as for Adults, Male/Female
Female: Lactating: Same as for Adults, Male/Female

Dietary supplement: Usual dose: 500 mg to 2 g 2-4 times/day

Mechanism of Action Moderates nerve and muscle performance via action potential excitation threshold regulation

Other Adverse Effects Frequency not defined:

Mild hypercalcemia (calcium: >10.5 mg/dL) may be asymptomatic or manifest itself as constipation, anorexia, nausea, and vomiting

More severe hypercalcemia (calcium: >12 mg/dL) is associated with confusion, delirium, stupor, and coma

Drug Interactions

Increased Effect/Toxicity: High doses of calcium with thiazide diuretics may result in milk-alkali syndrome and hypercalcemia; monitor response. Calcium salts may decrease T_4 absorption; separate dose from levothyroxine by at least 4 hours. Calcium acetate may potentiate digoxin toxicity.

Decreased Effect: Absorption of tetracycline, atenolol (and potentially other beta-blockers), iron, quinolone antibiotics, alendronate, sodium fluoride, and zinc absorption may be significantly decreased; space administration times. Effects of calcium channel blockers (eg, verapamil) effects may be diminished. Polystyrene sulfonate's potassium-binding ability may be reduced; avoid concurrent administration.

Drug Uptake Absorption: Requires vitamin D

Pregnancy Risk Factor C

Generic Available No

Calcium Disodium Versenate® *see* Edetate Calcium Disodium *on page 428*

Calcium Glubionate (KAL see um gloo BYE oh nate)

U.S. Brand Names Neo-Calglucon® [OTC]

Mexican Brand Names Calcium-Sandoz®

Pharmacologic Category Calcium Salt

Use Adjunct in prevention of postmenopausal osteoporosis; treatment and prevention of calcium depletion

(Continued)

Calcium Glubionate *(Continued)*

Local Anesthetic/Vasoconstrictor Precautions No information available to require special precautions

Effects on Dental Treatment No effects or complications reported

Dosage Oral:

Recommended daily allowance (RDA) (in terms of elemental calcium):

<6 months: 360 mg/day

6-12 months: 540 mg/day

1-10 years: 800 mg/day

10-18 years: 1200 mg/day

Adults: 800 mg/day

Syrup is a hyperosmolar solution; dosage is in terms of calcium glubionate

Neonatal hypocalcemia: 1200 mg/kg/day in 4-6 divided doses

Maintenance: Children: 600-2000 mg/kg/day in 4 divided doses up to a maximum of 9 g/day

Adults: 6-18 g/day in divided doses

Mechanism of Action As dietary supplement, used to prevent or treat negative calcium balance; in osteoporosis, it helps to prevent or decrease the rate of bone loss. The calcium in calcium salts moderates nerve and muscle performance and allows normal cardiac function.

Other Adverse Effects Frequency not defined:

Central nervous system: Dizziness, headache, mental confusion

Endocrine & metabolic: Hypercalcemia, hypomagnesemia, hypophosphatemia, milk-alkali syndrome

Gastrointestinal: GI irritation, diarrhea, constipation, xerostomia

Renal: Hypercalciuria

Note: Mild hypercalcemia (calcium: >10.5 mg/dL) may be asymptomatic or manifest itself as constipation, anorexia, nausea, and vomiting. More severe hypercalcemia (calcium: >12 mg/dL) is associated with confusion, delirium, stupor, and coma.

Drug Interactions

Increased Effect/Toxicity: High doses of calcium with thiazide diuretics may result in milk-alkali syndrome and hypercalcemia; monitor response. Calcium salts may decrease T_4 absorption; separate dose from levothyroxine by at least 4 hours. Calcium acetate may potentiate digoxin toxicity.

Decreased Effect: Absorption of tetracycline, atenolol (and potentially other beta-blockers), iron, quinolone antibiotics, alendronate, sodium fluoride, and zinc absorption may be significantly decreased; space administration times. Effects of calcium channel blockers (eg, verapamil) effects may be diminished. Polystyrene sulfonate's potassium-binding ability may be reduced; avoid concurrent administration.

Drug Uptake Absorption: Requires vitamin D; minimal unless chronic, high doses are given; calcium is absorbed in soluble, ionized form; solubility of calcium is increased in an acid environment

Pregnancy Risk Factor C

Generic Available No

Calcium Gluceptate (KAL see um gloo SEP tate)

Pharmacologic Category Calcium Salt

Use Treatment of cardiac disturbances of hyperkalemia, hypocalcemia, or calcium channel blocker toxicity; cardiac resuscitation when epinephrine fails to improve myocardial contractions; treatment of hypermagnesemia and hypocalcemia

Local Anesthetic/Vasoconstrictor Precautions No information available to require special precautions

Effects on Dental Treatment No effects or complications reported

Dosage I.V. (dose expressed in mg of calcium gluceptate):

Cardiac resuscitation in the presence of hypocalcemia, hyperkalemia, magnesium toxicity, or calcium channel blocker toxicity:

Children: 110 mg/kg/dose

Adults: 1.1-1.5 g (5-7 mL)

Hypocalcemia:

Children: 200-500 mg/kg/day divided every 6 hours

Adults: 500 mg to 1.1 g/dose as needed

After citrated blood administration: Children and Adults: 0.4 mEq/100 mL blood infused

Mechanism of Action Moderates nerve and muscle performance via action potential excitation threshold regulation

Drug Interactions

Increased Effect/Toxicity: High doses of calcium with thiazide diuretics may result in milk-alkali syndrome and hypercalcemia; monitor response. Calcium may potentiate digoxin toxicity.

Decreased Effect: Effects of calcium channel blockers (eg, verapamil) effects may be diminished.

Drug Uptake Absorption: I.M. and I.V. calcium salts are absorbed directly into the bloodstream

Pregnancy Risk Factor C

Generic Available Yes

Calcium Gluconate (KAL see um GLOO koe nate)

U.S. Brand Names Calfort®; Cal-G®

Pharmacologic Category Calcium Salt; Electrolyte Supplement, Oral; Electrolyte Supplement, Parenteral

Use Treatment and prevention of hypocalcemia; treatment of tetany, cardiac disturbances of hyperkalemia, cardiac resuscitation when epinephrine fails to improve myocardial contractions, hypocalcemia, or calcium channel blocker toxicity; calcium supplementation

Local Anesthetic/Vasoconstrictor Precautions No information available to require special precautions

Effects on Dental Treatment No effects or complications reported

Dosage Dosage is in terms of **elemental** calcium:

Dietary Reference Intake:

0-6 months: 210 mg/day
7-12 months: 270 mg/day
1-3 years: 500 mg/day
4-8 years: 800 mg/day
Adults, Male/Female:
9-18 years: 1300 mg/day
19-50 years: 1000 mg/day
≥51 years: 1200 mg/day
Female: Pregnancy: Same as for Adults, Male/Female
Female: Lactating: Same as for Adults, Male/Female

Dosage expressed in terms of **calcium gluconate**

Hypocalcemia: I.V.:
Neonates: 200-800 mg/kg/day as a continuous infusion or in 4 divided doses
Infants and Children: 200-500 mg/kg/day as a continuous infusion or in 4 divided doses
Adults: 2-15 g/24 hours as a continuous infusion or in divided doses

Hypocalcemia: Oral:
Children: 200-500 mg/kg/day divided every 6 hours
Adults: 500 mg to 2 g 2-4 times/day
Osteoporosis/bone loss: Oral: 1000-1500 mg in divided doses/day

Hypocalcemia secondary to citrated blood infusion: I.V.: Give 0.45 mEq **elemental** calcium for each 100 mL citrated blood infused

Hypocalcemic tetany: I.V.:
Neonates: 100-200 mg/kg/dose, may follow with 500 mg/kg/day in 3-4 divided doses or as an infusion
Infants and Children: 100-200 mg/kg/dose (0.5-0.7 mEq/kg/dose) over 5-10 minutes; may repeat every 6-8 hours **or** follow with an infusion of 500 mg/kg/day
Adults: 1-3 g (4.5-16 mEq) may be administered until therapeutic response occurs

Calcium antagonist toxicity, magnesium intoxication or cardiac arrest in the presence of hyperkalemia or hypocalcemia: Calcium chloride is recommended calcium salt: I.V.:
Infants and Children: 100 mg/kg/dose (maximum: 3 g/dose)
Adults: 500-800 mg; maximum: 3 g/dose

Maintenance electrolyte requirements for total parenteral nutrition: I.V.: Daily requirements: Adults: 8-16 mEq/1000 kcal/24 hours

Dosing adjustment in renal impairment: Cl_{cr} <25 mL/minute: Dosage adjustments may be necessary depending on the serum calcium levels

Mechanism of Action As dietary supplement, used to prevent or treat negative calcium balance; in osteoporosis, it helps to prevent or decrease the rate of bone loss. The calcium in calcium salts moderates nerve and muscle performance and allows normal cardiac function.

Drug Interactions

Increased Effect/Toxicity: High doses of calcium with thiazide diuretics may result in milk-alkali syndrome and hypercalcemia; monitor response. Oral administration of calcium salts may decrease T_4 absorption; separate dose from levothyroxine by at least 4 hours. Calcium acetate may potentiate digoxin toxicity.

Decreased Effect: Absorption of tetracycline, atenolol (and potentially other beta-blockers), iron, quinolone antibiotics, alendronate, sodium fluoride, and zinc absorption may be significantly decreased by oral calcium administration; space administration times. Effects of calcium channel blockers (eg, verapamil) effects may be diminished. Polystyrene sulfonate's potassium-binding ability may be reduced; avoid concurrent oral administration.

Drug Uptake Absorption: I.M. and I.V. calcium salts are absorbed directly into the bloodstream; absorption from the GI tract requires vitamin D; calcium is absorbed in

(Continued)

Calcium Gluconate *(Continued)*

soluble, ionized form; solubility of calcium is increased in an acid environment (except calcium lactate)

Pregnancy Risk Factor C

Generic Available Yes

Calcium Lactate (KAL see um LAK tate)

U.S. Brand Names Calbon®; Cal-Lac®; Ridactate®

Pharmacologic Category Calcium Salt

Use Adjunct in prevention of postmenopausal osteoporosis; treatment and prevention of calcium depletion

Local Anesthetic/Vasoconstrictor Precautions No information available to require special precautions

Effects on Dental Treatment No effects or complications reported

Dosage Oral (in terms of calcium lactate)

Dietary Reference Intake (in terms of elemental calcium):

0-6 months: 210 mg/day
7-12 months: 270 mg/day
1-3 years: 500 mg/day
4-8 years: 800 mg/day
Adults, Male/Female:
9-18 years: 1300 mg/day
19-50 years: 1000 mg/day
≥51 years: 1200 mg/day
Female: Pregnancy: Same as Adults, Male/Female
Female: Lactating: Same as Adults, Male/Female

Children: 500 mg/kg/day divided every 6-8 hours; maximum daily dose: 9 g

Adults: 1.5-3 g divided every 8 hours

Mechanism of Action As dietary supplement, used to prevent or treat negative calcium balance; in osteoporosis, it helps to prevent or decrease the rate of bone loss. The calcium in calcium salts moderates nerve and muscle performance and allows normal cardiac function.

Drug Interactions

Increased Effect/Toxicity: High doses of calcium with thiazide diuretics may result in milk-alkali syndrome and hypercalcemia; monitor response. Calcium salts may decrease T_4 absorption; separate dose from levothyroxine by at least 4 hours. Calcium acetate may potentiate digoxin toxicity.

Decreased Effect: Absorption of tetracycline, atenolol (and potentially other beta-blockers), iron, quinolone antibiotics, alendronate, sodium fluoride, and zinc absorption may be significantly decreased; space administration times. Effects of calcium channel blockers (eg, verapamil) effects may be diminished. Polystyrene sulfonate's potassium-binding ability may be reduced; avoid concurrent administration.

Drug Uptake Absorption: From the GI tract requires vitamin D

Pregnancy Risk Factor C

Generic Available Yes

Calcium Phosphate, Tribasic (KAL see um FOS fate tri BAY sik)

U.S. Brand Names Posture® [OTC]

Pharmacologic Category Calcium Salt

Synonyms Tricalcium Phosphate

Use Adjunct in prevention of postmenopausal osteoporosis; treatment and prevention of calcium depletion

Local Anesthetic/Vasoconstrictor Precautions No information available to require special precautions

Effects on Dental Treatment No effects or complications reported

Dosage Oral (dosage is in terms of elemental calcium):

Dietary Reference Intake:

0-6 months: 210 mg/day
7-12 months: 270 mg/day
1-3 years: 500 mg/day
4-8 years: 800 mg/day
Adults, Male/Female:
9-18 years: 1300 mg/day
19-50 years: 1000 mg/day
≥51 years: 1200 mg/day
Female: Pregnancy: Same as for Adults, Male/Female
Female: Lactating: Same as for Adults, Male/Female

Prevention of osteoporosis:
Children: 45-65 mg/kg/day
Adults: 1-2 g/day

Mechanism of Action As dietary supplement, used to prevent or treat negative calcium balance; in osteoporosis, it helps to prevent or decrease the rate of bone loss. The calcium in calcium salts moderates nerve and muscle performance and allows normal cardiac function.

Drug Interactions

Increased Effect/Toxicity: High doses of calcium with thiazide diuretics may result in milk-alkali syndrome and hypercalcemia; monitor response. Calcium salts may decrease T_4 absorption; separate dose from levothyroxine by at least 4 hours. Calcium acetate may potentiate digoxin toxicity.

Decreased Effect: Absorption of tetracycline, atenolol (and potentially other beta-blockers), iron, quinolone antibiotics, alendronate, sodium fluoride, and zinc absorption may be significantly decreased; space administration times. Effects of calcium channel blockers (eg, verapamil) effects may be diminished. Polystyrene sulfonate's potassium-binding ability may be reduced; avoid concurrent administration.

Pregnancy Risk Factor C

Generic Available No

Calcium Polycarbophil (KAL see um pol i KAR boe fil)

U.S. Brand Names Equalactin® Chewable Tablet [OTC]; Fiberall® Chewable Tablet [OTC]; FiberCon® Tablet [OTC]; Fiber-Lax® Tablet [OTC]; Mitrolan® Chewable Tablet [OTC]

Pharmacologic Category Antidiarrheal; Laxative, Bulk-Producing

Use Treatment of constipation or diarrhea; calcium polycarbophil is supplied as the approved substitute whenever a bulk-forming laxative is ordered in a tablet, capsule, wafer, or other oral solid dosage form

Local Anesthetic/Vasoconstrictor Precautions No information available to require special precautions

Effects on Dental Treatment Oral medication should be given at least 1 hour prior to taking the bulk-producing laxative in order to prevent decreased absorption of medication.

Dosage Oral:

Children:

2-6 years: 500 mg (1 tablet) 1-2 times/day, up to 1.5 g/day

6-12 years: 500 mg (1 tablet) 1-3 times/day, up to 3 g/day

Adults: 1 g 4 times/day, up to 6 g/day

Mechanism of Action Restoring a more normal moisture level and providing bulk in the patient's intestinal tract

Other Adverse Effects 1% to 10%: Gastrointestinal: Abdominal fullness

Drug Interactions

Increased Effect/Toxicity: High doses of calcium with thiazide diuretics may result in milk-alkali syndrome and hypercalcemia; monitor response. Calcium salts may decrease T_4 absorption; separate dose from levothyroxine by at least 4 hours. Calcium acetate may potentiate digoxin toxicity.

Decreased Effect: Absorption of tetracycline, atenolol (and potentially other beta-blockers), iron, quinolone antibiotics, alendronate, sodium fluoride, and zinc absorption may be significantly decreased; space administration times. Effects of calcium channel blockers (eg, verapamil) effects may be diminished. Polystyrene sulfonate's potassium-binding ability may be reduced; avoid concurrent administration.

Pregnancy Risk Factor C

Generic Available Yes

Calderol® *see* Calcifediol *on page 198*

Caldesene® [OTC] *see* Undecylenic Acid and Derivatives *on page 1221*

Calfactant (cal FAC tant)

U.S. Brand Names Infasurf®

Pharmacologic Category Lung Surfactant

Use Prevention of respiratory distress syndrome (RDS) in premature infants at high risk for RDS and for the treatment ("rescue") of premature infants who develop RDS; decreases the incidence of RDS, mortality due to RDS, and air leaks associated with RDS

Local Anesthetic/Vasoconstrictor Precautions No information available to require special precautions

Effects on Dental Treatment No effects or complications reported

Dosage Should be administered intratracheally through a side-port adapter into the endotracheal tube; two attendants, one to instill the suspension, the other to monitor the patient and assist in positioning, facilitate the dosing; the dose (3 mL/kg) should be administered in two aliquots of 1.5 mL/kg each; after each aliquot is instilled, the infant should be positioned with either the right or the left side dependent; administration is made while ventilation is continued over 20-30 breaths for each aliquot, with small bursts timed only during the inspiratory cycles; a pause followed by evaluation of the respiratory status and repositioning should separate the two aliquots

Mechanism of Action Adsorbs rapidly to the surface of the air:liquid interface and modifies surface tension similarly to natural lung surfactant. A minimum surface

(Continued)

Calfactant *(Continued)*

tension of ≤3 mN/m is produced *in vitro* as measured on a pulsating bubble surfactometer. *Ex vivo*, restores the pressure volume mechanics and compliance of surfactant-deficient rat lungs. *In vivo*, improves lung compliance, respiratory gas exchange, and survival in preterm lambs with profound surfactant deficiency.

Other Adverse Effects >10%:

Cardiovascular: Bradycardia (34%), cyanosis (65%)

Respiratory: Airway obstruction (39%), reflux (21%), requirement for manual ventilation (16%), reintubation (1% to 10%)

Drug Uptake No human studies of absorption of calfactant have been performed

Generic Available No

Calfort® *see* Calcium Gluconate *on page 205*

Cal-G® *see* Calcium Gluconate *on page 205*

Cal-Lac® *see* Calcium Lactate *on page 206*

Calm-X® Oral [OTC] *see* DimenhyDRINATE *on page 396*

Cal-Plus® [OTC] *see* Calcium Carbonate *on page 201*

Caltrate® 600 [OTC] *see* Calcium Carbonate *on page 201*

Caltrate, Jr.® [OTC] *see* Calcium Carbonate *on page 201*

Campath® *see* Alemtuzumab *on page 48*

Campho-Phenique® [OTC] *see* Camphor and Phenol *on page 208*

Camphor and Phenol (KAM for & FEE nole)

U.S. Brand Names Campho-Phenique® [OTC]

Pharmacologic Category Topical Skin Product

Synonyms Phenol and Camphor

Use Relief of pain and for minor infections

Local Anesthetic/Vasoconstrictor Precautions No information available to require special precautions

Effects on Dental Treatment No effects or complications reported

Dosage Apply as needed

Pregnancy Risk Factor C

Generic Available Yes

Camptosar® *see* Irinotecan *on page 654*

Canasa™ *see* Mesalamine *on page 772*

Cancidas® *see* Caspofungin *on page 229*

Candesartan (kan de SAR tan)

U.S. Brand Names Atacand®

Canadian Brand Names Atacand®

Mexican Brand Names Atacand®

Pharmacologic Category Angiotensin II Receptor Blocker

Synonyms Candesartan Cilexetil

Use Alone or in combination with other antihypertensive agents in treating essential hypertension; may have an advantage over losartan due to minimal metabolism requirements and consequent use in mild to moderate hepatic impairment

Local Anesthetic/Vasoconstrictor Precautions No information available to require special precautions

Effects on Dental Treatment No effects or complications reported

Dosage Adults: Oral: Dosage must be individualized; BP response is dose-related over the range of 2-32 mg; the usual recommended starting dose of 16 mg once daily when it is used as monotherapy in patients who are not volume depleted; it can be administered once or twice daily with total daily doses ranging from 8-32 mg; larger doses do not appear to have a greater effect and there is relatively little experience with such doses; most of the antihypertensive effect is present within 2 weeks and maximal BP reduction is generally obtained within 4-6 weeks of treatment

No initial dosage adjustment is necessary for elderly patients (although higher concentrations (C_{max}) and AUC were observed in these populations), for patients with mildly impaired renal function, or for patients with mildly impaired hepatic function.

Mechanism of Action An angiotensin receptor antagonist; angiotensin II acts as a vasoconstrictor. In addition to causing direct vasoconstriction, angiotensin II also stimulates the release of aldosterone. Once aldosterone is released, sodium as well as water are reabsorbed. The end result is an elevation in BP. Candesartan binds to the AT1 angiotensin II receptor. This binding prevents angiotensin II from binding to the receptor thereby blocking the vasoconstriction and the aldosterone secreting effects of angiotensin II.

Other Adverse Effects May be associated with worsening of renal function in patients dependent on renin-angiotensin-aldosterone system. Frequency not defined:

Cardiovascular: Flushing, tachycardia, palpitations, angina, myocardial infarction,

Central nervous system: Dizziness, lightheadedness, drowsiness, headache, vertigo, anxiety, depression, somnolence, fever
Dermatologic: Angioedema, rash
Endocrine & metabolic: Hyperglycemia, hypertriglyceridemia
Genitourinary: Hyperuricemia, hematuria
Neuromuscular & skeletal: Back pain, increased CPK, weakness
Respiratory: Upper respiratory tract infection, bronchitis, epistaxis
Miscellaneous: Diaphoresis (increased)

Drug Interactions Not metabolized by cytochrome P450

Increased Effect/Toxicity: The risk of lithium toxicity may be increased by candesartan; monitor lithium levels. Concurrent use with potassium-sparing diuretics (amiloride, spironolactone, triamterene), potassium supplements, or trimethoprim (high-dose) may increase the risk of hyperkalemia.

Drug Uptake

Onset of action: 2-3 hours; Peak effect: 6-8 hours
Duration: >24 hours
Half-life, elimination (dose-dependent): 5-9 hours
Time to peak: 3-4 hours; AUC may be doubled with renal impairment and in the elderly

Pregnancy Risk Factor C/D (2nd and 3rd trimesters)

Generic Available No

Candesartan and Hydrochlorothiazide

(kan de SAR tan & hye droe klor oh THYE a zide)

U.S. Brand Names Atacand HCT™

Pharmacologic Category Angiotensin II Receptor Blocker Combination

Synonyms Candesartan Cilexetil and Hydrochlorothiazide

Use Treatment of hypertension; combination product should not be used for initial therapy

Local Anesthetic/Vasoconstrictor Precautions No information available to require special precautions

Effects on Dental Treatment No effects or complications reported

Dosage Adults: Oral: Replacement therapy: Combination product can be substituted for individual agents; maximum therapeutic effect would be expected within 4 weeks

Usual dosage range:
Candesartan: 8-32 mg/day, given once daily or twice daily in divided doses
Hydrochlorothiazide: 12.5-50 mg once daily

Mechanism of Action Candesartan: Candesartan is an angiotensin receptor antagonist. Angiotensin II acts as a vasoconstrictor. In addition to causing direct vasoconstriction, angiotensin II also stimulates the release of aldosterone. Once aldosterone is released, sodium as well as water are reabsorbed. The end result is an elevation in BP. Candesartan binds to the AT1 angiotensin II receptor. This binding prevents angiotensin II from binding to the receptor, thereby blocking the vasoconstriction and the aldosterone-secreting effects of angiotensin II.

Hydrochlorothiazide: Inhibits sodium reabsorption in the distal tubules causing increased excretion of sodium and water as well as potassium and hydrogen ions

Other Adverse Effects Reactions which follow have been reported with the combination product; refer to individual drug monographs for additional adverse reactions that may be expected from each agent.

1% to 10%:
Central nervous system: Dizziness (3%), headache (3%, placebo 5%)
Neuromuscular & skeletal: Back pain (3%)
Respiratory: Upper respiratory tract infection (4%)
Miscellaneous: Flu-like symptoms (2%)

Drug Interactions

Based on **candesartan** component: Not significantly metabolized by cytochrome P450 enzymes at therapeutic concentrations
Lithium: Risk of toxicity may be increased by candesartan; monitor lithium levels
NSAIDs: May decrease angiotensin II antagonist efficacy; effect has been seen with losartan, but may occur with other medications in this class; monitor BP
Potassium-sparing diuretics (amiloride, spironolactone, triamterene): Increased risk of hyperkalemia
Potassium supplements: May increase the risk of hyperkalemia
Trimethoprim (high dose): May increase the risk of hyperkalemia

Based on **hydrochlorothiazide** component:
ACTH, corticosteroids: May increase hypokalemia
Angiotensin-converting enzyme inhibitors: Increased hypotension if aggressively diuresed with a thiazide diuretic
Antidiabetic agents: May require dosage adjustment of oral agents and insulin; monitor
Barbiturates, narcotics: May potentiate orthostatic hypertension
Cholestyramine and colestipol resins: Decreased absorption of hydrochlorothiazide

(Continued)

Candesartan and Hydrochlorothiazide *(Continued)*

Cyclosporine and thiazides can increase the risk of gout or renal toxicity; avoid concurrent use
Digoxin: Toxicity can be exacerbated if a thiazide induces hypokalemia or hypomagnesemia
Lithium: Toxicity can occur by reducing renal excretion of lithium; monitor lithium concentration and adjust as needed
Neuromuscular blocking agents: Can prolong blockade; monitor serum potassium and neuromuscular status
Norepinephrine: Hydrochlorothiazide may decrease response to pressor amines; monitor
NSAIDs: May lead to decreased effect of thiazides; monitor

Drug Uptake

Candesartan:
- Onset of action: 2-3 hours
- Duration: >24 hours
- Half-life, elimination (dose-dependent): 5-9 hours
- Time to peak: 3-4 hours

Hydrochlorothiazide:
- Onset of action: Oral: ≤2 hours
- Duration: 6-12 hours
- Half-life, elimination: 5.6-14.8 hours

Pregnancy Risk Factor C/D (2nd and 3rd trimesters)

Generic Available No

Cantharidin (kan THAR e din)

U.S. Brand Names Verr-Canth™

Canadian Brand Names Canthacur®; Cantharone®

Pharmacologic Category Keratolytic Agent

Use Removal of ordinary and periungual warts

Local Anesthetic/Vasoconstrictor Precautions No information available to require special precautions

Effects on Dental Treatment No effects or complications reported

Dosage Apply directly to lesion, cover with nonporous tape, remove tape in 24 hours, reapply if necessary

Other Adverse Effects 1% to 10%:
- Cardiovascular: Syncope
- Central nervous system: Delirium, ataxia
- Dermatologic: Dermal irritation, dermal burns, acantholysis
- Gastrointestinal: GI hemorrhage, rectal bleeding, dysphagia
- Genitourinary: Priapism
- Hepatic: Fatty degeneration
- Neuromuscular & skeletal: Hyper-reflexia
- Ocular: Conjunctivitis, iritis, keratitis
- Renal: Proteinuria, hematuria
- Respiratory: Burning of oropharynx

Pregnancy Risk Factor C

Generic Available No

Cantil® *see* Mepenzolate Bromide *on page 760*
Capastat® Sulfate *see* Capreomycin *on page 212*

Capecitabine (ka pe SITE a been)

U.S. Brand Names Xeloda®

Canadian Brand Names Xeloda®

Mexican Brand Names Xeloda®

Pharmacologic Category Antineoplastic Agent, Antimetabolite

Use

Treatment of metastatic colorectal cancer
Treatment of metastatic breast cancer in combination with docetaxel after failure of prior anthracycline therapy
Monotherapy treatment of metastatic breast cancer resistant to both paclitaxel and an anthracycline-containing chemotherapy regimen or resistant to paclitaxel and for whom further anthracycline therapy is not indicated (eg, patients who have received cumulative doses of 400 mg/m² of doxorubicin or doxorubicin equivalents). Resistance is defined as progressive disease while on treatment, with or without an initial response, or relapse within 6 months of completing treatment with an anthracycline-containing adjuvant regimen.

Local Anesthetic/Vasoconstrictor Precautions No information available to require special precautions

Effects on Dental Treatment Relatively high incidence of stomatitis; oral candidiasis has been reported

Mechanism of Action A prodrug of fluorouracil; undergoes hydrolysis in the liver and tissues to form fluorouracil which is the active moiety; fluorouracil is a fluorinated pyrimidine antimetabolite that inhibits thymidylate synthetase, blocking the methylation of deoxyuridylic acid to thymidylic acid, interfering with DNA, and to a lesser degree, RNA synthesis. Fluorouracil appears to be phase specific for the G_1 and S phases of the cell cycle.

Other Adverse Effects Frequency derived from monotherapy trials:

>10%:

Cardiovascular: Edema (9% to 15%)

Central nervous system: Fatigue (~40%), fever (12% to 18%), pain (colorectal cancer: 12%)

Dermatologic: Palmar-plantar erythrodysesthesia (hand-and-foot syndrome) (~55%, may be dose limiting), dermatitis (27% to 37%)

Gastrointestinal: Diarrhea (~55%, may be dose limiting), mild to moderate nausea (43% to 53%), vomiting (27% to 37%), stomatitis (~25%), decreased appetite (colorectal cancer: 26%), anorexia (23%), abdominal pain (20% to 35%), constipation (~15%)

Hematologic: Lymphopenia (94%), anemia (72% to 80%; Grade 3/4: <1% to 3%), neutropenia (13% to 26%; Grade 3/4: 1% to 2%), thrombocytopenia (24%; Grade 3/4: 1% to 3%)

Hepatic: Increased bilirubin (22% to 48%)

Neuromuscular & skeletal: Paresthesia (21%)

Ocular: Eye irritation (~15%)

Respiratory: Dyspnea (colorectal cancer: 14%)

5% to 10%:

Cardiovascular: Venous thrombosis (colorectal cancer: 8%), chest pain (colorectal cancer: 6%)

Central nervous system: Headache (~10%), dizziness (~8%), insomnia (8%), mood alteration (colorectal cancer: 5%), depression (colorectal cancer: 5%)

Dermatologic: Nail disorders (7%), skin discoloration (colorectal cancer: 7%), alopecia (colorectal cancer: 6%)

Endocrine & metabolic: Dehydration (7%)

Gastrointestinal: Motility disorder (colorectal cancer: 10%), oral discomfort (colorectal cancer: 10%), dyspepsia (8%), upper GI inflammatory disorders (colorectal cancer: 8%), hemorrhage (colorectal cancer: 6%), ileus (colorectal cancer: 6%), taste disturbance (colorectal cancer: 6%)

Neuromuscular & skeletal: Back pain (colorectal cancer: 10%), myalgia (9%), neuropathy (colorectal cancer: 10%), arthralgia (colorectal cancer: 8%), limb pain (colorectal cancer: 6%)

Respiratory: Cough (7%), sore throat (2%), epistaxis (3%)

Ocular: Abnormal vision (colorectal cancer: 5%)

Miscellaneous: Viral infection (colorectal cancer: 5%)

<5%: Abdominal distension, angina, appetite increased, arthritis, ascites, asthma, ataxia, atrial fibrillation, bronchitis, bone pain, bradycardia, bronchopneumonia, bronchospasm, cachexia, cardiac arrest, cardiac failure, cardiomyopathy, cerebral vascular accident, cholestasis, colitis, confusion, conjunctivitis, deep vein thrombosis, diaphoresis increased, duodenitis, dysarthria, dysphagia, dysrhythmia, ecchymoses, EKG changes, encephalopathy, esophagitis, fibrosis, fungal infection, gastric ulcer, gastritis, gastroenteritis, GI hemorrhage, hematemesis, hemoptysis, hepatitis, hepatic failure, hepatic fibrosis, hoarseness, hot flushes, hypokalemia, hypomagnesemia, hypotension, hypersensitivity, hypertension, hypertriglyceridemia, idiopathic thrombocytopenia purpura, ileus, impaired balance, infections, influenza-like illness, intestinal obstruction (~1%), irritability, joint stiffness, keratoconjunctivitis, laryngitis, leukopenia, loss of consciousness, lymphedema, myocardial infarction, myocardial ischemia, myocarditis, necrotizing enterocolitis, nocturia, oral candidiasis, pericardial effusion, thrombocytopenic purpura, pancytopenia, photosensitivity reaction, pneumonia, proctalgia, pruritus, pulmonary embolism, radiation recall syndrome, renal impairment, respiratory distress, sedation, sepsis, skin ulceration, toxic dilation of intestine, tachycardia, thirst, thrombophlebitis, tremor, weight gain, ventricular extrasystoles, vertigo

Drug Interactions Increased Effect/Toxicity: Administration immediately before an aluminum hydroxide/magnesium hydroxide antacid increases the absorption of capecitabine. The concentration of capecitabine's active metabolite (5-fluorouracil) is increased and its toxicity may be enhanced by leucovorin. Deaths from severe enterocolitis, diarrhea, and dehydration have been reported in elderly patients receiving weekly leucovorin and fluorouracil. Response to warfarin may be increased by capecitabine; changes may occur days to months after starting or stopping capecitabine therapy. Capecitabine may increase serum concentration/effects of drugs metabolized by CYP2C9.

Drug Uptake

Absorption: Rapid and extensive

Half-life, elimination: 0.5-1 hour

Time to peak: 1.5 hours; peak fluorouracil level: 2 hours

Pregnancy Risk Factor D

(Continued)

Capecitabine *(Continued)*

Generic Available No

Capex™ *see* Fluocinolone *on page 512*

Capital® and Codeine *see* Acetaminophen and Codeine *on page 28*

Capitrol® *see* Chloroxine *on page 268*

Capoten® *see* Captopril *on page 213*

Capozide® *see* Captopril and Hydrochlorothiazide *on page 214*

Capreomycin (kap ree oh MYE sin)

Related Information

Nonviral Infectious Diseases *on page 1342*

U.S. Brand Names Capastat® Sulfate

Pharmacologic Category Antibiotic, Miscellaneous; Antitubercular Agent

Synonyms Capreomycin Sulfate

Use Treatment of tuberculosis in conjunction with at least one other antituberculosis agent

Local Anesthetic/Vasoconstrictor Precautions No information available to require special precautions

Effects on Dental Treatment No effects or complications reported

Dosage I.M.:

Children: 15-20 mg/kg/day, up to 1 g/day maximum

Adults: 15-30 mg/kg/day up to 1 g/day for 60-120 days, followed by 1 g 2-3 times/week

Mechanism of Action A cyclic polypeptide antimicrobial; administered as a mixture of capreomycin IA and capreomycin IB; mechanism is not well understood. Mycobacterial species that have become resistant to other agents are usually still sensitive to the action of capreomycin. However, significant cross-resistance with viomycin, kanamycin, and neomycin occurs.

Other Adverse Effects

>10%:

Renal: Nephrotoxicity (increased thirst, anorexia, nausea, vomiting, greatly increased or decreased frequency of urination)

Otic: Ototoxicity

1% to 10%:

Hematologic: Eosinophilia

Drug Interactions Increased Effect/Toxicity: May increase effect/duration of nondepolarizing neuromuscular blocking agents; additive toxicity (nephrotoxicity and ototoxicity), respiratory paralysis may occur with aminoglycosides (eg, streptomycin).

Drug Uptake

Absorption: Oral: Poor absorption necessitates parenteral administration

Half-life, elimination: 4-6 hours (dependent upon renal function; varies with creatinine clearance)

Time to peak: I.M.: ≤1 hour

Pregnancy Risk Factor C

Generic Available No

Capsaicin (kap SAY sin)

U.S. Brand Names Capsin® [OTC]; Capzasin-P® [OTC]; Dolorac™ [OTC]; No Pain-HP® [OTC]; R-Gel® [OTC]; Zostrix® [OTC]; Zostrix®-HP [OTC]

Canadian Brand Names Antiphogistine Rub A-535 Capsaicin; Zostrix®; Zostrix® H.P.

Pharmacologic Category Analgesic, Topical; Topical Skin Product

Use FDA approved for the topical treatment of pain associated with postherpetic neuralgia, rheumatoid arthritis, osteoarthritis, diabetic neuropathy, and postsurgical pain.

Unlabeled/Investigational: Treatment of pain associated with psoriasis, chronic neuralgias unresponsive to other forms of therapy, and intractable pruritus

Local Anesthetic/Vasoconstrictor Precautions No information available to require special precautions

Effects on Dental Treatment No effects or complications reported

Dosage Children ≥2 years and Adults: Topical: Apply to affected area at least 3-4 times/day; application frequency <3-4 times/day prevents the total depletion, inhibition of synthesis, and transport of substance P resulting in decreased clinical efficacy and increased local discomfort

Mechanism of Action Induces release of substance P, the principal chemomediator of pain impulses from the periphery to the CNS, from peripheral sensory neurons; after repeated application, capsaicin depletes the neuron of substance P and prevents reaccumulation

Other Adverse Effects

>10%: Local: Transient burning on application which usually diminishes with repeated use (≥30%)

1% to 10%:

Dermatologic: Itching, stinging sensation, erythema

Respiratory: Cough

Drug Uptake Data following the use of topical capsaicin in humans are lacking.

Onset of action: Topical: 14-28 days; Peak effect: 4-6 weeks of continuous therapy

Duration: Several hours

Pregnancy Risk Factor C

Generic Available Yes

Capsin® [OTC] *see* Capsaicin *on page 212*

Captopril (KAP toe pril)

Related Information

Cardiovascular Diseases *on page 1308*

U.S. Brand Names Capoten®

Canadian Brand Names Alti-Captopril; Apo®-Capto; Capoten™; Gen-Captopril; Novo-Captopril; Nu-Capto®; PMS-Captopril®

Mexican Brand Names Capitral®; Capoten®; Capotena; Captral®; Cardipril®; Cryopril; Ecapresan; Ecaten; Kenolan; Lenpryl; Precaptil; Romir

Pharmacologic Category Angiotensin-Converting Enzyme (ACE) Inhibitor

Synonyms ACE

Use Management of hypertension and treatment of CHF; left ventricular dysfunction after myocardial infarction (MI), diabetic nephropathy

Unlabeled/Investigational: Treatment of hypertensive crisis, rheumatoid arthritis; diagnosis of anatomic renal artery stenosis, hypertension secondary to scleroderma renal crisis; diagnosis of aldosteronism, idiopathic edema, Bartter's syndrome, postmyocardial infarction for prevention of ventricular failure; increase circulation in Raynaud's phenomenon, hypertension secondary to Takayasu's disease

Local Anesthetic/Vasoconstrictor Precautions No information available to require special precautions

Effects on Dental Treatment No effects or complications reported

Dosage Dosage must be titrated according to patient's response; use lowest effective dose.

Oral:

Children: Initial: 0.5 mg/kg/dose; titrate upward to maximum of 6 mg/kg/day in 2-4 divided doses

Older Children: Initial: 6.25-12.5 mg/dose every 12-24 hours; titrate upward to maximum of 6 mg/kg/day

Adolescents: Initial: 12.5-25 mg/dose given every 8-12 hours; increase by 25 mg/dose to maximum of 450 mg/day

Adults:

Hypertension:

Initial dose: 12.5-25 mg 2-3 times/day; may increase by 12.5-25 mg/dose at 1- to 2-week intervals up to 50 mg 3 times/day; add diuretic before further dosage increases

Maximum dose: 150 mg 3 times/day

Congestive heart failure:

Initial dose: 6.25-12.5 mg 3 times/day in conjunction with cardiac glycoside and diuretic therapy; initial dose depends upon patient's fluid/electrolyte status

Target dose: 50 mg 3 times/day

Maximum dose: 100 mg 3 times/day

Mechanism of Action Competitive inhibitor of angiotensin-converting enzyme (ACE); prevents conversion of angiotensin I to angiotensin II, a potent vasoconstrictor; results in lower levels of angiotensin II which causes an increase in plasma renin activity and a reduction in aldosterone secretion

Other Adverse Effects

1% to 10%:

Cardiovascular: Hypotension (1% to 3%), tachycardia (1%), chest pain (1%), palpitation (1%)

Dermatologic: Rash (maculopapular or urticarial) (4% to 7%), pruritus (2%); in patients with rash, a positive ANA and/or eosinophilia has been noted in 7% to 10%.

Endocrine & metabolic: Hyperkalemia (1% to 11%)

Hematologic: Neutropenia may occur in up to 4% of patients with renal insufficiency or collagen-vascular disease.

Renal: Proteinuria (1%), increased serum creatinine, worsening of renal function (may occur in patients with bilateral renal artery stenosis or hypovolemia)

Respiratory: Cough (<1% to 2%)

Miscellaneous: Hypersensitivity reactions (rash, pruritus, fever, arthralgia, and eosinophilia) have occurred in 4% to 7% of patients (depending on dose and renal function); dysgeusia - loss of taste or diminished perception (2% to 4%)

(Continued)

Captopril *(Continued)*

Frequency not defined:

Cardiovascular: Angioedema, cardiac arrest, cerebrovascular insufficiency, rhythm disturbances, orthostatic hypotension, syncope, flushing, pallor, angina, myocardial infarction, Raynaud's syndrome, CHF

Central nervous system: Ataxia, confusion, depression, nervousness, somnolence

Dermatologic: Bullous pemphigus, erythema multiforme, Stevens-Johnson syndrome, exfoliative dermatitis

Endocrine & metabolic: Serum transaminases, serum bilirubin, alkaline phosphatase increased; gynecomastia

Gastrointestinal: Pancreatitis, glossitis, dyspepsia

Genitourinary: Urinary frequency, impotence

Hematologic: Anemia, thrombocytopenia, pancytopenia, agranulocytosis, anemia

Hepatic: Jaundice, hepatitis, hepatic necrosis (rare), cholestasis, hyponatremia (symptomatic)

Neuromuscular & skeletal: Asthenia, myalgia, myasthenia

Ocular: Blurred vision

Renal: Renal insufficiency, renal failure, nephrotic syndrome, polyuria, oliguria

Respiratory: Bronchospasm, eosinophilic pneumonitis, rhinitis

Miscellaneous: Anaphylactoid reactions

Drug Interactions CYP2D6 enzyme substrate

Increased Effect/Toxicity: Potassium supplements, co-trimoxazole (high dose), angiotensin II receptor antagonists (candesartan, losartan, irbesartan, etc), or potassium-sparing diuretics (amiloride, spironolactone, triamterene) may result in elevated serum potassium levels when combined with captopril. ACE inhibitor effects may be increased by phenothiazines or probenecid (increases levels of captopril). ACE inhibitors may increase serum concentration/effects of digoxin, lithium, and sulfonlyureas. Diuretics have additive hypotensive effects with ACE inhibitors, and hypovolemia increases the potential for adverse renal effects of ACE inhibitors. In patients with compromised renal function, coadministration with nonsteroidal anti-inflammatory drugs may result in further deterioration of renal function. Allopurinol and ACE inhibitors may cause a higher risk of hypersensitivity reaction when taken concurrently.

Decreased Effect: Aspirin (high dose) may reduce the therapeutic effects of ACE inhibitors; at low dosages this does not appear to be significant. Rifampin may decrease the effect of ACE inhibitors. Antacids may decrease the bioavailability of ACE inhibitors (may be more likely to occur with captopril); separate administration times by 1-2 hours. NSAIDs, specifically indomethacin, may reduce the hypotensive effects of ACE inhibitors. More likely to occur in low renin or volume dependent hypertensive patients.

Drug Uptake

Onset of action: Maximal decrease in blood pressure 1-1.5 hours after dose

Absorption: 60% to 75%; food decreases absorption by 30% to 40%

Duration: Dose related, may require several weeks of therapy before full hypotensive effect is seen

Half-life, elimination (dependent upon renal and cardiac function): Adults: 1.9 hours; Congestive heart failure: 2.06 hours; Anuria: 20-40 hours

Time to peak: 1-2 hours

Pregnancy Risk Factor C/D (2nd and 3rd trimesters)

Generic Available Yes

Captopril and Hydrochlorothiazide

(KAP toe pril & hye droe klor oh THYE a zide)

Related Information

Cardiovascular Diseases *on page 1308*

U.S. Brand Names Capozide®

Canadian Brand Names Capozide®

Pharmacologic Category Antihypertensive Agent Combination

Synonyms Hydrochlorothiazide and Captopril

Use Management of hypertension and treatment of CHF

Local Anesthetic/Vasoconstrictor Precautions No information available to require special precautions

Effects on Dental Treatment No effects or complications reported

Dosage Adults: Oral:

Hypertension: Initial: 25 mg 2-3 times/day; may increase at 1- to 2-week intervals up to 150 mg 3 times/day (captopril dosages)

Congestive heart failure: 6.25-25 mg 3 times/day (maximum: 450 mg/day) (captopril dosages)

Mechanism of Action Captopril is a competitive inhibitor of angiotensin-converting enzyme (ACE); prevents conversion of angiotensin I to angiotensin II, a potent vasoconstrictor. This results in lower levels of angiotensin II which causes an increase in plasma renin activity and a reduction in aldosterone secretion. Hydrochlorothiazide inhibits sodium reabsorption in the distal tubules causing increased excretion of sodium and water as well as potassium and hydrogen ions.

Other Adverse Effects

Captopril:

1% to 10%:

Cardiovascular: Hypotension (1% to 3%), tachycardia (1%), chest pain (1%), palpitation (1%)

Dermatologic: Rash (maculopapular or urticarial) (4% to 7%), pruritus (2%); in patients with rash, a positive ANA and/or eosinophilia has been noted in 7% to 10%.

Endocrine & metabolic: Hyperkalemia (1% to 11%)

Hematologic: Neutropenia may occur in up to 4% of patients with renal insufficiency or collagen-vascular disease.

Renal: Proteinuria (1%), increased serum creatinine, worsening of renal function (may occur in patients with bilateral renal artery stenosis or hypovolemia)

Respiratory: Cough (<1% to 2%)

Miscellaneous: Hypersensitivity reactions (rash, pruritus, fever, arthralgia, and eosinophilia) have occurred in 4% to 7% of patients (depending on dose and renal function); dysgeusia - loss of taste or diminished perception (2% to 4%)

Frequency not defined:

Cardiovascular: Angioedema, cardiac arrest, cerebrovascular insufficiency, rhythm disturbances, orthostatic hypotension, syncope, flushing, pallor, angina, myocardial infarction, Raynaud's syndrome, CHF

Central nervous system: Ataxia, confusion, depression, nervousness, somnolence

Dermatologic: Bullous pemphigus, erythema multiforme, Stevens-Johnson syndrome, exfoliative dermatitis

Endocrine & metabolic: Increased serum transaminases, increased serum bilirubin, increased alkaline phosphatase, gynecomastia

Gastrointestinal: Pancreatitis, glossitis, dyspepsia

Genitourinary: Urinary frequency, impotence

Hematologic: Anemia, thrombocytopenia, pancytopenia, agranulocytosis, anemia

Hepatic: Jaundice, hepatitis, hepatic necrosis (rare), cholestasis, hyponatremia (symptomatic)

Neuromuscular & skeletal: Asthenia, myalgia, myasthenia

Ocular: Blurred vision

Renal: Renal insufficiency, renal failure, nephrotic syndrome, polyuria, oliguria

Respiratory: Bronchospasm, eosinophilic pneumonitis, rhinitis

Miscellaneous: Anaphylactoid reactions

Hydrochlorothiazide:

1% to 10%:

Cardiovascular: Orthostatic hypotension, hypotension

Dermatologic: Photosensitivity

Endocrine & metabolic: Hypokalemia

Gastrointestinal: Anorexia, epigastric distress

Contraindications Hypersensitivity to captopril, hydrochlorothiazide or any component of their formulation

Drug Interactions See Captopril *on page 213* and Hydrochlorothiazide *on page 595*

Drug Uptake See Captopril *on page 213* and Hydrochlorothiazide *on page 595*

Pregnancy Risk Factor C/D (2nd and 3rd trimesters)

Generic Available Yes

Capzasin-P® [OTC] *see* Capsaicin *on page 212*

Carac™ *see* Fluorouracil *on page 516*

Carafate® *see* Sucralfate *on page 1113*

Carbachol (KAR ba kole)

U.S. Brand Names Carbastat®; Carboptic®; Isopto® Carbachol; Miostat® Intraocular

Canadian Brand Names Carbastat®; Isopto® Carbachol; Miostat®

Pharmacologic Category Cholinergic Agonist; Ophthalmic Agent, Antiglaucoma; Ophthalmic Agent, Miotic

Synonyms Carbacholine; Carbamylcholine Chloride

Use Lowers intraocular pressure in the treatment of glaucoma; cause miosis during surgery

Local Anesthetic/Vasoconstrictor Precautions No information available to require special precautions

Effects on Dental Treatment Ophthalmic use of carbachol has no effect on dental treatment.

Dosage Adults:

Ophthalmic: Instill 1-2 drops up to 3 times/day

Intraocular: 0.5 mL instilled into anterior chamber before or after securing sutures

Mechanism of Action Synthetic direct-acting cholinergic agent that causes miosis by stimulating muscarinic receptors in the eye

(Continued)

Carbachol *(Continued)*

Other Adverse Effects 1% to 10%: Ocular: Blurred vision, eye pain

Drug Interactions NSAIDs may reduce carbachol's effect.

Drug Uptake

Ophthalmic instillation:

Onset of miositic effect: 10-20 minutes

Duration of reduction in IOP: 4-8 hours

Intraocular administration:

Onset of miositic effect: 2-5 minutes

Duration: 24 hours

Pregnancy Risk Factor C

Generic Available No

Carbamazepine (kar ba MAZ e peen)

Related Information

Dental Drug Interactions: Update on Drug Combinations Requiring Special Considerations *on page 1434*

U.S. Brand Names Carbatrol®; Epitol®; Tegretol®; Tegretol®-XR

Canadian Brand Names Apo®-Carbamazepine; Gen-Carbamazepine CR; Novo-Carbamaz; Nu-Carbamazepine®; PMS-Carbamazepine; Taro-Carbamazepin; Tegretol®

Mexican Brand Names Carbazep; Carbazina; Clostedal®; Neugeron; Tegretol®

Pharmacologic Category Anticonvulsant, Miscellaneous

Synonyms CBZ

Use

Dental: Relief of pain in trigeminal or glossopharyngeal neuralgia

Medical: Prophylaxis of partial seizures with complex symptomatology (psychomotor, temporal lobe), generalized tonic-clonic seizures (grand mal), mixed seizure patterns

Unlabeled/Investigational: Treatment of bipolar disorders and other affective disorders, resistant schizophrenia, ethanol withdrawal, restless leg syndrome, psychotic behavior associated with dementia, post-traumatic stress disorders

Local Anesthetic/Vasoconstrictor Precautions No information available to require special precautions

Effects on Dental Treatment Some patients may experience sore throat or mouth ulcers.

Dosage Oral (dosage must be adjusted according to patient's response and serum concentration):

Children:

<6 years: Initial: 5 mg/kg/day; dosage may be increased every 5-7 days to 10 mg/kg/day; then up to 20 mg/kg/day if necessary; administer in 2-4 divided doses

6-12 years: Initial: 100 mg twice daily or 10 mg/kg/day in 2 divided doses; increase by 100 mg/day at weekly intervals depending upon response; usual maintenance: 20-30 mg/kg/day in 2-4 divided doses (maximum dose: 1000 mg/day)

Children >12 years and Adults: 200 mg twice daily to start, increase by 200 mg/day at weekly intervals until therapeutic levels achieved; usual dose: 400-1200 mg/day in 2-4 divided doses; maximum dose: 12-15 years: 1000 mg/day, >15 years: 1200 mg/day; some patients have required up to 1.6-2.4 g/day

Trigeminal or glossopharyngeal neuralgia: Initial: 100 mg twice daily with food, gradually increasing in increments of 100 mg twice daily as needed; usual maintenance: 400-800 mg daily in 2 divided doses; maximum dose: 1200 mg/day

Elderly: 100 mg 1-2 times daily, increase in increments of 100 mg/day at weekly intervals until therapeutic level is achieved; usual dose: 400-1000 mg/day

Dosing adjustment in renal impairment: Cl_{cr} <10 mL/minute: Administer 75% of dose

Mechanism of Action In addition to anticonvulsant effects, carbamazepine has anticholinergic, antineuralgic, antidiuretic, muscle relaxant and antiarrhythmic properties; may depress activity in the nucleus ventralis of the thalamus or decrease synaptic transmission or decrease summation of temporal stimulation leading to neural discharge by limiting influx of sodium ions across cell membrane or other unknown mechanisms; stimulates the release of ADH and potentiates its action in promoting reabsorption of water; chemically related to tricyclic antidepressants

Other Adverse Effects Frequency not defined:

Cardiovascular: Edema, CHF, syncope, bradycardia, hypertension or hypotension, AV block, arrhythmias, thrombophlebitis, thromboembolism, lymphadenopathy

Central nervous system: Sedation, dizziness, fatigue, ataxia, confusion, headache, slurred speech, aseptic meningitis (case report)

Dermatologic: Rash, urticaria, toxic epidermal necrolysis, Stevens-Johnson syndrome, photosensitivity reaction, alterations in skin pigmentation, exfoliative dermatitis, erythema multiforme, purpura, alopecia

Endocrine & metabolic: Hyponatremia, SIADH, fever, chills

Gastrointestinal: Nausea, vomiting, gastric distress, abdominal pain, diarrhea, constipation, anorexia, pancreatitis

Genitourinary: Urinary retention, urinary frequency, azotemia, renal failure, impotence

Hematologic: Aplastic anemia, agranulocytosis, eosinophilia, leukopenia, pancytopenia, thrombocytopenia, bone marrow suppression, acute intermittent porphyria, leukocytosis

Hepatic: Hepatitis, abnormal LFTs, jaundice, hepatic failure

Neuromuscular & skeletal: Peripheral neuritis

Ocular: Blurred vision, nystagmus, lens opacities, conjunctivitis

Otic: Tinnitus, hyperacusis

Miscellaneous: Hypersensitivity (including multiorgan reactions, may include vasculitis, disorders mimicking lymphoma, eosinophilia, hepatosplenomegaly), diaphoresis

Contraindications Hypersensitivity to carbamazepine or any component of the formulation; may have cross-sensitivity with tricyclic antidepressants; marrow depression; MAO inhibitor use; pregnancy (may harm fetus)

Warnings/Precautions MAO inhibitors should be discontinued for a minimum of 14 days before carbamazepine is begun; administer with caution to patients with history of cardiac damage, hepatic or renal disease; potentially fatal blood cell abnormalities have been reported following treatment; patients with a previous history of adverse hematologic reaction to any drug may be at increased risk; early detection of hematologic change is important; advise patients of early signs and symptoms including fever, sore throat, mouth ulcers, infections, easy bruising, petechial or purpuric hemorrhage; carbamazepine is not effective in absence, myoclonic or akinetic seizures; exacerbation of certain seizure types have been seen after initiation of carbamazepine therapy in children with mixed seizure disorders. Elderly may have increased risk of SIADH-like syndrome. Carbamazepine has mild anticholinergic activity; use with caution in patients with increased intraocular pressure (monitor closely), or sensitivity to anticholinergic effects (urinary retention, constipation). Drug should be discontinued if there are any signs of hypersensitivity.

Drug Interactions CYP2C8 and 3A3/4 enzyme substrate; CYP1A2, 2C, and 3A3/4 inducer. **Note:** Carbamazepine (CBZ) is a heteroinducer. It induces its own metabolism as well as the metabolism of other drugs. If CBZ is added to a drug regimen, serum concentration may decrease. Conversely, if CBZ is part of an ongoing regimen and it is discontinued, elevated concentrations of the other drugs may result.

Acetaminophen: Carbamazepine may enhance hepatotoxic potential of acetaminophen; risk is greater in acetaminophen overdose

Antipsychotics: Carbamazepine may enhance the metabolism (decrease the efficacy) of antipsychotics; monitor for altered response; dose adjustment may be needed

Barbiturates: May reduce serum concentration of carbamazepine; monitor

Benzodiazepines: Serum concentrations and effect of benzodiazepines may be reduced by carbamazepine; monitor for decreased effect

Calcium channel blockers: Diltiazem and verapamil may increase carbamazepine levels, due to enzyme inhibition (see below); other calcium channel blockers (felodipine) may be decreased by carbamazepine due to enzyme induction

Chlorpromazine: **Note:** Carbamazepine suspension is incompatible with chlorpromazine solution. Schedule carbamazepine suspension at least 1-2 hours apart from other liquid medicinals.

Corticosteroids: Metabolism may be increased by carbamazepine

Cyclosporine (and other immunosuppressants): Carbamazepine may enhance the metabolism of immunosuppressants, decreasing its clinical effect; includes both cyclosporine and tacrolimus

CYP2C8/9 inhibitors: Serum levels and/or toxicity of carbamazepine may be increased; inhibitors include amiodarone, cimetidine, fluvoxamine, some NSAIDs, metronidazole, ritonavir, sulfonamides, troglitazone, valproic acid, and zafirlukast; monitor for increased effect/toxicity

CYP3A3/4 inhibitors: Serum level and/or toxicity of carbamazepine may be increased; inhibitors include amiodarone, cimetidine, clarithromycin, erythromycin, delavirdine, diltiazem, dirithromycin, disulfiram, fluoxetine, fluvoxamine, grapefruit juice, indinavir, itraconazole, ketoconazole, metronidazole, nefazodone, nevirapine, propoxyphene, quinine, quinupristin-dalfopristin, ritonavir, saquinavir, ticlopidine, verapamil, zafirlukast, zileuton; monitor for altered effects; a decrease in carbamazepine dosage may be required

Danazol: May increase serum concentration of carbamazepine; monitor

Doxycycline: Carbamazepine may enhance the metabolism of doxycycline, decreasing its clinical effect

Ethosuximide: Serum levels may be reduced by carbamazepine

Felbamate: May increase carbamazepine levels and toxicity (increased epoxide metabolite concentrations); carbamazepine may decrease felbamate levels due to enzyme induction

Immunosuppressants: Carbamazepine may enhance the metabolism of immunosuppressants, decreasing its clinical effect; includes both cyclosporine and tacrolimus

(Continued)

Carbamazepine *(Continued)*

Isoniazid: May increase the serum concentration and toxicity of carbamazepine; in addition, carbamazepine may increase the hepatic toxicity of isoniazid (INH)

Isotretinoin: May decrease the effect of carbamazepine

Lamotrigine: Increases the epoxide metabolite of carbamazepine resulting in toxicity; carbamazepine increases the metabolism of lamotrigine

Lithium: Neurotoxicity may result in patients receiving concurrent carbamazepine

Loxapine: May increase concentrations of epoxide metabolite and toxicity of carbamazepine

Methadone: Carbamazepine may enhance the metabolism of methadone resulting in methadone withdrawal

Methylphenidate: concurrent use of carbamazepine may reduce the therapeutic effect of methylphenidate; limited documentation; monitor for decreased effect

Neuromuscular blocking agents, nondepolarizing: Effects may be of shorter duration when administered to patients receiving carbamazepine

Oral contraceptives: Metabolism may be increased by carbamazepine, resulting in a loss of efficacy

Phenytoin: Carbamazepine levels may be decreased by phenytoin; metabolism may be altered by carbamazepine

SSRIs: Metabolism may be increased by carbamazepine (due to enzyme induction)

Theophylline: Serum levels may be reduced by carbamazepine

Thioridazine: **Note:** Carbamazepine suspension is incompatible with thioridazine liquid. Schedule carbamazepine suspension at least 1-2 hours apart from other liquid medicinals.

Thyroid: Serum levels may be reduced by carbamazepine

Tramadol: Tramadol's risk of seizures may be increased with TCAs (carbamazepine may be associated with similar risk due to chemical similarity to TCAs)

Tricyclic antidepressants: May increase serum concentration of carbamazepine; carbamazepine may decrease concentrations of tricyclics due to enzyme induction

Valproic acid: Serum levels may be reduced by carbamazepine; carbamazepine levels may also be altered by valproic acid

Warfarin: Carbamazepine may inhibit the hypoprothrombinemic effects of oral anticoagulants via increased metabolism; this combination should generally be avoided

Dietary/Ethanol/Herb Considerations

Ethanol: Avoid use; may increase CNS depression.

Food: Administer with food to reduce GI upset; food may increase serum concentration. Avoid grapefruit products; may increase serum concentration.

Herb/Nutraceutical: Avoid evening primrose; decreases seizure threshold. Avoid gotu kola, kava, SAMe, St John's wort, and valerian; may increase CNS depression.

Drug Uptake

Onset of action: Steady-state: Several days

Absorption: Slow from GI tract

Half-life, elimination: Initial: 18-55 hours; Multiple dosing: Children: 8-14 hours; Adults: 12-17 hours

Time to peak: Unpredictable, 4-8 hours

Pregnancy Risk Factor D

Breast-feeding Considerations May be taken while breast-feeding

Dosage Forms CAP, extended release: 200 mg, 300 mg. **SUSP, oral:** 100 mg/5 mL (450 mL). **TAB:** 200 mg. **TAB, chewable:** 100 mg. **TAB, extended release:** 100 mg, 200 mg, 400 mg

Generic Available Yes

Carbamide Peroxide (KAR ba mide per OKS ide)

Related Information

Oral Rinse Products *on page 1462*

U.S. Brand Names Auro® Ear Drops [OTC]; Debrox® Otic [OTC]; E•R•O Ear [OTC]; Gly-Oxide® Oral [OTC]; Mollifene® Ear Wax Removing Formula [OTC]; Murine® Ear Drops [OTC]; Orajel® Perioseptic® [OTC]; Proxigel® Oral [OTC]

Pharmacologic Category Otic Agent, Cerumenolytic

Synonyms Urea Peroxide

Use Dental: Relief of minor swelling of gums, oral mucosal surfaces, and lips including canker sores and dental irritation; emulsify and disperse ear wax

Local Anesthetic/Vasoconstrictor Precautions No information available to require special precautions

Effects on Dental Treatment No effects or complications reported

Dosage Children and Adults:

Gel: Gently massage on affected area 4 times/day; do not drink or rinse mouth for 5 minutes after use

Oral solution (should not be used for >7 days): Oral preparation should not be used in children <3 years of age; apply several drops undiluted on affected area 4 times/day after meals and at bedtime; expectorate after 2-3 minutes **or** place 10 drops onto tongue, mix with saliva, swish for several minutes, expectorate

Otic:

Children <12 years: Tilt head sideways and individualize the dose according to patient size; 3 drops (range: 1-5 drops) twice daily for up to 4 days, tip of applicator should not enter ear canal; keep drops in ear for several minutes by keeping head tilted and placing cotton in ear

Children ≥12 years and Adults: Tilt head sideways and instill 5-10 drops twice daily up to 4 days, tip of applicator should not enter ear canal; keep drops in ear for several minutes by keeping head tilted and placing cotton in ear

Mechanism of Action Releases hydrogen peroxide which serves as a source of nascent oxygen upon contact with catalase; deodorant action is probably due to inhibition of odor-causing bacteria; softens impacted cerumen due to its foaming action

Other Adverse Effects 1% to 10%:

Dermatologic: Rash

Local: Irritation, redness

Miscellaneous: Superinfections

Contraindications Otic preparation should not be used in patients with a perforated tympanic membrane; ear drainage, ear pain or rash in the ear; do not use otic preparation longer than 4 days; ophthalmic administration; oral preparation should not be used in children <3 years

Warnings/Precautions

Oral: With prolonged use of oral carbamide peroxide, there is a potential for overgrowth of opportunistic organisms; damage to periodontal tissues; delayed wound healing; should not be used for longer than 7 days

Otic: Do not use if ear drainage or discharge, ear pain, irritation, or rash in ear; should not be used for longer than 4 days

Drug Uptake Onset of action: ~24 hours

Pregnancy Risk Factor C

Dosage Forms GEl, oral: 10% (34 g). **SOLN, oral:** 10% (15 mL, 60 mL); 15% (13.3 mL). **SOLN, otic:** 6.5% (15 mL, 30 mL)

Generic Available Yes

Carbastat® *see* Carbachol *on page 215*

Carbatrol® *see* Carbamazepine *on page 216*

Carbaxefed DM RF *see* Carbinoxamine, Pseudoephedrine, and Dextromethorphan *on page 221*

Carbaxefed RF *see* Carbinoxamine and Pseudoephedrine *on page 221*

Carbenicillin (kar ben i SIL in)

U.S. Brand Names Geocillin®

Mexican Brand Names Carbecin

Pharmacologic Category Antibiotic, Penicillin

Synonyms Carbenicillin Indanyl Sodium; Carindacillin

Use Treatment of serious urinary tract infections and prostatitis caused by susceptible gram-negative aerobic bacilli or mixed aerobic-anaerobic bacterial infections excluding those secondary to *Klebsiella* sp and *Serratia marcescens*

Local Anesthetic/Vasoconstrictor Precautions No information available to require special precautions

Effects on Dental Treatment Prolonged use of penicillins may lead to development of oral candidiasis.

Dosage Oral:

Children: 30-50 mg/kg/day divided every 6 hours; maximum dose: 2-3 g/day

Adults: 1-2 tablets every 6 hours for urinary tract infections or 2 tablets every 6 hours for prostatitis

Mechanism of Action Inhibits bacterial cell wall synthesis by binding to one or more of the penicillin binding proteins (PBPs); which in turn inhibits the final transpeptidation step of peptidoglycan synthesis in bacterial cell walls, thus inhibiting cell wall biosynthesis. Bacteria eventually lyse due to ongoing activity of cell wall autolytic enzymes (autolysins and murein hydrolases) while cell wall assembly is arrested.

Other Adverse Effects

>10%: Gastrointestinal: Diarrhea

1% to 10%: Gastrointestinal: Nausea, bad taste, vomiting, flatulence, glossitis

Drug Interactions

Increased Effect/Toxicity: Increased bleeding effects if taken with high doses of heparin or oral anticoagulants. Aminoglycosides may be synergistic against selected organisms. Probenecid and disulfiram may increase levels of penicillins (carbenicillin). Effects of warfarin may be increased.

Decreased Effect: Decreased efficacy of oral contraceptives is possible with carbenicillin. Decreased effectiveness with tetracyclines.

Drug Uptake

Absorption: Oral: 30% to 40%

(Continued)

Carbenicillin *(Continued)*

Half-life, elimination:

Children: 0.8-1.8 hours

Adults: 1-1.5 hours; Renal Insufficiency: 10-20 hours

Time to peak (dependent on renal function): 0.5-2 hours; serum concentration following oral absorption are inadequate for treatment of systemic infections

Pregnancy Risk Factor B

Generic Available No

Carbidopa (kar bi DOE pa)

U.S. Brand Names Lodosyn®

Pharmacologic Category Anti-Parkinson's Agent, Dopamine Agonist

Use Given with levodopa in the treatment of parkinsonism to enable a lower dosage of levodopa to be used and a more rapid response to be obtained and to decrease side-effects; for details of administration and dosage, see Levodopa; has no effect without levodopa

Local Anesthetic/Vasoconstrictor Precautions No information available to require special precautions

Effects on Dental Treatment Dopaminergic therapy in Parkinson's disease includes the use of carbidopa in combination with levodopa. Carbidopa/levodopa combination is associated with orthostatic hypotension. Patients medicated with this drug combination should be carefully assisted from the chair and observed for signs of orthostatic hypotension.

Dosage Adults: Oral: 70-100 mg/day; maximum daily dose: 200 mg

Mechanism of Action A peripheral decarboxylase inhibitor with little or no pharmacological activity when given alone in usual doses; inhibits the peripheral decarboxylation of levodopa to dopamine; and as it does not cross the blood-brain barrier, unlike levodopa, effective brain concentrations of dopamine are produced with lower doses of levodopa. At the same time reduced peripheral formation of dopamine reduces peripheral side-effects, notably nausea and vomiting, and cardiac arrhythmias, although the dyskinesias and adverse mental effects associated with levodopa therapy tend to develop earlier.

Other Adverse Effects Associated with concomitant administration with levodopa:

>10%: Central nervous system: Anxiety, confusion, nervousness, mental depression

1% to 10%:

Cardiovascular: Orthostatic hypotension, palpitations, cardiac arrhythmias

Central nervous system: Memory loss, nervousness, insomnia, fatigue, hallucinations, ataxia, dystonic movements

Gastrointestinal: Nausea, vomiting, GI bleeding

Ocular: Blurred vision

Drug Interactions Interactions apply to carbidopa/levodopa combination therapy:

Antacids: Levodopa absorption may be increased; monitor

Anticholinergics: May reduce the efficacy of levodopa, possibly due to reduced GI absorption (also see tricyclic antidepressants); limited evidence of clinical significance; monitor

Antipsychotics: May inhibit the antiparkinsonian effects of levodopa via dopamine receptor blockade; use antipsychotics with low dopamine blockade (clozapine, olanzapine, quetiapine)

Benzodiazepines: May inhibit the antiparkinsonian effects of levodopa; monitor for reduced effect

Clonidine: May reduce the efficacy of levodopa; monitor

Dextromethorphan: Toxic reactions have occurred with dextromethorphan

Furazolidone: May increase the effect/toxicity of levodopa; hypertensive episodes have been reported; monitor

Iron salts: Binds levodopa and reduces its bioavailability; separate doses of iron and levodopa

Linezolid: Due to MAO inhibition (see note on MAO inhibitors), this agent is best avoided

MAO inhibitors: Concurrent use of levodopa with nonselective MAO inhibitors may result in hypertensive reactions via an increased storage and release of dopamine, norepinephrine, or both; use with carbidopa to minimize reactions if combination is necessary, otherwise avoid combination.

L-methionine: May inhibit levodopa's antiparkinsonian effects; monitor for reduced effect

Metoclopramide: May increase the absorption/effect of levodopa; hypertensive episodes have been reported. Levodopa antagonizes metoclopramide's effects on lower esophageal sphincter pressure. Avoid use of metoclopramide for reflux, monitor response to levodopa carefully if used.

Methyldopa: May potentiate the effects of levodopa; levodopa may increase the hypotensive response to methyldopa; monitor

Papaverine: May decrease the efficacy of levodopa; includes other similar agents (ethaverine); monitor

Penicillamine: May increase serum concentration of levodopa; monitor for increased effect

Phenytoin: May inhibit levodopa's antiparkinsonian effects; monitor for reduced effect

Pyridoxine: May inhibit levodopa's antiparkinsonian effects; monitor for reduced effect

Spiramycin: May inhibit levodopa's antiparkinsonian effects; monitor for reduced effect

Tacrine: May inhibit the effects of levodopa via enhanced cholinergic activity; monitor for reduced effect

Tricyclic antidepressants: May decrease the absorption (bioavailability) of levodopa; rare hypertensive episodes have also been attributed to this combination

Drug Uptake

Absorption: 40% to 70%; rapid but incomplete from GI tract

Half-life, elimination: 1-2 hours

Pregnancy Risk Factor C

Generic Available No

Carbinoxamine and Pseudoephedrine

(kar bi NOKS a meen & soo doe e FED rin)

U.S. Brand Names Andehist NR Drops; Carbaxefed RF; Hydro-Tussin™-CBX; Palgic®-D; Palgic®-DS; Rondec® Drops; Rondec® Tablets; Rondec-TR®

Pharmacologic Category Adrenergic Agonist Agent; Antihistamine, H_1 Blocker; Decongestant

Synonyms Pseudoephedrine and Carbinoxamine

Use Temporary relief of nasal congestion, running nose, sneezing, itching of nose or throat, and itchy, watery eyes due to the common cold, hay fever, or other respiratory allergies

Local Anesthetic/Vasoconstrictor Precautions Pseudoephedrine is a sympathomimetic which has potential to enhance vasoconstrictor effects of epinephrine; use local anesthetic with vasoconstrictor with caution

Effects on Dental Treatment 1% to 10%: Xerostomia; disappears with discontinuation

Dosage Oral:

- Children:
  - Drops: 1-18 months: 0.25-1 mL 4 times/day
  - Syrup:
    - 18 months to 6 years: 2.5 mL 3-4 times/day
    - >6 years: 5 mL 2-4 times/day
- Adults:
  - Liquid: 5 mL 4 times/day
  - Tablets: 1 tablet 4 times/day

Mechanism of Action Carbinoxamine competes with histamine for H_1-receptor sites on effector cells in the GI tract, blood vessels, and respiratory tract

Other Adverse Effects

- >10%:
  - Central nervous system: Slight to moderate drowsiness
  - Respiratory: Thickening of bronchial secretions
- 1% to 10%:
  - Central nervous system: Headache, fatigue, nervousness, dizziness
  - Gastrointestinal: Appetite increase, weight gain, nausea, diarrhea, abdominal pain, xerostomia
  - Neuromuscular & skeletal: Arthralgia
  - Respiratory: Pharyngitis

Drug Interactions Increased effect/toxicity with barbiturates, tricyclic antidepressants, MAO inhibitors, and ethanolamine antihistamines

Pregnancy Risk Factor C

Generic Available Yes

Carbinoxamine, Pseudoephedrine, and Dextromethorphan

(kar bi NOKS a meen, soo doe e FED rin, & deks troe meth OR fan)

U.S. Brand Names Andehist DM NR Drops; Carbaxefed DM RF; Rondec®-DM Drops

Pharmacologic Category Antihistamine/Decongestant/Antitussive

Synonyms Carbinoxamine, Dextromethorphan, and Pseudoephedrine; Dextromethorphan, Carbinoxamine, and Pseudoephedrine; Dextromethorphan, Pseudoephedrine, and Carbinoxamine; Pseudoephedrine, Carbinoxamine, and Dextromethorphan; Pseudoephedrine, Dextromethorphan, and Carbinoxamine

Use Relief of coughs and upper respiratory symptoms, including nasal congestion, associated with allergy or the common cold

Local Anesthetic/Vasoconstrictor Precautions Use with caution since pseudoephedrine is a sympathomimetic amine which could interact with epinephrine to cause a pressor response

(Continued)

Carbinoxamine, Pseudoephedrine, and Dextromethorphan *(Continued)*

Effects on Dental Treatment ≤10%: Tachycardia, palpitations, xerostomia; use vasoconstrictor with caution

Dosage

Infants: Drops:

1-3 months: 1/4 mL 4 times/day

3-6 months: 1/2 mL 4 times/day

6-9 months: 3/4 mL 4 times/day

9-18 months: 1 mL 4 times/day

Children 1½ to 6 years: Syrup: 2.5 mL 4 times/day

Children >6 years and Adults: Syrup: 5 mL 4 times/day

Mechanism of Action Carbinoxamine competes with histamine for H_1-receptor sites on effector cells in the GI tract, blood vessels, and respiratory tract; pseudoephedrine, a sympathomimetic amine and isomer of ephedrine, acts as a decongestant in respiratory tract mucous membranes with less vasoconstrictor action than ephedrine in normotensive individuals; dextromethorphan, a non-narcotic antitussive, increases cough threshold by its activity on the medulla oblongata.

Warnings/Precautions Research on chicken embryos exposed to concentrations of dextromethorphan relative to those typically taken by humans has shown to cause birth defects and fetal death; more study is needed, but it is suggested that pregnant women should be advised not to use dextromethorphan-containing medications

Pregnancy Risk Factor C

Generic Available Yes

Carbocaine® *see* Mepivacaine *on page 764*

Carbocaine® 2% with Neo-Cobefrin® *see* Mepivacaine and Levonordefrin *on page 765*

Carbocaine® 3% *see* Mepivacaine Dental Anesthetic *on page 767*

Carbol-Fuchsin Solution (kar bol-FOOK sin soe LOO shun)

U.S. Brand Names Castellani Paint Modified

Pharmacologic Category Antifungal Agent, Topical

Synonyms Castellani Paint

Use Treatment of superficial mycotic infections

Local Anesthetic/Vasoconstrictor Precautions No information available to require special precautions

Effects on Dental Treatment No effects or complications reported

Dosage Apply to affected area 2-4 times/day

Generic Available No

Carboplatin (KAR boe pla tin)

U.S. Brand Names Paraplatin®

Canadian Brand Names Paraplatin-AQ

Mexican Brand Names Blastocarb; Carboplat; Carbotec®; Paraplatin®

Pharmacologic Category Antineoplastic Agent, Alkylating Agent

Synonyms CBDCA

Use Initial treatment of ovarian cancer; secondary treatment of advanced ovarian cancer

Unlabeled/Investigational: Lung cancer, head and neck cancer, endometrial cancer, esophageal cancer, bladder cancer, breast cancer, cervical cancer, CNS tumors, germ cell tumors, osteogenic sarcoma, and high-dose therapy with stem cell/bone marrow support

Local Anesthetic/Vasoconstrictor Precautions No information available to require special precautions

Effects on Dental Treatment >10%: Stomatitis

Mechanism of Action Analogue of cisplatin which covalently binds to DNA; possible cross-linking and interference with the function of DNA

Other Adverse Effects

>10%:

Dermatologic: Alopecia (includes other agents in combination with carboplatin)

Endocrine & metabolic: Hypomagnesemia, hypokalemia, hyponatremia, hypocalcemia; less severe than those seen after cisplatin (usually asymptomatic)

Gastrointestinal: Nausea, vomiting

Hematologic: Myelosuppression is dose-related and is the dose-limiting toxicity; thrombocytopenia is the predominant manifestation, with a reported incidence of 37% in patients receiving 400 mg/m^2 as a single agent and 80% in patients receiving 520 mg/m^2; leukopenia has been reported in 27% to 38% of patients receiving carboplatin as a single agent

Nadir: ~21 days following a single dose

Hepatic: Increased alkaline phosphatase, AST (usually mild and reversible)

Otic: Hearing loss at high tones (above speech ranges) has been reported in up to 19% in one series; clinically important ototoxicity is not usually seen; routine audiometric testing is not recommended

Renal: Elevations in creatinine and BUN have been reported; most of them are mild and they are commonly reversible; considerably less nephrotoxic than cisplatin

1% to 10%: Neuromuscular & skeletal: Peripheral neuropathy (4% to 6%; up to 10% in older and/or previously-treated patients)

Drug Interactions Increased Effect/Toxicity: Nephrotoxic drugs, aminoglycosides increase risk of ototoxicity. When administered as sequential infusions, observational studies indicate a potential for increased toxicity when platinum derivatives (carboplatin, cisplatin) are administered before taxane derivatives (docetaxel, paclitaxel).

Drug Uptake Half-life, elimination: Terminal: 22-40 hours; Cl_{cr} >60 mL/minute: 2.5-5.9 hours

Pregnancy Risk Factor D

Generic Available No

Carboprost Tromethamine (KAR boe prost tro METH a meen)

U.S. Brand Names Hemabate™

Canadian Brand Names Hemabate™

Pharmacologic Category Abortifacient; Prostaglandin

Synonyms Carboprost

Use Termination of pregnancy

Unlabeled/Investigational: Hemorrhagic cystitis

Local Anesthetic/Vasoconstrictor Precautions No information available to require special precautions

Effects on Dental Treatment No effects or complications reported

Dosage Adults: I.M.:

Abortion: 250 mcg to start, 250 mcg at 1½-hour to 3½-hour intervals depending on uterine response; a 500 mcg dose may be given if uterine response is not adequate after several 250 mcg doses; do not exceed 12 mg total dose

Refractory postpartum uterine bleeding: Initial: 250 mcg; may repeat at 15- to 90-minute intervals to a total dose of 2 mg

Bladder irrigation for hemorrhagic cystitis **(refer to individual protocols)**: [0.4-1.0 mg/dL as solution] 50 mL instilled into bladder 4 times/day for 1 hour

Mechanism of Action A prostaglandin similar to prostaglandin F_2 alpha (dinoprost) except for the addition of a methyl group at the C-15 position; this substitution produces longer duration of activity than dinoprost. Carboprost stimulates uterine contractility which usually results in expulsion of the products of conception and is used to induce abortion between 13-20 weeks of pregnancy. Hemostasis at the placentation site is achieved through the myometrial contractions produced by carboprost.

Other Adverse Effects

>10%: Gastrointestinal: Nausea (33%)

1% to 10%:

- Cardiovascular: Flushing (7%)
- Central nervous system: Dizziness, headache
- Gastrointestinal: Stomach cramps

Drug Interactions Toxicity may be increased by oxytocic agents.

Pregnancy Risk Factor X

Generic Available No

Carboptic® *see* Carbachol *on page 215*

Carboxymethylcellulose (kar boks ee meth il SEL yoo lose)

U.S. Brand Names Cellufresh® [OTC]; Celluvisc® [OTC]

Canadian Brand Names Celluvisc™; Refresh Plus™; Refresh Tears™

Pharmacologic Category Ophthalmic Agent, Miscellaneous

Synonyms Carbose D; Carboxymethylcellulose Sodium

Use Preservative-free artificial tear substitute

Local Anesthetic/Vasoconstrictor Precautions No information available to require special precautions

Effects on Dental Treatment No effects or complications reported

Dosage Adults: Ophthalmic: Instill 1-2 drops into eye(s) 3-4 times/day

Generic Available Yes

Cardene® *see* NiCARdipine *on page 862*

Cardene® I.V. *see* NiCARdipine *on page 862*

Cardene® SR *see* NiCARdipine *on page 862*

Cardio-Green® *see* Indocyanine Green *on page 634*

Cardioquin® *see* Quinidine *on page 1034*

Cardizem® *see* Diltiazem *on page 394*

Cardizem® CD *see* Diltiazem *on page 394*

Cardizem® SR *see* Diltiazem *on page 394*
Cardura® *see* Doxazosin *on page 413*

Carisoprodol (kar i soe PROE dole)

Related Information

Carisoprodol and Aspirin *on page 224*

U.S. Brand Names Soma®

Canadian Brand Names Soma®

Pharmacologic Category Skeletal Muscle Relaxant

Synonyms Carisoprodate; Isobamate

Use

Dental: Treatment of muscle spasm associated with acute temporomandibular joint pain

Medical: Skeletal muscle relaxant

Local Anesthetic/Vasoconstrictor Precautions No information available to require special precautions

Effects on Dental Treatment No effects or complications reported

Dosage Adults: Oral: 350 mg 3-4 times/day; take last dose at bedtime; compound: 1-2 tablets 4 times/day

Mechanism of Action Precise mechanism is not yet clear, but many effects have been ascribed to its central depressant actions.

Other Adverse Effects

>10%: Central nervous system: Drowsiness

1% to 10%:

- Cardiovascular: Tachycardia, tightness in chest, flushing of face, syncope
- Central nervous system: Mental depression, allergic fever, dizziness, lightheadedness, headache, paradoxical CNS stimulation
- Dermatologic: Angioedema
- Gastrointestinal: Nausea, vomiting, stomach cramps
- Neuromuscular & skeletal: Trembling
- Ocular: Burning eyes
- Respiratory: Dyspnea
- Miscellaneous: Hiccups

<1%: Ataxia, rash, urticaria, erythema multiforme, aplastic anemia, leukopenia, eosinophilia, blurred vision

Contraindications Hypersensitivity to carisoprodol, meprobamate, or any component of their formulation; acute intermittent porphyria

Warnings/Precautions Use with caution in renal and hepatic dysfunction

Drug Interactions CYP2C19 enzyme substrate

Increased Toxicity: CNS depressants, phenothiazines

Dietary/Ethanol/Herb Considerations

Ethanol: Avoid use; may increase CNS depression.

Herb/Nutraceutical: Avoid gotu kola, kava, SAMe, St John's wort, and valerian; may increase CNS depression.

Drug Uptake

Onset of action: ≤30 minutes

Duration: 4-6 hours

Half-life, elimination: 8 hours

Time to peak: 4 hours

Pregnancy Risk Factor C

Dosage Forms TAB: 350 mg

Generic Available Yes

Carisoprodol and Aspirin (kar i soe PROE dole & AS pir in)

U.S. Brand Names Soma® Compound

Pharmacologic Category Skeletal Muscle Relaxant

Synonyms Aspirin and Carisoprodol

Use Skeletal muscle relaxant

Local Anesthetic/Vasoconstrictor Precautions No information available to require special precautions

Effects on Dental Treatment

Avoid aspirin, if possible, for 1 week prior to surgery due to possibility of postoperative bleeding.

Use with caution in impaired hepatic function; use with caution in patients with platelet and bleeding disorders, renal dysfunction, erosive gastritis, or peptic ulcer disease, previous nonreaction does not guarantee future safe taking of medication; do not use aspirin in children <16 years of age for chickenpox or flu symptoms due to the association with Reye's syndrome

Elderly are a high-risk population for adverse effects from nonsteroidal anti-inflammatory agents. As much as 60% of elderly with GI complications to NSAIDs can develop peptic ulceration and/or hemorrhage asymptomatically. Also, concomitant disease and drug use contribute to the risk for GI adverse effects. Use lowest effective dose for shortest period possible. Consider renal function decline with age. Use with caution in patients with history of asthma.

Dosage Adults: Oral: 1-2 tablets 4 times/day

Drug Interactions See Carisoprodol *on page 224* and Aspirin *on page 119*

Dietary/Ethanol/Herb Considerations

Ethanol: Avoid use; may enhance gastric mucosal irritation and increase CNS depression.

Herb/Nutraceutical: Avoid gotu kola, kava, SAMe, St John's wort, and valerian; may increase CNS depression.

Drug Uptake See Carisoprodol *on page 224* and Aspirin *on page 119*

Pregnancy Risk Factor C/D (full-dose aspirin in 3rd trimester)

Dosage Forms TAB: Carisoprodol 200 mg and aspirin 325 mg

Generic Available Yes

Carisoprodol, Aspirin, and Codeine

(kar i soe PROE dole, AS pir in, and KOE deen)

U.S. Brand Names Soma® Compound w/Codeine

Pharmacologic Category Skeletal Muscle Relaxant

Synonyms Aspirin, Carisoprodol, and Codeine; Codeine, Aspirin, and Carisoprodol

Use Skeletal muscle relaxant

Local Anesthetic/Vasoconstrictor Precautions No information available to require special precautions

Effects on Dental Treatment Avoid aspirin, if possible, for 1 week prior to surgery due to possibility of postoperative bleeding.

Restrictions C-III

Dosage Adults: Oral: 1 or 2 tablets 4 times/day

Dietary/Ethanol/Herb Considerations

Ethanol: Avoid use; may enhance gastric mucosal irritation and increase CNS depression.

Herb/Nutraceutical: Avoid gotu kola, kava, SAMe, St John's wort, and valerian; may increase CNS depression.

Drug Uptake See Carisoprodol *on page 224*, Aspirin *on page 119* and Codeine *on page 317*

Pregnancy Risk Factor C/D (full-dose aspirin in 3rd trimester)

Dosage Forms TAB: Carisoprodol 200 mg, aspirin 325 mg, and codeine 16 mg

Generic Available Yes

Carmol® [OTC] *see* Urea *on page 1221*

Carmol-HC® *see* Urea and Hydrocortisone *on page 1222*

Carmol® Scalp *see* Sulfacetamide Sodium *on page 1115*

Carmustine (kar MUS teen)

U.S. Brand Names BiCNU®; Gliadel®

Canadian Brand Names BiCNU®

Mexican Brand Names Bicnu®

Pharmacologic Category Antineoplastic Agent, Alkylating Agent

Synonyms BCNU

Use Treatment of brain tumors (glioblastoma, brainstem glioma, medulloblastoma, astrocytoma, ependymoma, and metastatic brain tumors), multiple myeloma, Hodgkin's disease non-Hodgkin's lymphomas, melanoma, lung cancer, colon cancer

Gliadel®: Adjunct to surgery in patients with recurrent glioblastoma multiforme

Local Anesthetic/Vasoconstrictor Precautions No information available to require special precautions

Effects on Dental Treatment No effects or complications reported

Mechanism of Action Interferes with the normal function of DNA by alkylation and cross-linking the strands of DNA, and by possible protein modification

Other Adverse Effects

>10%:

- Cardiovascular: Hypotension with high dose therapy, due to the alcohol content of the diluent
- Central nervous system: Dizziness, ataxia; Wafers: Seizures (54%) postoperatively
- Dermatologic: Pain and burning at the injection site (may be relieved by diluting the drug and infusing it through a fast-running dextrose or saline infusion); phlebitis
- Gastrointestinal: Severe nausea and vomiting, usually begins within 2-4 hours of drug administration and lasts for 4-6 hours. Patients should receive a prophylactic antiemetic regimen including a serotonin (5-HT_3) antagonist and dexamethasone
- Hematologic: Myelosuppression - cumulative, dose-related, delayed, thrombocytopenia is usually more common and more severe than leukopenia
  - Onset: 7-14 days
  - Nadir: 21-35 days
  - Recovery: 42-56 days

(Continued)

Carmustine *(Continued)*

Hepatic: Reversible increases in bilirubin, alkaline phosphatase, and SGOT occur in 20% to 25% of patients

Ocular: Ocular toxicities (transient conjunctival flushing and blurred vision), retinal hemorrhages

Respiratory: Interstitial fibrosis occurs in up to 50% of patients receiving a cumulative dose >1400 mg/m^2, or bone marrow transplantation doses; may be delayed up to 3 years; rare in patients receiving lower doses. A history of lung disease or concomitant bleomycin therapy may increase the risk of this reaction. Patients should have baseline and periodic pulmonary function tests, patients with forced vital capacity (FVC) or carbon monoxide diffusing capacity of the lungs (DLCO) <70% of predicted are at higher risk.

1% to 10%:

Central nervous system: Wafers: Amnesia, aphasia, ataxia, cerebral edema, confusion, convulsion, depression, diplopia, dizziness, headache, hemiplegia, hydrocephalus, insomnia, meningitis, somnolence, stupor

Dermatologic: Facial flushing, probably due to the alcohol diluent; alopecia

Gastrointestinal: Anorexia, constipation, diarrhea, stomatitis

Hematologic: Anemia

Drug Interactions Increased Toxicity: Carmustine given in combination with cimetidine is reported to cause bone marrow depression. Carmustine given in combination with etoposide is reported to cause severe hepatic dysfunction with hyperbilirubinemia, ascites, and thrombocytopenia.

Drug Uptake

Absorption: Highly lipid soluble

Half-life, elimination: Biphasic: Initial: 1.4 minutes; Secondary: 20 minutes (active metabolites: plasma half-life of 67 hours)

Pregnancy Risk Factor D

Generic Available No

Carnitor® *see* Levocarnitine *on page 698*

Carrington Antifungal [OTC] *see* Miconazole *on page 807*

Carteolol (KAR tee oh lole)

Related Information

Cardiovascular Diseases *on page 1308*

U.S. Brand Names Cartrol® Oral; Ocupress® Ophthalmic

Canadian Brand Names Cartrol® Oral; Ocupress® Ophthalmic

Pharmacologic Category Beta Blocker With Intrinsic Sympathomimetic Activity; Ophthalmic Agent, Antiglaucoma

Synonyms Carteolol Hydrochloride

Use Management of hypertension; treatment of chronic open-angle glaucoma and intraocular hypertension

Local Anesthetic/Vasoconstrictor Precautions No information available to require special precautions

Effects on Dental Treatment Noncardioselective beta-blockers (ie, propranolol, nadolol) enhance the pressor response to epinephrine, resulting in hypertension and bradycardia. This has not been reported for carteolol, a cardioselective beta-blocker. Therefore, local anesthetic with vasoconstrictor can be safely used in patients medicated with carteolol. Many nonsteroidal anti-inflammatory drugs such as ibuprofen and indomethacin can reduce the hypotensive effect of beta-blockers after 3 or more weeks of therapy with the NSAID. Short-term NSAID use (ie, 3 days) requires no special precautions in patients taking beta-blockers

Dosage Adults:

Oral: 2.5 mg as a single daily dose, with a maintenance dose normally 2.5-5 mg once daily; maximum daily dose: 10 mg; doses >10 mg do not increase response and may in fact decrease effect

Ophthalmic: Instill 1 drop in affected eye(s) twice daily

Mechanism of Action Competitively blocks beta$_1$-adrenergic receptors with little or no effect on beta$_2$-receptors except at high doses; exhibits membrane stabilizing and intrinsic sympathomimetic activity; has negative inotropic and chronotropic effects and can significantly slow AV nodal conduction

Other Adverse Effects

Ophthalmic:

>10%: Ocular: Conjunctival hyperemia

1% to 10%: Ocular: Anisocoria, corneal punctate keratitis, corneal staining, decreased corneal sensitivity, eye pain, vision disturbances

Systemic:

>10%:

Central nervous system: Drowsiness, insomnia

Endocrine & metabolic: Decreased sexual ability

1% to 10%:

Cardiovascular: Bradycardia, palpitations, edema, CHF, reduced peripheral circulation

Central nervous system: Mental depression

Gastrointestinal: Diarrhea or constipation, nausea, vomiting, stomach discomfort

Respiratory: Bronchospasm

Miscellaneous: Cold extremities

Drug Interactions

Increased Effect/Toxicity: Carteolol may increase the effects of other drugs which slow AV conduction (digoxin, verapamil, diltiazem), alpha-blockers (prazosin, terazosin), and alpha-adrenergic stimulants (epinephrine, phenylephrine). Carteolol may mask the tachycardia from hypoglycemia caused by insulin and oral hypoglycemics. In patients receiving concurrent therapy, the risk of hypertensive crisis is increased when either clonidine or the beta-blocker is withdrawn. Reserpine has been shown to enhance the effect of beta-blockers. Beta-blockers may increase the action or levels of disopyramide, nondepolarizing muscle relaxants, and theophylline although the effects are difficult to predict.

Decreased Effect: Decreased effect of beta-blockers with aluminum salts, barbiturates, calcium salts, cholestyramine, colestipol, NSAIDs, penicillins (ampicillin), rifampin, salicylates, and sulfinpyrazone due to decreased bioavailability and plasma concentrations. Beta-blockers may decrease the effect of sulfonylureas (possibly hyperglycemia). Nonselective beta-blockers blunt the effect of beta-2 adrenergic agonists (albuterol).

Drug Uptake

Onset of action: Oral: 1-1.5 hours

Absorption: Oral: 80%

Duration: 12 hours

Half-life, elimination: 6 hours

Time to peak: 2 hours

Pregnancy Risk Factor C (manufacturer); D (2nd and 3rd trimesters - expert analysis)

Generic Available Yes: Drops

Selected Readings

Foster CA and Aston SJ, "Propranolol-Epinephrine Interaction: A Potential Disaster," *Plast Reconstr Surg*, 1983, 72(1):74-8.

Wong DG, Spence JD, Lamki L, et al, "Effect of Nonsteroidal Anti-inflammatory Drugs on Control of Hypertension of Beta-Blockers and Diuretics," *Lancet*, 1986, 1(8488):997-1001.

Wynn RL, "Dental Nonsteroidal Anti-inflammatory Drugs and Prostaglandin-Based Drug Interactions, Part Two," *Gen Dent*, 1992, 40(2):104, 106, 108.

Wynn RL, "Epinephrine Interactions With Beta-Blockers," *Gen Dent*, 1994, 42(1):16, 18.

Cartia® XT *see* Diltiazem *on page 394*

Cartrol® Oral *see* Carteolol *on page 226*

Carvedilol (KAR ve dil ole)

Related Information

Cardiovascular Diseases *on page 1308*

U.S. Brand Names Coreg®

Canadian Brand Names Coreg™

Mexican Brand Names Dilatrend®

Pharmacologic Category Beta Blocker With Alpha-Blocking Activity

Use Management of hypertension; can be used alone or in combination with other agents, especially thiazide-type diuretics; mild to severe heart failure of ischemic or cardiomyopathic origin following standardized therapy.

Unlabeled/Investigational: Angina pectoris

Local Anesthetic/Vasoconstrictor Precautions Use with caution, epinephrine has interacted with noncardioselective beta-blockers to result in initial hypertensive episode followed by bradycardia

Effects on Dental Treatment Noncardioselective beta-blockers (ie, propranolol, nadolol) enhance the pressor response to epinephrine, resulting in hypertension and bradycardia. Many nonsteroidal anti-inflammatory drugs, such as ibuprofen and indomethacin, can reduce the hypotensive effect of beta-blockers after 3 or more weeks of therapy with the NSAID. Short-term NSAID use (ie, 3 days) requires no special precautions in patients taking beta-blockers.

Dosage Oral: Adults: Reduce dosage if heart rate drops to <55 beats/minute.

Hypertension: 6.25 mg twice daily; if tolerated, dose should be maintained for 1-2 weeks, then increased to 12.5 mg twice daily. Dosage may be increased to a maximum of 25 mg twice daily after 1-2 weeks. Maximum dose: 50 mg/day

Congestive heart failure: 3.125 mg twice daily for 2 weeks; if this dose is tolerated, may increase to 6.25 mg twice daily. Double the dose every 2 weeks to the highest dose tolerated by patient. (Prior to initiating therapy, other heart failure medications should be stabilized and fluid retention minimized.)

Maximum recommended dose:

Mild to moderate heart failure:

<85 kg: 25 mg twice daily

>85 kg: 50 mg twice daily

Severe heart failure: 25 mg twice daily

Angina pectoris (unlabeled use): 25-50 mg twice daily

Dosing adjustment in hepatic impairment: Use is contraindicated

(Continued)

Carvedilol *(Continued)*

Mechanism of Action As a racemic mixture, carvedilol has nonselective beta-adrenoreceptor and alpha-adrenergic blocking activity. No intrinsic sympathomimetic activity has been documented. Associated effects in hypertensive patients include reduction of cardiac output, exercise- or beta agonist-induced tachycardia, reduction of reflex orthostatic tachycardia, vasodilation, decreased peripheral vascular resistance (especially in standing position), decreased renal vascular resistance, reduced plasma renin activity, and increased levels of atrial natriuretic peptide. In CHF, associated effects include decreased pulmonary capillary wedge pressure, decreased pulmonary artery pressure, decreased heart rate, decreased systemic vascular resistance, increased stroke volume index, and decreased right arterial pressure (RAP).

Other Adverse Effects Note: Frequency ranges include data from hypertension and heart failure trials. Higher rates of adverse reactions have generally been noted in patients with CHF. However, the frequency of adverse effects associated with placebo is also increased in this population. Events occurring at a frequency > placebo in clinical trials.

>10%:

- Central nervous system: Dizziness (6% to 32%), fatigue (4% to 24%)
- Endocrine & metabolic: Hyperglycemia (5% to 12%), weight gain (10% to 12%)
- Gastrointestinal: Diarrhea (2% to 12%)
- Neuromuscular & skeletal: Weakness (11%)
- Respiratory: Upper respiratory tract infection (14% to 18%)

1% to 10%:

- Cardiovascular: Bradycardia (2% to 10%), hypotension (9% to 14%), hypertension (3%), AV block (3%), angina (2% to 6%), postural hypotension (2%), syncope (3% to 8%), dependent edema (4%), palpitations, peripheral edema (1% to 7%), generalized edema (5% to 6%)
- Central nervous system: Pain (9%), headache (5% to 8%), fever (3%), paresthesia (2%), somnolence (2%), insomnia (2%), malaise, hypesthesia, vertigo
- Endocrine & metabolic: Gout (6%), hypercholesterolemia (4%), dehydration (2%), hyperkalemia (3%), hypervolemia (2%), hypertriglyceridemia (1%), hyperuricemia, hypoglycemia, hyponatremia
- Gastrointestinal: Nausea (4% to 9%), vomiting (6%), melena, periodontitis
- Genitourinary: Urinary tract infection (2% to 3%), hematuria (3%), impotence
- Hematologic: Thrombocytopenia (1% to 2%), decreased prothrombin, purpura
- Hepatic: Increased transaminases, increased alkaline phosphatase
- Neuromuscular & skeletal: Back pain (2% to 7%), arthralgia (6%), myalgia (3%), muscle cramps
- Ocular: Blurred vision (3% to 5%)
- Renal: Increased BUN (6%), abnormal renal function, albuminuria, glycosuria, increased creatinine (3%), kidney failure
- Respiratory: Sinusitis (5%), bronchitis (5%), pharyngitis (2% to 3%), rhinitis (2%), increased cough (5%)
- Miscellaneous: Infection (2%), injury (3% to 6%), increased diaphoresis (3%), viral infection (2%), allergy, sudden death

Additional events from clinical trials in heart failure patients occurring at a frequency >2% but ≤ the frequency reported in patients receiving placebo: Asthenia, cardiac failure, flatulence, palpitation, arthritis, depression, anemia, coughing, rash, leg cramps, chest pain, dyspepsia.

Warnings/Precautions Initiate cautiously and monitor for possible deterioration in CHF. Adjustment of other medications (ACE inhibitors and/or diuretics) may be required. In severe chronic heart failure, trial patients were excluded if they had cardiac-related rales, ascites, or a serum creatinine >2.8 mg/dL. Discontinue therapy if any evidence of liver injury occurs. Use caution in patients with PVD (can aggravate arterial insufficiency). Use caution with concurrent use of beta-blockers and either verapamil or diltiazem; bradycardia or heart block can occur. Patients with bronchospastic disease should not receive beta-blockers. Use cautiously in diabetics because it can mask prominent hypoglycemic symptoms. Can mask signs of thyrotoxicosis. Use care with anesthetic agents that decrease myocardial function. Safety and efficacy in children <18 years of age have not been established.

Drug Interactions CYP1A2, 2E1, 2C9 (major), 2C19, 2D6 (major), 3A3/4 enzyme substrate

Increased Effect/Toxicity: Clonidine and cimetidine increase the serum concentration and effects of carvedilol. Carvedilol may increase the levels of cyclosporine. Carvedilol may increase the effects of other drugs which slow AV conduction (digoxin, verapamil, diltiazem), alpha-blockers (prazosin, terazosin), and alpha-adrenergic stimulants (epinephrine, phenylephrine). Carvedilol may mask the tachycardia from hypoglycemia caused by insulin and oral hypoglycemics. In patients receiving concurrent therapy, the risk of hypertensive crisis is increased when either clonidine or the beta-blocker is withdrawn. Reserpine has been shown to enhance the effect of beta-blockers. Beta-blockers may increase the action or levels of disopyramide, nondepolarizing muscle relaxants, and theophylline although the effects are difficult to predict.

Decreased Effect: Rifampin may reduce the plasma concentration of carvedilol by up to 70%. Decreased effect of beta-blockers has also occurred with aluminum salts, barbiturates, calcium salts, cholestyramine, colestipol, NSAIDs, penicillins (ampicillin), salicylates, and sulfinpyrazone due to decreased bioavailability and plasma concentrations. Beta-blockers may decrease the effect of sulfonylureas. Nonselective beta-blockers blunt the effect of beta-2 adrenergic agonists (albuterol).

Drug Uptake

Onset of action: 1-2 hours

Absorption: Rapid; food decreases the rate but not extent of absorption; administration with food minimizes risks of orthostatic hypotension

Half-life, elimination: 7-10 hours

Pregnancy Risk Factor C (manufacturer); D (2nd and 3rd trimesters - expert analysis)

Generic Available No

Selected Readings

Foster CA and Aston SJ, "Propranolol-Epinephrine Interaction: A Potential Disaster," *Plast Reconstr Surg*, 1983, 72(1):74-8.

Wong DG, Spence JD, Lamki L, et al, "Effect of Nonsteroidal Anti-inflammatory Drugs on Control of Hypertension of Beta-Blockers and Diuretics," *Lancet*, 1986, 1(8488):997-1001.

Wynn RL, "Dental Nonsteroidal Anti-inflammatory Drugs and Prostaglandin-Based Drug Interactions, Part Two," *Gen Dent*, 1992, 40(2):104, 106, 108.

Wynn RL, "Epinephrine Interactions With Beta-Blockers," *Gen Dent*, 1994, 42(1):16, 18.

Cascara Sagrada (kas KAR a sah GRAH dah)

Pharmacologic Category Laxative, Stimulant

Use Temporary relief of constipation; sometimes used with milk of magnesia ("black and white" mixture)

Local Anesthetic/Vasoconstrictor Precautions No information available to require special precautions

Effects on Dental Treatment No effects or complications reported

Dosage Cascara sagrada fluid extract is 5 times more potent than cascara sagrada aromatic fluid extract.

Oral (aromatic fluid extract):

Children 2-11 years: 2.5 mL/day (range: 1-3 mL) as needed

Children ≥12 years and Adults: 5 mL/day (range: 2-6 mL) as needed at bedtime (1 tablet as needed at bedtime)

Mechanism of Action Direct chemical irritation of the intestinal mucosa resulting in an increased rate of colonic motility and change in fluid and electrolyte secretion

Other Adverse Effects 1% to 10%:

Central nervous system: Faintness

Endocrine & metabolic: Electrolyte and fluid imbalance

Gastrointestinal: Abdominal cramps, nausea, diarrhea

Genitourinary: Discoloration of urine (reddish pink or brown)

Drug Interactions Decreases effect of oral anticoagulants

Drug Uptake

Onset of action: 6-10 hours

Absorption: Oral: Poorly from small intestine

Pregnancy Risk Factor C

Generic Available Yes

Casodex® *see* Bicalutamide *on page 164*

Caspofungin (kas poe FUN jin)

U.S. Brand Names Cancidas®

Mexican Brand Names Cancidas®

Pharmacologic Category Antifungal Agent, Parenteral

Synonyms Caspofungin Acetate

Use Treatment of invasive *Aspergillus* infection in patients who do not tolerate or do not respond to other antifungal therapies (including amphotericin B, lipid formulations of amphotericin B, or itraconazole); has not been studied as an initial therapy for aspergillosis

Local Anesthetic/Vasoconstrictor Precautions No information available to require special precautions

Effects on Dental Treatment No effects or complications reported

Dosage I.V.:

Children: Safety and efficacy in pediatric patients have not been established

Adults: *Aspergillus* infection (invasive):

Initial dose: 70 mg infused slowly (over 1 hour)

Subsequent dosing: 50 mg/day (infused over 1 hour)

Duration of treatment should be determined by patient status and clinical response (limited experience beyond 2 weeks of therapy); efficacy of 70 mg/day dose (in patients not responding to 50 mg/day) has not been adequately studied, although this dose appears to be well tolerated

Patients receiving carbamazepine, dexamethasone, efavirenz, nelfinavir, nevirapine, phenytoin, and rifampin (and possibly other enzyme inducers)

(Continued)

Caspofungin *(Continued)*

may require an increased daily dose of caspofungin (70 mg/day) if response to 50 mg/day is inadequate.

Mechanism of Action Inhibits synthesis of β(1,3)-D-glucan, an essential component of the cell wall of susceptible fungi. Highest activity in regions of active cell growth. Mammalian cells do not require β(1,3)-D-glucan, limiting potential toxicity.

Other Adverse Effects Note: Listing includes some reactions/frequencies noted during investigational use for indications other than *Aspergillus*.

>10%:

- Central nervous system: Headache (up to 11%), fever (3% to 26%)
- Hepatic: Increased serum alkaline phosphatase (3% to 11%), increased transaminases (up to 13%)
- Local: Infusion site reactions (2% to 12%), phlebitis (up to 16%)

1% to 10%:

- Cardiovascular: Flushing (3%), edema (up to 3%)
- Central nervous system: Fever (3%), headache, chills (up to 3%), pain (1% to 5%), paresthesia (1% to 3%)
- Dermatologic: Rash (<1% to 4%), pruritus (2% to 3%), erythema (1% to 2%)
- Endocrine & metabolic: Decreased serum potassium (3%)
- Gastrointestinal: Nausea (3% to 6%), vomiting (1% to 3%), abdominal pain, diarrhea (1% to 4%)
- Hematologic: Increased eosinophils (3%), decreased hemoglobin (3% to 12%), decreased neutrophils (2% to 3%), increased WBC (5% to 6%), anemia (up to 4%)
- Hepatic: Increased serum alkaline phosphatase (3%)
- Local: Infusion site reactions (3%), induration (up to 3%)
- Neuromuscular & skeletal: Myalgia (up to 3%)
- Renal: Proteinuria (5%), hematuria (2%), increased serum creatinine (<1% to 2%), increased urinary WBCs (up to 8%)
- Miscellaneous: Flu-like syndrome (3%)

Drug Interactions

Increased Effect/Toxicity: Concurrent administration of cyclosporine may increase caspofungin concentrations. In limited experience, a high frequency of elevated hepatic serum transaminases was observed.

Decreased Effect: Caspofungin may decrease blood concentrations of tacrolimus. In limited experience, some enzyme inducers decreased the serum concentration of caspofungin.

Drug Uptake Half-life, elimination: Beta: Initial: 9-11 hours; Terminal: 40-50 hours

Pregnancy Risk Factor C

Generic Available No

Castellani Paint Modified *see* Carbol-Fuchsin Solution *on page 222*

Castor Oil (KAS tor oyl)

U.S. Brand Names Emulsoil® [OTC]; Neoloid® [OTC]; Purge® [OTC]

Pharmacologic Category Laxative, Miscellaneous

Synonyms Oleum Ricini

Use Preparation for rectal or bowel examination or surgery; rarely used to relieve constipation; also applied to skin as emollient and protectant

Local Anesthetic/Vasoconstrictor Precautions No information available to require special precautions

Effects on Dental Treatment No effects or complications reported

Dosage Oral:

Liquid:

- Children 2-11 years: 5-15 mL as a single dose
- Children ≥12 years and Adults: 15-60 mL as a single dose

Emulsified:

- 36.4%:
  - Children <2 years: 5-15 mL/dose
  - Children 2-11 years: 7.5-30 mL/dose
  - Children ≥12 years and Adults: 30-60 mL/dose
- 60% to 67%:
  - Children <2 years: 1.25-5 mL
  - Children 2-12 years: 5-15 mL
  - Adults: 15-45 mL
- 95%, mix with 1/2 to 1 full glass liquid:
  - Children: 5-10 mL
  - Adults: 15-60 mL

Mechanism of Action Acts primarily in the small intestine; hydrolyzed to ricinoleic acid which reduces net absorption of fluid and electrolytes and stimulates peristalsis

Other Adverse Effects 1% to 10%:

- Central nervous system: Dizziness
- Endocrine & metabolic: Electrolyte disturbance

Gastrointestinal: Abdominal cramps, nausea, diarrhea

Drug Uptake Onset of action: Oral: 2-6 hours

Pregnancy Risk Factor X

Generic Available Yes

Cataflam® *see* Diclofenac *on page 378*
Catapres® *see* Clonidine *on page 308*
Catapres-TTS®-1 *see* Clonidine *on page 308*
Catapres-TTS®-2 *see* Clonidine *on page 308*
Catapres-TTS®-3 *see* Clonidine *on page 308*
Cathflo™ Activase® *see* Alteplase *on page 59*
Caverject® *see* Alprostadil *on page 58*
Ceclor® *see* Cefaclor *on page 231*
Ceclor® CD *see* Cefaclor *on page 231*
Cecon® [OTC] *see* Ascorbic Acid *on page 117*
Cedax® *see* Ceftibuten *on page 243*
CeeNU® *see* Lomustine *on page 724*

Cefaclor (SEF a klor)

U.S. Brand Names Ceclor®; Ceclor® CD

Canadian Brand Names Apo®-Cefaclor; Ceclor®; Novo-Cefaclor; Nu-Cefaclor; PMS-Cefaclor; Scheinpharm Cefaclor

Mexican Brand Names Ceclor®

Pharmacologic Category Antibiotic, Cephalosporin (Second Generation)

Use

Dental: An alternate antibiotic in treatment of orofacial infections in patients allergic to penicillins; susceptible bacteria including aerobic gram-positive bacteria and anaerobes

Medical: Infections caused by susceptible organisms including *Staphylococcus aureus* and *H. influenzae*; treatment of otitis media, sinusitis, and infections involving the respiratory tract, skin and skin structure, bone and joint, and urinary tract

Local Anesthetic/Vasoconstrictor Precautions No information available to require special precautions

Effects on Dental Treatment No effects or complications reported

Dosage Oral:

Children >1 month: 20-40 mg/kg/day divided every 8-12 hours; maximum dose: 2 g/day (total daily dose may be divided into two doses for treatment of otitis media or pharyngitis)

Adults: 250-500 mg every 8 hours

Extended release tablets: 500 mg every 12 hours for 7 days for acute bacterial exacerbations of secondary infections with chronic bronchitis or 375 mg every 12 hour for 10 days for pharyngitis or tonsillitis or for uncomplicated skin and skin structure infections

Dosing adjustment in renal impairment: Cl_{cr} <50 mL/minute: Administer 50% of dose

Hemodialysis: Moderately dialyzable (20% to 50%)

Mechanism of Action Inhibits bacterial cell wall synthesis by binding to one or more of the penicillin-binding proteins (PBPs) which in turn inhibits the final transpeptidation step of peptidoglycan synthesis in bacterial cell walls, thus inhibiting cell wall biosynthesis. Bacteria eventually lyse due to ongoing activity of cell wall autolytic enzymes (autolysins and murein hydrolases) while cell wall assembly is arrested.

Other Adverse Effects

1% to 10%:

Dermatologic: Rash (maculopapular, erythematous, or morbilliform) (1% to 2%)

Gastrointestinal: Diarrhea (2%)

Hematologic: Eosinophilia (2%)

Hepatic: Elevated transaminases (3%)

<1%: Anaphylaxis, urticaria, pruritus, angioedema, serum-sickness, arthralgia, hepatitis, cholestatic jaundice, Stevens-Johnson syndrome, nausea, vomiting, pseudomembranous colitis, vaginitis, hemolytic anemia, neutropenia, interstitial nephritis, CNS irritability, hyperactivity, agitation, nervousness, insomnia, confusion, dizziness, hallucinations, somnolence, seizures, prolonged PT

Reactions reported with other cephalosporins include fever, abdominal pain, superinfection, renal dysfunction, toxic nephropathy, hemorrhage, cholestasis

Contraindications Hypersensitivity to cefaclor, other cephalosporins, or any component of their formulation

Warnings/Precautions Modify dosage in patients with severe renal impairment; prolonged use may result in superinfection; a low incidence of cross-hypersensitivity to penicillins exists

Drug Interactions

Increased Effect: Probenecid may decrease cephalosporin elimination

(Continued)

Cefaclor *(Continued)*

Increased Toxicity: Furosemide, aminoglycosides may be a possible additive to nephrotoxicity

Dietary/Ethanol/Herb Considerations Administer with food to reduce GI upset; serum concentration may slightly decrease.

Drug Uptake

Absorption: Oral: Well absorbed, acid stable

Half-life, elimination: 0.5-1 hour; prolonged with renal impairment

Time to peak: Capsule: 60 minutes; Suspension: 45 minutes

Pregnancy Risk Factor B

Breast-feeding Considerations Theoretically, drug absorbed by nursing infant may change bowel flora or affect fever work-up result. **Note:** As a class, cephalosporins are used to treat infections in infants.

Dosage Forms CAP: 250 mg, 500 mg. **POWDER, oral suspension:** 125 mg/5 mL (75 mL, 150 mL); 187 mg/5 mL (50 mL, 100 mL); 250 mg/5 mL (75 mL, 150 mL); 375 mg/5 mL (50 mL, 100 mL). **TAB, extended release:** 375 mg, 500 mg

Generic Available Yes

Comments Patients allergic to penicillins can use a cephalosporin; the incidence of cross-reactivity between penicillins and cephalosporins is 1% when the allergic reaction to penicillin is delayed. Cefaclor is effective against anaerobic bacteria, but the sensitivity of alpha-hemolytic *Streptococcus* vary; approximately 10% of strains are resistant. Nearly 70% are intermediately sensitive. If the patient has a history of immediate reaction to penicillin, the incidence of cross-reactivity is 20%; cephalosporins are contraindicated in these patients.

Selected Readings Saxon A, Beall GN, Rohr AS, et al, "Immediate Hypersensitivity Reactions to Beta-Lactam Antibiotics," *Ann Intern Med*, 1987, 107(2):204-15.

Cefadroxil (sef a DROKS il)

Related Information

Antibiotic Prophylaxis, Preprocedural Guidelines for Dental Patients *on page 1344*

U.S. Brand Names Duricef®

Canadian Brand Names Apo®-Cefadroxil; Duricef™; Novo-Cefadroxil

Mexican Brand Names Cefamox; Duracef®

Pharmacologic Category Antibiotic, Cephalosporin (First Generation)

Synonyms Cefadroxil Monohydrate

Use

Dental: Alternative antibiotic for prevention of bacterial endocarditis. Individuals allergic to amoxicillin (penicillins) may receive cefadroxil provided they have not had an immediate, local, or systemic IgE-mediated anaphylactic allergic reaction to penicillin.

Medical: Treatment of susceptible bacterial infections, including those caused by group A beta-hemolytic *Streptococcus*

Local Anesthetic/Vasoconstrictor Precautions No information available to require special precautions

Effects on Dental Treatment No effects or complications reported

Dosage Oral:

Children: 30 mg/kg/day divided twice daily up to a maximum of 2 g/day

Prophylaxis: 50 mg/kg orally 1 hour before procedure with no follow-up dose needed

Adults: 1-2 g/day in 2 divided doses

Prophylaxis: 2 g 1 hour before procedure with no follow-up dose needed

Mechanism of Action Inhibits bacterial cell wall synthesis by binding to one or more of the penicillin-binding proteins (PBPs) which in turn inhibits the final transpeptidation step of peptidoglycan synthesis in bacterial cell walls, thus inhibiting cell wall biosynthesis. Bacteria eventually lyse due to ongoing activity of cell wall autolytic enzymes (autolysins and murein hydrolases) while cell wall assembly is arrested.

Other Adverse Effects

1% to 10%: Gastrointestinal: Diarrhea

<1%: Anaphylaxis, rash (maculopapular and erythematous), erythema multiforme, Stevens-Johnson syndrome, serum sickness, arthralgia, urticaria, pruritus, angioedema, pseudomembranous colitis, abdominal pain, dyspepsia, nausea, vomiting, elevated transaminases, cholestasis, vaginitis, neutropenia, agranulocytosis, thrombocytopenia, fever

Reactions reported with other cephalosporins include toxic epidermal necrolysis, abdominal pain, superinfection. renal dysfunction, toxic nephropathy, aplastic anemia, hemolytic anemia, hemorrhage, prolonged prothrombin time, increased BUN, increased creatinine, eosinophilia, pancytopenia, seizures

Contraindications Hypersensitivity to cefadroxil, other cephalosporins, or any component of their formulation

Warnings/Precautions Modify dosage in patients with severe renal impairment; prolonged use may result in superinfection; use with caution in patients with a history of penicillin allergy especially IgE-mediated reactions (eg, anaphylaxis, urticaria); may cause antibiotic-associated colitis or colitis secondary to *C. difficile*

Drug Interactions

Increased Effect: Probenecid may decrease cephalosporin elimination

Increased Toxicity: Furosemide, aminoglycosides may be a possible additive to nephrotoxicity

Dietary/Ethanol/Herb Considerations Food: Administration with food, infant formula, or cow's milk does **not** significantly affect absorption.

Drug Uptake

Absorption: Oral: Rapid and well absorbed from GI tract

Half-life, elimination: 1-2 hours; Renal failure: 20-24 hours

Time to peak: 70-90 minutes

Pregnancy Risk Factor B

Breast-feeding Considerations Theoretically, drug absorbed by nursing infant may change bowel flora or affect fever work-up result. **Note:** As a class, cephalosporins are used to treat infections in infants.

Dosage Forms CAP: 500 mg. **SUSP, oral:** 125 mg/5 mL, 250 mg/5 mL, 500 mg/5 mL (50 mL, 100 mL). **TAB:** 1 g

Generic Available Yes

Selected Readings

"Advisory Statement. Antibiotic Prophylaxis for Dental Patients With Total Joint Replacements. American Dental Association; American Academy of Orthopedic Surgeons," *J Am Dent Assoc*, 1997, 128(7):1004-8.

Dajani AS, Taubert KA, Wilson W, et al, "Prevention of Bacterial Endocarditis. Recommendations by the American Heart Association," *JAMA*, 1997, 277(22):1794-801.

Dajani AS, Taubert KA, Wilson W, et al, "Prevention of Bacterial Endocarditis: Recommendations by the American Heart Association," *J Am Dent Assoc*, 1997, 128(8):1142-51.

Donowitz GR and Mandell GL, "Drug Therapy. Beta-Lactam Antibiotics (1)," *N Engl J Med*, 1988, 318(7):419-26.

Donowitz GR and Mandell GL, "Drug Therapy. Beta-Lactam Antibiotics (2)," *N Engl J Med*, 1988, 318(8):490-500.

Gustaferro CA and Steckelberg JM, "Cephalosporin Antimicrobial Agents and Related Compounds," *Mayo Clin Proc*, 1991, 66(10):1064-73.

Cefadyl® *see* Cephapirin *on page 253*

Cefamandole (sef a MAN dole)

U.S. Brand Names Mandol®

Pharmacologic Category Antibiotic, Cephalosporin (Second Generation)

Synonyms Cefamandole Nafate

Use Treatment of susceptible bacterial infection; mainly respiratory tract, skin and skin structure, bone and joint, urinary tract and gynecologic, septicemia; surgical prophylaxis. Active against methicillin-sensitive staphylococci, many streptococci, and various gram-negative bacilli including *E. coli*, some *Klebsiella*, *P. mirabilis*, *H. influenzae*, and *Moraxella*.

Local Anesthetic/Vasoconstrictor Precautions No information available to require special precautions

Effects on Dental Treatment No effects or complications reported

Dosage I.M., I.V.:

Children: 100-150 mg/kg/day in divided doses every 4-6 hours

Adults: 4-12 g/24 hours divided every 4-6 hours or 500-1000 mg every 4-8 hours; maximum: 2 g/dose

Mechanism of Action Inhibits bacterial cell wall synthesis by binding to one or more of the penicillin-binding proteins (PBPs) which in turn inhibits the final transpeptidation step of peptidoglycan synthesis in bacterial cell walls, thus inhibiting cell wall biosynthesis. Bacteria eventually lyse due to ongoing activity of cell wall autolytic enzymes (autolysins and murein hydrolases) while cell wall assembly is arrested.

Other Adverse Effects Contains MTT side chain which may lead to increased risk of hypoprothrombinemia and bleeding.

1% to 10%:

Gastrointestinal: Diarrhea

Local: Thrombophlebitis

Reactions reported with other cephalosporins include toxic epidermal necrolysis, Stevens-Johnson syndrome, abdominal pain, superinfection, renal dysfunction, toxic nephropathy, aplastic anemia, hemolytic anemia, hemorrhage, pancytopenia, vaginitis, seizures

Drug Interactions Increased Effect/Toxicity: Increased cefamandole plasma concentrations when taken with probenecid. Aminoglycosides, furosemide when taken with cefamandole may increase nephrotoxicity. Increase in hypoprothrombinemic effect with warfarin or heparin and cefamandole.

Drug Uptake

Half-life, elimination: 30-60 minutes

Time to peak: I.M.: 1-2 hours; I.V.: ≤10 minutes

Pregnancy Risk Factor B

Generic Available No

Cefazolin (sef A zoe lin)

Related Information

Animal and Human Bites Guidelines *on page 1416*

Antibiotic Prophylaxis, Preprocedural Guidelines for Dental Patients *on page 1344*

U.S. Brand Names Ancef®; Kefzol®

Canadian Brand Names Ancef®; Kefzol®

Mexican Brand Names Cefamezin

Pharmacologic Category Antibiotic, Cephalosporin (First Generation)

Synonyms Cefazolin Sodium

Use

Dental: Alternative antibiotic for prevention of bacterial endocarditis when parenteral administration is needed. Individuals allergic to amoxicillin (penicillins) may receive cefazolin provided they have not had an immediate, local, or systemic IgE-mediated anaphylactic allergic reaction to penicillin. Alternate antibiotic for premedication in patients not allergic to penicillin who may be at potential increased risk of hematogenous total joint infection when parenteral administration is needed.

Medical: Treatment of gram-positive bacilli and cocci (except enterococcus); some gram-negative bacilli including *E. coli*, *Proteus*, and *Klebsiella* may be susceptible

Local Anesthetic/Vasoconstrictor Precautions No information available to require special precautions

Effects on Dental Treatment No effects or complications reported

Dosage I.M., I.V.:

Children >1 month: 25-100 mg/kg/day divided every 6-8 hours; maximum: 6 g/day

Adults: 250 mg to 2 g every 6-12 (usually 8) hours, depending on severity of infection; maximum dose: 12 g/day

Prophylaxis against bacterial endocarditis:

Infants and Children: 25 mg/kg 30 minutes before procedure; maximum dose: 1 g

Adults: 1 g 30 minutes before procedure

Dosing adjustment in renal impairment:

Cl_{cr} 10-30 mL/minute: Administer every 12 hours

Cl_{cr} <10 mL/minute: Administer every 24 hours

Hemodialysis: Moderately dialyzable (20% to 50%); administer dose postdialysis or administer supplemental dose of 0.5-1 g after dialysis

Peritoneal dialysis: Administer 0.5 g every 12 hours

Continuous arteriovenous or venovenous hemofiltration: Dose as for Cl_{cr} 10-30 mL/minute; removes 30 mg of cefazolin per liter of filtrate per day

Mechanism of Action Inhibits bacterial cell wall synthesis by binding to one or more of the penicillin-binding proteins (PBPs) which in turn inhibits the final transpeptidation step of peptidoglycan synthesis in bacterial cell walls, thus inhibiting cell wall biosynthesis. Bacteria eventually lyse due to ongoing activity of cell wall autolytic enzymes (autolysins and murein hydrolases) while cell wall assembly is arrested.

Other Adverse Effects

1% to 10%:

Gastrointestinal: Diarrhea

Local: Pain at injection site

<1%: Anaphylaxis, rash, pruritus, Stevens-Johnson syndrome, oral candidiasis, nausea, vomiting, abdominal cramps, anorexia, pseudomembranous colitis, eosinophilia, neutropenia, leukopenia, thrombocytopenia, thrombocytosis, elevated transaminases, phlebitis, vaginitis, fever, seizures

Other reactions with cephalosporins include toxic epidermal necrolysis, abdominal pain, cholestasis, superinfection, renal dysfunction, toxic nephropathy, aplastic anemia, hemolytic anemia, hemorrhage, prolonged prothrombin time, pancytopenia

Contraindications Hypersensitivity to cefazolin sodium, other cephalosporins, or any component of their formulation

Warnings/Precautions Modify dosage in patients with severe renal impairment; prolonged use may result in superinfection; use with caution in patients with a history of penicillin allergy especially IgE-mediated reactions (eg, anaphylaxis, urticaria); may cause antibiotic-associated colitis or colitis secondary to *C. difficile*

Drug Interactions

Increased Effect: High-dose probenecid decreases clearance

Increased Toxicity: Aminoglycosides increase nephrotoxic potential

Drug Uptake

Half-life, elimination: 90-150 minutes (increases with renal impairment)

Time to peak: I.M.: 0.5-2 hours; I.V.: ≤5 minutes

Pregnancy Risk Factor B

Breast-feeding Considerations Theoretically, drug absorbed by nursing infant may change bowel flora or affect fever work-up result. **Note:** As a class, cephalosporins are used to treat infections in infants.

Dosage Forms INF [premixed in D_5W, frozen] (Ancef®): 500 mg (50 mL); 1 g (50 mL). **Injection, powder for reconstitution** (Ancef®, Kefzol®): 500 mg, 1 g, 10 g, 20

g. **Injection, powder for reconstitution:** 500 mg, 1 g [with 50 mL D_5W in DUPLEX™ container]

Generic Available Yes

Selected Readings

"Advisory Statement. Antibiotic Prophylaxis for Dental Patients With Total Joint Replacements. American Dental Association; American Academy of Orthopedic Surgeons," *J Am Dent Assoc*, 1997, 128(7):1004-8.

Dajani AS, Taubert KA, Wilson W, et al, "Prevention of Bacterial Endocarditis. Recommendations by the American Heart Association," *JAMA*, 1997, 277(22):1794-801.

Dajani AS, Taubert KA, Wilson W, et al, "Prevention of Bacterial Endocarditis: Recommendations by the American Heart Association," *J Am Dent Assoc*, 1997, 128(8):1142-51.

Donowitz GR and Mandell GL, "Drug Therapy. Beta-Lactam Antibiotics (1)," *N Engl J Med*, 1988, 318(7):419-26.

Donowitz GR and Mandell GL, "Drug Therapy. Beta-Lactam Antibiotics (2)," *N Engl J Med*, 1988, 318(8):490-500.

Gustaferro CA and Steckelberg JM, "Cephalosporin Antimicrobial Agents and Related Compounds," *Mayo Clin Proc*, 1991, 66(10):1064-73.

Cefdinir (SEF di ner)

U.S. Brand Names Omnicef®

Canadian Brand Names Omnicef®

Pharmacologic Category Antibiotic, Cephalosporin (Third Generation)

Synonyms CFDN

Use Treatment of community-acquired pneumonia, acute exacerbations of chronic bronchitis, acute bacterial otitis media, acute maxillary sinusitis, pharyngitis/tonsillitis, and uncomplicated skin and skin structure infections.

Local Anesthetic/Vasoconstrictor Precautions No information available to require special precautions

Effects on Dental Treatment No effects or complications reported

Dosage Oral:

Children (otitis media with effusion): 7 mg/kg orally twice daily or 14 mg/kg orally once daily

Adults and Adolescent: 300 mg orally twice daily. An oral dose of 600 mg once daily has been used in streptococcal pharyngitis.

Mechanism of Action Inhibits bacterial cell wall synthesis by binding to one or more of the penicillin-binding proteins (PBPs) which in turn inhibits the final transpeptidation step of peptidoglycan synthesis in bacterial cell walls, thus inhibiting cell wall biosynthesis. Bacteria eventually lyse due to ongoing activity of cell wall autolytic enzymes (autolysins and murein hydrolases) while cell wall assembly is arrested.

Other Adverse Effects 1% to 10%

Dermatologic: Cutaneous moniliasis (1%)

Gastrointestinal: Diarrhea (8%), rash (3%), vomiting (1%), increased GGT (1%)

Other reactions with cephalosporins include dizziness, fever, headache, encephalopathy, asterixis, neuromuscular excitability, seizures, aplastic anemia, interstitial nephritis, toxic nephropathy, angioedema, hemorrhage, prolonged PT, serum-sickness reactions, and superinfection

Drug Interactions

Increased Effect/Toxicity: Probenecid increases the effects of cephalosporins by decreasing the renal elimination in those which are secreted by tubular secretion. Anticoagulant effects may be increased when administered with cephalosporins.

Decreased Effect: Coadministration with iron or antacids reduces the rate and extent of cefdinir absorption.

Drug Uptake Half-life, elimination: 100 minutes

Pregnancy Risk Factor B

Generic Available No

Cefditoren (sef de TOR en)

U.S. Brand Names Spectracef™

Pharmacologic Category Antibiotic, Cephalosporin

Synonyms Cefditoren Pivoxil

Use Treatment of acute bacterial exacerbation of chronic bronchitis (due to susceptible organisms including *Haemophilus influenzae, Haemophilus parainfluenzae, Streptococcus pneumoniae*-penicillin susceptible only, *Moraxella catarrhalis*); pharyngitis or tonsillitis (*Streptococcus pyogenes*); and uncomplicated skin and skin-structure infections (*Staphylococcus aureus*-not MRSA, *Streptococcus pyogenes*)

Local Anesthetic/Vasoconstrictor Precautions No information available to require special precautions

Effects on Dental Treatment No effects or complications reported

Dosage Oral:

Children ≥12 years and Adults:

Acute bacterial exacerbation of chronic bronchitis: 400 mg twice daily for 10 days

Pharyngitis, tonsillitis, uncomplicated skin and skin structure infections: 200 mg twice daily for 10 days

Elderly: Refer to adult dosing

(Continued)

Cefditoren *(Continued)*

Dosage adjustment in renal impairment:

Cl_{cr} 30-49 mL/minute: Maximum dose: 200 mg twice daily

Cl_{cr} <30 mL/minute: Maximum dose: 200 mg once daily

End-stage renal disease: Appropriate dosing not established

Mechanism of Action Inhibits bacterial cell wall synthesis by binding to one or more of the penicillin binding proteins (PBPs); which in turn inhibits the final transpeptidation step of peptidoglycan synthesis in bacterial cell walls, thus inhibiting cell wall biosynthesis; bacteria eventually lyse due to ongoing activity of cell wall autolytic enzymes (autolysins and murein hydrolases) while cell wall assembly is arrested

Other Adverse Effects

>10%: Gastrointestinal: Diarrhea (11% to 14%)

1% to 10%:

Central nervous system: Headache (2%)

Endocrine & metabolic: Glucose increased (1%)

Gastrointestinal: Nausea (4% to 6%), abdominal pain (2%), dyspepsia (1% to 2%), vomiting (1%)

Genitourinary: Vaginal moniliasis (3% to 6%)

Hematologic: Hematocrit decreased (2%)

Renal: Hematuria (3%), urinary white blood cells increased (2%)

<1%: Abnormal dreams, decreased serum albumin, allergic reaction, anorexia, increased appetite, BUN increased, decreased serum calcium, decreased serum chloride, increased serum cholesterol, coagulation time increased, constipation, diaphoresis, dizziness, eructation, eosinophils increased, fever, flatulence, fungal infection, gastritis, gastrointestinal disorder, hemoglobin decreased, hyperglycemia, inorganic phosphorus decreased, insomnia, leukopenia, lymphocytes increased, mouth ulceration, myalgia, nervousness, neutrophils decreased, oral moniliasis, pain, peripheral edema, pharyngitis, platelet count increased, positive direct Coombs' test, potassium increased, pseudomembranous colitis, proteinuria, pruritus, rash, rhinitis, SGOT increased, SGPT increased, sinusitis, somnolence, stomatitis, taste perversion, thrombocytopenia, urinary frequency, urticaria, vaginitis, weakness, weight loss, white blood cell increase/decrease, xerostomia

Additional adverse effects seen with cephalosporin antibiotics: Anaphylaxis, aplastic anemia, cholestasis, erythema multiforme, hemorrhage, hemolytic anemia, renal dysfunction, reversible hyperactivity, serum sickness-like reaction, Stevens-Johnson syndrome, toxic epidermal necrolysis, toxic nephropathy

Contraindications Hypersensitivity to cefditoren, other cephalosporins, milk protein, or any component of the formulation; carnitine deficiency

Warnings/Precautions Use with caution in patients with a history of penicillin allergy, especially IgE-mediated reactions (eg, anaphylaxis, urticaria); may cause antibiotic-associated colitis or colitis secondary to *C. difficile*. Use caution in patients with renal or hepatic impairment. Cefditoren causes renal excretion of carnitine, do not use in patients with carnitine deficiency; not for long-term therapy due to the possible development of carnitine deficiency over time. Cefditoren tablets contain sodium caseinate, which may cause hypersensitivity reactions in patients with milk protein hypersensitivity; this does not affect patients with lactose intolerance. Safety and efficacy have not been established in children <12 years of age.

Drug Interactions

Antacids: Aluminum- and magnesium-containing antacids decrease oral absorption; concomitant use should be avoided.

Histamine H_2 antagonists: Famotidine decreases oral absorption; concomitant use should be avoided.

Probenecid: Serum concentration of cefditoren may be increased.

Dietary/Ethanol/Herb Considerations Food: Administer with food; moderate- to high-fat meals increase bioavailability and maximum plasma concentration. Plasma carnitine levels are decreased during therapy (39% with 200 mg dosing, 63% with 400 mg dosing); Boiled milk, buttermilk, or yogurt may reduce diarrhea.

Drug Uptake

Half-life, elimination: 1.6 ± 0.4 hours

Time to peak: 1.5-3 hours

Pregnancy Risk Factor B

Dosage Forms **TAB:** 200 mg

Generic Available No

Cefepime (SEF e pim)

U.S. Brand Names Maxipime®

Canadian Brand Names Maxipime™

Mexican Brand Names Maxipime®

Pharmacologic Category Antibiotic, Cephalosporin (Fourth Generation)

Synonyms Cefepime Hydrochloride

Use Treatment of uncomplicated and complicated urinary tract infections, including pyelonephritis caused by typical urinary tract pathogens; monotherapy for febrile neutropenia; uncomplicated skin and skin structure infections caused by *Streptococcus pyogenes*; moderate to severe pneumonia caused by pneumococcus, *Pseudomonas aeruginosa*, and other gram-negative organisms; complicated intra-abdominal infections (in combination with metronidazole). Also active against methicillin-susceptible staphylococci, *Enterobacter* sp, and many other gram-negative bacilli.

Children 2 months to 16 years: Empiric therapy of febrile neutropenia patients, uncomplicated skin/soft tissue infections, pneumonia, and uncomplicated/complicated urinary tract infections.

Local Anesthetic/Vasoconstrictor Precautions No information available to require special precautions

Effects on Dental Treatment No effects or complications reported

Dosage I.V.:

Children: Unlabeled: 50 mg/kg every 8 hours; maximum dose: 2 g

Adults:

Most infections: 1-2 g every 12 hours for 5-10 days; higher doses or more frequent administration may be required in pseudomonal infections

Urinary tract infections, uncomplicated: 500 mg every 12 hours

Mechanism of Action Inhibits bacterial cell wall synthesis by binding to one or more of the penicillin-binding proteins (PBPs) which in turn inhibits the final transpeptidation step of peptidoglycan synthesis in bacterial cell walls, thus inhibiting cell wall biosynthesis. Bacterial eventually lyse due to ongoing activity of cell wall autolytic enzymes (autolysis and murein hydrolases) while cell wall assembly is arrested.

Other Adverse Effects

>10%: Hematologic: Positive Coombs' test without hemolysis

1% to 10%:

Central nervous system: Fever (1%), headache (1%)

Dermatologic: Rash, pruritus

Gastrointestinal: Diarrhea, nausea, vomiting

Local: Pain, erythema at injection site

Other reactions with cephalosporins include aplastic anemia, erythema multiforme, hemolytic anemia, hemorrhage, pancytopenia, prolonged PT, renal dysfunction, Stevens-Johnson syndrome, superinfection, toxic epidermal necrolysis, toxic nephropathy, vaginitis

Warnings/Precautions Modify dosage in patients with severe renal impairment; prolonged use may result in superinfection; a low incidence of cross-hypersensitivity to penicillins exists

Drug Interactions Increased Effect/Toxicity: High-dose probenecid decreases clearance and increases effect of cefepime. Aminoglycosides increase nephrotoxic potential when taken with cefepime.

Drug Uptake

Absorption: I.M.: Rapid and complete; T_{max}: 0.5-1.5 hours

Half-life, elimination: 2 hours

Time to peak: 0.5-1.5 hours

Pregnancy Risk Factor B

Generic Available No

Cefixime (sef IKS eem)

Related Information

Nonviral Infectious Diseases *on page 1342*

U.S. Brand Names Suprax®

Canadian Brand Names Suprax®

Mexican Brand Names Denvar; Novacef

Pharmacologic Category Antibiotic, Cephalosporin (Third Generation)

Use Treatment of urinary tract infections, otitis media, respiratory infections due to susceptible organisms including *S. pneumoniae* and *pyogenes*, *H. influenzae* and many *Enterobacteriaceae*; documented poor compliance with other oral antimicrobials; outpatient therapy of serious soft tissue or skeletal infections due to susceptible organisms; single-dose oral treatment of uncomplicated cervical/urethral gonorrhea due to *N. gonorrhoeae*

Local Anesthetic/Vasoconstrictor Precautions No information available to require special precautions

Effects on Dental Treatment No effects or complications reported

Dosage Oral:

Children: 8 mg/kg/day in 1-2 divided doses; maximum dose: 400 mg/day

Children >50 kg or >12 years and Adults: 400 mg/day in 1-2 divided doses

Uncomplicated cervical/urethral gonorrhea due to *N. gonorrhoeae*: 400 mg as a single dose

Mechanism of Action Inhibits bacterial cell wall synthesis by binding to one or more of the penicillin-binding proteins (PBPs) which in turn inhibits the final transpeptidation step of peptidoglycan synthesis in bacterial cell walls, thus inhibiting cell

(Continued)

Cefixime *(Continued)*

wall biosynthesis. Bacteria eventually lyse due to ongoing activity of cell wall autolytic enzymes (autolysins and murein hydrolases) while cell wall assembly is arrested.

Other Adverse Effects

>10%: Gastrointestinal: Diarrhea (16%)

1% to 10%: Gastrointestinal: Abdominal pain, nausea, dyspepsia, flatulence

Reactions reported with other cephalosporins include anaphylaxis, seizures, toxic epidermal necrolysis, renal dysfunction, toxic nephropathy, interstitial nephritis, cholestasis, aplastic anemia, hemolytic anemia, hemorrhage, pancytopenia, neutropenia, agranulocytosis, colitis, superinfection

Drug Interactions

Increased Effect/Toxicity: Probenecid increases cefixime concentration. Cefixime may increase carbamazepine. Furosemide, aminoglycosides may be a possible additive to nephrotoxicity.

Decreased Effect: Probenecid may decrease cephalosporin elimination.

Drug Uptake

Absorption: Oral: 40% to 50%

Half-life, elimination: 3-4 hours; Renal failure: ≤11.5 hours

Time to peak: 2-6 hours; peak is 15% to 50% higher for oral suspension versus tablets; presence of food delays time to peak

Pregnancy Risk Factor B

Generic Available No

Cefizox® *see* Ceftizoxime *on page 244*

Cefobid® *see* Cefoperazone *on page 238*

Cefol® Filmtab® *see* Vitamins, Multiple *on page 1246*

Cefonicid *Not Available in U.S.* (se FON i sid)

U.S. Brand Names Monocid® [DSC]

Mexican Brand Names Monocidur

Pharmacologic Category Antibiotic, Cephalosporin (Second Generation)

Synonyms Cefonicid Sodium

Use Treatment of susceptible bacterial infection; mainly respiratory tract, skin and skin structure, bone and joint, urinary tract and gynecologic, as well as, septicemia; second generation cephalosporin

Local Anesthetic/Vasoconstrictor Precautions No information available to require special precautions

Effects on Dental Treatment No effects or complications reported

Dosage Adults: I.M., I.V.: 0.5-2 g every 24 hours

Prophylaxis: Preop: 1 g/hour

Mechanism of Action Inhibits bacterial cell wall synthesis by binding to one or more of the penicillin-binding proteins (PBPs) which in turn inhibits the final transpeptidation step of peptidoglycan synthesis in bacterial cell walls, thus inhibiting cell wall biosynthesis. Bacteria eventually lyse due to ongoing activity of cell wall autolytic enzymes (autolysins and murein hydrolases) while cell wall assembly is arrested.

Other Adverse Effects

1% to 10%:

Hematologic: Increased eosinophils (3%), increased platelets (2%)

Hepatic: Altered LFTs (increased transaminases, LDH, alkaline phosphatase) (2%)

Local: Pain, burning at injection site (6%)

Reactions reported with other cephalosporins include anaphylaxis, seizures, Stevens-Johnson syndrome, toxic epidermal necrolysis, renal dysfunction, toxic nephropathy, cholestasis, aplastic anemia, hemolytic anemia, hemorrhage, pancytopenia, agranulocytosis, colitis, superinfection

Drug Interactions Increased Effect/Toxicity: Probenecid may decrease cephalosporin elimination. Furosemide, aminoglycosides in combination with cefonicid may result in additive nephrotoxicity.

Drug Uptake

Absorption: I.M.: Well absorbed

Half-life, elimination: 3.5-5.8 hours

Pregnancy Risk Factor B

Generic Available No

Cefoperazone (sef oh PER a zone)

U.S. Brand Names Cefobid®

Canadian Brand Names Cefobid®

Pharmacologic Category Antibiotic, Cephalosporin (Third Generation)

Synonyms Cefoperazone Sodium

Use Treatment of susceptible bacterial infection; mainly respiratory tract, skin and skin structure, bone and joint, urinary tract and gynecologic as well as septicemia.

Active against a variety of gram-negative bacilli, some gram-positive cocci, and has some activity against *Pseudomonas aeruginosa*.

Local Anesthetic/Vasoconstrictor Precautions No information available to require special precautions

Effects on Dental Treatment No effects or complications reported

Dosage I.M., I.V.:

Children: 100-150 mg/kg/day divided every 8-12 hours; up to 12 g/day

Adults: 2-4 g/day in divided doses every 12 hours; up to 12 g/day

Mechanism of Action Inhibits bacterial cell wall synthesis by binding to one or more of the penicillin-binding proteins (PBPs) which in turn inhibits the final transpeptidation step of peptidoglycan synthesis in bacterial cell walls, thus inhibiting cell wall biosynthesis. Bacteria eventually lyse due to ongoing activity of cell wall autolytic enzymes (autolysins and murein hydrolases) while cell wall assembly is arrested.

Other Adverse Effects Contains MTT side chain which may lead to increased risk of hypoprothrombinemia and bleeding.

1% to 10%:

Dermatologic: Rash (maculopapular or erythematous) (2%)

Gastrointestinal: Diarrhea (3%)

Hematologic: Decreased neutrophils (2%), decreased hemoglobin or hematocrit (5%), eosinophilia (10%)

Hepatic: Increased transaminases (5% to 10%)

Reactions reported with other cephalosporins include anaphylaxis, seizures, Stevens-Johnson syndrome, toxic epidermal necrolysis, renal dysfunction, toxic nephropathy, cholestasis, aplastic anemia, hemolytic anemia, pancytopenia, agranulocytosis, colitis, superinfection

Drug Interactions Increased Effect/Toxicity: Probenecid may decrease cephalosporin elimination resulting in increased levels. Furosemide, aminoglycosides in combination with cefoperazone may result in additive nephrotoxicity.

Drug Uptake

Half-life, elimination: 2 hours (increases with hepatic impairment or biliary obstruction)

Time to peak: I.M.: 1-2 hours; I.V.: 15-20 minutes (serum concentration 2-3 times the serum concentration following I.M. administration)

Pregnancy Risk Factor B

Generic Available No

Cefotan® *see* Cefotetan *on page 240*

Cefotaxime (sef oh TAKS eem)

U.S. Brand Names Claforan®

Canadian Brand Names Claforan®

Mexican Brand Names Alfotax; Benaxima; Biosint®; Cefaxim; Cefoclin; Cefradil®; Claforan®; Fotexina®; Taporin®; Viken

Pharmacologic Category Antibiotic, Cephalosporin (Third Generation)

Synonyms Cefotaxime Sodium

Use Treatment of susceptible infection in respiratory tract, skin and skin structure, bone and joint, urinary tract, gynecologic as well as septicemia, and documented or suspected meningitis. Active against most gram-negative bacilli (not *Pseudomonas*) and gram-positive cocci (not enterococcus). Active against many penicillin-resistant pneumococci.

Local Anesthetic/Vasoconstrictor Precautions No information available to require special precautions

Effects on Dental Treatment No effects or complications reported

Dosage

Infants and Children 1 month to 12 years: I.M., I.V.: <50 kg: 50-180 mg/kg/day in divided doses every 4-6 hours

Meningitis: 200 mg/kg/day in divided doses every 6 hours

Children >12 years and Adults:

Uncomplicated infections: I.M., I.V.: 1 g every 12 hours

Moderate/severe infections: I.M., I.V.: 1-2 g every 8 hours

Infections commonly needing higher doses (eg, septicemia): I.V.: 2 g every 6-8 hours

Life-threatening infections: I.V.: 2 g every 4 hours

Preop: I.M., I.V.: 1 g 30-90 minutes before surgery

C-section: 1 g as soon as the umbilical cord is clamped, then 1 g I.M., I.V. at 6- and 12-hour intervals

Dosing interval in renal impairment:

Cl_{cr} 10-50 mL/minute: Administer every 8-12 hours

Cl_{cr} <10 mL/minute: Administer every 24 hours

Hemodialysis: Moderately dialyzable

Dosing adjustment in hepatic impairment: Moderate dosage reduction is recommended in severe liver disease

Continuous arteriovenous or venovenous hemodiafiltration effects: Administer 1 g every 12 hour

(Continued)

Cefotaxime *(Continued)*

Mechanism of Action Inhibits bacterial cell wall synthesis by binding to one or more of the penicillin-binding proteins (PBPs) which in turn inhibits the final transpeptidation step of peptidoglycan synthesis in bacterial cell walls, thus inhibiting cell wall biosynthesis. Bacteria eventually lyse due to ongoing activity of cell wall autolytic enzymes (autolysins and murein hydrolases) while cell wall assembly is arrested.

Other Adverse Effects

1% to 10%:

- Dermatologic: Rash, pruritus
- Gastrointestinal: Diarrhea, nausea, vomiting, colitis
- Local: Pain at injection site

Reactions reported with other cephalosporins include agranulocytosis, aplastic anemia, cholestasis, hemolytic anemia, hemorrhage, pancytopenia, renal dysfunction, seizures, superinfection, toxic nephropathy.

Drug Interactions Increased Effect/Probenecid may decrease cephalosporin elimination resulting in increased levels. Furosemide, aminoglycosides in combination with cefotaxime may result in additive nephrotoxicity.

Drug Uptake

Half-life, elimination:

Cefotaxime: Premature neonates <1 week: 5-6 hours; Full-term neonates <1 week: 2-3.4 hours; Adults: 1-1.5 hours; prolonged with renal and/or hepatic impairment

Desacetylcefotaxime: 1.5-1.9 hours (prolonged with renal impairment)

Time to peak: I.M.: ~30 minutes

Pregnancy Risk Factor B

Generic Available Yes

Cefotetan (SEF oh tee tan)

Related Information

Animal and Human Bites Guidelines *on page 1416*

U.S. Brand Names Cefotan®

Canadian Brand Names Cefotan®

Pharmacologic Category Antibiotic, Cephalosporin (Second Generation)

Synonyms Cefotetan Disodium

Use Less active against staphylococci and streptococci than first generation cephalosporins, but active against anaerobes including *Bacteroides fragilis*; active against gram-negative enteric bacilli including *E. coli*, *Klebsiella*, and *Proteus*; used predominantly for respiratory tract, skin and skin structure, bone and joint, urinary tract and gynecologic as well as septicemia; surgical prophylaxis; intra-abdominal infections and other mixed infections

Local Anesthetic/Vasoconstrictor Precautions No information available to require special precautions

Effects on Dental Treatment No effects or complications reported

Dosage I.M., I.V.:

Children: 20-40 mg/kg/dose every 12 hours

Adults: 1-6 g/day in divided doses every 12 hours; usual dose: 1-2 g every 12 hours for 5-10 days; 1-2 g may be given every 24 hours for urinary tract infection

Dosing interval in renal impairment:

Cl_{cr} 10-30 mL/minute: Administer every 24 hours

Cl_{cr} <10 mL/minute: Administer every 48 hours

Hemodialysis: Slightly dialyzable (5% to 20%); administer ¼ the usual dose every 24 hours on days between dialysis; administer ½ the usual dose on the day of dialysis.

Continuous arteriovenous or venovenous hemodiafiltration effects: Administer 750 mg every 12 hours

Mechanism of Action Inhibits bacterial cell wall synthesis by binding to one or more of the penicillin-binding proteins (PBPs) which in turn inhibits the final transpeptidation step of peptidoglycan synthesis in bacterial cell walls, thus inhibiting cell wall biosynthesis. Bacteria eventually lyse due to ongoing activity of cell wall autolytic enzymes (autolysins and murein hydrolases) while cell wall assembly is arrested.

Other Adverse Effects Contains MTT side chain which may lead to increased risk of hypoprothrombinemia and bleeding.

1% to 10%:

- Gastrointestinal: Diarrhea (1.3%)
- Hepatic: Increased transaminases (1.2%)
- Miscellaneous: Hypersensitivity reactions (1.2%)

Reactions reported with other cephalosporins include seizures, Stevens-Johnson syndrome, toxic epidermal necrolysis, renal dysfunction, toxic nephropathy, cholestasis, aplastic anemia, hemolytic anemia, hemorrhage, pancytopenia, agranulocytosis, colitis, superinfection

Drug Interactions Increased Effect/Toxicity: Probenecid may decrease cephalosporin elimination. Furosemide, aminoglycosides in combination with cefotetan may result in additive nephrotoxicity. Effects of warfarin may be enhanced due to effects on GI flora.

Drug Uptake

Half-life, elimination: 3-5 hours

Time to peak: I.M.: 1.5-3 hours

Pregnancy Risk Factor B

Generic Available Yes

Cefoxitin (se FOKS i tin)

U.S. Brand Names Mefoxin®

Canadian Brand Names Mefoxin®

Pharmacologic Category Antibiotic, Cephalosporin (Second Generation)

Synonyms Cefoxitin Sodium

Use Less active against staphylococci and streptococci than first generation cephalosporins, but active against anaerobes including *Bacteroides fragilis*; active against gram-negative enteric bacilli including *E. coli*, *Klebsiella*, and *Proteus*; used predominantly for respiratory tract, skin and skin structure, bone and joint, urinary tract and gynecologic as well as septicemia; surgical prophylaxis; intra-abdominal infections and other mixed infections

Local Anesthetic/Vasoconstrictor Precautions No information available to require special precautions

Effects on Dental Treatment No effects or complications reported

Dosage I.M., I.V.:

Children >3 months:

Mild-moderate infection: 80-100 mg/kg/day in divided doses every 4-6 hours

Severe infection: 100-160 mg/kg/day in divided doses every 4-6 hours

Maximum dose: 12 g/day

Adults: 1-2 g every 6-8 hours (I.M. injection is painful); up to 12 g/day

Mechanism of Action Inhibits bacterial cell wall synthesis by binding to one or more of the penicillin-binding proteins (PBPs) which in turn inhibits the final transpeptidation step of peptidoglycan synthesis in bacterial cell walls, thus inhibiting cell wall biosynthesis. Bacteria eventually lyse due to ongoing activity of cell wall autolytic enzymes (autolysins and murein hydrolases) while cell wall assembly is arrested.

Other Adverse Effects

1% to 10%: Gastrointestinal: Diarrhea

Reactions reported with other cephalosporins include seizures, Stevens-Johnson syndrome, toxic epidermal necrolysis, erythema multiforme, urticaria, serum-sickness reactions, renal dysfunction, toxic nephropathy, cholestasis, aplastic anemia, hemolytic anemia, hemorrhage, pancytopenia, agranulocytosis, colitis, vaginitis, superinfection

Drug Interactions Increased Effect/Toxicity: Probenecid may decrease cephalosporin elimination. Furosemide, aminoglycosides in combination with cefoxitin may result in additive nephrotoxicity.

Drug Uptake

Half-life, elimination: 45-60 minutes (increases significantly with renal impairment)

Time to peak: I.M.: 20-30 minutes; I.V.: ≤5 minutes

Pregnancy Risk Factor B

Generic Available No

Cefpodoxime (sef pode OKS eem)

U.S. Brand Names Vantin®

Canadian Brand Names Vantin®

Mexican Brand Names Orelox®

Pharmacologic Category Antibiotic, Cephalosporin (Third Generation)

Synonyms Cefpodoxime Proxetil

Use Treatment of susceptible acute, community-acquired pneumonia caused by *S. pneumoniae* or nonbeta-lactamase producing *H. influenzae*; acute uncomplicated gonorrhea caused by *N. gonorrhoeae*; uncomplicated skin and skin structure infections caused by *S. aureus* or *S. pyogenes*; acute otitis media caused by *S. pneumoniae, H. influenzae*, or *M. catarrhalis*; pharyngitis or tonsillitis; and uncomplicated urinary tract infections caused by *E. coli*, *Klebsiella*, and *Proteus*

Local Anesthetic/Vasoconstrictor Precautions No information available to require special precautions

Effects on Dental Treatment No effects or complications reported

Dosage Oral:

Children >5 months to 12 years:

Acute otitis media: 10 mg/kg/day as a single dose or divided every 12 hours (400 mg/day)

Pharyngitis/tonsillitis: 10 mg/kg/day in 2 divided doses (maximum: 200 mg/day)

Children ≥13 years and Adults:

Acute community-acquired pneumonia and bacterial exacerbations of chronic bronchitis: 200 mg every 12 hours for 14 days and 10 days, respectively

Skin and skin structure: 400 mg every 12 hours for 7-14 days

(Continued)

Cefpodoxime *(Continued)*

Uncomplicated gonorrhea (male and female) and rectal gonococcal infections (female): 200 mg as a single dose

Pharyngitis/tonsillitis: 100 mg every 12 hours for 10 days

Uncomplicated urinary tract infection: 100 mg every 12 hours for 7 days

Mechanism of Action Inhibits bacterial cell wall synthesis by binding to one or more of the penicillin-binding proteins (PBPs) which in turn inhibits the final transpeptidation step of peptidoglycan synthesis in bacterial cell walls, thus inhibiting cell wall biosynthesis. Bacteria eventually lyse due to ongoing activity of cell wall autolytic enzymes (autolysins and murein hydrolases) while cell wall assembly is arrested.

Other Adverse Effects

>10%:

Dermatologic: Diaper rash (12%)

Gastrointestinal: Diarrhea in infants and toddlers (15%)

1% to 10%:

Central nervous system: Headache (1%)

Dermatologic: Rash (1%)

Gastrointestinal: Diarrhea (7%), nausea (4%), abdominal pain (2%), vomiting (1% to 2%)

Genitourinary: Vaginal infections (3%)

Reactions reported with other cephalosporins include seizures, Stevens-Johnson syndrome, toxic epidermal necrolysis, erythema multiforme, urticaria, serum-sickness reactions, renal dysfunction, interstitial nephritis toxic nephropathy, cholestasis, aplastic anemia, hemolytic anemia, hemorrhage, pancytopenia, agranulocytosis, colitis, vaginitis, superinfection

Drug Interactions

Increased Effect/Toxicity: Probenecid may decrease cephalosporin elimination. Furosemide, aminoglycosides in combination with cefpodoxime may result in additive nephrotoxicity.

Decreased Effect: Antacids and H_2-receptor antagonists reduce absorption and serum concentration of cefpodoxime.

Drug Uptake

Absorption: Rapid and well (50%), acid stable; enhanced in the presence of food or low gastric pH

Half-life, elimination: 2.2 hours; prolonged with renal impairment

Time to peak: ~1 hour

Pregnancy Risk Factor B

Generic Available No

Cefprozil (sef PROE zil)

U.S. Brand Names Cefzil®

Canadian Brand Names Cefzil®

Mexican Brand Names Procef®

Pharmacologic Category Antibiotic, Cephalosporin (Second Generation)

Use Infections causes by susceptible organisms including *S. pneumoniae*, *S. aureus*, *S. pyogenes*; treatment of otitis media and infections involving the respiratory tract and skin and skin structure

Local Anesthetic/Vasoconstrictor Precautions No information available to require special precautions

Effects on Dental Treatment No effects or complications reported

Dosage Oral:

Children >6 months to 12 years: 7.5-15 mg/kg every 12 hours for 10 days

Pharyngitis/tonsillitis:

Children 2-12 years: 15 mg/kg/day divided every 12 hours; maximum: 1 g/day

Children >13 years and Adults: 250-500 mg every 12-24 hours for 10-14 days

Mechanism of Action Inhibits bacterial cell wall synthesis by binding to one or more of the penicillin-binding proteins (PBPs) which in turn inhibits the final transpeptidation step of peptidoglycan synthesis in bacterial cell walls, thus inhibiting cell wall biosynthesis. Bacteria eventually lyse due to ongoing activity of cell wall autolytic enzymes (autolysins and murein hydrolases) while cell wall assembly is arrested.

Other Adverse Effects

1% to 10%:

Central nervous system: Dizziness (1%)

Dermatologic: Diaper rash (2%)

Gastrointestinal: Diarrhea (3%), nausea (4%), vomiting (1%), abdominal pain (1%)

Genitourinary: Vaginitis, genital pruritus (2%)

Hepatic: Increased transaminases (2%)

Miscellaneous: Superinfection

Reactions reported with other cephalosporins include seizures, toxic epidermal necrolysis, renal dysfunction, interstitial nephritis, toxic nephropathy, aplastic anemia, hemolytic anemia, hemorrhage, pancytopenia, agranulocytosis, colitis, vaginitis, superinfection

Drug Interactions Increased Effect/Toxicity: Probenecid may decrease cephalosporin elimination. Furosemide, aminoglycosides in combination with cefprozil may result in additive nephrotoxicity.

Drug Uptake

Absorption: Oral: Well absorbed (94%)
Half-life, elimination: 1.3 hours (normal renal function)
Time to peak: 1.5 hours (fasting state)

Pregnancy Risk Factor B

Generic Available No

Ceftazidime (SEF tay zi deem)

U.S. Brand Names Ceptaz®; Fortaz®; Tazicef®; Tazidime®

Canadian Brand Names Ceptaz®; Fortaz®; Tazidime®

Mexican Brand Names Ceftazim; Fortum; Izadima®; Tagal®; Taloken; Taxifur®; Waytrax

Pharmacologic Category Antibiotic, Cephalosporin (Third Generation)

Use Treatment of documented susceptible *Pseudomonas aeruginosa* infection; *Pseudomonas* infection in patients at risk of developing aminoglycoside-induced nephrotoxicity and/or ototoxicity; empiric therapy of febrile, granulocytopenic patients

Local Anesthetic/Vasoconstrictor Precautions No information available to require special precautions

Effects on Dental Treatment No effects or complications reported

Dosage I.M., I.V.:

Children 1 month to 12 years: 30-50 mg/kg/dose every 8 hours; maximum dose: 6 g/day
Adults: 1-2 g every 8-12 hours
  Urinary tract infections: 250-500 mg every 12 hours

Mechanism of Action Inhibits bacterial cell wall synthesis by binding to one or more of the penicillin-binding proteins (PBPs) which in turn inhibits the final transpeptidation step of peptidoglycan synthesis in bacterial cell walls, thus inhibiting cell wall biosynthesis. Bacteria eventually lyse due to ongoing activity of cell wall autolytic enzymes (autolysins and murein hydrolases) while cell wall assembly is arrested.

Other Adverse Effects

1% to 10%:
  Gastrointestinal: Diarrhea (1%)
  Local: Pain at injection site (1%)
  Miscellaneous: Hypersensitivity reactions (2%)

Reactions reported with other cephalosporins include seizures, urticaria, serum-sickness reactions, renal dysfunction, interstitial nephritis, toxic nephropathy, elevated BUN, elevated creatinine, cholestasis, aplastic anemia, hemolytic anemia, pancytopenia, agranulocytosis, colitis, prolonged PT, hemorrhage, superinfection

Drug Interactions Increased Effect/Toxicity: Probenecid may decrease cephalosporin elimination. Aminoglycosides: *in vitro* studies indicate additive or synergistic effect against some strains of Enterobacteriaceae and *Pseudomonas aeruginosa*. Furosemide, aminoglycosides in combination with ceftazidime may result in additive nephrotoxicity.

Drug Uptake

Half-life, elimination: 1-2 hours, prolonged with renal impairment; Neonates <23 days: 2.2-4.7 hours
Time to peak: I.M.: ≤1 hour

Pregnancy Risk Factor B

Generic Available No

Ceftibuten (sef TYE byoo ten)

Related Information

Oral Bacterial Infections *on page 1367*

U.S. Brand Names Cedax®

Mexican Brand Names Cedax®

Pharmacologic Category Antibiotic, Cephalosporin (Third Generation)

Use Oral cephalosporin for bronchitis, otitis media, and strep throat

Local Anesthetic/Vasoconstrictor Precautions No information available to require special precautions

Effects on Dental Treatment No effects or complications reported

Dosage Oral:

Children <12 years: 9 mg/kg/day for 10 days; maximum daily dose: 400 mg
Children ≥12 years and Adults: 400 mg once daily for 10 days; maximum: 400 mg

Mechanism of Action Inhibits bacterial cell wall synthesis by binding to one or more of the penicillin-binding proteins (PBPs) which in turn inhibits the final transpeptidation step of peptidoglycan synthesis in bacterial cell walls, thus inhibiting cell

(Continued)

Ceftibuten *(Continued)*

wall biosynthesis. Bacteria eventually lyse due to ongoing activity of cell wall autolytic enzymes (autolysins and murein hydrolases) while cell wall assembly is arrested.

Other Adverse Effects

1% to 10%:

Central nervous system: Headache (3%), dizziness (1%)

Gastrointestinal: Nausea (4%), diarrhea (3%), dyspepsia (2%), vomiting (1%), abdominal pain (1%)

Hematologic: Increased eosinophils (3%), decreased hemoglobin (2%), thrombocytosis

Hepatic: Increased ALT (1%), increased bilirubin (1%)

Renal: Increased BUN (4%)

Reactions reported with other cephalosporins include anaphylaxis, fever, paresthesia, pruritus, Stevens-Johnson syndrome, toxic epidermal necrolysis, erythema multiforme, angioedema, pseudomembranous colitis, hemolytic anemia, candidiasis, vaginitis, encephalopathy, asterixis, neuromuscular excitability, seizures, serum-sickness reactions, renal dysfunction, interstitial nephritis, toxic nephropathy, cholestasis, aplastic anemia, hemolytic anemia, pancytopenia, agranulocytosis, colitis, prolonged PT, hemorrhage, superinfection

Contraindications Hypersensitivity to ceftibuten, cephalosporins, or any component of their formulation

Warnings/Precautions Modify dosage in patients with severe renal impairment, prolonged use may result in superinfection; a low incidence of cross-hypersensitivity to penicillins exist

Drug Interactions Increased Effect/Toxicity: High-dose probenecid decreases clearance. Aminoglycosides in combination with ceftibuten may increase nephrotoxic potential.

Drug Uptake

Absorption: Rapid; food decreases peak concentrations, delays T_{max} and lowers AUC

Half-life, elimination: 2 hours

Time to peak: 2-3 hours

Pregnancy Risk Factor B

Generic Available No

Comments In clinical trials, ceftibuten once or twice daily was at least as effective as cefaclor or ciprofloxacin for treatment of acute bacterial exacerbations of bronchitis, as effective as amoxicillin/clavulanic acid or cefaclor for otitis media, as effective as penicillin for pharyngitis, and as effective as trimethoprim-sulfamethoxazole for urinary tract infections

Ceftin® *see* Cefuroxime *on page 246*

Ceftizoxime (sef ti ZOKS eem)

U.S. Brand Names Cefizox®

Canadian Brand Names Cefizox®

Mexican Brand Names Ultracef®

Pharmacologic Category Antibiotic, Cephalosporin (Third Generation)

Synonyms Ceftizoxime Sodium

Use Treatment of susceptible nonpseudomonal gram-negative rod infections or mixed gram-negative and anaerobic infections; predominantly respiratory tract, skin and skin structure, bone and joint, urinary tract and gynecologic, as well as septicemia

Local Anesthetic/Vasoconstrictor Precautions No information available to require special precautions

Effects on Dental Treatment No effects or complications reported

Dosage I.M., I.V.:

Children ≥6 months: 150-200 mg/kg/day divided every 6-8 hours (maximum of 12 g/24 hours)

Adults: 1-2 g every 8-12 hours, up to 2 g every 4 hours or 4 g every 8 hours for life-threatening infections

Mechanism of Action Inhibits bacterial cell wall synthesis by binding to one or more of the penicillin-binding proteins (PBPs) which in turn inhibits the final transpeptidation step of peptidoglycan synthesis in bacterial cell walls, thus inhibiting cell wall biosynthesis. Bacteria eventually lyse due to ongoing activity of cell wall autolytic enzymes (autolysins and murein hydrolases) while cell wall assembly is arrested.

Other Adverse Effects

1% to 10%:

Central nervous system: Fever

Dermatologic: Rash, pruritus

Hematologic: Eosinophilia, thrombocytosis

Hepatic: Elevated transaminases, alkaline phosphatase

Local: Pain, burning at injection site

Other reactions reported with cephalosporins include Stevens-Johnson syndrome, toxic epidermal necrolysis, erythema multiforme, pseudomembranous colitis, angioedema, hemolytic anemia, candidiasis, encephalopathy, asterixis, neuromuscular excitability, seizures, serum-sickness reactions, renal dysfunction, interstitial nephritis, toxic nephropathy, cholestasis, aplastic anemia, hemolytic anemia, pancytopenia, agranulocytosis, colitis, prolonged PT, hemorrhage, superinfection

Drug Interactions Increased Effect/Toxicity: Probenecid may decrease cephalosporin elimination. Furosemide, aminoglycosides in combination with ceftizoxime may result in additive nephrotoxicity.

Drug Uptake

Half-life, elimination: 1.6 hours; Cl_{cr}<10 mL/minute: 25 hours

Time to peak: I.M.: 0.5-1 hour

Pregnancy Risk Factor B

Generic Available No

Ceftriaxone (sef trye AKS one)

Related Information

Animal and Human Bites Guidelines *on page 1416*

Nonviral Infectious Diseases *on page 1342*

U.S. Brand Names Rocephin®

Canadian Brand Names Rocephin®

Mexican Brand Names Benaxona; Cefaxona®; Ceftrex®; Rocephin®; Tacex®; Terbac®; Triaken®

Pharmacologic Category Antibiotic, Cephalosporin (Third Generation)

Synonyms Ceftriaxone Sodium

Use Treatment of lower respiratory tract infections, skin and skin structure infections, bone and joint infections, intra-abdominal and urinary tract infections, sepsis and meningitis due to susceptible organisms; documented or suspected infection due to susceptible organisms in home care patients and patients without I.V. line access; treatment of documented or suspected gonococcal infection or chancroid; emergency room management of patients at high risk for bacteremia, periorbital or buccal cellulitis, salmonellosis or shigellosis, and pneumonia of unestablished etiology (<5 years of age); treatment of Lyme disease, depends on the stage of the disease (used in Stage II and Stage III, but not stage I; doxycycline is the drug of choice for Stage I)

Local Anesthetic/Vasoconstrictor Precautions No information available to require special precautions

Effects on Dental Treatment No effects or complications reported

Dosage I.M., I.V.:

Neonates:

- Postnatal age ≤7 days: 50 mg/kg/day given every 24 hours
- Postnatal age >7 days:
  - ≤2000 g: 50 mg/kg/day given every 24 hours
  - >2000 g: 50-75 mg/kg/day given every 24 hours
- Gonococcal prophylaxis: 25-50 mg/kg as a single dose (dose not to exceed 125 mg)
- Gonococcal infection: 25-50 mg/kg/day (maximum dose: 125 mg) given every 24 hours for 10-14 days

Infants and Children: 50-75 mg/kg/day in 1-2 divided doses every 12-24 hours; maximum: 2 g/24 hours

- Meningitis: 100 mg/kg/day divided every 12-24 hours, up to a maximum of 4 g/24 hours; loading dose of 75 mg/kg/dose may be given at start of therapy
- Otitis media: I.M.: 50 mg/kg as a single dose (maximum: 1 g)
- Uncomplicated gonococcal infections, sexual assault, and STD prophylaxis: I.M.: 125 mg as a single dose plus doxycycline
- Complicated gonococcal infections:
  - Infants: I.M., I.V.: 25-50 mg/kg/day in a single dose (maximum: 125 mg/dose); treat for 7 days for disseminated infection and 7-14 days for documented meningitis
  - <45 kg: 50 mg/kg/day once daily; maximum: 1 g/day; for ophthalmia, peritonitis, arthritis, or bacteremia: 50-100 mg/kg/day divided every 12-24 hours; maximum: 2 g/day for meningitis or endocarditis
  - >45 kg: 1 g/day once daily for disseminated gonococcal infections; 1-2 g dose every 12 hours for meningitis or endocarditis
- Acute epididymitis: I.M.: 250 mg in a single dose

Adults: 1-2 g every 12-24 hours (depending on the type and severity of infection); maximum dose: 2 g every 12 hours for treatment of meningitis

- Uncomplicated gonorrhea: I.M.: 250 mg as a single dose
- Surgical prophylaxis: 1 g 30 minutes to 2 hours before surgery

Hemodialysis: Not dialyzable (0% to 5%); administer dose postdialysis

Peritoneal dialysis: Administer 750 mg every 12 hours

Continuous arteriovenous or venovenous hemofiltration: Removes 10 mg of ceftriaxone per liter of filtrate per day

(Continued)

Ceftriaxone *(Continued)*

Mechanism of Action Inhibits bacterial cell wall synthesis by binding to one or more of the penicillin-binding proteins (PBPs) which in turn inhibits the final transpeptidation step of peptidoglycan synthesis in bacterial cell walls, thus inhibiting cell wall biosynthesis. Bacteria eventually lyse due to ongoing activity of cell wall autolytic enzymes (autolysins and murein hydrolases) while cell wall assembly is arrested.

Other Adverse Effects

1% to 10%:

Dermatologic: Rash (2%)

Gastrointestinal: Diarrhea (3%)

Hematologic: Eosinophilia (6%), thrombocytosis (5%), leukopenia (2%)

Hepatic: Elevated transaminases (3.1% to 3.3%)

Local: Pain, induration at injection site (I.V. 1%); warmth, tightness, induration (5% to 17%) following I.M. injection

Renal: Increased BUN (1%)

Reactions reported with other cephalosporins include angioedema, aplastic anemia, asterixis, cholestasis, colitis, encephalopathy, erythema multiforme, hemorrhage, interstitial nephritis, neuromuscular excitability, pancytopenia, paresthesia, pseudomembranous colitis, renal dysfunction, seizures, Stevens-Johnson syndrome, superinfection, toxic epidermal necrolysis, toxic nephropathy

Drug Interactions Increased Effect/Toxicity: Aminoglycosides may result in synergistic antibacterial activity. High-dose probenecid decreases clearance. Aminoglycosides increase nephrotoxic potential.

Drug Uptake

Absorption: I.M.: Well absorbed

Half-life, elimination (dependent on renal/hepatic function):

Normal: 5-9 hours

Neonates: Postnatal (1-4 days old): 16 hours; 9-30 days old: 9 hours

Time to peak: I.M.: 1-2 hours

Pregnancy Risk Factor B

Generic Available No

Cefuroxime (se fyoor OKS eem)

U.S. Brand Names Ceftin®; Kefurox®; Zinacef®

Canadian Brand Names Ceftin®; Kefurox®; Zinacef®

Mexican Brand Names Cefuracet®; Cetoxil®; Froxal®; Zinnat®

Pharmacologic Category Antibiotic, Cephalosporin (Second Generation)

Synonyms Cefuroxime Axetil; Cefuroxime Sodium

Use Treatment of infections caused by staphylococci, group B streptococci, *H. influenzae* (type A and B), *E. coli*, *Enterobacter*, *Salmonella*, and *Klebsiella*; treatment of susceptible infections of the lower respiratory tract, otitis media, urinary tract, skin and soft tissue, bone and joint, sepsis and gonorrhea

Local Anesthetic/Vasoconstrictor Precautions No information available to require special precautions

Effects on Dental Treatment No effects or complications reported

Dosage Cefuroxime axetil film-coated tablets and oral suspension are not bioequivalent and are not substitutable on a mg/mg basis.

Children ≥3 months:

Pharyngitis, tonsillitis: Oral:

Suspension: 20 mg/kg/day (maximum: 500 mg/day) in 2 divided doses

Tablet: 125 mg every 12 hours

Acute otitis media, impetigo: Oral:

Suspension: 30 mg/kg/day (maximum: 1 g/day) in 2 divided doses for 10 days

Tablet: 250 mg twice daily for 10 days

I.M., I.V.: 75-150 mg/kg/day divided every 8 hours; maximum dose: 6 g/day

Meningitis: Not recommended (doses of 200-240 mg/kg/day divided every 6-8 hours have been used); maximum dose: 9 g/day

Acute bacterial maxillary sinusitis:

Suspension: 30 mg/kg/day in 2 divided doses for 10 days; maximum dose: 1 g/day

Tablet: 250 mg twice daily for 10 days

Adults:

Oral: 250-500 mg twice daily; uncomplicated urinary tract infection: 125-250 mg every 12 hours

I.M., I.V.: 750 mg to 1.5 g/dose every 8 hours or 100-150 mg/kg/day in divided doses every 6-8 hours; maximum: 6 g/24 hours

Dosing adjustment in renal impairment:

Cl_{cr} 10-20 mL/minute: Administer every 12 hours

Cl_{cr} <10 mL/minute: Administer every 24 hours

Hemodialysis: Dialyzable (25%)

Continuous arteriovenous or venovenous hemodiafiltration effects: Dose as for Cl_{cr} 10-20 mL/minute

Mechanism of Action Inhibits bacterial cell wall synthesis by binding to one or more of the penicillin-binding proteins (PBPs) which in turn inhibits the final transpeptidation step of peptidoglycan synthesis in bacterial cell walls, thus inhibiting cell wall biosynthesis. Bacteria eventually lyse due to ongoing activity of cell wall autolytic enzymes (autolysins and murein hydrolases) while cell wall assembly is arrested.

Other Adverse Effects

1% to 10%:

Hematologic: Eosinophilia (7%), decreased hemoglobin and hematocrit (10%)

Hepatic: Increased transaminases (4%), increased alkaline phosphatase (2%)

Local: Thrombophlebitis (2%)

Reactions reported with other cephalosporins include agranulocytosis, aplastic anemia, asterixis, encephalopathy, hemorrhage, neuromuscular excitability, serum-sickness reactions, superinfection, toxic nephropathy

Drug Interactions

Increased Effect: High-dose probenecid decreases clearance.

Increased Toxicity: Aminoglycosides increase nephrotoxic potential.

Drug Uptake

Absorption: Oral (cefuroxime axetil): Increased when given with or shortly after food or infant formula

Half-life, elimination: Adults: 1-2 hours (increases with renal impairment); I.M.: 0.25-1 hour; I.V.: 2-3 minutes

Neonates: ≤3 days old : 5.1-5.8 hours; 6-14 days old: 2-4.2 hours; 3-4 weeks old: 1-1.5 hours

Time to peak: I.M.: ~15-60 minutes; I.V.: 2-3 minutes

Pregnancy Risk Factor B

Generic Available Yes

Cefzil® *see* Cefprozil *on page 242*
Celebrex® *see* Celecoxib *on page 247*

Celecoxib (ce le COX ib)

Related Information

Rheumatoid Arthritis and Osteoarthritis *on page 1340*

U.S. Brand Names Celebrex®

Canadian Brand Names Celebrex®

Mexican Brand Names Celebrex®

Pharmacologic Category Nonsteroidal Anti-inflammatory Drug (NSAID), COX-2 Selective

Use Relief of the signs and symptoms of osteoarthritis; relief of the signs and symptoms of rheumatoid arthritis in adults; decreasing intestinal polyps in familial adenomatous polyposis (FAP); management of acute pain; treatment of primary dysmenorrhea

Local Anesthetic/Vasoconstrictor Precautions No information available to require special precautions

Effects on Dental Treatment Nonselective NSAIDs are known to reversibly decrease platelet aggregation via mechanisms different than observed with aspirin. According to the manufacturer, celecoxib, at single dose up to 800 mg and multiple doses of 600 mg twice daily, had no effect on platelet aggregation or bleeding time. Comparative NSAIDs (naproxen 500 mg twice daily, ibuprofen 800 mg three times daily or diclofenac 75 mg twice daily) significantly reduced platelet aggregation and prolonged the bleeding times.

Dosage Oral:

Adults:

Acute pain or primary dysmenorrhea: Initial dose: 400 mg, followed by an additional 200 mg if needed on day 1; maintenance dose: 200 mg twice daily as needed

Familial adenomatous polyposis (FAP): 400 mg twice daily

Osteoarthritis: 200 mg/day as a single dose or in divided dose twice daily

Rheumatoid arthritis: 100-200 mg twice daily

Elderly: No specific adjustment is recommended; however, the AUC in elderly patients may be increased by 50% as compared to younger subjects. Use the lowest recommended dose in patients weighing <50 kg.

Dosing adjustment in renal impairment: No specific dosage adjustment is recommended; not recommended in patients with advanced renal disease

Dosing adjustment in hepatic impairment: Reduced dosage is recommended (AUC may be increased by 40% to 180%); decrease dose by 50% in patients with moderate hepatic impairment (Child-Pugh class II)

Mechanism of Action Inhibits prostaglandin synthesis by decreasing the activity of the enzyme, cyclo-oxygenase-2 (COX-2), which results in decreased formation of prostaglandin precursors. Celecoxib does not inhibit cyclo-oxygenase-1 (COX-1) at therapeutic concentrations.

Other Adverse Effects

>10%: Central nervous system: Headache (16%)

(Continued)

Celecoxib *(Continued)*

2% to 10%:
- Cardiovascular: Peripheral edema (2%)
- Central nervous system: Insomnia (2%), dizziness (2%)
- Dermatologic: Skin rash (2%)
- Gastrointestinal: Dyspepsia (9%), diarrhea (6%), abdominal pain (4%), nausea (4%), flatulence (2%)
- Neuromuscular & skeletal: Back pain (3%)
- Respiratory: Upper respiratory tract infection (8%), sinusitis (5%), pharyngitis (2%), rhinitis (2%)
- Miscellaneous: Accidental injury (3%)

0.1% to 2%:
- Cardiovascular: Hypertension (aggravated), chest pain, myocardial infarction, palpitation, tachycardia, facial edema
- Central nervous system: Migraine, vertigo, hypoesthesia, fatigue, fever, pain, hypotonia, anxiety, depression, nervousness, somnolence
- Dermatologic: Alopecia, dermatitis, photosensitivity, pruritus, rash (maculopapular), rash (erythematous), dry skin, urticaria
- Endocrine & metabolic: Hot flashes, diabetes mellitus, hyperglycemia, hypercholesterolemia, breast pain, dysmenorrhea, menstrual disturbances, hypokalemia
- Gastrointestinal: Constipation, tenesmus, diverticulitis, eructation, esophagitis, gastroenteritis, vomiting, gastroesophageal reflux, hemorrhoids, hiatal hernia, melena, stomatitis, anorexia, increased appetite, taste disturbance, xerostomia, tooth disorder, weight gain
- Genitourinary: Prostate disorder, vaginal bleeding, vaginitis, monilial vaginitis, dysuria, cystitis, urinary frequency, incontinence, urinary tract infection,
- Hematologic: Anemia, thrombocytopenia, ecchymosis
- Hepatic: Elevated transaminases, increased alkaline phosphatase
- Neuromuscular & skeletal: Leg cramps, increased CPK, neck stiffness, arthralgia, myalgia, bone disorder, fracture, synovitis, tendonitis, neuralgia, paresthesia, neuropathy, weakness
- Ocular: Glaucoma, blurred vision, cataract, conjunctivitis, eye pain
- Otic: Deafness, tinnitus, earache, otitis media
- Renal: Increased BUN, increased creatinine, albuminuria, hematuria, renal calculi
- Respiratory: Bronchitis, bronchospasm, cough, dyspnea, laryngitis, pneumonia, epistaxis
- Miscellaneous: Allergic reactions, flu-like syndrome, breast cancer, herpes infection, bacterial infection, moniliasis, viral infection, increased diaphoresis

Warnings/Precautions Gastrointestinal irritation, ulceration, bleeding, and perforation may occur with NSAIDs (it is unclear whether celecoxib is associated with rates of these events which are similar to nonselective NSAIDs). Use with caution in patients with a history of GI disease (bleeding or ulcers), use lowest dose for shortest time possible. Use with caution in patients with decreased renal function, hepatic disease, CHF, hypertension, or asthma. Anaphylactoid reactions may occur, even with no prior exposure to celecoxib. Use caution in patients with known or suspected deficiency of cytochrome P450 isoenzyme 2C9. Safety and efficacy have not been established in patients <18 years of age.

Drug Interactions CYP2C9 enzyme substrate, CYP2D6 enzyme inhibitor
- ACE inhibitors: Antihypertensive effect may be diminished by celecoxib.
- Aspirin: Low-dose aspirin may be used with celecoxib, however monitor for GI complications.
- CYP2C9 inhibitors (ie, amiodarone, fluoxetine, sulfonamides, ritonavir, zafirlukast): Theoretically, may result in significant increases in celecoxib concentrations.
- Fluconazole: Fluconazole increases celecoxib concentrations twofold. Lowest dose of celecoxib should be used.
- Lithium: Plasma levels of lithium are increased by ~17% when used with celecoxib. Monitor lithium levels closely when treatment with celecoxib is started or withdrawn.
- Loop diuretics (bumetanide, furosemide, torsemide): Natriuretic effect of furosemide and other loop diuretics may be decreased by celecoxib.
- Methotrexate: Severe bone marrow suppression, aplastic anemia, and GI toxicity have been reported with concomitant NSAID therapy. Selective COX-2 inhibitors appear to have a lower risk of this toxicity, however, caution is warranted.
- Thiazide diuretics: Natriuretic effects of thiazide diuretics may be decreased by celecoxib.
- Warfarin: Bleeding events and increased prothrombin time have been reported with concomitant use. Monitor closely, especially in the elderly.

Drug Uptake
- Half-life, elimination: 11 hours
- Time to peak: 3 hours

Pregnancy Risk Factor C/D (3rd trimester)

Generic Available No

Comments According to the manufacturer, two out of 5,285 patients (0.04%) experienced significant upper GI bleeding, at 14 and 32 days after initiation of dosing. Approximately 40% of the 5,285 patients were in studies that required them to be free of ulcers by endoscopy at entry into the study. As a result, the manufacturer stressed that it is unclear if the study population is representative of the general population. As of this printing, long-term studies comparing the incidence of serious upper GI adverse effects in patients taking celecoxib compared to other nonselective NSAIDs had not been reported. Celecoxib does not appear to inhibit platelet aggregation at recommended doses. Reports have shown that celecoxib does not generally affect platelet counts, prothrombin time or partial thromboplastin time (PTT).

Cross-reactivity, including bronchospasm, between aspirin and other NSAIDs has been reported in aspirin-sensitive patients. The manufacturer suggests that celecoxib should not be administered to patients with this type of aspirin sensitivity and should be used with caution in patients with pre-existing asthma.

The manufacturer studied the effect of celecoxib on the anticoagulant effect of warfarin and found no alteration of anticoagulant effect, as determined by prothrombin time, in patients taking 2 mg to 5 mg daily. However, the manufacturer has issued a caution when using celecoxib with warfarin since those patients are at increased risk of bleeding complications.

A literature report suggested that the enzyme COX-2 (cyclo-oxygenase type 2) is a major source of systemic prostacyclin biosynthesis in humans. Prostacyclin is involved in blood vessel dilation and inhibition of blood clotting. In view of the fact that celecoxib inhibits the COX-2 enzyme, prostacyclin production could be suppressed. The resultant effects on hemostasis are unknown at this time.

Recent news reports have noted an association between selective COX-2 inhibitors and increased cardiovascular risk. This was prompted by publication of a meta-analysis entitled "Risk of Cardiovascular Events Associated With Selective COX-2 Inhibitors" in the August 22, 2001, edition of the Journal of the American Medical Association (JAMA), viewable at http://jama.ama-assn.org/issues/v286n8/rfull/jsc10193.html. The researchers reanalyzed four previously published trials, assessing cardiovascular events in patients receiving either celecoxib or rofecoxib. They found an association between the use of COX-2 inhibitors and cardiovascular events (including myocardial infarction and ischemic stroke). The annualized myocardial infarction rate was found to be significantly higher in patients receiving celecoxib or rofecoxib than in the control (placebo) group from a recent meta-analysis of primary prevention trials. Although cause and effect cannot be established (these trials were originally designed to assess GI effects, not cardiovascular ones), the authors believe the available data raise a cautionary flag concerning the risk of cardiovascular events with the use of COX-2 inhibitors. The manufacturers of these agents, as well as other healthcare professionals, dispute the methods and validity of the study's conclusions. To date, the FDA has not required any change in the labeling of these agents. Further study is required before any potential risk may be defined.

Selected Readings

Everts B, Wahrborg P, Hedner T, "COX-2 Specific Inhibitors - The Emergence of a New Class of Analgesic and Anti-inflammatory Drugs," *Clin Rheumatol*, 2000, 19(5):331-43.

Jouzeau JY, Terlain B, Abid A, et al, "Cyclo-oxygenase Isoenzymes. How Recent Findings Affect Thinking About Nonsteroidal Anti-inflammatory Drugs," *Drugs*, 1997, 53(4):563-82.

Kaplan-Machlis B and Klostermeyer BS, "The Cyclo-oxygenase-2 Inhibitors: Safety and Effectiveness," *Ann Pharmacother*, 1999, 33(9):979-88.

Kurumbail RG, Stevens AM, Gierse JK, et al, "Structural Basis for Selective Inhibition of Cyclo-oxygenase-2 By Anti-inflammatory Agents," *Nature*, 1996, 384(6610):644-8.

Malmstrom K, Daniels S, Kotey P, et al, "Comparison of Rofecoxib and Celecoxib, two Cyclooxygenase-2 Inhibitors, in Postoperative Dental Pain: A Randomized Placebo- and Active-Comparator-Controlled Clinical Trial," *Clin Ther*, 1999, 21(10):1653-63.

McAdam BF, Catella-Lawson F, Mardini IA, et al, "Systemic Biosynthesis of Prostacyclin by Cyclo-oxygenase (COX)-2: The Human Pharmacology of a Selective Inhibitor of COX-2," *Proc Natl Acad Sci U S A*, 1999, 96(1):272-7.

Moore PA and Hersh EV, "Celecoxib and Rofecoxib. The Role of COX-2 Inhibitors in Dental Practice," *J Am Dent Assoc*, 2001, 132(4):451-6.

Needleman P and Isakson PC, "The Discovery and Function of COX-2," *J Rheumatol*, 1997, 24(S49):6-8.

Whelton A, Maurath CJ, Verburg KM, et al, "Renal Safety and Tolerability of Celecoxib, a Novel Cyclo-oxygenase-2 Inhibitor," *Am J Ther*, 2000, 7(3):159-75.

Wynn RL, "The New COX-2 Inhibitors: Celecoxib and Rofecoxib," *Home Health Care Consultant*, 2001, 8(10):24-31.

Wynn RL, "The New COX-2 Inhibitors: Rofecoxib (Vioxx®) and Celecoxib (Celebrex™)," *Gen Dent*, 2000, 48(1):16-20.

Wynn RL, "NSAIDS and Cardiovascular Effects, Celecoxib for Dental Pain, and a New Analgesic - Tramadol with Acetaminophen," *Gen Dent*, 2002, 50(3):218-222.

Celestone® *see* Betamethasone *on page 159*

Celestone® Phosphate *see* Betamethasone *on page 159*

Celestone® Soluspan® *see* Betamethasone *on page 159*

Celexa™ *see* Citalopram *on page 294*

CellCept® *see* Mycophenolate *on page 836*

Cellufresh® [OTC] *see* Carboxymethylcellulose *on page 223*

Cellulose, Oxidized (SEL yoo lose, OKS i dyzed)

U.S. Brand Names Oxycel®; Surgicel®

Pharmacologic Category Hemostatic Agent

Synonyms Absorbable Cotton

Use Temporary packing for the control of capillary, venous, or small arterial hemorrhage

Local Anesthetic/Vasoconstrictor Precautions No information available to require special precautions

Effects on Dental Treatment No effects or complications reported

Dosage Minimal amounts of an appropriate size are laid on the bleeding site

Other Adverse Effects 1% to 10%:

Central nervous system: Headache

Respiratory: Nasal burning or stinging, sneezing (rhinological procedures)

Miscellaneous: Encapsulation of fluid, foreign body reactions (with or without) infection

Contraindications Packing or wadding as a hemostatic agents; packing or implantation in fractures or laminectomies; control of hemorrhage from large arteries or on nonhemorrhagic serous oozing surfaces

Warnings/Precautions By swelling, oxidized cellulose may cause nerve damage by pressure in bony confine (ie, optic nerve and chiasm); always remove from these sites of application or do not use at all (see Contraindications); do not autoclave, do not moisten with water or saline (lessens hemostatic effect). Avoid wadding or packing tightly; do not use after application of $AgNO_3$ or other escharotic agents.

Dosage Forms PAD (Oxycel®): 3" x 3" (8 ply). **PLEDGET** (Oxycel®): 2" x 1" x 1". **STRIP:** (Oxycel®): 5" x 1/2" (4 ply), 18" x 2" (4 ply), 36" x 1/2" (4 ply); (Surgicel®): 1/2" x 2", 2" x 3", 2" x 14", 4" x 8"

Generic Available No

Cellulose, Oxidized Regenerated

(SEL yoo lose, OKS i dyzed re JEN er aye ted)

U.S. Brand Names Surgicel® Absorbable Hemostat

Pharmacologic Category Hemostatic Agent

Use

Dental: To control bleeding created during dental surgery

Medical: Hemostatic

Local Anesthetic/Vasoconstrictor Precautions No information available to require special precautions

Effects on Dental Treatment No effects or complications reported

Dosage Minimal amounts of the fabric strip are laid on the bleeding site or held firmly against the tissues until hemostasis occurs.

Mechanism of Action Cellulose, oxidized regenerated is saturated with blood at the bleeding site and swells into a brownish or black gelatinous mass which aids in the formation of a clot. When used in small amounts, it is absorbed from the sites of implantation with little or no tissue reaction.

Contraindications Packing or wadding (unless it is removed after hemostasis occurs); implantation in bone defects

Warnings/Precautions Autoclaving causes physical breakdown of the product. Closing the material in a contaminated wound without drainage may lead to complications. The material should not be moistened before insertion since the hemostatic effect is greater when applied dry. The material should not be impregnated with anti-infective agents. Its hemostatic effect is not enhanced by the addition of thrombin. The material may be left *in situ* when necessary but it is advisable to remove it once hemostasis is achieved.

Dosage Forms STRIP, knitted fabric: 1/2" x 2" envelopes

Generic Available No

Comments Oxidized regenerated cellulose is prepared by the controlled oxidation of regenerated cellulose. The fabric is white with a pale yellow cast and has a faint, caramel-like aroma. A slight discoloration may occur with age but this does not effect its hemostatic actions.

Cellulose Sodium Phosphate (sel yoo lose SOW dee um FOS fate)

U.S. Brand Names Calcibind®

Canadian Brand Names Calcibind®

Pharmacologic Category Urinary Tract Product

Synonyms CSP; Sodium Cellulose Phosphate

Use Adjunct to dietary restriction to reduce renal calculi formation in absorptive hypercalciuria type I

Local Anesthetic/Vasoconstrictor Precautions No information available to require special precautions

Effects on Dental Treatment No effects or complications reported

Dosage Adults: Oral: 5 g 3 times/day with meals; decrease dose to 5 g with main meal and 2.5 g with each of two other meals when urinary calcium declines to <150 mg/day

Pregnancy Risk Factor C
Generic Available No

Celluvisc® [OTC] *see* Carboxymethylcellulose *on page 223*
Celontin® *see* Methsuximide *on page 791*
Cenafed® [OTC] *see* Pseudoephedrine *on page 1022*
Cenafed® Plus Tablet [OTC] *see* Triprolidine and Pseudoephedrine *on page 1213*
Cena-K® *see* Potassium Chloride *on page 977*
Cenestin® *see* Estrogens, Conjugated (Synthetic) *on page 466*
Cenolate® *see* Sodium Ascorbate *on page 1093*
Cēpacol® Anesthetic Troches [OTC] *see* Cetylpyridinium and Benzocaine *on page 256*
Cēpacol® Mouthwash/Gargle [OTC] *see* Cetylpyridinium *on page 256*
Cēpastat® [OTC] *see* Phenol *on page 946*

Cephalexin (sef a LEKS in)

Related Information

Antibiotic Prophylaxis, Preprocedural Guidelines for Dental Patients *on page 1344*
Dental Drug Interactions: Update on Drug Combinations Requiring Special Considerations *on page 1434*
Oral Bacterial Infections *on page 1367*

U.S. Brand Names Biocef; Keflex®; Keftab®

Canadian Brand Names Apo®-Cephalex; Keftab®; Novo-Lexin®; Nu-Cephalex®; PMS-Cephalexin

Mexican Brand Names Ceporex; Naxifelar

Pharmacologic Category Antibiotic, Cephalosporin (First Generation)

Synonyms Cephalexin Hydrochloride; Cephalexin Monohydrate

Use Treatment of susceptible bacterial infections, including those caused by group A beta-hemolytic *Streptococcus*, *Staphylococcus*, *Klebsiella pneumoniae*, *E. coli*, *Proteus mirabilis*, and *Shigella*; predominantly used for lower respiratory tract, urinary tract, skin and soft tissue, and bone and joint; prophylaxis against bacterial endocarditis in high-risk patients undergoing surgical or dental procedures who are allergic to penicillin

Local Anesthetic/Vasoconstrictor Precautions No information available to require special precautions

Effects on Dental Treatment No effects or complications reported

Dosage Oral:

Children: 25-50 mg/kg/day every 6 hours; severe infections: 50-100 mg/kg/day in divided doses every 6 hours; maximum: 3 g/24 hours
Adults: 250-1000 mg every 6 hours; maximum: 4 g/day
Prophylaxis of bacterial endocarditis (dental, oral, respiratory tract, or esophageal procedures):
Children: 50 mg/kg 1 hour prior to procedure
Adults: 2 g 1 hour prior to procedure

Dosing adjustment in renal impairment: Adults:
Cl_{cr} 10-40 mL/minute: 250-500 mg every 8-12 hours
Cl_{cr} <10 mL/minute: 250 mg every 12-24 hours

Hemodialysis: Moderately dialyzable (20% to 50%)

Mechanism of Action Inhibits bacterial cell wall synthesis by binding to one or more of the penicillin-binding proteins (PBPs) which in turn inhibits the final transpeptidation step of peptidoglycan synthesis in bacterial cell walls, thus inhibiting cell wall biosynthesis. Bacteria eventually lyse due to ongoing activity of cell wall autolytic enzymes (autolysins and murein hydrolases) while cell wall assembly is arrested.

Other Adverse Effects

1% to 10%: Gastrointestinal: Diarrhea
<1%: Dizziness, fatigue, headache, rash, urticaria, angioedema, anaphylaxis, erythema multiforme, toxic epidermal necrolysis, Stevens-Johnson syndrome, serum-sickness reaction, nausea, vomiting, dyspepsia, gastritis, abdominal pain, pseudomembranous colitis, interstitial nephritis, agitation, hallucinations, confusion, arthralgia, eosinophilia, neutropenia, thrombocytopenia, anemia, increased transaminases, hepatitis, cholestasis
Other reactions with cephalosporins include anaphylaxis, vomiting, agranulocytosis, colitis, pancytopenia, aplastic anemia, hemolytic anemia, hemorrhage, prolonged PT, encephalopathy, asterixis, neuromuscular excitability, seizures, superinfection

Contraindications Hypersensitivity to cephalexin, other cephalosporins, or any component of their formulation

Warnings/Precautions Modify dosage in patients with severe renal impairment, prolonged use may result in superinfection; use with caution in patients with a history of penicillin allergy, especially IgE-mediated reactions (eg, anaphylaxis, urticaria); may cause antibiotic-associated colitis or colitis secondary to *C. difficile*
(Continued)

Cephalexin *(Continued)*

Drug Interactions

Increased Effect: High-dose probenecid decreases clearance

Increased Toxicity: Aminoglycosides increase nephrotoxic potential

Dietary/Ethanol/Herb Considerations Food: Administer with food to reduce GI upset; food may decrease serum concentration. Administer 1 hour before or 2 hours after meals to increase total absorption.

Drug Uptake

Absorption: Adults: Rapid; Children: Delayed in young children; may be decreased up to 50% in neonates

Duration: 6 hours

Half-life, elimination: Neonates: 5 hours old; Children 3-12 months: 2.5 hours; Adults: 0.5-1.2 hours; prolonged with renal impairment

Time to peak: Oral: ≤1 hour

Pregnancy Risk Factor B

Breast-feeding Considerations Theoretically, drug absorbed by nursing infant may change bowel flora or affect fever work-up result. **Note:** As a class, cephalosporins are used to treat infections in infants.

Dosage Forms CAP, as monohydrate: 250 mg, 500 mg. **POWDER, oral suspension, as monohydrate:** 125 mg/5 mL (5 mL unit dose, 60 mL, 100 mL, 200 mL); 250 mg/5 mL (5 mL unit dose, 100 mL, 200 mL). **TAB, as hydrochloride:** 500 mg. **TAB, as monohydrate:** 250 mg, 500 mg, 1 g.

Generic Available Yes

Comments Cephalexin is effective against anaerobic bacteria, but the sensitivity of alpha-hemolytic *Streptococcus* vary; approximately 10% of strains are resistant. Nearly 70% are intermediately sensitive. Patients allergic to penicillins can use a cephalosporin; the incidence of cross-reactivity between penicillins and cephalosporins is 1% when the allergic reaction to penicillin is delayed. If the patient has a history of immediate reaction to penicillin, the incidence of cross-reactivity is 20%; cephalosporins are contraindicated in these patients.

Selected Readings

"Advisory Statement. Antibiotic Prophylaxis for Dental Patients With Total Joint Replacements. American Dental Association; American Academy of Orthopedic Surgeons," *J Am Dent Assoc*, 1997, 128(7):1004-8.

Dajani AS, Taubert KA, Wilson W, et al, "Prevention of Bacterial Endocarditis. Recommendations by the American Heart Association," *JAMA* 1997, 277(22):1794-801.

Dajani AS, Taubert KA, Wilson W, et al, "Prevention of Bacterial Endocarditis: Recommendations by the American Heart Association," *J Am Dent Assoc* 1997, 128(8):1142-51.

Saxon A, Beall GN, Rohr AS, et al, "Immediate Hypersensitivity Reactions to Beta-Lactam Antibiotics," *Ann Intern Med*, 1987, 107(2):204-15.

Wynn RL, Bergman SA, Meiller TF, et al, "Antibiotics in Treating Oral-Facial Infections of Odontogenic Origin: An Update", *Gen Dent*, 2001, 49(3):238-40, 242, 244 passim.

Cephalothin (sef A loe thin)

Canadian Brand Names Ceporacin®

Pharmacologic Category Antibiotic, Cephalosporin (First Generation)

Synonyms Cephalothin Sodium

Use Treatment of susceptible bacterial infections, including those caused by group A beta-hemolytic *Streptococcus*; respiratory, genitourinary, GI, skin and soft tissue, bone and joint infections; septicemia; cephalexin is the oral equivalent

Local Anesthetic/Vasoconstrictor Precautions No information available to require special precautions

Effects on Dental Treatment No effects or complications reported

Dosage I.M., I.V.:

Children: 75-125 mg/kg/day divided every 4-6 hours; maximum dose: 10 g in a 24-hour period

Adults: 500 mg to 2 g every 4-6 hours

Mechanism of Action Inhibits bacterial cell wall synthesis by binding to one or more of the penicillin-binding proteins (PBPs) which in turn inhibits the final transpeptidation step of peptidoglycan synthesis in bacterial cell walls, thus inhibiting cell wall biosynthesis. Bacteria eventually lyse due to ongoing activity of cell wall autolytic enzymes (autolysins and murein hydrolases) while cell wall assembly is arrested.

Other Adverse Effects

1% to 10%: Gastrointestinal: Diarrhea, nausea, vomiting

Other reactions with cephalosporins include anaphylaxis, erythema multiforme, toxic epidermal necrolysis, Stevens-Johnson syndrome, dizziness, fever, headache, CNS irritability, seizures, decreased hemoglobin, neutropenia, leukopenia, agranulocytosis, pancytopenia, aplastic anemia, hemolytic anemia, interstitial nephritis, toxic nephropathy, vaginitis, angioedema, cholestasis, hemorrhage, prolonged PT, serum-sickness reactions, superinfection

Drug Interactions Increased Effect/Toxicity: Probenecid may decrease cephalosporin elimination. Aminoglycosides may increase nephrotoxic potential.

Drug Uptake

Half-life, elimination: 30-60 minutes

Time to peak: I.M.: ≤30 minutes; I.V.: ≤15 minutes

Pregnancy Risk Factor B

Generic Available Yes

Cephapirin (sef a PYE rin)

U.S. Brand Names Cefadyl®

Canadian Brand Names Cefadyl®

Pharmacologic Category Antibiotic, Cephalosporin (First Generation)

Synonyms Cephapirin Sodium

Use Treatment of infections when caused by susceptible strains including group A beta-hemolytic *Streptococcus*; used in serious respiratory, genitourinary, GI, skin and soft tissue, bone and joint infections; septicemia; endocarditis; identical to cephalothin

Local Anesthetic/Vasoconstrictor Precautions No information available to require special precautions

Effects on Dental Treatment No effects or complications reported

Dosage I.M., I.V.:

Children: 10-20 mg/kg/dose every 6 hours up to 4 g/24 hours

Adults: 500 mg to 1 g every 6 hours up to 12 g/day

Mechanism of Action Inhibits bacterial cell wall synthesis by binding to one or more of the penicillin-binding proteins (PBPs) which in turn inhibits the final transpeptidation step of peptidoglycan synthesis in bacterial cell walls, thus inhibiting cell wall biosynthesis. Bacteria eventually lyse due to ongoing activity of cell wall autolytic enzymes (autolysins and murein hydrolases) while cell wall assembly is arrested.

Other Adverse Effects

1% to 10%: Gastrointestinal: Diarrhea

Reactions reported with other cephalosporins include anaphylaxis, erythema multiforme, toxic epidermal necrolysis, Stevens-Johnson syndrome, dizziness, fever, headache, encephalopathy, asterixis, neuromuscular excitability, seizures, nausea, vomiting, pseudomembranous colitis, decreased hemoglobin, agranulocytosis, pancytopenia, aplastic anemia, hemolytic anemia, interstitial nephritis, toxic nephropathy, pain at injection site, vaginitis, angioedema, cholestasis, hemorrhage, prolonged PT, serum-sickness reactions, superinfection

Drug Interactions Increased Effect/Toxicity: High-dose probenecid decreases clearance of cephapirin. Aminoglycosides in combination with cephapirin may result in additive nephrotoxicity.

Drug Uptake

Half-life, elimination: 36-60 minutes

Time to peak: I.M.: ≤30 minutes; I.V.: ≤5 minutes

Pregnancy Risk Factor B

Generic Available No

Cephradine (SEF ra deen)

Related Information

Antibiotic Prophylaxis, Preprocedural Guidelines for Dental Patients *on page 1344*

U.S. Brand Names Velosef®

Mexican Brand Names Veracef

Pharmacologic Category Antibiotic, Cephalosporin (First Generation)

Use Treatment of infections when caused by susceptible strains in respiratory, genitourinary, GI, skin and soft tissue, bone and joint infections; treatment of susceptible gram-positive bacilli and cocci (never enterococcus); some gram-negative bacilli including *E. coli*, *Proteus*, and *Klebsiella* may be susceptible

Local Anesthetic/Vasoconstrictor Precautions No information available to require special precautions

Effects on Dental Treatment No effects or complications reported

Dosage Oral:

Children ≥9 months: 25-50 mg/kg/day in divided doses every 6 hours

Adults: 250-500 mg every 6-12 hours

Dosing adjustment in renal impairment: Adults:

Cl_{cr} 10-50 mL/minute: 250 mg every 6 hours

Cl_{cr} <10 mL/minute: 125 mg every 6 hours

Mechanism of Action Inhibits bacterial cell wall synthesis by binding to one or more of the penicillin-binding proteins (PBPs) which in turn inhibits the final transpeptidation step of peptidoglycan synthesis in bacterial cell walls, thus inhibiting cell wall biosynthesis. Bacteria eventually lyse due to ongoing activity of cell wall autolytic enzymes (autolysins and murein hydrolases) while cell wall assembly is arrested.

Other Adverse Effects

1% to 10%: Gastrointestinal: Diarrhea

<1% (Limited to important or life-threatening symptoms): Rash, nausea, vomiting, pseudomembranous colitis, increased BUN, increased creatinine

(Continued)

Cephradine *(Continued)*

Other reactions with cephalosporins include anaphylaxis, erythema multiforme, toxic epidermal necrolysis, Stevens-Johnson syndrome, dizziness, fever, headache, encephalopathy, asterixis, neuromuscular excitability, seizures, neutropenia, leukopenia, agranulocytosis, pancytopenia, aplastic anemia, hemolytic anemia, interstitial nephritis, toxic nephropathy, vaginitis, angioedema, cholestasis, hemorrhage, prolonged PT, serum-sickness reactions, superinfection

Contraindications Hypersensitivity to cephradine, cephalosporins, or any component of their formulation

Warnings/Precautions Prolonged use may result in superinfection; use with caution in patients with a history of colitis; reduce dose in patients with renal dysfunction; a low incidence of cross-hypersensitivity with penicillins exists

Drug Interactions Increased Effect: High-dose probenecid decreases clearance of cephradine. Aminoglycosides in combination with cephradine may result in additive nephrotoxicity.

Dietary/Ethanol/Herb Considerations Food: Administer with food to reduce GI upset; absorption is delayed but absorption unaffected; Boiled milk, buttermilk, or yogurt may reduce diarrhea.

Drug Uptake

Absorption: Well absorbed; oral is faster than I.M.

Half-life, elimination: 1-2 hours (prolonged in renal impairment)

Time to peak: Oral, I.M.: 1-2 hours

Pregnancy Risk Factor B

Breast-feeding Considerations Theoretically, drug absorbed by nursing infant may change bowel flora or affect fever work-up result. **Note:** As a class, cephalosporins are used to treat infections in infants.

Dosage Forms CAP: 250 mg, 500 mg. **POWDER, oral suspension:** 125 mg/5 mL (5 mL, 100 mL, 200 mL); 250 mg/5 mL (5 mL, 100 mL, 200 mL)

Generic Available Yes

Selected Readings

"Advisory Statement. Antibiotic Prophylaxis for Dental Patients With Total Joint Replacements. American Dental Association; American Academy of Orthopedic Surgeons," *J Am Dent Assoc*, 1997, 128(7):1004-8.

Donowitz GR and Mandell GL, "Drug Therapy. Beta-Lactam Antibiotics (1)," *N Engl J Med*, 1988, 318(7):419-26.

Donowitz GR and Mandell GL, "Drug Therapy. Beta-Lactam Antibiotics (2)," *N Engl J Med*, 1988, 318(8):490-500.

Gustaferro CA and Steckelberg JM, "Cephalosporin Antimicrobial Agents and Related Compounds," *Mayo Clin Proc*, 1991, 66(10):1064-73.

Ceptaz® *see* Ceftazidime *on page 243*

Cerebyx® *see* Fosphenytoin *on page 541*

Ceredase® *see* Alglucerase *on page 52*

Cerezyme® *see* Imiglucerase *on page 625*

Cerose-DM® [OTC] *see* Chlorpheniramine, Phenylephrine, and Dextromethorphan *on page 271*

Cerubidine® *see* DAUNOrubicin Hydrochloride *on page 353*

Cerumenex® *see* Triethanolamine Polypeptide Oleate-Condensate *on page 1204*

Cervidil® Vaginal Insert *see* Dinoprostone *on page 397*

Cetacaine® *see* Benzocaine, Butyl Aminobenzoate, Tetracaine, and Benzalkonium Chloride *on page 152*

Cetacort® *see* Hydrocortisone *on page 608*

Cetafen® [OTC] *see* Acetaminophen *on page 26*

Cetafen Extra® [OTC] *see* Acetaminophen *on page 26*

Cetamide® *see* Sulfacetamide Sodium *on page 1115*

Cetapred® *see* Sulfacetamide Sodium and Prednisolone *on page 1116*

Cetirizine (se TI ra zeen)

U.S. Brand Names Zyrtec®

Canadian Brand Names Apo®-Cetirizine; Reactine™

Mexican Brand Names Virlix®; Zyrtec®

Pharmacologic Category Antihistamine

Synonyms Cetirizine Hydrochloride; P-071; UCB-P071

Use Perennial and seasonal allergic rhinitis and other allergic symptoms including chronic idiopathic urticaria

Local Anesthetic/Vasoconstrictor Precautions No information available to require special precautions

Effects on Dental Treatment No effects or complications reported

Dosage Children ≥12 years and Adults: Oral: 5-10 mg once daily, depending upon symptom severity

Mechanism of Action Competes with histamine for H_1-receptor sites on effector cells in the GI tract, blood vessels, and respiratory tract

Other Adverse Effects

>10%: Central nervous system: Headache has been reported to occur in 10% to 12% of patients, drowsiness has been reported in as much as 26% of patients on high doses

1% to 10%:

Central nervous system: Somnolence, fatigue, dizziness

Gastrointestinal: Xerostomia

Contraindications Hypersensitivity to cetirizine, hydroxyzine, or any component of their formulation

Warnings/Precautions Cetirizine should be used cautiously in patients with hepatic or renal dysfunction, the elderly and in nursing mothers. Doses >10 mg/day may cause significant drowsiness.

Drug Interactions Increased toxicity with CNS depressants and anticholinergics

Drug Uptake

Onset of action: 15-30 minutes

Absorption: Oral: Rapid

Half-life, elimination: 8-11 hours

Time to peak: 0.5-1 hour

Pregnancy Risk Factor B

Generic Available No

Cetirizine and Pseudoephedrine

(se TI ra zeen & soo doe e FED rin)

U.S. Brand Names Zyrtec-D 12 Hour™

Pharmacologic Category Antihistamine/Decongestant Combination

Synonyms Cetirizine Hydrochloride and Pseudoephedrine Hydrochloride; Pseudoephedrine Hydrochloride and Cetirizine Hydrochloride

Use Treatment of symptoms of seasonal or perennial allergic rhinitis

Local Anesthetic/Vasoconstrictor Precautions No information available to require special precautions

Effects on Dental Treatment No effects or complications reported

Dosage Oral:

Children ≥12 years and Adults: Seasonal/perennial allergic rhinitis: 1 tablet twice daily

Elderly: Adjust dose according to renal dysfunction

Dosage adjustment in renal impairment: Cl_{cr} 11-31 mL/minute or if patient is on hemodialysis: 1 tablet once daily

Dosage adjustment in hepatic impairment: 1 tablet once daily

Mechanism of Action Cetirizine is an antihistamine and exhibits selective inhibition of H_1 receptors. Pseudoephedrine is a sympathomimetic and exerts a decongestant action on nasal mucosa.

Other Adverse Effects

Based on **cetirizine** component:

>10%: Central nervous system: Headache (10% to 12%), drowsiness (26% with high doses)

1% to 10%:

Central nervous system: Somnolence, fatigue, dizziness

Gastrointestinal: Xerostomia

Based on **pseudoephedrine** component

Frequency not defined:

Cardiovascular: Tachycardia, palpitations, arrhythmias

Central nervous system: Nervousness, transient stimulation, insomnia, excitability, dizziness, drowsiness, convulsions, hallucinations, headache

Gastrointestinal: Nausea, vomiting

Genitourinary: Dysuria

Neuromuscular & skeletal: Weakness, tremor

Respiratory: Dyspnea

Miscellaneous: Diaphoresis

Drug Uptake See Cetirizine *on page 254* and Pseudoephedrine *on page 1022*

Zyrtec-D 12 Hour™:

Half-life, elimination: Cetirizine: 7.9 hours; Pseudoephedrine: 6 hours

Time to peak: Cetirizine: 2.2 hours; Pseudoephedrine: 4.4 hours

Pregnancy Risk Factor C

Generic Available No

Cetrorelix (se troh REE liks)

U.S. Brand Names Cetrotide™

Pharmacologic Category Antigonadotropic Agent

Synonyms Cetrorelix Acetate

Use Inhibits premature luteinizing hormone (LH) surges in women undergoing controlled ovarian stimulation

Local Anesthetic/Vasoconstrictor Precautions No information available to require special precautions

Effects on Dental Treatment No effects or complications reported

(Continued)

Cetrorelix *(Continued)*

Dosage S.C.: Adults: Female: Used in conjunction with controlled ovarian stimulation therapy using gonadotropins (FSH, HMG):

Single-dose regimen: 3 mg given when serum estradiol levels show appropriate stimulation response, usually stimulation day 7 (range days 5-9). If hCG is not administered within 4 days, continue cetrorelix at 0.25 mg/day until hCG is administered

Multiple-dose regimen: Cetrorelix Acetate dose regimen: 0.25 mg morning or evening of stimulation day 5, or morning of stimulation day 6; continue until hCG is administered.

Mechanism of Action Competes with naturally occurring GnRH for binding on receptors of the pituitary. This delays luteinizing hormone surge, preventing ovulation until the follicles are of adequate size.

Other Adverse Effects 1% to 10%:

Central nervous system: Headache (1%)

Endocrine & metabolic: Ovarian hyperstimulation syndrome, WHO grade II or III (3%)

Gastrointestinal: Nausea (1%)

Hepatic: Increased ALT, AST, GGT, and alkaline phosphatase (1% to 2%)

Drug Uptake

Onset of action: 0.25 mg dose: 2 hours; 3 mg dose: 1 hour

Absorption: Rapid

Duration: 0.25 mg dose: 24 hours; 3 mg dose: 4 days

Half-life, elimination: 0.25 mg dose: 5 hours; 0.25 mg multiple dose: 20.6 hours; 3 mg dose: 62.8 hours

Time to peak: 0.25 mg dose: 1 hour; 3 mg dose: 1.5 hours

Pregnancy Risk Factor X

Generic Available No

Cetrotide™ *see* Cetrorelix *on page 255*

Cetylpyridinium (SEE til peer i DI nee um)

U.S. Brand Names Cēpacol® Mouthwash/Gargle [OTC]

Pharmacologic Category Local Anesthetic

Synonyms Cetylpyridinium Chloride

Use Antiseptic

Local Anesthetic/Vasoconstrictor Precautions No information available to require special precautions

Effects on Dental Treatment No effects or complications reported

Dosage Children >6 years and Adults: Oral: Rinse or gargle to freshen mouth; may be used before or after brushing; may be used every 2-3 hours

Pregnancy Risk Factor C

Dosage Forms MOUTHWASH, as chloride: 0.05% and alcohol 14% (120 mL, 180 mL, 720 mL, 960 mL)

Generic Available No

Cetylpyridinium and Benzocaine

(SEE til peer i DI nee um & BEN zoe kane)

U.S. Brand Names Cēpacol® Anesthetic Troches [OTC]

Pharmacologic Category Local Anesthetic

Synonyms Benzocaine and Cetylpyridinium Chloride; Cetylpyridinium Chloride and Benzocaine

Use Symptomatic relief of sore throat

Local Anesthetic/Vasoconstrictor Precautions No information available to require special precautions

Effects on Dental Treatment No effects or complications reported

Dosage Antiseptic/anesthetic: Oral: Dissolve in mouth as needed for sore throat

Pregnancy Risk Factor C

Dosage Forms TROCHE: Cetylpyridinium 1:1500 and benzocaine 10 mg (18s)

Generic Available Yes

Cevi-Bid® [OTC] *see* Ascorbic Acid *on page 117*

Cevimeline (se vi ME leen)

Related Information

Management of Patients Undergoing Cancer Therapy *on page 1402*

U.S. Brand Names Evoxac™

Canadian Brand Names Evoxac™

Pharmacologic Category Cholinergic Agonist

Synonyms Cevimeline Hydrochloride

Use Treatment of symptoms of xerostomia in patients with Sjögren's syndrome

Local Anesthetic/Vasoconstrictor Precautions No information available to require special precautions

Effects on Dental Treatment No effects or complications reported

Dosage Oral:

Adults: 30 mg 3 times/day

Dosage adjustment in renal/hepatic impairment: Not studied; no specific dosage adjustment is recommended

Elderly: No specific dosage adjustment is recommended; however, use caution when initiating due to potential for increased sensitivity

Mechanism of Action Binds to muscarinic (cholinergic) receptors, causing an increase in secretion of exocrine glands (including salivary glands)

Other Adverse Effects

>10%:

Central nervous system: Headache (14%; placebo 20%)

Gastrointestinal: Nausea (14%), diarrhea (10%)

Respiratory: Rhinitis (11%), sinusitis (12%), upper respiratory infection (11%)

Miscellaneous: Increased sweating (19%)

1% to 10%:

Cardiovascular: Peripheral edema, chest pain, edema, palpitation

Central nervous system: Dizziness (4%), fatigue (3%), pain (3%), insomnia (2%), anxiety (1%), fever, depression, migraine, hypoesthesia, vertigo

Dermatologic: Rash (4%; placebo 6%), pruritus, skin disorder, erythematous rash

Endocrine & metabolic: Hot flashes (2%)

Gastrointestinal: Dyspepsia (8%; placebo 9%), abdominal pain (8%), vomiting (5%), excessive salivation (2%), constipation, salivary gland pain, xerostomia, sialoadenitis, gastroesophageal reflux, flatulence, ulcerative stomatitis, eructation, increased amylase, anorexia, tooth disorder

Genitourinary: Urinary tract infection (6%), vaginitis, cystitis

Hematologic: Anemia

Local: Abscess

Neuromuscular & skeletal: back pain (5%), arthralgia (4%), skeletal pain (3%), rigors (1%), hypertonia, tremor, myalgia, hyporeflexia, leg cramps

Ocular: Conjunctivitis (4%), abnormal vision, eye pain, eye abnormality, xerophthalmia

Otic: Earache, otitis media

Respiratory: Coughing (6%), bronchitis (4%), pneumonia, epistaxis

Miscellaneous: Flu-like syndrome, infection, fungal infection, allergy, hiccups

<1% (limited to important or life-threatening symptoms): Syncope, malaise, substernal chest pain, abnormal ECG, hypertension, hypotension, arrhythmia, T-wave inversion, angina, myocardial infarction, pericarditis, pulmonary embolism, peripheral ischemia, thrombophlebitis, vasculitis, dysphagia, enterocolitis, gastric ulcer, gastrointestinal hemorrhage, ileus, melena, mucositis, esophageal stricture, esophagitis, peptic ulcer, stomatitis, tongue discoloration, tongue ulceration, hypothyroidism, thrombocytopenic purpura, thrombocytopenia, anemia, eosinophilia, granulocytopenia, leukopenia, leukocytosis, lymphadenopathy, cholelithiasis, increased transaminases, arthropathy, avascular necrosis (femoral head), bursitis, costochondritis, synovitis, tendonitis, tenosynovitis, coma, dyskinesia, dysphonia, aggravated multiple sclerosis, neuralgia, neuropathy, paresthesia, agitation, confusion, depersonalization, emotional lability, manic reaction, paranoia, somnolence, hyperkinesia, hallucination, fall, sepsis, bronchospasm, nasal ulcer, pleural effusion, pulmonary fibrosis, systemic lupus erythematosus, alopecia, dermatitis, eczema, photosensitivity reaction, dry skin, skin ulceration, bullous eruption, deafness, motion sickness, parosmia, taste perversion, blepharitis, cataract, corneal ulceration, diplopia, glaucoma, anterior chamber hemorrhage, retinal disorder, scleritis, tinnitus, epididymitis, menstrual disorder, genital pruritus, dysuria, hematuria, renal calculus, abnormal renal function, decreased urine flow, postural hypotension, aphasia, convulsions, paralysis, gingival hyperplasia, intestinal obstruction, bundle branch block, increased CPK, electrolyte abnormality, aggressive behavior, delirium, impotence, apnea, oliguria, urinary retention, lymphocytosis

Contraindications Hypersensitivity to cevimeline or any component of the formulation; uncontrolled asthma; narrow-angle glaucoma; acute iritis; other conditions where miosis is undesirable

Warnings/Precautions May alter cardiac conduction and/or heart rate; use caution in patients with significant cardiovascular disease, including angina, myocardial infarction, or conduction disturbances. Cevimeline has the potential to increase bronchial smooth muscle tone, airway resistance, and bronchial secretions; use with caution in patients with controlled asthma, COPD, or chronic bronchitis. May cause decreased visual acuity (particularly at night and in patients with central lens changes) and impaired depth perception. Patients should be cautioned about driving at night or performing hazardous activities in reduced lighting. May cause a variety of parasympathomimetic effects, which may be particularly dangerous in elderly patients; excessive sweating may lead to dehydration in some patients.

Use with caution in patients with a history of biliary stones or nephrolithiasis; cevimeline may induce smooth muscle spasms, precipitating cholangitis, cholecystitis, biliary obstruction, renal colic, or ureteral reflux in susceptible patients. Patients with a known or suspected deficiency of CYP2D6 may be at higher risk of adverse effects. Safety and efficacy have not been established in pediatric patients.

(Continued)

Cevimeline *(Continued)*

Drug Interactions CYP2D6 and CYP3A3/4 substrate

Increased Effect/Toxicity: Drugs which inhibit CYP2D6 (including amiodarone, fluoxetine, paroxetine, quinidine, ritonavir) or CYP3A3/4 (including diltiazem, erythromycin, itraconazole, ketoconazole, verapamil) may increase levels of cevimeline. The effects of other cholinergic agents may be increased during concurrent administration with cevimeline. Concurrent use of cevimeline and beta-blockers may increase the potential for conduction disturbances.

Decreased Effect: Anticholinergic agents (atropine, TCAs, phenothiazines) may antagonize the effects of cevimeline

Dietary/Ethanol/Herb Considerations Food: May be taken with food; boiled milk, buttermilk, or yogurt may reduce diarrhea.

Drug Uptake

Half-life, elimination: 5 hours

Time to peak: 1.5-2 hours

Pregnancy Risk Factor C

Dosage Forms CAP: 30 mg

Generic Available No

Comments May be taken with or without food; take with food if medicine causes upset stomach. May cause decreased visual acuity (particularly at night and in patients with central lens changes) and impaired depth perception; patients should be cautioned about driving at night or performing hazardous activities in reduced lighting.

C-Gram [OTC] *see* Ascorbic Acid *on page 117*

CharcoAid® [OTC] *see* Charcoal *on page 258*

Charcoal (CHAR kole)

U.S. Brand Names Actidose® [OTC]; Actidose-Aqua® [OTC]; CharcoAid® [OTC]; Charcocaps® [OTC]; Liqui-Char® [OTC]

Canadian Brand Names Charcadole®; Charcadole®, Aqueous; Charcadole® TFS

Pharmacologic Category Antidiarrheal; Antidote; Antiflatulent

Synonyms Activated Carbon; Activated Charcoal; Adsorbent Charcoal; Liquid Antidote; Medicinal Carbon; Medicinal Charcoal

Use Emergency treatment in poisoning by drugs and chemicals; repetitive doses for gastric dialysis in uremia to adsorb various waste products, and repetitive doses have proven useful to enhance the elimination of certain drugs (eg, theophylline, phenobarbital, and aspirin)

Local Anesthetic/Vasoconstrictor Precautions No information available to require special precautions

Effects on Dental Treatment No effects or complications reported

Dosage Oral:

Acute poisoning:

Charcoal with sorbitol: Single-dose:

Children 1-12 years: 1-2 g/kg/dose or 15-30 g or ~ 5-10 times the weight of the ingested poison; 1 g adsorbs 100-1000 mg of poison; the use of repeat oral charcoal with sorbitol doses is not recommended. In young children, sorbitol should be repeated no more than 1-2 times/day.

Adults: 30-100 g

Charcoal in water:

Single-dose:

Children 1-12 years: 15-30 g or 1-2 g/kg

Adults: 30-100 g or 1-2 g/kg

Multiple-dose:

Children 1-12 years: 20-60 g or 0.5-1 g/kg every 2-6 hours until clinical observations, serum drug concentration have returned to a subtherapeutic range, or charcoal stool apparent

Adults: 20-60 g or 0.5-1 g/kg every 2-6 hours

Gastric dialysis: Adults: 20-50 g every 6 hours for 1-2 days

Intestinal gas, diarrhea, GI distress: Adults: 520-975 mg after meals or at first sign of discomfort; repeat as needed to a maximum dose of 4.16 g/day

Mechanism of Action Adsorbs toxic substances or irritants, thus inhibiting GI absorption; adsorbs intestinal gas; the addition of sorbitol results in hyperosmotic laxative action causing catharsis

Other Adverse Effects >10%:

Gastrointestinal: Vomiting, diarrhea with sorbitol, constipation

Miscellaneous: Stools will turn black

Drug Interactions Decreases effect of ipecac syrup

Drug Uptake Absorption: Not absorbed from GI tract

Pregnancy Risk Factor C

Generic Available Yes

Charcocaps® [OTC] *see* Charcoal *on page 258*

Chealamide® *see* Edetate Disodium *on page 429*

Chenix® *see* Chenodiol *on page 259*

Chenodiol (kee noe DYE ole)

U.S. Brand Names Chenix®

Pharmacologic Category Bile Acid

Synonyms Chenodeoxycholic Acid

Use Orphan drug: Oral dissolution of cholesterol gallstones in selected patients

Local Anesthetic/Vasoconstrictor Precautions No information available to require special precautions

Effects on Dental Treatment No effects or complications reported

Dosage Adults: Oral: 13-16 mg/kg/day in 2 divided doses, starting with 250 mg twice daily the first 2 weeks and increasing by 250 mg/day each week thereafter until the recommended or maximum tolerated dose is achieved

Mechanism of Action Primary acid excreted into bile, normally constituting one-third of the total biliary bile acids; synthesis is regulated by the relative composition and flux of cholesterol and bile acids through the hepatocyte by a negative feedback effect on the rate-limiting enzymes for synthesis of cholesterol (HMG CoA reductase) and bile acids (cholesterol 7 alpha-hydroxyl).

Other Adverse Effects

>10%:

Gastrointestinal: Diarrhea (mild), biliary pain

Miscellaneous: Aminotransferase increases

1% to 10%:

Endocrine & metabolic: Increases in cholesterol and LDL cholesterol

Gastrointestinal: Dyspepsia

Contraindications Hypersensitivity to chenodiol or any component of the formulation; presence of known hepatocyte dysfunction or bile ductal abnormalities; a gallbladder confirmed as nonvisualizing after two consecutive single doses of dye; radiopaque stones; gallstone complications or compelling reasons for gallbladder surgery; inflammatory bowel disease or active gastric or duodenal ulcer; pregnancy

Warnings/Precautions Chenodiol is hepatotoxic in animal models including subhuman Primates; chenodiol should be discontinued if aminotransferases exceed 3 times the upper normal limit; chenodiol may contribute to colon cancer in otherwise susceptible individuals

Drug Interactions Decreased Effect: Antacids, cholestyramine, colestipol, and oral contraceptives

Pregnancy Risk Factor X

Generic Available No

Cheracol® *see* Guaifenesin and Codeine *on page 568*

Cheracol® D [OTC] *see* Guaifenesin and Dextromethorphan *on page 569*

Chibroxin® *see* Norfloxacin *on page 876*

Chiggerex® [OTC] *see* Benzocaine *on page 151*

Chiggertox® [OTC] *see* Benzocaine *on page 151*

Children's Advil® [OTC] *see* Ibuprofen *on page 621*

Children's Dimetapp® Elixir Cold & Allergy [OTC] *see* Brompheniramine and Pseudoephedrine *on page 180*

Children's Hold® [OTC] *see* Dextromethorphan *on page 372*

Children's Kaopectate® [OTC] *see* Attapulgite *on page 132*

Children's Motrin® [OTC] *see* Ibuprofen *on page 621*

Children's Nostril® *see* Phenylephrine *on page 950*

Children's Silfedrine® [OTC] *see* Pseudoephedrine *on page 1022*

Children's Sudafed® Cough & Cold [OTC] *see* Pseudoephedrine and Dextromethorphan *on page 1023*

Children's Sudafed® Nasal Decongestant [OTC] *see* Pseudoephedrine *on page 1022*

Children's Tylenol® Cold [OTC] *see* Acetaminophen, Chlorpheniramine, and Pseudoephedrine *on page 33*

Children's Tylenol® Sinus [OTC] *see* Acetaminophen and Pseudoephedrine *on page 30*

Chirocaine® *see* Levobupivacaine *on page 696*

Chlo-Amine® [OTC] *see* Chlorpheniramine *on page 268*

Chlorafed® [OTC] *see* Chlorpheniramine and Pseudoephedrine *on page 270*

Chloral Hydrate (KLOR al HYE drate)

U.S. Brand Names Aquachloral® Supprettes®

Canadian Brand Names PMS-Chloral Hydrate

Pharmacologic Category Hypnotic, Miscellaneous

Synonyms Chloral; Hydrated Chloral; Trichloroacetaldehyde Monohydrate

Use Short-term sedative and hypnotic for procedures

Local Anesthetic/Vasoconstrictor Precautions No information available to require special precautions

Effects on Dental Treatment No effects or complications reported

Restrictions C-IV

(Continued)

Chloral Hydrate *(Continued)*

Dosage

Children:

Sedation or anxiety: Oral, rectal: 5-15 mg/kg/dose every 8 hours (maximum: 500 mg/dose)

Prior to EEG: Oral, rectal: 20-25 mg/kg/dose, 30-60 minutes prior to EEG; may repeat in 30 minutes to maximum of 100 mg/kg or 2 g total

Hypnotic: Oral, rectal: 20-40 mg/kg/dose up to a maximum of 50 mg/kg/24 hours or 1 g/dose or 2 g/24 hours

Sedation during nonpainful procedure: Oral: 50-75 mg/kg/dose 30-60 minutes prior to procedure; may repeat 30 minutes after initial dose if needed, to a total maximum dose of 120 mg/kg or 1 g total

Adults: Oral, rectal:

Sedation, anxiety: 250 mg 3 times/day

Hypnotic: 500-1000 mg at bedtime or 30 minutes prior to procedure, not to exceed 2 g/24 hours

Dosing adjustment/comments in renal impairment: Cl_{cr} <50 mL/minute: Avoid use

Hemodialysis: Dialyzable (50% to 100%); supplemental dose is not necessary

Dosing adjustment/comments in hepatic impairment: Avoid use in patients with severe hepatic impairment

Mechanism of Action Unknown; CNS depressant effects are due to its active metabolite trichloroethanol

Other Adverse Effects Frequency not defined:

Central nervous system: Ataxia, disorientation, sedation, excitement (paradoxical), dizziness, fever, headache, confusion, lightheadedness, nightmares, hallucinations, drowsiness, "hangover" effect

Dermatologic: Rash, urticaria

Gastrointestinal: Gastric irritation, nausea, vomiting, diarrhea, flatulence

Hematologic: Leukopenia, eosinophilia, acute intermittent porphyria

Miscellaneous: Physical and psychological dependence may occur with prolonged use of large doses

Contraindications Hypersensitivity to chloral hydrate or any component of the formulation; hepatic or renal impairment; gastritis or ulcers; severe cardiac disease

Warnings/Precautions Use with caution in patients with porphyria; use with caution in neonates, drug may accumulate with repeated use, prolonged use in neonates associated with hyperbilirubinemia; tolerance to hypnotic effect develops, therefore, not recommended for use >2 weeks; taper dosage to avoid withdrawal with prolonged use; trichloroethanol (TCE), a metabolite of chloral hydrate, is a carcinogen in mice; there is no data in humans. Chloral hydrate is considered a second line hypnotic agent in the elderly. Recent interpretive guidelines from the Health Care Financing Administration (HCFA) discourage the use of chloral hydrate in residents of long-term care facilities.

Drug Interactions CYP2E1 enzyme substrate

CNS depressants: Sedative effects and/or respiratory depression with chloral hydrate may be additive with other CNS depressants; monitor for increased effect; includes sedatives, antidepressants, narcotic analgesics, and benzodiazepines

Furosemide: Diaphoresis, flushing, and hypertension have occurred in patients who received I.V. furosemide within 24 hours after administration of chloral hydrate; consider using a benzodiazepine

Phenytoin: Half-life may be decreased by chloral hydrate; limited documentation (small, single-dose study); monitor

Warfarin: Effect of oral anticoagulants may be increased by chloral hydrate; monitor INR; warfarin dosage may require adjustment. Chloral hydrate's metabolite may displace warfarin from its protein binding sites resulting in an increase in the hypoprothrombinemic response to warfarin.

Dietary/Ethanol/Herb Considerations

Ethanol: Avoid use; may increase CNS depression.

Food: Administer with chilled liquid to mask taste.

Herb/Nutraceutical: Avoid gotu kola, kava, melatonin, SAMe, St John's wort, and valerian; may increase CNS depression.

Drug Uptake

Absorption: Oral: Rapid; Rectal: Well absorbed

Duration: 4-8 hours

Half-life, elimination: Active metabolite: 8-11 hours

Time to peak: 0.5-1 hour

Pregnancy Risk Factor C

Breast-feeding Considerations May be taken while breast-feeding

Dosage Forms CAP: 500 mg. **SUPP, rectal:** 324 mg, 500 mg, 648 mg. **SYR:** 500 mg/5 mL (5 mL, 10 mL, 480 mL)

Generic Available Yes

Chlorambucil (klor AM byoo sil)

U.S. Brand Names Leukeran®

Canadian Brand Names Leukeran®

Mexican Brand Names Leukeran®

Pharmacologic Category Antineoplastic Agent, Alkylating Agent

Use Management of chronic lymphocytic leukemia, Hodgkin's and non-Hodgkin's lymphoma; breast and ovarian carcinoma; Waldenström's macroglobulinemia, testicular carcinoma, thrombocythemia, choriocarcinoma

Local Anesthetic/Vasoconstrictor Precautions No information available to require special precautions

Effects on Dental Treatment No effects or complications reported

Mechanism of Action Interferes with DNA replication and RNA transcription by alkylation and cross-linking the strands of DNA

Other Adverse Effects

>10%:
- Dermatologic: Skin rashes
- Hematologic: Myelosuppression (common, dose-limiting)
  - Onset: 7 days
  - Nadir: 14 days
  - Recovery: 28 days; may be prolonged to 6-8 weeks in some patients
- Hepatic: Transient elevations in liver enzymes

1% to 10%:
- Endocrine & metabolic: Hyperuricemia, menstrual cramps
- Gastrointestinal: Mild nausea or vomiting, diarrhea, stomatitis

Drug Interactions Patients may experience impaired immune response to vaccines; possible infection after administration of live vaccines in patients receiving immunosuppressants.

Drug Uptake

Absorption: 70% to 80%

Half-life, elimination: 90 minutes to 2 hours; phenylacetic acid mustard: 2.5 hours

Pregnancy Risk Factor D

Generic Available No

Chloramphenicol (klor am FEN i kole)

U.S. Brand Names Chloromycetin®; Chloroptic®; Ocu-Chlor®

Canadian Brand Names Chloromycetin®; Diochloram®; Pentamycetin®

Mexican Brand Names Cetina; Chloromycetin®; Clorafen®; Cloramfeni®; Cloran®; Clordil®; Paraxin; Quemicetina

Pharmacologic Category Antibiotic, Ophthalmic; Antibiotic, Otic; Antibiotic, Miscellaneous

Use Treatment of serious infections due to organisms resistant to other less toxic antibiotics or when its penetrability into the site of infection is clinically superior to other antibiotics to which the organism is sensitive; useful in infections caused by *Bacteroides*, *H. influenzae*, *Neisseria meningitidis*, *Salmonella*, and *Rickettsia*

Local Anesthetic/Vasoconstrictor Precautions No information available to require special precautions

Effects on Dental Treatment No effects or complications reported

Dosage

Meningitis: I.V.: Infants >30 days and Children: 50-100 mg/kg/day divided every 6 hours

Other infections: I.V.:
- Infants >30 days and Children: 50-75 mg/kg/day divided every 6 hours; maximum daily dose: 4 g/day
- Adults: 50-100 mg/kg/day in divided doses every 6 hours; maximum daily dose: 4 g/day

Ophthalmic: Children and Adults: Instill 1-2 drops 4-6 times/day or 1.25 cm (1/2" of ointment every 3-4 hours); increase interval between applications after 72 hours to 2-3 times/day; treatment should continue for ~7 days

Otic solution: Instill 2-3 drops into ear 3 times/day

Topical: Gently rub into the affected area 1-4 times/day

Mechanism of Action Reversibly binds to 50S ribosomal subunits of susceptible organisms preventing amino acids from being transferred to growing peptide chains thus inhibiting protein synthesis

Other Adverse Effects

Three (3) major toxicities associated with chloramphenicol include:
- Aplastic anemia, an idiosyncratic reaction which can occur with any route of administration; usually occurs 3 weeks to 12 months after initial exposure to chloramphenicol
- Bone marrow suppression is thought to be dose-related with serum concentrations >25 μg/mL and reversible once chloramphenicol is discontinued; anemia and neutropenia may occur during the first week of therapy
- Gray syndrome is characterized by circulatory collapse, cyanosis, acidosis, abdominal distention, myocardial depression, coma, and death; reaction

(Continued)

Chloramphenicol *(Continued)*

appears to be associated with serum levels ≥50 μg/mL; may result from drug accumulation in patients with impaired hepatic or renal function

Additional adverse reactions include allergic sensitization (with topical use), angioneurotic edema, urticaria, vesicular dermatitis, maculopapular dermatitis, conjunctival hyperemia (ocular use), ocular burning/stinging (ocular use)

Drug Interactions CYP2C9 enzyme inhibitor

Increased Effect/Toxicity: Chloramphenicol increases serum concentration of chlorpropamide, phenytoin, and oral anticoagulants.

Decreased Effect: Phenobarbital and rifampin may decrease serum concentration of chloramphenicol.

Drug Uptake

Half-life, elimination (increases with marked hepatic or combined renal/hepatic dysfunction): 1.6-3.3 hours; End-stage renal disease: 3-7 hours; Cirrhosis: 10-12 hours

Neonates: Postnatal: 1-2 days old: 24 hours; 10-16 days old: 10 hours

Time to peak: Oral: 0.5-3 hours

Pregnancy Risk Factor C

Generic Available Yes

Chloramphenicol and Prednisolone

(klor am FEN i kole & pred NIS oh lone)

U.S. Brand Names Chloroptic-P®

Pharmacologic Category Antibiotic, Ophthalmic; Corticosteroid, Ophthalmic

Synonyms Prednisolone and Chloramphenicol

Use Topical anti-infective and corticosteroid for treatment of ocular infections

Local Anesthetic/Vasoconstrictor Precautions No information available to require special precautions

Effects on Dental Treatment No effects or complications reported

Dosage Ophthalmic: Instill 1-2 drops in eye(s) 2-4 times/day

Drug Uptake See Chloramphenicol *on page 261* and Prednisolone *on page 988*

Pregnancy Risk Factor C

Generic Available No

Chloramphenicol, Polymyxin B, and Hydrocortisone

(klor am FEN i kole, pol i MIKS in bee, & hye droe KOR ti sone)

Pharmacologic Category Antibiotic, Ophthalmic; Corticosteroid, Ophthalmic

Synonyms Chloramphenicol, Hydrocortisone, and Polymyxin B; Hydrocortisone, Chloramphenicol, and Polymyxin B; Hydrocortisone, Polymyxin B, and Chloramphenicol; Polymyxin B, Chloramphenicol, and Hydrocortisone; Polymyxin B, Hydrocortisone, and Chloramphenicol

Use Topical anti-infective and corticosteroid for treatment of ocular infections

Local Anesthetic/Vasoconstrictor Precautions No information available to require special precautions

Effects on Dental Treatment No effects or complications reported

Dosage Apply 1/2" ribbon every 3-4 hours until improvement occurs

Drug Uptake See Chloramphenicol *on page 261*, Polymyxin B *on page 971* and Hydrocortisone *on page 608*

Pregnancy Risk Factor C

Generic Available No

Chloraseptic® [OTC] *see* Phenol *on page 946*

Chlordiazepoxide (klor dye az e POKS ide)

U.S. Brand Names Librium®

Canadian Brand Names Apo®-Chlordiazepoxide; Novo-Poxide

Pharmacologic Category Benzodiazepine

Synonyms Methaminodiazepoxide Hydrochloride

Use Approved for anxiety, may be useful for acute alcohol withdrawal symptoms

Local Anesthetic/Vasoconstrictor Precautions No information available to require special precautions

Effects on Dental Treatment >10%: Xerostomia; disappears with discontinuation

Restrictions C-IV

Dosage

Children:

- <6 years: Not recommended
- >6 years: Anxiety: Oral, I.M.: 0.5 mg/kg/24 hours divided every 6-8 hours

Adults:

- Anxiety:
  - Oral: 15-100 mg divided 3-4 times/day
  - I.M., I.V.: Initial: 50-100 mg followed by 25-50 mg 3-4 times/day as needed
- Preoperative anxiety: I.M.: 50-100 mg prior to surgery

Alcohol withdrawal symptoms: Oral, I.V.: 50-100 mg to start, dose may be repeated in 2-4 hours as necessary to a maximum of 300 mg/24 hours

Mechanism of Action An anxiolytic sedative that produces CNS depression at the subcortical level, except at high doses, whereby it works at the cortical level binding to stereospecific benzodiazepine receptors on the postsynaptic GABA neuron at several sites within the CNS, including the limbic system, reticular formation. Enhancement of the inhibitory effect of GABA on neuronal excitability results by increased neuronal membrane permeability to chloride ions. This shift in chloride ions results in hyperpolarization (a less excitable state) and stabilization.

Other Adverse Effects

>10%:

Central nervous system: Drowsiness, fatigue, ataxia, lightheadedness, memory impairment, dysarthria, irritability

Dermatologic: Rash

Endocrine & metabolic: Decreased libido, menstrual disorders

Gastrointestinal: Xerostomia, decreased salivation, increased or decreased appetite, weight gain or loss

Genitourinary: Micturition difficulties

1% to 10%:

Cardiovascular: Hypotension

Central nervous system: Confusion, dizziness, disinhibition, akathisia, increased libido

Dermatologic: Dermatitis

Gastrointestinal: Increased salivation

Genitourinary: Sexual dysfunction, incontinence

Neuromuscular & skeletal: Rigidity, tremor, muscle cramps

Otic: Tinnitus

Respiratory: Nasal congestion

Drug Interactions CYP3A3/4 enzyme substrate

Increased Effect/Toxicity: Chlordiazepoxide potentiates the CNS depressant effects of narcotic analgesics, barbiturates, phenothiazines, antihistamines, MAO inhibitors, sedative-hypnotics, and cyclic antidepressants. Serum concentrations/effects of chlordiazepoxide may be increased by inhibitors of CYP3A3/4, including cimetidine, ciprofloxacin, clarithromycin, clozapine, diltiazem, disulfiram, digoxin, erythromycin, ethanol, fluconazole, fluoxetine, fluvoxamine, isoniazid, itraconazole, ketoconazole, labetalol, levodopa, loxapine, metoprolol, metronidazole, miconazole, nefazodone, omeprazole, phenytoin, rifabutin, rifampin, troleandomycin, valproic acid, and verapamil.

Decreased Effect: Carbamazepine, rifampin, rifabutin may enhance the metabolism of chlordiazepoxide and decrease its therapeutic effect.

Drug Uptake

Absorption: I.M.: Results in lower peak plasma levels than oral

Duration: 2-7 days

Half-life, elimination: 6.6-25 hours; End-stage renal disease: 5-30 hours; Cirrhosis: 30-63 hours

Time to peak: Oral: ≤2 hours; I.M.: Results in lower peak plasma concentration than oral

Pregnancy Risk Factor D

Generic Available Yes

Chloresium® [OTC] *see* Chlorophyll *on page 265*

Chlorhexidine Gluconate (klor HEKS i deen GLOO koe nate)

Related Information

Dentin Hypersensitivity, High Caries Index, and Xerostomia *on page 1388*

Management of Patients Undergoing Cancer Therapy *on page 1402*

Oral Bacterial Infections *on page 1367*

Oral Nonviral Soft Tissue Ulcerations or Erosions *on page 1384*

Periodontal Diseases *on page 1375*

U.S. Brand Names Avagard™ [OTC]; BactoShield® [OTC]; Betasept® [OTC]; Biopatch® [OTC]; Chlorostat® [OTC]; Dyna-Hex® [OTC]; Exidine® Scrub [OTC]; Hibiclens® [OTC]; Hibistat® [OTC]; Peridex®; PerioChip®; PerioGard®; Stat Touch 2 [OTC]

Canadian Brand Names Hibidil® 1:2000; ORO-Clense; SpectroGram 2™

Pharmacologic Category Antibiotic, Oral Rinse; Antibiotic, Topical

Use

Dental:

Antimicrobial dental rinse; active against gram-positive and gram-negative organisms, facultative anaerobes, aerobes, and yeast

Chip, for periodontal pocket insertion; indicated as an adjunct to scaling and root planing procedures for reduction of pocket depth in patients with adult periodontitis; may be used as part of a periodontal maintenance program

Medical: Cleanser for surgical scrub and skin wounds, germicidal hand rinse; active against gram-positive and gram-negative organisms, facultative anaerobes, aerobes, and yeast

(Continued)

Chlorhexidine Gluconate *(Continued)*

Orphan drug: Peridex®: Oral mucositis with cytoreductive therapy when used for patients undergoing bone marrow transplant

Local Anesthetic/Vasoconstrictor Precautions No information available to require special precautions

Effects on Dental Treatment Swelling of face has been reported.

Dosage Periodontal chip: Adults: One chip is inserted into a periodontal pocket with a probing pocket depth ≥5 mm. Up to 8 chips may be inserted in a single visit. Treatment is recommended every 3 months in pockets with a remaining depth ≥5 mm. If dislodgment occurs 7 days or more after placement, the subject is considered to have had the full course of treatment. If dislodgment occurs within 48 hours, a new chip should be inserted.

Insertion of periodontal chip: Pocket should be isolated and surrounding area dried prior to chip insertion. The chip should be grasped using forceps with the rounded edges away from the forceps. The chip should be inserted into the periodontal pocket to its maximum depth. It may be maneuvered into position using the tips of the forceps or a flat instrument. The chip biodegrades completely and does not need to be removed. Patients should avoid dental floss at the site of PerioChip® insertion for 10 days after placement because flossing might dislodge the chip.

Mechanism of Action The bactericidal effect is a result of the binding of this cationic molecule to negatively charged bacterial cell walls and extramicrobial complexes. At low concentrations, this causes an alteration of bacterial cell osmotic equilibrium and leakage of potassium and phosphorous resulting in a bacteriostatic effect. At high concentrations of chlorhexidine, the cytoplasmic contents of the bacterial cell precipitate and result in cell death.

Other Adverse Effects

Oral:

>10%: Increase of tartar on teeth, changes in taste. Staining of oral surfaces (mucosa, teeth, dorsum of tongue) may be visible as soon as 1 week after therapy begins and is more pronounced when there is a heavy accumulation of unremoved plaque and when teeth fillings have rough surfaces. Stain does not have a clinically adverse effect but because removal may not be possible, patient with frontal restoration should be advised of the potential permanency of the stain.

1% to 10%: Gastrointestinal: Tongue irritation, oral irritation

<1%: Facial edema, nasal congestion, dyspnea

Topical: Skin erythema and roughness, dryness, sensitization, allergic reactions

Contraindications Hypersensitivity to chlorhexidine gluconate or any component of the formulation

Warnings/Precautions

Oral: Staining of oral surfaces (mucosa, teeth, tooth restorations, dorsum of tongue) may occur; may be visible as soon as 1 week after therapy begins and is more pronounced when there is a heavy accumulation of unremoved plaque and when teeth fillings have rough surfaces. Stain does not have a clinically adverse effect, but because removal may not be possible, patient with frontal restoration should be advised of the potential permanency of the stain.

Topical: For topical use only. Keep out of eyes and ears. May stain fabric. There have been case reports of anaphylaxis following chlorhexidine disinfection. Not for preoperative preparation of face or head; avoid contact with meninges.

Drug Uptake PerioChip® releases chlorhexidine *in vitro* in a biphasic manner, initially releasing approximately 40% of the chlorhexidine within the first 24 hours and then releasing the remaining chlorhexidine for 7-10 days.

Absorption: ~30% retained in the oral cavity following rinsing and slowly released into oral fluids; poorly absorbed

Duration: Antimicrobial protection: Topical hand sanitizer (Avagard™): 6 hours

Time to peak, plasma: Detectable levels not present after 12 hours

Pregnancy Risk Factor B

Dosage Forms **CHIP, periodontal pocket:** (PerioChip®): 2.5 mg. **DRESSING** [with chlorhexidine]: ¾" (1.9 cm) disk [1.5 mm center hole]; 1" (2.5 cm) disk [4 mm center hole, 7 mm center hole]. **FOAM, topical:** 4% (180 mL). **LIQ, topical:** 2% (118 mL, 946 mL, 3800 mL). **LIQ, topical** [with ethyl alcohol 61%]: 1% (88 mL, 500 mL). **LIQ, topical** [with isopropyl alcohol 2%]: 2% (120 mL, 240 mL, 360 mL, 480 mL, 960 mL, 3840 mL, 4000 mL). **LIQ, topical** [with isopropyl alcohol 4%]: 4% (15 mL, 120 mL, 240 mL, 480 mL, 960 mL, 4000 mL). **RINSE, oral** (Peridex®, PerioGard®): 0.12% (480 mL). **RINSE, topical:** 0.5% (120 mL, 240 mL). **SPONGE/BRUSH:** 4% (22 mL). **WIPE:** 0.5% (50s)

Generic Available Yes

Selected Readings

al-Tannir MA and Goodman HS, "A Review of Chlorhexidine and Its Use in Special Populations," *Spec Care Dentist*, 1994, 14(3):116-22.

Emerson D and Pierce C, "A Case of a Single Ingestion of 4% Hibiclens®," *Vet Hum Toxicol*, 1988, 30(6):583.

Ferretti GA, Brown AT, Raybould TP, et al, "Oral Antimicrobial Agents - Chlorhexidine," *NCI Monogr*, 1990, 9:51-5.

Greenstein G, Berman C, and Jaffin R, "Chlorhexidine. An Adjunct to Periodontal Therapy," *J Periodontol*, 1986, 57(6):370-7.
Johnson BT, "Uses of Chlorhexidine in Dentistry," *Gen Dent*, 1995, 43(2):126-32, 134-40.
Massano G, Ciocatto E, Rosabianca C, et al, "Striking Aminotransferase Rise After Chlorhexidine Self-Poisoning," *Lancet*, 1982, 1(8266):289.
Quinn MW and Bini RM, "Bradycardia Associated With Chlorhexidine Spray," *Arch Dis Child*, 1989, 64(6):892-3.
Yong D, Parker FC, and Foran SM, "Severe Allergic Reactions and Intra-Urethral Chlorhexidine Gluconate," *Med J Aust*, 1995, 162(5):257-8.
Yusof ZA, "Chlorhexidine Mouthwash: A Review of Its Pharmacological Activity, Clinical Effects, Uses and Abuses," *Dent J Malays*, 1988, 10(1):9-16.

Chloromag® *see* Magnesium Chloride *on page 739*
Chloromycetin® *see* Chloramphenicol *on page 261*

Chlorophyll (KLOR oh fil)

U.S. Brand Names Chloresium® [OTC]; Derifil® [OTC]; Nullo® [OTC]; PALS® [OTC]

Pharmacologic Category Gastrointestinal Agent, Miscellaneous; Topical Skin Product

Synonyms Chlorophyllin

Use Topically promotes normal healing, relieves pain and swelling, and reduces malodors in wounds, burns, surface ulcers, abrasions and skin irritations; used orally to control fecal and urinary odors in colostomy, ileostomy, or incontinence

Local Anesthetic/Vasoconstrictor Precautions No information available to require special precautions

Effects on Dental Treatment No effects or complications reported

Dosage

Oral: Children >12 years and Adults: 1-2 tablets/day; may increase to 3 tablets/day
Ostomy: Take tablets orally or place in the appliance

Topical: Apply generously and cover with gauze, linen, or other appropriate dressing; do not change dressings more often than every 48-72 hours

Other Adverse Effects 1% to 10%: Gastrointestinal: Mild diarrhea, green stools

Generic Available Yes

Chloroprocaine (klor oh PROE kane)

Related Information

Oral Pain *on page 1360*

U.S. Brand Names Nesacaine®; Nesacaine®-MPF

Canadian Brand Names Nesacaine®-CE

Pharmacologic Category Local Anesthetic

Synonyms Chloroprocaine Hydrochloride

Use Infiltration anesthesia and peripheral and epidural anesthesia

Local Anesthetic/Vasoconstrictor Precautions No information available to require special precautions

Effects on Dental Treatment No effects or complications reported

Dosage Dosage varies with anesthetic procedure, the area to be anesthetized, the vascularity of the tissues, depth of anesthesia required, degree of muscle relaxation required, and duration of anesthesia; range: 1.5-25 mL of 2% to 3% solution; single adult dose should not exceed 800 mg

Infiltration and peripheral nerve block: 1% to 2%

Infiltration, peripheral and central nerve block, including caudal and epidural block: 2% to 3%, without preservatives

Mechanism of Action Chloroprocaine HCl is benzoic acid, 4-amino-2-chloro-2-(diethylamino) ethyl ester monohydrochloride. Chloroprocaine is an ester-type local anesthetic, which stabilizes the neuronal membranes and prevents initiation and transmission of nerve impulses thereby affecting local anesthetic actions. Local anesthetics including chloroprocaine, reversibly prevent generation and conduction of electrical impulses in neurons by decreasing the transient increase in permeability to sodium. The differential sensitivity generally depends on the size of the fiber; small fibers are more sensitive than larger fibers and require a longer period for recovery. Sensory pain fibers are usually blocked first, followed by fibers that transmit sensations of temperature, touch, and deep pressure. High concentrations block sympathetic somatic sensory and somatic motor fibers. The spread of anesthesia depends upon the distribution of the solution. This is primarily dependent on the volume of drug injected.

Warnings/Precautions Use with caution in patients with cardiac disease, renal disease, and hyperthyroidism; convulsions and cardiac arrest have been reported presumably due to intravascular injection

Drug Interactions

Increased Effect/Toxicity: Avoid concurrent use of bupivacaine due to safety and efficacy concerns.

Decreased Effect: The para-aminobenzoic acid metabolite of chloroprocaine may decrease the efficacy of sulfonamide antibiotics.

Drug Uptake

Onset of action: 6-12 minutes
Duration: 30-60 minutes

(Continued)

Chloroprocaine *(Continued)*

Pregnancy Risk Factor C

Generic Available Yes

Selected Readings

Freeman DW and Arnold NI, "Paracervical Block With Low Doses of Chloroprocaine: Fetal and Maternal Effects," *JAMA*, 1975, 231(1):56-7.

Jankowsky EC, "Pharmacologic Aspects of Local Anesthetic Use," *Anesth Clin North Am*, 1990, 8:1-25.

Chloroptic® *see* Chloramphenicol *on page 261*

Chloroptic-P® *see* Chloramphenicol and Prednisolone *on page 262*

Chloroquine Phosphate (KLOR oh kwin)

U.S. Brand Names Aralen® Phosphate

Canadian Brand Names Aralen®

Pharmacologic Category Aminoquinoline (Antimalarial)

Synonyms Chloroquine

Use Suppression or chemoprophylaxis of malaria; treatment of uncomplicated or mild-moderate malaria; extraintestinal amebiasis; rheumatoid arthritis; discoid lupus erythematosus, scleroderma, pemphigus

Local Anesthetic/Vasoconstrictor Precautions No information available to require special precautions

Effects on Dental Treatment No effects or complications reported

Dosage Oral (**dosage expressed in terms of mg of base**):

Suppression or prophylaxis of malaria:

- Children: Administer 5 mg base/kg/week on the same day each week (not to exceed 300 mg base/dose); begin 1-2 weeks prior to exposure; continue for 4-6 weeks after leaving endemic area; if suppressive therapy is not begun prior to exposure, double the initial loading dose to 10 mg base/kg and give in 2 divided doses 6 hours apart, followed by the usual dosage regimen
- Adults: 300 mg/week (base) on the same day each week; begin 1-2 weeks prior to exposure; continue for 4-6 weeks after leaving endemic area; if suppressive therapy is not begun prior to exposure, double the initial loading dose to 600 mg base and give in 2 divided doses 6 hours apart, followed by the usual dosage regimen

Acute attack:

- Children: 10 mg/kg on day 1, followed by 5 mg/kg 6 hours later and 5 mg/kg on days 2 and 3
- Adults: 600 mg on day 1, followed by 300 mg 6 hours later, followed by 300 mg on days 2 and 3

Extraintestinal amebiasis:

- Children: 10 mg/kg once daily for 2-3 weeks (up to 300 mg base/day)
- Adults: 600 mg base/day for 2 days followed by 300 mg base/day for at least 2-3 weeks

Mechanism of Action Binds to and inhibits DNA and RNA polymerase; interferes with metabolism and hemoglobin utilization by parasites; inhibits prostaglandin effects; chloroquine concentrates within parasite acid vesicles and raises internal pH resulting in inhibition of parasite growth; may involve aggregates of ferriprotoporphyrin IX acting as chloroquine receptors causing membrane damage; may also interfere with nucleoprotein synthesis

Other Adverse Effects Frequency not defined:

- Cardiovascular: Hypotension (rare), EKG changes (rare)
- Central nervous system: Fatigue, personality changes, headache
- Dermatologic: Pruritus, hair bleaching, pleomorphic skin eruptions, alopecia, lichen planus eruptions, alopecia, mucosal pigmentary changes (blue-black)
- Gastrointestinal: Nausea, diarrhea, vomiting, anorexia, stomatitis
- Hematologic: Blood dyscrasias
- Ocular: Retinopathy (including irreversible changes in some patients long-term or high dose), blurred vision
- Otic: Nerve deafness, tinnitus

Drug Interactions

- Increased Effect/Toxicity: Chloroquine serum concentration may be elevated with concomitant cimetidine use.
- Decreased Effect: Decreased absorption if administered concomitantly with kaolin and magnesium trisilicate.

Drug Uptake

- Absorption: Oral: Rapid (~89%)
- Duration: Small amounts may be present in urine months following discontinuation of therapy
- Half-life, elimination: 3-5 days
- Time to peak: 1-2 hours

Pregnancy Risk Factor C

Generic Available Yes

Chlorostat® [OTC] *see* Chlorhexidine Gluconate *on page 263*

Chlorothiazide (klor oh THYE a zide)

Related Information
Cardiovascular Diseases *on page 1308*

U.S. Brand Names Diuril®

Canadian Brand Names Diuril®

Pharmacologic Category Diuretic, Thiazide

Use Management of mild to moderate hypertension, or edema associated with CHF, pregnancy, or nephrotic syndrome in patients unable to take oral hydrochlorothiazide, when a thiazide is the diuretic of choice

Local Anesthetic/Vasoconstrictor Precautions No information available to require special precautions

Effects on Dental Treatment No effects or complications reported

Dosage I.V. form not recommended for children and should only be used in adults if unable to take oral in emergency situations:

Children >6 months:
- Oral: 20 mg/kg/day in 2 divided doses
- I.V.: 4 mg/kg/day

Adults:
- Oral: 500 mg to 2 g/day divided in 1-2 doses
- I.V.: 100-500 mg/day

Elderly: Oral: 500 mg once daily **or** 1 g 3 times/week

Mechanism of Action Inhibits sodium reabsorption in the distal tubules causing increased excretion of sodium and water as well as potassium and hydrogen ions, magnesium, phosphate, calcium

Other Adverse Effects 1% to 10%:
Cardiovascular: Orthostatic hypotension
Dermatologic: Photosensitivity
Endocrine & metabolic: Hypokalemia
Gastrointestinal: Anorexia, epigastric distress

Warnings/Precautions Use with caution in severe renal disease. Electrolyte disturbances (hypokalemia, hypochloremic alkalosis, hyponatremia) can occur. Use with caution in severe hepatic dysfunction; hepatic encephalopathy can be caused by electrolyte disturbances. Gout can be precipitate in certain patients with a history of gout, a familial predisposition to gout, or chronic renal failure. Cautious use in diabetics; may see a change in glucose control. I.V. use is generally not recommended (but is available). Can cause SLE exacerbation or activation. Use with caution in patients with moderate or high cholesterol concentrations. Photosensitization may occur. Correct hypokalemia before initiating therapy.

Chemical similarities are present among sulfonamides, sulfonylureas, carbonic anhydrase inhibitors, thiazides, and loop diuretics (except ethacrynic acid). Use in patients with thiazide or sulfonamide allergy is specifically contraindicated in product labeling, however a risk of cross-reaction exists in patients with allergy to any of these compounds; avoid use when previous reaction has been severe.

Drug Interactions

Increased Effect/Toxicity: Increased effect of chlorothiazide with furosemide and other loop diuretics. Increased hypotension and/or renal adverse effects of ACE inhibitors may result in aggressively diuresed patients. Beta-blockers increase hyperglycemic effects of thiazides in Type 2 diabetes mellitus. Cyclosporine and thiazides can increase the risk of gout or renal toxicity. Digoxin toxicity can be exacerbated if a thiazide induces hypokalemia or hypomagnesemia. Lithium toxicity can occur with thiazides due to reduced renal excretion of lithium. Thiazides may prolong the duration of action with neuromuscular blocking agents.

Decreased Effect: Effects of oral hypoglycemics may be decreased. Decreased absorption of chlorothiazide with cholestyramine and colestipol. NSAIDs can decrease the efficacy of thiazides, reducing the diuretic and antihypertensive effects.

Drug Uptake
Onset of action: Oral: 2 hours
Absorption: Oral: Poor
Duration of diuretic action: Oral: 6-12 hours; I.V.: ~2 hours
Half-life, elimination: 1-2 hours
Time to peak: Oral: ~4 hours

Pregnancy Risk Factor C (manufacturer); D (expert analysis)

Generic Available Yes: Tablet

Chlorothiazide and Methyldopa
(klor oh THYE a zide & meth il DOE pa)

U.S. Brand Names Aldoclor®

Canadian Brand Names Aldoclor®

Pharmacologic Category Antihypertensive Agent Combination

Synonyms Methyldopa and Chlorothiazide

Use Treatment of hypertension

(Continued)

Chlorothiazide and Methyldopa *(Continued)*

Local Anesthetic/Vasoconstrictor Precautions No information available to require special precautions

Effects on Dental Treatment No effects or complications reported

Dosage Oral: 1 tablet 2-3 times/day for first 48 hours, then adjust

Drug Uptake See Chlorothiazide *on page 267* and Methyldopa *on page 793*

Pregnancy Risk Factor D

Generic Available No

Chlorothiazide and Reserpine (klor oh THYE a zide & re SER peen)

U.S. Brand Names Diupres®

Pharmacologic Category Antihypertensive Agent Combination

Synonyms Reserpine and Chlorothiazide

Use Management of hypertension

Local Anesthetic/Vasoconstrictor Precautions No information available to require special precautions

Effects on Dental Treatment No effects or complications reported

Dosage Oral: 1-2 tablets 1-2 times/day

Drug Uptake See Chlorothiazide *on page 267* and Reserpine *on page 1046*

Pregnancy Risk Factor D

Generic Available Yes

Chloroxine (klor OKS een)

U.S. Brand Names Capitrol®

Canadian Brand Names Capitrol®

Pharmacologic Category Topical Skin Product

Use Treatment of dandruff or seborrheic dermatitis of the scalp

Local Anesthetic/Vasoconstrictor Precautions No information available to require special precautions

Effects on Dental Treatment No effects or complications reported

Dosage Use twice weekly, massage into wet scalp, avoid contact with eyes, lather should remain on the scalp for ~ 3 minutes, then rinsed; application should be repeated and the scalp rinsed thoroughly

Pregnancy Risk Factor C

Generic Available No

Chlorphed®-LA Nasal [OTC] *see* Oxymetazoline *on page 907*

Chlorphenesin (klor FEN e sin)

U.S. Brand Names Maolate®

Canadian Brand Names Mycil®

Pharmacologic Category Skeletal Muscle Relaxant

Synonyms Chlorphenesin Carbamate

Use Adjunctive treatment of discomfort in short-term, acute, painful musculoskeletal conditions

Local Anesthetic/Vasoconstrictor Precautions No information available to require special precautions

Effects on Dental Treatment No effects or complications reported

Dosage Adults: Oral: 800 mg 3 times/day, then adjusted to lowest effective dosage, usually 400 mg 4 times/day for up to a maximum of 2 months

Other Adverse Effects Frequency not defined:
- Central nervous system: Drowsiness, confusion, insomnia, increased nervousness, dizziness, paradoxical stimulation, headache
- Gastrointestinal: Stomach cramps, nausea
- Hematologic: Leukopenia, thrombocytopenia, agranulocytosis, pancytopenia (rare)
- Miscellaneous: Anaphylactoid reactions, drug fever

Pregnancy Risk Factor C

Generic Available No

Chlorpheniramine (klor fen IR a meen)

Related Information

Oral Bacterial Infections *on page 1367*

U.S. Brand Names Aller-Chlor® [OTC]; Chlo-Amine® [OTC]; Chlor-Trimeton® [OTC]

Canadian Brand Names Chlor-Tripolon®

Pharmacologic Category Antihistamine

Synonyms Chlorpheniramine Maleate; CTM

Use Perennial and seasonal allergic rhinitis and other allergic symptoms including urticaria

Local Anesthetic/Vasoconstrictor Precautions No information available to require special precautions

Effects on Dental Treatment Chronic use of antihistamines will inhibit salivary flow, particularly in elderly patients; this may contribute to periodontal disease and oral discomfort.

Dosage

Children: Oral: 0.35 mg/kg/day in divided doses every 4-6 hours

2-6 years: 1 mg every 4-6 hours, not to exceed 6 mg in 24 hours

6-12 years: 2 mg every 4-6 hours, not to exceed 12 mg/day or sustained release 8 mg at bedtime

Children >12 years and Adults: Oral: 4 mg every 4-6 hours, not to exceed 24 mg/day or sustained release 8-12 mg every 8-12 hours, not to exceed 24 mg/day

Adults: Allergic reactions: I.M., I.V., S.C.: 10-20 mg as a single dose; maximum recommended dose: 40 mg/24 hours

Elderly: 4 mg once or twice daily. **Note:** Duration of action may be 36 hours or more when serum concentration are low.

Mechanism of Action Competes with histamine for H_1-receptor sites on effector cells in the GI tract, blood vessels, and respiratory tract

Other Adverse Effects

>10%:

Central nervous system: Slight to moderate drowsiness

Respiratory: Thickening of bronchial secretions

1% to 10%:

Central nervous system: Headache, excitability, fatigue, nervousness, dizziness

Gastrointestinal: Nausea, xerostomia, diarrhea, abdominal pain, appetite increase, weight gain

Genitourinary: Urinary retention

Neuromuscular & skeletal: Arthralgia, weakness

Ocular: Diplopia

Renal: Polyuria

Respiratory: Pharyngitis

Drug Interactions

Increased Effect/Toxicity: CNS depressants may increase the degree of sedation and respiratory depression with antihistamines. May increase the absorption of digoxin. Central and/or peripheral anticholinergic syndrome can occur when administered with amantadine, rimantadine, narcotic analgesics, phenothiazines and other antipsychotics (especially with high anticholinergic activity), tricyclic antidepressants, quinidine, disopyramide, procainamide, and antihistamines.

Decreased Effect: May increase gastric degradation of levodopa and decrease the amount of levodopa absorbed by delaying gastric emptying. Therapeutic effects of cholinergic agents (tacrine, donepezil) and neuroleptics may be antagonized.

Drug Uptake Half-life, elimination: 20-24 hours

Pregnancy Risk Factor B

Generic Available Yes

Chlorpheniramine and Acetaminophen

(klor fen IR a meen & a seet a MIN oh fen)

U.S. Brand Names Coricidin® [OTC]

Pharmacologic Category Antihistamine/Analgesic

Synonyms Acetaminophen and Chlorpheniramine

Use Symptomatic relief of congestion, headache, aches and pains of colds and flu

Local Anesthetic/Vasoconstrictor Precautions No information available to require special precautions

Effects on Dental Treatment Chronic use of antihistamines will inhibit salivary flow, particularly in elderly patients; this may contribute to periodontal disease and oral discomfort.

Dosage Adults: Oral: 2 tablets every 4 hours, up to 20/day

Drug Uptake See Chlorpheniramine *on page 268* and Acetaminophen *on page 26*

Generic Available Yes

Selected Readings

Botting RM, "Mechanism of Action of Acetaminophen: Is There a Cyclooxygenase 3?," *Clin Infect Dis*, 2000, Suppl 5:S202-10.

Dart RC, Kuffner EK, and Rumack BH, "Treatment of Pain or Fever with Paracetamol (Acetaminophen) in the Alcoholic Patient: A Systematic Review," *Am J Ther*, 2000, 7(2):123-34.

Grant JA and Weiler JM, "A Report of a Rare Immediate Reaction After Ingestion of Acetaminophen," *Ann Allergy Asthma Immunol*, 2001, 87(3):227-9.

Kwan D, Bartle WR, and Walker SE, "The Effects of Acetaminophen on Pharmacokinetics and Pharmacodynamics of Warfarin," *J Clin Pharmacol*, 1999, 39(1):68-75.

McClain CJ, Price S, Barve S, et al, "Acetaminophen Hepatotoxicity: An Update," *Curr Gastroenterol Rep*, 1999, 1(1):42-9.

Shek KL, Chan LN, and Nutescu E, "Warfarin-Acetaminophen Drug Interaction Revisited," *Pharmacotherapy*, 1999, 19(10):1153-8.

Tanaka E, Yamazaki K, and Misawa S, "Update: The Clinical Importance of Acetaminophen Hepatotoxicity in Nonalcoholic and Alcoholic Subjects," *J Clin Pharm Ther*, 2000, 25(5):325-32.

Chlorpheniramine and Phenylephrine

(klor fen IR a meen & fen il EF rin)

U.S. Brand Names Dallergy-D®; Ed A-Hist®; Histatab® Plus [OTC]; Histor-D®; Rolatuss® Plain; Ru-Tuss®

Pharmacologic Category Antihistamine/Decongestant Combination

Synonyms Phenylephrine and Chlorpheniramine

(Continued)

Chlorpheniramine and Phenylephrine *(Continued)*

Use Temporary relief of nasal congestion and eustachian tube congestion as well as runny nose, sneezing, itching of nose or throat, itchy and watery eyes

Local Anesthetic/Vasoconstrictor Precautions Use with caution since phenylephrine is a sympathomimetic amine which could interact with epinephrine to cause a pressor response

Effects on Dental Treatment

Chlorpheniramine: Prolonged use will cause significant xerostomia

Phenylephrine: Up to 10% of patients could experience tachycardia, palpitations, and xerostomia (prolonged use worsens); use vasoconstrictor with caution

Dosage Oral:

Children:

2-5 years: 2.5 mL every 4 hours

6-12 years: 5 mL every 4 hours

Adults: 10 mL every 4 hours

Drug Interactions See Chlorpheniramine *on page 268* and Phenylephrine *on page 950*

Drug Uptake See Chlorpheniramine *on page 268* and Phenylephrine *on page 950*

Pregnancy Risk Factor C

Generic Available Yes

Chlorpheniramine and Pseudoephedrine

(klor fen IR a meen & soo doe e FED rin)

U.S. Brand Names Allerest® Maximum Strength [OTC]; Anamine® [OTC]; Anaplex® [OTC]; Chlorafed® [OTC]; Chlor-Trimeton® Allergy/Decongestant [OTC]; Codimal-LA® [OTC]; Codimal-LA® Half [OTC]; Co-Pyronil® 2 Pulvules® [OTC]; Deconamine® [OTC]; Deconamine® SR [OTC]; Fedahist® [OTC]; Hayfebrol® [OTC]; Histalet® [OTC]; Klerist-D® [OTC]; Pseudo-Gest Plus® [OTC]; Rhinosyn® [OTC]; Rhinosyn-PD® [OTC]; Ryna® [OTC]; Sudafed® Cold & Allergy [OTC]

Pharmacologic Category Antihistamine/Decongestant Combination

Synonyms Pseudoephedrine and Chlorpheniramine

Use Relief of nasal congestion associated with the common cold, hay fever, and other allergies, sinusitis, eustachian tube blockage, and vasomotor and allergic rhinitis

Local Anesthetic/Vasoconstrictor Precautions Use with caution since pseudoephedrine is a sympathomimetic amine which could interact with epinephrine to cause a pressor response

Effects on Dental Treatment

Chlorpheniramine: Prolonged use will cause significant xerostomia

Pseudoephedrine: Up to 10% of patients could experience tachycardia, palpitations, and xerostomia (prolonged use worsens); use vasoconstrictor with caution

Dosage Oral:

Capsule: 1 capsule every 12 hours

Tablet: 1 tablet 3-4 times/day

Drug Interactions See Pseudoephedrine *on page 1022* and Chlorpheniramine *on page 268*

Drug Uptake See Chlorpheniramine *on page 268* and Pseudoephedrine *on page 1022*

Pregnancy Risk Factor C

Generic Available Yes

Chlorpheniramine, Ephedrine, Phenylephrine, and Carbetapentane

(klor fen IR a meen, e FED rin, fen il EF rin, & kar bay ta PEN tane)

U.S. Brand Names Rentamine® [OTC]; Rynatuss® [OTC]; Rynatuss® Pediatric Suspension [OTC]; Tri-Tannate Plus® [OTC]

Pharmacologic Category Antihistamine/Decongestant/Antitussive

Use Symptomatic relief of cough

Local Anesthetic/Vasoconstrictor Precautions

Ephedrine: Use vasoconstrictors with caution since ephedrine may enhance cardiostimulation and vasopressor effects of sympathomimetics

Phenylephrine: Use with caution since phenylephrine is a sympathomimetic amine which could interact with epinephrine to cause a pressor response

Effects on Dental Treatment

Chlorpheniramine: Prolonged use will cause significant xerostomia

Ephedrine: No effects or complications reported

Phenylephrine: Up to 10% of patients could experience tachycardia, palpitations, and xerostomia; use vasoconstrictor with caution

Dosage Children:

<2 years: Titrate dose individually

2-6 years: 2.5-5 mL every 12 hours

>6 years: 5-10 mL every 12 hours

Drug Interactions See Chlorpheniramine *on page 268*, Ephedrine *on page 437*, and Phenylephrine *on page 950*

Pregnancy Risk Factor C

Generic Available Yes: Liquid

Chlorpheniramine, Phenylephrine, and Codeine

(klor fen IR a meen, fen il EF rin, & KOE deen with poe TASS ee um EYE oh dide)

U.S. Brand Names Pediacof®; Pedituss®

Pharmacologic Category Antihistamine/Decongestant/Antitussive/Expectorant

Use Symptomatic relief of rhinitis, nasal congestion and cough due to colds or allergy

Local Anesthetic/Vasoconstrictor Precautions Use with caution since phenylephrine is a sympathomimetic amine which could interact with epinephrine to cause a pressor response

Effects on Dental Treatment

Chlorpheniramine: Prolonged use will cause significant xerostomia

Codeine: <1%: Xerostomia

Phenylephrine: Up to 10% of patients could experience tachycardia, palpitations, and xerostomia (prolonged use worsens); use vasoconstrictor with caution

Restrictions C-V

Dosage Children 6 months to 12 years: 1.25-10 mL every 4-6 hours

Drug Interactions See Chlorpheniramine *on page 268*, Phenylephrine *on page 950*, and Codeine *on page 317*

Generic Available No

Chlorpheniramine, Phenylephrine, and Dextromethorphan

(klor fen IR a meen, fen il EF rin, & deks troe meth OR fan)

U.S. Brand Names Cerose-DM® [OTC]

Pharmacologic Category Antihistamine/Decongestant/Antitussive

Use Temporary relief of cough due to minor throat and bronchial irritation; relieves nasal congestion, runny nose and sneezing

Local Anesthetic/Vasoconstrictor Precautions

Chlorpheniramine, Dextromethorphan: No information available to require special precautions

Phenylephrine: Use with caution since phenylephrine is a sympathomimetic amine which could interact with epinephrine to cause a pressor response

Effects on Dental Treatment

Chlorpheniramine: Prolonged use will cause significant xerostomia

Dextromethorphan: No effects or complications reported

Phenylephrine: Up to 10% of patients could experience tachycardia, palpitations, and xerostomia (prolonged use worsens); use vasoconstrictor with caution

Dosage Adults: Oral: 5-10 mL 4 times/day

Warnings/Precautions Research on chicken embryos exposed to concentrations of dextromethorphan relative to those typically taken by humans has shown to cause birth defects and fetal death; more study is needed, but it is suggested that pregnant women should be advised not to use dextromethorphan-containing medications

Drug Interactions See Chlorpheniramine *on page 268*, Dextromethorphan *on page 372*, and Phenylephrine *on page 950*

Drug Uptake See Chlorpheniramine *on page 268*, Phenylephrine *on page 950* and Dextromethorphan *on page 372*

Generic Available No

Chlorpheniramine, Phenylephrine, and Methscopolamine

(klor fen IR a meen, fen il EF rin, & meth skoe POL a meen)

U.S. Brand Names D.A.II™; Dallergy®; Dura-Vent®/DA; Extendryl; Extendryl JR; Extendryl SR

Pharmacologic Category Antihistamine/Decongestant/Anticholinergic

Use Treatment of upper respiratory symptoms such as respiratory congestion, allergic rhinitis, vasomotor rhinitis, sinusitis, and allergic skin reactions of urticaria and angioedema

Local Anesthetic/Vasoconstrictor Precautions Use with caution since phenylephrine is a sympathomimetic amine which could interact with epinephrine to cause a pressor response

Effects on Dental Treatment

Chlorpheniramine: Prolonged use will cause significant xerostomia

Methscopolamine: Anticholinergic side effects can cause a reduction of saliva production or secretion contributes to discomfort and dental disease (ie, caries, oral candidiasis and periodontal disease)

Phenylephrine: Up to 10% of patients could experience tachycardia, palpitations, and xerostomia; use vasoconstrictor with caution

(Continued)

Chlorpheniramine, Phenylephrine, and Methscopolamine *(Continued)*

Dosage

Children 6-11 years: Relief of respiratory symptoms: Oral:

D.A.II™: One tablet every 12 hours

D.A. Chewable®, Extendryl chewable tablet: One tablet every 4 hours; do not exceed 4 doses in 24 hours

Dallergy®: One-half caplet every 12 hours

Dura-Vent®/DA: One-half tablet every 12 hours

Extendryl JR: One capsule every 12 hours

Extendryl syrup: 2.5-5 mL, may repeat up to every 4 hours depending on age and body weight

Children ≥12 years and Adults: Relief of respiratory symptoms: Oral: **Note:** If disturbances in urination occur in patients without renal impairment, medication should be discontinued for 1-2 days and should then be restarted at a lower dose

D.A.II™: Two tablets every 12 hours

Dallergy®, Extendryl SR: 1 capsule every 12 hours

Dura-Vent®/DA: One tablet every 12 hours

D.A. Chewable®, Extendryl: 1-2 chewable tablets every 4 hours

Extendryl syrup: 5-10 mL every 3-4 hours (4 times/day)

Elderly: Use with caution, may have increased adverse reactions

Dosage adjustment in renal impairment: Use is not recommended

Mechanism of Action

Chlorpheniramine maleate: Antihistamine

Phenylephrine hydrochloride: Sympathomimetic agent (primarily alpha), decongestant

Methscopolamine nitrate: Derivative of scopolamine, antisecretory effects

Other Adverse Effects Frequency not defined:

Cardiovascular: Arrhythmias, bradycardia, cardiovascular collapse, flushing, hypotension, pallor, palpitation, tachycardia

Central nervous system: Anxiety, convulsions, CNS depression, dizziness, drowsiness, excitability, fear, giddiness, hallucinations, headache, insomnia, irritability, lassitude, restlessness, tension, tremor

Gastrointestinal: Constipation, dysphagia, gastric irritation, nausea, xerostomia

Genitourinary: Dysuria, urinary retention

Neuromuscular & skeletal: Weakness

Ocular: Blurred vision, mydriasis

Respiratory: Dry nose, dry throat, respiratory difficulty

Contraindications Hypersensitivity to chlorpheniramine, methscopolamine, phenylephrine, or any component of their formulation; severe hypertension; severe coronary artery disease; narrow angle glaucoma; urinary retention; peptic ulcer; hyperthyroidism; MAO inhibitors or beta blockers; during asthma exacerbation

Warnings/Precautions Use with caution in patients with hypertension, diabetes mellitus, ischemic heart disease, increased intraocular pressure, and prostatic hypertrophy. Elderly patients may be more likely to exhibit adverse reactions; use with caution in patients >40 years. May cause excitability in some patients, especially children. If disturbances in urination occur, discontinue medication for 1-2 days and restart at lower dosage. Safety and efficacy in children <6 years have not been established.

D.A.II® chewable tablets: Contain 7.5 mg phenylalanine/tablet

Drug Interactions

Increased Effect/Toxicity: Concomitant use of antihistamines, beta-adrenergic blockers, CNS depressants, and MAO inhibitors

Decreased Effect: Decreases effects of antihypertensive agents with concomitant use

Drug Uptake See Chlorpheniramine *on page 268*, Phenylephrine *on page 950* and Methscopolamine *on page 791*

Pregnancy Risk Factor C

Generic Available Yes

Chlorpheniramine, Phenylephrine, and Phenyltoloxamine

(klor fen IR a meen, fen il EF rin, & fen il tole LOKS a meen)

U.S. Brand Names Comhist®; Comhist® LA

Pharmacologic Category Antihistamine/Decongestant Combination

Use Symptomatic relief of rhinitis and nasal congestion due to colds or allergy

Local Anesthetic/Vasoconstrictor Precautions Use with caution since phenylephrine is a sympathomimetic amine which could interact with epinephrine to cause a pressor response

Effects on Dental Treatment

Chlorpheniramine: Prolonged use will cause significant xerostomia

Phenylephrine: Up to 10% of patients could experience tachycardia, palpitations, and xerostomia; use vasoconstrictor with caution

Dosage Oral: 1 capsule every 8-12 hours or 1-2 tablets 3 times/day

Drug Interactions See Chlorpheniramine *on page 268* and Phenylephrine *on page 950*

Pregnancy Risk Factor C

Generic Available No

Chlorpheniramine, Pseudoephedrine, and Codeine

(klor fen IR a meen, soo doe e FED rin, & KOE deen)

U.S. Brand Names Codehist® DH; Decohistine® DH; Dihistine® DH; Ryna-C®

Pharmacologic Category Antihistamine/Decongestant/Antitussive

Use Temporary relief of cough associated with minor throat or bronchial irritation or nasal congestion due to common cold, allergic rhinitis, or sinusitis

Local Anesthetic/Vasoconstrictor Precautions Use with caution since pseudoephedrine is a sympathomimetic amine which could interact with epinephrine to cause a pressor response

Effects on Dental Treatment

Chlorpheniramine: Prolonged use will cause significant xerostomia

Codeine: <1%: Xerostomia

Pseudoephedrine: Up to 10% of patients could experience tachycardia, palpitations, and xerostomia; use vasoconstrictor with caution

Restrictions C-V

Dosage Oral:

Children:

25-50 lb: 1.25-2.50 mL every 4-6 hours, up to 4 doses in 24-hour period

50-90 lb: 2.5-5 mL every 4-6 hours, up to 4 doses in 24-hour period

Adults: 10 mL every 4-6 hours, up to 4 doses in 24-hour period

Other Adverse Effects 1% to 10%:

Cardiovascular: Hypotension

Central nervous system: Sedation, dizziness, drowsiness, increased intracranial pressure

Gastrointestinal: Constipation, biliary tract spasm

Genitourinary: Urinary tract spasm

Miscellaneous: Physical or psychological dependence with continued use

Drug Interactions See Pseudoephedrine *on page 1022*, Codeine *on page 317*, and Chlorpheniramine *on page 268*

Drug Uptake See Chlorpheniramine *on page 268*, Pseudoephedrine *on page 1022* and Codeine *on page 317*

Pregnancy Risk Factor C

Generic Available Yes

Chlorpheniramine, Pyrilamine, and Phenylephrine

(klor fen IR a meen, pye RIL a meen, & fen il EF rin)

U.S. Brand Names Rhinatate®; R-Tannamine®; R-Tannate®; Rynatan® Pediatric Suspension; Tanoral®; Triotann®; Tri-Tannate®

Pharmacologic Category Antihistamine/Decongestant Combination

Use Symptomatic relief of nasal congestion associated with upper respiratory tract condition

Local Anesthetic/Vasoconstrictor Precautions Use with caution since phenylephrine is a sympathomimetic amine which could interact with epinephrine to cause a pressor response

Effects on Dental Treatment

Chlorpheniramine: Prolonged use will cause significant xerostomia

Phenylephrine: Up to 10% of patients could experience tachycardia, palpitations, and xerostomia; use vasoconstrictor with caution

Dosage Children:

<2 years: Titrate dose individually

2-6 years: 2.5-5 mL every 12 hours

>6 years: 5-10 mL every 12 hours

Drug Interactions See Phenylephrine *on page 950* and Chlorpheniramine *on page 268*

Drug Uptake See Chlorpheniramine *on page 268* and Phenylephrine *on page 950*

Pregnancy Risk Factor C

Generic Available Yes

ChlorproMAZINE (klor PROE ma zeen)

U.S. Brand Names Thorazine®

Canadian Brand Names Chlorpromanyl®; Largactil®

Mexican Brand Names Largactil®

Pharmacologic Category Antipsychotic Agent, Phenothiazine, Aliphatic

Synonyms Chlorpromazine Hydrochloride; CPZ

Use Control of mania; treatment of schizophrenia; control of nausea and vomiting; relief of restlessness and apprehension before surgery; acute intermittent porphyria; adjunct in the treatment of tetanus; intractable hiccups; combativeness

(Continued)

ChlorproMAZINE *(Continued)*

and/or explosive hyperexcitable behavior in children 1-12 years of age and in short-term treatment of hyperactive children

Unlabeled/Investigational: Management of psychotic disorders

Local Anesthetic/Vasoconstrictor Precautions Most pharmacology textbooks state that in presence of phenothiazines, systemic doses of epinephrine paradoxically decrease the blood pressure. This is the so called "epinephrine reversal" phenomenon. This has never been observed when epinephrine is given by infiltration as part of the anesthesia procedure.

Effects on Dental Treatment

Significant hypotension may occur, especially when the drug is administered parenterally; orthostatic hypotension is due to alpha-receptor blockade, the elderly are at greater risk for orthostatic hypotension.

Tardive dyskinesia: Prevalence rate may be 40% in elderly; development of the syndrome and the irreversible nature are proportional to duration and total cumulative dose over time. Extrapyramidal reactions are more common in elderly with up to 50% developing these reactions after 60 years of age; drug-induced **Parkinson's syndrome** occurs often; **Akathisia** is the most common extrapyramidal reaction in elderly.

Increased confusion, memory loss, psychotic behavior, and agitation frequently occur as a consequence of anticholinergic effects. Antipsychotic associated sedation in nonpsychotic patients is extremely unpleasant due to feelings of depersonalization, derealization, and dysphoria

Dosage

Children ≥6 months:

Schizophrenia/psychoses:

Oral: 0.5-1 mg/kg/dose every 4-6 hours; older children may require 200 mg/day or higher

I.M., I.V.: 0.5-1 mg/kg/dose every 6-8 hours

<5 years (22.7 kg): Maximum: 40 mg/day

5-12 years (22.7-45.5 kg): Maximum: 75 mg/day

Nausea and vomiting:

Oral: 0.5-1 mg/kg/dose every 4-6 hours as needed

I.M., I.V.: 0.5-1 mg/kg/dose every 6-8 hours

<5 years (22.7 kg): Maximum: 40 mg/day

5-12 years (22.7-45.5 kg): Maximum: 75 mg/day

Rectal: 1 mg/kg/dose every 6-8 hours as needed

Adults:

Schizophrenia/psychoses:

Oral: Range: 30-2000 mg/day in 1-4 divided doses, initiate at lower doses and titrate as needed; usual dose: 400-600 mg/day; some patients may require 1-2 g/day

I.M., I.V.: Initial: 25 mg, may repeat (25-50 mg) in 1-4 hours, gradually increase to a maximum of 400 mg/dose every 4-6 hours until patient is controlled; usual dose: 300-800 mg/day

Intractable hiccups: Oral, I.M.: 25-50 mg 3-4 times/day

Nausea and vomiting:

Oral: 10-25 mg every 4-6 hours

I.M., I.V.: 25-50 mg every 4-6 hours

Rectal: 50-100 mg every 6-8 hours

Elderly: Behavioral symptoms associated with dementia: Initial: 10-25 mg 1-2 times/day; increase at 4- to 7-day intervals by 10-25 mg/day. Increase dose intervals (bid, tid, etc) as necessary to control behavior response or side effects; maximum daily dose: 800 mg; gradual increases (titration) may prevent some side effects or decrease their severity.

Dosing adjustment/comments in hepatic impairment: Avoid use in severe hepatic dysfunction

Mechanism of Action Blocks postsynaptic mesolimbic dopaminergic receptors in the brain; exhibits a strong alpha-adrenergic blocking effect and depresses the release of hypothalamic and hypophyseal hormones; believed to depress the reticular-activating system, thus affecting basal metabolism, body temperature, wakefulness, vasomotor tone, and emesis

Other Adverse Effects Frequency not defined:

Cardiovascular: Postural hypotension, tachycardia, dizziness, nonspecific QT changes

Central nervous system: Drowsiness, dystonias, akathisia, pseudoparkinsonism, tardive dyskinesia, neuroleptic malignant syndrome, seizures

Dermatologic: Photosensitivity, dermatitis, skin pigmentation (slate gray)

Endocrine & metabolic: Lactation, breast engorgement, false-positive pregnancy test, amenorrhea, gynecomastia, hyper- or hypoglycemia

Gastrointestinal: Xerostomia, constipation, nausea

Genitourinary: Urinary retention, ejaculatory disorder, impotence

Hematologic: Agranulocytosis, eosinophilia, leukopenia, hemolytic anemia, aplastic anemia, thrombocytopenic purpura

Hepatic: Jaundice

Ocular: Blurred vision, corneal and lenticular changes, epithelial keratopathy, pigmentary retinopathy

Warnings/Precautions Safety in children <6 months of age has not been established; use with caution in patients with seizures, bone marrow depression, or severe liver disease

Drug Interactions CYP1A2, 2D6, and 3A3/4 enzyme substrate; CYP2D6 enzyme inhibitor

Aluminum salts: May decrease the absorption of phenothiazines; monitor

Amphetamines: Efficacy may be diminished by antipsychotics; in addition, amphetamines may increase psychotic symptoms; avoid concurrent use

Anticholinergics: May inhibit the therapeutic response to phenothiazines and excess anticholinergic effects may occur; includes benztropine, trihexyphenidyl, biperiden, and drugs with significant anticholinergic activity (TCAs, antihistamines, disopyramide)

Antihypertensives: Concurrent use of phenothiazines with an antihypertensive may produce additive hypotensive effects (particularly orthostasis)

Bromocriptine: Phenothiazines inhibit the ability of bromocriptine to lower serum prolactin concentrations

CNS depressants: Sedative effects may be additive with phenothiazines; monitor for increased effect; includes barbiturates, benzodiazepines, narcotic analgesics, ethanol and other sedative agents

CYP1A2 inhibitors: Metabolism of phenothiazines may be decreased; increasing clinical effect or toxicity. Inhibitors include cimetidine, ciprofloxacin, fluvoxamine, isoniazid, ritonavir, and zileuton

CYP2D6 inhibitors: Metabolism of phenothiazines may be decreased; increasing clinical effect or toxicity; inhibitors include amiodarone, cimetidine, delavirdine, fluoxetine, paroxetine, propafenone, quinidine, and ritonavir; monitor for increased effect/toxicity

CYP3A3/4 inhibitors: Serum level and/or toxicity of chlorpromazine may be increased; inhibitors include amiodarone, cimetidine, clarithromycin, erythromycin, delavirdine, diltiazem, dirithromycin, disulfiram, fluoxetine, fluvoxamine, grapefruit juice, indinavir, itraconazole, ketoconazole, metronidazole, nefazodone, nevirapine, propoxyphene, quinupristin-dalfopristin, ritonavir, saquinavir, verapamil, zafirlukast, zileuton; monitor for increased response

CYP2D6 substrates: Chlorpromazine may decrease the metabolism of drugs metabolized by CYP2D6 (in addition to drugs specifically mentioned in this listing)

Enzyme inducers: May enhance the hepatic metabolism of phenothiazines; larger doses may be required; includes rifampin, rifabutin, barbiturates, phenytoin, and cigarette smoking

Epinephrine: Chlorpromazine (and possibly other low potency antipsychotics) may diminish the pressor effects of epinephrine

Guanethidine and guanadrel: Antihypertensive effects may be inhibited by chlorpromazine

Levodopa: Chlorpromazine may inhibit the antiparkinsonian effect of levodopa; avoid this combination

Lithium: Chlorpromazine may produce neurotoxicity with lithium; this is a rare effect

Metoclopramide: May increase extrapyramidal symptoms (EPS) or risk.

Phenytoin: May reduce serum levels of phenothiazines; phenothiazines may increase phenytoin serum levels

Propranolol: Serum concentrations of phenothiazines may be increased; propranolol also increases phenothiazine concentrations

Polypeptide antibiotics: Rare cases of respiratory paralysis have been reported with concurrent use of phenothiazines

QT_c-prolonging agents: Effects on QT_c interval may be additive with phenothiazines, increasing the risk of malignant arrhythmias; includes type Ia antiarrhythmics, TCAs, and some quinolone antibiotics (sparfloxacin, moxifloxacin and gatifloxacin)

Sulfadoxine-pyrimethamine: May increase phenothiazine concentrations

Tricyclic antidepressants: Concurrent use may produce increased toxicity or altered therapeutic response

Trazodone: Phenothiazines and trazodone may produce additive hypotensive effects

Valproic acid: Serum levels may be increased by phenothiazines

Drug Uptake

Half-life, elimination: Biphasic: Initial: 2 hours; Terminal: 30 hours

Time to peak: Oral : 1-2 hours

Pregnancy Risk Factor C

Generic Available Yes

ChlorproPAMIDE (klor PROE pa mide)

Related Information

Endocrine Disorders and Pregnancy *on page 1331*

U.S. Brand Names Diabinese®

Canadian Brand Names Apo®-Chlorpropamide; Diabinese™

Mexican Brand Names Deavynfar; Diabinese®; Insogen®

(Continued)

ChlorproPAMIDE *(Continued)*

Pharmacologic Category Antidiabetic Agent, Sulfonylurea

Use Control blood sugar in adult onset, noninsulin-dependent diabetes (type 2)

Unlabeled/Investigational: Neurogenic diabetes insipidus

Local Anesthetic/Vasoconstrictor Precautions No information available to require special precautions

Effects on Dental Treatment Chlorpropamide-dependent diabetics (noninsulin dependent, Type 2) should be appointed for dental treatment in morning in order to minimize chance of stress-induced hypoglycemia.

Dosage Oral: The dosage of chlorpropamide is variable and should be individualized based upon the patient's response

Initial dose:

Adults: 250 mg/day in mild to moderate diabetes in middle-aged, stable diabetic

Elderly: 100-125 mg/day in older patients

Subsequent dosages may be increased or decreased by 50-125 mg/day at 3- to 5-day intervals

Maintenance dose: 100-250 mg/day; severe diabetics may require 500 mg/day; avoid doses >750 mg/day

Dosing adjustment/comments in renal impairment: Cl_{cr} <50 mL/minute: Avoid use

Hemodialysis: Removed with hemoperfusion

Peritoneal dialysis: Supplemental dose is not necessary

Dosing adjustment in hepatic impairment: Dosage reduction is recommended. Conservative initial and maintenance doses are recommended in patients with liver impairment because chlorpropamide undergoes extensive hepatic metabolism.

Mechanism of Action Stimulates insulin release from the pancreatic beta cells; reduces glucose output from the liver; insulin sensitivity is increased at peripheral target sites

Other Adverse Effects

>10%:

Central nervous system: Headache, dizziness

Endocrine & metabolic: Hypoglycemia (severe)

Gastrointestinal: Anorexia, constipation, heartburn, epigastric fullness, nausea, vomiting, diarrhea

1% to 10%: Dermatologic: Skin rash, urticaria, photosensitivity

Warnings/Precautions Patients should be properly instructed in the early detection and treatment of hypoglycemia; long half-life may complicate recovery from excess effects. Because of chlorpropamide's long half-life, duration of action, and the increased risk for hypoglycemia, it is not considered a hypoglycemic agent of choice in the elderly.

Chemical similarities are present among sulfonamides, sulfonylureas, carbonic anhydrase inhibitors, thiazides, and loop diuretics (except ethacrynic acid). Use in patients with sulfonylurea or sulfonamide allergy is specifically contraindicated in product labeling, however a risk of cross-reaction exists in patients with allergy to any of these compounds; avoid use when previous reaction has been severe.

Product labeling states oral hypoglycemic drugs may be associated with an increased cardiovascular mortality as compared to treatment with diet alone or diet plus insulin. Data to support this association are limited, and several studies, including a large prospective trial (UKPDS) have not supported an association.

Drug Interactions CYP3A3/4 enzyme substrate

Increased Effect/Toxicity: A possible interaction between chlorpropamide and fluoroquinolone antibiotics has been reported resulting in a potentiation of hypoglycemic action of chlorpropamide. Toxic potential is increased when given concomitantly with other highly protein bound drugs (ie, phenylbutazone, oral anticoagulants, hydantoins, salicylates, NSAIDs, beta-blockers, sulfonamides) - increase hypoglycemic effect. Phenylbutazone may increase hypoglycemic effects. Possible interactions between chlorpropamide and coumarin derivatives have been reported that may either potentiate or weaken the effects of coumarin derivatives.

Decreased Effect: Certain drugs tend to produce hyperglycemia and may lead to loss of control (ie, thiazides and other diuretics, corticosteroids, phenothiazines, thyroid products, estrogens, oral contraceptives, phenytoin, nicotinic acid, sympathomimetics, calcium channel blocking drugs, and isoniazid). Possible interactions between chlorpropamide and coumarin derivatives have been reported that may either potentiate or weaken the effects of coumarin derivatives.

Drug Uptake

Onset of action: Peak effect: ~6-8 hours

Half-life, elimination: 30-42 hours (increases with renal impairment or elderly)

End-stage renal disease: 50-200 hours

Time to peak: 3-4 hours

Pregnancy Risk Factor C

Generic Available Yes

Chlorthalidone (klor THAL i done)

Related Information

Cardiovascular Diseases *on page 1308*

U.S. Brand Names Thalitone®

Canadian Brand Names Apo®-Chlorthalidone

Mexican Brand Names Higroton

Pharmacologic Category Diuretic, Thiazide

Synonyms Hygroton® [DSC]

Use Management of mild to moderate hypertension, used alone or in combination with other agents; treatment of edema associated with CHF, nephrotic syndrome, or pregnancy. Recent studies have found chlorthalidone effective in the treatment of isolated systolic hypertension in the elderly.

Local Anesthetic/Vasoconstrictor Precautions No information available to require special precautions

Effects on Dental Treatment No effects or complications reported

Dosage Oral:

Children: 2 mg/kg/dose 3 times/week or 1-2 mg/kg/day

Adults: 25-100 mg/day or 100 mg 3 times/week

Elderly: Initial: 12.5-25 mg/day or every other day; there is little advantage to using doses >25 mg/day

Mechanism of Action Sulfonamide-derived diuretic that inhibits sodium and chloride reabsorption in the cortical-diluting segment of the ascending loop of Henle

Other Adverse Effects 1% to 10%:

Dermatologic: Photosensitivity

Endocrine & metabolic: Hypokalemia

Gastrointestinal: Anorexia, epigastric distress

Warnings/Precautions Use with caution in patients with hypokalemia, renal disease, hepatic disease, gout, lupus erythematosus, or diabetes mellitus. Use with caution in severe renal diseases. Correct hypokalemia before initiating therapy. Chemical similarities are present among sulfonamides, sulfonylureas, carbonic anhydrase inhibitors, thiazides, and loop diuretics (except ethacrynic acid). Use in patients with thiazide or sulfonamide allergy is specifically contraindicated in product labeling, however a risk of cross-reaction exists in patients with allergy to any of these compounds; avoid use when previous reaction has been severe.

Drug Interactions

Increased Effect/Toxicity: Increased effect of chlorthalidone with furosemide and other loop diuretics. Increased hypotension and/or renal adverse effects of ACE inhibitors may result in aggressively diuresed patients. Beta-blockers increase hyperglycemic effects of thiazides in Type 2 diabetes mellitus. Cyclosporine and thiazides can increase the risk of gout or renal toxicity. Digoxin toxicity can be exacerbated if a thiazide induces hypokalemia or hypomagnesemia. Lithium toxicity can occur with thiazides due to reduced renal excretion of lithium. Thiazides may prolong the duration of action with neuromuscular blocking agents.

Decreased Effect: Effects of oral hypoglycemics may be decreased. Decreased absorption of chlorthalidone with cholestyramine and colestipol. NSAIDs can decrease the efficacy of chlorthalidone, reducing the diuretic and antihypertensive effects.

Drug Uptake

Onset of action: Peak effect: 2-6 hours

Absorption: Oral: 65%

Half-life, elimination: 35-55 hours (may increase with renal impairment); Anuria: 81 hours

Time to peak: 2-6 hours

Pregnancy Risk Factor B (manufacturer); D (expert analysis)

Generic Available Yes

Chlor-Trimeton® [OTC] *see* Chlorpheniramine *on page 268*

Chlor-Trimeton® Allergy/Decongestant [OTC] *see* Chlorpheniramine and Pseudoephedrine *on page 270*

Chlorzoxazone (klor ZOKS a zone)

Related Information

Temporomandibular Dysfunction (TMD) *on page 1397*

U.S. Brand Names Parafon Forte® DSC

Canadian Brand Names Parafon Forte®; Strifon Forte®

Pharmacologic Category Skeletal Muscle Relaxant

Use

Dental: Treatment of muscle spasm with acute temporomandibular joint pain

Medical: Treatment of muscle spasm associated with acute painful musculoskeletal conditions

Local Anesthetic/Vasoconstrictor Precautions No information available to require special precautions

Effects on Dental Treatment No effects or complications reported

(Continued)

Chlorzoxazone *(Continued)*

Dosage Oral:
Children: 20 mg/kg/day or 600 mg/m²/day in 3-4 divided doses
Adults: 250-500 mg 3-4 times/day up to 750 mg 3-4 times/day

Mechanism of Action Acts on the spinal cord and subcortical levels by depressing polysynaptic reflexes

Other Adverse Effects Frequency not defined:
Central nervous system: Dizziness, drowsiness lightheadedness, paradoxical stimulation, malaise
Dermatologic: Rash, petechiae, ecchymoses (rare), angioneurotic edema
Gastrointestinal: Nausea, vomiting, stomach cramps
Genitourinary: Urine discoloration
Hepatic: Liver dysfunction
Miscellaneous: Anaphylaxis (very rare)

Contraindications Hypersensitivity to chlorzoxazone or any component of the formulation; impaired liver function

Drug Interactions CYP2E1 enzyme substrate
Increased Effect/Toxicity: CNS depressants

Dietary/Ethanol/Herb Considerations
Ethanol: Avoid use; may increase CNS depression.
Herb/Nutraceutical: Avoid gotu kola, kava, SAMe, St John's wort, and valerian; may increase CNS depression.

Drug Uptake
Onset of action: ~1 hour
Absorption: Readily absorbed
Duration: 6-12 hours

Pregnancy Risk Factor C

Dosage Forms CAPLET (Parafon Forte® DSC): 500 mg. **TAB:** 250 mg

Generic Available Yes

Cholac® *see* Lactulose *on page 682*
Cholan-HMB® [OTC] *see* Dehydrocholic Acid *on page 355*

Cholecalciferol (kole e kal SI fer ole)

U.S. Brand Names Delta-D®

Canadian Brand Names D-Vi-Sol®

Pharmacologic Category Vitamin D Analog

Synonyms D_3

Use Dietary supplement, treatment of vitamin D deficiency or prophylaxis of deficiency

Local Anesthetic/Vasoconstrictor Precautions No information available to require special precautions

Effects on Dental Treatment No effects or complications reported

Dosage Adults: Oral: 400-1000 units/day

Other Adverse Effects Frequency not defined:
Cardiovascular: Hypotension, cardiac arrhythmias, hypertension, arrhythmia
Central nervous system: Irritability, headache, somnolence, overt psychosis (rare)
Dermatologic: Pruritus
Endocrine & metabolic: Polydipsia
Gastrointestinal: Nausea, vomiting, anorexia, pancreatitis, metallic taste, xerostomia, constipation, weight loss
Genitourinary: Albuminuria, polyuria
Hepatic: Increased liver function test
Neuromuscular & skeletal: Bone pain, myalgia, weakness, muscle pain
Ocular: Conjunctivitis, photophobia
Renal: Azotemia, nephrocalcinosis

Drug Interactions Thiazide diuretics, cholestyramine, colestipol, corticosteroids, mineral oil, phenytoin, barbiturates, digitalis glycosides, antacids (magnesium)

Pregnancy Risk Factor C

Generic Available No

Comments Cholecalciferol 1 mg = 40,000 units of vitamin D activity

Cholera Vaccine (KOL er a vak SEEN)

Canadian Brand Names Mutacol Berna®

Pharmacologic Category Vaccine

Use The World Health Organization no longer recommends cholera vaccination for travel to or from cholera-endemic areas. Some countries may still require evidence of a complete primary series or a booster dose given within 6 months of arrival. Vaccination should not be considered as an alternative to continued careful selection of foods and water. Ideally, cholera and yellow fever vaccines should be administered at least 3 weeks apart.

Local Anesthetic/Vasoconstrictor Precautions No information available to require special precautions

Effects on Dental Treatment No effects or complications reported

Dosage
Children:
6 months to 4 years: Two 0.2 mL doses I.M./S.C. 1 week to 1 month apart; booster doses (0.2 mL I.M./S.C.) every 6 months
5-10 years: Two 0.3 mL doses I.M./S.C. or two 0.2 mL intradermal doses 1 week to 1 month apart; booster doses (0.3 mL I.M./S.C. or 0.2 mL I.D.) every 6 months
Children ≥10 years and Adults: Two 0.5 mL doses given I.M./S.C. or two 0.2 mL doses I.D. 1 week to 1 month apart; booster doses (0.5 mL I.M. or S.C. or 0.2 mL I.D.) every 6 months

Mechanism of Action Inactivated vaccine producing active immunization

Other Adverse Effects **All serious adverse reactions must be reported to the U.S. Department of Health and Human Services (DHHS) Vaccine Adverse Event Reporting System (VAERS) 1-800-822-7967.**
>10%:
Central nervous system: Malaise, fever, headache
Local: Pain, edema, tenderness, erythema, and induration at injection site

Drug Interactions Decreased effect with yellow fever vaccine; data suggests that giving both vaccines within 3 weeks of each other may decrease the response to both.

Pregnancy Risk Factor C

Generic Available No

Comments Inactivated bacteria vaccine

Cholestyramine Resin (koe LES tir a meen REZ in)

Related Information
Cardiovascular Diseases *on page 1308*

U.S. Brand Names LoCHOLEST®; LoCHOLEST® Light; Prevalite®; Questran®; Questran® Light

Canadian Brand Names Novo-Cholamine; Novo-Cholamine Light; PMS-Cholestyramine; Questran®; Questran® Light Sugar Free

Pharmacologic Category Antilipemic Agent, Bile Acid Sequestrant

Use Adjunct in the management of primary hypercholesterolemia; pruritus associated with elevated levels of bile acids; diarrhea associated with excess fecal bile acids; binding toxicologic agents; pseudomembraneous colitis

Local Anesthetic/Vasoconstrictor Precautions No information available to require special precautions

Effects on Dental Treatment No effects or complications reported

Dosage Oral (dosages are expressed in terms of anhydrous resin):
Powder:
Children: 240 mg/kg/day in 3 divided doses; need to titrate dose depending on indication
Adults: 4 g 1-6 times/day to a maximum of 16-32 g/day
Tablet: Adults: Initial: 4 g once or twice daily; maintenance: 8-16 g/day in 2 divided doses

Mechanism of Action Forms a nonabsorbable complex with bile acids in the intestine, releasing chloride ions in the process; inhibits enterohepatic reuptake of intestinal bile salts and thereby increases the fecal loss of bile salt-bound low density lipoprotein cholesterol

Other Adverse Effects
>10%: Gastrointestinal: Constipation, heartburn, nausea, vomiting, stomach pain
1% to 10%:
Central nervous system: Headache
Gastrointestinal: Belching, bloating, diarrhea

Drug Interactions
Cholestyramine can reduce the absorption of numerous medications when used concurrently. Give other medications 1 hour before or 4-6 hours after giving cholestyramine. Medications which may be affected include HMG-CoA reductase inhibitors, thiazide diuretics, propranolol (and potentially other beta-blockers), corticosteroids, thyroid hormones, digoxin, valproic acid, NSAIDs, loop diuretics, sulfonylureas, troglitazone (and potentially other agents in this class).
Warfarin and other oral anticoagulants: Hypoprothrombinemic effects may be reduced by cholestyramine. Separate administration times (as detailed above) and monitor INR closely when initiating or discontinuing.

Drug Uptake
Onset of action: Peak effect: 21 days

Pregnancy Risk Factor C

Generic Available Yes

Choline Magnesium Trisalicylate
(KOE leen mag NEE zhum trye sa LIS i late)

Related Information
Rheumatoid Arthritis and Osteoarthritis *on page 1340*
Temporomandibular Dysfunction (TMD) *on page 1397*

(Continued)

Choline Magnesium Trisalicylate *(Continued)*

U.S. Brand Names Tricosal®; Trilisate®

Canadian Brand Names Trilisate®

Pharmacologic Category Salicylate

Use Management of osteoarthritis, rheumatoid arthritis, and other arthritis; salicylate salts may not inhibit platelet aggregation and, therefore, should not be substituted for aspirin in the prophylaxis of thrombosis

Local Anesthetic/Vasoconstrictor Precautions No information available to require special precautions

Effects on Dental Treatment NSAID formulations are known to reversibly decrease platelet aggregation via mechanisms different than observed with aspirin. The dentist should be aware of the potential of abnormal coagulation. Caution should also be exercised in the use of NSAIDs in patients already on anticoagulant therapy with drugs such as warfarin (Coumadin®).

Dosage Oral (based on total salicylate content):

Children <37 kg: 50 mg/kg/day given in 2 divided doses

Adults: 500 mg to 1.5 g 2-3 times/day; usual maintenance dose: 1-4.5 g/day

Mechanism of Action Inhibits prostaglandin synthesis; acts on the hypothalamus heat-regulating center to reduce fever; blocks the generation of pain impulses

Other Adverse Effects

>10%: Gastrointestinal: Nausea, heartburn, stomach pains, heartburn, epigastric discomfort

1% to 10%:

- Central nervous system: Fatigue
- Dermatologic: Rash
- Gastrointestinal: Gastrointestinal ulceration
- Hematologic: Hemolytic anemia
- Neuromuscular & skeletal: Weakness
- Ocular: Hearing impairment, tinnitus
- Respiratory: Dyspnea
- Miscellaneous: Anaphylactic shock

Warnings/Precautions Use with caution in patients with CHF, dehydration, hypertension, decreased renal or hepatic function, history of GI disease, active GI ulceration or bleeding, or those receiving anticoagulants. Withhold for at least 4-6 half-lives prior to surgical or dental procedures.

Drug Interactions

Increased Effect/Toxicity: Choline magnesium trisalicylate may increase the hypoprothrombinemic effect of warfarin.

Decreased Effect: Antacids may decrease choline magnesium trisalicylate absorption/ salicylate concentrations.

Drug Uptake

Onset of action: Peak effect: ~2 hours

Absorption: Stomach and small intestines

Half-life, elimination: Dose-dependent ranging from 2-3 hours at low doses to 30 hours at high doses

Time to peak: ~2 hours

Pregnancy Risk Factor C/D (3rd trimester)

Generic Available Yes

Choline Salicylate (KOE leen sa LIS i late)

Related Information

Rheumatoid Arthritis and Osteoarthritis *on page 1340*
Temporomandibular Dysfunction (TMD) *on page 1397*

U.S. Brand Names Arthropan® [OTC]

Canadian Brand Names Teejel®

Pharmacologic Category Salicylate

Use Temporary relief of pain of rheumatoid arthritis, rheumatic fever, osteoarthritis, and other conditions for which oral salicylates are recommended; useful in patients in which there is difficulty in administering doses in a tablet or capsule dosage form, because of the liquid dosage form

Local Anesthetic/Vasoconstrictor Precautions No information available to require special precautions

Effects on Dental Treatment NSAID formulations are known to reversibly decrease platelet aggregation via mechanisms different than observed with aspirin. The dentist should be aware of the potential of abnormal coagulation. Caution should also be exercised in the use of NSAIDs in patients already on anticoagulant therapy with drugs such as warfarin (Coumadin®).

Dosage Children >12 years and Adults: Oral: 5 mL (870 mg) every 3-4 hours, if necessary, but not >6 doses in 24 hours

Rheumatoid arthritis: 870-1740 mg (5-10 mL) up to 4 times/day

Mechanism of Action Inhibits prostaglandin synthesis; acts on the hypothalamus heat-regulating center to reduce fever; blocks the generation of pain impulses

Other Adverse Effects

>10%: Gastrointestinal: Nausea, heartburn, stomach pains, dyspepsia, epigastric discomfort

1% to 10%:

Central nervous system: Fatigue
Dermatologic: Rash
Gastrointestinal: Gastrointestinal ulceration
Hematologic: Hemolytic anemia
Neuromuscular & skeletal: Weakness
Respiratory: Dyspnea
Miscellaneous: Anaphylactic shock

Warnings/Precautions Use with caution in patients with CHF, dehydration, hypertension, decreased renal or hepatic function, history of GI disease, active GI ulceration or bleeding, or those receiving anticoagulants. Withhold for at least 4-6 half-lives prior to surgical or dental procedures.

Drug Interactions

Increased Effect/Toxicity: May increase effect of warfarin

Decreased Effect: Decreased effect of salicylates with antacids; effect of ACE-inhibitors and diuretics may be decreased by concurrent therapy with NSAIDs.

Drug Uptake

Absorption: From the stomach and small intestine within ~2 hours
Half-life, elimination (dose-dependent): Low dose: 2-3 hours; High dose: 30 hours
Time to peak: 1-2 hours

Pregnancy Risk Factor C/D (3rd trimester)

Generic Available No

Chondroitin Sulfate-Sodium Hyaluronate

(kon DROY tin SUL fate-SOW de um hye al yoor ON ate)

U.S. Brand Names Viscoat®

Pharmacologic Category Ophthalmic Agent, Viscoelastic

Synonyms Sodium Hyaluronate-Chrondroitin Sulfate

Use Surgical aid in anterior segment procedures, protects corneal endothelium and coats intraocular lens thus protecting it

Local Anesthetic/Vasoconstrictor Precautions No information available to require special precautions

Effects on Dental Treatment No effects or complications reported

Dosage Carefully introduce (using a 27-gauge needle or cannula) into anterior chamber after thoroughly cleaning the chamber with a balanced salt solution

Mechanism of Action Functions as a tissue lubricant and is thought to play an important role in modulating the interactions between adjacent tissues

Other Adverse Effects 1% to 10%: Increased intraocular pressure (transient)

Drug Uptake Absorption: Intravitreous injection: diffusion occurs slowly

Pregnancy Risk Factor C

Generic Available No

Chooz® [OTC] *see* Calcium Carbonate *on page 201*
Chorex® *see* Chorionic Gonadotropin *on page 281*

Chorionic Gonadotropin (kor ee ON ik goe NAD oh troe pin)

U.S. Brand Names Chorex®; Novarel™; Pregnyl®; Profasi®

Canadian Brand Names A.P.L.®; Pregnyl®; Profasi® HP

Pharmacologic Category Gonadotropin; Ovulation Stimulator

Synonyms CG; hCG

Use Induces ovulation and pregnancy in anovulatory, infertile females; treatment of hypogonadotropic hypogonadism, prepubertal cryptorchidism

Local Anesthetic/Vasoconstrictor Precautions No information available to require special precautions

Effects on Dental Treatment No effects or complications reported

Dosage I.M.:

Children:

Prepubertal cryptorchidism (not due to anatomical obstruction): 4000 units 3 times/week for 3 weeks

or

5000 units every other day for 4 injections

or

15 injections of 500-1000 units over a period of 6 weeks

or

500 units 3 times per week for 4-6 weeks. If unsuccessful, start another course 1 month later, giving 1000 units/injection.

Hypogonadotropic hypogonadism in males: 500-1000 units 3 times/week for 3 weeks, followed by the same dose twice weekly for 3 weeks

or

1000-2000 units 3 times/week

or

(Continued)

Chorionic Gonadotropin *(Continued)*

4000 units 3 times/week for 6-9 months; reduce dose to 2000 units 3 times/week for an additional 3 months

Adults:

Use with menotropins to stimulate spermatogenesis: 5000 units 3 times/week for 4-6 months. With the beginning of menotropins therapy, hCG dose is continued at 2000 2 times/week.

Induction of ovulation and pregnancy: 5000-10,000 units one day following last dose of menotropins

Mechanism of Action Stimulates production of gonadal steroid hormones by causing production of androgen by the testis; as a substitute for luteinizing hormone (LH) to stimulate ovulation

Other Adverse Effects

>10%: Endocrine & metabolic: Ovarian cysts, uncomplicated ovarian enlargement, pelvic pain

1% to 10%:

Central nervous system: Mental depression, fatigue, headache, irritability, restlessness

Endocrine & metabolic: Enlargement of breasts, precocious puberty

Local: Pain at the injection site

Drug Uptake Half-life, elimination: Biphasic: Initial: 11 hours; Terminal: 23 hours

Chorionic Gonadotropin (Recombinant)

(kor ee ON ik goe NAD oh troe pin ree KOM be nant)

U.S. Brand Names Ovidrel®

Pharmacologic Category Gonadotropin; Ovulation Stimulator

Synonyms Choriogonadotropin Alfa; r-hCG

Use As part of an assisted reproductive technology (ART) program, induces ovulation in infertile females who have been pretreated with follicle stimulating hormones (FSH); induces ovulation and pregnancy in infertile females when the cause of infertility is functional

Local Anesthetic/Vasoconstrictor Precautions No information available to require special precautions

Effects on Dental Treatment No effects or complications reported

Dosage S.C.: Adults: Female: Assisted reproductive technologies (ART) and ovulation induction: 250 mcg given 1 day following the last dose of follicle stimulating agent. Use only after adequate follicular development has been determined. Hold treatment when there is an excessive ovarian response.

Mechanism of Action Luteinizing hormone analogue produced by recombinant DNA techniques; stimulates rupture of the ovarian follicle once follicular development has occurred.

Other Adverse Effects

2% to 10%:

Endocrine & metabolic: Ovarian cyst (3%), ovarian hyperstimulation (<2% to 3%)

Gastrointestinal: Abdominal pain (3% to 4%), nausea (3%), vomiting (3%)

Local: Injection site: Pain (8%), bruising (3% to 5%), reaction (<2% to 3%), inflammation (<2% to 2%)

Miscellaneous: Postoperative pain (5%)

<2%:

Cardiovascular: Cardiac arrhythmia, heart murmur

Central nervous system: Dizziness, emotional lability, fever, headache, insomnia, malaise

Dermatologic: Pruritus, rash

Endocrine & metabolic: Breast pain, hot flashes, hyperglycemia, intermenstrual bleeding, vaginal hemorrhage

Gastrointestinal: Abdominal enlargement, diarrhea, flatulence

Genitourinary: Cervical carcinoma, cervical lesion, dysuria, genital herpes, genital moniliasis, leukorrhea, urinary incontinence, urinary tract infection, vaginitis

Hematologic: Leukocytosis

Neuromuscular & skeletal: Back pain, paresthesias

Renal: Albuminuria

Respiratory: Cough, pharyngitis, upper respiratory tract infection

Miscellaneous: Ectopic pregnancy, hiccups

In addition, the following have been reported with menotropin therapy: Adnexal torsion, hemoperitoneum, mild to moderate ovarian enlargement, pulmonary and vascular complications. Ovarian neoplasms have also been reported (rare) with multiple drug regimens used for ovarian induction (relationship not established).

Drug Interactions Specific drug interaction studies have not been conducted.

Drug Uptake

Half-life, elimination: Initial: 4 hours; Terminal: 29 hours

Time to peak: 12-24 hours

Pregnancy Risk Factor X

Generic Available No

Chroma-Pak® *see* Trace Metals *on page 1186*

Chronulac® *see* Lactulose *on page 682*

Chymodiactin® *see* Chymopapain *on page 283*

Chymopapain (KYE moe pa pane)

U.S. Brand Names Chymodiactin®

Pharmacologic Category Enzyme

Use Alternative to surgery in patients with herniated lumbar intervertebral disks

Local Anesthetic/Vasoconstrictor Precautions No information available to require special precautions

Effects on Dental Treatment No effects or complications reported

Dosage Adults: 2000-4000 units/disc with a maximum cumulative dose not to exceed 8000 units for patients with multiple disc herniations

Mechanism of Action When injected into the disc center, causes hydrolysis of the mucal mucopolysaccharide protein complex into acid polysaccharide, polypeptides, and amino acids; subsequently, the water trapping properties of the nucleus pulposus are destroyed which permanently diminishes the pressure within the disc. The adjacent structures including the annulus fibrosus are not affected by chymopapain.

Other Adverse Effects

>10%: Neuromuscular & skeletal: Back pain

1% to 10%:

Central nervous system: Dizziness, headache

Gastrointestinal: Nausea

Neuromuscular & skeletal: Weakness in legs

Drug Interactions Avoid discography (with intradiscal radiographic contrast media)

Pregnancy Risk Factor C

Generic Available No

Ciclopirox (sye kloe PEER oks)

Related Information

Oral Fungal Infections *on page 1377*

U.S. Brand Names Loprox®; Penlac™

Canadian Brand Names Loprox®; Penlac™

Mexican Brand Names Loprox®

Pharmacologic Category Antifungal Agent, Topical

Synonyms Ciclopirox Olamine

Use Treatment of tinea pedis (athlete's foot), tinea cruris (jock itch), tinea corporis (ringworm), cutaneous candidiasis, and tinea versicolor (pityriasis)

Local Anesthetic/Vasoconstrictor Precautions No information available to require special precautions

Effects on Dental Treatment No effects or complications reported

Dosage Children >10 years and Adults:

Cream/lotion: Apply twice daily, gently massage into affected areas; if no improvement after 4 weeks of treatment, re-evaluate the diagnosis

Lacquer: Apply to affected nails daily (as a part of a comprehensive management program for onychomycosis)

Mechanism of Action Inhibiting transport of essential elements in the fungal cell causing problems in synthesis of DNA, RNA, and protein

Other Adverse Effects 1% to 10%:

Dermatologic: Pruritus

Local: Irritation, redness, burning, or pain

Drug Uptake

Absorption: <2% through intact skin

Half-life, elimination: 1.7 hours

Pregnancy Risk Factor B

Generic Available No

Cidofovir (si DOF o veer)

Related Information

Systemic Viral Diseases *on page 1354*

U.S. Brand Names Vistide®

Pharmacologic Category Antiviral Agent

Use Treatment of CMV retinitis in patients with acquired immunodeficiency syndrome (AIDS)

Local Anesthetic/Vasoconstrictor Precautions No information available to require special precautions

Effects on Dental Treatment No effects or complications reported

Dosage

Induction treatment: 5 mg/kg once weekly for 2 consecutive weeks

Maintenance treatment: 5 mg/kg administered once every 2 weeks

Probenecid must be administered orally with each dose of cidofovir

(Continued)

Cidofovir *(Continued)*

Probenecid dose: 2 g 3 hours prior to cidofovir dose, 1 g 2 hours and 8 hours after completion of the infusion; patients should also receive 1 L of normal saline I.V. prior to each infusion of cidofovir; saline should be infused over 1-2 hours

Mechanism of Action Cidofovir is converted to cidofovir diphosphate which is the active intracellular metabolite; cidofovir diphosphate suppresses CMV replication by selective inhibition of viral DNA synthesis. Incorporation of cidofovir into growing viral DNA chain results in reductions in the rate of viral DNA synthesis.

Other Adverse Effects

>10%:

Central nervous system: Infection, chills, fever, headache, amnesia, anxiety, confusion, seizures, insomnia

Dermatologic: Alopecia, rash, acne, skin discoloration

Gastrointestinal: Nausea, vomiting, diarrhea, anorexia, abdominal pain, constipation, dyspepsia, gastritis

Hematologic: Thrombocytopenia, neutropenia, anemia

Neuromuscular & skeletal: Weakness, paresthesia

Ocular: Amblyopia, conjunctivitis, ocular hypotony

Renal: Tubular damage, proteinuria, elevated creatinine

Respiratory: Asthma, bronchitis, coughing, dyspnea, pharyngitis

1% to 10%:

Cardiovascular: Hypotension, pallor, syncope, tachycardia

Central nervous system: Dizziness, hallucinations, depression, somnolence, malaise

Dermatologic: Pruritus, urticaria

Endocrine & metabolic: Hyperglycemia, hyperlipidemia, hypocalcemia, hypokalemia, dehydration

Gastrointestinal: Abnormal taste, stomatitis

Genitourinary: Glycosuria, urinary incontinence, urinary tract infections

Neuromuscular & skeletal: Skeletal pain

Ocular: Retinal detachment, iritis, uveitis, abnormal vision

Renal: Hematuria

Respiratory: Pneumonia, rhinitis, sinusitis

Miscellaneous: Diaphoresis, allergic reactions

Warnings/Precautions Dose-dependent nephrotoxicity is a major dose-limiting toxicity related to cidofovir. Cidofovir is not recommended for use in patients with creatinine >1.5 mg/dL or creatinine clearance <55 mL/minute; in these benefits, consideration should be made of potential benefits vs risks. Dose adjustment or discontinuation may be required for changes in renal function while on therapy; renal function secondary to cidofovir is not always reversible. Neutropenia and metabolic acidosis (Fanconi syndrome) have been reported; administration of cidofovir must be accompanied by oral probenecid and I.V. saline prehydration.

Drug Interactions Increased Effect/Toxicity: Drugs with nephrotoxic potential (eg, amphotericin B, aminoglycosides, foscarnet, and I.V. pentamidine) should be avoided during cidofovir therapy.

Drug Uptake Half-life, elimination, plasma: ~2.6 hours (nonintracellular) [based on a combination of cidofovir administered with probenecid]

Pregnancy Risk Factor C

Generic Available No

Comments Cidofovir preparation should be performed in a class two laminar flow biologic safety cabinet and personnel should be wearing surgical gloves and a closed front surgical gown with knit cuffs; appropriate safety equipment is recommended for preparation, administration, and disposal of cidofovir. If cidofovir contacts skin, wash and flush thoroughly with water.

Selected Readings Hitchcock MJ, Jaffe HS, Martin JC, et al, "Cidofovir, A New Agent With Potent Antiherpesvirus Activity," *Antiviral Chemistry & Chemotherapy*, 1996, 7:115-27.

Cilazapril *Not Available in U.S.* (sye LAY za pril)

Canadian Brand Names Inhibace®

Pharmacologic Category Angiotensin-Converting Enzyme (ACE) Inhibitor

Synonyms Cilazapril Monohydrate

Use Management of hypertension; treatment of CHF

Local Anesthetic/Vasoconstrictor Precautions No information available to require special precautions

Effects on Dental Treatment No effects or complications reported

Dosage Oral:

Hypertension: 2.5-5 mg once daily (maximum dose: 10 mg/day)

Congestive heart failure: Initial: 0.5 mg once daily; if tolerated, after 5 days increase to 1 mg/day (lowest maintenance dose); may increase to maximum of 2.5 mg once daily

Elderly: Initial: 1.25 mg once daily; titrate slowly as tolerated

Dosage adjustment in renal impairment:

Hypertension:

Cl_{cr} 10-40 mL/minute: Initial: 0.5 mg once daily (maximum dose: 2.5 mg once daily)

Cl_{cr} <10 mL/minute: 0.25-0.5 mg once or twice weekly

Congestive heart failure:

Cl_{cr} 10-40 mL/minute: Initial: 0.25-0.5 mg once daily (maximum dose: 2.5 mg once daily)

Cl_{cr} <10 mL/minute: 0.25-0.5 mg once or twice weekly

Dosage adjustment in hepatic impairment: Initial: ≤0.5 mg once daily (with caution)

Mechanism of Action Competitive inhibitor of angiotensin-converting enzyme (ACE); prevents conversion of angiotensin I to angiotensin II, a potent vasoconstrictor; results in lower levels of angiotensin II which causes an increase in plasma renin activity and a reduction in aldosterone secretion

Other Adverse Effects 1% to 10%:

Cardiovascular: Palpitation (up to 1%), hypotension (symptomatic, up to 1% in CHF patients), orthostatic hypotension (2%)

Central nervous system: Headache (3% to 5%), dizziness (3% to 8%), fatigue (2% to 3%)

Gastrointestinal: Nausea (1% to 3%)

Neuromuscular & skeletal: Weakness (0.3% to 2%)

Renal: Increased serum creatinine

Respiratory: Cough (2% in hypertension, up to 7.5% in CHF patients)

Drug Interactions

Increased Effect/Toxicity: Angiotensin II receptor antagonists (candesartan, irbesartan, losartan, etc), potassium supplements, potassium-sparing diuretics (amiloride, spironolactone, triamterene), or sulfamethoxazole/trimethoprim (high dose) may result in elevated serum potassium levels when combined with cilazapril. ACE inhibitor effects may be increased by phenothiazines or probenecid (increases levels of other ACE-inhibitors). ACE inhibitors may increase serum concentrations/effects of digoxin, lithium, and sulfonlyureas. Diuretics have additive hypotensive effects with ACE inhibitors, and hypovolemia increases the potential for adverse renal effects of ACE inhibitors. In patients with compromised renal function, coadministration with nonsteroidal anti-inflammatory drugs may result in further deterioration of renal function. Allopurinol and ACE inhibitors may cause a higher risk of hypersensitivity reaction when taken concurrently.

Decreased Effect: Antacids may decrease the bioavailability of ACE inhibitors (may be more likely to occur with captopril); separate administration times by 1-2 hours. Aspirin (high dose) may reduce the therapeutic effects of ACE inhibitors; at low dosages this does not appear to be significant. NSAIDs may attenuate hypertensive efficacy; effect has been seen with captopril and may occur with other ACE inhibitors; monitor BP; may increase adverse renal effects. Rifampin may decrease the effect of ACE inhibitors.

Drug Uptake

Onset: Antihypertensive: ~1 hour

Absorption: Rapid

Duration: Therapeutic effect: 24 hours

Half-life, elimination: Cilazaprilat: Terminal: 36-49 hours

Time to peak: 3-7 hours

Pregnancy Risk Factor Not assigned; C/D (2nd and 3rd trimesters) based on other ACE-inhibitors

Cilostazol (sil OH sta zol)

U.S. Brand Names Pletal®

Canadian Brand Names Pletal®

Pharmacologic Category Antiplatelet Agent; Phosphodiesterase Enzyme Inhibitor

Synonyms OPC13013

Use Symptomatic management of peripheral vascular disease, primarily intermittent claudication

Unlabeled/Investigational: Treatment of acute coronary syndromes and for graft patency improvement in percutaneous coronary interventions with or without stenting

Local Anesthetic/Vasoconstrictor Precautions No information available to require special precautions

Effects on Dental Treatment Tongue edema has been observed (according to manufacturer); if a patient is to undergo elective surgery and an antiplatelet effect is not desired, a medical consult is suggested to consider reduction or discontinuation of cilostazol dose prior to surgery.

Dosage Adults: Oral: 100 mg twice daily taken at least one-half hour before or 2 hours after breakfast and dinner; dosage should be reduced to 50 mg twice daily during concurrent therapy with inhibitors of CYP3A4 or CYP2C19 (see Drug Interactions)

(Continued)

Cilostazol *(Continued)*

Mechanism of Action Cilostazol and its metabolites are inhibitors of phosphodiesterase III. As a result, cyclic AMP is increased leading to inhibition of platelet aggregation and vasodilation. Other effects of phosphodiesterase III inhibition include increased cardiac contractility, accelerated A-V nodal conduction, increased ventricular automaticity, heart rate, and coronary blood flow.

Other Adverse Effects

>10%:

- Central nervous system: Headache (27% to 34%)
- Gastrointestinal: Abnormal stools (12% to 15%), diarrhea (12% to 19%)
- Miscellaneous: Infection (10% to 14%)

2% to 10%:

- Cardiovascular: Peripheral edema (7% to 9%), palpitation (5% to 10%), tachycardia (4%)
- Central nervous system: Dizziness (9% to 10%)
- Gastrointestinal: Dyspepsia (6%), nausea (6% to 7%), abdominal pain (4% to 5%), flatulence (2% to 3%)
- Neuromuscular & skeletal: Back pain (6% to 7%), myalgia (2% to 3%)
- Respiratory: Rhinitis (7% to 12%), pharyngitis (7% to 10%), cough (3% to 4%)

<2%: Chills, facial edema, fever, edema, malaise, nuchal rigidity, pelvic pain, retroperitoneal hemorrhage, cerebral infarction/ischemia, CHF, cardiac arrest, hemorrhage, hypotension, myocardial infarction/ischemia, postural hypotension, ventricular arrhythmia, supraventricular arrhythmia, syncope, anorexia, cholelithiasis, colitis, duodenitis, peptic ulcer, duodenal ulcer, esophagitis, esophageal hemorrhage, gastritis, hematemesis, melena, tongue edema, diabetes mellitus, anemia, ecchymosis, polycythemia, purpura, increased creatinine, gout, hyperlipidemia, hyperuricemia, arthralgia, bone pain, bursitis, anxiety, insomnia, neuralgia, dry skin, urticaria, amblyopia, blindness, conjunctivitis, diplopia, retinal hemorrhage, cystitis, albuminuria, vaginitis, vaginal hemorrhage, urinary frequency

Contraindications Hypersensitivity to cilostazol or any component of the formulation; heart failure (of any severity)

Warnings/Precautions Use with caution in patients receiving platelet aggregation inhibitors (effects are unknown), hepatic impairment (not studied). Use with caution in patients receiving inhibitors of CYP3A4 (such as ketoconazole or erythromycin) or inhibitors of CYP2C19 (such as omeprazole); use with caution in severe underlying heart disease; use is not recommended in nursing mothers

Drug Interactions CYP2C19 (minor) and 3A3/4 (major) enzyme substrate

Increased Effect/Toxicity: Cilostazol serum concentration may be increased by erythromycin, diltiazem, and omeprazole. Increased concentrations of cilostazol may be anticipated during concurrent therapy with other inhibitors of CYP3A4 (ie, clarithromycin, ketoconazole, itraconazole, fluconazole, miconazole, fluvoxamine, fluoxetine, nefazodone, and sertraline) or inhibitors of CYP2C19. Aspirin-induced inhibition of platelet aggregation is potentiated by concurrent cilostazol. The effect on platelet aggregation with other antiplatelet drugs is unknown.

Drug Uptake

Onset of action: 2-4 weeks; may require up to 12 weeks

Half-life, elimination: 11-13 hours

Pregnancy Risk Factor C

Generic Available No

Ciloxan® *see* Ciprofloxacin *on page 288*

Cimetidine (sye MET i deen)

Related Information

Dental Drug Interactions: Update on Drug Combinations Requiring Special Considerations *on page 1434*

Gastrointestinal Disorders *on page 1326*

U.S. Brand Names Tagamet®; Tagamet® HB [OTC]

Canadian Brand Names Apo®-Cimetidine; Gen-Cimetidine; Novo-Cimetidine; Nu-Cimet®; PMS-Cimetidine; Tagamet®; Tagamet® HB

Mexican Brand Names Blocan; Cimetase®; Cimetigal; Columina; Tagamet®; Ulcedine; Zymerol

Pharmacologic Category Histamine H_2 Antagonist

Use Short-term treatment of active duodenal ulcers and benign gastric ulcers; long-term prophylaxis of duodenal ulcer; gastric hypersecretory states; gastroesophageal reflux; prevention of upper GI bleeding in critically ill patients.

Unlabeled/Investigational: Part of a multidrug regimen for *H. pylori* eradication to reduce the risk of duodenal ulcer recurrence

Local Anesthetic/Vasoconstrictor Precautions No information available to require special precautions

Effects on Dental Treatment No effects or complications reported

Dosage

Children: Oral, I.M., I.V.: 20-40 mg/kg/day in divided doses every 6 hours

Adults: Short-term treatment of active ulcers:

Oral: 300 mg 4 times/day or 800 mg at bedtime or 400 mg twice daily for up to 8 weeks

I.M., I.V.: 300 mg every 6 hours or 37.5 mg/hour by continuous infusion; I.V. dosage should be adjusted to maintain an intragastric pH ≥5

Patients with an active bleed: Give cimetidine as a continuous infusion (see above)

Duodenal ulcer prophylaxis: Oral: 400-800 mg at bedtime

Gastric hypersecretory conditions: Oral, I.M., I.V.: 300-600 mg every 6 hours; dosage not to exceed 2.4 g/day

Mechanism of Action Competitive inhibition of histamine at H_2-receptors of the gastric parietal cells resulting in reduced gastric acid secretion, gastric volume and hydrogen ion concentration reduced

Other Adverse Effects 1% to 10%:

Central nervous system: Headache, dizziness, agitation, drowsiness

Gastrointestinal: Diarrhea, nausea, vomiting

Drug Interactions CYP3A3/4 enzyme substrate; CYP1A2, 2C9, 2C18, 2C19, 2D6, and 3A3/4 enzyme inhibitor

Increased Effect/Toxicity: Cimetidine increases warfarin's effect in a dose-related manner. Cimetidine may increase serum concentration of alfentanil, amiodarone, benzodiazepines (except lorazepam, oxazepam, temazepam), beta-blockers (except atenolol, betaxolol, bisoprolol, nadolol, penbutolol), calcium channel blockers, carbamazepine, cisapride (avoid concurrent use), citalopram, flecainide, lidocaine, melphalan, meperidine, metronidazole, moricizine, paroxetine, phenytoin, procainamide, propafenone, quinidine, quinolone antibiotics, tacrine, TCAs, theophylline, and triamterene. Cimetidine increases carmustine's myelotoxicity; avoid concurrent use.

Decreased Effect: Ketoconazole, fluconazole, itraconazole (especially capsule) decrease serum concentration; avoid concurrent use with H_2 antagonists. Delavirdine's absorption is decreased; avoid concurrent use with H_2 antagonists.

Drug Uptake

Onset of action: 1 hour

Duration: 6 hours

Half-life, elimination: Neonates: 3.6 hours; Children: 1.4 hours; Adults: Normal renal function: 2 hours

Time to peak: Oral: 1-2 hours

Pregnancy Risk Factor B

Generic Available Yes

Cinobac® Pulvules® *see* Cinoxacin *on page 287*

Cinoxacin (sin OKS a sin)

U.S. Brand Names Cinobac® Pulvules®

Canadian Brand Names Cinobac®

Mexican Brand Names Gugecin

Pharmacologic Category Antibiotic, Quinolone

Use Treatment of urinary tract infections

Local Anesthetic/Vasoconstrictor Precautions No information available to require special precautions

Effects on Dental Treatment No effects or complications reported

Dosage Children >12 years and Adults: 1 g/day in 2-4 doses for 7-14 days

Mechanism of Action Inhibits microbial synthesis of DNA with resultant problems in protein synthesis

Other Adverse Effects 1% to 10%:

Central nervous system: Headache, dizziness

Gastrointestinal: Heartburn, abdominal pain, GI bleeding, belching, flatulence, anorexia, nausea

Drug Interactions

Increased Effect/Toxicity: Quinolones may cause increased levels of azlocillin, cyclosporine, and caffeine/theophylline. Azlocillin, cimetidine, loop diuretics (furosemide, torsemide), and probenecid increase quinolone levels (decreased renal secretion). An increased incidence of seizures may occur with foscarnet or NSAIDs. The hypoprothrombinemic effect of warfarin is enhanced by some quinolone antibiotics.

Decreased Effect: Metal cations (magnesium, aluminum, iron, and zinc) bind quinolones in the GI tract and inhibit absorption (by up to 98%). Due to electrolyte content, antacids, electrolyte supplements, sucralfate, quinapril, and some didanosine formulations should be avoided. Levofloxacin should be administered 4 hours before or 8 hours (a minimum of 2 hours before and 2 hours after) after these agents. Antineoplastic agents may decrease the absorption of quinolones.

Drug Uptake

Absorption: Oral: Rapid and complete; food decreases peak levels by 30% but not extent of absorption

Half-life, elimination: 1.5 hours (increases with renal impairment)

Time to peak: 2-3 hours

Pregnancy Risk Factor B

(Continued)

Cinoxacin *(Continued)*

Generic Available Yes

Cipro® *see* Ciprofloxacin *on page 288*

Ciprofloxacin (sip roe FLOKS a sin)

Related Information

Antibiotic Prophylaxis, Preprocedural Guidelines for Dental Patients *on page 1344*

Nonviral Infectious Diseases *on page 1342*

U.S. Brand Names Ciloxan®; Cipro®

Canadian Brand Names Ciloxan®; Cipro®

Mexican Brand Names Cimogal; Ciprobiotic®; Ciproflox®; Ciprofur®; Ciproxina®; Italnik®; Kenzoflex; Microrgan®; Mitroken®; Nivoflox®; Novoquin®; Opthaflox; Quinoflox®; Sophixin®; Suiflox®; Zipra®

Pharmacologic Category Antibiotic, Ophthalmic; Antibiotic, Quinolone

Synonyms Ciprofloxacin Hydrochloride

Use

Dental: Useful as a single agent or in combination with metronidazole in the treatment of periodontitis associated with the presence of *Actinobacillus actinomycetemcomitans*, (AA) as well as enteric rods/pseudomonads

Medical: Treatment of documented or suspected infections of the lower respiratory tract, sinuses, skin and skin structure, bone/joints, and urinary tract (including prostatitis) due to susceptible bacterial strains; especially indicated for pseudomonal infections and those due to multidrug-resistant gram-negative organisms, chronic bacterial prostatitis, infectious diarrhea, complicated gram-negative and anaerobic intra-abdominal infections (with metronidazole) due to *E. coli* (enteropathic strains), *B. fragilis, P. mirabilis, K. pneumoniae, P. aeruginosa, Campylobacter jejuni* or *Shigella*; approved for acute sinusitis caused by *H. influenzae* or *M. catarrhalis*; also used in treatment of typhoid fever due to *Salmonella typhi* (although eradication of the chronic typhoid carrier state has not been proven), osteomyelitis when parenteral therapy is not feasible, acute uncomplicated cystitis in females, to reduce incidence or progression of disease following exposure to aerolized *Bacillus anthracis*, febrile neutropenia (with piperacillin), and sexually-transmitted diseases such as uncomplicated cervical and urethral gonorrhea due to *Neisseria gonorrhoeae*; used ophthalmologically for superficial ocular infections (corneal ulcers, conjunctivitis) due to susceptible strains

Local Anesthetic/Vasoconstrictor Precautions No information available to require special precautions

Effects on Dental Treatment <1%: Painful oral mucosa, oral candidiasis, oral ulceration, xerostomia

Dosage

Children (see Warnings/Precautions):

Oral: 20-30 mg/kg/day in 2 divided doses; maximum: 1.5 g/day

Cystic fibrosis: 20-40 mg/kg/day divided every 12 hours

Anthrax:

Inhalational (postexposure prophylaxis): 10-15 mg/kg/dose every 12 hours for 60 days; maximum: 500 mg/dose

Cutaneous (treatment): 10-15 mg/kg every 12 hours for 60 days; amoxicillin 80 mg/kg/day divided every 8 hours is an option for completion of treatment after clinical improvement. **Note:** In the presence of systemic involvement, extensive edema, lesions on head/neck, refer to I.V. dosing for treatment of inhalational/GI/oropharyngeal anthrax

I.V.: 15-20 mg/kg/day divided every 12 hours

Cystic fibrosis: 15-30 mg/kg/day divided every 8-12 hours

Anthrax:

Inhalational (postexposure prophylaxis): 10 mg/kg/dose every 12 hours; do **not** exceed 400 mg/dose (800 mg/day)

Inhalational/GI/oropharyngeal (treatment): Initial: 10-15 mg/kg every 12 hours for 60 days (maximum: 500 mg/dose); switch to oral therapy when clinically appropriate; refer to Adults dosing for notes on combined therapy and duration

Adults: Oral:

Urinary tract infection: 250-500 mg every 12 hours for 7-10 days, depending on severity of infection and susceptibility

Cystitis, uncomplicated (in females): 100 mg or 250 mg every 12 hours for 3 days

Lower respiratory tract, skin/skin structure infections: 500-750 mg twice daily for 7-14 days depending on severity and susceptibility

Bone/joint infections: 500-750 mg twice daily for 4-6 weeks, depending on severity and susceptibility

Infectious diarrhea: 500 mg every 12 hours for 5-7 days

Typhoid fever: 500 mg every 12 hours for 10 days

Urethral/cervical gonococcal infections: 500 mg as a single dose (CDC recommends concomitant doxycycline or azithromycin due to developing resistance; avoid use in Asian or Western Pacific travelers)

Disseminated gonococcal infection: 500 mg twice daily to complete 7 days of therapy (initial treatment with ceftriaxone 1 g I.M./I.V. daily for 24-48 hours after improvement begins)

Chancroid: 500 mg twice daily for 3 days

Mild to moderate sinusitis: 500 mg every 12 hours for 10 days

Chronic bacterial prostatitis: 500 mg every 12 hours for 28 days

Anthrax:

Inhalational (postexposure prophylaxis): 500 mg every 12 hours for 60 days

Cutaneous (treatment): 500 mg every 12 hours for 60 days. **Note:** In the presence of systemic involvement, extensive edema, lesions on head/neck, refer to I.V. dosing for treatment of inhalational/GI/oropharyngeal anthrax

Adults: I.V.:

Lower respiratory tract, skin/skin structure infection, or bone/ joint infections:

Mild to moderate: 400 mg every 12 hours for 7-14 days

Severe or complicated: 400 mg every 8 hours for 7-14 days

Nosocomial pneumonia (mild to moderate to severe): 400 mg every 8 hours

Prostatitis (chronic, bacterial): 400 mg every 12 hours

Sinusitis (acute): 400 mg every 12 hours

Urinary tract infection:

Mild to moderate: 200 mg every 12 hours for 7-10 days

Severe or complicated: 400 mg every 12 hours for 7-10 days

Febrile neutropenia (with piperacillin): 400 mg every 8 hours for 7-14 days

Intra-abdominal infection (with metronidazole): 400 mg every 12 hours

Anthrax:

Inhalational (postexposure prophylaxis): 400 mg every 12 hours

Inhalational/GI/oropharyngeal (treatment): 400 mg every 12 hours. **Note:** Initial treatment should include two or more agents predicted to be effective (per CDC recommendations). Agents suggested for use in conjunction with ciprofloxacin or doxycycline include rifampin, vancomycin, imipenem, penicillin, ampicillin, chloramphenicol, clindamycin, and clarithromycin. May switch to oral antimicrobial therapy when clinically appropriate. Continue combined therapy for 60 days.

Elderly: No adjustment needed in patients with normal renal function

Ophthalmic:

Solution: Children >1 year and Adults: Instill 1-2 drops in eye(s) every 2 hours while awake for 2 days and 1-2 drops every 4 hours while awake for the next 5 days

Ointment: Children >2 years and Adults: Apply a 1/2" ribbon into the conjunctival sac 3 times/day for the first 2 days, followed by a 1/2" ribbon applied twice daily for the next 5 days

Dosing adjustment in renal impairment:

Cl_{cr} 30-50 mL/minute: Oral: 250-500 mg every 12 hours

Cl_{cr} 5-29 mL/minute:

Oral: 250-500 mg every 18 hours

I.V.: 200-400 mg every 18-24 hours

Dialysis: Only small amounts of ciprofloxacin are removed by hemo- or peritoneal dialysis (<10%); usual dose: 250-500 mg every 24 hours following dialysis

Continuous arteriovenous or venovenous hemodiafiltration effects: Administer 200-400 mg I.V. every 12 hours

Mechanism of Action Inhibits DNA-gyrase in susceptible organisms; inhibits relaxation of supercoiled DNA and promotes breakage of double-stranded DNA

Other Adverse Effects

1% to 10%:

Central nervous system: Headache (1%), restlessness (1%)

Dermatologic: Rash (1%)

Gastrointestinal: Nausea (5%), diarrhea (2%), vomiting (2%), abdominal pain (2%)

Hepatic: Elevated ALT/AST (2%)

Renal: Elevated serum creatinine (1%)

<1% and postmarketing reports (limited to important or life-threatening): Dizziness, confusion, seizures, anemia, increased liver enzymes, tremor, arthralgia, ruptured tendons, acute renal failure, palpitations, syncope, hypertension, angina pectoris, myocardial infarction, cardiopulmonary arrest, nightmares, hallucinations, drowsiness, gastrointestinal bleeding, cholestatic jaundice, joint pain, dyspnea, photosensitivity, edema, allergic reactions, visual disturbance, pseudomembranous colitis, agranulocytosis, prolongation of PT, erythema multiforme, Stevens-Johnson syndrome, toxic epidermal necrolysis

Contraindications Hypersensitivity to ciprofloxacin, other quinolones, or any component of their formulation

Warnings/Precautions Not recommended in children <18 years of age (exception - postexposure treatment of inhalational anthrax); has caused transient arthropathy in children. CNS stimulation may occur (tremor, restlessness, confusion, and very

(Continued)

Ciprofloxacin *(Continued)*

rarely hallucinations or seizures). Use with caution in patients with known or suspected CNS disorder. Green discoloration of teeth in newborns has been reported; prolonged use may result in superinfection. Tendon inflammation and/or rupture have been reported with ciprofloxacin and other quinolone antibiotics. Discontinue at first sign of tendon inflammation or pain.

Severe hypersensitivity reactions, including anaphylaxis, have occurred with quinolone therapy. If an allergic reaction occurs (itching, urticaria, dyspnea, facial edema, loss of consciousness, tingling, cardiovascular collapse), discontinue drug immediately. Quinolones may exacerbate myasthenia gravis, use with caution (rare, potentially life-threatening weakness of respiratory muscles may occur).

Drug Interactions CYP1A2 enzyme inhibitor

Aluminum/magnesium products, didanosine, quinapril, and sucralfate may decrease absorption of ciprofloxacin by ≥90% if administered concurrently. Administer ciprofloxacin at least 4 hours and preferably 6 hours after the dose of these agents or change to an H_2 antagonist or omeprazole.

Calcium, iron, zinc, and multivitamins with minerals products may decrease absorption of ciprofloxacin significantly if administered concurrently. Administer ciprofloxacin 2 hours before dose or at least 2 hours after the dose of these agents.

Caffeine and theophylline → CNS stimulation when concurrent with ciprofloxacin.

Antineoplastic agents may decrease the absorption of quinolones.

Cimetidine, and other H_2 antagonists may inhibit renal elimination of quinolones. No effect on bioavailability demonstrated with ciprofloxacin.

Cyclosporine: Ciprofloxacin may increase serum concentration.

Foscarnet has been associated with an increased risk of seizures with some quinolones.

Loop diuretics: Serum levels of some quinolones are increased by loop diuretic administration. May diminish renal excretion.

NSAIDs: The CNS stimulating effect of some quinolones may be enhanced, resulting in neuroexcitation and/or seizures.

Probenecid: Blocks renal secretion of quinolones, increasing concentrations.

Warfarin: The hypoprothrombinemic effect of warfarin is enhanced by ciprofloxacin; monitor INR closely during therapy.

Dietary/Ethanol/Herb Considerations

Food: Administer with food to reduce GI upset (manufacturer recommends administration 2 hours after meals). Food decreases rate, but not extent of absorption. Limit dairy products; may decrease absorption. Administration with caffeine may increase caffeine levels; restrict caffeine intake if excessive cardiac or CNS stimulation occurs.

Enteral feedings may decrease plasma concentrations of ciprofloxacin probably by >30% inhibition of absorption. Ciprofloxacin should not be administered with enteral feedings. The feeding would need to be discontinued for 1-2 hours prior to and after ciprofloxacin administration. Nasogastric administration produces a greater loss of ciprofloxacin bioavailability than does nasoduodenal administration.

Oral multivitamins, and mineral supplements: Absorption of ciprofloxacin is decreased by divalent and trivalent cations. The manufacturer states that the usual dietary intake of calcium has not been shown to interfere with ciprofloxacin absorption. These products may be taken 6 hours before or 2 hours following a dose of ciprofloxacin.

Herb/Nutraceutical: Avoid dong quai and St John's wort; may increase photosensitization.

Drug Uptake

Absorption: Oral: Rapid from GI tract (~50% to 85%)

Half-life, elimination: Children: 2.5 hours; Adults: 3-5 hours (normal renal function)

Time to peak: Oral: T_{max}: 0.5-2 hours

Pregnancy Risk Factor C

Breast-feeding Considerations Not compatible; can resume breast-feeding 48 hours after the last dose. Theoretically, may affect cartilage in weight-bearing joints.

Dosage Forms INF [in D_5W]: 400 mg (200 mL). **INF** [in NS or D_5W]: 200 mg (100 mL). **INJ:** 200 mg (20 mL); 400 mg (40 mL). **OINT, ophthalmic:** 3.33 mg/g [0.3% base] (3.5 g). **SOLN, ophthalmic:** 3.33 mg/g [0.3% base] (2.5 mL, 5 mL. 10 mL). **SUSP, oral:** 250 mg/5 mL (100 mL); 500 mg/5 mL (100 mL). **TAB:** 100 mg, 250 mg, 500 mg, 750 mg

Generic Available No

Selected Readings

Rams TE and Slots J, "Antibiotics in Periodontal Therapy: An Update," *Compendium*, 1992, 13(12):1130, 1132, 1134.

Wynn RL, Bergman SA, Meiller TF, et al, "Antibiotics in Treating Oral-Facial Infections of Odontogenic Origin: An Update", *Gen Dent*, 2001, 49(3):238-40, 242, 244 passim.

Ciprofloxacin and Hydrocortisone

(sip roe FLOKS a sin & hye droe KOR ti sone)

U.S. Brand Names Cipro® HC Otic

Canadian Brand Names Cipro® HC

Pharmacologic Category Antibiotic/Corticosteroid, Otic

Synonyms Hydrocortisone and Ciprofloxacin

Use Treatment of acute otitis externa, sometimes known as "swimmer's ear"

Local Anesthetic/Vasoconstrictor Precautions No information available to require special precautions

Effects on Dental Treatment No effects or complications reported

Dosage Children >1 year and Adults: Otic: The recommended dosage for all patients is 3 drops of the suspension in the affected ear twice daily for 7 days; twice-daily dosing schedule is more convenient for patients than that of existing treatments with hydrocortisone, which are typically administered 3-4 times/day; a twice-daily dosage schedule may be especially helpful for parents and caregivers of young children

Drug Uptake See Hydrocortisone *on page 608* and Ciprofloxacin *on page 288*

Generic Available No

Cipro® HC Otic *see* Ciprofloxacin and Hydrocortisone *on page 290*

Cisapride (SIS a pride)

Related Information

Endocrine Disorders and Pregnancy *on page 1331*

U.S. Brand Names Propulsid®

Mexican Brand Names Enteropride; Kinestase®; Unamol

Pharmacologic Category Gastrointestinal Agent, Prokinetic

Use Treatment of nocturnal symptoms of gastroesophageal reflux disease (GERD); has demonstrated effectiveness for gastroparesis, refractory constipation, and nonulcer dyspepsia

Local Anesthetic/Vasoconstrictor Precautions No information available to require special precautions

Effects on Dental Treatment No effects or complications reported

Restrictions Available in U.S. via limited-access protocol only

Dosage Oral:

Children: 0.15-0.3 mg/kg/dose 3-4 times/day; maximum: 10 mg/dose

Adults: Initial: 10 mg 4 times/day at least 15 minutes before meals and at bedtime; in some patients the dosage will need to be increased to 20 mg to obtain a satisfactory result

Mechanism of Action Enhances the release of acetylcholine at the myenteric plexus. *In vitro* studies have shown cisapride to have serotonin-4 receptor agonistic properties which may increase GI motility and cardiac rate; increases lower esophageal sphincter pressure and lower esophageal peristalsis; accelerates gastric emptying of both liquids and solids

Other Adverse Effects

>5%:

- Central nervous system: Headache
- Dermatologic: Rash
- Gastrointestinal: Diarrhea, GI cramping, dyspepsia, flatulence, nausea, xerostomia
- Respiratory: Rhinitis

<5%:

- Cardiovascular: Tachycardia
- Central nervous system: Extrapyramidal effects, somnolence, fatigue, seizures, insomnia, anxiety
- Hematologic: Thrombocytopenia, increased LFTs, pancytopenia, leukopenia, granulocytopenia, aplastic anemia
- Respiratory: Sinusitis, coughing, upper respiratory tract infection, increased incidence of viral infection

Contraindications Hypersensitivity to cisapride or any component of the formulation; GI hemorrhage, mechanical obstruction, GI perforation, or other situations when GI motility stimulation is dangerous

Serious cardiac arrhythmias including ventricular tachycardia, ventricular fibrillation, torsade de pointes, and QT prolongation have been reported in patients taking cisapride with other drugs that inhibit CYP3A4. Some of these events have been fatal. Concomitant oral or I.V. administration of the following drugs with cisapride may lead to elevated cisapride blood levels and is contraindicated:

- Antibiotics: Oral or I.V. erythromycin, clarithromycin, troleandomycin
- Antidepressants: Nefazodone
- Antifungals: Oral or I.V. fluconazole, itraconazole, miconazole, oral ketoconazole
- Protease inhibitors: Indinavir, ritonavir

Cisapride is also contraindicated for patients with history of prolonged electrocardiographic QT intervals, known family history of congenital long QT syndrome; clinically significant bradycardia, renal failure, history of ventricular arrhythmias, ischemic heart disease, and CHF; uncorrected electrolyte disorders (hypokalemia, hypomagnesemia); respiratory failure; and concomitant medications known to prolong the QT interval and increase the risk of arrhythmia, such as certain antiarrhythmics, certain antipsychotics, certain antidepressants, bepridil, sparfloxacin,

(Continued)

Cisapride *(Continued)*

and terodiline. The preceding list of drugs is not comprehensive. Cisapride should not be used in patients with uncorrected hypokalemia or hypomagnesemia, or who might experience rapid reduction of plasma potassium such as those administered potassium-wasting diuretics and/or insulin in acute settings.

A 12-lead EKG should be performed prior to administration of cisapride. Treatment with cisapride should not be initiated if the QT_c value exceeds 450 milliseconds. Serum electrolytes (potassium, calcium, and magnesium) and creatinine should be assessed prior to administration of cisapride and whenever conditions develop that may affect electrolyte balance or renal function.

Warnings/Precautions **Serious cardiac arrhythmias including ventricular tachycardia, ventricular fibrillation, torsade de pointes, and QT prolongation have been reported in patients taking this drug.** Many of these patients also took drugs expected to increase cisapride blood levels by inhibiting the CYP3A4 enzymes that metabolize cisapride. These drugs include clarithromycin, erythromycin, troleandomycin, nefazodone, fluconazole, itraconazole, ketoconazole, indinavir and ritonavir. Some of these events have been fatal. Cisapride is contraindicated in patients taking any of these drugs. **QT prolongation, torsade de pointes (sometimes with syncope), cardiac arrest and sudden death have been reported in patients taking cisapride without the above-mentioned contraindicated drugs.** Most patients had disorders that may have predisposed them to arrhythmias with cisapride. Cisapride is contraindicated for those patients with: history of prolonged electrocardiographic QT intervals; renal failure; history of ventricular arrhythmias, ischemic heart disease, and CHF; uncorrected electrolyte disorders (hypokalemia, hypomagnesemia); respiratory failure; and concomitant medications known to prolong the QT interval and increase the risk of arrhythmia, such as certain antiarrhythmics, including those of Class 1A (such as quinidine and procainamide) and Class III (such as sotalol); tricyclic antidepressants (such as amitriptyline); certain tetracyclic antidepressants (such as maprotiline); certain antipsychotic medications (such as certain phenothiazines and sertindole), bepridil, sparfloxacin and terodiline. (The preceding lists of drugs are not comprehensive.) Recommended doses of cisapride should not be exceeded.

Potential benefits should be weighed against risks prior administration of cisapride to patients who have or may develop prolongation of cardiac conduction intervals, particularly QT_c. These include patients with conditions that could predispose them to the development of serious arrhythmias, such as multiple organ failure, COPD, apnea and advanced cancer. Cisapride should not be used in patients with uncorrected hypokalemia or hypomagnesemia, such as those with severe dehydration, vomiting or malnutrition, or those taking potassium-wasting diuretics. Cisapride should not be used in patients who might experience rapid reduction of plasma potassium, such as those administered potassium-wasting diuretics and/or insulin in acute settings.

Drug Interactions CYP3A3/4 enzyme substrate

Increased Effect/Toxicity: Cisapride may increase blood levels of warfarin, diazepam, cimetidine, ranitidine, and CNS depressants. The risk of cisapride-induced malignant arrhythmias may be increased by azole antifungals (fluconazole, itraconazole, ketoconazole, miconazole), antiarrhythmics (Class Ia; quinidine, procainamide, and Class III; amiodarone, sotalol), bepridil, cimetidine, maprotiline, macrolide antibiotics (erythromycin, clarithromycin, troleandomycin), molindone, nefazodone, protease inhibitors (amprenavir, indinavir, nelfinavir, ritonavir), phenothiazines (eg, prochlorperazine, promethazine), sertindole, tricyclic antidepressants (eg amitriptyline), and some quinolone antibiotics (sparfloxacin, gatifloxacin, moxifloxacin). Cardiovascular disease or electrolyte imbalances (potentially due to diuretic therapy) increase the risk of malignant arrhythmias.

Decreased Effect: Cisapride may decrease the effect of atropine and digoxin.

Drug Uptake

Onset of action: 0.5-1 hour

Half-life, elimination: 6-12 hours

Pregnancy Risk Factor C

Generic Available No

Cisplatin (SIS pla tin)

U.S. Brand Names Platinol®; Platinol®-AQ

Canadian Brand Names Platinol®-AQ

Mexican Brand Names Blastolem; Medsaplatin; Niyaplat; Platinol®; Tecnoplatin®

Pharmacologic Category Antineoplastic Agent, Alkylating Agent

Synonyms CDDP

Use Management of metastatic testicular or ovarian carcinoma, advanced bladder cancer, osteosarcoma, Hodgkin's and non-Hodgkin's lymphoma, head or neck cancer, cervical cancer, lung cancer, brain tumors, neuroblastoma; used alone or in combination with other agents

Local Anesthetic/Vasoconstrictor Precautions No information available to require special precautions

Effects on Dental Treatment No effects or complications reported

Mechanism of Action Inhibits DNA synthesis by the formation of DNA cross-links; denatures the double helix; covalently binds to DNA bases and disrupts DNA function; may also bind to proteins; the *cis*-isomer is 14 times more cytotoxic than the *trans*-isomer; both forms cross-link DNA but cis-platinum is less easily recognized by cell enzymes and, therefore, not repaired. Cisplatin can also bind two adjacent guanines on the same strand of DNA producing intrastrand cross-linking and breakage

Other Adverse Effects

>10%:

Central nervous system: Neurotoxicity (Peripheral neuropathy is dose- and duration-dependent. The mechanism is through axonal degeneration with subsequent damage to the long sensory nerves. Toxicity can first be noted at cumulative doses of 200 mg/m^2, with measurable toxicity at cumulative doses >350 mg/m^2. This process is irreversible and progressive with continued therapy.)

Dermatologic: Mild alopecia

Gastrointestinal: **Highly emetogenic** (Cisplatin is one of the most emetogenic agents used in cancer chemotherapy. Nausea and vomiting occur in 76% to 100% of patients and are dose-related. Prophylactic antiemetics should always be prescribed; nausea and vomiting may last up to 1 week after therapy.)

Hematologic: Myelosuppressive: Mild with moderate doses, mild to moderate with high-dose therapy

WBC: Mild

Platelets: Mild

Onset: 10 days

Nadir: 14-23 days

Recovery: 21-39 days

Renal: Nephrotoxicity (Related to elimination, protein binding, and uptake of cisplatin. Two types of nephrotoxicity: Acute renal failure and chronic renal insufficiency.)

Acute renal failure and azotemia are dose-dependent and can be minimized with proper administration and prophylaxis. Damage to the proximal tubules by unbound cisplatin is suspected to cause the toxicity. It is manifested as increased BUN/creatinine, oliguria, protein wasting, and potassium, calcium, and magnesium wasting.

Chronic renal dysfunction can develop in patients receiving multiple courses of cisplatin. Slow release of tissue-bound cisplatin may contribute to chronic nephrotoxicity. Manifestations of toxicity are varied, and can include sodium and water wasting, nephropathy, hyperuricemia, decreased Cl_{cr}, and magnesium wasting.

Recommendations for minimizing nephrotoxicity include:

Prepare cisplatin in saline-containing vehicles

Infuse dose over 24 hours

Vigorous hydration (125-150 mL/hour) before, during, and after cisplatin administration

Simultaneous administration of either mannitol or furosemide

Pretreatment with amifostine

Avoidance of other nephrotoxic agents (aminoglycosides, amphotericin, etc)

Otic: Ototoxicity: Ototoxicity (Occurs in 10% to 30%, and is manifested as high frequency hearing loss. Baseline audiography should be performed. Ototoxicity is especially pronounced in children.)

Hepatic: Elevation of liver enzymes

1% to 10%:

Local: Extravasation (May cause thrombophlebitis and tissue damage if infiltrated; may use sodium thiosulfate as antidote, but consult hospital policy for guidelines.)

Irritant chemotherapy

Drug Interactions

Increased Effect/Toxicity: Cisplatin and ethacrynic acid have resulted in severe ototoxicity in animals. Delayed bleomycin elimination with decreased glomerular filtration rate. When administered as sequential infusions, observational studies indicate a potential for increased toxicity when platinum derivatives (carboplatin, cisplatin) are administered before taxane derivatives (docetaxel, paclitaxel).

Decreased Effect: Sodium thiosulfate theoretically inactivates drug systemically; has been used clinically to reduce systemic toxicity with intraperitoneal administration of cisplatin.

Drug Uptake Half-life, elimination: Initial: 20-30 minutes; Beta: 1 hour; Terminal: ~24 hours; Secondary half-life: 44-73 hours

Pregnancy Risk Factor D

Generic Available Yes

Comments Sodium content (10 mg): 35.4 mg (1.54 mEq)

Citalopram (sye TAL oh pram)

U.S. Brand Names Celexa™

Canadian Brand Names Celexa®

Mexican Brand Names Seropram®

Pharmacologic Category Antidepressant, Selective Serotonin Reuptake Inhibitor

Synonyms Citalopram Hydrobromide; Nitalapram

Use Treatment of dementia, smoking cessation, ethanol abuse, obsessive-compulsive disorder (OCD) in children, diabetic neuropathy

Local Anesthetic/Vasoconstrictor Precautions Although caution should be used in patients taking tricyclic antidepressants, no interactions have been reported with vasoconstrictors and citalopram, a nontricyclic antidepressant which acts to increase serotonin

Effects on Dental Treatment >10%: Xerostomia; premarketing trials reported abnormal taste

Dosage Oral:

Children and Adolescents: OCD (unlabeled use): 10-40 mg/day

Adults: Depression: Initial: 20 mg/day, generally with an increase to 40 mg/day; doses of more than 40 mg are not usually necessary. Should a dose increase be necessary, it should occur in 20 mg increments at intervals of no <1 week. Maximum dose: 60 mg/day; reduce dosage in elderly or those with hepatic impairment.

Mechanism of Action Inhibits CNS neuronal reuptake of serotonin, which enhances serotonergic activity. Activity as an antidepressant has been presumed to be associated with this effect. Has limited or no affinity for histamine, dopamine, acetylcholine (muscarinic), GABA, benzodiazepine, and adrenergic (alpha- and beta-) receptors. Antagonism of these receptors is believed to be associated with sedative, anticholinergic and cardiovascular adverse effects of tricyclic antidepressants.

Other Adverse Effects

>10%:

- Central nervous system: Somnolence, insomnia
- Gastrointestinal: Nausea, xerostomia
- Miscellaneous: Diaphoresis

<10%:

- Central nervous system: Anxiety, anorexia, agitation, yawning
- Dermatologic: Rash, pruritus
- Endocrine & metabolic: Sexual dysfunction
- Gastrointestinal: Diarrhea, dyspepsia, vomiting, abdominal pain, weight gain
- Neuromuscular & skeletal: Tremor, arthralgia, myalgia
- Respiratory: Cough, rhinitis, sinusitis

Drug Interactions CYP2C19 and 3A3/4 enzyme substrate; CYP2D6, 1A2, and 2C19 enzyme inhibitor (weak)

MAO inhibitors: Citalopram should not be used with nonselective MAO inhibitors (phenelzine, isocarboxazid) or other drugs with MAO inhibition (linezolid); fatal reactions have been reported. Wait 5 weeks after stopping citalopram before starting a nonselective MAO inhibitor and 2 weeks after stopping an MAO inhibitor before starting citalopram. Concurrent selegiline has been associated with mania, hypertension, or serotonin syndrome (risk may be reduced relative to nonselective MAO inhibitors).

Combined used of SSRIs and amphetamines, buspirone, meperidine, nefazodone, serotonin agonists (such as sumatriptan), sibutramine, other SSRIs, sympathomimetics, tramadol, and venlafaxine may increase the risk of serotonin syndrome. Risk of hyponatremia may increase with concurrent use of loop diuretics (bumetanide, furosemide, torsemide). Citalopram may increase the hypoprothrombinemic response to warfarin. Inhibitors of CYP3A3/4 or CYP2C19 may increase serum concentration/effects of citalopram.

Combined use of sumatriptan (and other serotonin agonists) may result in toxicity; weakness, hyper-reflexia, and incoordination have been observed with sumatriptan and SSRIs. In addition, concurrent use may theoretically increase the risk of serotonin syndrome; includes sumatriptan, naratriptan, rizatriptan, and zolmitriptan.

Drug Uptake No pharmacokinetic information is available concerning patients with severe renal impairment.

Onset of action: >2 weeks

Half-life, elimination: 24-48 hours; Average: 35 hours (doubles with hepatic impairment; AUC and half-life increases in the elderly)

Time to peak: 1-6 hours; Average: ≤4 hours

Mild to moderate renal impairment may reduce clearance

Pregnancy Risk Factor C

Generic Available No

Comments Problems with SSRI-induced bruxism have been reported and may preclude their use; clinicians attempting to evaluate any patient with bruxism or involuntary muscle movement, who is simultaneously being treated with an SSRI drug, should be aware of the potential association.

Selected Readings Gerber PE and Lynd LD, "Selective Serotonin Reuptake Inhibitor-induced Movement Disorders," *Ann Pharmacother*, 1998, 32(6):692-8.

Citanest® Forte *see* Prilocaine With Epinephrine *on page 993*

Citanest® Plain *see* Prilocaine *on page 992*

Citracal® [OTC] *see* Calcium Citrate *on page 203*

Citric Acid Bladder Mixture (SI trik AS id BLAD dur MIKS chur)

U.S. Brand Names Renacidin®

Pharmacologic Category Urinary Tract Product

Synonyms Citric Acid and d-gluconic Acid Irrigant; Hemiacidrin

Use Preparing solutions for irrigating indwelling urethral catheters; to dissolve or prevent formation of calcifications

Orphan drug: Treatment of renal and bladder calculi of the apatite or struvite type

Local Anesthetic/Vasoconstrictor Precautions No information available to require special precautions

Effects on Dental Treatment No effects or complications reported

Dosage 30-60 mL of 10% (sterile) solution 2-3 times/day by means of a rubber syringe

Pregnancy Risk Factor C

Generic Available Yes

Citrucel® [OTC] *see* Methylcellulose *on page 793*

Cladribine (KLA dri been)

U.S. Brand Names Leustatin™

Canadian Brand Names Leustatin®

Pharmacologic Category Antineoplastic Agent, Antimetabolite

Synonyms 2-CdA; 2-Chlorodeoxyadenosine

Use Hairy cell and chronic lymphocytic leukemias

Local Anesthetic/Vasoconstrictor Precautions No information available to require special precautions

Effects on Dental Treatment No effects or complications reported

Mechanism of Action A purine nucleoside analogue; prodrug which is activated via phosphorylation by deoxycytidine kinase to a 5′-triphosphate derivative. This active form incorporates into susceptible cells and into DNA to result in the breakage of DNA strand and shutdown of DNA synthesis and also results in a depletion of nicotinamide adenine dinucleotide and adenosine triphosphate (ATP). The induction of strand breaks results in a drop in the cofactor nicotinamide adenine dinucleotide and disruption of cell metabolism. ATP is depleted to deprive cells of an important source of energy. Cladribine is able to kill resting as well as dividing cells, unlike most other cytotoxic drugs.

Other Adverse Effects

>10%:

- Allergic: Fever (70%), chills (18%); skin reactions (erythema, itching) at the catheter site (18%)
- Central nervous system: Fatigue (17%), headache (13%)
- Dermatologic: Rash
- Hematologic: Myelosuppression, common, dose-limiting; leukopenia (70%); anemia (37%); thrombocytopenia (12%)
  - Nadir: 5-10 days
  - Recovery: 4-8 weeks

1% to 10%:

- Cardiovascular: Edema, tachycardia
- Central nervous system: Dizziness; pains; chills; malaise; severe infections, possibly related to thrombocytopenia
- Dermatologic: Pruritus, erythema
- Gastrointestinal: Nausea, mild to moderate, usually not seen at doses <0.3 mg/kg/day; constipation; abdominal pain
- Neuromuscular & skeletal: Myalgia, arthralgia, weakness
- Renal: Renal failure at high (>0.3 mg/kg/day) doses
- Miscellaneous: Diaphoresis, delayed herpes zoster infections, tumor lysis syndrome

Drug Uptake Half-life, elimination: Biphasic: Alpha: 25 minutes; Beta: 6.7 hours; Terminal, mean: 5.4 hours

Pregnancy Risk Factor D

Generic Available Yes

Claforan® *see* Cefotaxime *on page 239*

Clarinex® *see* Desloratadine *on page 360*

Clarithromycin (kla RITH roe mye sin)

Related Information

Antibiotic Prophylaxis, Preprocedural Guidelines for Dental Patients *on page 1344*
Gastrointestinal Disorders *on page 1326*
Oral Bacterial Infections *on page 1367*
Respiratory Diseases *on page 1328*

U.S. Brand Names Biaxin®; Biaxin® XL

Canadian Brand Names Biaxin®

Mexican Brand Names Adel®; Klaricid; Mabicrol®

Pharmacologic Category Antibiotic, Macrolide

Synonyms Cla

Use

Dental: Alternate antibiotic in the treatment of common orofacial infections caused by aerobic gram-positive cocci and susceptible anaerobes; alternate antibiotic for the prevention of bacterial endocarditis in patients undergoing dental procedures

Medical:

Adults:

Pharyngitis/tonsillitis due to susceptible *S. pyogenes*

Acute maxillary sinusitis and acute exacerbation of chronic bronchitis due to susceptible *H. influenzae, M. catarrhalis,* or *S. pneumoniae*;

Pneumonia due to susceptible *H. influenzae, Mycoplasma pneumoniae, S. pneumoniae,* or *Chlamydia pneumoniae* (TWAR);

Uncomplicated skin/skin structure infections due to susceptible *S. aureus, S. pyogenes*;

Disseminated mycobacterial infections due to *M. avium* or *M. intracellulare*

Prevention of disseminated mycobacterial infections due to *M. avium* complex (MAC) disease (eg, patients with advanced HIV infection)

Duodenal ulcer disease due to *H. pylori* in regimens with other drugs including amoxicillin and lansoprazole or omeprazole, ranitidine bismuth citrate, bismuth subsalicylate, tetracycline and/or an H_2 antagonist

Alternate antibiotic for prophylaxis of bacterial endocarditis in patients who are allergic to penicillin and undergoing surgical or dental procedures

Children:

Pharyngitis/tonsillitis, acute maxillary sinusitis, uncomplicated skin/skin structure infections, and mycobacterial infections due to the above organisms

Acute otitis media (*H. influenzae, M. catarrhalis,* or *S. pneumoniae*)

Prevention of disseminated mycobacterial infections due to MAC disease in patients with advanced HIV infection

Local Anesthetic/Vasoconstrictor Precautions No information available to require special precautions

Effects on Dental Treatment No effects or complications reported

Dosage Oral:

Children ≥6 months: 15 mg/kg/day divided every 12 hours for 10 days

Mycobacterial infection (prevention and treatment): 7.5 mg/kg twice daily, up to 500 mg twice daily

Prophylaxis of bacterial endocarditis: 15 mg/kg 1 hour before procedure (maximum dose: 500 mg)

Adults:

Usual dose: 250-500 mg every 12 hours **or** 1000 mg (two 500 mg extended release tablets) once daily for for 7-14 days

Upper respiratory tract: 250-500 mg every 12 hours for 10-14 days

Pharyngitis/tonsillitis: 250 mg every 12 hours for 10 days

Acute maxillary sinusitis: 500 mg every 12 hours **or** 1000 mg (two 500 mg extended release tablets) once daily for 14 days

Lower respiratory tract: 250-500 mg every 12 hours for 7-14 days

Acute exacerbation of chronic bronchitis due to:

M. catarrhalis and *S. pneumoniae*: 250 mg every 12 hours **or** 1000 mg (two 500 mg extended release tablets) once daily for 7-14 days

H. influenzae: 500 mg every 12 hours for 7-14 days

Pneumonia due to:

C. pneumoniae, M. pneumoniae, and *S. pneumoniae*: 250 mg every 12 hours for 7-14 days **or** 1000 mg (two 500 mg extended release tablets) once daily for 7 days

H. influenzae: 250 mg every 12 hours for 7 days **or** 1000 mg (two 500 mg extended release tablets) once daily for 7 days

Mycobacterial infection (prevention and treatment): 500 mg twice daily (use with other antimycobacterial drugs, eg, ethambutol, clofazimine, or rifampin)

Prophylaxis of bacterial endocarditis: 500 mg 1 hour prior to procedure

Uncomplicated skin and skin structure: 250 mg every 12 hours for 7-14 days

Helicobacter pylori: Combination regimen with bismuth subsalicylate, tetracycline, clarithromycin, and an H_2-receptor antagonist; or combination of omeprazole and clarithromycin; 250 mg twice daily to 500 mg 3 times/day

Dosing adjustment in renal impairment:

Cl_{cr} <30 mL/minute: Half the normal dose or double the dosing interval

In combination with ranitidine bismuth citrate: If Cl_{cr} <25 mL/minute, clarithromycin use is contraindicated

In combination with ritonavir:

Cl_{cr} 30-60 mL/minute: Decrease clarithromycin dose by 50%

Cl_{cr} <30 mL/minute: Decrease clarithromycin dose by 75%

Dosing adjustment in hepatic impairment: No dosing adjustment is needed in patients with normal renal function

Elderly: Pharmacokinetics are similar to those in younger adults; may have age-related reductions in renal function; monitor and adjust dose if necessary

Mechanism of Action Exerts its antibacterial action by binding to 50S ribosomal subunit resulting in inhibition of protein synthesis; the 14-OH metabolite is twice as active as the parent compound.

Other Adverse Effects

1% to 10%:

Central nervous system: Headache (adults and children 2%)

Dermatologic: Rash (children 3%)

Gastrointestinal: Diarrhea (adults 6%, children 6%); vomiting (children 6%); nausea (adults 3%); abnormal taste (adults 7%); heartburn (adults 2%); abdominal pain (adults 2%, children 3%)

Hepatic: Elevated prothrombin time (1%)

Renal: Elevated BUN (4%)

<1% (Limited to important or life-threatening): Ventricular tachycardia, QT prolongation, torsade de pointes, *Clostridium difficile* colitis, leukopenia, thrombocytopenia; elevated AST, alkaline phosphatase, and bilirubin; elevated serum creatinine, dyspnea, neutropenia, manic behavior, tremor, psychosis, vertigo, hepatitis, jaundice, hepatic dysfunction, hypoglycemia, anaphylaxis, Stevens-Johnson syndrome, toxic epidermal necrolysis, anxiety, hallucinations, anorexia, vomiting, tongue discoloration, glossitis, dizziness, neuromuscular blockade (case reports)

Contraindications Hypersensitivity to clarithromycin, erythromycin, any macrolide antibiotic, or any component of their formulations; use with pimozide, astemizole, cisapride, terfenadine; combination with ranitidine bismuth citrate should not be used in patients with history of acute porphyria or Cl_{cr} <25 mL/minute

Warnings/Precautions Dosage adjustment required with severe renal impairment, decreased dosage or prolonged dosing interval may be appropriate; antibiotic-associated colitis has been reported with use of clarithromycin. Macrolides (including clarithromycin) have been associated with rare QT prolongation and ventricular arrhythmias, including torsade de pointes. Safety and efficacy in children <6 months of age have not been established.

Drug Interactions CYP3A3/4 enzyme substrate; CYP1A2 and 3A3/4 enzyme inhibitor

Alfentanil (and possibly other narcotic analgesics): Serum levels may be increased by clarithromycin; monitor for increased effect.

Antipsychotic agents (particularly mesoridazine and thioridazine): Risk of QT_c prolongation and malignant arrhythmias may be increased.

Astemizole: Concomitant use is contraindicated; may lead to QT_c prolongation or torsade de pointes.

Benzodiazepines (those metabolized by CYP3A3/4, including alprazolam and triazolam): Serum levels may be increased by clarithromycin; somnolence and confusion have been reported.

Bromocriptine: Serum levels may be increased by clarithromycin; monitor for increased effect.

Buspirone: Serum levels may be increased by clarithromycin; monitor.

Calcium channel blockers (felodipine, verapamil, and potentially others metabolized by CYP3A3/4): Serum levels may be increased by clarithromycin; monitor.

Carbamazepine: Serum levels may be increased by clarithromycin; monitor.

Cilostazol: Serum levels may be increased by clarithromycin; monitor.

Cisapride: Serum levels may be increased by clarithromycin; serious arrhythmias have occurred; concurrent use contraindicated.

Clindamycin (and lincomycin): Use with clarithromycin may result in pharmacologic antagonism; manufacturer recommends avoiding this combination.

Clozapine: Serum levels may be increased by clarithromycin; monitor.

Colchicine: serum levels/toxicity may be increased by clarithromycin; monitor.

Cyclosporine: Serum levels may be increased by clarithromycin; monitor serum levels.

Delavirdine: Serum levels may be increased by clarithromycin; monitor.

Digoxin: Serum levels may be increased by clarithromycin; digoxin toxicity and potentially fatal arrhythmias have been reported; monitor digoxin levels.

Disopyramide: Serum levels may be increased by clarithromycin; in addition, QT_c prolongation and risk of malignant arrhythmia may be increased; avoid combination.

Ergot alkaloids: Concurrent use may lead to acute ergot toxicity (severe peripheral vasospasm and dysesthesia).

Fluconazole: Increases clarithromycin levels and AUC by ~25%

(Continued)

Clarithromycin *(Continued)*

HMG-CoA reductase inhibitors (atorvastatin, lovastatin, and simvastatin); Clarithromycin may increase serum levels of "statins" metabolized by CYP3A3/4, increasing the risk of myopathy/rhabdomyolysis (does not include fluvastatin and pravastatin).

Loratadine: Serum levels may be increased by clarithromycin; monitor.

Methylprednisolone: Serum levels may be increased by clarithromycin; monitor.

Neuromuscular-blocking agents: May be potentiated by clarithromycin (case reports).

Phenytoin: Serum levels may be increased by clarithromycin; other evidence suggested phenytoin levels may be decreased in some patients; monitor.

Pimozide: Serum levels may be increased, leading to malignant arrhythmias; concomitant use is contraindicated.

Protease inhibitors (amprenavir, nelfinavir, and ritonavir): May increase serum levels of clarithromycin.

QT_c-prolonging agents: Concomitant use may increase the risk of malignant arrhythmias.

Quinidine: Serum levels may be increased by clarithromycin; in addition, the risk of QT_c prolongation and malignant arrhythmias may be increased during concurrent use.

Quinolone antibiotics (sparfloxacin, gatifloxacin, or moxifloxacin): Concurrent use may increase the risk of malignant arrhythmias.

Rifabutin: Serum levels may be increased by clarithromycin; monitor.

Sildenafil: Serum levels may be increased by clarithromycin; monitor.

Tacrolimus: Serum levels may be increased by clarithromycin; monitor serum concentration.

Terfenadine: Serum levels may be increased by clarithromycin, may lead to QT_c prolongation and malignant arrhythmias, including torsade de pointes; concomitant use is contraindicated.

Theophylline: Serum levels may be increased by clarithromycin; monitor.

Valproic acid (and derivatives): Serum levels may be increased by clarithromycin; monitor.

Vinblastine (and vincristine): Serum levels may be increased by clarithromycin.

Warfarin: Effects may be potentiated; monitor INR closely and adjust warfarin dose as needed or choose another antibiotic

Zafirlukast: Serum levels may be decreased by clarithromycin; monitor.

Zidovudine: Peak levels (but not AUC) of zidovudine may be increased; other studies suggest levels may be decreased.

Zopiclone: Serum levels may be increased by clarithromycin; monitor.

Dietary/Ethanol/Herb Considerations

Ethanol: Use with caution; may increase CNS depression.

Administer with food or milk to reduce GI upset; extended release tablets should be taken with food; food or milk delays absorption but total absorption unaffected. Buttermilk, boiled milk, or yogurt may reduce diarrhea.

Herb/Nutraceutical: Avoid St John's wort; may decrease serum concentration.

Drug Uptake

Absorption: Rapid; highly stable in the presence of gastric acid (unlike erythromycin); food delays but does not affect extent of absorption

Half-life, elimination: 3-4 hours with a 250 mg dose; 5-7 hours with a 500 mg dose

Time to peak: Oral: 2-4 hours

Pregnancy Risk Factor C

Breast-feeding Considerations Erythromycins may be taken while breast-feeding.

Dosage Forms GRAN, oral suspension: 125 mg/5 mL (50 mL, 100 mL); 187.5 mg/5 mL (100 mL); 250 mg/5 mL (50 mL, 100 mL). **TAB, film coated:** 250 mg, 500 mg. **TAB, film coated, extended release:** 500 mg

Generic Available No

Comments *Helicobacter pylori* induced gastric ulcers: Combination regimen with bismuth subsalicylate, tetracycline, clarithromycin, and an H_2-receptor antagonist; or combination of omeprazole and clarithromycin. Adult dosage: Oral: 250 mg twice daily to 500 mg 3 times/day.

Selected Readings

Amsden GW, "Erythromycin, Clarithromycin, and Azithromycin: Are the Differences Real?" *Clin Ther*, 1996, 18(1):56-72.

Dajani AS, Taubert KA, Wilson W, et al, "Prevention of Bacterial Endocarditis. Recommendations by the American Heart Association," *JAMA* 1997, 277(22):1794-801.

Dajani AS, Taubert KA, Wilson W, et al, "Prevention of Bacterial Endocarditis: Recommendations by the American Heart Association," *J Am Dent Assoc* 1997, 128(8):1142-51.

"Pimozide (Orap) Contraindicated With Clarithromycin (Biaxin®) and Other Macrolide Antibiotics," *FDA Medical Bulletin*, October 1996, 26 (3).

Wynn RL, "New Erythromycins," *Gen Dent*, 1996, 44(4):304-7.

Wynn RL, Bergman SA, Meiller TF, et al, "Antibiotics in Treating Oral-Facial Infections of Odontogenic Origin: An Update", *Gen Dent*, 2001, 49(3):238-40, 242, 244 passim.

Claritin® *see* Loratadine *on page 728*

Claritin-D® 12-Hour *see* Loratadine and Pseudoephedrine *on page 729*

Claritin-D® 24-Hour *see* Loratadine and Pseudoephedrine *on page 729*

Claritin® RediTabs® *see* Loratadine *on page 728*
Clear Eyes® [OTC] *see* Naphazoline *on page 847*
Clear Eyes® ACR [OTC] *see* Naphazoline *on page 847*
Clear Tussin® 30 *see* Guaifenesin and Dextromethorphan *on page 569*

Clemastine (KLEM as teen)

U.S. Brand Names Antihist-1® [OTC]; Tavist®; Tavist®-1 [OTC]

Mexican Brand Names Tavist®

Pharmacologic Category Antihistamine

Synonyms Clemastine Fumarate

Use Perennial and seasonal allergic rhinitis and other allergic symptoms including urticaria

Local Anesthetic/Vasoconstrictor Precautions No information available to require special precautions

Effects on Dental Treatment No effects or complications reported

Dosage Oral:

Children: <12 years: 0.4-1 mg twice daily

Children >12 years and Adults: 1.34 mg twice daily to 2.68 mg 3 times/day; do not exceed 8.04 mg/day; lower doses should be considered in patients >60 years

Mechanism of Action Competes with histamine for H_1-receptor sites on effector cells in the GI tract, blood vessels, and respiratory tract

Other Adverse Effects

>10%:

Central nervous system: Slight to moderate drowsiness

Respiratory: Thickening of bronchial secretions

1% to 10%:

Central nervous system: Headache, fatigue, nervousness, increased dizziness

Gastrointestinal: Appetite increase, weight gain, nausea, diarrhea, abdominal pain, xerostomia

Neuromuscular & skeletal: Arthralgia

Respiratory: Pharyngitis

Drug Interactions

Increased Effect/Toxicity: CNS depressants may increase the degree of sedation and respiratory depression with antihistamines. May increase the absorption of digoxin. Central and/or peripheral anticholinergic syndrome can occur when administered with amantadine, rimantadine, narcotic analgesics, phenothiazines and other antipsychotics (especially with high anticholinergic activity), tricyclic antidepressants, quinidine, disopyramide, procainamide, and antihistamines.

Decreased Effect: May increase gastric degradation of levodopa and decrease the amount of levodopa absorbed by delaying gastric emptying. Therapeutic effects of cholinergic agents (tacrine, donepezil) and neuroleptics may be antagonized.

Drug Uptake

Onset of action: Peak effect: Therapeutic: 5-7 hours

Absorption: Almost complete

Duration: 8-16 hours

Pregnancy Risk Factor B

Generic Available Yes

Cleocin® *see* Clindamycin *on page 300*
Cleocin 3® *see* Clindamycin *on page 300*
Cleocin HCl® *see* Clindamycin *on page 300*
Cleocin T® *see* Clindamycin *on page 300*

Clidinium and Chlordiazepoxide

(kli DI nee um & klor dye az e POKS ide)

U.S. Brand Names Librax®

Canadian Brand Names Apo®-Chlorax; Librax®

Pharmacologic Category Antispasmodic Agent, Gastrointestinal; Benzodiazepine

Synonyms Chlordiazepoxide and Clidinium

Use Adjunct treatment of peptic ulcer, treatment of irritable bowel syndrome

Local Anesthetic/Vasoconstrictor Precautions No information available to require special precautions

Effects on Dental Treatment No effects or complications reported

Dosage Oral: 1-2 capsules 3-4 times/day, before meals or food and at bedtime

Other Adverse Effects 1% to 10%:

Central nervous system: Drowsiness ataxia, confusion, anticholinergic side effects

Gastrointestinal: Dry mouth, constipation, nausea

Drug Interactions Additive effects may result from concomitant benzodiazepine and/or anticholinergic therapy.

Pregnancy Risk Factor D

Generic Available Yes

Comments After extended therapy, abrupt discontinuation should be avoided and a gradual dose tapering schedule followed

Climara® *see* Estradiol *on page 457*
Clinac™ BPO *see* Benzoyl Peroxide *on page 153*
Clinda-Derm® *see* Clindamycin *on page 300*

Clindamycin (klin da MYE sin)

Related Information

Animal and Human Bites Guidelines *on page 1416*
Antibiotic Prophylaxis, Preprocedural Guidelines for Dental Patients *on page 1344*
Cardiovascular Diseases *on page 1308*
Oral Bacterial Infections *on page 1367*
Periodontal Diseases *on page 1375*

U.S. Brand Names Cleocin®; Cleocin 3®; Cleocin HCl®; Cleocin T®; Clinda-Derm®; Clindets® Pledgets; C/T/S®

Canadian Brand Names Alti-Clindamycin; Dalacin® C

Mexican Brand Names Clindazyn®; Cutaclin®; Dalacin C®; Dalacin T®; Dalacin V®; Galecin®; Klyndaken

Pharmacologic Category Antibiotic, Miscellaneous

Synonyms Clindamycin Hydrochloride; Clindamycin Phosphate

Use

Dental: Alternate antibiotic, when amoxicillin cannot be used, for the standard regimen for prevention of bacterial endocarditis in patients undergoing dental procedures; alternate antibiotic in the treatment of common oral-facial infections caused by aerobic gram-positive cocci and susceptible anaerobes; alternate antibiotic for prophylaxis for dental patients with total joint replacement

Medical: Treatment against aerobic and anaerobic streptococci (except enterococci), most staphylococci, *Bacteroides* sp and *Actinomyces*; used topically in treatment of severe acne, vaginally for *Gardnerella vaginalis*, alternate treatment for toxoplasmosis

Local Anesthetic/Vasoconstrictor Precautions No information available to require special precautions

Effects on Dental Treatment No effects or complications reported

Dosage Avoid in neonates (contains benzyl alcohol)

Infants and Children:
- Oral: 8-20 mg/kg/day as hydrochloride; 8-25 mg/kg/day as palmitate in 3-4 divided doses; minimum dose of palmitate: 37.5 mg 3 times/day
- I.M., I.V.:
  - <1 month: 15-20 mg/kg/day
  - >1 month: 20-40 mg/kg/day in 3-4 divided doses

Children: Prevention of bacterial endocarditis: Oral: 20 mg/kg 1 hour before procedure with no follow-up dose needed; for patients allergic to penicillin and unable to take oral medications: 20 mg/kg I.V. within 30 minutes before procedure

Children and Adults: Topical: Apply a thin film twice daily

Adults:
- Oral: 150-450 mg/dose every 6-8 hours; maximum dose: 1.8 g/day
- Prevention of bacterial endocarditis in patients unable to take amoxicillin: Oral: 600 mg 1 hour before procedure with no follow-up dose needed; for patients allergic to penicillin and unable to take oral medications: 600 mg I.V. within 30 minutes before procedure
- I.M., I.V.: 1.2-1.8 g/day in 2-4 divided doses; maximum dose: 4.8 g/day
- Pelvic inflammatory disease: I.V.: 900 mg every 8 hours with gentamicin 2 mg/kg, then 1.5 mg/kg every 8 hours; continue after discharge with doxycycline 100 mg twice daily to complete 14 days of total therapy
- *Pneumocystis carinii* pneumonia:
  - Oral: 300-450 mg 4 times/day with primaquine
  - I.M., I.V.: 1200-2400 mg/day with pyrimethamine
  - I.V.: 600 mg 4 times/day with primaquine
- Bacterial vaginosis:
  - Oral: 300 mg twice daily for 7 days
  - Intravaginal:
    - Suppositories: Insert one ovule (100 mg clindamycin) daily into vagina at bedtime for 3 days
    - Cream: One full applicator inserted intravaginally once daily before bedtime for 3 or 7 consecutive days

Dosing adjustment in hepatic impairment: Adjustment recommended in patients with severe hepatic disease

Mechanism of Action Reversibly binds to 50S ribosomal subunits preventing peptide bond formation thus inhibiting bacterial protein synthesis; bacteriostatic or bactericidal depending on drug concentration, infection site, and organism

Other Adverse Effects

Systemic:

>10%: Gastrointestinal: Diarrhea, abdominal pain

1% to 10%:
- Cardiovascular: Hypotension
- Dermatologic: Urticaria, rashes, Stevens-Johnson syndrome

Gastrointestinal: Pseudomembranous colitis, nausea, vomiting
Local: Thrombophlebitis, sterile abscess at I.M. injection site
Miscellaneous: Fungal overgrowth, hypersensitivity
<1% (Limited to important or life-threatening symptoms): Renal dysfunction (rare), neutropenia, granulocytopenia, thrombocytopenia, polyarthritis

Topical:
>10%: Dermatologic: Dryness, scaliness, or peeling of skin (lotion)
1% to 10%:
Dermatologic: Contact dermatitis, irritation
Gastrointestinal: Diarrhea (mild), abdominal pain
Miscellaneous: Hypersensitivity
<1% (Limited to important or life-threatening symptoms): Pseudomembranous colitis, nausea, vomiting, diarrhea (severe)

Vaginal:
>10%: Genitourinary: Vaginitis or vulvovaginal pruritus (from *Candida albicans*), painful intercourse
1% to 10%:
Central nervous system: Dizziness, headache
Gastrointestinal: Diarrhea, nausea, vomiting, stomach cramps

Contraindications Hypersensitivity to clindamycin or any component of the formulation; previous pseudomembranous colitis; hepatic impairment

Warnings/Precautions Dosage adjustment may be necessary in patients with severe hepatic dysfunction; can cause severe and possibly fatal colitis; use with caution in patients with a history of pseudomembranous colitis; discontinue drug if significant diarrhea, abdominal cramps, or passage of blood and mucus occurs

Drug Interactions CYP3A3/4 enzyme substrate
Increased duration of neuromuscular blockade from tubocurarine, pancuronium

Dietary/Ethanol/Herb Considerations
Food: Oral form may be taken with food but may delay peak concentration.
Herb/Nutraceutical: Avoid St John's wort; may decrease serum concentration.

Drug Uptake
Absorption: Oral: 90% rapidly from GI tract; Topical: ~10%
Half-life, elimination: Neonates: Premature: 8.7 hours; Full-term: 3.6 hours; Adults: 1.6-5.3 hours, average: 2-3 hours
Time to peak: Oral: ≤1 hour; I.M.: 1-3 hours

Pregnancy Risk Factor B

Breast-feeding Considerations May be taken while breast-feeding

Dosage Forms CAP, as hydrochloride: 75 mg, 150 mg, 300 mg. **CRM, vaginal:** 2% (40 g). **GEL, as phosphate:** 1% [10 mg/g] (7.5 g, 30 g). **GRAN, oral solution, as palmitate:** 75 mg/5 mL (100 mL). **INF, as phosphate** [in D_5W]: 300 mg (50 mL); 600 mg (50 mL). **INJ, as phosphate:** 150 mg/mL (2 mL, 4 mL, 6 mL, 50 mL, 60 mL). **LOTION:** 1% [10 mg/mL] (60 mL) **PLEDGET:** 1%. **SOLN, topical, as phosphate:** 1% [10 mg/mL] (30 mL, 60 mL, 480 mL). **SUPP, vaginal:** 2.5 g

Generic Available Yes

Comments Clindamycin has not been shown to interfere with oral contraceptive activity; however, it reduces GI microflora, thus, oral contraceptive users should be advised to use additional methods of birth control. About 1% of clindamycin users develop pseudomembranous colitis. Symptoms may occur 2-9 days after initiation of therapy; however, it has never occurred with the 1-dose regimen of clindamycin used to prevent bacterial endocarditis.

Selected Readings

"Advisory Statement. Antibiotic Prophylaxis for Dental Patients With Total Joint Replacements. American Dental Association; American Academy of Orthopedic Surgeons," *J Am Dent Assoc*, 1997, 128(7):1004-8.

Dajani AS, Taubert KA, Wilson W, et al, "Prevention of Bacterial Endocarditis. Recommendations by the American Heart Association," *JAMA* 1997, 277(22):1794-801.

Dajani AS, Taubert KA, Wilson W, et al, "Prevention of Bacterial Endocarditis: Recommendations by the American Heart Association," *J Am Dent Assoc* 1997, 128(8):1142-51.

Wynn RL, "Clindamycin: An Often Forgotten but Important Antibiotic," *AGD Impact*, 1994, 22:10.

Wynn RL and Bergman SA, "Antibiotics and Their Use in the Treatment of Orofacial Infections, Part I," *Gen Dent*, 1994, 42(5):398, 400, 402.

Wynn RL and Bergman SA, "Antibiotics and Their Use in the Treatment of Orofacial Infections, Part II," *Gen Dent*, 1994, 42(6):498-502.

Wynn RL, Bergman SA, Meiller TF, et al, "Antibiotics in Treating Oral-Facial Infections of Odontogenic Origin: An Update", *Gen Dent*, 2001, 49(3):238-40, 242, 244 passim.

Clindamycin and Benzoyl Peroxide

(klin da MYE sin & BEN zoe il peer OKS ide)

U.S. Brand Names BenzaClin™

Pharmacologic Category Topical Skin Product; Topical Skin Product, Acne

Synonyms Benzoyl Peroxide and Clindamycin

Use Topical treatment of acne vulgaris

Local Anesthetic/Vasoconstrictor Precautions No information available to require special precautions

Effects on Dental Treatment No effects or complications reported

Dosage Topical: Children ≥12 years and Adults: Acne: Apply twice daily (morning and evening) to affected areas after skin has been cleansed and dried

(Continued)

Clindamycin and Benzoyl Peroxide *(Continued)*

Mechanism of Action Clindamycin and benzoyl peroxide have activity against *Propionibacterium acnes in vitro.* This organism has been associated with acne vulgaris. Benzoyl peroxide releases free-radical oxygen which oxidizes bacterial proteins in the sebaceous follicles decreasing the number of anaerobic bacteria and decreasing irritating-type free fatty acids. Clindamycin reversibly binds to 50S ribosomal subunits preventing peptide bond formation thus inhibiting bacterial protein synthesis; bacteriostatic or bactericidal depending on drug concentration, infection site, and organism.

Other Adverse Effects

>10%: Dermatologic: Dry skin (12%)

1% to 10%: Dermatologic: Pruritus (2%), peeling (2%), erythema (1%), sunburn (1%)

Contraindications Hypersensitivity to benzoyl peroxide, lincomycin, clindamycin, or any component of their formulation; history of regional enteritis, ulcerative colitis, or antibiotic-associated colitis; concurrent use of erythromycin and clindamycin; breast-feeding

Drug Interactions

Increased Effect/Toxicity: Tretinoin may cause increased adverse events with concurrent use.

Decreased Effect: Erythromycin may antagonize clindamycin's effects.

Drug Uptake See Clindamycin *on page 300* and Benzoyl Peroxide *on page 153*

Pregnancy Risk Factor C

Generic Available No

Comments Skin should be clean and dry before applying; avoid applying to inside nose, mouth, eyes, and mucous membranes

Clindets® Pledgets *see* Clindamycin *on page 300*
Clinoril® *see* Sulindac *on page 1125*

Clioquinol (klye oh KWIN ole)

U.S. Brand Names Vioform® [OTC]

Mexican Brand Names Vioformo®

Pharmacologic Category Antifungal Agent, Topical

Synonyms Iodochlorhydroxyquin

Use Used topically in the treatment of tinea pedis, tinea cruris, and skin infections caused by dermatophytic fungi (ring worm)

Local Anesthetic/Vasoconstrictor Precautions No information available to require special precautions

Effects on Dental Treatment No effects or complications reported

Dosage Children and Adults: Topical: Apply 2-3 times/day; do not use for longer than 7 days

Mechanism of Action Chelates bacterial surface and trace metals needed for bacterial growth

Other Adverse Effects 1% to 10%:

Dermatologic: Skin irritation, rash

Neuromuscular & skeletal: Peripheral neuropathy

Ocular: Optic atrophy

Drug Uptake

Absorption: Occlusive dressing: ≤40% absorbed during a 12-hour period; enhanced under diapers

Half-life, elimination: 11-14 hours

Pregnancy Risk Factor C

Generic Available No

Clobazam *Not Available in U.S.* (KLOE ba zam)

Canadian Brand Names Alti-Clobazam; Frisium®; Novo-Clobazam; PMS-Clobazam

Pharmacologic Category Benzodiazepine

Use Adjunctive treatment of epilepsy

Unlabeled/Investigational: Monotherapy for epilepsy or intermittent seizures

Local Anesthetic/Vasoconstrictor Precautions No information available to require special precautions

Effects on Dental Treatment No effects or complications reported

Dosage Oral:

Children:

<2 years: Initial 0.5-1 mg/kg/day

2-16 years: Initial: 5 mg/day; may be increased (no more frequently than every 5 days) to a maximum of 40 mg/day

Adults: Initial: 5-15 mg/day; dosage may be gradually adjusted (based on tolerance and seizure control) to a maximum of 80 mg/day

Note: Daily doses of up to 30 mg may be taken as a single dose at bedtime; higher doses should be divided.

Dosage adjustment in hepatic impairment: Avoid use in severe hepatic impairment. Use lower doses in mild-moderate impairment and monitor closely.

Mechanism of Action Clobazam is a 1,5 benzodiazepine which binds to stereospecific benzodiazepine receptors on the postsynaptic GABA neuron at several sites within the CNS, including the limbic system, reticular formation. Enhancement of the inhibitory effect of GABA on neuronal excitability results by increased neuronal membrane permeability to chloride ions. This shift in chloride ions results in hyperpolarization (a less excitable state) and stabilization.

Other Adverse Effects

Central nervous system: Drowsiness (17%), ataxia (4%), dizziness (2%), behavior disorder (1%), confusion, depression, lethargy, slurred speech, tremor, anterograde amnesia. In addition, paradoxical reactions (including excitation, agitation, hallucinations, and psychosis) are known to occur with benzodiazepines.

Dermatologic: Rash, pruritus, urticaria

Gastrointestinal: Weight gain (2%); Dose-related: Xerostomia, constipation, nausea

Hematologic: Decreased WBCs and other hematologic abnormalities have been rarely associated with benzodiazepines

Neuromuscular & skeletal: Muscle spasm

Ocular: Blurred vision (1%)

Drug Interactions Possible CYP3A3/4 enzyme substrate (not defined)

Increased Effect/Toxicity: Benzodiazepines potentiate the CNS depressant effects of narcotic analgesics, barbiturates, phenothiazines, ethanol, antihistamines, MAO inhibitors, sedative-hypnotics, and cyclic antidepressants. Serum levels and/or effects of benzodiazepines may be increased by inhibitors of CYP3A3/4, including amiodarone, amprenavir, cimetidine, clarithromycin, erythromycin, delavirdine, diltiazem, dirithromycin, disulfiram, fluoxetine, fluvoxamine, grapefruit juice, indinavir, itraconazole, ketoconazole, nefazodone, nevirapine, propoxyphene, quinupristin-dalfopristin, ritonavir, saquinavir, verapamil, zafirlukast, zileuton.

Decreased Effect: Carbamazepine, rifampin, rifabutin may enhance the metabolism of benzodiazepines and decrease therapeutic effect.

Drug Uptake

Absorption: Rapid

Half-life, elimination: 18 hours; N-desmethyl (active): 42 hours

Time to peak: 15 minutes to 4 hours

Pregnancy Risk Factor Not assigned; similar agents rated D. Contraindicated in 1st trimester (per manufacturer).

Generic Available Yes

Comments Clobazam is a 1,5 benzodiazepine; other benzodiazepines are typically 1,4 substituted.

Clobetasol (kloe BAY ta sol)

Related Information

Oral Nonviral Soft Tissue Ulcerations or Erosions *on page 1384*

U.S. Brand Names Cormax®; Olux™; Temovate®

Canadian Brand Names Alti-Clobetasol; Dermovate®; Gen-Clobetasol; Novo-Clobetasol®

Mexican Brand Names Dermatovate®

Pharmacologic Category Corticosteroid, Topical

Synonyms Clobetasol Propionate

Use Short-term relief of inflammation of moderate to severe corticosteroid-responsive dermatosis (very high potency topical corticosteroid)

Local Anesthetic/Vasoconstrictor Precautions No information available to require special precautions

Effects on Dental Treatment No effects or complications reported

Dosage

Children: Use in children <12 years of age is **not** recommended

Adults: Topical:

Apply twice daily for up to 2 weeks with no more than 50 g/week. Therapy should be discontinued when control is achieved; if no improvement is seen, reassessment of diagnosis may be necessary.

Foam: Scalp: Apply to affected scalp twice daily for up to 2 weeks (≤50 g/week)

Mechanism of Action Stimulates the synthesis of enzymes needed to decrease inflammation, suppress mitotic activity, and cause vasoconstriction

Other Adverse Effects 1% to 10%:

Dermatologic: Erythema, papular rashes

Local: Itching, burning, dryness, irritation

Drug Uptake Absorption: Percutaneous absorption variable and dependent upon many factors including vehicle used, integrity of epidermis, dose, and use of occlusive dressings

Pregnancy Risk Factor C

Generic Available Yes

Clocort® Maximum Strength *see* Hydrocortisone *on page 608*

Clocortolone (kloe KOR toe lone)

U.S. Brand Names Cloderm®

Canadian Brand Names Cloderm®

Pharmacologic Category Corticosteroid, Topical

Synonyms Clocortolone Pivalate

Use Inflammation of corticosteroid-responsive dermatoses (medium potency topical corticosteroid)

Local Anesthetic/Vasoconstrictor Precautions No information available to require special precautions

Effects on Dental Treatment No effects or complications reported

Dosage Adults: Apply sparingly and gently; rub into affected area from 1-4 times/day
Therapy should be discontinued when control is achieved; if no improvement is seen, reassessment of diagnosis may be necessary.

Mechanism of Action Stimulates the synthesis of enzymes needed to decrease inflammation, suppress mitotic activity, and cause vasoconstriction

Other Adverse Effects 1% to 10%:
Dermatologic: Itching, erythema
Local: Burning, dryness, irritation, papular rashes

Drug Uptake Absorption: Percutaneous absorption is variable and dependent upon many factors including vehicle used, integrity of epidermis, dose, and use of occlusive dressings; small amounts enter circulatory system via skin

Pregnancy Risk Factor C

Generic Available No

Cloderm® *see* Clocortolone *on page 304*

Clofazimine (kloe FA zi meen)

U.S. Brand Names Lamprene®

Canadian Brand Names Lamprene®

Pharmacologic Category Leprostatic Agent

Synonyms Clofazimine Palmitate

Use Orphan drug: Treatment of dapsone-resistant leprosy; multibacillary dapsone-sensitive leprosy; erythema nodosum leprosum; *Mycobacterium avium-intracellulare* (MAI) infections

Local Anesthetic/Vasoconstrictor Precautions No information available to require special precautions

Effects on Dental Treatment No effects or complications reported

Dosage Oral:
Children: Leprosy: 1 mg/kg/day every 24 hours in combination with dapsone and rifampin
Adults:
Dapsone-resistant leprosy: 100 mg/day in combination with one or more antileprosy drugs for 3 years; then alone 100 mg/day
Dapsone-sensitive multibacillary leprosy: 100 mg/day in combination with two or more antileprosy drugs for at least 2 years and continue until negative skin smears are obtained, then institute single drug therapy with appropriate agent
Erythema nodosum leprosum: 100-200 mg/day for up to 3 months or longer then taper dose to 100 mg/day when possible
Pyoderma gangrenosum: 300-400 mg/day for up to 12 months

Mechanism of Action Binds preferentially to mycobacterial DNA to inhibit mycobacterial growth; also has some anti-inflammatory activity through an unknown mechanism

Other Adverse Effects
>10%:
Dermatologic: Dry skin
Gastrointestinal: Abdominal pain, nausea, vomiting, diarrhea
Miscellaneous: Pink to brownish-black discoloration of the skin and conjunctiva
1% to 10%:
Dermatologic: Rash, pruritus
Endocrine & metabolic: Elevated blood sugar
Gastrointestinal: Fecal discoloration
Genitourinary: Discoloration of urine
Ocular: Irritation of the eyes
Miscellaneous: Discoloration of sputum, sweat

Drug Interactions Decreased effect with dapsone (unconfirmed)

Drug Uptake
Absorption: Oral: 45% to 70% absorbed slowly
Half-life, elimination: Terminal: 8 days; Tissue: 70 days
Time to peak: 1-6 hours with chronic therapy

Pregnancy Risk Factor C

Generic Available No

Clofibrate (kloe FYE brate)

U.S. Brand Names Atromid-S®

Pharmacologic Category Antilipemic Agent, Fibric Acid

Use Adjunct to dietary therapy in the management of hyperlipidemias associated with high triglyceride levels (types III, IV, V); primarily lowers triglycerides and very low density lipoprotein

Local Anesthetic/Vasoconstrictor Precautions No information available to require special precautions

Effects on Dental Treatment No effects or complications reported

Dosage Adults: Oral: 500 mg 4 times/day; some patients may respond to lower doses

Mechanism of Action Mechanism is unclear but thought to reduce cholesterol synthesis and triglyceride hepatic-vascular transference

Other Adverse Effects

Frequency not defined.

Common: Gastrointestinal: Nausea, diarrhea

Less common:

Central nervous system: Headache, dizziness, fatigue

Gastrointestinal: Vomiting, loose stools, heartburn, flatulence, abdominal distress, epigastric pain

Neuromuscular & skeletal: Muscle cramping, aching, weakness, myalgia

Frequency unknown:

Central nervous system: Fever

Cardiovascular: Chest pain, cardiac arrhythmias

Dermatologic: Rash, urticaria, pruritus, alopecia, toxic epidermal necrolysis, erythema multiforme, Stevens-Johnson syndrome; dry, brittle hair

Endocrine & metabolic: Polyphagia, gynecomastia, hyperkalemia

Gastrointestinal: Stomatitis, gallstones, pancreatitis, gastritis, peptic ulcer, weight gain

Genitourinary: Impotence, decreased libido

Hematologic: Leukopenia, anemia, eosinophilia, agranulocytosis, thrombocytopenic purpura

Hepatic: Increased liver function test, hepatomegaly, jaundice

Local: Thrombophlebitis

Neuromuscular & skeletal: Myalgia, myopathy, myositis, arthralgia, rhabdomyolysis, increased creatinine phosphokinase (CPK), rheumatoid arthritis, tremor

Ocular: Photophobic

Renal: Dysuria, hematuria, proteinuria, renal toxicity (allergic), rhabdomyolysis-induced renal failure

Miscellaneous: Flu-like syndrome, increased diaphoresis, systemic lupus erythematosus

Drug Interactions CYP3A3/4 enzyme substrate

Increased Effect/Toxicity: Clofibrate may increase effects of warfarin, insulin, and sulfonylureas. Clofibrate's levels may be increased with probenecid. HMG-CoA reductase inhibitors (atorvastatin, cerivastatin, fluvastatin, lovastatin, pravastatin, simvastatin) may increase the risk of myopathy and rhabdomyolysis. The manufacturer warns against the concomitant use. However, combination therapy with statins has been used in some patients with resistant hyperlipidemias (with great caution).

Decreased Effect: Rifampin (and potentially other inducers of CYP3A4) may reduce blood levels of clofibrate.

Drug Uptake

Absorption: Complete; intestinal transformation is required to activate the drug

Half-life, elimination: 6-24 hours (increases significantly with renal impairment); Anuria: 110 hours

Time to peak: 3-6 hours

Pregnancy Risk Factor C

Generic Available Yes

Clomid® *see* ClomiPHENE *on page 305*

ClomiPHENE (KLOE mi feen)

U.S. Brand Names Clomid®; Milophene®; Serophene®

Canadian Brand Names Clomid®; Milophene®; Serophene®

Mexican Brand Names Omifin

Pharmacologic Category Ovulation Stimulator

Synonyms Clomiphene Citrate

Use Treatment of ovulatory failure in patients desiring pregnancy

Unlabeled/Investigational: Male infertility

Local Anesthetic/Vasoconstrictor Precautions No information available to require special precautions

Effects on Dental Treatment No effects or complications reported

Dosage Adults: Oral:

(Continued)

ClomiPHENE *(Continued)*

Males (infertility): 25 mg/day for 25 days with 5 days rest, or 100 mg every Monday, Wednesday, Friday

Females (ovulatory failure): Oral: 50 mg/day for 5 days (first course); start the regimen on or about the fifth day of cycle; if ovulation occurs do not increase dosage; if not, increase next course to 100 mg/day for 5 days. Three courses of therapy are an adequate therapeutic trial. Further treatment is not recommended in patients who do not exhibit ovulation.

Mechanism of Action Induces ovulation by stimulating the release of pituitary gonadotropins

Other Adverse Effects

>10%: Endocrine & metabolic: Hot flashes, ovarian enlargement

1% to 10%:

- Cardiovascular: Thromboembolism
- Central nervous system: Mental depression, headache
- Endocrine & metabolic: Breast enlargement (males), breast discomfort (females), abnormal menstrual flow, ovarian cyst formation, ovarian enlargement, premenstrual syndrome, uterine fibroid enlargement
- Gastrointestinal: Distention, bloating, nausea, vomiting
- Hepatic: Hepatotoxicity
- Ocular: Blurring of vision, diplopia, floaters, after-images, phosphenes, photophobia, scotoma

Drug Interactions Decreased Effect: Decreased response with danazol; clomiphene decreases estradiol response

Drug Uptake Half-life, elimination: 5-7 days

Pregnancy Risk Factor X

Generic Available Yes

ClomiPRAMINE (kloe MI pra meen)

U.S. Brand Names Anafranil®

Canadian Brand Names Anafranil®; Apo®-Clomipramine; Gen-Clomipramine; Novo-Clopramine

Mexican Brand Names Anafranil®

Pharmacologic Category Antidepressant, Tricyclic (Tertiary Amine)

Synonyms Clomipramine Hydrochloride

Use Treatment of obsessive-compulsive disorder (OCD)

Unlabeled/Investigational: Depression, panic attacks, chronic pain

Local Anesthetic/Vasoconstrictor Precautions Use with caution; epinephrine, norepinephrine and levonordefrin have been shown to have an increased pressor response in combination with TCAs

Effects on Dental Treatment

>10%: Xerostomia

Long-term treatment with TCAs such as clomipramine increases the risk of caries by reducing salivation and salivary buffer capacity.

Dosage Oral: Initial:

Children: 25 mg/day and gradually increase, as tolerated, to a maximum of 3 mg/kg/day or 200 mg/day, whichever is smaller

Adults: 25 mg/day and gradually increase, as tolerated, to 100 mg/day the first 2 weeks, may then be increased to a total of 250 mg/day maximum

Mechanism of Action Clomipramine appears to affect serotonin uptake while its active metabolite, desmethylclomipramine, affects norepinephrine uptake

Other Adverse Effects

>10%:

- Central nervous system: Dizziness, drowsiness, headache, insomnia, nervousness
- Endocrine & metabolic: Libido changes
- Gastrointestinal: Xerostomia, constipation, increased appetite, nausea, weight gain, dyspepsia, anorexia, abdominal pain
- Neuromuscular & skeletal: Fatigue, tremor, myoclonus
- Miscellaneous: Increased diaphoresis

1% to 10%:

- Cardiovascular: Hypotension, palpitations, tachycardia
- Central nervous system: Confusion, hypertonia, sleep disorder, yawning, speech disorder, abnormal dreaming, paresthesia, memory impairment, anxiety, twitching, impaired coordination, agitation, migraine, depersonalization, emotional lability, flushing, fever
- Dermatologic: Rash, pruritus, dermatitis
- Gastrointestinal: Diarrhea, vomiting
- Genitourinary: Difficult urination
- Ocular: Blurred vision, eye pain

Drug Interactions CYP1A2, 2C19, 2D6, and 3A3/4 enzyme substrate; CYP2D6 enzyme inhibitor

Increased Effect/Toxicity: Clomipramine increases the effects of amphetamines, anticholinergics, lithium, other CNS depressants (sedatives, hypnotics), chlorpropamide, tolazamide, phenothiazines, and warfarin. When used with MAO inhibitors or other serotonergic drugs, serotonin syndrome may occur. Clomipramine serum concentration/toxicity may be increased by SSRIs (to varying degrees), cimetidine, indinavir, methylphenidate, ritonavir, quinidine, diltiazem, phenothiazines, and verapamil. Pressor response to I.V. epinephrine, norepinephrine, and phenylephrine may be enhanced in patients receiving TCAs (**Note:** Effect is unlikely with epinephrine or levonordefrin dosages typically administered as infiltration in combination with local anesthetics). Combined use of beta-agonists or drugs which prolong QT_c (including quinidine, procainamide, disopyramide, cisapride, sparfloxacin, gatifloxacin, moxifloxacin) with TCAs may predispose patients to cardiac arrhythmias.

Decreased Effect: Clomipramine serum concentration/effect may be decreased by carbamazepine, cholestyramine, colestipol, phenobarbital, and rifampin. Clomipramine inhibits the antihypertensive response to bethanidine, clonidine, debrisoquin, guanadrel, guanethidine, guanabenz, and guanfacine.

Drug Uptake

Onset of action: Usually >2 weeks to therapeutic effect

Absorption: Oral: Rapid

Half-life, elimination: 20-30 hours

Pregnancy Risk Factor C

Generic Available Yes

Selected Readings

Boakes AJ, Laurence DR, Teoh PC, et al, "Interactions Between Sympathomimetic Amines and Antidepressant Agents in Man," *Br Med J*, 1973, 1(849):311-5.

Friedlander AH, Mahler ME, "Major Depressive Disorder. Psychopathology, Medical Management, and Dental Implications," *J Am Dent Assoc*, 201, 132(5):629-38.

Ganzberg S, "Psychoactive Drugs," *ADA Guide to Dental Therapeutics*, 2nd ed, Chicago, IL: ADA Publishing, a Division of ADA Business Enterprises, Inc, 2000, 376-405.

Jastak JT and Yagiela JA, "Vasoconstrictors and Local Anesthesia: A Review and Rationale for Use," *J Am Dent Assoc*, 1983, 107(4):623-30.

Mitchell JR, "Guanethidine and Related Agents. III Antagonism by Drugs Which Inhibit the Norepinephrine Pump in Man," *J Clin Invest*, 1970, 49(8):1596-604.

Rundegren J, van Dijken J, Mörnstad H, et al, "Oral Conditions in Patients Receiving Long-Term Treatment With Cyclic Antidepressant Drugs," *Swed Dent J*, 1985, 9(2):55-64.

Yagiela JA, "Adverse Drug Interactions in Dental Practice: Interactions Associated With Vasoconstrictors. Part V of a Series," *J Am Dent Assoc*, 1999, 130(5):701-9.

Clonazepam (kloe NA ze pam)

U.S. Brand Names Klonopin™

Canadian Brand Names Alti-Clonazepam; Apo®-Clonazepam; Clonapam; Gen-Clonazepam; Klonopin™; Novo-Clonazepam; Nu-Clonazepam; PMS-Clonazepam; Rho-Clonazepam; Rivotril®

Mexican Brand Names Kenoket; Rivotril®

Pharmacologic Category Benzodiazepine

Use Alone or as an adjunct in the treatment of petit mal variant (Lennox-Gastaut), akinetic, and myoclonic seizures; petit mal (absence) seizures unresponsive to succimides; panic disorder with or without agoraphobia

Unlabeled/Investigational: Restless legs syndrome, neuralgia, multifocal tic disorder, parkinsonian dysarthria, acute manic episodes, and adjunct therapy for schizophrenia

Local Anesthetic/Vasoconstrictor Precautions No information available to require special precautions

Effects on Dental Treatment No effects or complications reported

Restrictions C-IV

Dosage Oral:

Children <10 years or 30 kg: Seizure disorders:

Initial daily dose: 0.01-0.03 mg/kg/day (maximum: 0.05 mg/kg/day) given in 2-3 divided doses; increase by no more than 0.5 mg every third day until seizures are controlled or adverse effects seen

Usual maintenance dose: 0.1-0.2 mg/kg/day divided 3 times/day, not to exceed 0.2 mg/kg/day

Adults:

Seizure disorders:

Initial daily dose not to exceed 1.5 mg given in 3 divided doses; may increase by 0.5-1 mg every third day until seizures are controlled or adverse effects seen (maximum: 20 mg/day)

Usual maintenance dose: 0.05-0.2 mg/kg; do not exceed 20 mg/day

Panic disorder: 0.25 mg twice daily; increase in increments of 0.125-0.25 mg twice daily every 3 days; target dose: 1 mg/day (maximum: 4 mg/day)

Elderly: Initiate with low doses and observe closely

Hemodialysis: Supplemental dose is not necessary

Mechanism of Action The exact mechanism is unknown, but believed to be related to its ability to enhance the activity of GABA; suppresses the spike-and-wave discharge in absence seizures by depressing nerve transmission in the motor cortex

(Continued)

Clonazepam *(Continued)*

Other Adverse Effects

>10%: Central nervous system: Drowsiness

1% to 10%:

Central nervous system: Dizziness, abnormal coordination, ataxia, dysarthria, depression, memory disturbance, fatigue

Dermatologic: Dermatitis, allergic reactions

Endocrine & metabolic: Decreased libido

Gastrointestinal: Anorexia, constipation, diarrhea, xerostomia

Respiratory: Upper respiratory tract infection, sinusitis, rhinitis, coughing

Drug Interactions CYP3A3/4 enzyme substrate

Increased Effect/Toxicity: Combined use of clonazepam and valproic acid has been associated with absence seizures. Clonazepam potentiates the CNS depressant effects of narcotic analgesics, barbiturates, phenothiazines, antihistamines, MAO inhibitors, sedative-hypnotics, and cyclic antidepressants. Serum levels and/or toxicity of clonazepam may be increased by inhibitors of CYP3A3/4, including cimetidine, ciprofloxacin, clarithromycin, clozapine, delavirdine, diltiazem, disulfiram, digoxin, erythromycin, ethanol, fluconazole, fluoxetine, fluvoxamine, indinavir, isoniazid, itraconazole, ketoconazole, loxapine, metoprolol, metronidazole, miconazole, nefazodone, nevirapine, quinupristin/dalfopristin, omeprazole, phenytoin, rifabutin, rifampin, ritonavir, saquinavir, troleandomycin, verapamil, zafirlukast, and zileuton.

Decreased Effect: The combined use of clonazepam and valproic acid has been associated with absence seizures. Carbamazepine, rifampin, rifabutin may enhance the metabolism of clonazepam and decrease its therapeutic effect.

Drug Uptake

Onset of action: 20-60 minutes

Duration: Infants and young children: 6-8 hours; Adults: ≤12 hours

Absorption: Oral: Well absorbed

Half-life, elimination: Children: 22-33 hours; Adults: 19-50 hours

Time to peak: Oral: 1-3 hours; Steady-state: 5-7 days

Pregnancy Risk Factor D

Generic Available Yes

Clonidine (KLOE ni deen)

Related Information

Cardiovascular Diseases *on page 1308*

U.S. Brand Names Catapres®; Catapres-TTS®-1; Catapres-TTS®-2; Catapres-TTS®-3; Duraclon™

Canadian Brand Names Apo®-Clonidine; Carapres®; Dixarit®; Novo-Clonidine®; Nu-Clonidine®

Mexican Brand Names Catapresan-100®

Pharmacologic Category Alpha$_2$-Adrenergic Agonist

Synonyms Clonidine Hydrochloride

Use Management of mild to moderate hypertension; either used alone or in combination with other antihypertensives

Orphan drug: Duraclon™: For continuous epidural administration as adjunctive therapy with intraspinal opiates for treatment of cancer pain in patients tolerant to or unresponsive to intraspinal opiates

Unlabeled/Investigational: Heroin or nicotine withdrawal; severe pain; dysmenorrhea; vasomotor symptoms associated with menopause; ethanol dependence; prophylaxis of migraines; glaucoma; diabetes-associated diarrhea; impulse control disorder, attention-deficit/hyperactivity disorder (ADHD), clozapine-induced sialorrhea

Local Anesthetic/Vasoconstrictor Precautions No information available to require special precautions

Effects on Dental Treatment >10%: Significant xerostomia

Dosage

Children:

Oral:

Hypertension: Initial: 5-10 mcg/kg/day in divided doses every 8-12 hours; increase gradually at 5- to 7-day intervals to 25 mcg/kg/day in divided doses every 6 hours; maximum: 0.9 mg/day

Clonidine tolerance test (test of growth hormone release from pituitary): 0.15 mg/m^2 or 4 mcg/kg as single dose

ADHD (unlabeled use): Initial: 0.05 mg/day; increase every 3-7 days by 0.05 mg/day to 3-5 mcg/kg/day given in divided doses 3-4 times/day (maximum dose: 0.3-0.4 mg/day)

Epidural infusion: Pain management: Reserved for patients with severe intractable pain, unresponsive to other analgesics or epidural or spinal opiates: Initial: 0.5 mcg/kg/hour; adjust with caution, based on clinical effect

Adults:

Oral:

Acute hypertension (urgency): Initial 0.1-0.2 mg; may be followed by additional doses of 0.1 mg every hour, if necessary, to a maximum total dose of 0.6 mg

Hypertension: Initial dose: 0.1 mg twice daily, usual maintenance dose: 0.2-1.2 mg/day in 2-4 divided doses; maximum recommended dose: 2.4 mg/day

Nicotine withdrawal symptoms: 0.1 mg twice daily to maximum of 0.4 mg/day for 3-4 weeks

Transdermal: Hypertension: Apply once every 7 days; for initial therapy start with 0.1 mg and increase by 0.1 mg at 1- to 2-week intervals; dosages >0.6 mg do not improve efficacy

Epidural infusion: Pain management: Starting dose: 30 mcg/hour; titrate as required for relief of pain or presence of side effects; minimal experience with doses >40 mcg/hour; should be considered an adjunct to intraspinal opiate therapy

Elderly: Initial: 0.1 mg once daily at bedtime, increase gradually as needed

Dosing adjustment in renal impairment: Cl_{cr} <10 mL/minute: Administer 50% to 75% of normal dose initially

Dialysis: Not dialyzable (0% to 5%) via hemo- or peritoneal dialysis; supplemental dose not necessary

Mechanism of Action Stimulates alpha$_2$-adrenoceptors in the brain stem, thus activating an inhibitory neuron, resulting in reduced sympathetic outflow from the CNS, producing a decrease in peripheral resistance, renal vascular resistance, heart rate, and BP; epidural clonidine may produce pain relief at spinal presynaptic and postjunctional alpha$_2$-adrenoceptors by preventing pain signal transmission; pain relief occurs only for the body regions innervated by the spinal segments where analgesic concentrations of clonidine exist

Other Adverse Effects Incidence of adverse events is not always reported.

>10%:

Central nervous system: Drowsiness (35% oral, 12% transdermal), dizziness (16% oral, 2% transdermal)

Dermatologic: Transient localized skin reactions characterized by pruritus, and erythema (15% to 50% transdermal)

Gastrointestinal: Dry mouth (40% oral, 25% transdermal)

1% to 10%:

Cardiovascular: Orthostatic hypotension (3% oral)

Central nervous system: Headache (1% oral, 5% transdermal), sedation (3% transdermal), fatigue (6% transdermal), lethargy (3% transdermal), insomnia (2% transdermal), nervousness (3% oral, 1% transdermal), mental depression (1% oral)

Dermatologic: Rash (1% oral), allergic contact sensitivity (5% transdermal), localized vesiculation (7%), hyperpigmentation (5% at application site), edema (3%), excoriation (3%), burning (3%), throbbing, blanching (1%), papules (1%), and generalized macular rash (1%) has occurred in patients receiving transdermal clonidine.

Endocrine & metabolic: Sodium and water retention, sexual dysfunction (3% oral, 2% transdermal), impotence (3% oral, 2% transdermal), weakness (10% transdermal)

Gastrointestinal: Nausea (5% oral, 1% transdermal), vomiting (5% oral), anorexia and malaise (1% oral), constipation (10% oral, 1% transdermal), dry throat (2% transdermal), taste disturbance (1% transdermal), weight gain (1% oral)

Genitourinary: Nocturia (1% oral)

Hepatic: Liver function test (mild abnormalities, 1% oral)

Miscellaneous: Withdrawal syndrome (1% oral)

Drug Interactions

Increased Effect/Toxicity: Concurrent use with antipsychotics (especially low potency), narcotic analgesics, or nitroprusside may produce additive hypotensive effects. Clonidine may decrease the symptoms of hypoglycemia with oral hypoglycemic agents or insulin. Alcohol, barbiturates, and other CNS depressants may have additive CNS effects when combined with clonidine. Epidural clonidine may prolong the sensory and motor blockade of local anesthetics. Clonidine may increase cyclosporine (and perhaps tacrolimus) serum concentration. Beta-blockers may potentiate bradycardia in patients receiving clonidine and may increase the rebound hypertension of withdrawal. Tricyclic antidepressants may also enhance the hypertensive response associated with abrupt clonidine withdrawal.

Decreased Effect: Tricyclic antidepressants (TCAs) antagonize the hypotensive effects of clonidine.

Drug Uptake

Onset of action: Oral: 0.5-1 hour; T_{max}: 2-4 hours

Duration: 6-10 hours

Half-life, elimination: Adults: 6-20 hours; Renal impairment: 18-41 hours

Time to peak: 2-4 hours

Pregnancy Risk Factor C

Generic Available Yes: Tablet

Clonidine and Chlorthalidone (KLOE ni deen & klor THAL i done)

U.S. Brand Names Combipres®

Pharmacologic Category Antihypertensive Agent Combination

Synonyms Chlorthalidone and Clonidine

Use Management of mild to moderate hypertension

Local Anesthetic/Vasoconstrictor Precautions No information available to require special precautions

Effects on Dental Treatment No effects or complications reported

Dosage Oral: 1 tablet 1-2 times/day

Drug Uptake See Clonidine *on page 308* and Chlorthalidone *on page 277*

Pregnancy Risk Factor C

Generic Available Yes

Clopidogrel (kloh PID oh grel)

Related Information

Cardiovascular Diseases *on page 1308*

U.S. Brand Names Plavix®

Canadian Brand Names Plavix™

Pharmacologic Category Antiplatelet Agent

Synonyms Clopidogrel Bisulfate

Use Reduce atherosclerotic events (myocardial infarction, stroke, vascular deaths) in patients with atherosclerosis documented by recent myocardial infarction, recent stroke, or established peripheral arterial disease; prevention of thrombotic complications after coronary stenting

In aspirin-allergic patients, prevention of coronary artery bypass graft closure (saphenous vein)

Local Anesthetic/Vasoconstrictor Precautions No information available to require special precautions

Effects on Dental Treatment If a patient is to undergo elective surgery and an antiplatelet effect is not desired, clopidogrel should be discontinued 7 days prior to surgery.

Dosage Oral:

Adults: 75 mg once daily

Prevention of coronary artery bypass graft closure (saphenous vein): Aspirin-allergic patients (unlabeled use): Loading dose: 300 mg 6 hours following procedure; maintenance: 50-100 mg/day

Mechanism of Action Blocks the ADP receptors, which prevent fibrinogen binding at that site and thereby reduce the possibility of platelet adhesion and aggregation

Other Adverse Effects As with all drugs which may affect hemostasis, bleeding is associated with clopidogrel. Hemorrhage may occur at virtually any site. Risk is dependent on multiple variables, including the concurrent use of multiple agents which alter hemostasis and patient susceptibility.

>10%: Gastrointestinal: The overall incidence of gastrointestinal events (including abdominal pain, vomiting, dyspepsia, gastritis and constipation) has been documented to be 27% compared to 30% in patients receiving aspirin.

3% to 10%:

- Cardiovascular: Chest pain (8%), edema (4%), hypertension (4%)
- Central nervous system: Headache (3% to 8%), dizziness (2% to 6%), depression (4%), fatigue (3%), general pain (6%)
- Dermatologic: Rash (4%), pruritus (3%)
- Endocrine & metabolic: Hypercholesterolemia (4%)
- Gastrointestinal: Abdominal pain (2% to 6%), dyspepsia (2% to 5%), diarrhea (2% to 5%), nausea (3%)
- Genitourinary: Urinary tract infection (3%)
- Hematologic: Purpura (5%), epistaxis (3%)
- Hepatic: Liver function test abnormalities (<3%; discontinued in 0.11%)
- Neuromuscular & skeletal: Arthralgia (6%), back pain (6%)
- Respiratory: Dyspnea (5%), rhinitis (4%), bronchitis (4%), coughing (3%), upper respiratory infections (9%)
- Miscellaneous: Flu-like syndrome (8%)

1% to 3%: Anemia, anxiety, arthritis, atrial fibrillation, cardiac failure, cataract, conjunctivitis, constipation, cystitis, eczema, fever, GI hemorrhage, gout, hematoma, hyperuricemia, insomnia, leg cramps, neuralgia, palpitation, paresthesia, syncope, vertigo, vomiting, weakness

Contraindications Hypersensitivity to clopidogrel or any component of the formulation; active pathological bleeding such as PUD or intracranial hemorrhage; coagulation disorders

Warnings/Precautions Use with caution in patients who may be at risk of increased bleeding. Consider discontinuing 7 days before elective surgery. Use caution in mixing with other antiplatelet drugs. Use with caution in patients with severe liver disease (experience is limited). Cases of thrombotic thrombocytopenic purpura (usually occurring within the first 2 weeks of therapy) have been reported.

Drug Interactions CYP2C9 enzyme inhibitor (high concentrations - *in vitro*)

Anticoagulants or other antiplatelet agents may increase the risk of bleeding. Use with heparin in acute coronary syndrome is clinically accepted.

Aspirin: Clopidogrel may increase the antiplatelet effect of aspirin; bleeding time is not prolonged relative to clopidogrel alone. Concurrent use is accepted in clinical practice (particularly in ACS treatment).

CYP2C9 substrates (including amiodarone, cisapride, cyclosporine, diltiazem, fluvastatin, irbesartan, losartan, oral hypoglycemics, paclitaxel, phenytoin, quinidine, sildenafil, tamoxifen, torsemide, verapamil, and many NSAIDs) may have increased blood levels during concomitant therapy with clopidogrel. However, these combinations have not been investigated. Use caution during concomitant administration.

Drotrecogin alfa may increase the risk of bleeding.

NSAIDs: Concurrent use with clopidogrel may increase GI effects, including GI blood loss. NSAID use was excluded in ACS trial (CURE).

Thrombolytics may increase the risk of bleeding.

Warfarin metabolism may be decreased due to clopidogrel inhibition of CYP2C9. Hypoprothrombinemic effects may be increased; monitor INR carefully during initiation or withdrawal.

Drug Uptake

Onset of action: Inhibition of platelet aggregation detected: 2 hours after 400 mg administered; after second day of treatment with 50-100 mg/day

Peak effect: 50-100 mg/day: Bleeding time: 5-6 days; Platelet function: 3-7 days

Half-life, elimination: ~8 hours (carboxylic acid derivative)

Time to peak: Oral: ~1 hour

Pregnancy Risk Factor B

Generic Available No

Selected Readings Wynn RL, "Clopidogrel (Plavix): Dental Considerations of an Antiplatelet Drug," *Gen Dent*, 2001, 49(6):564-8.

Clorazepate (klor AZ e pate)

U.S. Brand Names Tranxene®

Canadian Brand Names Apo®-Clorazepate; Novo-Clopate®; Tranxene®

Mexican Brand Names Tranxene®

Pharmacologic Category Benzodiazepine

Synonyms Clorazepate Dipotassium

Use Treatment of generalized anxiety and panic disorders; management of alcohol withdrawal; adjunct anticonvulsant in management of partial seizures

Local Anesthetic/Vasoconstrictor Precautions No information available to require special precautions

Effects on Dental Treatment Many patients will experience drowsiness and xerostomia while taking clorazepate which will disappear with cessation of drug therapy. Orthostatic hypotension is possible. It is suggested that narcotic analgesics not be given for pain control to patients taking clorazepate due to enhanced sedation.

Restrictions C-IV

Dosage Oral:

Children 9-12 years: Anticonvulsant: Initial: 3.75-7.5 mg/dose twice daily; increase dose by 3.75 mg at weekly intervals, not to exceed 60 mg/day in 2-3 divided doses

Children >12 years and Adults: Anticonvulsant: Initial: Up to 7.5 mg/dose 2-3 times/day; increase dose by 7.5 mg at weekly intervals; not to exceed 90 mg/day

Adults:

Anxiety: 7.5-15 mg 2-4 times/day, or given as single dose of 11.25 or 22.5 mg at bedtime

Alcohol withdrawal: Initial: 30 mg, then 15 mg 2-4 times/day on first day; maximum daily dose: 90 mg; gradually decrease dose over subsequent days

Mechanism of Action Binds to stereospecific benzodiazepine receptors on the postsynaptic GABA (gamma aminobutyric acid) neuron at several sites within the CNS, including the limbic system, reticular formation. Enhancement of the inhibitory effect of GABA on neuronal excitability results by increased neuronal membrane permeability to chloride ions. This shift in chloride ions results in hyperpolarization (a less excitable state) and stabilization.

Other Adverse Effects Frequency not defined:

Cardiovascular: Hypotension

Central nervous system: Drowsiness, fatigue, ataxia, lightheadedness, memory impairment, insomnia, anxiety, headache, depression, slurred speech, confusion, nervousness, dizziness, irritability

Dermatologic: Rash

Endocrine & metabolic: Decreased libido

Gastrointestinal: Xerostomia, constipation, diarrhea, decreased salivation, nausea, vomiting, increased or decreased appetite

Neuromuscular & skeletal: Dysarthria, tremor

Ocular: Blurred vision, diplopia

Drug Interactions CYP3A3/4 enzyme substrate

Increased Effect/Toxicity: Clorazepate potentiates the CNS depressant effects of narcotic analgesics, barbiturates, phenothiazines, antihistamines, MAO inhibitors,

(Continued)

Clorazepate *(Continued)*

sedative-hypnotics, and cyclic antidepressants. Serum concentrations/toxicity of clorazepate may be increased by inhibitors of CYP3A3/4, including amprenavir, cimetidine, ciprofloxacin, clarithromycin, clozapine, diltiazem, disulfiram, digoxin, erythromycin, ethanol, fluconazole, fluoxetine, fluvoxamine, isoniazid, itraconazole, ketoconazole, labetalol, levodopa, loxapine, metoprolol, metronidazole, miconazole, nefazodone, nelfinavir, omeprazole, phenytoin, rifabutin, rifampin, ritonavir, troleandomycin, valproic acid, and verapamil.

Decreased Effect: Carbamazepine, rifampin, rifabutin may enhance the metabolism of clorazepate and decrease its therapeutic effect.

Drug Uptake

Onset of action: ~1 hour

Duration: Variable, 8-24 hours

Half-life, elimination: Adults: Desmethyldiazepam: 48-96 hours; Oxazepam: 6-8 hours

Time to peak: Oral: ≤1 hour

Pregnancy Risk Factor D

Generic Available Yes

Clorpactin® WCS-90 [OTC] *see* Oxychlorosene *on page 901*

Clotrimazole (kloe TRIM a zole)

Related Information

Oral Fungal Infections *on page 1377*

U.S. Brand Names Cruex® [OTC]; Gyne-Lotrimin® [OTC]; Gyne-Lotrimin® 3 [OTC]; Gynix® [OTC]; Lotrimin®; Lotrimin® AF [OTC]; Mycelex®; Mycelex®-3; Mycelex®-7 [OTC]; Mycelex® Twin Pack [OTC]; Trivagizole 3™

Canadian Brand Names Canesten® Topical, Canesten® Vaginal; Clotrimaderm; Scheinpharm™ Clotrimazole; Trivagizole-3®

Mexican Brand Names Candimon®; Lotrimin®

Pharmacologic Category Antifungal Agent, Oral Nonabsorbed; Antifungal Agent, Topical; Antifungal Agent, Vaginal

Use

Dental: Treatment of susceptible fungal infections, including oropharyngeal candidiasis; limited data suggests that the use of clotrimazole troches may be effective for prophylaxis against oropharyngeal candidiasis in neutropenic patients

Medical: Treatment of susceptible fungal infections including dermatophytoses, superficial mycoses, and cutaneous candidiasis, as well as vulvovaginal candidiasis

Local Anesthetic/Vasoconstrictor Precautions No information available to require special precautions

Effects on Dental Treatment No effects or complications reported

Dosage

Children >3 years and Adults:

Oral:

Prophylaxis: 10 mg troche dissolved 3 times/day for the duration of chemotherapy or until steroids are reduced to maintenance levels

Treatment: 10 mg troche dissolved slowly 5 times/day for 14 consecutive days

Topical (cream, lotion, solution): Apply twice daily; if no improvement occurs after 4 weeks of therapy, re-evaluate diagnosis

Children >12 years and Adults:

Vaginal:

Cream:

1%: Insert 1 applicatorful vaginal cream daily (preferably at bedtime) for 7 consecutive days

2%: Insert 1 applicatorful vaginal cream daily (preferably at bedtime) for 3 consecutive days

Tablet: Insert 100 mg/day for 7 days or 500 mg single dose

Topical (cream, lotion, solution): Apply to affected area twice daily (morning and evening) for 7 consecutive days

Mechanism of Action Binds to phospholipids in the fungal cell membrane altering cell wall permeability resulting in loss of essential intracellular elements

Other Adverse Effects

Oral:

>10%: Hepatic: Abnormal LFTs

1% to 10%:

Gastrointestinal: Nausea and vomiting may occur in patients on clotrimazole troches

Local: Mild burning, irritation, stinging to skin or vaginal area

Vaginal:

1% to 10%: Genitourinary: Vulvar/vaginal burning

<1% (Limited to important or life-threatening): Vulvar itching, soreness, edema, or discharge; polyuria; burning or itching of penis of sexual partner

Contraindications Hypersensitivity to clotrimazole or any component of the formulation

Warnings/Precautions Clotrimazole should not be used for treatment of systemic fungal infection; safety and effectiveness of troches in children <3 years of age have not been established; when using topical formulation, avoid contact with eyes.

Drug Interactions CYP3A3/4 and 3A5-7 enzyme inhibitor

Drug Uptake

Absorption: Oral (troche): Poor; Topical (cream, lotion): Negligible through intact skin

Duration: ≤3 hours

Time to peak:

Oral topical: Salivary levels occur within 3 hours following 30 minutes of dissolution time

Vaginal cream: High vaginal levels: 8-24 hours

Vaginal tablet: High vaginal levels: 1-2 days

Pregnancy Risk Factor B (topical); C (troches)

Dosage Forms COMBO PACK: Vaginal tablet 100 mg (7s) and vaginal cream 1% (7 g); vaginal tablet 200 mg (3s) and vaginal cream 1%; vaginal tablet 500 mg (1s) and vaginal cream 1% (7 g). **CRM** (Lotrimin®, Mycelex®): 1% (15 g, 30 g, 45 g, 90 g). **CRM, vaginal:** 1% (45 g, 90 g); (Mycelex®-3, Trivagizole 3™): 2% (25 g). **LOTION** (Lotrimin®): 1% (30 mL). **SOLN, topical** (Lotrimin®, Mycelex®): 1% (10 mL, 30 mL). **TAB, vaginal:** 100 mg (7s); 500 mg (1s). **TROCHE** (Mycelex®): 10 mg

Generic Available Yes

Cloxacillin (kloks a SIL in)

U.S. Brand Names Cloxapen®

Canadian Brand Names Apo®-Cloxi; Novo-Cloxin®; Nu-Cloxi®

Pharmacologic Category Antibiotic, Penicillin

Synonyms Cloxacillin Sodium

Use Treatment of susceptible bacterial infections, notably penicillinase-producing staphylococci causing respiratory tract, skin and skin structure, bone and joint, urinary tract infections

Local Anesthetic/Vasoconstrictor Precautions No information available to require special precautions

Effects on Dental Treatment Prolonged use of penicillins may lead to development of oral candidiasis.

Dosage Oral:

Children >1 month (<20 kg): 50-100 mg/kg/day in divided doses every 6 hours; up to a maximum of 4 g/day

Children (>20 kg) and Adults: 250-500 mg every 6 hours for at least 7 days

Hemodialysis: Not dialyzable (0% to 5%)

Mechanism of Action Inhibits bacterial cell wall synthesis by binding to one or more of the penicillin-binding proteins (PBPs) which in turn inhibits the final transpeptidation step of peptidoglycan synthesis in bacterial cell walls, thus inhibiting cell wall biosynthesis. Bacteria eventually lyse due to ongoing activity of cell wall autolytic enzymes (autolysins and murein hydrolases) while cell wall assembly is arrested.

Other Adverse Effects

1% to 10%: Gastrointestinal: Nausea, diarrhea, abdominal pain

<1%: Fever, seizures with extremely high doses and/or renal failure, rash (maculopapular to exfoliative), vomiting, pseudomembranous colitis, vaginitis, eosinophilia, leukopenia, neutropenia, thrombocytopenia, agranulocytosis, anemia, hemolytic anemia, prolonged PT, hepatotoxicity, transient elevated LFTs, hematuria, interstitial nephritis, increased BUN/creatinine, serum sickness-like reactions, hypersensitivity

Contraindications Hypersensitivity to cloxacillin, other penicillins, or any component of their formulation

Warnings/Precautions Monitor PT if patient concurrently on warfarin, elimination of drug is slow in renally impaired; use with caution in patients allergic to cephalosporins due to a low incidence of cross-hypersensitivity

Drug Interactions

Oral contraceptive efficacy may be reduced.

Probenecid, disulfiram may increase levels of penicillins (cloxacillin).

Warfarin's effects may be increased

Dietary/Ethanol/Herb Considerations Food: Administer on an empty stomach.

Drug Uptake

Absorption: Oral: ~50%

Half-life, elimination: 0.5-1.5 hours; prolonged with renal impairment and in neonates

Time to peak: 0.5-2 hours

Pregnancy Risk Factor B

Dosage Forms CAP: 250 mg, 500 mg. **POWDER, oral suspension:** 125 mg/5 mL (100 mL, 200 mL)

Generic Available Yes

(Continued)

Cloxacillin *(Continued)*

Comments Although cloxacillin is a penicillin antibiotic indicated for infections caused by penicillinase-secreting staph, amoxicillin with clavulanic acid is considered the drug of choice for these types of orofacial infections

Cloxapen® *see* Cloxacillin *on page 313*

Clozapine (KLOE za peen)

U.S. Brand Names Clozaril®

Canadian Brand Names Clozaril®

Mexican Brand Names Clopsine®; Leponex®

Pharmacologic Category Antipsychotic Agent, Dibenzodiazepine

Use Treatment of refractory schizophrenia

Unlabeled/Investigational: Schizoaffective disorder, bipolar disorder, childhood psychosis

Local Anesthetic/Vasoconstrictor Precautions Most pharmacology textbooks state that in presence of phenothiazines, systemic doses of epinephrine paradoxically decrease the blood pressure. This is the so called "epinephrine reversal" phenomenon. This has never been observed when epinephrine is given by infiltration as part of the anesthesia procedure.

Effects on Dental Treatment Many patients may experience orthostatic hypotension with clozapine; precautions should be taken; do not use atropine-like drugs for xerostomia in patients taking clozapine due to significant potentiation.

Dosage Oral: If dosing is interrupted for >48 hours, therapy must be reinitiated at 12.5-25 mg/day; may be increased more rapidly than with initial titration:

Children and Adolescents: Childhood psychosis (unlabeled use): Initial: 25 mg/day; increase to a target dose of 25-400 mg/day

Adults: Schizophrenia: Initial: 25 mg once or twice daily; increased, as tolerated to a target dose of 300-450 mg/day after 2-4 weeks, but may require doses as high as 600-900 mg/day

Elderly: Schizophrenia: Dose selection and titration should be cautious

In the event of planned termination of clozapine, gradual reduction in dose over a 1- to 2-week period is recommended. If conditions warrant abrupt discontinuation (leukopenia), monitor patient for psychosis and cholinergic rebound (headache, nausea, vomiting, diarrhea).

Mechanism of Action A weak dopamine$_1$ and dopamine$_2$ receptor blocker; blocks the serotonin$_2$, alpha-adrenergic, and histamine H_1 CNS receptors

Other Adverse Effects

>10%:
- Cardiovascular: Tachycardia
- Central nervous system: Drowsiness, dizziness
- Gastrointestinal: Constipation, weight gain, diarrhea, sialorrhea
- Genitourinary: Urinary incontinence

1% to 10%:
- Cardiovascular: EKG changes, hypertension, hypotension, syncope
- Central nervous system: Akathisia, seizures, headache, nightmares, akinesia, confusion, insomnia, fatigue, myoclonic jerks
- Dermatologic: Rash
- Gastrointestinal: Abdominal discomfort, heartburn, xerostomia, nausea, vomiting
- Hematologic: Eosinophilia, leukopenia
- Neuromuscular & skeletal: Tremor
- Miscellaneous: Diaphoresis (increased), fever

Drug Interactions CYP1A2, 2C (minor), 2D6 (minor), 2E1, 3A3/4 enzyme substrate

Anticholinergics: Clozapine has potent anticholinergic effects. May potentiate the effects of anticholinergic agents.

Antihypertensives: Clozapine may potentiate the hypotensive effects of antihypertensive agents.

Benzodiazepines: In combination with clozapine may produce respiratory depression and hypotension, especially during the first few weeks of therapy; monitor for altered response

Carbamazepine: A case of neuroleptic malignant syndrome has been reported in combination with clozapine; in addition, carbamazepine may alter clozapine levels (see enzyme inducers); monitor

CYP enzyme inducers: Metabolism of clozapine may be increased, decreasing its therapeutic effect; potential inducers include phenobarbital, phenytoin, carbamazepine, rifampin, rifabutin, and cigarette smoking (nicotine)

CYP1A2 inhibitors: Serum level and/or toxicity of clozapine may be increased; inhibitors include caffeine, cimetidine, ciprofloxacin, fluvoxamine, isoniazid, ritonavir, and zileuton; monitor for altered effects; a decrease in clozapine dosage may be required

CYP2D6 inhibitors: Serum levels and/or toxicity of clozapine may be increased; inhibitors include amiodarone, cimetidine, delavirdine, fluoxetine, paroxetine, propafenone, quinidine, and ritonavir; monitor for increased effect/toxicity

CYP2E1 inhibitors: Serum level and/or toxicity of clozapine may be increased; inhibitors include disulfiram and ritonavir; monitor for altered effects; a decrease in clozapine dosage may be required

CYP3A3/4 inhibitors: Serum level and/or toxicity of clozapine may be increased; inhibitors include amiodarone, cimetidine, clarithromycin, erythromycin, delavirdine, diltiazem, dirithromycin, disulfiram, fluoxetine, fluvoxamine, grapefruit juice, indinavir, itraconazole, ketoconazole, metronidazole, nefazodone, nevirapine, propoxyphene, quinupristin-dalfopristin, ritonavir, saquinavir, verapamil, zafirlukast, zileuton; monitor for altered effects; a decrease in clozapine dosage may be required

Epinephrine: Clozapine may reverse the pressor effect of epinephrine; use should be avoided in the treatment of drug-induced hypotension.

Metoclopramide: May increase extrapyramidal symptoms (EPS) or risk.

Risperidone: Effects and/or toxicity may be increased when combined with clozapine; monitor

Valproic acid: May cause reductions in clozapine concentrations; monitor for altered response

Drug Uptake

Half-life, elimination: 12 hours (range: 4-66 hours)

Time to peak: 2.5 hours

Pregnancy Risk Factor B

Generic Available Yes

Clozaril® *see* Clozapine *on page 314*

Coal Tar (KOLE tar)

U.S. Brand Names Denorex® [OTC]; DHS® Tar [OTC]; Duplex® T [OTC]; Estar® [OTC]; Fototar® [OTC]; Neutrogena® T/Derm; Oxipor® VHC [OTC]; Pentrax® [OTC]; Polytar® [OTC]; psoriGel® [OTC]; Tegrin® Dandruff Shampoo [OTC]; T/Gel® [OTC]; Zetar® [OTC]

Canadian Brand Names Balnetar®; Estar®; SpectroTar Skin Wash™; Targel®; Zetar®

Pharmacologic Category Topical Skin Product

Synonyms Crude Coal Tar; LCD; Pix Carbonis

Use Topically for controlling dandruff, seborrheic dermatitis, or psoriasis

Local Anesthetic/Vasoconstrictor Precautions No information available to require special precautions

Effects on Dental Treatment No effects or complications reported

Dosage Children and Adults: Topical:

Bath: Add appropriate amount to bath water, for adults usually 60-90 mL of a 5% to 20% solution or 15-25 mL of 30% lotion; soak 5-20 minutes, then pat dry; use once daily to 3 days

Shampoo: Rub shampoo onto wet hair and scalp, rinse thoroughly; repeat; leave on 5 minutes; rinse thoroughly; apply twice weekly for the first 2 weeks then once weekly or more often if needed

Skin: Apply to the affected area 1-4 times/day; decrease frequency to 2-3 times/week once condition has been controlled

Scalp psoriasis: Tar oil bath or coal tar solution may be painted sparingly to the lesions 3-12 hours before each shampoo

Psoriasis of the body, arms, legs: Apply at bedtime; if thick scales are present, use product with salicylic acid and apply several times during the day

Other Adverse Effects 1% to 10%: Dermatologic: Dermatitis, folliculitis

Pregnancy Risk Factor C

Generic Available Yes

Comments Avoid exposure to sunlight for 24 hours after use; may stain clothing and skin

Coal Tar and Salicylic Acid (KOLE tar & sal i SIL ik AS id)

U.S. Brand Names Neutrogena® T/Sal [OTC]; P & S Plus® [OTC]; X-Seb™ T [OTC]

Canadian Brand Names Sebcur/T®

Pharmacologic Category Topical Skin Product

Synonyms Salicylic Acid and Coal Tar

Use Seborrheal dermatitis; dandruff

Local Anesthetic/Vasoconstrictor Precautions No information available to require special precautions

Effects on Dental Treatment No effects or complications reported

Dosage Use as shampoo twice weekly

Drug Uptake See Coal Tar *on page 315* and Salicylic Acid *on page 1072*

Pregnancy Risk Factor C

Generic Available Yes

Coal Tar, Lanolin, and Mineral Oil

(KOLE tar, LAN oh lin, & MIN er al oyl)

U.S. Brand Names Balnetar® [OTC]

Canadian Brand Names Balnetar®

(Continued)

Coal Tar, Lanolin, and Mineral Oil *(Continued)*

Pharmacologic Category Topical Skin Product

Synonyms Coal Tar, Mineral Oil, and Lanolin; Lanolin, Coal Tar, and Mineral Oil; Lanolin, Mineral Oil, and Coal Tar; Mineral Oil, Coal Tar, and Lanolin; Mineral Oil, Lanolin, and Coal Tar

Use Psoriasis; seborrheic dermatitis; atopic dermatitis; eczematoid dermatitis

Local Anesthetic/Vasoconstrictor Precautions No information available to require special precautions

Effects on Dental Treatment No effects or complications reported

Dosage Add to bath water, soak for 5-20 minutes then pat dry

Generic Available No

Cocaine (koe KANE)

Pharmacologic Category Local Anesthetic

Synonyms Cocaine Hydrochloride

Use Topical anesthesia (ester derivative) for mucous membranes

Local Anesthetic/Vasoconstrictor Precautions Although plain local anesthetic is not contraindicated, vasoconstrictor is absolutely contraindicated in any patient under the influence of or within 2 hours of cocaine use

Effects on Dental Treatment See Comments

Restrictions C-II

Dosage Dosage depends on the area to be anesthetized, tissue vascularity, technique of anesthesia, and individual patient tolerance; use the lowest dose necessary to produce adequate anesthesia should be used, not to exceed 1 mg/kg. Use reduced dosages for children, elderly, or debilitated patients.

Topical application (ear, nose, throat, bronchoscopy): Concentrations of 1% to 4% are used; concentrations >4% are not recommended because of potential for increased incidence and severity of systemic toxic reactions

Mechanism of Action Blocks both the initiation and conduction of nerve impulses by decreasing the neuronal membrane's permeability to sodium ions, which results in inhibition of depolarization with resultant blockade of conduction; interferes with the uptake of norepinephrine by adrenergic nerve terminals producing vasoconstriction

Other Adverse Effects

>10%:

- Central nervous system: CNS stimulation
- Gastrointestinal: Loss of taste perception
- Respiratory: Rhinitis, nasal congestion
- Miscellaneous: Loss of smell

1% to 10%:

- Cardiovascular: Heart rate (decreased) with low doses, tachycardia with moderate doses, hypertension, cardiomyopathy, cardiac arrhythmias, myocarditis, QRS prolongation, Raynaud's phenomenon, cerebral vasculitis, thrombosis, fibrillation (atrial), flutter (atrial), sinus bradycardia, CHF, pulmonary hypertension, sinus tachycardia, tachycardia (supraventricular), arrhythmias (ventricular), vasoconstriction
- Central nervous system: Fever, nervousness, restlessness, euphoria, excitation, headache, psychosis, hallucinations, agitation, seizures, slurred speech, hyperthermia, dystonic reactions, cerebral vascular accident, vasculitis, clonic-tonic reactions, paranoia, sympathetic storm
- Dermatologic: Skin infarction, pruritus, madarosis
- Gastrointestinal: Nausea, anorexia, colonic ischemia, spontaneous bowel perforation
- Genitourinary: Priapism, uterine rupture
- Hematologic: Thrombocytopenia
- Neuromuscular & skeletal: Chorea (extrapyramidal), paresthesia, tremors, fasciculations
- Ocular: Mydriasis (peak effect at 45 minutes; may last up to 12 hours), sloughing of the corneal epithelium, ulceration of the cornea, iritis, mydriasis, chemosis
- Renal: Myoglobinuria, necrotizing vasculitis
- Respiratory: Tachypnea, nasal mucosa damage (when snorting), hyposmia, bronchiolitis obliterans organizing pneumonia
- Miscellaneous: "Washed-out" syndrome

Drug Interactions CYP3A3/4 enzyme substrate

Increased Effect/Toxicity: Increased toxicity with MAO inhibitors. Use with epinephrine may cause extreme hypertension and/or cardiac arrhythmias.

Beta-blockers potentiate cocaine-induced coronary vasoconstriction (potentiate alpha-adrenergic effect of cocaine); avoid concurrent use.

Drug Uptake Following topical administration to mucosa:

Onset of action: ≤1 minute

Absorption: Well absorbed through mucous membranes; limited by drug-induced vasoconstriction; enhanced by inflammation

Duration: ≥30 minutes, dose dependent; cocaine metabolites may appear in urine of neonates up to 5 days after birth due to maternal cocaine use shortly before birth

Half-life, elimination: 75 minutes

Time to peak: ≤5 minutes

Pregnancy Risk Factor C/X (nonmedicinal use)

Generic Available Yes

Comments The cocaine user, regardless of how the cocaine was administered, presents the potential of life-threatening situation in the dental operatory. The patient under the influence of cocaine could be compared to a car going 100 miles per hour. Blood pressure is elevated and heart rate is likely increased. The use of a local anesthetic with epinephrine in such a patient may result in a medical emergency. Such patients can be identified by their jitteriness, irritability, talkativeness, tremors, and short abrupt speech patterns. These same signs and symptoms may also be seen in a normal dental patient with preoperative dental anxiety; therefore, the dentist must be particularly alert in order to identify the potential cocaine abuser. If a patient is suspected, they should never be given a local anesthetic with vasoconstrictor for fear of exacerbating the cocaine-induced sympathetic response. Life-threatening episodes of cardiac arrhythmias and hypertensive crises have been reported when local anesthetic with vasoconstrictor was administered to a patient under the influence of cocaine. No local anesthetic used by any dentist can interfere with, nor test positive by cocaine in any urine testing screen. Therefore, the dentist does not need to be concerned with any false drug use accusations associated with dental anesthesia.

Codafed® Expectorant *see* Guaifenesin, Pseudoephedrine, and Codeine *on page 570*

Codehist® DH *see* Chlorpheniramine, Pseudoephedrine, and Codeine *on page 273*

Codeine (KOE deen)

Related Information

Dental Drug Interactions: Update on Drug Combinations Requiring Special Considerations *on page 1434*

Oral Pain *on page 1360*

Pharmacologic Category Analgesic, Narcotic; Antitussive

Synonyms Codeine Phosphate; Codeine Sulfate; Methylmorphine

Use Treatment of mild to moderate pain; antitussive in lower doses; dextromethorphan has equivalent antitussive activity but has much lower toxicity in accidental overdose

Local Anesthetic/Vasoconstrictor Precautions No information available to require special precautions

Effects on Dental Treatment <1%: Xerostomia

Restrictions C-II

Dosage

Analgesic: **Note:** Doses should be titrated to appropriate analgesic effect and side effects; when changing routes of administration, note that oral dose is $^2/_3$ as effective as parenteral dose

- Children: Oral, I.M., S.C.: 0.5-1 mg/kg/dose every 4-6 hours as needed; maximum: 60 mg/dose
- Adults: Oral, I.M., I.V., S.C.: 30 mg/dose; range: 15-60 mg every 4-6 hours as needed

Antitussive: Oral (for nonproductive cough):

- Children: 1-1.5 mg/kg/day in divided doses every 4-6 hours as needed: Alternative dose according to age:
  - 2-6 years: 2.5-5 mg every 4-6 hours as needed; maximum: 30 mg/day
  - 6-12 years: 5-10 mg every 4-6 hours as needed; maximum: 60 mg/day
- Adults: 10-20 mg/dose every 4-6 hours as needed; maximum: 120 mg/day

Dosing adjustment in renal impairment:

Cl_{cr} 10-50 mL/minute: Administer 75% of dose

Cl_{cr} <10 mL/minute: Administer 50% of dose

Dosing adjustment in hepatic impairment: Probably necessary

Mechanism of Action Binds to opiate receptors (mu and kappa subtypes) in the CNS, causing inhibition of ascending pain pathways, altering the perception of and response to pain; causes cough supression by direct central action in the medulla; produces generalized CNS depression

Other Adverse Effects

>10%:

- Central nervous system: Drowsiness
- Gastrointestinal: Constipation

1% to 10%:

- Cardiovascular: Tachycardia or bradycardia, hypotension
- Central nervous system: Dizziness, lightheadedness, false feeling of well being, malaise, headache, restlessness, paradoxical CNS stimulation, confusion
- Dermatologic: Rash, urticaria
- Gastrointestinal: Anorexia, nausea, vomiting, xerostomia
- Genitourinary: Decreased urination, ureteral spasm

(Continued)

Codeine *(Continued)*

Hepatic: Increased LFTs
Local: Burning at injection site
Neuromuscular & skeletal: Weakness
Ocular: Blurred vision
Respiratory: Dyspnea
Miscellaneous: Histamine release

<1%: Convulsions, hallucinations, mental depression, nightmares, insomnia, paralytic ileus, biliary spasm, stomach cramps, muscle rigidity, trembling

Frequency not defined: Increased AST, ALT

Contraindications Hypersensitivity to codeine or any component of the formulation; pregnancy (prolonged use or high doses at term)

Warnings/Precautions Use with caution in patients with hypersensitivity reactions to other phenanthrene derivative opioid agonists (morphine, hydrocodone, hydromorphone, levorphanol, oxycodone, oxymorphone); respiratory diseases including asthma, emphysema, COPD, or severe liver or renal insufficiency; some preparations contain sulfites which may cause allergic reactions; tolerance or drug dependence may result from extended use

Not recommended for use for cough control in patients with a productive cough; not recommended as an antitussive for children <2 years of age; the elderly may be particularly susceptible to the CNS depressant and confusion as well as constipating effects of narcotics

Not approved for I.V. administration (although this route has been used clinically). If given I.V., must be given slowly and the patient should be lying down. Rapid I.V. administration of narcotics may increase the incidence of serious adverse effects, in part due to limited opportunity to assess response prior to administration of the full dose. Access to respiratory support should be immediately available.

Drug Interactions CYP2D6 and 3A3/4 enzyme substrate; CYP2D6 enzyme inhibitor

Increased Toxicity: CNS depressants, phenothiazines, TCAs, other narcotic analgesics, guanabenz, MAO inhibitors, neuromuscular blockers

Decreased effect with cigarette smoking

Dietary/Ethanol/Herb Considerations

Ethanol: Avoid or limit use; may increase CNS depression.

Food: Administer with food to reduce GI upset.

Herb/Nutraceutical: Avoid gotu kola, kava, SAMe, and valerian; may increase CNS depression. Avoid St John's wort; may decrease serum concentration and increase CNS depression.

Drug Uptake

Onset of action: Analgesia: 30-45 minutes; Oral: 0.5-1 hour; I.M.: 10-30 minutes
Peak effect: Oral: 1-1.5 hours; I.M.: 0.5-1 hour
Absorption: Oral: Adequate
Duration: 4-6 hours
Half-life, elimination: 2.5-3.5 hours
Time to peak: 1-2 hours

Pregnancy Risk Factor C/D (prolonged use or high doses at term)

Breast-feeding Considerations May be taken while breast-feeding

Dosage Forms **INJ, as phosphate:** 30 mg (1 mL, 2 mL); 60 mg (1 mL, 2 mL). **SOLN, oral, as phosphate:** 15 mg/5 mL. **TAB, as phosphate, soluble:** 30 mg, 60 mg. **TAB, as sulfate:** 15 mg, 30 mg, 60 mg. **TAB, soluble, as sulfate:** 15 mg, 30 mg, 60 mg

Generic Available Yes

Comments It is recommended that codeine not be used as the sole entity for analgesia because of moderate efficacy along with relatively high incidence of nausea, sedation, and constipation. In addition, codeine has some narcotic addiction liability. Codeine in combination with acetaminophen or aspirin is recommended. Maximum effective analgesic dose of codeine is 60 mg (1 grain). Beyond 60 mg increases respiratory depression only.

Selected Readings

Desjardins PJ, Cooper SA, Gallegos TL, et al, "The Relative Analgesic Efficacy of Propiram Fumarate, Codeine, Aspirin, and Placebo in Postimpaction Dental Pain," *J Clin Pharmacol*, 1984, 24(1):35-42.

Forbes JA, Keller CK, Smith JW, et al, "Analgesic Effect of Naproxen Sodium, Codeine, a Naproxen-Codeine Combination and Aspirin on the Postoperative Pain of Oral Surgery," *Pharmacotherapy*, 1986, 6(5):211-8.

Codiclear® DH *see* Hydrocodone and Guaifenesin *on page 603*

Codimal-LA® [OTC] *see* Chlorpheniramine and Pseudoephedrine *on page 270*

Codimal-LA® Half [OTC] *see* Chlorpheniramine and Pseudoephedrine *on page 270*

Cogentin® *see* Benztropine *on page 155*

Co-Gesic® *see* Hydrocodone and Acetaminophen *on page 598*

Cognex® *see* Tacrine *on page 1127*

Colace® [OTC] *see* Docusate *on page 407*

Colchicine (KOL chi seen)

Mexican Brand Names Colchiquim

Pharmacologic Category Colchicine

Use Treatment of acute gouty arthritis attacks and in prevention of recurrences of such attacks; management of familial Mediterranean fever

Primary biliary cirrhosis

Local Anesthetic/Vasoconstrictor Precautions No information available to require special precautions

Effects on Dental Treatment No effects or complications reported

Dosage

Prophylaxis of familial Mediterranean fever: Oral:

Children:

≤5 years: 0.5 mg/day

>5 years: 1-1.5 mg/day in 2-3 divided doses

Adults: 1-2 mg/day in 2-3 divided doses

Gouty arthritis, acute attacks: Adults:

Oral: Initial: 0.5-1.2 mg, then 0.5-0.6 mg every 1-2 hours or 1-1.2 mg every 2 hours until relief or GI side effects (nausea, vomiting, or diarrhea) occur to a maximum total dose of 8 mg; wait 3 days before initiating another course of therapy

I.V.: Initial: 1-3 mg, then 0.5 mg every 6 hours until response, not to exceed 4 mg/day; if pain recurs, it may be necessary to administer a daily dose of 1-2 mg for several days, however, do not give more colchicine by any route for at least 7 days after a full course of I.V. therapy (4 mg), transfer to oral colchicine in a dose similar to that being given I.V.

Gouty arthritis, prophylaxis of recurrent attacks: Adults: Oral: 0.5-0.6 mg/day or every other day

Mechanism of Action Decreases leukocyte motility, decreases phagocytosis in joints and lactic acid production, thereby reducing the deposition of urate crystals that perpetuates the inflammatory response

Other Adverse Effects

>10%: Gastrointestinal: Nausea, vomiting, diarrhea, abdominal pain

1% to 10%:

Dermatologic: Alopecia

Gastrointestinal: Anorexia

Drug Interactions

Increased Effect/Toxicity: Increased toxicity may be seen when taken with sympathomimetic agents or CNS depressant (effects are enhanced). Alkalizing agents potentiate effects of colchicine.

Decreased Effect: Vitamin B_{12} absorption may be decreased with colchicine. Acidifying agents inhibit action of colchicine.

Drug Uptake

Onset of action: Oral: Pain relief: ~12 hours if adequately dosed; I.V.: 6-12 hours

Half-life, elimination: 12-30 minutes; End-stage renal disease: 45 minutes

Time to peak: Oral: 0.5-2 hours, declining for the next 2 hours before increasing again due to enterohepatic recycling

Pregnancy Risk Factor C (oral); D (parenteral)

Generic Available Yes

Colchicine and Probenecid (KOL chi seen & proe BEN e sid)

Pharmacologic Category Antigout Agent; Anti-inflammatory Agent; Uricosuric Agent

Synonyms ColBenemid® [DSC]; Probenecid and Colchicine

Use Treatment of chronic gouty arthritis when complicated by frequent, recurrent acute attacks of gout

Local Anesthetic/Vasoconstrictor Precautions No information available to require special precautions

Effects on Dental Treatment No effects or complications reported

Dosage Adults: Oral: 1 tablet daily for 1 week, then 1 tablet twice daily thereafter

Other Adverse Effects 1% to 10%:

Cardiovascular: Flushing

Central nervous system: Headache, dizziness

Dermatologic: Rash, alopecia

Gastrointestinal: Anorexia, nausea, vomiting, diarrhea, abdominal pain

Hematologic: Anemia, leukopenia, aplastic anemia, agranulocytosis

Hepatic: Hepatic necrosis, hepatotoxicity

Neuromuscular & skeletal: Peripheral neuritis, myopathy

Renal: Nephrotic syndrome, uric acid stones, polyuria

Miscellaneous: Hypersensitivity reactions

Drug Uptake See Colchicine *on page 319* and Probenecid *on page 996*

Pregnancy Risk Factor C

Generic Available Yes

Comments Do not initiate therapy until an acute gouty attack has subsided

Colesevelam (koh le SEV a lam)

U.S. Brand Names WelChol™

Canadian Brand Names WelChol™

Pharmacologic Category Antilipemic Agent, Bile Acid Sequestrant

Use Adjunctive therapy to diet and exercise in the management of elevated LDL in primary hypercholesterolemia (Fredrickson type IIa) when used alone or in combination with an HMG-CoA reductase inhibitor

Local Anesthetic/Vasoconstrictor Precautions No information available to require special precautions

Effects on Dental Treatment No effects or complications reported

Dosage Adult: Oral:

Monotherapy: 3 tablets twice daily with meals or 6 tablets once daily with a meal; maximum dose: 7 tablets/day

Combination therapy with an HMG-CoA reductase inhibitor: 4-6 tablets daily; maximum dose: 6 tablets/day

Mechanism of Action Binds bile acids including glycocholic acid in the intestine, impeding their reabsorption; increases the fecal loss of bile salt-bound LDL-C

Other Adverse Effects

>10%: Gastrointestinal: Constipation (11%)

2% to 10%:

- Gastrointestinal: Dyspepsia (8%)
- Neuromuscular & skeletal: Weakness (4%), myalgia (2%)
- Respiratory: Pharyngitis (3%)

Incidence ≤ placebo: Infection, headache, pain, back pain, abdominal pain, flu syndrome, flatulence, diarrhea, nausea, sinusitis, rhinitis, cough

Drug Interactions

Decreased Effect: Sustained-release verapamil AUC and C_{max} were reduced. Clinical significance unknown.

Digoxin, lovastatin, metoprolol, quinidine, valproic acid, or warfarin absorption was not significantly affected with concurrent administration.

Clinical effects of atorvastatin, lovastatin, and simvastatin were not changed by concurrent administration.

Drug Uptake

Absorption: Not significantly absorbed

Time to peak: Therapeutic: ~2 weeks

Pregnancy Risk Factor B

Generic Available No

Colestid® *see* Colestipol *on page 320*

Colestipol (koe LES ti pole)

Related Information

Cardiovascular Diseases *on page 1308*

U.S. Brand Names Colestid®

Canadian Brand Names Colestid®

Pharmacologic Category Antilipemic Agent, Bile Acid Sequestrant

Synonyms Colestipol Hydrochloride

Use Adjunct in management of primary hypercholesterolemia; regression of arteriolosclerosis; relief of pruritus associated with elevated levels of bile acids; possibly used to decrease plasma half-life of digoxin in toxicity

Local Anesthetic/Vasoconstrictor Precautions No information available to require special precautions

Effects on Dental Treatment No effects or complications reported

Dosage Adults: Oral: 5-30 g/day in divided doses 2-4 times/day

Mechanism of Action Binds with bile acids to form an insoluble complex that is eliminated in feces; it thereby increases the fecal loss of bile acid-bound low density lipoprotein cholesterol

Other Adverse Effects

>10%: Gastrointestinal: Constipation

1% to 10%:

- Central nervous system: Headache, dizziness, anxiety, vertigo, drowsiness, fatigue
- Gastrointestinal: Abdominal pain and distention, belching, flatulence, nausea, vomiting, diarrhea

Drug Interactions Decreased Effect: Colestipol can reduce the absorption of numerous medications when used concurrently. Give other medications 1 hour before or 4 hours after giving colestipol. Medications which may be affected include HMG-CoA reductase inhibitors, thiazide diuretics, propranolol (and potentially other beta-blockers), corticosteroids, thyroid hormones, digoxin, valproic acid, NSAIDs, loop diuretics, sulfonylureas, troglitazone (and potentially other agents in this class - pioglitazone and rosiglitazone). Absorption of warfarin and other oral anticoagulants is reduced by cholestyramine and possibly by colestipol; separate administration times (as detailed above).

Pregnancy Risk Factor C

Generic Available No

Colfosceril Palmitate (kole FOS er il PALM i tate)

U.S. Brand Names Exosurf Neonatal®

Canadian Brand Names Exosurf® Neonatal

Mexican Brand Names Exosurf®

Pharmacologic Category Lung Surfactant

Synonyms Dipalmitoylphosphatidylcholine; DPPC; Synthetic Lung Surfactant

Use Neonatal respiratory distress syndrome (RDS):

Prophylactic therapy: Infants at risk for developing RDS with body weight <1350 g; infants with evidence of pulmonary immaturity with body weight >1350 g

Rescue therapy: Treatment of infants with RDS based on respiratory distress not attributable to any other causes and chest radiographic findings consistent with RDS

Local Anesthetic/Vasoconstrictor Precautions No information available to require special precautions

Effects on Dental Treatment No effects or complications reported

Dosage For intratracheal use only

Prophylactic treatment: Give 5 mL/kg (as two 2.5 mL/kg half-doses) as soon as possible; the second and third doses should be administered at 12 and 24 hours later to those infants remaining on ventilators

Rescue treatment: Give 5 mL/kg (as two 2.5 mL/kg half-doses) as soon as the diagnosis of RDS is made; the second 5 mL/kg (as two 2.5 mL/kg half-doses) dose should be administered 12 hours later

Mechanism of Action Replaces deficient or ineffective endogenous lung surfactant in neonates with respiratory distress syndrome (RDS) or in neonates at risk of developing RDS; reduces surface tension and stabilizes the alveoli from collapsing

Other Adverse Effects 1% to 10%: Respiratory: Pulmonary hemorrhage, apnea, mucous plugging, decrease in transcutaneous O_2 >20%

Drug Uptake Absorption: Intratracheal: Absorbed from alveolus

Generic Available No

Colgate Total® Toothpaste *see* Triclosan and Fluoride *on page 1203*

Colistimethate (koe lis ti METH ate)

U.S. Brand Names Coly-Mycin® M

Canadian Brand Names Coly-Mycin® M

Pharmacologic Category Antibiotic, Miscellaneous

Synonyms Colistimethate Sodium

Use Treatment of infections due to sensitive strains of certain gram-negative bacilli

Local Anesthetic/Vasoconstrictor Precautions No information available to require special precautions

Effects on Dental Treatment No effects or complications reported

Dosage Children and Adults: I.M., I.V.: 2.5-5 mg/kg/day in 2-4 divided doses

Mechanism of Action Hydrolyzed to colistin, which acts as a cationic detergent which damages the bacterial cytoplasmic membrane causing leaking of intracellular substances and cell death

Other Adverse Effects 1% to 10%:

Central nervous system: Vertigo, slurring of speech

Dermatologic: Urticaria

Gastrointestinal: GI upset

Renal: Decreased urine output

Respiratory: Respiratory arrest

Drug Interactions Increased Effect/Toxicity: Other nephrotoxic drugs and neuromuscular blocking agents

Drug Uptake

Half-life, elimination: 1.5-8 hours; Anuria: ≤2-3 days

Time to peak: ~2 hours

Pregnancy Risk Factor B

Generic Available No

Colistin (koe LIS tin)

Pharmacologic Category Antibiotic, Miscellaneous; Antidiarrheal

Synonyms Polymyxin E

Use Treatment of diarrhea in infants and children caused by susceptible organisms, especially *E. coli* and *Shigella*

Local Anesthetic/Vasoconstrictor Precautions No information available to require special precautions

Effects on Dental Treatment No effects or complications reported

Dosage Diarrhea: Children: Oral: 5-15 mg/kg/day in 3 divided doses given every 8 hours

Mechanism of Action A polypeptide antibiotic that binds to and damages the bacterial cell membrane

(Continued)

Colistin *(Continued)*

Other Adverse Effects Frequency not defined:
Gastrointestinal: Nausea, vomiting
Neuromuscular & skeletal: Neuromuscular blockade
Renal: Nephrotoxicity
Respiratory: Respiratory arrest
Miscellaneous: Hypersensitivity reactions, superinfections

Drug Uptake
Absorption: Oral: Adults: Slightly absorbed from GI tract; Infants: Unpredictable
Half-life, elimination: 2.8-4.8 hours (increases with renal insufficiency); Anuria: 48-72 hours

Colistin, Neomycin, and Hydrocortisone

(koe LIS tin, nee oh MYE sin & hye droe KOR ti sone)

U.S. Brand Names Coly-Mycin® S Otic; Cortisporin®-TC Otic

Pharmacologic Category Antibiotic/Corticosteroid, Otic

Synonyms Hydrocortisone, Colistin, and Neomycin; Neomycin, Colistin, and Hydrocortisone

Use Treatment of superficial and susceptible bacterial infections of the external auditory canal; for treatment of susceptible bacterial infections of mastoidectomy and fenestration cavities

Local Anesthetic/Vasoconstrictor Precautions No information available to require special precautions

Effects on Dental Treatment No effects or complications reported

Dosage
Children: 3 drops in affected ear 3-4 times/day
Adults: 4 drops in affected ear 3-4 times/day

Pregnancy Risk Factor C

Generic Available No

CollaCote® *see* Collagen, Absorbable *on page 322*

Collagen, Absorbable (KOL la jen, ab SORB able)

U.S. Brand Names CollaCote®; CollaPlug®; CollaTape®

Pharmacologic Category Hemostatic Agent

Use
Dental: To control bleeding created during dental surgery
Medical: Hemostatic

Local Anesthetic/Vasoconstrictor Precautions No information available to require special precautions

Effects on Dental Treatment No effects or complications reported

Dosage Children and Adults: A sufficiently large dressing should be selected so as to completely cover the oral wound.

Mechanism of Action The highly porous sponge structure absorbs blood and wound exudate. The collagen component causes aggregation of platelets which bind to collagen fibrils. The aggregated platelets degranulate, releasing coagulation factors that promote the formation of fibrin.

Warnings/Precautions Should not be used on infected or contaminated wounds

Breast-feeding Considerations May be taken while breast-feeding

Dosage Forms DRESSING, wound: 3/8" x 3/4"; 3/4" x 1 1/2"; 1" x 3"

Generic Available Yes

Comments The dressing should be applied over the wound and held in place with moderate pressure. The period of time necessary to apply pressure will vary with the degree of bleeding. In general, 2-5 minutes should be sufficient to achieve hemostasis. At the end of the procedure, the dressing can be removed, replaced or left *in situ*, any excess dressing should be removed prior to wound closure.

Collagenase (KOL la je nase)

U.S. Brand Names Plaquase®; Santyl®

Canadian Brand Names Santyl®

Pharmacologic Category Enzyme, Topical Debridement

Use Promotes debridement of necrotic tissue in dermal ulcers and severe burns
Orphan drug: Injection: Treatment of Peyronie's disease; treatment of Dupytren's disease

Local Anesthetic/Vasoconstrictor Precautions No information available to require special precautions

Effects on Dental Treatment No effects or complications reported

Dosage Topical: Apply once daily

Mechanism of Action Collagenase is an enzyme derived from the fermentation of *Clostridium histolyticum* and differs from other proteolytic enzymes in that its enzymatic action has a high specificity for native and denatured collagen. Collagenase will not attack collagen in healthy tissue or newly formed granulation tissue. In addition, it does not act on fat, fibrin, keratin, or muscle.

Other Adverse Effects 1% to 10%: Local: Irritation

Drug Interactions Enzymatic activity is inhibited by detergents, benzalkonium chloride, hexachlorophene, nitrofurazone, tincture of iodine, and heavy metal ions (silver and mercury).

Pregnancy Risk Factor C

Generic Available No

CollaPlug® *see* Collagen, Absorbable *on page 322*

CollaTape® *see* Collagen, Absorbable *on page 322*

Collyrium Fresh® [OTC] *see* Tetrahydrozoline *on page 1150*

Colo-Fresh™ [OTC] *see* Bismuth *on page 167*

Coly-Mycin® M *see* Colistimethate *on page 321*

Coly-Mycin® S Otic *see* Colistin, Neomycin, and Hydrocortisone *on page 322*

Colyte® *see* Polyethylene Glycol-Electrolyte Solution *on page 970*

Combination Hormonal Contraceptives

(KOM bi na tion HOR mo nal kon tra SEP tivs)

U.S. Brand Names Alesse®; Apri®; Aviane™; Brevicon®; Cryselle™; Cyclessa®; Demulen®; Desogen®; Enpresse™; Estrostep® 21; Estrostep® Fe; femhrt®; Jenest™-28; Kariva™; Lessina™; Levlen®; Levlite™; Levora®; Loestrin®; Loestrin® Fe; Lo/Ovral®; Low-Ogestrel®; Microgestin™ Fe; Mircette®; Modicon®; Necon® 0.5/35; Necon® 1/35; Necon® 10/11; Nordette®; Norinyl® 1+35; Nortrel™; NuvaRing®; Ogestrel®; Ortho-Cept®; Ortho-Cyclen®; Ortho Evra™; Ortho-Novum®; Ortho Tri-Cyclen®; Ovcon®; Ovral®; PREVEN™; Tri-Levlen®; Tri-Norinyl®; Triphasil®; Trivora®; Yasmin®; Zovia™

Pharmacologic Category Contraceptive; Estrogen and Progestin Combination

Synonyms Ethinyl Estradiol and Desogestrel; Ethinyl Estradiol and Drospirenone; Ethinyl Estradiol and Ethynodiol Diacetate; Ethinyl Estradiol and Etonogestrel; Ethinyl Estradiol and Levonorgestrel; Ethinyl Estradiol and Norelgestromin; Ethinyl Estradiol and Norethindrone Acetate; Ethinyl Estradiol and Norgestimate; Ethinyl Estradiol and Norgestrel

Use Labeled indications are product specific and may include the following: Prevention of pregnancy; postcoital contraception; treatment of acne; moderate to severe vasomotor symptoms associated with menopause; prevention of osteoporosis

Unlabeled/Investigational: Treatment of hypermenorrhea, endometriosis, female hypogonadism

Local Anesthetic/Vasoconstrictor Precautions No information available to require special precautions

Effects on Dental Treatment No effects or complications reported

Dosage

Children ≥15 years and Adults: Female: Oral: Acne (Estrostep®, Ortho Tri-Cyclen®): Refer to dosing for contraception

Adults: Female: Contraception: Oral: (Abbreviated/refer to package insert):

- Schedule 1 (Sunday starter): Dose begins on first Sunday after onset of menstruation; if the menstrual period starts on Sunday, take first tablet that very same day. With a Sunday start, an additional method of contraception should be used until after the first 7 days of consecutive administration:
  - For 21-tablet package: 1 tablet/day for 21 consecutive days, followed by 7 days off of the medication; a new course begins on the 8th day after the last tablet is taken
  - For 28-tablet package: 1 tablet/day without interruption
- Schedule 2 (Day-1 starter): Dose starts on first day of menstrual cycle taking 1 tablet/day:
  - For 21-tablet package: 1 tablet/day for 21 consecutive days, followed by 7 days off of the medication; a new course begins on the 8th day after the last tablet is taken
  - For 28-tablet package: 1 tablet/day without interruption
- Missed doses **monophasic formulations** (refer to package insert for complete information):
  - One dose missed: Take as soon as remembered or take 2 tablets next day
  - Two consecutive doses missed in the first 2 weeks: Take 2 tablets as soon as remembered or 2 tablets next 2 days. An additional method of contraception should be used for 7 days after missed dose.
  - Two consecutive doses missed in week 3 or three consecutive doses missed at any time: An additional method of contraception must be used for 7 days after a missed dose.
- Missed doses **biphasic/triphasic formulations** (refer to package insert for complete information):
  - One dose missed: Take as soon as remembered or take 2 tablets next day.
  - Two consecutive doses missed in week 1 or week 2 of the pack: Take 2 tablets as soon as remembered and 2 tablets the next day. Resume taking 1 tablet/day until the pack is empty. An additional method of contraception should be used for 7 days after a missed dose.
  - Two consecutive doses missed in week 3 of the pack: An additional method of contraception must be used for 7 days after a missed dose.

(Continued)

Combination Hormonal Contraceptives *(Continued)*

Three or more consecutive doses missed: An additional method of contraception must be used for 7 days after a missed dose.

Topical patch: (Abbreviated labeling/refer to package insert): Apply one patch each week for 3 weeks (21 total days); followed by one week that is patch-free. Each patch should be applied on the same day each week ("patch change day") and only one patch should be worn at a time. No more than 7 days should pass during the patch-free interval.

If a patch becomes partially or completely detached for <24 hours: Try to reapply to same place, or replace with a new patch immediately. Do not reapply if patch is no longer sticky, if it is sticking to itself or another surface, or if it has material sticking to it.

If a patch becomes partially or completely detached for >24 hours (or time period is unknown): Apply a new patch and use this day of the week as the new "patch change day" from this point on. **An additional method of contraception (nonhormonal) should be used until after the first 7 days of consecutive administration.**

Vaginal ring: (Abbreviated labeling/refer to package insert): One ring, inserted vaginally and left in place for 3 consecutive weeks, then removed for 1 week. A new ring is inserted 7 days after the last was removed (even if bleeding is not complete) and should be inserted at ~ the same time of day the ring was removed the previous week.

If the ring is accidentally removed from the vagina at anytime during the 3-week period of use, it may be rinsed with cool or luke-warm water (not hot) and reinserted as soon as possible. If the ring is not reinserted within 3 hours, contraceptive effectiveness will be decreased. **An additional form of contraception should be used until the ring has been inserted for 7 continuous days.*** If the ring has been removed for longer than 1 week, pregnancy must be ruled out prior to restarting therapy. **An additional form of contraception should be used for the following 7 days.***

If the ring has been left in place for >3 weeks, a new ring should be inserted following a 1-week (ring-free) interval. Pregnancy must be ruled out prior to insertion and **an additional form of contraception should be used for the following 7 days.***

*Note: Diaphragms may interfere with proper ring placement, and therefore, are not recommended for use as an additional form of contraception.

Adults: Female: Postcoital contraception: Oral:

Ethinyl estradiol 0.03 mg and norgestrel 0.3 mg formulation: 4 tablets within 72 hours of unprotected intercourse and 4 tablets 12 hours after first dose

Ethinyl estradiol 0.05 mg and norgestrel 0.5 mg formulation: 2 tablets within 72 hours of unprotected intercourse and 2 tablets 12 hours after first dose

PREVEN™: Initial: 2 tablets as soon as possible (but within 72 hours of unprotected intercourse), followed by a second dose of 2 tablets 12 hours later.

Adults: Female: Moderate to severe vasomotor symptoms associated with menopause: Oral: femhrt® 1/5: 1 tablet/day; patients should be re-evaluated at 3- to 6-month intervals to determine if treatment is still necessary

Adults: Female: Prevention of osteoporosis: Oral: femhrt® 1/5: 1 tablet/day

Mechanism of Action Combination hormonal contraceptives inhibit ovulation via a negative feedback mechanism on the hypothalamus, which alters the normal pattern of gonadotropin secretion of a follicle-stimulating hormone (FSH) and luteinizing hormone by the anterior pituitary. The follicular phase FSH and midcycle surge of gonadotropins are inhibited. In addition, combination hormonal contraceptives produce alterations in the genital tract, including changes in the cervical mucus, rendering it unfavorable for sperm penetration even if ovulation occurs. Changes in the endometrium may also occur, producing an unfavorable environment for nidation. Combination hormonal contraceptive drugs may alter the tubal transport of the ova through the fallopian tubes. Progestational agents may also alter sperm fertility. Drospirenone is a spironolactone analogue with antimineralocorticoid and antiandrogenic activity.

Other Adverse Effects Adverse reactions associated with oral combination hormonal contraceptive agents are also likely to appear with vaginally-administered rings and topically-administered patches (frequency difficult to anticipate).

Cardiovascular: Arterial thromboembolism, cerebral hemorrhage, cerebral thrombosis, edema, hypertension, mesenteric thrombosis, myocardial infarction

Central nervous system: Depression, dizziness, headache, migraine, nervousness, premenstrual syndrome, stroke

Dermatologic: Acne, erythema multiforme, erythema nodosum, hirsutism, loss of scalp hair, melasma (may persist), rash (allergic)

Endocrine & metabolic: Amenorrhea, breakthrough bleeding, breast enlargement, breast secretion, breast tenderness, carbohydrate intolerance, lactation decreased (postpartum), glucose tolerance decreased, libido changes, menstrual flow changes, sex hormone-binding globulins (SHBG) increased, spotting, temporary infertility (following discontinuation), thyroid-binding globulin increased, triglycerides increased

Gastrointestinal: Abdominal cramps, appetite changes, bloating, colitis, gallbladder disease, nausea, vomiting, weight gain/loss
Genitourinary: Cervical erosion changes, cervical secretion changes, cystitis-like syndrome, vaginal candidiasis, vaginitis
Hematologic: Antithrombin III decreased, folate levels decreased, hemolytic uremic syndrome, norepinephrine-induced platelet aggregability increased, porphyria, prothrombin increased; factors VII, VIII, IX, and X increased
Hepatic: Benign liver tumors, Budd-Chiari syndrome, cholestasis, cholestatic jaundice, hepatic adenomas, jaundice
Local: Thrombophlebitis
Ocular: Cataracts, change in corneal curvature (steepening), contact lens intolerance, optic neuritis, retinal thrombosis
Renal: Impaired renal function
Respiratory: Pulmonary thromboembolism
Miscellaneous: Hemorrhagic eruption
Vaginal ring: Coital problems, device expulsion, emotional lability, foreign body sensation, vaginal discomfort

9% to 22%: Topical patch:
Central nervous system: Headache
Dermatologic: Application site reaction
Endocrine & metabolic: Breast symptoms
Gastrointestinal: Abdominal pain, nausea
Genitourinary: Menstrual cramps
Respiratory: Upper respiratory infection

Contraindications Hypersensitivity to ethinyl estradiol, desogestrel, drosperinone, ethynodiol diacetate, etonogestrel, levonorgestrel, norelgestromin, norethindrone acetate, norgestimate, norgestrel, or any component of the formulation; thrombophlebitis or thromboembolic disorders (current or history of), cerebral vascular disease, coronary artery disease, valvular heart disease with complications, severe hypertension; diabetes mellitus with vascular involvement; severe headache with focal neurological symptoms; known or suspected breast carcinoma, endometrial cancer, estrogen-dependent neoplasms, undiagnosed abnormal genital bleeding; hepatic dysfunction or tumor, cholestatic jaundice of pregnancy, jaundice with prior combination hormonal contraceptive use; major surgery with prolonged immobilization; heavy smoking (≥15 cigarettes/day) in patients >35 years of age; pregnancy

Ethinyl estradiol/drosperinone should not be used in patients with renal or adrenal insufficiency

Warnings/Precautions Combination hormonal contraceptives do not protect against HIV infection or other sexually-transmitted diseases. The risk of cardiovascular side effects increases in women who smoke cigarettes, especially those who are >35 years of age; women who use combination hormonal contraceptives should be strongly advised not to smoke. Combination hormonal contraceptives may lead to increased risk of myocardial infarction, use with caution in patients with risk factors for coronary artery disease. May increase the risk of thromboembolism. Combination hormonal contraceptives may have a dose-related risk of vascular disease, hypertension, and gallbladder disease. Women with hypertension should be encouraged to use a nonhormonal form of contraception. The use of combination hormonal contraceptives has been associated with a slight increase in frequency of breast cancer, however, studies are not consistent. Combination hormonal contraceptives may cause glucose intolerance. Retinal thrombosis has been reported (rarely). Use with caution in patients with renal disease, conditions that may be aggravated by fluid retention, depression, or history of migraine. Not for use prior to menarche.

Drospirenone has antimineralocorticoid activity that may lead to hyperkalemia in patients with renal insufficiency, hepatic dysfunction, or adrenal insufficiency. Use caution with medications that may increase serum potassium.

Combination hormonal contraceptives in the form of vaginally-administered rings or topically-administered patches may have similar adverse effects associated with oral contraceptive products. The topical patch may be less effective in patients weighing ≥90 kg (198 lbs) and an increased incidence of pregnancy has been reported in this population; consider another form of contraception.

Acne: For use only in females ≥15 years, who also desire oral contraceptive therapy, are unresponsive to topical treatments, and have no contraindications to oral contraceptive use; treatment must continue for at least 6 months.

Vasomotor symptoms associated with menopause and prevention of osteoporosis: For use only in postmenopausal women with an intact uterus

Drug Interactions

Cytochrome P450 effect:

Desogestrel: CYP2C9 and CYP2C19 enzyme substrate
Drospirenone: CYP3A4 enzyme substrate; CYP1A1, CYP2C9, CYP2C19, and CYP3A4 enzyme inhibitor (weak)
Ethinyl estradiol, etonogestrel, levonorgestrel, and norgestrel: CYP3A4 enzyme substrates

(Continued)

Combination Hormonal Contraceptives *(Continued)*

Drug interactions:

ACE inhibitors: Potential for hyperkalemia with ethinyl estradiol/drosperinone; monitor serum potassium during first cycle

Acetaminophen: May increase plasma concentration of synthetic estrogens, possibly by inhibiting conjugation. Combination hormonal contraceptives may also decrease the plasma concentration of acetaminophen.

Acitretin: Interferes with the contraceptive effect of microdosed progestin-containing "minipill" preparations. The effect on other progestational contraceptives (eg, implants, injectables) is unknown.

Aldosterone antagonists: Potential for hyperkalemia with ethinyl estradiol/drosperinone; monitor serum potassium during first cycle

Aminoglutethimide: May increase CYP metabolism of progestins leading to possible decrease in contraceptive effectiveness. Use of a nonhormonal contraceptive product is recommended.

Angiotensin II receptor antagonists: Potential for hyperkalemia with ethinyl estradiol/drosperinone; monitor serum potassium during first cycle

Antibiotics (ampicillin, tetracycline): Pregnancy has been reported following concomitant use, however pharmacokinetic studies have not shown consistent effects with these antibiotics on plasma concentrations of synthetic steroids. Use of a nonhormonal contraceptive product is recommended.

Anticoagulants: Combination hormonal contraceptives may increase or decrease the effects of coumarin derivatives. Combination hormonal contraceptives may also increase risk of thromboembolic disorders

Anticonvulsants (carbamazepine, felbamate, phenobarbital, phenytoin, topiramate): Increase the metabolism of ethinyl estradiol and/or some progestins, leading to possible decrease in contraceptive effectiveness. Use of a nonhormonal contraceptive product is recommended.

Ascorbic acid (vitamin C): Doses of ascorbic acid (1 g/day) have been reported to increase plasma concentration of synthetic estrogens by ~47%, possibly by inhibiting conjugation; clinical implications are unclear.

Atorvastatin: Atorvastatin increases the AUC for norethindrone and ethinyl estradiol.

Benzodiazepines: Combination hormonal contraceptives may decrease the clearance of some benzodiazepines (alprazolam, chlordiazepoxide, diazepam) and increase the clearance of others (lorazepam, oxazepam, temazepam)

Clofibric acid: Combination hormonal contraceptives may increase the clearance of clofibric acid.

Cyclosporine: Combination hormonal contraceptives may inhibit the metabolism of cyclosporine, leading to increased plasma concentrations; monitor cyclosporine levels

Griseofulvin: Griseofulvin may induce the metabolism of combination hormonal contraceptives causing menstrual changes; pregnancies have been reported. Use of barrier form of contraception is suggested while on griseofulvin therapy.

Heparin: Potential for hyperkalemia with ethinyl estradiol/drosperinone; monitor serum potassium during first cycle

Morphine: Combination hormonal contraceptives may increase the clearance of morphine.

NSAIDs: Potential for hyperkalemia with ethinyl estradiol/drosperinone when taken daily, long term; monitor serum potassium during first cycle

Non-nucleoside reverse transcriptase inhibitors (NNRTIs): Nevirapine may decrease plasma levels of combination hormonal contraceptives; use of a nonhormonal contraceptive product is recommended. No data for delavirdine; incomplete data for efavirenz

Potassium-sparing diuretics: Potential for hyperkalemia with ethinyl estradiol/drosperinone; monitor serum potassium during first cycle

Prednisolone: Ethinyl estradiol may inhibit the metabolism of prednisolone, leading to increased plasma concentrations.

Protease inhibitors: Amprenavir, lopinavir, nelfinavir, and ritonavir have been shown to decrease plasma levels of combination hormonal contraceptives; use of a nonhormonal contraceptive product is recommended. Indinavir has been shown to increase plasma levels of combination hormonal contraceptives. No data for saquinavir.

Repaglinide: Increased level of ethinyl estradiol (combined with levonorgestrel) with concurrent use

Rifampin: Rifampin increases the metabolism of ethinyl estradiol and some progestins (norethindrone) resulting in decreased contraceptive effectiveness and increased menstrual irregularities. Use of a nonhormonal contraceptive product is recommended.

Salicylic acid: Combination hormonal contraceptives may increase the clearance of salicylic acid.

Selegiline: Combination hormonal contraceptives may increase the serum concentration of selegiline.

Theophylline: Ethinyl estradiol may inhibit the metabolism of theophylline, leading to increased plasma concentrations.

Tricyclic antidepressants (amitriptyline, imipramine, nortriptyline): Metabolism may be inhibited by combination hormonal contraceptives, increasing plasma levels of antidepressant; use caution.

Troglitazone: Troglitazone decreases the serum concentrations of ethinyl estradiol and norethindrone by ~30% leading to possible reduction in contraceptive effectiveness

Drug Uptake

Absorption:

Topical patch: Absorption is therapeutically equivalent when applied to the abdomen, buttock, upper outer arm, and upper torso

Ethinyl estradiol: Rapid; reaches plateau by ~48 hours

Norelgestromin: Rapid; reaches plateau by ~48 hours

Duration: Intravaginal ring: Serum levels (contraceptive effectiveness) decrease after 3 weeks of continuous use

Pregnancy Risk Factor X

CombiPatch™ *see* Estradiol and Norethindrone *on page 459*

Combipres® *see* Clonidine and Chlorthalidone *on page 310*

Combivent® *see* Ipratropium and Albuterol *on page 652*

Combivir® *see* Zidovudine and Lamivudine *on page 1258*

Comhist® *see* Chlorpheniramine, Phenylephrine, and Phenyltoloxamine *on page 272*

Comhist® LA *see* Chlorpheniramine, Phenylephrine, and Phenyltoloxamine *on page 272*

Compazine® *see* Prochlorperazine *on page 999*

Compound W® [OTC] *see* Salicylic Acid *on page 1072*

Compoz® Gel Caps [OTC] *see* DiphenhydrAMINE *on page 398*

Compoz® Nighttime Sleep Aid [OTC] *see* DiphenhydrAMINE *on page 398*

Compro™ *see* Prochlorperazine *on page 999*

Comtan® *see* Entacapone *on page 436*

Comtrex® Allergy-Sinus [OTC] *see* Acetaminophen, Chlorpheniramine, and Pseudoephedrine *on page 33*

Comtrex® Non-Drowsy Cough and Cold [OTC] *see* Acetaminophen, Dextromethorphan, and Pseudoephedrine *on page 34*

Concerta™ *see* Methylphenidate *on page 795*

Condylox® *see* Podofilox *on page 968*

Congess® Jr *see* Guaifenesin and Pseudoephedrine *on page 570*

Congess® Sr *see* Guaifenesin and Pseudoephedrine *on page 570*

Congestac® *see* Guaifenesin and Pseudoephedrine *on page 570*

Constilac® *see* Lactulose *on page 682*

Constulose® *see* Lactulose *on page 682*

Contac® Severe Cold and Flu/Non-Drowsy [OTC] *see* Acetaminophen, Dextromethorphan, and Pseudoephedrine *on page 34*

Copaxone® *see* Glatiramer Acetate *on page 556*

Co-Pyronil® 2 Pulvules® [OTC] *see* Chlorpheniramine and Pseudoephedrine *on page 270*

Cordarone® *see* Amiodarone *on page 72*

Cordran® *see* Flurandrenolide *on page 521*

Cordran® SP *see* Flurandrenolide *on page 521*

Coreg® *see* Carvedilol *on page 227*

Corgard® *see* Nadolol *on page 839*

Coricidin® [OTC] *see* Chlorpheniramine and Acetaminophen *on page 269*

Corlopam® *see* Fenoldopam *on page 491*

Cormax® *see* Clobetasol *on page 303*

Cortaid® Maximum Strength [OTC] *see* Hydrocortisone *on page 608*

Cortaid® With Aloe [OTC] *see* Hydrocortisone *on page 608*

Cortatrigen® Otic *see* Neomycin, Polymyxin B, and Hydrocortisone *on page 857*

Cort-Dome® *see* Hydrocortisone *on page 608*

Cortef® *see* Hydrocortisone *on page 608*

Cortef® Feminine Itch *see* Hydrocortisone *on page 608*

Cortenema® *see* Hydrocortisone *on page 608*

Corticaine® *see* Dibucaine and Hydrocortisone *on page 376*

Corticaine® *see* Hydrocortisone *on page 608*

Corticotropin (kor ti koe TROE pin)

U.S. Brand Names Acthar®; H.P. Acthar® Gel

Pharmacologic Category Corticosteroid, Systemic

Synonyms ACTH; Adrenocorticotropic Hormone; Corticotropin, Repository

Use Acute exacerbations of multiple sclerosis; diagnostic aid in adrenocortical insufficiency, severe muscle weakness in myasthenia gravis; cosyntropin is preferred

(Continued)

Corticotropin *(Continued)*

over corticotropin for diagnostic test of adrenocortical insufficiency (cosyntropin is less allergenic and test is shorter in duration)

Local Anesthetic/Vasoconstrictor Precautions No information available to require special precautions

Effects on Dental Treatment No effects or complications reported

Dosage Injection has a rapid onset and duration of activity of ~ 2 hours; repository injection has slower onset, but may sustain effects for ≤3 days.

Children:

Anti-inflammatory/immunosuppressant:

I.M., I.V., S.C. (aqueous): 1.6 units/kg/day or 50 units/m²/day divided every 6-8 hours

I.M. (gel): 0.8 units/kg/day or 25 units/m²/day divided every 12-24 hours

Infantile spasms: Various regimens have been used. Some neurologists recommend low-dose ACTH (5-40 units/day) for short periods (1-6 weeks), while others recommend larger doses of ACTH (40-160 units/day) for long periods of treatment (3-12 months). Well designed comparative dosing studies are needed. Example of low dose regimen:

Initial: I.M. (gel): 20 units/day for 2 weeks, if patient responds, taper and discontinue; if patient does not respond, increase dose to 30 units/day for 4 weeks then taper and discontinue

I.M. usual dose (gel): 20-40 units/day or 5-8 units/kg/day in 1-2 divided doses; range: 5-160 units/day

Oral prednisone (2 mg/kg/day) was as effective as I.M. ACTH gel (20 units/day) in controlling infantile spasms

Adults: Acute exacerbation of multiple sclerosis: I.M.: 80-120 units/day for 2-3 weeks

Diagnostic purposes: I.V.: 10-25 units in 500 mL 5% dextrose in water infused over 8 hours

Repository injection: I.M., S.C.: 40-80 units every 24-72 hours

Mechanism of Action Stimulates the adrenal cortex to secrete adrenal steroids (including hydrocortisone, cortisone), androgenic substances, and a small amount of aldosterone

Other Adverse Effects

>10%:

Central nervous system: Insomnia, nervousness

Gastrointestinal: Increased appetite, indigestion

1% to 10%:

Dermatologic: Hirsutism

Endocrine & metabolic: Diabetes mellitus

Neuromuscular & skeletal: Arthralgia

Ocular: Cataracts

Respiratory: Epistaxis

Drug Interactions Decreased Effect: Can antagonize the effect of anticholinesterases (eg, neostigmine) in patients with myasthenia gravis; decreased corticotropin levels with barbiturates

Pregnancy Risk Factor C

Generic Available Yes

Cortifoam® *see* Hydrocortisone *on page 608*

Cortisone Acetate (KOR ti sone AS e tate)

Related Information

Respiratory Diseases *on page 1328*

Canadian Brand Names Cortone®

Pharmacologic Category Corticosteroid, Systemic

Synonyms Compound E

Use Management of adrenocortical insufficiency

Local Anesthetic/Vasoconstrictor Precautions No information available to require special precautions

Effects on Dental Treatment A compromised immune response may occur if patient has been taking systemic cortisone. The need for corticosteroid coverage in these patients should be considered before any dental treatment; consult with physician.

Dosage If possible, administer glucocorticoids before 9 AM to minimize adrenocortical suppression; dosing depends upon the condition being treated and the response of the patient; supplemental doses may be warranted during times of stress in the course of withdrawing therapy

Children:

Anti-inflammatory or immunosuppressive:

Oral: 2.5-10 mg/kg/day **or** 20-300 mg/m²/day in divided doses every 6-8 hours

I.M.: 1-5 mg/kg/day **or** 14-375 mg/m²/day in divided doses every 12-24 hours

Physiologic replacement:

Oral: 0.5-0.75 mg/kg/day **or** 20-25 mg/m²/day in divided doses every 8 hours

I.M.: 0.25-0.35 mg/kg/day once daily **or** 12.5 mg/m²/day

Stress coverage for surgery: I.M.: 1 and 2 days before preanesthesia, and 1-3 days after surgery: 50-62.5 mg/m²/day; 4 days after surgery: 31-50 mg/m²/day; 5 days after surgery, resume presurgical corticosteroid dose.

Adults: Oral, I.M.: 25-300 mg/day in divided doses every 12-24 hours

Mechanism of Action Decreases inflammation by suppression of migration of polymorphonuclear leukocytes and reversal of increased capillary permeability

Other Adverse Effects In chronic, long-term use, may result in cushingoid appearance, osteoporosis, muscle weakness (proximal), and suppression of the adrenal-hypothalmic pituitary axis.

>10%:

Central nervous system: Insomnia, nervousness
Gastrointestinal: Increased appetite, indigestion

1% to 10%:

Central nervous system: Dizziness or lightheadedness, headache
Dermatologic: Hirsutism, hypopigmentation
Endocrine & metabolic: Diabetes mellitus
Neuromuscular & skeletal: Arthralgia
Ocular: Cataracts, glaucoma
Respiratory: Epistaxis
Miscellaneous: Sweating

Drug Interactions CYP3A3/4 enzyme substrate

Increased Effect/Toxicity: Estrogens may increase cortisone effects. Cortisone may increase ulcerogenic potential of NSAIDs, and may increase potassium deletion due to diuretics.

Decreased Effect: Enzyme inducers (barbiturates, phenytoin, rifampin) may decrease cortisone effects. Effect of live virus vaccines may be decreased. Anticholinesterase agents may decrease effect of cortisone. Cortisone may decrease effects of warfarin and salicylates.

Drug Uptake

Onset of action: Peak effect: Oral: ~2 hours; I.M.: 20-48 hours
Absorption: Slow
Duration: 30-36 hours
Half-life, elimination: 0.5-2 hours; End-stage renal disease: 3.5 hours
Time to peak: Oral: ≤2 hours; I.M.: 20-48 hours

Pregnancy Risk Factor D

Generic Available Yes

Cortisporin® *see* Neomycin, Polymyxin B, and Hydrocortisone *on page 857*

Cortisporin® Ointment *see* Bacitracin, Neomycin, Polymyxin B, and Hydrocortisone *on page 141*

Cortisporin® Ophthalmic Suspension *see* Neomycin, Polymyxin B, and Hydrocortisone *on page 857*

Cortisporin®-TC Otic *see* Colistin, Neomycin, and Hydrocortisone *on page 322*

Cortizone®-5 [OTC] *see* Hydrocortisone *on page 608*

Cortizone®-10 [OTC] *see* Hydrocortisone *on page 608*

Cortrosyn® *see* Cosyntropin *on page 329*

Corvert® *see* Ibutilide *on page 623*

Cosmegen® *see* Dactinomycin *on page 345*

Cosyntropin (koe sin TROE pin)

U.S. Brand Names Cortrosyn®

Canadian Brand Names Cortrosyn®

Pharmacologic Category Diagnostic Agent

Synonyms Synacthen; Tetracosactide

Use Diagnostic test to differentiate primary adrenal from secondary (pituitary) adrenocortical insufficiency

Local Anesthetic/Vasoconstrictor Precautions No information available to require special precautions

Effects on Dental Treatment No effects or complications reported

Dosage

Adrenocortical insufficiency: I.M., I.V. (over 2 minutes): Peak plasma cortisol concentrations usually occur 45-60 minutes after cosyntropin administration

Children <2 years: 0.125 mg
Children >2 years and Adults: 0.25 mg

When greater cortisol stimulation is needed, an I.V. infusion may be used:

Children >2 years and Adults: 0.25 mg administered at 0.04 mg/hour over 6 hours

Congenital adrenal hyperplasia evaluation: 1 mg/m²/dose up to a maximum of 1 mg

Mechanism of Action Stimulates the adrenal cortex to secrete adrenal steroids (including hydrocortisone, cortisone), androgenic substances, and a small amount of aldosterone

Other Adverse Effects 1% to 10%:

Cardiovascular: Flushing

(Continued)

Cosyntropin *(Continued)*

Central nervous system: Mild fever
Dermatologic: Pruritus
Gastrointestinal: Chronic pancreatitis

Drug Interactions Decreased Effect: May decrease effect of anticholinesterases in patients with myasthenia gravis; nondepolarizing neuromuscular blockers, phenytoin and barbiturates may decrease effect of cosyntropin

Drug Uptake Time to peak: ≤1 hour; plasma cortisol levels rise within 5 minutes of I.M. or IVP administration

Pregnancy Risk Factor C

Generic Available No

Coumadin® *see* Warfarin *on page 1250*

Covera-HS® *see* Verapamil *on page 1236*

Cozaar® *see* Losartan *on page 732*

Creon® *see* Pancrelipase *on page 914*

Creo-Terpin® [OTC] *see* Dextromethorphan *on page 372*

Cresylate® *see* m-Cresyl Acetate *on page 747*

Crinone® *see* Progesterone *on page 1003*

Critic-Aid Skin Care® [OTC] *see* Zinc Oxide *on page 1260*

Crixivan® *see* Indinavir *on page 633*

Crolom® *see* Cromolyn Sodium *on page 330*

Cromolyn Sodium (KROE moe lin SOW dee um)

Related Information

Respiratory Diseases *on page 1328*

U.S. Brand Names Crolom®; Gastrocrom®; Intal®; Nasalcrom® [OTC]; Opticrom®

Canadian Brand Names Apo®-Cromolyn; Intal®; Nalcrom®; Nu-Cromolyn; Opticrom®

Pharmacologic Category Mast Cell Stabilizer

Synonyms Cromoglycic Acid; Disodium Cromoglycate; DSCG

Use Adjunct in the prophylaxis of allergic disorders, including rhinitis, giant papillary conjunctivitis, and asthma; inhalation product may be used for prevention of exercise-induced bronchospasm; systemic mastocytosis, food allergy, and treatment of inflammatory bowel disease; **cromolyn is a prophylactic drug with no benefit for acute situations**

Local Anesthetic/Vasoconstrictor Precautions No information available to require special precautions

Effects on Dental Treatment No effects or complications reported

Dosage

Oral:
- Systemic mastocytosis:
  - Neonates and preterm Infants: Not recommended
  - Infants and Children <2 years: 20 mg/kg/day in 4 divided doses; may increase in patients 6 months to 2 years of age if benefits not seen after 2-3 weeks; do not exceed 30 mg/kg/day
  - Children 2-12 years: 100 mg 4 times/day; not to exceed 40 mg/kg/day
  - Children >12 years and Adults: 200 mg 4 times/day
- Food allergy and inflammatory bowel disease:
  - Children <2 years: Not recommended
  - Children 2-12 years: Initial dose: 100 mg 4 times/day; may double the dose if effect is not satisfactory within 2-3 weeks; not to exceed 40 mg/kg/day
  - Children >12 years and Adults: Initial dose: 200 mg 4 times/day; may double the dose if effect is not satisfactory within 2-3 weeks; up to 400 mg 4 times/day
  - Once desired effect is achieved, dose may be tapered to lowest effective dose

Inhalation:
- For chronic control of asthma, taper frequency to the lowest effective dose (ie, 4 times/day to 3 times/day to twice daily):
  - Nebulization solution: Children >2 years and Adults: Initial: 20 mg 4 times/day; usual dose: 20 mg 3-4 times/day
- Metered spray:
  - Children 5-12 years: Initial: 2 inhalations 4 times/day; usual dose: 1-2 inhalations 3-4 times/day
  - Children ≥12 years and Adults: Initial: 2 inhalations 4 times/day; usual dose: 2-4 inhalations 3-4 times/day
- Prevention of allergen- or exercise-induced bronchospasm: Administer 10-15 minutes prior to exercise or allergen exposure but no longer than 1 hour before:
  - Nebulization solution: Children >2 years and Adults: Single dose of 20 mg
  - Metered spray: Children >5 years and Adults: Single dose of 2 inhalations

Ophthalmic: Children >4 years and Adults: 1-2 drops in each eye 4-6 times/day

Nasal: Allergic rhinitis (treatment and prophylaxis): Children ≥2 years and Adults: 1 spray into each nostril 3-4 times/day; may be increased to 6 times/day (symptomatic relief may require 2-4 weeks)

Mechanism of Action Prevents the mast cell release of histamine, leukotrienes and slow-reacting substance of anaphylaxis by inhibiting degranulation after contact with antigens

Other Adverse Effects

Inhalation:

>10%: Gastrointestinal: Unpleasant taste in mouth

Nasal:

>10%: Respiratory: Increase in sneezing, burning, stinging, or irritation inside of nose

1% to 10%:

Central nervous system: Headache
Gastrointestinal: Unpleasant taste
Respiratory: Hoarseness, coughing, postnasal drip

Ophthalmic:

>10%: Ocular: Burning or stinging of eye

1% to 10%: Ocular: Dryness or puffiness around the eye, watering or itching of eye

Systemic:

>10%:

Central nervous system: Headache
Gastrointestinal: Diarrhea

1% to 10%:

Central nervous system: Insomnia
Dermatologic: Rash
Gastrointestinal: Abdominal pain, nausea
Neuromuscular: Myalgia

Drug Interactions Isoproterenol

Drug Uptake

Absorption: Inhalation: Well absorbed; ~8% reaches the lungs; Oral: 0.5% to 2%
Half-life, elimination: 80-90 minutes
Time to peak: Inhalation: ≤15 minutes

Pregnancy Risk Factor B

Generic Available Yes: Solution for inhalation, Ophthalmic drops

Crotamiton (kroe TAM i tonn)

U.S. Brand Names Eurax® Topical

Mexican Brand Names Eurax®

Pharmacologic Category Scabicidal Agent

Use Treatment of scabies and symptomatic treatment of pruritus

Local Anesthetic/Vasoconstrictor Precautions No information available to require special precautions

Effects on Dental Treatment No effects or complications reported

Dosage Topical:

Scabicide: Children and Adults: Wash thoroughly and scrub away loose scales, then towel dry; apply a thin layer and massage drug onto skin of the entire body from the neck to the toes (with special attention to skin folds, creases, and interdigital spaces). Repeat application in 24 hours. Take a cleansing bath 48 hours after the final application. Treatment may be repeated after 7-10 days if live mites are still present.

Pruritus: Massage into affected areas until medication is completely absorbed; repeat as necessary

Mechanism of Action Unknown; has scabicidal activity against *Sarcoptes scabiei*

Pregnancy Risk Factor C

Generic Available No

Cruex® [OTC] *see* Clotrimazole *on page 312*
Cryselle™ *see* Combination Hormonal Contraceptives *on page 323*
Crystamine® *see* Cyanocobalamin *on page 331*
Crysti 1000® *see* Cyanocobalamin *on page 331*
Crystodigin® [DSC] *see* Digitoxin ***Not Available in U.S.*** *on page 388*
C/T/S® *see* Clindamycin *on page 300*
Cuprimine® *see* Penicillamine *on page 927*
Curosurf® *see* Poractant Alfa *on page 973*
Cutivate™ *see* Fluticasone *on page 525*

Cyanocobalamin (sye an oh koe BAL a min)

U.S. Brand Names Crystamine®; Crysti 1000®; Cyanoject®; Cyomin®; Ener-B®; Nascobal®

Canadian Brand Names Bedoz; Scheinpharm B12

Pharmacologic Category Vitamin, Water Soluble

Synonyms Vitamin B_{12}

Use

Dental: Vitamin B_{12} deficiency
(Continued)

Cyanocobalamin *(Continued)*

Medical: Treatment of pernicious anemia; increased B_{12} requirements due to pregnancy, thyrotoxicosis, hemorrhage, malignancy, liver or kidney disease

Local Anesthetic/Vasoconstrictor Precautions No information available to require special precautions

Effects on Dental Treatment No effects or complications reported

Dosage

Recommended daily allowance (RDA):
- Children: 0.3-2 mcg
- Adults: 2 mcg

Nutritional deficiency:
- Intranasal gel: 500 mcg once weekly
- Oral: 25-250 mcg/day

Anemias: I.M. or deep S.C. (oral is not generally recommended due to poor absorption and I.V. is not recommended due to more rapid elimination):
- Pernicious anemia, congenital (if evidence of neurologic involvement): 1000 mcg/day for at least 2 weeks; maintenance: 50-100 mcg/month or 100 mcg for 6-7 days; if there is clinical improvement, give 100 mcg every other day for 7 doses, then every 3-4 days for 2-3 weeks; follow with 100 mcg/month for life. Administer with folic acid if needed.
  - Children: 30-50 mcg/day for 2 or more weeks (to a total dose of 1000-5000 mcg), then follow with 100 mcg/month as maintenance dosage
  - Adults: 100 mcg/day for 6-7 days; if improvement, administer same dose on alternate days for 7 doses; then every 3-4 days for 2-3 weeks; once hematologic values have returned to normal, maintenance dosage: 100 mcg/month. **Note:** Use only parenteral therapy as oral therapy is not dependable.
- Hematologic remission (without evidence of nervous system involvement): Intranasal gel: 500 mcg once weekly

Vitamin B_{12} deficiency:
- Children:
  - Neurologic signs: 100 mcg/day for 10-15 days (total dose of 1-1.5 mg), then once or twice weekly for several months; may taper to 60 mcg every month
  - Hematologic signs: 10-50 mcg/day for 5-10 days, followed by 100-250 mcg/dose every 2-4 weeks
- Adults: Initial: 30 mcg/day for 5-10 days; maintenance: 100-200 mcg/month

Schilling test: I.M.: 1000 mcg

Mechanism of Action Coenzyme for various metabolic functions, including fat and carbohydrate metabolism and protein synthesis, used in cell replication and hematopoiesis

Other Adverse Effects

1% to 10%:
- Central nervous system: Headache (2% to 11%), anxiety, dizziness, pain, nervousness, hypoesthesia
- Dermatologic: Itching
- Gastrointestinal: Sore throat, nausea and vomiting, dyspepsia, diarrhea
- Neuromuscular & skeletal: Weakness (1% to 4%), back pain, arthritis, myalgia, paresthesia, abnormal gait
- Respiratory: Dyspnea, rhinitis

<1%: Peripheral vascular thrombosis, urticaria, anaphylaxis, CHF, pulmonary edema

Contraindications Hypersensitivity to cyanocobalamin, cobalt, or any component of their formulation; hereditary optic nerve atrophy; Leber's disease

Warnings/Precautions I.M. route used to treat pernicious anemia; vitamin B_{12} deficiency for >3 months results in irreversible degenerative CNS lesions; treatment of vitamin B_{12} megaloblastic anemia may result in severe hypokalemia, sometimes, fatal, when anemia corrects due to cellular potassium requirements. B_{12} deficiency masks signs of polycythemia vera; vegetarian diets may result in B_{12} deficiency; pernicious anemia occurs more often in gastric carcinoma than in general population.

Drug Interactions Decreased Effect: Neomycin, colchicine, anticonvulsants may decrease absorption; chloramphenicol may decrease B_{12} effects

Dietary/Ethanol/Herb Considerations Ethanol decreases B_{12} absorption.

Drug Uptake Absorption: Absorbed from the terminal ileum in the presence of calcium; for absorption to occur gastric "intrinsic factor" must be present to transfer the compound across the intestinal mucosa

Pregnancy Risk Factor A/C (dose exceeding RDA recommendation); C (nasal gel)

Dosage Forms GEL, intranasal (Nascobal®): 500 mcg/0.1 mL (5 mL). **INJ:** 100 mcg/mL (1 mL, 10 mL, 30 mL); 1000 mcg/mL (1 mL, 10 mL, 30 mL). **TAB [OTC]:** 25 mcg, 50 mcg, 100 mcg, 250 mcg, 500 mcg, 1000 mcg

Generic Available Yes

Cyanoject® *see* Cyanocobalamin *on page 331*

Cyclandelate (sye KLAN de late)

Pharmacologic Category Vasodilator

Use Considered as "possibly effective" for adjunctive therapy in peripheral vascular disease and possibly senility due to cerebrovascular disease or multi-infarct dementia; migraine prophylaxis, vertigo, tinnitus, and visual disturbances secondary to cerebrovascular insufficiency and diabetic peripheral polyneuropathy

Local Anesthetic/Vasoconstrictor Precautions No information available to require special precautions

Effects on Dental Treatment No effects or complications reported

Dosage Adults: Oral: Initial: 1.2-1.6 g/day in divided doses before meals and at bedtime until response; maintenance therapy: 400-800 mg/day in 2-4 divided doses; start with lowest dose in elderly due to hypotensive potential; decrease dose by 200 mg decrements to achieve minimal maintenance dose; improvement can usually be seen over weeks of therapy and prolonged use; short courses of therapy are usually ineffective and not recommended

Mechanism of Action Cyclandelate, 3,3,5-trimethylcyclohexyl mandelate is a vasodilator that exerts a direct, papaverine-like action on smooth muscles, particularly that found within the blood vessels. Animal data indicate that cyclandelate also has antispasmodic properties; exhibits no adrenergic stimulation or blocking action; action exceeds that of papaverine; mild calcium channel blocking agent, may benefit in mild hypercalcemia; calcium channel blocking activity may explain some of its pharmacologic effects (enhanced blood flow) and inhibition of platelet aggregation.

Drug Interactions May enhance action of drugs causing vasodilation/hypotension

Pregnancy Risk Factor C

Generic Available Yes

Cyclessa® *see* Combination Hormonal Contraceptives *on page 323*

Cyclizine (SYE kli zeen)

U.S. Brand Names Marezine® [OTC]

Pharmacologic Category Antihistamine

Synonyms Cyclizine Hydrochloride; Cyclizine Lactate

Use Prevention and treatment of nausea, vomiting, and vertigo associated with motion sickness; control of postoperative nausea and vomiting

Local Anesthetic/Vasoconstrictor Precautions No information available to require special precautions

Effects on Dental Treatment >10%: Xerostomia

Dosage

Children 6-12 years:

- Oral: 25 mg up to 3 times/day
- I.M.: Not recommended

Adults:

- Oral: 50 mg taken 30 minutes before departure, may repeat in 4-6 hours if needed, up to 200 mg/day
- I.M.: 50 mg every 4-6 hours as needed

Mechanism of Action A piperazine derivative with properties of histamines; mechanism in inhibiting the symptoms of motion sickness is not known. It may have effects directly on the labyrinthine apparatus and central actions on the labyrinthine apparatus and on the chemoreceptor trigger zone. Cyclizine exerts a central anticholinergic action.

Other Adverse Effects

>10%:

- Central nervous system: Drowsiness
- Gastrointestinal: Xerostomia

1% to 10%:

- Central nervous system: Headache
- Dermatologic: Dermatitis
- Gastrointestinal: Nausea
- Genitourinary: Urinary retention
- Ocular: Diplopia
- Renal: Polyuria

Drug Interactions Increased effect/toxicity with CNS depressants

Pregnancy Risk Factor B

Generic Available No

Cyclobenzaprine (sye kloe BEN za preen)

Related Information

Temporomandibular Dysfunction (TMD) *on page 1397*

U.S. Brand Names Flexeril®

Canadian Brand Names Apo®-Cyclobenzaprine; Flexeril®; Flexitec; Gen-Cyclobenzaprine; Novo-Cycloprine®; Nu-Cyclobenzaprine

Pharmacologic Category Skeletal Muscle Relaxant

Synonyms Cyclobenzaprine Hydrochloride

(Continued)

Cyclobenzaprine *(Continued)*

Use

Dental: Treatment of muscle spasm associated with acute temporomandibular joint pain

Medical: Treatment of muscle spasm associated with acute painful musculoskeletal conditions; supportive therapy in tetanus

Local Anesthetic/Vasoconstrictor Precautions No information available to require special precautions

Effects on Dental Treatment >10%: Xerostomia

Dosage Oral: **Note:** Do not use longer than 2-3 weeks

Children: Dosage has not been established

Adults: 20-40 mg/day in 2-4 divided doses; maximum dose: 60 mg/day

Mechanism of Action Centrally-acting skeletal muscle relaxant pharmacologically related to tricyclic antidepressants; reduces tonic somatic motor activity influencing both alpha and gamma motor neurons

Other Adverse Effects

>10%:

- Central nervous system: Drowsiness, dizziness, lightheadedness
- Gastrointestinal: Xerostomia

1% to 10%:

- Cardiovascular: Edema of the face/lips, syncope
- Gastrointestinal: Bloated feeling
- Genitourinary: Problems in urinating, polyuria
- Hepatic: Hepatitis
- Neuromuscular & skeletal: Problems in speaking, muscle weakness
- Ocular: Blurred vision
- Otic: Tinnitus

<1%: Tachycardia, hypotension, arrhythmia, headache, fatigue, nervousness, confusion, ataxia, rash, dermatitis, dyspepsia, nausea, constipation, stomach cramps, unpleasant taste

Contraindications Hypersensitivity to cyclobenzaprine or any component of the formulation; concomitant use with or within 14 days of MAO inhibitors; hyperthyroidism; CHF or arrhythmias

Warnings/Precautions Cyclobenzaprine shares the toxic potentials of the tricyclic antidepressants and the usual precautions of tricyclic antidepressant therapy should be observed; use with caution in patients with urinary hesitancy or angle-closure glaucoma

Drug Interactions CYP1A2, 2D6, and 3A3/4 enzyme substrate

Increased Toxicity: Do not use concomitantly or within 14 days after MAO inhibitors. Because of similarities to the tricyclic antidepressants, may have additive toxicities. Use caution with other anticholinergics due to additive anticholinergic action of cyclobenzaprine. Effects of barbiturates and other CNS depressants may be enhanced.

Dietary/Ethanol/Herb Considerations

Ethanol: Avoid use; may increase CNS depression.

Herb/Nutraceutical: Avoid gotu kola, kava, SAMe, and valerian; may increase CNS depression. Avoid St John's wort; may decrease serum concentration and increase CNS depression.

Drug Uptake

Onset of action: ~1 hour

Absorption: Oral: Completely

Duration: 8 to >24 hours

Half-life, elimination: 1-3 days

Time to peak: 3-8 hours

Pregnancy Risk Factor B

Dosage Forms TAB: 10 mg

Generic Available Yes

Cyclocort® *see* Amcinonide *on page 65*

Cyclogyl® *see* Cyclopentolate *on page 334*

Cyclomydril® *see* Cyclopentolate and Phenylephrine *on page 335*

Cyclopentolate (sye kloe PEN toe late)

U.S. Brand Names AK-Pentolate®; Cyclogyl®; I-Pentolate®

Canadian Brand Names Cyclogyl®; Diopentolate®

Pharmacologic Category Anticholinergic Agent, Ophthalmic

Synonyms Cyclopentolate Hydrochloride

Use Diagnostic procedures requiring mydriasis and cycloplegia

Local Anesthetic/Vasoconstrictor Precautions No information available to require special precautions

Effects on Dental Treatment No effects or complications reported

Dosage

Children: Instill 1 drop of 0.5%, 1%, or 2% in eye followed by 1 drop of 0.5% or 1% in 5 minutes, if necessary

Adults: Instill 1 drop of 1% followed by another drop in 5 minutes; 2% solution in heavily pigmented iris

Mechanism of Action Prevents the muscle of the ciliary body and the sphincter muscle of the iris from responding to cholinergic stimulation, causing mydriasis and cycloplegia

Other Adverse Effects 1% to 10%:

Cardiovascular: Tachycardia

Central nervous system: Restlessness, hallucinations, psychosis, hyperactivity, seizures, incoherent speech, ataxia

Dermatologic: Burning sensation

Ocular: Increase in intraocular pressure, loss of visual accommodation

Miscellaneous: Allergic reaction

Drug Interactions Carbachol and/or cholinesterase inhibitor effects may be decreased with concurrent use.

Drug Uptake

Onset of action: Peak effect: Cycloplegia: 25-75 minutes; Mydriasis: 30-60 minutes

Duration: ≤24 hours

Pregnancy Risk Factor C

Generic Available Yes

Comments Pilocarpine ophthalmic drops applied after the examination may reduce recovery time to 3-6 hours

Cyclopentolate and Phenylephrine

(sye kloe PEN toe late & fen il EF rin)

U.S. Brand Names Cyclomydril®

Pharmacologic Category Ophthalmic Agent, Antiglaucoma

Synonyms Phenylephrine and Cyclopentolate

Use Induce mydriasis greater than that produced with cyclopentolate HCl alone

Local Anesthetic/Vasoconstrictor Precautions No information available to require special precautions

Effects on Dental Treatment No effects or complications reported

Dosage Ophthalmic: Neonates, Infants, Children, and Adults: Instill 1 drop into the eye every 5-10 minutes, for up to 3 doses, approximately 40-50 minutes before the examination

Drug Uptake See Cyclopentolate *on page 334* and Phenylephrine *on page 950*

Pregnancy Risk Factor C

Generic Available No

Cyclophosphamide (sye kloe FOS fa mide)

U.S. Brand Names Cytoxan®; Neosar®

Canadian Brand Names Cytoxan®; Procytox®

Mexican Brand Names Genoxal; Ledoxina

Pharmacologic Category Antineoplastic Agent, Alkylating Agent

Synonyms CPM; CTX; CYT; NSC-26271

Use Treatment of Hodgkin's and non-Hodgkin's lymphoma, Burkitt's lymphoma, chronic lymphocytic leukemia, chronic granulocytic leukemia, AML, ALL, mycosis fungoides, breast cancer, multiple myeloma, neuroblastoma, retinoblastoma, rhabdomyosarcoma, Ewing's sarcoma; testicular, endometrium and ovarian, and lung cancer, and as a conditioning regimen for BMT; prophylaxis of rejection for kidney, heart, liver, and BMT transplants, severe rheumatoid disorders, nephrotic syndrome, Wegener's granulomatosis, idiopathic pulmonary hemosideroses, myasthenia gravis, multiple sclerosis, systemic lupus erythematosus, lupus nephritis, autoimmune hemolytic anemia, idiopathic thrombocytic purpura, macroglobulinemia, and antibody-induced pure red cell aplasia

Local Anesthetic/Vasoconstrictor Precautions No information available to require special precautions

Effects on Dental Treatment No effects or complications reported

Dosage See individual protocols.

Children: I.V.:

SLE: 500-750 mg/m^2 every month; maximum dose: 1 g/m^2

JRA/vasculitis: 10 mg/kg every 2 weeks

Children and Adults:

Nephrotic syndrome: Oral: 2-3 mg/kg/day every day for up to 12 weeks when corticosteroids are unsuccessful

Mechanism of Action Interferes with the normal function of DNA by alkylation and cross-linking the strands of DNA, and by possible protein modification; cyclophosphamide also possesses potent immunosuppressive activity; note that cyclophosphamide must be metabolized to its active form in the liver

Other Adverse Effects

>10%:

Dermatologic: Alopecia (40% to 60%) but hair will usually regrow although it may be a different color and/or texture. Hair loss usually begins 3-6 weeks after the start of therapy.

(Continued)

Cyclophosphamide *(Continued)*

Endocrine & metabolic: Fertility: May cause sterility; interferes with oogenesis and spermatogenesis; may be irreversible in some patients; gonadal suppression (amenorrhea)

Gastrointestinal: Nausea and vomiting occur more frequently with larger doses, usually beginning 6-10 hours after administration; anorexia, diarrhea, mucositis, and stomatitis are also seen

Genitourinary: Severe, potentially fatal acute hemorrhagic cystitis or urinary fibrosis, believed to be a result of chemical irritation of the bladder by acrolein, a cyclophosphamide metabolite, occurs in 7% to 12% of patients and has been reported in up to 40% of patients in some series. Patients should be encouraged to drink plenty of fluids (3-4 L/day) during therapy, void frequently, and avoid taking the drug at night. With large I.V. doses, I.V. hydration is usually recommended. The use of mesna and/or continuous bladder irrigation is rarely needed for doses <2 g/m^2.

Hematologic: Thrombocytopenia and anemia are less common than leukopenia
- Onset: 7 days
- Nadir: 10-14 days
- Recovery: 21 days

1% to 10%:

Central nervous system: Headache

Dermatologic: Skin rash, facial flushing

Renal: SIADH may occur, usually with doses >50 mg/kg (or 1 g/m^2); renal tubular necrosis, which usually resolves with discontinuation of the drug, is also reported

Respiratory: Nasal congestion occurs when I.V. doses are administered too rapidly (large doses via 30-60 minute infusion); patients experience runny eyes, rhinorrhea, sinus congestion, and sneezing during or immediately after the infusion. If needed, a decongestant or decongestant/antihistamine (eg, pseudoephedrine or pseudoephedrine/triprolidine) can be used to prevent or relieve these symptoms.

Drug Interactions CYP2B6, 2D6, and 3A3/4 enzyme substrate

Increased Effect/Toxicity: Allopurinol may cause an increase in bone marrow depression and may result in significant elevations of cyclophosphamide cytotoxic metabolites. Cyclophosphamide reduces serum pseudocholinesterase concentrations and may prolong the neuromuscular blocking activity of succinylcholine; use with caution with halothane, nitrous oxide, and succinylcholine. Chloramphenicol causes prolonged cyclophosphamide half-life and increased toxicity. Doxorubicin: Cyclophosphamide may enhance cardiac toxicity of anthracyclines. Phenobarbital and phenytoin induce hepatic enzymes and cause a more rapid production of cyclophosphamide metabolites with a concurrent decrease in the serum half-life of the parent compound. Tetrahydrocannabinol results in enhanced immunosuppression in animal studies. Thiazide diuretics: Leukopenia may be prolonged.

Decreased Effect: May decrease digoxin serum concentration. Cimetidine inhibits hepatic metabolism of drugs and may decrease the activation of cyclophosphamide.

Drug Uptake

Absorption: Oral: Well absorbed

Half-life, elimination: 4-8 hours

Time to peak: Oral: ~1 hour

Pregnancy Risk Factor D

Generic Available Yes

CycloSERINE (sye kloe SER een)

Related Information

Nonviral Infectious Diseases *on page 1342*

U.S. Brand Names Seromycin® Pulvules®

Pharmacologic Category Antibiotic, Miscellaneous; Antitubercular Agent

Use Adjunctive treatment in pulmonary or extrapulmonary tuberculosis; treatment of acute urinary tract infections caused by *E. coli* or *Enterobacter* sp when less toxic conventional therapy has failed or is contraindicated

Local Anesthetic/Vasoconstrictor Precautions No information available to require special precautions

Effects on Dental Treatment No effects or complications reported

Dosage Some of the neurotoxic effects may be relieved or prevented by the concomitant administration of pyridoxine

Tuberculosis: Oral:

Children: 10-20 mg/kg/day in 2 divided doses up to 1000 mg/day for 18-24 months

Adults: Initial: 250 mg every 12 hours for 14 days, then give 500 mg to 1 g/day in 2 divided doses for 18-24 months (maximum daily dose: 1 g)

Mechanism of Action Inhibits bacterial cell wall synthesis by competing with amino acid (D-alanine) for incorporation into the bacterial cell wall; bacteriostatic or bactericidal

Other Adverse Effects Frequency not defined:

Cardiovascular: Cardiac arrhythmias

Central nervous system: Drowsiness, headache, dizziness, vertigo, seizures, confusion, psychosis, paresis, coma

Dermatologic: Rash

Endocrine & metabolic: Vitamin B_{12} deficiency

Hematologic: Folate deficiency

Hepatic: Liver enzymes increased

Neuromuscular & skeletal: Tremor

Drug Interactions Increased Effect/Toxicity: Isoniazid and ethionamide increase toxicity of cycloserine. Cycloserine inhibits the hepatic metabolism of phenytoin and may increase risk of epileptic seizures.

Drug Uptake

Absorption: Oral: ~70% to 90% from the GI tract

Half-life, elimination (dependent on renal function): 10 hours

Time to peak: Oral: 3-4 hours

Pregnancy Risk Factor C

Generic Available No

CycloSPORINE (SYE kloe spor een)

U.S. Brand Names Gengraf™; Neoral®; Sandimmune®

Canadian Brand Names Neoral®; Sandimmune® I.V.

Mexican Brand Names Consupren; Sandimmun Neoral®

Pharmacologic Category Immunosuppressant Agent

Synonyms CSA; CyA; Cyclosporin A

Use Prophylaxis of organ rejection in kidney, liver, and heart transplants, has been used with azathioprine and/or corticosteroids; severe, active rheumatoid arthritis (RA) not responsive to methotrexate alone; severe, recalcitrant plaque psoriasis in nonimmunocompromised adults unresponsive to or unable to tolerate other systemic therapy

Unlabeled/Investigational: Short-term, high-dose cyclosporine as a modulator of multidrug resistance in cancer treatment; allogenic bone marrow transplants for prevention and treatment of graft-versus-host disease; also used in some cases of severe autoimmune disease (ie, SLE, myasthenia gravis) that are resistant to corticosteroids and other therapy; focal segmental glomerulosclerosis

Local Anesthetic/Vasoconstrictor Precautions No information available to require special precautions

Effects on Dental Treatment Gingival hypertrophy

Dosage Neoral® and Sandimmune® are not bioequivalent and cannot be used interchangeably.

Children: Transplant: Refer to adult dosing; children may require, and are able to tolerate, larger doses than adults

Adults:

Newly-transplanted patients: Adjunct therapy with corticosteroids is recommended. Initial dose should be given 4-12 hours prior to transplant or may be given postoperatively; adjust initial dose to achieve desired plasma concentration

Oral: Dose is dependent upon type of transplant and formulation:

Cyclosporine (modified):

Renal: 9 ± 3 mg/kg/day, divided twice daily

Liver: 8 ± 4 mg/kg/day, divided twice daily

Heart: 7 ± 3 mg/kg/day, divided twice daily

Cyclosporine (nonmodified): Initial dose: 15 mg/kg/day as a single dose (range 14-18 mg/kg); lower doses of 10-14 mg/kg/day have been used for renal transplants. Continue initial dose daily for 1-2 weeks; taper by 5% per week to a maintenance dose of 5-10 mg/kg/day; some renal transplant patients may be dosed as low as 3 mg/kg/day

When using the nonmodified formulation, cyclosporine levels may increase in liver transplant patients when the T-tube is closed; dose may need decreased

I.V.: Cyclosporine (nonmodified): Initial dose: 5-6 mg/kg/day as a single dose ($^1/_3$ the oral dose), infused over 2-6 hours; use should be limited to patients unable to take capsules or oral solution; patients should be switched to an oral dosage form as soon as possible

Conversion to cyclosporine (modified) from cyclosporine (nonmodified): Start with daily dose previously used and adjust to obtain preconversion cyclosporine trough concentration. Plasma concentrations should be monitored every 4-7 days and dose adjusted as necessary, until desired trough level is obtained. When transferring patients with previously poor absorption of cyclosporine (nonmodified), monitor trough levels at least twice weekly (especially if initial dose exceeds 10 mg/kg/day); high plasma concentrations are likely to occur.

Rheumatoid arthritis: Oral: Cyclosporine (modified): Initial dose: 2.5 mg/kg/day, divided twice daily; salicylates, NSAIDs, and oral glucocorticoids may be

(Continued)

CycloSPORINE *(Continued)*

continued (refer to Drug Interactions); dose may be increased by 0.5-0.75 mg/kg/day if insufficient response is seen after 8 weeks of treatment; additional dosage increases may be made again at 12 weeks (maximum dose: 4 mg/kg/day). Discontinue if no benefit is seen by 16 weeks of therapy.

Note: Increase the frequency of BP monitoring after each alteration in dosage of cyclosporine. Cyclosporine dosage should be decreased by 25% to 50% in patients with no history of hypertension who develop sustained hypertension during therapy and, if hypertension persists, treatment with cyclosporine should be discontinued.

Psoriasis: Oral: Cyclosporine (modified): Initial dose: 2.5 mg/kg/day, divided twice daily; dose may be increased by 0.5 mg/kg/day if insufficient response is seen after 4 weeks of treatment. Additional dosage increases may be made every 2 weeks if needed; (maximum dose: 4 mg/kg/day). Discontinue if no benefit is seen by 6 weeks of therapy. Once patients are adequately controlled, the dose should be decreased to the lowest effective dose. Doses lower than 2.5 mg/kg/day may be effective. Treatment longer than 1 year is not recommended.

Note: Increase the frequency of BP monitoring after each alteration in dosage of cyclosporine. Cyclosporine dosage should be decreased by 25% to 50% in patients with no history of hypertension who develop sustained hypertension during therapy and, if hypertension persists, treatment with cyclosporine should be discontinued.

Focal segmental glomerulosclerosis: Initial: 3 mg/kg/day divided every 12 hours

Autoimmune diseases: 1-3 mg/kg/day

Dosage adjustment in renal impairment: For severe psoriasis:

Serum creatinine levels ≥25% above pretreatment levels: Take another sample within 2 weeks; if the level remains ≥25% above pretreatment levels, decrease dosage of cyclosporine (modified) by 25% to 50%. If 2 dosage adjustments do not reverse the increase in serum creatinine levels, treatment should be discontinued.

Serum creatinine levels ≥50% above pretreatment levels: Decrease cyclosporine dosage by 25% to 50%. If 2 dosage adjustments do not reverse the increase in serum creatinine levels, treatment should be discontinued.

Hemodialysis/peritoneal dialysis: Supplemental dose is not necessary.

Dosage adjustment in hepatic impairment: Probably necessary; monitor levels closely

Mechanism of Action Inhibition of production and release of interleukin II and inhibits interleukin II-induced activation of resting T-lymphocytes

Other Adverse Effects Adverse reactions reported with kidney, liver, and heart transplantation, unless otherwise noted. Although percentage is reported for specific condition, reaction may occur in anyone taking cyclosporine. Reactions reported for rheumatoid arthritis (RA) are based on cyclosporine (modified) 2.5 mg/kg/day versus placebo.

>10%:

- Cardiovascular: Hypertension (13% to 53%; psoriasis 25% to 27%)
- Central nervous system: Headache (2% to 15%; RA 17%, psoriasis 14% to 16%)
- Dermatologic: Hirsutism (21% to 45%), hypertrichosis (RA 19%)
- Endocrine & metabolic: Increased triglycerides (psoriasis 15%), female reproductive disorder (psoriasis 8% to 11%)
- Gastrointestinal: Nausea (RA 23%), diarrhea (RA 12%), gum hyperplasia (4% to 16%), abdominal discomfort (RA 15%), dyspepsia (RA 12%)
- Neuromuscular & skeletal: Tremor (12% to 55%)
- Renal: Renal dysfunction/nephropathy (25% to 38%; RA 10%, psoriasis 21%), creatinine elevation ≥50% (RA 24%), increased creatinine (psoriasis 16% to 20%)
- Respiratory: Upper respiratory infection (psoriasis 8% to 11%)
- Miscellaneous: Infection (psoriasis 24% to 25%)

Kidney, liver, and heart transplant only (≤2% unless otherwise noted):

- Cardiovascular: Flushes (<1% to 4%), myocardial infarction
- Central nervous system: Convulsions (1% to 5%), anxiety, confusion, fever, lethargy
- Dermatologic: Acne (1% to 6%), brittle fingernails, hair breaking, pruritus
- Endocrine & metabolic: Gynecomastia (<1% to 4%), hyperglycemia
- Gastrointestinal: Nausea (2% to 10%), vomiting (2% to 10%), diarrhea (3% to 8%), abdominal discomfort (<1% to 7%), cramps (0% to 4%), anorexia, constipation, gastritis, mouth sores, pancreatitis, swallowing difficulty, upper GI bleed, weight loss
- Hematologic: Leukopenia (<1% to 6%), anemia, thrombocytopenia
- Hepatic: Hepatotoxicity (<1% to 7%)
- Neuromuscular & skeletal: Paresthesia (1% to 3%), joint pain, muscle pain, tingling, weakness
- Ocular: Conjunctivitis, visual disturbance
- Otic: Hearing loss, tinnitus
- Renal: Hematuria
- Respiratory: Sinusitis (<1% to 7%)

Miscellaneous: Lymphoma (<1% to 6%), allergic reactions, hiccups, night sweats

Rheumatoid arthritis only (1% to <3% unless otherwise noted):

Cardiovascular: Hypertension (8%), edema (5%), chest pain (4%), arrhythmia (2%), abnormal heart sounds, cardiac failure, myocardial infarction, peripheral ischemia

Central nervous system: Dizziness (8%), pain (6%), insomnia (4%), depression (3%), migraine (2%), anxiety, hypoesthesia, emotional lability, impaired concentration, malaise, nervousness, paranoia, somnolence, vertigo

Dermatologic: Purpura (3%), abnormal pigmentation, angioedema, cellulitis, dermatitis, dry skin, eczema, folliculitis, nail disorder, pruritus, skin disorder, urticaria

Endocrine & metabolic: Menstrual disorder (3%), breast fibroadenosis, breast pain, diabetes mellitus, goiter, hot flashes, hyperkalemia, hyperuricemia, hypoglycemia, libido increased/decreased

Gastrointestinal: Vomiting (9%), flatulence (5%), gingivitis (4%), gum hyperplasia (2%), constipation, xerostomia, dysphagia, enanthema, eructation, esophagitis, gastric ulcer, gastritis, gastroenteritis, gingival bleeding, glossitis, peptic ulcer, salivary gland enlargement, taste perversion, tongue disorder, tooth disorder, weight loss/gain

Genitourinary: Leukorrhea (1%), abnormal urine, micturition urgency, nocturia, polyuria, pyelonephritis, urinary incontinence, uterine hemorrhage

Hematologic: Anemia, leukopenia

Hepatic: Bilirubinemia

Neuromuscular & skeletal: Paresthesia (8%), tremor (8%), leg cramps/muscle contractions (2%), arthralgia, bone fracture, joint dislocation, myalgia, neuropathy, stiffness, synovial cyst, tendon disorder, weakness

Ocular: Abnormal vision, cataract, conjunctivitis, eye pain

Otic: Tinnitus, deafness, vestibular disorder

Renal: Increased BUN, hematuria, renal abscess

Respiratory: Cough (5%), dyspnea (5%), sinusitis (4%), abnormal chest sounds, bronchospasm, epistaxis

Miscellaneous: Infection (9%), abscess, allergy, bacterial infection, carcinoma, fungal infection, herpes simplex, herpes zoster, lymphadenopathy, moniliasis, diaphoresis increased, tonsillitis, viral infection

Psoriasis only (1% to <3% unless otherwise noted):

Cardiovascular: Chest pain, flushes

Central nervous system: Psychiatric events (4% to 5%), pain (3% to 4%), dizziness, fever, insomnia, nervousness, vertigo

Dermatologic: Hypertrichosis (5% to 7%), acne, dry skin, folliculitis, keratosis, pruritus, rash, skin malignancies

Endocrine & metabolic: Hot flashes

Gastrointestinal: Nausea (5% to 6%), diarrhea (5% to 6%), gum hyperplasia (4% to 6%), abdominal discomfort (3% to 6%), dyspepsia (2% to 3%), abdominal distention, appetite increased, constipation, gingival bleeding

Genitourinary: Micturition increased

Hematologic: Bleeding disorder, clotting disorder, platelet disorder, red blood cell disorder

Hepatic: Hyperbilirubinemia

Neuromuscular & skeletal: Paresthesia (5% to 7%), arthralgia (1% to 6%)

Ocular: Abnormal vision

Respiratory: Bronchospasm (5%), cough (5%), dyspnea (5%), rhinitis (5%), respiratory infection

Miscellaneous: Flu-like symptoms (8% to 10%)

Contraindications Hypersensitivity to cyclosporine or any component of the formulation

In treatment for rheumatoid arthritis and psoriasis: Abnormal renal function; uncontrolled hypertension; malignancies; concomitant treatment with PUVA or UVB therapy, methotrexate, other immunosuppressive agents, coal tar, or radiation therapy

Drug Interactions CYP3A3/4 enzyme substrate; CYP3A3/4 enzyme inhibitor

Increased Effect/Toxicity:

Drugs that increase cyclosporine concentrations: Allopurinol, metoclopramide, nicardipine, octreotide

CYP3A3/4 inhibitors: Serum level and/or toxicity of cyclosporine may be increased. Inhibitors include amiodarone, bromocriptine, cimetidine, clarithromycin, danazol, erythromycin, delavirdine, diltiazem, disulfiram, fluconazole, fluoxetine, fluvoxamine, indinavir, itraconazole, ketoconazole, nefazodone, nevirapine, propoxyphene, quinupristin-dalfopristin, ritonavir, saquinavir, verapamil, zafirlukast, zileuton.

Drugs that enhance nephrotoxicity of cyclosporine: Aminoglycosides, amphotericin B, acyclovir, cimetidine, ketoconazole, lovastatin, melphalan, NSAIDs, ranitidine, trimethoprim and sulfamethoxazole, tacrolimus

Cyclosporine increases toxicity of: Digoxin, diuretics, methotrexate, nifedipine

(Continued)

CycloSPORINE *(Continued)*

Voriconazole: Cyclosporine serum concentrations may be increased; monitor serum concentrations and renal function. Decrease cyclosporine dosage by 50% when initiating voriconazole.

Decreased Effect:

Drugs that decrease cyclosporine concentrations: Carbamazepine, nafcillin, phenobarbital, phenytoin, rifampin, isoniazid, ticlopidine

Cyclosporine decreases effect of: Live vaccines

Drug Uptake

Absorption: Oral:

Cyclosporine (nonmodified): Erratically and incompletely absorbed; dependent on presence of food, bile acids, and GI motility; larger oral doses are needed in pediatrics due to shorter bowel length and limited intestinal absorption

Cyclosporine (modified): Erratically and incompletely absorbed; increased absorption, up to 30% when compared to cyclosporine (nonmodified); absorption less dependent on food, bile acids, or GI motility when compared to cyclosporine (nonmodified)

Half-life, elimination: Oral: May be prolonged in patients with hepatic dysfunction and lower in pediatric patients due to the higher metabolism rate

Cyclosporine (nonmodified): Biphasic: Alpha: 1.4 hours; Terminal: 19 hours (range: 10-27 hours)

Cyclosporine (modified): Biphasic: Terminal: 8.4 hours (range: 5-18 hours)

Time to peak: Oral:

Cyclosporine (nonmodified): 2-6 hours; some patients have a second peak at 5-6 hours

Cyclosporine (modified): Renal transplant: 1.5-2 hours

Pregnancy Risk Factor C

Generic Available Yes

Comments Cyclosporine serum levels are likely to be increased with clarithromycin or erythromycin administration. Toxic cyclosporine concentrations and renal toxicity may result. Clarithromycin inhibits the CYP3A4 enzyme which metabolizes cyclosporine. Azithromycin (Zithromax®) and dirithromycin (Dynabac®) are unlikely to interact with cyclosporine.

Selected Readings

Ferrari SL, Goffin E, Mourad M, et al, "The Interaction Between Clarithromycin and Cyclosporine in Kidney Transplant Recipients," *Transplantation*, 1994, 58(6):725-7.

Harnett JD, Parfrey PS, Paul MD, et al, "Erythromycin-Cyclosporine Interaction in Renal Transplant Recipients," *Transplantation*, 1987, 43(2):316-8.

Cycofed® Pediatric *see* Guaifenesin, Pseudoephedrine, and Codeine *on page 570*

Cyklokapron® *see* Tranexamic Acid *on page 1190*

Cylert® *see* Pemoline *on page 925*

Cylex® [OTC] *see* Benzocaine *on page 151*

Cyomin® *see* Cyanocobalamin *on page 331*

Cyproheptadine (si proe HEP ta deen)

U.S. Brand Names Periactin®

Canadian Brand Names Periactin®

Mexican Brand Names Viternum®

Pharmacologic Category Antihistamine

Synonyms Cyproheptadine Hydrochloride

Use Perennial and seasonal allergic rhinitis and other allergic symptoms including urticaria; its off-labeled uses have included appetite stimulation, blepharospasm, cluster headaches, migraine headaches, Nelson's syndrome, pruritus, schizophrenia, spinal cord damage associated spasticity, and tardive dyskinesia

Local Anesthetic/Vasoconstrictor Precautions No information available to require special precautions

Effects on Dental Treatment No effects or complications reported

Dosage Oral:

Children: 0.25 mg/kg/day in 2-3 divided doses or 8 mg/m^2/day in 2-3 divided doses

2-6 years: 2 mg every 8-12 hours (not to exceed 12 mg/day)

7-14 years: 4 mg every 8-12 hours (not to exceed 16 mg/day)

Adults: 4-20 mg/day divided every 8 hours (not to exceed 0.5 mg/kg/day) in patients with significant hepatic dysfunction

Mechanism of Action A potent antihistamine and serotonin antagonist, competes with histamine for H_1-receptor sites on effector cells in the GI tract, blood vessels, and respiratory tract

Other Adverse Effects

>10%:

Central nervous system: Slight to moderate drowsiness

Respiratory: Thickening of bronchial secretions

1% to 10%:

Central nervous system: Headache, fatigue, nervousness, dizziness

Gastrointestinal: Appetite stimulation, nausea, diarrhea, abdominal pain, xerostomia

Neuromuscular & skeletal: Arthralgia
Respiratory: Pharyngitis

Drug Interactions Increased Effect/Toxicity: May potentiate the effect of CNS depressants; MAO inhibitors may cause hallucinations

Pregnancy Risk Factor B

Generic Available Yes

Cystadane® *see* Betaine Anhydrous *on page 158*

Cystagon® *see* Cysteamine *on page 341*

Cysteamine (sis TEE a meen)

U.S. Brand Names Cystagon®

Pharmacologic Category Anticystine Agent; Urinary Tract Product

Synonyms Cysteamine Bitartrate

Use Orphan drug: Treatment of nephropathic cystinosis

Local Anesthetic/Vasoconstrictor Precautions No information available to require special precautions

Effects on Dental Treatment No effects or complications reported

Dosage Initiate therapy with 1/4 to 1/8 of maintenance dose; titrate slowly upward over 4-6 weeks

Children <12 years: Oral: Maintenance: 1.3 g/m^2/day divided into 4 doses

Children >12 years and Adults (>110 lb): 2 g/day in 4 divided doses; dosage may in increased to 1.95 g/m^2/day if cystine levels are <1 nmol/1/2 cystine/mg protein, although intolerance and incidence of adverse events may be increased

Mechanism of Action Reacts with cystine in the lysosome to convert it to cysteine and to a cysteine-cysteamine mixed disulfide, both of which can then exit the lysosome in patients with cystinosis, an inherited defect of lysosomal transport

Other Adverse Effects

>5%:

- Central nervous system: Fever, lethargy (11%)
- Dermatologic: Rash (7%)
- Gastrointestinal: Vomiting (35%), anorexia (31%), diarrhea (16%)

<5%:

- Cardiovascular: Hypertension
- Central nervous system: Somnolence, encephalopathy, headache, seizures, ataxia, confusion, dizziness, jitteriness, nervousness, impaired cognition, emotional changes, hallucinations, nightmares
- Dermatologic: Urticaria
- Endocrine & metabolic: Dehydration
- Gastrointestinal: Bad breath, abdominal pain, dyspepsia, constipation, gastroenteritis, duodenitis, duodenal ulceration
- Hematologic: Anemia, leukopenia
- Hepatic: Abnormal LFTs
- Neuromuscular & skeletal: Tremor, hyperkinesia
- Otic: Decreased hearing

Pregnancy Risk Factor C

Generic Available No

Cysteine (SIS teen)

Pharmacologic Category Dietary Supplement

Synonyms Cysteine Hydrochloride

Use Total parenteral nutrition of infants as an additive to meet the I.V. amino acid requirements

Local Anesthetic/Vasoconstrictor Precautions No information available to require special precautions

Effects on Dental Treatment No effects or complications reported

Dosage Combine 500 mg of cysteine with 12.5 g of amino acid, then dilute with 50% dextrose

Mechanism of Action A sulfur-containing amino acid synthesized from methionine via the transulfuration pathway; precursor of the tripeptide glutathione and also of taurine. Newborn infants have a relative deficiency of the enzyme necessary to affect this conversion. Cysteine may be considered an essential amino acid in infants.

Other Adverse Effects Frequency not defined:

- Central nervous system: Fever
- Endocrine & metabolic: Metabolic acidosis
- Gastrointestinal: Nausea
- Renal: Elevated BUN, azotemia

Generic Available Yes

Cystospaz® *see* Hyoscyamine *on page 617*

Cystospaz-M® *see* Hyoscyamine *on page 617*

Cytadren® *see* Aminoglutethimide *on page 69*

Cytarabine (sye TARE a been)

U.S. Brand Names Cytosar-U®

Canadian Brand Names Cytosar®

Mexican Brand Names Laracit®

Pharmacologic Category Antineoplastic Agent, Antimetabolite

Synonyms Arabinosylcytosine; Ara-C; Cytarabine Hydrochloride; Cytosine Arabinosine Hydrochloride

Use Ara-C is one of the most active agents in leukemia; also active against lymphoma, meningeal leukemia, and meningeal lymphoma; has little use in the treatment of solid tumors

Local Anesthetic/Vasoconstrictor Precautions No information available to require special precautions

Effects on Dental Treatment No effects or complications reported

Mechanism of Action Inhibition of DNA synthesis; cell cycle-specific for the S phase of cell division; cytosine gains entry into cells by a carrier process, and then must be converted to its active compound; cytosine acts as an analog and is incorporated into DNA; however, the primary action is inhibition of DNA polymerase resulting in decreased DNA synthesis and repair; degree of its cytotoxicity correlates linearly with its incorporation into DNA; therefore, incorporation into the DNA is responsible for drug activity and toxicity

Other Adverse Effects

>10%:

- Central nervous system: Fever (>80%)
- Dermatologic: Alopecia
- Gastrointestinal: Nausea, vomiting, diarrhea, and mucositis which subside quickly after discontinuing the drug; GI effects may be more pronounced with divided I.V. bolus doses than with continuous infusion
- Hematologic: Myelosuppression; neutropenia and thrombocytopenia are severe, anemia may also occur
  - Onset: 4-7 days
  - Nadir: 14-18 days
  - Recovery: 21-28 days
- Hepatic: Hepatic dysfunction, mild jaundice, and acute increases in transaminases can be produced
- Ocular: Tearing, ocular pain, foreign body sensation, photophobia, and blurred vision may occur with high-dose therapy; ophthalmic corticosteroids usually prevent or relieve the condition

1% to 10%:

- Cardiovascular: Thrombophlebitis, cardiomegaly
- Central nervous system: Dizziness, headache, somnolence, confusion, malaise; a severe cerebellar toxicity occurs in about 8% of patients receiving a high dose (>36-48 g/m²/cycle); it is irreversible or fatal in about 1%
- Dermatologic: Skin freckling, itching, cellulitis at injection site; rash, pain, erythema, and skin sloughing of the palmar and plantar surfaces may occur with high-dose therapy. Prophylactic topical steroids and/or skin moisturizers may be useful.
- Genitourinary: Urinary retention
- Neuromuscular & skeletal: Myalgia, bone pain
- Respiratory: Syndrome of sudden respiratory distress, including tachypnea, hypoxemia, interstitial and alveolar infiltrates progressing to pulmonary edema, pneumonia

Drug Interactions

Increased Effect/Toxicity: Alkylating agents and radiation, purine analogs, and methotrexate when coadministered with cytarabine result in increased toxic effects.

Decreased Effect: Decreases effect of gentamicin, flucytosine, digoxin oral tablet absorption

Drug Uptake

Absorption: Because high concentrations of cytidine deaminase are in the GI mucosa and liver, 3- to 10-fold higher doses than I.V. would need to be given orally; therefore, the oral route is not used

Half-life, elimination: Initial: 7-20 minutes; Terminal: 0.5-2.6 hours

Pregnancy Risk Factor D

Generic Available Yes

Cytarabine (Liposomal) (sye TARE a been lip po SOE mal)

U.S. Brand Names DepoCyt™

Canadian Brand Names DepoCyt™

Pharmacologic Category Antineoplastic Agent, Antimetabolite

Use Intrathecal treatment of lymphomatous meningitis

Local Anesthetic/Vasoconstrictor Precautions No information available to require special precautions

Effects on Dental Treatment No effects or complications reported

Mechanism of Action This is a sustained-release formulation of the active ingredient cytarabine, which acts through inhibition of DNA synthesis; cell cycle-specific for the S phase of cell division; cytosine gains entry into cells by a carrier process, and then must be converted to its active compound; cytosine acts as an analog and is incorporated into DNA; however, the primary action is inhibition of DNA polymerase resulting in decreased DNA synthesis and repair; degree of its cytotoxicity correlates linearly with its incorporation into DNA; therefore, incorporation into the DNA is responsible for drug activity and toxicity

Other Adverse Effects Chemical arachnoiditis is commonly observed, and may include neck pain, neck rigidity, headache, fever, nausea, vomiting, and back pain. It may occur in up to 100% of cycles without dexamethasone prophylaxis. The incidence is reduced to 33% when dexamethasone is used concurrently.

>10%:
- Central nervous system: Headache (28%), confusion (14%), somnolence (12%), fever (11%), pain (11%)
- Gastrointestinal: Vomiting (12%), nausea (11%)

1% to 10%:
- Cardiovascular: Peripheral edema (7%)
- Gastrointestinal: Constipation (7%)
- Genitourinary: Incontinence (3%)
- Hematologic: Neutropenia (9%), thrombocytopenia (8%), anemia (1%)
- Neuromuscular & skeletal: Back pain (7%), weakness (19%), abnormal gait (4%)

Contraindications Hypersensitivity to cytarabine or any component of the formulation; active meningeal infection

Warnings/Precautions The U.S. Food and Drug Administration (FDA) currently recommends that procedures for proper handling and disposal of antineoplastic agents be considered. The incidence and severity of chemical arachnoiditis is reduced by coadministration with dexamethasone. May cause neurotoxicity. Blockage to CSF flow may increase the risk of neurotoxicity. Safety and use in pediatric patients have not been established.

Drug Interactions The limited systemic exposure minimizes the potential for interaction between liposomal cytarabine and other medications. No formal studies of interactions with other medications have been conducted.

Drug Uptake

Absorption: Systemic exposure following intrathecal administration is negligible, since the transfer rate from CSF to plasma is slow.

Half-life, elimination: CSF: 100-263 hours

Time to peak: CSF: ~5 hours

Pregnancy Risk Factor D

Generic Available No

Cytomel® *see* Liothyronine *on page 715*

Cytosar-U® *see* Cytarabine *on page 342*

Cytotec® *see* Misoprostol *on page 820*

Cytovene® *see* Ganciclovir *on page 547*

Cytoxan® *see* Cyclophosphamide *on page 335*

Dacarbazine (da KAR ba zeen)

U.S. Brand Names DTIC-Dome®

Canadian Brand Names DTIC®

Pharmacologic Category Antineoplastic Agent, Alkylating Agent

Synonyms DIC; Dimethyl Triazeno Imidazol Carboxamide; DTIC; Imidazole Carboxamide

Use Singly or in various combination therapy in treatment of malignant melanoma, Hodgkin's disease, soft-tissue sarcomas (fibrosarcomas, rhabdomyosarcoma), islet cell carcinoma, medullary carcinoma of the thyroid, and neuroblastoma

Local Anesthetic/Vasoconstrictor Precautions No information available to require special precautions

Effects on Dental Treatment No effects or complications reported

Mechanism of Action Alkylating agent which forms methylcarbonium ions that attack nucleophilic groups in DNA; cross-links strands of DNA resulting in the inhibition of DNA, RNA, and protein synthesis, but the exact mechanism of action is still unclear; originally developed as a purine antimetabolite, but it does not interfere with purine synthesis; metabolism by the host is necessary for activation of dacarbazine, then the methylated species acts by alkylation of nucleic acids; dacarbazine is active in all phases of the cell cycle

Other Adverse Effects

>10%:
- Gastrointestinal: Nausea and vomiting (>90%), can be severe and dose-limiting; nausea and vomiting decrease on successive days when DTIC is given daily for 5 days
- Hematologic: Myelosuppression, leukopenia, thrombocytopenia - dose-limiting
  - Onset: 5-7 days
  - Nadir: 7-10 days

(Continued)

Dacarbazine *(Continued)*

Recovery: 21-28 days

Local: Pain on infusion, may be minimized by administration through a central line, or by administration as a short infusion (eg, 1-2 hours as opposed to bolus injection)

1% to 10%:

Dermatologic: Alopecia, rash, photosensitivity

Gastrointestinal: Anorexia, metallic taste

Miscellaneous: Flu-like syndrome (fever, myalgias, malaise)

Drug Interactions Increased Effect/Toxicity: Metabolism may be increased by drugs that induce hepatic enzymes (carbamazepine, phenytoin, phenobarbital, and rifampin), potentially leading to decreased efficacy. Patients may experience impaired immune response to vaccines; possible infection after administration of live vaccines in patients receiving immunosuppressants.

Drug Uptake

Onset of action: I.V.: 18-24 days

Absorption: Oral administration demonstrates slow and variable absorption; I.V. administration preferred

Half-life, elimination: Biphasic: Initial: 20-40 minutes; Terminal: 5 hours

Pregnancy Risk Factor C

Generic Available Yes

Daclizumab (dac KLYE zue mab)

U.S. Brand Names Zenapax®

Canadian Brand Names Zenapax®

Pharmacologic Category Immunosuppressant Agent

Use Prevention of rejection of kidney transplants

Local Anesthetic/Vasoconstrictor Precautions No information available to require special precautions

Effects on Dental Treatment No effects or complications reported

Dosage Daclizumab is used adjunctively with other immunosuppressants (eg, cyclosporine, corticosteroids, mycophenolate mofetil, and azathioprine): I.V.:

Children: Use same weight-based dose as adults

Adults:

Immunoprophylaxis against acute renal allograft rejection: 1 mg/kg infused over 15 minutes within 24 hours before transplantation (day 0), then every 14 days for 4 doses

Treatment of graft-versus-host disease (limited data): 0.5-1.5 mg/kg, repeat same dosage for transient response. Repeat doses have been administered 11-48 days following the initial dose.

Mechanism of Action Inhibits the binding of IL-2 to the high affinity IL-2 receptor, thus suppressing T cell activity against allografts. Its active ingredient, daclizumab, a humanized monoclonal antibody, binds to the alpha subunit of the high affinity interleukin-2 receptor (IL-2R) which is expressed on activated T cells.

Other Adverse Effects Although reported adverse events are frequent, when daclizumab is compared with placebo the incidence of adverse effects is similar between the two groups. Many of the adverse effects reported during clinical trial use of daclizumab may be related to the patient population, transplant procedure, and concurrent transplant medications.

≥2%:

Cardiovascular: Bleeding, hypertension, hypotension, tachycardia, thrombosis, edema

Central nervous system: Headache, tremor, dizziness, prickly sensation, fatigue, fever

Dermatologic: Acne, hirsutism, increased diaphoresis, pruritus

Endocrine & metabolic: Dehydration, diabetes mellitus

Gastrointestinal: Abdominal pain or distension, constipation, diarrhea, dyspepsia, epigastric pain, flatulence, gastritis, nausea, vomiting

Genitourinary: Dysuria, oliguria, hematuria, renal dysfunction

Neuromuscular & skeletal: Back pain, leg cramps, musculoskeletal pain

Ocular: Blurred vision

Respiratory: Atelectasis, coughing, dyspnea, hypoxia, pharyngitis, pleural effusion, rhinitis

Miscellaneous: Infectious complications

Drug Uptake

Volume of central compartment: 2.5 L

Volume of peripheral compartment: 3.4 L

Half-life, elimination (estimated): Terminal: 20 days (480 hours)

Pregnancy Risk Factor C

Generic Available No

Dactinomycin (dak ti noe MYE sin)

U.S. Brand Names Cosmegen®

Canadian Brand Names Cosmegen®

Mexican Brand Names Ac-De®

Pharmacologic Category Antineoplastic Agent, Antibiotic

Synonyms ACT; Actinomycin D

Use Management, either alone or in combination with other treatment modalities of Wilms' tumor, rhabdomyosarcoma, neuroblastoma, retinoblastoma, Ewing's sarcoma, trophoblastic neoplasms, testicular carcinoma, sarcoma botryoides, and other malignancies

Local Anesthetic/Vasoconstrictor Precautions No information available to require special precautions

Effects on Dental Treatment No effects or complications reported

Mechanism of Action Binds to the guanine portion of DNA intercalating between guanine and cytosine base pairs inhibiting DNA and RNA synthesis and protein synthesis; product of *Streptomyces parvullus* (a yeast species)

Other Adverse Effects

>10%:

Central nervous system: Unusual fatigue, malaise, fever

Dermatologic: Alopecia (reversible), skin eruptions, acne, increased pigmentation of previously irradiated skin, cheilitis

Endocrine & metabolic: Hypocalcemia

Gastrointestinal: **Highly emetogenic** (severe nausea and vomiting occur in most patients and persist for up to 24 hours); stomatitis, anorexia, abdominal pain, esophagitis, diarrhea, dysphagia, GI ulceration, pharyngitis

Time course of nausea/vomiting: Onset: 2-5 hours; Duration: 4-24 hours

Hematologic: Myelosuppressive: Dose-limiting toxicity; anemia, aplastic anemia, agranulocytosis, pancytopenia, leukopenia, thrombocytopenia, reticulopenia

WBC: Moderate

Platelets: Moderate

Onset (days): 7

Nadir (days): 14-21

Recovery (days): 21-28

Hepatic: Liver toxicity, ascites, hepatomegaly, hepatitis

Local: Extravasation (an irritant and should be administered through a rapidly running I.V. line; extravasation can lead to tissue necrosis, pain, and ulceration)

Vesicant chemotherapy

1% to 10%: Gastrointestinal: Mucositis

Drug Interactions Increased Effect/Toxicity: Potentiates the effects of radiation therapy; radiation may cause skin erythema which may become severe. Also associated with GI toxicity.

Drug Uptake

Half-life, elimination: 36 hours

Time to peak: I.V.: 2-5 minutes

Pregnancy Risk Factor C

Generic Available No

D.A.II™ *see* Chlorpheniramine, Phenylephrine, and Methscopolamine *on page 271*

Dairy Ease® [OTC] *see* Lactase *on page 681*

Dakin's Solution *see* Sodium Hypochlorite Solution *on page 1097*

Dalalone® *see* Dexamethasone *on page 363*

Dalalone D.P.® *see* Dexamethasone *on page 363*

Dalalone L.A.® *see* Dexamethasone *on page 363*

Dalgan® *see* Dezocine *on page 373*

Dallergy® *see* Chlorpheniramine, Phenylephrine, and Methscopolamine *on page 271*

Dallergy-D® *see* Chlorpheniramine and Phenylephrine *on page 269*

Dalmane® *see* Flurazepam *on page 522*

Dalteparin (dal TE pa rin)

U.S. Brand Names Fragmin®

Canadian Brand Names Fragmin®

Pharmacologic Category Low Molecular Weight Heparin

Use Prevention of deep vein thrombosis which may lead to pulmonary embolism, in patients requiring abdominal surgery who are at risk for thromboembolism complications (ie, patients >40 years of age, obese, patients with malignancy, history of deep vein thrombosis or pulmonary embolism, and surgical procedures requiring general anesthesia and lasting longer than 30 minutes)

Local Anesthetic/Vasoconstrictor Precautions No information available to require special precautions

Effects on Dental Treatment No effects or complications reported

Dosage Adults: S.C.:

Low-moderate risk patients: 2500 units 1-2 hours prior to surgery, then once daily for 5-10 days postoperatively

(Continued)

Dalteparin *(Continued)*

High risk patients: 5000 units 1-2 hours prior to surgery and then once daily for 5-10 days postoperatively

Mechanism of Action Low molecular weight heparin analog with a molecular weight of 4000-6000 daltons; the commercial product contains 3% to 15% heparin with a molecular weight <3000 daltons, 65% to 78% with a molecular weight of 3000-8000 daltons and 14% to 26% with a molecular weight >8000 daltons; while dalteparin has been shown to inhibit both factor Xa and factor IIa (thrombin), the antithrombotic effect of dalteparin is characterized by a higher ratio of antifactor Xa to antifactor IIa activity (ratio = 4)

Other Adverse Effects 1% to 10%

Hematologic: Bleeding (2.7% to 4.6%), wound hematoma (0.1% to 3.4%)

Local: Pain at injection site (up to 12%), injection site hematoma (0.2% to 7.1%)

Warnings/Precautions Use with caution in patients with pre-existing thrombocytopenia, recent childbirth, subacute bacterial endocarditis, peptic ulcer disease, pericarditis or pericardial effusion, liver or renal function impairment, recent lumbar puncture, vasculitis, concurrent use of aspirin (increased bleeding risk), previous hypersensitivity to heparin, heparin-associated thrombocytopenia. Patients should be observed closely for bleeding if dalteparin is administered during or immediately following diagnostic lumbar puncture, epidural anesthesia, or spinal anesthesia. If thromboembolism develops despite dalteparin prophylaxis, dalteparin should be discontinued and appropriate treatment should be initiated.

Drug Interactions The risk of bleeding with dalteparin may be increased by drugs which affect platelet function (eg, aspirin, NSAIDs, dipyridamole, ticlopidine, clopidogrel), oral anticoagulants, and thrombolytic agents. Although the risk of bleeding may be increased during concurrent warfarin therapy, dalteparin is commonly continued during the initiation of warfarin therapy to assure anticoagulation and to protect against possible transient hypercoagulability.

Drug Uptake

Onset of action: 1-2 hours

Duration: >12 hours

Half-life, elimination: 2-5 hours (route dependent)

Time to peak: 4 hours

Pregnancy Risk Factor B

Generic Available No

Danaparoid (da NAP a roid)

U.S. Brand Names Orgaran®

Canadian Brand Names Orgaran®

Pharmacologic Category Anticoagulant

Synonyms Danaparoid Sodium

Use Prophylaxis of postoperative deep vein thrombosis (DVT) following elective hip replacement surgery

Unlabeled/Investigational: Systemic anticoagulation for patients with heparin-induced thrombocytopenia: factor Xa inhibition is used to monitor degree of anticoagulation if necessary

Local Anesthetic/Vasoconstrictor Precautions No information available to require special precautions

Effects on Dental Treatment No effects or complications reported

Dosage S.C.:

Children: Safety and effectiveness have not been established.

Adults:

Prevention of DVT following hip replacement: S.C.: 750 anti-Xa units twice daily; beginning 1-4 hours before surgery and then not sooner than 2 hours after surgery and every 12 hours until the risk of DVT has diminished. The average duration of therapy is 7-10 days.

Adults: Treatment (unlabeled uses): Based on diagnosis/indication: See table on following page.

Dosing adjustment in elderly and severe renal impairment: Adjustment may be necessary. Patients with serum creatinine levels ≥2.0 mg/dL should be carefully monitored.

Hemodialysis: See table on following page.

Mechanism of Action Prevents fibrin formation in coagulation pathway via thrombin generation inhibition by anti-Xa and anti-IIa effects.

Other Adverse Effects As with all anticoagulants, bleeding is the major adverse effect of danaparoid. Hemorrhage may occur at virtually any site. Risk is dependent on multiple variables.

>10%:

Central nervous system: Fever (22%)

Gastrointestinal: Nausea (4% to 14%), constipation (4% to 11%)

1% to 10%:

Cardiovascular: Peripheral edema (3%), edema (3%)

Central nervous system: Insomnia (3%), headache (3%), asthenia (2%), dizziness (2%), pain (9%)
Dermatologic: Rash (2% to 5%), pruritus (4%)
Gastrointestinal: Vomiting (3%)
Genitourinary: Urinary tract infection (3% to 4%), urinary retention (2%)
Hematologic: Anemia (2%)
Local: Injection site pain (8% to 14%), injection site hematoma (5%)
Neuromuscular & skeletal: Joint disorder (3%)
Miscellaneous: Infection (2%)

Adult Danaparoid Treatment Dosing Regimens (Not FDA Approved)

	Body Weight (kg)	I.V. Bolus aFXaU	Long–Term Infusion aFXaU	Level of aFXaU/mL	Monitoring
Deep Vein Thrombosis OR Acute Pulmonary Embolism	<55 55-90 >90	1250 2500 3750	400 units/h over 4 h then 300 units/h over 4 h, then 150-200 units/h maintenance dose	0.5-0.8	Days 1-3 daily, then every alternate day
Deep Vein Thrombosis OR Pulmonary Embolism >5 d old	<90 >90	1250 1250	S.C.: 3 x 750/d S.C.: 3 x 1250/d	<0.5	Not necessary
Embolectomy	<90 >90 and high risk	2500 preoperatively 2500 preoperatively	S.C.: 2 x 1250/d postoperatively 150-200 units/ hour I.V.; perioperative arterial irrigation, if necessary: 750 units/20 mL NaCl	<0.4 0.5-0.8	Not necessary Days 1-3 daily, then every alternate day
Peripheral Arterial Bypass		2500 preoperatively	150-200 units/h	0.5-0.8	Days 1-3 daily, then every alternate day
Cardiac Catheter	<90 >90	2500 preoperatively 3750 preoperatively			
Surgery (excluding vascular)			S.C.: 750, 1-4 h preoperatively S.C.: 750, 2-5 h postoperatively, then 2 x 750/d	<0.35	Not necessary

Hemodialysis With Danaparoid Sodium

Dialysis on alternate days	**Dosage prior to dialysis in aFXaU (dosage for body wt <55 kg)**	
First dialysis	3750 (<55 kg 2500)	
Second dialysis	3750 (<55 kg 2000)	
Further dialysis:		
aFXa level before dialysis (eg, day 5)	**Bolus before next dialysis, aFXaU (eg, day 7)**	**aFXa level during dialysis**
<0.3	3000 (<55 kg 2000)	0.5-0.8
0.3-0.35	2500 (<55 kg 2000)	
0.35-0.4	2000 (<55 kg 1500)	
>0.4	No bolus; if fibrin strands occur, 1500 aFXaU I.V.	
Monitoring: 30 minutes before dialysis and after 4 hours of dialysis		
Daily Dialysis		
First dialysis	3750 (<55 kg 2500)	
Second dialysis	2500 (<55 kg 2000)	
Further dialyses	See above	
As with "dialysis on alternate days", always take the aFXa activity preceding the previous dialysis as a basis for the current dosage.		

Warnings/Precautions Do not administer intramuscularly; use with extreme caution in patients with a history of bacterial endocarditis, hemorrhagic stroke,

(Continued)

Danaparoid *(Continued)*

recent CNS or ophthalmological surgery, bleeding diathesis, uncontrolled arterial hypertension, or a history of recent GI ulceration and hemorrhage. Danaparoid shows a low cross-sensitivity with antiplatelet antibodies in individuals with type II heparin-induced thrombocytopenia. This product contains sodium sulfite which may cause allergic-type reactions, including anaphylactic symptoms and life-threatening asthmatic episodes in susceptible people; this is seen more frequently in asthmatics.

Carefully monitor patients receiving low molecular weight heparins or heparinoids. These drugs, when used concurrently with spinal or epidural anesthesia or spinal puncture, may cause bleeding or hematomas within the spinal column. Increased pressure on the spinal cord may result in permanent paralysis if not detected and treated immediately.

Note: Danaparoid is **not** effectively antagonized by protamine sulfate. No other antidote is available, so extreme caution is needed in monitoring dose given and resulting Xa inhibition effect.

Drug Interactions The risk of hemorrhage associated with danaparoid may be increased with thrombolytic agents, oral anticoagulants (warfarin) and drugs which affect platelet function (eg, aspirin, NSAIDs, dipyridamole, ticlopidine, clopidogrel).

Drug Uptake

Onset of action: S.C.: Maximum antifactor Xa and antithrombin (antifactor IIa) activities in 2-5 hours

Half-life, Plasma, elimination: Mean: Terminal: ~24 hours

Pregnancy Risk Factor B

Generic Available No

Danazol (DA na zole)

U.S. Brand Names Danocrine®

Canadian Brand Names Cyclomen®; Danocrine®

Mexican Brand Names Ladogal; Norciden; Zoldan-A

Pharmacologic Category Androgen

Use Treatment of endometriosis, fibrocystic breast disease, and hereditary angioedema

Local Anesthetic/Vasoconstrictor Precautions No information available to require special precautions

Effects on Dental Treatment No effects or complications reported

Dosage Adults: Oral:

Female: Endometriosis: Initial: 200-400 mg/day in 2 divided doses for mild disease; individualize dosage. Usual maintenance dose: 800 mg/day in 2 divided doses to achieve amenorrhea and rapid response to painful symptoms. Continue therapy uninterrupted for 3-6 months (up to 9 months).

Female: Fibrocystic breast disease: Range: 100-400 mg/day in 2 divided doses

Male/Female: Hereditary angioedema: Initial: 200 mg 2-3 times/day; after favorable response, decrease the dosage by 50% or less at intervals of 1-3 months or longer if the frequency of attacks dictates. If an attack occurs, increase the dosage by up to 200 mg/day.

Mechanism of Action Suppresses pituitary output of follicle-stimulating hormone and luteinizing hormone that causes regression and atrophy of normal and ectopic endometrial tissue; decreases rate of growth of abnormal breast tissue; reduces attacks associated with hereditary angioedema by increasing levels of C4 component of complement

Other Adverse Effects Frequency not defined:

Cardiovascular: Benign intracranial hypertension (rare), edema, flushing, hypertension, diaphoresis

Central nervous system: Anxiety (rare), chills (rare), convulsions (rare), depression, dizziness, emotional lability, fainting, fever (rare), Guillain-Barré syndrome, headache, nervousness, sleep disorders, tremor

Dermatologic: Acne, hair loss, mild hirsutism, maculopapular rash, papular rash, petechial rash, pruritus, purpuric rash, seborrhea, Stevens-Johnson syndrome (rare), photosensitivity (rare), urticaria, vesicular rash

Endocrine & metabolic: Amenorrhea (which may continue post therapy), breast size reduction, clitoris hypertrophy, glucose intolerance, HDL decreased, LDL increased, libido changes, nipple discharge, menstrual disturbances (spotting, altered timing of cycle), semen abnormalities (changes in volume, viscosity, sperm count/motility), spermatogenesis reduction

Gastrointestinal: Appetite changes (rare), bleeding gums (rare), constipation, gastroenteritis, nausea, pancreatitis (rare), vomiting, weight gain

Genitourinary: Vaginal dryness, vaginal irritation, pelvic pain

Hematologic: Eosinophilia, erythrocytosis (reversible), leukocytosis, leukopenia, platelet count increased, polycythemia, RBC increased, thrombocytopenia

Hepatic: Cholestatic jaundice, hepatic adenoma, jaundice, liver enzymes (elevated), malignant tumors (after prolonged use), peliosis hepatis

Neuromuscular & skeletal: Back pain, carpal tunnel syndrome (rare), extremity pain, joint lockup, joint pain, joint swelling, muscle cramps, neck pain, paresthesias, spasms, weakness

Ocular: Cataracts (rare), visual disturbances

Renal: Hematuria

Respiratory: Nasal congestion (rare)

Miscellaneous: Voice change (hoarseness, sore throat, instability, deepening of pitch)

Drug Interactions CYP3A3/4 enzyme inhibitor

Increased Effect/Toxicity: Danazol may increase serum concentration of carbamazepine, cyclosporine, tacrolimus, and warfarin leading to toxicity; dosage adjustment may be needed; monitor. Concomitant use of danazol and HMG-CoA reductase inhibitors may lead to severe myopathy or rhabdomyolysis. Danazol may enhance the glucose-lowering effect of hypoglycemic agents.

Decreased Effect: Danazol may decrease effectiveness of hormonal contraceptives. Nonhormonal birth control methods are recommended.

Drug Uptake

Onset of action: Therapeutic: ~4 weeks

Half-life, elimination: 4.5 hours (variable)

Time to peak: ≤2 hours

Pregnancy Risk Factor X

Generic Available Yes

Danocrine® *see* Danazol *on page 348*

Dantrium® *see* Dantrolene *on page 349*

Dantrolene (DAN troe leen)

U.S. Brand Names Dantrium®

Canadian Brand Names Dantrium®

Pharmacologic Category Skeletal Muscle Relaxant

Synonyms Dantrolene Sodium

Use Treatment of spasticity associated with spinal cord injury, stroke, cerebral palsy, or multiple sclerosis; also used as treatment of malignant hyperthermia

Unlabeled/Investigational: Neuroleptic malignant syndrome (NMS)

Local Anesthetic/Vasoconstrictor Precautions No information available to require special precautions

Effects on Dental Treatment No effects or complications reported

Dosage

Spasticity: Oral:

Children: Initial: 0.5 mg/kg/dose twice daily, increase frequency to 3-4 times/day at 4- to 7-day intervals, then increase dose by 0.5 mg/kg to a maximum of 3 mg/kg/dose 2-4 times/day up to 400 mg/day

Adults: 25 mg/day to start, increase frequency to 2-4 times/day, then increase dose by 25 mg every 4-7 days to a maximum of 100 mg 2-4 times/day or 400 mg/day

Malignant hyperthermia: Children and Adults:

Preoperative prophylaxis:

Oral: 4-8 mg/kg/day in 4 divided doses, begin 1-2 days prior to surgery with last dose 3-4 hours prior to surgery

I.V.: 2.5 mg/kg ~1¼ hours prior to anesthesia and infused over 1 hour with additional doses as needed and individualized

Crisis: I.V.: 2.5 mg/kg; may repeat dose up to cumulative dose of 10 mg/kg; if physiologic and metabolic abnormalities reappear, repeat regimen

Postcrisis follow-up: Oral: 4-8 mg/kg/day in 4 divided doses for 1-3 days; I.V. dantrolene may be used when oral therapy is not practical; individualize dosage beginning with 1 mg/kg or more as the clinical situation dictates

Neuroleptic malignant syndrome (unlabeled use): I.V.: 1 mg/kg; may repeat dose up to maximum cumulative dose of 10 mg/kg, then switch to oral dosage

Mechanism of Action Acts directly on skeletal muscle by interfering with release of calcium ion from the sarcoplasmic reticulum; prevents or reduces the increase in myoplasmic calcium ion concentration that activates the acute catabolic processes associated with malignant hyperthermia

Other Adverse Effects

>10%:

Central nervous system: Drowsiness, dizziness, lightheadedness, fatigue

Dermatologic: Rash

Gastrointestinal: Diarrhea (mild), vomiting

Neuromuscular & skeletal: Muscle weakness

1% to 10%:

Cardiovascular: Pleural effusion with pericarditis

Central nervous system: Chills, fever, headache, insomnia, nervousness, mental depression

Gastrointestinal: Diarrhea (severe), constipation, anorexia, stomach cramps

Ocular: Blurred vision

Respiratory: Respiratory depression

(Continued)

Dantrolene *(Continued)*

Drug Interactions Increased toxicity with estrogens (hepatotoxicity), CNS depressants (sedation), MAO inhibitors, phenothiazines, clindamycin (increased neuromuscular blockade), verapamil (hyperkalemia and cardiac depression), warfarin, clofibrate, and tolbutamide.

Drug Uptake
Absorption: Slow and incomplete from GI tract
Half-life, elimination: 8.7 hours

Pregnancy Risk Factor C

Generic Available No

Dapiprazole (DA pi pray zole)

U.S. Brand Names Rēv-Eyes™

Pharmacologic Category Alpha$_1$ Blocker, Ophthalmic

Synonyms Dapiprazole Hydrochloride

Use Reverse dilation due to drugs (adrenergic or parasympathomimetic) after eye exams

Local Anesthetic/Vasoconstrictor Precautions No information available to require special precautions

Effects on Dental Treatment No effects or complications reported

Dosage Adults: Administer 2 drops followed 5 minutes later by an additional 2 drops applied to the conjunctiva of each eye; should not be used more frequently than once a week in the same patient

Mechanism of Action A selective alpha-adrenergic blocking agent, exerting effects primarily on alpha$_1$-adrenoceptors; induces miosis via relaxation of the smooth dilator (radial) muscle of the iris, which causes pupillary constriction. It is devoid of cholinergic effects. Dapiprazole also partially reverses the cycloplegia induced with parasympatholytic agents such as tropicamide. Although the drug has no significant effect on the ciliary muscle *per se*, it may increase accommodative amplitude, therefore relieving the symptoms of paralysis of accommodation.

Other Adverse Effects
>10%:
Central nervous system: Headache
Ocular: Conjunctival injection, burning sensation in the eyes, lid edema, ptosis, lid erythema, chemosis, itching, punctate keratitis, corneal edema, photophobia
1% to 10%: Ocular: Dry eyes, blurring of vision, tearing of eye

Pregnancy Risk Factor B

Generic Available No

Dapsone (DAP sone)

Related Information
HIV Infection and AIDS *on page 1334*

Canadian Brand Names Avlosulfon®

Mexican Brand Names Dapsoderm-X®

Pharmacologic Category Antibiotic, Miscellaneous

Synonyms Diaminodiphenylsulfone

Use Treatment of leprosy and dermatitis herpetiformis (infections caused by *Mycobacterium leprae*), alternative agent for *Pneumocystis carinii* pneumonia prophylaxis (given alone) and treatment (given with trimethoprim)

Local Anesthetic/Vasoconstrictor Precautions No information available to require special precautions

Effects on Dental Treatment No effects or complications reported

Dosage Oral:
Leprosy:
Children: 1-2 mg/kg/24 hours, up to a maximum of 100 mg/day
Adults: 50-100 mg/day for 3-10 years
Dermatitis herpetiformis: Adults: Start at 50 mg/day, increase to 300 mg/day, or higher to achieve full control, reduce dosage to minimum level as soon as possible
Prophylaxis of *Pneumocystis carinii* pneumonia: Children >1 month: 1 mg/kg/day; maximum: 100 mg
Treatment of *Pneumocystis carinii* pneumonia: Adults: 100 mg/day in combination with trimethoprim (20 mg/kg/day) for 21 days

Mechanism of Action A sulfone antimicrobial; mechanism of the sulfones is similar to that of the sulfonamides. Sulfonamides are competitive antagonists of para-aminobenzoic acid (PABA) and prevent normal bacterial utilization of PABA for the synthesis of folic acid.

Other Adverse Effects
>10%:
Hematologic: Hemolytic anemia, methemoglobinemia with cyanosis
Dermatologic: Skin rash
1% to 10%:
Central nervous system: Reactional states

Hematologic: Dose-related hemolysis,

Drug Interactions CYP2C9, 2E1, and 3A3/4 enzyme substrate

Increased Effect/Toxicity: Folic acid antagonists (methotrexate) may increase the risk of hematologic reactions of dapsone; probenecid decreases dapsone excretion; trimethoprim with dapsone may increase toxic effects of both drugs Dapsone levels may be increased by protease inhibitors (amprenavir, nelfinavir, ritonavir).

Decreased Effect: Para-aminobenzoic acid and rifampin levels are decreased when given with dapsone.

Drug Uptake

Absorption: Oral: Well absorbed

Half-life, elimination: 30 hours (range: 10-50 hours)

Pregnancy Risk Factor C

Generic Available Yes

Daranide® *see* Dichlorphenamide *on page 377*
Daraprim® *see* Pyrimethamine *on page 1028*

Darbepoetin Alfa (dar be POE e tin AL fa)

U.S. Brand Names Aranesp™

Pharmacologic Category Colony Stimulating Factor; Growth Factor; Recombinant Human Erythropoietin

Synonyms Erythropoiesis Stimulating Protein

Use Treatment of anemia associated with chronic renal failure, including patients on dialysis (end-stage renal disease) and patients not on dialysis

Local Anesthetic/Vasoconstrictor Precautions No information available to require special precautions

Effects on Dental Treatment No effects or complications reported

Dosage I.V., S.C.:

Correction of anemia:

Initial: 0.45 mcg/kg once weekly; dosage should be titrated to limit increases in hemoglobin to <1 g/dL over any 2-week interval, with a target concentration of <12 g/dL.

Maintenance: Titrated to hematologic response. Some patients may require doses <0.45 mcg/kg once weekly. Selected patients may be managed by administering S.C. doses every 2 weeks.

Conversion from epoetin alfa to darbepoetin alfa: Initial: Estimate dosage based on weekly epoetin alfa dosage. See table.

Conversion From Epoetin Alfa to Darbepoetin Alfa

Previous Dosage of Epoetin Alfa (units/week)	Darbopoetin Alfa Dosage (mcg/week)
<2500	6.25
2500-4999	12.5
5000-10,999	25
11,000-17,999	40
18,000-33,999	60
34,000-89,999	100
≥90,000	200

Note: In patients receiving epoetin alfa 2-3 times per week, darbepoetin alfa is administered once weekly. In patients receiving epoetin alfa once weekly, darbepoetin alfa is administered once every 2 weeks.

Dosage adjustment: It is recommended that the dosage of darbepoetin should be decreased if the hemoglobin increases >1 g/dL in any 2-week period. If the increase in hemoglobin is <1 g/dL over 4 weeks and iron stores are adequate, increase by ~25% of the previous dose. Further increases may be made at 4-week intervals. If the hemoglobin is increasing and approaches the target value of 12 g/dL, decrease weekly dosage by ~25%. If hemoglobin exceeds the target value, hold dose until hemoglobin is <12 g/dL and reduce dose by 25%.

Elderly: Refer to adult dosing.

Dosage adjustment in renal impairment: Dosage requirements for patients with chronic renal failure who do not require dialysis may be lower than in dialysis patients. Monitor patients closely during the time period in which a dialysis regimen is initiated, dosage requirement may increase.

Mechanism of Action Induces erythropoiesis by stimulating the division and differentiation of committed erythroid progenitor cells; induces the release of reticulocytes from the bone marrow into the bloodstream, where they mature to erythrocytes. There is a dose response relationship with this effect. This results in an increase in reticulocyte counts followed by a rise in hematocrit and hemoglobin levels. When administered S.C. or I.V., darbepoetin's half-life is ~3 times that of epoetin alfa concentrations.

(Continued)

Darbepoetin Alfa *(Continued)*

Other Adverse Effects Note: Frequency of adverse events cited may be, in part, a reflection of population in which the drug is used and/or associated with dialysis procedures.

>10%:

Cardiovascular: Hypertension (23%), hypotension (22%), peripheral edema (11%), arrhythmia (10%)

Central nervous system: Headache (16%)

Gastrointestinal: Diarrhea (16%), vomiting (15%), nausea (14%), abdominal pain (12%)

Neuromuscular & skeletal: Myalgia (21%), arthralgia (11%), limb pain (10%)

Respiratory: Upper respiratory infection (14%), dyspnea (12%), cough (10%)

Miscellaneous: Infection (27%)

1% to 10%:

Cardiovascular: Angina/chest pain (6% to 8%), fluid overload (6%), CHF (6%), myocardial infarction (2%)

Central nervous system: Fatigue (9%), fever (9%), dizziness (8%), seizure (1%), stroke (1%), transient ischemic attack (1%)

Dermatologic: Pruritus (8%)

Gastrointestinal: Constipation (5%)

Local: Injection site pain (7%)

Neuromuscular & skeletal: Back pain (8%), weakness (5%)

Respiratory: Bronchitis (6%)

Miscellaneous: Vascular access thrombosis (8%, annualized rate 0.22 events per patient year), vascular access infection (6%), influenza-like symptoms (6%), vascular access hemorrhage (6%)

Drug Uptake

Onset of action: Increased hemoglobin levels not generally observed until 2-6 weeks after initiating treatment

Absorption: S.C.: Slow

Half-life, elimination: Terminal: I.V.: 21 hours, S.C.: 49 hours; half-life of darbepoetin alfa is ~3 times as long as epoetin alfa

Time to peak: S.C.: 34 hours (range: 24-72 hours)

Pregnancy Risk Factor C

Generic Available No

Daricon® *see* Oxyphencyclimine *on page 909*
Darvocet-N® 50 *see* Propoxyphene and Acetaminophen *on page 1013*
Darvocet-N® 100 *see* Propoxyphene and Acetaminophen *on page 1013*
Darvon® *see* Propoxyphene *on page 1013*
Darvon® Compound-65 Pulvules® *see* Propoxyphene and Aspirin *on page 1015*
Darvon-N® *see* Propoxyphene *on page 1013*

DAUNOrubicin Citrate (Liposomal)

(daw noe ROO bi sin SI trate lip po SOE mal)

U.S. Brand Names DaunoXome®

Pharmacologic Category Antineoplastic Agent, Anthracycline

Use Advanced HIV-associated Kaposi's sarcoma; first-line cytotoxic therapy for advanced HIV-associated Kaposi's sarcoma

Local Anesthetic/Vasoconstrictor Precautions No information available to require special precautions

Effects on Dental Treatment No effects or complications reported

Mechanism of Action Liposomes have been shown to penetrate solid tumors more effectively, possibly because of their small size and longer circulation time. Once in tissues, daunorubicin is released. Daunorubicin inhibits DNA and RNA synthesis by intercalation between DNA base pairs and by steric obstruction; and intercalates at points of local uncoiling of the double helix. Although the exact mechanism is unclear, it appears that direct binding to DNA (intercalation) and inhibition of DNA repair (topoisomerase II inhibition) result in blockade of DNA and RNA synthesis and fragmentation of DNA; see Daunorubicin Hydrochloride *on page 353.*

Other Adverse Effects

>10%:

Central nervous system: Fatigue (51%), headache (28%), neuropathy (13%)

Hematologic: Myelosuppression, neutropenia (51%), thrombocytopenia, anemia
- Onset: 7 days
- Nadir: 14 days
- Recovery: 21 days

Gastrointestinal: Abdominal pain, vomiting, anorexia (23%); diarrhea (38%); nausea (55%)

Respiratory: Cough (28%), dyspnea (26%), rhinitis

1% to 10%:

Allergic: Allergic reactions (24%)

Cardiovascular: Hypertension, palpitations, syncope, tachycardia, chest pain, edema

Dermatologic: Alopecia (8%), pruritus (7%)
Endocrine & metabolic: Hot flashes
Gastrointestinal: Constipation (7%), stomatitis (10%)
Neuromuscular & skeletal: Arthralgia (7%), myalgia (7%)
Ocular: Conjunctivitis, eye pain (5%)
Respiratory: Sinusitis

Contraindications Hypersensitivity to daunorubicin citrate or any component of the formulation

Warnings/Precautions

The U.S. Food and Drug Administration (FDA) currently recommends that procedures for proper handling and disposal of antineoplastic agents be considered.

The primary toxicity is myelosuppression, especially off the granulocytic series, which may be severe, with much less marked effects on platelets and erythroid series. Potential cardiac toxicity, particularly in patients who have received prior anthracyclines or who have pre-existing cardiac disease, may occur. See Daunorubicin Hydrochloride *on page 353*.

Although grade 3-4 injection site inflammation has been reported in patients treated with the liposomal daunorubicin, no instances of local tissue necrosis were observed with extravasation.

Reduce dosage in patients with impaired hepatic function. Hyperuricemia can be induced secondary to rapid lysis of leukemic cells. As a precaution, administer allopurinol prior to initiating antileukemic therapy.

Drug Interactions Patients may experience impaired immune response to vaccines; possible infection after administration of live vaccines in patients receiving immunosuppressants. Incompatible with sodium bicarbonate and 5-FU, heparin, dexamethasone

Drug Uptake Half-life, elimination: 4.4 hours; Terminal: 3-5 hours

Pregnancy Risk Factor D

Generic Available No

DAUNOrubicin Hydrochloride

(daw noe ROO bi sin hye droe KLOR ide)

U.S. Brand Names Cerubidine®

Canadian Brand Names Cerubidine®

Mexican Brand Names Rubilem®; Trixilem

Pharmacologic Category Antineoplastic Agent, Anthracycline

Synonyms Daunomycin; DNR; Rubidomycin Hydrochloride

Use In combination with other agents in the treatment of leukemias (ALL, AML)

Local Anesthetic/Vasoconstrictor Precautions No information available to require special precautions

Effects on Dental Treatment No effects or complications reported

Mechanism of Action Inhibition of DNA and RNA synthesis, by intercalating between DNA base pairs and by steric obstruction; is not cell cycle-specific for the S phase of cell division; daunomycin is preferred over doxorubicin for the treatment of ANLL because of its dose-limiting toxicity (myelosuppression) is not of concern in the therapy of this disease; has less mucositis associated with its use

Other Adverse Effects

>10%:

Cardiovascular: Transient EKG abnormalities (supraventricular tachycardia, S-T wave changes, atrial or ventricular extrasystoles); generally asymptomatic and self-limiting. Congestive heart failure, dose-related, may be delayed for 7-8 years after treatment. Cumulative dose, radiation therapy, age, and use of cyclophosphamide all increase the risk. Recommended maximum cumulative doses:
- No risk factors: 550-600 mg/m^2
- Concurrent radiation: 450 mg/m^2
- Regardless of cumulative dose, if the left ventricular ejection fraction is <30% to 40%, the drug is usually not given

Dermatologic: Alopecia, radiation recall
Gastrointestinal: Mild nausea or vomiting, stomatitis
Genitourinary: Discoloration of urine (red)
Hematologic: Myelosuppression, primarily leukopenia; thrombocytopenia and anemia
- Onset: 7 days
- Nadir: 10-14 days
- Recovery: 21-28 days

1% to 10%:

Dermatologic: Skin "flare" at injection site; discoloration of saliva, sweat, or tears
Endocrine & metabolic: Hyperuricemia
Gastrointestinal: GI ulceration, diarrhea

Warnings/Precautions The U.S. Food and Drug Administration (FDA) currently recommends that procedures for proper handling and disposal of antineoplastic agents be considered. I.V. use only, severe local tissue necrosis will result if extravasation occurs; reduce dose in patients with impaired hepatic, renal, or biliary function; severe myelosuppression is possible when used in therapeutic doses.

(Continued)

DAUNOrubicin Hydrochloride *(Continued)*

Total cumulative dose should take into account previous or concomitant treatment with cardiotoxic agents or irradiation of chest.

Irreversible myocardial toxicity may occur as total dosage approaches:
- 550 mg/m² in adults
- 400 mg/m² in patients receiving chest radiation
- 300 mg/m² in children >2 years of age or
- 10 mg/kg in children <2 years; this may occur during therapy or several months after therapy

Drug Interactions Patients may experience impaired immune response to vaccines; possible infection after administration of live vaccines in patients receiving immunosuppressants.

Drug Uptake Half-life, elimination: Initial: 2 minutes; Elimination: 14-20 hours; Terminal: 18.5 hours; Daunorubicinol plasma: 24-48 hours

Pregnancy Risk Factor D

Generic Available Yes

DaunoXome® *see* DAUNOrubicin Citrate (Liposomal) *on page 352*
1-Day™ [OTC] *see* Tioconazole *on page 1172*
Daypro™ *see* Oxaprozin *on page 895*
DC 240® Softgels® [OTC] *see* Docusate *on page 407*
DDAVP® *see* Desmopressin Acetate *on page 361*
Debacterol® *see* Sulfonated Phenolics in Aqueous Solution *on page 1124*
Debrisan® [OTC] *see* Dextranomer *on page 370*
Debrox® Otic [OTC] *see* Carbamide Peroxide *on page 218*
Decadron® *see* Dexamethasone *on page 363*
Decadron®-LA *see* Dexamethasone *on page 363*
Decadron® Phosphate *see* Dexamethasone *on page 363*
Deca-Durabolin® *see* Nandrolone *on page 846*
Decaject® *see* Dexamethasone *on page 363*
Decaject-LA® *see* Dexamethasone *on page 363*
Decaspray® *see* Dexamethasone *on page 363*
Declomycin® *see* Demeclocycline *on page 357*
Decofed® [OTC] *see* Pseudoephedrine *on page 1022*
Decohistine® DH *see* Chlorpheniramine, Pseudoephedrine, and Codeine *on page 273*
Decohistine® Expectorant *see* Guaifenesin, Pseudoephedrine, and Codeine *on page 570*
Deconamine® [OTC] *see* Chlorpheniramine and Pseudoephedrine *on page 270*
Deconamine® SR [OTC] *see* Chlorpheniramine and Pseudoephedrine *on page 270*
Deconsal® II *see* Guaifenesin and Pseudoephedrine *on page 570*
Deconsal® Sprinkle® *see* Guaifenesin and Phenylephrine *on page 569*
Defen-LA® *see* Guaifenesin and Pseudoephedrine *on page 570*

Deferoxamine (de fer OKS a meen)

U.S. Brand Names Desferal®

Canadian Brand Names Desferal®

Pharmacologic Category Antidote

Synonyms Deferoxamine Mesylate

Use Acute iron intoxication when serum iron is >450-500 µg/dL or when clinical signs of significant iron toxicity exist; chronic iron overload secondary to multiple transfusions; diagnostic test for iron overload; iron overload secondary to congenital anemias; hemochromatosis; removal of corneal rust rings following surgical removal of foreign bodies

Unlabeled/Investigational: Treatment of aluminum accumulation in renal failure; treatment of aluminum-induced bone disease

Local Anesthetic/Vasoconstrictor Precautions No information available to require special precautions

Effects on Dental Treatment No effects or complications reported

Dosage

Children and Adults:

Acute iron toxicity: I.V. route is used when severe toxicity is evidenced by systemic symptoms (coma, shock, metabolic acidosis, or severe GI bleeding) or potentially severe intoxications (serum iron level >500 µg/dL). When severe symptoms are not present, the I.M. route may be preferred; however, the use of deferoxamine in situations where the serum iron concentration is <500 µg/dL or when severe toxicity is not evident is a subject of some clinical debate.

Dose: For the first 1000 mg, infuse at 15 mg/kg/hour (although rates up to 40-50 mg/kg/hour have been given in patients with massive iron intoxication); may be followed by 500 mg every 4 hours for up to 2 doses; subsequent doses of 500 mg have been administered every 4-12 hours

Maximum recommended dose: 6 g/day (however, doses as high as 16-37 g have been administered)

Children:

Chronic iron overload: S.C.: 20-40 mg/kg/day over 8-12 hours (via a portable, controlled infusion device)

Aluminum-induced bone disease: 20-40 mg/kg every hemodialysis treatment, frequency dependent on clinical status of the patient

Adults: Chronic iron overload:

I.M.: 500-1000 mg/day; in addition, 2000 mg should be given with each unit of blood transfused (administer separately from blood)

I.V.: 2 g after each unit of blood infusion at 15 mg/kg/hour

S.C.: 1-2 g every day over 8-24 hours

Dosing adjustment in renal impairment: Cl_{cr} <10 mL/minute: Administer 50% of dose

Has been used investigationally as a single 40 mg/kg I.V. dose over 2 hours, to promote mobilization of aluminum from tissue stores as an aid in the diagnosis of aluminum-associated osteodystrophy

Mechanism of Action Complexes with trivalent ions (ferric ions) to form ferrioxamine, which are removed by the kidneys

Other Adverse Effects Frequency not defined:

Cardiovascular: Flushing, hypotension, tachycardia, shock, edema

Central nervous system: Convulsions, fever, dizziness, neuropathy, paresthesia, seizures, exacerbation of aluminum-related encephalopathy (dialysis), headache, CNS depression, coma, aphasia, agitation

Dermatologic: Erythema, urticaria, pruritus, rash, cutaneous wheal formation

Endocrine & metabolic: Hypocalcemia

Gastrointestinal: Abdominal discomfort, diarrhea, nausea

Genitourinary: Dysuria

Hematologic: Thrombocytopenia, leukopenia

Local: Pain and induration at injection site

Neuromuscular & skeletal: Leg cramps

Ocular: Blurred vision, visual loss, scotoma, visual field defects, impaired vision, optic neuritis, cataracts, retinal pigmentary abnormalities

Otic: Hearing loss, tinnitus

Renal: Renal impairment, acute renal failure

Respiratory: Acute respiratory distress syndrome (with dyspnea, cyanosis)

Miscellaneous: Anaphylaxis

Drug Interactions Increased Toxicity: May cause loss of consciousness when administered with prochlorperazine; concomitant treatment with vitamin C (>500 mg/day) has been associated with cardiac impairment.

Drug Uptake

Absorption: Oral: <15%

Half-life, elimination: Parent drug: 6.1 hours; Ferrioxamine: 5.8 hours

Pregnancy Risk Factor C

Generic Available No

Dehydrocholic Acid (dee hye droe KOE lik AS id)

U.S. Brand Names Cholan-HMB® [OTC]

Pharmacologic Category Bile Acid; Laxative, Hydrocholeretic

Use Relief of constipation; adjunct to various biliary tract conditions

Local Anesthetic/Vasoconstrictor Precautions No information available to require special precautions

Effects on Dental Treatment No effects or complications reported

Dosage Children >12 years and Adults: 250-500 mg 2-3 times/day after meals up to 1.5 g/day

Other Adverse Effects 1% to 10%:

Endocrine & metabolic: Dehydration

Gastrointestinal: Diarrhea, abdominal cramps

Pregnancy Risk Factor C

Generic Available Yes

Del Aqua® *see* Benzoyl Peroxide *on page 153*

Delatestryl® *see* Testosterone *on page 1143*

Delavirdine (de la VIR deen)

Related Information

HIV Infection and AIDS *on page 1334*

U.S. Brand Names Rescriptor®

Canadian Brand Names Rescriptor®

Mexican Brand Names Rescriptor®

Pharmacologic Category Antiretroviral Agent, Reverse Transcriptase Inhibitor (Non-nucleoside)

Synonyms U-90152S

Use Treatment of HIV-1 infection in combination with appropriate antiretrovirals

(Continued)

Delavirdine *(Continued)*

Local Anesthetic/Vasoconstrictor Precautions No information available to require special precautions

Effects on Dental Treatment No effects or complications reported

Dosage Adults: Oral: 400 mg 3 times/day

Mechanism of Action Binds directly to reverse transcriptase, blocking RNA-dependent and DNA-dependent DNA polymerase activities

Other Adverse Effects

>10%: Dermatologic: Rash (3.2% required discontinuation)

1% to 10%:

Central nervous system: Headache, fatigue

Dermatologic: Pruritus

Gastrointestinal: Nausea, diarrhea, vomiting

Metabolic: Increased ALT (SGPT), increased AST (SGOT)

Drug Interactions CYP2D6 and 3A3/4 enzyme substrate; CYP2D6 and 3A3/4 enzyme inhibitor

Increased Effect/Toxicity: Delavirdine concentrations may be increased by clarithromycin, ketoconazole, and fluoxetine. Delavirdine increases plasma concentrations of alprazolam, amiodarone, amphetamines, amprenavir, astemizole, bepridil, calcium channel blockers (dihydropyridine-type), cisapride, clarithromycin, dapsone, dexamethasone, ergot alkaloids, flecainide, HMG-CoA reductase inhibitors, indinavir, methadone, midazolam, pimozide, propafenone, quinidine, rifabutin, saquinavir, sildenafil, terfenadine, triazolam, and warfarin.

Decreased Effect: Decreased plasma concentrations of delavirdine with carbamazepine, dexamethasone, phenobarbital, phenytoin, rifabutin, rifampin, didanosine, and saquinavir. Decreased absorption of delavirdine with antacids, histamine-2 receptor antagonists, proton pump inhibitors (omeprazole, lansoprazole), and didanosine. Delavirdine decreases plasma concentrations of didanosine.

Drug Uptake

Absorption: Rapid; AUC may be higher in females

Half-life, elimination: 2-11 hours

Time to peak, plasma: 1 hour

Pregnancy Risk Factor C

Generic Available No

Delcort® *see* Hydrocortisone *on page 608*

Delestrogen® *see* Estradiol *on page 457*

Delfen® [OTC] *see* Nonoxynol 9 *on page 874*

Del-Mycin® *see* Erythromycin, Topical *on page 454*

Delsym® [OTC] *see* Dextromethorphan *on page 372*

Delta-Cortef® *see* PrednisoLONE *on page 988*

Delta-D® *see* Cholecalciferol *on page 278*

Deltasone® *see* PredniSONE *on page 990*

Delta-Tritex® *see* Triamcinolone *on page 1197*

Demadex® *see* Torsemide *on page 1185*

Demecarium (dem e KARE ee um)

U.S. Brand Names Humorsol®

Canadian Brand Names Humorsol®

Pharmacologic Category Cholinergic Agonist; Ophthalmic Agent, Antiglaucoma; Ophthalmic Agent, Miotic

Synonyms Demecarium Bromide

Use Management of chronic simple glaucoma, chronic and acute angle-closure glaucoma; strabismus

Local Anesthetic/Vasoconstrictor Precautions No information available to require special precautions

Effects on Dental Treatment No effects or complications reported

Dosage Children and Adults: Ophthalmic:

Glaucoma: Instill 1 drop into eyes twice weekly to a maximum dosage of 1 or 2 drops twice daily for up to 4 months

Strabismus:

Diagnosis: Instill 1 drop daily for 2 weeks, then 1 drop every 2 days for 2-3 weeks. If eyes become straighter, an accommodative factor is demonstrated.

Therapy: Instill not more than 1 drop at a time in both eyes every day for 2-3 weeks. Then reduce dosage to 1 drop every other day for 3-4 weeks and re-evaluate. Continue at 1 drop every 2 days to 1 drop twice a week and evaluate the patient's condition every 4-12 weeks. If improvement continues, reduce dose to 1 drop once a week and eventually off of medication. Discontinue therapy after 4 months if control of the condition still requires 1 drop every 2 days.

Mechanism of Action Cholinesterase inhibitor (anticholinesterase) which causes acetylcholine to accumulate at cholinergic receptor sites and produces effects equivalent to excessive stimulation of cholinergic receptors. Demecarium mainly acts by inhibiting true (erythrocyte) cholinesterase and causes a reduction in intraocular pressure due to facilitation of outflow of aqueous humor; the reduction is likely to be particularly marked in eyes in which the pressure is elevated.

Other Adverse Effects 1% to 10%: Ocular: Stinging, burning eyes, myopia, visual blurring

Pregnancy Risk Factor C

Generic Available No

Demeclocycline (dem e kloe SYE kleen)

U.S. Brand Names Declomycin®

Canadian Brand Names Declomycin®

Mexican Brand Names Ledermicina

Pharmacologic Category Antibiotic, Tetracycline Derivative

Synonyms Demeclocycline Hydrochloride; Demethylchlortetracycline

Use Treatment of susceptible bacterial infections (acne, gonorrhea, pertussis and urinary tract infections) caused by both gram-negative and gram-positive organisms; used when penicillin is contraindicated (other agents are preferred); treatment of chronic syndrome of inappropriate secretion of antidiuretic hormone (SIADH)

Local Anesthetic/Vasoconstrictor Precautions No information available to require special precautions

Effects on Dental Treatment Tetracyclines are not recommended for use during pregnancy or in children ≤8 years of age since they have been reported to cause enamel hypoplasia and permanent teeth discoloration. The use of tetracyclines should only be used in these patients if other agents are contraindicated or alternative antimicrobials will not eradicate the organism. Long-term use associated with oral candidiasis.

Dosage Oral:

Children ≥8 years: 8-12 mg/kg/day divided every 6-12 hours

Adults: 150 mg 4 times/day or 300 mg twice daily

- Uncomplicated gonorrhea (penicillin sensitive): 600 mg stat, 300 mg every 12 hours for 4 days (3 g total)
- SIADH: 900-1200 mg/day or 13-15 mg/kg/day divided every 6-8 hours initially, then decrease to 0.6-0.9 g/day

Mechanism of Action Inhibits protein synthesis by binding with the 30S and possibly the 50S ribosomal subunit(s) of susceptible bacteria; may also cause alterations in the cytoplasmic membrane; inhibits the action of ADH in patients with chronic SIADH

Other Adverse Effects

>10%:

- Central nervous system: Dizziness, lightheadedness, unsteadiness
- Dermatologic: Photosensitivity
- Gastrointestinal: Nausea, diarrhea
- Miscellaneous: Discoloration of teeth in children

1% to 10%:

- Dermatologic: Photosensitivity
- Endocrine & metabolic: Diabetes insipidus syndrome
- Gastrointestinal: Nausea, diarrhea, hypertrophy of the papilla, pancreatitis
- Hepatic: Hepatotoxicity
- Miscellaneous: Superinfections (fungal overgrowth)

Drug Interactions

Increased Effect/Toxicity: Increased effect of warfarin, digoxin when taken with demeclocycline.

Decreased Effect: Decreased effect with antacids (aluminum, calcium, zinc, or magnesium), bismuth salts, sodium bicarbonate, barbiturates, carbamazepine, and hydantoins. Decreased effect of oral contraceptives, penicillins.

Drug Uptake

Onset of diuretic effect in SIADH: Several days

Absorption: ~50% to 80% from GI tract; food (especially dairy products) reduces absorption

Half-life, elimination: Renal Impairment: 10-17 hours

Time to peak: Oral: 3-6 hours

Pregnancy Risk Factor D

Generic Available No

Demerol® *see* Meperidine *on page 760*

Demser® *see* Metyrosine *on page 806*

Demulen® *see* Combination Hormonal Contraceptives *on page 323*

Denavir™ *see* Penciclovir *on page 926*

Denileukin Diftitox (de ne LU kin DEFT e tox)

U.S. Brand Names ONTAK®

Pharmacologic Category Antineoplastic Agent, Miscellaneous

Use Treatment of patients with persistent or recurrent cutaneous T-cell lymphoma whose malignant cells express the CD25 component of the IL-2 receptor

(Continued)

Denileukin Diftitox *(Continued)*

Local Anesthetic/Vasoconstrictor Precautions No information available to require special precautions

Effects on Dental Treatment No effects or complications reported

Mechanism of Action Denileukin diftitox is a fusion protein (a combination of amino acid sequences from diphtheria toxin and interleukin-2) which selectively delivers the cytotoxic activity of diphtheria toxin to targeted cells. It interacts with the high-affinity IL-2 receptor on the surface of malignant cells to inhibit intracellular protein synthesis, rapidly leading to cell death.

Other Adverse Effects The occurrence of adverse events diminishes after the first two treatment courses. Infusion-related hypersensitivity reactions have been reported in 69% of patients. Reactions are variable, but may include hypotension, back pain, dyspnea, vasodilation, rash, chest pain, tachycardia, dysphagia, syncope or anaphylaxis. In addition, a flu-like syndrome, beginning several hours to days following infusion, occurred in 91% of patients.

In 27% of patients, vascular leak syndrome occurred, characterized by hypotension, edema, or hypoalbuminemia. The syndrome usually developed within the first 2 weeks of infusion. Six percent of patients who developed this syndrome required hospitalization. The symptoms may persist or even worsen despite cessation of denileukin diftitox.

Severe (Grade 3 and 4) reactions which occurred with an incidence over 10% included: Chills/fever (22%), asthenia (22%), infection (24%), pain (13%), nausea/vomiting (14%), hypoalbuminemia (14%), transaminase elevation (15%), edema (15%), dyspnea (14%), and rash (13%).

The following list of symptoms reported during treatment includes all levels of severity:

>10%:

- Cardiovascular: Edema (47%), hypotension (36%), chest pain (24%), vasodilation (22%), tachycardia (12%)
- Central nervous system: Fever/chills (81%), headache (26%), pain (48%), dizziness (22%), nervousness (11%)
- Dermatologic: Rash (34%), pruritus (20%)
- Endocrine & metabolic: Hypoalbuminemia (83%), hypocalcemia (17%), weight loss (14%)
- Gastrointestinal: Nausea/vomiting (64%), anorexia (36%), diarrhea (29%)
- Hematologic: Decreased lymphocyte count (34%), anemia (18%)
- Hepatic: Increased transaminases (61%)
- Neuromuscular & skeletal: Asthenia (66%), myalgia (17%)
- Respiratory: Dyspnea (29%), increased cough (26%), pharyngitis (17%), rhinitis (13%)
- Miscellaneous: Hypersensitivity (69%), infection (48%), vascular leak syndrome (27%), increased diaphoresis (10%), paresthesia (13%)

1% to 10%:

- Cardiovascular: Hypertension (6%), arrhythmias (6%), myocardial infarction (1%)
- Central nervous system: Insomnia (9%), confusion (8%)
- Endocrine & metabolic: Dehydration (9%), hypokalemia (6%), hyperthyroidism (<5%), hypothyroidism (<5%)
- Gastrointestinal: Constipation (9%), dyspepsia (7%), dysphagia (6%), pancreatitis (<5%)
- Genitourinary: Hematuria (10%), albuminuria (10%), pyuria (10%)
- Hematologic: Thrombotic events (7%), thrombocytopenia (8%), leukopenia (6%)
- Local: Injection site reaction (8%), anaphylaxis (1%)
- Neuromuscular & skeletal: Arthralgia (8%)
- Renal: Increased creatinine (7%), acute renal insufficiency (<5%), microscopic hematuria (<5%)
- Respiratory: Lung disorder (8%)

Contraindications Hypersensitivity to denileukin diftitox, diphtheria toxin, interleukin-2, or any component their formulation

Warnings/Precautions Acute hypersensitivity reactions, including anaphylaxis, may occur; most events occur during or within 24 hours of the first dose of a treatment cycle. Has been associated with a delayed-onset vascular leak syndrome, which may be severe. The onset of symptoms of vascular leak syndrome usually occurred within the first 2 weeks of infusion and may persist or worsen after cessation of denileukin diftitox. Pre-existing low serum albumin levels may predict or predispose to vascular leak syndrome. Denileukin diftitox may impair immune function. Use with caution in patients with pre-existing cardiovascular disease and in patients >65 years of age.

Drug Interactions Limited information; denileukin diftitox does not appear to have an effect on cytochrome P450 enzymes.

Drug Uptake Half-life, elimination: Initial: 2-5 minutes; Terminal: 70-80 minutes

Pregnancy Risk Factor C

Generic Available No

Denorex® [OTC] *see* Coal Tar *on page 315*

DentiPatch® *see* Lidocaine Transoral *on page 713*
Depacon® *see* Valproic Acid and Derivatives *on page 1227*
Depakene® *see* Valproic Acid and Derivatives *on page 1227*
Depakote® Delayed Release *see* Valproic Acid and Derivatives *on page 1227*
Depakote® ER *see* Valproic Acid and Derivatives *on page 1227*
Depakote® Sprinkle® *see* Valproic Acid and Derivatives *on page 1227*
Depen® *see* Penicillamine *on page 927*
depMedalone® *see* MethylPREDNISolone *on page 797*
DepoCyt™ *see* Cytarabine (Liposomal) *on page 342*
Depo®-Estradiol *see* Estradiol *on page 457*
Depoject® *see* MethylPREDNISolone *on page 797*
Depo-Medrol® *see* MethylPREDNISolone *on page 797*
Deponit® Patch *see* Nitroglycerin *on page 871*
Depopred® *see* MethylPREDNISolone *on page 797*
Depo-Provera® *see* MedroxyPROGESTERone Acetate *on page 753*
Depo-Testadiol® *see* Estradiol and Testosterone *on page 461*
Depotestogen® *see* Estradiol and Testosterone *on page 461*
Depo®-Testosterone *see* Testosterone *on page 1143*
Deproist® Expectorant With Codeine *see* Guaifenesin, Pseudoephedrine, and Codeine *on page 570*
Derifil® [OTC] *see* Chlorophyll *on page 265*
Dermacort® *see* Hydrocortisone *on page 608*
Dermaflex® Gel *see* Lidocaine *on page 706*
Derma-Smoothe/FS® *see* Fluocinolone *on page 512*
Dermatop® *see* Prednicarbate *on page 987*
DermiCort® *see* Hydrocortisone *on page 608*
Dermolate® [OTC] *see* Hydrocortisone *on page 608*
Dermtex® HC With Aloe *see* Hydrocortisone *on page 608*
Desferal® *see* Deferoxamine *on page 354*

Desipramine (des IP ra meen)

U.S. Brand Names Norpramin®

Canadian Brand Names Alti-Desipramine; Apo®-Desipramine; Norpramin®; Novo-Desipramine; Nu-Desipramine; PMS-Desipramine

Pharmacologic Category Antidepressant, Tricyclic (Secondary Amine)

Synonyms Desipramine Hydrochloride; Desmethylimipramine Hydrochloride

Use Treatment of various forms of depression, often in conjunction with psychotherapy; analgesic adjunct in chronic pain, peripheral neuropathies

Unlabeled/Investigational: Analgesic adjunct in chronic pain; peripheral neuropathies; substance-related disorders; attention-deficit/hyperactivity disorder (ADHD)

Local Anesthetic/Vasoconstrictor Precautions Use with caution; epinephrine, norepinephrine and levonordefrin have been shown to have an increased pressor response in combination TCAs

Effects on Dental Treatment

>10%: Xerostomia

Long-term treatment with TCAs increases the risk of caries by reducing salivation and salivary buffer capacity.

Dosage Oral:

Children 6-12 years: 10-30 mg/day or 1-5 mg/kg/day in divided doses; do not exceed 5 mg/kg/day

Adolescents: Initial: 25-50 mg/day; gradually increase to 100 mg/day in single or divided doses; maximum: 150 mg/day

Adults: Initial: 75 mg/day in divided doses; increase gradually to 150-200 mg/day in divided or single dose; maximum: 300 mg/day

Elderly: Initial: 10-25 mg/day; increase by 10-25 mg every 3 days for inpatients and every week for outpatients if tolerated; usual maintenance dose: 75-100 mg/day, but doses up to 300 mg/day may be necessary

Mechanism of Action Traditionally believed to increase the synaptic concentration of norepinephrine in the CNS by inhibition of reuptake by the presynaptic neuronal membrane. However, additional receptor effects have been found including desensitization of adenyl cyclase, down regulation of beta-adrenergic receptors, and down regulation of serotonin receptors.

Other Adverse Effects Frequency not defined:

Cardiovascular: Arrhythmias, hypotension, hypertension, palpitations, heart block, tachycardia

Central nervous system: Dizziness, drowsiness, headache, confusion, delirium, hallucinations, nervousness, restlessness, parkinsonian syndrome, insomnia, disorientation, anxiety, agitation, hypomania, exacerbation of psychosis, incoordination, seizures, extrapyramidal symptoms

Dermatologic: Alopecia, photosensitivity, skin rash, urticaria

Endocrine & metabolic: Breast enlargement, galactorrhea, SIADH

(Continued)

Desipramine *(Continued)*

Gastrointestinal: Xerostomia, decreased lower esophageal sphincter tone may cause GE reflux, constipation, nausea, unpleasant taste, weight gain/loss, anorexia, abdominal cramps, diarrhea, heartburn

Genitourinary: Difficult urination, sexual dysfunction, testicular edema

Hematologic: Agranulocytosis, eosinophilia, purpura, thrombocytopenia

Hepatic: Cholestatic jaundice, increased liver enzyme

Neuromuscular & skeletal: Fine muscle tremors, weakness, numbness, tingling, paresthesia of extremities, ataxia

Ocular: Blurred vision, disturbances of accommodation, mydriasis, increased intraocular pressure

Miscellaneous: Diaphoresis (excessive), allergic reactions

Drug Interactions CYP1A2 and 2D6 enzyme substrate; CYP2D6 inhibitor

Increased Effect/Toxicity: Desipramine increases the effects of amphetamines, anticholinergics, other CNS depressants (sedatives, hypnotics) chlorpropamide, tolazamide, and warfarin. When used with MAO inhibitors, serotonin syndrome may occur. The SSRIs (to varying degrees), cimetidine, indinavir, methylphenidate, ritonavir (and other protease inhibitors), quinidine, diltiazem, and verapamil inhibit the metabolism of TCAs and clinical toxicity may result. Use of lithium with a TCA may increase the risk for neurotoxicity. Phenothiazines may increase concentration of some TCAs and TCAs may increase concentration of phenothiazines. Pressor response to I.V. epinephrine, norepinephrine, and phenylephrine may be enhanced in patients receiving TCAs (**Note:** Effect is unlikely with epinephrine or levonordefrin dosages typically administered as infiltration in combination with local anesthetics). Combined use of beta-agonists or drugs which prolong QT_c (including quinidine, procainamide, disopyramide, cisapride, sparfloxacin, gatifloxacin, moxifloxacin) with TCAs may predispose patients to cardiac arrhythmias.

Decreased Effect: Desipramine's serum concentration/effect may be decreased by carbamazepine, cholestyramine, colestipol, phenobarbital, and rifampin. Desipramine inhibits the antihypertensive effect of to bethanidine, clonidine, debrisoquin, guanadrel, guanethidine, guanabenz, or guanfacine.

Drug Uptake

Onset of action: 1-3 weeks; Maximum antidepressant effect: >2 weeks

Absorption: Well absorbed (90%) from GI tract

Half-life, elimination: Adults: 12-57 hours, 7-60 hours

Time to peak, plasma: 4-6 hours

Pregnancy Risk Factor C

Generic Available Yes

Selected Readings

Boakes AJ, Laurence DR, Teoh PC, et al, "Interactions Between Sympathomimetic Amines and Antidepressant Agents in Man," *Br Med J*, 1973, 1(849):311-5.

Friedlander AH, Mahler ME, "Major Depressive Disorder. Psychopathology, Medical Management, and Dental Implications," *J Am Dent Assoc*, 201, 132(5):629-38.

Ganzberg S, "Psychoactive Drugs," *ADA Guide to Dental Therapeutics*, 2nd ed, Chicago, IL: ADA Publishing, a Division of ADA Business Enterprises, Inc, 2000, 376-405.

Jastak JT and Yagiela JA, "Vasoconstrictors and Local Anesthesia: A Review and Rationale for Use," *J Am Dent Assoc*, 1983, 107(4):623-30.

Mitchell JR, "Guanethidine and Related Agents. III Antagonism by Drugs Which Inhibit the Norepinephrine Pump in Man," *J Clin Invest*, 1970, 49(8):1596-604.

Rundegren J, van Dijken J, Mörnstad H, et al, "Oral Conditions in Patients Receiving Long-Term Treatment With Cyclic Antidepressant Drugs," *Swed Dent J*, 1985, 9(2):55-64.

Yagiela JA, "Adverse Drug Interactions in Dental Practice: Interactions Associated With Vasoconstrictors. Part V of a Series," *J Am Dent Assoc*, 1999, 130(5):701-9.

Desitin® [OTC] *see* Zinc Oxide *on page 1260*

Desitin® [OTC] *see* Zinc Oxide, Cod Liver Oil, and Talc *on page 1261*

Desitin® Creamy [OTC] *see* Zinc Oxide *on page 1260*

Desloratadine (des lor AT a deen)

U.S. Brand Names Clarinex®

Pharmacologic Category Antihistamine, Nonsedating

Use Relief of nasal and non-nasal symptoms of seasonal allergic rhinitis (SAR) and perennial allergic rhinitis (PAR); treatment of chronic idiopathic urticaria (CIU)

Local Anesthetic/Vasoconstrictor Precautions No information available to require special precautions

Effects on Dental Treatment No effects or complications reported

Dosage Oral:

Adults and Children ≥12 years: 5 mg once daily

Dosage adjustment in renal/hepatic impairment: 5 mg every other day

Mechanism of Action Desloratadine, a major metabolite of loratadine, is a long-acting tricyclic antihistamine with selective peripheral histamine H_1 receptor antagonistic activity and additional anti-inflammatory properties.

Other Adverse Effects

>10%: Central nervous system: Headache (14%)

1% to 10%:

Central nervous system: Fatigue (2% to 5%), somnolence (2%), dizziness (4%)

Endocrine & metabolic: Dysmenorrhea (2%)
Gastrointestinal: Dry mouth (3%), nausea (5%), dyspepsia (3%)
Neuromuscular & skeletal: Myalgia (3%)
Respiratory: Pharyngitis (3% to 4%)

Drug Interactions Increased Effect/Toxicity: With concurrent use of desloratadine and erythromycin or ketoconazole, the C_{max} and AUC of desloratadine and its metabolite are increased; however, no clinically-significant changes in the safety profile of desloratadine were observed in clinical studies.

Drug Uptake
Half-life, elimination: 27 hours
Time to peak: 3 hours

Pregnancy Risk Factor C

Generic Available No

Desmopressin Acetate (des moe PRES in)

U.S. Brand Names DDAVP®; Stimate™

Canadian Brand Names DDAVP®; Octostim®

Mexican Brand Names Minirin

Pharmacologic Category Vasopressin Analog, Synthetic

Synonyms 1-Deamino-8-D-Arginine Vasopressin; Desmopressin

Use Treatment of diabetes insipidus and controlling bleeding in mild hemophilia, von Willebrand disease, and thrombocytopenia (eg, uremia)

Local Anesthetic/Vasoconstrictor Precautions No information available to require special precautions

Effects on Dental Treatment No effects or complications reported

Dosage
Children:
Diabetes insipidus:
Intranasal (using 100 mcg/mL nasal solution): 3 months to 12 years: Initial: 5 mcg/day (0.05 mL/day) divided 1-2 times/day; range: 5-30 mcg/day (0.05-0.3 mL/day) divided 1-2 times/day; adjust morning and evening doses separately for an adequate diurnal rhythm of water turnover; doses <10 mcg should be administered using the rhinal tube system
Oral: ≥4 years: Initial: 0.05 mg twice daily; total daily dose should be increased or decreased as needed to obtain adequate antidiuresis (range: 0.1-1.2 mg divided 2-3 times/day)
Hemophilia A and von Willebrand disease (type I):
I.V.: >3 months: 0.3 mcg/kg by slow infusion; may repeat dose if needed; begin 30 minutes before procedure
Intranasal: ≥11 months: Refer to adult dosing.
Nocturnal enuresis:
Intranasal (using 100 mcg/mL nasal solution): ≥6 years: Initial: 20 mcg (0.2 mL) at bedtime; range: 10-40 mcg; it is recommended that 1/2 of the dose be given in each nostril
Oral: 0.2 mg at bedtime; dose may be titrated up to 0.6 mg to achieve desired response. Patients previously on intranasal therapy can begin oral tablets 24 hours after the last intranasal dose.
Children ≥12 years and Adults:
Diabetes insipidus:
I.V., S.C.: 2-4 mcg/day (0.5-1 mL) in 2 divided doses or 1/10 of the maintenance intranasal dose
Intranasal (using 100 mcg/mL nasal solution): 10-40 mcg/day (0.1-0.4 mL) divided 1-3 times/day; adjust morning and evening doses separately for an adequate diurnal rhythm of water turnover. **Note:** The nasal spray pump can only deliver doses of 10 mcg (0.1 mL) or multiples of 10 mcg (0.1 mL); if doses other than this are needed, the rhinal tube delivery system is preferred.
Oral: Initial: 0.05 mg twice daily; total daily dose should be increased or decreased as needed to obtain adequate antidiuresis (range: 0.1-1.2 mg divided 2-3 times/day)
Hemophilia A and mild to moderate von Willebrand disease (type I):
I.V.: 0.3 mcg/kg by slow infusion, begin 30 minutes before procedure
Intranasal: Using high concentration spray (1.5 mg/mL): <50 kg: 150 mcg (1 spray); >50 kg: 300 mcg (1 spray each nostril); repeat use is determined by the patient's clinical condition and laboratory work; if using preoperatively, administer 2 hours before surgery

Mechanism of Action Enhances reabsorption of water in the kidneys by increasing cellular permeability of the collecting ducts; possibly causes smooth muscle constriction with resultant vasoconstriction; raises plasma concentrations of von Willebrand factor and factor VIII

Other Adverse Effects 1% to 10%:
Cardiovascular: Facial flushing
Central nervous system: Headache, dizziness
Gastrointestinal: Nausea, abdominal cramps
Genitourinary: Vulval pain
Local: Pain at the injection site
(Continued)

Desmopressin Acetate *(Continued)*

Respiratory: Nasal congestion

Drug Interactions

Increased Effect/Toxicity: Chlorpropamide, fludrocortisone may increase ADH response.

Decreased Effect: Demeclocycline and lithium may decrease ADH response.

Drug Uptake

Half-life, elimination: Terminal: 1.25 hours

Nasal: Absorption: Slow; 10% to 20%

Intranasal:

Onset of ADH effects: ≤1 hour

Time to peak: 1-5 hours

Duration: 5-21 hours

I.V. infusion:

Onset of increased factor VIII activity: 15-30 minutes

Time to peak: 1.5-3 hours

Pregnancy Risk Factor B

Generic Available Yes

Desogen® *see* Combination Hormonal Contraceptives *on page 323*

Desonide (DES oh nide)

U.S. Brand Names DesOwen®; Tridesilon®

Canadian Brand Names Desocort®; Scheinpharm Desonide

Mexican Brand Names Desowen®

Pharmacologic Category Corticosteroid, Topical

Use Adjunctive therapy for inflammation in acute and chronic corticosteroid responsive dermatosis (low potency corticosteroid)

Local Anesthetic/Vasoconstrictor Precautions No information available to require special precautions

Effects on Dental Treatment No effects or complications reported

Dosage Children and Adults: Topical: Apply 2-4 times/day sparingly

Therapy should be discontinued when control is achieved; if no improvement is seen, reassessment of diagnosis may be necessary.

Mechanism of Action Stimulates the synthesis of enzymes needed to decrease inflammation, suppress mitotic activity, and cause vasoconstriction

Drug Uptake

Onset of action: ~7 days

Absorption: Extensive from scalp, face, axilla and scrotum; adequate through epidermis on appendages; absorption can be increased with occlusion or the addition of penetrants (eg, urea, DMSO)

Pregnancy Risk Factor C

Generic Available Yes

DesOwen® *see* Desonide *on page 362*

Desoximetasone (des oks i MET a sone)

U.S. Brand Names Topicort®; Topicort®-LP

Canadian Brand Names Taro-Desoximetasone; Topicort®

Pharmacologic Category Corticosteroid, Topical

Use Relieves inflammation and pruritic symptoms of corticosteroid-responsive dermatosis [medium to high potency topical corticosteroid]

Local Anesthetic/Vasoconstrictor Precautions No information available to require special precautions

Effects on Dental Treatment No effects or complications reported

Dosage Topical:

Children: Apply sparingly in a very thin film to affected area 1-2 times/day

Adults: Apply sparingly in a thin film twice daily

Therapy should be discontinued when control is achieved; if no improvement is seen, reassessment of diagnosis may be necessary.

Mechanism of Action Stimulates the synthesis of enzymes needed to decrease inflammation, suppress mitotic activity, and cause vasoconstriction

Drug Uptake Absorption: Topical: Extensive from the scalp, face, axilla, and scrotum and adequate through epidermis on appendages; absorption can be increased with occlusion or the addition of penetrants

Pregnancy Risk Factor C

Generic Available Yes

Desoxyn® *see* Methamphetamine *on page 779*
Desoxyn® Gradumet® *see* Methamphetamine *on page 779*
Desquam-E™ *see* Benzoyl Peroxide *on page 153*
Desquam-X® *see* Benzoyl Peroxide *on page 153*
Desyrel® *see* Trazodone *on page 1193*
Detane® [OTC] *see* Benzocaine *on page 151*

Detrol™ *see* Tolterodine *on page 1181*
Detrol® LA *see* Tolterodine *on page 1181*
Dexacidin® *see* Neomycin, Polymyxin B, and Dexamethasone *on page 856*
Dexacort® Phosphate Turbinaire® *see* Dexamethasone *on page 363*

Dexamethasone (deks a METH a sone)

Related Information
Dental Office Emergencies *on page 1418*
Neomycin, Polymyxin B, and Dexamethasone *on page 856*
Oral Nonviral Soft Tissue Ulcerations or Erosions *on page 1384*
Respiratory Diseases *on page 1328*

U.S. Brand Names AK-Dex®; Baldex®; Dalalone®; Dalalone D.P.®; Dalalone L.A.®; Decadron®; Decadron®-LA; Decadron® Phosphate; Decaject®; Decaject-LA®; Decaspray®; Dexacort® Phosphate Turbinaire®; Dexasone®; Dexasone® L.A.; Dexone®; Dexone® LA; Hexadrol®; Hexadrol® Phosphate; Maxidex®; Solurex®; Solurex L.A.®

Canadian Brand Names Decadron®; Dexasone®; Diodex®; Hexadrol® Phosphate; Maxidex®; PMS-Dexamethasone

Mexican Brand Names Alin; Alin Depot; Decadron®; Decadronal®; Decorex; Dexagrin®; Dibasona; Indarzona®

Pharmacologic Category Corticosteroid, Nasal; Corticosteroid, Ophthalmic; Corticosteroid, Systemic; Corticosteroid, Topical

Synonyms Dexamethasone Acetate; Dexamethasone Sodium Phosphate

Use
Dental: Treatment of a variety of oral diseases of allergic, inflammatory or autoimmune origin
Medical: Systemically and locally for chronic swelling, allergic, hematologic, neoplastic, and autoimmune diseases; may be used in management of cerebral edema, septic shock, as a diagnostic agent, antiemetic
General indicator consistent with depression; diagnosis of Cushing's syndrome

Local Anesthetic/Vasoconstrictor Precautions No information available to require special precautions

Effects on Dental Treatment No effects or complications reported

Dosage
Children:
- Antiemetic (prior to chemotherapy): I.V. (should be given as sodium phosphate): 10 mg/m^2/dose (maximum: 20 mg) for first dose then 5 mg/m^2/dose every 6 hours as needed
- Anti-inflammatory immunosuppressant: Oral, I.M., I.V. (injections should be given as sodium phosphate): 0.08-0.3 mg/kg/day **or** 2.5-10 mg/m^2/day in divided doses every 6-12 hours
- Extubation or airway edema: Oral, I.M., I.V. (injections should be given as sodium phosphate): 0.5-2 mg/kg/day in divided doses every 6 hours beginning 24 hours prior to extubation and continuing for 4-6 doses afterwards
- Cerebral edema: I.V. (should be given as sodium phosphate): Loading dose: 1-2 mg/kg/dose as a single dose; maintenance: 1-1.5 mg/kg/day (maximum: 16 mg/day) in divided doses every 4-6 hours for 5 days then taper for 5 days, then discontinue
- Bacterial meningitis in infants and children >2 months: I.V. (should be given as sodium phosphate): 0.6 mg/kg/day in 4 divided doses every 6 hours for the first 4 days of antibiotic treatment; start dexamethasone at the time of the first dose of antibiotic
- Physiologic replacement: Oral, I.M., I.V.: 0.03-0.15 mg/kg/day or 0.6-0.75 mg/m^2/day in divided doses every 6-12 hours

Adults:
- Antiemetic:
  - Prophylaxis: Oral, I.V.: 10-20 mg 15-30 minutes before treatment on each treatment day
    - Continuous infusion regimen: Oral or I.V.: 10 mg every 12 hours on each treatment day
    - Mildly emetogenic therapy: Oral, I.M., I.V.: 4 mg every 4-6 hours
  - Delayed nausea/vomiting: Oral:
    - 8 mg every 12 hours for 2 days; then
    - 4 mg every 12 hours for 2 days **or**
    - 20 mg 1 hour before chemotherapy; then
    - 10 mg 12 hours after chemotherapy; then
    - 8 mg every 12 hours for 4 doses; then
    - 4 mg every 12 hours for 4 doses
- Anti-inflammatory:
  - Oral, I.M., I.V. (injections should be given as sodium phosphate): 0.75-9 mg/day in divided doses every 6-12 hours
  - I.M. (as acetate): 8-16 mg; may repeat in 1-3 weeks
  - Intralesional (as acetate): 0.8-1.6 mg
  - Intra-articular/soft tissue (as acetate): 4-16 mg; may repeat in 1-3 weeks
  - Intra-articular, intralesional, or soft tissue (as sodium phosphate): 0.4-6 mg/day

(Continued)

Dexamethasone *(Continued)*

Ophthalmic:

Ointment: Apply thin coating into conjunctival sac 3-4 times/day; gradually taper dose to discontinue

Suspension: Instill 2 drops into conjunctival sac every hour during the day and every other hour during the night; gradually reduce dose to every 3-4 hours, then to 3-4 times/day

Topical: Apply 1-4 times/day. Therapy should be discontinued when control is achieved; if no improvement is seen, reassessment of diagnosis may be necessary.

Chemotherapy: Oral, I.V.: 40 mg every day for 4 days, repeated every 4 weeks (VAD regimen)

Cerebral edema: I.V. 10 mg stat, 4 mg I.M./I.V. (should be given as sodium phosphate) every 6 hours until response is maximized, then switch to oral regimen, then taper off if appropriate; dosage may be reduced after 24 days and gradually discontinued over 5-7 days

Dexamethasone suppression test (depression indicator) or diagnosis for Cushing's syndrome (unlabeled uses): Oral: 1 mg at 11 PM, draw blood at 8 AM the following day for plasma cortisol determination

Physiological replacement: Oral, I.M., I.V. (should be given as sodium phosphate): 0.03-0.15 mg/kg/day **OR** 0.6-0.75 mg/m^2/day in divided doses every 6-12 hours

Treatment of shock:

Addisonian crisis/shock (ie, adrenal insufficiency/responsive to steroid therapy): I.V. (given as sodium phosphate): 4-10 mg as a single dose, which may be repeated if necessary

Unresponsive shock (ie, unresponsive to steroid therapy): I.V. (given as sodium phosphate): 1-6 mg/kg as a single I.V. dose or up to 40 mg initially followed by repeat doses every 2-6 hours while shock persists

Hemodialysis: Supplemental dose is not necessary

Peritoneal dialysis: Supplemental dose is not necessary

Mechanism of Action Decreases inflammation by suppression of migration of polymorphonuclear leukocytes and reversal of increased capillary permeability; suppresses normal immune response

Other Adverse Effects

Systemic:

>10%:

Central nervous system: Insomnia, nervousness

Gastrointestinal: Increased appetite, indigestion

1% to 10%:

Dermatologic: Hirsutism

Endocrine & metabolic: Diabetes mellitus

Neuromuscular & skeletal: Arthralgia

Ocular: Cataracts

Respiratory: Epistaxis

<1% and/or case reports: Seizures, mood swings, headache, delirium, hallucinations, euphoria, skin atrophy, bruising, hyperpigmentation, acne, amenorrhea, sodium and water retention, Cushing's syndrome, hyperglycemia, bone growth suppression, abdominal distention, ulcerative esophagitis, pancreatitis, muscle wasting, hypersensitivity reactions

Topical: <1%: Itching, dryness, folliculitis, hypertrichosis, acneiform eruptions, hypopigmentation, perioral dermatitis, allergic contact dermatitis, skin maceration, skin atrophy, striae; miliaria, local burning, irritation; secondary infection

Contraindications Hypersensitivity to dexamethasone or any component of the formulation; active untreated infections; ophthalmic use in viral, fungal, or tuberculosis diseases of the eye

Warnings/Precautions Fatalities have occurred due to adrenal insufficiency in asthmatic patients during and after transfer from systemic corticosteroids to aerosol steroids; aerosol steroids do **not** provide the systemic steroid needed to treat patients having trauma, surgery, or infections; use with caution in patients with hypothyroidism, cirrhosis, hypertension, CHF, ulcerative colitis, thromboembolic disorders. Corticosteroids should be used with caution in patients with diabetes, osteoporosis, peptic ulcer, glaucoma, cataracts, or tuberculosis. Use caution in hepatic impairment. Because of the risk of adverse effects, systemic corticosteroids should be used cautiously in the elderly in the smallest possible dose and for the shortest possible time.

Controlled clinical studies have shown that inhaled and intranasal corticosteroids may cause a reduction in growth velocity in pediatric patients. Growth velocity provides a means of comparing the rate of growth among children of the same age.

In studies involving inhaled corticosteroids, the average reduction in growth velocity was approximately 1 cm (about 1/3 of an inch) per year. It appears that the reduction is related to dose and how long the child takes the drug.

FDA's Pulmonary and Allergy Drugs and Metabolic and Endocrine Drugs advisory committees discussed this issue at a July 1998 meeting. They recommended that the agency develop classwide labeling to inform healthcare providers so they would understand this potential side effect and monitor growth routinely in pediatric patients who are treated with inhaled corticosteroids, intranasal corticosteroids or both.

Long-term effects of this reduction in growth velocity on final adult height are unknown. Likewise, it also has not yet been determined whether patients' growth will "catch up" if treatment in discontinued. Drug manufacturers will continue to monitor these drugs to learn more about long-term effects. Children are prescribed inhaled corticosteroids to treat asthma. Intranasal corticosteroids are generally used to prevent and treat allergy-related nasal symptoms.

Patients are advised not to stop using their inhaled or intranasal corticosteroids without first speaking to their healthcare providers about the benefits of these drugs compared to their risks.

Drug Interactions CYP3A3/4 enzyme substrate; CYP3A3/4 enzyme inducer; CYP3A3/4 enzyme inhibitor

Increased Effect: Salmeterol: The addition of salmeterol has been demonstrated to improve response to inhaled corticosteroids (as compared to increasing steroid dosage).

Decreased Effect: Barbiturates, phenytoin, rifampin may decrease dexamethasone effects; dexamethasone decreases effect of salicylates, vaccines, toxoids

Dietary/Ethanol/Herb Considerations

Ethanol: Avoid use; may enhance gastric mucosal irritation.

Food: Administer with food to reduce GI upset. Limit caffeine. Interferes with calcium absorption; may require increased intake of calcium, folate, phosphorus. potassium, pyridoxine, vitamin C, and vitamin D.

Herb/Nutraceutical: Avoid cat's claw and echinacea due to immunostimulant properties.

Drug Uptake

Onset of action: Acetate: Prompt

Absorption: Rapid and complete

Duration: ≤72 hours

Half-life, elimination (dependent on renal function): 1.8-3.5 hours; Biological: 36-54 hours

Time to peak: Oral: 1-2 hours; I.M.: ~8 hours

Pregnancy Risk Factor C

Dosage Forms AERO, topical: 0.04% (25 g). **CONC, oral:** 0.5 mg/0.5 mL (30 mL). **CRM, as sodium phosphate:** 0.1% (15 g, 30 g). **ELIX:** 0.5 mg/5 mL (5 mL, 20 mL, 100 mL, 120 mL, 237 mL, 240 mL, 500 mL). **INJ, suspension, as acetate:** 8 mg/mL (1 mL, 5 mL); 16 mg/mL (1 mL, 5 mL). **INJ, as sodium phosphate:** 4 mg/mL (1 mL, 5 mL, 10 mL, 25 mL, 30 mL); 10 mg/mL (1 mL, 10 mL); 20 mg/mL (5 mL); 24 mg/mL (5 mL, 10 mL). **OINT, ophthalmic, as sodium phosphate:** 0.05% (3.5 g). **SOLN, oral:** 0.5 mg/5 mL (5 mL, 20 mL, 500 mL). **SUSP, ophthalmic, as sodium phosphate:** 0.1% (5 mL, 15 mL). **TAB:** 0.25 mg, 0.5 mg, 0.75 mg, 1 mg, 1.5 mg, 2 mg, 4 mg, 6 mg. **TAB** [therapeutic pack]: 6 x 1.5 mg; 8 x 0.75 mg

Generic Available Yes

Dexasone® *see* Dexamethasone *on page 363*

Dexasone® L.A. *see* Dexamethasone *on page 363*

Dexasporin® *see* Neomycin, Polymyxin B, and Dexamethasone *on page 856*

Dexbrompheniramine and Pseudoephedrine

(deks brom fen EER a meen & soo doe e FED rin)

U.S. Brand Names Brompheril® [OTC]; Disobrom® [OTC]; Disophrol® Chronotabs® [OTC]; Drixomed®; Drixoral® Cold & Allergy [OTC]; Histrodrix®; Resporal®

Canadian Brand Names Drixoral®

Pharmacologic Category Antihistamine/Decongestant Combination

Synonyms Pseudoephedrine and Dexbrompheniramine

Use Relief of symptoms of upper respiratory mucosal congestion in seasonal and perennial nasal allergies, acute rhinitis, rhinosinusitis and eustachian tube blockage

Local Anesthetic/Vasoconstrictor Precautions Use with caution since pseudoephedrine is a sympathomimetic amine which could interact with epinephrine to cause a pressor response

Effects on Dental Treatment ≤10%: Tachycardia, palpitations, xerostomia; use vasoconstrictor with caution

Dosage Children >12 years and Adults: Oral: 1 tablet every 12 hours, may require 1 tablet every 8 hours

Pregnancy Risk Factor B

Generic Available Yes

Dexchlorpheniramine (deks klor fen EER a meen)

U.S. Brand Names Polaramine®

Canadian Brand Names Polaramine®

Pharmacologic Category Antihistamine

Synonyms Dexchlorpheniramine Maleate

(Continued)

Dexchlorpheniramine *(Continued)*

Use Perennial and seasonal allergic rhinitis and other allergic symptoms including urticaria

Local Anesthetic/Vasoconstrictor Precautions No information available to require special precautions

Effects on Dental Treatment ≤10%: Significant xerostomia and drowsiness; disappears with discontinuation

Dosage Oral:

Children:

2-5 years: 0.5 mg every 4-6 hours (do not use timed release)

6-11 years: 1 mg every 4-6 hours or 4 mg timed release at bedtime

Adults: 2 mg every 4-6 hours or 4-6 mg timed release at bedtime or every 8-10 hours

Mechanism of Action Competes with histamine for H_1-receptor sites on effector cells in the GI tract, blood vessels, and respiratory tract

Other Adverse Effects

>10%:

Central nervous system: Slight to moderate drowsiness

Respiratory: Thickening of bronchial secretions

1% to 10%:

Central nervous system: Headache, fatigue, nervousness, dizziness

Gastrointestinal: Appetite increase, weight gain, nausea, diarrhea, abdominal pain, xerostomia

Neuromuscular & skeletal: Arthralgia

Respiratory: Pharyngitis

Drug Interactions

Increased Effect/Toxicity: CNS depressants may increase the degree of sedation and respiratory depression with antihistamines. May increase the absorption of digoxin. Central and/or peripheral anticholinergic syndrome can occur when administered with amantadine, rimantadine, narcotic analgesics, phenothiazines and other antipsychotics (especially with high anticholinergic activity), tricyclic antidepressants, quinidine, disopyramide, procainamide, and antihistamines.

Decreased Effect: May increase gastric degradation of levodopa and decrease the amount of levodopa absorbed by delaying gastric emptying; therapeutic effects of cholinergic agents (tacrine, donepezil) and neuroleptics may be antagonized.

Drug Uptake

Onset of action: ~1 hour

Absorption: Well absorbed from GI tract

Duration: 3-6 hours

Pregnancy Risk Factor B

Generic Available Yes

Dexedrine® *see* Dextroamphetamine *on page 370*

Dexferrum® *see* Iron Dextran Complex *on page 655*

Dexmedetomidine (deks MED e toe mi deen)

U.S. Brand Names Precedex™

Canadian Brand Names Precedex™

Pharmacologic Category $Alpha_2$-Adrenergic Agonist; Sedative

Synonyms Dexmedetomidine Hydrochloride

Use Sedation of initially intubated and mechanically ventilated patients during treatment in an intensive care setting; duration of infusion should not exceed 24 hours

Unlabeled/Investigational: Unlabeled uses include premedication prior to anesthesia induction with thiopental; relief of pain and reduction of opioid dose following laparoscopic tubal ligation; as an adjunct anesthetic in ophthalmic surgery; treatment of shivering; premedication to attenuate the cardiostimulatory and postanesthetic delirium of ketamine

Local Anesthetic/Vasoconstrictor Precautions No information available to require special precautions

Effects on Dental Treatment No effects or complications reported

Dosage Individualized and titrated to desired clinical effect

Adults: I.V.: Solution must be diluted prior to administration. Initial: Loading infusion of 1 mcg/kg over 10 minutes, followed by a maintenance infusion of 0.2-0.7 mcg/kg/hour; not indicated for infusions lasting >24 hours

Elderly (>65 years of age): Dosage reduction may need to be considered. No specific guidelines available. Dose selections should be cautious, at the low end of dosage range; titration should be slower, allowing adequate time to evaluate response.

Dosage adjustment in hepatic impairment: Dosage reduction may need to be considered; no specific guidelines available.

Mechanism of Action A relatively selective $alpha_2$ receptor agonist; stimulation of this receptor subtype within the CNS causes sedation. It has not been associated with respiratory depression within the recommended dosage range. At high dosages or following rapid bolus administration, it may cause $alpha_1$ and $alpha_2$ stimulation.

Other Adverse Effects

>10%:

Cardiovascular: Hypotension (30%)

Gastrointestinal: Nausea (11%)

1% to 10%:

Cardiovascular: Bradycardia (8%), atrial fibrillation (7%)

Central nervous system: Pain (3%)

Hematologic: Anemia (3%), leukocytosis (2%)

Renal: Oliguria (2%)

Respiratory: Hypoxia (6%), pulmonary edema (2%), pleural effusion (3%)

Miscellaneous: Infection (2%), thirst (2%)

Drug Interactions CYP2A6 enzyme substrate

Increased Effect/Toxicity: Possible enhanced effects and pharmacodynamic interaction with sedatives, hypnotics, opioids, and anesthetics; monitor and decrease the dose as necessary of each agent and/or dexmedetomidine. Enhanced effects may occur with sevoflurane, isoflurane, propofol, alfentanil, and midazolam. Hypotension and/or bradycardia may be increased by vasodilators and heart rate-lowering agents.

Drug Uptake

Onset of action: Rapid

Half-life, elimination: 6 minutes; Terminal: 2 hours

Pregnancy Risk Factor C

Generic Available No

Comments Must be administered using a controlled infusion device. Patients must be in a monitored intensive care setting. Solution should be diluted in 0.9% sodium chloride prior to administration (2 mL dexmedetomidine diluted in 48 mL 0.9% sodium chloride to a total volume of 50 mL). To minimize the risk of bradycardia or hypotension, loading dose should be infused over ≤10 minutes. Must be titrated to clinical effect with adequate monitoring of sedation. It is not necessary to discontinue the infusion prior to extubation provided the infusion does not exceed 24 hours. Heart rate, blood pressure, and degree of sedation should be monitored.

Dexmethylphenidate (dex meth il FEN i date)

U.S. Brand Names Focalin™

Pharmacologic Category Central Nervous System Stimulant

Synonyms Dexmethylphenidate Hydrochloride

Use Treatment of attention-deficit/hyperactivity disorder (ADHD)

Local Anesthetic/Vasoconstrictor Precautions No information available to require special precautions

Effects on Dental Treatment No effects or complications reported

Restrictions C-II

Dosage Oral: Children ≥6 years and Adults: Treatment of ADHD: Initial: 2.5 mg twice daily in patients not currently taking methylphenidate; dosage may be adjusted in 2.5-5 mg increments at weekly intervals (maximum dose: 20 mg/day); doses should be taken at least 4 hours apart

When switching from methylphenidate to dexmethylphenidate, the starting dose of dexmethylphenidate should be half that of methylphenidate (maximum dose: 20 mg/day)

Safety and efficacy for long-term use of dexmethylphenidate have not yet been established. Patients should be re-evaluated at appropriate intervals to assess continued need of the medication.

Dose reductions and discontinuation: Reduce dose or discontinue in patients with paradoxical aggravation. Discontinue if no improvement is seen after one month of treatment.

Mechanism of Action The more active, *d-threo*-enantiomer, of racemic methylphenidate; it is a CNS stimulant which blocks the reuptake of norepinephrine and dopamine, and increases their release into the extraneuronal space.

Other Adverse Effects

>10%: Gastrointestinal: Abdominal pain (15%)

1% to 10%:

Central nervous system: Fever (5%)

Gastrointestinal: Nausea (9%), anorexia (6%)

Adverse effects seen with **methylphenidate** (frequency not defined):

Cardiovascular: Angina, cardiac arrhythmias, cerebral arteritis, cerebral occlusion, hypertension, hypotension, palpitations, pulse increase/decrease, tachycardia

Central nervous system: Depression, dizziness, drowsiness, fever, headache, insomnia, nervousness, neuroleptic malignant syndrome (NMS), Tourette's syndrome, toxic psychosis

Dermatologic: Erythema multiforme, exfoliative dermatitis, hair loss, rash, urticaria

Endocrine & metabolic: Growth retardation

(Continued)

Dexmethylphenidate *(Continued)*

Gastrointestinal: Abdominal pain, anorexia, nausea, vomiting, weight loss
Hematologic: Anemia, leukopenia, thrombocytopenic purpura
Hepatic: Abnormal liver function tests, hepatic coma, transaminase elevation
Neuromuscular & skeletal: Arthralgia, dyskinesia
Ocular: Blurred vision
Renal: Necrotizing vasculitis
Respiratory: Cough increased, pharyngitis, sinusitis, upper respiratory tract infection
Miscellaneous: Hypersensitivity reactions

Warnings/Precautions Recommended to be used as part of a comprehensive treatment program for ADHD. Use with caution in patients with bipolar disorder, diabetes mellitus, cardiovascular disease, hyperthyroidism, seizure disorders, insomnia, porphyria, or hypertension. Use caution in patients with history of ethanol or drug abuse. May exacerbate symptoms of behavior and thought disorder in psychotic patients. Do not use to treat severe depression or fatigue states. Potential for drug dependency exists - avoid abrupt discontinuation in patients who have received for prolonged periods. Visual disturbances have been reported with methylphenidate (rare). Stimulant use has been associated with growth suppression. Stimulants may unmask tics in individuals with coexisting Tourette's syndrome. Safety and efficacy in children <6 years of age not established.

Drug Interactions

Increased Effect/Toxicity: Methylphenidate may cause hypertensive effects when used in combination with MAO inhibitors or drugs with MAO-inhibiting activity (linezolid). Risk may be less with selegiline (MAO type B selective at low doses); it is best to avoid this combination. NMS has been reported in a patient receiving methylphenidate and venlafaxine. Methylphenidate may increase levels of phenytoin, phenobarbital, TCAs, and warfarin. Increased toxicity with clonidine and sibutramine.

Decreased Effect: Effectiveness of antihypertensive agents may be decreased. Carbamazepine may decrease the effect of methylphenidate.

Drug Uptake

Absorption: Rapid
Half-life, elimination: 2.2 hours
Time to peak: Fasting: 1-1.5 hours

Pregnancy Risk Factor C

Generic Available No

Dexone® *see* Dexamethasone *on page 363*
Dexone® LA *see* Dexamethasone *on page 363*

Dexpanthenol (deks PAN the nole)

U.S. Brand Names Ilopan®; Panthoderm® Cream [OTC]

Pharmacologic Category Gastrointestinal Agent, Stimulant

Synonyms Pantothenyl Alcohol

Use Prophylactic use to minimize paralytic ileus, treatment of postoperative distention

Local Anesthetic/Vasoconstrictor Precautions No information available to require special precautions

Effects on Dental Treatment No effects or complications reported

Dosage

Children and Adults: Relief of itching and aid in skin healing: Topical: Apply to affected area 1-2 times/day

Adults:
- Relief of gas retention: Oral: 2-3 tablets 3 times/day
- Prevention of postoperative ileus: I.M.: 250-500 mg stat, repeat in 2 hours, followed by doses every 6 hours until danger passes
- Paralyzed ileus: I.M.: 500 mg stat, repeat in 2 hours, followed by doses every 6 hours, if needed

Mechanism of Action A pantothenic acid B vitamin analog that is converted to coenzyme A internally; coenzyme A is essential to normal fatty acid synthesis, amino acid synthesis and acetylation of choline in the production of the neurotransmitter, acetylcholine

Drug Interactions Increases/prolongs effect of succinylcholine; do not administer within 1 hour.

Drug Uptake Absorption: Well absorbed

Pregnancy Risk Factor C

Generic Available Yes: Injection

Dexrazoxane (deks ray ZOKS ane)

U.S. Brand Names Zinecard®

Canadian Brand Names Zinecard™

Pharmacologic Category Cardioprotectant

Synonyms ICRF-187

Use Reduction of the incidence and severity of cardiomyopathy associated with doxorubicin administration in women with metastatic breast cancer who have received a cumulative doxorubicin dose of 300 mg/m^2 and who would benefit from continuing therapy with doxorubicin. It is not recommended for use with the initiation of doxorubicin therapy.

Local Anesthetic/Vasoconstrictor Precautions No information available to require special precautions

Effects on Dental Treatment No effects or complications reported

Dosage Adults: I.V.: The recommended dosage ratio of dexrazoxane:doxorubicin is 10:1 (eg, 500 mg/m^2 dexrazoxane:50 mg/m^2 doxorubicin). Administer the reconstituted solution by slow I.V. push or rapid I.V. infusion from a bag. After completing the infusion, and prior to a total elapsed time of 30 minutes (from the beginning of the dexrazoxane infusion), give the I.V. injection of doxorubicin.

Mechanism of Action Derivative of EDTA and potent intracellular chelating agent. The mechanism of cardioprotectant activity is not fully understood. Appears to be converted intracellularly to a ring-opened chelating agent that interferes with iron-mediated free radical generation thought to be responsible, in part, for anthracycline-induced cardiomyopathy.

Other Adverse Effects Adverse reactions are likely attributable to the FAC regimen, with the exception of pain on injection that was observed mainly with dexrazoxane. Patients receiving FAC with dexrazoxane experienced more severe leukopenia, granulocytopenia, and thrombocytopenia at nadir than those receiving FAC without dexrazoxane; but recovery counts were similar.

1% to 10%: Dermatologic: Urticaria, recall skin reaction, extravasation

Drug Interactions Concurrent use with the initiation of FAC therapy is not recommended; may interfere with the antitumor efficacy of the regimen.

Drug Uptake Half-life, elimination: 2.1-2.5 hours

Pregnancy Risk Factor C

Generic Available No

Dextran (DEKS tran)

U.S. Brand Names Gentran®; LMD®; Macrodex®; Rheomacrodex®

Canadian Brand Names Gentran®

Mexican Brand Names Alpha-Dextrano"40"; Rheomacrodex®

Pharmacologic Category Plasma Volume Expander

Synonyms Dextran 40; Dextran 70; Dextran, High Molecular Weight; Dextran, Low Molecular Weight

Use Blood volume expander used in treatment of shock or impending shock when blood or blood products are not available; dextran 40 is also used as a priming fluid in cardiopulmonary bypass and for prophylaxis of venous thrombosis and pulmonary embolism in surgical procedures associated with a high risk of thromboembolic complications

Local Anesthetic/Vasoconstrictor Precautions No information available to require special precautions

Effects on Dental Treatment No effects or complications reported

Dosage I.V. (requires an infusion pump): Dose and infusion rate are dependent upon the patient's fluid status and must be individualized:

Volume expansion/shock:

Children: Total dose should not exceed 20 mL/kg during first 24 hours

Adults: 500-1000 mL at a rate of 20-40 mL/minute; maximum daily dose: 20 mL/kg for first 24 hours; 10 mL/kg/day thereafter; therapy should not be continued beyond 5 days

Pump prime (Dextran 40): Varies with the volume of the pump oxygenator; generally, the 10% solution is added in a dose of 1-2 g/kg

Prophylaxis of venous thrombosis/pulmonary embolism (Dextran 40): Begin during surgical procedure and give 50-100 g on the day of surgery; an additional 50 g (500 mL) should be administered every 2-3 days during the period of risk (up to 2 weeks postoperatively); usual maximum infusion rate for nonemergency use: 4 mL/minute

Mechanism of Action Produces plasma volume expansion by virtue of its highly colloidal starch structure, similar to albumin

Drug Uptake Onset of volume-expanding effect: I.V. infusion: Within minutes to 1 hour, depending upon the molecular weight polysaccharide administered

Pregnancy Risk Factor C

Generic Available No

Comments Dextran 40 is known as low molecular weight dextran (LMD®) and has an average molecular weight of 40,000; dextran 75 has an average molecular weight of 75,000

Dextran 1 (DEKS tran won)

U.S. Brand Names Promit®

Pharmacologic Category Plasma Volume Expander

Use Prophylaxis of serious anaphylactic reactions to I.V. infusion of dextran

(Continued)

Dextran 1 *(Continued)*

Local Anesthetic/Vasoconstrictor Precautions No information available to require special precautions

Effects on Dental Treatment No effects or complications reported

Dosage I.V. (time between dextran 1 and dextran solution should not exceed 15 minutes):

Children: 0.3 mL/kg 1-2 minutes before I.V. infusion of dextran

Adults: 20 mL 1-2 minutes before I.V. infusion of dextran

Mechanism of Action Binds to dextran-reactive immunoglobulin without bridge formation and no formation of large immune complexes

Pregnancy Risk Factor C

Generic Available No

Dextranomer (deks TRAN oh mer)

U.S. Brand Names Debrisan® [OTC]

Mexican Brand Names Debrisan®

Pharmacologic Category Topical Skin Product

Use Clean exudative ulcers and wounds such as venous stasis ulcers, decubitus ulcers, and infected traumatic and surgical wounds; no controlled studies have found dextranomer to be more effective than conventional therapy

Local Anesthetic/Vasoconstrictor Precautions No information available to require special precautions

Effects on Dental Treatment No effects or complications reported

Dosage Debride and clean wound prior to application; apply to affected area once or twice daily in a 1/4" layer; apply a dressing and seal on all four sides; removal should be done by irrigation

Mechanism of Action A network of dextran-sucrose beads possessing a great many exposed hydroxy groups; when this network is applied to an exudative wound surface, the exudate is drawn by capillary forces generated by the swelling of the beads, with vacuum forces producing an upward flow of exudate into the network

Other Adverse Effects 1% to 10%:

Local: Transitory pain, blistering

Dermatologic: Maceration may occur, erythema

Hematologic: Bleeding

Pregnancy Risk Factor C

Generic Available No

Dextroamphetamine (deks troe am FET a meen)

Related Information

Dextroamphetamine and Amphetamine *on page 371*

U.S. Brand Names Dexedrine®

Canadian Brand Names Dexedrine®

Pharmacologic Category Stimulant

Synonyms Dextroamphetamine Sulfate

Use Narcolepsy; attention-deficit/hyperactivity disorder (ADHD)

Unlabeled/Investigational: Exogenous obesity; depression; abnormal behavioral syndrome in children (minimal brain dysfunction)

Local Anesthetic/Vasoconstrictor Precautions Use vasoconstriction with caution in patients taking dextroamphetamine. Amphetamines enhance the sympathomimetic response of epinephrine and norepinephrine leading to potential hypertension and cardiotoxicity.

Effects on Dental Treatment Up to 10% of patients taking dextroamphetamines may present with hypertension. The use of local anesthetic without vasoconstrictor is recommended in these patients.

Restrictions C-II

Dosage Oral:

Children:

- Narcolepsy: 6-12 years: Initial: 5 mg/day; may increase at 5 mg increments in weekly intervals until side effects appear (maximum dose: 60 mg/day)
- ADHD:
  - 3-5 years: Initial: 2.5 mg/day given every morning; increase by 2.5 mg/day in weekly intervals until optimal response is obtained; usual range: 0.1-0.5 mg/kg/dose every morning with maximum of 40 mg/day
  - ≥6 years: 5 mg once or twice daily; increase in increments of 5 mg/day at weekly intervals until optimal response is obtained; usual range: 0.1-0.5 mg/kg/dose every morning (5-20 mg/day) with maximum of 40 mg/day

Children >12 years and Adults:

- Narcolepsy: Initial: 10 mg/day, may increase at 10 mg increments in weekly intervals until side effects appear; maximum: 60 mg/day
- Exogenous obesity (unlabeled use): 5-30 mg/day in divided doses of 5-10 mg 30-60 minutes before meals

Mechanism of Action Blocks reuptake of dopamine and norepinephrine from the synapse, thus increases the amount of circulating dopamine and norepinephrine in cerebral cortex to reticular activating system; inhibits the action of monoamine oxidase and causes catecholamines to be released. Peripheral actions include elevated BP, weak bronchodilator, and respiratory stimulant action.

Other Adverse Effects Frequency not defined:

Cardiovascular: Palpitations, tachycardia, hypertension, cardiomyopathy

Central nervous system: Overstimulation, euphoria, dyskinesia, dysphoria, exacerbation of motor and phonic tics, restlessness, insomnia, dizziness, headache, psychosis, Tourette's syndrome

Dermatologic: Rash, urticaria

Endocrine & metabolic: Changes in libido

Gastrointestinal: Diarrhea, constipation, anorexia, weight loss, xerostomia, unpleasant taste

Genitourinary: Impotence

Neuromuscular & skeletal: Tremor

Drug Interactions

Increased Effect/Toxicity: Dextroamphetamine may precipitate hypertensive crisis or serotonin syndrome in patients receiving MAO inhibitors (selegiline >10 mg/day, isocarboxazid, phenelzine, tranylcypromine, furazolidone). Serotonin syndrome has also been associated with combinations of amphetamines and SSRIs; these combinations should be avoided. TCAs may enhance the effects of amphetamines. Large doses of antacids or urinary alkalinizers increase the half-life and duration of action of amphetamines. May precipitate arrhythmias in patients receiving general anesthetics.

Decreased Effect: Amphetamines inhibit the antihypertensive response to guanethidine and guanadrel. Urinary acidifiers decrease the half-life and duration of action of amphetamines.

Drug Uptake

Onset of action: 1-1.5 hours

Half-life, elimination: Adults: 10-13 hours

Time to peak: Immediate release tablet: ~3 hours

Pregnancy Risk Factor C

Generic Available Yes

Dextroamphetamine and Amphetamine

(deks troe am FET a meen & am FET a meen)

U.S. Brand Names Adderall®; Adderall XR™

Pharmacologic Category Stimulant

Synonyms Amphetamine and Dextroamphetamine

Use Attention-deficit/hyperactivity disorder (ADHD); narcolepsy

Unlabeled/Investigational: Short-term adjunct to exogenous obesity

Local Anesthetic/Vasoconstrictor Precautions Use vasoconstriction with caution in patients taking dextroamphetamine. Amphetamines enhance the sympathomimetic response of epinephrine and norepinephrine leading to potential hypertension and cardiotoxicity.

Effects on Dental Treatment Up to 10% of patients taking dextroamphetamines may present with hypertension. The use of local anesthetic without vasoconstrictor is recommended in these patients.

Restrictions C-II

Dosage Oral:

Narcolepsy:

Children:

6-12 years: 5 mg/day, increase by 5 mg at weekly intervals

>12 years: 10 mg/day, increase by 10 mg at weekly intervals

Adults: 5-60 mg/day in 2-3 divided doses

Attention deficit/hyperactivity disorder: Children:

3-5 years: 2.5 mg/day, increase by 2.5 mg at weekly intervals

>6 years: 5 mg/day, increase by 5 mg at weekly intervals not to exceed 40 mg/day

Short-term adjunct to exogenous obesity: Children >12 years and Adults: 5-30 mg/day in divided doses

Mechanism of Action Blocks reuptake of dopamine and norepinephrine from the synapse, thus increases the amount of circulating dopamine and norepinephrine in cerebral cortex to reticular activating system; inhibits the action of monoamine oxidase and causes catecholamines to be released. Peripheral actions include elevated BP, weak bronchodilator, and respiratory stimulant action.

Other Adverse Effects Also see Dextroamphetamine *on page 370*

As reported with Adderall XR™:

>10%:

Central nervous system: Insomnia (1% to 17%)

Gastrointestinal: Appetite decreased (22%), abdominal pain (14%)

1% to 10%:

Central nervous system: Emotional lability (1% to 9%), nervousness (6%), fever (4%), dizziness (2%), weakness (2%)

Gastrointestinal: Vomiting (7%), nausea (5%), anorexia (3%), diarrhea (2%), dyspepsia (2%), weight loss (1%)

(Continued)

Dextroamphetamine and Amphetamine *(Continued)*

Miscellaneous: Infection (2% to 4%)

The following have been reported with amphetamine use.

Frequency not defined:

Cardiovascular: Palpitations, tachycardia, hypertension, cardiomyopathy

Central nervous system: Overstimulation, euphoria, dyskinesia, dysphoria, exacerbation of motor and phonic tics, restlessness, insomnia, headache, psychosis, exacerbation of Tourette's syndrome

Dermatologic: Rash, urticaria

Endocrine & metabolic: Changes in libido

Gastrointestinal: Constipation, xerostomia, unpleasant taste

Genitourinary: Impotence

Neuromuscular & skeletal: Tremor

Drug Interactions Amphetamine: CYP2D6 enzyme substrate

Increased Effect/Toxicity: Dextroamphetamine and amphetamine may precipitate hypertensive crisis or serotonin syndrome in patients receiving MAO inhibitors (selegiline >10 mg/day, isocarboxazid, phenelzine, tranylcypromine, furazolidone). Serotonin syndrome has also been associated with combinations of amphetamines and SSRIs; these combinations should be avoided. TCAs may enhance the effects of amphetamines, potentially leading to hypertensive crisis. Large doses of antacids or urinary alkalinizers increase the half-life and duration of action of amphetamines. May precipitate arrhythmias in patients receiving general anesthetics. Inhibitors of CYP2D6 may increase the effects of amphetamines (includes amiodarone, cimetidine, delavirdine, fluoxetine, paroxetine, propafenone, quinidine, and ritonavir).

Decreased Effect: Amphetamines inhibit the antihypertensive response to guanethidine and guanadrel. Urinary acidifiers decrease the half-life and duration of action of amphetamines. Enzyme inducers (barbiturates, carbamazepine, phenytoin, and rifampin) may decrease serum concentration of amphetamines.

Drug Uptake

Half-life, elimination:

Adderall®: 3 hours

Adderall XR™: ~7 hours

Amphetamine: Adults: 13 hours

Also see Dextroamphetamine *on page 370*

Pregnancy Risk Factor C

Generic Available Yes: Tablet

Dextromethorphan (deks troe meth OR fan)

Related Information

Acetaminophen, Dextromethorphan, and Pseudoephedrine *on page 34*

Guaifenesin, Pseudoephedrine, and Dextromethorphan *on page 571*

U.S. Brand Names Benylin DM® [OTC]; Benylin® Pediatric [OTC]; Children's Hold® [OTC]; Creo-Terpin® [OTC]; Delsym® [OTC]; Drixoral® Cough Liquid Caps [OTC]; Hold® DM [OTC]; Pertussin® CS [OTC]; Pertussin® ES [OTC]; Robitussin® Cough Calmers [OTC]; Robitussin® Pediatric [OTC]; Scot-Tussin DM® Cough Chasers [OTC]; Silphen DM® [OTC]; St. Joseph® Cough Suppressant [OTC]; Sucrets® Cough Calmers [OTC]; Suppress® [OTC]; Trocal® [OTC]; Vicks Formula 44® [OTC]; Vicks Formula 44® Pediatric Formula [OTC]

Mexican Brand Names Athos®; Bekidiba Dex®; Neopulmonier®; Romilar®

Pharmacologic Category Antitussive

Use Symptomatic relief of coughs caused by minor viral upper respiratory tract infections or inhaled irritants; most effective for a chronic nonproductive cough

Unlabeled/Investigational: *N*-methyl-D-aspartate (NMDA) antagonist in cerebral injury

Local Anesthetic/Vasoconstrictor Precautions No information available to require special precautions

Effects on Dental Treatment No effects or complications reported

Dosage Oral:

Children:

<2 years: Use only as directed by a physician

2-6 years (syrup): 2.5-7.5 mg every 4-8 hours; extended release is 15 mg twice daily (maximum: 30 mg/24 hours)

6-12 years: 5-10 mg every 4 hours or 15 mg every 6-8 hours; extended release is 30 mg twice daily (maximum: 60 mg/24 hours)

Children >12 years and Adults: 10-30 mg every 4-8 hours or 30 mg every 6-8 hours; extended release is 60 mg twice daily (maximum: 120 mg/24 hours)

Mechanism of Action Chemical relative of morphine lacking narcotic properties except in overdose; controls cough by depressing the medullary cough center

Warnings/Precautions Research on chicken embryos exposed to concentrations of dextromethorphan relative to those typically taken by humans has shown to cause birth defects and fetal death; more study is needed, but it is suggested that pregnant women should be advised not to use dextromethorphan-containing medications

Drug Interactions CYP2D6, 2E1, 3A3/4 enzyme substrate

May increase effect/toxicity of MAO inhibitors

Drug Uptake

Onset of antitussive action: 15-30 minutes

Duration: ≤6 hours

Pregnancy Risk Factor C

Generic Available Yes

Dey-Lute® Isoetharine *see* Isoetharine *on page 658*

Dezocine (DEZ oh seen)

U.S. Brand Names Dalgan®

Canadian Brand Names Dalgan®

Pharmacologic Category Analgesic, Narcotic

Use Relief of moderate to severe postoperative, acute renal and ureteral colic, and cancer pain

Local Anesthetic/Vasoconstrictor Precautions No information available to require special precautions

Effects on Dental Treatment No effects or complications reported

Dosage Adults (not recommended for patients <18 years):

I.M.: Initial: 5-20 mg; may be repeated every 3-6 hours as needed; maximum: 120 mg/day and 20 mg/dose

I.V.: Initial: 2.5-10 mg; may be repeated every 2-4 hours as needed

Mechanism of Action Binds to opiate receptors in the CNS, causing inhibition of ascending pain pathways, altering the perception of and response to pain; produces generalized CNS depression; it is a mixed agonist-antagonist that appears to bind selectively to CNS μ and Δ opiate receptors

Other Adverse Effects 1% to 10%:

Central nervous system: Sedation, dizziness, vertigo

Gastrointestinal: Nausea, vomiting

Local: Injection site reactions

Drug Interactions Additive effect with CNS depressants

Drug Uptake

Onset of analgesic effect: 15-30 minutes; Peak effect: 1 hour

Duration of analgesic effect: 4-6 hours

Half-life, elimination: 2.6-2.8 hours

Pregnancy Risk Factor C

Generic Available No

Selected Readings "Drugs for Pain," *Med Lett Drugs Ther*, 1998, 40(1033):79-84.

DHC® *see* Hydrocodone and Acetaminophen *on page 598*

DHC Plus® *see* Dihydrocodeine Compound *on page 392*

D.H.E. 45® *see* Dihydroergotamine *on page 393*

DHS® Tar [OTC] *see* Coal Tar *on page 315*

DHS Zinc® [OTC] *see* Pyrithione Zinc *on page 1029*

DHT™ *see* Dihydrotachysterol *on page 394*

Diaβeta® *see* GlyBURIDE *on page 560*

Diabetic Tussin® DM [OTC] *see* Guaifenesin and Dextromethorphan *on page 569*

Diabetic Tussin® EX [OTC] *see* Guaifenesin *on page 568*

Diabinese® *see* ChlorproPAMIDE *on page 275*

Dialume® [OTC] *see* Aluminum Hydroxide *on page 61*

Diamox® *see* AcetaZOLAMIDE *on page 35*

Diamox Sequels® *see* AcetaZOLAMIDE *on page 35*

Diaparene® [OTC] *see* Methylbenzethonium Chloride *on page 793*

Diar-Aid® [OTC] *see* Loperamide *on page 725*

Diasorb® [OTC] *see* Attapulgite *on page 132*

Diastat® Rectal Delivery System *see* Diazepam *on page 373*

Diazepam (dye AZ e pam)

Related Information

Dental Drug Interactions: Update on Drug Combinations Requiring Special Considerations *on page 1434*

Dental Office Emergencies *on page 1418*

Patients Requiring Sedation *on page 1400*

Temporomandibular Dysfunction (TMD) *on page 1397*

U.S. Brand Names Diastat® Rectal Delivery System; Diazepam Intensol®; Valium®

Canadian Brand Names Apo®-Diazepam; Diastat®; Diazemuls®; Valium®; Vivol®

Mexican Brand Names Alboral®; Diatex; Ortopsique®; Pacitran®; Valium®

Pharmacologic Category Benzodiazepine

Use

Dental: Oral medication for preoperative dental anxiety; sedative component in I.V. conscious sedation in oral surgery patients; skeletal muscle relaxant

(Continued)

Diazepam *(Continued)*

Medical: Management of anxiety disorders, ethanol withdrawal symptoms; skeletal muscle relaxant; treatment of convulsive disorders

Orphan drug: Viscous solution for rectal administration: Management of selected, refractory epilepsy patients on stable regimens of antiepileptic drugs (AEDs) requiring intermittent use of diazepam to control episodes of increased seizure activity

Unlabeled/Investigational: Panic disorders; preoperative sedation, light anesthesia, amnesia

Local Anesthetic/Vasoconstrictor Precautions No information available to require special precautions

Effects on Dental Treatment >10%: Xerostomia, changes in salivation

Restrictions C-IV

Dosage Oral absorption is more reliable than I.M.

Children:

Conscious sedation for procedures: Oral: 0.2-0.3 mg/kg (maximum: 10 mg) 45-60 minutes prior to procedure

Sedation/muscle relaxant/anxiety:

Oral: 0.12-0.8 mg/kg/day in divided doses every 6-8 hours

I.M., I.V.: 0.04-0.3 mg/kg/dose every 2-4 hours to a maximum of 0.6 mg/kg within an 8-hour period if needed

Status epilepticus:

Infants 30 days to 5 years: I.V.: 0.05-0.3 mg/kg/dose given over 2-3 minutes, every 15-30 minutes to a maximum total dose of 5 mg; repeat in 2-4 hours as needed **or** 0.2-0.5 mg/dose every 2-5 minutes to a maximum total dose of 5 mg

>5 years: I.V.: 0.05-0.3 mg/kg/dose given over 2-3 minutes every 15-30 minutes to a maximum total dose of 10 mg; repeat in 2-4 hours as needed **or** 1 mg/dose given over 2-3 minutes, every 2-5 minutes to a maximum total dose of 10 mg

Rectal: 0.5 mg/kg, then 0.25 mg/kg in 10 minutes if needed

Anticonvulsant (acute treatment): Rectal gel formulation:

Infants <6 months: Not recommended

Children <2 years: Safety and efficacy have not been studied

Children 2-5 years: 0.5 mg/kg

Children 6-11 years: 0.3 mg/kg

Children ≥12 years and Adults: 0.2 mg/kg

Note: Dosage should be rounded upward to the next available dose, 2.5, 5, 10, 15, and 20 mg/dose; dose may be repeated in 4-12 hours if needed; do not use more than 5 times per month or more than once every 5 days

Adolescents: Conscious sedation for procedures:

Oral: 10 mg

I.V.: 5 mg, may repeat with $^1/_2$ dose if needed

Adults:

Anxiety/sedation/skeletal muscle relaxant:

Oral: 2-10 mg 2-4 times/day

I.M., I.V.: 2-10 mg, may repeat in 3-4 hours if needed

Status epilepticus: I.V.: 5-10 mg every 10-20 minutes, up to 30 mg in an 8-hour period; may repeat in 2-4 hours if necessary

Rapid tranquilization of agitated patient (administer every 30-60 minutes): Oral: 5-10 mg; average total dose for tranquilization: 20-60 mg

Elderly: Oral: Initial:

Anxiety: 1-2 mg 1-2 times/day; increase gradually as needed, rarely need to use >10 mg/day (watch for hypotension and excessive sedation)

Skeletal muscle relaxant: 2-5 mg 2-4 times/day

Hemodialysis: Not dialyzable (0% to 5%); supplemental dose is not necessary

Dosing adjustment in hepatic impairment: Reduce dose by 50% in cirrhosis and avoid in severe/acute liver disease

Mechanism of Action Binds to stereospecific benzodiazepine receptors on the postsynaptic GABA (gamma-aminobutyric acid) neuron at several sites within the CNS, including the limbic system, reticular formation. Enhancement of the inhibitory effect of GABA on neuronal excitability results by increased neuronal membrane permeability to chloride ions. This shift in chloride ions results in hyperpolarization (a less excitable state) and stabilization.

Other Adverse Effects Frequency not defined:

Cardiovascular: Hypotension

Central nervous system: Drowsiness, ataxia, amnesia, slurred speech, paradoxical excitement or rage, fatigue, insomnia, memory impairment, headache, anxiety, depression, vertigo, confusion

Dermatologic: Rash

Endocrine & metabolic: Changes in libido

Gastrointestinal: Changes in salivation, constipation, nausea

Genitourinary: Incontinence, urinary retention

Hepatic: Jaundice

Local: Phlebitis, pain with injection

Neuromuscular & skeletal: Dysarthria, tremor

Ocular: Blurred vision, diplopia

Respiratory: Decrease in respiratory rate, apnea

Contraindications Hypersensitivity to diazepam or any component of the formulation (cross-sensitivity with other benzodiazepines may exist); narrow-angle glaucoma; children <6 months of age (oral) or <30 days of age (parenteral); pregnancy

Warnings/Precautions Use with caution in patients receiving other CNS depressants, patients with low albumin, hepatic dysfunction, and in the elderly and young infants. Due to its long-acting metabolite, diazepam is not considered a drug of choice in the elderly; long-acting benzodiazepines have been associated with falls in the elderly.

Drug Interactions CYP2B6, 2C8/9, 2C19, 3A3/4, 3A5-7 enzyme substrate; CYP2C19 and 3A3/4 enzyme inhibitor

CNS depressants: Sedative effects and/or respiratory depression may be additive with CNS depressants; includes barbiturates, narcotic analgesics, and other sedative agents; monitor for increased effect

CYP1A2 inhibitors: Metabolism of diazepam may be decreased; increasing clinical effect or toxicity; inhibitors include cimetidine, ciprofloxacin, fluvoxamine, isoniazid, ritonavir, and zileuton.

CYP2C8/9 inhibitors: Serum levels and/or toxicity of diazepam may be increased; inhibitors include amiodarone, cimetidine, fluvoxamine, some NSAIDs, metronidazole, ritonavir, sulfonamides, troglitazone, valproic acid, and zafirlukast; monitor for increased sedation

Enzyme inducers: Metabolism of some benzodiazepines may be increased, decreasing their therapeutic effect; consider using an alternative sedative/hypnotic agent; potential inducers include phenobarbital, phenytoin, carbamazepine, rifampin, and rifabutin

Levodopa: Therapeutic effects may be diminished in some patients following the addition of a benzodiazepine; limited/inconsistent data

Oral contraceptives: May decrease the clearance of some benzodiazepines (those which undergo oxidative metabolism); monitor for increased benzodiazepine effect

Theophylline: May partially antagonize some of the effects of benzodiazepines; monitor for decreased response; may require higher doses for sedation

Dietary/Ethanol/Herb Considerations

Ethanol: Avoid use; may increase CNS depression.

Food: May be taken with food but may increase serum concentration. Avoid grapefruit products; may increase serum concentration/toxicity.

Herb/Nutraceutical: Avoid gotu kola, kava, SAMe, and valerian; may increase CNS depression. Avoid St John's wort; may decrease serum concentration and increase CNS depression. Melatonin may enhance diazepam activity; use cautiously.

Drug Uptake

Onset of action: Almost immediate

Absorption: Oral: 85% to 100%, more reliable than I.M.

Duration: I.V.: Status epilepticus: 20-30 minutes

Half-life, elimination: Parent drug: Adults: 20-50 hours; increased half-life in neonates, elderly, and those with severe hepatic disorders; Active major metabolite (desmethyldiazepam): 50-100 hours; may be prolonged in neonates

Pregnancy Risk Factor D

Breast-feeding Considerations Not compatible

Dosage Forms CONC, oral (Diazepam Intensol®): 5 mg/mL (30 mL). **GEL, rectal** [delivery system; twin pack] (Diastat®): Adult rectal tip (6 cm): 5 mg/mL (10 mg, 15 mg, 20 mg); pediatric rectal tip (4.4 cm): 5 mg/mL (2.5 mg, 5 mg, 10 mg). **INJ:** 5 mg/mL (1 mL, 2 mL, 5 mL, 10 mL). **SOLN, oral:** 5 mg/5 mL (5 mL, 10 mL, 500 mL). **TAB:** 2 mg, 5 mg, 10 mg

Generic Available Yes

Diazepam Intensol® *see* Diazepam *on page 373*

Diazoxide (dye az OKS ide)

U.S. Brand Names Hyperstat® I.V.; Proglycem®

Canadian Brand Names Hyperstat® I.V.; Proglycem®

Mexican Brand Names Hyperstat I.V.®; Sefulken; Sefulken®

Pharmacologic Category Antihypertensive; Antihypoglycemic Agent

Use

Oral: Hypoglycemia related to islet cell adenoma, carcinoma, hyperplasia, or adenomatosis, nesidioblastosis, leucine sensitivity, or extrapancreatic malignancy

I.V.: Emergency lowering of BP

Local Anesthetic/Vasoconstrictor Precautions No information available to require special precautions

Effects on Dental Treatment No effects or complications reported

(Continued)

Diazoxide *(Continued)*

Dosage

Hypertension: Children and Adults: I.V.: 1-3 mg/kg up to a maximum of 150 mg in a single injection; repeat dose in 5-15 minutes until BP adequately reduced; repeat administration at intervals of 4-24 hours; monitor the BP closely; do not use longer than 10 days

Hyperinsulinemic hypoglycemia: Oral: **Note:** Use lower dose listed as initial dose
Children and Adults: 3-8 mg/kg/day in divided doses every 8-12 hours

Mechanism of Action Inhibits insulin release from the pancreas; produces direct smooth muscle relaxation of the peripheral arterioles which results in decrease in BP and reflex increase in heart rate and cardiac output

Other Adverse Effects 1% to 10%:

Cardiovascular: Hypotension
Central nervous system: Dizziness
Gastrointestinal: Nausea, vomiting
Neuromuscular & skeletal: Weakness

Drug Interactions

Increased Effect/Toxicity: Diuretics and hypotensive agents may potentiate diazoxide adverse effects. Diazoxide may decrease warfarin protein binding.

Decreased Effect: Diazoxide may increase phenytoin metabolism or free fraction.

Drug Uptake

Onset of action: Hyperglycemic: Oral: ~1 hour
Peak effect: Hypotensive: I.V.: ~5 minutes

Duration: Hyperglycemic: Oral: Normal renal function: 8 hours; Hypotensive: I.V.: ~3-12 hours

Half-life, elimination: Children: 9-24 hours; Adults: 20-36 hours; End-stage renal disease: >30 hours

Pregnancy Risk Factor C

Generic Available No

Dibent® *see* Dicyclomine *on page 382*

Dibenzyline® *see* Phenoxybenzamine *on page 947*

Dibucaine (DYE byoo kane)

U.S. Brand Names Nupercainal® [OTC]

Pharmacologic Category Local Anesthetic

Use

Dental: Amide derivative local anesthetic for minor skin conditions

Medical: Fast, temporary relief of pain and itching due to hemorrhoids, minor burns

Local Anesthetic/Vasoconstrictor Precautions No information available to require special precautions

Effects on Dental Treatment No effects or complications reported

Dosage Children and Adults: Topical: Apply gently to the affected areas; ≤30 g for adults or 7.5 g for children should be used in any 24-hour period

Mechanism of Action Local anesthetics bind selectively to the intracellular surface of sodium channels to block influx of sodium into the axon. As a result, depolarization necessary for action potential propagation and subsequent nerve function is prevented. The block at the sodium channel is reversible. When drug diffuses away from the axon, sodium channel function is restored and nerve propagation returns.

Other Adverse Effects 1% to 10%:

Dermatologic: Angioedema, contact dermatitis
Local: Burning

Contraindications Hypersensitivity to dibucaine, amide-type anesthetics, or any component of their formulation; ophthalmic use

Warnings/Precautions Avoid use in sensitive individuals

Drug Uptake

Onset of action: ~15 minutes

Absorption: Poor through intact skin; well absorbed through mucous membranes and excoriated skin

Duration: 2-4 hours

Pregnancy Risk Factor C

Breast-feeding Considerations No data reported; topical administration is probably compatible.

Dosage Forms CRM: 0.5% (45 g). **OINT:** 1% (30 g, 60 g, 454 g)

Generic Available Yes

Dibucaine and Hydrocortisone

(DYE byoo kane & hye droe KOR ti sone)

U.S. Brand Names Corticaine®

Pharmacologic Category Corticosteroid, Topical (Low Potency); Local Anesthetic, Topical

Synonyms Hydrocortisone and Dibucaine

Use Relief of the inflammatory and pruritic manifestations of corticosteroid-responsive dermatoses and for external anal itching

Local Anesthetic/Vasoconstrictor Precautions No information available to require special precautions

Effects on Dental Treatment No effects or complications reported

Dosage Topical: Apply to affected areas 2-4 times/day

Therapy should be discontinued when control is achieved; if no improvement is seen, reassessment of diagnosis may be necessary.

Dicarbosil® [OTC] *see* Calcium Carbonate *on page 201*

Dichlorodifluoromethane and Trichloromonofluoromethane

(dye klor oh dye flor oh METH ane & tri klor oh mon oh flor oh METH ane)

Related Information

Temporomandibular Dysfunction (TMD) *on page 1397*

U.S. Brand Names Fluori-Methane®

Pharmacologic Category Analgesic, Topical

Synonyms Trichloromonofluoromethane and Dichlorodifluoromethane

Use

Dental: Topical application in the management of myofascial pain, restricted motion, and muscle spasm

Medical: For the control of pain associated with injections

Local Anesthetic/Vasoconstrictor Precautions No information available to require special precautions

Effects on Dental Treatment No effects or complications reported

Dosage Invert bottle over treatment area ~ 12" away from site of application; open dispenseal spring valve completely, allowing liquid to flow in a stream from the bottle. The rate of spraying is ~ 10 cm/second and should be continued until entire muscle has been covered.

Contraindications Hypersensitivity to dichlorofluoromethane and/or trichloromonofluoromethane or any component of the formulation; vascular impairment of the extremities

Warnings/Precautions For external use only; care should be taken to minimize inhalation of vapors, especially with application to head and neck; avoid contact with eyes; should not be applied to the point of frost formation

Dosage Forms AERO, topical: Dichlorodifluoromethane 15% and trichloromonofluoromethane 85% (103 mL)

Generic Available No

Comments Dichlorodifluoromethane and trichloromonofluoromethane are not classified as carcinogens; based on animal studies and human experience, these fluorocarbons pose no hazard to man relative to systemic toxicity, carcinogenicity, mutagenicity, or teratogenicity when occupational exposures are <1000 ppm over an 8-hour time weighted average.

Dichlorphenamide (dye klor FEN a mide)

U.S. Brand Names Daranide®

Canadian Brand Names Daranide®

Pharmacologic Category Carbonic Anhydrase Inhibitor; Diuretic, Carbonic Anhydrase Inhibitor; Ophthalmic Agent, Antiglaucoma

Synonyms Diclofenamide

Use Adjunct in treatment of open-angle glaucoma and perioperative treatment for angle-closure glaucoma

Local Anesthetic/Vasoconstrictor Precautions No information available to require special precautions

Effects on Dental Treatment No effects or complications reported

Dosage Adults: Oral: 100-200 mg to start followed by 100 mg every 12 hours until desired response is obtained; maintenance dose: 25-50 mg 1-3 times/day

Other Adverse Effects

>10%:
- Central nervous system: Fatigue, malaise
- Gastrointestinal: Diarrhea, anorexia, metallic taste
- Genitourinary: Polyuria
- Renal: Polyuria

1% to 10%:
- Central nervous system: Mental depression, somnolence
- Renal: Renal calculi

Warnings/Precautions Chemical similarities are present among sulfonamides, sulfonylureas, carbonic anhydrase inhibitors, thiazides, and loop diuretics (except ethacrynic acid). In patients with allergy to one of these compounds, a risk of cross-reaction exists; avoid use when previous reaction has been severe.

Drug Interactions Increased lithium excretion and altered excretion of other drugs by alkalinization of the urine.

Pregnancy Risk Factor C

Generic Available No

Diclofenac (dye KLOE fen ak)

Related Information

Rheumatoid Arthritis and Osteoarthritis *on page 1340*
Temporomandibular Dysfunction (TMD) *on page 1397*

U.S. Brand Names Cataflam®; Solaraze™; Voltaren®; Voltaren®-XR

Canadian Brand Names Apo®-Diclo; Apo®-Diclo SR; Cataflam®; Diclotec; Novo-Difenac®; Novo-Difenac K; Novo-Difenac-SR®; Nu-Diclo; Nu-Diclo-SR; PMS-Diclofenac; PMS-Diclofenac SR; Riva-Diclofenac; Riva-Diclofenac-K; Voltaren®; Voltaren Ophtha®; Voltaren Rapide®

Mexican Brand Names 3-A Ofteno®; Artrenac; Cataflam®; Clonodifen®; Deflox®; Dicloran®; Dolaren®; Dolflam®; Dolo Pangavit-D; Fustaren®; Galedol; Lifenac®; Lifenal; Liroken; Logesic; Merxil®; Selectofen®; Volfenac Gel®; Volfenac Retard®; Voltaren®

Pharmacologic Category Nonsteroidal Anti-inflammatory Drug (NSAID)

Synonyms Diclofenac Potassium; Diclofenac Sodium

Use

Immediate-release tablets: Acute treatment of mild to moderate pain; ankylosing spondylitis; primary dysmenorrhea; acute and chronic treatment of rheumatoid arthritis, osteoarthritis

Delayed-release tablets: Acute and chronic treatment of rheumatoid arthritis, osteoarthritis, ankylosing spondylitis

Extended-release tablets: Chronic treatment of osteoarthritis, rheumatoid arthritis

Ophthalmic solution: Postoperative inflammation following cataract extraction; temporary relief of pain and photophobia in patients undergoing corneal refractive surgery

Topical gel: Actinic keratosis (AK) in conjunction with sun avoidance

Unlabeled/Investigational: Juvenile rheumatoid arthritis

Local Anesthetic/Vasoconstrictor Precautions No information available to require special precautions

Effects on Dental Treatment NSAID formulations are known to reversibly decrease platelet aggregation via mechanisms different than observed with aspirin. The dentist should be aware of the potential of abnormal coagulation. Caution should also be exercised in the use of NSAIDs in patients already on anticoagulant therapy with drugs such as warfarin (Coumadin®).

Dosage

Adults:

Oral:

Analgesia/primary dysmenorrhea: Starting dose: 50 mg 3 times/day; maximum dose: 150 mg/day

Rheumatoid arthritis: 150-200 mg/day in 2-4 divided doses (100 mg/day of sustained release product)

Osteoarthritis: 100-150 mg/day in 2-3 divided doses (100-200 mg/day of sustained release product)

Ankylosing spondylitis: 100-125 mg/day in 4-5 divided doses

Ophthalmic:

Cataract surgery: Instill 1 drop into affected eye 4 times/day beginning 24 hours after cataract surgery and continuing for 2 weeks

Corneal refractive surgery: Instill 1-2 drops into affected eye within the hour prior to surgery, within 15 minutes following surgery, and then continue for 4 times/day, up to 3 days

Topical: Apply gel to lesion area twice daily for 60-90 days

Dosage adjustment in renal impairment: Monitor closely in patients with significant renal impairment

Elderly: No specific dosing recommendations; elderly may demonstrate adverse effects at lower doses than younger adults, and >60% may develop asymptomatic peptic ulceration with or without hemorrhage; monitor renal function

Mechanism of Action Inhibits prostaglandin synthesis by decreasing the activity of the enzyme, cyclo-oxygenase, which results in decreased formation of prostaglandin precursors. Mechanism of action for the treatment of AK has not been established.

Other Adverse Effects

>10%:

Local: Application site reactions (gel): Pruritus (31% to 52%), rash (35% to 46%), contact dermatitis (19% to 33%), dry skin (25% to 27%), pain (15% to 26%), exfoliation (6% to 24%), paresthesia (8% to 20%)

Ocular: Ophthalmic drops (incidence may be dependent upon indication): Lacrimation (30%), keratitis (28%), elevated IOP (15%), transient burning/stinging (15%)

1% to 10%:

Central nervous system: Headache (7%), dizziness (3%)

Dermatologic: Pruritus (1% to 3%), rash (1% to 3%)

Endocrine & metabolic: Fluid retention (1% to 3%)

Gastrointestinal: Abdominal cramps (3% to 9%), abdominal pain (3% to 9%), constipation (3% to 9%), diarrhea (3% to 9%), flatulence (3% to 9%), indigestion (3% to 9%), nausea (3% to 9%), abdominal distention (1% to 3%), peptic ulcer/GI bleed (0.6% to 2%)

Hepatic: Increased ALT/AST (2%)

Local: Application site reactions (gel): Edema (4%)

Ocular: Ophthalmic drops: Abnormal vision, acute elevated IOP, blurred vision, conjunctivitis, corneal deposits, corneal edema, corneal opacity, corneal lesions, discharge, eyelid swelling, injection, iritis, irritation, itching, lacrimation disorder, ocular allergy

Otic: Tinnitus (1% to 3%)

Contraindications Hypersensitivity to diclofenac, any component of the formulation, aspirin or other nonsteroidal anti-inflammatory drugs (NSAIDs), including patients who experience bronchospasm, asthma, rhinitis, or urticaria following NSAID or aspirin; porphyria; pregnancy (3rd trimester)

Warnings/Precautions Use with caution in patients with CHF, dehydration, hypertension, decreased renal or hepatic function, history of GI disease, active GI ulceration or bleeding, or those receiving anticoagulants. Anaphylactoid reactions have been reported with NSAID use, even without prior exposure; may be more common in patients with the aspirin triad. Use with caution in patients with pre-existing asthma. Rare cases of severe hepatic reactions (including necrosis, jaundice, fulminant hepatitis) have been reported. Vision changes (including changes in color) have been rarely reported with oral diclofenac. Topical gel should not be applied to the eyes, open wounds, infected areas, or to exfoliative dermatitis. Monitor patients for 1 year following application of ophthalmic drops for corneal refractive procedures. Patients using ophthalmic drops should not wear soft contact lenses. Ophthalmic drops may slow/delay healing or prolong bleeding time following surgery. Elderly are at a high risk for adverse effects from nonsteroidal anti-inflammatory agents. As many as 60% of elderly can develop peptic ulceration and/or hemorrhage asymptomatically.

Use lowest effective dose for shortest period possible. Use of NSAIDs can compromise existing renal function especially when Cl_{cr} is <30 mL/minute. CNS adverse effects such as confusion, agitation, and hallucination are generally seen in overdose or high-dose situations; however, elderly may demonstrate these adverse effects at lower doses than younger adults. Withhold for at least 4-6 half-lives prior to surgical or dental procedures.

Drug Interactions CYP2C8 and 2C9 enzyme substrate; CYP2C9 enzyme inhibitor

ACE inhibitors: Antihypertensive effects may be decreased by concurrent therapy with NSAIDs; monitor BP

Angiotensin II antagonists: Antihypertensive effects may be decreased by concurrent therapy with NSAIDs; monitor BP

Anticoagulants (warfarin, heparin, LMWHs) in combination with NSAIDs can cause increased risk of bleeding.

Other antiplatelet drugs (ticlopidine, clopidogrel, aspirin, abciximab, dipyridamole, eptifibatide, tirofiban) can cause an increased risk of bleeding.

Cholestyramine and colestipol reduce the bioavailability of diclofenac; separate administration times.

Corticosteroids may increase the risk of GI ulceration; avoid concurrent use.

Cyclosporine: NSAIDs may increase serum creatinine, potassium, BP, and cyclosporine levels; monitor cyclosporine levels and renal function carefully.

Gentamicin and amikacin serum concentrations are increased by indomethacin in premature infants. Results may apply to other aminoglycosides and NSAIDs.

Hydralazine's antihypertensive effect is decreased; avoid concurrent use.

Lithium levels can be increased; avoid concurrent use if possible or monitor lithium levels and adjust dose. Sulindac may have the least effect. When NSAID is stopped, lithium will need adjustment again.

Loop diuretics efficacy (diuretic and antihypertensive effect) is reduced. Indomethacin reduces this efficacy, however, it may be anticipated with any NSAID.

Methotrexate: Severe bone marrow suppression, aplastic anemia, and GI toxicity have been reported with concomitant NSAID therapy. Avoid use during moderate or high-dose methotrexate (increased and prolonged methotrexate levels). NSAID use during low-dose treatment of rheumatoid arthritis has not been fully evaluated; extreme caution is warranted.

Thiazides antihypertensive effects are decreased; avoid concurrent use.

Verapamil plasma concentration is decreased by diclofenac; avoid concurrent use.

Warfarin's INRs may be increased by piroxicam. Other NSAIDs may have the same effect depending on dose and duration. Monitor INR closely. Use the lowest dose of NSAIDs possible and for the briefest duration.

Drug Uptake

Onset of action: Cataflam® has a more rapid onset of action than does the sodium salt (Voltaren®), because it is absorbed in the stomach instead of the duodenum.

Absorption: Topical: 10% (gel)

Half-life, elimination: 2 hours

Time to peak: Cataflam®: ≤1 hour; Voltaren®: ≤2 hours

Pregnancy Risk Factor B/D (3rd trimester)

(Continued)

Diclofenac *(Continued)*

Generic Available Yes

Diclofenac and Misoprostol (dye KLOE fen ak & mye soe PROST ole)

Related Information

Rheumatoid Arthritis and Osteoarthritis *on page 1340*

U.S. Brand Names Arthrotec®

Canadian Brand Names Arthrotec®

Pharmacologic Category Nonsteroidal Anti-inflammatory Drug (NSAID); Prostaglandin

Synonyms Misoprostol and Diclofenac

Use The diclofenac component is indicated for the treatment of osteoarthritis and rheumatoid arthritis; the misoprostol component is indicated for the prophylaxis of NSAID-induced gastric and duodenal ulceration

Local Anesthetic/Vasoconstrictor Precautions No information available to require special precautions

Effects on Dental Treatment No effects or complications reported

Dosage Oral:

Adults:

Arthrotec® 50:

Osteoarthritis: 1 tablet 2-3 times/day

Rheumatoid arthritis: 1 tablet 3-4 times/day

For both regimens, if not tolerated by patient, the dose may be reduced to 1 tablet twice daily

Arthrotec® 75:

Patients who cannot tolerate full daily Arthrotec® 50 regimens: 1 tablet twice daily

Note: The use of these tablets may not be as effective at preventing GI ulceration

Elderly: No specific dosage adjustment is recommended; may require reduced dosage due to lower body weight; monitor renal function

Mechanism of Action See Diclofenac *on page 378* and Misoprostol *on page 820*

Other Adverse Effects Also see Diclofenac *on page 378* and Misoprostol *on page 820*

>10%: Gastrointestinal: Abdominal pain (21%), diarrhea (19%), nausea (11%), dyspepsia (14%)

1% to 10%:

Endocrine & metabolic: Elevated transaminase levels

Gastrointestinal: Flatulence (9%)

Hematologic: Anemia

Miscellaneous: Anaphylactic reactions

Warnings/Precautions Use in premenopausal women (warn about risk with pregnancy and advise use of effective contraception); withhold for at least 4-6 half-lives prior to surgical or dental procedures

Drug Interactions

Increased effect/toxicity: Aspirin (shared toxicity), digoxin (elevated digoxin levels), warfarin (synergistic bleeding potential), cyclosporine (increased nephrotoxicity), lithium (increased lithium levels)

Decreased effects: Aspirin (displaces diclofenac from binding sites), antihypertensive agents (decreased BP control), antacids (may decrease absorption)

ACE inhibitors: Antihypertensive effects may be decreased by concurrent therapy with NSAIDs; monitor BP

Angiotensin II antagonists: Antihypertensive effects may be decreased by concurrent therapy with NSAIDs; monitor BP

Methotrexate: Severe bone marrow suppression, aplastic anemia, and GI toxicity have been reported with concomitant NSAID therapy. Avoid use during moderate or high-dose methotrexate (increased and prolonged methotrexate levels). NSAID use during low-dose treatment of rheumatoid arthritis has not been fully evaluated; extreme caution is warranted.

Drug Uptake See Diclofenac *on page 378* and Misoprostol *on page 820*

Pregnancy Risk Factor X

Generic Available No

Dicloxacillin (dye kloks a SIL in)

Related Information

Oral Bacterial Infections *on page 1367*

U.S. Brand Names Dycill®; Pathocil®

Canadian Brand Names Dycill®; Pathocil®

Mexican Brand Names Brispen; Cilpen®; Ditterolina®; Posipen

Pharmacologic Category Antibiotic, Penicillin

Synonyms Dicloxacillin Sodium

Use

Dental: Treatment of susceptible orofacial infections, notably penicillinase-producing staph

Medical: Treatment of systemic infections in the medical patient such as pneumonia, skin and soft tissue infections, and osteomyelitis caused by penicillinase-producing staphylococci

Local Anesthetic/Vasoconstrictor Precautions No information available to require special precautions

Effects on Dental Treatment Prolonged use of penicillins may lead to development of oral candidiasis.

Dosage Oral:

Use in newborns not recommended

Children <40 kg: 12.5-25 mg/kg/day divided every 6 hours; doses of 50-100 mg/kg/day in divided doses every 6 hours have been used for therapy of osteomyelitis

Children >40 kg and Adults: 125-250 mg every 6 hours

Hemodialysis: Not dialyzable (0% to 5%); supplemental dosage not necessary

Peritoneal dialysis: Supplemental dosage not necessary

Continuous arteriovenous or venovenous hemofiltration: Supplemental dosage not necessary

Mechanism of Action Inhibits bacterial cell wall synthesis by binding to one or more of the penicillin binding proteins (PBPs); which in turn inhibits the final transpeptidation step of peptidoglycan synthesis in bacterial cell walls, thus inhibiting cell wall biosynthesis. Bacteria eventually lyse due to ongoing activity of cell wall autolytic enzymes (autolysins and murein hydrolases) while cell wall assembly is arrested.

Other Adverse Effects

1% to 10%: Gastrointestinal: Nausea, diarrhea, abdominal pain

<1%: Fever, seizures with extremely high doses and/or renal failure, rash (maculopapular to exfoliative), vomiting, pseudomembranous colitis, vaginitis, eosinophilia, leukopenia, neutropenia, thrombocytopenia, agranulocytosis, anemia, hemolytic anemia, prolonged PT, hepatotoxicity, transient elevated LFTs, hematuria, interstitial nephritis, increased BUN/creatinine, serum sickness-like reactions, hypersensitivity

Contraindications Hypersensitivity to dicloxacillin, penicillin, or any component of their formulation

Warnings/Precautions Monitor PT if patient concurrently on warfarin; elimination of drug is slow in neonates; use with caution in patients allergic to cephalosporins; bad taste of suspension may make compliance difficult

Drug Interactions

Oral contraceptive efficacy may be reduced.

Probenecid, disulfiram may increase levels of penicillins (dicloxacillin).

Warfarin: Concurrent use may decrease effect of warfarin

Dietary/Ethanol/Herb Considerations Food: Administer on an empty stomach; food decreases absorption rate and serum concentration.

Drug Uptake

Absorption: 35% to 76% from GI tract; food decreases rate and extent of absorption

Half-life, elimination: 0.6-0.8 hours (prolonged with renal impairment)

Time to peak: 0.5-2 hours

Pregnancy Risk Factor B

Dosage Forms CAP, as sodium: 125 mg, 250 mg, 500 mg. **SUSP, powder for, as sodium, oral:** 62.5 mg/5 mL (80 mL, 100 mL, 200 mL)

Generic Available Yes

Comments Although dicloxacillin is a penicillin antibiotic indicated for infections caused by penicillinase secreting staph, amoxicillin with clavulanic acid is considered the drug of choice for these types of orofacial infections

Dicumarol (dye KOO ma role)

Related Information

Cardiovascular Diseases *on page 1308*

Pharmacologic Category Anticoagulant, Coumarin Derivative

Synonyms Bishydroxycoumarin

Use Prophylaxis and treatment of thromboembolic disorders

Local Anesthetic/Vasoconstrictor Precautions No information available to require special precautions

Effects on Dental Treatment Signs of dicumarol overdose may first appear as bleeding from gingival tissue; consultation with prescribing physician is advisable prior to surgery to determine temporary dose reduction or withdrawal of medication.

Dosage Adults: Oral: 25-200 mg/day based on prothrombin time (PT) determinations

Mechanism of Action Interferes with hepatic synthesis of vitamin K-dependent coagulation factors (II, VII, IX, X)

Other Adverse Effects 1% to 10%:

Dermatologic: Skin lesions, alopecia, skin necrosis

Gastrointestinal: Anorexia, nausea, vomiting, stomach cramps, diarrhea

(Continued)

Dicumarol *(Continued)*

Hematologic: Hemorrhage; leukopenia, unrecognized bleeding sites (eg, colon cancer) may be uncovered by anticoagulation

Respiratory: Hemoptysis

Drug Interactions

May accentuate toxicities of oral hypoglycemics and anticonvulsants.

Drugs which decrease prothrombin time: Antacids, antihistamines, phenobarbital, carbamazepine, cholestyramine, meprobamate, glutethimide, ethchlorvynol, oral contraceptives, ranitidine, chloral hydrate, diuretics.

Drugs which increase prothrombin time: Allopurinol, amiodarone, cimetidine, clofibrate, dextran, diazoxide, diflunisal, diuretics, disulfiram, fenoprofen, ibuprofen, indomethacin, influenza virus vaccine, methyldopa, methylphenidate, MAO inhibitors, naproxen, nortriptyline, phenytoin, propylthiouracil, salicylates, quinidine, quinine, ranitidine, tolbutamide, thyroid drugs, sulindac, co-trimoxazole.

Pregnancy Risk Factor D

Generic Available Yes

Dicyclomine (dye SYE kloe meen)

U.S. Brand Names Antispas®; Bentyl®; Byclomine®; Dibent®; Di-Spaz®; Or-Tyl®

Canadian Brand Names Bentylol®; Formulex®; Lomine

Pharmacologic Category Anticholinergic Agent

Synonyms Dicyclomine Hydrochloride; Dicycloverine Hydrochloride

Use Treatment of functional disturbances of GI motility such as irritable bowel syndrome

Unlabeled/Investigational: Urinary incontinence

Local Anesthetic/Vasoconstrictor Precautions No information available to require special precautions

Effects on Dental Treatment >10%: Xerostomia

Dosage

Oral:

Children: 10 mg/dose 3-4 times/day

Adults: Begin with 80 mg/day in 4 equally divided doses, then increase up to 160 mg/day

I.M. **(should not be used I.V.)**: Adults: 80 mg/day in 4 divided doses (20 mg/dose)

Mechanism of Action Blocks the action of acetylcholine at parasympathetic sites in smooth muscle, secretory glands and the CNS

Other Adverse Effects Adverse reactions are included here that have been reported for pharmacologically similar drugs with anticholinergic/antispasmodic action. Frequency not defined:

Cardiovascular: Syncope, tachycardia, palpitations

Central nervous system: Dizziness, lightheadedness, tingling, headache, drowsiness, nervousness, numbness, mental confusion and/or excitement, dyskinesia, lethargy, speech disturbance, insomnia

Dermatologic: Rash, urticaria, itching, and other dermal manifestations; severe allergic reaction or drug idiosyncrasies including anaphylaxis

Endocrine & metabolic: Suppression of lactation

Gastrointestinal: Xerostomia, nausea, vomiting, constipation, bloated feeling, abdominal pain, taste loss, anorexia

Genitourinary: Urinary hesitancy, urinary retention, impotence

Neuromuscular & skeletal: Weakness

Ocular: Blurred vision, diplopia, mydriasis, cycloplegia, increased ocular tension

Respiratory: Dyspnea, apnea, asphyxia, nasal stuffiness or congestion, sneezing, throat congestion

Miscellaneous: Decreased diaphoresis

Drug Interactions

Increased Effect/Toxicity: Dicyclomine taken with anticholinergics, amantadine, narcotic analgesics, Type I antiarrhythmics, antihistamines, phenothiazines, tricyclic antidepressants may result in increased toxicity.

Decreased effect with phenothiazines, anti-Parkinson's drugs, haloperidol, sustained release dosage forms, and with antacids.

Drug Uptake

Onset of action: 1-2 hours

Absorption: Oral: Well absorbed

Duration: ≤4 hours

Half-life, elimination: Initial: 1.8 hours; Terminal: 9-10 hours

Pregnancy Risk Factor B

Generic Available Yes

Didanosine (dye DAN oh seen)

Related Information

HIV Infection and AIDS *on page 1334*

U.S. Brand Names Videx®; Videx® EC

Canadian Brand Names Videx®

Mexican Brand Names Videx®

Pharmacologic Category Antiretroviral Agent, Reverse Transcriptase Inhibitor (Nucleoside)

Synonyms ddI; Dideoxyinosine

Use Treatment of advanced HIV infection in patients who are intolerant of zidovudine therapy or who have demonstrated significant clinical or immunologic deterioration during zidovudine therapy

Local Anesthetic/Vasoconstrictor Precautions No information available to require special precautions

Effects on Dental Treatment No effects or complications reported

Dosage Treatment of HIV infection: Oral (administer on an empty stomach):

Children: 180 mg/m²/day divided every 12 hours **or** dosing is based on body surface area (m²) as follows:

- BSA ≤0.4 m²: 25 mg twice daily (tablets)
- BSA 0.5-0.7 m²: 50 mg twice daily (tablets)
- BSA 0.8-1.0 m²: 75 mg twice daily (tablets)
- BSA 1.1-1.4 m²: 100 mg twice daily (tablets)
- Children <1 year should receive 1 tablet per dose and children >1 year should receive 2-4 tablets per dose for adequate buffering and absorption; tablets should be chewed or dispersed

Adults: Dosing based on patient weight:

Note: Preferred dosing frequency is twice daily for didanosine tablets

Tablets:
- <60 kg: 125 mg twice daily or 250 mg once daily
- ≥60 kg: 200 mg twice daily or 400 mg once daily

Note: Adults should receive 2-4 tablets per dose for adequate buffering and absorption; tablets should be chewed or dispersed; didanosine has also been used as 300 mg once daily

Buffered Powder:
- <60 kg: 167 mg twice daily
- ≥60 kg; 250 mg twice daily

Sustained release capsule:
- <60 kg: 250 mg once daily
- ≥60 kg; 400 mg once daily

Dosage adjustment in renal impairment: Dosing based on patient weight, creatinine clearance, and dosage form:

Tablet = Chewable/dispersible buffered tablet; 2 tablets must be taken with each dose; different strengths of tablets may be combined to yield the recommended dose

Solution = Buffered powder for oral solution

Dosing for patients ≥60 kg:

Cl_{cr} ≥60 mL/minute:
- Tablet: 400 mg once daily or 200 mg twice daily
- Solution: 250 mg twice daily
- Sustained release capsule: 400 mg once daily

Cl_{cr} 30-59 mL/minute:
- Tablet: 200 mg once daily or 100 mg twice daily
- Solution: 100 mg twice daily
- Sustained release capsule: 200 mg once daily

Cl_{cr} 10-29 mL/minute:
- Tablet: 150 mg once daily
- Solution: 167 mg once daily
- Sustained release capsule: 125 mg once daily

Cl_{cr} <10 mL/minute:
- Tablet: 100 mg once daily
- Solution: 100 mg once daily
- Sustained release capsule: 125 mg once daily

Dosing for patients <60 kg:

Cl_{cr} ≥60 mL/minute:
- Tablet: 250 mg once daily or 125 mg twice daily
- Solution: 167 mg twice daily
- Sustained release capsule: 250 mg once daily

Cl_{cr} 30-59 mL/minute:
- Tablet: 150 mg once daily or 75 mg twice daily
- Solution: 100 mg twice daily
- Sustained release capsule: 125 mg once daily

Cl_{cr} 10-29 mL/minute:
- Tablet: 100 mg once daily
- Solution: 100 mg once daily
- Sustained release capsule: 125 mg once daily

Cl_{cr} <10 mL/minute:
- Tablet: 75 mg once daily
- Solution: 100 mg once daily
- Sustained release capsule: Use alternate formulation

Hemodialysis: Removed by hemodialysis (40% to 60%)

(Continued)

Didanosine *(Continued)*

Dosing adjustment in hepatic impairment: Should be considered; monitor for toxicity

Elderly patients have a higher frequency of pancreatitis (10% versus 5% in younger patients); monitor renal function and dose accordingly

Mechanism of Action A purine nucleoside analogue and the deamination product of dideoxyadenosine (ddA), inhibits HIV replication *in vitro* in both T cells and monocytes; is converted within the cell to the mono-, di-, and triphosphates of ddA which act as substrate and inhibitor of HIV reverse transcriptase substrate and inhibitor of HIV reverse transcriptase, thereby blocking viral DNA synthesis and suppressing HIV replication

Other Adverse Effects As reported in monotherapy studies; risk of toxicity may increase when combined with other agents.

>10%:

Gastrointestinal: Increased amylase (15% to 17%), abdominal pain (7% to 13%), diarrhea (19% to 28%)

Neuromuscular & skeletal: Peripheral neuropathy (17% to 20%)

1% to 10%:

Dermatologic: Rash, pruritus

Endocrine & metabolic: Increased uric acid

Gastrointestinal: Pancreatitis; patients >65 years of age had a higher frequency of pancreatitis than younger patients

Hepatic: Increased SGOT, increased SGPT, increased alkaline phosphatase

Drug Interactions

Increased Effect/Toxicity: Concomitant administration of other drugs which have the potential to cause peripheral neuropathy or pancreatitis may increase the risk of these toxicities Allopurinol may increase didanosine concentration; avoid concurrent use. Concomitant use of antacids with buffered tablet or pediatric didanosine solution may potentiate adverse effects of aluminum- or magnesium-containing antacids. Ganciclovir may increase didanosine concentration; monitor. Hydroxyurea may precipitate didanosine-induced pancreatitis if added to therapy; concomitant use is not recommended.

Decreased Effect: Didanosine buffered tablets and buffered pediatric solution may decrease absorption of quinolones or tetracyclines (administer 2 hours prior to didanosine buffered formulations). Didanosine should be held during PCP treatment with pentamidine. Didanosine may decrease levels of indinavir. Drugs whose absorption depends on the level of acidity in the stomach such as ketoconazole, itraconazole, and dapsone should be administered at least 2 hours prior to the buffered formulations of didanosine (not affected by sustained release capsules). Methadone may decrease didanosine concentrations.

Drug Uptake

Absorption: Subject to degradation by acidic pH of stomach; some formulations are buffered to resist acidic pH; ≤50% reduction in peak plasma concentration is observed in presence of food. Sustained release capsules contain enteric-coated beadlets which dissolve in the small intestine.

Half-life, elimination:

Children and Adolescents: 0.8 hour

Adults: Normal renal function: 1.5 hours; however, its active metabolite ddATP has an intracellular half-life >12 hours *in vitro*; Impaired renal function: 2.5-5 hours

Time to peak: Buffered tablets: 0.67 hours; sustained release capsules: 2 hours

Pregnancy Risk Factor B

Generic Available No

Didrex® *see* Benzphetamine *on page 154*

Didronel® *see* Etidronate Disodium *on page 478*

Diethylpropion (dye eth il PROE pee on)

U.S. Brand Names Tenuate®; Tenuate® Dospan®

Canadian Brand Names Tenuate®; Tenuate® Dospan®

Mexican Brand Names Ifa Norex®; Neobes®

Pharmacologic Category Anorexiant

Synonyms Amfepramone; Diethylpropion Hydrochloride

Use Short-term adjunct in exogenous obesity

Unlabeled/Investigational: Migraine

Local Anesthetic/Vasoconstrictor Precautions Use vasoconstrictor with caution in patients taking diethylpropion. Amphetamine-like drugs such as diethylpropion enhance the sympathomimetic response of epinephrine and norepinephrine leading to potential hypertension and cardiotoxicity.

Effects on Dental Treatment Up to 10% of patients may present with hypertension. The use of local anesthetic without vasoconstrictor is recommended in these patients.

Restrictions C-IV

Dosage Adults: Oral:

Tablet: 25 mg 3 times/day before meals or food

Tablet, controlled release: 75 mg at midmorning

Mechanism of Action Used as an anorexiant agent possessing pharmacological and chemical properties similar to those of amphetamines; mechanism in reducing appetite appears to be secondary to CNS effects, specifically stimulation of the hypothalamus to release catecholamines into the CNS; anorexiant effects are mediated via norepinephrine and dopamine metabolism. An increase in physical activity and metabolic effects (inhibition of lipogenesis and enhancement of lipolysis) may also contribute to weight loss.

Other Adverse Effects Frequency not defined:

Cardiovascular: Hypertension, palpitations, tachycardia, chest pain, T-wave changes, arrhythmias, pulmonary hypertension, valvulopathy

Central nervous system: Euphoria, nervousness, insomnia, restlessness, dizziness, anxiety, headache, agitation, confusion, mental depression, psychosis, CVA, seizure

Dermatologic: Alopecia, urticaria, skin rash, ecchymosis, erythema

Endocrine & metabolic: Changes in libido, gynecomastia, menstrual irregularities, porphyria

Gastrointestinal: Nausea, vomiting, abdominal cramps, constipation, xerostomia, metallic taste

Genitourinary: Impotence

Hematologic: Bone marrow depression, agranulocytosis, leukopenia

Neuromuscular & skeletal: Tremor

Ocular: Blurred vision, mydriasis

Drug Interactions

Increased Effect/Toxicity: Concurrent use or use within 14 days following the administration of a MAO inhibitor is contraindicated (hypertensive crisis). Concurrent use of sibutramine and diethylpropion is contraindicated (severe hypertension, tachycardia). Concurrent use with TCAs may result in enhanced toxicity. Concurrent use with other anorectic agents may cause serious cardiac problems and is contraindicated.

Decreased Effect: Diethylpropion may displace guanethidine from the neuron and antagonize its antihypertensive effects; discontinue diethylpropion or use alternative antihypertensive.

Drug Uptake

Onset of action: 1 hour

Duration: 12-24 hours

Pregnancy Risk Factor B

Generic Available Yes

Diethylstilbestrol (dye eth il stil BES trole)

U.S. Brand Names Stilphostrol®

Canadian Brand Names Honvol®; Stilbestrol

Mexican Brand Names Honvan®

Pharmacologic Category Estrogen Derivative

Synonyms DES; Diethylstilbestrol Diphosphate Sodium; Stilbestrol

Use Palliative treatment of inoperable metastatic prostatic carcinoma and postmenopausal, inoperable, progressing breast cancer

Local Anesthetic/Vasoconstrictor Precautions No information available to require special precautions

Effects on Dental Treatment No effects or complications reported

Dosage Adults:

Male:

Prostate carcinoma (inoperable, progressing): Oral: 1-3 mg/day

Diphosphate: Inoperable progressing prostate cancer:

Oral: 50 mg 3 times/day; increase up to 200 mg or more 3 times/day; maximum daily dose: 1 g

I.V.: Give 0.5 g, dissolved in 250 mL of saline or D_5W, administer slowly the first 10-15 minutes then adjust rate so that the entire amount is given in 1 hour; repeat for ≥5 days depending on patient response, then repeat 0.25-0.5 g 1-2 times for 1 week or change to oral therapy

Female: Postmenopausal inoperable, progressing breast carcinoma: Oral: 15 mg/day

Mechanism of Action Competes with estrogenic and androgenic compounds for binding onto tumor cells and thereby inhibits their effects on tumor growth

Other Adverse Effects

>10%:

Cardiovascular: Peripheral edema

Endocrine & metabolic: Enlargement of breasts (female and male), breast tenderness

Gastrointestinal: Nausea, anorexia, bloating

1% to 10%:

Central nervous system: Headache, migraine headache

Endocrine & metabolic: Increased libido (female), decreased libido (male)

Gastrointestinal: Vomiting, diarrhea

(Continued)

Diethylstilbestrol *(Continued)*

Drug Interactions
Increased Effect: Corticosteroids, TCAs, succinylcholine
Decreased Effect: Barbiturates, phenytoin, and rifampin may decrease steroids; oral anticoagulants

Pregnancy Risk Factor X

Generic Available No

Difenoxin and Atropine (dye fen OKS in & A troe peen)

U.S. Brand Names Motofen®

Pharmacologic Category Antidiarrheal

Synonyms Atropine and Difenoxin

Use Treatment of diarrhea

Local Anesthetic/Vasoconstrictor Precautions No information available to require special precautions

Effects on Dental Treatment No effects or complications reported

Restrictions C-IV

Dosage Adults: Oral: Initial: 2 tablets, then 1 tablet after each loose stool; 1 tablet every 3-4 hours, up to 8 tablets in a 24-hour period; if no improvement after 48 hours, continued administration is not indicated

Other Adverse Effects 1% to 10%:
Central nervous system: Dizziness, drowsiness, lightheadedness, headache
Gastrointestinal: Nausea, vomiting, xerostomia, epigastric distress

Drug Interactions Increased Effect/Toxicity: May potentiate action of barbiturates, tranquilizers, and narcotics. Difenoxin has the potential to prolong biological half-life of drugs for which the rate of elimination is dependent on the microsomal drug metabolizing enzyme system. Concurrent use with MAO inhibitors may precipitate hypertensive crisis.

Pregnancy Risk Factor C

Generic Available No

Differin® *see* Adapalene *on page 42*

Diflorasone (dye FLOR a sone)

U.S. Brand Names Maxiflor®; Psorcon™; Psorcon™ E

Canadian Brand Names Florone®; Psorcon™

Pharmacologic Category Corticosteroid, Topical

Synonyms Diflorasone Diacetate

Use Relieves inflammation and pruritic symptoms of corticosteroid-responsive dermatosis (high to very high potency topical corticosteroid)
Maxiflor®: High potency topical corticosteroid
Psorcon™: Very high potency topical corticosteroid

Local Anesthetic/Vasoconstrictor Precautions No information available to require special precautions

Effects on Dental Treatment No effects or complications reported

Dosage Topical: Apply ointment sparingly 1-3 times/day; apply cream sparingly 2-4 times/day
Therapy should be discontinued when control is achieved; if no improvement is seen, reassessment of diagnosis may be necessary.

Mechanism of Action Decreases inflammation by suppression of migration of polymorphonuclear leukocytes and reversal of increased capillary permeability

Drug Uptake Absorption: Topical: Negligible, around 1% reaches dermal layers or systemic circulation; occlusive dressings increase absorption percutaneously

Pregnancy Risk Factor C

Generic Available Yes

Diflucan® *see* Fluconazole *on page 506*

Diflunisal (dye FLOO ni sal)

Related Information
Dental Drug Interactions: Update on Drug Combinations Requiring Special Considerations *on page 1434*
Oral Pain *on page 1360*
Rheumatoid Arthritis and Osteoarthritis *on page 1340*
Temporomandibular Dysfunction (TMD) *on page 1397*

U.S. Brand Names Dolobid®

Canadian Brand Names Apo®-Diflunisal; Novo-Diflunisal; Nu-Diflunisal

Mexican Brand Names Dolobid®

Pharmacologic Category Nonsteroidal Anti-inflammatory Drug (NSAID)

Use
Dental: Treatment of postoperative pain
Medical: Management of pain and inflammatory disorders usually including rheumatoid arthritis and osteoarthritis

Local Anesthetic/Vasoconstrictor Precautions No information available to require special precautions

Effects on Dental Treatment NSAID formulations are known to reversibly decrease platelet aggregation via mechanisms different than observed with aspirin. The dentist should be aware of the potential of abnormal coagulation. Caution should also be exercised in the use of NSAIDs in patients already on anticoagulant therapy with drugs such as warfarin (Coumadin®).

Dosage Adults: Oral:

Pain: Initial: 500-1000 mg followed by 250-500 mg every 8-12 hours; maximum daily dose: 1.5 g

Inflammatory condition: 500-1000 mg/day in 2 divided doses; maximum daily dose: 1.5 g

Dosing adjustment in renal impairment: Cl_{cr} <50 mL/minute: Administer 50% of normal dose

Mechanism of Action Inhibits prostaglandin synthesis by decreasing the activity of the enzyme, cyclooxygenase, which results in decreased formation of prostaglandin precursors

Other Adverse Effects

>10%:

Central nervous system: Headache
Endocrine & metabolic: Fluid retention

1% to 10%:

Cardiovascular: Angina pectoris, arrhythmias
Central nervous system: Dizziness
Dermatologic: Rash
Gastrointestinal: GI ulceration
Genitourinary: Vaginal bleeding
Otic: Tinnitus

<1%: Chest pain, vasculitis, tachycardia, convulsions, hallucinations, mental depression, drowsiness, nervousness, insomnia, toxic epidermal necrolysis, urticaria, exfoliative dermatitis, itching, erythema multiforme, Stevens-Johnson syndrome, angioedema, stomatitis, esophagitis or gastritis, cystitis, hemolytic anemia, agranulocytosis, thrombocytopenia, hepatitis, peripheral neuropathy, trembling, weakness, blurred vision, change in vision, decreased hearing, interstitial nephritis, nephrotic syndrome, renal impairment, wheezing, dyspnea, anaphylaxis, diaphoresis (increased)

Contraindications Hypersensitivity to diflunisal or any component of the formulation; potential cross-sensitivity with other nonsteroidal anti-inflammatory agents including aspirin; active GI bleeding; pregnancy (3rd trimester)

Warnings/Precautions Ophthalmologic effects; peripheral edema; possibility of Reye's syndrome; use with caution in patients with CHF, dehydration, hypertension, decreased renal or hepatic function, history of GI disease, active GI ulceration or bleeding, or those receiving anticoagulants; withhold for at least 4-6 half-lives prior to surgical or dental procedures

Drug Interactions

ACE inhibitors: Antihypertensive effects may be decreased by concurrent therapy with NSAIDs; monitor BP

Angiotensin II antagonists: Antihypertensive effects may be decreased by concurrent therapy with NSAIDs; monitor BP

Antacids: Decreased effect (may decrease absorption)

Increased effect/toxicity: Digoxin, anticoagulants, phenytoin, sulfonylureas, sulfonamides, lithium, hydrochlorothiazide, acetaminophen (levels)

Methotrexate: Severe bone marrow suppression, aplastic anemia, and GI toxicity have been reported with concomitant NSAID therapy. Avoid use during moderate or high-dose methotrexate (increased and prolonged methotrexate levels). NSAID use during low-dose treatment of rheumatoid arthritis has not been fully evaluated; extreme caution is warranted.

Dietary/Ethanol/Herb Considerations

Ethanol: Avoid use; may enhance gastric mucosal irritation.

Food: Administer with food or milk to reduce GI upset. Avoid excessive amounts of fruit juices, vitamin C or salicylate-containing foods (curry powder, prunes, raisins, tea, or licorice).

Herb/Nutraceutical: Avoid cat's claw, dong quai, evening primrose, feverfew, garlic, ginger, ginkgo biloba, ginseng, green tea, horse chestnut, and red clover due to additional antiplatelet activity. Avoid kava and valerian; may enhance benzodiazepine activity. Limit licorice due to salicylate content.

Drug Uptake

Onset of action: Analgesic: ~1 hour
Absorption: Well absorbed
Duration: 8-12 hours
Half-life, elimination: 8-12 hours; prolonged with renal impairment
Time to peak: 2-3 hours

Pregnancy Risk Factor C (1st and 2nd trimesters); D (3rd trimester)

Breast-feeding Considerations Diflunisal is excreted in breast milk, however, there is no specific data regarding use during lactation

(Continued)

Diflunisal *(Continued)*

Dosage Forms TAB: 250 mg, 500 mg

Generic Available Yes

Comments The advantage of diflunisal as a pain reliever is its 12-hour duration of effect. In many cases, this long effect will ensure a full night sleep during the postoperative pain period.

Selected Readings

Ahmad N, Grad HA, Haas DA, et al, "The Efficacy of Nonopioid Analgesics for Postoperative Dental Pain: A Meta-Analysis," *Anesth Prog*, 1997, 44(4):119-26.

Brooks PM and Day RO, "Nonsteroidal Anti-inflammatory Drugs - Differences and Similarities," *N Engl J Med*, 1991, 324(24):1716-25.

Dionne R, "Additive Analgesia Without Opioid Side Effects," *Compend Contin Educ Dent*, 2000, 21(7):572-4, 576-7.

Dionne RA, "New Approaches to Preventing and Treating Postoperative Pain," *J Am Dent Assoc*, 1992, 123(6):26-34.

Dionne RA and Berthold CW, "Therapeutic Uses of Nonsteroidal Anti-Inflammatory Drugs in Dentistry," *Crit Rev Oral Biol Med*, 2001, 12(4):315-30.

Forbes JA, Calderazzo JP, Bowser MW, et al, "A 12-Hour Evaluation of the Analgesic Efficacy of Diflunisal, Aspirin, and Placebo in Postoperative Dental Pain," *J Clin Pharmacol*, 1982, 22(2-3):89-96.

Gobetti JP, "Controlling Dental Pain," *J Am Dent Assoc*, 1992, 123(6):47-52.

Nguyen AM, Graham DY, Gage T, et al, "Nonsteroidal Anti-Inflammatory Drug Use in Dentistry: Gastrointestinal Implications," *Gen Dent*, 1999, 47(6):590-6.

Digibind® *see* Digoxin Immune Fab *on page 391*

DigiFab™ *see* Digoxin Immune Fab *on page 391*

Digitoxin *Not Available in U.S.* (di ji TOKS in)

Related Information

Cardiovascular Diseases *on page 1308*

U.S. Brand Names Crystodigin® [DSC]

Canadian Brand Names Digitaline®

Pharmacologic Category Antiarrhythmic Agent, Class IV

Use Treatment of CHF and to slow the ventricular rate in tachyarrhythmias such as atrial fibrillation, atrial flutter, and supraventricular tachycardia (paroxysmal atrial tachycardia); cardiogenic shock

Local Anesthetic/Vasoconstrictor Precautions Use vasoconstrictors with caution due to risk of cardiac arrhythmias with digitoxin.

Effects on Dental Treatment Sensitive gag reflex may cause difficulty in taking a dental impression.

Restrictions Not available in U.S.

Dosage Oral:

Children: Doses are very individualized; **when recommended**, digitalizing dose is as follows:

- <1 year: 0.045 mg/kg
- 1-2 years: 0.04 mg/kg
- >2 years: 0.03 mg/kg (equivalent to 0.75 mg/mm^2)
- Maintenance: ~$^1/_{10}$ of the digitalizing dose

Adults:

- Rapid loading dose: Initial: 0.6 mg, followed by 0.4 mg, then 0.2 mg at intervals of 4-6 hours
- Slow loading dose: Initial: 0.2 mg twice daily for 4 days, followed by maintenance dose
- Maintenance: 0.05-0.3 mg/day
- Most common dose: 0.15 mg/day

Mechanism of Action Most potent of the digitalis glycosides; binds to and inhibits magnesium and adenosine triphosphate-dependent sodium and potassium ATPase, thereby increasing the influx of calcium ions from extracellular to intracellular cytoplasm, due to the inhibition of sodium and potassium ion movement across the myocardial membranes; this increase in calcium ions results in a potentiation of the activity of the contractile heart muscle fibers and an increase in the force of myocardial contraction (positive inotropic effect). Digitalis may also increase intracellular entry of calcium via slow calcium channel influx; stimulates release and blocks re-uptake of norepinephrine and decreases conduction throughout the S-A and A-V nodes.

Other Adverse Effects 1% to 10%: Gastrointestinal: Abdominal pain, anorexia, nausea, vomiting

Effects reported for digoxin may also alter response/levels of digitoxin. Frequency not defined (incidence not always reported):

Cardiovascular: Heart block; first-, second- (Wenckebach), or third-degree heart block; asystole; atrial tachycardia with block; AV dissociation; accelerated junctional rhythm; ventricular tachycardia or ventricular fibrillation; PR prolongation; ST segment depression

Central nervous system: Visual disturbances (blurred or yellow vision), headache (3%), weakness, dizziness (5%), apathy, confusion, mental disturbances (4%), anxiety, depression, delirium, hallucinations, fever

Dermatologic: Maculopapular rash (2%), erythematous, scarlatiniform, papular, vesicular or bullous rashes, urticaria, pruritus, facial, angioneurotic or laryngeal edema, shedding of fingernails or toenails, alopecia

Children are more likely to experience cardiac arrhythmias as a sign of excessive dosing. The most common are conduction disturbances or tachyarrhythmias (atrial tachycardia with or without block) and junctional tachycardia. Ventricular tachyarrhythmias are less common. In infants, sinus bradycardia may be a sign of digoxin toxicity. Any arrhythmia seen in a child on digoxin should be considered as digoxin toxicity. The gastrointestinal and central nervous system symptoms are not frequently seen in children.

Drug Interactions Effects reported for digoxin may also alter response/levels of digitoxin:

Increased Effect/Toxicity: Beta-blocking agents (propranolol), verapamil, and diltiazem may have additive effects on heart rate. Carvedilol has additive effects on heart rate and inhibits the metabolism of digoxin and possibly digitoxin. Digoxin levels may be increased by amiodarone (reduce digoxin dose 50%), bepridil, cyclosporine, diltiazem, indomethacin, itraconazole, some macrolides (erythromycin, clarithromycin), methimazole, nitrendipine, propafenone, propylthiouracil, quinidine (reduce digoxin dose 33% to 50% on initiation), tetracyclines, and verapamil. Moricizine may increase the toxicity of digoxin (mechanism undefined). Spironolactone may interfere with some digoxin assays, but may also increase blood levels directly. Succinylcholine administration to patients on digoxin has been associated with an increased risk of arrhythmias. Rare cases of acute digoxin toxicity have been associated with parenteral calcium (bolus) administration. The following medications have been associated with increased digoxin blood levels which appear to be of limited clinical significance: Famciclovir, flecainide, ibuprofen, fluoxetine, nefazodone, cimetidine, famotidine, ranitidine, omeprazole, trimethoprim.

Decreased Effect: Amiloride and spironolactone may reduce the inotropic response to digoxin. Cholestyramine, colestipol, kaolin-pectin, and metoclopramide may reduce digoxin absorption. Levothyroxine (and other thyroid supplements) may decrease digoxin blood levels. Penicillamine has been associated with reductions in digoxin blood levels The following reported interactions appear to be of limited clinical significance: Aminoglutethimide, aminosalicylic acid, aluminum-containing antacids, sucralfate, sulfasalazine, neomycin, ticlopidine.

Drug Uptake

Onset of action: Oral: 1-4 hours; Peak effect: 8-12 hours

Absorption: 90% to 100%

Duration: 2 weeks

Half-life, elimination: 7-8 days

Time to peak: 8-12 hours

Pregnancy Risk Factor C

Generic Available No

Digoxin (di JOKS in)

Related Information

Cardiovascular Diseases *on page 1308*

U.S. Brand Names Lanoxicaps®; Lanoxin®

Canadian Brand Names Lanoxicaps®; Lanoxin®

Mexican Brand Names Lanoxin®; Mapluxin®

Pharmacologic Category Antiarrhythmic Agent, Class IV; Cardiac Glycoside

Use Treatment of CHF and to slow the ventricular rate in tachyarrhythmias such as atrial fibrillation, atrial flutter, and supraventricular tachycardia (paroxysmal atrial tachycardia); cardiogenic shock

Dosage Recommendations for Digoxin

Age	Total Digitalizing Dose** (mcg/kg*)		Daily Maintenance Dose*** (mcg/kg*)	
	P.O.	I.V. or I.M.	P.O.	I.V. or I.M.
Preterm infant*	20-30	15-25	5-7.5	4-6
Full-term infant*	25-35	20-30	6-10	5-8
1 month - 2 years*	35-60	30-50	10-15	7.5-12
2-5 years*	30-40	25-35	7.5-10	6-9
5-10 years*	20-35	15-30	5-10	4-8
>10 years*	10-15	8-12	2.5-5	2-3
Adults	0.75-1.5 mg	0.5-1 mg	0.125-0.5 mg	0.1-0.4 mg

*Based on lean body weight and normal renal function for age. Decrease dose in patients with ↓ renal function; digitalizing dose often not recommended in infants and children.

**Give one-half of the total digitalizing dose (TDD) in the initial dose, then give one-quarter of the TDD in each of two subsequent doses at 8- to 12-hour intervals. Obtain EKG 6 hours after each dose to assess potential toxicity.

***Divided every 12 hours in infants and children <10 years of age. Given once daily to children >10 years of age and adults.

(Continued)

Digoxin *(Continued)*

Local Anesthetic/Vasoconstrictor Precautions Use vasoconstrictor with caution due to risk of cardiac arrhythmias with digoxin

Effects on Dental Treatment Sensitive gag reflex may cause difficulty in taking a dental impression.

Dosage When changing from oral (tablets or liquid) or I.M. to I.V. therapy, dosage should be reduced by 20% to 25%. See table on previous page.

Mechanism of Action

Congestive heart failure: Inhibition of the sodium/potassium ATPase pump which acts to increase the intracellular sodium-calcium exchange to increase intracellular calcium leading to increased contractility

Supraventricular arrhythmias: Direct suppression of the A-V node conduction to increase effective refractory period and decrease conduction velocity - positive inotropic effect, enhanced vagal tone, and decreased ventricular rate to fast atrial arrhythmias. Atrial fibrillation may decrease sensitivity and increase tolerance to higher serum digoxin concentrations.

Other Adverse Effects Frequency not defined (incidence not always reported):

Cardiovascular: Heart block; first-, second- (Wenckebach), or third-degree heart block; asystole; atrial tachycardia with block; AV dissociation; accelerated junctional rhythm; ventricular tachycardia or ventricular fibrillation; PR prolongation; ST segment depression

Central nervous system: Visual disturbances (blurred or yellow vision), headache (3%), weakness, dizziness (5%), apathy, confusion, mental disturbances (4%), anxiety, depression, delirium, hallucinations, fever

Dermatologic: Maculopapular rash (2%), erythematous, scarlatiniform, papular, vesicular or bullous rashes, urticaria, pruritus, facial, angioneurotic or laryngeal edema, shedding of fingernails or toenails, alopecia

Gastrointestinal: Nausea (3%), vomiting (2%), diarrhea (3%), abdominal pain

Children are more likely to experience cardiac arrhythmias as a sign of excessive dosing. The most common are conduction disturbances or tachyarrhythmias (atrial tachycardia with or without block) and junctional tachycardia. Ventricular tachyarrhythmias are less common. In infants, sinus bradycardia may be a sign of digoxin toxicity. Any arrhythmia seen in a child on digoxin should be considered as digoxin toxicity. The gastrointestinal and central nervous system symptoms are not frequently seen in children.

Drug Interactions

Increased Effect/Toxicity: Beta-blocking agents (propranolol), verapamil, and diltiazem may have additive effects on heart rate. Carvedilol has additive effects on heart rate and inhibits the metabolism of digoxin. Digoxin levels may be increased by amiodarone (reduce digoxin dose 50%), bepridil, cyclosporine, diltiazem, indomethacin, itraconazole, some macrolides (erythromycin, clarithromycin), methimazole, nitrendipine, propafenone, propylthiouracil, quinidine (reduce digoxin dose 33% to 50% on initiation), tetracyclines, and verapamil. Moricizine may increase the toxicity of digoxin (mechanism undefined). Spironolactone may interfere with some digoxin assays, but may also increase blood levels directly. Succinylcholine administration to patients on digoxin has been associated with an increased risk of arrhythmias. Rare cases of acute digoxin toxicity have been associated with parenteral calcium (bolus) administration. The following medications have been associated with increased digoxin blood levels which appear to be of limited clinical significance: Famciclovir, flecainide, ibuprofen, fluoxetine, nefazodone, cimetidine, famotidine, ranitidine, omeprazole, trimethoprim.

Decreased Effect: Amiloride and spironolactone may reduce the inotropic response to digoxin. Cholestyramine, colestipol, kaolin-pectin, and metoclopramide may reduce digoxin absorption. Levothyroxine (and other thyroid supplements) may decrease digoxin blood levels. Penicillamine has been associated with reductions in digoxin blood levels The following reported interactions appear to be of limited clinical significance: Aminoglutethimide, aminosalicylic acid, aluminum-containing antacids, sucralfate, sulfasalazine, neomycin, ticlopidine.

Drug Uptake

Onset of action: Oral: 1-2 hours; I.V.: 5-30 minutes

Peak effect: Oral: 2-8 hours; I.V.: 1-4 hours

Absorption: By passive nonsaturable diffusion in the upper small intestine; food may delay, but does not affect extent of absorption

Duration: Adults: 3-4 days both drugs

Half-life, elimination: Parent drug: 38 hours; Metabolites: Digoxigenin: 4 hours; Monodigitoxoside: 3-12 hours

Half-life, elimination (age, renal and cardiac function dependent):

Neonates: Premature: 61-170 hours; Full-term: 35-45 hours

Infants: 18-25 hours

Children: 35 hours

Adults: 38-48 hours

Adults, anephric: 4-6 days

Time to peak: Oral: ~1 hour; I.V.: 1-4 hours

Pregnancy Risk Factor C

Generic Available Yes: Injection, tablet

Digoxin Immune Fab (di JOKS in i MYUN fab)

U.S. Brand Names Digibind®; DigiFab™

Canadian Brand Names Digibind®

Pharmacologic Category Antidote

Synonyms Antidigoxin Fab Fragments, Ovine

Use Treatment of life-threatening or potentially life-threatening digoxin intoxication, including:

- Acute digoxin ingestion (ie, >10 mg in adults or >4 mg in children)
- Chronic ingestions leading to steady-state digoxin concentrations > 6 ng/mL in adults or >4 ng/mL in children
- Manifestations of digoxin toxicity due to overdose (life-threatening ventricular arrhythmias, progressive bradycardia, second- or third-degree heart block not responsive to atropine, serum potassium >5 mEq/L in adults or >6 mEq in children)

Local Anesthetic/Vasoconstrictor Precautions No information available to require special precautions

Effects on Dental Treatment No effects or complications reported

Dosage Each vial of Digibind® 38 mg or DigiFab™ 40 mg will bind ~0.5 mg of digoxin or digitoxin.

Estimation of the dose is based on the body burden of digitalis. This may be calculated if the amount ingested is known or the postdistribution serum drug level is known (round dose to the nearest whole vial). See table.

Digoxin Immune Fab

Tablets Ingested (0.25 mg)	Fab Dose (vials)
5	2
10	4
25	10
50	20
75	30
100	40
150	60
200	80

Fab dose based on serum drug level postdistribution:

Digoxin: No. of vials = level (ng/mL) x body weight (kg) divided by 100

Digitoxin: No. of vials = digitoxin (ng/mL) x body weight (kg) divided by 1000

If neither amount ingested nor drug level are known, dose empirically as follows:

For acute toxicity: 20 vials, administered in 2 divided doses to decrease the possibility of a febrile reaction, and to avoid fluid overload in small children.

For chronic toxicity: 6 vials; for infants and small children (≤20kg), a single vial may be sufficient

Mechanism of Action Digoxin immune antigen-binding fragments (Fab) are specific antibodies for the treatment of digitalis intoxication in carefully selected patients; binds with molecules of digoxin or digitoxin and then is excreted by the kidneys and removed from the body.

Other Adverse Effects Frequency not defined:

Cardiovascular: Effects (due to withdrawal of digitalis) include exacerbation of low cardiac output states and CHF, rapid ventricular response in patients with atrial fibrillation; postural hypotension

Endocrine & metabolic: Hypokalemia

Local: Phlebitis

Miscellaneous: Allergic reactions, serum sickness

Contraindications Hypersensitivity to sheep products

Drug Interactions Digoxin: Following administration of digoxin immune Fab, serum digoxin levels are markedly increased due to bound complexes (may be clinically misleading, since bound complex cannot interact with receptors).

Drug Uptake

Onset of action: I.V.: 2-30 minutes

Half-life, elimination: 15-20 hours (increases with renal impairment)

Pregnancy Risk Factor C

Generic Available No

Dihistine® DH *see* Chlorpheniramine, Pseudoephedrine, and Codeine *on page 273*

Dihistine® Expectorant *see* Guaifenesin, Pseudoephedrine, and Codeine *on page 570*

Dihydrex® *see* DiphenhydrAMINE *on page 398*

Dihydrocodeine Compound (dye hye droe KOE deen KOM pound)

Related Information

Oral Pain *on page 1360*

U.S. Brand Names DHC Plus®; Synalgos®-DC

Pharmacologic Category Analgesic, Narcotic

Use

Dental: Management of postoperative pain

Medical: Management of mild to moderate pain from medical conditions

Local Anesthetic/Vasoconstrictor Precautions No information available to require special precautions

Effects on Dental Treatment

Use with caution in patients with platelet and bleeding disorders, renal dysfunction, erosive gastritis, or peptic ulcer disease, previous nonreaction does not guarantee future safe taking of medication; use with caution in impaired hepatic function; do not use aspirin in children <16 years of age for chickenpox or flu symptoms due to the association with Reye's syndrome

Avoid aspirin, if possible, for 1 week prior to surgery due to possibility of postoperative bleeding

Elderly are a high-risk population for adverse effects from nonsteroidal anti-inflammatory agents. As much as 60% of elderly with GI complications to NSAIDs can develop peptic ulceration and/or hemorrhage asymptomatically. Also, concomitant disease and drug use contribute to the risk for GI adverse effects. Use lowest effective dose for shortest period possible. Consider renal function decline with age. Use with caution in patients with history of asthma.

Restrictions C-III

Dosage Oral:

Adults: 1-2 capsules every 4-6 hours as needed for pain

Elderly: Initial dosing should be cautious (low end of dosing range); refer to Adult dosing.

Mechanism of Action Dihydrocodeine binds to opiate receptors (mu and kappa subtypes) in the CNS causing inhibition of ascending pain pathways, altering the perception of and response to pain; produces generalized CNS depression; causes cough suppression by direct central action in the medulla; produces generalized CNS depression

Acetaminophen inhibits the synthesis of prostaglandins in the CNS and peripherally blocks pain impulse generation; produces antipyresis from inhibition of hypothalamic heat-regulating center

Aspirin inhibits prostaglandin synthesis by decreasing the activity of the enzyme, cyclooxygenase, which results in decreased formation of prostaglandin precursors acts on the hypothalamic heat-regulating center to reduce fever, blocks thromboxane synthetase action which prevents formation of the platelet-aggregating substance thromboxane A_2

Other Adverse Effects

>10%:

- Central nervous system: Lightheadedness, dizziness, drowsiness, sedation
- Dermatologic: Pruritus, skin reactions
- Gastrointestinal: Nausea, vomiting, constipation

1% to 10%:

- Cardiovascular: Hypotension, palpitations, bradycardia, peripheral vasodilation
- Central nervous system: Increased intracranial pressure
- Endocrine & metabolic: Antidiuretic hormone release
- Gastrointestinal: Biliary tract spasm
- Genitourinary: Urinary tract spasm
- Ocular: Miosis
- Respiratory: Respiratory depression
- Miscellaneous: Histamine release, physical and psychological dependence with prolonged use

Contraindications Hypersensitivity to dihydrocodeine or any component of the formulation; pregnancy (prolonged use or high doses at term)

Warnings/Precautions Use with caution in patients with hypersensitivity reactions to other phenanthrene derivative opioid agonists (morphine, hydrocodone, hydromorphone, levorphanol, oxycodone, oxymorphone); respiratory diseases including asthma, emphysema, COPD, or severe liver or renal insufficiency; some preparations contain sulfites which may cause allergic reactions; dextromethorphan has equivalent antitussive activity but has much lower toxicity in accidental overdose; tolerance of drug dependence may result from extended use

Drug Interactions CYP2D6 enzyme substrate

MAO inhibitors may increase adverse symptoms

Dietary/Ethanol/Herb Considerations

Ethanol: Avoid use; may increase CNS depression.

Food: Administer with food. Fruit, fluids, and fiber may reduce constipation.

Herb/Nutraceutical: Avoid gotu kola, kava, SAMe, St John's wort, and valerian; may increase CNS depression.

Drug Uptake

Onset of action: 10-30 minutes

Duration: Oral: 4-6 hours

Half-life, elimination: 3.8 hours

Time to peak: 30-60 minutes

Pregnancy Risk Factor B/D (prolonged use or high doses at term)

Breast-feeding Considerations

Acetaminophen: May be taken while breast-feeding.

Aspirin: Use cautiously due to potential adverse effects in nursing infants.

Dosage Forms CAP: (DHC Plus®): Dihydrocodeine 16 mg, acetaminophen 356.4 mg, and caffeine 30 mg; (Synalgos®-DC): Dihydrocodeine 16 mg, aspirin 356.4 mg, and caffeine 30 mg

Generic Available Yes

Comments Dihydrocodeine products, as with other narcotic analgesics, are recommended only for acute dosing (ie, 3 days or less). The most common adverse effect you will see in your dental patients from dihydrocodeine is nausea, followed by sedation and constipation. Dihydrocodeine has narcotic addiction liability, especially when given long-term. Dihydrocodeine with aspirin could have anticoagulant effects and could possibly affect bleeding times. Dihydrocodeine with acetaminophen should be used with caution in patients with alcoholic liver disease.

Selected Readings "Drugs for Pain," *Med Lett Drugs Ther*, 1998, 40(1033):79-84.

Dihydroergotamine (dye hye droe er GOT a meen)

U.S. Brand Names D.H.E. 45®; Migranal® Nasal Spray

Canadian Brand Names Migranal®

Pharmacologic Category Ergot Derivative

Synonyms DHE; Dihydroergotamine Mesylate

Use

Injection: Aborts or prevents vascular headaches; also as an adjunct for DVT prophylaxis for hip surgery, for orthostatic hypotension, xerostomia secondary to antidepressant use, and pelvic congestion with pain;

Nasal spray: Acute treatment of migraine headaches with or without aura; is not indicated for prophylactic therapy or for the management of hemiplegic or basilar migraine

Unlabeled/Investigational: Adjunct for DVT prophylaxis for hip surgery, for orthostatic hypotension, xerostomia secondary to antidepressant use, and pelvic congestion with pain

Local Anesthetic/Vasoconstrictor Precautions No information available to require special precautions

Effects on Dental Treatment ~1%: Xerostomia

Dosage Adults:

I.M.: 1 mg at first sign of headache; repeat hourly to a maximum dose of 3 mg total

I.V.: Up to 2 mg maximum dose for faster effects; maximum dose: 6 mg/week

Mechanism of Action Ergot alkaloid alpha-adrenergic blocker directly stimulates vascular smooth muscle to vasoconstrict peripheral and cerebral vessels; also has effects on serotonin receptors

Other Adverse Effects

>10%: Nasal spray: Respiratory: Rhinitis (26%)

Cardiovascular: Localized edema, peripheral vascular effects (numbness and tingling of fingers and toes)

1% to 10%: Nasal spray:

Cardiovascular: Precordial distress and pain, transient tachycardia or bradycardia

Central nervous system: Dizziness (4%), somnolence (3%)

Endocrine & metabolic: Hot flashes (1%)

Gastrointestinal: Nausea (10%), taste disturbance (8%), vomiting (4%), diarrhea (2%)

Local: Application site reaction (6%)

Neuromuscular & skeletal: Weakness (1%), stiffness (1%)

Respiratory: Pharyngitis (3%)

Drug Interactions CYP3A enzyme inhibitor

Increased Effect/Toxicity: Concurrent use of protease inhibitors (amprenavir, nelfinavir, and ritonavir) may increase toxicity of dihydroergotamine (use is contraindicated). Increased effect of heparin. Increased toxicity with erythromycin, clarithromycin, nitroglycerin, propranolol, and troleandomycin. Potential for serotonin syndrome if combined with other serotonergic drugs.

Drug Uptake

Onset of action: 15-30 minutes

Duration: 3-4 hours

Half-life, elimination: 1.3-3.9 hours

Time to peak: I.M.: 15-30 minutes

Pregnancy Risk Factor X

Generic Available No

Dihydrotachysterol (dye hye droe tak IS ter ole)

U.S. Brand Names DHT™; Hytakerol®

Canadian Brand Names Hytakerol®

Pharmacologic Category Vitamin D Analog

Synonyms Dichysterol

Use Treatment of hypocalcemia associated with hypoparathyroidism; prophylaxis of hypocalcemic tetany following thyroid surgery

Local Anesthetic/Vasoconstrictor Precautions No information available to require special precautions

Effects on Dental Treatment No effects or complications reported

Dosage Oral:

Hypoparathyroidism:

Young Children: Initial: 1-5 mg/day for 4 days, then 0.1-0.5 mg/day

Older Children and Adults: Initial: 0.8-2.4 mg/day for several days followed by maintenance doses of 0.2-1 mg/day

Nutritional rickets: 0.5 mg as a single dose or 13-50 mcg/day until healing occurs

Renal osteodystrophy: Maintenance: 0.25-0.6 mg/24 hours adjusted as necessary to achieve normal serum calcium levels and promote bone healing

Mechanism of Action Synthetic analogue of vitamin D with a faster onset of action; stimulates calcium and phosphate absorption from the small intestine, promotes secretion of calcium from bone to blood; promotes renal tubule resorption of phosphate

Other Adverse Effects

>10%:

Endocrine & metabolic: Hypercalcemia

Renal: Elevated serum creatinine, hypercalciuria

1% to 10%:

Cardiovascular: Hypotension, cardiac arrhythmias, hypertension

Central nervous system: Irritability, headache

Dermatologic: Pruritus

Endocrine & metabolic: Polydipsia, hypermagnesemia

Gastrointestinal: Nausea, vomiting, constipation, anorexia, pancreatitis, metallic taste

Genitourinary: Polyuria

Neuromuscular & skeletal: Myalgia, bone pain

Ocular: Conjunctivitis, photophobia

Drug Interactions

Increased Effect/Toxicity: Thiazide diuretics may increase calcium levels.

Decreased effect/levels of vitamin D if taken with cholestyramine, colestipol, or mineral oil. Phenytoin and phenobarbital may inhibit activation leading to decreased effectiveness.

Drug Uptake

Onset of action: Peak effect: Calcium: 2-4 weeks

Duration: ≤9 weeks

Absorption: Well absorbed

Pregnancy Risk Factor A/D (dose exceeding RDA recommendation)

Generic Available No

Dihydroxyaluminum Sodium Carbonate

(dye hye DROKS i a LOO mi num SOW dee um KAR bun ate)

Pharmacologic Category Antacid

Use Symptomatic relief of upset stomach associated with hyperacidity

Local Anesthetic/Vasoconstrictor Precautions No information available to require special precautions

Effects on Dental Treatment No effects or complications reported

Dosage Oral: Chew 1-2 tablets as needed

Dilacor® XR *see* Diltiazem *on page 394*

Dilantin® *see* Phenytoin *on page 951*

Dilatrate®-SR *see* Isosorbide Dinitrate *on page 661*

Dilaudid® *see* Hydromorphone *on page 611*

Dilaudid-5® *see* Hydromorphone *on page 611*

Dilaudid-HP® *see* Hydromorphone *on page 611*

Dilor® *see* Dyphylline *on page 426*

Diltia® XT *see* Diltiazem *on page 394*

Diltiazem (dil TYE a zem)

Related Information

Calcium Channel Blockers and Gingival Hyperplasia *on page 1432*

Cardiovascular Diseases *on page 1308*

Enalapril and Diltiazem *on page 433*

U.S. Brand Names Cardizem®; Cardizem® CD; Cardizem® SR; Cartia® XT; Dilacor® XR; Diltia® XT; Tiamate®; Tiazac®

Canadian Brand Names Alti-Diltiazem; Alti-Diltiazem CD; Apo®-Diltiaz; Apo®-Diltiaz CD; Apo®-Diltiaz SR; Cardizem®; Cardizem® CD; Cardizem® SR; Gen-Diltiazem; Gen-Diltiazem SR; Novo-Diltazem; Novo-Diltazem SR; Nu-Diltiaz; Nu-Diltiaz-CD; Rhoxal-diltiazem SR; Syn-Diltiazem®; Tiazac®

Mexican Brand Names Angiotrofin; Angiotrofin A.P.; Angiotrofin Retard; Presoken; Presoquim; Tilazem

Pharmacologic Category Calcium Channel Blocker

Synonyms Diltiazem Hydrochloride

Use

Capsule: Essential hypertension (alone or in combination) - sustained release only; chronic stable angina or angina from coronary artery spasm

Injection: Atrial fibrillation or atrial flutter; paroxysmal supraventricular tachycardia (PSVT)

Unlabeled/Investigational: Therapy of Duchenne muscular dystrophy

Local Anesthetic/Vasoconstrictor Precautions No information available to require special precautions

Effects on Dental Treatment ~1%: Gingival hyperplasia (fewer reports with diltiazem than with other CCBs); usually disappears with discontinuation (consultation with physician is suggested)

Dosage Adults:

Oral: 30-120 mg 3-4 times/day; dosage should be increased gradually, at 1- to 2-day intervals until optimum response is obtained; usual maintenance dose: 240-360 mg/day

Sustained-release capsules:

Cardizem® SR: Initial: 60-120 mg twice daily; adjust to maximum antihypertensive effect (usually within 14 days); usual range: 240-360 mg/day

Cardizem® CD, Tiazac®: Hypertension: Total daily dose of short-acting administered once daily or initially 180 or 240 mg once daily; adjust to maximum effect (usually within 14 days); maximum: 360 mg/day; usual range: 240-360 mg/day

Cardizem® CD: Angina: Initial: 120-180 mg once daily; maximum: 480 mg once/day

Dilacor® XR:

Hypertension: 180-240 mg once daily; maximum: 540 mg/day; usual range: 180-480 mg/day; use lower dose in elderly

Angina: Initial: 120 mg/day; titrate slowly over 7-14 days up to 480 mg/day, as needed

Note: Hypertensive or anginal patients treated with other formulations of diltiazem sustained release can be safely switched to Dilacor® XR at the nearest equivalent total daily dose; subsequent titration may be needed

I.V. (requires an infusion pump): See table.

Diltiazem — I.V. Dosage and Administration

Initial Bolus Dose	0.25 mg/kg actual body weight over 2 minutes (average adult dose: 20 mg)
Repeat Bolus Dose: May be administered after 15 minutes if the response is inadequate	0.35 mg/kg actual body weight over 2 minutes (average adult dose: 25 mg)
Continuous Infusion: Infusions >24 hours or infusion rates >15 mg/hour are not recommended due to potential accumulation of metabolites and increased toxicity.	Initial infusion rate of 10 mg/hour; rate may be increased in 5 mg/hour increments up to 15 mg/hour, as needed; some patients may respond to an initial rate of 5 mg/hour

If Cardizem® injectable is administered by continuous infusion for >24 hours, the possibility of decreased diltiazem clearance, prolonged elimination half-life, and increased diltiazem and/or diltiazem metabolite plasma concentrations should be considered

Conversion from I.V. diltiazem to oral diltiazem: Start oral ~ 3 hours after bolus dose

Oral dose (mg/day) is ~ equal to [rate (mg/hour) x 3 + 3] x 10

3 mg/hour = 120 mg/day
5 mg/hour = 180 mg/day
7 mg/hour = 240 mg/day
11 mg/hour = 360 mg/day (maximum recommended dose)

Mechanism of Action Inhibits calcium ion from entering the "slow channels" or select voltage-sensitive areas of vascular smooth muscle and myocardium during depolarization, producing a relaxation of coronary vascular smooth muscle and coronary vasodilation; increases myocardial oxygen delivery in patients with vasospastic angina

Other Adverse Effects

>10%: Gastrointestinal: Gingival hyperplasia (21%)
(Continued)

Diltiazem *(Continued)*

1% to 10%:

Cardiovascular: Sinus bradycardia (2% to 6%), first-degree AV block (2% to 8%), EKG abnormality (4%), peripheral edema (dose-related 5% to 8%), flushing (2% to 3%), hypotension (1%), palpitations (1%)

Central nervous system: Dizziness (3% to 7%), headache (5% to 12%), somnolence (1%), insomnia (1%)

Dermatological: Rash (1% to 2%)

Gastrointestinal: Nausea (1% to 2%), constipation (2%), dyspepsia (1%)

Neuromuscular & skeletal: Weakness (3% to 5%)

Renal: Polyuria (1%)

Warnings/Precautions Concomitant use with beta-blockers or digoxin can result in conduction disturbances. Avoid concurrent I.V. use of diltiazem and a beta-blocker - monitor closely when I.V. diltiazem is used. Use caution in left ventricular dysfunction and CHF (can exacerbate condition). Symptomatic hypotension can occur. Use with caution in hepatic or renal dysfunction.

Drug Interactions CYP3A3/4 enzyme substrate; CYP1A2, 2D6, and 3A3/4 enzyme inhibitor

Increased Effect/Toxicity: Diltiazem effects may be additive with amiodarone, beta-blockers, or digoxin, which may lead to bradycardia, other conduction delays, and decreased cardiac output. Serum concentrations/toxicity of diltiazem may be increased by inhibitors of CYP3A3/4, including amprenavir, cimetidine, ciprofloxacin, clarithromycin, clozapine, diltiazem, disulfiram, digoxin, erythromycin, fluconazole, fluoxetine, fluvoxamine, isoniazid, itraconazole, ketoconazole, labetalol, levodopa, loxapine, metoprolol, metronidazole, miconazole, nefazodone, nelfinavir, omeprazole, phenytoin, rifabutin, rifampin, ritonavir, troleandomycin, valproic acid, and verapamil. Diltiazem may increase serum concentration/toxicity of alfentanil (possibly fentanyl and sufentanil), some benzodiazepines (specifically midazolam and triazolam), carbamazepine, cisapride (QT prolongation, arrhythmia), cyclosporine, digoxin, HMG-CoA reductase inhibitors (atorvastatin, lovastatin, simvastatin), lithium (neurotoxicity), midazolam, moricizine, and tacrolimus.

Decreased Effect: Rifampin markedly reduces diltiazem serum concentration resulting in decreased diltiazem effect. Coadministration with other cytochrome P450 enzyme inducers should be avoided (includes phenytoin, barbiturates, and carbamazepine).

Drug Uptake

Onset of action: Oral: 30-60 minutes (including sustained release)

Absorption: 80% to 90%

Half-life, elimination: 4-6 hours, may increase with renal impairment; 5-7 hours with sustained release

Time to peak: Short-acting tablets: 2-3 hours; Sustained release: 6-11 hours

Pregnancy Risk Factor C

Generic Available Yes

Dimacol® Caplets [OTC] *see* Guaifenesin, Pseudoephedrine, and Dextromethorphan *on page 571*

DimenhyDRINATE (dye men HYE dri nate)

U.S. Brand Names Calm-X® Oral [OTC]; Dimetabs® Oral [OTC]; Dramamine® Oral [OTC]; Dymenate® [OTC]; Hydrate®; TripTone® Caplets® [OTC]

Canadian Brand Names Apo®-Dimenhydrinate; Gravol®

Mexican Brand Names Dramamine®; Vomisin®

Pharmacologic Category Antihistamine

Use Treatment and prevention of nausea, vertigo, and vomiting associated with motion sickness

Local Anesthetic/Vasoconstrictor Precautions No information available to require special precautions

Effects on Dental Treatment ≤10%: Significant xerostomia and drowsiness; disappears with discontinuation

Dosage

Children:

Oral:

2-5 years: 12.5-25 mg every 6-8 hours, maximum: 75 mg/day

6-12 years: 25-50 mg every 6-8 hours, maximum: 150 mg/day

I.M.: 1.25 mg/kg or 37.5 mg/m² 4 times/day, not to exceed 300 mg/day

Adults: Oral, I.M., I.V.: 50-100 mg every 4-6 hours, not to exceed 400 mg/day

Mechanism of Action Competes with histamine for H_1-receptor sites on effector cells in the GI tract, blood vessels, and respiratory tract; blocks chemoreceptor trigger zone, diminishes vestibular stimulation, and depresses labyrinthine function through its central anticholinergic activity

Other Adverse Effects

>10%:

Central nervous system: Slight to moderate drowsiness

Respiratory: Thickening of bronchial secretions

1% to 10%:

Central nervous system: Headache, fatigue, nervousness, dizziness

Gastrointestinal: Appetite increase, weight gain, nausea, diarrhea, abdominal pain, xerostomia

Neuromuscular & skeletal: Arthralgia

Respiratory: Pharyngitis

Drug Interactions

Increased Effect/Toxicity: CNS depressants may increase the degree of sedation and respiratory depression with antihistamines. Digoxin absorption may be increased. Central and/or peripheral anticholinergic syndrome can occur when administered with amantadine, rimantadine, narcotic analgesics, phenothiazines and other antipsychotics (especially with high anticholinergic activity), tricyclic antidepressants, quinidine, disopyramide, procainamide, and antihistamines.

Decreased Effect: May increase gastric degradation of levodopa and decrease the amount of levodopa absorbed by delaying gastric emptying; therapeutic effects of cholinergic agents (tacrine, donepezil) and neuroleptics may be antagonized.

Drug Uptake

Onset of action: Oral: 15-30 minutes

Absorption: Oral: Well absorbed

Pregnancy Risk Factor B

Generic Available Yes

Dimercaprol (dye mer KAP role)

U.S. Brand Names BAL in Oil®

Pharmacologic Category Antidote

Synonyms BAL; British Anti-Lewisite; Dithioglycerol

Use Antidote to gold, arsenic, and mercury poisoning; adjunct to edetate calcium disodium in lead poisoning

Local Anesthetic/Vasoconstrictor Precautions No information available to require special precautions

Effects on Dental Treatment No effects or complications reported

Dosage Children and Adults: Deep I.M.:

Mild arsenic and gold poisoning: 2.5 mg/kg/dose every 6 hours for 2 days, then every 12 hours on the third day, and once daily thereafter for 10 days

Severe arsenic and gold poisoning: 3 mg/kg/dose every 4 hours for 2 days then every 6 hours on the third day, then every 12 hours thereafter for 10 days

Mercury poisoning: Initial: 5 mg/kg followed by 2.5 mg/kg/dose 1-2 times/day for 10 days

Lead poisoning (use with edetate calcium disodium):

Mild: 3 mg/kg/dose every 4 hours for 5-7 days

Severe and acute encephalopathy: 4 mg/kg/dose initially alone then every 4 hours in combination of edetate calcium disodium

Mechanism of Action Sulfhydryl group combines with ions of various heavy metals to form relatively stable, nontoxic, soluble chelates which are excreted in urine

Other Adverse Effects

>10%:

Cardiovascular: Hypertension, tachycardia (dose-related)

Central nervous system: Convulsions, headache

1% to 10%: Gastrointestinal: Nausea, vomiting

Drug Interactions Increased Effect/Toxicity: Toxic complexes with iron, cadmium, selenium, or uranium

Drug Uptake Time to peak: 0.5-1 hour

Pregnancy Risk Factor C

Generic Available No

Dimetabs® Oral [OTC] *see* DimenhyDRINATE *on page 396*

Dimetapp® Decongestant Liqui-Gels® [OTC] *see* Pseudoephedrine *on page 1022*

Dinoprostone (dye noe PROST one)

U.S. Brand Names Cervidil® Vaginal Insert; Prepidil® Vaginal Gel; Prostin E_2® Vaginal Suppository

Canadian Brand Names Cervidil™; Prepidil®; Prostin® E2

Mexican Brand Names Prepidil®; Propess®

Pharmacologic Category Abortifacient; Prostaglandin

Synonyms PGE_2; Prostaglandin E_2

Use

Gel: Promote cervical ripening prior to labor induction; usage for gel include any patient undergoing induction of labor with an unripe cervix, most commonly for pre-eclampsia, eclampsia, postdates, diabetes, intrauterine growth retardation, and chronic hypertension

Suppositories: Terminate pregnancy from 12th through 28th week of gestation; evacuate uterus in cases of missed abortion or intrauterine fetal death; manage benign hydatidiform mole

Vaginal insert: Initiation and/or cervical ripening in patients at or near term in whom there is a medical or obstetrical indication for the induction of labor

(Continued)

Dinoprostone *(Continued)*

Local Anesthetic/Vasoconstrictor Precautions No information available to require special precautions

Effects on Dental Treatment No effects or complications reported

Dosage

Abortifacient: Insert 1 suppository high in vagina, repeat at 3- to 5-hour intervals until abortion occurs up to 240 mg (maximum dose); continued administration for longer than 2 days is not advisable

Cervical ripening:
- Gel:
  - Intracervical: 0.25-1 mg
  - Intravaginal: 2.5 mg
- Suppositories: Intracervical: 2-3 mg

Mechanism of Action A synthetic prostaglandin E_2 abortifacient that stimulates uterine contractions similar to those seen during natural labor

Other Adverse Effects

>10%:
- Central nervous system: Headache
- Gastrointestinal: Vomiting, diarrhea, nausea

1% to 10%:
- Cardiovascular: Bradycardia
- Central nervous system: Fever
- Endocrine & metabolic: Uterine hypertonus, increased uterine pain
- Neuromuscular & skeletal: Back pain
- Respiratory: Wheezing, dyspnea, coughing, bronchospasm

Drug Interactions Increases effect of oxytocics

Drug Uptake

Onset of action (uterine contractions): Within 10 minutes

Absorption: Vaginal: Slow

Duration: ≤2-3 hours

Pregnancy Risk Factor C

Generic Available No

Diocto® [OTC] *see* Docusate *on page 407*

Diocto C® [OTC] *see* Docusate and Casanthranol *on page 407*

Diotame® [OTC] *see* Bismuth *on page 167*

Diovan® *see* Valsartan *on page 1230*

Diovan HCT® *see* Valsartan and Hydrochlorothiazide *on page 1231*

Dipentum® *see* Olsalazine *on page 886*

Diphenacen-50® *see* DiphenhydrAMINE *on page 398*

Diphenatol® *see* Diphenoxylate and Atropine *on page 400*

Diphen® Cough [OTC] *see* DiphenhydrAMINE *on page 398*

Diphenhist [OTC] *see* DiphenhydrAMINE *on page 398*

DiphenhydrAMINE (dye fen HYE dra meen)

Related Information

Dental Office Emergencies *on page 1418*

Diphenhydramine and Pseudoephedrine *on page 400*

Management of Patients Undergoing Cancer Therapy *on page 1402*

Oral Nonviral Soft Tissue Ulcerations or Erosions *on page 1384*

Oral Viral Infections *on page 1380*

U.S. Brand Names AllerMax® [OTC]; Banophen® [OTC]; Benadryl® [OTC]; Bydramine® Cough Syrup [OTC]; Compoz® Gel Caps [OTC]; Compoz® Nighttime Sleep Aid [OTC]; Dihydrex®; Diphenacen-50®; Diphen® Cough [OTC]; Diphenhist [OTC]; Dormin® [OTC]; Genahist®; Hyrexin-50®; Maximum Strength Nytol® [OTC]; Miles Nervine® [OTC]; Nordryl®; Nytol® [OTC]; Siladryl® [OTC]; Silphen® Cough [OTC]; Sleep-eze 3® Oral [OTC]; Sleepinal® [OTC]; Sleepwell 2-nite® [OTC]; Sominex® [OTC]; Tusstat®; Twilite® [OTC]; Uni-Bent® Cough Syrup; 40 Winks® [OTC]

Canadian Brand Names Allerdryl®; Allernix; Benadryl®; Nytol™; Nytol™ Extra Strength; PMS-Diphenhydramine

Pharmacologic Category Antihistamine

Synonyms Diphenhydramine Hydrochloride

Use Symptomatic relief of allergic symptoms caused by histamine release which include nasal allergies and allergic dermatosis; can be used for mild nighttime sedation; prevention of motion sickness and as an antitussive; has antinauseant and topical anesthetic properties; treatment of antipsychotic-induced extrapyramidal symptoms

Local Anesthetic/Vasoconstrictor Precautions No information available to require special precautions

Effects on Dental Treatment Chronic use of antihistamines will inhibit salivary flow, particularly in elderly patients; may contribute to periodontal disease and oral discomfort.

Dosage

Children:

Oral, I.M., I.V.:

Treatment of moderate to severe allergic reactions: 5 mg/kg/day or 150 mg/m²/day in divided doses every 6-8 hours, not to exceed 300 mg/day

Minor allergic rhinitis or motion sickness:

2 to <6 years: 6.25 mg every 4-6 hours; maximum: 37.5 mg/day

6 to <12 years: 12.5-25 mg every 4-6 hours; maximum: 150 mg/day

≥12 years: 25-50 mg every 4-6 hours; maximum: 300 mg/day

Night-time sleep aid: 30 minutes before bedtime:

2 to <12 years: 1 mg/kg/dose; maximum: 50 mg/dose

≥12 years: 50 mg

Oral: Antitussive:

2 to <6 years: 6.25 mg every 4 hours; maximum 37.5 mg/day

6 to <12 years: 12.5 mg every 4 hours; maximum 75 mg/day

≥12 years: 25 mg every 4 hours; maximum 150 mg/day

I.M., I.V.: Treatment of dystonic reactions: 0.5-1 mg/kg/dose

Adults:

Oral: 25-50 mg every 6-8 hours

Minor allergic rhinitis or motion sickness: 25-50 mg every 4-6 hours; maximum: 300 mg/day

Moderate to severe allergic reactions: 25-50 mg every 4 hours, not to exceed 400 mg/day

Nighttime sleep aid: 50 mg at bedtime

I.M., I.V.: 10-50 mg in a single dose every 2-4 hours, not to exceed 400 mg/day

Dystonic reaction: 50 mg in a single dose; may repeat in 20-30 minutes if necessary

Topical: For external application, not longer than 7 days

Mechanism of Action Competes with histamine for H_1-receptor sites on effector cells in the GI tract, blood vessels, and respiratory tract; anticholinergic and sedative effects are also seen

Other Adverse Effects Frequency not defined:

Cardiovascular: Hypotension, palpitations, tachycardia

Central nervous system: Sedation, sleepiness, dizziness, disturbed coordination, headache, fatigue, nervousness, paradoxical excitement, insomnia, euphoria, confusion

Dermatologic: Photosensitivity, rash, angioedema, urticaria

Gastrointestinal: Nausea, vomiting, diarrhea, abdominal pain, xerostomia, appetite increase, weight gain, dry mucous membranes, anorexia

Genitourinary: Urinary retention, urinary frequency, difficult urination

Hematologic: Hemolytic anemia, thrombocytopenia, agranulocytosis

Neuromuscular & skeletal: Tremor, paresthesia

Ocular: blurred vision

Respiratory: Thickening of bronchial secretions

Contraindications Hypersensitivity to diphenhydramine or any component of the formulation; acute asthma; neonates

Warnings/Precautions Use with caution in patients with angle-closure glaucoma, peptic ulcer, urinary tract obstruction, hyperthyroidism; some preparations contain sodium bisulfite; syrup contains alcohol; diphenhydramine has high sedative and anticholinergic properties, so it may not be considered the antihistamine of choice for prolonged use in the elderly

Drug Interactions CYP2D6 enzyme substrate

Amantadine, rimantadine: Central and/or peripheral anticholinergic syndrome can occur when administered with amantadine or rimantadine

Anticholinergic agents: Central and/or peripheral anticholinergic syndrome can occur when administered with narcotic analgesics, phenothiazines and other antipsychotics (especially with high anticholinergic activity), tricyclic antidepressants, quinidine and some other antiarrhythmics, and antihistamines

Atenolol: Drugs with high anticholinergic activity may increase the bioavailability of atenolol (and possibly other beta-blockers); monitor for increased effect

Cholinergic agents: Drugs with high anticholinergic activity may antagonize the therapeutic effect of cholinergic agents; includes donepezil, rivastigmine, and tacrine

CNS depressants: Sedative effects may be additive with CNS depressants; includes benzodiazepines, barbiturates, narcotic analgesics, and other sedative agents; monitor for increased effect

Digoxin: Drugs with high anticholinergic activity may decrease gastric degradation and increase the amount of digoxin absorbed by delaying gastric emptying

Ethanol: Syrup should not be given to patients taking drugs that can cause disulfiram reactions (ie, metronidazole, chlorpropamide) due to high alcohol content

Levodopa: Drugs with high anticholinergic activity may increase gastric degradation and decrease the amount of levodopa absorbed by delaying gastric emptying

Neuroleptics: Drugs with high anticholinergic activity may antagonize the therapeutic effects of neuroleptics

(Continued)

DiphenhydrAMINE *(Continued)*

Dietary/Ethanol/Herb Considerations

Ethanol: Avoid use; may increase CNS depression.

Food: May be taken with food

Herb/Nutraceutical: Avoid gotu kola, kava, SAMe, St John's wort, and valerian; may increase CNS depression.

Drug Uptake

Onset of action: Maximum sedative effect: 1-3 hours; I.V.: More rapid

Absorption: Oral: 40% to 60% reaches systemic circulation due to first-pass metabolism

Duration: 4-7 hours; Maximum sedative effect: 1-3 hours

Half-life, elimination: Elderly: 13.5 hours; Adults: 2-8 hours

Time to peak: 2-4 hours

Pregnancy Risk Factor B

Breast-feeding Considerations Infants may be more sensitive to the effects of antihistamines.

Dosage Forms CAP: 25 mg, 50 mg. **CRM:** 1%, 2%. **ELIX:** 12.5 mg/5 mL (5 mL, 10 mL, 20 mL, 120 mL, 480 mL, 3780 mL). **INJ:** 10 mg/mL (10 mL, 30 mL); 50 mg/mL (1 mL, 10 mL). **LIQ:** 6.25/5 mL. **LOTION:** 1% (75 mL). **SPRAY, topical:** 1% (60 mL), 2%. **SYR:** 12.5 mg/5 mL (5 mL, 120 mL, 240 mL, 480 mL, 3780 mL). **TAB:** 25 mg, 50 mg. **TAB, chewable:** 12.5 mg

Generic Available Yes

Comments 25-50 mg of diphenhydramine orally every 4-6 hours can be used to treat mild dermatologic manifestations of allergic reactions to penicillin and other antibiotics. Diphenhydramine is not recommended as local anesthetic for either infiltration route or nerve block since the vehicle has caused local necrosis upon injection. A 50:50 mixture of diphenhydramine liquid (12.5 mg/5 mL) in Kaopectate® or Maalox® is used as a local application for recurrent aphthous ulcers; swish 1 tablespoonful for 2 minutes 4 times/day.

Diphenhydramine and Pseudoephedrine

(dye fen HYE dra meen & soo doe e FED rin)

U.S. Brand Names Actifed® Allergy (Night) [OTC]; Banophen® Decongestant [OTC]; Benadryl® Decongestant Allergy [OTC]

Pharmacologic Category Antihistamine/Decongestant Combination

Synonyms Pseudoephedrine and Diphenhydramine

Use Relief of symptoms of upper respiratory mucosal congestion in seasonal and perennial nasal allergies, acute rhinitis, rhinosinusitis, and eustachian tube blockage

Local Anesthetic/Vasoconstrictor Precautions Use with caution since pseudoephedrine is a sympathomimetic amine which could interact with epinephrine to cause a pressor response

Effects on Dental Treatment Chronic use of antihistamines will inhibit salivary flow, particularly in elderly patients; may contribute to periodontal disease and oral discomfort.

Dosage Adults: Oral: 1 capsule or tablet every 4-6 hours, up to 4/day

Other Adverse Effects See Diphenhydramine *on page 398* and Pseudoephedrine *on page 1022*

Drug Interactions See Diphenhydramine *on page 398* and Pseudoephedrine *on page 1022*

Generic Available Yes

Diphenoxylate and Atropine

(dye fen OKS i late & A troe peen)

U.S. Brand Names Diphenatol®; Lomocot®; Lomotil®; Lonox®

Canadian Brand Names Lomotil®

Pharmacologic Category Antidiarrheal

Synonyms Atropine and Diphenoxylate

Use Treatment of diarrhea

Local Anesthetic/Vasoconstrictor Precautions No information available to require special precautions

Effects on Dental Treatment ≤10%: Significant xerostomia and drowsiness; disappears with discontinuation

Restrictions C-V

Dosage Oral:

Children (use with caution in young children due to variable responses): Liquid: 0.3-0.4 mg of diphenoxylate/kg/day in 2-4 divided doses **or**

<2 years: Not recommended

2-5 years: 2 mg of diphenoxylate 3 times/day

5-8 years: 2 mg of diphenoxylate 4 times/day

8-12 years: 2 mg of diphenoxylate 5 times/day

Adults: 15-20 mg/day of diphenoxylate in 3-4 divided doses; maintenance: 5-15 mg/day in 2-3 divided doses

Mechanism of Action Diphenoxylate inhibits excessive GI motility and GI propulsion; commercial preparations contain a subtherapeutic amount of atropine to discourage abuse

Other Adverse Effects 1% to 10%:

Central nervous system: Nervousness, restlessness, dizziness, drowsiness, headache, mental depression

Gastrointestinal: Paralytic ileus, xerostomia

Genitourinary: Urinary retention and dysuria

Ocular: Blurred vision

Respiratory: Respiratory depression

Drug Interactions Increased Effect/Toxicity: MAO inhibitors (hypertensive crisis), CNS depressants when taken with diphenoxylate may result in increased adverse effects, antimuscarinics (paralytic ileus); may prolong half-life of drugs metabolized in liver.

Drug Uptake

See Atropine *on page 130*

Diphenoxylate:

Onset of action: Antidiarrheal: 45-60 minutes; Peak effect: Antidiarrheal: ~2 hours

Duration: Antidiarrheal: 3-4 hours

Absorption: Well absorbed

Half-life, elimination: Diphenoxylate: 2.5 hours

Time to peak: 2 hours

Pregnancy Risk Factor C

Generic Available Yes

Dipivefrin (dye PI ve frin)

U.S. Brand Names AKPro®; Propine®

Canadian Brand Names Ophtho-Dipivefrin™; PMS-Dipivefrin; Propine®

Pharmacologic Category Alpha/Beta Agonist; Ophthalmic Agent, Antiglaucoma; Ophthalmic Agent, Vasoconstrictor

Synonyms Dipivalyl Epinephrine; Dipivefrin Hydrochloride; DPE

Use Reduces elevated intraocular pressure in chronic open-angle glaucoma; also used in treatment of ocular hypertension, low tension, and secondary glaucomas

Local Anesthetic/Vasoconstrictor Precautions No information available to require special precautions

Effects on Dental Treatment No effects or complications reported

Dosage Adults: Ophthalmic: Instill 1 drop every 12 hours into the eyes

Mechanism of Action Dipivefrin is a prodrug of epinephrine which is the active agent that stimulates alpha- and/or beta-adrenergic receptors increasing aqueous humor outflow

Other Adverse Effects 1% to 10%:

Central nervous system: Headache

Local: Burning, stinging

Ocular: Ocular congestion, photophobia, mydriasis, blurred vision, ocular pain, bulbar conjunctival follicles, blepharoconjunctivitis, cystoid macular edema

Drug Interactions Increased or synergistic effect when used with other agents to lower intraocular pressure.

Drug Uptake

Onset of ocular pressure effect: ≤30 minutes

Absorption: Rapid into the aqueous humor

Duration: ≥12 hours

Onset of mydriasitic effect: ≤30 minutes

Absorption: Rapid into the aqueous humor

Duration: Several hours

Pregnancy Risk Factor B

Generic Available Yes

Diprivan® *see* Propofol *on page 1011*

Diprolene® *see* Betamethasone *on page 159*

Diprolene® AF *see* Betamethasone *on page 159*

Diprosone® *see* Betamethasone *on page 159*

Dipyridamole (dye peer ID a mole)

U.S. Brand Names Persantine®

Canadian Brand Names Apo®-Dipyridamole FC; Novo-Dipiradol; Persantine®

Mexican Brand Names Dirinol; Lodimol; Trompersantin

Pharmacologic Category Antiplatelet Agent; Vasodilator

Use Maintains patency after surgical grafting procedures including coronary artery bypass; used with warfarin to decrease thrombosis in patients after artificial heart valve replacement; used with aspirin in prevention of coronary artery thrombosis; in combination with aspirin or warfarin to prevent other thromboembolic disorders. Dipyridamole may also be given 2 days prior to open heart surgery to prevent

(Continued)

Dipyridamole *(Continued)*

platelet activation by extracorporeal bypass pump and as a diagnostic agent in CAD.

Unlabeled/Investigational Treatment of proteinuria in pediatric renal disease

Local Anesthetic/Vasoconstrictor Precautions No information available to require special precautions

Effects on Dental Treatment No effects or complications reported

Dosage

Oral:

Children: 3-6 mg/kg/day in 3 divided doses

Doses of 4-10 mg/kg/day have been used investigationally to treat proteinuria in pediatric renal disease

Adults: 75-400 mg/day in 3-4 divided doses

I.V.: 0.14 mg/kg/minute for 4 minutes; maximum dose: 60 mg

Mechanism of Action Inhibits the activity of adenosine deaminase and phosphodiesterase, which causes an accumulation of adenosine, adenine nucleotides, and cyclic AMP; these mediators then inhibit platelet aggregation and may cause vasodilation; may also stimulate release of prostacyclin or PGD_2; causes coronary vasodilation

Other Adverse Effects

>10%:

Cardiovascular: Exacerbation of angina pectoris (20% I.V.)

Central nervous system: Dizziness (14% oral), headache (12% I.V.)

1% to 10%:

Cardiovascular: Hypotension (5%), hypertension (2%), BP lability (2%), EKG abnormalities (ST-T changes, extrasystoles), chest pain, tachycardia (3% I.V.)

Central nervous system: Headache (2% I.V.), flushing (3% I.V.), fatigue (1% I.V.)

Dermatologic: Rash (2% oral)

Gastrointestinal: Abdominal distress (6% oral), nausea (5% I.V.)

Neuromuscular & skeletal: Paresthesia (1% I.V.)

Respiratory: Dyspnea (3% I.V.)

Drug Interactions

Increased Effect/Toxicity: Dipyridamole enhances the risk of bleeding with aspirin (and other antiplatelet agents), heparin, low-molecular weight heparins, and warfarin. Adenosine blood levels and pharmacologic effects are increased with dipyridamole; consider reduced doses of adenosine.

Decreased Effect: Decreased vasodilation from I.V. dipyridamole when given to patients taking theophylline. Theophylline may reduce the pharmacologic effects of dipyridamole (hold theophylline preparations for 36-48 hours before dipyridamole facilitated stress test).

Drug Uptake

Absorption: Readily, but variable

Half-life, elimination: Terminal: 10-12 hours

Time to peak: 2-2.5 hours

Pregnancy Risk Factor B

Generic Available Yes

Dirithromycin (dye RITH roe mye sin)

U.S. Brand Names Dynabac®

Pharmacologic Category Antibiotic, Macrolide

Use Treatment of mild to moderate upper and lower respiratory tract infections, infections of the skin and skin structure, and sexually transmitted diseases due to susceptible strains

Local Anesthetic/Vasoconstrictor Precautions No information available to require special precautions

Effects on Dental Treatment No effects or complications reported

Dosage Adults: Oral: 500 mg once daily for 7-14 days (14 days required for treatment of community-acquired pneumonia due to *Legionella*, *Mycoplasma*, or *S. pneumoniae*; 10 days is recommended for treatment of *S. pyogenes* pharyngitis/tonsillitis)

Mechanism of Action After being converted during intestinal absorption to its active form, erthromycylamine, dirithromycin inhibits protein synthesis by binding to the 50S ribosomal subunits of susceptible microorganisms

Other Adverse Effects 1% to 10%:

Central nervous system: Headache, dizziness, vertigo, insomnia

Dermatologic: Rash, pruritus, urticaria

Endocrine & metabolic: Hyperkalemia, increased CPK

Gastrointestinal: Abdominal pain, nausea, diarrhea, vomiting, heartburn, flatulence

Hematologic: Thrombocytosis, eosinophilia, segmented neutrophils

Neuromuscular & skeletal: Weakness, pain

Respiratory: Increased cough, dyspnea

Contraindications Hypersensitivity to dirithromycin, any macrolide, or any component of their formulation; the FDA has issued a contraindication with pimozide (Orap®), clarithromycin, and other macrolide antibiotics

Warnings/Precautions Contrary to potential serious consequences with other macrolides (eg, cardiac arrhythmias), the combination of terfenadine and dirithromycin has not shown alteration of terfenadine metabolism; however, caution should be taken during coadministration of dirithromycin and terfenadine

Drug Interactions CYP3A3/4 enzyme inhibitor

Increased Effect/Toxicity: Absorption of dirithromycin is slightly enhanced with concomitant antacids and H_2 antagonists. Dirithromycin may, like erythromycin, increase the effect of alfentanil, anticoagulants, bromocriptine, carbamazepine, cyclosporine, digoxin, disopyramide, ergots, methylprednisolone, cisapride, astemizole, and triazolam.

Interactions with nonsedating antihistamines (eg, astemizole and terfenadine) or theophylline are not known to occur; however, caution is advised with coadministration.

Drug Uptake

Absorption: Rapid; nonenzymatically hydrolyzed to erythromycylamine; T_{max}: 4 hours

Half-life, elimination: 8 hours (range: 2-36 hours)

Pregnancy Risk Factor C

Generic Available No

Selected Readings "Pimozide (Orap) Contraindicated With Clarithromycin (Biaxin®) and Other Macrolide Antibiotics," *FDA Medical Bulletin*, October 1996, 26(3).

Disalcid® *see* Salsalate *on page 1074*

Disobrom® [OTC] *see* Dexbrompheniramine and Pseudoephedrine *on page 365*

Disophrol® Chronotabs® [OTC] *see* Dexbrompheniramine and Pseudoephedrine *on page 365*

Disopyramide (dye soe PEER a mide)

Related Information

Cardiovascular Diseases *on page 1308*

U.S. Brand Names Norpace®; Norpace® CR

Canadian Brand Names Norpace®; Rythmodan®; Rythmodan®-LA

Mexican Brand Names Dimodan

Pharmacologic Category Antiarrhythmic Agent, Class Ia

Synonyms Disopyramide Phosphate

Use Suppression and prevention of unifocal and multifocal premature, ventricular premature complexes, coupled ventricular tachycardia; effective in the conversion of atrial fibrillation, atrial flutter, and paroxysmal atrial tachycardia to normal sinus rhythm and prevention of the reoccurrence of these arrhythmias after conversion by other methods

Local Anesthetic/Vasoconstrictor Precautions No information available to require special precautions

Effects on Dental Treatment No effects or complications reported

Dosage Oral:

Children:
- <1 year: 10-30 mg/kg/24 hours in 4 divided doses
- 1-4 years: 10-20 mg/kg/24 hours in 4 divided doses
- 4-12 years: 10-15 mg/kg/24 hours in 4 divided doses
- 12-18 years: 6-15 mg/kg/24 hours in 4 divided doses

Adults:
- <50 kg: 100 mg every 6 hours or 200 mg every 12 hours (controlled release)
- >50 kg: 150 mg every 6 hours or 300 mg every 12 hours (controlled release); if no response, may increase to 200 mg every 6 hours; maximum dose required for patients with severe refractory ventricular tachycardia is 400 mg every 6 hours

Mechanism of Action Class IA antiarrhythmic: Decreases myocardial excitability and conduction velocity; reduces disparity in refractory between normal and infarcted myocardium; possesses anticholinergic, peripheral vasoconstrictive, and negative inotropic effects

Other Adverse Effects The most common adverse effects are related to cholinergic blockade. The most serious adverse effects of disopyramide are hypotension and CHF.

>10%:
- Gastrointestinal: Xerostomia (32%), constipation (11%)
- Genitourinary: Urinary hesitancy (14% to 23%)

1% to 10%:
- Cardiovascular: Congestive heart failure, hypotension, cardiac conduction disturbance, edema, syncope, chest pain
- Central nervous system: Fatigue, headache, malaise, dizziness, nervousness
- Dermatologic: Rash, generalized dermatoses, pruritus
- Endocrine & metabolic: Hypokalemia, elevated cholesterol, elevated triglycerides
- Gastrointestinal: Dry throat, nausea, abdominal distension, flatulence, abdominal bloating, anorexia, diarrhea, vomiting, weight gain
- Genitourinary: Urinary retention, urinary frequency, urinary urgency, impotence (1% to 3%)

(Continued)

Disopyramide *(Continued)*

Neuromuscular & skeletal: Muscle weakness, muscular pain
Ocular: Blurred vision, dry eyes
Respiratory: Dyspnea

Drug Interactions CYP3A3/4 enzyme substrate

Increased Effect/Toxicity: Disopyramide may increase the effects/toxicity of anticholinergics, beta-blockers, flecainide, procainamide, quinidine, or propafenone. Digoxin and quinidine serum concentration may be increased by disopyramide. Erythromycin and clarithromycin may increase disopyramide serum concentration, increasing toxicity (widening QT interval).

Disopyramide effect/toxicity may be additive with drugs which may prolong the QT interval - amiodarone, amitriptyline, astemizole, bepridil, cisapride (use is contraindicated), disopyramide, erythromycin, haloperidol, imipramine, pimozide, quinidine, sotalol, and thioridazine. In addition concurrent use with sparfloxacin, gatifloxacin, and moxifloxacin may result in additional prolongation of the QT interval; concurrent use is contraindicated.

Decreased Effect: Hepatic microsomal enzyme inducing agents (eg, phenytoin, phenobarbital, rifampin) may increase metabolism of disopyramide leading to a decreased effect. Anticoagulants may have decreased prothrombin times after discontinuation of disopyramide.

Drug Uptake

Onset of action: 0.5-3.5 hours
Absorption: 60% to 83%
Duration: 1.5-8.5 hours
Half-life, elimination: Adults: 4-10 hours (increases with hepatic or renal impairment)

Pregnancy Risk Factor C

Generic Available Yes

Disotate® *see* Edetate Disodium *on page 429*

Di-Spaz® *see* Dicyclomine *on page 382*

Disulfiram (dye SUL fi ram)

U.S. Brand Names Antabuse®

Canadian Brand Names Antabuse®

Pharmacologic Category Aldehyde Dehydrogenase Inhibitor

Use Management of chronic alcoholism

Local Anesthetic/Vasoconstrictor Precautions No information available to require special precautions

Effects on Dental Treatment No effects or complications reported

Dosage Adults: Oral: Do not administer until the patient has abstained from alcohol for at least 12 hours

Initial: 500 mg/day as a single dose for 1-2 weeks; maximum daily dose is 500 mg
Average maintenance dose: 250 mg/day; range: 125-500 mg; duration of therapy is to continue until the patient is fully recovered socially and a basis for permanent self control has been established; maintenance therapy may be required for months or even years

Mechanism of Action A thiuram derivative which interferes with aldehyde dehydrogenase; when taken concomitantly with ethanol, there is an increase in serum acetaldehyde levels. High acetaldehyde causes uncomfortable symptoms including flushing, nausea, thirst, palpitations, chest pain, vertigo, and hypotension. This reaction is the basis for disulfiram use in postwithdrawal long-term care of alcoholism.

Other Adverse Effects Frequency not defined:

Central nervous system: Drowsiness, headache, fatigue, psychosis
Dermatologic: Rash, acneiform eruptions, allergic dermatitis
Gastrointestinal: Metallic or garlic-like aftertaste
Genitourinary: Impotence
Hepatic: Hepatitis (cholestatic and fulminant), hepatic failure (multiple case reports)
Neuromuscular & skeletal: Peripheral neuritis, polyneuritis, peripheral neuropathy
Ocular: Optic neuritis

Drug Interactions CYP2C9 and 2E1 enzyme inhibitor, both disulfiram and diethyldithiocarbamate (disulfiram metabolite) are CYP3A3/4 inhibitors

Increased Effect/Toxicity: Disulfiram may increase serum concentration of benzodiazepines that undergo oxidative metabolism (all but oxazepam, lorazepam, temazepam). Disulfiram increases phenytoin and theophylline serum concentration; toxicity may occur. Disulfiram inhibits the metabolism of warfarin resulting in an increased hypoprothrombinemic response. Disulfiram results in severe ethanol intolerance (Antabuse® reaction) secondary to disulfiram's ability to inhibit aldehyde dehydrogenase; this combination should be avoided. Combined use with isoniazid, metronidazole, or MAO inhibitors may result in adverse CNS effects; this combination should be avoided. Some pharmaceutic dosage forms include ethanol, including elixirs and I.V. trimethoprim-sulfamethoxazole (contains 10% ethanol as a solubilizing agent); these may inadvertently provoke an Antabuse® reaction.

Drug Uptake

Absorption: Rapid from GI tract

Duration: May persist for 1-2 weeks after last dose

Time to peak: 12 hours

Pregnancy Risk Factor C

Generic Available Yes

Ditropan® *see* Oxybutynin *on page 900*

Ditropan® XL *see* Oxybutynin *on page 900*

Diupres® *see* Chlorothiazide and Reserpine *on page 268*

Diuril® *see* Chlorothiazide *on page 267*

Dizmiss® [OTC] *see* Meclizine *on page 750*

Doan's®, Original [OTC] *see* Magnesium Salicylate *on page 742*

DOBUTamine (doe BYOO ta meen)

U.S. Brand Names Dobutrex®

Canadian Brand Names Dobutrex®

Mexican Brand Names Dobuject; Dobutrex®; Oxiken

Pharmacologic Category Adrenergic Agonist Agent

Synonyms Dobutamine Hydrochloride

Use Short-term management of patients with cardiac decompensation

Unlabeled/Investigational: Postive inotropic agent for use in myocardial dysfunction of sepsis

Local Anesthetic/Vasoconstrictor Precautions No information available to require special precautions

Effects on Dental Treatment No effects or complications reported

Dosage I.V. infusion:

Children: 2.5-15 mcg/kg/minute, titrate to desired response

Adults: 2.5-15 mcg/kg/minute; maximum: 40 mcg/kg/minute, titrate to desired response

Infusion Rates of Various Dilutions of Dobutamine

Desired Delivery Rate (mcg/kg/minute)	Infusion Rate (mL/kg/minute)	
	500 mcg/mL*	1000 mcg/mL**
2.5	0.005	0.0025
5.0	0.01	0.005
7.5	0.015	0.0075
10.0	0.02	0.01
12.5	0.025	0.0125
15.0	0.03	0.015

* 500 mg per liter or 250 mg per 500 mL of diluent.

**1000 mg per liter or 250 mg per 250 mL of diluent.

Mechanism of Action Stimulates $beta_1$-adrenergic receptors, causing increased contractility and heart rate, with little effect on $beta_2$- or alpha-receptors

Other Adverse Effects Incidence of adverse events is not always reported.

Cardiovascular: Increased heart rate, increased BP, increased ventricular ectopic activity, hypotension, premature ventricular beats (5%, dose-related), anginal pain (1% to 3%), nonspecific chest pain (1% to 3%), palpitations (1% to 3%)

Central nervous system: Fever (1% to 3%), headache (1% to 3%), paresthesia

Endocrine & metabolic: Slight decrease in serum potassium

Gastrointestinal: Nausea (1% to 3%)

Hematologic: Thrombocytopenia (isolated cases)

Local: Phlebitis, local inflammatory changes and pain from infiltration, cutaneous necrosis (isolated cases)

Neuromuscular & skeletal: Mild leg cramps

Respiratory: Shortness of breath (1% to 3%)

Drug Interactions

Increased Effect/Toxicity: General anesthetics (eg, halothane or cyclopropane) and usual doses of dobutamine have resulted in ventricular arrhythmias in animals. Bretylium and may potentiate dobutamine's effects. Beta-blockers (nonselective ones) may increase hypertensive effect; avoid concurrent use. Cocaine may cause malignant arrhythmias. Guanethidine, MAO inhibitors, methyldopa, reserpine, and tricyclic antidepressants can increase the pressor response to sympathomimetics.

Decreased Effect: Beta-adrenergic blockers may decrease effect of dobutamine and increase risk of severe hypotension.

Drug Uptake

Onset of action: I.V.: 1-10 minutes; Peak effect: 10-20 minutes

Half-life, elimination: 2 minutes

Pregnancy Risk Factor B

Generic Available Yes

Dobutrex® *see* DOBUTamine *on page 405*

Docetaxel (doe se TAKS el)

U.S. Brand Names Taxotere®

Canadian Brand Names Taxotere®

Mexican Brand Names Taxotere®

Pharmacologic Category Antineoplastic Agent, Natural Source (Plant) Derivative

Use FDA-approved: Treatment of patients with locally advanced or metastatic breast cancer who have progressed during anthracycline-based therapy or have relapsed during anthracycline-based adjuvant therapy

Unlabeled/Investigational: Treatment of nonsmall cell lung cancer, gastric, pancreatic, head and neck, ovarian, soft tissue sarcoma, and melanoma

Local Anesthetic/Vasoconstrictor Precautions No information available to require special precautions

Effects on Dental Treatment No effects or complications reported

Dosage Adults: I.V.: 60-100 mg/m^2 administered over 1 hour every 3 weeks

Mechanism of Action Semisynthetic agent prepared from a noncytotoxic precursor which is extracted from the needles of the European Yew *Taxus baccata*. Docetaxel differs structurally from the prototype taxoid, paclitaxel, by substitutions at the C-10 and C-5 positions. It is an antimicrotubule agent, but exhibits a unique mechanism of action. Unlike other antimicrotubule agents that induce microtubule disassembly (eg, vinca alkaloids and colchicine), docetaxel promotes the assembly of microtubules from tubulin dimers, and inhibits the depolymerization of tubulin which leads to bundles of microtubules in the cell.

Other Adverse Effects

>10%:

Allergic: Angioedema, rash, flushing, fever, hypotension (30%); patients should be premedicated with dexamethasone starting the day before docetaxel administration

Dermatologic: Alopecia (80%); nail banding, onycholysis (28%); hypo- or hyperpigmentation (28%)

Endocrine & metabolic: Fluid retention, including peripheral edema, pleural effusions, and ascites (17% to 70%), may be more common at cumulative doses ≥400 mg/m^2

Gastrointestinal: Mucositis (45%), may be dose-limiting; mild to moderate nausea and vomiting (40% to 80%), diarrhea (25%)

Hematologic: Myelosuppression, neutropenia, thrombocytopenia, anemia

- Onset: 4-7 days
- Nadir: 5-9 days
- Recovery: 21 days

Hepatic: Increased transaminase levels (18%)

Neuromuscular & skeletal: Peripheral neuropathies (13%)

1% to 10%:

Cardiovascular: Myocardial infarction

Dermatologic: Rash and skin eruptions (6%)

Gastrointestinal: GI perforation, neutropenic enterocolitis

Hepatic: Increased bilirubin (9%)

Neuromuscular & skeletal: Paresthesia, dysesthesia, pain/burning sensation (7%), may be related to prior cisplatin therapy and/or high (500-700 mg/m^2) cumulative doses of docetaxel

Drug Interactions CYP3A3/4 enzyme substrate

Increased Effect/Toxicity: Increased toxicity with cytochrome P450 substrate agents. Possibility of an inhibition of metabolism of docetaxel in patients treated with ketoconazole, erythromycin, terfenadine, astemizole, or cyclosporine. When administered as sequential infusions, observational studies indicate a potential for increased toxicity when platinum derivatives (carboplatin, cisplatin) are administered before taxane derivatives (docetaxel, paclitaxel).

Drug Uptake

Administered by I.V. infusion; exhibits linear pharmacokinetics at the recommended dosage range

Half-life, elimination; α, β, and γ phases are 4 minutes, 36 minutes, and 11.1 hours, respectively

Pregnancy Risk Factor D

Generic Available No

Docosanol (doe KOE san ole)

U.S. Brand Names Abreva™ [OTC]

Pharmacologic Category Antiviral Agent, Topical

Synonyms Behenyl Alcohol; *n*-Docosanol

Use Treatment of herpes simplex of the face or lips

Local Anesthetic/Vasoconstrictor Precautions No information available to require special precautions

Effects on Dental Treatment No effects or complications reported

Dosage Children ≥12 years and Adults: Topical: Apply 5 times/day to affected area of face or lips. Start at first sign of cold sore or fever blister and continue until healed.

Mechanism of Action Prevents viral entry and replication at the cellular level

Other Adverse Effects Limited information; headache reported (frequency similar to placebo)

Contraindications Hypersensitivity to docosanol or any component of the formulation

Warnings/Precautions For external use only. Do not apply to inside of mouth or around eyes. Not for use in children <12 years of age.

Generic Available No

Comments Wash hands before and after applying cream. Begin treatment at first tingle of cold sore or fever blister. Rub into area gently, but completely. Do not apply directly to inside of mouth or around eyes. Contact healthcare provider if sore gets worse or does not heal within 10 days. Do not share this product with others, may spread infection. Notify healthcare professional if pregnant or breast-feeding.

Docusate (DOK yoo sate)

U.S. Brand Names Colace® [OTC]; DC 240® Softgels® [OTC]; Diocto® [OTC]; DOS® Softgel® [OTC]; D-S-S® [OTC]; Ex-Lax® Stool Softener [OTC]; Modane® Soft [OTC]; Regulax SS® [OTC]; Surfak® [OTC]

Canadian Brand Names Albert® Docusate; Colace®; Colax-C®; PMS-Docusate Calcium; PMS-Docusate Sodium; Regulex®; Selax®; Soflax™

Pharmacologic Category Stool Softener

Synonyms Dioctyl Calcium Sulfosuccinate; Dioctyl Sodium Sulfosuccinate; Docusate Calcium; Docusate Potassium; Docusate Sodium; DOSS; DSS

Use Stool softener in patients who should avoid straining during defecation and constipation associated with hard, dry stools; prophylaxis for straining (Valsalva) following myocardial infarction. A safe agent to be used in elderly; some evidence that doses <200 mg are ineffective; stool softeners are unnecessary if stool is well hydrated or "mushy" and soft; shown to be ineffective used long-term.

Unlabeled/Investigational Ceruminolytic

Local Anesthetic/Vasoconstrictor Precautions No information available to require special precautions

Effects on Dental Treatment No effects or complications reported

Dosage Docusate salts are interchangeable; the amount of sodium, calcium, or potassium per dosage unit is clinically insignificant

Children <3 years: Oral: 10-40 mg/day in 1-4 divided doses

Children: Oral:

- 3-6 years: 20-60 mg/day in 1-4 divided doses
- 6-12 years: 40-150 mg/day in 1-4 divided doses

Adolescents and Adults: Oral: 50-500 mg/day in 1-4 divided doses

Older Children and Adults: Rectal: Add 50-100 mg of docusate liquid to enema fluid (saline or water); give as retention or flushing enema

Mechanism of Action Reduces surface tension of the oil-water interface of the stool resulting in enhanced incorporation of water and fat allowing for stool softening

Other Adverse Effects 1% to 10%:

Gastrointestinal: Intestinal obstruction, diarrhea, abdominal cramping

Miscellaneous: Throat irritation

Drug Interactions

Increased Toxicity with mineral oil, phenolphthalein.

Decreased Effect: High doses decrease effect of warfarin.

Drug Uptake Onset of action: 12-72 hours

Pregnancy Risk Factor C

Generic Available Yes

Docusate and Casanthranol (DOK yoo sate & ka SAN thra nole)

U.S. Brand Names Diocto C® [OTC]; Doxidan® [OTC]; Genasoft® Plus [OTC]; Peri-Colace® [OTC]; Silace-C® [OTC]

Canadian Brand Names Peri-Colace®

Pharmacologic Category Laxative/Stool Softener

Synonyms Casanthranol and Docusate; DSS With Casanthranol

Use Treatment of constipation generally associated with dry, hard stools and decreased intestinal motility

Local Anesthetic/Vasoconstrictor Precautions No information available to require special precautions

Effects on Dental Treatment No effects or complications reported

Dosage Oral:

Children: 5-15 mL of syrup at bedtime or 1 capsule at bedtime

Adults: 1-2 capsules or 15-30 mL syrup at bedtime, may be increased to 2 capsules or 30 mL twice daily or 3 capsules at bedtime

Other Adverse Effects 1% to 10%:

Dermatologic: Rash

(Continued)

Docusate and Casanthranol *(Continued)*

Gastrointestinal: Intestinal obstruction, diarrhea, abdominal cramping, throat irritation

Pregnancy Risk Factor C

Generic Available Yes

Dofetilide (doe FET il ide)

U.S. Brand Names Tikosyn™

Canadian Brand Names Tikosyn™

Pharmacologic Category Antiarrhythmic Agent, Class III

Use Maintenance of normal sinus rhythm in patients with atrial fibrillation/atrial flutter of greater than 1-week duration who have been converted to normal sinus rhythm. It is indicated for the conversion of atrial fibrillation and atrial flutter to normal sinus rhythm.

Local Anesthetic/Vasoconstrictor Precautions No information available to require special precautions

Effects on Dental Treatment No effects or complications reported

Dosage

Adults: Oral:

Note: QT_c must be determined prior to first dose

Initial: 500 mcg orally twice daily. Initial dosage must be adjusted in patients with estimated Cl_{cr} <60 mL/minute. Dofetilide may be initiated at lower doses than recommended based on physician discretion.

Modification of dosage in response to initial dose:

QT_c interval should be measured 2-3 hours after the initial dose. If the QT_c >15% of baseline, or if the QT_c is >500 msec (550 msec in patients with ventricular conduction abnormalities), dofetilide should be adjusted. If the starting dose is 500 mcg twice daily, then adjust to 250 mcg twice daily. If the starting dose was 250 mcg twice daily, then adjust to 125 mcg twice daily. If the starting dose was 125 mcg twice daily, then adjust to 125 mcg every day.

Continued monitoring for doses 2-5:

QT_c interval must be determined 2-3 hours after each subsequent dose of dofetilide for in-hospital doses 2-5. If the measured QT_c is >500 msec (550 msec in patients with ventricular conduction abnormalities) dofetilide should be stopped.

Mechanism of Action Vaughan Williams class III antiarrhythmic activity. Blockade of the cardiac ion channel carrying the rapid component of the delayed rectifier potassium current. Dofetilide has no effect on sodium channels, adrenergic alpha-receptors, or adrenergic beta-receptors. It increases the monophasic action potential duration due to delayed repolarization. The increase in the QT interval is a function of prolongation of both effective and functional refractory periods in the His-Purkinje system and the ventricles. Changes in cardiac conduction velocity and sinus node function have not been observed in patients with or without structural heart disease. PR and QRS width remain the same in patients with pre-existing heart block and or sick sinus syndrome.

Other Adverse Effects

Supraventricular arrhythmia patients (incidence > placebo)

>10%: Central nervous system: Headache (11%)

2% to 10%:

Central nervous system: Dizziness (8%), insomnia (4%)

Cardiovascular: Ventricular tachycardia (2.6% to 3.7%), chest pain (10%), torsade de pointes (3.3% in CHF patients and 0.9% in patients with a recent MI; up to 10.5% in patients receiving doses in excess of those recommended). Torsade de pointes occurs most frequently within the first 3 days of therapy.

Dermatologic: Rash (3%)

Gastrointestinal: Nausea (5%), diarrhea (3%), abdominal pain (3%)

Neuromuscular & skeletal: Back pain (3%)

Respiratory: Dyspnea (6%), respiratory tract infection (7%)

Miscellaneous: Flu syndrome (4%)

<2%:

Central nervous system: CVA, facial paralysis, flaccid paralysis, migraine, paralysis

Cardiovascular: AV block (0.4% to 1.5%), ventricular fibrillation (0% to 0.4%), bundle branch block, heart block, edema, heart arrest, myocardial infarct, sudden death, syncope

Dermatologic: Angioedema

Gastrointestinal: Liver damage

Neuromuscular & skeletal: Paresthesia

Respiratory: Cough

>2% (incidence ≤ placebo): Anxiety, pain, angina, atrial fibrillation, hypertension, palpitation, supraventricular tachycardia, peripheral edema, urinary tract infection, weakness, arthralgia, diaphoresis

Drug Interactions CYP3A3/4 enzyme substrate (minor)

Increased Effect/Toxicity: Dofetilide concentrations are increased by cimetidine, verapamil, ketoconazole, and trimethoprim (concurrent use of these agents is contraindicated). Dofetilide levels may also be increased by renal cationic transport inhibitors (including triamterene, metformin, amiloride, and megestrol) or inhibitors of cytochrome P450 isoenzyme 3A3/4 (including amiodarone, azole antifungal agents, clarithromycin, cannabinoids, diltiazem, erythromycin, nefazodone, norfloxacin, protease inhibitors, quinidine, serotonin reuptake inhibitors, verapamil, and zafirlukast). Diuretics and other drugs which may deplete potassium and/or magnesium (aminoglycoside antibiotics, amphotericin, cyclosporine) may increase dofetilide's toxicity (torsade de pointes). **Note:** If dofetilide needs to be discontinued to allow dosing of other potentially interacting drug(s), a washout period of at least two days is needed before starting the other drug(s).

Drug Uptake

Absorption: >90%

Half-life, elimination: 10 hours

Time to peak: 2-3 hours (fasting)

Pregnancy Risk Factor C

Generic Available No

Comments The major dose-related toxicity is torsade de pointes. Treatment should be symptomatic and supportive. Watch for excessive prolongation of the QT interval in overdose situations. Continuous cardiac monitoring is necessary. A charcoal slurry is helpful when given early (15 minutes) after the overdose. Isoproterenol infusion into anesthetized dogs with cardiac pacing corrects the atrial and ventricular effective refractory periods caused by dofetilide. General treatment measures, override pacing, and magnesium therapy appear to be effective in the management of dofetilide-induced torsade de pointes.

Selected Readings

Buxton AE, Lee KL, Fisher JD, et al, "A Randomized Study of the Prevention of Sudden Death in Patients With Coronary Artery Disease," *N Engl J Med*, 1999, 341(25):1882-90.

Prystowsky EN, Benson DW Jr, Fuster V, et al, "Management of Patients With Atrial Fibrillation: A Statement for Healthcare Professionals. From the Subcommittee on Electrocardiography and Electrophysiology, American Heart Association," *Circulation*, 1996, 93(6):1262-77.

Wynn RL, "Atrial Fibrillation: Medications and Dental Considerations," *Gen Dent*, 1999, 47(6):548-51.

Dolacet® *see* Hydrocodone and Acetaminophen *on page 598*

Dolasetron (dol A se tron)

U.S. Brand Names Anzemet®

Canadian Brand Names Anzemet®

Mexican Brand Names Anzemet®

Pharmacologic Category Selective 5-HT_3 Receptor Antagonist

Synonyms Dolasetron Mesylate

Use

Oral: The prevention of nausea and vomiting associated with moderately-emetogenic cancer chemotherapy, including initial and repeat courses; the prevention of postoperative nausea and vomiting.

Parenteral: The prevention of nausea and vomiting associated with initial and repeat courses of emetogenic cancer chemotherapy, including high dose cisplatin; the prevention of postoperative nausea and vomiting; as with other antiemetics, routine prophylaxis is not recommended for patients in whom there is little expectation that nausea and/or vomiting will occur postoperatively; in patients where nausea and/or vomiting must be avoided postoperatively, injection is recommended even where the incidence of postoperative nausea and/or vomiting is low; the treatment of postoperative nausea and/or vomiting

Local Anesthetic/Vasoconstrictor Precautions No information available to require special precautions

Effects on Dental Treatment No effects or complications reported

Dosage

Oral:

Prevention of cancer chemotherapy-induced nausea and vomiting:

Children (2-16 years): 1.8 mg/kg given within 1 hour before chemotherapy, up to a maximum of 100 mg; safety and effectiveness in pediatric patients under 2 years of age have not been established

Adults: 100 mg given within 1 hour before chemotherapy

Use in the elderly, renal failure patients, or hepatically impaired patients: No dosage adjustment is recommended

Prevention of postoperative nausea and vomiting:

Children (2-16 years): 1.2 mg/kg given within 2 hours before surgery, up to a maximum of 100 mg; safety and effectiveness in pediatric patients under 2 years of age have not been established

Adults: 100 mg within 2 hours before surgery

Use in the elderly, renal failure patients, or hepatically impaired patients: No dosage adjustment is recommended

I.V.:

Prevention of cancer chemotherapy-induced nausea and vomiting

Adults: From clinical trials, the dose is 1.8 mg/kg given as a single dose ~ 30 minutes before chemotherapy; alternatively, for most patients, a fixed dose of 100 mg can be administered over 30 seconds.

(Continued)

Dolasetron *(Continued)*

Children (2-16 years): 1.8 mg/kg given as a single dose ~ 30 minutes before chemotherapy, up to a maximum of 100 mg; safety and effectiveness in pediatric patients under 2 years of age have not been established.

Injection mixed in apple or apple-grape juice may be used for oral dosing of pediatric patients. When injection is administered orally, the recommended dosage in pediatric patients 2 to 16 years of age is 1.8 mg/kg up to a maximum 100 mg dose given within 1 hour before chemotherapy. The diluted product may be kept up to 2 hours at room temperature before use.

Use in the elderly, in renal failure patients, or in hepatically impaired patients: No dosage adjustment is recommended.

Prevention of postoperative nausea and/or vomiting

Adults: 12.5 mg given as a single dose ~ 15 minutes before the cessation of anesthesia (prevention) or as soon as nausea or vomiting presents (treatment).

Children (2-16 years): 0.35 mg/kg, with a maximum dose of 12.5 mg, given as a single dose ~ 15 minutes before the cessation of anesthesia or as soon as nausea or vomiting presents. Safety and effectiveness in pediatric patients under 2 years of age have not been established. Injection mixed in apple or apple-grape juice may be used for oral dosing of pediatric patients; dosage in pediatric patients 2 to 16 years is 1.2 mg/kg up to a maximum 100-mg dose given before surgery.

Mechanism of Action Selective serotonin receptor (5-HT_3) antagonist, blocking serotonin both peripherally (primary site of action) and centrally at the chemoreceptor trigger zone

Other Adverse Effects

>10%:

Central nervous system: Headache (31%), dizziness, lightheadedness (23%)

Gastrointestinal: Loose stools/diarrhea (50%); increased appetite (27%); taste alterations (12%)

1% to 10%:

Cardiovascular: Hypertension, hypotension (6%), EKG abnormalities, prolonged P-R, QRS, and QT_c intervals

Central nervous system: Sedation (8%), slow movement (3%), nervousness (3%), fatigue (2%), listlessness, grogginess

Gastrointestinal: Nausea (6%), constipation (3%), diarrhea, abdominal pain, flatulence

Hepatic: Mild elevations of serum aminotransferases (7%)

Local: Pain at injection site (1%)

Neuromuscular & skeletal: Paresthesia

Ocular: Visual disturbances (mostly blurred vision) (9%); photosensitivity (2%)

Drug Interactions CYP2D6 and 3A3/4 enzyme substrate

Increased Effect/Toxicity: Increased blood levels of active metabolite may occur during concurrent administration of cimetidine and atenolol. Inhibitors of this isoenzyme may increase blood levels of active metabolite. Due to the potential to potentiate QT_c prolongation, drugs which may prolong QT interval directly (eg, antiarrhythmics) or by causing alterations in electrolytes (eg, diuretics) should be used with caution.

Decreased Effect: Blood levels of active metabolite are decreased during coadministration of rifampin.

Drug Uptake Half-life, elimination: Dolasetron: 10 minutes; MDL 74,156: 8 hours

Pregnancy Risk Factor B

Generic Available No

Comments A single I.V. dose of dolasetron mesylate (1.8 or 2.4 mg/kg) has comparable safety and efficacy to a single 32 mg I.V. dose of ondansetron in patients receiving cisplatin chemotherapy.

Dolobid® *see* Diflunisal *on page 386*

Dolophine® *see* Methadone *on page 778*

Dolorac™ [OTC] *see* Capsaicin *on page 212*

Domeboro® [OTC] *see* Aluminum Sulfate and Calcium Acetate *on page 63*

Donepezil (doh NEP e zil)

U.S. Brand Names Aricept®

Canadian Brand Names Aricept®

Mexican Brand Names Eranz®

Pharmacologic Category Acetylcholinesterase Inhibitor (Central)

Synonyms E2020

Use Treatment of mild to moderate dementia of the Alzheimer's type

Unlabeled/Investigational: Attention-deficit/hyperactivity disorder (ADHD)

Local Anesthetic/Vasoconstrictor Precautions No information available to require special precautions

Effects on Dental Treatment No effects or complications reported

Dosage Oral:

Children: ADHD (unlabeled use): 5 mg/day

Adults: Dementia of Alzheimer's type: Initial: 5 mg/day at bedtime; may increase to 10 mg/day at bedtime after 4-6 weeks

Mechanism of Action Alzheimer's disease is characterized by cholinergic deficiency in the cortex and basal forebrain, which contributes to cognitive deficits. Donepezil reversibly and noncompetitively inhibits centrally-active acetylcholinesterase, the enzyme responsible for hydrolysis of acetylcholine. This appears to result in increased concentrations of acetylcholine available for synaptic transmission in the CNS. There is no evidence that donepezil alters the course of the underlying dementing process.

Other Adverse Effects

>10%:

Central nervous system: Headache

Gastrointestinal: Nausea, diarrhea

1% to 10%:

Cardiovascular: Syncope, chest pain, hypertension, atrial fibrillation, hypotension, hot flashes

Central nervous system: Abnormal dreams, depression, dizziness, fatigue, insomnia, somnolence

Dermatologic: Bruising

Gastrointestinal: Anorexia, vomiting, weight loss, fecal incontinence, GI bleeding, bloating, epigastric pain

Genitourinary: Frequent urination

Neuromuscular & skeletal: Muscle cramps, arthritis, body pain

Warnings/Precautions Use with caution in patients with sick sinus syndrome or other supraventricular cardiac conduction abnormalities, in patients with seizures or asthma; avoid use in nursing mothers

Drug Interactions CYP2D6 and 3A3/4 enzyme substrate

Increased Effect/Toxicity: Ketoconazole and quinidine inhibit donepezil's metabolism *in vitro* and may increase toxicity. A synergistic effect may be seen with concurrent administration of succinylcholine or cholinergic agonists (bethanechol).

Decreased Effect: Donepezil levels may be decreased by enzyme inducers (phenytoin, carbamazepine, dexamethasone, rifampin, and phenobarbital). Anticholinergic agents (benztropine) may inhibit the effects of donepezil.

Drug Uptake

Absorption: Well absorbed

Duration: May be prolonged, particularly in elderly

Half-life, elimination, plasma: 70 hours

Time to peak, plasma: 3-4 hours

Pregnancy Risk Factor C

Generic Available No

Donnapectolin-PG® *see* Hyoscyamine, Atropine, Scopolamine, Kaolin, Pectin, and Opium *on page 619*

Donnatal® *see* Hyoscyamine, Atropine, Scopolamine, and Phenobarbital *on page 618*

Dopar® *see* Levodopa *on page 699*

Dopram® *see* Doxapram *on page 413*

Doral® *see* Quazepam *on page 1029*

Dormin® [OTC] *see* DiphenhydrAMINE *on page 398*

Dornase Alfa (DOOR nase AL fa)

U.S. Brand Names Pulmozyme®

Canadian Brand Names Pulmozyme™

Mexican Brand Names Pulmozyme®

Pharmacologic Category Enzyme

Synonyms DNase; Recombinant Human Deoxyribonuclease

Use Management of cystic fibrosis patients to reduce the frequency of respiratory infections that require parenteral antibiotics, and to improve pulmonary function

Unlabeled/Investigational: Treatment of chronic bronchitis

Local Anesthetic/Vasoconstrictor Precautions No information available to require special precautions

Effects on Dental Treatment No effects or complications reported

Dosage Children >5 years and Adults: Inhalation: 2.5 mg once daily through selected nebulizers in conjunction with a Pulmo-Aide® or a Pari-Proneb® compressor

Mechanism of Action The hallmark of cystic fibrosis lung disease is the presence of abundant, purulent airway secretions composed primarily of highly polymerized DNA. The principal source of this DNA is the nuclei of degenerating neutrophils, which is present in large concentrations in infected lung secretions. The presence of this DNA produces a viscous mucous that may contribute to the decreased mucociliary transport and persistent infections that are commonly seen in this population. Dornase alfa is a deoxyribonuclease (DNA) enzyme produced by recombinant gene technology. Dornase selectively cleaves DNA, thus reducing

(Continued)

Dornase Alfa *(Continued)*

mucous viscosity and as a result, airflow in the lung is improved and the risk of bacterial infection may be decreased.

Other Adverse Effects

>10%:

Respiratory: Pharyngitis

Miscellaneous: Voice alteration

1% to 10%:

Cardiovascular: Chest pain

Dermatologic: Rash

Ocular: Conjunctivitis

Respiratory: Laryngitis, cough, dyspnea, hemoptysis, rhinitis, hoarse throat, wheezing

Drug Interactions Dornase alfa can be effectively and safely used in conjunction with standard CF therapies including oral, inhaled, and parenteral antibiotics, bronchodilators, enzyme supplements, vitamins, oral and inhaled corticosteroids, and analgesics. No formal drug interaction studies have been performed.

Drug Uptake

Onset of action: Nebulization: Enzyme levels are measured in sputum in ~15 minutes

Duration: Rapidly declines

Pregnancy Risk Factor B

Generic Available No

Doryx® *see* Doxycycline *on page 418*

Dorzolamide (dor ZOLE a mide)

U.S. Brand Names Trusopt®

Canadian Brand Names Trusopt®

Mexican Brand Names Trusopt®

Pharmacologic Category Carbonic Anhydrase Inhibitor; Ophthalmic Agent, Antiglaucoma

Synonyms Dorzolamide Hydrochloride

Use Lower intraocular pressure in the treatment of glaucoma

Local Anesthetic/Vasoconstrictor Precautions No information available to require special precautions

Effects on Dental Treatment No effects or complications reported

Dosage Adults: Glaucoma: Instill 1 drop in the affected eye(s) 3 times/day

Mechanism of Action Reversible inhibition of the enzyme carbonic anhydrase resulting in reduction of hydrogen ion secretion at renal tubule and an increased renal excretion of sodium, potassium, bicarbonate, and water to decrease production of aqueous humor; also inhibits carbonic anhydrase in CNS to retard abnormal and excessive discharge from CNS neurons

Other Adverse Effects

>10%:

Gastrointestinal: Bitter taste following administration (25%)

Ocular: Burning, stinging or discomfort immediately following administration (33%); superficial punctate keratitis (10% to 15%); signs and symptoms of ocular allergic reaction (10%)

5% to 10% Ocular: Blurred vision, conjunctivitis, lid reactions, tearing, dryness, photophobia

Warnings/Precautions Although administered topically, systemic absorption occurs. Same types of adverse reactions attributed to sulfonamides may occur with topical administration. Chemical similarities are present among sulfonamides, sulfonylureas, carbonic anhydrase inhibitors, thiazides, and loop diuretics (except ethacrynic acid). In patients with allergy to one of these compounds, a risk of cross-reaction exists; avoid use when previous reaction has been severe. Because dorzolamide and its metabolite are excreted predominantly by the kidney, it is not recommended for use in patients with severe renal impairment (Cl_{cr} <30 mL/minute); use with caution in patients with hepatic impairment. Local ocular adverse effects (conjunctivitis and lid reactions) were reported with chronic administration. Many resolved with discontinuation of drug therapy. If such reactions occur, discontinue dorzolamide. There is a potential for an additive effect in patients receiving an oral carbonic anhydrase inhibitor and dorzolamide. The concomitant administration of dorzolamide and oral carbonic anhydrase inhibitors is not recommended. Choriodal detachment has been reported after filtration procedures. Benzalkonium chloride is the preservative in dorzolamide which may be absorbed by soft contact lenses. Dorzolamide should not be administered while wearing soft contact lenses.

Drug Interactions Salicylate use may result in carbonic anhydrase inhibitor accumulation and toxicity including CNS depression and metabolic acidosis.

Drug Uptake

Absorption: Topical: Reaches systemic circulation where it accumulates in RBCs during chronic dosing as a result of binding to CA-11

Duration: 8-12 hours

Half-life, elimination: Terminal RBC: 147 days; washes out of RBCs nonlinearly, resulting in a rapid decline of drug concentration initially, followed by a slower elimination phase with a half-life of about 4 months

Time to peak: 2 hours

Pregnancy Risk Factor C

Generic Available No

DOS® Softgel® [OTC] *see* Docusate *on page 407*

Dostinex® *see* Cabergoline *on page 197*

Dovonex® *see* Calcipotriene *on page 199*

Doxapram (DOKS a pram)

U.S. Brand Names Dopram®

Canadian Brand Names Dopram®

Pharmacologic Category Respiratory Stimulant; Stimulant

Synonyms Doxapram Hydrochloride

Use Respiratory and CNS stimulant for respiratory depression secondary to anesthesia, drug-induced CNS depression; acute hypercapnia secondary to COPD

Local Anesthetic/Vasoconstrictor Precautions No information available to require special precautions

Effects on Dental Treatment No effects or complications reported

Dosage Contains a significant amount of benzyl alcohol (0.9%); I.V.: Adults:

Respiratory depression following anesthesia:

Intermittent injection: Initial: 0.5-1 mg/kg; may repeat at 5-minute intervals (only in patients who demonstrate initial response); maximum total dose: 2 mg/kg

I.V. infusion: Initial: 5 mg/minute until adequate response or adverse effects seen; decrease to 1-3 mg/minute; maximum total dose: 4 mg/kg

Drug-induced CNS depression:

Intermittent injection: Initial: 1-2 mg/kg, repeat after 5 minutes; may repeat at 1-2 hour intervals (until sustained consciousness); maximum 3 g/day

I.V. infusion: Initial: Bolus dose of 2 mg/kg, repeat after 5 minutes. If no response, wait 1-2 hours and repeat. If some stimulation is noted, initiate infusion at 1-3 mg/minute (depending on size of patient/depth of CNS depression); suspend infusion if patient begins to awaken. Infusion should not be continued for >2 hours. May reinstitute infusion as described above, including bolus, after rest interval of 30 minutes to 2 hours; maximum: 3 g/day

Acute hypercapnia secondary to COPD: I.V. infusion: Initial: Initiate infusion at 1-2 mg/minute (depending on size of patient/depth of CNS depression); may increase to maximum rate of 3 mg/minute; infusion should not be continued for >2 hours. Monitor arterial blood gases prior to initiation of infusion and at 30-minute intervals during the infusion (to identify possible development of acidosis/CO_2 retention). Additional infusions are not recommended (per manufacturer).

Hemodialysis: Not dialyzable

Mechanism of Action Stimulates respiration through action on respiratory center in medulla or indirectly on peripheral carotid chemoreceptors

Other Adverse Effects

1% to 10%:

Cardiovascular: Angina, ectopic beats, hypotension, palpitations, tachycardia, vasoconstriction

Central nervous system: Headache

Gastrointestinal: Nausea, vomiting

Respiratory: Dyspnea

Drug Interactions Increased Effect/Toxicity: Increased BP with sympathomimetics and MAO inhibitors. Halothane, cyclopropane, and enflurane may sensitize the myocardium to catecholamine and epinephrine which is released at the initiation of doxapram, hence, separate discontinuation of anesthetics and start of doxapram until the volatile agent has been excreted.

Drug Uptake

Onset of respiratory stimulating effect: I.V.: 20-40 seconds

Duration: 5-12 minutes

Half-life, elimination, mean: Adults: 3.4 hours

Time to peak: 1-2 minutes

Pregnancy Risk Factor B

Generic Available Yes

Comments Initial studies suggest a therapeutic range of at least 1.5 mg/L; toxicity becomes frequent at serum levels >5 mg/L

Doxazosin (doks AYE zoe sin)

Related Information

Cardiovascular Diseases *on page 1308*

U.S. Brand Names Cardura®

Canadian Brand Names Apo®-Doxazosin; Cardura-1™; Cardura-2™; Cardura-4™; Gen-Doxazosin; Novo-Doxazosin

Mexican Brand Names Cardura®

Pharmacologic Category Alpha$_1$ Blocker

(Continued)

Doxazosin *(Continued)*

Use Treatment of hypertension alone or in conjunction with diuretics, cardiac glycosides, ACE inhibitors, or calcium antagonists (particularly appropriate for those with hypertension and other cardiovascular risk factors such as hypercholesterolemia and diabetes mellitus); treatment of urinary outflow obstruction and/or obstructive and irritative symptoms associated with benign prostatic hyperplasia (BPH), particularly useful in patients with troublesome symptoms who are unable or unwilling to undergo invasive procedures, but who require rapid symptomatic relief

Local Anesthetic/Vasoconstrictor Precautions No information available to require special precautions

Effects on Dental Treatment No effects or complications reported

Dosage Oral:

Adults: 1 mg once daily in morning or evening; may be increased to 2 mg once daily. Thereafter titrate upwards, if needed, over several weeks, balancing therapeutic benefit with doxazosin-induced postural hypotension

Hypertension: Maximum dose: 16 mg/day

BPH: Maximum dose: 8 mg/day

Elderly: Initial: 0.5 mg once daily

Mechanism of Action Competitively inhibits postsynaptic alpha-adrenergic receptors which results in vasodilation of veins and arterioles and a decrease in total peripheral resistance and BP; approximately 50% as potent on a weight by weight basis as prazosin

Other Adverse Effects

>10%: Central nervous system: Dizziness (16% to 19%), headache (10% to 14%)

1% to 10%:

Cardiovascular: Orthostatic hypotension (dose-related; 0.3% up to 10%), edema (3% to 4%), hypotension (2%), palpitation (1% to 2%), chest pain (1% to 2%), arrhythmia (1%), syncope (2%), flushing (1%)

Central nervous system: Fatigue (8% to 12%), somnolence (3% to 5%), nervousness (2%), pain (2%), vertigo (2%), insomnia (1%), anxiety (1%), paresthesia (1%), movement disorder (1%), ataxia (1%), hypertonia (1%), depression (1%), weakness (1%)

Dermatologic: Rash (1%), pruritus (1%)

Endocrine & metabolic: Sexual dysfunction (2%)

Gastrointestinal: Abdominal pain (2%), diarrhea (2%), dyspepsia (1% to 2%), nausea (2% to 3%), xerostomia (1% to 2%), constipation (1%), flatulence (1%)

Genitourinary: Urinary tract infection (1%), impotence (1%), polyuria (2%), incontinence (1%)

Neuromuscular & skeletal: Back pain (2%), arthritis (1%), muscle weakness (1%), myalgia (1%), muscle cramps (1%)

Ocular: Abnormal vision (1% to 2%), conjunctivitis (1%)

Otic: Tinnitus (1%)

Respiratory: Rhinitis (3%), dyspnea (1% to 3%), respiratory disorder (1%), epistaxis (1%)

Miscellaneous: Flu-like syndrome (1%), increased diaphoresis (1%)

Drug Interactions

Increased Effect/Toxicity: Increased hypotensive effect with beta-blockers, diuretics, ACE inhibitors, calcium channel blockers, and other antihypertensive medications.

Decreased Effect: NSAIDs decrease hypotensive effect.

Drug Uptake Not significantly affected by increased age

Duration: >24 hours

Half-life, elimination: 22 hours

Time to peak: 2-3 hours

Pregnancy Risk Factor C

Generic Available Yes

Doxepin (DOKS e pin)

U.S. Brand Names Sinequan®; Zonalon® Cream

Canadian Brand Names Alti-Doxepin; Apo®-Doxepin; Novo-Doxepin; Sinequan™; Zonalon

Pharmacologic Category Antidepressant, Tricyclic (Tertiary Amine); Topical Skin Product

Synonyms Doxepin Hydrochloride

Use

Oral: Depression

Topical: Short-term (<8 days) management of moderate pruritus in adults with atopic dermatitis or lichen simplex chronicus

Unlabeled/Investigational: Analgesic for certain chronic and neuropathic pain; anxiety

Local Anesthetic/Vasoconstrictor Precautions Use with caution; epinephrine, norepinephrine and levonordefrin have been shown to have an increased pressor response in combination with TCAs

Effects on Dental Treatment

>10%: Xerostomia

Long-term treatment with TCAs increases the risk of caries by reducing salivation and salivary buffer capacity.

Dosage

Oral (entire daily dose may be given at bedtime):

Depression or anxiety (unlabeled use):

Children: 1-3 mg/kg/day in single or divided doses

Adolescents: Initial: 25-50 mg/day in single or divided doses; gradually increase to 100 mg/day

Adults: Initial: 30-150 mg/day at bedtime or in 2-3 divided doses; may gradually increase up to 300 mg/day; single dose should not exceed 150 mg; select patients may respond to 25-50 mg/day

Elderly: Use a lower dose and adjust gradually

Dosing adjustment in hepatic impairment: Use a lower dose and adjust gradually

Topical: Adults: Apply a thin film 4 times/day with at least 3- to 4-hour interval between applications. **Note:** Low-dose (25-50 mg) oral administration has also been used to treat pruritus, but systemic effects are increased.

Mechanism of Action Increases the synaptic concentration of serotonin and/or norepinephrine in the CNS by inhibition of their reuptake by the presynaptic neuronal membrane.

Other Adverse Effects Frequency not defined:

Cardiovascular: Hypotension, hypertension, tachycardia

Central nervous system: Drowsiness, dizziness, headache, disorientation, ataxia, confusion, seizure

Dermatologic: Alopecia, photosensitivity, rash, pruritus

Endocrine & metabolic: Breast enlargement, galactorrhea, SIADH, increase or decrease in blood sugar, increased or decreased libido

Gastrointestinal: Xerostomia, constipation, vomiting, indigestion, anorexia, aphthous stomatitis, nausea, unpleasant taste, weight gain, diarrhea, trouble with gums, decreased lower esophageal sphincter tone may cause GE reflux

Genitourinary: Urinary retention, testicular edema

Hematologic: Agranulocytosis, leukopenia, eosinophilia, thrombocytopenia, purpura

Neuromuscular & skeletal: Weakness, tremors, numbness, paresthesia, extrapyramidal symptoms, tardive dyskinesia

Ocular: Blurred vision

Otic: Tinnitus

Miscellaneous: Diaphoresis (excessive), allergic reactions

Drug Interactions CYP2D6 enzyme substrate

Increased Effect/Toxicity: Doxepin increases the effects of amphetamines, anticholinergics, other CNS depressants (sedatives, hypnotics), chlorpropamide, tolazamide, and warfarin. When used with MAO inhibitors, hyperpyrexia, hypertension, tachycardia, confusion, seizures, and **deaths have been reported** (serotonin syndrome). The SSRIs (to varying degrees), cimetidine, indinavir, methylphenidate, ritonavir, quinidine, diltiazem, and verapamil inhibit the metabolism of TCAs and clinical toxicity may result. Use of lithium with a TCA may increase the risk for neurotoxicity. Phenothiazines may increase concentration of some TCAs and TCAs may increase concentration of phenothiazines. Pressor response to I.V. epinephrine, norepinephrine, and phenylephrine may be enhanced in patients receiving TCAs (**Note:** Effect is unlikely with epinephrine or levonordefrin dosages typically administered as infiltration in combination with local anesthetics). Combined use of beta-agonists or drugs which prolong QT_c (including quinidine, procainamide, disopyramide, cisapride, sparfloxacin, gatifloxacin, moxifloxacin) with TCAs may predispose patients to cardiac arrhythmias.

Decreased Effect: Carbamazepine, phenobarbital, and rifampin may increase the metabolism of doxepin resulting in decreased effect of doxepin. Doxepin inhibits the antihypertensive response to bethanidine, clonidine, debrisoquin, guanadrel, guanethidine, guanabenz, and guanfacine. Cholestyramine and colestipol may bind TCAs and reduce their absorption.

Drug Uptake

Onset of action: Peak effect: Antidepressant: Usually >2 weeks; Anxiolytic: may occur sooner

Half-life, elimination: Adults: 6-8 hours

Pregnancy Risk Factor C

Generic Available Yes: Oral

Selected Readings

Friedlander AH, Mahler ME, "Major Depressive Disorder. Psychopathology, Medical Management, and Dental Implications," *J Am Dent Assoc*, 201, 132(5):629-38.

Ganzberg S, "Psychoactive Drugs," *ADA Guide to Dental Therapeutics*, 2nd ed, Chicago, IL: ADA Publishing, a Division of ADA Business Enterprises, Inc, 2000, 376-405.

Jastak JT and Yagiela JA, "Vasoconstrictors and Local Anesthesia: A Review and Rationale for Use," *J Am Dent Assoc*, 1983, 107(4):623-30.

Mitchell JR, "Guanethidine and Related Agents. III Antagonism by Drugs Which Inhibit the Norepinephrine Pump in Man," *J Clin Invest*, 1970, 49(8):1596-604.

(Continued)

Doxepin *(Continued)*

Rundegren J, van Dijken J, Mörnstad H, et al, "Oral Conditions in Patients Receiving Long-Term Treatment With Cyclic Antidepressant Drugs," *Swed Dent J*, 1985, 9(2):55-64.
Yagiela JA, "Adverse Drug Interactions in Dental Practice: Interactions Associated With Vasoconstrictors. Part V of a Series," *J Am Dent Assoc*, 1999, 130(5):701-9.

Doxercalciferol (dox er kal si FEER ole)

U.S. Brand Names Hectorol®

Canadian Brand Names Hectorol®

Pharmacologic Category Vitamin D Analog

Use Reduction of elevated intact parathyroid hormone (iPTH) in the management of secondary hyperparathyroidism in patients on chronic hemodialysis.

Local Anesthetic/Vasoconstrictor Precautions No information available to require special precautions

Effects on Dental Treatment No effects or complications reported

Dosage Adults: Oral:

If the iPTH >400 pg/mL, then the initial dose is 10 mcg 3 times/week at dialysis. The dose is adjusted at 8-week intervals based upon the iPTH levels.

If the iPTH level is decreased by 50% and >300 pg/mL, then the dose can be increased to 12.5 mcg 3 times/week for 8 more weeks. This titration process can continue at 8-week intervals up to a maximum dose of 20 mcg 3 times/week. Each increase should be by 2.5 mcg/dose.

If the iPTH is between 150-300 pg/mL, maintain the current dose.

If the iPTH is <100 pg/mL, then suspend the drug for 1 week. Resume doxercalciferol at a reduced dose. Decrease each dose (not weekly dose) by at least 2.5 mcg.

Mechanism of Action Metabolized to the active form of vitamin D which controls the intestinal absorption of dietary calcium, the tubular reabsorption of calcium by the kidneys, and in conjunction with PTH, the mobilization of calcium from the skeleton.

Other Adverse Effects

>10%:

- Central nervous system: Headache (28%), malaise (28%), dizziness (11.5%)
- Cardiovascular: Edema (34.4%)
- Gastrointestinal: Nausea/vomiting (34%)
- Respiratory: Dyspnea (11.5%)

1% to 10%:

- Central nervous system: Sleep disorder (3.3%)
- Cardiovascular: Bradycardia (6.6%)
- Gastrointestinal: Anorexia (4.9%), constipation (3.3%), dyspepsia (4.9%)
- Dermatologic: Pruritus (8.2%)
- Neuromuscular & skeletal: Arthralgia (4.9%)
- Miscellaneous: Abscess (3.3%)

Some of the signs and symptoms of hypercalcemia include anorexia, nausea, vomiting, constipation, polyuria, weakness, fatigue, confusion, stupor, and coma.

Contraindications History of hypercalcemia or evidence of vitamin D toxicity; hyperphosphatemia should be corrected before initiating therapy.

Warnings/Precautions Other forms of vitamin D should be discontinued when doxercalciferol is started. Overdose from vitamin D is dangerous and needs to be avoided. Careful dosage titration and monitoring can minimize risk. Hyperphosphatemia exacerbates secondary hyperparathyroidism, diminishing the effect of doxercalciferol. Hyperphosphatemia needs to be corrected for best results. Use with caution in patients with hepatic impairment. Safety and efficacy have not been established in pediatrics.

Drug Interactions

Increased Effect/Toxicity: Doxercalciferol toxicity may be increased by concurrent use of other vitamin D supplements or magnesium-containing antacids and supplements.

Decreased Effect: Absorption of doxercalciferol is reduced with mineral oil and cholestyramine.

Drug Uptake Half-life, elimination: Active metabolite: 32-37 hours, ≤96 hours

Pregnancy Risk Factor B

Generic Available No

Doxidan® [OTC] *see* Docusate and Casanthranol *on page 407*

Doxil® *see* DOXOrubicin (Liposomal) *on page 417*

DOXOrubicin (doks oh ROO bi sin)

U.S. Brand Names Adriamycin PFS®; Adriamycin RDF®; Rubex®

Canadian Brand Names Adriamycin®; Caelyx®

Mexican Brand Names Adriblastina®; Caelyx®; Doxolem; Doxotec®

Pharmacologic Category Antineoplastic Agent, Anthracycline

Synonyms ADR; Doxorubicin Hydrochloride; Hydroxydaunomycin Hydrochloride

Use Treatment of various solid tumors including ovarian, breast, and bladder tumors; various lymphomas and leukemias (ANL, ALL), soft tissue sarcomas, neuroblastoma, osteosarcoma

Local Anesthetic/Vasoconstrictor Precautions No information available to require special precautions

Effects on Dental Treatment No effects or complications reported

Mechanism of Action Works through inhibition of topoisomerase-II at the point of DNA cleavage; a second mechanism of action is the production of free radicals (the hydroxy radical OH) by doxorubicin, which in turn can destroy DNA and cancerous cells. Doxorubicin is also a very powerful iron chelator, equal to deferoxamine. The iron-doxorubicin complex can bind DNA and cell membranes rapidly and produce free radicals that immediately cleave the DNA and cell membranes. Inhibits DNA and RNA synthesis by intercalating between DNA base pairs and by steric obstruction; active throughout entire cell cycle.

Other Adverse Effects

>10%:

Cardiovascular: Transient EKG abnormalities (supraventricular tachycardia, S-T wave changes, atrial or ventricular extrasystoles); generally asymptomatic and self-limiting. Congestive heart failure, dose-related, may be delayed for 7-8 years after treatment. Cumulative dose, radiation therapy, age, and use of cyclophosphamide all increase the risk. Recommended maximum cumulative doses:

No risk factors: 550 mg/m²

Concurrent radiation: 450 mg/m²

Regardless of cumulative dose, if the left ventricular ejection fraction is <30% to 40%, the drug is usually not given

Dermatologic: Alopecia, radiation recall

Gastrointestinal: Nausea, vomiting, stomatitis, GI ulceration, anorexia, diarrhea

Genitourinary: Discoloration of urine, mild dysuria, urinary frequency, hematuria, bladder spasms, cystitis following bladder instillation

Hematologic: Myelosuppression, primarily leukopenia (75%); thrombocytopenia and anemia

Onset: 7 days

Nadir: 10-14 days

Recovery: 21-28 days

1% to 10%:

Dermatologic: Skin "flare" at injection site; discoloration of saliva, sweat, or tears

Endocrine & metabolic: Hyperuricemia

Drug Interactions CYP3A3/4 enzyme substrate; CYP2D6 enzyme inhibitor

Increased Effect/Toxicity: Allopurinol may enhance the antitumor activity of doxorubicin (animal data only). Cyclosporine may increase doxorubicin levels, enhancing hematologic toxicity or may induce coma or seizures. Cyclophosphamide enhances the cardiac toxicity of doxorubicin by producing additional myocardial cell damage. Mercaptopurine increases doxorubicin toxicities. Streptozocin greatly enhances leukopenia and thrombocytopenia. Verapamil alters the cellular distribution of doxorubicin and may result in increased cell toxicity by inhibition of the P-glycoprotein pump. Paclitaxel reduces doxorubicin clearance and increases toxicity if administered prior to doxorubicin. High doses of progesterone enhance toxicity (neutropenia and thrombocytopenia). Based on mouse studies, cardiotoxicity may be enhanced by verapamil. Concurrent therapy with actinomycin-D may result in recall pneumonitis following radiation.

Decreased Effect: Doxorubicin may decrease plasma concentrations and effectiveness of digoxin and phenytoin. Phenobarbital increases elimination (decreases effect) of doxorubicin.

Drug Uptake

Absorption: Oral: Poor (<50%)

Half-life, elimination:

Doxorubicin: 1-3 hours; Metabolites: 3-3.5 hours

Terminal: 17-30 hours

Triphasic: Primary: 30 minutes

Male: 54 hours; female: 35 hours

Pregnancy Risk Factor D

Generic Available Yes

DOXOrubicin (Liposomal) (doks oh ROO bi sin lip pah SOW mal)

U.S. Brand Names Doxil®

Canadian Brand Names Doxil®

Pharmacologic Category Antineoplastic Agent, Anthracycline

Synonyms Doxorubicin Hydrochloride (Liposomal)

Use Treatment of AIDS-related Kaposi's sarcoma in patients with disease that has progressed on prior combination chemotherapy or in patients who are intolerant to such therapy; treatment of metastatic carcinoma of the ovary in patients with disease that is refractory to both paclitaxel and platinum-based regimens

Unlabeled/Investigational: Breast cancer and solid tumors

(Continued)

DOXOrubicin (Liposomal) *(Continued)*

Local Anesthetic/Vasoconstrictor Precautions No information available to require special precautions

Effects on Dental Treatment No effects or complications reported

Mechanism of Action Doxil® is doxorubicin hydrochloride encapsulated in long-circulating STEALTH® liposomes. Liposomes are microscopic vesicles composed of a phospholipid bilayer that are capable of encapsulating active drugs. Doxorubicin works through inhibition of topoisomerase-II at the point of DNA cleavage. A second mechanism of action is the production of free radicals (the hydroxy radical OH) by doxorubicin, which in turn can destroy DNA and cancerous cells. Doxorubicin is also a very powerful iron chelator, equal to deferoxamine. The iron-doxorubicin complex can bind DNA and cell membranes rapidly and produce free radicals that immediately cleave the DNA and cell membranes. Inhibits DNA and RNA synthesis by intercalating between DNA base pairs and by steric obstruction; active throughout entire cell cycle.

Other Adverse Effects

>10%:

- Gastrointestinal: Nausea (18%)
- Hematologic: Myelosuppression, leukopenia (60% to 80%), thrombocytopenia (6% to 24%), anemia (6% to 53%)
  - Onset: 7 days
  - Nadir: 10-14 days
  - Recovery: 21-28 days

1% to 10%:

- Cardiovascular: Arrhythmias, pericardial effusion, tachycardia, cardiomyopathy, CHF (1%)
- Dermatologic: Hyperpigmentation of nail beds; erythematous streaking of vein; alopecia (9%)
- Gastrointestinal: Vomiting (8%), mucositis (7%)
- Miscellaneous: Infusion-related reactions (bronchospasm, chest tightness, chills, dyspnea, facial edema, flushing, headache, hypotension, pruritus) have occurred (up to 10%)

Drug Interactions

CYP3A3/4 enzyme substrate; CYP2D6 enzyme inhibitor

Increased Effect/Toxicity: No formal drug interaction studies have been conducted with doxorubicin hydrochloride liposome injection; however, it may interact with drugs known to interact with the conventional formulation of doxorubicin hydrochloride. Allopurinol may enhance the antitumor activity of doxorubicin (animal data only). Cyclosporine may induce coma or seizures. Cyclophosphamide enhances the cardiac toxicity of doxorubicin by producing additional myocardial cell damage. Mercaptopurine increases toxicities. Streptozocin greatly enhances leukopenia and thrombocytopenia. Verapamil alters the cellular distribution of doxorubicin and may result in increased cell toxicity by inhibition of the P-glycoprotein pump.

Decreased Effect: No formal drug interaction studies have been conducted with doxorubicin hydrochloride liposome injection; however, it may interact with drugs known to interact with the conventional formulation of doxorubicin hydrochloride. Doxorubicin may decrease plasma concentrations and effectiveness of digoxin and phenytoin. Phenobarbital increases elimination (decreases effect) of doxorubicin.

Pregnancy Risk Factor D

Generic Available No

Doxy-100™ *see* Doxycycline *on page 418*

Doxycycline (doks i SYE kleen)

Related Information

Animal and Human Bites Guidelines *on page 1416*
Nonviral Infectious Diseases *on page 1342*
Periodontal Diseases *on page 1375*

U.S. Brand Names Adoxa™; Doryx®; Doxy-100™; Monodox®; Periostat®; Vibramycin®; Vibra-Tabs®

Canadian Brand Names Apo®-Doxy; Apo®-Doxy Tabs; Doxycin; Doxytec; Novo-Doxylin; Nu-Doxycycline; Vibra-Tabs™

Mexican Brand Names Vibramicina®

Pharmacologic Category Antibiotic, Tetracycline Derivative

Synonyms Doxycycline Calcium; Doxycycline Hyclate; Doxycycline Monohydrate

Use

Dental: Treatment of periodontitis associated with presence of *Actinobacillus actinomycetemcomitans* AA; Atridox™ is indicated for the treatment of chronic adult periodontitis for gain in clinical attachment, reduction in probing depth, and reduction in bleeding on probing; Periostat® is indicated for use as an adjunct to scaling and root planing to promote attachment level gain and to reduce pocket depth in adult periodontitis (systemic levels are subinhibitory against bacteria)

Medical: Principally in the treatment of infections caused by susceptible *Rickettsia*, *Chlamydia*, and *Mycoplasma* along with uncommon susceptible gram-negative and gram-positive organisms; alternative to mefloquine for malaria prophylaxis; treatment for syphilis in penicillin-allergic patients; often active against vancomycin-resistant enterococci; used for community-acquired pneumonia and other common infections due to susceptible organisms; anthrax due to *Bacillus anthracis*, including inhalational anthrax (postexposure), to reduce the incidence or progression of disease following exposure to aerolized *Bacillus anthracis*

Unlabeled/Investigational: Sclerosing agent for pleural effusion injection

Local Anesthetic/Vasoconstrictor Precautions No information available to require special precautions

Effects on Dental Treatment Opportunistic "superinfection" with *Candida albicans*; tetracyclines are not recommended for use during pregnancy or in children ≤8 years of age since they have been reported to cause enamel hypoplasia and permanent teeth discoloration. The use of tetracyclines should only be used in these patients if other agents are contraindicated or alternative antimicrobials will not eradicate the organism. Long-term use associated with oral candidiasis.

Dosage

Children:

Anthrax: Doxycycline should be used in children if antibiotic susceptibility testing, exhaustion of drug supplies, or allergic reaction preclude use of penicillin or ciprofloxacin. For treatment, the consensus recommendation does not include a loading dose for doxycycline.

Inhalational (postexposure prophylaxis) (*MMWR*, 2001, 50:889-893): Oral, I.V. (use oral route when possible):

≤8 years: 2.2 mg/kg every 12 hours for 60 days

>8 years and ≤45 kg: 2.2 mg/kg every 12 hours for 60 days

>8 years and >45 kg: 100 mg every 12 hours for 60 days

Cutaneous (treatment): Oral: See dosing for "Inhalational (postexposure prophylaxis)"

Note: In the presence of systemic involvement, extensive edema, and/or lesions on head/neck, doxycycline should initially be administered I.V.

Inhalational/GI/oropharyngeal (treatment): I.V.: Refer to dosing for inhalational anthrax (postexposure prophylaxis); switch to oral therapy when clinically appropriate; refer to Adults dosing for "Note" on combined therapy and duration

Children ≥8 years (<45 kg): Oral, I.V.: 2-5 mg/kg/day in 1-2 divided doses, not to exceed 200 mg/day

Children >8 years (>45 kg) and Adults: Oral, I.V.: 100-200 mg/day in 1-2 divided doses

Acute gonococcal infection (PID) in combination with another antibiotic: 100 mg every 12 hours until improved, followed by 100 mg orally twice daily to complete 14 days

Community-acquired pneumonia: 100 mg twice daily

Lyme disease: Oral: 100 mg twice daily for 14-21 days

Early syphilis: 200 mg/day in divided doses for 14 days

Late syphilis: 200 mg/day in divided doses for 28 days

Uncomplicated chlamydial infections: 100 mg twice daily for ≥7 days

Endometritis, salpingitis, parametritis, or peritonitis: 100 mg I.V. twice daily with cefoxitin 2 g every 6 hours for 4 days and for ≥48 hours after patient improves; then continue with oral therapy 100 mg twice daily to complete a 10- to 14-day course of therapy

Sclerosing agent for pleural effusion injection (unlabeled use): 500 mg as a single dose in 30-50 mL of NS or SWI

Periodontitis: Oral (Periostat®): 20 mg twice daily as an adjunct following scaling and root planing; may be administered for up to 9 months. Safety beyond 12 months of treatment and efficacy beyond 9 months of treatment have not been established.

Adults:

Anthrax:

Inhalational (postexposure prophylaxis): Oral, I.V. (use oral route when possible): 100 mg every 12 hours for 60 days (*MMWR*, 2001, 50:889-93); **Note:** Preliminary recommendation, FDA review and update is anticipated.

Cutaneous (treatment): Oral: 100 mg every 12 hours for 60 days. **Note:** In the presence of systemic involvement, extensive edema, lesions on head/neck, refer to I.V. dosing for treatment of inhalational/GI/oropharyngeal anthrax

Inhalational/GI/oropharyngeal (treatment): I.V.: Initial: 100 mg every 12 hours; switch to oral therapy when clinically appropriate; some recommend initial loading dose of 200 mg, followed by 100 mg every 8-12 hours (*JAMA*, 1997, 278:399-411). **Note:** Initial treatment should include two or more agents predicted to be effective (per CDC recommendations). Agents suggested for use in conjunction with doxycycline or ciprofloxacin include rifampin, vancomycin, imipenem, penicillin, ampicillin, chloramphenicol, clindamycin, and clarithromycin. May switch to oral antimicrobial therapy when clinically appropriate. Continue combined therapy for 60 days

(Continued)

Doxycycline *(Continued)*

Dosing adjustment in renal impairment: Cl_{cr} <10 mL/minute: 100 mg every 24 hours

Dialysis: Not dialyzable; 0% to 5% by hemo- and peritoneal methods or by continuous arteriovenous or venovenous hemofiltration: No supplemental dosage necessary

Mechanism of Action Inhibits protein synthesis by binding with the 30S and possibly the 50S ribosomal subunit(s) of susceptible bacteria; may also cause alterations in the cytoplasmic membrane

Periostat® capsules (proposed mechanism): Has been shown to inhibit collagenase activity *in vitro*. Also has been noted to reduce elevated collagenase activity in the gingival crevicular fluid of patients with periodontal disease. Systemic levels do not reach inhibitory concentrations against bacteria.

Other Adverse Effects Frequency not defined:

Cardiovascular: Intracranial hypertension, pericarditis

Dermatologic: Angioneurotic edema, exfoliative dermatitis (rare), photosensitivity, rash, urticaria

Endocrine & metabolic: Brown/black discoloration of thyroid gland (no dysfunction reported)

Gastrointestinal: Anorexia, diarrhea, dysphagia, enterocolitis, esophagitis (rare), esophageal ulcerations (rare), glossitis, inflammatory lesions in anogenital region, tooth discoloration (children)

Hematologic: Eosinophilia, hemolytic anemia, neutropenia, thrombocytopenia

Renal: Increased BUN

Miscellaneous: Anaphylactoid purpura, anaphylaxis, bulging fontanels (infants), SLE exacerbation

Adverse effects in clinical trials with Periostat® occurring at a frequency greater than placebo included common cold, nausea, dyspepsia, joint pain, diarrhea, rash, menstrual cramp, acid indigestion, pain, and bronchitis.

Contraindications Hypersensitivity to doxycycline, tetracycline, or any component of their formulation; children <8 years of age, except in treatment of anthrax (including inhalational anthrax postexposure prophylaxis); severe hepatic dysfunction; pregnancy

Warnings/Precautions Use of tetracyclines during tooth development may cause permanent discoloration of the teeth and enamel hypoplasia; prolonged use may result in superinfection; photosensitivity reaction may occur with this drug; avoid prolonged exposure to sunlight or tanning equipment. Do not administer to children ≤8 years of age.

Periostat®: Effectiveness has not been established in patients with coexistent oral candidiasis; use with caution in patients with a history or predisposition to oral candidiasis

Drug Interactions CYP3A3/4 inhibitor

Antacids (containing aluminum, calcium, or magnesium): Decreased absorption of tetracyclines

Anticoagulants: Tetracyclines may decrease plasma thrombin activity; monitor

Barbiturates: Decreased half-life of doxycycline

Carbamazepine: Decreased half-life of doxycycline

Iron-containing products: Decreased absorption of tetracyclines

Methoxyflurane: Concomitant use may cause fatal renal toxicity.

Oral contraceptives: Tetracyclines decrease contraceptive effect.

Phenytoin: Decreased half-life of doxycycline

Dietary/Ethanol/Herb Considerations

Ethanol: Avoid or limit use (<3 drinks/day); chronic ingestion may decrease serum concentration.

Food: Administer with food due to GI intolerance; may decrease absorption up to 20%. Of currently available tetracyclines, doxycycline has the least affinity for calcium; may decrease absorption of amino acids, calcium, iron, magnesium, and zinc. Administration with calcium or iron may decrease doxycycline absorption. Boiled milk, buttermilk, or yogurt may reduce diarrhea.

Herb/Nutraceutical: Avoid dong quai; may cause additional photosensitization. Avoid St John's wort; may decrease serum concentration and cause additional photosensitization.

Drug Uptake

Absorption: Almost completely from the GI tract; food or milk may reduce by 20%

Half-life, elimination: 12-15 hours; Multiple dose: Usually 22-24 ; End-stage renal disease: 18-25 hours

Time to peak: 1.5-4 hours

Pregnancy Risk Factor D

Breast-feeding Considerations Not recommended

Dosage Forms CAP, as hyclate (Vibramycin®): 50 mg, 100 mg. **CAP, as monohydrate** (Monodox®): 50 mg, 100 mg. **CAP, coated pellets, as hyclate** (Doryx®): 100 mg. **INJ, powder for reconstitution, as hyclate** (Doxy-100™): 100 mg. **POWDER, oral suspension, as monohydrate** (Vibramycin®): 25 mg/5 mL (60 mL). **SYR, as**

calcium (Vibramycin®): 50 mg/5 mL (480 mL). **TAB, as hyclate:** (Periostat®): 20 mg; (Vibra-Tabs®): 100 mg. **TAB, as monohydrate** (Adoxa™): 50 mg, 100 mg

Generic Available Yes

Comments To enhance awareness of all options for the treatment of anthrax, the FDA, on October 18, 2001, announced the plans to review and revise labeling for several antibiotics which may be of value in treating exposure/infection by *Bacillus anthracis*. In addition, interim guidelines concerning treatment have been issued by the Centers for Disease Control (CDC), available at http://www.cdc.gov/mmwr/preview/mmwrhtml/mm5041a2.htm.

On October 30, 2001, the FDA suggested revisions in product labeling concerning the dosing regimen for the treatment of anthrax, including cutaneous and inhalation anthrax (postexposure). These revisions have been incorporated into this monograph.

The FDA notification is intended to remind healthcare professionals that doxycycline is currently approved for the treatment of all forms of anthrax.

Refer to http://www.fda.gov/OHRMS/DOCKETS/98fr/cd01156.pdf (last accessed November 1, 2001) and "Update: Investigation of Bioterrorism-Related Anthrax and Interim Guidelines for Exposure Management and Antimicrobial Therapy, October 2001," *MMWR*, October 26, 2001, 50(42):909-19, viewable at http:www.cdc.gov/mmwr/preview/mmwrhtml/mm5042a1.htm (last accessed October 26, 2001).

Doxycycline Hyclate Periodontal Extended-Release Liquid (doks i SYE kleen HI klayt per ee oh DON tal)

U.S. Brand Names Atridox™

Pharmacologic Category Antibiotic, Tetracycline Derivative

Use Dental: Treatment of periodontitis associated with presence of *Actinobacillus actinomycetemcomitans* (AA)

Atridox™ gel is indicated for the treatment of adult periodontitis for a gain in clinical attachment, reduction in probing depth, and reduction in bleeding on probing.

Local Anesthetic/Vasoconstrictor Precautions No information available to require special precautions

Effects on Dental Treatment Mechanical oral hygiene procedures (ie, toothbrushing, flossing) should be avoided in any treated area for 7 days.

Dosage Adults: Subgingival application: Dose depends on size, shape and number of pockets treated. Contains 50 mg doxycycline per 500 mg of formulation in each final blended syringe product. Application may be repeated four months after initial treatment.

Atridox™ subgingival controlled-release product: The delivery system consists of 2 separate syringes in a single pouch. Syringe A contains 450 mg of a bioabsorbable polymer gel; syringe B contains doxycycline hyclate 50 mg. To prepare for instillation, couple syringe A to syringe B. Inject contents of syringe A (purple stripe) into syringe B, then push contents back into syringe A. Repeat this mixing cycle at a rate of one cycle per second for 100 cycles. If syringes are stored prior to use (a maximum of 3 days), repeat mixing cycle 10 times before use. After appropriate mixing, contents should be in syringe A. Holding syringes vertically, with syringe A at the bottom, pull back on the syringe A plunger, allowing contents to flow down barrel for several seconds. Uncouple syringes and attach enclosed blunt cannula to syringe A. Local anesthesia is not required for placement. Cannula tip may be bent to resemble periodontal probe and used to explore pocket. Express product from syringe until pocket is filled. To separate tip from formulation, turn tip towards the tooth and press against tooth surface to achieve separation. An appropriate dental instrument may be used to pack gel into the pocket. Pockets may be covered with either Coe-pak™ or Octyldent™ dental adhesive.

Mechanism of Action Inhibits protein synthesis by binding with the 30S and possibly the 50S ribosomal subunit(s) of susceptible bacteria; may also cause alterations in the cytoplasmic membrane; inhibits collagenase *in vitro* and has been shown to inhibit collagenase in the gingival crevicular fluid in adults with periodontitis

Other Adverse Effects

>10%: Discoloration of teeth in children

<1%: Gastrointestinal: Nausea, diarrhea

Rare adverse effects of tetracyclines: Glossitis, vomiting, dysphagia, hepatotoxicity, esophageal ulceration (if capsule forms are taken before lying down), rash, anaphylaxis, exfoliative dermatitis, photosensitivity, exacerbations of SLE, hemolytic anemia, neutropenia and thrombocytopenia

Doxycycline periodontal gel (Atridox™): The adverse effects reported in clinical trials were similar in incidence between doxycycline-containing product and vehicle alone. In addition, these effects were comparable to standard therapies including scaling and root planing or oral hygiene.

Events associated with application reported with an incidence >1% included: gum discomfort (18%), toothache (14%), periodontal abscess (10%), tooth sensitivity (8%), broken tooth (5%), tooth mobility (2%), endodontic abscess (2%)

(Continued)

Doxycycline Hyclate Periodontal Extended-Release Liquid *(Continued)*

and jaw pain (1%). Systemic adverse events included headache (27%), muscle aches (7%), diarrhea (3%), upset stomach (4%), and nausea (2%). Although there is no known relationship between doxycycline and hypertension, unspecified essential hypertension was noted in 1.6% of the doxycycline gel group, as compared to 0.2% in the vehicle group. Allergic reactions to the vehicle were also reported in two patients.

Contraindications Hypersensitivity to doxycycline, tetracycline, or any component of their formulation; children <8 years of age; severe hepatic dysfunction

Warnings/Precautions Do not use during pregnancy; use of tetracyclines during tooth development may cause permanent discoloration of the teeth and enamel hypoplasia; prolonged use may result in superinfection, including oral or vaginal candidiasis; photosensitivity reaction may occur with this drug; avoid prolonged exposure to sunlight or tanning equipment

Specific warnings for doxycycline gel (Atridox™): Has not been evaluated or tested in immunocompromised patients, patients with oral candidiasis, in conditions characterized by severe periodontal defects with little remaining periodontium, or in regeneration of alveolar bone. Use may result in overgrowth of nonsusceptible organisms, including fungi. Effects of treatment >6 months have not been evaluated.

Drug Interactions Iron and bismuth subsalicylate may decrease doxycycline bioavailability; barbiturates, phenytoin, and carbamazepine decrease doxycycline's half-life; increased effect of warfarin. Concurrent use of tetracycline may render oral contraceptives less effective. Concurrent use of tetracycline and Penthrane® has been reported to result in fatal renal toxicity.

Dietary/Ethanol/Herb Considerations Food: May be taken with food or milk.

Drug Uptake Systemic absorption from dental subgingival gel may occur, but is limited by the slow rate of dissolution from this formulation over 7 days.

Pregnancy Risk Factor D

Dosage Forms GEL, subgingival (Atridox™): 50 mg in each 500 mg of blended formulation [doxycycline syringe (50 mg)]

Generic Available No

Doxycycline Subantimicrobial

(doks i SYE kleen sub an tee mye CRO bee al)

U.S. Brand Names Periostat®

Pharmacologic Category Antibiotic, Tetracycline Derivative

Use Dental: Treatment of periodontitis associated with presence of *Actinobacillus actinomycetemcomitans* (AA)

Periostat® is indicated for use as an adjunct to scaling and root planing to promote attachment level gain and to reduce pocket depth in adult periodontitis (systemic levels are subinhibitory against bacteria)

Local Anesthetic/Vasoconstrictor Precautions No information available to require special precautions

Effects on Dental Treatment No effects or complications reported with subantimicrobial doses of doxycycline.

Dosage Adults: Oral: Dental: As adjunctive treatment for periodontitis: 20 mg twice daily at least 1 hour before or 2 hours after morning and evening meals for up to 9 months

Mechanism of Action Periostat® (proposed mechanism of action): Has been shown to inhibit collagenase activity *in vitro*. Also has been noted to reduce elevated collagenase activity in the gingival crevicular fluid of patients with periodontal disease. Systemic levels do not reach inhibitory concentrations against bacteria.

Dosage Forms TAB: 20 mg

Selected Readings

Golub LM, Ciancio S, Ramamurthy NS, et al, "Low-Dose Doxycycline Therapy: Effect on Gingival and Crevicular Fluid Collagenase Activity in Humans," *J Periodontal Res*, 1990, 25(6):321-30.

Golub LM, Lee HM, Greenwald RA, et al, "A Matrix Metalloproteinase Inhibitor Reduces Bone-Type Collagen Degradation Fragments and Specific Collagenases in Gingival Crevicular Fluid During Adult Periodontitis," *Inflamm Res*, 1997, 46(8):310-9.

Golub LM, Sorsa T, Lee HM, et al, "Doxycycline Inhibits Neutrophil (PMN)-Type Matrix Metalloproteinases in Human Adult Periodontitis Gingiva," *J Clin Periodontol*, 1995, 22(2):100-9.

Rams TE and Slots J, "Antibiotics in Periodontal Therapy: An Update," *Compendium*, 1992, 13(12):1130, 1132, 1134.

Dramamine® II [OTC] *see* Meclizine *on page 750*

Dramamine® Oral [OTC] *see* DimenhyDRINATE *on page 396*

Dri-Ear® Otic [OTC] *see* Boric Acid *on page 171*

Drisdol® *see* Ergocalciferol *on page 446*

Dristan® Long Lasting Nasal [OTC] *see* Oxymetazoline *on page 907*

Dristan® Sinus Caplets *see* Pseudoephedrine and Ibuprofen *on page 1024*

Drithocreme® *see* Anthralin *on page 102*

Drithocreme® HP 1% *see* Anthralin *on page 102*

Dritho-Scalp® *see* Anthralin *on page 102*

Drixomed® *see* Dexbrompheniramine and Pseudoephedrine *on page 365*

Drixoral® Cold & Allergy [OTC] *see* Dexbrompheniramine and Pseudoephedrine *on page 365*

Drixoral® Cough Liquid Caps [OTC] *see* Dextromethorphan *on page 372*

Dronabinol (droe NAB i nol)

Related Information

Chemical Dependency and Smoking Cessation *on page 1410*

U.S. Brand Names Marinol®

Canadian Brand Names Marinol®

Pharmacologic Category Antiemetic

Synonyms Tetrahydrocannabinol; THC

Use When conventional antiemetics fail to relieve the nausea and vomiting associated with cancer chemotherapy, AIDS-related anorexia

Local Anesthetic/Vasoconstrictor Precautions No information available to require special precautions

Effects on Dental Treatment No effects or complications reported

Restrictions C-III

Dosage Oral:

Children: NCI protocol recommends 5 mg/m^2 starting 6-8 hours before chemotherapy and every 4-6 hours after to be continued for 12 hours after chemotherapy is discontinued

Adults: 5 mg/m^2 1-3 hours before chemotherapy, then give 5 mg/m^2/dose every 2-4 hours after chemotherapy for a total of 4-6 doses/day; dose may be increased up to a maximum of 15 mg/m^2/dose if needed (dosage may be increased by 2.5 mg/m^2 increments)

Appetite stimulant (AIDS-related): Initial: 2.5 mg twice daily (before lunch and dinner); titrate up to a maximum of 20 mg/day

Mechanism of Action Not well defined, probably inhibits the vomiting center in the medulla oblongata

Other Adverse Effects

>10%:

Central nervous system: Drowsiness (48%), sedation (53%), confusion (30%), dizziness (21%), detachment, anxiety, difficulty concentrating, mood change

Gastrointestinal: Increased appetite (may be troublesome when used as an antiemetic), xerostomia (38% to 50%)

1% to 10%:

Cardiovascular: Orthostatic hypotension, tachycardia

Central nervous system: Ataxia (4%), depression (7%), headache, vertigo, hallucinations (5%), memory lapse (4%)

Neuromuscular & skeletal: Paresthesia, weakness

Drug Interactions CYP2C18 and 3A3/4 enzyme substrate

Increased toxicity (drowsiness) with barbiturates and benzodiazepines

Drug Uptake

Absorption: Oral: Erratic, 90% to 95%; ~10% to 20% of dose gets into systemic circulation

Half-life, elimination: THC: 19-24 hours; THC metabolites: 49-53 hours

Time to peak: 2-3 hours

Pregnancy Risk Factor C

Generic Available No

Droperidol (droe PER i dole)

U.S. Brand Names Inapsine®

Pharmacologic Category Antiemetic; Antipsychotic Agent, Butyrophenone

Use Antiemetic in surgical and diagnostic procedures; preoperative medication in patients when other treatments are ineffective or inappropriate

Local Anesthetic/Vasoconstrictor Precautions Manufacturer's information states that droperidol may block vasopressor activity of epinephrine. This has not been observed during use of epinephrine as a vasoconstrictor in local anesthesia.

Effects on Dental Treatment See Warnings/Precautions

Dosage Titrate carefully to desired effect

Children 2-12 years: Nausea and vomiting: I.M., I.V.: 0.05-0.06 mg/kg (maximum initial dose: 0.1 mg/kg); additional doses may be repeated to achieve effect; administer additional doses with caution

Adults: Nausea and vomiting: I.M., I.V.: Initial: 2.5 mg; additional doses of 1.25 mg may be administered to achieve desired effect; administer additional doses with caution

Mechanism of Action Butyrophenone derivative that produces tranquilization, sedation, and an antiemetic effect; other effects include alpha-adrenergic blockade, peripheral vascular dilation, and reduction of the pressor effect of epinephrine resulting in hypotension and decreased peripheral vascular resistance; may also reduce pulmonary artery pressure

(Continued)

Droperidol *(Continued)*

Other Adverse Effects EKG changes, retinal pigmentation are more common than with chlorpromazine. Relative to other neuroleptics, droperidol has a low potency of cholinergic blockade.

>10%:

Cardiovascular: QT_c prolongation (dose-dependent)

Central nervous system: Restlessness, anxiety, extrapyramidal symptoms, dystonic reactions, pseudoparkinsonian signs and symptoms, tardive dyskinesia, seizures, altered central temperature regulation, akathisia

Endocrine & metabolic: Swelling of breasts

Gastrointestinal: Weight gain, constipation

1% to 10%:

Cardiovascular: Hypotension (especially orthostatic), tachycardia, abnormal T waves with prolonged ventricular repolarization

Central nervous system: Hallucinations, sedation, drowsiness, persistent tardive dyskinesia

Gastrointestinal: Nausea, vomiting

Genitourinary: Dysuria

Warnings/Precautions

Safety in children <6 months of age has not been established; use with caution in patients with seizures, bone marrow suppression, or severe liver disease

Significant hypotension may occur, especially when the drug is administered parenterally; injection contains benzyl alcohol; injection also contains sulfites which may cause allergic reaction

Tardive dyskinesia: Prevalence rate may be 40% in elderly; development of the syndrome and the irreversible nature are proportional to duration and total cumulative dose over time. May be reversible if diagnosed early in therapy.

Extrapyramidal reactions are more common in elderly with up to 50% developing these reactions after 60 years of age. Drug-induced **Parkinson's syndrome** occurs often. **Akathisia** is the most common extrapyramidal symptom in elderly.

Increased confusion, memory loss, psychotic behavior, and agitation frequently occur as a consequence of anticholinergic effects

Orthostatic hypotension is due to alpha-receptor blockade, the elderly are at greater risk for orthostatic hypotension

Antipsychotic associated sedation in nonpsychotic patients is extremely unpleasant due to feelings of depersonalization, derealization, and dysphoria

Life-threatening arrhythmias have occurred at therapeutic doses of antipsychotics

Drug Interactions

CNS depressants: Sedative effects may be additive with other CNS depressants; monitor for increased effect; includes benzodiazepines, barbiturates, antipsychotics, ethanol, opiates, and other sedative medications

Cyclobenzaprine: Droperidol and cyclobenzaprine may have an additive effect on prolonging the QT interval; based on limited documentation; monitor

Inhalation anesthetics: Droperidol in combination with certain forms of induction anesthesia may produce peripheral vasodilitation and hypotension

Metoclopramide: May increase extrapyramidal symptoms (EPS) or risk.

Potassium- or magnesium-depleting agents: May increase the risk of serious arrhythmias with droperidol; includes many diuretics, aminoglycosides, cyclosporine, supraphysiologic doses of corticosteroids with mineralocorticoid effects, laxatives, and amphotericin B; monitor serum potassium and magnesium levels closely.

Propofol: An increased incidence of postoperative nausea and vomiting have been reported following coadministration

QT_c-prolonging agents: May result in additive effects on cardiac conduction, potentially resulting in malignant or lethal arrhythmias; concurrent use is contraindicated. Includes cisapride, Class I and Class III antiarrhythmics (amiodarone, dofetilide, procainamide, quinidine, sotalol), pimozide, some quinolone antibiotics (moxifloxacin, sparfloxacin, gatifloxacin), tricyclic antidepressants, and some phenothiazines (mesoridazine, thioridazine).

Drug Uptake Following parenteral administration:

Duration: Parenteral: 2-4 hours, ≤12 hours

Half-life, elimination: Adults: 2.3 hours

Time to peak: ≤30 minutes

Pregnancy Risk Factor C

Generic Available Yes

Drotrecogin Alfa (dro TRE coe jin AL fa)

U.S. Brand Names Xigris™

Pharmacologic Category Protein C (Activated)

Synonyms Activated Protein C, Human, Recombinant; Drotrecogin Alfa, Activated; Protein C (Activated), Human, Recombinant

Use Reduction of mortality from severe sepsis (associated with organ dysfunction) in adults at high risk of death (based on APACHE II score ≥25)

Local Anesthetic/Vasoconstrictor Precautions No information available to require special precautions

Effects on Dental Treatment No effects or complications reported

Dosage I.V.: Adults: 24 mcg/kg/hour for a total of 96 hours; stop infusion **immediately** if clinically-important bleeding is identified

Mechanism of Action Inhibits factors Va and VIIIa, limiting thrombotic effects. Additional *in vitro* data suggest inhibition of plasminogen activator inhibitor-1 (PAF-1) resulting in profibrinolytic activity, inhibition of macrophage production of tumor necrosis factor, blocking of leukocyte adhesion, and limitation of thrombin-induced inflammatory responses. Relative contribution of effects on the reduction of mortality from sepsis is not completely understood.

Other Adverse Effects As with all drugs which may affect hemostasis, bleeding is the major adverse effect associated with drotrecogin alfa. Hemorrhage may occur at virtually any site. Risk is dependent on multiple variables, including the dosage administered, concurrent use of multiple agents which alter hemostasis, and patient predisposition.

>10%:

Dermatologic: Bruising

Gastrointestinal: Gastrointestinal bleeding

1% to 10%: Hematologic: Bleeding (serious 2.4% during infusion vs 3.5% during 28-day study period)

Drug Interactions Increased Effect/Toxicity: Concurrent use of antiplatelet agents, including aspirin (>650 mg/day, recent use within 7 days), cilostazol, clopidogrel, dipyridamole, ticlopidine, NSAIDs, or glycoprotein IIb/IIIa antagonists (recent use within 7 days) may increase risk of bleeding. Concurrent use of low molecular weight heparins or heparin at therapeutic rates of infusion may increase the risk of bleeding. However, the use of low-dose prophylactic heparin does not appear to affect safety. Recent use of thrombolytic agents (within 3 days) may increase the risk of bleeding. Recent use of warfarin (within 7 days or elevation of INR ≥3) may increase the risk of bleeding. Other drugs which interfere with coagulation may increase risk of bleeding (including antithrombin III, danaparoid, direct thrombin inhibitors)

Drug Uptake

Duration: Plasma nondetectable within 2 hours of discontinuation

Half-life, elimination: 1.6 hours

Pregnancy Risk Factor C

Generic Available No

Droxia™ *see* Hydroxyurea *on page 615*

Dr Scholl's Athlete's Foot [OTC] *see* Tolnaftate *on page 1181*

Dr Scholl's® Disk [OTC] *see* Salicylic Acid *on page 1072*

Dr Scholl's Maximum Strength Tritin [OTC] *see* Tolnaftate *on page 1181*

Dr Scholl's® Wart Remover [OTC] *see* Salicylic Acid *on page 1072*

D-S-S® [OTC] *see* Docusate *on page 407*

DTIC-Dome® *see* Dacarbazine *on page 343*

Dulcolax® [OTC] *see* Bisacodyl *on page 166*

Dull-C® [OTC] *see* Ascorbic Acid *on page 117*

DuoCet™ *see* Hydrocodone and Acetaminophen *on page 598*

Duo-Cyp® *see* Estradiol and Testosterone *on page 461*

DuoFilm® [OTC] *see* Salicylic Acid *on page 1072*

Duogen (Tentative Brand Name) *see* Dutasteride *on page 425*

DuoNeb™ *see* Ipratropium and Albuterol *on page 652*

DuoPlant® [OTC] *see* Salicylic Acid *on page 1072*

Duphalac® *see* Lactulose *on page 682*

Duplex® T [OTC] *see* Coal Tar *on page 315*

Duraclon™ *see* Clonidine *on page 308*

Duragesic® *see* Fentanyl *on page 493*

Duralone® *see* MethylPREDNISolone *on page 797*

Duramist® Plus [OTC] *see* Oxymetazoline *on page 907*

Duramorph® *see* Morphine Sulfate *on page 829*

Duranest® *see* Etidocaine With Epinephrine *on page 477*

Duration® Nasal [OTC] *see* Oxymetazoline *on page 907*

Duratuss™ *see* Guaifenesin and Pseudoephedrine *on page 570*

Duratuss-G® *see* Guaifenesin *on page 568*

Duratuss® HD *see* Hydrocodone, Pseudoephedrine, and Guaifenesin *on page 608*

Dura-Vent®/DA *see* Chlorpheniramine, Phenylephrine, and Methscopolamine *on page 271*

Duricef® *see* Cefadroxil *on page 232*

Dutasteride (doo TAS teer ide)

U.S. Brand Names Duogen (Tentative Brand Name)

Pharmacologic Category Antiandrogen

(Continued)

Dutasteride *(Continued)*

Use Treatment of symptomatic benign prostatic hyperplasia (BPH)

Unlabeled/Investigational: Treatment of male pattern baldness

Local Anesthetic/Vasoconstrictor Precautions No information available to require special precautions

Effects on Dental Treatment No effects or complications reported

Dosage Oral:

Adults: Male: 0.5 mg once daily

Dosage adjustment in hepatic impairment: Use caution; no specific adjustments recommended

Mechanism of Action A 4-azo analog of testosterone which is a competitive, selective inhibitor of both reproductive tissues (type 2) and skin and hepatic (type 1) 5α-reductase, resulting in inhibition of the conversion of testosterone to dihydrotestosterone and markedly suppresses serum dihydrotestosterone levels

Other Adverse Effects

>10%: Endocrine & metabolic: Serum testosterone increased, thyroid-stimulating hormone increased

1% to 10%: Endocrine & metabolic: Impotence (5%), libido decreased (3%), ejaculation disorders (2%), gynecomastia (including breast tenderness, breast enlargement) (1% to 2%)

Drug Interactions CYP3A3/4 enzyme substrate

Increased Effect/Toxicity: Diltiazem, verapamil, and other CYP3A3/4 inhibitors increase dutasteride levels because of CYP3A3/4 inhibition.

Drug Uptake

Absorption: Via skin when handling capsules

Half-life, elimination: Terminal: 5 weeks

Time to peak: 2-3 hours

Pregnancy Risk Factor X

Generic Available No

Dyazide® *see* Hydrochlorothiazide and Triamterene *on page 597*

Dycill® *see* Dicloxacillin *on page 380*

Dymenate® [OTC] *see* DimenhyDRINATE *on page 396*

Dynabac® *see* Dirithromycin *on page 402*

Dynacin® *see* Minocycline *on page 816*

DynaCirc® *see* Isradipine *on page 665*

DynaCirc® CR *see* Isradipine *on page 665*

Dyna-Hex® [OTC] *see* Chlorhexidine Gluconate *on page 263*

Dyphylline (DYE fi lin)

U.S. Brand Names Dilor®; Lufyllin®

Canadian Brand Names Dilor®; Lufyllin®

Pharmacologic Category Theophylline Derivative

Synonyms Dihydroxypropyl Theophylline

Use Bronchodilator in reversible airway obstruction due to asthma or COPD

Local Anesthetic/Vasoconstrictor Precautions No information available to require special precautions

Effects on Dental Treatment Do not prescribe any erythromycin product to patients taking theophylline products. Erythromycin will delay the normal metabolic inactivation of theophyllines leading to increased blood levels; this has resulted in nausea, vomiting and CNS restlessness.

Dosage

Children: I.M.: 4.4-6.6 mg/kg/day in divided doses

Adults:

Oral: Up to 15 mg/kg 4 times/day, individualize dosage

I.M.: 250-500 mg, do not exceed total dosage of 15 mg/kg every 6 hours

Other Adverse Effects Uncommon at serum theophylline concentrations ≤20 mcg/mL

1% to 10%:

Cardiovascular: Tachycardia

Central nervous system: Nervousness, restlessness

Gastrointestinal: Nausea, vomiting

Drug Interactions

Increased Effect/Toxicity: Dyphylline may decrease the effects of phenytoin, lithium, and neuromuscular blocking agents. Dyphylline may have synergistic toxicity with sympathomimetics. Cimetidine, ranitidine, allopurinol, beta-blockers (nonspecific), erythromycin, influenza virus vaccine, corticosteroids, ephedrine, quinolones, thyroid hormones, oral contraceptives, amiodarone, troleandomycin, clindamycin, carbamazepine, isoniazid, loop diuretics, and lincomycin may increase dyphylline concentrations. Tetracyclines may enhance dyphylline toxicity.

Decreased Effect: Cigarette and marijuana smoking, rifampin, barbiturates, hydantoins, ketoconazole, sulfinpyrazone, sympathomimetics, isoniazid, loop diuretics, carbamazepine, and aminoglutethimide may decrease dyphylline concentrations. Dyphylline may antagonize benzodiazepine's sedative action.

Pregnancy Risk Factor C

Generic Available Yes

Comments This drug is rarely used today. Requires a special laboratory measuring procedure rather than the standard theophylline assay. Saliva levels are approximately equal to 60% of plasma levels; charcoal-broiled foods may increase elimination, reducing half-life by 50%; cigarette smoking may require an increase of dosage by 50% to 100%. Because different salts of theophylline have different theophylline content, various salts are not equivalent.

Dyrenium® *see* Triamterene *on page 1200*

Easprin® *see* Aspirin *on page 119*

Echothiophate Iodide (ek oh THYE oh fate EYE oh dide)

U.S. Brand Names Phospholine Iodide®

Canadian Brand Names Phospholine Iodide®

Pharmacologic Category Ophthalmic Agent, Antiglaucoma; Ophthalmic Agent, Miotic

Synonyms Ecostigmine Iodide

Use Reverses toxic CNS effects caused by anticholinergic drugs; used as miotic in treatment of glaucoma; accommodative esotropia

Local Anesthetic/Vasoconstrictor Precautions No information available to require special precautions

Effects on Dental Treatment No effects or complications reported

Dosage Adults:

Ophthalmic: Glaucoma: Instill 1 drop twice daily into eyes with 1 dose just prior to bedtime; some patients have been treated with 1 dose daily or every other day

Accommodative esotropia:

Diagnosis: Instill 1 drop of 0.125% once daily into both eyes at bedtime for 2-3 weeks

Treatment: Use lowest concentration and frequency which gives satisfactory response, with a maximum dose of 0.125% once daily, although more intensive therapy may be used for short periods of time

Mechanism of Action Produces miosis and changes in accommodation by inhibiting cholinesterase, thereby preventing the breakdown of acetylcholine; acetylcholine is, therefore, allowed to continuously stimulate the iris and ciliary muscles of the eye

Other Adverse Effects 1% to 10%: Ocular: Stinging, burning eyes, myopia, visual blurring

Drug Uptake

Onset of action: Miosis: 10-30 minutes; Intraocular pressure decrease: 4-8 hours

Peak effect: Intraocular pressure decrease: 24 hours

Duration: 1-4 weeks

Pregnancy Risk Factor C

Generic Available No

EC-Naprosyn® *see* Naproxen *on page 848*

E-Complex-600® [OTC] *see* Vitamin E *on page 1245*

Econazole (e KONE a zole)

U.S. Brand Names Spectazole™

Canadian Brand Names Ecostatin®; Spectazole™

Mexican Brand Names Micostyl; Pevaryl Lipogel®

Pharmacologic Category Antifungal Agent, Topical

Synonyms Econazole Nitrate

Use Topical treatment of tinea pedis (athlete's foot), tinea cruris (jock itch), tinea corporis (ringworm), tinea versicolor, and cutaneous candidiasis

Local Anesthetic/Vasoconstrictor Precautions No information available to require special precautions

Effects on Dental Treatment No effects or complications reported

Dosage Children and Adults: Topical:

Tinea pedis, tinea cruris, tinea corporis, tinea versicolor: Apply sufficient amount to cover affected areas once daily

Cutaneous candidiasis: Apply sufficient quantity twice daily (morning and evening)

Duration of treatment: Candidal infections and tinea cruris, versicolor, and corporis should be treated for 2 weeks and tinea pedis for 1 month; occasionally, longer treatment periods may be required

Mechanism of Action Alters fungal cell wall membrane permeability; may interfere with RNA and protein synthesis, and lipid metabolism

Other Adverse Effects 1% to 10%: Genitourinary: Vulvar/vaginal burning

Drug Uptake Absorption: Topical: <10%

Pregnancy Risk Factor C

Generic Available No

Econopred® *see* PrednisoLONE *on page 988*
Econopred® Plus *see* PrednisoLONE *on page 988*
Ecotrin® [OTC] *see* Aspirin *on page 119*
Ecotrin® Low Adult Strength [OTC] *see* Aspirin *on page 119*
Ecotrin® Maximum Strength [OTC] *see* Aspirin *on page 119*
Ed A-Hist® *see* Chlorpheniramine and Phenylephrine *on page 269*
Edecrin® [DSC] *see* Ethacrynic Acid *on page 471*

Edetate Calcium Disodium (ED e tate KAL see um dye SOW dee um)

U.S. Brand Names Calcium Disodium Versenate®

Pharmacologic Category Chelating Agent

Synonyms Calcium Disodium Edetate; Calcium EDTA

Use Treatment of acute and chronic lead poisoning; used as an aid in the diagnosis of lead poisoning

Local Anesthetic/Vasoconstrictor Precautions No information available to require special precautions

Effects on Dental Treatment No effects or complications reported

Dosage Several regimens have been recommended:

Diagnosis of lead poisoning: Mobilization test (not recommended by AAP guidelines): I.M., I.V.:

Children: 500 mg/m^2/dose, (maximum dose: 1 g) as a single dose or divided into 2 doses

Adults: 500 mg/m^2/dose

Note: Urine is collected for 24 hours after first EDTA dose and analyzed for lead content; if the ratio of mcg of lead in urine to mg calcium EDTA given is >1, then test is considered positive; for convenience, an 8-hour urine collection may be done after a single 50 mg/kg I.M. (maximum dose: 1 g) or 500 mg/m^2 I.V. dose; a positive test occurs if the ratio of lead excretion to mg calcium EDTA >0.5-0.6.

Treatment of lead poisoning: Children and Adults (each regimen is specific for route):

Symptoms of lead encephalopathy and/or blood lead level >70 mcg/dL: Treat 5 days; give in conjunction with dimercaprol; wait a minimum of 2 days with no treatment before considering a repeat course:

I.M.: 250 mg/m^2/dose every 4 hours

I.V.: 50 mg/kg/day as 24-hour continuous I.V. infusion **or** 1-1.5 g/m^2 I.V. as either an 8- to 24-hour infusion or divided into 2 doses every 12 hours

Symptomatic lead poisoning **without** encephalopathy **or** asymptomatic with blood lead level >70 mcg/dL: Treat 3-5 days; treatment with dimercaprol is recommended until the blood lead level concentration <50 mcg/dL:

I.M.: 167 mg/m^2 every 4 hours

I.V.: 1 g/m^2 as an 8- to 24-hour infusion or divided every 12 hours

Asymptomatic **children** with blood lead level 45-69 mcg/dL: I.V.: 25 mg/kg/day for 5 days as an 8- to 24-hour infusion or divided into 2 doses every 12 hours

Depending upon the blood lead level, additional courses may be necessary; repeat at least 2-4 days and preferably 2-4 weeks apart

Adults with lead nephropathy: An alternative dosing regimen reflecting the reduction in renal clearance is based upon the serum creatinine (see table):

Alternative Dosing Regimen for Adults With Lead Nephropathy

Serum Creatinine (mg/dL)	Ca EDTA dosage
≤2	1 g/m^2/day for 5 days
2-3	500 mg/m^2/day for 5 days
3-4	500 mg/m^2/dose every 48 hours for 3 doses
>4	500 mg/m^2/week

Repeat these regimens monthly until lead excretion is reduced toward normal.

Mechanism of Action Calcium is displaced by divalent and trivalent heavy metals, forming a nonionizing soluble complex that is excreted in urine

Other Adverse Effects Frequency not defined:

Cardiovascular: Hypotension, arrhythmias, EKG changes
Central nervous system: Fever, headache, chills
Dermatologic: Skin lesions, cheilosis
Endocrine & metabolic: Hypercalcemia, zinc deficiency
Gastrointestinal: GI upset, anorexia, nausea, vomiting
Hematologic: Transient marrow suppression, anemia
Hepatic: Mild increase in LFTs
Local: Pain at injection site following I.M. injection, thrombophlebitis following I.V. infusion (when concentration >5 mg/mL)
Neuromuscular & skeletal: Arthralgia, tremor, numbness, paresthesia
Ocular: Lacrimation

Renal: Renal tubular necrosis, proteinuria, microscopic hematuria
Respiratory: Sneezing, nasal congestion
Miscellaneous: Zinc deficiency

Contraindications Severe renal disease, anuria

Drug Interactions Decreased Effect: Do not use simultaneously with zinc insulin preparations; do not mix in the same syringe with dimercaprol.

Drug Uptake
Onset of action: Chelation of lead: I.V.: 1 hour
Absorption: I.M., S.C.: Well absorbed
Half-life, elimination, plasma: I.M.: 1.5 hours; I.V.: 20 minutes

Pregnancy Risk Factor B

Generic Available No

Edetate Disodium (ED e tate dye SOW dee um)

U.S. Brand Names Chealamide®; Disotate®; Endrate®

Pharmacologic Category Chelating Agent

Synonyms Edathamil Disodium; EDTA; Sodium Edetate

Use Emergency treatment of hypercalcemia; control digitalis-induced cardiac dysrhythmias (ventricular arrhythmias)

Local Anesthetic/Vasoconstrictor Precautions No information available to require special precautions

Effects on Dental Treatment No effects or complications reported

Dosage Hypercalcemia: I.V.:
Children: 40-70 mg/kg/day slow infusion over 3-4 hours or more to a maximum of 3 g/24 hours; administer for 5 days and allow 5 days between courses of therapy
Adults: 50 mg/kg/day over 3 or more hours to a maximum of 3 g/24 hours; a suggested regimen of 5 days followed by 2 days without drug and repeated courses up to 15 total doses

Mechanism of Action Chelates with divalent or trivalent metals to form a soluble complex that is then eliminated in urine

Other Adverse Effects Rapid I.V. administration or excessive doses may cause a sudden drop in serum calcium concentration which may lead to hypocalcemic tetany, seizures, arrhythmias, and death from respiratory arrest. Do **not** exceed recommended dosage and rate of administration.
1% to 10%: Gastrointestinal: Nausea, vomiting, abdominal cramps, diarrhea

Contraindications Severe renal failure or anuria

Drug Interactions Increased effect of insulin (edetate disodium may decrease blood glucose concentrations and reduce insulin requirements in diabetic patients treated with insulin).

Drug Uptake
Half-life, elimination: 20-60 minutes
Time to peak: I.V.: 24-48 hours

Pregnancy Risk Factor C

Generic Available Yes

Comments Sodium content of 1 g: 5.4 mEq

Edex® *see* Alprostadil *on page 58*
ED-SPAZ® *see* Hyoscyamine *on page 617*
E.E.S.® *see* Erythromycin *on page 450*

Efavirenz (e FAV e renz)

Related Information
HIV Infection and AIDS *on page 1334*

U.S. Brand Names Sustiva®

Canadian Brand Names Sustiva®

Pharmacologic Category Antiretroviral Agent, Reverse Transcriptase Inhibitor (Non-nucleoside)

Use Treatment of HIV-1 infections in combination with at least two other antiretroviral agents; also has some activity against hepatitis B virus and herpes viruses

Local Anesthetic/Vasoconstrictor Precautions No information available to require special precautions

Effects on Dental Treatment <2%: Xerostomia and taste disturbance

Dosage Oral: Dosing at bedtime is recommended to limit CNS effects; should not be used as single-agent therapy
Children: Dosage is based on body weight
10 kg to <15 kg: 200 mg
15 kg to <20 kg: 250 mg
20 kg to <25 kg: 300 mg
25 kg to <32.5 kg: 350 mg
32.5 kg to <40 kg: 400 mg
≥40 kg: 600 mg
Adults: 600 mg once daily
(Continued)

Efavirenz *(Continued)*

Mechanism of Action As a non-nucleoside reverse transcriptase inhibitor, efavirenz has activity against HIV-1 by binding to reverse transcriptase. It consequently blocks the RNA-dependent and DNA-dependent DNA polymerase activities including HIV-1 replication. It does not require intracellular phosphorylation for antiviral activity.

Other Adverse Effects

>10%:

Central nervous system: Dizziness* (2% to 28%), depression (1% to 16%), insomnia (6% to 16%), anxiety (1% to 11%), pain* (1% to 13%)

Dermatologic: Rash* (NCI grade 1: 9% to 11%; NCI grade 2: 15% to 32%)

Endocrine & metabolic: HDL increased (25% to 35%), total cholesterol increased (20% to 40%)

Gastrointestinal: Diarrhea* (3% to 14%), nausea* (2% to 12%)

1% to 10%

Central nervous system: Impaired concentration (2% to 8%), headache* (2% to 7%), somnolence (2% to 7%), fatigue (2% to 7%), abnormal dreams (1% to 6%), nervousness (2% to 6%), severe depression (2%), hallucinations (1%)

Dermatologic: Pruritus (1% to 9%), diaphoresis increased (1% to 2%)

Gastrointestinal: Vomiting* (6% to 7%), dyspepsia (3%), abdominal pain (1% to 3%), anorexia (1% to 2%)

*Adverse effect reported in ≥10% of patients 3-16 years of age

Drug Interactions CYP2B6 and CYP2D6 enzyme substrate; CYP2B6, CYP2C19, 2C9, 3A3/4 enzyme inhibitor; CYP3A4 enzyme inducer

Amprenavir: AUC of amprenavir may be decreased by 36%.

Anticonvulsants (carbamazepine, phenytoin, phenobarbital): Serum concentrations of anticonvulsant and/or efavirenz may be decreased; monitor.

Antifungal agents: Specific drug interaction studies have not been conducted with itraconazole, ketoconazole; decreased serum concentrations of antifungal may occur. Fluconazole may increase serum concentrations of efavirenz.

Astemizole: Toxicity is significantly increased by efavirenz; concurrent use is contraindicated.

Benzodiazepines: Toxicity of some benzodiazepines may be increased by efavirenz; concurrent use of midazolam and triazolam is contraindicated.

Cisapride: Toxicity is significantly increased by efavirenz; concurrent use is contraindicated.

Clarithromycin: Serum concentrations of clarithromycin are decreased by efavirenz, clinical significance unknown; rash reported with concomitant use (46%); azithromycin or other alternative agent should be considered.

Ergot alkaloids (dihydroergotamine, ergotamine, ergonovine, methylergonovine): Toxicity is significantly increased by efavirenz; concurrent use is contraindicated.

Estrogens (ethinyl estradiol): Serum concentrations of ethinyl estradiol. are increased by efavirenz; clinical significance not known, barrier contraception is recommended.

Indinavir: AUC of indinavir is decreased by 31%; dose of indinavir should be increased.

Methadone: Serum concentrations of methadone are decreased by efavirenz; stable patients should be monitored for withdrawal.

Nelfinavir: AUC of nelfinavir is increased by 20%.

Rifabutin: Serum concentrations of rifabutin are decreased by efavirenz; rifabutin dose should be increased.

Rifampin: Serum concentrations of efavirenz are decreased by rifampin.

Ritonavir: AUC of both agents are increased by ~20%; associated with increased adverse effects and laboratory abnormalities; monitoring of liver enzymes is recommended.

Saquinavir: AUC of saquinavir is decreased by ~60%; do not use saquinavir as sole protease inhibitor.

St John's wort: Specific drug interaction studies have not been conducted; serum concentrations of efavirenz are expected to significantly decrease.

Warfarin: Serum concentrations of warfarin may be increased or decreased; monitor.

Drug Uptake

Absorption: Increased 50% by fatty meals

Half-life, elimination: Single dose: 52-76 hours; Multiple doses: 40-55 hours

Time to peak: 3-8 hours

Pregnancy Risk Factor C

Generic Available No

Effer-K™ *see* Potassium Bicarbonate and Potassium Citrate, Effervescent *on page 976*

Effexor® *see* Venlafaxine *on page 1235*

Effexor® XR *see* Venlafaxine *on page 1235*

Efidac/24® [OTC] *see* Pseudoephedrine *on page 1022*

Eflornithine (ee FLOR ni theen)

U.S. Brand Names Vaniqa™

Pharmacologic Category Antiprotozoal; Topical Skin Product

Synonyms DFMO; Eflornithine Hydrochloride

Use Cream: Females ≥12 years: Reduce unwanted hair from face and adjacent areas under the chin

Orphan drug: Injection: Treatment of meningoencephalitic stage of *Trypanosoma brucei gambiense* infection (sleeping sickness)

Local Anesthetic/Vasoconstrictor Precautions No information available to require special precautions

Effects on Dental Treatment No effects or complications reported

Dosage

Children ≥12 years and Adults: Females: Topical: Apply thin layer of cream to affected areas of face and adjacent chin twice daily, at least 8 hours apart

Adults: I.V. infusion: 100 mg/kg/dose given every 6 hours (over at least 45 minutes) for 14 days

Mechanism of Action Exerts antitumor and antiprotozoal effects through specific, irreversible ("suicide") inhibition of the enzyme ornithine decarboxylase (ODC) which is the rate-limiting enzyme in the biosynthesis of putrescine, spermine, and spermidine, the major polyamines in nucleated cells. Polyamines are necessary for the synthesis of DNA, RNA, and proteins and are, therefore, necessary for cell growth and differentiation. Although many microorganisms and higher plants are able to produce polyamines from alternate biochemical pathways, all mammalian cells depend on ornithine decarboxylase to produce polyamines. Eflornithine inhibits ODC and rapidly depletes animal cells of putrescine and spermidine; the concentration of spermine remains the same or may even increase. Rapidly dividing cells appear to most susceptible to the effects of eflornithine. Topically, the inhibition of ODC in the skin leads to a decreased rate of hair growth.

Other Adverse Effects

Injection:
- >10%: Hematologic (reversible): Anemia (55%), leukopenia (37%), thrombocytopenia (14%)
- 1% to 10%:
  - Central nervous system: Seizures (may be due to the disease) (8%), dizziness
  - Dermatologic: Alopecia
  - Gastrointestinal: Vomiting, diarrhea
  - Hematologic: Eosinophilia
  - Otic: Hearing impairment

Topical:
- >10%: Dermatologic: Acne (11% to 21%), pseudofolliculitis barbae (5% to 15%)
- 1% to 10%:
  - Central nervous system: Headache (4% to 5%), dizziness (1%), vertigo (0.3% to 1%)
  - Dermatologic: Pruritus (3% to 4%), burning skin (2% to 4%), tingling skin (1% to 4%), dry skin (2% to 3%), rash (1% to 3%), facial edema (0.3% to 3%), alopecia (1% to 2%), skin irritation (1% to 2%), erythema (0% to 2%), ingrown hair (0.3% to 2%), folliculitis (0% to 1%)
  - Gastrointestinal: Dyspepsia (2%), anorexia (0.7% to 2%)

Drug Interactions Cream: Possible interactions with other topical products have not been studied.

Drug Uptake

Absorption: Well absorbed from GI tract; Topical: <1%

Half-life, elimination: I.V.: 3-3.5 hours; Topical: 8 hours (apparent)

Pregnancy Risk Factor C

Generic Available No

Efudex® *see* Fluorouracil *on page 516*
ELA-Max® [OTC] *see* Lidocaine *on page 706*
Elavil® *see* Amitriptyline *on page 75*
Eldecort® *see* Hydrocortisone *on page 608*
Eldepryl® *see* Selegiline *on page 1079*
Eldercaps® [OTC] *see* Vitamins, Multiple *on page 1246*
Eldopaque® [OTC] *see* Hydroquinone *on page 611*
Eldopaque Forte® *see* Hydroquinone *on page 611*
Eldoquin® [OTC] *see* Hydroquinone *on page 611*
Eldoquin® Forte® *see* Hydroquinone *on page 611*
Elidel® *see* Pimecrolimus *on page 958*
Eligard™ *see* Leuprolide Acetate *on page 692*
Elimite™ *see* Permethrin *on page 940*
Elixophyllin® *see* Theophylline *on page 1152*
Ellence™ *see* Epirubicin *on page 441*
Elmiron® *see* Pentosan Polysulfate Sodium *on page 936*
Elocon® *see* Mometasone Furoate *on page 827*

Elspar® *see* Asparaginase *on page 118*
Emcyt® *see* Estramustine *on page 462*
Emetrol® [OTC] *see* Phosphorated Carbohydrate Solution *on page 953*
Emgel™ *see* Erythromycin, Topical *on page 454*
Emko® [OTC] *see* Nonoxynol 9 *on page 874*
EMLA® *see* Lidocaine and Prilocaine *on page 711*
Empirin® With Codeine *see* Aspirin and Codeine *on page 122*
EmTet® *see* Tetracycline *on page 1147*
Emulsoil® [OTC] *see* Castor Oil *on page 230*
E-Mycin® *see* Erythromycin *on page 450*

Enalapril (e NAL a pril)

Related Information

Cardiovascular Diseases *on page 1308*
Enalapril and Diltiazem *on page 433*
Enalapril and Felodipine *on page 433*

U.S. Brand Names Vasotec®; Vasotec® I.V.

Canadian Brand Names Vasotec®; Vasotec® I.V.

Mexican Brand Names Enaladil; Feliberal®; Glioten; Kenopril; Norpril®; Palane®; Pulsol®; Renitec

Pharmacologic Category Angiotensin-Converting Enzyme (ACE) Inhibitor

Synonyms Enalaprilat; Enalapril Maleate

Use Management of mild to severe hypertension; treatment of CHF, left ventricular dysfunction after myocardial infarction

Unlabeled/Investigational: Hypertensive crisis, diabetic nephropathy, rheumatoid arthritis, diagnosis of anatomic renal artery stenosis, hypertension secondary to scleroderma renal crisis, diagnosis of aldosteronism, idiopathic edema, Bartter's syndrome, postmyocardial infarction for prevention of ventricular failure; severe CHF in infants, neonatal hypertension, acute pulmonary edema

Local Anesthetic/Vasoconstrictor Precautions No information available to require special precautions

Effects on Dental Treatment No effects or complications reported

Dosage Use lower listed initial dose in patients with hyponatremia, hypovolemia, severe CHF, decreased renal function, or in those receiving diuretics.

Oral: **Enalapril**: Children 1 month to 16 years: Hypertension: Initial: 0.08 mg/kg (up to 5 mg) once daily; adjust dosage based on patient response; doses >0.58 mg/kg (40 mg) have not been evaluated in pediatric patients

Investigational: Congestive heart failure: Initial oral doses of **enalapril**: 0.1 mg/kg/day increasing as needed over 2 weeks to 0.5 mg/kg/day have been used in infants

Investigational: Neonatal hypertension: I.V. doses of **enalaprilat**: 5-10 mcg/kg/dose administered every 8-24 hours have been used; monitor patients carefully; select patients may require higher doses

Adults:

Oral: **Enalapril**

Hypertension: 2.5-5 mg/day then increase as required, usual therapeutic dose for hypertension: 10-40 mg/day in 1-2 divided doses. **Note:** Initiate with 2.5 mg if patient is taking a diuretic which cannot be discontinued. May add a diuretic if BP cannot be controlled with enalapril alone.

Heart failure: As standard therapy alone or with diuretics, beta-blockers, and digoxin, initiate with 2.5 mg once or twice daily (usual range: 5-20 mg/day in 2 divided doses; target: 40 mg)

Asymptomatic left ventricular dysfunction: 2.5 mg twice daily, titrated as tolerated to 20 mg/day

I.V.: **Enalaprilat**

Hypertension: 1.25 mg/dose, given over 5 minutes every 6 hours; doses as high as 5 mg/dose every 6 hours have been tolerated for up to 36 hours. **Note:** If patients are concomitantly receiving diuretic therapy, begin with 0.625 mg I.V. over 5 minutes; if the effect is not adequate after 1 hour, repeat the dose and administer 1.25 mg at 6-hour intervals thereafter; if adequate, administer 0.625 mg I.V. every 6 hours.

Heart failure: Avoid I.V. administration in patients with unstable heart failure or those suffering acute myocardial infarction.

Conversion from I.V. to oral therapy if not concurrently on diuretics: 5 mg once daily; subsequent titration as needed; if concurrently receiving diuretics and responding to 0.625 mg I.V. every 6 hours, initiate with 2.5 mg/day.

Mechanism of Action Competitive inhibitor of angiotensin-converting enzyme (ACE); prevents conversion of angiotensin I to angiotensin II, a potent vasoconstrictor; results in lower levels of angiotensin II which causes an increase in plasma renin activity and a reduction in aldosterone secretion

Other Adverse Effects Frequency ranges include data from hypertension and heart failure trials. Higher rates of adverse reactions have generally been noted in patients with CHF. However, the frequency of adverse effects associated with placebo is also increased in this population.

1% to 10%:
Cardiovascular: Hypotension (0.9% to 7%), chest pain (2%), syncope (0.5% to 2%), orthostasis (2%), orthostatic hypotension (2%)
Central nervous system: Headache (2% to 5%), dizziness (4% to 8%), fatigue (2% to 3%), weakness (2%)
Dermatologic: Rash (2%) Gastrointestinal: Abnormal taste, abdominal pain, vomiting, nausea, diarrhea, anorexia, constipation
Neuromuscular & skeletal: Weakness
Renal: Increased serum creatinine (0.2% to 20%), worsening of renal function (in patients with bilateral renal artery stenosis or hypovolemia)
Respiratory (1% to 2%): Bronchitis, cough, dyspnea

Drug Interactions CYP3A3/4 enzyme substrate

Increased Effect/Toxicity: Potassium supplements, co-trimoxazole (high dose), angiotensin II receptor antagonists (candesartan, losartan, irbesartan, etc), or potassium-sparing diuretics (amiloride, spironolactone, triamterene) may result in elevated serum potassium levels when combined with enalapril. ACE inhibitor effects may be increased by phenothiazines or probenecid (increases levels of captopril). ACE inhibitors may increase serum concentration/effects of digoxin, lithium, and sulfonlyureas. Diuretics have additive hypotensive effects with ACE inhibitors, and hypovolemia increases the potential for adverse renal effects of ACE inhibitors. In patients with compromised renal function, coadministration with nonsteroidal anti-inflammatory drugs may result in further deterioration of renal function. Allopurinol and ACE inhibitors may cause a higher risk of hypersensitivity reaction when taken concurrently.

Decreased Effect: Aspirin (high dose) may reduce the therapeutic effects of ACE inhibitors; at low dosages this does not appear to be significant. Rifampin may decrease the effect of ACE inhibitors. Antacids may decrease the bioavailability of ACE inhibitors (may be more likely to occur with captopril); separate administration times by 1-2 hours. NSAIDs, specifically indomethacin, may reduce the hypotensive effects of ACE inhibitors. More likely to occur in low renin or volume dependent hypertensive patients.

Drug Uptake

Onset of action: Oral: ~1 hour
Absorption: Oral: 55% to 75%
Duration: Oral: 12-24 hours
Half-life, elimination:
Enalapril: Adults: 2 hours; CHF: 3.4-5.8 hours
Enalaprilat: Infants 6 weeks to 8 months: 6-10 hours; Adults: 35-38 hours
Time to peak: Oral: Enalapril: 0.5-1.5 hours; Enalaprilat (active): 3-4.5 hours

Pregnancy Risk Factor C/D (2nd and 3rd trimesters)

Generic Available Yes

Enalapril and Diltiazem (e NAL a pril & dil TYE a zem)

U.S. Brand Names Teczem®

Canadian Brand Names Teczem®

Pharmacologic Category Antihypertensive Agent Combination

Synonyms Diltiazem and Enalapril

Use Combination drug for treatment of hypertension

Local Anesthetic/Vasoconstrictor Precautions No information available to require special precautions

Effects on Dental Treatment ~1%: Gingival hyperplasia (fewer reports with felodipine than with other CCBs); disappears with discontinuation (consultation with physician is suggested)

Dosage Adults: Oral: One tablet daily, if further BP control is required, increase dosage to two tablets daily

Drug Uptake See Enalapril *on page 432* and Diltiazem *on page 394*

Pregnancy Risk Factor C/D (2nd and 3rd trimesters)

Generic Available No

Enalapril and Felodipine (e NAL a pril & fe LOE di peen)

U.S. Brand Names Lexxel™

Canadian Brand Names Lexxel™

Pharmacologic Category Antihypertensive Agent Combination

Synonyms Felodipine and Enalapril

Use Treatment of hypertension

Local Anesthetic/Vasoconstrictor Precautions No information available to require special precautions

Effects on Dental Treatment ~1%: Gingival hyperplasia (fewer reports with felodipine than with other CCBs); disappears with discontinuation (consultation with physician is suggested)

Dosage Adults: Oral: 1 tablet daily

Mechanism of Action See Enalapril *on page 432* and Felodipine *on page 489*

Other Adverse Effects See Enalapril *on page 432* and Felodipine *on page 489*

Drug Interactions See Enalapril *on page 432* and Felodipine *on page 489*

(Continued)

Enalapril and Felodipine *(Continued)*

Drug Uptake See Enalapril *on page 432* and Felodipine *on page 489*
Pregnancy Risk Factor C/D (2nd and 3rd trimesters)
Generic Available No

Enalapril and Hydrochlorothiazide

(e NAL a pril & hye droe klor oh THYE a zide)

Related Information
Cardiovascular Diseases *on page 1308*
U.S. Brand Names Vaseretic® 5-12.5; Vaseretic® 10-25
Canadian Brand Names Vaseretic®
Pharmacologic Category Antihypertensive Agent Combination
Synonyms Hydrochlorothiazide and Enalapril
Use Treatment of hypertension
Local Anesthetic/Vasoconstrictor Precautions No information available to require special precautions
Effects on Dental Treatment No effects or complications reported
Dosage Oral: Dose is individualized
Drug Uptake See Enalapril *on page 432* and Hydrochlorothiazide *on page 595*
Pregnancy Risk Factor C/D (2nd and 3rd trimesters)
Generic Available No

Enbrel® *see* Etanercept *on page 470*
Encare® [OTC] *see* Nonoxynol 9 *on page 874*
Endal® *see* Guaifenesin and Phenylephrine *on page 569*
End Lice® [OTC] *see* Pyrethrins *on page 1026*
Endocet® *see* Oxycodone and Acetaminophen *on page 903*
Endocodone™ *see* Oxycodone *on page 901*
Endodan® *see* Oxycodone and Aspirin *on page 905*
Endrate® *see* Edetate Disodium *on page 429*
Enduron® *see* Methyclothiazide *on page 792*
Enduronyl® *see* Methyclothiazide and Deserpidine *on page 793*
Enduronyl® Forte *see* Methyclothiazide and Deserpidine *on page 793*
Ener-B® *see* Cyanocobalamin *on page 331*
Engerix-B® *see* Hepatitis B Vaccine *on page 584*
Enisyl® [OTC] *see* Lysine *on page 738*

Enoxaparin (ee noks a PA rin)

U.S. Brand Names Lovenox®
Canadian Brand Names Lovenox®
Mexican Brand Names Clexane®
Pharmacologic Category Low Molecular Weight Heparin
Synonyms Enoxaparin Sodium
Use

Prevention of deep vein thrombosis following hip or knee replacement surgery or abdominal surgery in patients at risk for thromboembolic complications (high-risk patients include those with one or more of the following risk factors: >40 years of age, obese, general anesthesia lasting >30 minutes, malignancy, history of deep vein thrombosis or pulmonary embolism)

Prevention of deep vein thrombosis in medical patients at risk for thromboembolic complications due to severely restricted mobility during acute illness

Inpatient treatment of acute deep vein thrombosis with and without pulmonary embolism when administered in conjunction with warfarin sodium

Outpatient treatment of acute deep vein thrombosis without pulmonary embolism when administered in conjunction with warfarin sodium

Prevention of ischemic complications of unstable angina and non-Q wave myocardial infarction (when administered with aspirin)

Local Anesthetic/Vasoconstrictor Precautions No information available to require special precautions
Effects on Dental Treatment No effects or complications reported
Dosage S.C.:

Children: Prophylaxis of DVT following abdominal, hip replacement or knee replacement surgery: Safety and effectiveness have not been established. Few studies have been conducted; the Fifth American College of Chest Physicians Consensus Conference on Antithrombotic Therapy (Michelson, 1998) recommends low molecular weight heparin as an alternative to heparin therapy in children ≥2 months with DVT or pulmonary embolism; the following initial doses and titration schedule, based on therapeutic antifactor Xa levels of 0.5-1 unit/mL, are recommended. **Note:** For treatment of DVT or pulmonary embolism in children ≥2 months of age, enoxaparin should be continued for 5-10 days and oral anticoagulation should be overlapped for 4-5 days (Michelson, 1998)

Infants >2 months and Children ≤18 years: Prophylaxis: Initial: 0.5 mg/kg every 12 hours; treatment: Initial: 1 mg/kg every 12 hours

Dosage titration:

Antifactor Xa <0.35 units/mL: Increase dose by 25%; repeat antifactor Xa level 4 hour after next dose

Antifactor Xa 0.35-0.49 units/mL: Increase dose by 10%; repeat antifactor Xa level 4 hour after next dose

Antifactor Xa 0.5-1 unit/mL: Keep same dosage; repeat antifactor Xa level next day, then 1 week later (4 hour after dose)

Antifactor Xa 1.1-1.5 units/mL: Decrease dose by 20%; repeat antifactor Xa level before next dose

Antifactor Xa 1.6-2 units/mL: Hold dose for 3 hour and decrease dose by 30%; repeat antifactor Xa level before next dose, then 4 hour after next dose

Antifactor Xa >2 units/mL: Hold all doses until antifactor Xa is 0.5 units/mL, then decrease dose by 40%; repeat antifactor Xa level before next dose and every 12 hour until antifactor Xa <0.5 units/mL

Adults:

DVT prophylaxis in hip replacement:

30 mg twice daily: First dose within 12-24 hours after surgery and every 12 hours until risk of deep vein thrombosis has diminished or the patient is adequately anticoagulated on warfarin. Average duration of therapy: 7-10 days.

40 mg once daily: First dose within 9-15 hours before surgery and daily until risk of deep vein thrombosis has diminished or the patient is adequately anticoagulated on warfarin. Average duration of therapy: 7-10 days unless warfarin is not given concurrently, then 40 mg S.C. once daily should be continued for 3 more weeks (4 weeks total).

DVT prophylaxis in knee replacement: 30 mg twice daily: First dose within 12-24 hours after surgery and every 12 hours until risk of deep vein thrombosis has diminished. Average duration of therapy: 7-10 days; maximum course: 14 days.

DVT prophylaxis in high-risk patients undergoing abdominal surgery: 40 mg once daily, with initial dose given 2 hours prior to surgery; usual duration: 7-10 days and up to 12 days has been tolerated in clinical trials.

DVT prophylaxis in medical patients with severely restricted mobility during acute illness: 40 mg once daily; usual duration: 6-11 days; up to 14 days was used in clinical trial

Treatment of acute proximal DVT: Start warfarin within 72 hours and continue enoxaparin until INR is between 2.0 and 3.0 (usually 7 days).

Inpatient treatment of DVT with or without pulmonary embolism: 1 mg/kg/dose every 12 hours or 1.5 mg/kg once daily.

Outpatient treatment of DVT without pulmonary embolism: 1 mg/kg/dose every 12 hours.

Prevention of ischemic complications with unstable angina or non-Q-wave myocardial infarction: 1 mg/kg twice daily in conjunction with oral aspirin therapy (100-325 mg once daily); treatment should be continued for a minimum of 2 days and continued until clinical stabilization (usually 2-8 days).

Elderly: Increased incidence of bleeding with doses of 1.5 mg/kg/day or 1 mg/kg every 12 hours; injection-associated bleeding and serious adverse reactions are also increased in the elderly. Careful attention should be paid to elderly patients <45 kg.

Dosing adjustment in renal impairment: Total clearance is lower and elimination is delayed in patients with renal failure; adjustment may be necessary in elderly and patients with severe renal impairment.

Hemodialysis: Supplemental dose is not necessary.

Peritoneal dialysis: Significant drug removal is unlikely based on physiochemical characteristics.

Mechanism of Action Standard heparin consists of components with molecular weights ranging from 4000 to 30,000 daltons with a mean of 16,000 daltons. Heparin acts as an anticoagulant by enhancing the inhibition rate of clotting proteases by antithrombin III impairing normal hemostasis and inhibition of factor Xa. Low molecular weight heparins have a small effect on the activated partial thromboplastin time and strongly inhibit factor Xa. Enoxaparin is derived from porcine heparin that undergoes benzylation followed by alkaline depolymerization. The average molecular weight of enoxaparin is 4500 daltons which is distributed as (≤20%) 2000 daltons, (≥68%) 2000-8000 daltons, and (≤15%) >8000 daltons. Enoxaparin has a higher ratio of antifactor Xa to antifactor IIa activity than unfractionated heparin.

Other Adverse Effects As with all anticoagulants, bleeding is the major adverse effect of enoxaparin. Hemorrhage may occur at virtually any site. Risk is dependent on multiple variables. At the recommended doses, single injections of enoxaparin do not significantly influence platelet aggregation or affect global clotting time (ie, PT or aPTT).

1% to 10%:

Central nervous system: Fever (5% to 8%), confusion, pain

Dermatologic: Erythema, bruising

Gastrointestinal: Nausea (3%), diarrhea

(Continued)

Enoxaparin *(Continued)*

Hematologic: Hemorrhage (5% to 13%), thrombocytopenia (2%), hypochromic anemia (2%)
Hepatic: Increased ALT/AST
Local: Injection site hematoma (9%), local reactions (irritation, pain, ecchymosis, erythema)

Warnings/Precautions Do not administer intramuscularly; use with extreme caution in patients with a history of heparin-induced thrombocytopenia; bacterial endocarditis, hemorrhagic stroke, recent CNS or ophthalmological surgery, bleeding diathesis, uncontrolled arterial hypertension, or a history of recent GI ulceration and hemorrhage. Elderly and patients with renal insufficiency may show delayed elimination of enoxaparin; avoid use in lactation.

Drug Interactions Increased Effect/Toxicity: Risk of bleeding with enoxaparin may be increased with thrombolytic agents, oral anticoagulants (warfarin), drugs which affect platelet function (eg, aspirin, NSAIDs, dipyridamole, ticlopidine, clopidogrel, and IIb/IIIa antagonists). Although the risk of bleeding may be increased during concurrent therapy with warfarin, enoxaparin is commonly continued during the initiation of warfarin therapy to assure anticoagulation and to protect against possible transient hypercoagulability. Some cephalosporins and penicillins may block platelet aggregation, theoretically increasing the risk of bleeding.

Drug Uptake

Onset of action: Maximum antifactor Xa and antithrombin (antifactor IIa) activities occur 3-5 hours after S.C. administration
Duration: Following a 40 mg dose, significant antifactor Xa activity persists in plasma for ~12 hours
Half-life, elimination, plasma: Low molecular weight heparin is 2-4 times longer than standard heparin independent of the dose

Pregnancy Risk Factor B

Generic Available No

Enpresse™ *see* Combination Hormonal Contraceptives *on page 323*

Entacapone (en TA ka pone)

U.S. Brand Names Comtan®

Canadian Brand Names Comtan®

Pharmacologic Category Anti-Parkinson's Agent, COMT Inhibitor

Use Adjunct to levodopa/carbidopa therapy in patients with idiopathic Parkinson's disease who experience "wearing-off" symptoms at the end of a dosing interval

Local Anesthetic/Vasoconstrictor Precautions No information available to require special precautions

Effects on Dental Treatment Dopaminergic therapy in Parkinson's disease (ie, treatment with levodopa) is associated with orthostatic hypotension. Entacapone enhances levodopa bioavailability and may increase the occurrence of hypotension/syncope in the dental patient. The patient should be carefully assisted from the chair and observed for signs of orthostatic hypotension.

Dosage

Adults: Oral: 200 mg dose, up to a maximum of 8 times/day; maximum daily dose: 1600 mg/day. Always administer with levodopa/carbidopa. To optimize therapy the levodopa/carbidopa dosage must be reduced, usually by 25%. This reduction is usually necessary when the patient is taking >800 mg of levodopa daily.

Mechanism of Action In the presence of a decarboxylase inhibitor such as carbidopa, catechol-O-methyltransferase (COMT) becomes the major metabolizing enzyme for levodopa. Entacapone inhibits COMT peripherally and alters the pharmacokinetics of levodopa. Serum concentrations of levodopa become more sustained when entacapone is used with levodopa/carbidopa combinations.

Other Adverse Effects

>10%:
Gastrointestinal: Nausea (14%)
Neuromuscular & skeletal: Dyskinesia (25%), placebo (15%)

1% to 10%:
Cardiovascular: Orthostatic hypotension (4%), syncope (1%)
Central nervous system: Dizziness (8%), fatigue (6%), hallucinations (4%), anxiety (2%), somnolence (2%), agitation (1%)
Dermatologic: Purpura (2%)
Gastrointestinal: Diarrhea (10%), abdominal pain (8%), constipation (6%), vomiting (4%), xerostomia (3%), dyspepsia (2%), flatulence (2%), gastritis (1%), taste perversion (1%)
Genitourinary: Brown-orange urine discoloration (10%)
Neuromuscular & skeletal: Hyperkinesia (10%), hypokinesia (9%), back pain (4%), weakness (2%)
Respiratory: Dyspnea (3%)
Miscellaneous: Increased diaphoresis (2%), bacterial infection (1%)

Note: Approximately 14% of the 603 patients given entacapone in the double-blind, placebo-controlled trials discontinued treatment due to adverse events compared to 9% of the 400 patients who received placebo.

Contraindications Hypersensitivity to entacapone or any of component of the formulation

Warnings/Precautions May increase risk of orthostatic hypotension and syncope. May cause diarrhea, hallucinations; may cause or exacerbate dyskinesia. This drug should be slowly withdrawn if discontinuation is needed. Use caution in patients with hepatic impairment and renal impairment (nephrotoxicity has been described in animal models). Other drugs metabolized by COMT (isoproterenol, epinephrine, norepinephrine, dopamine, dobutamine, alpha-methyldopa, apomorphine, isoetherine and bitolterol) should be used cautiously. Increases in heart rate, arrhythmias, and changes in BP could occur when used concurrently. A syndrome resembling neuroleptic malignant syndrome (hyperpyrexia, confusion) has rarely occurred in patients receiving entacapone. Entacapone has been associated with cases of rhabdomyolysis. Fibrotic complications (retroperitoneal or pulmonary fibrosis) associated with ergot alkaloids have been reported in patients receiving entacapone along with pergolide or bromocriptine.

Drug Interactions CYP1A2, 2A6, 2C9, 2C19, 2D6, 2E1, 3A3/4 enzyme inhibitor; these effects are seen only at concentrations higher than those achieved at recommended dosing.

Increased Effect/Toxicity: Cardiac effects with drugs metabolized by COMT (eg, epinephrine, isoproterenol, dopamine, apomorphine, bitolterol, dobutamine, methyldopa) increased other CNS depressants; nonselective MAO inhibitors are not recommended; chelates iron. Caution with drugs that interfere with glucuronidation, intestinal, biliary excretion, intestinal beta-glucuronidase (eg, probenecid, cholestyramine, erythromycin, chloramphenicol, rifampicin, ampicillin).

Decreased Effect: Entacapone is an iron chelator and an iron supplement should not be administered concurrently with this medicine.

Drug Uptake

Onset of action: Rapid

Absorption: Rapid

Half-life, elimination: B-phase: 0.4-0.7 hour; Y-phase: 2.4 hours

Time to peak: 1 hour

Pregnancy Risk Factor C

Generic Available No

Entertainer's Secret® [OTC] *see* Saliva Substitute *on page 1073*

Entex® PSE *see* Guaifenesin and Pseudoephedrine *on page 570*

Entocort™ EC *see* Budesonide *on page 180*

Entsol® [OTC] *see* Sodium Chloride *on page 1094*

Entsol® Mist [OTC] *see* Sodium Chloride *on page 1094*

Entsol® Single Use [OTC] *see* Sodium Chloride *on page 1094*

Enulose® *see* Lactulose *on page 682*

Enzone® *see* Pramoxine and Hydrocortisone *on page 984*

Ephedrine (e FED rin)

U.S. Brand Names Kondon's Nasal® [OTC]; Pretz-D® [OTC]

Pharmacologic Category Alpha/Beta Agonist

Synonyms Ephedrine Sulfate

Use Treatment of bronchial asthma, nasal congestion, acute bronchospasm, idiopathic orthostatic hypotension

Local Anesthetic/Vasoconstrictor Precautions Use vasoconstrictors with caution since ephedrine may enhance cardiostimulation and vasopressor effects of sympathomimetics such as epinephrine

Effects on Dental Treatment No effects or complications reported

Dosage

Children:

Oral, S.C.: 3 mg/kg/day or 25-100 mg/m²/day in 4-6 divided doses every 4-6 hours

I.M., slow I.V. push: 0.2-0.3 mg/kg/dose every 4-6 hours

Adults:

Oral: 25-50 mg every 3-4 hours as needed

I.M., S.C.: 25-50 mg, parenteral adult dose should not exceed 150 mg in 24 hours

I.V.: 5-25 mg/dose slow I.V. push repeated after 5-10 minutes as needed, then every 3-4 hours not to exceed 150 mg/24 hours

Mechanism of Action Releases tissue stores of epinephrine and thereby produces an alpha- and beta-adrenergic stimulation; longer-acting and less potent than epinephrine

Other Adverse Effects Frequency not defined:

Cardiovascular: Hypertension, tachycardia, palpitations, elevation or depression of BP, unusual pallor, chest pain, arrhythmias

Central nervous system: CNS stimulating effects, nervousness, anxiety, apprehension, fear, tension, agitation, excitation, restlessness, irritability, insomnia, hyperactivity, dizziness, headache

Gastrointestinal: Xerostomia, nausea, anorexia, GI upset, vomiting

Genitourinary: Painful urination

(Continued)

Ephedrine *(Continued)*

Neuromuscular & skeletal: Trembling, tremor (more common in the elderly), weakness

Respiratory: Dyspnea

Miscellaneous: Diaphoresis (increased)

Drug Interactions

Increased Effect/Toxicity: Increased (toxic) cardiac stimulation with other sympathomimetic agents, theophylline, cardiac glycosides, or general anesthetics. Increased BP with atropine or MAO inhibitors.

Decreased Effect: Alpha- and beta-adrenergic blocking agents decrease ephedrine vasopressor effects.

Drug Uptake

Onset of action: Oral: Bronchodilation: 0.25-1 hour

Duration: Oral: 3-6 hours

Half-life, elimination: 2.5-3.6 hours

Pregnancy Risk Factor C

Generic Available Yes

Epifoam® *see* Pramoxine and Hydrocortisone *on page 984*

Epifrin® *see* Epinephrine *on page 438*

E-Pilo-x® *see* Pilocarpine and Epinephrine *on page 956*

Epinal® *see* Epinephryl Borate *on page 441*

Epinephrine (ep i NEF rin)

Related Information

Dental Drug Interactions: Update on Drug Combinations Requiring Special Considerations *on page 1434*

Dental Office Emergencies *on page 1418*

Respiratory Diseases *on page 1328*

U.S. Brand Names Adrenalin® (Dental); Sus-Phrine® (Dental)

Pharmacologic Category Adrenergic Agonist Agent; Alpha/Beta Agonist; Antidote; Bronchodilator; Vasoconstrictor

Use Dental: Emergency drug for treatment of anaphylactic reactions; used as vasoconstrictor to prolong local anesthesia

Local Anesthetic/Vasoconstrictor Precautions No information available to require special precautions

Effects on Dental Treatment No effects or complications reported

Dosage Hypersensitivity reaction:

Children: S.C.: 0.01 mg/kg every 15 minutes for 2 doses then every 4 hours as needed (single doses not to exceed 0.5 mg)

Adults: I.M., S.C.: 0.2-0.5 mg every 20 minutes to 4 hours (single dose maximum: 1 mg)

Mechanism of Action Stimulates alpha-, beta$_1$-, and beta$_2$-adrenergic receptors resulting in relaxation of smooth muscle of the bronchial tree, cardiac stimulation, and dilation of skeletal muscle vasculature; small doses can cause vasodilation via beta$_2$-vascular receptors; large doses may produce constriction of skeletal and vascular smooth muscle; decreases production of aqueous humor and increases aqueous outflow; dilates the pupil by contracting the dilator muscle

Contraindications Hypersensitivity to epinephrine or any component of the formulation; cardiac arrhythmias; angle-closure glaucoma

Warnings/Precautions Use with caution in elderly patients, patients with diabetes mellitus, cardiovascular diseases (angina, tachycardia, myocardial infarction), thyroid disease, or cerebral arteriosclerosis, Parkinson's; some products contain sulfites as antioxidants. Rapid I.V. infusion may cause death from cerebrovascular hemorrhage or cardiac arrhythmias. Oral inhalation of epinephrine is **not** the preferred route of administration.

Drug Interactions Increased cardiac irritability if administered concurrently with halogenated inhalational anesthetics, beta-blocking agents, alpha-blocking agents

Dietary/Ethanol/Herb Considerations

Food: Avoid caffeine.

Herb/Nutraceutical: Avoid ephedra, ginseng, and yohimbe; may cause CNS stimulation. Ginger is a positive inotrope and could affect inotropic agents.

Pregnancy Risk Factor C

Breast-feeding Considerations Usual infiltration doses of epinephrine given to nursing mothers has not been shown to affect the health of the nursing infant.

Dosage Forms INJ: (Adrenalin®): 1 mg/mL [1:1000] (1 mL, 30 mL). **INJ, suspension for:** (Sus-Phrine®): 5 mg/mL [1:200] (0.3 mL, 5 mL)

Generic Available Yes

Epinephrine (ep i NEF rin)

Related Information

Dental Drug Interactions: Update on Drug Combinations Requiring Special Considerations *on page 1434*

Dental Office Emergencies *on page 1418*

Epinephrine *on page 438*
Respiratory Diseases *on page 1328*

U.S. Brand Names Adrenalin®; AsthmaHaler®; Bronitin®; Epifrin®; EpiPen® Auto-Injector; EpiPen® Jr Auto-Injector; Glaucon®; Primatene® Mist [OTC]; Sus-Phrine®

Canadian Brand Names Adrenalin®; Epipen®; Epipen® Jr.; Vaponefrin®

Pharmacologic Category Alpha/Beta Agonist; Antidote; Ophthalmic Agent, Antiglaucoma

Synonyms Adrenaline; Epinephrine Bitartrate; Epinephrine Hydrochloride

Use Treatment of bronchospasms, anaphylactic reactions, cardiac arrest, management of open-angle (chronic simple) glaucoma

Unlabeled/Investigational: ACLS guidelines: Ventricular fibrillation (VF) or pulseless ventricular tachycardia (VT) unresponsive to initial defibrillatory shocks; pulseless electrical activity, asystole, hypotension unresponsive to volume resuscitation; symptomatic bradycardia or heart block unresponsive to atropine or pacing

Local Anesthetic/Vasoconstrictor Precautions No information available to require special precautions

Effects on Dental Treatment No effects or complications reported

Dosage

Bronchodilator:

Children: S.C.: 10 mcg/kg (0.01 mL/kg of 1:1000) (single doses not to exceed 0.5 mg); injection suspension (1:200): 0.005 mL/kg/dose (0.025 mg/kg/dose) to a maximum of 0.15 mL (0.75 mg for single dose) every 8-12 hours

Adults:

I.M., S.C. (1:1000): 0.1-0.5 mg every 10-15 minutes to 4 hours

Suspension (1:200) S.C.: 0.1-0.3 mL (0.5-1.5 mg)

I.V.: 0.1-0.25 mg (single dose maximum: 1 mg)

Cardiac arrest:

Children: Asystole or pulseless arrest:

I.V., intraosseous: First dose: 0.01 mg/kg (0.1 mL/kg of a 1:10,000 solution); subsequent doses: 0.1 mg/kg (0.1 mL/kg of a 1:1000 solution); doses as high as 0.2 mg/kg may be effective; repeat every 3-5 minutes

Intratracheal: 0.1 mg/kg (0.1 mL/kg of a 1:1000 solution); doses as high as 0.2 mg/kg may be effective

Adults: Asystole:

I.V.: 1 mg every 3-5 minutes; if this approach fails, alternative regimens include: Intermediate: 2-5 mg every 3-5 minutes; Escalating: 1 mg, 3 mg, 5 mg at 3-minute intervals; High: 0.1 mg/kg every 3-5 minutes

Intratracheal: Although optimal dose is unknown, doses of 2-2.5 times the I.V. dose may be needed

Bradycardia: Children:

I.V.: 0.01 mg/kg (0.1 mL/kg of 1:10,000 solution) every 3-5 minutes as needed (maximum: 1 mg/10 mL)

Intratracheal: 0.1 mg/kg (0.1 mL/kg of 1:1000 solution every 3-5 minutes); doses as high as 0.2 mg/kg may be effective

Refractory hypotension (refractory to dopamine/dobutamine): I.V. infusion administration requires the use of an infusion pump:

Children: Infusion rate 0.1-4 mcg/kg/minute

Adults: I.V. infusion: 1 mg in 250 mL NS/D_5W at 0.1-1 mcg/kg/minute; titrate to desired effect

Hypersensitivity reaction:

Children: S.C.: 0.01 mg/kg every 15 minutes for 2 doses then every 4 hours as needed (single doses not to exceed 0.5 mg)

Adults: I.M., S.C.: 0.2-0.5 mg every 20 minutes to 4 hours (single dose maximum: 1 mg)

Nebulization:

Children <2 years: 0.25 mL of 1:1000 diluted in 3 mL NS with treatments ordered individually

Children >2 years and Adolescents: 0.5 mL of 1:1000 concentration diluted in 3 mL NS

Children >2 years and Adults (racemic epinephrine):

<10 kg: 2 mL of 1:8 dilution over 15 minutes every 1-4 hours
10-15 kg: 2 mL of 1:6 dilution over 15 minutes every 1-4 hours
15-20 kg: 2 mL of 1:4 dilution over 15 minutes every 1-4 hours
>20 kg: 2 mL of 1:3 dilution over 15 minutes every 1-4 hours

Adults: Instill 8-15 drops into nebulizer reservoirs; administer 1-3 inhalations 4-6 times/day

Ophthalmic: Instill 1-2 drops in eye(s) once or twice daily

Intranasal: Children ≥6 years and Adults: Apply locally as drops or spray or with sterile swab

Mechanism of Action Stimulates alpha-, $beta_1$-, and $beta_2$-adrenergic receptors resulting in relaxation of smooth muscle of the bronchial tree, cardiac stimulation, and dilation of skeletal muscle vasculature; small doses can cause vasodilation via $beta_2$-vascular receptors; large doses may produce constriction of skeletal and

(Continued)

Epinephrine *(Continued)*

vascular smooth muscle; decreases production of aqueous humor and increases aqueous outflow; dilates the pupil by contracting the dilator muscle

Other Adverse Effects Frequency not defined:

Cardiovascular: Tachycardia (parenteral), pounding heartbeat, flushing, hypertension, pallor, chest pain, increased myocardial oxygen consumption, cardiac arrhythmias, sudden death, angina, vasoconstriction

Central nervous system: Nervousness, anxiety, restlessness, headache, dizziness, lightheadedness, insomnia

Gastrointestinal: Nausea, vomiting, xerostomia,dry throat

Genitourinary: Acute urinary retention in patients with bladder outflow obstruction

Neuromuscular & skeletal: Weakness, trembling

Ocular: Precipitation or or exacerbation of narrow-angle glaucoma, transient stinging, burning, eye pain, allergic lid reaction, ocular irritation

Renal: Decreased renal and splanchnic blood flow

Respiratory: Wheezing, dyspnea

Miscellaneous: Diaphoresis (increased)

Contraindications Hypersensitivity to epinephrine or any component of the formulation; cardiac arrhythmias, angle-closure glaucoma

Warnings/Precautions Use with caution in elderly patients, patients with diabetes mellitus, cardiovascular diseases (angina, tachycardia, myocardial infarction), thyroid disease, or cerebral arteriosclerosis, Parkinson's; some products contain sulfites as antioxidants. Rapid I.V. infusion may cause death from cerebrovascular hemorrhage or cardiac arrhythmias. Oral inhalation of epinephrine is **not** the preferred route of administration.

Drug Interactions

Increased Effect/Toxicity: Increased cardiac irritability if administered concurrently with halogenated inhalation anesthetics, beta-blocking agents, or alpha-blocking agents.

Decreased Effect: Decreased bronchodilation with β-blockers. Decreases antihypertensive effects of methyldopa or guanethidine.

Drug Uptake

Onset of action: Bronchodilation: S.C.: ~5-10 minutes; Inhalation: ~1 minute; Conjunctival instillation: IOP declines ~1 hour

Peak effect: Conjunctival instillation: 4-8 hours

Absorption: Oral: Rapid; metabolized in the GI tract and liver; pharmacologically active concentrations are not achieved

Duration: Conjunctival instillation: Ocular effect: 12-24 hours

Pregnancy Risk Factor C

Generic Available Yes

Epinephrine, Racemic (ep i NEF rin, ra SEE mik)

U.S. Brand Names AsthmaNefrin®; microNefrin®; S-2®; Vaponefrin®

Pharmacologic Category Alpha/Beta Agonist; Vasoconstrictor

Local Anesthetic/Vasoconstrictor Precautions No information available to require special precautions

Effects on Dental Treatment No effects or complications reported

Drug Uptake

Onset of action: Bronchodilation: S.C.: 5-10 minutes; Inhalation: ~1 minute

Dosage Forms INH, solution for, oral: (AsthmaNefrin®, microNefrin®, S-2®): Racepinephrine 2.25% [epinephrine base 1.125%] (7.5 mL, 15 mL, 30 mL)

Generic Available Yes

Epinephrine, Racemic and Aluminum Potassium Sulfate

(ep i NEF rin, ra SEE mik and a LOO mi num poe TASS ee um SUL fate)

U.S. Brand Names Van R Gingibraid®

Pharmacologic Category Adrenergic Agonist Agent; Alpha/Beta Agonist; Astringent; Vasoconstrictor

Use Dental: Gingival retraction

Local Anesthetic/Vasoconstrictor Precautions No information available to require special precautions

Effects on Dental Treatment Tissue retraction around base of the tooth (therapeutic effect)

Dosage Pass the impregnated yarn around the neck of the tooth and place into gingival sulcus; normal tissue moisture, water, or gingival retraction solutions activate impregnated yarn. Limit use to one quadrant of the mouth at a time; recommended use is for 3-8 minutes in the mouth.

Mechanism of Action Epinephrine stimulates $alpha_1$ adrenergic receptors to cause vasoconstriction in blood vessels in gingiva; aluminum potassium sulfate, precipitates tissue and blood proteins

Contraindications Hypersensitivity to epinephrine or any component of the formulation; cardiovascular disease; hyperthyroidism; diabetes; application to areas of heavy or deep bleeding or over exposed bone

Warnings/Precautions Caution should be exercised whenever using gingival retraction cords with epinephrine since it delivers vasoconstrictor doses of racemic epinephrine to patients; the general medical history should be thoroughly evaluated before using in any patient

Dosage Forms YARN, saturated in solution of 8% racemic epinephrine and 7% aluminum potassium sulfate: Type "0e": 0.20 ±0.10 mg epinephrine/inch; Type "1e": 0.40 ±0.20 mg epinephrine/inch; Type "2e": 0.60 ±0.20 mg epinephrine/inch

Generic Available No

Epinephryl Borate (ep i NEF ril BOR ate)

U.S. Brand Names Epinal®

Pharmacologic Category Adrenergic Agonist Agent

Use Reduces elevated intraocular pressure in chronic open-angle glaucoma

Local Anesthetic/Vasoconstrictor Precautions No information available to require special precautions

Effects on Dental Treatment No effects or complications reported

Dosage Adults: Ophthalmic: Instill 1 drop into the eyes once or twice daily

Generic Available No

EpiPen® Auto-Injector *see* Epinephrine *on page 438*

EpiPen® Jr Auto-Injector *see* Epinephrine *on page 438*

Epirubicin (ep i ROO bi sin)

U.S. Brand Names Ellence™

Canadian Brand Names Ellence™; Pharmorubicin®

Mexican Brand Names Epilem®; Farmorubicin®

Pharmacologic Category Antineoplastic Agent, Anthracycline

Use As a component of adjuvant therapy following primary resection of primary breast cancer in patients with evidence of axillary node tumor involvement

Local Anesthetic/Vasoconstrictor Precautions No information available to require special precautions

Effects on Dental Treatment No effects or complications reported

Mechanism of Action An anthracycline cytotoxic agent; precise mechanism of its cytotoxic and antiproliferative effect has not been elucidated. Epirubicin is known to inhibit DNA and RNA synthesis by steric obstruction after intercalating between DNA base pairs; active throughout entire cell cycle. Intercalation triggers DNA cleavage by topoisomerase II, resulting in cytocidal activity. Epirubicin also inhibits DNA helicase, and generates cytotoxic free radicals.

Other Adverse Effects

Vesicant chemotherapy. Epirubicin infiltration can cause severe inflammation, tissue necrosis, and ulceration. If the drug is infiltrated, consult institutional policy, apply ice to the area, and elevate the limb. Can have ongoing tissue destruction secondary to propagation of free radicals; may require debridement.

Grade 3 and 4 leukopenia may occur in 1.5% to 58.6% of patients, depending on the protocol and dosage of epirubicin. Grade 3 or 4 gastrointestinal toxicity was noted to occur in 22% to 25% of patients.

>10%:
- Central nervous system: Lethargy (1% to 46%)
- Dermatologic: Alopecia (69% to 95%)
- Endocrine & metabolic: Amenorrhea (69% to 72%), hot flashes (5% to 39%)
- Gastrointestinal: Nausea, vomiting (83% to 92%), mucositis (9% to 59%), diarrhea (7% to 25%)
- Hematologic: Leukopenia (49% to 80%), neutropenia (54% to 80%), anemia (13% to 72%), thrombocytopenia (5% to 49%)
- Local: Injection site reactions (3% to 20%)
- Ocular: Conjunctivitis (1% to 15%)
- Miscellaneous: Infection (15% to 21%)

1% to 10%:
- Cardiovascular: Congestive heart failure (0.4% to 1.5%), decreased LVEF (asymptomatic) (1.4% to 1.8%)
- Central nervous system: Fever (1% to 5%)
- Dermatologic: Rash (1% to 9%), skin changes (0.7% to 5%)
- Gastrointestinal: Anorexia (2% to 3%)

Other reactions (percentage not specified): Acute myelogenous leukemia (0.2% at 3 years), acute lymphoid leukemia, increased transaminases, radiation recall, skin and nail hyperpigmentation, photosensitivity reaction, hypersensitivity, anaphylaxis, urticaria, premature menopause in women

Contraindications Hypersensitivity to epirubicin, other anthracyclines, anthracenediones, or any component of their formulation; baseline neutrophil count <1500 cells/mm^3; severe myocardial insufficiency; recent myocardial infarction; previous treatment with anthracyclines up to the maximum cumulative dose; severe hepatic dysfunction

Drug Interactions No systematic evaluation of the potential for interaction with inhibitors or inducers of cytochrome P450 isoenzymes has been performed. Cimetidine increased the blood levels of epirubicin (AUC increased by 50%).

(Continued)

Epirubicin *(Continued)*

Drug Uptake Half-life, elimination, triphasic: Terminal, mean: 33 hours

Pregnancy Risk Factor D

Generic Available No

Epitol® *see* Carbamazepine *on page 216*

Epivir® *see* Lamivudine *on page 683*

Epivir-HBV® *see* Lamivudine *on page 683*

Epoetin Alfa (e POE e tin AL fa)

U.S. Brand Names Epogen®; Procrit®

Canadian Brand Names Eprex®

Mexican Brand Names Epomax®; Eprex®

Pharmacologic Category Colony Stimulating Factor

Synonyms EPO; Erythropoietin; *r*HuEPO-α

Use

Treatment of anemia related to zidovudine therapy in HIV-infected patients; in patients when the endogenous erythropoietin level is ≤500 mU/mL and the dose of zidovudine is ≤4200 mg/week

Treatment of anemia in cancer patients on chemotherapy; in patients with nonmyeloid malignancies where anemia is caused by the effect of the concomitantly administered chemotherapy; to decrease the need for transfusions in patients who will be receiving chemotherapy for a minimum of 2 months

Reduction of allogeneic block transfusion in surgery patients scheduled to undergo elective, noncardiac, nonvascular surgery

Orphan drug: Epogen®: Treatment of anemia associated with end-stage renal disease; treatment of anemia associated with HIV infection or HIV treatment

Unlabeled/Investigational: Anemia associated with rheumatic disease; hypogenerative anemia of Rh hemolytic disease; sickle cell anemia; acute renal failure; Gaucher's disease; Castleman's disease; paroxysmal nocturnal hemoglobinuria

Local Anesthetic/Vasoconstrictor Precautions No information available to require special precautions

Effects on Dental Treatment No effects or complications reported

Dosage

Individuals with anemia due to iron deficiency, sickle cell disease, autoimmune hemolytic anemia, and bleeding, generally have appropriate endogenous EPO levels to drive erythropoiesis and would not ordinarily be candidates for EPO therapy.

In patients on dialysis, epoetin alfa usually has been administered as an IVP 3 times/week. While the administration is independent of the dialysis procedure, it may be administered into the venous line at the end of the dialysis procedure to obviate the need for additional venous access; in patients with CRF not on dialysis, epoetin alfa may be given either as an IVP or S.C. injection.

Children and Adults: Dosing recommendations:

Dosing schedules need to be individualized and careful monitoring of patients receiving the drug is mandatory

*r*HuEPO-α may be ineffective if other factors such as iron or B_{12}/folate deficiency limit marrow response

IVP, S.C.:

Chronic renal failure patients:

Initial dose: 50-100 units/kg 3 times/week

Dose should be reduced when the hematocrit reaches the target range of 30% to 36% or a hematocrit increase >4% points over any 2-week period

Dose should be held if the hematocrit exceeds 36% and until the hematocrit decreases to the target range (30% to 36%).

Dose should be increased not more frequently than once a month, unless clinically indicated. After any dose adjustment, the hematocrit should be determined twice weekly for at least 2-6 weeks. If a hematocrit increase of 5-6 points is not achieved after a 8-week period and iron stores are adequate, the dose may be incrementally increased. Further increases may be made at 4-6 week intervals until the desired response is obtained.

Maintenance dose: Should be individualized to maintain the hematocrit within the 30% to 33% target range. The median maintenance dose in phase III studies in chronic renal failure patients on dialysis was 75 units/kg 3 times/week (range 12.5-525 units/kg 3 times/week).

Epoetin doses of 75-150 units/kg/week have been shown to maintain hematocrits of 36% to 38% for up to 6 months in patients with chronic renal failure not requiring dialysis

Zidovudine-treated HIV patients: Prior to beginning epoetin alfa, serum erythropoietin levels should be determined. Available evidence suggest that patients receiving zidovudine with endogenous serum erythropoietin levels >500 mU/mL are unlikely to respond to therapy with epoetin alfa.

Initial dose: For patients with serum erythropoietin levels <500 mU/mL who are receiving a dose of zidovudine ≤4,200 mg/week: 100 units/kg 3 times/week for 8 weeks.

Dose should be held if the hematocrit is >40% until the hematocrit drops to 36%. The dose should be reduced by 25% when the treatment is resumed and then titrated to maintain the desired hematocrit.

Dose should be reduced if the initial dose of epoetin alfa includes a rapid rise in hematocrit (>4% points in any 2-week period).

Increase dose by 50-100 units/kg if the response is not satisfactory in terms of reducing transfusion requirements or increasing hematocrit after 8 weeks of therapy. Response should be evaluated every 4-8 weeks thereafter and the dose adjusted and the dose adjusted accordingly by 50-100 units/kg increments 3 times/week. If patients have not responded satisfactorily to a dose of 300 units/kg 3 times/week, it is unlikely that they will respond to higher doses.

Maintenance dose: Dose should be titrated to maintain target hematocrit range: 36% to 40%

Cancer patients on chemotherapy: Although no specific serum erythropoietin level can be stipulated above which patients would be unlikely to respond to epoetin alfa therapy, treatment of patients with grossly elevated serum erythropoietin levels (>200 mU/mL) is not recommended

Initial dose: 150 units/kg 3 times/week

Increase dose: Response should be evaluated every 8 weeks thereafter and the dose adjusted and the dose adjusted accordingly by 50-100 units/kg increments 3 times/week up to 300 units/kg 3 times/week if the response is not satisfactory. If patients have not responded satisfactorily to a dose of 300 units/kg 3 times/week, it is unlikely that they will respond to higher doses.

Dose should be held if the hematocrit is >40% until the hematocrit drops to 36%. The dose should be reduced by 25% when the treatment is resumed and then titrated to maintain the desired hematocrit.

Dose should be reduced if the initial dose of epoetin alfa includes a rapid rise in hematocrit (>4% points in any 2-week period), the dose should be reduced

Maintenance dose: Dose should be titrated to maintain target hematocrit range: 36% to 40%

Mechanism of Action Induces erythropoiesis by stimulating the division and differentiation of committed erythroid progenitor cells; induces the release of reticulocytes from the bone marrow into the blood stream, where they mature to erythrocytes. There is a dose response relationship with this effect. This results in an increase in reticulocyte counts followed by a rise in hematocrit and hemoglobin levels.

Other Adverse Effects

>10%:

Cardiovascular: Hypertension

Central nervous system: Fatigue, headache, fever

1% to 10%:

Cardiovascular: Edema, chest pain

Central nervous system: Seizures

Gastrointestinal: Nausea, vomiting, diarrhea

Hematologic: Clotted access

Neuromuscular & skeletal: Arthralgias, asthenia

Drug Uptake

Onset of action: Several days; Peak effect: 2-3 weeks

Half-life, elimination: Circulating: 4-13 hours with chronic renal failure; 20% shorter with normal renal function

Time to peak: S.C.: 2-8 hours

Pregnancy Risk Factor C

Generic Available No

Comments Epogen® reimbursement hotline number for information regarding coverage of epoetin alfa is 1-800-2-PAY-EPO. ProCrit™ reimbursement hotline is 1-800-441-1366.

Epogen® *see* Epoetin Alfa *on page 442*

Epoprostenol (e poe PROST en ole)

U.S. Brand Names Flolan®

Canadian Brand Names Flolan®

Pharmacologic Category Prostaglandin

Synonyms Epoprostenol Sodium; PGI_2; PGX; Prostacyclin

Use

Orphan drug: Treatment of primary pulmonary hypertension; treatment of secondary pulmonary hypertension due to intrinsic precapillary pulmonary vascular disease

Unlabeled/Investigational: Other potential uses include pulmonary hypertension associated with ARDS, SLE, or CHF; neonatal pulmonary hypertension; cardiopulmonary bypass surgery; hemodialysis; atherosclerosis; peripheral vascular disorders; and neonatal purpura fulminans

(Continued)

Epoprostenol *(Continued)*

Local Anesthetic/Vasoconstrictor Precautions No information available to require special precautions

Effects on Dental Treatment No effects or complications reported

Dosage I.V.: The drug is administered by continuous I.V. infusion via a central venous catheter using an ambulatory infusion pump; during dose ranging it may be administered peripherally (see table for preparation).

Preparation of Infusion

To make 100 mL of solution with concentration:	Directions
3000 ng/mL	Dissolve one 0.5 mg vial with 5 mL supplied diluent, withdraw 3 mL, and add to sufficient diluent to make a total of 100 mL.
5000 ng/mL	Dissolve one 0.5 mg vial with 5 mL supplied diluent, withdraw entire vial contents, and add a sufficient volume of diluent to make a total of 100 mL.
10,000 ng/mL	Dissolve two 0.5 mg vials each with 5 mL supplied diluent, withdraw entire vial contents, and add a sufficient volume of diluent to make a total of 100 mL.
15,000 ng/mL	Dissolve one 1.5 mg vial with 5 mL supplied diluent, withdraw entire vial contents, and add a sufficient volume of diluent to make a total of 100 mL.

Acute dose ranging: The initial infusion rate should be 2 ng/kg/minute by continuous I.V. and increased in increments of 2 ng/kg/minute every 15 minutes or longer until dose-limiting effects are elicited (such as chest pain, anxiety, dizziness, changes in heart rate, dyspnea, nausea, vomiting, headache, hypotension and/or flushing)

Continuous chronic infusion: Initial: 4 ng/kg/minute **less** than the maximum-tolerated infusion rate determined during acute dose ranging.

If maximum-tolerated infusion rate is <5 ng/kg/minute the chronic infusion rate should be $\frac{1}{2}$ the maximum-tolerated acute infusion rate

Dosage adjustments: Dose adjustments in the chronic infusion rate should be based on persistence, recurrence or worsening of patient symptoms of pulmonary hypertension

If symptoms persist or recur after improving, the infusion rate should be increased by 1-2 ng/kg/minute increments, every 15 minutes or greater; following establishment of a new chronic infusion rate, the patient should be observed and vital signs monitored.

Mechanism of Action Strong vasodilator of all vascular beds and potent endogenous inhibitor of platelet aggregation; reduction in platelet aggregation results from epoprostenol's activation of intracellular adenylate cyclase and the resultant increase in cyclic adenosine monophosphate concentrations within the platelets; capable of decreasing thrombogenesis and platelet clumping in the lungs by inhibiting platelet aggregation

Other Adverse Effects

>10%:

Central nervous system: Fever, chills, anxiety, nervousness, dizziness, headache, hyperesthesia, pain
Cardiovascular: Flushing, tachycardia, syncope, heart failure
Gastrointestinal: Diarrhea, nausea, vomiting
Neuromuscular & skeletal: Jaw pain, myalgia, tremor, paresthesia
Respiratory: Hypoxia
Miscellaneous: Sepsis, flu-like symptoms

1% to 10%:

Cardiovascular: Bradycardia, chest pain pectoris, edema, arrhythmias, pallor, cyanosis, palpitations, cerebrovascular accident, myocardial ischemia, chest pain
Central nervous system: Seizures, confusion, depression, insomnia, muscle weakness
Dermatologic: Pruritus, rash
Endocrine & metabolic: Hypokalemia, weight change
Gastrointestinal: Abdominal pain, anorexia, constipation
Hematologic: Hemorrhage
Hepatic: Ascites
Neuromuscular & skeletal: Arthralgias, bone pain
Hematologic: Disseminated intravascular coagulation
Ocular: Amblyopia
Respiratory: Cough increase, dyspnea, epistaxis, pleural effusion
Miscellaneous: Sweating

Drug Interactions Increased Effect/Toxicity: The hypotensive effects of epoprostenol may be exacerbated by other vasodilators, diuretics, or by using acetate in dialysis fluids. Patients treated with anticoagulants (heparins, warfarin, thrombin

Ergonovine *(Continued)*

Use Prevention and treatment of postpartum and postabortion hemorrhage caused by uterine atony or subinvolution

Unlabeled/Investigational: Migraine headaches, diagnostically to identify Prinzmetal's angina

Local Anesthetic/Vasoconstrictor Precautions No information available to require special precautions

Effects on Dental Treatment No effects or complications reported

Dosage Adults:

Oral: 1-2 tablets (0.2-0.4 mg) every 6-12 hours for up to 48 hours

I.M., I.V. (I.V. should be reserved for emergency use only): 0.2 mg, repeat dose in 2-4 hours as needed

Mechanism of Action Ergot alkaloid alpha-adrenergic agonist directly stimulates vascular smooth muscle to vasoconstrict peripheral and cerebral vessels; may also have antagonist effects on serotonin

Other Adverse Effects

>10%:

- Cardiovascular: Hypertension (especially with rapid I.V. administration)
- Central nervous system: Headache
- Endocrine and metabolic: Uterine cramping

1% to 10%:

- Cardiovascular: Bradycardia
- Central nervous system: Dizziness
- Gastrointestinal: Stomach pain, nausea, vomiting diarrhea, unpleasant taste
- Otic: Tinnitus
- Respiratory: Nasal congestion
- Miscellaneous: Sweating

Drug Interactions

- 5-HT_1 receptor antagonists (sumatriptan): Avoid use within 24 hours (per manufacturer)
- Macrolide antibiotics: Erythromycin, clarithromycin, and troleandomycin may increase levels of ergot alkaloids, resulting in toxicity (ischemia, vasospasm)
- Propranolol: Rare toxicity (peripheral vasoconstriction) reported; monitor
- Ritonavir, amprenavir, and nelfinavir increase blood levels of ergot alkaloids; avoid concurrent use
- Sibutramine: May cause serotonin syndrome; avoid concurrent use
- SSRIs: Rarely, weakness and incoordination have been noted when used concurrently with 5-HT_1 agonists; monitor
- Vasoconstrictors: Effects may be increased

Drug Uptake

Onset of action: Oral: 5-15 minutes; I.M.: 2-5 minutes

Duration: I.M.: Uterine effect: 3 hours; I.V.: ~45 minutes

Pregnancy Risk Factor X

Generic Available No

Ergotamine (er GOT a meen)

U.S. Brand Names Cafergot®; Ergomar®; Wigraine®

Canadian Brand Names Cafergor®; Ergomar®

Mexican Brand Names Ergocaf; Sydolil

Pharmacologic Category Ergot Derivative

Synonyms Ergotamine Tartrate; Ergotamine Tartrate and Caffeine

Use Abort or prevent vascular headaches, such as migraine or cluster

Local Anesthetic/Vasoconstrictor Precautions No information available to require special precautions

Effects on Dental Treatment >10%: Xerostomia

Dosage Adults:

Oral:

- Cafergot®: 2 tablets at onset of attack; then 1 tablet every 30 minutes as neede maximum: 6 tablets per attack; do not exceed 10 tablets/week
- Ergostat®: 1 tablet under tongue at first sign, then 1 tablet every 30 minutes, tablets/24 hours, 5 tablets/week

Rectal (Cafergot® suppositories, Wigraine® suppositories, Cafatine® suppositories 1 at first sign of an attack; follow with second dose after 1 hour, if neede maximum dose: 2 per attack; do not exceed 5/week

Mechanism of Action Has partial agonist and/or antagonist activity agai tryptaminergic, dopaminergic and alpha-adrenergic receptors depending upon th site; is a highly active uterine stimulant; it causes constriction of peripheral a cranial blood vessels and produces depression of central vasomotor centers

Other Adverse Effects

>10%:

- Cardiovascular: Tachycardia, bradycardia, arterial spasm, claudication and v constriction; rebound headache may occur with sudden withdrawal of the in patients on prolonged therapy; localized edema, peripheral vascular ef (numbness and tingling of fingers and toes)

inhibitors) or antiplatelet agents (ticlopidine, clopidogrel, IIb/IIIa antagonists, aspirin) and epoprostenol should be monitored for increased bleeding risk.

Drug Uptake Half-life, elimination: 2.7-6 minutes; Continuous infusion: ~15 minutes

Pregnancy Risk Factor B

Generic Available No

Eprosartan (ep roe SAR tan)

U.S. Brand Names Teveten®

Pharmacologic Category Angiotensin II Receptor Blocker

Use For use in the management of essential hypertension

Local Anesthetic/Vasoconstrictor Precautions No information available to require special precautions

Effects on Dental Treatment No effects or complications reported

Dosage Oral: 400-800 mg once daily, or 200-400 mg twice daily

Mechanism of Action Angiotensin II is formed from angiotensin I in a reaction catalyzed by angiotensin-converting enzyme (ACE, kininase II). Angiotensin II is the principal pressor agent of the renin-angiotensin system, with effects that include vasoconstriction, stimulation of synthesis and release of aldosterone, cardiac stimulation, and renal reabsorption of sodium. Eprosartan blocks the vasoconstrictor and aldosterone-secreting effects of angiotensin II by selectively blocking the binding of angiotensin II to the AT1 receptor in many tissues, such as vascular smooth muscle and the adrenal gland. Its action is therefore independent of the pathways for angiotensin II synthesis. Blockade of the renin-angiotensin system with ACE inhibitors, which inhibit the biosynthesis of angiotensin II from angiotensin I, is widely used in the treatment of hypertension. ACE inhibitors also inhibit the degradation of bradykinin, a reaction also catalyzed by ACE. Because eprosartan does not inhibit ACE (kininase II), it does not affect the response to bradykinin. Whether this difference has clinical relevance is not yet known. Eprosartan does not bind to or block other hormone receptors or ion channels known to be important in cardiovascular regulation.

Other Adverse Effects

1% to 10%:

- Central nervous system: Fatigue (2%), depression (1%)
- Endocrine & metabolic: Hypertriglyceridemia (1%)
- Gastrointestinal: Abdominal pain (2%)
- Genitourinary: Urinary tract infection (1%)
- Respiratory: Upper respiratory tract infection (8%), rhinitis (4%), pharyngitis (4%), cough (4%)
- Miscellaneous: Viral infection (2%), injury (2%)

Drug Interactions Increased Effect/Toxicity: May increase risk of lithium toxicity; may increase risk of hyperkalemia with potassium-sparing diuretics (eg, amiloride, potassium, spironolactone, triamterene), potassium supplements, or high doses of trimethoprim

Drug Uptake

Half-life, elimination: Terminal: 5-9 hours

Time to peak: Fasting: 1-2 hours

Pregnancy Risk Factor C (1st trimester); D (2nd and 3rd trimesters)

Generic Available No

Eptifibatide (ep TIF i ba tide)

Related Information

Cardiovascular Diseases *on page 1308*

U.S. Brand Names Integrilin®

Canadian Brand Names Integrilin™

Pharmacologic Category Antiplatelet Agent, Glycoprotein IIb/IIIa Inhibitor

Synonyms Intrifiban

Use Treatment of patients with acute coronary syndrome (UA/NQMI), including patients who are to be managed medically and those undergoing percutaneous coronary intervention (PCI including PTCA; intracoronary stenting)

Local Anesthetic/Vasoconstrictor Precautions No information available to require special precautions

Effects on Dental Treatment Bleeding may occur while patient is medicated with eptifibatide. Platelet function is restored in about 4 hours following discontinuation.

Dosage I.V.: Adults:

Acute coronary syndrome: Bolus of 180 mcg/kg (maximum: 22.6 mg) over 1-2 minutes, begun as soon as possible following diagnosis, followed by a continuous infusion of 2 mcg/kg/minute (maximum: 15 mg/hour) until hospital discharge or initiation of CABG surgery, up to 72 hours. Concurrent aspirin (160-325 mg initially and daily thereafter) and heparin therapy (target aPTT 50-70 seconds) are recommended.

Percutaneous coronary intervention (PCI): Bolus of 180 mcg/kg (maximum: 22.6 mg) administered immediately before the initiation of PCI, followed by a continuous infusion of 2 mcg/kg/minute (maximum: 15 mg/hour). A second 180 mcg/kg bolus (maximum: 22.6 mg) should be administered 10 minutes after the first

(Continued)

Eptifibatide *(Continued)*

bolus. Infusion should be continued until hospital discharge or for up to 18-24 hours, whichever comes first; minimum of 12 hours of infusion is recommended. Concurrent aspirin (160-325 mg 1-24 hours before PCI and daily thereafter) and heparin therapy (ACT 200-300 seconds during PCI) are recommended. Heparin infusion after PCI is discouraged. In patients who undergo coronary artery bypass graft surgery, discontinue infusion prior to surgery.

Dosing adjustment in renal impairment:

Acute coronary syndrome: S_{cr} >2 mg/dL and <4 mg/dL: Use 180 mcg/kg bolus (maximum: 22.6 mg) and 1 mcg/kg/minute infusion (maximum: 7.5 mg/hour)

Percutaneous coronary intervention (PCI): Adults: S_{cr} >2 mg/dL and <4 mg/dL: Use 180 mcg/kg bolus (maximum: 22.6 mg) administered immediately before the initiation of PCI and followed by a continuous infusion of 1 mcg/kg/minute (maximum: 7.5 mg/hour). A second 180 mcg/kg (maximum: 22.6 mg) bolus should be administered 10 minutes after the first bolus.

Mechanism of Action Eptifibatide is a cyclic heptapeptide which blocks the glycoprotein IIb/IIa receptor, the binding site for fibrinogen, von Willebrand factor, and other ligands. Inhibition of binding at this final common receptor reversibly blocks platelet aggregation and prevents thrombosis.

Other Adverse Effects Bleeding is the major drug-related adverse effect. Major bleeding was reported in 4.4% to 10.8%; minor bleeding was reported in 10.5% to 14.2%; requirement for transfusion was reported in 5.5% to 12.8%. Incidence of bleeding is also related to heparin intensity (aPTT goal 50-70 seconds). Patients weighing <70 kg may have an increased risk of major bleeding.

1% to 10%: Hematologic: Thrombocytopenia (1.2% to 3.2%)

Frequency not defined:
- Cardiovascular: Hypotension
- Local: Injection site reaction
- Neuromuscular & skeletal: Back pain

Drug Interactions Increased Effect/Toxicity: Eptifibatide effect may be increased by other drugs which affect hemostasis include thrombolytics, oral anticoagulants, nonsteroidal anti-inflammatory agents, dipyridamole, heparin, low molecular weight heparins, ticlopidine, and clopidogrel. Avoid concomitant use of other IIb/IIIa inhibitors. Cephalosporins which contain the MTT side chain may theoretically increase the risk of hemorrhage. Use with aspirin and heparin may increase bleeding over aspirin and heparin alone. However, aspirin and heparin were used concurrently in the majority of patients in the major clinical studies of eptifibatide.

Drug Uptake
- Onset of action: ≤1 hour
- Duration: Platelet function restored ~4 hours following discontinuation
- Half-life, elimination: 2.5 hours

Pregnancy Risk Factor B

Generic Available No

Equagesic® *see* Aspirin and Meprobamate *on page 124*
Equalactin® Chewable Tablet [OTC] *see* Calcium Polycarbophil *on page 207*
Equanil® *see* Meprobamate *on page 768*
Equilet® [OTC] *see* Calcium Carbonate *on page 201*
Ergamisol® *see* Levamisole *on page 694*

Ergocalciferol (er goe kal SIF e role)

U.S. Brand Names Calciferol™; Drisdol®

Canadian Brand Names Drisdol®; Ostoforte®

Pharmacologic Category Vitamin D Analog

Synonyms Activated Ergosterol; Viosterol; Vitamin D_2

Use Treatment of refractory rickets, hypophosphatemia, hypoparathyroidism

Local Anesthetic/Vasoconstrictor Precautions No information available to require special precautions

Effects on Dental Treatment No effects or complications reported

Dosage Oral dosing is preferred

Dietary supplementation (each mcg = 40 USP units):
- Healthy Children: 10 mcg/day (400 units)
- Adults: 10 mcg/day (400 units)

Renal failure:
- Children: 100-1000 mcg/day (4000-40,000 units)
- Adults: 500 mcg/day (20,000 units)

Hypoparathyroidism:
- Children: 1.25-5 mg/day (50,000-200,000 units) and calcium supplements
- Adults: 625 mcg to 5 mg/day (25,000-200,000 units) and calcium supplements

Vitamin D-dependent rickets:
- Children: 75-125 mcg/day (3000-5000 units); maximum: 1500 mcg/day
- Adults: 250 mcg to 1.5 mg/day (10,000-60,000 units)

Nutritional rickets and osteomalacia:
- Children and Adults (with normal absorption): 25-125 mcg/day (1000-5000 units)

- Children with malabsorption: 250-625 mcg/day (10,000-25,000 units)
- Adults with malabsorption: 250-7500 mcg (10,000-300,000 units)

Vitamin D-resistant rickets:
- Children: Initial: 1000-2000 mcg/day (40,000-80,000 units) with phosphate supplements; daily dosage is increased at 3- to 4-month intervals in 250-500 mcg (10,000-20,000 units) increments
- Adults: 250-1500 mcg/day (10,000-60,000 units) with phosphate supplements

Mechanism of Action Stimulates calcium and phosphate absorption from the small intestine, promotes secretion of calcium from bone to blood; promotes renal tubule phosphate resorption

Other Adverse Effects Frequency not defined:
- Cardiovascular: Hypotension, cardiac arrhythmias, hypertension
- Central nervous system: Irritability, headache
- Dermatologic: Pruritus
- Endocrine & metabolic: Polydipsia, hypermagnesemia
- Gastrointestinal: Nausea, vomiting, constipation, anorexia, pancreatitis, metallic taste
- Genitourinary: Polyuria
- Neuromuscular & skeletal: Myalgia, bone pain
- Ocular: Conjunctivitis, photophobia

Drug Interactions
- Increased Effect/Toxicity: Thiazide diuretics may increase vitamin D effects. Cardiac glycosides may increase toxicity.
- Decreased Effect: Cholestyramine, colestipol, mineral oil may decrease oral absorption.

Drug Uptake
- Absorption: Readily; requires bile
- Time to peak: ~1 month following daily doses

Pregnancy Risk Factor A/C (dose exceeding RDA recommendation)

Generic Available Yes

Ergoloid Mesylates (ER goe loid MES i lates)

U.S. Brand Names Germinal®; Hydergine®; Hydergine® LC

Canadian Brand Names Hydergine®

Pharmacologic Category Ergot Derivative

Synonyms Dihydroergotoxine; Dihydrogenated Ergot Alkaloids

Use Treatment of cerebrovascular insufficiency in primary progressive dementia, Alzheimer's dementia, and senile onset

Local Anesthetic/Vasoconstrictor Precautions No information available to require special precautions

Effects on Dental Treatment No effects or complications reported

Dosage Adults: Oral: 1 mg 3 times/day up to 4.5-12 mg/day; up to 6 months of therapy may be necessary

Mechanism of Action Ergoloid mesylates do not have the vasoconstrictor effects of the natural ergot alkaloids; exact mechanism in dementia is unknown; originally classed as peripheral and cerebral vasodilator, now considered a "metabolic enhancer"; there is no specific evidence which clearly establishes the mechanism by which ergoloid mesylate preparations produce mental effects, nor is there conclusive evidence that the drug particularly affects cerebral arteriosclerosis or cerebrovascular insufficiency

Other Adverse Effects 1% to 10%:
- Gastrointestinal: Transient nausea
- Miscellaneous: Sublingual irritation

Drug Interactions Increased Effect/Toxicity: Avoid use of 5-HT_1 receptor antagonists (sumatriptan) within 24 hours (per manufacturer). Macrolide antibiotics (erythromycin, clarithromycin, and troleandomycin) and protease inhibitors (ritonavir, amprenavir, and nelfinavir) may increase levels of ergot alkaloids, resulting in toxicity (ischemia, vasospasm). Rare toxicity (peripheral vasoconstriction) reported with propranolol. Concurrent use with sibutramine may cause serotonin syndrome; avoid concurrent use. Rarely, weakness and incoordination have been noted when used concurrently with 5-HT_1 agonists or SSRIs. Effects of dopamine or vasoconstrictors may be increased.

Drug Uptake
- Absorption: Rapid yet incomplete
- Half-life, elimination: 3.5 hours
- Time to peak: ~1 hour

Pregnancy Risk Factor C

Generic Available Yes

Ergomar® *see* Ergotamine *on page 448*

Ergonovine (er goe NOE veen)

U.S. Brand Names Ergotrate® Maleate Injection

Pharmacologic Category Ergot Derivative

Synonyms Ergometrine Maleate; Ergonovine Maleate

(Continued)

Central nervous system: Drowsiness, dizziness
Gastrointestinal: Nausea, vomiting, diarrhea, xerostomia
1% to 10%:
Cardiovascular: Transient tachycardia or bradycardia
Neuromuscular & skeletal: Weakness in the legs, abdominal or muscle pain, muscle pains in the extremities, paresthesia

Drug Interactions
5-HT_1 receptor antagonists (sumatriptan): Avoid use within 24 hours (per manufacturer)
Macrolide antibiotics: Erythromycin, clarithromycin, and troleandomycin may increase levels of ergot alkaloids, resulting in toxicity (ischemia, vasospasm)
Propranolol: Rare toxicity (peripheral vasoconstriction) reported; monitor
Ritonavir, amprenavir, and nelfinavir increase blood levels of ergot alkaloids; avoid concurrent use
Sibutramine: May cause serotonin syndrome; avoid concurrent use
SSRIs: Rarely, weakness and incoordination have been noted when used concurrently with 5-HT_1 agonists; monitor
Vasoconstrictors: Effects may be increased

Drug Uptake
Absorption: Oral, rectal: Erratic; enhanced by caffeine coadministration
Time to peak: 0.5-3 hours following coadministration with caffeine

Pregnancy Risk Factor X

Generic Available Yes

Ergotrate® Maleate Injection *see* Ergonovine *on page 447*
E•R•O Ear [OTC] *see* Carbamide Peroxide *on page 218*

Ertapenem (er ta PEN em)

U.S. Brand Names Invanz™

Pharmacologic Category Antibiotic, Carbapenem

Synonyms Ertapenem Sodium; L-749,345; MK-0826

Use Treatment of moderate-severe, complicated intra-abdominal infections, skin and skin structure infections, pyelonephritis, acute pelvic infections, and community-acquired pneumonia. Antibacterial coverage includes aerobic gram-positive organisms, aerobic gram-negative organisms, anaerobic organisms.

Methicillin-resistant *Staphylococcus*, *Enterococcus* spp, penicillin-resistant strains of *Streptococcus pneumoniae*, beta-lactamase-positive strains of *Haemophilus influenzae* are **resistant** to ertapenem, as are most *Pseudomonas aeruginosa*.

Local Anesthetic/Vasoconstrictor Precautions No information available to require special precautions

Effects on Dental Treatment No effects or complications reported

Dosage Adults: I.V., I.M.: **Note:** I.V. therapy may be administered for up to 14 days; I.M. for up to 7 days
Intra-abdominal infection: 1 g/day for 5-14 days
Skin and skin structure infections: 1 g/day for 7-14 days
Community-acquired pneumonia: 1 g/day; duration of total antibiotic treatment: 10-14 days
Urinary tract infections/pyelonephritis: 1 g/day; duration of total antibiotic treatment: 10-14 days
Acute pelvic infections: 1 g/day for 3-10 days
Elderly: Refer to adult dosing.
Dosage adjustment in renal impairment: Cl_{cr} <30 mL/minute: 500 mg/day
Hemodialysis: When the daily dose is given within 6 hours prior to hemodialysis, a supplementary dose of 150 mg is required following hemodialysis.
Dosage adjustment in hepatic impairment: Adjustments cannot be recommended (lack of experience and research in this patient population).

Mechanism of Action Inhibits bacterial cell wall synthesis by binding to one or more of the penicillin binding proteins; which in turn inhibits the final transpeptidation step of peptidoglycan synthesis in bacterial cell walls, thus inhibiting cell wall biosynthesis. Bacteria eventually lyse due to ongoing activity of cell wall autolytic enzymes (autolysins and murein hydrolases) while cell wall assembly is arrested.

Other Adverse Effects 1% to 10%:
Cardiovascular: Swelling/edema (3%), chest pain (1%), hypertension (0.7% to 2%), hypotension (1% to 2%), tachycardia (1% to 2%)
Central nervous system: Headache (6% to 7%), altered mental status (ie, agitation, confusion, disorientation, decreased mental acuity, changed mental status, somnolence, stupor) (3% to 5%), fever (2% to 5%), insomnia (3%), dizziness (2%), fatigue (1%), anxiety (0.8% to 1%)
Dermatologic: Rash (2% to 3%), pruritus (1% to 2%), erythema (1% to 2%)
Gastrointestinal: Diarrhea (9% to 10%), nausea (6% to 9%), abdominal pain (4%), vomiting (4%), constipation (3% to 4%), acid regurgitation (1% to 2%), dyspepsia (1%), oral candidiasis (0.1% to 1%)
Genitourinary: Vaginitis (1% to 3%)
Hematologic: Platelet count increased (4% to 7%), eosinophils increased (1% to 2%)
(Continued)

Ertapenem *(Continued)*

Hepatic: Hepatic enzyme elevations (7% to 9%), alkaline phosphatase increase (4% to 7%)

Local: Infused vein complications (5% to 7%), phlebitis/thrombophlebitis (1.5% to 2%), extravasation (0.7% to 2%)

Neuromuscular & skeletal: Leg pain (0.4% to 1%)

Respiratory: Dyspnea (1% to 3%), cough (1% to 2%), pharyngitis (0.7% to 1%), rales/rhonchi (0.5% to 1%), respiratory distress (0.2% to 1%)

Drug Interactions Probenecid: Reduces renal clearance of ertapenem; small increase in half-life. Use not recommended to extend ertapenem's half-life.

Drug Uptake

Absorption: I.M.: Almost complete

Half-life, elimination: 4 hours

Time to peak: I.M.: 2.3 hours

Pregnancy Risk Factor B

Generic Available No

Eryc® *see* Erythromycin *on page 450*

Erycette® *see* Erythromycin, Topical *on page 454*

EryDerm® Topical *see* Erythromycin, Topical *on page 454*

Erygel® *see* Erythromycin, Topical *on page 454*

Erymax® *see* Erythromycin, Topical *on page 454*

EryPed® *see* Erythromycin *on page 450*

Ery-Tab® *see* Erythromycin *on page 450*

Erythrocin® *see* Erythromycin *on page 450*

Erythromycin (er ith roe MYE sin)

Related Information

Cardiovascular Diseases *on page 1308*

Dental Drug Interactions: Update on Drug Combinations Requiring Special Considerations *on page 1434*

Oral Bacterial Infections *on page 1367*

Oral Viral Infections *on page 1380*

Respiratory Diseases *on page 1328*

U.S. Brand Names E.E.S.®; E-Mycin®; Eryc®; EryPed®; Ery-Tab®; Erythrocin®; PCE®

Canadian Brand Names Apo®-Erythro Base; Apo®-Erythro E-C; Apo®-Erythro-ES; Apo®-Erythro-S; Diomycin®; EES®; Erybid™; Eryc®; Erythrocin®; Erythrocin™ I.V.; Erythromid®; Ilosone®; Novo-Rythro Encap; Nu-Erythromycin-S; PCE®; PMS-Erythromycin

Mexican Brand Names Eritroquim; Ilosone®; Latotryd®; Lauricin; Lauritran®; Lederpax; Luritran®; Optomicin®; Pantomicina®; Procephal®; Tromigal

Pharmacologic Category Antibiotic, Macrolide

Synonyms Erythromycin Base; Erythromycin Estolate; Erythromycin Ethylsuccinate; Erythromycin Gluceptate; Erythromycin Lactobionate; Erythromycin Stearate

Use

Dental: An alternative to penicillin VK for treating orofacial infections

Medical: Treatment of susceptible bacterial infections including *S. pyogenes*, some *S. pneumoniae*, some *S. aureus*, *M. pneumoniae*, *Legionella pneumophila*, diphtheria, pertussis, chancroid, *Chlamydia*, erythrasma, *N. gonorrhoeae*, *E. histolytica*, syphilis and nongonococcal urethritis, and *Campylobacter* gastroenteritis; used in conjunction with neomycin for decontaminating the bowel

Unlabeled/Investigational: Treatment of gastroparesis

Local Anesthetic/Vasoconstrictor Precautions No information available to require special precautions

Effects on Dental Treatment 1% to 10%: Oral candidiasis

Dosage

Infants and Children (**Note:** 400 mg ethylsuccinate = 250 mg base, stearate, or estolate salts):

- Oral: 30-50 mg/kg/day divided every 6-8 hours; may double doses in severe infections
- Orofacial infections: Base and ethylsuccinate: 30-50 mg/kg/day divided every 6-8 hours; do not exceed 2 g /day
- Preop bowel preparation: 20 mg/kg erythromycin base at 1, 2, and 11 PM on the day before surgery combined with mechanical cleansing of the large intestine and oral neomycin
- I.V.: Lactobionate: 20-40 mg/kg/day divided every 6 hours

Adults:

- Oral:
  - Base: 250-500 mg every 6-12 hours for at least 7 days
  - Ethylsuccinate: 400-800 mg every 6-12 hours for at least 7 days
  - Orofacial infections: Stearate or base: 250-500 mg every 6 hours for at least 7 days; Ethylsuccinate: 400-800 mg every 6 hours for at least 7 days

Preop bowel preparation: 1 g erythromycin base at 1, 2, and 11 PM on the day before surgery combined with mechanical cleansing of the large intestine and oral neomycin

I.V.: Lactobionate: 15-20 mg/kg/day divided every 6 hours or 500 mg to 1 g every 6 hours, or given as a continuous infusion over 24 hours (maximum: 4 g/24 hours)

Children and Adults: Ophthalmic: Instill 1/2" (1.25 cm) 2-8 times/day depending on the severity of the infection

Dialysis: Slightly dialyzable (5% to 20%); no supplemental dosage necessary in hemo or peritoneal dialysis or in continuous arteriovenous or venovenous hemofiltration

Erythromycin has been used as a prokinetic agent to improve gastric emptying time and intestinal motility. In adults, 200 mg was infused I.V. initially followed by 250 mg orally 3 times/day 30 minutes before meals. In children, erythromycin 3 mg/kg I.V. has been infused over 60 minutes initially followed by 20 mg/kg/day orally in 3-4 divided doses before meals or before meals and at bedtime

Mechanism of Action Inhibits RNA-dependent protein synthesis at the chain elongation step; binds to the 50S ribosomal subunit resulting in blockage of transpeptidation

Other Adverse Effects

Cardiovascular: Ventricular arrhythmias, QT_c prolongation, torsade de pointes (rare), ventricular tachycardia (rare)

Central nervous system: Headache (8%), pain (2%), fever, seizures

Dermatitis: Rash (3%), pruritus (1%)

Gastrointestinal: Abdominal pain (8%), cramping, nausea (8%), oral candidiasis, vomiting (3%), diarrhea (7%), dyspepsia (2%), flatulence (2%), anorexia, pseudomembranous colitis, hypertrophic pyloric stenosis (including cases in infants or IHPS), pancreatitis

Hematologic: Eosinophilia (1%)

Hepatic: Cholestatic jaundice (most common with estolate), increased LFTs (2%)

Local: Phlebitis at the injection site, thrombophlebitis (frequency not defined)

Neuromuscular & skeletal: Weakness (2%)

Respiratory: Dyspnea (1%), cough (3%)

Miscellaneous: Hypersensitivity reactions, allergic reactions

Contraindications Hypersensitivity to erythromycin or any component of the formulation; pre-existing liver disease (erythromycin estolate); concomitant use with pimozide, terfenadine, astemizole, or cisapride; hepatic impairment

Warnings/Precautions Hepatic impairment with or without jaundice has occurred, it may be accompanied by malaise, nausea, vomiting, abdominal colic, and fever; discontinue use if these occur; avoid using erythromycin lactobionate in neonates since formulations may contain benzyl alcohol which is associated with toxicity in neonates; observe for superinfections. Macrolides have been associated with rare QT_c prolongation and ventricular arrhythmias, including torsade de pointes.

Drug Interactions CYP3A3/4 and CYP2B6 (minor) enzyme substrate; CYP1A2 and 3A3/4 enzyme inhibitor

Alfentanil (and possibly other narcotic analgesics): Serum levels may be increased by erythromycin; monitor for increased effect.

Antipsychotic agents (particularly mesoridazine and thioridazine): Risk of QT_c prolongation and malignant arrhythmias may be increased.

Astemizole: Concomitant use is contraindicated; may lead to QT_c prolongation or torsade de pointes.

Benzodiazepines (those metabolized by CYP3A3/4, including alprazolam and triazolam): Serum levels may be increased by erythromycin; somnolence and confusion have been reported.

Bromocriptine: Serum levels may be increased by erythromycin; monitor for increased effect.

Buspirone: Serum levels may be increased by erythromycin; monitor.

Calcium channel blockers (felodipine, verapamil, and potentially others metabolized by CYP3A3/4): Serum levels may be increased by erythromycin; monitor.

Carbamazepine: Serum levels may be increased by erythromycin; monitor.

Cilostazol: Serum levels may be increased by erythromycin.

Cisapride: Serum levels may be increased by erythromycin; serious arrhythmias have occurred; concurrent use contraindicated.

Clindamycin (and lincomycin): Use with erythromycin may result in pharmacologic antagonism; manufacturer recommends avoiding this combination.

Clozapine: Serum levels may be increased by erythromycin; monitor.

Colchicine: serum levels/toxicity may be increased by erythromycin; monitor.

Cyclosporine: Serum levels may be increased by erythromycin; monitor serum levels.

Delavirdine: Serum levels of erythromycin may be increased; also, serum levels of delavirdine may increased by erythromycin (low risk); monitor.

Digoxin: Serum levels may be increased by erythromycin; monitor digoxin levels.

Disopyramide: Serum levels may be increased by erythromycin; in addition, QT_c prolongation and risk of malignant arrhythmia may be increased; avoid combination.

(Continued)

Erythromycin *(Continued)*

Ergot alkaloids: Concurrent use may lead to acute ergot toxicity (severe peripheral vasospasm and dysesthesia).

HMG-CoA reductase inhibitors (atorvastatin, lovastatin, and simvastatin); Erythromycin may increase serum levels of "statins" metabolized by CYP3A3/4, increasing the risk of myopathy/rhabdomyolysis (does not include fluvastatin and pravastatin).

Loratadine: Serum levels may be increased by erythromycin; monitor.

Methylprednisolone: Serum levels may be increased by erythromycin; monitor.

Neuromuscular-blocking agents: May be potentiated by erythromycin (case reports).

Phenytoin: Serum levels may be increased by erythromycin; other evidence suggested phenytoin levels may be decreased in some patients; monitor.

Pimozide: Serum levels may be increased, leading to malignant arrhythmias; concomitant use is contraindicated.

Protease inhibitors (amprenavir, nelfinavir, and ritonavir): May increase serum levels of erythromycin.

QT_c-prolonging agents: Concomitant use may increase the risk of malignant arrhythmias.

Quinidine: Serum levels may be increased by erythromycin; in addition, the risk of QT_c prolongation and malignant arrhythmias may be increased during concurrent use.

Quinolone antibiotics (sparfloxacin, gatifloxacin, and moxifloxacin): Concurrent use may increase the risk of malignant arrhythmias.

Rifabutin: Serum levels may be increased by erythromycin; monitor.

Sildenafil: Serum levels may be increased by erythromycin; consider reduction in sildenafil dosage.

Tacrolimus: Serum levels may be increased by erythromycin; monitor serum concentration.

Terfenadine: Serum levels may be increased by erythromycin, may lead to QT_c prolongation and malignant arrhythmias, including torsade de pointes; concomitant use is contraindicated.

Theophylline: Serum levels may be increased by erythromycin; monitor.

Valproic acid (and derivatives): Serum levels may be increased by erythromycin; monitor.

Vinblastine (and vincristine): Serum levels may be increased by erythromycin.

Warfarin: Effects may be potentiated; monitor INR closely and adjust warfarin dose as needed or choose another antibiotic.

Zafirlukast: Serum levels may be decreased by erythromycin; monitor.

Zopiclone: Serum levels may be increased by erythromycin; monitor.

Dietary/Ethanol/Herb Considerations

Ethanol: Avoid use; ethanol effects may be enhanced and absorption of erythromycin may be decreased.

Food increases absorption and may alter serum concentration. Avoid milk and acidic beverages 1 hour before or after a dose. Ethylsuccinate, estolate, and enteric-coated products are **not** affected by food; ethylsuccinate may be better absorbed with food.

Herb/Nutraceutical: Avoid St John's wort; may decrease serum concentration.

Drug Uptake

Absorption: Variable but better with salt forms than with base form; 18% to 45% absorbed orally; due to differences in absorption, **200 mg erythromycin ethylsuccinate produces the same serum concentration as 125 mg of erythromycin base** hours for the ethylsuccinate

Half-life, elimination: Peak effect: 1.5-2 hours; End-stage renal disease: 5-6 hours

Time to peak: 4 hours for the base; Ethylsuccinate: 0.5-2.5 hours; delayed in presence of food due to differences in absorption

Pregnancy Risk Factor B

Breast-feeding Considerations May be taken while breast-feeding

Dosage Forms CAP, as estolate: 250 mg. **CAP, delayed release, as base:** 250 mg. **CAP, delayed release, enteric-coated pellets, as base** (Eryc®): 250 mg. **DROPS, oral, as ethylsuccinate** (EryPed®): 100 mg/2.5 mL (50 mL). **GRAN, oral suspension, as ethylsuccinate** (EryPed®): 200 mg/5 mL, 400 mg/5 mL (60 mL, 100 mL, 200 mL). **INJ, as gluceptate:** 1000 mg (30 mL). **INJ, powder for reconstitution, as lactobionate:** 500 mg, 1000 mg. **OINT, ophthalmic, as base:** 0.55 mg (3.5 g). **POWDER, oral suspension, as ethylsuccinate** (E.E.S.®): 200 mg/5 mL (100 mL, 200 mL). **SUSP, oral, as estolate:** 125 mg/5 mL (120 mL, 200 mL, 480 mL); 250 mg/5 mL (150 mL, 200 mL, 480 mL). **SUSP, oral, as ethylsuccinate** (E.E.S.®, EryPed®): 200 mg/5 mL (5 mL, 100 mL, 200 mL, 480 mL); 400 mg/5 mL (5 mL, 60 mL, 100 mL, 200 mL, 480 mL). **TAB, as ethylsuccinate** (E.E.S.®): 400 mg. **TAB, chewable, as ethylsuccinate** (EryPed®): 200 mg. **TAB, delayed release, as base:** 333 mg. **TAB, enteric coated, as base** (E-Mycin®, Ery-Tab®): 250 mg, 333 mg, 500 mg. **TAB, film coated, as base:** 250 mg, 500 mg. **TAB, film coated, as stearate** (Erythrocin®): 250 mg, 500 mg. **TAB, polymer-coated particles, as base** (PCE®): 333 mg, 500 mg

Generic Available Yes

Comments Many patients cannot tolerate erythromycin because of abdominal pain and nausea; the mechanism of this adverse effect appears to be the motilin agonistic properties of erythromycin in the GI tract. For these patients, clindamycin is indicated as the alternative antibiotic for treatment of orofacial infections.

Erythromycin has been used as a prokinetic agent to improve gastric emptying time and intestinal motility. In adults, 200 mg was infused I.V. initially followed by 250 mg orally 3 times/day 30 minutes before meals. In children, erythromycin 3 mg/kg I.V. has been infused over 60 minutes initially followed by 20 mg/kg/day orally in 3-4 divided doses before meals or before meals and at bedtime.

HMG-CoA reductase inhibitors, also known as the statins, effectively decrease the hepatic cholesterol biosynthesis resulting in the reduction of blood LDL-cholesterol concentrations. The AUC of atorvastatin (Lipitor®) was increased 33% by erythromycin administration. Combination of erythromycin and lovastatin (Mevacor®) has been associated with rhabdomyolysis (Ayanian, et al). The administration of erythromycin with cerivastatin (Baycol®) produced a 50% increase in area under the concentration curve for cerivastatin. The mechanism of erythromycin is inhibiting the CYP3A4 metabolism of atorvastatin, lovastatin, and cerivastatin. Simvastatin (Zocor®) would likely be affected in a similar manner by the coadministration of erythromycin. Clarithromycin (Biaxin®) may exert a similar effect as erythromycin on atorvastatin, lovastatin, cerivastatin, and simvastatin. Erythromycin 3 times/day had no effect on pravastatin (Pravachol®) plasma concentrations (Bottorff, et al).

Selected Readings

Ayanian JZ, Fuchs CS, and Stone RM, "Lovastatin and Rhabdomyolysis," *Ann Intern Med*, 1988, 109(8):682-3.

"Pimozide (Orap) Contraindicated With Clarithromycin (Biaxin®) and Other Macrolide Antibiotics," *FDA Medical Bulletin*, October 1996, 26(3).

Wynn RL and Bergman SA, "Antibiotics and Their Use in the Treatment of Orofacial Infections, Part I," *Gen Dent*, 1994, 42(5):398, 400, 402.

Wynn RL and Bergman SA, "Antibiotics and Their Use in the Treatment of Orofacial Infections, Part II," *Gen Dent*, 1994, 42(6):498-502.

Wynn RL, "Current Concepts of the Erythromycins," *Gen Dent*, 1991, 39(6):408,10-1.

Erythromycin and Benzoyl Peroxide

(er ith roe MYE sin & BEN zoe il per OKS ide)

U.S. Brand Names Benzamycin®

Pharmacologic Category Topical Skin Product; Topical Skin Product, Acne

Synonyms Benzoyl Peroxide and Erythromycin

Use Topical control of acne vulgaris

Local Anesthetic/Vasoconstrictor Precautions No information available to require special precautions

Effects on Dental Treatment No effects or complications reported

Dosage Apply twice daily, morning and evening

Drug Uptake See Erythromycin *on page 450* and Benzoyl Peroxide *on page 153*

Pregnancy Risk Factor C

Generic Available No

Erythromycin and Sulfisoxazole

(er ith roe MYE sin & sul fi SOKS a zole)

U.S. Brand Names Eryzole®; Pediazole®

Canadian Brand Names Pediazole®

Pharmacologic Category Antibiotic, Macrolide; Antibiotic, Macrolide Combination; Antibiotic, Sulfonamide Derivative

Synonyms Sulfisoxazole and Erythromycin

Use Treatment of susceptible bacterial infections of the upper and lower respiratory tract, otitis media in children caused by susceptible strains of *Haemophilus influenzae*, and other infections in patients allergic to penicillin

Local Anesthetic/Vasoconstrictor Precautions No information available to require special precautions

Effects on Dental Treatment No effects or complications reported

Dosage Oral (dosage recommendation is based on the product's erythromycin content):

Children ≥2 months: 50 mg/kg/day erythromycin and 150 mg/kg/day sulfisoxazole in divided doses every 6 hours; not to exceed 2 g erythromycin/day or 6 g sulfisoxazole/day for 10 days

Adults: 400 mg erythromycin and 1200 mg sulfisoxazole every 6 hours

Mechanism of Action Erythromycin inhibits bacterial protein synthesis; sulfisoxazole competitively inhibits bacterial synthesis of folic acid from para-aminobenzoic acid

Other Adverse Effects Frequency not defined:

Cardiovascular: Ventricular arrhythmias,

Central nervous system: Headache, fever

Dermatologic: Rash, Stevens-Johnson syndrome, toxic epidermal necrolysis

Gastrointestinal: Abdominal pain, cramping, nausea, vomiting, oral candidiasis, hypertrophic pyloric stenosis, diarrhea, pseudomembranous colitis

Hematologic: Agranulocytosis, aplastic anemia, eosinophilia

(Continued)

Erythromycin and Sulfisoxazole *(Continued)*

Hepatic: Hepatic necrosis, cholestatic jaundice
Local: Phlebitis at the injection site, thrombophlebitis
Renal: Toxic nephrosis, crystalluria
Miscellaneous: Hypersensitivity reactions

Warnings/Precautions Use with caution in patients with impaired renal or hepatic function, G6PD deficiency (hemolysis may occur). Chemical similarities are present among sulfonamides, sulfonylureas, carbonic anhydrase inhibitors, thiazides, and loop diuretics (except ethacrynic acid). In patients with allergy to one of these compounds, a risk of cross-reaction exists; avoid use when previous reaction has been severe.

Drug Interactions See Erythromycin *on page 450* and Sulfisoxazole *on page 1123*

Drug Uptake
Erythromycin ethylsuccinate:
Absorption: Well absorbed
Half-life, elimination: 1-1.5 hours
Sulfisoxazole acetyl:
Absorption: Readily absorbed
Half-life, elimination: 6 hours (increases with renal impairment)

Pregnancy Risk Factor C

Generic Available Yes

Erythromycin, Topical (er ith roe MYE sin TOP i kal)

U.S. Brand Names Akne-Mycin®; A/T/S®; Del-Mycin®; Emgel™; Erycette®; EryDerm® Topical; Erygel®; Erymax®; E-Solve-2®; ETS-2%®; Ilotycin®; Romycin®; Staticin®; Theramycin Z®; T-Stat®

Pharmacologic Category Antibiotic, Ophthalmic; Antibiotic, Topical; Topical Skin Product; Topical Skin Product, Acne

Use Topical treatment of acne vulgaris

Local Anesthetic/Vasoconstrictor Precautions No information available to require special precautions

Effects on Dental Treatment No effects or complications reported

Dosage
Neonates:
Ophthalmic: Prophylaxis of neonatal gonococcal or chlamydial conjunctivitis: 0.5-1 cm ribbon of ointment should be instilled into each conjunctival sac
Children and Adults:
Ophthalmic: Instill one or more times daily depending on the severity of the infection
Topical: Apply 2% solution over the affected area twice daily after the skin has been thoroughly washed and patted dry

Other Adverse Effects 1% to 10%: Dermatologic: Erythema, desquamation, dryness, pruritus

Pregnancy Risk Factor B

Generic Available Yes

Eryzole® *see* Erythromycin and Sulfisoxazole *on page 453*
Esclim® *see* Estradiol *on page 457*
Esgic® *see* Butalbital, Acetaminophen, and Caffeine *on page 192*
Esgic-Plus™ *see* Butalbital, Acetaminophen, and Caffeine *on page 192*
Esidrix® *see* Hydrochlorothiazide *on page 595*
Eskalith® *see* Lithium *on page 722*
Eskalith CR® *see* Lithium *on page 722*

Esmolol (ES moe lol)

U.S. Brand Names Brevibloc®

Canadian Brand Names Brevibloc®

Mexican Brand Names Brevibloc®

Pharmacologic Category Antiarrhythmic Agent, Class II; Beta Blocker, $Beta_1$ Selective

Synonyms Esmolol Hydrochloride

Use Treatment of supraventricular tachycardia, atrial fibrillation/flutter (primarily to control ventricular rate), and hypertension (especially perioperatively)

Local Anesthetic/Vasoconstrictor Precautions No information available to require special precautions

Effects on Dental Treatment No effects or complications reported

Dosage I.V. infusion requires an infusion pump (must be adjusted to individual response and tolerance):
Children: A limited amount of information regarding esmolol use in pediatric patients is currently available. Some centers have utilized doses of 100-500 mcg/kg given over 1 minute for control of supraventricular tachycardias.

Loading doses of 500 mcg/kg/minute over 1 minute with maximal doses of 50-250 mcg/kg/minute (mean = 173) have been used in addition to nitroprusside to treat postoperative hypertension after coarctation of aorta repair.

Adults:

Intraoperative tachycardia and/or hypertension (immediate control): Initial bolus: 80 mg (~1 mg/kg) over 30 seconds, followed by a 150 mcg/kg/minute infusion, if necessary. Adjust infusion rate as needed to maintain desired heart rate and/or BP, up to 300 mcg/kg/minute.

Supraventricular tachycardia or gradual control of postoperative tachycardia/hypertension: Loading dose: 500 mcg/kg over 1 minute; follow with a 50 mcg/kg/minute infusion for 4 minutes; response to this initial infusion rate may be a rough indication of the responsiveness of the ventricular rate.

Infusion may be continued at 50 mcg/kg/minute or, if the response is inadequate, titrated upward in 50 mcg/kg/minute increments (increased no more frequently than every 4 minutes) to a maximum of 200 mcg/kg/minute.

To achieve more rapid response, following the initial loading dose and 50 mcg/kg/minute infusion, rebolus with a second 500 mcg/kg loading dose over 1 minute, and increase the maintenance infusion to 100 mcg/kg/minute for 4 minutes. If necessary, a third (and final) 500 mcg/kg loading dose may be administered, prior to increasing to an infusion rate of 150 mcg/minute. After 4 minutes of the 150 mcg/kg/minute infusion, the infusion rate may be increased to a maximum rate of 200 mcg/kg/minute (without a bolus dose).

Usual dosage range (SVT): 50-200 mcg/kg/minute with average dose of 100 mcg/kg/minute. For control of postoperative hypertension, as many as one-third of patients may require higher doses (250-300 mcg/kg/minute) to control BP; the safety of doses >300 mcg/kg/minute has not been studied.

Esmolol: Hemodynamic effects of beta-blockade return to baseline within 20-30 minutes after discontinuing esmolol infusions.

Guidelines for withdrawal of therapy:

Transfer to alternative antiarrhythmic drug (propranolol, digoxin, verapamil).

Infusion should be reduced by 50% 30 minutes following the first dose of the alternative agent.

Following the second dose of the alternative drug, patient's response should be monitored and if control is adequate for the first hours, esmolol may be discontinued.

Dialysis: Not removed by hemo- or peritoneal dialysis; supplemental dose is not necessary.

Mechanism of Action Class II antiarrhythmic: Competitively blocks response to $beta_1$-adrenergic stimulation with little or no effect of $beta_2$-receptors except at high doses, no intrinsic sympathomimetic activity, no membrane stabilizing activity

Other Adverse Effects

>10%:

Cardiovascular: Asymptomatic hypotension (25%), symptomatic hypotension (12%)

Miscellaneous: Diaphoresis (10%)

1% to 10%:

Cardiovascular: Peripheral ischemia (1%)

Central nervous system: Dizziness (3%), somnolence (3%), confusion (2%), headache (2%), agitation (2%), fatigue (1%)

Gastrointestinal: Nausea (7%), vomiting (1%)

Local: Pain on injection (8%)

Contraindications Hypersensitivity to esmolol, other beta-blockers, or any component of the formulation; sinus bradycardia or heart block; uncompensated CHF; cardiogenic shock

Drug Interactions

Increased Effect/Toxicity: Esmolol may increase the effect/toxicity of verapamil, and may increase potential for hypertensive crisis after or during withdrawal of either agent when combined with clonidine. Esmolol may extend the effect of neuromuscular blocking agents (succinylcholine). Esmolol may increase digoxin serum concentration by 10% to 20% and may increase theophylline concentrations. Morphine may increase esmolol blood concentrations.

Decreased effect of beta-blockers with aluminum salts, barbiturates, calcium salts, cholestyramine, colestipol, NSAIDs, penicillins (ampicillin), rifampin, salicylates, and sulfinpyrazone due to decreased bioavailability and plasma concentrations. Beta-blockers may decrease the effect of sulfonylureas. Xanthines (eg, theophylline, caffeine) may decrease effects of esmolol.

Drug Uptake

Onset of action: Beta-blockade: I.V.: 2-10 minutes (quickest when loading doses are administered)

Duration: 10-30 minutes; prolonged following higher cumulative doses, extended duration of use

Half-life, elimination: Adults: 9 minutes

Pregnancy Risk Factor C (manufacturer); D (2nd and 3rd trimesters - expert analysis)

Generic Available No

(Continued)

Esmolol *(Continued)*

Selected Readings

Foster CA and Aston SJ, "Propranolol-Epinephrine Interaction: A Potential Disaster," *Plast Reconstr Surg*, 1983, 72(1):74-8.

Wong DG, Spence JD, Lamki L, et al, "Effect of Nonsteroidal Anti-inflammatory Drugs on Control of Hypertension of Beta-Blockers and Diuretics," *Lancet*, 1986, 1(8488):997-1001.

Wynn RL, "Dental Nonsteroidal Anti-inflammatory Drugs and Prostaglandin-Based Drug Interactions, Part Two," *Gen Dent*, 1992, 40(2):104, 106, 108.

Wynn RL, "Epinephrine Interactions With Beta-Blockers," *Gen Dent*, 1994, 42(1):16, 18.

E-Solve-2® *see* Erythromycin, Topical *on page 454*

Esomeprazole (es oh ME pray zol)

U.S. Brand Names Nexium™

Pharmacologic Category Proton Pump Inhibitor

Synonyms Esomeprazole Magnesium

Use Short-term (4-8 weeks) treatment of erosive esophagitis; maintaining symptom resolution and healing of erosive esophagitis; treatment of symptomatic gastroesophageal reflux disease; as part of a multidrug regimen for *Helicobacter pylori* eradication in patients with duodenal ulcer disease (active or history of within the past 5 years)

Local Anesthetic/Vasoconstrictor Precautions No information available to require special precautions

Effects on Dental Treatment No effects or complications reported

Dosage Note: Delayed-release capsules should be swallowed whole and taken at least 1 hour before eating

Children: Safety and efficacy have not been established in pediatric patients

Adults: Oral:

Erosive esophagitis (healing): 20-40 mg once daily for 4-8 weeks; maintenance: 20 mg once daily

Symptomatic GERD: 20 mg once daily for 4 weeks

Helicobacter pylori eradication: 40 mg once daily; requires combination therapy

Mechanism of Action Proton pump inhibitor suppresses gastric acid secretion by inhibition of the H^+/K^+-ATPase in the gastric parietal cell

Other Adverse Effects 1% to 10%:

Central nervous system: Headache (4% to 6%)

Gastrointestinal: Diarrhea (4%), nausea, flatulence, abdominal pain (4%), constipation, xerostomia

Contraindications Hypersensitivity to esomeprazole, lansoprazole, omeprazole, rabeprazole, or any component of their formulation

Drug Interactions CYP2C19 and 3A3/4 enzyme substrate

Increased Effect/Toxicity: Increases serum concentration of diazepam, digoxin, and penicillins

Decreased Effect: Decreases absorption of dapsone, iron, itraconazole, ketoconazole and other drugs where an acidic stomach is required for absorption

Drug Uptake

Half-life, elimination: 1-1.5 hours

Time to peak: 1.5 hours

Pregnancy Risk Factor B

Generic Available No

Esoterica® Facial [OTC] *see* Hydroquinone *on page 611*

Esoterica® Regular [OTC] *see* Hydroquinone *on page 611*

Esoterica® Sensitive Skin Formula [OTC] *see* Hydroquinone *on page 611*

Esoterica® Sunscreen [OTC] *see* Hydroquinone *on page 611*

Estar® [OTC] *see* Coal Tar *on page 315*

Estazolam (es TA zoe lam)

U.S. Brand Names ProSom™

Mexican Brand Names Tasedan

Pharmacologic Category Benzodiazepine

Use Short-term management of insomnia; there has been little experience with this drug in the elderly, but because of its lack of active metabolites, it is a reasonable choice when a benzodiazepine hypnotic is indicated

Local Anesthetic/Vasoconstrictor Precautions No information available to require special precautions

Effects on Dental Treatment ≤10%: Significant xerostomia; disappears with discontinuation

Restrictions C-IV

Dosage Adults: Oral: 1 mg at bedtime, some patients may require 2 mg; start at doses of 0.5 mg in debilitated or small elderly patients

Mechanism of Action Benzodiazepines may exert their pharmacologic effect through potentiation of the inhibitory activity of GABA. Benzodiazepines do not alter the synthesis, release, reuptake, or enzymatic degradation of GABA. Binds to stereospecific benzodiazepine receptors on the postsynaptic GABA neuron at several sites within the CNS, including the limbic system, reticular formation.

Enhancement of the inhibitory effect of GABA on neuronal excitability results by increased neuronal membrane permeability to chloride ions. This shift in chloride ions results in hyperpolarization (a less excitable state) and stabilization.

Other Adverse Effects

>10%:

Central nervous system: Somnolence

Neuromuscular & skeletal: Weakness

1% to 10%:

Cardiovascular: Flushing, palpitations

Central nervous system: Anxiety, confusion, dizziness, hypokinesia, abnormal coordination, hangover effect, agitation, amnesia, apathy, emotional lability, euphoria, hostility, seizure, sleep disorder, stupor, twitch

Dermatologic: Dermatitis, pruritus, rash, urticaria

Gastrointestinal: Xerostomia, constipation, decreased appetite, flatulence, gastritis, increased appetite, perverse taste

Genitourinary: Frequent urination, menstrual cramps, urinary hesitancy, urinary frequency, vaginal discharge/itching

Neuromuscular & skeletal: Paresthesia

Otic: Photophobia, eye pain, eye swelling

Respiratory: Cough, dyspnea, asthma, rhinitis, sinusitis

Miscellaneous: Diaphoresis

Drug Interactions CYP3A3/4 enzyme substrate

Increased Effect/Toxicity: Serum levels and/or toxicity of estazolam may be increased by cimetidine, ciprofloxacin, clarithromycin, clozapine, CNS depressants, diltiazem, disulfiram, digoxin, erythromycin, fluconazole, fluoxetine, fluvoxamine, isoniazid, itraconazole, ketoconazole, labetalol, levodopa, loxapine, metoprolol, metronidazole, miconazole, nefazodone, omeprazole, phenytoin, rifabutin, rifampin, troleandomycin, valproic acid, and verapamil.

Decreased Effect: Carbamazepine, rifampin, rifabutin may enhance the metabolism of estazolam and decrease its therapeutic effect.

Drug Uptake Studies have shown that the elderly are more sensitive to the effects of benzodiazepines as compared to younger adults

Onset of action: ~1 hour

Duration: Variable

Half-life, elimination: 10-24 hours (no significant changes in the elderly)

Time to peak: 0.5-1.6 hours

Pregnancy Risk Factor X

Generic Available Yes

Estinyl® *see* Ethinyl Estradiol *on page 474*

Estrace® *see* Estradiol *on page 457*

Estraderm® *see* Estradiol *on page 457*

Estradiol (es tra DYE ole)

Related Information

Endocrine Disorders and Pregnancy *on page 1331*

U.S. Brand Names Alora®; Climara®; Delestrogen®; Depo®-Estradiol; Esclim®; Estrace®; Estraderm®; Estring®; Gynodiol™; Vagifem®; Vivelle®; Vivelle-Dot®

Canadian Brand Names Climara®; Delestrogen®; Depo®-Estradiol; Estrace®; Estraderm®; Estring®; Estrogel®; Oesclim®; Vagifem®; Vivelle®

Mexican Brand Names Climaderm; Estraderm TTS®; Ginedisc®; Oestrogel; Systen

Pharmacologic Category Estrogen Derivative

Synonyms Estradiol Cypionate; Estradiol Hemihydrate; Estradiol Transdermal; Estradiol Valerate

Use Treatment of moderate to severe vasomotor symptoms associated with menopause; treatment of vulvar and vaginal atrophy; hypoestrogenism (due to hypogonadism, castration, or primary ovarian failure); prostatic cancer (palliation), breast cancer (palliation), osteoporosis (prophylactic); abnormal uterine bleeding due to hormonal imbalance; postmenopausal urogenital symptoms of the lower urinary tract (urinary urgency, dysuria)

Local Anesthetic/Vasoconstrictor Precautions No information available to require special precautions

Effects on Dental Treatment No effects or complications reported

Dosage All dosage needs to be adjusted based upon the patient's response

Oral:

Prostate cancer (androgen-dependent, inoperable, progressing): 10 mg 3 times/day for at least 3 months

Breast cancer (inoperable, progressing in appropriately selected patients): 10 mg 3 times/day for at least 3 months

Osteoporosis prophylaxis in postmenopausal females: 0.5 mg/day in a cyclic regimen (3 weeks on and 1 week off)

Female hypoestrogenism (due to hypogonadism, castration, or primary ovarian failure): 1-2 mg/day; titrate as necessary to control symptoms using minimal effective dose for maintenance therapy

(Continued)

Estradiol *(Continued)*

Treatment of moderate to severe vasomotor symptoms associated with menopause: 1-2 mg/day, adjusted as necessary to limit symptoms; administration should be cyclic (3 weeks on, 1 week off). Patients should be re-evaluated at 3- to 6-month intervals to determine if treatment is still necessary.

I.M.

Prostate cancer: Valerate: ≥30 mg or more every 1-2 weeks

Moderate to severe vasomotor symptoms associated with menopause:

Cypionate: 1-5 mg every 3-4 weeks

Valerate: 10-20 mg every 4 weeks

Female hypoestrogenism (due to hypogonadism):

Cypionate: 1.5-2 mg monthly

Valerate: 10-20 mg every 4 weeks

Transdermal: Indicated dose may be used continuously in patients without an intact uterus. May be given continuously or cyclically (3 weeks on, 1 week off) in patients with an intact uterus. When changing patients from oral to transdermal therapy, start transdermal patch 1 week after discontinuing oral hormone (may begin sooner if symptoms reappear within 1 week):

Once-weekly patch:

Moderate to severe vasomotor symptoms associated with menopause (Climara®): Apply 0.025 mg/day patch once weekly. Adjust dose as necessary to control symptoms. Patients should be re-evaluated at 3- to 6-month intervals to determine if treatment is still necessary.

Osteoporosis prophylaxis in postmenopausal women (Climara®): Apply patch once weekly; minimum effective dose 0.025 mg/day; adjust response to therapy by biochemical markers and bone mineral density

Twice-weekly patch:

Moderate to severe vasomotor symptoms associated with menopause, vulvar/vaginal atrophy, female hypogonadism: Titrate to lowest dose possible to control symptoms, adjusting initial dose after the first month of therapy; re-evaluate therapy at 3- to 6-month intervals to taper or discontinue medication:

Alora®, Esclim®, Estraderm®, Vivelle-Dot™: Apply 0.05 mg patch twice weekly

Vivelle®: Apply 0.0375 mg patch twice weekly

Prevention of osteoporosis in postmenopausal women:

Estraderm®: Apply 0.05 mg patch twice weekly

Vivelle®: Apply 0.025 mg patch twice weekly, adjust dose as necessary

Vaginal cream: Vulvar and vaginal atrophy: Insert 2-4 g/day intravaginally for 2 weeks, then gradually reduce to ½ the initial dose for 2 weeks, followed by a maintenance dose of 1 g 1-3 times/week

Vaginal ring: Postmenopausal vaginal atrophy, urogenital symptoms: Estring®: Following insertion, Estring® should remain in place for 90 days

Vaginal tablets: Atrophic vaginitis: Vagifem®: Initial: Insert 1 tablet once daily for 2 weeks; maintenance: Insert 1 tablet twice weekly; attempts to discontinue or taper medication should be made at 3- to 6-month intervals

Dosing adjustment in hepatic impairment:

Mild to moderate liver impairment: Dosage reduction of estrogens is recommended

Severe liver impairment: **Not recommended**

Mechanism of Action Increases synthesis of DNA, RNA, and various proteins in target tissues; reduces the release of gonadotropin-releasing hormone from the hypothalamus and FSH and LH release from the pituitary; it is the principle intracellular human estrogen, more potent than estrone and estriol at the receptor level and it is the primary estrogen secreted prior to menopause. Following menopause, estrone and estrone sulfate are more highly produced. Estrogens modulate the pituitary secretion of gonadotropins, luteinizing hormone, and follicle-stimulating hormone through a negative feedback system; estrogen replacement reduces elevated levels of these hormones in postmenopausal women.

Other Adverse Effects Frequency not defined:

Cardiovascular: Edema, hypertension, venous thromboembolism

Central nervous system: Dizziness, headache, mental depression, migraine

Dermatologic: Chloasma, erythema multiforme, erythema nodosum, hemorrhagic eruption, hirsutism, loss of scalp hair, melasma

Endocrine & metabolic: Breast enlargement, breast tenderness, changes in libido, increased thyroid-binding globulin, increased total thyroid hormone (T_4), increased serum triglycerides/phospholipids, increased HDL-cholesterol, decreased LDL-cholesterol, impaired glucose tolerance, hypercalcemia

Gastrointestinal: Abdominal cramps, bloating, cholecystitis, cholelithiasis, gallbladder disease, nausea, pancreatitis, vomiting, weight gain/loss

Genitourinary: Alterations in frequency and flow of menses, changes in cervical secretions, endometrial cancer, increased size of uterine leiomyomata, vaginal candidiasis

Vaginal: Trauma from applicator insertion may occur in women with severely atrophic vaginal mucosa

Hematologic: Aggravation of porphyria, decreased antithrombin III and antifactor Xa, increased levels of fibrinogen, increased platelet aggregability and platelet count; increased prothrombin and factors VII, VIII, IX, X

Hepatic: Cholestatic jaundice

Local: Transdermal patches: Burning, erythema, irritation, pruritus, rash

Neuromuscular & skeletal: Chorea

Ocular: Intolerance to contact lenses, steeping of corneal curvature

Respiratory: Pulmonary thromboembolism

Miscellaneous: Carbohydrate intolerance

Drug Interactions CYP1A2 and 3A3/4 enzyme substrate; CYP1A2 enzyme inhibitor

Anticoagulants: Increase potential for thromboembolic events

Corticosteroids: Estrogens may enhance the effects of hydrocortisone and prednisone

Enzyme inducers: May increase the metabolism of estradiol resulting in decreased effect; includes carbamazepine, phenobarbital, phenytoin, primidone, rifabutin, and rifampin

Drug Uptake

Absorption: Oral, topical: Well absorbed

Half-life, elimination: 50-60 minutes

Pregnancy Risk Factor X

Generic Available Yes

Estradiol and Norethindrone (es tra DYE ole & nor eth IN drone)

U.S. Brand Names Activella™; CombiPatch™

Pharmacologic Category Estrogen Derivative

Synonyms Norethindrone and Estradiol

Use For use in women with an intact uterus

Tablet: Treatment of moderate to severe vasomotor symptoms associated with menopause; treatment of vulvar and vaginal atrophy; prophylaxis for postmenopausal osteoporosis

Transdermal patch: Treatment of moderate to severe vasomotor symptoms associated with menopause; treatment of vulvar and vaginal atrophy; treatment of hypoestrogenism due to hypogonadism, castration, or primary ovarian failure

Local Anesthetic/Vasoconstrictor Precautions No information available to require special precautions

Effects on Dental Treatment No effects or complications reported

Dosage Adults:

Oral: 1 tablet daily

Transdermal patch:

Continuous combined regimen: Apply one patch twice weekly

Continuous sequential regimen: Apply estradiol-only patch for first 14 days of cycle, followed by one Combi-Patch® applied twice weekly for the remaining 14 days of a 28-day cycle

Other Adverse Effects Frequency not defined:

Cardiovascular: Altered BP, cardiovascular accident, edema, venous thromboembolism

Central nervous system: Dizziness, fatigue, headache, insomnia, mental depression, migraine, nervousness

Dermatologic: Chloasma, erythema multiforme, erythema nodosum, hemorrhagic eruption, hirsutism, itching, loss of scalp hair, melasma, pruritus, skin rash

Endocrine & metabolic: Breast enlargement, breast tenderness, breast pain, changes in libido

Gastrointestinal: Abdominal pain, bloating, changes in appetite, flatulence, gallbladder disease, nausea, pancreatitis, vomiting, weight gain/loss

Genitourinary: Alterations in frequency and flow of menses, changes in cervical secretions, cystitis-like syndrome, increased size of uterine leiomyomata, premenstrual-like syndrome, vaginal candidiasis, vaginitis

Hematologic: Aggravation of porphyria

Hepatic: Cholestatic jaundice

Local: Application site reaction (transdermal patch)

Neuromuscular & skeletal: Arthralgia, back pain, chorea, myalgia, weakness

Ocular: Intolerance to contact lenses, steeping of corneal curvature

Respiratory: Pharyngitis, pulmonary thromboembolism, rhinitis

Miscellaneous: Allergic reactions, carbohydrate intolerance, flu-like syndrome

Drug Uptake Absorption: Well absorbed

Activella:™

Half-life, elimination: Estradiol: 12-14 hours; Norethindrone: 8-11 hours

Time to peak: Estradiol: 5-8 hours See Estradiol *on page 457* and Norethindrone *on page 876*

Pregnancy Risk Factor X

Generic Available No

Estradiol and Norgestimate (es tra DYE ole & nor JES ti mate)

U.S. Brand Names Ortho-Prefest®

Pharmacologic Category Estrogen and Progestin Combination

Synonyms Estradiol and NGM; Norgestimate and Estradiol

Use Women with an intact uterus: Treatment of moderate to severe vasomotor symptoms associated with menopause; treatment of atrophic vaginitis; prevention of osteoporosis

Local Anesthetic/Vasoconstrictor Precautions No information available to require special precautions

Effects on Dental Treatment No effects or complications reported

Dosage Oral: Adults: Females with an intact uterus:

Treatment of menopausal symptoms, atrophic vaginitis: Treatment is cyclical and consists of the following: One tablet of estradiol 1 mg (pink tablet) once daily for 3 days, followed by 1 tablet of estradiol 1 mg and norgestimate 0.09 mg (white tablet) once daily for 3 days; repeat sequence continuously. **Note:** This dose may not be the lowest effective combination for these indications. In case of a missed tablet, restart therapy with next available tablet in sequence (taking only 1 tablet each day).

Prevention of osteoporosis: See "Treatment of menopausal symptoms"

Mechanism of Action Estrogens are responsible for the development and maintenance of the female reproductive system and secondary sexual characteristics. Estradiol is the principle intracellular human estrogen and is more potent than estrone and estriol at the receptor level; it is the primary estrogen secreted prior to menopause. Following menopause, estrone and estrone sulfate are more highly produced. Estrogens modulate the pituitary secretion of gonadotropins, luteinizing hormone, and follicle-stimulating hormone through a negative feedback system; estrogen replacement reduces elevated levels of these hormones in postmenopausal women.

Progestins inhibit gonadotropin production which then prevents follicular maturation and ovulation. In women with adequate estrogen, progestins transform a proliferative endometrium into a secretory endometrium; when administered with estradiol, reduces the incidence of endometrial hyperplasia and risk of adenocarcinoma.

Other Adverse Effects

>10:
- Central nervous system: Headache (23%)
- Endocrine & metabolic: Breast pain (16%)
- Gastrointestinal: Abdominal pain (12%)
- Neuromuscular & skeletal: Back pain (12%)
- Respiratory: Upper respiratory tract infection (21%)
- Miscellaneous: Flu-like symptoms (11%)

1% to 10%:
- Central nervous system: Fatigue (6%), pain (6%), depression (5%), dizziness (5%)
- Endocrine & metabolic: Vaginal bleeding (9%), dysmenorrhea (8%), vaginitis (7%)
- Gastrointestinal: Nausea (6%), flatulence (5%)
- Neuromuscular & skeletal: Arthralgia (9%), myalgia (5%)
- Respiratory: Sinusitis (8%), pharyngitis (7%), coughing (5%)
- Miscellaneous: Viral infection (6%)

Additional adverse effects associated with **estrogens**. Frequency not defined:
- Cardiovascular: Edema
- Central nervous system: Migraine
- Dermatologic: Chloasma, melasma, erythema multiforme, hemorrhagic eruptions, loss of scalp hair, hirsutism
- Endocrine & metabolic: Breast tenderness, breast enlargement, galactorrhea, decreased carbohydrate tolerance, changes in libido
- Gastrointestinal: Abdominal cramps, bloating, gallbladder disease, vomiting, weight gain/loss
- Genitourinary: Changes in vaginal bleeding, abnormal withdrawal bleeding/flow, breakthrough bleeding, spotting, increase in size of uterine leiomyomata, vaginal candidiasis, changes in cervical secretion
- Hematologic: Porphyria
- Hepatic: Cholestatic jaundice
- Neuromuscular & skeletal: Chorea
- Ocular: Steepening of corneal curvature, intolerance to contact lenses

Drug Interactions

Increased Effect/Toxicity: Acetaminophen and ascorbic acid may increase plasma concentrations of estrogen component. Atorvastatin and indinavir increase plasma concentrations of estrogen/progestin combinations. Estrogen/progestin combinations increase the plasma concentrations of alprazolam, chlordiazepoxide, cyclosporine, diazepam, prednisolone, selegiline, theophylline, tricyclic antidepressants. Estrogen/progestin combinations may increase (or decrease) the effects of coumarin derivatives.

Decreased Effect: Estrogen/progestin combinations may decrease plasma concentrations of acetaminophen, clofibric acid, lorazepam, morphine, oxazepam, salicylic acid, temazepam. Estrogen/progestin levels decreased by aminoglutethimide, amprenavir, anticonvulsants, griseofulvin, lopinavir, nelfinavir, nevirapine, rifampin, and ritonavir. Estrogen/progestin combinations may decrease (or increase) the effects of coumarin derivatives.

Drug Uptake Half-life, elimination: Estradiol: 16 hours; 17-deacetylnorgestimate: 37 hours See Estradiol *on page 457*

Pregnancy Risk Factor X

Generic Available No

Estradiol and Testosterone (es tra DYE ole & tes TOS ter one)

U.S. Brand Names Depo-Testadiol®; Depotestogen®; Duo-Cyp®; Valertest No.1®

Canadian Brand Names Climacteron®

Pharmacologic Category Estrogen Derivative

Synonyms Estradiol Cypionate and Testosterone Cypionate; Estradiol Valerate and Testosterone Enanthate; Testosterone and Estradiol

Use Vasomotor symptoms associated with menopause; postpartum breast engorgement

Local Anesthetic/Vasoconstrictor Precautions No information available to require special precautions

Effects on Dental Treatment No effects or complications reported

Dosage Adults: All dosage needs to be adjusted based upon the patient's response

Other Adverse Effects Frequency not defined:

- Cardiovascular: Hypertension, edema, thromboembolism, myocardial infarction
- Central nervous system: Stroke, depression, dizziness, anxiety, headache, migraine
- Dermatologic: Chloasma, melasma, rash
- Endocrine & metabolic: Alterations in frequency and flow of menses, breast tenderness or enlargement, decreased glucose tolerance, increased triglycerides and LDL
- Gastrointestinal: Nausea, GI distress
- Hepatic: Cholestatic jaundice
- Miscellaneous: Increased susceptibility to *Candida* infection

Drug Uptake See Estradiol *on page 457* and Testosterone *on page 1143*

Pregnancy Risk Factor X

Generic Available No

Estradiol Cypionate and Medroxyprogesterone Acetate

(es tra DYE ole sip pe OH nate & me DROKS ee proe JES te rone AS e tate)

U.S. Brand Names Lunelle™

Pharmacologic Category Contraceptive

Synonyms E_2C and MPA; Medroxyprogesterone Acetate and Estradiol Cypionate

Use Prevention of pregnancy

Local Anesthetic/Vasoconstrictor Precautions No information available to require special precautions

Effects on Dental Treatment Since this is a combination estrogen-progesterone product, when prescribing antibiotics, patient must be warned to use additional methods of birth control if on hormonal contraceptives.

Dosage Adults: Female: I.M.: 0.5 mL

- First dose: Within first 5 days of menstrual period or within 5 days of a complete first trimester abortion; do not administer <4 weeks postpartum **if not breast-feeding** or <6 weeks postpartum **if breast-feeding**
- Maintenance dose: Monthly, every 28-30 days following previous injection; do not exceed 33 days; pregnancy must be ruled out if >33 days have past between injections; bleeding episodes cannot be used to guide injection schedule; shortening schedule may lead to menstrual pattern changes
- Switching from other forms of contraception: First injection should be given within 7 days of last active oral contraceptive pill; when switching from other methods, timing of injection should ensure continuous contraceptive coverage
- Elderly: Not intended for use in postmenopausal women

Mechanism of Action Inhibits secretion of gonadotropins, leading to prevention of follicular maturation and ovulation. Also leads to thickening and reduction in volume of cervical mucus (decreases sperm penetration) and thinning of endometrium (reduces possibility of implantation).

Other Adverse Effects Frequency not defined:

- Cardiovascular: Arterial thromboembolism, cerebral hemorrhage, cerebral thrombosis, edema, hypertension, mesenteric thrombosis, myocardial infarction
- Central nervous system: Dizziness, emotional lability, headache, mental depression, migraine, nervousness, premenstrual syndrome
- Dermatologic: Acne, alopecia, erythema multiforme, erythema nodosum, hirsutism, melasma, rash (allergic)
- Endocrine & metabolic: Amenorrhea, breast enlargement, breast secretion, breast tenderness/pain, decreased lactation (immediately postpartum), decreased

(Continued)

Estradiol Cypionate and Medroxyprogesterone Acetate *(Continued)*

libido/libido changes, dysmenorrhea, menorrhagia, metrorrhagia, temporary infertility following discontinuation

Gastrointestinal: Abdominal pain, appetite changes, enlarged abdomen, colitis, gallbladder disease, nausea, weight gain/loss (weight gain was the most common reason for discontinuing medication)

Genitourinary: Cervical changes, cystitis-like syndrome, vaginal moniliasis, vaginitis, vulvovaginal disorder

Hematologic: Hemolytic uremic syndrome, hemorrhagic eruption, porphyria

Hepatic: Budd-Chiari syndrome, hepatic adenoma, benign hepatic tumor

Local: Thrombophlebitis

Neuromuscular & skeletal: Weakness

Ocular: Cataracts, intolerance to contact lenses, retinal thrombosis

Renal: Impaired renal function

Respiratory: Pulmonary thromboembolism

Miscellaneous: Anaphylaxis, carbohydrate intolerance

Drug Interactions Ethinyl estradiol is a CYP1A2, 3A3/4, and 3A5-7 enzyme substrate.

Increased Effect/Toxicity: Estradiol may inhibit metabolism of cyclosporine, prednisolone, and theophylline, leading to increased plasma concentrations.

Decreased Effect: Estradiol may decrease plasma concentrations of acetaminophen, clofibrate, morphine, salicylic acid, and temazepam. Enzyme inducers (carbamazepine, phenobarbital, phenytoin, and rifampin) may increase the metabolism of estradiol, resulting in decreased effect, leading to pregnancy. Griseofulvin, penicillins, and tetracyclines have been shown to alter pharmacokinetics of oral contraceptives leading to pregnancy; effects are not consistent with synthetic steroids. Aminoglutethimide and phenylbutazone may decrease contraceptive effectiveness and increase menstrual irregularities. St John's wort may induce hepatic enzymes resulting in decreased effect of contraceptive and breakthrough bleeding.

Drug Uptake

Absorption: Prolonged

Half-life, elimination: Mean: 17 β-estradiol: 8.4 days; MPA: 14.7 days

Time to peak: 17 β-estradiol: 1-7 days; MPA: 1-10 days

Pregnancy Risk Factor X

Estramustine (es tra MUS teen)

U.S. Brand Names Emcyt®

Canadian Brand Names Emcyt®

Pharmacologic Category Antineoplastic Agent, Alkylating Agent

Synonyms Estramustine Phosphate Sodium

Use Palliative treatment of prostatic carcinoma (progressive or metastatic)

Local Anesthetic/Vasoconstrictor Precautions No information available to require special precautions

Effects on Dental Treatment No effects or complications reported

Mechanism of Action Mechanism is not completely clear, thought to act as an alkylating agent and as estrogen

Other Adverse Effects

>10%:

- Cardiovascular: Impaired arterial circulation; ischemic heart disease; venous thromboembolism; cardiac decompensation (58%), about 50% of complications occur within the first 2 months of therapy, 85% occur within the first year; edema
- Endocrine & metabolic: Sodium and water retention, gynecomastia, breast tenderness, decreased libido
- Gastrointestinal: Nausea, vomiting, may be dose-limiting
- Hematologic: Thrombocytopenia
- Local: Thrombophlebitis (nearly 100% with I.V. administration)
- Respiratory: Dyspnea

1% to 10%:

- Cardiovascular: Myocardial infarction
- Central nervous system: Insomnia, lethargy
- Gastrointestinal: Diarrhea, anorexia, flatulence
- Hematologic: Leukopenia
- Hepatic: Increases in serum transaminases, jaundice
- Neuromuscular & skeletal: Leg cramps
- Respiratory: Pulmonary embolism

Drug Interactions Decreased Effect: Calcium-rich drugs may impair oral absorption.

Drug Uptake

Absorption: Oral: Well absorbed (75%)

Half-life, elimination: Terminal: 20-24 hours

Time to peak: 2-3 hours

Pregnancy Risk Factor C

Generic Available No

Estratab® *see* Estrogens, Esterified *on page 467*

Estratest® *see* Estrogens and Methyltestosterone *on page 463*

Estratest® H.S. *see* Estrogens and Methyltestosterone *on page 463*

Estring® *see* Estradiol *on page 457*

Estrogens and Methyltestosterone

(ES troe jenz & meth il tes TOS te rone)

Related Information

Endocrine Disorders and Pregnancy *on page 1331*

U.S. Brand Names Estratest®; Estratest® H.S.

Canadian Brand Names Estratest®

Pharmacologic Category Estrogen Derivative

Synonyms Conjugated Estrogen and Methyltestosterone; Esterified Estrogen and Methyltestosterone

Use Atrophic vaginitis; hypogonadism; primary ovarian failure; vasomotor symptoms of menopause; prostatic carcinoma; osteoporosis prophylactic

Local Anesthetic/Vasoconstrictor Precautions No information available to require special precautions

Effects on Dental Treatment No effects or complications reported

Dosage Adults: Female: Oral: Lowest dose that will control symptoms should be chosen, normally given 3 weeks on and 1 week off

Mechanism of Action Conjugated estrogens: Combination of the sodium salts of the sulfate esters of estrogenic substances, representing the average composition of material obtained from pregnant mare's urine. The primary preparation utilized is Premarin®; however, other generic products are available. Premarin® contains 50% to 65% estrone sodium sulfate, 20% to 35% equilin sodium sulfate, and 17 alpha-dihydroequilin, together with smaller amounts of 17 alpha-estradiol, equilenin, and 17 alpha-dihydroequilenin, all as salts of the sulfate ester. Estrogens are important for developing secondary sex characteristics and promote growth in development of the vagina, uterus, fallopian tubes, and enlargement of the breast. Eventually, they stimulate and limit linear skeletal growth, and have widespread effects on metabolism such as transporting proteins and electrolyte balance. Conjugates activate estrogen receptors (DNA protein complex) located in estrogen-responsive tissues. Once activated, regulate transcription of certain genes leading to observed effects.

Testosterone: It has been reported that androgens increase protein anabolism and decrease protein catabolism; increases synthesis of DNA, RNA, and various proteins in target tissues; however, nitrogen balance is only improved when androgen therapy is accompanied by adequate caloric and protein intake. Testosterone and related androgens cause retention of phosphorous, potassium, sodium, and nitrogen, and decrease renal excretion of calcium. Production of red blood cells secondary to erythropoietic factor stimulation has been reported with androgen administration.

Other Adverse Effects 1% to 10%:

Cardiovascular: Increase in BP, edema, thromboembolic disorder

Central nervous system: Depression, headache

Dermatologic: Chloasma, melasma

Endocrine & metabolic: Breast tenderness, change in menstrual flow, hypercalcemia

Gastrointestinal: Nausea, vomiting

Hepatic: Cholestatic jaundice

Drug Uptake

Conjugated estrogens:

- Absorption: Readily absorbed from GI tract

Testosterone:

- Duration of therapeutic effect: Depends upon route of administration and which testosterone ester used; slow absorption extends duration of activity; I.M. administration usually lasts for 2-4 weeks
- Absorption: I.M.: Absorbed slowly allowing for dosing intervals of 2-4 weeks
- Half-life, elimination: I.M.: ~8 days

See Estrogens, Conjugated *on page 463* and Methyltestosterone *on page 799*

Pregnancy Risk Factor X

Generic Available No

Estrogens, Conjugated (ES troe jenz KON joo gate ed, EE kwine)

Related Information

Dental Drug Interactions: Update on Drug Combinations Requiring Special Considerations *on page 1434*

Endocrine Disorders and Pregnancy *on page 1331*

U.S. Brand Names Premarin®

(Continued)

Estrogens, Conjugated *(Continued)*

Canadian Brand Names Cenestin; C.E.S.®; Congest; PMS-Conjugated Estrogens; Premarin®

Pharmacologic Category Estrogen Derivative

Synonyms C.E.S.; Estrogenic Substances, Conjugated

Use Treatment of moderate to severe vasomotor symptoms associated with menopause; treatment of vulvar and vaginal atrophy; hypoestrogenism (due to hypogonadism, castration, or primary ovarian failure); prostatic cancer (palliation); breast cancer (palliation); osteoporosis (prophylactic)

Unlabeled/Investigational: Uremic bleeding; abnormal uterine bleeding

Local Anesthetic/Vasoconstrictor Precautions No information available to require special precautions

Effects on Dental Treatment No effects or complications reported

Dosage Adults:

Male and Female:

Breast cancer palliation, metastatic disease in selected patients: Oral: 10 mg 3 times/day for at least 3 months

Uremic bleeding: I.V.: 0.6 mg/kg/day for 5 days

Male: Androgen-dependent prostate cancer: Oral: 1.25-2.5 mg 3 times/day

Female:

Prevention of osteoporosis in postmenopausal women: Oral: 0.625 mg/day, cyclically* or daily, depending on medical assessment of patient

Moderate to severe vasomotor symptoms: Oral: 0.625 mg/day; lowest dose that will control symptoms should be used. Medication should be discontinued as soon as possible. May be given cyclically* or daily, depending on medical assessment of patient

Vulvar and vaginal atrophy:

Oral: 0.3-1.25 mg (or more) daily, depending on tissue response of the patient; lowest dose that will control symptoms should be used. Medication should be discontinued as soon as possible. May be given cyclically* or daily, depending on medical assessment of patient.

Vaginal cream: Intravaginal: ½ to 2 g/day given cyclically*

Female hypogonadism: Oral: 0.3-0.625 mg/day given cyclically*; adjust dose in response to symptoms and endometrium response; progestin treatment should be added to maintain bone mineral density

Female castration, primary ovarian failure: Oral: 1.25 mg/day given cyclically*; adjust according to severity of symptoms and patient response. For maintenance, adjust to the lowest effective dose.

Abnormal uterine bleeding:

Acute/heavy bleeding:

Oral: 1.25 mg, may repeat every 4 hours for 24 hours, followed by 1.25 mg once daily for 7-10 days

I.V.: 25 mg, may repeat every 4 hours up to 3 doses

Note: Oral/I.V.: Treatment should be followed by a low-dose oral contraceptive; medroxyprogesterone acetate along with or following estrogen therapy can also be given

Nonacute/lesser bleeding: Oral: 1.25 mg once daily for 7-10 days

***Cyclic administration:** Either 3 weeks on, 1 week off **or** 25 days on, 5 days off

Mechanism of Action Contains a mixture of estrone sulfate, equilin sulfate, 17 alpha-dihydroequilin, 17 alpha-estradiol and 17 beta-dihydroequilin; estrogens are responsible for the development and maintenance of the female reproductive system and secondary sexual characteristics. Estradiol is the principle intracellular human estrogen and is more potent than estrone and estriol at the receptor level; it is the primary estrogen secreted prior to menopause. Following menopause, estrone and estrone sulfate are more highly produced. Estrogens modulate the pituitary secretion of gonadotropins, luteinizing hormone, and follicle-stimulating hormone through a negative feedback system; estrogen replacement reduces elevated levels of these hormones in postmenopausal women.

Other Adverse Effects Frequency not defined:

Cardiovascular: Edema, hypertension, venous thromboembolism

Central nervous system: Dizziness, headache, mental depression, migraine

Dermatologic: Chloasma, erythema multiforme, erythema nodosum, hemorrhagic eruption, hirsutism, loss of scalp hair, melasma

Endocrine & metabolic: Breast enlargement, breast tenderness, changes in libido, increased thyroid-binding globulin, increased total thyroid hormone (T_4), increased serum triglycerides/phospholipids, increased HDL-cholesterol, decreased LDL-cholesterol, impaired glucose tolerance, hypercalcemia

Gastrointestinal: Abdominal cramps, bloating, cholecystitis, cholelithiasis, gallbladder disease, nausea, pancreatitis, vomiting, weight gain/loss

Genitourinary: Alterations in frequency and flow of menses, changes in cervical secretions, endometrial cancer, increased size of uterine leiomyomata, vaginal candidiasis

Hematologic: Aggravation of porphyria, decreased antithrombin III and antifactor Xa, increased levels of fibrinogen, increased platelet aggregability and platelet count; increased prothrombin and factors VII, VIII, IX, X

Hepatic: Cholestatic jaundice
Neuromuscular & skeletal: Chorea
Ocular: Intolerance to contact lenses, steeping of corneal curvature
Respiratory: Pulmonary thromboembolism
Miscellaneous: Carbohydrate intolerance

Drug Interactions May be a substrate for cytochrome isoenzymes (profile not defined)

Increased Effect/Toxicity: Hydrocortisone taken with estrogen may cause corticosteroid-induced toxicity. Increased potential for thromboembolic events with anticoagulants.

Decreased Effect: Rifampin, nelfinavir, and ritonavir decrease estradiol serum concentration. Anticonvulsants which are enzyme inducers (barbiturates, carbamazepine, phenobarbital, phenytoin, primidone) may potentially decrease estrogen levels.

Drug Uptake Absorption: Well absorbed

Pregnancy Risk Factor X

Generic Available No

Estrogens (Conjugated) and Medroxyprogesterone

(ES troe jenz KON joo gate ed & me DROKS ee proe JES te rone)

Related Information

Endocrine Disorders and Pregnancy *on page 1331*

U.S. Brand Names Premphase®; Prempro™

Canadian Brand Names Premphase®; Prempro™

Pharmacologic Category Estrogen Derivative

Synonyms Medroxyprogesterone and Estrogens (Conjugated); MPA and Estrogens (Conjugated)

Use Women with an intact uterus for the treatment of moderate to severe vasomotor symptoms associated with the menopause; treatment of atrophic vaginitis; primary ovarian failure; osteoporosis prophylactic

Local Anesthetic/Vasoconstrictor Precautions No information available to require special precautions

Effects on Dental Treatment No effects or complications reported

Dosage Oral: Adults:

Treatment of moderate to severe vasomotor symptoms associated with menopause or treatment of atrophic vaginitis in females with an intact uterus:

- Premphase®: One maroon conjugated estrogen 0.625 mg tablet daily on days 1 through 14 and one light blue conjugated estrogen 0.625 mg/MPA 5 mg tablet daily on days 15 through 28; re-evaluate patients at 3- and 6-month intervals to determine if treatment is still necessary; monitor patients for signs of endometrial cancer; rule out malignancy if unexplained vaginal bleeding occurs
- Prempro™: One conjugated estrogen 0.625 mg/MPA 2.5 mg tablet daily; re-evaluate at 3-and 6-month intervals to determine if therapy is still needed; dose may be increased to one conjugated estrogen 0.625 mg/MPA 5 mg tablet daily in patients with bleeding or spotting, once malignancy has been ruled out

Osteoporosis prophylaxis in females with an intact uterus:

- Premphase®: One maroon conjugated estrogen 0.625 tablet daily on days 1 through 14 and one light blue conjugated estrogen 0.625 mg/MPA 5 mg tablet daily on days 15 through 28; monitor patients for signs of endometrial cancer; rule out malignancy if unexplained vaginal bleeding occurs
- Prempro™: One conjugated estrogen 0.625 mg/MPA 2.5 mg tablet daily; dose may be increased to one conjugated estrogen 0.625 mg/MPA 5 mg tablet daily; in patients with bleeding or spotting, once malignancy has been ruled out

Mechanism of Action Conjugated estrogens contain a mixture of estrone sulfate, equilin sulfate, 17 alpha-dihydroequilin, 17 alpha-estradiol, and 17 beta-dihydroequilin. Estrogens are responsible for the development and maintenance of the female reproductive system and secondary sexual characteristics. Estradiol is the principle intracellular human estrogen and is more potent than estrone and estriol at the receptor level; it is the primary estrogen secreted prior to menopause. Following menopause, estrone and estrone sulfate are more highly produced. Estrogens modulate the pituitary secretion of gonadotropins, luteinizing hormone, and follicle-stimulating hormone through a negative feedback system; estrogen replacement reduces elevated levels of these hormones in postmenopausal women.

MPA inhibits gonadotropin production which then prevents follicular maturation and ovulation. In women with adequate estrogen, MPA transforms a proliferative endometrium into a secretory endometrium; when administered with conjugated estrogens, reduces the incidence of endometrial hyperplasia and risk of adenocarcinoma.

Other Adverse Effects

>10%:

Central nervous system: Headache (28% to 37%), pain (11% to 13%), depression (6% to 11%)

Endocrine & metabolic: Breast pain (32% to 38%), dysmenorrhea (8% to 13%)

(Continued)

Estrogens (Conjugated) and Medroxyprogesterone *(Continued)*

Gastrointestinal: Abdominal pain (16% to 23%), nausea (9% to 11%)
Neuromuscular & skeletal: Back pain (13% to 16%)
Respiratory: Pharyngitis (11% to 13%)
Miscellaneous: Infection (16% to 18%), flu-like syndrome (10% to 13%)

1% to 10%:
Cardiovascular: Peripheral edema (3% to 4%)
Central nervous system: Dizziness (3% to 5%)
Dermatologic: Pruritus (5% to 10%), rash (4% to 6%)
Endocrine & metabolic: Leukorrhea (5% to 9%)
Gastrointestinal: Flatulence (8% to 9%), diarrhea (5% to 6%), dyspepsia (5% to 6%)
Genitourinary: Vaginitis (5% to 7%), cervical changes (4% to 5%), vaginal hemorrhage (1% to 3%)
Neuromuscular & skeletal: Weakness (6% to 10%), arthralgia (7% to 9%), leg cramps (3% to 5%), hypertonia (3% to 4%)
Respiratory: Sinusitis (7% to 8%), rhinitis (6% to 8%)

Additional adverse effects reported with conjugated estrogens and/or progestins: Abdominal cramps, acne, abnormal uterine bleeding, aggravation of porphyria, amenorrhea, anaphylactoid reactions, anaphylaxis, antifactor Xa decreased, antithrombin III decreased, appetite changes, bloating, breast enlargement, breast tenderness, cerebral embolism, cerebral thrombosis, chloasma, cholestatic jaundice, cholecystitis, cholelithiasis, chorea, contact lens intolerance, cystitis-like syndrome, decreased carbohydrate tolerance; factors VII, VIII, IX, X, XII, VII-X complex, and II-VII-X complex increased; endometrial hyperplasia, erythema multiforme, erythema nodosum, galactorrhea, hemorrhagic eruption, fatigue, fibrinogen increased, impaired glucose tolerance, HDL-cholesterol increased, hirsutism, hypertension, increase in size of uterine leiomyomata, gallbladder disease, insomnia, LDL-cholesterol decreased, libido changes, loss of scalp hair, melasma, migraine, nervousness, optic neuritis, pancreatitis, platelet aggregability and platelet count increased, premenstrual like syndrome, PT and PTT accelerated, pulmonary embolism, pyrexia, retinal thrombosis, somnolence, steepening of corneal curvature, thrombophlebitis, thyroid-binding globulin increased, total thyroid hormone (T_4) increased, triglycerides increased, urticaria, vaginal candidiasis, vomiting, weight gain/loss

Contraindications Hypersensitivity to conjugated estrogens, medroxyprogesterone (MPA), or any component of their formulation; undiagnosed abnormal vaginal bleeding; history of or current thrombophlebitis or thromboembolic disorders; known or suspected pregnancy; carcinoma of the breast; estrogen-dependent tumor; hepatic dysfunction or disease

Drug Interactions Estrogen may induce and is a substrate for CYP isoenzymes; estradiol is a CYP1A2 enzyme inhibitor

Increased Effect/Toxicity: Hydrocortisone taken with estrogen may cause corticosteroid-induced toxicity. Increased potential for thromboembolic events with anticoagulants.

Decreased Effect: Conjugated estrogens: Anticonvulsants which are enzyme inducers (barbiturates, carbamazepine, phenobarbital, phenytoin, primidone) may potentially decrease estrogen levels. Rifampin, nelfinavir, and ritonavir decrease estradiol serum concentration. MPA: Aminoglutethimide: May decrease effects by increasing hepatic metabolism

Drug Uptake
Absorption: Well absorbed
Half-life, elimination: Conjugated estrogens: 10-24 hours; MPA: 38-46 hours
Time to peak: Conjugated estrogens: 4-10 hours; MPA: 2-4 hours
See Estrogens, Conjugated *on page 463* and Medroxyprogesterone Acetate *on page 753*

Pregnancy Risk Factor X

Generic Available No

Estrogens, Conjugated (Synthetic)

(ES troe jenz, KON joo gate ed, aye, sin THET ik)

Related Information
Endocrine Disorders and Pregnancy *on page 1331*

U.S. Brand Names Cenestin®

Canadian Brand Names Cenestin™

Pharmacologic Category Estrogen Derivative

Synonyms Estrogens, Conjugated, A (Synthetic)

Use Treatment of moderate to severe vasomotor symptoms of menopause

Local Anesthetic/Vasoconstrictor Precautions No information available to require special precautions

Effects on Dental Treatment No effects or complications reported

Dosage Adolescents and Adults: Moderate to severe vasomotor symptoms: Oral: 0.625 mg/day; may be titrated up to 1.25 mg/day. Attempts to discontinue medication should be made at 3- to 6-month intervals.

Mechanism of Action Increases the synthesis of DNA, RNA, and various proteins in target tissues; reduces the release of gonadotropin-releasing hormone from the hypothalamus; reduces FSH and LH release from the pituitary

Other Adverse Effects

>10%:

Cardiovascular: Palpitation (21%), peripheral edema (10%)

Central nervous system; Headache (68%), insomnia (42%), paresthesia (33%), nervousness (28%), depression (28%), pain (11%), dizziness (11%)

Endocrine & metabolic: Breast pain (29%), menorrhagia (14%)

Gastrointestinal: Abdominal pain (28%), flatulence (29%), nausea (18%), dyspepsia (10%)

Musculoskeletal: Myalgia (28%), arthralgia (25%), back pain (14%)

Miscellaneous: Weakness (33%), infection (14%)

1% to 10%:

Central nervous system: Hypertonia (6%), fever (1%)

Gastrointestinal: Vomiting (7%), constipation (6%), diarrhea (6%)

Musculoskeletal: Leg cramps (10%)

Respiratory: Pharyngitis (8%), rhinitis (8%), cough (6%)

Additional adverse reactions associated with estrogen therapy: Increase in BP, hypercalcemia, thromboembolic disorder, myocardial infarction, hypertension, anxiety, stroke, chorea chloasma, melasma, rash, erythema multiforme, erythema nodosum, alopecia, hirsutism, breast tumors, amenorrhea, alterations in frequency and flow of menses, changes in cervical secretions, pancreatitis, decreased glucose tolerance, weight gain/loss, increased triglycerides and LDL, GI distress, cholestatic jaundice, aggravation of porphyria, breast tenderness, breast enlargement, changes in libido, intolerance to contact lenses, changes in corneal curvature, increased susceptibility to *Candida* infection

Drug Interactions

Increased Effect/Toxicity: Specific drug interactions have not been conducted for the synthetic preparation, however the following interactions have been noted for conjugated estrogens. Hydrocortisone increases corticosteroid toxic potential. Increased potential for thromboembolic events with anticoagulants.

Decreased Effect: Specific drug interactions have not been conducted for the synthetic preparation, however the following interactions have been noted for conjugated estrogens. Rifampin decreases estrogen serum concentration (other enzyme inducers may share this effect).

Drug Uptake Absorption: Readily absorbed from GI tract; peak concentrations in 4-16 hours

Pregnancy Risk Factor X

Generic Available No

Comments Not biologically equivalent to conjugated estrogens from equine source. Contains 9 unique estrogenic compounds (equine source contains at least 10 active estrogenic compounds).

Estrogens, Esterified (ES troe jenz, es TER i fied)

Related Information

Dental Drug Interactions: Update on Drug Combinations Requiring Special Considerations *on page 1434*

Endocrine Disorders and Pregnancy *on page 1331*

U.S. Brand Names Estratab®; Menest®

Canadian Brand Names Estratab®; Menest®

Pharmacologic Category Estrogen Derivative

Synonyms Esterified Estrogens

Use Atrophic vaginitis; hypogonadism; primary ovarian failure; vasomotor symptoms of menopause; prostatic carcinoma; osteoporosis prophylactic

Local Anesthetic/Vasoconstrictor Precautions No information available to require special precautions

Effects on Dental Treatment No effects or complications reported

Dosage Adults: Oral:

Male: Prostate cancer (inoperable, progressing): 1.25-2.5 mg 3 times/day

Female:

Hypogonadism: 2.5-7.5 mg/day for 20 days, off 10 days and repeat until menses occur

Moderate to severe vasomotor symptoms: 0.3-1.25 mg/day

Breast cancer (inoperable, progressing): 10 mg 3 times/day for at least 3 months

Mechanism of Action Primary effects on the interphase DNA-protein complex (chromatin) by binding to a receptor (usually located in the cytoplasm of a target cell) and initiating translocation of the hormone-receptor complex to the nucleus. Esterified estrogens contain a mixture of estrogenic substances; the principle component is estrone. Preparations contain 75% to 85% sodium estrone sulfate and 6% to 15% sodium equilin sulfate such that the total is not <90%. Estrogens

(Continued)

Estrogens, Esterified *(Continued)*

are responsible for the development and maintenance of the female reproductive system and secondary sexual characteristics. Estradiol is the principle intracellular human estrogen and is more potent than estrone and estriol at the receptor level; it is the primary estrogen secreted prior to menopause. In males and following menopause in females, estrone and estrone sulfate are more highly produced. Estrogens modulate the pituitary secretion of gonadotropins, luteinizing hormone, and follicle-stimulating hormone through a negative feedback system; estrogen replacement reduces elevated levels of these hormones.

Other Adverse Effects Frequency not defined:

Cardiovascular: Edema, hypertension, venous thromboembolism

Central nervous system: Dizziness, headache, mental depression, migraine

Dermatologic: Chloasma, erythema multiforme, erythema nodosum, hemorrhagic eruption, hirsutism, loss of scalp hair, melasma

Endocrine & metabolic: Breast enlargement, breast tenderness, changes in libido, increased thyroid-binding globulin, increased total thyroid hormone (T_4), increased serum triglycerides/phospholipids, increased HDL cholesterol, decreased LDL cholesterol, impaired glucose tolerance, hypercalcemia

Gastrointestinal: Abdominal cramps, bloating, cholecystitis, cholelithiasis, gallbladder disease, nausea, pancreatitis, vomiting, weight gain/loss

Genitourinary: Alterations in frequency and flow of menses, changes in cervical secretions, endometrial cancer, increased size of uterine leiomyomata, vaginal candidiasis

Hematologic: Aggravation of porphyria, decreased antithrombin III and antifactor Xa, increased levels of fibrinogen, increased platelet aggregability and platelet count; increased prothrombin and factors VII, VIII, IX, X

Hepatic: Cholestatic jaundice

Neuromuscular & skeletal: Chorea

Ocular: Intolerance to contact lenses, steeping of corneal curvature

Respiratory: Pulmonary thromboembolism

Miscellaneous: Carbohydrate intolerance

Drug Interactions May induce and is a substrate for cytochrome isoenzymes (profile not defined); estradiol is a CYP1A2 enzyme inhibitor

Increased Effect/Toxicity: Hydrocortisone taken with estrogen may cause corticosteroid-induced toxicity. Increased potential for thromboembolic events with anticoagulants.

Decreased Effect: Rifampin, nelfinavir, and ritonavir decrease estradiol serum concentration. Anticonvulsants which are enzyme inducers (barbiturates, carbamazepine, phenobarbital, phenytoin, primidone) may potentially decrease estrogen levels.

Drug Uptake Absorption: Readily

Pregnancy Risk Factor X

Generic Available No

Estrone (ES trone)

Related Information

Endocrine Disorders and Pregnancy *on page 1331*

U.S. Brand Names Kestrone®

Canadian Brand Names Oestrilin

Pharmacologic Category Estrogen Derivative

Synonyms Estrogenic Substance Aqueous

Use Hypogonadism; primary ovarian failure; vasomotor symptoms of menopause; prostatic carcinoma; inoperable breast cancer, kraurosis vulvae, abnormal uterine bleeding due to hormone imbalance

Local Anesthetic/Vasoconstrictor Precautions No information available to require special precautions

Effects on Dental Treatment No effects or complications reported

Dosage Adults: I.M.:

Male: Prostatic carcinoma: 2-4 mg 2-3 times/week

Female:

- Senile vaginitis and kraurosis vulvae: 0.1-0.5 mg 2-3 times/week
- Breast cancer (inoperable, progressing): 5 mg 3 or more times/week
- Primary ovarian failure, hypogonadism: 0.1-1 mg/week, up to 2 mg/week in single or divided doses
- Abnormal uterine bleeding: 2.5 mg/day for several days

Mechanism of Action A natural ovarian estrogenic hormone available as an aqueous mixture of water insoluble estrone and water soluble estrone potassium sulfate; all estrogens, including estrone, act in a similar manner; there is no evidence that there are biological differences among various estrogen preparations other than their ability to bind to cellular receptors inside the target cells.

Other Adverse Effects

>10%:

- Cardiovascular: Peripheral edema
- Endocrine & metabolic: Enlargement of breasts, breast tenderness

Gastrointestinal: Nausea, anorexia, bloating

1% to 10%:

Central nervous system: Headache

Endocrine & metabolic: Increased libido

Gastrointestinal: Vomiting, diarrhea

Drug Interactions

Increased Effect/Toxicity: Hydrocortisone taken with estrogen may cause corticosteroid-induced toxicity. Increased potential for thromboembolic events with anticoagulants. Estrone may increase the effect of carbamazepine, tricyclic antidepressants, and corticosteroids. Increased thromboembolic potential when estrone is taken with oral anticoagulants.

Decreased Effect: Rifampin decreases estrogen serum concentration.

Drug Uptake Absorption: Readily absorbed from the GI tract

Pregnancy Risk Factor X

Generic Available Yes

Estropipate (ES troe pih pate)

Related Information

Endocrine Disorders and Pregnancy *on page 1331*

U.S. Brand Names Ogen®; Ortho-Est®

Canadian Brand Names Ogen®

Mexican Brand Names Ogen®

Pharmacologic Category Estrogen Derivative

Synonyms Piperazine Estrone Sulfate

Use Atrophic vaginitis; hypogonadism; primary ovarian failure; vasomotor symptoms of menopause; osteoporosis prophylactic

Local Anesthetic/Vasoconstrictor Precautions No information available to require special precautions

Effects on Dental Treatment No effects or complications reported

Dosage Adults: Female:

Moderate to severe vasomotor symptoms: Oral: 0.625-5 mg/day

Hypogonadism or primary ovarian failure: Oral: 1.25-7.5 mg/day for 3 weeks followed by an 8- to 10-day rest period

Osteoporosis prevention: Oral: 0.625 mg/day for 25 days of a 31-day cycle

Atrophic vaginitis or kraurosis vulvae: Vaginal: Instill 2-4 g/day 3 weeks on and 1 week off

Mechanism of Action Crystalline estrone that has been solubilized as the sulfate and stabilized with piperazine. Primary effects on the interphase DNA-protein complex (chromatin) by binding to a receptor (usually located in the cytoplasm of a target cell) and initiating translocation of the hormone receptor complex to the nucleus. Estrogens are responsible for the development and maintenance of the female reproductive system and secondary sexual characteristics. Estradiol is the principle intracellular human estrogen and is more potent than estrone and estriol at the receptor level; it is the primary estrogen secreted prior to menopause. In males and following menopause in females, estrone and estrone sulfate are more highly produced. Estrogens modulate the pituitary secretion of gonadotropins, luteinizing hormone, and follicle-stimulating hormone through a negative feedback system; estrogen replacement reduces elevated levels of these hormones. Estropipate is prepared from purified crystalline estrone that has been solubilized as the sulfate and stabilized with piperazine.

Other Adverse Effects Frequency not defined:

Cardiovascular: Edema, hypertension, venous thromboembolism

Central nervous system: Dizziness, headache, mental depression, migraine

Dermatologic: Chloasma, erythema multiforme, erythema nodosum, hemorrhagic eruption, hirsutism, loss of scalp hair, melasma

Endocrine & metabolic: Breast enlargement, breast tenderness, changes in libido, increased thyroid-binding globulin, increased total thyroid hormone (T_4), increased serum triglycerides/phospholipids, increased HDL cholesterol, decreased LDL cholesterol, impaired glucose tolerance, hypercalcemia

Gastrointestinal: Abdominal cramps, bloating, cholecystitis, cholelithiasis, gallbladder disease, nausea, pancreatitis, vomiting, weight gain/loss

Genitourinary: Alterations in frequency and flow of menses, changes in cervical secretions, endometrial cancer, increased size of uterine leiomyomata, vaginal candidiasis

Hematologic: Aggravation of porphyria, decreased antithrombin III and antifactor Xa, increased levels of fibrinogen, increased platelet aggregability and platelet count; increased prothrombin and factors VII, VIII, IX, X

Hepatic: Cholestatic jaundice

Neuromuscular & skeletal: Chorea

Ocular: Intolerance to contact lenses, steeping of corneal curvature

Respiratory: Pulmonary thromboembolism

Miscellaneous: Carbohydrate intolerance

(Continued)

Estropipate *(Continued)*

Drug Interactions

Increased Effect/Toxicity: Hydrocortisone taken with estrogen may cause corticosteroid-induced toxicity. Increased potential for thromboembolic events with anticoagulants.

Decreased Effect: Rifampin, nelfinavir, and ritonavir decrease estradiol serum concentration. Anticonvulsants which are enzyme inducers (barbiturates, carbamazepine, phenobarbital, phenytoin, primidone) may potentially decrease estrogen levels.

Drug Uptake Absorption: Well absorbed

Pregnancy Risk Factor X

Generic Available Yes

Estrostep® 21 *see* Combination Hormonal Contraceptives *on page 323*
Estrostep® Fe *see* Combination Hormonal Contraceptives *on page 323*

Etanercept (et a NER cept)

Related Information

Rheumatoid Arthritis and Osteoarthritis *on page 1340*

U.S. Brand Names Enbrel®

Pharmacologic Category Antirheumatic, Disease Modifying

Use Reduction in signs and symptoms of moderately to severely active rheumatoid arthritis, moderately to severely active polyarticular juvenile arthritis, or psoriatic arthritis in patients who have had an inadequate response to one or more disease-modifying antirheumatic drugs (DMARDs)

Unlabeled/Investigational: Crohn's disease

Local Anesthetic/Vasoconstrictor Precautions No information available to require special precautions

Effects on Dental Treatment No effects or complications reported

Dosage

Children 4-17 years: Juvenile rheumatoid arthritis: S.C.: 0.4 mg/kg (maximum: 25 mg dose) twice weekly; doses should be separated by 72-96 hours

Adult: Rheumatoid arthritis, psoriatic arthritis: S.C.: 25 mg given twice weekly; doses should be separated by 72-96 hours; if the physician determines that it is appropriate, patients may self-inject after proper training in injection technique

Elderly: Although greater sensitivity of some elderly patients cannot be ruled out, no overall differences in safety or effectiveness were observed

Mechanism of Action Etanercept is a recombinant DNA-derived protein composed of tumor necrosis factor receptor (TNFR) linked to the Fc portion of human IgG1. Etanercept binds tumor necrosis factor (TNF) and blocks its interaction with cell surface receptors. TNF plays an important role in the inflammatory processes of rheumatoid arthritis (RA) and the resulting joint pathology.

Other Adverse Effects Events reported include those >3% with incidence higher than placebo.

>10%:

- Central nervous system: Headache (17%)
- Local: Injection site reaction (37%)
- Respiratory: Respiratory tract infection (38%), upper respiratory tract infection (29%), rhinitis (12%)
- Miscellaneous: Infection (35%), positive ANA (11%), positive antidouble stranded DNA antibodies (15% by RIA, 3% by *Crithidia lucilae* assay)

≥3% to 10%:

- Central nervous system: Dizziness (7%)
- Dermatologic: Rash (5%)
- Gastrointestinal: Abdominal pain (5%), dyspepsia (4%), nausea (9%), vomiting (3%)
- Neuromuscular & skeletal: Weakness (5%)
- Respiratory: Pharyngitis (7%), respiratory disorder (5%), sinusitis (3%), cough (6%)

<3%: Alopecia, cerebral ischemia, cholecystitis, deep vein thrombosis, depression, dyspnea, gastrointestinal hemorrhage, heart failure, infection (serious), malignancies, membranous glomerulopathy, myocardial infarction, myocardial ischemia, pancreatitis, polymyositis, pulmonary embolism, thrombophlebitis, vasculitis (cutaneous)

Pediatric patients (JRA): The percentages of patients reporting abdominal pain (17%) and vomiting (14.5%) was higher than in adult RA. Two patients developed varicella infection associated with aseptic meningitis which resolved without complications (see Warnings/Precautions).

Warnings/Precautions Etanercept may affect defenses against infections and malignancies. Safety and efficacy in patients with immunosuppression or chronic infections have not been evaluated. Rare cases of tuberculosis have been reported. Discontinue administration if patient develops a serious infection. Do not start drug administration in patients with an active infection. Use caution in patients predisposed to infection, such as poorly-controlled diabetes.

Use caution in patients with pre-existing or recent-onset demyelinating CNS disorders (rare cases described in postmarketing experience). Use caution in patients with a history of significant hematologic abnormalities; has been associated with pancytopenia and aplastic anemia (rare cases in postmarketing experience). Patients must be advised to seek medical attention if they develop signs and symptoms suggestive of blood dyscrasias. Discontinue if significant hematologic abnormalities are confirmed.

Impact on the development and course of malignancies is not fully defined. Treatment may result in the formation of autoimmune antibodies; cases of autoimmune disease have not been described. Non-neutralizing antibodies to etanercept may also be formed. No correlation of antibody development to clinical response or adverse events has been observed. The long-term immunogenicity, carcinogenic potential, or effect on fertility are unknown. No evidence of mutagenic activity has been observed *in vitro* or *in vivo*. The safety of etanercept has not been studied in children <4 years of age.

Allergic reactions may occur (<0.2%), but anaphylaxis has not been observed. If an anaphylactic reaction or other serious allergic reaction occurs, administration of etanercept should be discontinued immediately and appropriate therapy initiated.

Patients should be brought up to date with all immunizations before initiating therapy. No data are available concerning the effects of etanercept on vaccination. Live vaccines should not be given concurrently. No data are available concerning secondary transmission of live vaccines in patients receiving etanercept. Patients with a significant exposure to varicella virus should temporarily discontinue etanercept. Treatment with varicella zoster immune globulin should be considered.

Drug Interactions Specific drug interaction studies have not been conducted.

Drug Uptake

Onset of action: ~2-3 weeks

Half-life, elimination: 115 hours (range: 98-300 hours)

Time to peak: 72 hours (range: 48-96 hours)

Pregnancy Risk Factor B

Generic Available No

Ethacrynic Acid (eth a KRIN ik AS id)

Related Information

Cardiovascular Diseases *on page 1308*

U.S. Brand Names Edecrin® [DSC]

Canadian Brand Names Edecrin®

Pharmacologic Category Diuretic, Loop

Synonyms Ethacrynate Sodium

Use Management of edema associated with CHF; hepatic cirrhosis or renal disease; short-term management of ascites due to malignancy, idiopathic edema, and lymphedema

Local Anesthetic/Vasoconstrictor Precautions No information available to require special precautions

Effects on Dental Treatment No effects or complications reported

Dosage I.V. formulation should be diluted in D_5W or NS (1 mg/mL) and infused over several minutes

Children:

- Oral: 1 mg/kg/dose once daily; increase at intervals of 2-3 days as needed, to a maximum of 3 mg/kg/day
- I.V.: 1 mg/kg/dose, (maximum: 50 mg/dose); repeat doses not routinely recommended; however, if indicated, repeat doses every 8-12 hours

Adults:

- Oral: 50-100 mg/day in 1-2 divided doses; may increase in increments of 25-50 mg at intervals of several days to a maximum of 400 mg/24 hours
- I.V.: 0.5-1 mg/kg/dose (maximum: 100 mg/dose); repeat doses not routinely recommended; however, if indicated, repeat doses every 8-12 hours

Mechanism of Action Inhibits reabsorption of sodium and chloride in the ascending loop of Henle and distal renal tubule, interfering with the chloride-binding cotransport system, thus causing increased excretion of water, sodium, chloride, magnesium, and calcium

Other Adverse Effects Frequency not defined:

Central nervous system: Headache, fatigue, apprehension, confusion, fever, chills, encephalopathy (patients with pre-existing liver disease); vertigo

Dermatologic: Skin rash, Henoch-Schönlein purpura (in patient with rheumatic heart disease)

Endocrine & metabolic: Hyponatremia, hyperglycemia, variations in phosphorus, CO_2 content, bicarbonate, and calcium; reversible hyperuricemia, gout, hyperglycemia, hypoglycemia (occurred in two uremic patients who received doses above those recommended)

Gastrointestinal: Anorexia, malaise, abdominal discomfort or pain, dysphagia, nausea, vomiting, and diarrhea, gastrointestinal bleeding, acute pancreatitis (rare)

Genitourinary: Hematuria

(Continued)

Ethacrynic Acid *(Continued)*

Hepatic: Jaundice, abnormal LFTs
Hematology: Agranulocytosis, severe neutropenia, thrombocytopenia
Local: Thrombophlebitis (with I.V. use), local irritation and pain,
Ocular: Blurred vision
Otic: Deafness, tinnitus, temporary or permanent deafness
Renal: Increased serum creatinine

Drug Interactions

Increased Effect/Toxicity: Ethacrynic acid-induced hypokalemia may predispose to digoxin toxicity and may increase the risk of arrhythmia with drugs which may prolong QT interval, including type Ia and type III antiarrhythmic agents, cisapride, terfenadine, and some quinolones (sparfloxacin, gatifloxacin, and moxifloxacin). The risk of toxicity from lithium and salicylates (high dose) may be increased by loop diuretics. Hypotensive effects and/or adverse renal effects of ACE inhibitors and NSAIDs are potentiated by ethacrynic acid-induced hypovolemia. The effects of peripheral adrenergic-blocking drugs or ganglionic blockers may be increased by ethacrynic acid. May increase the risk of ototoxicity with other ototoxic agents (aminoglycosides, cis-platinum), especially in patients with renal dysfunction; synergistic diuretic effects occur with thiazide-type diuretics. Diuretics tend to be synergistic with other antihypertensive agents, and hypotension may occur. Nephrotoxicity has been associated with concomitant use of cephaloridine or cephalexin.

Decreased Effect: Probenecid decreases diuretic effects of ethacrynic acid. Glucose tolerance may be decreased by loop diuretics, requiring adjustment of hypoglycemic agents. Cholestyramine or colestipol may reduce bioavailability of ethacrynic acid. Indomethacin (and other NSAIDs) may reduce natriuretic and hypotensive effects of diuretics.

Drug Uptake

Onset of action: Diuresis: Oral: ~30 minutes; I.V.: 5 minutes
Absorption: Oral: Rapid
Duration: Oral: 12 hours; I.V.: 2 hours
Half-life, elimination: 2-4 hours
Time to peak: Oral: 2 hours; I.V.: 30 minutes

Pregnancy Risk Factor B

Generic Available No

Ethambutol (e THAM byoo tole)

Related Information

Nonviral Infectious Diseases *on page 1342*

U.S. Brand Names Myambutol®

Canadian Brand Names Etibi®; Myambutol®

Pharmacologic Category Antitubercular Agent

Synonyms Ethambutol Hydrochloride

Use Treatment of tuberculosis and other mycobacterial diseases in conjunction with other antituberculosis agents

Local Anesthetic/Vasoconstrictor Precautions No information available to require special precautions

Effects on Dental Treatment No effects or complications reported

Dosage Ethambutol is generally not recommended in children whose visual acuity cannot be monitored (<6 years of age). However, ethambutol should be considered for all children with organisms resistant to other drugs, when susceptibility to ethambutol has been demonstrated, or susceptibility is likely. **Note:** A four-drug regimen (isoniazid, rifampin, pyrazinamide, and either streptomycin or ethambutol) is preferred for the initial, empiric treatment of TB. When the drug susceptibility results are available, the regimen should be altered as appropriate.

Oral:

Patients with tuberculosis and without HIV infection:

OPTION 1: Isoniazid resistance rate <4%: Administer daily isoniazid, rifampin, and pyrazinamide for 8 weeks followed by isoniazid and rifampin daily or directly observed therapy (DOT) 2-3 times/week for 16 weeks. If isoniazid resistance rate is not documented, ethambutol or streptomycin should also be administered until susceptibility to isoniazid or rifampin is demonstrated. Continue treatment for at least 6 months or 3 months beyond culture conversion.

OPTION 2: Administer daily isoniazid, rifampin, pyrazinamide, and either streptomycin or ethambutol for 2 weeks followed by DOT 2 times/week administration of the same drugs for 6 weeks, and subsequently, with isoniazid and rifampin DOT 2 times/week administration for 16 weeks

OPTION 3: Administer isoniazid, rifampin, pyrazinamide, and either ethambutol or streptomycin by DOT 3 times/week for 6 months

Patients with TB and with HIV infection: Administer any of the above OPTIONS 1, 2 or 3; however, treatment should be continued for a total of 9 months and at least 6 months beyond culture conversion

Note: Some experts recommend that the duration of therapy should be extended to 9 months for patients with disseminated disease, miliary disease, disease involving the bones or joints, or tuberculosis lymphadenitis

Children and Adults:

Daily therapy: 15-25 mg/kg/day (maximum: 2.5 g/day)

Directly observed therapy (DOT): Twice weekly: 50 mg/kg (maximum: 2.5 g)

DOT: 3 times/week: 25-30 mg/kg (maximum: 2.5 g)

Adults: Treatment of disseminated *Mycobacterium avium* complex (MAC) in patients with advanced HIV infection: 15 mg/kg ethambutol in combination with azithromycin 600 mg daily

Mechanism of Action Suppresses mycobacteria multiplication by interfering with RNA synthesis

Other Adverse Effects Frequency not defined:

Central nervous system: Headache, confusion, disorientation, malaise, mental confusion, fever

Dermatologic: Rash, pruritus

Endocrine & metabolic: Acute gout or hyperuricemia

Gastrointestinal: Abdominal pain, anorexia, nausea, vomiting

Hepatic: Abnormal LFTs

Neuromuscular & skeletal: Peripheral neuritis

Ocular: Optic neuritis; symptoms may include decreased acuity, scotoma, color blindness, or visual defects (usually reversible with discontinuation, irreversible blindness has been described)

Miscellaneous: Anaphylaxis

Drug Interactions Absorption is decreased when taken with aluminum salts.

Drug Uptake

Absorption: Oral: ~80%

Half-life, elimination: 2.5-3.6 hours; End-stage renal disease: 7-15 hours

Time to peak: 2-4 hours

Pregnancy Risk Factor B

Generic Available No

Ethamolin® *see* Ethanolamine Oleate *on page 473*

Ethanolamine Oleate (ETH a nol a meen OH lee ate)

U.S. Brand Names Ethamolin®

Pharmacologic Category Sclerosing Agent

Synonyms Monoethanolamine

Use Orphan drug: Sclerosing agent used for bleeding esophageal varices

Local Anesthetic/Vasoconstrictor Precautions No information available to require special precautions

Effects on Dental Treatment No effects or complications reported

Dosage Adults: 1.5-5 mL per varix, up to 20 mL total or 0.4 mL/kg; patients with severe hepatic dysfunction should receive less than recommended maximum dose

Mechanism of Action Derived from oleic acid and similar in physical properties to sodium morrhuate; however, the exact mechanism of the hemostatic effect used in endoscopic injection sclerotherapy is not known. Intravenously injected ethanolamine oleate produces a sterile inflammatory response resulting in fibrosis and occlusion of the vein; a dose-related extravascular inflammatory reaction occurs when the drug diffuses through the venous wall. Autopsy results indicate that variceal obliteration occurs secondary to mural necrosis and fibrosis. Thrombosis appears to be a transient reaction.

Other Adverse Effects 1% to 10%:

Central nervous system: Pyrexia (1.8%)

Gastrointestinal: Esophageal ulcer (2%), esophageal stricture (1.3%)

Neuromuscular & skeletal: Retrosternal pain

Respiratory: Pleural effusion (2%), pneumonia (1.2%)

Miscellaneous: Retrosternal pain (1.6%)

Pregnancy Risk Factor C

Generic Available No

Ethaverine (eth AV er een)

U.S. Brand Names Ethavex-100®

Pharmacologic Category Vasodilator

Synonyms Ethaverine Hydrochloride

Use Peripheral and cerebral vascular insufficiency associated with arterial spasm

Local Anesthetic/Vasoconstrictor Precautions No information available to require special precautions

Effects on Dental Treatment No effects or complications reported

Dosage Adults: Oral: 100 mg 3 times/day

Other Adverse Effects Frequency not defined:

Cardiovascular: Tachycardia, hypotension

Central nervous system: Depression, dizziness, vertigo, drowsiness, sedation, lethargy, headache, xerostomia

Dermatologic: Pruritus, flushing of the face

(Continued)

Ethaverine *(Continued)*

Gastrointestinal: Nausea, constipation
Hepatic: Hepatic hypersensitivity
Miscellaneous: Diaphoresis

Generic Available Yes

Ethavex-100® *see* Ethaverine *on page 473*

Ethchlorvynol (eth klor VI nole)

U.S. Brand Names Placidyl®

Pharmacologic Category Hypnotic, Miscellaneous

Use Short-term management of insomnia

Local Anesthetic/Vasoconstrictor Precautions No information available to require special precautions

Effects on Dental Treatment No effects or complications reported

Restrictions C-IV

Dosage Adults: Oral: 500-1000 mg at bedtime

Mechanism of Action Unknown; causes nonspecific depression of the reticular activating system

Other Adverse Effects Frequency not defined:
Cardiovascular: Hypotension, syncope
Central nervous system: Dizziness, facial numbness, mild hangover, excitement, ataxia, hysteria, prolonged hypnosis, mild stimulation, giddiness
Dermatologic: Rash, urticaria
Gastrointestinal: Indigestion, nausea, stomach pain, unpleasant aftertaste, vomiting
Hematologic: Thrombocytopenia
Hepatic: Cholestatic jaundice
Neuromuscular & skeletal: Weakness (severe)
Ocular: Blurred vision

Drug Interactions
Increased toxicity (CNS depression) with CNS depressants.
Decreased Effect: May inhibit the hypoprothrombinemic response to warfarin via an unknown mechanism; monitor for altered anticoagulant effect or consider using a benzodiazepine.

Drug Uptake
Onset of action: 15-60 minutes
Absorption: Rapidly
Duration: 5 hours
Half-life, elimination: 10-20 hours
Time to peak: 2 hours

Pregnancy Risk Factor C

Generic Available No

Ethinyl Estradiol (ETH in il es tra DYE ole)

Related Information
Endocrine Disorders and Pregnancy *on page 1331*

U.S. Brand Names Estinyl®

Pharmacologic Category Estrogen Derivative

Use Hypogonadism; primary ovarian failure; vasomotor symptoms of menopause; prostatic carcinoma; breast cancer

Local Anesthetic/Vasoconstrictor Precautions No information available to require special precautions

Effects on Dental Treatment No effects or complications reported

Dosage Adults: Oral:
Male: Prostatic cancer (inoperable, progressing): 0.15-2 mg/day for palliation
Female:
Hypogonadism: 0.05 mg 1-3 times/day for 2 weeks of a theoretical menstrual cycle followed by progesterone for 3-6 months
Vasomotor symptoms: 0.02-0.05 mg for 21 days, off 7 days and repeat
Breast cancer (inoperable, progressing): 1 mg 3 times/day for palliation

Mechanism of Action Estrogens are responsible for the development and maintenance of the female reproductive system and secondary sexual characteristics. Estradiol is the principle intracellular human estrogen and is more potent than estrone and estriol at the receptor level; it is the primary estrogen secreted prior to menopause. In males and following menopause in females, estrone and estrone sulfate are more highly produced. Estrogens modulate the pituitary secretion of gonadotropins, luteinizing hormone, and follicle-stimulating hormone through a negative feedback system; estrogen replacement reduces elevated levels of these hormones; increases the synthesis of DNA, RNA, and various proteins in target tissues. Ethinyl estradiol is a synthetic derivative of estradiol. The addition of the ethinyl group prevents rapid degradation by the liver.

Other Adverse Effects Frequency not defined:
Cardiovascular: Edema, hypertension, venous thromboembolism
Central nervous system: Dizziness, headache, mental depression, migraine

Dermatologic: Chloasma, erythema multiforme, erythema nodosum, hemorrhagic eruption, hirsutism, loss of scalp hair, melasma

Endocrine & metabolic: Breast enlargement, breast tenderness, changes in libido, increased thyroid-binding globulin, increased total thyroid hormone (T_4), increased serum triglycerides/phospholipids, increased HDL-cholesterol, decreased LDL-cholesterol, impaired glucose tolerance, hypercalcemia

Gastrointestinal: Abdominal cramps, bloating, cholecystitis, cholelithiasis, gallbladder disease, nausea, pancreatitis, vomiting, weight gain/loss

Genitourinary: Alterations in frequency and flow of menses, changes in cervical secretions, endometrial cancer, increased size of uterine leiomyomata, vaginal candidiasis

Hematologic: Aggravation of porphyria, decreased antithrombin III and antifactor Xa, increased levels of fibrinogen, increased platelet aggregability and platelet count; increased prothrombin and factors VII, VIII, IX, X

Hepatic: Cholestatic jaundice

Neuromuscular & skeletal: Chorea

Ocular: Intolerance to contact lenses, steeping of corneal curvature

Respiratory: Pulmonary thromboembolism

Miscellaneous: Carbohydrate intolerance

Drug Interactions CYP3A3/4 and 3A5-7 enzyme substrate; CYP1A2, 2C19, and 3A3/4 (weak) enzyme inhibitor

Increased Effect/Toxicity: Hydrocortisone taken with estrogen may cause corticosteroid-induced toxicity. Increased potential for thromboembolic events with anticoagulants.

Decreased Effect: Rifampin, nelfinavir, and ritonavir decrease estradiol serum concentration. Anticonvulsants which are enzyme inducers (barbiturates, carbamazepine, phenobarbital, phenytoin, primidone) may potentially decrease estrogen levels.

Drug Uptake

Absorption: Oral: Rapid and complete

Half-life, elimination: ~8-25 hours

Time to peak: Initial: 2-3 hours; Secondary: 12 hours

Pregnancy Risk Factor X

Generic Available No

Ethionamide (e thye on AM ide)

Related Information

Nonviral Infectious Diseases *on page 1342*

U.S. Brand Names Trecator®-SC

Canadian Brand Names Trecator®-SC

Pharmacologic Category Antitubercular Agent

Use Treatment of tuberculosis and other mycobacterial diseases, in conjunction with other antituberculosis agents, when first-line agents have failed or resistance has been demonstrated

Local Anesthetic/Vasoconstrictor Precautions No information available to require special precautions

Effects on Dental Treatment No effects or complications reported

Dosage Oral:

Children: 15-20 mg/kg/day in 2 divided doses, not to exceed 1 g/day

Adults: 500-1000 mg/day in 1-3 divided doses

Mechanism of Action Inhibits peptide synthesis

Other Adverse Effects Frequency not defined:

Cardiovascular: Postural hypotension

Central nervous system: Psychiatric disturbances, drowsiness, dizziness, seizures, headache

Dermatologic: Rash, alopecia

Endocrine & metabolic: Hypothyroidism or goiter, hypoglycemia, gynecomastia

Gastrointestinal: Metallic taste, diarrhea, anorexia, nausea, vomiting, stomatitis, abdominal pain

Hematologic: Thrombocytopenia

Hepatic: Hepatitis (5%), jaundice

Neuromuscular & skeletal: Peripheral neuritis, weakness (common)

Ocular: Optic neuritis, blurred vision

Respiratory: Olfactory disturbances

Drug Interactions Increased effect/toxicity with cycloserine and isoniazid; increased hepatotoxicity with rifampin

Drug Uptake

Absorption: Rapid

Half-life, elimination: 2-3 hours

Time to peak: ~3 hours

Pregnancy Risk Factor C

Generic Available No

Ethmozine® *see* Moricizine *on page 828*

Ethosuximide (eth oh SUKS i mide)

U.S. Brand Names Zarontin®

Canadian Brand Names Zarontin®

Pharmacologic Category Anticonvulsant, Succinimide

Use Management of absence (petit mal) seizures, myoclonic seizures, and akinetic epilepsy; considered to be drug of choice for simple absence seizures

Local Anesthetic/Vasoconstrictor Precautions No information available to require special precautions

Effects on Dental Treatment No effects or complications reported

Dosage Oral:

Children 3-6 years: Initial: 250 mg/day (or 15 mg/kg/day) in 2 divided doses; increase every 4-7 days; usual maintenance dose: 15-40 mg/kg/day in 2 divided doses

Children >6 years and Adults: Initial: 250 mg twice daily; increase by 250 mg as needed every 4-7 days up to 1.5 g/day in 2 divided doses; usual maintenance dose: 20-40 mg/kg/day in 2 divided doses

Dosing comment in renal/hepatic dysfunction: Use with caution.

Mechanism of Action Increases the seizure threshold and suppresses paroxysmal spike-and-wave pattern in absence seizures; depresses nerve transmission in the motor cortex

Other Adverse Effects Frequency not defined:

Central nervous system: Ataxia, drowsiness, sedation, dizziness, lethargy, euphoria, headache, irritability, hyperactivity, fatigue, night terrors, disturbance in sleep, inability to concentrate, aggressiveness, mental depression (with cases of overt suicidal intentions), paranoid psychosis

Dermatologic: Stevens-Johnson syndrome, SLE, rash, hirsutism

Endocrine & metabolic: Increased libido

Gastrointestinal: Weight loss, gastric upset, cramps, epigastric pain, diarrhea, nausea, vomiting, anorexia, abdominal pain, gum hypertrophy, tongue swelling

Genitourinary: Vaginal bleeding, microscopic hematuria

Hematologic: Leukopenia, agranulocytosis, pancytopenia, eosinophilia

Ocular: Myopia

Miscellaneous: Hiccups

Drug Interactions CYP3A3/4 enzyme substrate; CYP3A3/4 enzyme inducer

Increased Effect/Toxicity: Isoniazid may inhibit hepatic metabolism of ethosuximide with a resultant increase in ethosuximide serum concentration. Ethosuximide may elevate phenytoin levels. Valproate acid has been reported to both increase and decrease ethosuximide levels.

Decreased Effect: Enzyme inducers (phenobarbital, rifampin, phenytoin, valproic acid) may decrease levels of ethosuximide.

Drug Uptake

Half-life, elimination: Children: 30 hours; Adults: 50-60 hours

Time to peak: Capsule: ~2-4 hours; Syrup: <2-4 hours

Pregnancy Risk Factor C

Generic Available Yes

Ethotoin (ETH oh toyn)

U.S. Brand Names Peganone®

Canadian Brand Names Peganone®

Pharmacologic Category Anticonvulsant, Hydantoin

Synonyms Ethylphenylhydantoin

Use Generalized tonic-clonic or complex-partial seizures

Local Anesthetic/Vasoconstrictor Precautions No information available to require special precautions

Effects on Dental Treatment No effects or complications reported

Dosage Oral:

Children: 30-60 mg/kg/day or 250 mg twice daily, may be increased up to 2-3 g/day

Adults: 250 mg 4 times/day after meals, may be increased up to 3 g/day in divided doses 4 times/day

Other Adverse Effects

>10%:

Central nervous system: Psychiatric changes, slurred speech, trembling, dizziness, drowsiness

Gastrointestinal: Constipation, nausea, vomiting

Neuromuscular & skeletal: Trembling

1% to 10%:

Central nervous system: Drowsiness, headache, insomnia

Dermatologic: Skin rash

Gastrointestinal: Anorexia, weight loss

Hematologic: Leukopenia

Hepatic: Hepatitis

Renal: Increase in serum creatinine

Drug Interactions Drug interactions for ethotoin not specifically evaluated, but extrapolated from phenytoin (CYP2C9 and 2C19 enzyme substrate; CYP1A2, 3A3/4, and 3A5-7 enzyme inducer). Also see Phenytoin *on page 951*

Pregnancy Risk Factor D

Generic Available No

Ethyl Chloride (ETH il KLOR ide)

Pharmacologic Category Local Anesthetic

Synonyms Chloroethane

Use Local anesthetic in minor operative procedures and to relieve pain caused by insect stings and burns, and irritation caused by myofascial and visceral pain syndromes

Local Anesthetic/Vasoconstrictor Precautions No information available to require special precautions

Effects on Dental Treatment No effects or complications reported

Dosage varies with use.

Other Adverse Effects 1% to 10%: Mucous membrane irritation, freezing may alter skin pigment

Pregnancy Risk Factor C

Generic Available Yes

Comments Spray for a few seconds to the point of frost formation when the tissue becomes white; avoid prolonged spraying of skin beyond this point

Ethyl Chloride and Dichlorotetrafluoroethane

(ETH il KLOR ide & dye klor oh te tra floo or oh ETH ane)

U.S. Brand Names Fluro-Ethyl®

Pharmacologic Category Local Anesthetic

Synonyms Dichlorotetrafluoroethane and Ethyl Chloride

Use Topical refrigerant anesthetic to control pain associated with minor surgical procedures, dermabrasion, injections, contusions, and minor strains

Local Anesthetic/Vasoconstrictor Precautions No information available to require special precautions

Effects on Dental Treatment No effects or complications reported

Dosage Press gently on side of spray valve allowing the liquid to emerge as a fine mist ~ 2" to 4" from site of application

Pregnancy Risk Factor C

Generic Available No

Ethyol® *see* Amifostine *on page 66*

Etidocaine With Epinephrine (e TI doe kane)

Related Information

Oral Pain *on page 1360*

U.S. Brand Names Duranest®

Canadian Brand Names Duranest®

Pharmacologic Category Local Anesthetic

Synonyms Etidocaine Hydrochloride

Use Dental: An amide-type local anesthetic for local infiltration anesthesia; injection near nerve trunks to produce nerve block

Local Anesthetic/Vasoconstrictor Precautions No information available to require special precautions

Effects on Dental Treatment No effects or complications reported

Dosage

Children <10 years: Dosage has not been established

Children >10 years and Adults: Dental infiltration and nerve block: 15-75 mg (1-5 mL) as a 1.5% solution; up to a maximum of 5.5 mg/kg of body weight but not to exceed 400 mg/injection of etidocaine hydrochloride with epinephrine 1:200,000. The effective anesthetic dose varies with procedure, intensity of anesthesia

# of Cartridges (1.8 mL)	Etidocaine (1.5%) (mg)	Epinephrine 1:200,000 (mg)
1	27	0.009
2	54	0.018
3	81	0.027
4	108	0.036
5	135	0.045
6	162	0.054
7	189	0.063
8	216	0.072
9	243	0.081
10	270	0.090

(Continued)

Etidocaine With Epinephrine *(Continued)*

needed, duration of anesthesia required, and physical condition of the patient. Always use the lowest effective dose along with careful aspiration.

The numbers of dental carpules (1.8 mL) in the table provide the indicated amounts of etidocaine hydrochloride 1.5% and epinephrine 1:200,000.

Note: Doses of etidocaine hydrochloride with epinephrine cited from USP Dispensing Information (USP DI), 17th ed, The United States Pharmacopeial Convention, Inc, Rockville, MD, 1997, 136.

Mechanism of Action Local anesthetics bind selectively to the intracellular surface of sodium channels to block influx of sodium into the axon. As a result, depolarization necessary for action potential propagation and subsequent nerve function is prevented. Local anesthetics reversibly prevent generation and conduction of electrical impulses in neurons by decreasing the transient increase in permeability to sodium. The differential sensitivity generally depends on the size of the fiber; small fibers are more sensitive than larger fibers and require a longer period for recovery. Sensory pain fibers are usually blocked first, followed by fibers that transmit sensations of temperature, touch, and deep pressure. High concentrations block sympathetic somatic sensory and somatic motor fibers. The spread of anesthesia depends upon the distribution of the solution. This is primarily dependent on the site of administration and volume of drug injected. The block at the sodium channel is reversible. When drug diffuses away from the axon, sodium channel function is restored and nerve propagation is subsequently restored.

Epinephrine prolongs the duration of the anesthetic actions of etidocaine by causing vasoconstriction (alpha adrenergic receptor agonist) of the vasculature surrounding the nerve axons. This prevents the diffusion of lidocaine away from the nerves resulting in a longer retention in the axon.

Other Adverse Effects Frequency not defined:

Cardiovascular: Myocardial depression, hypotension, bradycardia, cardiovascular collapse

Central nervous system: Anxiety, restlessness, disorientation, confusion, seizures, drowsiness, unconsciousness, chills

Dermatologic: Urticaria, nausea, vomiting

Local: Transient stinging or burning at injection site

Neuromuscular & skeletal: Tremor

Ocular: Blurred vision

Otic: Tinnitus

Respiratory: Respiratory arrest

Miscellaneous: Anaphylactoid reactions, shivering

Contraindications Hypersensitivity to etidocaine, other amide local anesthetics, or any component of their formulation; heart block; severe hemorrhage; severe hypotension

Warnings/Precautions Should be avoided in patients with uncontrolled hyperthyroidism. Should be used in minimal amounts in patients with significant cardiovascular problems (because of epinephrine component). Aspirate the syringe after tissue penetration and before injection to minimize chance of direct vascular injection.

Drug Interactions Due to epinephrine component, use with tricyclic antidepressants or MAO inhibitors could result in increased pressor response; use with nonselective beta-blockers (ie, propranolol) could result in serious hypertension and reflex bradycardia.

Drug Uptake

Onset of action: Maxillary infiltration and inferior alveolar nerve block: 3-5 minutes

Absorption: Rapid

Duration: 5-10 hours after infiltration or nerve block

Half-life, elimination: 2.7 hours

Pregnancy Risk Factor B

Breast-feeding Considerations Usual infiltration doses of etidocaine hydrochloride with epinephrine given to nursing mothers has not been shown to affect the health of the nursing infant.

Dosage Forms INJ: 1% [10 mg/mL] (30 mL). **INJ, with epinephrine 1:200,000:** 1% [10 mg/mL] (30 mL); 1.5% [15 mg/mL] (20 mL)

Generic Available No

Selected Readings

Ayoub ST and Coleman AE, "A Review of Local Anesthetics," *Gen Dent*, 1992, 40(4):285-7, 289-90.

Jastak JT and Yagiela JA, "Vasoconstrictors and Local Anesthesia: A Review and Rationale for Use," *J Am Dent Assoc*, 1983, 107(4):623-30.

MacKenzie TA and Young ER, "Local Anesthetic Update," *Anesth Prog*, 1993, 40(2):29-34.

Wynn RL, "Epinephrine Interactions With Beta-Blockers," *Gen Dent*, 1994, 42(1):16, 18.

Wynn RL, "Recent Research on Mechanisms of Local Anesthetics," *Gen Dent*, 1995, 43(4):316-8.

Yagiela JA, "Local Anesthetics," *Anesth Prog*, 1991, 38(4-5):128-41.

Etidronate Disodium (e ti DROE nate dye SOW dee um)

U.S. Brand Names Didronel®

Canadian Brand Names Didronel®

Pharmacologic Category Bisphosphonate Derivative

Synonyms EHDP; Sodium Etidronate

Use Symptomatic treatment of Paget's disease and heterotopic ossification due to spinal cord injury or after total hip replacement, hypercalcemia associated with malignancy

Local Anesthetic/Vasoconstrictor Precautions No information available to require special precautions

Effects on Dental Treatment No effects or complications reported

Dosage Adults:

Paget's disease: Oral: 5 mg/kg/day given every day for ≤6 months; may give 10 mg/kg/day for up to 3 months; daily dose may be divided if adverse GI effects occur

Heterotopic ossification with spinal cord injury: 20 mg/kg/day for 2 weeks, then 10 mg/kg/day for 10 weeks (this dosage has been used in children, however, treatment >1 year has been associated with a rachitic syndrome)

Hypercalcemia associated with malignancy:

I.V. (Dilute dose in at least 250 mL NS): 7.5 mg/kg/day for 3 days; there should be at least 7 days between courses of treatment

Oral: Start 20 mg/kg/day on the last day of infusion and continue for 30-90 days

Mechanism of Action Decreases bone resorption by inhibiting osteocystic osteolysis; decreases mineral release and matrix or collagen breakdown in bone

Other Adverse Effects

>10%: Neuromuscular & skeletal: Bone pain (10% to 20%, Paget's)

1% to 10%:

Central nervous system: Fever (9%), convulsions (3%)

Endocrine & metabolic: Hypophosphatemia (3%), hypomagnesemia (3%), fluid overload (6%), hypercalcemia of malignancy

Gastrointestinal: Diarrhea and nausea (7% to 30%, dose-related), constipation (3%), abnormal taste (3%)

Hepatic: LFT changes (3%)

Respiratory: Dyspnea (3%)

Renal: Increased serum creatinine (10%)

Drug Interactions Foscarnet and plicamycin may have additive hypocalcemic effect.

Drug Uptake

Onset of action: 1-3 months

Absorption: Dose-dependent

Duration: Can persist for 12 months without continuous therapy

Pregnancy Risk Factor B (oral); C (parenteral)

Generic Available No

Etodine® [OTC] *see* Povidone-Iodine *on page 982*

Etodolac (ee toe DOE lak)

Related Information

Rheumatoid Arthritis and Osteoarthritis *on page 1340*
Temporomandibular Dysfunction (TMD) *on page 1397*

U.S. Brand Names Lodine®; Lodine® XL

Canadian Brand Names Apo®-Etodolac; Gen-Etodolac; Lodine®; Utradol™

Mexican Brand Names Lodine® Retard

Pharmacologic Category Nonsteroidal Anti-inflammatory Drug (NSAID)

Synonyms Etodolic Acid

Use

Dental: Management of postoperative pain

Medical: Acute and long-term use in the management of signs and symptoms of osteoarthritis and management of pain, not approved for use in rheumatoid arthritis

Local Anesthetic/Vasoconstrictor Precautions No information available to require special precautions

Effects on Dental Treatment NSAID formulations are known to reversibly decrease platelet aggregation via mechanisms different than observed with aspirin. The dentist should be aware of the potential of abnormal coagulation. Caution should also be exercised in the use of NSAIDs in patients already on anticoagulant therapy with drugs such as warfarin (Coumadin®).

Dosage Adults: Oral: Single dose of 76-100 mg is comparable to the analgesic effect of aspirin 650 mg; in patients ≥65 years, no substantial differences in the pharmacokinetics or side-effects profile were seen compared with the general population

Acute pain: 200-400 mg every 6-8 hours, as needed, not to exceed total daily doses of 1200 mg; for patients weighing <60 kg, total daily dose should not exceed 20 mg/kg/day; extended release dose: 1 tablet daily

Mechanism of Action Inhibits prostaglandin synthesis by decreasing the activity of the enzyme, cyclo-oxygenase, which results in decreased formation of prostaglandin precursors

Other Adverse Effects

1% to 10%:

Central nervous system: Depression (1% to 3%)

Dermatologic: Rash (1% to 3%), pruritus (1% to 3%)

(Continued)

Etodolac *(Continued)*

Gastrointestinal: Abdominal cramps (3% to 9%), nausea (3% to 9%), vomiting (1% to 3%), dyspepsia (10%), diarrhea (3% to 9%), constipation (1% to 3%), flatulence (3% to 9%), melena (1% to 3%), gastritis (1% to 3%)

Genitourinary: Polyuria (1% to 3%)

Neuromuscular & skeletal: Weakness (3% to 9%)

Ocular: Blurred vision (1% to 3%)

Otic: Tinnitus (1% to 3%)

<1%: Congestive heart failure, hypertension, arrhythmia, tachycardia, confusion, hallucinations, aseptic meningitis, mental depression, drowsiness, insomnia, urticaria, erythema multiforme, toxic epidermal necrolysis, Stevens-Johnson syndrome, angioedema, polydipsia, hot flashes, GI ulceration, cystitis, agranulocytosis, anemia, hemolytic anemia, bone marrow suppression, leukopenia, thrombocytopenia, hepatitis, peripheral neuropathy, toxic amblyopia, blurred vision, conjunctivitis, dry eyes, decreased hearing, acute renal failure, allergic rhinitis, dyspnea, epistaxis, anorexia, stomatitis

Contraindications Hypersensitivity to etodolac, aspirin, other NSAIDs, or any component of their formulation; active gastric/duodenal ulcer disease; pregnancy (3rd trimester)

Warnings/Precautions Use with caution in patients with CHF, hypertension, dehydration, decreased renal or hepatic function, history of GI disease (bleeding or ulcers), or those receiving anticoagulants. Elderly are at a high risk for adverse effects from nonsteroidal anti-inflammatory agents. As much as 60% of elderly can develop peptic ulceration and/or hemorrhage asymptomatically.

Use lowest effective dose for shortest period possible. Use of NSAIDs can compromise existing renal function especially when Cl_{cr} is <30 mL/minute. CNS adverse effects such as confusion, agitation, and hallucination are generally seen in overdose or high-dose situations; however, elderly may demonstrate these adverse effects at lower doses than younger adults. Withhold for at least 4-6 half-lives prior to surgical or dental procedures.

Drug Interactions

ACE inhibitors: Antihypertensive effects may be decreased by concurrent therapy with NSAIDs; monitor BP.

Angiotensin II antagonists: Antihypertensive effects may be decreased by concurrent therapy with NSAIDs; monitor BP.

Anticoagulants (warfarin, heparin, LMWHs) in combination with NSAIDs can cause increased risk of bleeding.

Other antiplatelet drugs (ticlopidine, clopidogrel, aspirin, abciximab, dipyridamole, eptifibatide, tirofiban) can cause an increased risk of bleeding.

Cholestyramine and colestipol reduce the bioavailability of some NSAIDs; separate administration times.

Corticosteroids may increase the risk of GI ulceration; avoid concurrent use.

Cyclosporine: NSAIDs may increase serum creatinine, potassium, BP, and cyclosporine levels; monitor cyclosporine levels and renal function carefully.

Hydralazine's antihypertensive effect is decreased; avoid concurrent use.

Lithium levels can be increased; avoid concurrent use if possible or monitor lithium levels and adjust dose. Sulindac may have the least effect. When NSAID is stopped, lithium will need adjustment again.

Loop diuretics efficacy (diuretic and antihypertensive effect) is reduced. Indomethacin reduces this efficacy, however, it may be anticipated with any NSAID.

Methotrexate: Severe bone marrow suppression, aplastic anemia, and GI toxicity have been reported with concomitant NSAID therapy. Avoid use during moderate or high-dose methotrexate (increased and prolonged methotrexate levels). NSAID use during low-dose treatment of rheumatoid arthritis has not been fully evaluated; extreme caution is warranted.

Thiazides antihypertensive effects are decreased; avoid concurrent use.

Verapamil plasma concentration is decreased by some NSAIDs; avoid concurrent use.

Warfarin's INRs may be increased by piroxicam. Other NSAIDs may have the same effect depending on dose and duration. Monitor INR closely. Use the lowest dose of NSAIDs possible and for the briefest duration.

Dietary/Ethanol/Herb Considerations

Ethanol: Avoid use; may enhance gastric mucosal irritation.

Food: Administer with food or milk to reduce GI upset; may decrease peak serum concentration. Avoid garlic, ginger, and green tea.

Herb/Nutraceutical: Avoid cat's claw, dong quai, evening primrose, feverfew, garlic, ginger, ginkgo biloba, ginseng, green tea, horse chestnut, and red clover due to additional antiplatelet activity. Avoid kava and valerian; may enhance benzodiazepine activity.

Drug Uptake

Onset of action: 0.5 hours following single dose of 200-400 mg; Analgesic: 2-4 hours; Maximum anti-inflammatory effect: A few days

Absorption: Well absorbed

Duration: 4-6 hours

Half-life, elimination: 7 hours
Time to peak: 1 hour

Pregnancy Risk Factor C/D (3rd trimester)

Dosage Forms CAP (Lodine®): 200 mg, 300 mg. **TAB** (Lodine®): 400 mg, 500 mg. **TAB, extended release** (Lodine® XL): 400 mg, 500 mg, 600 mg

Generic Available Yes

Selected Readings

Brooks PM and Day RO, "Nonsteroidal Anti-inflammatory Drugs - Differences and Similarities," *N Engl J Med*, 1991, 324(24):1716-25.

Tucker PW, Smith JR, and Adams DF, "A Comparison of 2 Analgesic Regimens for the Control of Postoperative Periodontal Discomfort," *J Periodontol*, 1996, 67(2):125-9.

Etomidate (e TOM i date)

U.S. Brand Names Amidate®

Canadian Brand Names Amidate®

Pharmacologic Category General Anesthetic

Use Induction of general anesthesia

Unlabeled/Investigational: Sedation for diagnosis of seizure foci

Local Anesthetic/Vasoconstrictor Precautions No information available to require special precautions

Effects on Dental Treatment No effects or complications reported

Dosage Children >10 years and Adults: I.V.: 0.2-0.6 mg/kg over a period of 30-60 seconds for induction of anesthesia

Mechanism of Action Ultrashort-acting nonbarbiturate hypnotic used for the induction of anesthesia; chemically, it is a carboxylated imidazole and has been shown to produce a rapid induction of anesthesia with minimal cardiovascular and respiratory effects; produces EEG burst suppression at high doses

Other Adverse Effects

>10%:
- Endocrine & metabolic: Adrenal suppression
- Gastrointestinal: Nausea, vomiting on emergence from anesthesia
- Local: Pain at injection site (30% to 80%)
- Neuromuscular & skeletal: Myoclonus (33%), transient skeletal movements, uncontrolled eye movements
- Ocular: Uncontrolled eye movements

1% to 10%: Hiccups

Warnings/Precautions Consider exogenous corticosteroid replacement in patients undergoing severe stress

Drug Interactions Increased Effect/Toxicity: Fentanyl decreases etomidate elimination. Verapamil may increase the anesthetic and respiratory depressant effects of etomidate.

Drug Uptake

Onset of action: 30-60 seconds; Peak effect: 1 minute
Duration: 3-5 minutes; terminated by redistribution
Half-life, elimination: Terminal: 2.6 hours

Pregnancy Risk Factor C

Generic Available Yes

Etopophos® *see* Etoposide Phosphate *on page 482*

Etoposide (e toe POE side)

U.S. Brand Names Toposar®; VePesid®

Canadian Brand Names VePesid®

Mexican Brand Names Etopos®; Lastet; Medsaposide; Serozide®; VePesid®; Vp-Tec®

Pharmacologic Category Antineoplastic Agent, Podophyllotoxin Derivative

Synonyms Epipodophyllotoxin; VP-16; VP-16-213

Use Treatment of lymphomas, ANLL, lung, testicular, bladder, and prostate carcinoma, hepatoma, rhabdomyosarcoma, uterine carcinoma, neuroblastoma, mycosis fungoides, Kaposi's sarcoma, histiocytosis, gestational trophoblastic disease, Ewing's sarcoma, Wilms' tumor, and brain tumors

Local Anesthetic/Vasoconstrictor Precautions No information available to require special precautions

Effects on Dental Treatment No effects or complications reported

Mechanism of Action Does not inhibit microtubular assembly; has been shown to delay transit of cells through the S phase and arrest cells in late S or early G_2 phase; may inhibit mitochondrial transport at the NADH dehydrogenase level or inhibit uptake of nucleosides into HeLa cells; etoposide is a topoisomerase II (an enzyme which breaks and repairs DNA); inhibitor and appears to cause DNA strand breaks

Other Adverse Effects

>10%:
- Cardiovascular: Hypotension if the drug is infused too fast
- Dermatologic: Alopecia (22% to 93%)
- Endocrine & metabolic: Ovarian failure (38%), amenorrhea

(Continued)

Etoposide *(Continued)*

Gastrointestinal: Mild to moderate nausea and vomiting; mucositis, especially at high doses; anorexia (10% to 13%)
Hematologic: Myelosuppression, leukopenia (91%), thrombocytopenia (41%), anemia
Onset: 5-7 days
Nadir: 7-14 days
Recovery: 21-28 days
1% to 10%:
Gastrointestinal: Stomatitis (1% to 6%), diarrhea (1% to 13%), abdominal pain
Neuromuscular & skeletal: Peripheral neuropathies (0.7% to 2%)

Drug Interactions CYP3A3/4 enzyme substrate

Increased Effect/Toxicity: The effects of etoposide may be increased by calcium antagonists (increased effects noted *in vitro*). Cyclosporine may increase the levels of etoposide. Etoposide may increase the effects/toxicity of methotrexate and warfarin. There have been reports of frequent hepatic dysfunction with hyperbilirubinemia, ascites, and thrombocytopenia when etoposide is combined with carmustine.

Drug Uptake

Absorption: Oral: 25% to 75%; significant inter- and intrapatient variation
Half-life, elimination: Terminal: 4-15 hours; Children: Normal renal/hepatic function: 6-8 hours
Time to peak: Oral: 1-1.5 hours

Pregnancy Risk Factor D

Generic Available Yes

Etoposide Phosphate (e toe POE side FOS fate)

U.S. Brand Names Etopophos®

Pharmacologic Category Antineoplastic Agent, Podophyllotoxin Derivative

Use Treatment of refractory testicular tumors and small cell lung cancer

Local Anesthetic/Vasoconstrictor Precautions No information available to require special precautions

Effects on Dental Treatment No effects or complications reported

Mechanism of Action Etoposide phosphate is converted *in vivo* to the active moiety, etoposide, by dephosphorylation. Etoposide inhibits mitotic activity; inhibits cells from entering prophase; inhibits DNA synthesis. Initially thought to be mitotic inhibitors similar to podophyllotoxin, but actually have no effect on microtubule assembly. However, later shown to induce DNA strand breakage and inhibition of topoisomerase II (an enzyme which breaks and repairs DNA); etoposide acts in late S or early G2 phases.

Other Adverse Effects Based on **etoposide**:

>10%:
Cardiovascular: Hypotension if the drug is infused too fast
Dermatologic: Alopecia (22% to 93%)
Endocrine & metabolic: Ovarian failure (38%), amenorrhea
Gastrointestinal: Mild to moderate nausea and vomiting; mucositis, especially at high doses; anorexia (10% to 13%)
Hematologic: Myelosuppression, leukopenia (91%), thrombocytopenia (41%), anemia
Onset: 5-7 days
Nadir: 7-14 days
Recovery: 21-28 days
1% to 10%:
Gastrointestinal: Stomatitis (1% to 6%), diarrhea (1% to 13%), abdominal pain
Neuromuscular & skeletal: Peripheral neuropathies (0.7% to 2%)

Drug Interactions Increased Effect/Toxicity: Etoposide taken with warfarin may result in prolongation of bleeding times. Alteration of MTX transport has been found as a slow efflux of MTX and its polyglutamated form out of the cell, leading to intercellular accumulation of MTX. Calcium antagonists increase the rate of VP-16-induced DNA damage and cytotoxicity *in vitro*. Use with carmustine has shown reports of frequent hepatic dysfunction with hyperbilirubinemia, ascites, and thrombocytopenia. Cyclosporine may cause additive cytotoxic effects on tumor cells.

Drug Uptake Half-life, elimination: Terminal: 4-15 hours; Children: 6-8 hours

Pregnancy Risk Factor D

Generic Available No

Etrafon® *see* Amitriptyline and Perphenazine *on page 77*
ETS-2%® *see* Erythromycin, Topical *on page 454*
Eudal®-SR *see* Guaifenesin and Pseudoephedrine *on page 570*
Eulexin® *see* Flutamide *on page 525*
Eurax® Topical *see* Crotamiton *on page 331*
Evalose® *see* Lactulose *on page 682*
Evista® *see* Raloxifene *on page 1039*

E-Vitamin® [OTC] *see* Vitamin E *on page 1245*

Evoxac™ *see* Cevimeline *on page 256*

Exact® Acne Medication [OTC] *see* Benzoyl Peroxide *on page 153*

Excedrin® Extra Strength [OTC] *see* Acetaminophen, Aspirin, and Caffeine *on page 33*

Excedrin® Migraine [OTC] *see* Acetaminophen, Aspirin, and Caffeine *on page 33*

Excedrin® P.M. [OTC] *see* Acetaminophen and Diphenhydramine *on page 30*

Exelderm® *see* Sulconazole *on page 1114*

Exelon® *see* Rivastigmine *on page 1062*

Exemestane (ex e MES tane)

U.S. Brand Names Aromasin®

Canadian Brand Names Aromasin®

Pharmacologic Category Antineoplastic Agent, Miscellaneous

Use Treatment of advanced breast cancer in postmenopausal women whose disease has progressed following tamoxifen therapy

Local Anesthetic/Vasoconstrictor Precautions No information available to require special precautions

Effects on Dental Treatment No effects or complications reported

Mechanism of Action An irreversible, steroidal aromatase inactivator; prevents conversion of androgens to estrogens by tying up the enzyme aromatase; lowers circulating estrogens in breast cancers where growth is estrogen-dependent

Other Adverse Effects

>10%:

Central nervous system: Fatigue (22%), pain (13%), depression (13%), insomnia (11%), anxiety (10%)

Endocrine & metabolic: Hot flashes (13%)

Gastrointestinal: Nausea (18%)

1% to 10%:

Cardiovascular: Edema (7%), hypertension (5%), chest pain

Central nervous system: Dizziness (8%), headache (8%), fever (5%), hypoesthesia, confusion

Dermatologic: Rash, itching, alopecia

Gastrointestinal: Vomiting (7%), abdominal pain (6%), anorexia (6%), constipation (5%), diarrhea (4%), increased appetite (3%), dyspepsia

Genitourinary: Urinary tract infection

Neuromuscular & skeletal: Weakness, paresthesia, pathological fracture, arthralgia

Respiratory: Dyspnea (10%), cough (6%), bronchitis, sinusitis, pharyngitis, rhinitis

Miscellaneous: Influenza-like symptoms (6%), diaphoresis (6%), lymphedema, infection

A dose-dependent decrease in sex hormone-binding globulin has been observed with daily doses of 25 mg or more. Serum luteinizing hormone and follicle-stimulating hormone levels have increased with this medicine.

Contraindications Hypersensitivity to exemestane or any component of the formulation; pregnancy or lactation

Warnings/Precautions Not indicated for premenopausal women; not to be given with estrogen-containing agents. Use with caution in hepatic impairment or renal insufficiency.

Drug Interactions CYP3A3/4 enzyme substrate

Increased Effect/Toxicity: Although exemestane is a CYP3A4 substrate, ketoconazole, a CYP3A4 inhibitor, did not change the pharmacokinetics of exemestane. No other potential drug interactions have been evaluated.

Drug Uptake

Absorption: Rapid

Half-life, elimination: 24 hours

Time to peak: Women with breast cancer: 1.2 hours

Pregnancy Risk Factor D

Generic Available No

Exidine® Scrub [OTC] *see* Chlorhexidine Gluconate *on page 263*

ex-lax® *see* Senna *on page 1081*

ex-lax® Maximum Relief *see* Senna *on page 1081*

Ex-Lax® Stool Softener [OTC] *see* Docusate *on page 407*

Exosurf Neonatal® *see* Colfosceril Palmitate *on page 321*

Extendryl *see* Chlorpheniramine, Phenylephrine, and Methscopolamine *on page 271*

Extendryl JR *see* Chlorpheniramine, Phenylephrine, and Methscopolamine *on page 271*

Extendryl SR *see* Chlorpheniramine, Phenylephrine, and Methscopolamine *on page 271*

Extra Action Cough Syrup [OTC] *see* Guaifenesin and Dextromethorphan *on page 569*

Extra Strength Doan's® [OTC] *see* Magnesium Salicylate *on page 742*

Eyesine® [OTC] *see* Tetrahydrozoline *on page 1150*
Ezide® *see* Hydrochlorothiazide *on page 595*

Factor IX Complex (Human) (FAK ter nyne KOM pleks HYU man)

U.S. Brand Names AlphaNine® SD; BeneFix™; Hemonyne®; Konȳne® 80; Profilnine® SD; Proplex® T

Pharmacologic Category Antihemophilic Agent; Blood Product Derivative

Synonyms Prothrombin Complex Concentrate

Use

Control bleeding in patients with factor IX deficiency (hemophilia B or Christmas disease) **Note:** Factor IX concentrate containing **only** factor IX is also available and preferable for this indication.

Prevention/control of bleeding in hemophilia A patients with inhibitors to factor VIII

Prevention/control of bleeding in patients with factor VII deficiency

Emergency correction of the coagulopathy of warfarin excess in critical situations.

Local Anesthetic/Vasoconstrictor Precautions No information available to require special precautions

Effects on Dental Treatment No effects or complications reported

Dosage Children and Adults: Dosage is expressed in units of factor IX activity and must be individualized. I.V. only:

Formula for units required to raise blood level %:

Total blood volume (mL blood/kg) = 70 mL/kg (adults), 80 mL/kg (children)

Plasma volume = total blood volume (mL) x [1 - Hct (in decimals)]

For example, for a 70 kg adult with a Hct = 40%: Plasma volume = [70 kg x 70 mL/kg] x [1 - 0.4] = 2940 mL

To calculate number of units needed to increase level to desired range (highly individualized and dependent on patient's condition): Number of units = desired level increase [desired level - actual level] x plasma volume (in mL)

For example, for a 100% level in the above patient who has an actual level of 20%: Number of units needed = [1 (for a 100% level) - 0.2] x 2940 mL = 2352 units

As a general rule, the level of factor IX required for treatment of different conditions is listed below:

Minor Spontaneous Hemorrhage, Prophylaxis:

- Desired levels of factor IX for hemostasis: 15% to 25%
- Initial loading dose to achieve desired level: <20-30 units/kg
- Frequency of dosing: Once; repeated in 24 hours if necessary
- Duration of treatment: Once; repeated if necessary

Major Trauma or Surgery:

- Desired levels of factor IX for hemostasis: 25% to 50%
- Initial loading dose to achieve desired level: <75 units/kg
- Frequency of dosing: Every 18-30 hours, depending on half-life and measured factor IX levels
- Duration of treatment: Up to 10 days, depending upon nature of insult

Factor VIII inhibitor patients: 75 units/kg/dose; may be given every 6-12 hours

Anticoagulant overdosage: I.V.: 15 units/kg

Mechanism of Action Replaces deficient clotting factor including factor X; hemophilia B, or Christmas disease, is an X-linked recessively inherited disorder of blood coagulation characterized by insufficient or abnormal synthesis of the clotting protein factor IX. Factor IX is a vitamin K-dependent coagulation factor which is synthesized in the liver. Factor IX is activated by factor XIa in the intrinsic coagulation pathway. Activated factor IX (IXa), in combination with factor VII:C activates factor X to Xa, resulting ultimately in the conversion of prothrombin to thrombin and the formation of a fibrin clot. The infusion of exogenous factor IX to replace the deficiency present in hemophilia B temporarily restores hemostasis.

Other Adverse Effects 1% to 10%:

Central nervous system: Fever, headache, chills

Neuromuscular & skeletal: Tingling

Miscellaneous: Following rapid administration: Transient fever

Drug Interactions Do not coadminister with aminocaproic acid; may increase risk for thrombosis.

Drug Uptake Half-life, elimination:

VII component: Cleared rapidly from the serum in two phases; initial: 4-6 hours; terminal: 22.5 hours

IX component: 24 hours

Pregnancy Risk Factor C

Generic Available No

Comments Factor VII and IX units are listed per vial and per lot to lot variation

Factor VIIa, Recombinant (FAK ter SEV en ree KOM be nant)

U.S. Brand Names Novo-Seven®

Pharmacologic Category Antihemophilic Agent; Blood Product Derivative

Synonyms Coagulation Factor VIIa; rFVIIa

Use Treatment of bleeding episodes in patients with hemophilia A or B when inhibitors to factor VIII or factor IX are present

Local Anesthetic/Vasoconstrictor Precautions No information available to require special precautions

Effects on Dental Treatment No effects or complications reported

Dosage Children and Adults: I.V. administration only: 90 mcg/kg every 2 hours until hemostasis is achieved or until the treatment is judged ineffective. The dose and interval may be adjusted based upon the severity of bleeding and the degree of hemostasis achieved. The duration of therapy following hemostasis has not been fully established; for patients experiencing severe bleeds, dosing should be continued at 3- to 6-hour intervals after hemostasis has been achieved and the duration of dosing should be minimized.

In clinical trials, dosages have ranged from 35-120 mcg/kg and a decision on the final therapeutic dosages was reached within 8 hours in the majority of patients

Mechanism of Action Recombinant factor VIIa, a vitamin K-dependent glycoprotein, promotes hemostasis by activating the extrinsic pathway of the coagulation cascade. It replaces deficient activated coagulation factor VII, which complexes with tissue factor and may activate coagulation factor X to Xa and factor IX to IXa. When complexed with other factors, coagulation factor Xa converts prothrombin to thrombin, a key step in the formation of a fibrin-platelet hemostatic plug

Other Adverse Effects 1% to 10%:

Cardiovascular: Hypertension

Hematologic: Hemorrhage, decreased plasma fibrinogen

Musculoskeletal: Hemarthrosis

Warnings/Precautions Patients should be monitored for signs and symptoms of activation of the coagulation system or thrombosis. Thrombotic events may be increased in patients with disseminated intravascular coagulation (DIC), advanced atherosclerotic disease, sepsis or crush injury. Decreased dosage or discontinuation is warranted in confirmed DIC. Efficacy with prolonged infusions and data evaluating this agent's long-term adverse effects are limited.

Drug Uptake Half-life, elimination: 2.3 hours (1.7-2.7)

Pregnancy Risk Factor C

Generic Available No

Famciclovir (fam SYE kloe veer)

Related Information

Systemic Viral Diseases *on page 1354*

U.S. Brand Names Famvir™

Canadian Brand Names Famvir®

Pharmacologic Category Antiviral Agent

Use Management of acute herpes zoster (shingles); treatment of recurrent mucocutaneous herpes simplex infections in HIV-infected patients

Local Anesthetic/Vasoconstrictor Precautions No information available to require special precautions

Effects on Dental Treatment No effects or complications reported

Dosage Adults: Oral:

Acute herpes zoster: 500 mg every 8 hours for 7 days

Recurrent herpes simplex in immunocompetent patients: 125 mg twice daily for 5 days

Mechanism of Action After undergoing rapid biotransformation to the active compound, penciclovir, famciclovir is phosphorylated by viral thymidine kinase in HSV-1, HSV-2, and VZV-infected cells to a monophosphate form; this is then converted to penciclovir triphosphate and competes with deoxyguanosine triphosphate to inhibit HSV-2 polymerase (ie, herpes viral DNA synthesis/replication is selectively inhibited)

Other Adverse Effects 1% to 10%:

Central nervous system: Fatigue (4% to 6%), fever (1% to 3%), dizziness (3% to 5%), somnolence (1% to 2%), headache

Dermatologic: Pruritus (1% to 4%)

Gastrointestinal: Diarrhea (4% to 8%), vomiting (1% to 5%), constipation (1% to 5%), anorexia (1% to 3%), abdominal pain (1% to 4%), nausea

Neuromuscular & skeletal: Paresthesia (1% to 3%)

Respiratory: Sinusitis/pharyngitis (2%)

Drug Interactions Increased Effect/Toxicity:

Cimetidine: Penciclovir AUC may increase due to impaired metabolism.

Digoxin: C_{max} of digoxin increases by ~19%.

Probenecid: Penciclovir serum concentration significantly increase.

Theophylline: Penciclovir AUC/C_{max} may increase and renal clearance decrease, although not clinically significant.

Drug Uptake

Absorption: Food decreases the maximum peak concentration and delays time to peak; AUC remains the same

Half-life, elimination: Penciclovir: 2-3 hours (10, 20, and 7 hours in HSV-1, HSV-2, and VZV-infected cells); linearly decreased with reductions in renal failure

Time to peak: 0.9 hours; C_{max} and T_{max} are decreased and prolonged with noncompensated hepatic impairment

(Continued)

Famciclovir *(Continued)*

Pregnancy Risk Factor B

Generic Available No

Famotidine (fa MOE ti deen)

Related Information

Gastrointestinal Disorders *on page 1326*

U.S. Brand Names Mylanta AR® [DSC]; Pepcid®; Pepcid® AC [OTC]; Pepcid RPD™

Canadian Brand Names Alti-Famotidine; Apo®-Famotidine; Gen-Famotidine; Novo-Famotidine; Nu-Famotidine; Pepcid®; Pepcid AC®; Pepcid® I.V.; Rhoxal-famotidine; Ulcidine®

Mexican Brand Names Durater; Famoxal; Farmotex®; Pepcidine®; Sigafam

Pharmacologic Category Histamine H_2 Antagonist

Use

Pepcid®: Therapy and treatment of duodenal ulcer, gastric ulcer, control gastric pH in critically ill patients, symptomatic relief in gastritis, gastroesophageal reflux, active benign ulcer, and pathological hypersecretory conditions

Pepcid® AC: Relief of heartburn, acid indigestion, and sour stomach

Unlabeled/Investigational: Part of a multidrug regimen for *H. pylori* eradication to reduce the risk of duodenal ulcer recurrence

Local Anesthetic/Vasoconstrictor Precautions No information available to require special precautions

Effects on Dental Treatment No effects or complications reported

Dosage

Children: 1-16 years: Treatment duration and dose should be individualized

Peptic ulcer:

Oral: 0.5 mg/kg/day at bedtime or divided twice daily (maximum dose: 40 mg/day); doses of up to 1 mg/kg/day have been used in clinical studies

I.V.: 0.25 mg/kg every 12 hours (maximum dose: 40 mg/day); doses of up to 0.5 mg/kg have been used in clinical studies

GERD: Oral: 1 mg/kg/day divided twice daily (maximum dose: 40 mg twice daily); doses of up to 2 mg/kg/day have been used in clinical studies

Adults:

Duodenal ulcer: Oral: Acute therapy: 40 mg/day at bedtime for 4-8 weeks; maintenance therapy: 20 mg/day at bedtime

Gastric ulcer: Oral: Acute therapy: 40 mg/day at bedtime

Hypersecretory conditions: Oral: Initial: 20 mg every 6 hours, may increase in increments up to 160 mg every 6 hours

GERD: Oral: 20 mg twice daily for 6 weeks

Esophagitis and accompanying symptoms due to GERD: Oral: 20 mg or 40 mg twice daily for up to 12 weeks

Patients unable to take oral medication: I.V.: 20 mg every 12 hours

Heartburn, indigestion, sour stomach: Pepcid® AC [OTC]: Oral: 10 mg every 12 hours; dose may be taken 15-60 minutes before eating foods known to cause heartburn

Dosing adjustment in renal impairment:

Cl_{cr} <50 mL/minute: Manufacturer recommendation: Administer 50% of dose **or** increase the dosing interval to every 36-48 hours (to limit potential CNS adverse effects).

Cl_{cr} <10 mL/minute: Administer 50% of dose **or** increase dosing interval to every 36-48 hours.

Mechanism of Action Competitive inhibition of histamine at H_2-receptors of the gastric parietal cells, which inhibits gastric acid secretion

Other Adverse Effects 1% to 10%:

Central nervous system: Dizziness (1%), headache (5%)

Gastrointestinal: Constipation (1%), diarrhea (2%)

Drug Interactions

Cefpodoxime: Histamine H_2 antagonists may decrease the absorption of cefpodoxime; separate oral doses by at least 2 hours. Risk: Moderate

Cefuroxime: Histamine H_2 antagonists may decrease the absorption of cefuroxime; separate oral doses by at least 2 hours. Risk: Moderate

Cyclosporine: Histamine H_2 antagonists may increase the serum concentration of cyclosporine; monitor

Delavirdine: Delavirdine's absorption is decreased; avoid concurrent use with H_2 antagonists

Itraconazole: Histamine H_2 antagonists may decrease the absorption of itraconazole; monitor

Ketoconazole: Histamine H_2 antagonists may decrease the absorption of ketoconazole; monitor

Drug Uptake

Onset of GI effect: Oral: ≤1 hour

Duration: 10-12 hours

Half-life, elimination: 2.5-3.5 hours (increases with renal impairment); Oliguria: 20 hours

Time to peak: Oral: ~1-3 hours

Pregnancy Risk Factor B

Generic Available Yes

Famotidine, Calcium Carbonate, and Magnesium Hydroxide

(fa MOE ti deen, KAL see um KAR bun ate, & mag NEE zhum hye DROKS ide)

U.S. Brand Names Pepcid® Complete [OTC]

Pharmacologic Category Antacid; Histamine H_2 Antagonist

Synonyms Calcium Carbonate, Magnesium Hydroxide, and Famotidine; Magnesium Hydroxide, Famotidine, and Calcium Carbonate

Use Relief of heartburn due to acid indigestion

Local Anesthetic/Vasoconstrictor Precautions No information available to require special precautions

Effects on Dental Treatment No effects or complications reported

Dosage Children ≥12 years and Adults: Relief of heartburn due to acid indigestion: Oral: Pepcid® Complete: 1 tablet as needed; ≤2 tablets in 24 hours; do **not** swallow whole, chew tablet completely before swallowing; do not use for longer than 14 days (see Comments for dosing ranges for individual ingredients)

Mechanism of Action

Famotidine: H_2 antagonist

Calcium carbonate: Antacid

Magnesium hydroxide: Antacid

Other Adverse Effects See Famotidine *on page 486*, Calcium Carbonate *on page 201*, and Magnesium Hydroxide *on page 741*

Warnings/Precautions See Famotidine *on page 486*, Calcium Carbonate *on page 201*, and Magnesium Hydroxide *on page 741*

Drug Interactions See Famotidine *on page 486*, Calcium Carbonate *on page 201*, and Magnesium Hydroxide *on page 741*

Drug Uptake See Famotidine *on page 486*, Calcium Carbonate *on page 201*, and Magnesium Hydroxide *on page 741*

Comments Presented in dosage field is the specific OTC labeling for the indicated product. Dosing ranges of the individual ingredients include:

Adults:

Famotidine: Duodenal/gastric ulcer: 40 mg/day at bedtime

Calcium carbonate: Antacid: ≤3 g/day of elemental calcium

Magnesium hydroxide: Antacid: Approximately ≤5 g/day of magnesium hydroxide

Healthcare providers should also refer to the individual monographs for more specific information.

Famvir™ *see* Famciclovir *on page 485*

Fansidar® *see* Sulfadoxine and Pyrimethamine *on page 1118*

Fareston® *see* Toremifene *on page 1184*

Faslodex® *see* Fulvestrant *on page 543*

Fat Emulsion (fat e MUL shun)

U.S. Brand Names Intralipid®; Liposyn®; Nutrilipid®; Soyacal®

Canadian Brand Names Intralipid®

Mexican Brand Names Lipocin; Lyposyn

Pharmacologic Category Caloric Agent

Synonyms Intravenous Fat Emulsion

Use Source of calories and essential fatty acids for patients requiring parenteral nutrition of extended duration

Local Anesthetic/Vasoconstrictor Precautions No information available to require special precautions

Effects on Dental Treatment No effects or complications reported

Dosage Fat emulsion should not exceed 60% of the total daily calories

Children: Initial dose: 0.5-1 g/kg/day, increase by 0.5 g/kg/day to a maximum of 3-4 g/kg/day; maximum rate of infusion: 0.25 g/kg/hour (1.25 mL/kg/hour of 20% solution)

Adolescents and Adults: Initial dose: 1 g/kg/day, increase by 0.5-1 g/kg/day to a maximum of 2.5 g/kg/day of 10% and 3 g/kg/day of 20%; maximum rate of infusion: 0.25 g/kg/hour (1.25 mL/kg/hour of 20% solution); do not exceed 50 mL/hour (20%) or 100 mL/hour (10%)

Note: At the onset of therapy, the patient should be observed for any immediate allergic reactions such as dyspnea, cyanosis, and fever. Slower initial rates of infusion may be used for the first 10-15 minutes of the infusion (eg, 0.1 mL/minute of 10% or 0.05 mL/minute of 20% solution).

Prevention of fatty acid deficiency (8% to 10% of total caloric intake): 0.5-1 g/kg/24 hours

Children: 5-10 mL/kg/day at 0.1 mL/minute then up to 100 mL/hour

Adults: 500 mL twice weekly at rate of 1 mL/minute for 30 minutes, then increase to 500 mL over 4-6 hours

Can be used in both children and adults on a daily basis as a caloric source in TPN

(Continued)

Fat Emulsion *(Continued)*

Other Adverse Effects Frequency not defined:
- Cardiovascular: Cyanosis, flushing, chest pain
- Central nervous system: Headache, dizziness
- Endocrine & metabolic: Hyperlipemia
- Gastrointestinal: Nausea, vomiting, diarrhea
- Hematologic: Hypercoagulability, thrombocytopenia in neonates (rare)
- Hepatic: Hepatomegaly
- Local: Thrombophlebitis
- Respiratory: Dyspnea
- Miscellaneous: Sepsis, diaphoresis

Drug Uptake Half-life, elimination: 0.5-1 hour

Pregnancy Risk Factor B/C

Generic Available Yes

Fedahist® [OTC] *see* Chlorpheniramine and Pseudoephedrine *on page 270*

Fedahist® Expectorant [OTC] *see* Guaifenesin and Pseudoephedrine *on page 570*

Feen-A-Mint® [OTC] *see* Bisacodyl *on page 166*

Feiba VH Immuno® *see* Anti-inhibitor Coagulant Complex *on page 107*

Felbamate (FEL ba mate)

U.S. Brand Names Felbatol®

Pharmacologic Category Anticonvulsant, Miscellaneous

Use Not as a first-line antiepileptic treatment; only in those patients who respond inadequately to alternative treatments and whose epilepsy is so severe that a substantial risk of aplastic anemia and/or liver failure is deemed acceptable in light of the benefits conferred by its use. Patient must be fully advised of risk and has signed written informed consent. Felbamate can be used as either monotherapy or adjunctive therapy in the treatment of partial seizures (with and without generalization) and in adults with epilepsy.

Orphan drug: Adjunctive therapy in the treatment of partial and generalized seizures associated with Lennox-Gastaut syndrome in children

Local Anesthetic/Vasoconstrictor Precautions No information available to require special precautions

Effects on Dental Treatment No effects or complications reported

Dosage Anticonvulsant:

Monotherapy: Children >14 years and Adults:

Initial: 1200 mg/day in divided doses 3 or 4 times/day; titrate previously untreated patients under close clinical supervision, increasing the dosage in 600 mg increments every 2 weeks to 2400 mg/day based on clinical response and thereafter to 3600 mg/day as clinically indicated

Conversion to monotherapy: Initiate at 1200 mg/day in divided doses 3 or 4 times/day, reduce the dosage of the concomitant anticonvulsant(s) by 20% to 33% at the initiation of felbamate therapy; at week 2, increase the felbamate dosage to 2400 mg/day while reducing the dosage of the other anticonvulsant(s) up to an additional 33% of their original dosage; at week 3, increase the felbamate dosage up to 3600 mg/day and continue to reduce the dosage of the other anticonvulsant(s) as clinically indicated

Adjunctive therapy: Children with Lennox-Gastaut and ages 2-14 years:

Week 1:
- Felbamate: 15 mg/kg/day divided 3-4 times/day
- Concomitant anticonvulsant(s): Reduce original dosage by 20% to 30%

Week 2:
- Felbamate: 30 mg/kg/day divided 3-4 times/day
- Concomitant anticonvulsant(s): Reduce original dosage up to an additional 33%

Week 3:
- Felbamate: 45 mg/kg/day divided 3-4 times/day
- Concomitant anticonvulsant(s): Reduce dosage as clinically indicated

Adjunctive therapy: Children >14 years and Adults:

Week 1:
- Felbamate: 1200 mg/day initial dose
- Concomitant anticonvulsant(s): Reduce original dosage by 20% to 33%

Week 2:
- Felbamate: 2400 mg/day (therapeutic range)
- Concomitant anticonvulsant(s): Reduce original dosage by up to an additional 33%

Week 3:
- Felbamate: 3600 mg/day (therapeutic range)
- Concomitant anticonvulsant(s): Reduce original dosage as clinically indicated

Mechanism of Action Mechanism of action is unknown but has properties in common with other marketed anticonvulsants; has weak inhibitory effects on

GABA-receptor binding, benzodiazepine receptor binding, and is devoid of activity at the MK-801 receptor binding site of the NMDA receptor-ionophore complex.

Other Adverse Effects

>10%:

Central nervous system: Somnolence, headache, fatigue, dizziness

Gastrointestinal: Nausea, anorexia, vomiting, constipation

1% to 10%:

Cardiovascular: Chest pain, palpitations, tachycardia

Central nervous system: Depression or behavior changes, nervousness, anxiety, ataxia, stupor, malaise, agitation, psychological disturbances, aggressive reaction

Dermatologic: Skin rash, acne, pruritus

Gastrointestinal: Xerostomia, diarrhea, abdominal pain, weight gain, taste perversion

Neuromuscular & skeletal: Tremor, abnormal gait, paresthesia, myalgia

Ocular: Diplopia, abnormal vision

Respiratory: Sinusitis, pharyngitis

Miscellaneous: ALT increase

Drug Interactions CYP2C19 enzyme inhibitor

Increased Effect/Toxicity: Felbamate increases serum phenytoin, phenobarbital, and valproic acid concentrations which may result in toxicity; consider decreasing phenytoin or phenobarbital dosage by 25%. A decrease in valproic acid dosage may also be necessary.

Decreased Effect: Carbamazepine, phenytoin may decrease serum felbamate concentrations. Felbamate may decrease carbamazepine levels and increase levels of the active metabolite of carbamazepine (10,11-epoxide) resulting in carbamazepine toxicity; monitor for signs of carbamazepine toxicity (dizziness, ataxia, nystagmus, drowsiness).

Drug Uptake

Absorption: Oral: Rapid and almost complete; tablet absorption unaffected by food.

Half-life, elimination: 20-23 hours (average)

Time to peak: ~3 hours

Pregnancy Risk Factor C

Generic Available No

Comments Monotherapy has not been associated with gingival hyperplasia, impaired concentration, weight gain, or abnormal thinking

Felbatol® *see* Felbamate *on page 488*

Feldene® *see* Piroxicam *on page 965*

Felodipine (fe LOE di peen)

Related Information

Calcium Channel Blockers and Gingival Hyperplasia *on page 1432*

Cardiovascular Diseases *on page 1308*

Enalapril and Felodipine *on page 433*

U.S. Brand Names Plendil®

Canadian Brand Names Plendil®; Renedil®

Mexican Brand Names Logimax; Munobal; Plendil®

Pharmacologic Category Calcium Channel Blocker

Use Treatment of hypertension, CHF

Local Anesthetic/Vasoconstrictor Precautions No information available to require special precautions

Effects on Dental Treatment ~1%: Gingival hyperplasia (fewer reports with felodipine than with other CCBs); disappears with discontinuation (consultation with physician is suggested)

Dosage Adults: Oral: 5-10 mg once daily; increase by 5 mg at 2-week intervals, as needed, to a maximum of 20 mg/day (Elderly: Begin with 2.5 mg/day)

Dosing adjustment/comments in hepatic impairment: May require lower dosages (initial: 2.5 mg/day); monitor BP

Mechanism of Action Inhibits calcium ions from entering the select voltage-sensitive areas or "slow channels" of vascular smooth muscle and myocardium during depolarization, producing a relaxation of coronary vascular smooth muscle and coronary vasodilation; increases myocardial oxygen delivery in patients with vasospastic angina

Other Adverse Effects

>10%: Central nervous system: Headache (11% to 15%)

2% to 20%: Cardiovascular: Peripheral edema (2% to 17%), tachycardia (0.4% to 2.5%), flushing (4% to 7%)

Gastrointestinal: Gingival hyperplasia

Drug Interactions CYP3A3/4 enzyme substrate

Increased Effect/Toxicity: Inhibitors of CYP3A4, including azole antifungals (ketoconazole, itraconazole) and erythromycin, may inhibit calcium channel blocker metabolism, increasing the effects of felodipine. Beta-blockers may have increased pharmacokinetic or pharmacodynamic interactions with felodipine. Cyclosporine increases felodipine's serum concentration.

(Continued)

Felodipine *(Continued)*

Decreased Effect: Felodipine may decrease pharmacologic actions of theophylline. Calcium may reduce the calcium channel blocker's effects, particularly hypotension. Carbamazepine significantly reduces felodipine's bioavailability; avoid this combination. Nafcillin decreases plasma concentration of felodipine; avoid this combination. Rifampin increases the metabolism of felodipine. Felodipine may decrease pharmacologic actions of theophylline.

Drug Uptake

Onset of action: 2-5 hours
Absorption: 100%; absolute: 20% due to first-pass effect
Duration: 16-24 hours
Half-life, elimination: 11-16 hours

Pregnancy Risk Factor C

Generic Available No

Selected Readings

Lombardi T, Fiore-Donno G, Belser U, et al, "Felodipine-Induced Gingival Hyperplasia: A Clinical and Histologic Study," *J Oral Pathol Med*, 1991, 20(2):89-92.

Young PC, Turiansky GW, Sau P, et al, "Felodipine-Induced Gingival Hyperplasia," *Cutis*, 1998, 62(1):41-3.

Femara® *see* Letrozole *on page 690*
femhrt® *see* Combination Hormonal Contraceptives *on page 323*
Femilax™ [OTC] *see* Bisacodyl *on page 166*
Femiron® [OTC] *see* Ferrous Fumarate *on page 497*
Fenesin™ *see* Guaifenesin *on page 568*
Fenesin™ DM *see* Guaifenesin and Dextromethorphan *on page 569*

Fenofibrate (fen oh FYE brate)

U.S. Brand Names TriCor®

Canadian Brand Names Apo®-Fenofibrate; Apo®-Feno-Micro; Gen-Fenofibrate Micro; Lipidil Micro®; Lipidil Supra®; Nu-Fenofibrate; PMS-Fenofibrate Micro; TriCor®

Mexican Brand Names Controlip®; Lipidil®

Pharmacologic Category Antilipemic Agent, Fibric Acid

Synonyms Procetofene; Proctofene

Use

Adjunct to dietary therapy for the treatment of adults with very high elevations of serum triglyceride levels (types IV and V hyperlipidemia) who are at risk of pancreatitis and who do not respond adequately to a determined dietary effort; its efficacy can be enhanced by combination with other hypolipidemic agents that have a different mechanism of action; safety and efficacy may be greater than that of clofibrate

Treatment of hypercholesterolemia as adjunctive therapy to diet for the reduction of low-density lipoprotein cholesterol (LDL-C), total cholesterol (Total-C), triglycerides, and apolipoprotein B (Apo B) in adult patients with primary hypercholesterolemia or mixed dyslipidemia (Fredrickson types IIa and IIb)

Local Anesthetic/Vasoconstrictor Precautions No information available to require special precautions

Effects on Dental Treatment No effects or complications reported

Dosage As of September, 2001, a tablet formulation became available which will replace the capsules, as soon as existing supply is exhausted.

Oral:

Children >10 years: 5 mg/kg/day

Adults:

- Hypertriglyceridemia: Initial:
  - Capsule: 67 mg/day with meals, up to 200 mg/day
  - Tablet: 54 mg/day with meals, up to 160 mg/day
- Hypercholesterolemia or mixed hyperlipidemia: Initial:
  - Capsule: 200 mg/day with meals
  - Tablet: 160 mg/day with meals

Elderly: Initial: 67 mg/day (capsule) or 54 mg/day (tablet)

Dosage adjustment in renal impairment: Decrease dose or increase dosing interval for patients with renal failure: Initial: 67 mg/day (capsule) or 54 mg/day (tablet)

Mechanism of Action Fenofibric acid is believed to increase VLDL catabolism by enhancing the synthesis of lipoprotein lipase; as a result of a decrease in VLDL levels, total plasma triglycerides are reduced by 30% to 60%; modest increase in HDL occurs in some hypertriglyceridemic patients

Other Adverse Effects

1% to 10%:

- Gastrointestinal: Abdominal pain (5%), constipation (2%)
- Hepatic: Abnormal liver function test (7%), creatine phosphokinase increased (3%), ALT increased (3%), AST increased (3%)
- Neuromuscular & skeletal: Back pain (3%)
- Respiratory: Respiratory disorder (6%), rhinitis (2%)

Frequency not defined:

Cardiovascular: Angina pectoris, arrhythmias, atrial fibrillation, cardiovascular disorder, chest pain, coronary artery disorder, edema, electrocardiogram abnormality, extrasystoles, hypertension, hypotension, migraine, myocardial infarction, palpitations, peripheral edema, peripheral vascular disorder, phlebitis, tachycardia, varicose veins, vasodilatation

Central nervous system: Anxiety, depression, dizziness, fever, insomnia, malaise, nervousness, neuralgia, pain, somnolence, vertigo

Dermatologic: Acne, alopecia, bruising, contact dermatitis, eczema, fungal dermatitis, maculopapular rash, nail disorder, photosensitivity reaction, pruritus, skin disorder, skin ulcer, urticaria

Endocrine & metabolic: Diabetes mellitus, gout, gynecomastia, hypoglycemia, hyperuricemia

Gastrointestinal: Anorexia, appetite increased, colitis, diarrhea, xerostomia, duodenal ulcer, dyspepsia, eructation, esophagitis, flatulence, gastroenteritis, gastritis, gastrointestinal disorder, nausea, peptic ulcer, rectal disorder, rectal hemorrhage, tooth disorder, vomiting, weight gain/loss

Genitourinary: Cystitis, dysuria, prostatic disorder, libido decreased, pregnancy (unintended), urinary frequency, urolithiasis, vaginal moniliasis

Hematologic: Anemia, eosinophilia, leukopenia, lymphadenopathy, thrombocytopenia

Hepatic: Cholelithiasis, cholecystitis, fatty liver deposits

Neuromuscular & skeletal: Arthralgia, arthritis, arthrosis, bursitis, hypertonia, joint disorder, leg cramps, myalgia, myasthenia, myositis, paresthesia, tenosynovitis

Ocular: Abnormal vision, amblyopia, cataract, conjunctivitis, eye disorder, refraction disorder

Otic: Ear pain, otitis media

Renal: Creatinine increased, kidney function abnormality

Respiratory: Asthma, bronchitis, cough increased, dyspnea, laryngitis, pharyngitis, pneumonia, sinusitis

Miscellaneous: Accidental injury, allergic reaction, cyst, diaphoresis, herpes simplex, herpes zoster, infection

Drug Interactions

Increased Effect/Toxicity: The hypolipidemic effect of fenofibrate is increased when used with cholestyramine or colestipol. Fenofibrate may increase the effect of chlorpropamide and warfarin. Concurrent use of fenofibrate with HMG-CoA reductase inhibitors (atorvastatin, cerivastatin, fluvastatin, lovastatin, pravastatin, simvastatin) may increase the risk of myopathy and rhabdomyolysis. The manufacturer warns against concomitant use. However, combination therapy with statins has been used in some patients with resistant hyperlipidemias (with great caution).

Decreased Effect: Rifampin (and potentially other enzyme inducers) may decrease levels of fenofibrate.

Drug Uptake

Absorption: 60% to 90% when given with meals

Half-life, elimination: Fenofibrate: 21 hours (30 hours in elderly, 44-54 hours in hepatic impairment)

Time to peak: 4-6 hours

Pregnancy Risk Factor C

Generic Available No

Fenoldopam (fe NOL doe pam)

U.S. Brand Names Corlopam®

Canadian Brand Names Corlopam®

Pharmacologic Category Dopamine Agonist

Synonyms Fenoldopam Mesylate

Use Investigational in U.S.: Severe hypertension; CHF

Local Anesthetic/Vasoconstrictor Precautions No information available to require special precautions

Effects on Dental Treatment No effects or complications reported

Dosage

Oral: 100 mg 2-4 times daily

I.V.: Severe hypertension: Initial: 0.1 mcg/kg/minute; may be increased in increments of 0.05-0.2 mcg/kg/minute; maximal infusion rate: 1.6 mcg/kg/minute

Mechanism of Action A selective postsynaptic dopamine agonist (D_1-receptors) which exerts hypotensive effects by decreasing peripheral vasculature resistance with increased renal blood flow, diuresis, and natriuresis; 6 times as potent as dopamine in producing renal vasodilitation; has minimal adrenergic effects

Other Adverse Effects Frequency not defined:

Cardiovascular: Fibrillation (atrial), hypotension, edema, tachycardia, facial flushing, asymptomatic T wave flattening on EKG, flutter (atrial), chest pain, angina

Central nervous system: Headache, dizziness

Gastrointestinal: Nausea, vomiting, diarrhea

Ocular: Intraocular pressure (increased)

(Continued)

Fenoldopam *(Continued)*

Contraindications Hypersensitivity to fenoldopam or any component of the formulation

Warnings/Precautions Use with caution in patients with cirrhosis, unstable angina or glaucoma

Drug Interactions Increased Effect/Toxicity: Concurrent acetaminophen may increase fenoldopam levels (30% to 70%). Beta-blockers increase the risk of hypotension.

Drug Uptake

Onset of action: I.V.: 10 minutes
Absorption: Oral: Good
Duration: Oral: 2-4 hours; I.V.: 1 hour
Half-life, elimination: I.V.: 9.8 minutes
Time to peak: 1 hour

Generic Available No

Fenoprofen (fen oh PROE fen)

Related Information

Rheumatoid Arthritis and Osteoarthritis *on page 1340*
Temporomandibular Dysfunction (TMD) *on page 1397*

U.S. Brand Names Nalfon®

Canadian Brand Names Nalfon®

Pharmacologic Category Nonsteroidal Anti-inflammatory Drug (NSAID)

Synonyms Fenoprofen Calcium

Use Symptomatic treatment of acute and chronic rheumatoid arthritis and osteoarthritis; relief of mild to moderate pain

Local Anesthetic/Vasoconstrictor Precautions No information available to require special precautions

Effects on Dental Treatment NSAID formulations are known to reversibly decrease platelet aggregation via mechanisms different than observed with aspirin. The dentist should be aware of the potential of abnormal coagulation. Caution should also be exercised in the use of NSAIDs in patients already on anticoagulant therapy with drugs such as warfarin (Coumadin®).

Dosage Adults: Oral:

Rheumatoid arthritis: 300-600 mg 3-4 times/day up to 3.2 g/day
Mild to moderate pain: 200 mg every 4-6 hours as needed

Mechanism of Action Inhibits prostaglandin synthesis by decreasing the activity of the enzyme, cyclo-oxygenase, which results in decreased formation of prostaglandin precursors

Other Adverse Effects

>10%:

- Central nervous system: Dizziness (7% to 15%), somnolence (9% to 15%)
- Gastrointestinal: Abdominal cramps (2% to 4%), heartburn, indigestion, nausea (8% to 14%), dyspepsia (10% to 14%), flatulence (14%), anorexia (14%), constipation (7% to 14%), occult blood in stool (14%), vomiting (3% to 14%), diarrhea (2% to 14%)

1% to 10%:

- Central nervous system: Headache (9%)
- Dermatologic: Itching
- Endocrine & metabolic: Fluid retention

Warnings/Precautions Use with caution in patients with CHF, hypertension, decreased renal or hepatic function, history of GI disease (bleeding or ulcers), or those receiving anticoagulants. Elderly are at a high risk for adverse effects from nonsteroidal anti-inflammatory agents. As much as 60% of elderly can develop peptic ulceration and/or hemorrhage asymptomatically.

Use lowest effective dose for shortest period possible. Use of NSAIDs can compromise existing renal function especially when Cl_{cr} is <30 mL/minute. CNS adverse effects such as confusion, agitation, and hallucination are generally seen in overdose or high-dose situations; however, elderly may demonstrate these adverse effects at lower doses than younger adults. Withhold for at least 4-6 half-lives prior to surgical or dental procedures.

Drug Interactions

ACE inhibitors: Antihypertensive effects may be decreased by concurrent therapy with NSAIDs; monitor BP.

Angiotensin II antagonists: Antihypertensive effects may be decreased by concurrent therapy with NSAIDs; monitor BP.

Anticoagulants (warfarin, heparin, LMWHs) in combination with NSAIDs can cause increased risk of bleeding.

Other antiplatelet drugs (ticlopidine, clopidogrel, aspirin, abciximab, dipyridamole, eptifibatide, tirofiban) can cause an increased risk of bleeding.

Cholestyramine and colestipol reduce the bioavailability of diclofenac; separate administration times.

Corticosteroids may increase the risk of GI ulceration; avoid concurrent use.

Cyclosporine: NSAIDs may increase serum creatinine, potassium, BP, and cyclosporine levels; monitor cyclosporine levels and renal function carefully.

Gentamicin and amikacin serum concentrations are increased by indomethacin in premature infants. Results may apply to other aminoglycosides and NSAIDs.

Hydralazine's antihypertensive effect is decreased; avoid concurrent use.

Lithium levels can be increased; avoid concurrent use if possible or monitor lithium levels and adjust dose. Sulindac may have the least effect. When NSAID is stopped, lithium will need adjustment again.

Loop diuretics efficacy (diuretic and antihypertensive effect) is reduced. Indomethacin reduces this efficacy, however, it may be anticipated with any NSAID.

Methotrexate: Severe bone marrow suppression, aplastic anemia, and GI toxicity have been reported with concomitant NSAID therapy. Avoid use during moderate or high-dose methotrexate (increased and prolonged methotrexate levels). NSAID use during low-dose treatment of rheumatoid arthritis has not been fully evaluated; extreme caution is warranted.

Verapamil plasma concentration is decreased by diclofenac; avoid concurrent use.

Warfarin's INRs may be increased by piroxicam. Other NSAIDs may have the same effect depending on dose and duration. Monitor INR closely. Use the lowest dose of NSAIDs possible and for the briefest duration.

Drug Uptake

Onset of action: A few days

Absorption: Rapid; 80%

Half-life, elimination: 2.5-3 hours

Time to peak: ~2 hours

Pregnancy Risk Factor B/D (3rd trimester)

Generic Available Yes

Fenoterol *Not Available in U.S.* (fen oh TER ole)

Canadian Brand Names Berotec®

Pharmacologic Category $Beta_2$ Agonist

Synonyms Fenoterol Hydrobromide

Use Treatment and prevention of symptoms of reversible obstructive pulmonary disease (including asthma and acute bronchospasm), chronic bronchitis, emphysema

Local Anesthetic/Vasoconstrictor Precautions No information available to require special precautions

Effects on Dental Treatment No effects or complications reported

Dosage Inhalation: Children ≥12 years of age and Adults:

MDI:

- Acute treatment: 1 puff initially; may repeat in 5 minutes; if relief is not evident, additional doses and/or other therapy may be necessary
- Intermittent/long-term treatment: 1-2 puffs 3-4 times/day (maximum of 8 puffs/24 hours)

Solution: 0.5-1 mg (up to maximum of 2.5 mg)

Mechanism of Action Relaxes bronchial smooth muscle by action on $beta_2$ receptors with little effect on heart rate.

Other Adverse Effects Frequency of most effects may be dose-related, approximate frequencies noted below. In the treatment of acute bronchospasm (high-dose nebulization), symptoms of headache (up to 12%), tremor (32%), and tachycardia (up to 21%) are frequently noted.

1% to 10%:

- Cardiovascular: Palpitations, tachycardia
- Central nervous system: Headache, dizziness, nervousness
- Neuromuscular & skeletal: Tremor, muscle cramps
- Respiratory: Pharyngeal irritation, cough

Drug Interactions

Increased Effect/Toxicity: When used with inhaled ipratropium, an increased duration of bronchodilation may occur. Cardiovascular effects are potentiated in patients also receiving MAO inhibitors, tricyclic antidepressants, and sympathomimetic agents (eg, amphetamine, dopamine, dobutamine). Fenoterol may increase the risk of malignant arrhythmias with inhaled anesthetics (eg, enflurane, halothane). Concurrent use with diuretics may increase the risk of hypokalemia.

Decreased Effect: Decreased effect with nonselective beta-adrenergic blockers (eg, propranolol)

Drug Uptake

Onset of action: 5 minutes

Peak effect: 30-60 minutes

Duration: 3-4 hours (≤6-8 hours)

Pregnancy Risk Factor Not available; similar agents rated C

Fentanyl (FEN ta nil)

U.S. Brand Names Actiq®; Duragesic®; Sublimaze®

Canadian Brand Names Actiq®; Duragesic®

Mexican Brand Names Durogesic; Fentanest

(Continued)

Fentanyl *(Continued)*

Pharmacologic Category Analgesic, Narcotic; General Anesthetic

Synonyms Fentanyl Citrate

Use

Dental: Adjunct in preoperative I.V. conscious sedation in patients undergoing dental surgery

Medical: Sedation, relief of pain, preoperative medication, adjunct to general or regional anesthesia, management of chronic pain (transdermal product)

Actiq® is indicated only for management of breakthrough cancer pain in patients who are tolerant to and currently receiving opioid therapy for persistent cancer pain.

Local Anesthetic/Vasoconstrictor Precautions No information available to require special precautions

Effects on Dental Treatment No effects or complications reported

Restrictions C-II

Dosage Doses should be titrated to appropriate effects; wide range of doses, dependent upon desired degree of analgesia/anesthesia

Children 1-12 years:

Sedation for minor procedures/analgesia: I.M., I.V.: 1-2 mcg/kg/dose; may repeat at 30- to 60-minute intervals. **Note:** Children 18-36 months of age may require 2-3 mcg/kg/dose

Continuous sedation/analgesia: Initial I.V. bolus: 1-2 mcg/kg then 1 mcg/kg/hour; titrate upward; usual: 1-3 mcg/kg/hour

Pain control: Transdermal: Not recommended

Children >12 years and Adults: Sedation for minor procedures/analgesia: I.M., I.V.: 0.5-1 mcg/kg/dose; higher doses are used for major procedures

Adults:

Preoperative sedation, adjunct to regional anesthesia, postoperative pain: I.M., I.V.: 50-100 mcg/dose

Continuous sedation/analgesia (including ICU settings): Initial I.V. bolus: 25-50 mcg; then 1 mcg/kg/hour; titrate upward; usual: 1-3 mcg/kg/hour

Adjunct to general anesthesia: I.M., I.V.: 2-50 mcg/kg

General anesthesia without additional anesthetic agents: I.V. 50-100 mcg/kg with O_2 and skeletal muscle relaxant

Breakthrough cancer pain: Adults: Transmucosal: Actiq® dosing should be individually titrated to provide adequate analgesia with minimal side effects. It is indicated only for management of breakthrough cancer pain in patients who are tolerant to and currently receiving opioid therapy for persistent cancer pain. An initial starting dose of 200 mcg should be used for the treatment of breakthrough cancer pain. Patients should be monitored closely in order to determine the proper dose. If redosing for the same episode is necessary, the second dose may be started 15 minutes after completion of the first dose. Dosing should be titrated so that the patient's pain can be treated with one single dose. Generally, 1-2 days is required to determine the proper dose of analgesia with limited side effects. Once the dose has been determined, consumption should be limited to 4 units/day or less. Patients needing more than 4 units/day should have the dose of their long-term opioid re-evaluated. If signs of excessive opioid effects occur before a dose is complete, the unit should be removed from the patients mouth immediately, and subsequent doses decreased.

Pain control: Adults: Transdermal: Initial: 25 mcg/hour system; if currently receiving opiates, convert to fentanyl equivalent and administer equianalgesic dosage titrated to minimize the adverse effects and provide analgesia. To convert patients from oral or parenteral opioids to Duragesic®, the previous 24-hour analgesic requirement should be calculated. This analgesic requirement should be converted to the equianalgesic oral morphine dose.

See tables.

Equianalgesic Doses of Opioid Agonists

Drug	Equianalgesic Dose (mg)	
	I.M.	P.O.
Codeine	130	200
Hydromorphone	1.5	7.5
Levorphanol	2	4
Meperidine	75	—
Methadone	10	20
Morphine	10	60
Oxycodone	15	30
Oxymorphone	1	10 (PR)

From *N Engl J Med*, 1985, 313:84-95.

Corresponding Doses of Oral/Intramuscular Morphine and Duragesic™

P.O. 24-Hour Morphine (mg/d)	I.M. 24-Hour Morphine (mg/d)	Duragesic™ Dose (mcg/h)
45-134	8-22	25
135-224	28-37	50
225-314	38-52	75
315-404	53-67	100
405-494	68-82	125
495-584	83-97	150
585-674	98-112	175
675-764	113-127	200
765-854	128-142	225
855-944	143-157	250
945-1034	158-172	275
1035-1124	173-187	300

Product information, Duragesic™ — Janssen Pharmaceutica, January, 1991.

The dosage should not be titrated more frequently than every 3 days after the initial dose or every 6 days thereafter. The majority of patients are controlled on every 72-hour administration, however, a small number of patients require every 48-hour administration.

Elderly >65 years: Transmucosal: Actiq®: Dose should be reduced to 2.5-5 mcg/kg; elderly have been found to be twice as sensitive as younger patients to the effects of fentanyl. Patients in this age group generally require smaller doses of Actiq® than younger patients

Dosing adjustment in renal impairment:

Cl_{cr} 10-50 mL/minute: Administer at 75% of normal dose

Cl_{cr}<10 mL/minute: Administer at 50% of normal dose

Dosing adjustment in renal/hepatic impairment: Actiq®: Although fentanyl kinetics may be altered in renal/hepatic disease, Actiq® can be used successfully in the management of breakthrough cancer pain. Doses should be titrated to reach clinical effect with careful monitoring of patients with severe renal/hepatic disease.

Mechanism of Action Binds to opiate receptors (mu and kappa subtypes) in the CNS causing inhibition of ascending pain pathways, altering the perception of and response to pain; produces generalized CNS depression

Other Adverse Effects

>10%:

Cardiovascular: Hypotension, bradycardia

Central nervous system: CNS depression, drowsiness, sedation

Gastrointestinal: Nausea, vomiting, constipation

Respiratory: Respiratory depression

1% to 10%:

Cardiovascular: Cardiac arrhythmias, orthostatic hypotension

Central nervous system: Confusion

Gastrointestinal: Biliary tract spasm

Ocular: Miosis

<1%: ADH release, bronchospasm, circulatory depression, CNS excitation or delirium, cold/clammy skin, convulsions, dysesthesia, erythema, itching, laryngospasm, paradoxical dizziness, physical and psychological dependence with prolonged use, pruritus, rash, urinary tract spasm, urticaria

Postmarketing and/or case reports: Blurred vision, edema, tachycardia, weight loss

Contraindications Hypersensitivity to fentanyl or any component of the formulation; increased intracranial pressure; severe respiratory depression; severe liver or renal insufficiency; pregnancy (prolonged use or high doses near term)

Actiq® must not be used in patients who are intolerant to opioids. Patients are considered opioid-tolerant if they are taking at least 60 mg morphine/day, 50 mcg transdermal fentanyl/hour, or an equivalent dose of another opioid for ≥1 week.

Warnings/Precautions Fentanyl shares the toxic potentials of opiate agonists, and precautions of opiate agonist therapy should be observed; use with caution in patients with bradycardia; rapid I.V. infusion may result in skeletal muscle and chest wall rigidity leading to impaired ventilation leading to respiratory distress leading to apnea, bronchoconstriction, laryngospasm; inject slowly over 3-5 minutes; nondepolarizing skeletal muscle relaxant may be required. Tolerance of drug dependence may result from extended use.

Actiq® should be used only for the care of cancer patients and is intended for use by specialists who are knowledgeable in treating cancer pain. Actiq® preparations contain an amount of medication that can be fatal to children. Keep all units out of the reach of children and discard any open units properly. Patients and caregivers

(Continued)

Fentanyl *(Continued)*

should be counseled on the dangers to children including the risk of exposure to partially-consumed units. Safety and efficacy have not been established in children <16 years of age.

Topical patches: Serum fentanyl concentrations may increase approximately one-third for patients with a body temperature of 40°C secondary to a temperature-dependent increase in fentanyl release from the system and increased skin permeability. Patients who experience adverse reactions should be monitored for at least 12 hours after removal of the patch.

The elderly may be particularly susceptible to the CNS depressant and constipating effects of narcotics

Drug Interactions CYP3A3/4 enzyme substrate

CNS depressants: Increased sedation with CNS depressants, phenothiazines

CYP3A3/4 inducers (including carbamazepine, phenytoin, phenobarbital, rifampin): May decrease serum concentration of fentanyl by increasing metabolism.

CYP3A3/4 inhibitors (including erythromycin, clarithromycin, ketoconazole, itraconazole, protease inhibitors): May increase serum concentration of fentanyl.

MAO inhibitors: Not recommended to use Actiq® within 14 days. Severe and unpredictable potentiation by MAO Inhibitors has been reported with opioid analgesics.

Dietary/Ethanol/Herb Considerations

Ethanol: Avoid use; may increase CNS depression.

Food: Glucose may cause hyperglycemia.

Herb/Nutraceutical: Avoid gotu kola, kava, SAMe, and valerian; may increase CNS depression. Avoid St John's wort; may decrease serum concentration.

Drug Uptake

Onset of action (respiratory depressant effect may last longer than analgesic effect): I.M.: Analgesia: 7-15 minutes; I.V.: Analgesia: Almost immediate; Transmucosal (lozenge): 5-15 minutes with a maximum reduction in activity/apprehension

Absorption: Transmucosal: Rapid, ~25% from the buccal mucosa; 75% swallowed with saliva and slowly absorbed from gastrointestinal tract

Duration: I.M.: 1-2 hours; I.V.: 0.5-1 hour; Transmucosal: Related to blood level of drug

Half-life, elimination: 2-4 hours; Transmucosal: 6.6 hours (range: 5-15 hours)

Time to peak: Transmucosal: Analgesic: 20-30 minutes

Pregnancy Risk Factor B/D (prolonged use or high doses at term)

Breast-feeding Considerations Not contraindicated

Dosage Forms INJ [preservative free]: 0.05 mg/mL (2 mL, 5 mL, 10 mL, 20 mL, 30 mL, 50 mL). **LOZ, oral transmucosal** (Actiq®): 200 mcg, 400 mcg, 600 mcg, 800 mcg, 1200 mcg, 1600 mcg. **TRANSDERMAL SYSTEM:** 25 mcg/hour [10 cm^2]; 50 mcg/hour [20 cm^2]; 75 mcg/hour [30 cm^2]; 100 mcg/hour [40 cm^2] (5s)

Generic Available Yes: Injection only

Comments Transdermal fentanyl should not be used as a pain reliever in dentistry due to danger of hypoventilation

Selected Readings Dionne RA, Yagiela JA, Moore PA, et al, "Comparing Efficacy and Safety of Four Intravenous Sedation Regimens in Dental Outpatients," *Am Dent Assoc*, 2001, 132(6):740-51.

Feosol® [OTC] *see* Ferrous Sulfate *on page 498*

Feostat® [OTC] *see* Ferrous Fumarate *on page 497*

Feracid® *see* Glutamic Acid *on page 560*

Feratab® [OTC] *see* Ferrous Sulfate *on page 498*

Fergon® [OTC] *see* Ferrous Gluconate *on page 498*

Fer-In-Sol® [OTC] *see* Ferrous Sulfate *on page 498*

Fer-Iron® [OTC] *see* Ferrous Sulfate *on page 498*

Fero-Grad 500® [OTC] *see* Ferrous Sulfate and Ascorbic Acid *on page 499*

Ferric Gluconate (FER ik GLOO koe nate)

U.S. Brand Names Ferrlecit®

Pharmacologic Category Iron Salt

Synonyms Sodium Ferric Gluconate

Use Repletion of total body iron content in patients with iron deficiency anemia who are undergoing hemodialysis in conjunction with erythropoietin therapy

Local Anesthetic/Vasoconstrictor Precautions No information available to require special precautions

Effects on Dental Treatment Do not prescribe tetracyclines simultaneously with iron since GI tract absorption of both tetracycline and iron may be inhibited.

Dosage Adults:

Test dose (recommended): 2 mL diluted in 50 mL 0.9% sodium chloride over 60 minutes

Repletion of iron in hemodialysis patients: I.V.: 125 mg (10 mL) in 100 mL 0.9% sodium chloride over 1 hour during hemodialysis. Most patients will require a cumulative dose of 1 g elemental iron over ~ 8 sequential dialysis treatments to achieve a favorable response.

Mechanism of Action Supplies a source to elemental iron necessary to the function of hemoglobin, myoglobin, and specific enzyme systems; allows transport of oxygen via hemoglobin

Other Adverse Effects Major adverse reactions include hypotension and hypersensitivity reactions. Hypersensitivity reactions have included pruritus, chest pain, hypotension, nausea, abdominal pain, flank pain, fatigue, and rash.

Frequency not defined:
Cardiovascular: Hypotension (serious hypotension in 1%), chest pain, hypertension, syncope, tachycardia, angina, myocardial infarction, pulmonary edema, hypovolemia, peripheral edema
Central nervous system: Headache, fatigue, fever, malaise, dizziness, paresthesia, insomnia, agitation, somnolence, pain
Dermatologic: Pruritus, rash
Endocrine & metabolic: Hyperkalemia, hypoglycemia, hypokalemia
Gastrointestinal: Abdominal pain, nausea, vomiting, diarrhea, rectal disorder, dyspepsia, flatulence, melena, epigastric pain
Genitourinary: Urinary tract infection
Hematologic: Anemia, abnormal erythrocytes, lymphadenopathy
Local: Injection site reactions, injection site pain
Neuromuscular & skeletal: Weakness, back pain, leg cramps, myalgia, arthralgia, paresthesia, groin pain
Ocular: Blurred vision, conjunctivitis
Respiratory: Dyspnea, cough, rhinitis, upper respiratory infection, pneumonia
Miscellaneous: Hypersensitivity reactions, infection, rigors, chills, flu-like syndrome, sepsis, carcinoma, increased diaphoresis

Contraindications Hypersensitivity to ferric gluconate or any component of the formulation; anemia not caused by iron deficiency; heart failure (of any severity); iron overload

Drug Interactions Decreased Effect: Chloramphenicol may decrease effect of ferric gluconate injection; ferric gluconate injection may decrease the absorption of oral iron.

Drug Uptake Pharmacokinetic studies have not been conducted. The total body iron content normally ranges from 2-4 g of elemental iron.
Half-life, elimination: Bound: 1 hour

Pregnancy Risk Factor B

Generic Available No

Comments Contains benzyl alcohol 9 mg/mL

Ferrlecit® *see* Ferric Gluconate *on page 496*
Ferro-Sequels® [OTC] *see* Ferrous Fumarate *on page 497*

Ferrous Fumarate (FER us FYOO ma rate)

U.S. Brand Names Femiron® [OTC]; Feostat® [OTC]; Ferro-Sequels® [OTC]; Hemocyte® [OTC]; Ircon® [OTC]; Nephro-Fer™ [OTC]; Span-FF®

Canadian Brand Names Palafer®

Mexican Brand Names Ferval®

Pharmacologic Category Iron Salt

Use Prevention and treatment of iron deficiency anemias

Local Anesthetic/Vasoconstrictor Precautions No information available to require special precautions

Effects on Dental Treatment Do not prescribe tetracyclines simultaneously with iron since GI tract absorption of both tetracycline and iron may be inhibited.

Dosage Oral **(dose expressed in terms of elemental iron):**
Children:
- Severe iron deficiency anemia: 4-6 mg Fe/kg/day in 3 divided doses
- Mild to moderate iron deficiency anemia: 3 mg Fe/kg/day in 1-2 divided doses
- Prophylaxis: 1-2 mg Fe/kg/day

Adults:
- Iron deficiency: 60-100 mg twice daily up to 60 mg 2 times/day
- Prophylaxis: 60-100 mg/day
- To avoid GI upset, start with a single daily dose and increase by 1 tablet/day each week or as tolerated until desired daily dose is achieved

Elderly: 200 mg 3-4 times/day

Mechanism of Action Replaces iron found in hemoglobin, myoglobin, and enzymes; allows the transportation of oxygen via hemoglobin

Other Adverse Effects
>10%: Gastrointestinal: Stomach cramping, constipation, nausea, vomiting, dark stools
1% to 10%:
- Gastrointestinal: Heartburn, diarrhea, staining of teeth
- Genitourinary: Discoloration of urine

(Continued)

Ferrous Fumarate *(Continued)*

Drug Interactions

Increased Effect/Toxicity: Concurrent administration of ≥200 mg vitamin C per 30 mg elemental iron increases absorption of oral iron.

Decreased Effect: Absorption of oral preparation of iron and tetracyclines are decreased when both of these drugs are given together. Absorption of fluoroquinolones, levodopa, methyldopa, and penicillamine may be decreased due to formation of a ferric ion-quinolone complex. Concurrent administration of antacids, H_2 blockers (cimetidine), or proton pump inhibitors may decrease iron absorption. Response to iron therapy may be delayed by chloramphenicol.

Drug Uptake

Onset of hematologic response: Red blood cell form and color changes within 3-10 days

Peak effect: Reticulocytosis: 5-10 days; hemoglobin values increase within 2-4 weeks

Absorption: Oral: Iron is absorbed in the duodenum and upper jejunum; 10% absorbed (increased to 20% to 30% with iron deficiency); food and achlorhydria decreases absorption

Pregnancy Risk Factor A

Generic Available Yes

Ferrous Gluconate (FER us GLOO koe nate)

U.S. Brand Names Fergon® [OTC]

Canadian Brand Names Apo®-Ferrous Gluconate

Pharmacologic Category Iron Salt

Use Prevention and treatment of iron deficiency anemias

Local Anesthetic/Vasoconstrictor Precautions No information available to require special precautions

Effects on Dental Treatment Do not prescribe tetracyclines simultaneously with iron since GI tract absorption of both tetracycline and iron may be inhibited.

Dosage Oral **(dose expressed in terms of elemental iron):**

Children:

Severe iron deficiency anemia: 4-6 mg Fe/kg/day in 3 divided doses

Mild to moderate iron deficiency anemia: 3 mg Fe/kg/day in 1-2 divided doses

Prophylaxis: 1-2 mg Fe/kg/day

Adults:

Iron deficiency: 60 mg twice daily up to 60 mg 4 times/day

Prophylaxis: 60 mg/day

Mechanism of Action Replaces iron found in hemoglobin, myoglobin, and enzymes; allows the transportation of oxygen via hemoglobin

Other Adverse Effects

>10%: Gastrointestinal: Stomach cramping, constipation, nausea, vomiting, dark stools

1% to 10%:

Gastrointestinal: Heartburn, diarrhea, staining of teeth

Genitourinary: Discoloration of urine

Drug Interactions

Increased Effect/Toxicity: Concurrent administration of ≥200 mg vitamin C per 30 mg elemental iron increases absorption of oral iron.

Decreased Effect: Absorption of oral preparation of iron and tetracyclines are decreased when both of these drugs are given together. Absorption of fluoroquinolones, levodopa, methyldopa, and penicillamine may be decreased due to formation of a ferric ion-quinolone complex. Concurrent administration of antacids, H_2 blockers (cimetidine), or proton pump inhibitors may decrease iron absorption. Response to iron therapy may be delayed by chloramphenicol.

Drug Uptake Onset of action: Red blood cells form and color changes within 3-10 days; peak reticulocytosis occurs in 5-10 days; hemoglobin values increase within 2-4 weeks

Pregnancy Risk Factor A

Generic Available Yes

Ferrous Sulfate (FER us SUL fate)

U.S. Brand Names Feosol® [OTC]; Feratab® [OTC]; Fer-In-Sol® [OTC]; Fer-Iron® [OTC]; Slow FE® [OTC]

Canadian Brand Names Apo®-Ferrous Sulfate; Fer-In-Sol®; Ferodan™

Mexican Brand Names Hemobion®

Pharmacologic Category Iron Salt

Synonyms $FeSO_4$

Use Prevention and treatment of iron deficiency anemias

Local Anesthetic/Vasoconstrictor Precautions No information available to require special precautions

Effects on Dental Treatment Do not prescribe tetracyclines simultaneously with iron since GI tract absorption of both tetracycline and iron may be inhibited.

Dosage Oral:
Children **(dose expressed in terms of elemental iron)**:
Severe iron deficiency anemia: 4-6 mg Fe/kg/day in 3 divided doses
Mild to moderate iron deficiency anemia: 3 mg Fe/kg/day in 1-2 divided doses
Prophylaxis: 1-2 mg Fe/kg/day up to a maximum of 15 mg/day
Adults **(dose expressed in terms of ferrous sulfate)**:
Iron deficiency: 300 mg twice daily up to 300 mg 4 times/day or 250 mg (extended release) 1-2 times/day
Prophylaxis: 300 mg/day

Mechanism of Action Replaces iron, found in hemoglobin, myoglobin, and other enzymes; allows the transportation of oxygen via hemoglobin

Other Adverse Effects
>10%: Gastrointestinal: GI irritation, epigastric pain, nausea, dark stool, vomiting, stomach cramping, constipation
1% to 10%:
Gastrointestinal: Heartburn, diarrhea
Genitourinary: Discoloration of urine
Miscellaneous: Liquid preparations may temporarily stain the teeth

Drug Interactions
Increased Effect/Toxicity: Concurrent administration of ≥200 mg vitamin C per 30 mg elemental iron increases absorption of oral iron.
Decreased Effect: Absorption of oral preparation of iron and tetracyclines are decreased when both of these drugs are given together. Absorption of fluoroquinolones, levodopa, methyldopa, and penicillamine may be decreased due to formation of a ferric ion-quinolone complex. Concurrent administration of antacids, H_2 blockers (cimetidine), or proton pump inhibitors may decrease iron absorption. Response to iron therapy may be delayed by chloramphenicol.

Drug Uptake
Onset of action: Red blood cell form and color changes within 3-10 days; peak reticulocytosis occurs in 5-10 days; hemoglobin values increase within 2-4 weeks
Absorption: Oral: Iron is absorbed in the duodenum and upper jejunum; 10% absorbed (increases to 20% to 30% with iron deficiency); food and achlorhydria decreases absorption

Pregnancy Risk Factor A

Generic Available Yes

Ferrous Sulfate and Ascorbic Acid

(FER us SUL fate & a SKOR bik AS id)

U.S. Brand Names Fero-Grad 500® [OTC]

Pharmacologic Category Iron Salt; Vitamin

Synonyms Ascorbic Acid and Ferrous Sulfate

Use Treatment of iron deficiency in nonpregnant adults; treatment and prevention of iron deficiency in pregnant adults

Local Anesthetic/Vasoconstrictor Precautions No information available to require special precautions

Effects on Dental Treatment Do not prescribe tetracyclines simultaneously with iron since GI tract absorption of both tetracycline and iron may be inhibited.

Dosage Adults: Oral: 1 tablet daily

Other Adverse Effects Based on **ferrous sulfate** component:
>10%: Gastrointestinal: GI irritation, epigastric pain, nausea, dark stool, vomiting, stomach cramping, constipation
1% to 10%:
Gastrointestinal: Heartburn, diarrhea
Genitourinary: Discoloration of urine
Miscellaneous: Liquid preparations may temporarily stain the teeth

Drug Interactions
Increased Effect/Toxicity: Concurrent administration of ≥200 mg vitamin C per 30 mg elemental iron increases absorption of oral iron.
Decreased Effect: Absorption of oral preparation of iron and tetracyclines are decreased when both of these drugs are given together. Absorption of quinolones may be decreased due to formation of a ferric ion-quinolone complex when given concurrently. Concurrent administration of antacids and H_2 blockers (cimetidine) may decrease iron absorption. Iron may decrease absorption of levodopa, methyldopa, penicillamine when given at the same time. Response to iron therapy may be delayed by chloramphenicol.

Drug Uptake See Ferrous Sulfate *on page 498* and Ascorbic Acid *on page 117*

Generic Available No

Ferrous Sulfate, Ascorbic Acid, and Vitamin B Complex

(FER us SUL fate, a SKOR bik AS id, & VYE ta min bee KOM pleks)

U.S. Brand Names Iberet®-Liquid [OTC]; Iberet®-Liquid 500 [OTC]

Pharmacologic Category Iron Salt; Vitamin

Use Conditions of iron deficiency with an increased needed for B-complex vitamins and vitamin C

(Continued)

Ferrous Sulfate, Ascorbic Acid, and Vitamin B Complex *(Continued)*

Local Anesthetic/Vasoconstrictor Precautions No information available to require special precautions

Effects on Dental Treatment Do not prescribe tetracyclines simultaneously with iron since GI tract absorption of both tetracycline and iron may be inhibited.

Dosage Oral:

Children 1-3 years: 5 mL twice daily after meals
Children >4 years and Adults: 10 mL 3 times/day after meals

Other Adverse Effects Based on **ferrous sulfate** component:

>10%: Gastrointestinal: GI irritation, epigastric pain, nausea, dark stool, vomiting, stomach cramping, constipation

1% to 10%:

- Gastrointestinal: Heartburn, diarrhea
- Genitourinary: Discoloration of urine
- Miscellaneous: Liquid preparations may temporarily stain the teeth

Drug Interactions Decreased Effect: Absorption of oral preparation of iron and tetracyclines are decreased when both of these drugs are given together. Absorption of quinolones may be decreased due to formation of a ferric ion-quinolone complex when given concurrently. Concurrent administration of antacids and H_2 blockers (cimetidine) may decrease iron absorption. Iron may decrease absorption of levodopa, methyldopa, penicillamine when given at the same time. Response to iron therapy may be delayed by chloramphenicol.

Drug Uptake See Ferrous Sulfate *on page 498*, Vitamin B Complex *on page 1244*, and Ascorbic Acid *on page 117*

Generic Available No

Ferrous Sulfate, Ascorbic Acid, Vitamin B Complex, and Folic Acid

(FER us SUL fate, a SKOR bik AS id, VYE ta min bee KOM pleks, & FOE lik AS id)

U.S. Brand Names Iberet-Folic-500®

Pharmacologic Category Vitamin

Use Treatment of iron deficiency and prevention of concomitant folic acid deficiency where there is an associated deficient intake or increased need for B-complex vitamins

Local Anesthetic/Vasoconstrictor Precautions No information available to require special precautions

Effects on Dental Treatment Do not prescribe tetracyclines simultaneously with iron since GI tract absorption of both tetracycline and iron may be inhibited.

Dosage Adults: Oral: 1 tablet daily

Other Adverse Effects Based on **ferrous sulfate** component:

>10%: Gastrointestinal: GI irritation, epigastric pain, nausea, dark stool, vomiting, stomach cramping, constipation

1% to 10%:

- Gastrointestinal: Heartburn, diarrhea
- Genitourinary: Discoloration of urine
- Miscellaneous: Liquid preparations may temporarily stain the teeth

Drug Interactions Decreased Effect: Absorption of oral preparation of iron and tetracyclines are decreased when both of these drugs are given together. Absorption of quinolones may be decreased due to formation of a ferric ion-quinolone complex when given concurrently. Concurrent administration of antacids and H_2 blockers (cimetidine) may decrease iron absorption. Iron may decrease absorption of levodopa, methyldopa, penicillamine when given at the same time. Response to iron therapy may be delayed by chloramphenicol.

Drug Uptake See Ferrous Sulfate *on page 498*, Vitamin B Complex *on page 1244*, Ascorbic Acid *on page 117*, and Folic Acid *on page 530*

Pregnancy Risk Factor A

Generic Available Yes

Fertinex® *see* Follitropins *on page 531*
Fertinex® *see* Urofollitropin *on page 1222*
Feverall® [OTC] *see* Acetaminophen *on page 26*

Fexofenadine (feks oh FEN a deen)

U.S. Brand Names Allegra®

Canadian Brand Names Allegra®

Mexican Brand Names Allegra®

Pharmacologic Category Antihistamine, Nonsedating

Synonyms Fexofenadine Hydrochloride

Use Nonsedating antihistamine indicated for the relief of seasonal allergic rhinitis and chronic idiopathic urticaria

Local Anesthetic/Vasoconstrictor Precautions No information available to require special precautions

Effects on Dental Treatment No effects or complications reported

Dosage Oral:

Children 6-11 years: 30 mg twice daily (once daily in children with impaired renal function)

Children ≥12 years and Adults:

Seasonal allergic rhinitis: 60 mg twice daily **or** 180 mg once daily

Chronic idiopathic urticaria: 60 mg twice daily

Dosing adjustment in renal impairment: Recommended initial doses of 60 mg once daily

Mechanism of Action An active metabolite of terfenadine, also competes with histamine for H_1-receptor sites on effector cells in the GI tract, blood vessels, and respiratory tract; it appears that fexofenadine does not cross the blood brain barrier to any appreciable degree, resulting in a reduced potential for sedation

Other Adverse Effects

>10%: Central nervous system: Headache 11% (with once-daily dosing)

1% to 10%:

Central nervous system: Fever (2%), dizziness (2%), pain (2%), drowsiness (1% to 2%), fatigue (1%)

Endocrine & metabolic: Dysmenorrhea (2%)

Gastrointestinal: Nausea (2%), dyspepsia (1%)

Neuromuscular & skeletal: Back pain (2% to 3%)

Otic: Otitis media (3%)

Respiratory: Cough (4%), upper respiratory tract infection (4%), sinusitis (2%)

Miscellaneous: Viral infection (3%)

Drug Interactions CYP2D6 enzyme inhibitor (weak)

Increased Effect/Toxicity: Erythromycin and ketoconazole increased the levels of fexofenadine; however, no increase in adverse events or QT_c intervals was noted. The effect of other macrolide agents or azoles has not been investigated.

Decreased Effect: Aluminum- and magnesium-containing antacids decrease plasma concentrations of fexofenadine; separate administration is recommended.

Drug Uptake

Onset of action: 1 hour

Duration of antihistaminic effect: ≤12 hours

Half-life, elimination: 14.4 hours

Time to peak: ~2.6 hours after oral administration

Pregnancy Risk Factor C

Generic Available No

Selected Readings

"Fexofenadine," *Med Lett Drugs Ther*, 1996, 38(986):95-6.

Markham A and Wagstaff AJ, "Fexofenadine," *Drugs*, 1998, 55(2):269-74 (discussion 275-6).

Simons FE, Bergman JN, Watson WT, et al, "The Clinical Pharmacology of Fexofenadine in Children," *J Allergy Clin Immunol*, 1996, 98(6 Pt 1):1062-4.

Fexofenadine and Pseudoephedrine

(feks oh FEN a deen & soo doe e FED rin)

U.S. Brand Names Allegra-D®

Canadian Brand Names Allegra-D®

Pharmacologic Category Antihistamine/Decongestant Combination

Synonyms Pseudoephedrine and Fexofenadine

Use Relief of symptoms associated with seasonal allergic rhinitis in adults and children 12 years of age and older. Symptoms treated effectively include sneezing, rhinorrhea, itchy nose/palate/ and/or throat, itchy/watery/red eyes, and nasal congestion.

Local Anesthetic/Vasoconstrictor Precautions Pseudoephedrine component: Use with caution since pseudoephedrine is a sympathomimetic amine which could interact with epinephrine to cause a pressor response

Effects on Dental Treatment Pseudoephedrine component: Up to 10% of patients could experience tachycardia, palpitations, and xerostomia; use vasoconstrictor with caution.

Dosage Oral: Adults: One tablet twice daily for adults and children 12 years of age and older. It is recommended that the administration with food should be avoided. A dose of one tablet once daily is recommended as the starting dose in patients with decreased renal function.

Drug Uptake See Fexofenadine *on page 500*, Pseudoephedrine *on page 1022*

Pregnancy Risk Factor C

Generic Available No

Fiberall® Chewable Tablet [OTC] *see* Calcium Polycarbophil *on page 207*

Fiberall® Powder [OTC] *see* Psyllium *on page 1025*

Fiberall® Wafer [OTC] *see* Psyllium *on page 1025*

FiberCon® Tablet [OTC] *see* Calcium Polycarbophil *on page 207*

Fiber-Lax® Tablet [OTC] *see* Calcium Polycarbophil *on page 207*

Fibrin Sealant Kit (FI brin SEEL ent kit)

U.S. Brand Names Tisseel® VH Fibrin Sealant Kit

Canadian Brand Names Tisseel® VH Fibrin Sealant Kit

Pharmacologic Category Hemostatic Agent

Synonyms FS

Use Adjunct to hemostasis in cardiopulmonary bypass surgery and splenic injury (due to blunt or penetrating trauma to the abdomen) when the control of bleeding by conventional surgical techniques is ineffective or impractical; adjunctive sealant for closure of colostomies; hemostatic agent in heparinized patients undergoing cardiopulmonary bypass

Local Anesthetic/Vasoconstrictor Precautions No information available to require special precautions

Effects on Dental Treatment No effects or complications reported

Dosage Adjunct to hemostasis: Adults: Apply topically; actual dose is based on size of surface to be covered:

Maximum area to be sealed: 4 cm^2
  Required size of Tisseel® VH kit: 0.5 mL
Maximum area to be sealed: 8 cm^2
  Required size of Tisseel® VH kit: 1 mL
Maximum area to be sealed: 16 cm^2
  Required size of Tisseel® VH kit: 2 mL
Maximum area to be sealed: 40 cm^2
  Required size of Tisseel® VH kit: 5 mL

Apply in thin layers to avoid excess formation of granulation tissue and slow absorption of the sealant. Following application, hold the sealed parts in the desired position for 3-5 minutes. To prevent sealant from adhering to gloves or surgical instruments, wet them with saline prior to contact.

Mechanism of Action Formation of a biodegradable adhesive is done by duplicating the last step of the coagulation cascade, the formation of fibrin from fibrinogen. Fibrinogen is the main component of the sealant solution. The solution also contains thrombin, which transforms fibrinogen from the sealer protein solution into fibrin, and fibrinolysis inhibitor (aprotinin), which prevents the premature degradation of fibrin. When mixed as directed, a viscous solution forms that sets into an elastic coagulum.

Other Adverse Effects No adverse events were reported in clinical trials. Anaphylactoid or anaphylactic reactions have occurred with other plasma-derived products.

Drug Interactions Decreased Effect: Local concentrations/applications of alcohol, heavy-metal ions, iodine; oxycellulose preparations

Drug Uptake Onset of action: Final prepared sealant reaches 70% strength in ~10 minutes, full strength in ~2 hours

Pregnancy Risk Factor C

Filgrastim (fil GRA stim)

U.S. Brand Names Neupogen®

Canadian Brand Names Neupogen®

Mexican Brand Names Neupogen®

Pharmacologic Category Colony Stimulating Factor

Synonyms G-CSF; Granulocyte Colony Stimulating Factor

Use To reduce the duration of neutropenia and the associated risk of infection in patients with nonmyeloid malignancies receiving myelosuppressive chemotherapeutic regimens associated with a significant incidence of severe neutropenia with fever; it has also been used in AIDS patients on zidovudine and in patients with noncancer chemotherapy-induced neutropenia

Local Anesthetic/Vasoconstrictor Precautions No information available to require special precautions

Effects on Dental Treatment No effects or complications reported

Dosage Children and Adults: administered S.C. or I.V. as a single daily infusion over 20-30 minutes

Myelosuppressive chemotherapy: 5 mcg/kg/day S.C. or I.V. Doses may be increased in increments of 5 mcg/kg for each chemotherapy cycle, according to the duration and severity of the absolute neutrophil count (ANC) nadir. In phase III trials, efficacy was observed at doses of 4-6 mcg/kg/day. Discontinue therapy if the ANC count is >10,000/mm^3 after the ANC nadir has occurred following the expected chemotherapy-induced neutrophil nadir. Some cancer centers are stopping therapy at an ANC of 2500. Duration of therapy needed to attenuate chemotherapy-induced neutropenia may be dependent on the myelosuppressive potential of the chemotherapy regimen employed. Duration of therapy in clinical studies has ranged from 2 weeks to 3 years.

Bone marrow transplant patients: 10 mcg/kg/day as an I.V. infusion of 4 or 24 hours or as continuous 24-hour S.C. infusion. Administer first dose at least 24 hours after cytotoxic chemotherapy and at least 24 hours after bone marrow infusion. See table on following page.

Severe chronic neutropenia:
  Congenital neutropenia: 6 mcg/kg twice daily S.C.

Filgrastim Dose Based on Neutrophil Response

Absolute Neutrophil Count (ANC)	Filgrastim Dose Adjustment
When ANC >1000/mm^3 for 3 consecutive days	Reduce to 5 mcg/kg/day
If ANC remains >1000/mm^3 for 3 more consecutive days	Discontinue filgrastim
If ANC decreases to <1000/mm^3	Resume at 5 mcg/kg/day

If ANC decreases <1000/mm^3 during the 5 mcg/kg/day dose, increase dose to 10 mcg/kg/day and follow the above steps in the table.

Idiopathic/cyclic neutropenia: 5 mcg/kg/day S.C.

Chronic daily administration is required to maintain clinical benefit. Adjust dose based on the patients' clinical course as well as ANC. In phase III studies, the target ANC was 1,500-10,000/mm^3. Reduce the dose of the ANC if persistently >10,000/mm^3.

Premature discontinuation of G-CSF therapy prior to the time of recovery from the expected neutrophil is generally not recommended. A transient increase in neutrophil counts is typically seen 1-2 days after initiation of therapy.

Mechanism of Action Stimulates the production, maturation, and activation of neutrophils, G-CSF activates neutrophils to increase both their migration and cytotoxicity. Natural proteins which stimulate hematopoietic stem cells to proliferate, prolong cell survival, stimulate cell differentiation, and stimulate functional activity of mature cells. CSFs are produced by a wide variety of cell types. Specific mechanisms of action are not yet fully understood, but possibly work by a second-messenger pathway with resultant protein production. See table.

Proliferation / Differentiation	G-CSF (Filgrastim)	GM-CSF (Sargramostim)
Neutrophils	Yes	Yes
Eosinophils	No	Yes
Macrophages	No	Yes
Neutrophil migration	Enhanced	Inhibited

Other Adverse Effects

>10%:

Cardiovascular: Chest pain

Central nervous system: Fever

Dermatologic: Alopecia

Endocrine & metabolic: Fluid retention

Gastrointestinal: Nausea, vomiting, diarrhea, mucositis; splenomegaly - up to 33% of patients with cyclic neutropenia/congenital agranulocytosis receiving filgrastim for ≥14 days; rare in other patients

Neuromuscular & skeletal: Bone pain (24%), commonly in the lower back, posterior iliac crest, and sternum

1% to 10%:

Cardiovascular: S-T segment depression (3%)

Central nervous system: Headache

Dermatologic: Rash

Gastrointestinal: Anorexia, constipation, sore throat

Hematologic: Leukocytosis

Local: Pain at injection site

Neuromuscular & skeletal: Weakness

Respiratory: Dyspnea, cough

Drug Interactions Drugs which may potentiate the release of neutrophils (eg, lithium) should be used with caution.

Drug Uptake

Onset of action: ~24 hours; plateaus in 3-5 days;

Peak effect: Plasma levels maintained for ≤12 hours

Absorption: S.C.: 100%

Duration: ANC decreases by 50% within 2 days after discontinuing G-CSF; white counts return to the normal range in 4-7 days

Half-life, elimination: 1.8-3.5 hours

Time to peak: S.C.: 2-6 hours

Pregnancy Risk Factor C

Generic Available No

Comments Reimbursement hotline: 1-800-28-AMGEN

Finasteride (fi NAS teer ide)

U.S. Brand Names Propecia®; Proscar®

Canadian Brand Names Propecia®; Proscar®

Mexican Brand Names Propeshia®; Proscar®

Pharmacologic Category Antiandrogen

(Continued)

Finasteride *(Continued)*

Use Early data indicate that finasteride is useful in the treatment of symptomatic benign prostatic hyperplasia (BPH); male pattern baldness or androgenetic alopecia

Unlabeled/Investigational: Adjuvant monotherapy after radical prostatectomy in the treatment of prostatic cancer; female hirsutism

Local Anesthetic/Vasoconstrictor Precautions No information available to require special precautions

Effects on Dental Treatment No effects or complications reported

Dosage Adults: Male: Oral:

Benign prostatic hyperplasia: 5 mg/day as a single dose; clinical responses occur within 12 weeks to 6 months of initiation of therapy; long-term administration is recommended for maximal response

Male pattern baldness: 1 mg daily

Mechanism of Action Finasteride is a 4-azo analog of testosterone and is a competitive inhibitor of both tissue and hepatic 5-alpha reductase. This results in inhibition of the conversion of testosterone to dihydrotestosterone and markedly suppresses serum dihydrotestosterone levels; depending on dose and duration, serum testosterone concentrations may or may not increase. Testosterone-dependent processes such as fertility, muscle strength, potency, and libido are not affected by finasteride.

Other Adverse Effects 1% to 10%:

Endocrine & metabolic: Libido decreased

Genitourinary: <4% incidence of erectile dysfunction, decreased volume of ejaculate

Drug Interactions CYP3A3/4 enzyme substrate

Drug Uptake

Onset of action: 3-6 months of ongoing therapy

Absorption: May be reduced with food

Duration:

After a single oral dose as small as 0.5 mg: 65% depression of plasma dihydrotestosterone levels persists 5-7 days

After 6 months of treatment with 5 mg/day: Circulating dihydrotestosterone levels are reduced to castrate levels without significant effects on circulating testosterone; levels return to normal within 14 days of discontinuation of treatment

Half-life, elimination: Parent drug: ~5-17 hours (mean: 1.9 fasting, 4.2 with breakfast); Elderly: 8 hours; Adults: 6 hours (3-16); rate decreased in elderly, but no dosage adjustment needed

Time to peak: Oral: 2-6 hours

Pregnancy Risk Factor X

Generic Available No

Finevin™ *see* Azelaic Acid *on page 136*

Fioricet® *see* Butalbital, Acetaminophen, and Caffeine *on page 192*

Fioricet® with Codeine *see* Butalbital, Acetaminophen, Caffeine, and Codeine *on page 192*

Fiorinal® *see* Butalbital, Aspirin, and Caffeine *on page 194*

Fiorinal® With Codeine *see* Butalbital, Aspirin, Caffeine, and Codeine *on page 194*

Flagyl® *see* Metronidazole *on page 804*

Flagyl ER® *see* Metronidazole *on page 804*

Flarex® *see* Fluorometholone *on page 515*

Flatulex® [OTC] *see* Simethicone *on page 1088*

Flavoxate (fla VOKS ate)

U.S. Brand Names Urispas®

Canadian Brand Names Urispas®

Mexican Brand Names Bladuril®

Pharmacologic Category Antispasmodic Agent, Urinary

Synonyms Flavoxate Hydrochloride

Use Antispasmodic to provide symptomatic relief of dysuria, nocturia, suprapubic pain, urgency, and incontinence due to detrusor instability and hyper-reflexia in elderly with cystitis, urethritis, urethrocystitis, urethrotrigonitis, and prostatitis

Local Anesthetic/Vasoconstrictor Precautions No information available to require special precautions

Effects on Dental Treatment >10%: Xerostomia

Dosage Children >12 years and Adults: Oral: 100-200 mg 3-4 times/day; reduce the dose when symptoms improve

Mechanism of Action Synthetic antispasmodic with similar actions to that of propantheline; it exerts a direct relaxant effect on smooth muscles via phosphodiesterase inhibition, providing relief to a variety of smooth muscle spasms; it is especially useful for the treatment of bladder spasticity, whereby it produces an increase in urinary capacity

Other Adverse Effects Frequency not defined:
- Cardiovascular: Tachycardia, palpitations
- Central nervous system: Drowsiness, confusion (especially in the elderly), nervousness, fatigue, vertigo, headache, hyperpyrexia
- Dermatologic: Rash. urticaria
- Gastrointestinal: Constipation, nausea, vomiting, xerostomia, dry throat
- Genitourinary: Dysuria
- Hematologic: Leukopenia
- Ocular: Increased intraocular pressure, blurred vision

Drug Uptake Onset of action: 55-60 minutes

Pregnancy Risk Factor B

Generic Available No

Flecainide (fle KAY nide)

Related Information

Cardiovascular Diseases *on page 1308*

U.S. Brand Names Tambocor™

Canadian Brand Names Tambocor™

Mexican Brand Names Tambocor®

Pharmacologic Category Antiarrhythmic Agent, Class Ic

Synonyms Flecainide Acetate

Use Prevention and suppression of documented life-threatening ventricular arrhythmias (ie, sustained ventricular tachycardia); controlling symptomatic, disabling supraventricular tachycardias in patients without structural heart disease in whom other agents fail

Local Anesthetic/Vasoconstrictor Precautions No information available to require special precautions

Effects on Dental Treatment No effects or complications reported

Dosage Oral:
- Children:
  - Initial: 3 mg/kg/day or 50-100 mg/m²/day in 3 divided doses
  - Usual: 3-6 mg/kg/day or 100-150 mg/m²/day in 3 divided doses; up to 11 mg/kg/day or 200 mg/m²/day for uncontrolled patients with subtherapeutic levels
- Adults:
  - Life-threatening ventricular arrhythmias:
    - Initial: 100 mg every 12 hours
    - Increase by 50-100 mg/day (given in 2 doses/day) every 4 days; maximum: 400 mg/day
    - For patients receiving 400 mg/day who are not controlled and have trough concentrations <0.6 μg/mL, dosage may be increased to 600 mg/day
  - Prevention of paroxysmal supraventricular arrhythmias in patients with disabling symptoms but no structural heart disease:
    - Initial: 50 mg every 12 hours
    - Increase by 50 mg twice daily at 4-day intervals; maximum: 300 mg/day

Mechanism of Action Class IC antiarrhythmic; slows conduction in cardiac tissue by altering transport of ions across cell membranes; causes slight prolongation of refractory periods; decreases the rate of rise of the action potential without affecting its duration; increases electrical stimulation threshold of ventricle, His-Purkinje system; possesses local anesthetic and moderate negative inotropic effects

Other Adverse Effects
- >10%:
  - Central nervous system: Dizziness (19% to 30%)
  - Ocular: Visual disturbances (16%)
  - Respiratory: Dyspnea (~10%)
- 1% to 10%:
  - Cardiovascular: Palpitations (6%), chest pain (5%), edema (3.5%), tachycardia (1% to 3%), proarrhythmic (4% to 12%), sinus node dysfunction (1.2%)
  - Central nervous system: Headache (4% to 10%), fatigue (8%), nervousness (5%) additional symptoms occurring at a frequency between 1% and 3%: fever, malaise, hypoesthesia, paresis, ataxia, vertigo, syncope, somnolence, tinnitus, anxiety, insomnia, depression
  - Dermatologic: Rash (1% to 3%)
  - Gastrointestinal: Nausea (9%), constipation (1%), abdominal pain (3%), anorexia (1% to 3%), diarrhea (0.7% to 3%)
  - Neuromuscular & skeletal: Tremor (5%), weakness (5%), paresthesias (1%)
  - Ocular: Diplopia (1% to 3%), blurred vision

Drug Interactions CYP2D6 enzyme substrate

Increased Effect/Toxicity: Flecainide concentrations may be increased by amiodarone (reduce flecainide 25% to 33%), amprenavir, cimetidine, digoxin, propranolol, quinidine, and ritonavir. Beta-adrenergic blockers, disopyramide, verapamil may enhance flecainide's negative inotropic effects. Alkalinizing agents (ie, high-dose antacids, cimetidine, carbonic anhydrase inhibitors, sodium bicarbonate) may decrease flecainide clearance, potentially increasing toxicity. Propranolol blood levels are increased by flecainide.

Decreased Effect: Smoking and acid urine increase flecainide clearance.

(Continued)

Flecainide *(Continued)*

Drug Uptake

Absorption: Oral: Rapid

Half-life, elimination: Infants: 11-12 hours; Children: 8 hours; Adults: 7-22 hours, increased with congestive heart failure or renal dysfunction; End-stage renal disease: 19-26 hours

Time to peak: ~1.5-3 hours

Pregnancy Risk Factor C

Generic Available No

Fleet® Babylax® [OTC] *see* Glycerin *on page 562*
Fleet® Bisacodyl Enema [OTC] *see* Bisacodyl *on page 166*
Fleet® Enema [OTC] *see* Sodium Phosphates *on page 1098*
Fleet® Pain Relief [OTC] *see* Pramoxine *on page 984*
Fleet® Phospho®-Soda [OTC] *see* Sodium Phosphates *on page 1098*
Fleet® Stimulant Laxative [OTC] *see* Bisacodyl *on page 166*
Flexeril® *see* Cyclobenzaprine *on page 333*
Flolan® *see* Epoprostenol *on page 443*
Flomax® *see* Tamsulosin *on page 1132*
Flonase® *see* Fluticasone *on page 525*
Florical® [OTC] *see* Calcium Carbonate *on page 201*
Florinef® *see* Fludrocortisone Acetate *on page 510*
Floropryl® *see* Isoflurophate *on page 658*
Flovent® *see* Fluticasone *on page 525*
Flovent® Rotadisk® *see* Fluticasone *on page 525*
Floxin® *see* Ofloxacin *on page 883*

Floxuridine (floks YOOR i deen)

U.S. Brand Names FUDR®

Canadian Brand Names FUDR®

Pharmacologic Category Antineoplastic Agent, Antimetabolite

Synonyms Fluorodeoxyuridine; FUDR

Use Palliative management of carcinomas of head, neck, and brain as well as liver, gallbladder, and bile ducts

Local Anesthetic/Vasoconstrictor Precautions No information available to require special

Effects on Dental Treatment No effects or complications reported

Mechanism of Action Mechanism of action and pharmacokinetics are very similar to 5-FU; FUDR® is the deoxyribonucleotide of 5-FU. Inhibits DNA and RNA synthesis via formation of carbonium ions; cross-links strands of DNA, causing an imbalance of growth and cell death.

Other Adverse Effects

>10%:

Gastrointestinal: Stomatitis, diarrhea; may be dose-limiting

Hematologic: Myelosuppression, may be dose-limiting; leukopenia, thrombocytopenia, anemia

1% to 10%:

Dermatologic: Alopecia, photosensitivity, hyperpigmentation of the skin, localized erythema, dermatitis

Gastrointestinal: Anorexia

Hepatic: Biliary sclerosis, cholecystitis, jaundice

Drug Interactions

Increased Effect/Toxicity: Any form of therapy which adds to the stress of the patient, interferes with nutrition, or depresses bone marrow function will increase the toxicity of floxuridine. Pentostatin and floxuridine administered together has resulted in fatal pulmonary toxicity.

Decreased Effect: Patients may experience impaired immune response to vaccines; possible infection after administration of live vaccines in patients receiving immunosuppressants.

Pregnancy Risk Factor D

Generic Available No

Fluconazole (floo KOE na zole)

Related Information

Oral Fungal Infections *on page 1377*

U.S. Brand Names Diflucan®

Canadian Brand Names Apo®-Fluconazole; Diflucan™

Mexican Brand Names Afungil®; Diflucan®; Neofomiral®; Oxifungol; Zonal

Pharmacologic Category Antifungal Agent, Oral; Antifungal Agent, Parenteral

Use Oral fluconazole should be used in persons able to tolerate oral medications; parenteral fluconazole should be reserved for patients who are both unable to take oral medications and are unable to tolerate amphotericin B (eg, due to hypersensitivity or renal insufficiency)

Dental: Treatment of susceptible fungal infections in the oral cavity including candidiasis, oral thrush, and chronic mucocutaneous candidiasis; treatment of esophageal and oropharyngeal candidiasis caused by *Candida* species; treatment of severe, chronic mucocutaneous candidiasis caused by *Candida* species

Medical: Vaginal candidiasis unresponsive to nystatin or clotrimazole; treatment of hepatosplenic candidiasis; treatment of other *Candida* infections in persons unable to tolerate amphotericin B; treatment of cryptococcal infections; secondary prophylaxis for cryptococcal meningitis in persons with AIDS; antifungal prophylaxis in allogeneic bone marrow transplant recipients

Local Anesthetic/Vasoconstrictor Precautions No information available to require special precautions

Effects on Dental Treatment No effects or complications reported

Dosage The daily dose of fluconazole is the same for oral and I.V. administration

Neonates: First 2 weeks of life, especially premature neonates: Same dose as older children every 72 hours

Children: Once-daily dosing by indication: See table.

Fluconazole — Once-Daily Dosing — Children

Indication	Day 1	Daily Therapy	Minimum Duration of Therapy
Oropharyngeal candidiasis	6 mg/kg	3 mg/kg	2 weeks
Esophageal candidiasis	6 mg/kg	3-12 mg/kg	3 weeks and for at least 2 weeks following resolution of symptoms
Systemic candidiasis	—	6-12 mg/kg	4 weeks
Cryptococcal meningitis acute	12 mg/kg	6-12 mg/kg	10-12 weeks after CSF culture becomes negative
relapse suppression	6 mg/kg	6 mg/kg	N/A

N/A = Not applicable

Adults: Oral, I.V.: Once-daily dosing by indication: See table.

Fluconazole — Once-Daily Dosing — Adults

Indication	Day 1	Daily Therapy	Minimum Duration of Therapy
Oropharyngeal candidiasis	200 mg	100 mg	2 weeks
Esophageal candidiasis	200 mg	100 mg	3 weeks and for at least 2 weeks following resolution of symptoms
Prevention of candidiasis in bone marrow transplant	400 mg	400 mg	3 days before neutropenia 1 week after neutrophils >1000 cells/mm^3
Candidiasis UTIs, peritonitis	50-200 mg	50-200 mg	N/A
Systemic candidiasis	400 mg	200 mg	4 weeks
Cryptococcal meningitis acute	400 mg	200 mg	10-12 weeks after CSF culture becomes negative
relapse suppression	200 mg	200 mg	N/A
Vaginal candidiasis	150 mg	Single dose	N/A

NA = Not applicable

Dosing adjustment/interval in renal impairment:

No adjustment for vaginal candidiasis single-dose therapy

For multiple dosing, administer usual load then adjust daily doses

Cl_{cr} 11-50 mL/minute: Administer 50% of recommended dose or administer every 48 hours

Hemodialysis: One dose after each dialysis

Continuous arteriovenous or venovenous hemodiafiltration effects: Dose as for Cl_{cr} 10-50 mL/minute

(Continued)

Fluconazole *(Continued)*

Mechanism of Action Interferes with cytochrome P450 activity, decreasing ergosterol synthesis (principal sterol in fungal cell membrane) and inhibiting cell membrane formation

Other Adverse Effects Frequency not defined:

Cardiovascular: Pallor, angioedema

Central nervous system: Headache (2% to 13%), seizures, dizziness

Dermatologic: Rash (2%), alopecia, toxic epidermal necrolysis, Stevens-Johnson syndrome

Endocrine & metabolic: Hypertriglyceridemia, hypokalemia

Gastrointestinal: Nausea (4% to 7%), vomiting (2%), abdominal pain (2% to 6%), diarrhea (2% to 3%), taste perversion

Hematologic: Leukopenia, thrombocytopenia

Hepatic: Hepatic failure (rare), hepatitis, cholestasis, jaundice, increased ALT/AST, increased alkaline phosphatase

Respiratory: Dyspnea

Miscellaneous: Anaphylactic reactions (rare)

Contraindications Hypersensitivity to fluconazole, other azoles, or any component of their formulation; concomitant administration with terfenadine, cisapride, or astemizole

Warnings/Precautions Should be used with caution in patients with renal and hepatic dysfunction or previous hepatotoxicity from other azole derivatives. Patients who develop abnormal LFTs during fluconazole therapy should be monitored closely and discontinued if symptoms consistent with liver disease develop. **Should be used with caution in patients receiving cisapride or astemizole.**

Drug Interactions CYP2C9 enzyme inducer; CYP2C9, 2C18, and 2C19 enzyme inhibitor and CYP3A3/4 enzyme inhibitor (weak)

Alprazolam, triazolam, midazolam, and diazepam serum concentration are increased; consider a benzodiazepine not metabolized by CYP3A3/4 or another antifungal that is metabolized by CYP3A3/4.

Calcium channel blockers may have increased serum concentration; consider another agent instead of a calcium channel blocker, another antifungal, or reduce the dose of the calcium channel blocker. Monitor BP.

Losartan's active metabolite is reduced in concentration; consider another antihypertensive agent unaffected by the azole antifungals, another antifungal, or monitor BP closely.

HMG-CoA reductase inhibitors (except pravastatin and fluvastatin) have increased serum concentration; switch to pravastatin/fluvastatin or monitor for development of myopathy.

Caffeine's metabolism is decreased; monitor for tachycardia, nervousness, and anxiety.

Cisapride's serum concentration is increased which may lead to malignant arrhythmias; concurrent use is contraindicated.

Tacrolimus's serum concentration is increased; monitor tacrolimus's serum concentration and renal function.

Cyclosporine's serum concentration is increased; monitor cyclosporine's serum concentration and renal function.

Rifampin decreases fluconazole's serum concentration; monitor infection status.

Warfarin's effects are increased; monitor INR and adjust warfarin's dose as needed.

Phenytoin's serum concentration is increased; monitor phenytoin levels and adjust dose as needed.

Dietary/Ethanol/Herb Considerations Food: Administer with food to reduce GI upset.

Drug Uptake

Absorption: >90%

Half-life, elimination (dependent on renal function): 25-30 hours

Time to peak: Oral: 2-4 hours

Pregnancy Risk Factor C

Breast-feeding Considerations Probably safe (not absorbed orally)

Dosage Forms INJ: 2 mg/mL (100 mL, 200 mL). **POWDER, oral suspension:** 10 mg/mL (35 mL); 40 mg/mL (35 mL). **TAB:** 50 mg, 100 mg, 150 mg, 200 mg

Generic Available No

Flucytosine (floo SYE toe seen)

U.S. Brand Names Ancobon®

Canadian Brand Names Ancobon®

Pharmacologic Category Antifungal Agent, Oral

Synonyms 5-FC; 5-Flurocytosine

Use Adjunctive treatment of susceptible fungal infections (usually *Candida* or *Cryptococcus*); in combination with amphotericin B, fluconazole, or itraconazole; synergy with amphotericin B for fungal infections (*Aspergillus*)

Local Anesthetic/Vasoconstrictor Precautions No information available to require special precautions

Effects on Dental Treatment No effects or complications reported

Dosage Children and Adults: Oral: 50-150 mg/kg/day in divided doses every 6 hours

Mechanism of Action Penetrates fungal cells and is converted to fluorouracil which competes with uracil interfering with fungal RNA and protein synthesis

Other Adverse Effects Frequency not defined:

Central nervous system: Confusion, headache, hallucinations, dizziness, drowsiness, psychosis, parkinsonism, ataxia, sedation
Dermatologic: Rash, photosensitivity, pruritus, urticaria
Endocrine & metabolic: Temporary growth failure, hypoglycemia, hypokalemia
Gastrointestinal: Nausea, vomiting, diarrhea, abdominal pain, loss of appetite
Hematologic: Bone marrow suppression, anemia, leukopenia, thrombocytopenia
Hepatic: Elevated liver enzymes, hepatitis, jaundice, azotemia
Neuromuscular & skeletal: Peripheral neuropathy, paresthesia, weakness
Otic: Hearing loss
Renal: Elevated BUN and serum creatinine, renal failure
Respiratory: Respiratory arrest
Miscellaneous: Anaphylaxis

Drug Interactions Increased effect with amphotericin B; amphotericin B-induced renal dysfunction may predispose patient to flucytosine accumulation and myelosuppression.

Drug Uptake

Absorption: Oral: 75% to 90%
Half-life, elimination: 3-8 hours; Anuria: ≤200 hours; End-stage renal disease: 75-200 hours
Time to peak: ~2-6 hours

Pregnancy Risk Factor C

Generic Available No

Fludara® *see* Fludarabine *on page 509*

Fludarabine (floo DARE a been)

U.S. Brand Names Fludara®

Canadian Brand Names Fludara®

Mexican Brand Names Fludara®

Pharmacologic Category Antineoplastic Agent, Antimetabolite

Synonyms Fludarabine Phosphate

Use Salvage therapy of non-Hodgkin's lymphoma and acute leukemias

Orphan drug: Treatment of chronic lymphocytic leukemia (CLL), including refractory CLL

Local Anesthetic/Vasoconstrictor Precautions No information available to require special precautions

Effects on Dental Treatment No effects or complications reported

Mechanism of Action Fludarabine is analogous to that of Ara-C and Ara-A. Following systemic administration, FAMP is rapidly dephosphorylated to 2-fluoro-Ara-A. 2-Fluoro-Ara-A enters the cell by a carrier-mediated transport process, then is phosphorylated intracellularly by deoxycytidine kinase to form the active metabolite 2-fluoro-Ara-ATP. 2-Fluoro-Ara-ATP inhibits DNA synthesis by inhibition of DNA polymerase and ribonucleotide reductase.

Other Adverse Effects

>10%:

Cardiovascular: Edema
Central nervous system: Fatigue, somnolence (30%), chills, pain
Dermatologic: Rash
Hematologic: Myelosuppression, dose-limiting toxicity, primarily leukopenia and thrombocytopenia
Nadir: 10-14 days
Recovery: 5-7 weeks
Neuromuscular & skeletal: Paresthesia, myalgia, weakness

1% to 10%:

Cardiovascular: Congestive heart failure
Central nervous system: Malaise, headache
Dermatologic: Alopecia
Endocrine & metabolic: Hyperglycemia
Gastrointestinal: Anorexia, stomatitis (1.5%), diarrhea (1.8%), mild nausea/vomiting (3% to 10%)
Hematologic: Eosinophilia, hemolytic anemia, may be dose-limiting, possibly fatal in some patients

Drug Interactions Increased Effect/Toxicity: Cytarabine when administered with or prior to a fludarabine dose competes for deoxycytidine kinase decreasing the metabolism of F-ara-A to the active F-ara-ATP (inhibits the antineoplastic effect of fludarabine); however, administering fludarabine prior to cytarabine may stimulate activation of cytarabine.

Drug Uptake Half-life, elimination: 2-fluoro-vidarabine: 9 hours

Pregnancy Risk Factor D

Generic Available No

Fludrocortisone Acetate (floo droe KOR ti sone)

U.S. Brand Names Florinef®

Canadian Brand Names Florinef®

Pharmacologic Category Corticosteroid, Systemic

Synonyms Fludrocortisone; Fluohydrisone Acetate; Fluohydrocortisone Acetate; 9α-Fluorohydrocortisone Acetate

Use Partial replacement therapy for primary and secondary adrenocortical insufficiency in Addison's disease; treatment of salt-losing adrenogenital syndrome

Local Anesthetic/Vasoconstrictor Precautions No information available to require special precautions

Effects on Dental Treatment No effects or complications reported

Dosage Adults: Oral: 0.1-0.2 mg/day with ranges of 0.1 mg 3 times/week to 0.2 mg/day

Mechanism of Action Promotes increased reabsorption of sodium and loss of potassium from renal distal tubules

Other Adverse Effects 1% to 10%:

Cardiovascular: Hypertension, edema, CHF
Central nervous system: Convulsions, headache, dizziness
Dermatologic: Acne, rash, bruising
Endocrine & metabolic: Hypokalemic alkalosis, suppression of growth, hyperglycemia, HPA suppression
Gastrointestinal: Peptic ulcer
Neuromuscular & skeletal: Muscle weakness
Ocular: Cataracts
Miscellaneous: Diaphoresis

Drug Interactions Decreased Effect: May decrease salicylate levels; anticholinesterases effects are antagonized; corticosteroid effects decreased by rifampin, barbiturates, and hydantoins.

Drug Uptake

Absorption: Rapid and complete
Half-life, elimination: Plasma: 30-35 minutes; Biological: 18-36 hours
Time to peak: ~1.7 hours

Pregnancy Risk Factor C

Generic Available No

Flumadine® *see* Rimantadine *on page 1055*

Flumazenil (FLOO may ze nil)

Related Information

Dental Office Emergencies *on page 1418*

U.S. Brand Names Romazicon™

Canadian Brand Names Anexate®; Romazicon™

Mexican Brand Names Lanexat®

Pharmacologic Category Antidote

Use Benzodiazepine antagonist - reverses sedative effects of benzodiazepines used in general anesthesia; for management of benzodiazepine overdose; flumazenil does **not** antagonize the CNS effects of other GABA agonists (such as ethanol, barbiturates, or general anesthetics), **does not** reverse narcotics

Local Anesthetic/Vasoconstrictor Precautions No information available to require special precautions

Effects on Dental Treatment No effects or complications reported

Dosage See table on following page.

Resedation: Repeated doses may be given at 20-minute intervals as needed; repeat treatment doses of 1 mg (at a rate of 0.5 mg/minute) should be given at any time and ≤3 mg should be given in any hour. After intoxication with high doses of benzodiazepines, the duration of a single dose of flumazenil is not expected to exceed 1 hour; if desired, the period of wakefulness may be prolonged with repeated low I.V. doses of flumazenil, or by an infusion of 0.1-0.4 mg/hour. Most patients with benzodiazepine overdose will respond to a cumulative dose of 1-3 mg and doses >3 mg do not reliably produce additional effects. Rarely, patients with a partial response at 3 mg may require additional titration up to a total dose of 5 mg. **If a patient has not responded 5 minutes after receiving a cumulative dose of 5 mg, the major cause of sedation is not likely to be due to benzodiazepines.**

Mechanism of Action Antagonizes the effect of benzodiazepines on the GABA/benzodiazepine receptor complex. Flumazenil is benzodiazepine specific and does not antagonize other nonbenzodiazepine GABA agonists (including ethanol, barbiturates, general anesthetics); flumazenil does not reverse the effects of opiates

Other Adverse Effects

>10%: Gastrointestinal: Vomiting, nausea

1% to 10%:

Cardiovascular: Palpitations
Central nervous system: Headache, anxiety, nervousness, insomnia, abnormal

crying, euphoria, depression, agitation, dizziness, emotional lability, ataxia, depersonalization, increased tears, dysphoria, paranoia

Endocrine & metabolic: Hot flashes

Gastrointestinal: Xerostomia

Local: Pain at injection site

Neuromuscular & skeletal: Tremor, weakness, paresthesia

Ocular: Abnormal vision, blurred vision

Respiratory: Dyspnea, hyperventilation

Miscellaneous: Diaphoresis

Flumazenil

Pediatric Dosage (Further studies are needed.)	
Pediatric dosage for **reversal of conscious sedation:** Intravenously through a freely running intravenous infusion into a large vein to minimize pain at the injection site	
Initial dose	0.01 mg/kg over 15 seconds (maximum dose of 0.2 mg)
Repeat doses	0.005-0.01 mg/kg (maximum dose of 0.2 mg) repeated at 1-minute intervals
Maximum total cumulative dose	1 mg
Pediatric dosage for **management of benzodiazepine overdose:** Intravenously through a freely running intravenous infusion into a large vein to minimize pain at the injection site	
Initial dose	0.01 mg/kg (maximum dose: 0.2 mg)
Repeat doses	0.01 mg/kg (maximum dose of 0.2 mg) repeated at 1-minute intervals
Maximum total cumulative dose	1 mg
In place of repeat bolus doses, follow-up continuous infusions of 0.005-0.01 mg/kg/hour have been used; further studies are needed	
Adult Dosage	
Adult dosage for **reversal of conscious sedation:** Intravenously through a freely running intravenous infusion into a large vein to minimize pain at the injection site	
Initial dose	0.2 mg intravenously over 15 seconds
Repeat doses	If desired level of consciousness is not obtained, 0.2 mg may be repeated at 1-minute intervals
Maximum total cumulative dose	1 mg (usual dose: 0.6-1 mg) **In the event of resedation:** repeat doses may be given at 20-minute intervals with maximum of 1 mg/dose and 3 mg/hour
Adult dosage for **suspected benzodiazepine overdose:** Intravenously through a freely running intravenous infusion into a large vein to minimize pain at the injection site	
Initial dose	0.2 mg intravenously over 30 seconds
Repeat doses	0.5 mg over 30 seconds repeated at 1-minute intervals
Maximum total cumulative dose	3 mg (usual dose: 1-3 mg) Patients with a partial response at 3 mg may require additional titration up to a total dose of 5 mg. If a patient has not responded 5 minutes after cumulative dose of 5 mg, the major cause of sedation is not likely due to benzodiazepines. **In the event of resedation:** may repeat doses at 20-minute intervals with maximum of 1 mg/dose and 3 mg/hour

Drug Interactions Increased Effect/Toxicity: Use with caution in overdosage involving mixed drug overdose. Toxic effects may emerge (especially with cyclic antidepressants) with the reversal of the benzodiazepine effect by flumazenil.

Benzodiazepines: Flumazenil may precipitate acute withdrawal reaction, including seizures, in patients who are habituated.

Drug Uptake

Onset of action: 1-3 minutes; 80% response within 3 minutes

Duration (dose-dependent): Resedation usually within 1 hour; duration related to benzodiazepine plasma concentrations; reversal effects of flumazenil may wear off before effects of benzodiazepine

Half-life, elimination: Adults: Alpha: 7-15 minutes; Terminal: 41-79 minutes

Time to peak: 6-10 minutes

Pregnancy Risk Factor C

Generic Available No

Flunisolide (floo NIS oh lide)

Related Information

Respiratory Diseases *on page 1328*

(Continued)

Flunisolide *(Continued)*

U.S. Brand Names AeroBid®; AeroBid®-M; Nasalide®; Nasarel®

Canadian Brand Names Alti-Flunisolide; Apo®-Flunisolide; Nasalide®; Rhinalar®

Pharmacologic Category Corticosteroid, Inhalant (Oral); Corticosteroid, Nasal

Use Steroid-dependent asthma; nasal solution is used for seasonal or perennial rhinitis

Local Anesthetic/Vasoconstrictor Precautions No information available to require special precautions

Effects on Dental Treatment No effects or complications reported

Dosage

Children >6 years:

Oral inhalation: 2 inhalations twice daily (morning and evening) up to 4 inhalations/day

Nasal: 1 spray each nostril twice daily (morning and evening), not to exceed 4 sprays/day each nostril

Adults:

Oral inhalation: 2 inhalations twice daily (morning and evening) up to 8 inhalations/day maximum

Nasal: 2 sprays each nostril twice daily (morning and evening); maximum dose: 8 sprays/day in each nostril

Mechanism of Action Decreases inflammation by suppression of migration of polymorphonuclear leukocytes and reversal of increased capillary permeability; does not depress hypothalamus

Other Adverse Effects

>10%:

Cardiovascular: Pounding heartbeat

Central nervous system: Dizziness, headache, nervousness

Dermatologic: Itching, rash

Endocrine & metabolic: Adrenal suppression, menstrual problems

Gastrointestinal: GI irritation, anorexia, sore throat, bitter taste

Local: Nasal burning, *Candida* infections of the nose or pharynx, atrophic rhinitis

Respiratory: Sneezing, coughing, upper respiratory tract infection, bronchitis, nasal congestion, nasal dryness

Miscellaneous: Increased susceptibility to infections

1% to 10%:

Central nervous system: Insomnia, psychic changes

Dermatologic: Acne, urticaria

Gastrointestinal: Increase in appetite, xerostomia, dry throat, loss of taste perception

Ocular: Cataracts

Respiratory: Epistaxis

Miscellaneous: Diaphoresis, loss of smell

Drug Interactions Increased Effect/Toxicity: Expect interactions similar to other corticosteroids. Salmeterol: The addition of salmeterol has been demonstrated to improve response to inhaled corticosteroids (as compared to increasing steroid dosage).

Drug Uptake

Absorption: Nasal inhalation: ~50%

Half-life, elimination: 1.8 hours

Pregnancy Risk Factor C

Generic Available No

Fluocinolone (floo oh SIN oh lone)

U.S. Brand Names Capex™; Derma-Smoothe/FS®; FS Shampoo® [DSC]; Synalar®

Canadian Brand Names Capex®; Derma-Smoothe/FS®; Fluoderm; Synalar®

Mexican Brand Names Synalar®

Pharmacologic Category Corticosteroid, Topical

Synonyms Fluocinolone Acetonide

Use Relief of susceptible inflammatory dermatosis [low, medium, high potency topical corticosteroid]; psoriasis of the scalp; atopic dermatitis in children ≥2 years of age

Local Anesthetic/Vasoconstrictor Precautions No information available to require special precautions

Effects on Dental Treatment No effects or complications reported

Dosage Topical: Therapy should be discontinued when control is achieved; if no improvement is seen, reassessment of diagnosis may be necessary.

Children ≥2 years: Atopic dermatitis (Derma-Smoothe/FS®): Moisten skin; apply to affected area twice daily; do not use >4 weeks

Children and Adults: Corticosteroid-responsive dermatoses: Cream, lotion, ointment, solution: Apply a thin layer to affected area 2-4 times/day; may use occlusive dressings to manage psoriasis or recalcitrant conditions

Adults:

Atopic dermatitis (Derma-Smoothe/FS®): Apply thin film to affected area 3 times/day

Scalp psoriasis (Derma-Smoothe/FS®): Massage thoroughly into wet or dampened hair/scalp; cover with shower cap. Leave on overnight (or for at least 4 hours). Remove by washing hair with shampoo and rinsing thoroughly.

Seborrheic dermatitis of the scalp (Capex™): Apply no more than 1 ounce to scalp once daily; work into lather and allow to remain on scalp for ~5 minutes. Remove from hair and scalp by rinsing thoroughly with water.

Mechanism of Action A synthetic corticosteroid which differs structurally from triamcinolone acetonide in the presence of an additional fluorine atom in the 6-alpha position on the steroid nucleus. The mechanism of action for all topical corticosteroids is not well defined, however, is believed to be a combination of anti-inflammatory, antipruritic, and vasoconstrictive properties.

Other Adverse Effects Frequency not defined:

Dermatologic: Acneiform eruptions, allergic contact dermatitis, burning sensation, dryness, folliculitis, hypertrichosis, hypopigmentation, irritation, itching, miliaria, skin atrophy, striae

Endocrine & metabolic: Cushing's syndrome, HPA axis suppression

Miscellaneous: Secondary infection

Drug Uptake Absorption: Dependent on strength of preparation, amount applied,and nature of skin at application site; ranges from ~1% in thick stratum corneum areas (palms, soles, elbows, etc) to 36% in areas of thinnest stratum corneum (face, eyelids, etc); increased in areas of skin damage, inflammation, or occlusion

Pregnancy Risk Factor C

Generic Available Yes (except oil, shampoo)

Fluocinolone, Hydroquinone, and Tretinoin *Not Available in U.S.* (floo oh SIN oh lone, HYE droe kwin one, & TRET i noyn)

U.S. Brand Names Tri-Luma™

Pharmacologic Category Corticosteroid, Topical; Depigmenting Agent; Retinoic Acid Derivative

Synonyms Hydroquinone, Fluocinolone Acetonide, and Tretinoin; Tretinoin, Fluocinolone Acetonide, and Hydroquinone

Use Short-term treatment of moderate to severe melasma of the face

Local Anesthetic/Vasoconstrictor Precautions No information available to require special precautions

Effects on Dental Treatment No effects or complications reported

Dosage Topical: Adults: Melasma: Apply a thin film once daily to hyperpigmented areas of melasma (including 1/2 inch of normal-appearing surrounding skin). Apply 30 minutes prior to bedtime; not indicated for use beyond 8 weeks. Do not use occlusive dressings.

Mechanism of Action Not clearly defined; hydroquinone may interrupt melanin synthesis (tyrosine-tyrosinase pathway); reduces hyperpigmentation

Other Adverse Effects

>10%

Dermatologic: Erythema (41%), desquamation (38%), burning (18%), dry skin (14%), pruritus (11%)

1% to 10%

Cardiovascular: Telangiectasia (3%)

Central nervous system: Paresthesia (3%), hyperesthesia (2%)

Dermatologic: Acne (5%), pigmentation change (2%), irritation (2%), papules (1%), rash (1%), rosacea (1%), vesicles (1%)

Gastrointestinal: Xerostomia (1%)

Drug Interactions Increased Effect/Toxicity: Avoid soaps/cosmetic preparations which are medicated, abrasive, irritating, or any product with strong drying effects (including alcohol, astringent, benzoyl peroxide, resorcinol, salicylic acid, sulfur). Drugs with photosensitizing effects should also be avoided (eg, tetracyclines, thiazides, fluoroquinolones, phenothiazines, sulfonamides).

Drug Uptake Absorption: Minimal

Pregnancy Risk Factor C

Generic Available No

Fluocinonide (floo oh SIN oh nide)

Related Information

Oral Nonviral Soft Tissue Ulcerations or Erosions *on page 1384*

U.S. Brand Names Lidex®; Lidex-E®

Canadian Brand Names Lidemol®; Lidex®; Lyderm®; Lydonide; Tiamol®; Topsyn®

Mexican Brand Names Topsyn®

Pharmacologic Category Corticosteroid, Topical

Use Anti-inflammatory, antipruritic, relief of inflammatory and pruritic manifestations [high potency topical corticosteroid]

Local Anesthetic/Vasoconstrictor Precautions No information available to require special precautions

Effects on Dental Treatment No effects or complications reported

(Continued)

Fluocinonide *(Continued)*

Dosage Children and Adults: Topical: Apply thin layer to affected area 2-4 times/day depending on the severity of the condition

Therapy should be discontinued when control is achieved; if no improvement is seen, reassessment of diagnosis may be necessary.

Mechanism of Action Fluorinated topical corticosteroid considered to be of high potency. The mechanism of action for all topical corticosteroids is not well defined, however, is felt to be a combination of three important properties: anti-inflammatory activity, immunosuppressive properties, and antiproliferative actions.

Other Adverse Effects Frequency not defined:

Cardiovascular: Intracranial hypertension

Dermatologic: Acne, hypopigmentation, allergic dermatitis, maceration of the skin, skin atrophy, striae, miliaria, telangiectasia, folliculitis, hypertrichosis

Endocrine & metabolic: HPA suppression, Cushing's syndrome, growth retardation

Local: Burning, itching, irritation, dryness, folliculitis, hypertrichosis

Miscellaneous: Secondary infection

Drug Uptake Absorption: Dependent on amount applied and nature of skin at application site; ranges from ~1% in areas of thick stratum corneum (palms, soles, elbows, etc) to 36% in areas of thin stratum corneum (face, eyelids, etc); absorption is increased in areas of skin damage, inflammation, or occlusion

Pregnancy Risk Factor C

Generic Available Yes

Fluogen® *see* Influenza Virus Vaccine *on page 637*

Fluoracaine® *see* Proparacaine and Fluorescein *on page 1010*

Fluoride (FLOR ide)

Related Information

Dentin Hypersensitivity, High Caries Index, and Xerostomia *on page 1388*

Management of Patients Undergoing Cancer Therapy *on page 1402*

U.S. Brand Names ACT® [OTC]; Fluorigard® [OTC]; Fluorinse®; Fluoritab®; Flura-Drops®; Flura-Loz®; Gel-Kam®; Gel-Tin® [OTC]; Karidium®; Karigel®; Karigel®-N; Luride®; Luride® Lozi-Tab®; Luride®-SF Lozi-Tabs®; Minute-Gel®; Pediaflor®; Pharmaflur®; Phos-Flur®; Point-Two®; PreviDent®; PreviDent® 5000 Plus™; Stop® [OTC]; Thera-Flur®; Thera-Flur-N®

Canadian Brand Names Fluor-A-Day®; Fluotic®

Mexican Brand Names Audifluor®

Pharmacologic Category Dietary Supplement

Synonyms Acidulated Phosphate Fluoride; Sodium Fluoride; Stannous Fluoride

Use Dental: Prevention of dental caries

Local Anesthetic/Vasoconstrictor Precautions No information available to require special precautions

Effects on Dental Treatment No effects or complications reported

Dosage Oral:

Recommended daily fluoride supplement (2.2 mg of sodium fluoride is equivalent to 1 mg of fluoride ion): See table.

Fluoride Ion

Fluoride Content of Drinking Water	Daily Dose, Oral (mg)
<0.3 ppm	
Birth - 6 months	None
6 months - 3 years	0.25
3-6 years	0.5
6-16 years	1.0
0.3-0.6 ppm	
Birth - 6 months	0
6 months - 3 years	0
3-6 years	0.25
6-16 years	0.5

Table from: Recommeded dosage schedule of The American Dental Association, The American Academy of Pediatric Dentistry, and The American Academy of Pediatrics

Dental rinse or gel:

Adults: 10 mL rinse or apply to teeth and spit daily after brushing

Children 6-12 years: 5-10 mL rinse or apply to teeth and spit daily after brushing

Mechanism of Action Promotes remineralization of decalcified enamel; inhibits the cariogenic microbial process in dental plaque; increases tooth resistance to acid dissolution

Other Adverse Effects <1%: Rash, nausea, vomiting, products containing stannous fluoride may stain the teeth

Contraindications Hypersensitivity to fluoride, tartrazine, or any component of their formulation; when fluoride content of drinking water exceeds 0.7 ppm; low sodium or sodium-free diets; 1 mg tablets in children <3 years of age or when drinking water fluoride content is ≥0.3 ppm; 1 mg/5 mL rinse (as supplement) in children <6 years of age

Warnings/Precautions Prolonged ingestion with excessive doses may result in dental fluorosis and osseous changes; do **not** exceed recommended dosage; some products contain tartrazine

Drug Interactions Decreased Effect/Absorption with magnesium-, aluminum-, and calcium-containing products

Dietary/Ethanol/Herb Considerations Food: Do not administer with milk; do **not** allow eating or drinking for 30 minutes after use.

Drug Uptake

Absorption: Rapid and complete from GI tract; calcium, iron, or magnesium may delay absorption

Time to peak: 30-60 minutes

Pregnancy Risk Factor C

Dosage Forms Fluoride ion content listed in brackets: **CRM, oral topical, as sodium** (PreviDent® 5000 Plus™): 1.1% (51 g). **DROPS, oral, as sodium:** (Fluoritab®, Flura-Drops®): 0.55 mg/drop (22.8 mL, 24 mL); (Karidium®): 0.275 mg/drop (30 mL, 60 mL); (Luride®, Pediaflor®): 1.1 mg/mL [0.5 mg/mL] (50 mL) **GEL, oral topical, acidulated phosphate fluoride** (Minute-Gel®): 1.23% (480 mL). **GEL, oral topical, sodium fluoride** (Karigel®, Karigel®-N, PreviDent®): 1.1% [0.5%] (24 g, 30 g, 60 g, 120 g, 130 g, 250 g). **GEL, oral topical, stannous fluoride** (Gel Kam®): 0.4% [0.1%] (60 g, 65 g, 105 g, 120 g). **LOZ, as sodium** (Flura-Loz®): 2.2 mg [1 mg]. **RINSE, oral, as sodium:** 0.05% [0.02%] (90 mL, 180 mL, 300 mL, 360 mL, 480 mL); (Fluorinse®, Point-Two®): 0.2% [0.09%] (240 mL, 480 mL, 3780 mL); (PreviDent®): 0.2% (250 mL). **SOLN, oral, as sodium** (Phos-Flur®): 0.44 mg/mL [0.2 mg/mL] (250 mL, 500 mL, 3780 mL). **TAB, as sodium** (Flura®, Karidium®): 2.2 mg [1 mg]. **TAB, chewable:** (Fluoritab®, Luride® Lozi-Tabs®, Pharmaflur®): 1.1 mg [0.5 mg]; (Fluoritab®, Karidium®, Luride® Lozi-Tabs®, Luride®-SF Lozi-Tabs®, Pharmaflur®): 2.2 mg [1 mg]

Generic Available Yes

Comments Neutral pH fluoride preparations are preferred in patients with oral mucositis to reduce tissue irritation; long-term use of acidulated fluorides has been associated with enamel demineralization and damage to porcelain crowns

Selected Readings Wynn RC, "Fluoride: After 50 Years, a Clearer Picture of Its Mechanism," *Gen Dent*, 2002, 50(2):118-22, 124, 126.

Fluorigard® [OTC] *see* Fluoride *on page 514*

Fluori-Methane® *see* Dichlorodifluoromethane and Trichloromonofluoromethane *on page 377*

Fluorinse® *see* Fluoride *on page 514*

Fluoritab® *see* Fluoride *on page 514*

Fluorometholone (flure oh METH oh lone)

U.S. Brand Names Flarex®; Fluor-Op®; FML®; FML® Forte

Canadian Brand Names Flarex®; FML®; FML Forte®

Pharmacologic Category Corticosteroid, Ophthalmic

Use Inflammatory conditions of the eye, including keratitis, iritis, cyclitis, and conjunctivitis

Local Anesthetic/Vasoconstrictor Precautions No information available to require special precautions

Effects on Dental Treatment No effects or complications reported

Dosage Children >2 years and Adults: Ophthalmic: Re-evaluate therapy if improvement is not seen within 2 days; use care not to discontinue prematurely; in chronic conditions, gradually decrease dosing frequency prior to discontinuing treatment

Ointment: Apply small amount (~1/2 inch ribbon) to conjunctival sac every 4 hours in severe cases; 1-3 times/day in mild to moderate cases

Solution: Instill 1-2 drops into conjunctival sac every hour during day, every 2 hours at night until favorable response is obtained, then use 1 drop every 4 hours; for mild to moderate inflammation, instill 1-2 drops into conjunctival sac 2-4 times/day

Mechanism of Action Decreases inflammation by suppression of migration of polymorphonuclear leukocytes and reversal of increased capillary permeability

Other Adverse Effects Frequency not defined:

Ocular: Anterior uveitis, burning upon application, cataract formation, conjunctival hyperemia, conjunctivitis, corneal ulcers, glaucoma with optic nerve damage, perforation of the globe, secondary ocular infection (bacterial, fungal, viral), intraocular pressure elevation, visual acuity and field defects, keratitis, mydriasis, stinging upon application, delayed wound healing

Miscellaneous: Systemic hypercorticoidism (rare) and taste perversion have also been reported

(Continued)

Fluorometholone *(Continued)*

Drug Uptake Absorption: Into aqueous humor with slight systemic absorption
Pregnancy Risk Factor C
Generic Available No

Fluor-Op® *see* Fluorometholone *on page 515*
Fluoroplex® *see* Fluorouracil *on page 516*

Fluorouracil (flure oh YOOR a sil)

U.S. Brand Names Adrucil®; Carac™; Efudex®; Fluoroplex®
Canadian Brand Names Adrucil®; Efudex®
Mexican Brand Names Efudix
Pharmacologic Category Antineoplastic Agent, Antimetabolite
Synonyms 5-Fluorouracil; 5-FU
Use Treatment of carcinomas of the breast, colon, head and neck, pancreas, rectum, or stomach; topically for the management of actinic or solar keratoses and superficial basal cell carcinomas
Local Anesthetic/Vasoconstrictor Precautions No information available to require special precautions
Effects on Dental Treatment No effects or complications reported
Dosage Adults:
Actinic keratoses: Topical:
Carac™: Apply thin film to lesions once daily for up to 4 weeks, as tolerated
Efudex®: Apply cream or solution to lesions twice daily for 2-4 weeks; complete healing may not be evident for 1-2 months following treatment
Fluoroplex®: Apply to lesions twice daily for 2-6 weeks
Basal cell carcinoma: Topical: Efudex®: Apply 5% cream or solution to affected lesions twice daily for 3-6 weeks; treatment may be continued for up to 10-12 weeks
Mechanism of Action A pyrimidine antimetabolite that interferes with DNA synthesis by blocking the methylation of deoxyuricytic acid; 5-FU rapidly enters the cell and is activated to the nucleotide level; there it inhibits thymidylate synthetase (TS), or is incorporated into RNA (most evident during the GI phase of the cell cycle). The reduced folate cofactor is required for tight binding to occur between the 5-FdUMP and TS.
Other Adverse Effects Toxicity depends on route and duration of treatment
I.V.:
Cardiovascular: Angina, myocardial ischemia, nail changes
Central nervous system: Acute cerebellar syndrome, confusion, disorientation, euphoria, headache, nystagmus
Dermatologic: Alopecia, dermatitis, dry skin, fissuring, palmar-plantar erythrodysesthesia syndrome, pruritic maculopapular rash, photosensitivity, vein pigmentations
Gastrointestinal: Anorexia, bleeding, diarrhea, esophagopharyngitis, nausea, sloughing, stomatitis, ulceration, vomiting
Hematologic: Agranulocytosis, anemia, leukopenia, pancytopenia, thrombocytopenia
Myelosuppression:
Onset: 7-10 days
Nadir: 9-14 days
Recovery: 21-28 days
Local: Thrombophlebitis
Ocular: Lacrimation, lacrimal duct stenosis, photophobia, visual changes
Respiratory: Epistaxis
Miscellaneous: Anaphylaxis, generalized allergic reactions, loss of nails
Topical:
Central nervous system: Headache, telangiectasia
Dermatologic: Photosensitivity, pruritus, rash, scarring
Hematologic: Leukocytosis
Local: Allergic contact dermatitis, burning, crusting, dryness, edema, erosion, erythema, hyperpigmentation, irritation, pain, soreness, ulceration
Ocular: Eye irritation (burning, watering, sensitivity, stinging, itching)
Miscellaneous: Birth defects, miscarriage
Drug Interactions
Increased Effect/Toxicity: Leucovorin increases the folate pool and, in certain tumors, may promote TS inhibition and increase 5-FU activity. Leucovorin must be given before or with the 5-FU to prime the cells; it is not used as a rescue agent in this case. Allopurinol inhibits thymidine phosphorylase (an enzyme that activates 5-FU). The antitumor effect of 5-FU appears to be unaltered, but the toxicity is increased. Cimetidine results in increased plasma concentrations of 5-FU due to drug metabolism inhibition and reduction of liver blood flow induced by cimetidine.
Decreased Effect: Methotrexate: This interaction is schedule dependent; **5-FU should be given following MTX, not prior to.** If 5-FU is given first: 5-FU inhibits

the TS binding and thus the reduced folate pool is not depleted, thereby negating the effect of MTX.

Drug Uptake

Absorption: Oral: Erratic and rarely used

Duration: ~3 weeks

Half-life, elimination: Biphasic: Initial: 6-20 minutes; doses of 400-600 mg/m^2 produce drug concentrations above the threshold for cytotoxicity for normal tissue and remain there for 6 hours; 2 metabolites, FdUMP and FUTP, have prolonged half-lives depending on the type of tissue; the clinical effect of these metabolites has not been determined

Pregnancy Risk Factor D (injection); X (topical)

Generic Available Yes: Injection

Fluoxetine (floo OKS e teen)

U.S. Brand Names Prozac®; Prozac® Weekly™; Sarafem™

Canadian Brand Names Alti-Fluoxetine; Apo®-Fluoxetine; Gen-Fluoxetine; Novo-Fluoxetine; Nu-Fluoxetine; PMS-Fluoxetine; Prozac®; Rhoxal-fluoxetine; Scheinpharm™ Fluoxetine

Mexican Brand Names Fluoxac®; Prozac®; Siquial®

Pharmacologic Category Antidepressant, Selective Serotonin Reuptake Inhibitor

Synonyms Fluoxetine Hydrochloride

Use Treatment of major depression; geriatric depression; treatment of binge-eating and vomiting in patients with moderate-to-severe bulimia nervosa; obsessive-compulsive disorder (OCD); premenstrual dysphoric disorder (PMDD)

Unlabeled/Investigational: Selective mutism

Local Anesthetic/Vasoconstrictor Precautions Although caution should be used in patients taking tricyclic antidepressants, no interactions have been reported with vasoconstrictors and fluoxetine, a nontricyclic antidepressant which acts to increase serotonin

Effects on Dental Treatment >10%: Xerostomia

Dosage Oral:

Children:

<5 years: No dosing information available

5-18 years: Initial: 5-10 mg/day; titrate upwards as needed (usual maximum dose: 60 mg/day)

Adults: 20 mg/day in the morning; may increase after several weeks by 20 mg/day increments; maximum: 80 mg/day; doses >20 mg should be divided into morning and noon doses. **Note:** Lower doses of 5-10 mg/day have been used for initial treatment.

Usual dosage range:

Bulimia nervosa: 60-80 mg/day

Depression: 20-40 mg/day; patients maintained on Prozac® 20 mg/day may be changed to Prozac® Weekly™ 90 mg/week, starting dose 7 days after the last 20 mg/day dose

Obesity: 20-60 mg/day

OCD: 40-80 mg/day

PMDD (Sarafem™): 20 mg/day

Elderly: Depression: Some patients may require an initial dose of 10 mg/day with dosage increases of 10 and 20 mg every several weeks as tolerated; should not be taken at night unless patient experiences sedation

Dosing adjustment in renal impairment:

Single dose studies: Pharmacokinetics of fluoxetine and norfluoxetine were similar among subjects with all levels of impaired renal function, including anephric patients on chronic hemodialysis

Chronic administration: Additional accumulation of fluoxetine or norfluoxetine may occur in patients with severely impaired renal function

Hemodialysis: Not removed by hemodialysis

Dosing adjustment in hepatic impairment: Elimination half-life of fluoxetine is prolonged in patients with hepatic impairment; a lower or less frequent dose of fluoxetine should be used in these patients

Cirrhosis patients: Administer a lower dose or less frequent dosing interval

Compensated cirrhosis without ascites: Administer 50% of normal dose

Mechanism of Action Inhibits CNS neuron serotonin uptake; minimal or no effect on reuptake of norepinephrine or dopamine; does not significantly bind to alpha-adrenergic, histamine or cholinergic receptors; may therefore be useful in patients at risk from sedation, hypotension, and anticholinergic effects of tricyclic antidepressants

Other Adverse Effects Predominant adverse effects are CNS and GI

>10%:

Central nervous system: Headache, nervousness (7% to 14%), insomnia (9% to 24%), anxiety, drowsiness

Gastrointestinal: Nausea, diarrhea, xerostomia, anorexia

Neuromuscular & skeletal: Weakness, tremor

1% to 10%:

Cardiovascular: Vasodilation, palpitation, hypertension

(Continued)

Fluoxetine *(Continued)*

Central nervous system: Amnesia, confusion, emotional lability, sleep disorder, dizziness, agitation, yawning, pain, fever, abnormal dreams

Dermatologic: Rash, pruritus

Systemic events, possibly related to vasculitis (including lupus-like syndrome), have occurred rarely in patients with rash; may include lung, kidney, and/or hepatic involvement. Death has been reported.

Endocrine & metabolic: SIADH, hypoglycemia, hyponatremia (elderly or volume-depleted patients)

Gastrointestinal: Dyspepsia, increased appetite, constipation, vomiting, flatulence, weight gain/loss, abdominal pain, dyspepsia

Genitourinary: Sexual dysfunction, urinary frequency

Ocular: Abnormal vision

Respiratory: Pharyngitis

Miscellaneous: Diaphoresis, fever, flu syndrome, infection, abnormal thinking

Warnings/Precautions Potential for severe reaction when used with MAO inhibitors - serotonin syndrome (hyperthermia, muscular rigidity, mental status changes/agitation, autonomic instability) may occur. Fluoxetine may elevate plasma concentrations of thioridazine and increase the risk of QT_c interval prolongation. This may lead to serious ventricular arrhythmias such as torsade de pointes-type arrhythmias and sudden death. Fluoxetine use has been associated with occurrences of significant rash and allergic events, including vasculitis, lupus-like syndrome, laryngospasm, anaphylactoid reactions, and pulmonary inflammatory disease. May precipitate a shift to mania or hypomania in patients with bipolar disease. May cause insomnia, anxiety, nervousness or anorexia. Use with caution in patients where weight loss is undesirable. May impair cognitive or motor performance - caution operating hazardous machinery or driving. Use caution in patients with depression, particularly if suicidal risk may be present. Use caution in patients with a previous seizure disorder or condition predisposing to seizures such as brain damage, alcoholism, or concurrent therapy with other drugs which lower the seizure threshold. Use with caution in patients with hepatic or renal dysfunction and in elderly patients. May cause hyponatremia/SIADH. May increase the risks associated with electroconvulsive treatment. Use with caution in patients at risk of bleeding or receiving concurrent anticoagulant therapy - may cause impairment in platelet function. May alter glycemic control in patients with diabetes. Due to the long half-life of fluoxetine and its metabolites, the effects and interactions noted may persist for prolonged periods following discontinuation. May cause or exacerbate sexual dysfunction.

Drug Interactions CYP2D6 (minor) and CYP3A3/4 enzyme substrate; CYP2C9 enzyme inducer; CYP1A2 (high dose), 2C9, 2C19, 2D6, and 3A3/4 enzyme inhibitor

MAO inhibitors: Fluoxetine should not be used with nonselective MAO inhibitors (phenelzine, isocarboxazid) or other drugs with MAO inhibition (linezolid); fatal reactions have been reported. Wait 5 weeks after stopping fluoxetine before starting a nonselective MAO inhibitor and 2 weeks after stopping an MAO inhibitor before starting fluoxetine. Concurrent selegiline has been associated with mania, hypertension, or serotonin syndrome (risk may be reduced relative to nonselective MAO inhibitors).

Phenothiazines: Fluoxetine may inhibit the metabolism of thioridazine or mesoridazine, resulting in increased plasma concentrations and increasing the risk of QT_c interval prolongation. This may lead to serious ventricular arrhythmias, such as torsade de pointes-type arrhythmias and sudden death. Do not use together. Wait at least 5 weeks after discontinuing fluoxetine prior to starting thioridazine.

Combined used of SSRIs and amphetamines, buspirone, meperidine, nefazodone, serotonin agonists (such as sumatriptan), sibutramine, other SSRIs, sympathomimetics, tramadol, and venlafaxine may increase the risk of serotonin syndrome. Fluoxetine may increase serum concentration/effects of benzodiazepines (alprazolam and diazepam), beta-blockers (except atenolol or nadolol), carbamazepine, carvedilol, clozapine, cyclosporine (and possibly tacrolimus), dextromethorphan, digoxin, haloperidol, HMG-CoA reductase inhibitors (lovastatin and simvastatin - increasing the risk of rhabdomyolysis), phenytoin, propafenone, trazodone, tricyclic antidepressants, and valproic acid. Concurrent lithium may increase risk of nephrotoxicity. Risk of hyponatremia may increase with concurrent use of loop diuretics (bumetanide, furosemide, torsemide). Fluoxetine may increase the hypoprothrombinemic response to warfarin.

Combined use of sumatriptan (and other serotonin agonists) may result in toxicity; weakness, hyper-reflexia, and incoordination have been observed with sumatriptan and SSRIs. In addition, concurrent use may theoretically increase the risk of serotonin syndrome; includes sumatriptan, naratriptan, rizatriptan, and zolmitriptan.

Drug Uptake

Absorption: Oral: Well absorbed; delayed 1-2 hours with weekly formulation

Half-life, elimination: Adults: Parent drug: 2-3 days; Metabolite (norfluoxetine): 4-16 days due to long half-life; resolution of adverse reactions after discontinuation may be slow

Time to peak: 4-8 hours

Note: Weekly formulation results in greater fluctuations between peak and trough concentrations of fluoxetine and norfluoxetine compared to once-daily dosing (24% daily/164% weekly; 17% daily/43% weekly, respectively). Trough concentrations are 76% lower for fluoxetine and 47% lower for norfluoxetine than the concentrations maintained by 20 mg once-daily dosing. Steady-state fluoxetine concentrations are ~50% lower following the once-weekly regimen compared to 20 mg once daily.

Pregnancy Risk Factor C

Generic Available No (except 90 mg capsule)

Comments Problems with SSRI-induced bruxism have been reported and may preclude their use; clinicians attempting to evaluate any patient with bruxism or involuntary muscle movement, who is simultaneously being treated with an SSRI drug, should be aware of this potential association.

EKG may reveal S-T segment depression; not shown to be teratogenic in rodents; 15-60 mg/day, buspirone and cyproheptadine, may be useful in treatment of sexual dysfunction during treatment with a selective serotonin reuptake inhibitor.

Weekly capsules are a delayed release formulation containing enteric-coated pellets of fluoxetine hydrochloride, equivalent to 90 mg fluoxetine. Therapeutic equivalence of weekly formulation with daily formulation for delaying time to relapse has not been established.

Selected Readings

Friedlander AH and Mahler ME, "Major Depressive Disorder. Psychopathology, Medical Management, and Dental Implications," *J Am Dent Assoc*, 2001, 132(5):629-38.

Gerber PE and Lynd LD, "Selective Serotonin Reuptake Inhibitor-induced Movement Disorders," *Ann Pharmacother*, 1998, 32(6):692-8.

Wynn RL, "New Antidepressant Medications," *Gen Dent*, 1997, 45(1):24-8.

Fluoxymesterone (floo oks i MES te rone)

U.S. Brand Names Halotestin®

Canadian Brand Names Halotestin®

Mexican Brand Names Stenox

Pharmacologic Category Androgen

Use Replacement of endogenous testicular hormone; in females, used as palliative treatment of breast cancer, postpartum breast engorgement

Unlabeled/Investigational: Stimulation of erythropoiesis, angioneurotic edema

Local Anesthetic/Vasoconstrictor Precautions No information available to require special precautions

Effects on Dental Treatment No effects or complications reported

Restrictions C-III

Dosage Adults: Oral:

Male:
- Hypogonadism: 5-20 mg/day
- Delayed puberty: 2.5-20 mg/day for 4-6 months

Female:
- Inoperable breast carcinoma: 10-40 mg/day in divided doses for 1-3 months
- Breast engorgement: 2.5 mg after delivery, 5-10 mg/day in divided doses for 4-5 days

Mechanism of Action Synthetic androgenic anabolic hormone responsible for the normal growth and development of male sex hormones and development of male sex organs and maintenance of secondary sex characteristics; synthetic testosterone derivative with significant androgen activity; stimulates RNA polymerase activity resulting in an increase in protein production; increases bone development; halogenated derivative of testosterone with up to 5 times the activity of methyltestosterone

Other Adverse Effects

>10%:
- Male: Priapism
- Female: Menstrual problems (amenorrhea), virilism, breast soreness
- Cardiovascular: Edema
- Dermatologic: Acne

1% to 10%:
- Male: Prostatic carcinoma, hirsutism (increase in pubic hair growth), impotence, testicular atrophy
- Cardiovascular: Edema
- Gastrointestinal: GI irritation, nausea, vomiting
- Genitourinary: Prostatic hyperplasia
- Hepatic: Hepatic dysfunction

Drug Interactions

Increased Effect/Toxicity: Fluoxymesterone may suppress clotting factors II, V, VII, and X; therefore, bleeding may occur in patients on anticoagulant therapy May

(Continued)

Fluoxymesterone *(Continued)*

elevate cyclosporine serum concentration. May enhance hypoglycemic effect of insulin therapy; may decrease blood glucose concentrations and insulin requirements in patients with diabetes. Lithium may potentiate EPS and other CNS effect. May potentiate the effects of narcotics including respiratory depression

Decreased Effect: May decrease barbiturate levels and fluphenazine effectiveness

Drug Uptake

Absorption: Oral: Rapid

Half-life, elimination: 10-100 minutes

Pregnancy Risk Factor X

Generic Available Yes

Fluphenazine (floo FEN a zeen)

U.S. Brand Names Permitil®; Prolixin®; Prolixin Decanoate®; Prolixin Enanthate®

Canadian Brand Names Apo®-Fluphenazine; Modecate®; Moditen® Enanthate; Moditen® HCl; PMS-Fluphenazine Decanoate; Rho®-Fluphenazine Decanoate

Pharmacologic Category Antipsychotic Agent, Phenothiazine, Piperazine

Synonyms Fluphenazine Decanoate; Fluphenazine Enanthate; Fluphenazine Hydrochloride

Use Management of manifestations of psychotic disorders and schizophrenia; depot formulation may offer improved outcome in individuals with psychosis who are nonadherent with oral antipsychotics

Unlabeled/Investigational: Pervasive developmental disorder

Local Anesthetic/Vasoconstrictor Precautions Most pharmacology textbooks state that in presence of phenothiazines, systemic doses of epinephrine paradoxically decrease the blood pressure. This is the so called "epinephrine reversal" phenomenon. This has never been observed when epinephrine is given by infiltration as part of the anesthesia procedure.

Effects on Dental Treatment Orthostatic hypotension and nasal congestion possible in dental patients. Since the drug is a dopamine antagonist, extrapyramidal symptoms of the TMJ a possibility.

Dosage

Children: Oral: Childhood-onset pervasive developmental disorder (unlabeled use): 0.04 mg/kg/day

Adults: Psychoses:

- Oral: 0.5-10 mg/day in divided doses at 6- to 8-hour intervals; some patients may require up to 40 mg/day
- I.M.: 2.5-10 mg/day in divided doses at 6- to 8-hour intervals (parenteral dose is $^1/_3$ to $^1/_2$ the oral dose for the hydrochloride salts)
- I.M. (decanoate): 12.5 mg every 2 weeks
  - Conversion from hydrochloride to decanoate I.M. 0.5 mL (12.5 mg) decanoate every 3 weeks is ~ equivalent to 10 mg hydrochloride/day
- I.M. (enanthate): 12.5-25 mg every 2 weeks

Hemodialysis: Not dialyzable (0% to 5%)

Mechanism of Action Blocks postsynaptic mesolimbic dopaminergic D_1 and D_2 receptors in the brain; exhibits a strong alpha-adrenergic blocking and anticholinergic effect, depresses the release of hypothalamic and hypophyseal hormones; believed to depress the reticular activating system thus affecting basal metabolism, body temperature, wakefulness, vasomotor tone, and emesis

Other Adverse Effects Frequency not defined:

Cardiovascular: Hypotension, tachycardia, fluctuations in BP, hypertension, arrhythmias, edema

Central nervous system: Parkinsonian symptoms, akathisia, dystonias, tardive dyskinesia, dizziness, hyper-reflexia, headache, cerebral edema, drowsiness, lethargy, restlessness, excitement, bizarre dreams, EEG changes, depression, seizures, NMS, altered central temperature regulation

Dermatologic: Increased sensitivity to sun, rash, skin pigmentation, itching, erythema, urticaria, seborrhea, eczema, dermatitis

Endocrine & metabolic: Changes in menstrual cycle, breast pain, amenorrhea, galactorrhea, gynecomastia, changes in libido, elevated prolactin, SIADH

Gastrointestinal: Weight gain, loss of appetite, salivation, xerostomia, constipation, paralytic ileus, laryngeal edema

Genitourinary: Ejaculatory disturbances, impotence, polyuria, bladder paralysis, enuresis

Hematologic: Agranulocytosis, leukopenia, thrombocytopenia, nonthrombocytopenic purpura, eosinophilia, pancytopenia

Hepatic: Cholestatic jaundice, hepatotoxicity

Neuromuscular & skeletal: Trembling of fingers, SLE, facial hemispasm

Ocular: Pigmentary retinopathy, cornea and lens changes, blurred vision, glaucoma

Respiratory: Nasal congestion, asthma

Drug Interactions CYP2D6 enzyme substrate; CYP2D6 enzyme inhibitor

Aluminum salts: May decrease the absorption of phenothiazines; monitor

Amphetamines: Efficacy may be diminished by antipsychotics; in addition, amphetamines may increase psychotic symptoms. Avoid concurrent use

Anticholinergics: May inhibit the therapeutic response to phenothiazines and excess anticholinergic effects may occur; includes benztropine, trihexyphenidyl, biperiden, and drugs with significant anticholinergic activity (TCAs, antihistamines, disopyramide)

Antihypertensives: Concurrent use of phenothiazines with an antihypertensive may produce additive hypotensive effects (particularly orthostasis)

Bromocriptine: Phenothiazines inhibit the ability of bromocriptine to lower serum prolactin concentrations

CNS depressants: Sedative effects may be additive with phenothiazines; monitor for increased effect; includes barbiturates, benzodiazepines, narcotic analgesics, ethanol, and other sedative agents

CYP2D6 inhibitors: Metabolism of phenothiazines may be decreased; increasing clinical effect or toxicity; inhibitors include amiodarone, cimetidine, delavirdine, fluoxetine, paroxetine, propafenone, quinidine, and ritonavir; monitor for increased effect/toxicity

Enzyme inducers: May enhance the hepatic metabolism of phenothiazines; larger doses may be required; includes rifampin, rifabutin, barbiturates, phenytoin, and cigarette smoking

Epinephrine: Chlorpromazine (and possibly other low potency antipsychotics) may diminish the pressor effects of epinephrine

Guanethidine and guanadrel: Antihypertensive effects may be inhibited by phenothiazines

Levodopa: Phenothiazines may inhibit the antiparkinsonian effect of levodopa; avoid this combination

Lithium: Phenothiazines may produce neurotoxicity with lithium; this is a rare effect

Metoclopramide: May increase extrapyramidal symptoms (EPS) or risk.

Phenytoin: May reduce serum levels of phenothiazines; phenothiazines may increase phenytoin serum levels

Propranolol: Serum concentrations of phenothiazines may be increased; propranolol also increases phenothiazine concentrations

Polypeptide antibiotics: Rare cases of respiratory paralysis have been reported with concurrent use of phenothiazines

QT_c-prolonging agents: Effects on QT_c interval may be additive with phenothiazines, increasing the risk of malignant arrhythmias; includes type Ia antiarrhythmics, TCAs, and some quinolone antibiotics (sparfloxacin, moxifloxacin and gatifloxacin)

Sulfadoxine-pyrimethamine: May increase phenothiazine concentrations

Tricyclic antidepressants: Concurrent use may produce increased toxicity or altered therapeutic response

Trazodone: Phenothiazines and trazodone may produce additive hypotensive effects

Valproic acid: Serum levels may be increased by phenothiazines

Drug Uptake

Onset of action: I.M., S.C. (derivative dependent): Hydrochloride salt: ~1 hour

Peak effect: Neuroleptic: Decanoate: 48-96 hours

Duration: Hydrochloride salt: 6-8 hours; Decanoate (lasts the longest): 24-72 hours

Half-life, elimination (derivative dependent): Enanthate: 84-96 hours; Hydrochloride: 33 hours; Decanoate: 163-232 hours

Pregnancy Risk Factor C

Generic Available Yes

Flura-Drops® *see* Fluoride *on page 514*

Flura-Loz® *see* Fluoride *on page 514*

Flurandrenolide (flure an DREN oh lide)

U.S. Brand Names Cordran®; Cordran® SP

Canadian Brand Names Cordran®

Pharmacologic Category Corticosteroid, Topical

Synonyms Flurandrenolone

Use Inflammation of corticosteroid-responsive dermatoses [medium potency topical corticosteroid]

Local Anesthetic/Vasoconstrictor Precautions No information available to require special precautions

Effects on Dental Treatment No effects or complications reported

Dosage Topical:

Children:

Ointment, cream: Apply sparingly 1-2 times/day

Tape: Apply once daily

Adults: Cream, lotion, ointment: Apply sparingly 2-3 times/day

Therapy should be discontinued when control is achieved; if no improvement is seen, reassessment of diagnosis may be necessary.

Mechanism of Action Decreases inflammation by suppression of migration of polymorphonuclear leukocytes and reversal of increased capillary permeability

Other Adverse Effects Frequency not defined:

Cardiovascular: Intracranial hypertension

(Continued)

Flurandrenolide *(Continued)*

Dermatologic: Itching, dry skin, folliculitis, hypertrichosis, acneiform eruptions, hyperpigmentation, perioral dermatitis, allergic contact dermatitis, skin atrophy, striae, miliaria, acne, maceration of the skin

Endocrine & metabolic: Cushing's syndrome, growth retardation, HPA suppression

Local: Burning, irritation

Miscellaneous: Secondary infection

Drug Uptake Absorption: Adequate with intact skin; repeated applications lead to depot effects on skin, potentially resulting in enhanced percutaneous absorption

Pregnancy Risk Factor C

Generic Available Yes

Flurazepam (flure AZ e pam)

U.S. Brand Names Dalmane®

Canadian Brand Names Apo®-Flurazepam; Dalmane®; Somnol®

Pharmacologic Category Benzodiazepine

Synonyms Flurazepam Hydrochloride

Use Short-term treatment of insomnia

Local Anesthetic/Vasoconstrictor Precautions No information available to require special precautions

Effects on Dental Treatment >10%: Xerostomia

Restrictions C-IV

Dosage Oral:

Children: Insomnia: >15 years: 15 mg at bedtime

Adults: Insomnia: 15-30 mg at bedtime

Elderly: Insomnia: Oral: 15 mg at bedtime; avoid use if possible

Mechanism of Action Binds to stereospecific benzodiazepine receptors on the postsynaptic GABA (gamma-aminobutyric acid) neuron at several sites within the CNS, including the limbic system, reticular formation. Enhancement of the inhibitory effect of GABA on neuronal excitability results by increased neuronal membrane permeability to chloride ions. This shift in chloride ions results in hyperpolarization (a less excitable state) and stabilization.

Other Adverse Effects Frequency not defined:

Cardiovascular: Palpitations, chest pain

Central nervous system: Drowsiness, ataxia, lightheadedness, memory impairment, depression, headache, hangover effect, confusion, nervousness, dizziness, falling, apprehension, irritability, euphoria, slurred speech, restlessness, hallucinations, paradoxical reactions, talkativeness

Dermatologic: Rash, pruritus

Gastrointestinal: Xerostomia, constipation, increased/excessive salivation, heartburn, upset stomach, nausea, vomiting, diarrhea, increased or decreased appetite, bitter taste, weight gain/loss

Hematologic: Granulocytopenia, euphoria

Hepatic: Elevated AST/ALT, total bilirubin, alkaline phosphatase, cholestatic jaundice

Neuromuscular & skeletal: Dysarthria, body/joint pain, reflex slowing, weakness

Ocular: Blurred vision, burning eyes, difficulty focusing

Otic: Tinnitus

Respiratory: Apnea, dyspnea

Miscellaneous: Diaphoresis, drug dependence

Drug Interactions CYP2D6 and CYP3A3/4 enzyme substrate

Increased Effect/Toxicity: Serum levels and response to flurazepam may be increased by amprenavir, cimetidine, ciprofloxacin, clarithromycin, clozapine, CNS depressants, diltiazem, disulfiram, digoxin, erythromycin, fluconazole, fluoxetine, fluvoxamine, isoniazid, itraconazole, ketoconazole, labetalol, levodopa, loxapine, metoprolol, metronidazole, miconazole, nefazodone, nelfinavir, omeprazole, phenytoin, rifabutin, rifampin, ritonavir, troleandomycin, valproic acid, and verapamil.

Decreased Effect: Carbamazepine, rifampin, and rifabutin may enhance the metabolism of flurazepam and decrease its therapeutic effect; consider using an alternative sedative/hypnotic agent.

Drug Uptake

Onset of action: Hypnotic: 15-20 minutes; Peak effect: 3-6 hours

Duration: 7-8 hours

Half-life, elimination: Desalkylflurazepam:

- Adults: Single dose: 74-90 hours; multiple dose: 111-113 hours
- Elderly (61-85 years): Single dose: 120-160 hours; multiple dose: 126-158 hours

Pregnancy Risk Factor X

Generic Available Yes

Flurbiprofen (flure BI proe fen)

Related Information

Dental Drug Interactions: Update on Drug Combinations Requiring Special Considerations *on page 1434*

Rheumatoid Arthritis and Osteoarthritis *on page 1340*
Temporomandibular Dysfunction (TMD) *on page 1397*

U.S. Brand Names Ansaid® Oral; Ocufen® Ophthalmic

Canadian Brand Names Alti-Flurbiprofen; Ansaid®; Apo®-Flurbiprofen; Froben®; Froben-SR®; Novo-Flurprofen; Nu-Flurprofen; Ocufen™

Mexican Brand Names Ansaid®

Pharmacologic Category Nonsteroidal Anti-inflammatory Drug (NSAID)

Synonyms Flurbiprofen Sodium

Use

Dental: Management of postoperative pain

Medical:

Oral: Acute or long-term treatment of signs and symptoms of rheumatoid arthritis and osteoarthritis

Ophthalmic: Inhibition of intraoperative miosis; prevention and management of postoperative ocular inflammation and postoperative cystoid macular edema remains to be determined

Local Anesthetic/Vasoconstrictor Precautions No information available to require special precautions

Effects on Dental Treatment

<1%: Xerostomia

NSAID formulations are known to reversibly decrease platelet aggregation via mechanisms different than observed with aspirin. The dentist should be aware of the potential of abnormal coagulation. Caution should also be exercised in the use of NSAIDs in patients already on anticoagulant therapy with drugs such as warfarin (Coumadin®).

Dosage

Oral: Rheumatoid arthritis and osteoarthritis: 200-300 mg/day in 2-, 3-, or 4 divided doses

Ophthalmic: Instill 1 drop every 30 minutes, 2 hours prior to surgery (total of 4 drops to each affected eye)

Mechanism of Action Inhibits prostaglandin synthesis by decreasing the activity of the enzyme, cyclo-oxygenase, which results in decreased formation of prostaglandin precursors

Other Adverse Effects

Ophthalmic:

>10%: Ocular: Slowing of corneal wound healing, mild ocular stinging, itching and burning eyes, ocular irritation

1% to 10%: Ocular: Eye redness

Oral:

Cardiovascular: Congestive heart failure, hypertension, arrhythmias, tachycardia, angioedema

Central nervous system: Headache (3% to 9%), nervousness, dizziness (1% to 10%), confusion, hallucinations, aseptic meningitis, mental depression, drowsiness, insomnia

Dermatologic: Itching, rash, urticaria, erythema multiforme, toxic epidermal necrolysis, Stevens-Johnson syndrome

Endocrine & metabolic: Fluid retention (3% to 9%), polydipsia, hot flashes

Gastrointestinal: Vomiting (1% to 3%), diarrhea (3% to 9%), constipation (1% to 3%), flatulence (1% to 3%), abdominal cramps (3% to 9%), heartburn, indigestion, nausea (3% to 9%), dyspepsia (3% to 9%), gastritis, GI ulceration, stomatitis (<1%)

Genitourinary: Urinary tract infection (3% to 9%), cystitis, polyuria

Hematologic: Agranulocytosis, anemia, hemolytic anemia, bone marrow suppression, leukopenia, thrombocytopenia

Hepatic: Increased LFTs (1% to 3%), hepatitis

Neuromuscular & skeletal: Peripheral neuropathy

Ocular: Toxic amblyopia, blurred vision, conjunctivitis, dry eyes,

Otic: Decreased hearing, tinnitus

Renal: Acute renal failure

Respiratory: Dyspnea, allergic rhinitis, epistaxis

Contraindications Hypersensitivity to flurbiprofen or any component of the formulation; dendritic keratitis; pregnancy (3rd trimester)

Warnings/Precautions Use with caution in patients with CHF, hypertension, dehydration, decreased renal or hepatic function, history of GI disease (bleeding or ulcers), or those receiving anticoagulants. Elderly are at a high risk for adverse effects from nonsteroidal anti-inflammatory agents. As much as 60% of elderly can develop peptic ulceration and/or hemorrhage asymptomatically.

Use lowest effective dose for shortest period possible. Use of NSAIDs can compromise existing renal function especially when Cl_{cr} is <30 mL/minute. CNS adverse effects such as confusion, agitation, and hallucination are generally seen in overdose or high-dose situations; however, elderly may demonstrate these adverse effects at lower doses than younger adults. Withhold for at least 4-6 half-lives prior to surgical or dental procedures. Ophthalmic solution contains thimerosal.

Drug Interactions CYP2C9 enzyme substrate; CYP2C9 enzyme inhibitor

(Continued)

Flurbiprofen *(Continued)*

ACE inhibitors: Antihypertensive effects may be decreased by concurrent therapy with NSAIDs; monitor BP.

Angiotensin II antagonists: Antihypertensive effects may be decreased by concurrent therapy with NSAIDs; monitor BP.

Anticoagulants (warfarin, heparin, LMWHs) in combination with NSAIDs can cause increased risk of bleeding.

Other antiplatelet drugs (ticlopidine, clopidogrel, aspirin, abciximab, dipyridamole, eptifibatide, tirofiban) can cause an increased risk of bleeding.

Loop diuretics efficacy (diuretic and antihypertensive effect) is reduced. Indomethacin reduces this efficacy, however, it may be anticipated with any NSAID.

Cholestyramine and colestipol reduce the bioavailability of some NSAIDs; separate administration times.

Corticosteroids may increase the risk of GI ulceration; avoid concurrent use.

Cyclosporine: NSAIDs may increase serum creatinine, potassium, BP, and cyclosporine levels; monitor cyclosporine levels and renal function carefully.

Gentamicin and amikacin serum concentrations are increased by indomethacin in premature infants. Results may apply to other aminoglycosides and NSAIDs.

Hydralazine's antihypertensive effect is decreased; avoid concurrent use.

Lithium levels can be increased; avoid concurrent use if possible or monitor lithium levels and adjust dose. Sulindac may have the least effect. When NSAID is stopped, lithium will need adjustment again.

Methotrexate: Severe bone marrow suppression, aplastic anemia, and GI toxicity have been reported with concomitant NSAID therapy. Avoid use during moderate or high-dose methotrexate (increased and prolonged methotrexate levels). NSAID use during low-dose treatment of rheumatoid arthritis has not been fully evaluated; extreme caution is warranted.

Thiazides antihypertensive effects are decreased; avoid concurrent use.

Warfarin's INRs may be increased by piroxicam. Other NSAIDs may have the same effect depending on dose and duration. Monitor INR closely. Use the lowest dose of NSAIDs possible and for the briefest duration.

Verapamil plasma concentration is decreased by some NSAIDs; avoid concurrent use.

Dietary/Ethanol/Herb Considerations

Ethanol: Avoid use; may enhance gastric mucosal irritation.

Food: Administer with food or milk to reduce GI upset; may decrease rate but not extent of absorption. Avoid garlic, ginger, and green tea.

Herb/Nutraceutical: Avoid cat's claw, dong quai, evening primrose, feverfew, garlic, ginger, ginkgo biloba, ginseng, green tea, horse chestnut, and red clover due to additional antiplatelet activity.

Drug Uptake

Onset of action: 1-2 hours

Half-life, elimination: 5.7 hours

Time to peak: 1.5 hours

Pregnancy Risk Factor C/D (3rd trimester)

Dosage Forms SOLN, ophthalmic (Ocufen®): 0.03% (2.5 mL, 5 mL, 10 mL). **TAB** (Ansaid®): 50 mg, 100 mg

Generic Available Yes

Comments Flurbiprofen is a chiral NSAID with the S-(+) enantiomer possessing most of the beneficial anti-inflammatory activity; both the S-(+) and R-(-) enantiomers possess analgesic activity. All flurbiprofen preparations are marketed as the racemic mixture (equal parts of each enantiomer). Flurbiprofen may be effective in the treatment of periodontal disease. Animal studies have shown flurbiprofen in topical form to be effective in reducing loss of attachment and bone loss. Flurbiprofen as with other NSAIDs can be administered preoperatively in the patient undergoing dental surgery in order to delay the onset and severity of postoperative pain. Doses which have been used are 100 mg twice daily the day before procedure, and 50-100 mg 30 minutes before the procedure.

Selected Readings

Ahmad N, Grad HA, Haas DA, et al, "The Efficacy of Nonopioid Analgesics for Postoperative Dental Pain: A Meta-Analysis," *Anesth Prog*, 1997, 44(4):119-26.

Bragger U, Muhle T, Fourmousis I, et al, "Effect of the NSAID Flurbiprofen on Remodeling After Periodontal Surgery," *J Periodontal Res*, 1997, 32(7):575-82.

Cooper SA and Kupperman A, "The Analgesic Efficacy of Flurbiprofen Compared to Acetaminophen With Codeine," *J Clin Dent*, 1991, 2(3):70-4.

Dionne R, "Additive Analgesia Without Opioid Side Effects," *Compend Contin Educ Dent*, 2000, 21(7):572-4, 576-7.

Dionne RA, "Suppression of Dental Pain by the Preoperative Administration of Flurbiprofen," *Am J Med*, 1986, 80(3A):41-9.

Dionne RA and Berthold CW, "Therapeutic Uses of Nonsteroidal Anti-Inflammatory Drugs in Dentistry," *Crit Rev Oral Biol Med*, 2001, 12(4):315-30.

Dionne RA, Snyder J, and Hargreaves KM, "Analgesic Efficacy of Flurbiprofen in Comparison With Acetaminophen, Acetaminophen Plus Codeine, and Placebo After Impacted Third Molar Removal," *J Oral Maxillofac Surg*, 1994, 52(9):919-24.

Forbes JA, Yorio CC, Selinger LR, et al, "An Evaluation of Flurbiprofen, Aspirin, and Placebo in Postoperative Oral Surgery Pain," *Pharmacotherapy*, 1989, 9(2):66-73.

Gallardo F and Rossi E, "Analgesic Efficacy of Flurbiprofen as Compared to Acetaminophen and Placebo After Periodontal Surgery," *J Periodontol*, 1990, 61(4):224-7.

Jeffcoat MK, Reddy MS, Haigh S, et al, "A Comparison of Topical Ketorolac, Systemic Flurbiprofen, and Placebo for the Inhibition of Bone Loss in Adult Periodontitis," *J Periodontol*, 1995, 66(5):329-38.

Jeffcoat MK, Reddy MS, Wang IC, et al, "The Effect of Systemic Flurbiprofen on Bone Supporting Dental Implants," *J Am Dent Assoc*, 1995, 126(3):305-11.

Malmberg AB and Yaksh TL, "Antinociception Produced by Spinal Delivery of the S and R Enantiomers of Flurbiprofen in the Formalin Test," *Eur J Pharmacol*, 1994, 256(2):205-9.

Nguyen AM, Graham DY, Gage T, et al, "Nonsteroidal Anti-Inflammatory Drug Use in Dentistry: Gastrointestinal Implications," *Gen Dent*, 1999, 47(6):590-6.

Fluro-Ethyl® *see* Ethyl Chloride and Dichlorotetrafluoroethane *on page 477*

FluShield® *see* Influenza Virus Vaccine *on page 637*

Flutamide (FLOO ta mide)

U.S. Brand Names Eulexin®

Canadian Brand Names Apo®-Flutamide; Euflex®; Eulexin®; Novo-Flutamide; PMS-Flutamide

Mexican Brand Names Eulexin®; Fluken; Flulem

Pharmacologic Category Antiandrogen

Use In combination therapy with LHRH agonist analogues in treatment of metastatic prostatic carcinoma. A study has shown that the addition of flutamide to leuprolide therapy in patients with advanced prostatic cancer increased median actuarial survival time to 34.9 months versus 27.9 months with leuprolide alone. To achieve benefit to combination therapy, both drugs need to be started simultaneously.

Unlabeled/Investigational: Female hirsutism

Local Anesthetic/Vasoconstrictor Precautions No information available to require special precautions

Effects on Dental Treatment No effects or complications reported

Dosage Oral: Adults:

Prostatic carcinoma: 2 capsules every 8 hours for a total daily dose of 750 mg

Female hirsutism: 250 mg daily

Mechanism of Action Nonsteroidal antiandrogen that inhibits androgen uptake or inhibits binding of androgen in target tissues

Other Adverse Effects

>10%:

- Endocrine & metabolic: Gynecomastia, hot flashes, breast tenderness, galactorrhea (9% to 42%); impotence; decreased libido; tumor flare
- Gastrointestinal: Nausea, vomiting (11% to 12%)
- Hepatic: Increased AST (SGOT) and LDH levels, transient, mild

1% to 10%:

- Cardiovascular: Hypertension (1%), edema
- Central nervous system: Drowsiness, confusion, depression, anxiety, nervousness, headache, dizziness, insomnia
- Dermatologic: Pruritus, ecchymosis, photosensitivity, herpes zoster
- Gastrointestinal: Anorexia, increased appetite, constipation, indigestion, upset stomach (4% to 6%); diarrhea
- Hematologic: Anemia (6%), leukopenia (3%), thrombocytopenia (1%)
- Neuromuscular & skeletal: Weakness (1%)

Contraindications Hypersensitivity to flutamide or any component of the formulation; severe hepatic impairment; pregnancy

Drug Interactions CYP3A3/4 enzyme substrate

May increased effects of warfarin

Drug Uptake

Absorption: Rapid and complete

Half-life, elimination: 5-6 hours

Pregnancy Risk Factor D

Generic Available Yes

Comments To achieve benefit to combination therapy, both drugs need to be started simultaneously

Flutex® *see* Triamcinolone *on page 1197*

Fluticasone (floo TIK a sone)

Related Information

Respiratory Diseases *on page 1328*

U.S. Brand Names Cutivate™; Flonase®; Flovent®; Flovent® Rotadisk®

Canadian Brand Names Cutivate™; Flonase®; Flovent®

Mexican Brand Names Cutivate®; Flixonase®; Flixotide®

Pharmacologic Category Corticosteroid, Inhalant (Oral); Corticosteroid, Nasal; Corticosteroid, Topical; Corticosteroid, Topical (Medium Potency)

Synonyms Fluticasone Propionate

Use

Inhalation: Maintenance treatment of asthma as prophylactic therapy. It is also indicated for patients requiring oral corticosteroid therapy for asthma to assist in total discontinuation or reduction of total oral dose. NOT indicated for the relief of acute bronchospasm.

Intranasal: Management of seasonal and perennial allergic rhinitis and nonallergic rhinitis in patients ≥4 years of age

(Continued)

Fluticasone *(Continued)*

Topical: Relief of inflammation and pruritus associated with corticosteroid-responsive dermatoses [medium potency topical corticosteroid]

Local Anesthetic/Vasoconstrictor Precautions No information available to require special precautions

Effects on Dental Treatment Localized infections with *Candida albicans* or *Aspergillus niger* have occurred frequently in the mouth and pharynx with repetitive use of oral inhaler of corticosteroids. These infections may require treatment with appropriate antifungal therapy or discontinuance of treatment with corticosteroid inhaler.

Dosage

Children:

Asthma: Inhalation, oral:

Flovent®: Children ≥12 years: Refer to Adult dosing

Flovent® Diskus® and Rotadisk®: Note: Titrate to the lowest effective dose once asthma stability is achieved; children previously maintained on Flovent® Rotadisk® may require dosage adjustments when transferred to Flovent® Diskus®

Children ≥4-11 years: Dosing based on previous therapy

Bronchodilator alone: Recommended starting dose: 50 mcg twice daily; highest recommended dose: 100 mcg twice daily

Inhaled corticosteroids: Recommended starting dose: 50 mcg twice daily; highest recommended dose: 100 mcg twice daily; a higher starting dose may be considered in patients previously requiring higher doses of inhaled corticosteroids

Children ≥11 years: Refer to Adult dosing

Inflammation/pruritus associated with corticosteroid-responsive dermatoses: Topical: Children >3 months: Apply sparingly in a thin film twice daily; therapy should be discontinued when control is achieved. If no improvement is seen within 2 weeks, reassessment of diagnosis may be necessary. Safety and efficacy for use in pediatric patients >4 weeks have not been established.

Rhinitis: Intranasal: Children ≥4 years and Adolescents: Initial: 1 spray (50 mcg/spray) per nostril once daily; patients not adequately responding or patients with more severe symptoms may use 2 sprays (100 mcg) per nostril. Depending on response, dosage may be reduced to 100 mcg daily. Total daily dosage should not exceed 2 sprays in each nostril (200 mcg)/day. Dosing should be at regular intervals.

Adults:

Asthma: Inhalation, oral: Note: Titrate to the lowest effective dose once asthma stability is achieved

Flovent®: Dosing based on previous therapy

Bronchodilator alone: Recommended starting dose: 88 mcg twice daily; highest recommended dose: 440 mcg twice daily

Inhaled corticosteroids: Recommended starting dose: 88-220 mcg twice daily; highest recommended dose: 440 mcg twice daily; a higher starting dose may be considered in patients previously requiring higher doses of inhaled corticosteroids

Oral corticosteroids: Recommended starting dose: 880 mcg twice daily; highest recommended dose: 880 mcg twice daily; starting dose is patient dependent. In patients on chronic oral corticosteroids therapy, reduce prednisone dose no faster than 2.5 mg/day on a weekly basis; begin taper after ≥1 week of fluticasone therapy

Flovent® Diskus® and Rotadisk®: Dosing based on previous therapy

Bronchodilator alone: Recommended starting dose 100 mcg twice daily; highest recommended dose: 500 mcg twice daily

Inhaled corticosteroids: 100-250 mcg twice daily; highest recommended dose: 500 mcg twice daily; a higher starting dose may be considered in patients previously requiring higher doses of inhaled corticosteroids

Oral corticosteroids: 500-1000 mcg twice daily; highest recommended dose: 1000 mcg twice daily; starting dose is patient dependent. In patients on chronic oral corticosteroids therapy, reduce prednisone dose no faster than 2.5 mg/day on a weekly basis; begin taper after ≥1 week of fluticasone therapy

Inflammation/pruritus associated with corticosteroid-responsive dermatoses: Topical: Apply sparingly in a thin film twice daily; therapy should be discontinued when control is achieved. If no improvement is seen within 2 weeks, reassessment of diagnosis may be necessary.

Rhinitis: Intranasal: Initial: 2 sprays (50 mcg/spray) per nostril once daily; may also be divided into 100 mcg twice a day. After the first few days, dosage may be reduced to 1 spray per nostril once daily for maintenance therapy. Dosing should be at regular intervals.

Dosage adjustment in hepatic impairment: Fluticasone is primarily cleared in the liver. Fluticasone plasma concentrations may be increased in patients with hepatic impairment, use with caution; monitor.

Mechanism of Action Fluticasone belongs to a new group of corticosteroids which utilizes a fluorocarbothioate ester linkage at the 17 carbon position; extremely potent vasoconstrictive and anti-inflammatory activity; has a weak HPA inhibitory potency when applied topically, which gives the drug a high therapeutic index. The effectiveness of inhaled fluticasone is due to its direct local effect. The mechanism of action for all topical corticosteroids is believed to be a combination of three important properties: anti-inflammatory activity, immunosuppressive properties, and antiproliferative actions.

Other Adverse Effects

Oral inhalation: Frequency depends upon population studied and dosing used. Reactions reported are representative of multiple oral formulations.

>3%:

Central nervous system: Headache (2% to 22%), fever (1% to 7%)

Gastrointestinal: Nausea/vomiting (1% to 8%), viral GI infection (3% to 5%), diarrhea (1% to 4%), GI discomfort/pain (1% to 4%)

Neuromuscular & skeletal: Muscle injury (1% to 5%), musculoskeletal pain (1% to 5%), back problems (<1% to 4%)

Respiratory: Upper respiratory tract infection (14% to 22%), throat irritation (3% to 22%), nasal congestion (4% to 16%), pharyngitis (6% to 14%), oral candidiasis (<1% to 11%), sinusitis/sinus infection (3% to 10%), rhinitis (1% to 9%), influenza (3% to 8%), bronchitis (1% to 8%), dysphonia (<1% to 8%), upper respiratory inflammation (5%), allergic rhinitis (3% to 5%), cough (1% to 5%), nasal discharge (1% to 5%), viral respiratory infection (1% to 5%)

Miscellaneous: Viral infection (2% to 5%)

1% to 3%:

Cardiovascular: Chest symptoms, edema, palpitations, swelling

Central nervous system: Dizziness, fatigue, malaise, migraine, mood disorders, nervousness, paralysis of cranial nerves, pain, sleep disorders, giddiness

Dermatologic: Acne, dermatitis/dermatosis, eczema, folliculitis, fungal skin infection, photodermatitis, pruritus, skin rash, urticaria, viral skin infection

Endocrine & metabolic: Dysmenorrhea, fluid disturbances, goiter, uric acid metabolism disorder

Gastrointestinal: Abdominal discomfort/pain, appetite disturbances, colitis, dyspepsia, gastroenteritis, gastrointestinal infections, mouth/tongue disorder, oral erythema, oral rash, oral ulcerations, stomach disorder, viral gastroenteritis, weight gain

Genitourinary: Urinary tract infection

Hematologic: Hematoma

Hepatic: Cholecystitis

Local: Irritation from inhalant

Neuromuscular & skeletal: Arthralgia/articular rheumatism, limb pain, muscle cramps/spasms, musculoskeletal inflammation

Ocular: Blepharoconjunctivitis, conjunctivitis, irritation, keratitis

Otic: Earache, ear polyps, otitis

Respiratory: Chest congestion, dyspnea, epistaxis, laryngitis, lower respiratory infections, mouth irritation, nasal pain, nasopharyngitis, nose/throat polyps, oropharyngeal plaques, sneezing, throat constriction

Miscellaneous: Bacterial infections, burns, contusion, cysts, dental discomfort/pain, dental problems, fungal infections, lumps, masses, pressure-induced disorders, postoperative complications, soft tissue injury, tonsillitis, tooth decay, wounds/lacerations

Drug Uptake

Absorption: Cream: 5% (increases with inflammation); Oral inhalation: Primarily via lungs, minimal absorption from GI tract due to presystemic metabolism

Half-life, elimination: I.V.: 8 hours

Pregnancy Risk Factor C

Generic Available No

Fluvastatin (FLOO va sta tin)

Related Information

Cardiovascular Diseases *on page 1308*

U.S. Brand Names Lescol®; Lescol® XL

Canadian Brand Names Lescol®

Mexican Brand Names Canef®; Lescol®

Pharmacologic Category Antilipemic Agent, HMG-CoA Reductase Inhibitor

Use To be used as a component of multiple risk factor intervention in patients at risk for atherosclerosis vascular disease due to hypercholesterolemia

Adjunct to dietary therapy to reduce elevated total cholesterol (total-C), LDL-C, triglyceride, and apolipoprotein B (apo-B) levels and to increase HDL-C in primary hypercholesterolemia and mixed dyslipidemia (Fredrickson types IIa and IIb); to slow the progression of coronary atherosclerosis in patients with coronary heart disease

Local Anesthetic/Vasoconstrictor Precautions No information available to require special precautions

Effects on Dental Treatment No effects or complications reported

Dosage Adults: Oral:

(Continued)

Fluvastatin *(Continued)*

Patients requiring ≥25% decrease in LDL-C: 40 mg capsule or 80 mg extended release tablet once daily in the evening; may also use 40 mg capsule twice daily

Patients requiring < 25% decrease in LDL-C: 20 mg capsule once daily in the evening

Note: Dosing range: 20-80 mg/day; adjust dose based on response to therapy; maximum response occurs within 4-6 weeks

Mechanism of Action Acts by competitively inhibiting 3-hydroxyl-3-methylglutaryl-coenzyme A (HMG-CoA) reductase, the enzyme that catalyzes the reduction of HMG-CoA to mevalonate; this is an early rate-limiting step in cholesterol biosynthesis. HDL is increased while total, LDL and VLDL cholesterols, apolipoprotein B, and plasma triglycerides are decreased

Other Adverse Effects As reported with fluvastatin capsules; in general, adverse reactions reported with fluvastatin extended release tablet were similar, but the incidence was less.

1% to 10%:

- Central nervous system: Headache (9%), fatigue (3%), insomnia (3%)
- Gastrointestinal: Dyspepsia (8%), diarrhea (5%), abdominal pain (5%), nausea (3%)
- Genitourinary: Urinary tract infection (2%)
- Neuromuscular & skeletal: Myalgia (5%)
- Respiratory: Sinusitis (3%), bronchitis (2%)

Warnings/Precautions Secondary causes of hyperlipidemia should be ruled out prior to therapy. Liver function must be monitored by periodic laboratory assessment. Rhabdomyolysis with acute renal failure has occurred with fluvastatin and other HMG-CoA reductase inhibitors. Risk may be increased with concurrent use of other drugs which may cause rhabdomyolysis (including gemfibrozil, fibric acid derivatives, or niacin at doses ≥1 g/day). Temporarily discontinue in any patient experiencing an acute or serious condition predisposing to renal failure secondary to rhabdomyolysis. Use caution in patients with previous liver disease or heavy ethanol use. Treatment in patients <18 years of age is not recommended.

Drug Interactions CYP2C9 enzyme substrate; CYP2C9, 2C18, and 2C19 enzyme inhibitor

Increased Effect/Toxicity: Cimetidine, omeprazole, ranitidine, and ritonavir may increase fluvastatin blood levels. Clofibrate, erythromycin, gemfibrozil, fenofibrate, and niacin may increase the risk of myopathy and rhabdomyolysis. Anticoagulant effect of warfarin may be increased by fluvastatin. Cholestyramine effect will be additive with fluvastatin if administration times are separated. Fluvastatin may increase C_{max} and decrease clearance of digoxin.

Decreased Effect: Administration of cholestyramine at the same time with fluvastatin reduces absorption and clinical effect of fluvastatin. Separate administration times by at least 4 hours. Rifampin and rifabutin may decrease fluvastatin blood levels.

Drug Uptake Half-life, elimination: 1.2 hours

Pregnancy Risk Factor X

Generic Available No

Fluvirin® *see* Influenza Virus Vaccine *on page 637*

Fluvoxamine (floo VOKS ah meen)

U.S. Brand Names Luvox®

Canadian Brand Names Alti-Fluvoxamine; Apo®-Fluvoxamine; Gen-Fluvoxamine; Luvox®; Novo-Fluvoxamine; Nu-Fluvoxamine; PMS-Fluvoxamine

Mexican Brand Names Luvox®

Pharmacologic Category Antidepressant, Selective Serotonin Reuptake Inhibitor

Use Treatment of obsessive-compulsive disorder (OCD) in children ≥8 years of age and adults

Unlabeled/Investigational: Treatment of major depression; panic disorder; anxiety disorders in children

Local Anesthetic/Vasoconstrictor Precautions Although caution should be used in patients taking tricyclic antidepressants, no interactions have been reported with vasoconstrictors and fluvoxamine, a nontricyclic antidepressant which acts to increase serotonin

Effects on Dental Treatment No effects or complications reported

Dosage Oral: A total daily dose of >50 mg should be given in 2 divided doses.

Children 8-17 years: Initial: 25 mg at bedtime; adjust in 25 mg increments at 4- to 7-day intervals, as tolerated, to maximum therapeutic benefit: Range: 50-200 mg/day

Maximum: Children: 8-11 years: 200 mg/day, adolescents: 300 mg/day; lower doses may be effective in female versus male patients

Adults: Initial: 50 mg at bedtime; adjust in 50 mg increments at 4- to 7-day intervals; usual dose range: 100-300 mg/day; divide total daily dose into 2 doses; administer larger portion at bedtime

Elderly: Reduce dose, titrate slowly

Dosage adjustment in hepatic impairment: Reduce dose, titrate slowly

Mechanism of Action Inhibits CNS neuron serotonin uptake; minimal or no effect on reuptake of norepinephrine or dopamine; does not significantly bind to alpha-adrenergic, histamine or cholinergic receptors

Other Adverse Effects

>10%:

Central nervous system: Headache (22%), somnolence (22%), insomnia (21%), nervousness (12%), dizziness (11%)

Gastrointestinal: Nausea (40%), diarrhea (11%), xerostomia (14%)

Neuromuscular & skeletal: Weakness (14%)

1% to 10%:

Cardiovascular: Palpitations

Central nervous system: Somnolence, mania, hypomania, vertigo, abnormal thinking, agitation, anxiety, malaise, amnesia, yawning, hypertonia, CNS stimulation, depression

Endocrine & metabolic: Decreased libido

Gastrointestinal: Abdominal pain, vomiting, dyspepsia, constipation, abnormal taste, anorexia, flatulence, weight gain

Genitourinary: Delayed ejaculation, impotence, anorgasmia, urinary frequency, urinary retention

Neuromuscular & skeletal: Tremors

Ocular: Blurred vision

Respiratory: Dyspnea

Miscellaneous: Diaphoresis

Drug Interactions CYP1A2 enzyme substrate; CYP1A2, 2C9, 2C19, 2D6, and 3A3/4 enzyme inhibitor

MAO inhibitors: Fluvoxamine should not be used with nonselective MAO inhibitors (phenelzine, isocarboxazid) and drugs with MAO inhibitor properties (linezolid); fatal reactions have been reported. Wait 5 weeks after stopping fluvoxamine before starting a nonselective MAO inhibitor and 2 weeks after stopping an MAO inhibitor before starting fluvoxamine. Concurrent selegiline has been associated with mania, hypertension, or serotonin syndrome (risk may be reduced relative to nonselective MAO inhibitors).

Phenothiazines: Fluvoxamine may inhibit the metabolism of thioridazine or mesoridazine, resulting in increased plasma concentrations and increasing the risk of QT_c interval prolongation. This may lead to serious ventricular arrhythmias, such as torsade de pointes-type arrhythmias and sudden death. Do not use together. Wait at least 5 weeks after discontinuing fluvoxamine prior to starting thioridazine.

Combined used of SSRIs and amphetamines, buspirone, meperidine, nefazodone, serotonin agonists (such as sumatriptan), sibutramine, other SSRIs, sympathomimetics, tramadol, and venlafaxine may increase the risk of serotonin syndrome. Fluvoxamine may increase serum concentration/effects of benzodiazepines (alprazolam and diazepam), beta-blockers (except atenolol or nadolol), carbamazepine, carvedilol, clozapine, cyclosporin (and possibly tacrolimus), dextromethorphan, digoxin, haloperidol, HMG-CoA reductase inhibitors (lovastatin and simvastatin - increasing the risk of rhabdomyolysis), mexiletine, phenytoin, propafenone, quinidine, tacrine, theophylline, trazodone, tricyclic antidepressants, and valproic acid. Concurrent lithium may increase risk of nephrotoxicity. Risk of hyponatremia may increase with concurrent use of loop diuretics (bumetanide, furosemide, torsemide). Fluvoxamine may increase the hypoprothrombinemic response to warfarin.

Combined use of sumatriptan (and other serotonin agonists) may result in toxicity; weakness, hyper-reflexia, and incoordination have been observed with sumatriptan and SSRIs. In addition, concurrent use may theoretically increase the risk of serotonin syndrome; includes sumatriptan, naratriptan, rizatriptan, and zolmitriptan.

Drug Uptake

Onset of action: Therapeutic: >2 weeks

Absorption: Steady-state plasma concentrations have been noted to be 2-3 times higher in children than those in adolescents; female children demonstrated a significantly higher AUC than males

Half-life, elimination, plasma: ~15 hours

Time to peak, plasma: 3-8 hours

Pregnancy Risk Factor C

Generic Available Yes

Comments Problems with SSRI-induced bruxism have been reported and may preclude their use; clinicians attempting to evaluate any patient with bruxism or involuntary muscle movement, who is simultaneously being treated with an SSRI drug, should be aware of the potential association.

Selected Readings

Friedlander AH, Mahler ME, "Major Depressive Disorder. Psychopathology, Medical Management, and Dental Implications," *J Am Dent Assoc*, 2001, 132(5):629-38.

Gerber PE and Lynd LD, "Selective Serotonin Reuptake Inhibitor-induced Movement Disorders," *Ann Pharmacother*, 1998, 32(6):692-8.

Wynn RL, "New Antidepressant Medications," *Gen Dent*, 1997, 45(1):24-8.

Fluzone® *see* Influenza Virus Vaccine *on page 637*
FML® *see* Fluorometholone *on page 515*
FML® Forte *see* Fluorometholone *on page 515*
FML-S® *see* Sulfacetamide Sodium and Fluorometholone *on page 1115*
Focalin™ *see* Dexmethylphenidate *on page 367*
Foille® [OTC] *see* Benzocaine *on page 151*
Foille® Medicated First Aid [OTC] *see* Benzocaine *on page 151*
Foille® Plus [OTC] *see* Benzocaine *on page 151*

Folic Acid (FOE lik AS id)

U.S. Brand Names Folvite®
Canadian Brand Names Apo®-Folic
Mexican Brand Names A.f. Valdecasas®; Flynoken®; Folitab
Pharmacologic Category Vitamin
Synonyms Folacin; Folate; Pteroylglutamic Acid
Use
Dental: Treatment of megaloblastic and macrocytic anemias due to folate deficiency
Medical: Dietary supplement in prevention of neural tube defects
Local Anesthetic/Vasoconstrictor Precautions No information available to require special precautions
Effects on Dental Treatment No effects or complications reported
Dosage Oral, I.M., I.V., S.C.:
Children: Initial: 1 mg/day
Deficiency: 0.5-1 mg/day
Maintenance dose:
<4 years: Up to 0.3 mg/day
>4 years: 0.4 mg/day
Adults: Initial: 1 mg/day
Deficiency: 1-3 mg/day
Maintenance dose: 0.5 mg/day
Women of childbearing age, pregnant, and lactating women: 0.8 mg/day
Mechanism of Action Necessary for formation of a number of coenzymes in many metabolic systems, particularly for purine and pyrimidine synthesis; required for nucleoprotein synthesis and maintenance in erythropoiesis; stimulates WBC and platelet production in folate deficiency anemia
Other Adverse Effects Frequency not defined:
Cardiovascular: Slight flushing
Central nervous system: General malaise
Dermatologic: Pruritus, rash
Respiratory: Bronchospasm
Miscellaneous: Allergic reaction
Contraindications Pernicious, aplastic, or normocytic anemias
Warnings/Precautions Doses >0.1 mg/day may obscure pernicious anemia with continuing irreversible nerve damage progression. Resistance to treatment may occur with depressed hematopoiesis, alcoholism, deficiencies of other vitamins. Injection contains benzyl alcohol (1.5%) as preservative (use care in administration to neonates).
Drug Interactions Decreased Effect: In folate-deficient patients, folic acid therapy (>15 mg/day) may increase phenytoin metabolism. Phenytoin, primidone, para-aminosalicylic acid, and sulfasalazine may decrease serum folate concentrations and cause deficiency. Oral contraceptives may also impair folate metabolism producing depletion, but the effect is unlikely to cause anemia or megaloblastic changes. Concurrent administration of chloramphenicol and folic acid may result in antagonism of the hematopoietic response to folic acid; dihydrofolate reductase inhibitors (eg, methotrexate, trimethoprim) may interfere with folic acid utilization.
Drug Uptake
Absorption: In the proximal part of the small intestine
Time to peak: Oral: 0.5-1 hour
Pregnancy Risk Factor A/C (dose exceeding RDA recommendation)
Breast-feeding Considerations May be taken while breast-feeding
Dosage Forms INJ: 5 mg/mL (10 mL); (Folvite®): 5 mg/mL (10 mL). **TAB:** 0.4 mg, 0.8 mg, 1 mg; (Folvite®): 1 mg
Generic Available Yes

Folic Acid, Cyanocobalamin, and Pyridoxine

(FOE lik AS id, sye an oh koe BAL a min, & peer i DOKS een)
U.S. Brand Names Foltx™
Pharmacologic Category Vitamin
Synonyms Cyanocobalamin, Folic Acid, and Pyridoxine; Folacin, Vitamin B_{12}, and Vitamin B_6; Pyridoxine, Folic Acid, and Cyanocobalamin
Use Nutritional supplement in end-stage renal failure, dialysis, hyperhomocysteinemia, homocystinuria, malabsorption syndromes, dietary deficiencies

Local Anesthetic/Vasoconstrictor Precautions No information available to require special precautions

Effects on Dental Treatment No effects or complications reported

Dosage Oral: Adults: 1 tablet daily

Drug Interactions See Folic Acid *on page 530*, Cyanocobalamin *on page 331* and Pyridoxine *on page 1027*

Drug Uptake See Folic Acid *on page 530*, Cyanocobalamin *on page 331*, and Pyridoxine *on page 1027*

Follistim® *see* Follitropins *on page 531*

Follitropins (foe li TRO pins)

U.S. Brand Names Bravelle™; Fertinex®; Follistim®; Gonal-F®

Canadian Brand Names Gonal-F®; Puregon™

Mexican Brand Names Gonal-F®; Puregon®

Pharmacologic Category Gonadotropin; Ovulation Stimulator

Synonyms Follitropin Alfa; Follitropin Alpha; Follitropin Beta; Recombinant Human Follicle Stimulating Hormone; rFSH-alpha; rFSH-beta; rhFSH-alpha; rhFSH-beta; Urofollitropin

Use

Urofollitropin (Fertinex®):

Polycystic ovary syndrome: Administered sequentially with hCG for the stimulation of follicular recruitment and development and the induction of ovulation in patients with polycystic ovary syndrome and infertility, who have failed to respond or conceive following adequate clomiphene citrate therapy

Follicle stimulation: Stimulation of the development of multiple follicles in ovulatory patients undergoing assisted reproductive technologies such as *in vitro* fertilization

Follitropin alfa (Gonal-F®) / follitropin beta (Follistim®):

Ovulation induction: Induction of ovulation and pregnancy in anovulatory infertile patients in whom the cause of infertility is functional and not caused by primary ovarian failure

Orphan drug: Induction of spermatogenesis in adult males with primary and secondary hypogonadotropic hypogonadism in whom the cause of infertility is not due to primary testicular failure

Local Anesthetic/Vasoconstrictor Precautions No information available to require special precautions

Effects on Dental Treatment No effects or complications reported

Dosage

Urofollitropin (Fertinex®): Adults: S.C.:

Polycystic ovary syndrome: Initial recommended dose of the first cycle: 75 international units/day; consider dose adjustment after 5-7 days; additional dose adjustments may be considered based on individual patient response. The dose should not be increased more than twice in any cycle or by >75 international units per adjustment. To complete follicular development and affect ovulation in the absence of an endogenous LH surge, give 5000-10,000 units hCG, 1 day after the last dose of urofollitropin. Withhold hCG if serum estradiol is >2000 pg/mL.

Individualize the initial dose administered in subsequent cycles for each patient based on her response in the preceding cycle. Doses of >300 int. units of FSH/day are not routinely recommended. As in the initial cycle, 5000-10,000 units of hCG must be given 1 day after the last dose of urofollitropin to complete follicular development and induce ovulation.

Give the lowest dose consistent with the expectation of good results. Over the course of treatment, doses may range between 75-300 int. units/day depending on individual patient response. Administer urofollitropin until adequate follicular development as indicated by serum estradiol and vaginal ultrasonography. A response is generally evident after 5-7 days.

Encourage the couple to have intercourse daily, beginning on the day prior to the administration of hCG until ovulation becomes apparent from the indices employed for determination of progestational activity. Take care to ensure insemination.

Follicle stimulation: For Assisted Reproductive Technologies, initiate therapy with urofollitropin in the early follicular phase (cycle day 2 or 3) at a dose of 150 int. units/day, until sufficient follicular development is attained. In most cases, therapy should not exceed 10 days.

Follitropin alfa (Gonal-F®): Adults: S.C.:

Ovulation induction: Female: Initial recommended dose of the first cycle: 75 international units/day. Consider dose adjustment after 5-7 days; additional dose adjustments of up to 37.5 int. units may be considered after 14 days. Further dose increases of the same magnitude can be made, if necessary, every 7 days. To complete follicular development and affect ovulation in the absence of an endogenous LH surge, give 5000-10,000 units hCG, 1 day after the last dose of follitropin alfa. Withhold hCG if serum estradiol is >2000 pg/mL.

Individualize the initial dose administered in subsequent cycles for each patient based on her response in the preceding cycle. Doses of >300 int. units of

(Continued)

Follitropins *(Continued)*

FSH/day are not routinely recommended. As in the initial cycle, 5000-10,000 units of hCG must be given 1 day after the last dose of urofollitropin to complete follicular development and induce ovulation.

Give the lowest dose consistent with the expectation of good results. Over the course of treatment, doses may range between 75-300 int. units/day depending on individual patient response. Administer urofollitropin until adequate follicular development as indicated by serum estradiol and vaginal ultrasonography. A response is generally evident after 5-7 days.

Encourage the couple to have intercourse daily, beginning on the day prior to the administration of hCG until ovulation becomes apparent from the indices employed for determination of progestational activity. Take care to ensure insemination.

Follicle stimulation: Female: Initiate therapy with follitropin alfa in the early follicular phase (cycle day 2 or 3) at a dose of 150 int. units/day, until sufficient follicular development is attained. In most cases, therapy should not exceed 10 days.

In patients undergoing Assisted Reproductive Technologies, whose endogenous gonadotropin levels are suppressed, initiate follitropin alfa at a dose of 225 int. units/day. Continue treatment until adequate follicular development is indicated as determined by ultrasound in combination with measurement of serum estradiol levels. Consider adjustments to dose after 5 days based on the patient's response; adjust subsequent dosage every 3-5 days by ≤75-150 int. units additionally at each adjustment. Doses >450 int. units/day are not recommended. Once adequate follicular development is evident, administer hCG (5000-10,000 units) to induce final follicular maturation in preparation for oocyte.

Spermatogenesis induction: Male: Therapy should begin with hCG pretreatment until serum testosterone is in normal range, then 150 int. units 3 times/week with hCG 3 times/week; continue with lowest dose needed to induce spermatogenesis (maximum dose: 300 int. units 3 times/week); may be given for up to 18 months

Follitropin beta (Follistim®): Adults: S.C. or I.M.:

Ovulation induction: Stepwise approach: Initiate therapy with 75 int. units/day for up to 14 days. Increase by 37.5 int. units at weekly intervals until follicular growth or serum estradiol levels indicate an adequate response. The maximum, individualized, daily dose that has been safely used for ovulation induction in patients during clinical trials is 300 international units. Treat the patient until ultrasonic visualizations or serum estradiol determinations indicate preovulatory conditions greater than or equal to normal values followed by 5000-10,000 units hCG.

During treatment and during a 2-week post-treatment period, examine patients at least every other day for signs of excessive ovarian stimulation. Discontinue follitropin beta administration if the ovaries become abnormally enlarged or abdominal pain occurs.

Encourage the couple to have intercourse daily, beginning on the day prior to the administration of hCG until ovulation becomes apparent from the indices employed for determination of progestational activity. Take care to ensure insemination.

Follicle stimulation: A starting dose of 150-225 int. units of follitropin beta is recommended for at least the first 4 days of treatment. The dose may be adjusted for the individual patient based upon their ovarian response. Daily maintenance doses ranging from 75-300 int. units for 6-12 days are usually sufficient, although longer treatment may be necessary. However, maintenance doses of up to 375-600 int. units may be necessary according to individual response. The maximum daily dose used in clinical studies is 600 international units. When a sufficient number of follicles of adequate size are present, the final maturation of the follicles is induced by administering hCG at a dose of 5000-10,000 int. units. Oocyte retrieval is performed 34-36 hours later. Withhold hCG in cases where the ovaries are abnormally enlarged on the last day of follitropin beta therapy.

Mechanism of Action Urofollitropin is a preparation of highly purified follicle-stimulating hormone (FSH) extracted from the urine of postmenopausal women. Follitropin alfa and follitropin beta are human FSH preparations of recombinant DNA origin. Follitropins stimulate ovarian follicular growth in women who do not have primary ovarian failure, and stimulate spermatogenesis in men with hypogonadotrophic hypogonadism. FSH is required for normal follicular growth, maturation, gonadal steroid production, and spermatogenesis.

Other Adverse Effects

2% to 10%:

Central nervous system: Headache, dizziness, fever

Dermatologic: Acne (male), dermoid cyst (male), dry skin, body rash, hair loss, hives

Endocrine & metabolic: Ovarian hyperstimulation syndrome, adnexal torsion, mild to moderate ovarian enlargement, abdominal pain, ovarian cysts, breast tenderness, gynecomastia (male)

Gastrointestinal: Nausea, vomiting, diarrhea, abdominal cramps, bloating, flatulence, dyspepsia

Genitourinary: Urinary tract infection, menstrual disorder, intermenstrual bleeding, dysmenorrhea, cervical lesion

Local: Pain, rash, swelling, or irritation at the site of injection

Neuromuscular & skeletal: Back pain, varicose veins (male)

Respiratory: Exacerbation of asthma, sinusitis, pharyngitis

Miscellaneous: Febrile reactions accompanied by chills, musculoskeletal, joint pains, malaise, headache, and fatigue; flu-like symptoms

Contraindications Hypersensitivity to follitropins or any component of the formulation; high levels of FSH indicating primary ovarian failure; uncontrolled thyroid or adrenal dysfunction; presence of any cause of infertility other than anovulation; tumor of the ovary, breast, uterus, hypothalamus, or pituitary gland; abnormal vaginal bleeding of undetermined origin; ovarian cysts or enlargement not due to polycystic ovary syndrome; pregnancy

Warnings/Precautions These medications should only be used by physicians who are thoroughly familiar with infertility problems and their management. To minimize risks, use only at the lowest effective dose. Monitor ovarian response with serum estradiol and vaginal ultrasound on a regular basis.

Ovarian enlargement which may be accompanied by abdominal distention or abdominal pain, occurs in ~20% of those treated with urofollitropin and hCG, and generally regresses without treatment within 2-3 weeks. Ovarian hyperstimulation syndrome, characterized by severe ovarian enlargement, abdominal pain/distention, nausea, vomiting, diarrhea, dyspnea, and oliguria, and may be accompanied by ascites, pleural effusion, hypovolemia, electrolyte imbalance, hemoperitoneum, and thromboembolic events is reported in about 6% of patients. If hyperstimulation occurs, stop treatment and hospitalize patient. This syndrome develops rapidly within 24 hours to several days and generally occurs during the 7-10 days immediately following treatment. Hemoconcentration associated with fluid loss into the abdominal cavity has occurred and should be assessed by fluid intake & output, weight, hematocrit, serum & urinary electrolytes, urine specific gravity, BUN and creatinine, and abdominal girth. Determinations should be performed daily or more often if the need arises. Treatment is primarily symptomatic and consists of bed rest, fluid and electrolyte replacement and analgesics. The ascitic, pleural and pericardial fluids should never be removed because of the potential danger of injury.

Serious pulmonary conditions (atelectasis, acute respiratory distress syndrome and exacerbation of asthma) have been reported. Thromboembolic events, both in association with and separate from ovarian hyperstimulation syndrome, have been reported.

Multiple pregnancies have been associated with these medications, including triplet and quintuplet gestations. Advise patient of the potential risk of multiple births before starting the treatment.

Drug Uptake

Onset of effect: Peak effect: Spermatogenesis, median: 165 days (range: 25-327 days); follicle development: Within cycle

Absorption: Rate limited: I.M., S.C.: Slower than elimination rate

Half-life, elimination:

Mean: S.C.: Follitropin alfa: 24-32 hours; Follitropin beta: ~30 hours

Mean terminal: Multiple dosing: I.M. follitropin alfa, S.C. Follitropin beta: ~30 hours

Time to peak:

Follitropin alfa: S.C.: 16 hours; I.M.: 25 hours

Follitropin beta: I.M.: 27 hours

Urofollitropin: S.C.: 15 hours; I.M.: 10 hours

Pregnancy Risk Factor X

Generic Available No

Foltx™ *see* Folic Acid, Cyanocobalamin, and Pyridoxine *on page 530*

Folvite® *see* Folic Acid *on page 530*

Fomepizole (foe ME pi zole)

U.S. Brand Names Antizol®

Pharmacologic Category Antidote

Synonyms 4-Methylpyrazole; 4-MP

Use

Orphan drug: Treatment of methanol or ethylene glycol poisoning alone or in combination with hemodialysis

Unlabeled/Investigational: Known or suspected propylene glycol toxicity

Local Anesthetic/Vasoconstrictor Precautions No information available to require special precautions

(Continued)

Fomepizole *(Continued)*

Effects on Dental Treatment No effects or complications reported

Dosage Oral: 15 mg/kg followed by 5 mg/kg in 12 hours and then 10 mg/kg every 12 hours until levels of toxin are not present

One other protocol (from France) suggests an infusion of 10-20 mg/kg before dialysis and I.V. infusion of 1-1.5 mg/kg/hour during hemodialysis

META (methylpyrazole for toxic alcohol) study in U.S. (investigational): Loading I.V. dose of 15 mg/kg followed by 10 mg/kg I.V. every 12 hours for 48 hours; continue treatment until methanol or ethylene glycol levels are <20 mg/dL; supplemental doses required during dialysis; contact your local poison center regarding this study

Mechanism of Action Fomepizole competitively inhibits alcohol dehydrogenase, an enzyme which catalyzes the metabolism of ethanol, ethylene glycol, and methanol to their toxic metabolites. Ethylene glycol is metabolized to glycoaldehyde, then oxidized to glycolate, glyoxylate, and oxalate. Glycolate and oxalate are responsible for metabolic acidosis and renal damage. Methanol is metabolized to formaldehyde, then oxidized to formic acid. Formic acid is responsible for metabolic acidosis and visual disturbances.

Other Adverse Effects

>10%:

- Central nervous system: Headache (14%)
- Gastrointestinal: Nausea (11%)

1% to 10% (≤3% unless otherwise noted):

- Cardiovascular: Bradycardia, facial flush, hypotension, phlebosclerosis, shock, tachycardia
- Central nervous system: Dizziness (6%), increased drowsiness (6%), agitation, anxiety, lightheadedness, seizure, vertigo
- Dermatologic: Rash
- Gastrointestinal: Bad/metallic taste (6%), abdominal pain, decreased appetite, diarrhea, heartburn, vomiting
- Hematologic: Anemia, disseminated intravascular coagulation, eosinophilia, lymphangitis
- Hepatic: Increased LFTs
- Local: Application site reaction, inflammation at the injection site, pain during injection, phlebitis
- Neuromuscular & skeletal: Backache
- Ocular: Nystagmus, transient blurred vision, visual disturbances
- Renal: Anuria
- Respiratory: Abnormal smell, hiccups, pharyngitis
- Miscellaneous: Multiorgan failure, speech disturbances

Drug Interactions CYP450 mixed enzyme inducer; Specific drug interaction studies have not been conducted. Metabolism may be affected by (or affect the metabolism of) other medications that are metabolized via the CYP450 enzyme system.

Drug Uptake

Absorption: Oral: Readily absorbed

Half-life, elimination: Has not been calculated; varies with dose

Time to peak: 1.5-2 hours

Pregnancy Risk Factor C

Generic Available No

Selected Readings

Borron SW and Baud FJ, "Intravenous 4-Methylpyrazole as an Antidote for Diethylene Glycol and Triethylene Glycol Poisoning: A Case Report," *Vet Hum Toxicol*, 1997, 37(1): 26-8.

Brent J, McMartin K, Phillips S, et al, "4-Methylpyrazole (Fomepizole) Therapy of Ethylene Glycol Poisoning: Preliminary Results of the Meta Trial," *J Toxicol Clin Toxicol*, 1997, 35(5):507.

Brent J, McMartin K, Phillips SP, et al, "4-Methylpyrazole (Fomepizole) Therapy of Methanol Poisoning: Preliminary Results of the Meta Trial," *J Toxicol Clin Toxicol*, 1997, 35(5):507.

Hung O, Kaplan J, Hoffman R, et al, "Improved Understanding of the Ethanol-Chloral Hydrate Interaction Using 4-MP," *J Toxicol Clin Toxicol*, 1997, 35(5):507-8.

Jacobsen D and McMartin KE, "Antidotes for Methanol and Ethylene Glycol Poisoning," *J Toxicol Clin Toxicol*, 1997, 35(2):127-43.

Jacobsen D and McMartin K, "4-Methylpyrazole - Present Status," *J Toxicol Clin Toxicol*, 1996, 34(4):379-81.

Jacobsen D, Ostensen J, Bredesen L, et al, "4-Methylpyrazole (4-MP) Is Effectively Removed by Haemodialysis in the Pig Model," *Hum Exp Toxicol*, 1996, 15(6):494-6.

Jacobsen D, Sebastian CS, Barron SK, et al, "Effects of 4-Methylpyrazole, Methanol/Ethylene Glycol Antidote in Healthy Humans," *J Emerg Med*, 1990, 8(4):455-61.

Jobard E, Harry P, Turcant A, et al, "4-Methylpyrazole and Hemodialysis in Ethylene Glycol Poisoning," *J Toxicol Clin Toxicol*, 1996, 34(4):373-7.

McMartin KE and Heath A, "Treatment of Ethylene Glycol Poisoning With Intravenous 4-Methylpyrazole," *N Engl J Med*, 1989, 320(2):125.

Fomivirsen (foe MI vir sen)

Related Information

Systemic Viral Diseases *on page 1354*

U.S. Brand Names Vitravene™

Canadian Brand Names Vitravene™

Pharmacologic Category Antiviral Agent, Ophthalmic

Synonyms Fomivirsen Sodium

Use Treatment of cytomegalovirus (CMV) retinitis; CMV can affect one or both eyes in patients with acquired immunodeficiency syndrome (AIDS) who cannot take other treatment(s) for CMV retinitis or who did not respond to other treatments for CMV retinitis; the diagnosis should be made after a comprehensive eye exam, including indirect ophthalmoscopy

Local Anesthetic/Vasoconstrictor Precautions No information available to require special precautions

Effects on Dental Treatment No effects or complications reported

Dosage Treatment consists of two phases:

Phase I (induction phase): One injection (6.6 mg) every other week for 2 doses

Phase II (maintenance phase): One injection (6.6 mg) once every 4 weeks

Mechanism of Action Inhibits synthesis of viral protein by binding to mRNA which blocks replication of cytomegalovirus through an antisense mechanism

Other Adverse Effects

5% to 10%:

- Central nervous system: Fever, headache
- Gastrointestinal: Abdominal pain, diarrhea, nausea, vomiting
- Hematologic: Anemia
- Neuromuscular & skeletal: Asthenia
- Ocular: Uveitis, abnormal vision, anterior chamber inflammation, blurred vision, cataract, conjunctival hemorrhage, decreased visual acuity, loss of color vision, eye pain, increased intraocular pressure, photophobia, retinal detachment, retinal edema, retinal hemorrhage, retinal pigment changes, vitreitis
- Respiratory: Pneumonia, sinusitis
- Miscellaneous: Systemic CMV, sepsis, infection

2% to 5%:

- Cardiovascular: Chest pain
- Central nervous system: Confusion, depression, dizziness, neuropathy, pain
- Endocrine & metabolic: Dehydration
- Gastrointestinal: Abnormal LFTs, pancreatitis, anorexia, weight loss
- Hematologic: Thrombocytopenia, lymphoma
- Neuromuscular & skeletal: Back pain, cachexia
- Ocular: Application site reaction, conjunctival hyperemia, conjunctivitis, corneal edema, decreased peripheral vision, eye irritation, keratic precipitates, optic neuritis, photopsia, retinal vascular disease, visual field defect, vitreous hemorrhage, vitreous opacity
- Renal: Kidney failure
- Respiratory: Bronchitis, dyspnea, cough
- Miscellaneous: Allergic reaction, flu-like syndrome, diaphoresis (increased)

Warnings/Precautions Only works in the eye in which it is injected and does not treat CMV elsewhere in the body. Because CMV may be in other parts of the body and not only in the treated eye, a physician should monitor patient for CMV in the untreated eye or CMV elsewhere in the body (eg, pneumonitis, colitis); not recommended if there has been treatment within the last 2-4 weeks with cidofovir because of the increased risk of eye inflammation

Drug Interactions Drug interactions between fomivirsen and other medications have not been studied.

Drug Uptake Pharmacokinetic studies have not been conducted in humans.

Generic Available No

Fondaparinux (fon da PARE i nuks)

U.S. Brand Names Arixtra®

Pharmacologic Category Factor Xa Inhibitor

Synonyms Fondaparinux Sodium

Use Prophylaxis of deep vein thrombosis (DVT) in patients undergoing surgery for hip fracture or hip or knee replacement

Unlabeled/Investigational: Treatment of DVT

Local Anesthetic/Vasoconstrictor Precautions No information available to require special precautions

Effects on Dental Treatment No effects or complications reported

Dosage S.C.:

Adults: ≥50 kg: Usual dose: 2.5 mg once daily. **Note:** Initiate dose after hemostasis has been established, 6-8 hours postoperatively.

Elderly: Use caution, elimination may be prolonged; assess renal function before initiating therapy

Dosage adjustment in renal impairment:

Cl_{cr} 30-50 mL/minute: Use caution

Cl_{cr} <30 mL/minute: Contraindicated

Mechanism of Action Fondaparinux is a synthetic pentasaccharide that causes an antithrombin III-mediated selective inhibition of factor Xa. Neutralization of factor Xa interrupts the blood coagulation cascade and inhibits thrombin formation and thrombus development.

Other Adverse Effects As with all anticoagulants, bleeding is the major adverse effect. Hemorrhage may occur at any site. Risk appears to be increased by a

(Continued)

Fondaparinux *(Continued)*

number of factors including renal dysfunction, age (>75 years), and weight (<50 kg).

>10%:
- Central nervous system: Fever (14%)
- Gastrointestinal: Nausea (11%)
- Hematologic: Anemia (20%)

1% to 10%:
- Cardiovascular: Edema (9%), hypotension (4%), confusion (3%)
- Central nervous system: Insomnia (5%), dizziness (4%), headache (2%), pain (2%)
- Dermatologic: Rash (8%), purpura (4%), bullous eruption (3%)
- Endocrine & metabolic: Hypokalemia (4%)
- Gastrointestinal: Constipation (9%), vomiting (6%), diarrhea (3%), dyspepsia (2%)
- Genitourinary: Urinary tract infection (4%), urinary retention (3%)
- Hematologic: Moderate thrombocytopenia (50,000-100,000/mm^3: 3%), major bleeding (2% to 3%), minor bleeding (3% to 4%), hematoma (3%)
- Hepatic: SGOT increased (2%), SGPT increased (3%)
- Local: Injection site reaction (bleeding, rash, pruritus)
- Miscellaneous: Wound drainage increased (5%)

Drug Interactions Increased Effect/Toxicity: Anticoagulants, antiplatelet agents, drotrecogin alfa, nonsteroidal anti-inflammatory agents, salicylates and thrombolytic agents may enhance the anticoagulant effect and/or increase the risk of bleeding.

Drug Uptake
- Absorption: Rapid and complete
- Half-life, elimination: 17-21 hours; increases with worsening renal function
- Time to peak: 2-3 hours

Pregnancy Risk Factor B

Generic Available No

Foradil® Aerolizer™ *see* Formoterol *on page 536*

Formoterol (for MOH te rol)

U.S. Brand Names Foradil® Aerolizer™

Canadian Brand Names Foradil®; Oxeze® Turbuhaler®

Mexican Brand Names Foradil®; Oxis®

Pharmacologic Category Beta$_2$ Agonist

Synonyms Formoterol Fumarate

Use Maintenance treatment of asthma and prevention of bronchospasm in patients ≥5 years of age with reversible obstructive airway disease, including patients with symptoms of nocturnal asthma, who require regular treatment with inhaled, short-acting beta$_2$ agonists; prevention of exercise-induced bronchospasm in patients ≥12 years of age

Local Anesthetic/Vasoconstrictor Precautions No information available to require special precautions

Effects on Dental Treatment No effects or complications reported

Dosage Inhalation:
- Children ≥5 years and Adults: Asthma maintenance: 12 mcg capsule every 12 hours
- Children ≥12 years and Adults: Exercise-induced bronchospasm: 12 mcg capsule at least 15 minutes before exercise on an "as needed" basis; additional doses should not be used for another 12 hours. **Note:** If already using for asthma maintenance then should not use additional doses for exercise-induced bronchospasm.

Mechanism of Action Relaxes bronchial smooth muscle by selective action on beta$_2$ receptors with little effect on heart rate. Formoterol has a long-acting effect.

Other Adverse Effects Children are more likely to have infection, inflammation, abdominal pain, nausea, and dyspepsia.

>10%: Miscellaneous: Viral infection (17%)

1% to 10%:
- Cardiovascular: Chest pain (2%)
- Central nervous system: Tremor (2%), dizziness (2%), insomnia (2%), dysphonia (1%)
- Dermatologic: Rash (1%)
- Respiratory: Bronchitis (5%), infection (3%), dyspnea (2%), tonsillitis (1%)

Contraindications Hypersensitivity to adrenergic amines, formoterol, or any component of their formulation; need for acute bronchodilation; use with or within 2 weeks of MAO inhibitor

Drug Interactions CYP2A6, CYP2C9, CYP2C19, CYP2D6 enzyme substrate

Increased Effect/Toxicity: Adrenergic agonists, antidepressants (tricyclic), beta blockers, corticosteroids, diuretics, drugs that prolong QT$_c$ interval, MAO inhibitors, theophylline derivatives

Drug Uptake

Absorption: Rapidly into plasma

Duration: Improvement in FEV_1 observed for 12 hours in most patients

Half-life, elimination: ~10-14 hours

Time to peak: Maximum improvement in FEV_1 in 1-3 hours

Pregnancy Risk Factor C

Generic Available No

Fortaz® *see* Ceftazidime *on page 243*

Fortovase® *see* Saquinavir *on page 1075*

Fosamax® *see* Alendronate *on page 49*

Foscarnet (fos KAR net)

Related Information

Systemic Viral Diseases *on page 1354*

U.S. Brand Names Foscavir®

Canadian Brand Names Foscavir®

Pharmacologic Category Antiviral Agent

Synonyms PFA; Phosphonoformate; Phosphonoformic Acid

Use Approved indications in adult patients:

Herpesvirus infections suspected to be caused by acyclovir (HSV, VZV) or ganciclovir (CMV) resistant strains (this occurs almost exclusively in persons with advanced AIDS who have received prolonged treatment for a herpesvirus infection)

CMV retinitis in persons with AIDS

Other CMV infections in persons unable to tolerate ganciclovir

Local Anesthetic/Vasoconstrictor Precautions No information available to require special precautions

Effects on Dental Treatment No effects or complications reported

Dosage

Adolescents and Adults: I.V.:

Induction treatment: 60 mg/kg/dose every 8 hours for 14-21 days

Maintenance therapy: 90-120 mg/kg/day as a single infusion

See tables.

Induction Dosing of Foscarnet in Patients with Abnormal Renal Function

Cl_{cr} (mL/min/kg)	HSV Equivalent to 40 mg/kg every 12 hours	HSV Equivalent to 40 mg/kg every 8 hours	CMV Equivalent to 60 mg/kg every 8 hours	CMV Equivalent to 90 mg/kg every 12 hours
<0.4	Not recommended	Not recommended	Not recommended	Not recommended
≥0.4-0.5	20 mg/kg every 24 hours	35 mg/kg every 24 hours	50 mg/kg every 24 hours	50 mg/kg every 24 hours
>0.5-0.6	25 mg/kg every 24 hours	40 mg/kg every 24 hours	60 mg/kg every 24 hours	60 mg/kg every 24 hours
>0.6-0.8	35 mg/kg every 24 hours	25 mg/kg every 12 hours	40 mg/kg every 12 hours	80 mg/kg every 24 hours
>0.8-1.0	20 mg/kg every 12 hours	35 mg/kg every 12 hours	50 mg/kg every 12 hours	50 mg/kg every 12 hours
>1.0-1.4	30 mg/kg every 12 hours	30 mg/kg every 8 hours	45 mg/kg every 8 hours	70 mg/kg every 12 hours
>1.4	40 mg/kg every 12 hours	40 mg/kg every 8 hours	60 mg/kg every 8 hours	90 mg/kg every 12 hours

Maintenance Dosing of Foscarnet in Patients with Abnormal Renal Function

Cl_{cr} (mL/min/kg)	CMV Equivalent to 90 mg/kg every 24 hours	CMV Equivalent to 120 mg/kg every 24 hours
<0.4	Not recommended	Not recommended
≥0.4-0.5	50 mg/kg every 48 hours	65 mg/kg every 48 hours
>0.5-0.6	60 mg/kg every 48 hours	80 mg/kg every 48 hours
>0.6-0.8	80 mg/kg every 48 hours	105 mg/kg every 48 hours
>0.8-1.0	50 mg/kg every 24 hours	65 mg/kg every 24 hours
>1.0-1.4	70 mg/kg every 24 hours	90 mg/kg every 24 hours
>1.4	90 mg/kg every 24 hours	120 mg/kg every 24 hours

(Continued)

Foscarnet *(Continued)*

Mechanism of Action Pyrophosphate analogue which acts as a noncompetitive inhibitor of many viral RNA and DNA polymerases as well as HIV reverse transcriptase. Inhibitory effects occur at concentrations which do not affect host cellular DNA polymerases; however, some human cell growth suppression has been observed with high *in vitro* concentrations. Similar to ganciclovir, foscarnet is a virostatic agent. Foscarnet does not require activation by thymidine kinase.

Other Adverse Effects

>10%:

- Central nervous system: Fever (65%), headache (26%), seizures (10%)
- Gastrointestinal: Nausea (47%), diarrhea (30%), vomiting
- Hematologic: Anemia (33%)
- Renal: Abnormal renal function/decreased creatinine clearance (27%)

1% to 10%:

- Central nervous system: Fatigue, malaise, dizziness, hypoesthesia, depression/confusion/anxiety (≥5%)
- Dermatologic: Rash
- Endocrine & metabolic: Electrolyte imbalance (especially potassium, calcium, magnesium, and phosphorus)
- Gastrointestinal: Anorexia
- Hematologic: Granulocytopenia, leukopenia (≥5%), thrombocytopenia, thrombosis
- Local: Injection site pain
- Neuromuscular & skeletal: Paresthesia, involuntary muscle contractions, rigors, neuropathy (peripheral), weakness
- Ocular: Vision abnormalities
- Respiratory: Coughing, dyspnea (≥5%)
- Miscellaneous: Sepsis, diaphoresis (increased)

Drug Interactions Increased Effect/Toxicity: Concurrent use with ciprofloxacin (or other fluoroquinolone) increases seizure potential. Acute renal failure (reversible) has been reported with cyclosporine due most likely to a synergistic toxic effect. Nephrotoxic drugs (amphotericin B, I.V. pentamidine, aminoglycosides, etc) should be avoided, if possible, to minimize additive renal risk with foscarnet. Concurrent use of pentamidine also increases the potential for hypocalcemia. Protease inhibitors (ritonavir, saquinavir) have been associated with an increased risk of renal impairment during concurrent use of foscarnet

Drug Uptake

Absorption: Oral: Poor; I.V. therapy required for treatment of viral infections in AIDS patients

Half-life, elimination: ~3 hours

Pregnancy Risk Factor C

Generic Available No

Foscavir® *see* Foscarnet *on page 537*

Fosfomycin (fos foe MYE sin)

U.S. Brand Names Monurol™

Canadian Brand Names Monurol™

Mexican Brand Names Fosfocil®; Monurol®

Pharmacologic Category Antibiotic, Miscellaneous

Synonyms Fosfomycin Tromethamine

Use A single oral dose in the treatment of uncomplicated urinary tract infections in women due to susceptible strains of *E. coli* and *Enterococcus*; multiple doses have been investigated for complicated urinary tract infections in men; may have an advantage over other agents since it maintains high concentration in the urine for up to 48 hours

Local Anesthetic/Vasoconstrictor Precautions No information available to require special precautions

Effects on Dental Treatment No effects or complications reported

Dosage Adults: Urinary tract infections: Oral:

Female: Single dose of 3 g in 4 oz of water

Male: 3 g once daily for 2-3 days for complicated urinary tract infections

Mechanism of Action As a phosphonic acid derivative, fosfomycin inhibits bacterial wall synthesis (bactericidal) by inactivating the enzyme, pyruvyl transferase, which is critical in the synthesis of cell walls by bacteria; the tromethamine salt is preferable to the calcium salt due to its superior absorption; many gram-positive and gram-negative organisms are inhibited staphylococci, pneumococci, *E. coli, Salmonella, Shigella, H. influenzae, Neisseria* spp, and some strains of *P. aeruginosa*, indole-negative *Proteus*, and *Providencia*; *B. fragilis*, and anaerobic gram-negative cocci are resistant; *in vitro* synergism occurs with penicillins, cephalosporins, aminoglycosides, erythromycin, and tetracyclines.

Other Adverse Effects >1%:

Central nervous system: Headache

Dermatologic: Rash

Gastrointestinal: Diarrhea (2% to 8%), nausea, vomiting, epigastric discomfort, anorexia

Drug Interactions Decreased Effect: Antacids or calcium salts may cause precipitate formation and decrease fosfomycin absorption. Increased GI motility due to metoclopramide may lower fosfomycin tromethamine serum concentration and urinary excretion. This drug interaction possibly could be extrapolated to other medications which increase GI motility.

Drug Uptake

Absorption: Well absorbed

Half-life, elimination: 4-8 hours (increases with renal failure); Cl_{cr} <10 mL/minute: 50 hours

Time to peak: 2 hours

Pregnancy Risk Factor B

Generic Available No

Fosinopril (foe SIN oh pril)

Related Information

Cardiovascular Diseases *on page 1308*

U.S. Brand Names Monopril®

Canadian Brand Names Monopril™

Pharmacologic Category Angiotensin-Converting Enzyme (ACE) Inhibitor

Use Treatment of hypertension, either alone or in combination with other antihypertensive agents; CHF

Local Anesthetic/Vasoconstrictor Precautions No information available to require special precautions

Effects on Dental Treatment No effects or complications reported

Dosage Adults: Oral:

Hypertension: Initial: 10 mg/day; increase to a maximum dose of 80 mg/day; most patients are maintained on 20-40 mg/day; may need to divide the dose into two if trough effect is inadequate; discontinue the diuretic, if possible 2-3 days before initiation of therapy; resume diuretic therapy carefully, if needed.

Heart failure: Initial: 10 mg/day (5 mg if renal dysfunction present) and increase, as needed, to a maximum of 40 mg once daily over several weeks; usual dose: 20-40 mg/day; if hypotension, orthostasis, or azotemia occur during titration, consider decreasing concomitant diuretic dose, if any

Mechanism of Action Competitive inhibitor of angiotensin-converting enzyme (ACE); prevents conversion of angiotensin I to angiotensin II, a potent vasoconstrictor; results in lower levels of angiotensin II which causes an increase in plasma renin activity and a reduction in aldosterone secretion; a CNS mechanism may also be involved in hypotensive effect as angiotensin II increases adrenergic outflow from CNS; vasoactive kallikreins may be decreased in conversion to active hormones by ACE inhibitors, thus reducing BP

Other Adverse Effects Note: Frequency ranges include data from hypertension and heart failure trials. Higher rates of adverse reactions have generally been noted in patients with CHF. However, the frequency of adverse effects associated with placebo is also increased in this population.

>10%: Central nervous system: Dizziness (2% to 12%)

1% to 10%:

- Cardiovascular: Orthostatic hypotension (1% to 2%), palpitation (1%)
- Central nervous system: Dizziness (1% to 2%; up to 12% in CHF patients), headache (3%), weakness (1%), fatigue (1% to 2%)
- Endocrine & metabolic: Hyperkalemia (2.6%)
- Gastrointestinal: Diarrhea (2%), nausea/vomiting (1.2% to 2.2%)
- Hepatic: Increased transaminases
- Neuromuscular & skeletal: Musculoskeletal pain (<1% to 3%), noncardiac chest pain (<1% to 2%)
- Renal: Increased serum creatinine, worsening of renal function (in patients with bilateral renal artery stenosis or hypovolemia)
- Respiratory: Cough (2% to 10%)
- Miscellaneous: Upper respiratory infection (2%)

>1% but ≤ frequency in patients receiving placebo: Sexual dysfunction, fever, flu-like syndrome, dyspnea, rash, headache, insomnia

Other events reported with ACE inhibitors: Neutropenia, agranulocytosis, eosinophilic pneumonitis, cardiac arrest, pancytopenia, hemolytic anemia, anemia, aplastic anemia, thrombocytopenia, acute renal failure, hepatic failure, jaundice, symptomatic hyponatremia, bullous pemphigus, exfoliative dermatitis, Stevens-Johnson syndrome. In addition, a syndrome which may include fever, myalgia, arthralgia, interstitial nephritis, vasculitis, rash, eosinophilia and positive ANA, and elevated ESR has been reported for other ACE inhibitors.

Drug Interactions

Increased Effect/Toxicity: Potassium supplements, co-trimoxazole (high dose), angiotensin II receptor antagonists (candesartan, losartan, irbesartan, etc), or potassium-sparing diuretics (amiloride, spironolactone, triamterene) may result in elevated serum potassium levels when combined with fosinopril. ACE inhibitor

(Continued)

Fosinopril *(Continued)*

effects may be increased by phenothiazines or probenecid (increases levels of captopril). ACE inhibitors may increase serum concentration/effects of digoxin, lithium, and sulfonlyureas. Diuretics have additive hypotensive effects with ACE inhibitors, and hypovolemia increases the potential for adverse renal effects of ACE inhibitors. In patients with compromised renal function, coadministration with nonsteroidal anti-inflammatory drugs may result in further deterioration of renal function. Allopurinol and ACE inhibitors may cause a higher risk of hypersensitivity reaction when taken concurrently.

Decreased Effect: Aspirin (high dose) may reduce the therapeutic effects of ACE inhibitors; at low dosages this does not appear to be significant. Rifampin may decrease the effect of ACE inhibitors. Antacids may decrease the bioavailability of ACE inhibitors (may be more likely to occur with captopril); separate administration times by 1-2 hours. NSAIDs, specifically indomethacin, may reduce the hypotensive effects of ACE inhibitors. More likely to occur in low renin or volume dependent hypertensive patients.

Drug Uptake

Onset of action: 1 hour

Absorption: 36%

Duration: 24 hours

Half-life, elimination: Fosinoprilat: 12 hours

Time to peak: ~3 hours

Pregnancy Risk Factor C/D (2nd and 3rd trimesters)

Generic Available No

Fosinopril and Hydrochlorothiazide

(foe SIN oh pril & hye droe klor oh THYE a zide)

U.S. Brand Names Monopril-HCT®

Canadian Brand Names Monopril-HCT®

Pharmacologic Category Antihypertensive Agent Combination

Synonyms Hydrochlorothiazide and Fosinopril

Use Treatment of hypertension; not indicated for first-line treatment

Local Anesthetic/Vasoconstrictor Precautions No information available to require special precautions

Effects on Dental Treatment No effects or complications reported

Dosage A patient whose BP is not adequately controlled with fosinopril or hydrochlorothiazide monotherapy may be switched to combination therapy; **not** for initial treatment.

Oral: Adults: Hypertension: Fosinopril 10-80 mg per day, hydrochlorothiazide 12.5-50 mg per day

Mechanism of Action Fosinopril is a competitive inhibitor of angiotensin-converting enzyme (ACE); prevents conversion of angiotensin I to angiotensin II, a potent vasoconstrictor; results in lower levels of angiotensin II which causes an increase in plasma renin activity and a reduction in aldosterone secretion; a CNS mechanism may also be involved in hypotensive effect as angiotensin II increases adrenergic outflow from CNS; vasoactive kallikreins may be decreased in conversion to active hormones by ACE inhibitors, thus reducing BP. Hydrochlorothiazide inhibits sodium reabsorption in the distal tubules causing increased excretion of sodium and water as well as potassium and hydrogen ions.

Other Adverse Effects

2% to 10%:

Central nervous system: Headache (7%, less than placebo), fatigue (4%), dizziness (3%), orthostatic hypotension (2%)

Neuromuscular & skeletal: Musculoskeletal pain (2%)

Respiratory: Cough (6%), upper respiratory infection (2%, less than placebo)

<2%: Abdominal pain, angioedema, breast mass, BUN elevation (similar to placebo), chest pain, creatinine elevation (similar to placebo), depression, diarrhea, dyspepsia, dysuria, edema, eosinophilia, esophagitis, fever, flushing, gastritis, gout, heartburn, hepatic necrosis, leukopenia, libido change, liver function test elevations (transaminases, LDH, alkaline phosphatase, serum bilirubin), muscle cramps, myalgia, nausea, neutropenia, numbness, paresthesia, pharyngitis, pruritus, rash, rhinitis, sexual dysfunction, sinus congestion, somnolence, syncope, tinnitus, urinary frequency, urinary tract infection, viral infection, vomiting, weakness

Other adverse events reported with **ACE inhibitors**: Aplastic anemia, bullous pemphigus, cardiac arrest, cholestatic jaundice, exfoliative dermatitis, hemolytic anemia, hyperkalemia, pancreatitis, pancytopenia, photosensitivity; syndrome that may include one or more of arthralgia/arthritis, vasculitis, serositis, myalgia, fever, rash or other dermopathy, positive ANA titer, leukocytosis, eosinophilia, and elevated ESR; thrombocytopenia

Other adverse events reported with **hydrochlorothiazide**: Agranulocytosis, anaphylactic reactions, anorexia, blurred vision (transient), constipation, cramping, glucosuria, hemolytic anemia, hyperglycemia, hyperuricemia, hypokalemia, jaundice (intrahepatic cholestatic), lightheadedness, muscle spasm, necrotizing angiitis, pancreatitis, photosensitivity, pneumonitis, pulmonary edema, purpura, respiratory distress, restlessness, sialadenitis, SLE, Stevens-Johnson syndrome, urticaria, vertigo, xanthopsia

Contraindications

Based on **fosinopril** component: Hypersensitivity to fosinopril or any component of the formulation; angioedema related to previous treatment with an ACE inhibitor; bilateral renal artery stenosis; primary hyperaldosteronism; pregnancy (2nd and 3rd trimesters)

Based on **hydrochlorothiazide** component: Hypersensitivity to hydrochlorothiazide, thiazides, sulfonamide-derived drugs, or any component of their formulation; anuria; renal decompensation; pregnancy. Chemical similarities are present among sulfonamides, sulfonylureas, carbonic anhydrase inhibitors, thiazides, and loop diuretics (except ethacrynic acid). Use in patients with sulfonamide allergy is specifically contraindicated in product labeling, however a risk of cross-reaction exists in patients with allergy to any of these compounds; avoid use when previous reaction has been severe.

Drug Interactions

Increased Effect/Toxicity: $Alpha_1$ blockers, diuretics increase hypotension. Beta blockers may increase hyperglycemic effect. Cyclosporine may increase risk of gout or renal toxicity. Risk of lithium toxicity may be increased. Mercaptopurine may increase risk of neutropenia. Digoxin and neuromuscular-blocking agents: Effects may be increased with hypokalemia. Potassium-sparing diuretics, potassium supplements, trimethoprim may increase risk of hyperkalemia.

Decreased Effect: Aspirin, NSAIDs may decrease antihypertensive effect. Antacids, cholestyramine, colestipol may decrease absorption.

Drug Uptake

Onset of action: Fosinopril: 1 hour; Hydrochlorothiazide: ≤2 hours
Duration: Fosinopril: 24 hours; Hydrochlorothiazide: 6-12 hours
Half-life, elimination: Fosinopril: 12 hours; Hydrochlorothiazide: 5.6-14.8 hours
Time to peak: Fosinopril:~3 hours; Hydrochlorothiazide: 1-2.5 hours

Pregnancy Risk Factor C (1st trimester)/D (2nd and 3rd trimester)

Generic Available No

Fosphenytoin (FOS fen i toyn)

U.S. Brand Names Cerebyx®

Canadian Brand Names Cerebyx®

Pharmacologic Category Anticonvulsant, Hydantoin

Synonyms Fosphenytoin Sodium

Use Indicated for short-term parenteral administration when other means of phenytoin administration are unavailable, inappropriate or deemed less advantageous; the safety and effectiveness of fosphenytoin in this use has not been systematically evaluated for >5 days; may be used for the control of generalized convulsive status epilepticus and prevention and treatment of seizures occurring during neurosurgery

Local Anesthetic/Vasoconstrictor Precautions No information available to require special precautions

Effects on Dental Treatment No effects or complications reported

Dosage The dose, concentration in solutions, and infusion rates for fosphenytoin are expressed as phenytoin sodium equivalents; fosphenytoin should always be prescribed and dispensed in phenytoin sodium equivalents.

Children 5-18 years: I.V.: A limited number of children have been studied. Seven children received a single I.V. loading dose of fosphenytoin 10-20 mg **PE**/kg for the treatment of acute generalized convulsive status epilepticus (Pellock, 1996). Some centers are using the phenytoin dosing guidelines in children and dosing fosphenytoin using **PE** doses equal to the phenytoin doses (ie, phenytoin 1 mg = fosphenytoin 1 mg **PE**). Further pediatric studies are needed.

Adults:

Status epilepticus: I.V.: Loading dose: Phenytoin equivalent: 15-20 mg/kg I.V. administered at 100-150 mg/minute

Nonemergent loading and maintenance dosing: I.V. or I.M.:

Loading dose: Phenytoin equivalent: 10-20 mg/kg I.V. or I.M. (maximum I.V. rate: 150 mg/minute)

Initial daily maintenance dose: Phenytoin equivalent: 4-6 mg/kg/day I.V. or I.M.

I.M. or I.V. substitution for oral phenytoin therapy: May be substituted for oral phenytoin sodium at the same total daily dose, however, Dilantin® capsules are ~90% bioavailable by the oral route; phenytoin, supplied as fosphenytoin, is 100% bioavailable by both the I.M. and I.V. routes; for this reason, plasma phenytoin concentrations may increase when I.M. or I.V. fosphenytoin is substituted for oral phenytoin sodium therapy; in clinical trials I.M. fosphenytoin was administered as a single daily dose utilizing either 1 or 2 injection sites; some patients may require more frequent dosing

Dosing adjustments in renal/hepatic impairment: Phenytoin clearance may be substantially reduced in cirrhosis and plasma concentration monitoring with dose adjustment advisable; free phenytoin levels should be monitored closely in

(Continued)

Fosphenytoin *(Continued)*

patients with renal or hepatic disease or in those with hypoalbuminemia; furthermore, fosphenytoin clearance to phenytoin may be increased without a similar increase in phenytoin in these patients leading to increase frequency and severity of adverse events

Mechanism of Action Diphosphate ester salt of phenytoin which acts as a water soluble prodrug of phenytoin; after administration, plasma esterases convert fosphenytoin to phosphate, formaldehyde and phenytoin as the active moiety; phenytoin works by stabilizing neuronal membranes and decreasing seizure activity by increasing efflux or decreasing influx of sodium ions across cell membranes in the motor cortex during generation of nerve impulses

Other Adverse Effects The more important adverse clinical events caused by I.V. use of fosphenytoin or phenytoin are cardiovascular collapse and/or CNS depression. Hypotension can occur when either drug is administered rapidly by I.V.; do not exceed rate of 150 mg phenytoin equivalent/minute.

Frequency not defined: Pain upon injection, sensory paresthesia (long-term treatment), nephrotic syndrome

>10%:

Central nervous system: Dizziness (31%), somnolence (21%), ataxia (11%)
Dermatologic: Pruritus (49%)
Ocular: Nystagmus (44%)

1% to 10%:

Cardiovascular: Hypotension (8%), vasodilation (>1%), tachycardia (2%)
Central nervous system: Stupor (8%), incoordination (4%), paresthesia (4%), choreoathetosis (4%), tremor (3%), agitation (3%)
Gastrointestinal: Nausea (>5%), vomiting (2%)
Ocular: Blurred vision (2%), diplopia (3%)

Warnings/Precautions Doses of fosphenytoin are expressed as their phenytoin sodium equivalent; antiepileptic drugs should not be abruptly discontinued; hypotension may occur, especially after I.V. administration at high doses and high rates of administration, administration of phenytoin has been associated with atrial and ventricular conduction depression and ventricular fibrillation, careful cardiac monitoring is needed when administering I.V. loading doses of fosphenytoin; use with caution in patients with hypotension and severe myocardial insufficiency; discontinue if skin rash or lymphadenopathy occurs; acute hepatotoxicity associated with a hypersensitivity syndrome characterized by fever, skin eruptions and lymphadenopathy has been reported to occur within the first 2 months of treatment

Drug Interactions CYP2C9 and 2C19 enzyme substrate; CYP1A2, 2B6, 2C, 2C9, 2C18, 2C19, 2D6, 3A3/4, and 3A5-7 enzyme inducer

Increased Effect/Toxicity: Phenytoin may increase phenobarbital and primidone levels. Protein binding of phenytoin can be affected by valproic acid or salicylates. Serum phenytoin concentrations may be increased by cimetidine, felbamate, ethosuximide, methsuximide, chloramphenicol, disulfiram, fluconazole, omeprazole, isoniazid, trimethoprim, or sulfonamides.

Decreased Effect: No drugs are known to interfere with the conversion of fosphenytoin to phenytoin. Phenytoin may decrease the serum concentration or effectiveness of valproic acid, ethosuximide, felbamate, benzodiazepines, carbamazepine, lamotrigine, primidone, warfarin, oral contraceptives, corticosteroids, cyclosporine, theophylline, chloramphenicol, rifampin, doxycycline, quinidine, mexiletine, disopyramide, dopamine, or nondepolarizing skeletal muscle relaxants. Serum phenytoin concentrations may be decreased by rifampin, cisplatin, vinblastine, bleomycin, and folic acid.

Drug Uptake Fosphenytoin is a prodrug of phenytoin and its anticonvulsant effects are attributable to phenytoin. See Phenytoin *on page 951*

Onset of action: May be more rapid due to more rapid infusion

Conversion to phenytoin: Following I.V. administration conversion half-life is 15 minutes; following I.M. administration peak phenytoin levels are reached in 3 hours

Half-life, elimination: Variable (kinetics of phenytoin are saturable); mean: 12-29 hours

Pregnancy Risk Factor D

Generic Available No

Fostex® 10% BPO [OTC] *see* Benzoyl Peroxide *on page 153*

Fototar® [OTC] *see* Coal Tar *on page 315*

Fragmin® *see* Dalteparin *on page 345*

Freezone® [OTC] *see* Salicylic Acid *on page 1072*

Frova™ *see* Frovatriptan *on page 542*

Frovatriptan (froe va TRIP tan)

U.S. Brand Names Frova™

Pharmacologic Category Antimigraine Agent; Serotonin 5-$HT_{1B, 1D}$ Receptor Agonist

Synonyms Frovatriptan Succinate

Use Acute treatment of migraine with or without aura in adults

Local Anesthetic/Vasoconstrictor Precautions No information available to require special precautions

Effects on Dental Treatment No effects or complications reported

Dosage Oral:

Adults: Migraine: 2.5 mg; if headache recurs, a second dose may be given if first dose provided some relief and at least 2 hours have elapsed since the first dose (maximum daily dose: 7.5 mg)

Dosage adjustment in hepatic impairment: No adjustment necessary in mild to moderate hepatic impairment; use with caution in severe impairment

Mechanism of Action Selective agonist for serotonin (5-HT_{1B} and 5-HT_{1D} receptor) in cranial arteries to cause vasoconstriction and reduces sterile inflammation associated with antidromic neuronal transmission correlating with relief of migraine.

Other Adverse Effects 1% to 10%:

Cardiovascular: Chest pain (2%), flushing (4%), palpitation (1%)

Central nervous system: Dizziness (8%), fatigue (5%), headache (4%), hot or cold sensation (3%), anxiety (1%), dysesthesia (1%), hypoesthesia (1%), insomnia (1%), pain (1%)

Gastrointestinal: Hyposalivation (3%), dyspepsia (2%), abdominal pain (1%), diarrhea (1%), vomiting (1%)

Neuromuscular & skeletal: Paresthesia (4%), skeletal pain (3%)

Ocular: Visual abnormalities (1%)

Otic: Tinnitus (1%)

Respiratory: Rhinitis (1%), sinusitis (1%)

Miscellaneous: Diaphoresis (1%)

Drug Interactions CYP1A2 enzyme substrate

CYP1A2 inducers: May decrease serum concentrations of frovatriptan (eg, carbamazepine, phenobarbital, phenytoin, ritonavir)

CYP1A2 inhibitors: May increase serum concentrations of frovatriptan (eg, cimetidine, ciprofloxacin, erythromycin)

Ergot derivatives: Ergot derivatives may cause prolonged vasospastic reactions, creating additive toxicity with frovatriptan. Do not use within 24 hours of each other.

Estrogens (oral contraceptives): Estradiol may increase serum concentrations of frovatriptan

Propranolol: Propranolol may increase serum concentrations of frovatriptan

Selective serotonin reuptake inhibitors (SSRIs): Frovatriptan may increase SSRI toxicity (eg, weakness, hyper-reflexia, incoordination)

Serotonin agonists: May exhibit additive toxicity with other serotonin agonists (eg, antidepressants, dextromethorphan, tramadol), leading to serotonin syndrome.

Drug Uptake

Half-life, elimination: 26 hours

Time to peak: 2-4 hours

Pregnancy Risk Factor C

Generic Available No

FS Shampoo® [DSC] *see* Fluocinolone *on page 512*

FUDR® *see* Floxuridine *on page 506*

Fulvestrant (fool VES trant)

U.S. Brand Names Faslodex®

Pharmacologic Category Antineoplastic Agent, Estrogen Receptor Antagonist

Synonyms ICI 182,780

Use Treatment of hormone receptor positive metastatic breast cancer in postmenopausal women with disease progression following antiestrogen therapy.

Local Anesthetic/Vasoconstrictor Precautions No information available to require special precautions

Effects on Dental Treatment No effects or complications reported

Dosage I.M.:

Adults (postmenopausal women): 250 mg at 1-month intervals

Dosage adjustment in hepatic impairment: Use in moderate to severe hepatic impairment has not been evaluated; use caution.

Mechanism of Action Steroidal compound which competitively binds to estrogen receptors on tumors and other tissue targets, producing a nuclear complex that decreases DNA synthesis and inhibits estrogen effects; has no estrogen-receptor agonist activity; causes down-regulation of estrogen receptors and inhibits tumor growth

Other Adverse Effects

>10%:

Cardiovascular: Vasodilation (18%)

Central nervous system: Pain (19%), headache (15%)

Gastrointestinal: Nausea (26%), vomiting (13%), constipation (13%), diarrhea (12%), abdominal pain (12%)

Local: Injection site reaction (11%)

Neuromuscular & skeletal: Weakness (23%), bone pain (16%), back pain (14%)

(Continued)

Fulvestrant *(Continued)*

Respiratory: Pharyngitis (16%), dyspnea (15%)

1% to 10%:

Cardiovascular: Edema (9%), chest pain (7%)

Central nervous system: Dizziness (7%), insomnia (7%), paresthesia (6%), fever (6%), depression (6%), anxiety (5%)

Dermatologic: Rash (7%)

Gastrointestinal: Anorexia (9%)

Genitourinary: Pelvic pain (10%), urinary tract infection (6%)

Hematologic: Anemia (5%)

Neuromuscular and skeletal: Arthritis (3%)

Respiratory: Cough (10%)

Miscellaneous: Increased diaphoresis (5%)

Drug Interactions CYP3A3/4 enzyme substrate; relative contribution not defined

Specific interactions studies have not been conducted.

Increased Effect/Toxicity: Serum concentration and/or toxicity may be increased by CYP3A3/4 inhibitors: Amiodarone, cimetidine, clarithromycin, erythromycin, delavirdine, diltiazem, dirithromycin, disulfiram, fluoxetine, fluvoxamine, indinavir, itraconazole, ketoconazole, nefazodone, nevirapine, propoxyphene, quinupristin-dalfopristin, ritonavir, saquinavir, verapamil, zafirlukast, zileuton

Decreased Effect: Serum concentration may be increased by enzyme-inducing agents, decreasing therapeutic effect; potential inducers include phenobarbital, phenytoin, carbamazepine, rifampin, and rifabutin. However, a clinical study with rifampin did not demonstrate an effect on fulvestrant pharmacokinetics.

Drug Uptake

Duration: I.M.: Plasma levels maintained for at least 1 month

Half-life, elimination: ~40 days

Time to peak: I.M.: ~7 days

Pregnancy Risk Factor D

Generic Available No

Fulvicin® P/G *see* Griseofulvin *on page 567*

Fulvicin-U/F® *see* Griseofulvin *on page 567*

Fungizone® *see* Amphotericin B (Conventional) *on page 91*

Fungoid® Tincture [OTC] *see* Miconazole *on page 807*

Furacin® *see* Nitrofurazone *on page 870*

Furadantin® *see* Nitrofurantoin *on page 870*

Furazolidone (fyoor a ZOE li done)

U.S. Brand Names Furoxone®

Canadian Brand Names Furoxone®

Mexican Brand Names Furoxona®; Fuxol; Salmocide®

Pharmacologic Category Antiprotozoal

Use Treatment of bacterial or protozoal diarrhea and enteritis caused by susceptible organisms *Giardia lamblia* and *Vibrio cholerae*

Local Anesthetic/Vasoconstrictor Precautions No information available to require special precautions

Effects on Dental Treatment No effects or complications reported

Dosage Oral:

Children >1 month: 5-8 mg/kg/day in 4 divided doses for 7 days, not to exceed 400 mg/day or 8.8 mg/kg/day

Adults: 100 mg 4 times/day for 7 days

Mechanism of Action Inhibits several vital enzymatic reactions causing antibacterial and antiprotozoal action

Other Adverse Effects

>10%: Genitourinary: Discoloration of urine (dark yellow to brown)

1% to 10%:

Central nervous system: Headache

Gastrointestinal: Abdominal pain, diarrhea, nausea, vomiting

Drug Interactions Increased Effect/Toxicity: Increased effect with sympathomimetic amines, tricyclic antidepressants, tyramine-containing foods, MAO inhibitors, meperidine, anorexiants, dextromethorphan, fluoxetine, paroxetine, sertraline, and trazodone. Increased effect/toxicity of levodopa.

Drug Uptake Absorption: Oral: Poor

Pregnancy Risk Factor C

Generic Available No

Furosemide (fyoor OH se mide)

Related Information

Cardiovascular Diseases *on page 1308*

U.S. Brand Names Lasix®

Canadian Brand Names Apo®-Furosemide; Lasix®; Lasix® Special

Mexican Brand Names Edenol; Henexal; Lasix®; Selectofur®; Zafimida®

Pharmacologic Category Diuretic, Loop

Synonyms Frusemide

Use Management of edema associated with CHF and hepatic or renal disease; used alone or in combination with antihypertensives in treatment of hypertension

Local Anesthetic/Vasoconstrictor Precautions No information available to require special precautions

Effects on Dental Treatment No effects or complications reported

Dosage

Children:

Oral: 1-2 mg/kg/dose increased in increments of 1 mg/kg/dose with each succeeding dose until a satisfactory effect is achieved to a maximum of 6 mg/kg/dose no more frequently than 6 hours

I.M., I.V.: 1 mg/kg/dose, increasing by each succeeding dose at 1 mg/kg/dose at intervals of 6-12 hours until a satisfactory response up to 6 mg/kg/dose

Adults:

Oral: 20-80 mg/dose initially increased in increments of 20-40 mg/dose at intervals of 6-8 hours; usual maintenance dose interval is twice daily or every day

I.M., I.V.: 20-40 mg/dose, may be repeated in 1-2 hours as needed and increased by 20 mg/dose with each succeeding dose up to 1000 mg/day; usual dosing interval: 6-12 hours

Continuous I.V. infusion: Initial I.V. bolus dose of 0.1 mg/kg followed by continuous I.V. infusion doses of 0.1 mg/kg/hour doubled every 2 hours to a maximum of 0.4 mg/kg/hour if urine output is <1 mL/kg/hour have been found to be effective and result in a lower daily requirement of furosemide than with intermittent dosing. Other studies have used 20-160 mg/hour continuous I.V. infusion

Elderly: Oral, I.M., I.V.: Initial: 20 mg/day; increase slowly to desired response

Mechanism of Action Inhibits reabsorption of sodium and chloride in the ascending loop of Henle and distal renal tubule, interfering with the chloride-binding cotransport system, thus causing increased excretion of water, sodium, chloride, magnesium, and calcium

Other Adverse Effects Frequency not defined:

Cardiovascular: Orthostatic hypotension, necrotizing angiitis, thrombophlebitis, chronic aortitis, acute hypotension, sudden death from cardiac arrest (with I.V. or I.M. administration)

Central nervous system: Paresthesias, vertigo, dizziness, lightheadedness, headache, blurred vision, xanthopsia , fever, restlessness

Dermatologic: Exfoliative dermatitis, erythema multiforme, purpura, photosensitivity, urticaria, rash, pruritus, cutaneous vasculitis

Endocrine & metabolic: Hyperglycemia, hyperuricemia, hypokalemia, hypochloremia, metabolic alkalosis, hypocalcemia, hypomagnesemia, gout, hypernatremia

Gastrointestinal: Nausea, vomiting, anorexia, oral and gastric irritation, cramping, diarrhea, constipation, pancreatitis, intrahepatic cholestatic jaundice, ischemia hepatitis

Genitourinary: Urinary bladder spasm, urinary frequency

Hematological: Aplastic anemia (rare), thrombocytopenia, agranulocytosis (rare), hemolytic anemia, leukopenia, anemia, purpura

Neuromuscular & skeletal: Muscle spasm, weakness

Otic: Hearing impairment (reversible or permanent with rapid I.V. or I.M. administration), tinnitus, reversible deafness (with rapid I.V. or I.M. administration)

Renal: Vasculitis, allergic interstitial nephritis, glycosuria, fall in glomerular filtration rate and renal blood flow (due to overdiuresis), transient rise in BUN

Miscellaneous: Anaphylaxis (rare), exacerbate or activate systemic lupus erythematosus

Warnings/Precautions Adjust dose to avoid dehydration. In cirrhosis, avoid electrolyte and acid/base imbalances that might lead to hepatic encephalopathy. Ototoxicity is associated with rapid I.V. administration, renal impairment, excessive doses, and concurrent use of other ototoxins. Hypersensitivity reactions can rarely occur. Monitor fluid status and renal function in an attempt to prevent oliguria, azotemia, and reversible increases in BUN and creatinine. Close medical supervision of aggressive diuresis required. Monitor closely for electrolyte imbalances particularly hypokalemia. Watch for and correct electrolyte disturbances. Coadministration of antihypertensives may increase the risk of hypotension. Avoid use of medications in which the toxicity is enhanced by hypokalemia (including quinolones with QT prolongation).

Chemical similarities are present among sulfonamides, sulfonylureas, carbonic anhydrase inhibitors, thiazides, and loop diuretics (except ethacrynic acid). Use in patients with sulfonylurea allergy is specifically contraindicated in product labeling, however a risk of cross-reaction exists in patients with allergy to any of these compounds; avoid use when previous reaction has been severe.

Drug Interactions

Increased Effect/Toxicity: Furosemide-induced hypokalemia may predispose to digoxin toxicity and may increase the risk of arrhythmia with drugs which may prolong QT interval, including type Ia and type III antiarrhythmic agents, cisapride, terfenadine, and some quinolones (sparfloxacin, gatifloxacin, and moxifloxacin). The risk of toxicity from lithium and salicylates (high dose) may be

(Continued)

Furosemide *(Continued)*

increased by loop diuretics. Hypotensive effects and/or adverse renal effects of ACE inhibitors and NSAIDs are potentiated by furosemide-induced hypovolemia. The effects of peripheral adrenergic-blocking drugs or ganglionic blockers may be increased by furosemide. Furosemide may increase the risk of ototoxicity with other ototoxic agents (aminoglycosides, cis-platinum), especially in patients with renal dysfunction. Synergistic diuretic effects occur with thiazide-type diuretics. Diuretics tend to be synergistic with other antihypertensive agents, and hypotension may occur.

Decreased Effect: Indomethacin, aspirin, phenobarbital, phenytoin, and NSAIDs may reduce natriuretic and hypotensive effects of furosemide. Colestipol, cholestyramine, and sucralfate may reduce the effect of furosemide; separate administration by 2 hours. Furosemide may antagonize the effect of skeletal muscle relaxants (tubocurarine). Glucose tolerance may be decreased by furosemide, requiring an adjustment in the dose of hypoglycemic agents. Metformin may decrease furosemide concentrations.

Drug Uptake

Onset of action: Oral: 30-60 minutes; I.M.: 30 minutes; I.V.: ≤5 minutes
Absorption: Oral: 60% to 67%
Duration: Oral: 6-8 hours; I.V.: 2 hours
Half-life, elimination: 0.5-1.1 hours; End-stage renal disease: 9 hours
Time to peak: Oral: 1-2 hours

Pregnancy Risk Factor C

Generic Available Yes

Furoxone® *see* Furazolidone *on page 544*

Gabapentin (GA ba pen tin)

U.S. Brand Names Neurontin®

Canadian Brand Names Neurontin™

Mexican Brand Names Neurontin®

Pharmacologic Category Anticonvulsant, Miscellaneous

Use

Dental: Treatment of oral-facial neuropathic pain

Medical: Adjunct for treatment of partial seizures with and without secondary generalized seizures in patients >12 years of age with epilepsy; adjunct for treatment of partial seizures in pediatric patients 3-12 years of age

Unlabeled/Investigational: Bipolar disorder, chronic pain, social phobia

Local Anesthetic/Vasoconstrictor Precautions No information available to require special precautions

Effects on Dental Treatment No effects or complications reported

Dosage

Children: Anticonvulsant: Oral

Children 3-12 years: Initial: 10-15 mg/kg/day in 3 divided doses; titrate to effective dose over ~3 days; dosages of up to 50 mg/kg/day have been tolerated in clinical studies

Children 3-4 years: Effective dose: 40 mg/kg/day in 3 divided doses

Children ≥5-12 years: Effective dose: 25-35 mg/kg/day in 3 divided doses

Note: If gabapentin is discontinued or if another anticonvulsant is added to therapy, it should be done slowly over a minimum of 1 week

Children >12 years: Refer to Adult dosing

Adults:

Anticonvulsant: Oral:

Initial: 300 mg 3 times/day, if necessary the dose may be increased up to 1800 mg/day

Maintenance: 900-1800 mg/day administered in 3 divided doses; doses of up to 2400 mg/day have been tolerated in long-term clinical studies; up to 3600 mg/day has been tolerated in short-term studies

Note: If gabapentin is discontinued or if another anticonvulsant is added to therapy, it should be done slowly over a minimum of 1 week

Pain: Oral: 300-1800 mg/day given in 3 divided doses has been the most common dosage range

Bipolar disorder: Oral: 300-3000 mg/day given in 3 divided doses

Neuropathic pain (titrate dose): 300 mg once a day on day 1; 300 mg twice a day on day 2; and 300 mg three times a day on day 3; thereafter, the dose can be increased using increments of 300 mg per day given in three divided doses; maximum dose of 1800mg/day

Mechanism of Action Exact mechanism of action is not known, but does have properties in common with other anticonvulsants; although structurally related to GABA, it does not interact with GABA receptors

Other Adverse Effects As reported in patients >12 years of age, unless otherwise noted

>10%:

Central nervous system: Somnolence (20%), dizziness (17%), ataxia (12%), fatigue (11% in adults)

Miscellaneous: Viral infection (11% in children 3-12 years)

1% to 10%:

Cardiovascular: Peripheral edema (2%)

Central nervous system: Fever (10% in children 3-12 years), hostility (8% in children 3-12 years), somnolence (8% in children 3-12 years), emotional lability (4% to 6% in children 3-12 years), fatigue (3% in children 3-12 years), abnormal thinking (2% in children and adults), amnesia (2%), depression (2%), dizziness (2% in children 3-12 years), dysarthria (2%), nervousness (2%), abnormal coordination (1%), twitching (1%)

Dermatologic: Pruritus (1%)

Gastrointestinal: Nausea/vomiting (8% in children 3-12 years), weight gain (3% in adults and children), dyspepsia (2%), dry throat (2%), xerostomia (2%), appetite stimulation (1%), constipation (1%), dental abnormalities (1%)

Genitourinary: Impotence (1%)

Hematologic: Leukopenia (1%), decreased WBC (1%)

Neuromuscular & skeletal: Tremor (7%), hyperkinesia (3% to 5% in children 3-12 years), back pain (2%), myalgia (2%)

Ocular: Nystagmus (8%), diplopia (6%), blurred vision (4%)

Respiratory: Rhinitis (4%), bronchitis (3% in children 3-12 years), pharyngitis (3%), coughing (2%), respiratory infection (2% in children 3-12 years)

Warnings/Precautions Avoid abrupt withdrawal, may precipitate seizures; may be associated with a slight incidence (0.6%) of status epilepticus and sudden deaths (0.0038 deaths/patient year); use cautiously in patients with severe renal dysfunction; rat studies demonstrated an association with pancreatic adenocarcinoma in male rats; clinical implication unknown. May cause CNS depression, which may impair physical or mental abilities. Patients must be cautioned about performing tasks which require mental alertness (ie, operating machinery or driving). Effects with other sedative drugs or ethanol may be potentiated. Pediatric patients (3-12 years of age) have shown increased incidence of CNS-related adverse effects, including emotional lability, hostility, thought disorder, and hyperkinesia. Safety and efficacy in children <3 years of age have not been established.

Drug Interactions

Increased Effect/Toxicity: Cimetidine may increased gabapentin levels. Gabapentin may increase peak concentrations of norethindrone.

Decreased Effect: Gabapentin does not modify plasma concentrations of standard anticonvulsant medications (eg, valproic acid, carbamazepine, phenytoin, or phenobarbital). Antacids reduce the bioavailability of gabapentin by 20%.

Drug Uptake

Absorption: Oral: 50% to 60%

Half-life, elimination: 5-7 hours

Pregnancy Risk Factor C

Generic Available No

Selected Readings

Laird MA and Gidal BE, "Use of Gabapentin in the Treatment of Neuropathic Pain," *Ann Pharmacother*, 2000, 34(6):802-7.

Rose MA and Kam PCA, "Gabapentin: Pharmacology and Its Use in Pain Management," *Anaesthesia*, 2002, 57:451-62.

Rosenberg JM, Harrell C, Ristic H, et al, "The Effect of Gabapentin on Neuropathic Pain," *Clin J Pain*, 1997, 13(3):251-5.

Rowbotham M, Harden N, Stacey B, et al, "Gabapentin for the Treatment of Postherpetic Neuralgia: A Randomized Controlled Trial," *JAMA*, 1998, 280(21):1837-42.

Gabitril® *see* Tiagabine *on page 1165*

Gamimune® N *see* Immune Globulin, Intravenous *on page 630*

Gammagard® S/D *see* Immune Globulin, Intravenous *on page 630*

Gammar®-P I.V. *see* Immune Globulin, Intravenous *on page 630*

Ganciclovir (gan SYE kloe veer)

Related Information

Systemic Viral Diseases *on page 1354*

U.S. Brand Names Cytovene®; Vitrasert®

Canadian Brand Names Cytovene®; Vitrasert®

Mexican Brand Names Cymevene

Pharmacologic Category Antiviral Agent

Synonyms DHPG Sodium; GCV Sodium; Nordeoxyguanosine

Use Treatment of CMV retinitis in immunocompromised individuals, including patients with acquired immunodeficiency syndrome; treatment of CMV pneumonia in marrow transplant recipients AIDS patients and organ transplant recipients with CMV colitis, pneumonitis, and multiorgan involvement; bone marrow transplant patients when given in combination with IVIG or CMV hyperimmune globulin

Oral: Alternative to the I.V. formulation for maintenance treatment of CMV retinitis in immunocompromised patients, including patients with AIDS, in whom retinitis is stable following appropriate induction therapy and for whom the risk of more rapid progression is balanced by the benefit associated with avoiding daily I.V. infusions

Local Anesthetic/Vasoconstrictor Precautions No information available to require special precautions

(Continued)

Ganciclovir *(Continued)*

Effects on Dental Treatment No effects or complications reported

Dosage

CMV retinitis: Slow I.V. infusion (dosing is based on total body weight):

Children >3 months and Adults:

Induction therapy: 5 mg/kg/dose every 12 hours for 14-21 days followed by maintenance therapy

Maintenance therapy: 5 mg/kg/day as a single daily dose for 7 days/week or 6 mg/kg/day for 5 days/week

CMV retinitis: Oral: 1000 mg 3 times/day with food **or** 500 mg 6 times/day with food

Prevention of CMV disease in patients with advanced HIV infection and normal renal function: Oral: 1000 mg 3 times/day with food

Prevention of CMV disease in transplant patients: Same initial and maintenance dose as CMV retinitis except duration of initial course is 7-14 days, duration of maintenance therapy is dependent on clinical condition and degree of immunosuppression

Intravitreal implant: One implant for 5- to 8-month period; following depletion of ganciclovir, as evidenced by progression of retinitis, implant may be removed and replaced

Elderly: Refer to adult dosing; in general, dose selection should be cautious, reflecting greater frequency of organ impairment

Mechanism of Action Ganciclovir is phosphorylated to a substrate which competitively inhibits the binding of deoxyguanosine triphosphate to DNA polymerase resulting in inhibition of viral DNA synthesis

Other Adverse Effects

>10%:

Central nervous system: Fever (38% to 48%)

Dermatologic: Rash (oral: 15%, I.V.: 10%)

Gastrointestinal: Abdominal pain (17% to 19%), diarrhea (40%), nausea (25%), anorexia (15%), vomiting (13%)

Hematologic: Anemia (20% to 25%), leukopenia (30% to 40%)

1% to 10%:

Central nervous system: Confusion, neuropathy (8% to 9%), headache (4%)

Dermatologic: Pruritus (5%)

Hematologic: Thrombocytopenia (6%), neutropenia with ANC <500/mm^3 (oral: 5%, I.V.: 14%)

Neuromuscular & skeletal: Paresthesia (6% to 10%), weakness (6%)

Miscellaneous: Sepsis (oral: 4%, I.V.: 15%)

Drug Interactions

Increased Effect/Toxicity: Immunosuppressive agents may increase hematologic toxicity of ganciclovir. Imipenem/cilastatin may increase seizure potential. Oral ganciclovir increases blood levels of zidovudine, although zidovudine decreases steady-state levels of ganciclovir. Since both drugs have the potential to cause neutropenia and anemia, some patients may not tolerate concomitant therapy with these drugs at full dosage. Didanosine levels are increased with concurrent ganciclovir. Other nephrotoxic drugs (eg, amphotericin and cyclosporine) may have additive nephrotoxicity with ganciclovir.

Decreased Effect: A decrease in blood levels of ganciclovir AUC may occur when used with didanosine.

Drug Uptake Half-life, elimination: 1.7-5.8 hours (increases with impaired renal function); End-stage renal disease: 5-28 hours

Pregnancy Risk Factor C

Generic Available No

Ganirelix (ga ni REL ix)

U.S. Brand Names Antagon®

Canadian Brand Names Antagon®

Pharmacologic Category Antigonadotropic Agent

Synonyms Ganirelix Acetate

Use Inhibits premature luteinizing hormone (LH) surges in women undergoing controlled ovarian hyperstimulation in fertility clinics.

Local Anesthetic/Vasoconstrictor Precautions No information available to require special precautions

Effects on Dental Treatment No effects or complications reported

Dosage Adult: S.C.: 250 mcg/day during the early to midfollicular phase after initiating follicle-stimulating hormone; treatment should be continued daily until the day of chorionic gonadotropin administration

Mechanism of Action Competitively blocks the gonadotropin-release hormone receptors on the pituitary gonadotroph and transduction pathway. This suppresses gonadotropin secretion and luteinizing hormone secretion preventing ovulation until the follicles are of adequate size.

Other Adverse Effects 1% to 10%:

Central nervous system: Headache (3%)

Endocrine & metabolic: Ovarian hyperstimulation syndrome (2.4%)

Gastrointestinal: Abdominal pain (4.8%), nausea (1.1%), and abdominal pain (1%)
Genitourinary: Vaginal bleeding (1.8%)
Local: Injection site reaction (1.1%)

Contraindications Hypersensitivity to ganirelix, gonadotropin-releasing hormone or any other analog, or any component of their formulation; known or suspected pregnancy

Warnings/Precautions Should only be prescribed by fertility specialists. The packaging contains natural rubber latex (may cause allergic reactions). Pregnancy must be excluded before starting medication.

Drug Uptake
Absorption: S.C.: Rapid
Half-life, elimination: 16.2 hours
Time to peak: 1.1 hours

Pregnancy Risk Factor X

Generic Available No

Gantanol® *see* Sulfamethoxazole *on page 1119*
Gantrisin® *see* SulfiSOXAZOLE *on page 1123*
Garamycin® *see* Gentamicin *on page 554*
Gastrocrom® *see* Cromolyn Sodium *on page 330*
Gas-X® [OTC] *see* Simethicone *on page 1088*

Gatifloxacin (ga ti FLOKS a sin)

Related Information
Oral Bacterial Infections *on page 1367*
Respiratory Diseases *on page 1328*

U.S. Brand Names Tequin®

Canadian Brand Names Tequin®

Pharmacologic Category Antibiotic, Quinolone

Use Treatment of the following infections when caused by susceptible bacteria: Acute bacterial exacerbation of chronic bronchitis due to *S. pneumoniae, H. influenzae, H. parainfluenzae, M. catarrhalis*, or *S. aureus*; acute sinusitis due to *S. pneumoniae, H. influenzae*; community acquired pneumonia due to *S. pneumoniae, H. influenzae, H. parainfluenzae, M. catarrhalis, S. aureus, M. pneumoniae, C. pneumoniae*, or *L. pneumophilia*; uncomplicated urinary tract infections (cystitis) due to *E. coli, K. pneumoniae*, or *P. mirabilis*; complicated urinary tract infections due to *E. coli, K. pneumoniae*, or *P. mirabilis*; pyelonephritis due to *E. coli*; uncomplicated urethral and cervical gonorrhea; acute, uncomplicated rectal infections in women due to *N. gonorrhoeae*

Local Anesthetic/Vasoconstrictor Precautions No information available to require special precautions

Effects on Dental Treatment No effects or complications reported

Dosage Adult: Oral, I.V.:
Acute bacterial exacerbation of chronic bronchitis; 400 mg every 24 hours for 7-10 days
Acute sinusitis: 400 mg every 24 hours for 10 days
Community acquired pneumonia: 400 mg every 24 hours for 7-14 days
Uncomplicated urinary tract infections (cystitis): 200-400 mg every 24 hours for 3 days
Complicated urinary tract infections: 400 mg every 24 hours for 7-10 days
Acute pyelonephritis: 400 mg every 24 hours for 7-10 days
Uncomplicated urethral gonorrhea in men, cervical or rectal gonorrhea in women: 400 mg single dose

Dosage adjustment in renal impairment: Creatinine clearance <40 mL/minute (or patients on hemodialysis/CAPD) should receive an initial dose of 400 mg, followed by a subsequent dose of 200 mg every 24 hours. Patients receiving single-dose or 3-day therapy for appropriate indications do not require dosage adjustment. Administer after hemodialysis.

Dosage adjustment in hepatic impairment: No dosage adjustment is required in mild-moderate hepatic disease. No data are available in severe hepatic impairment (Child-Pugh Class C).

Elderly: No dosage adjustment is required based on age, however, assessment of renal function is particularly important in this population.

Mechanism of Action Gatifloxacin is a DNA gyrase inhibitor, and also inhibits topoisomerase IV. DNA gyrase (topoisomerase II) is an essential bacterial enzyme that maintains the superhelical structure of DNA. DNA gyrase is required for DNA replication and transcription, DNA repair, recombination, and transposition; inhibition is bactericidal.

Other Adverse Effects
3% to 10%:
Central nervous system: Headache (3%), dizziness (3%)
Gastrointestinal: Nausea (8%), diarrhea (4%)
Genitourinary: Vaginitis (6%)
Local: Injection site reactions (5%)

(Continued)

Gatifloxacin *(Continued)*

0.1% to 3%: Abdominal pain, abnormal dreams, abnormal vision, agitation, allergic reaction, anorexia, anxiety, back pain, chest pain, chills, confusion, constipation, diaphoresis, dyspepsia, dyspnea, dysuria, elevated alkaline phosphatase, elevated serum transaminases, fever, flatulence, gastritis, glossitis, hematuria, hypertension, increased serum amylase, increased serum bilirubin, insomnia, mouth ulceration, nervousness, oral candidiasis, palpitation, paresthesia, peripheral edema, pharyngitis, pruritus, rash, stomatitis, taste perversion, tinnitus, tremor, vasodilation, vertigo, vomiting

Contraindications Hypersensitivity to gatifloxacin, other quinolone antibiotics, or any component of their formulation; known prolongation of QT interval, uncorrected hypokalemia, or concurrent administration of other medications known to prolong the QT interval (including Class Ia and Class III antiarrhythmics, cisapride, erythromycin, antipsychotics, and tricyclic antidepressants)

Warnings/Precautions Use with caution in patients with significant bradycardia or acute myocardial ischemia. Safety and effectiveness in pediatric patients (<18 years of age) have not been established. Experience in immature animals has resulted in permanent arthropathy. Use with caution in individuals at risk of seizures (CNS disorders or concurrent therapy with medications which may lower seizure threshold). Discontinue in patients who experience significant CNS adverse effects (dizziness, hallucinations, suicidal ideation or actions). Use caution in renal dysfunction (dosage adjustment required) and in severe hepatic insufficiency (no data available). Use caution in patients with diabetes - glucose regulation may be altered.

Severe hypersensitivity reactions, including anaphylaxis, have occurred with quinolone therapy. If an allergic reaction occurs (itching, urticaria, dyspnea or facial edema, loss of consciousness, tingling, cardiovascular collapse) discontinue drug immediately. Prolonged use may result in superinfection; pseudomembranous colitis may occur and should be considered in all patients who present with diarrhea. Tendon inflammation and/or rupture has been reported with other quinolone antibiotics. This has not been reported for gatifloxacin. Discontinue at first sign of tendon inflammation or pain.

Drug Interactions

Increased Effect/Toxicity: Drugs which prolong QT interval (including Class Ia and Class III antiarrhythmics, erythromycin, cisapride, antipsychotics, and cyclic antidepressants) are contraindicated with gatifloxacin. Drugs which may induce bradycardia (eg, beta-blockers, amiodarone) should be avoided, Probenecid, loop diuretics, and cimetidine (possibly other H_2 antagonists) may increase the serum concentration of gatifloxacin (based on experience with other quinolones). Digoxin levels may be increased in some patients by gatifloxacin. NSAIDs and foscarnet have been associated with an increased risk of seizures with some quinolones (not reported with gatifloxacin). The hypoprothrombinemic effect of warfarin is enhanced by some quinolone antibiotics. Monitoring of the INR during concurrent therapy is recommended by the manufacturer. Gatifloxacin may alter glucose control in patients receiving hypoglycemic agents with or without insulin.

Decreased Effect: Metal cations (magnesium, aluminum, iron, and zinc) inhibit intestinal absorption of gatifloxacin (by up to 98%). Antacids, electrolyte supplements, sucralfate, quinapril, and some didanosine formulations should be avoided. Gatifloxacin should be administered 4 hours before or 8 hours after these agents. Calcium carbonate was not found to alter the absorption of gatifloxacin. Antineoplastic agents, H_2 antagonists, and proton pump inhibitors may also decrease absorption of some quinolones. Gatifloxacin may alter glucose control in patients receiving hypoglycemic agents with or without insulin.

Drug Uptake

Absorption: Oral: Well absorbed

Half-life, elimination: 7.1-13.9 hours; ESRD/CAPD: 30-40 hours

Time to peak: Oral: 1 hour

Pregnancy Risk Factor C

Generic Available No

Gaviscon® Extra Strength [OTC] *see* Aluminum Hydroxide and Magnesium Carbonate *on page 62*

Gaviscon® Liquid [OTC] *see* Aluminum Hydroxide and Magnesium Carbonate *on page 62*

Gaviscon® Tablet [OTC] *see* Aluminum Hydroxide and Magnesium Trisilicate *on page 63*

Gee Gee® [OTC] *see* Guaifenesin *on page 568*

Gelatin, Absorbable (JEL a tin, ab SORB a ble)

U.S. Brand Names Gelfilm®; Gelfoam®

Pharmacologic Category Hemostatic Agent

Synonyms Absorbable Gelatin Sponge

Use

Dental: Adjunct to provide hemostasis in oral and dental surgery

Medical: In medicine, adjunct to provide hemostasis in surgery; open prostatic surgery

Local Anesthetic/Vasoconstrictor Precautions No information available to require special precautions

Effects on Dental Treatment No effects or complications reported

Dosage Hemostasis: Apply packs or sponges dry or saturated with sodium chloride. When applied dry, hold in place with moderate pressure. When applied wet, squeeze to remove air bubbles. The powder is applied as a paste prepared by adding ~ 4 mL of sterile saline solution to the powder.

Other Adverse Effects 1% to 10%: Local: Infection and abscess formation

Contraindications Closure of skin incisions (may interfere with the healing of skin edges)

Warnings/Precautions Do not sterilize by heat; do not use in the presence of infection

Dosage Forms PACK: Size 2 cm (40 cm x 2 cm) (1s); size 6 cm (40 cm x 6 cm) (6s). **PACK, dental:** Size 2 (10 mm x 20 mm x 7 mm) (15s); size 4 (20 mm x 20 mm x 7 mm) (15s)

Generic Available No

Gelatin, Pectin, and Methylcellulose

(JEL a tin, PEK tin, & meth il SEL yoo lose)

U.S. Brand Names Orabase® Plain [OTC]

Pharmacologic Category Topical Skin Product

Use Temporary relief from minor oral irritations

Local Anesthetic/Vasoconstrictor Precautions No information available to require special precautions

Effects on Dental Treatment No effects or complications reported

Dosage Press small dabs into place until the involved area is coated with a thin film; do not try to spread onto area; may be used as often as needed

Generic Available No

Gelfilm® *see* Gelatin, Absorbable *on page 550*
Gelfoam® *see* Gelatin, Absorbable *on page 550*
Gel-Kam® *see* Fluoride *on page 514*
Gel-Tin® [OTC] *see* Fluoride *on page 514*
Gelucast® *see* Zinc Gelatin *on page 1260*

Gemcitabine (jem SIT a been)

U.S. Brand Names Gemzar®

Canadian Brand Names Gemzar®

Mexican Brand Names Gemzar®

Pharmacologic Category Antineoplastic Agent, Antimetabolite

Synonyms Gemcitabine Hydrochloride

Use Treatment of patients with inoperable pancreatic cancer; in combination with cisplatin for the first-line treatment of patients with inoperable, locally advanced (stage IIIA or IIIB) or metastatic (stage IV) nonsmall cell lung cancer

Local Anesthetic/Vasoconstrictor Precautions No information available to require special precautions

Effects on Dental Treatment No effects or complications reported

Mechanism of Action Nucleoside analogue that primarily kills cells undergoing DNA synthesis (S-phase) and blocks the progression of cells through the G1/S-phase boundary

Other Adverse Effects

>10%:

- Central nervous system: Fatigue, fever (40%), lethargy, pain (10% to 48%), somnolence (5% to 11%)
- Dermatologic: Alopecia (15%); mild to moderate rashes (5% to 32%)
- Endocrine & metabolic: Increased serum transaminase levels (~66%), mild, transient
- Gastrointestinal: Mild nausea, vomiting, anorexia (20% to 70%); stomatitis (10% to 14%)
- Hematologic: Myelosuppression (20% to 30%), primarily leukopenia, may be dose-limiting
- Neuromuscular & skeletal: Weakness (15% to 25%)
- Renal: Proteinuria, hematuria (45%), elevation of BUN
- Respiratory: Mild to moderate dyspnea (10% to 23%)
- Miscellaneous: Flu-like syndrome (myalgia, fever, chills, fatigue) (20% to 100%), may be dose-limiting

1% to 10%:

- Dermatologic: Pruritus (8%)
- Gastrointestinal: Mild diarrhea (7%), constipation (6%)
- Hematologic: Thrombocytopenia (~10%), anemia (6%)
- Hepatic: Elevated bilirubin (10%)

(Continued)

Gemcitabine *(Continued)*

Neuromuscular & skeletal: Paresthesia (2% to 10%), peripheral neuropathies (paresthesias, decreased tendon reflexes) (3.5%)
Respiratory: Severe dyspnea (3%)
Miscellaneous: Allergic reactions (4%), mild, usually edema, bronchospasm

Warnings/Precautions The U.S. Food & Drug Administration (FDA) recommends that procedures for proper handling and disposal of antineoplastic agents be considered. Prolongation of the infusion time >60 minutes and more frequent than weekly dosing have been shown to increase toxicity. Gemcitabine can suppress bone marrow function manifested by leukopenia, thrombocytopenia and anemia, and myelosuppression is usually the dose-limiting ototoxicity. The incidence of fever is 41% and gemcitabine may cause fever in the absence of clinical infection. Rash has been reported in 30% of patients - typically a macular or finely granular maculopapular pruritic eruption of mild-moderate severity involving the trunk and extremities. Gemcitabine should be used with caution in patients with pre-existing renal impairment (mild proteinuria and hematuria were commonly reported; hemolytic uremic syndrome has been reported) and hepatic impairment (associated with transient elevations of serum transaminases in $^2/_3$ of patients - but no evidence of increasing hepatic toxicity).

Drug Interactions No confirmed interactions have been reported. No specific drug interaction studies have been conducted.

Drug Uptake
Half-life, elimination: Infusion time: ≤1 hour: 32-94 minutes; Infusion time: 3-4 hours: 4-10.5 hours
Time to peak: 30 minutes

Pregnancy Risk Factor D

Generic Available No

Gemfibrozil (jem FI broe zil)

Related Information
Cardiovascular Diseases *on page 1308*

U.S. Brand Names Lopid®

Canadian Brand Names Apo®-Gemfibrozil; Gen-Gemfibrozil; Lopid®; Novo-Gemfibrozil; Nu-Gemfibrozil; PMS-Gemfibrozil

Mexican Brand Names Lopid®

Pharmacologic Category Antilipemic Agent, Fibric Acid

Synonyms CI-719

Use Treatment of hypertriglyceridemia in types IV and V hyperlipidemia for patients who are at greater risk for pancreatitis and who have not responded to dietary intervention

Local Anesthetic/Vasoconstrictor Precautions No information available to require special precautions

Effects on Dental Treatment No effects or complications reported

Dosage
Adults: Oral: 1200 mg/day in 2 divided doses, 30 minutes before breakfast and dinner
Hemodialysis: Not removed by hemodialysis; supplemental dose is not necessary

Mechanism of Action The exact mechanism of action of gemfibrozil is unknown, however, several theories exist regarding the VLDL effect; it can inhibit lipolysis and decrease subsequent hepatic fatty acid uptake as well as inhibit hepatic secretion of VLDL; together these actions decrease serum VLDL levels; increases HDL cholesterol; the mechanism behind HDL elevation is currently unknown

Other Adverse Effects
>10% Gastrointestinal: Dyspepsia (20%)
1% to 10%:
Central nervous system: Fatigue (4%), vertigo (2%), headache (1%)
Dermatologic: Eczema (2%), rash (2%)
Gastrointestinal: Abdominal pain (10%), diarrhea (7%), nausea/vomiting (3%), constipation (1%)

Drug Interactions CYP3A3/4 enzyme substrate
Increased Effect/Toxicity: Gemfibrozil may potentiate the effects of bexarotene (avoid concurrent use), sulfonylureas (including glyburide, chlorpropamide), and warfarin. HMG-CoA reductase inhibitors (atorvastatin, fluvastatin, lovastatin, pravastatin, simvastatin) may increase the risk of myopathy and rhabdomyolysis. The manufacturer warns against the concurrent use of lovastatin. However, combination therapy with statins has been used in some patients with resistant hyperlipidemias (with great caution).
Decreased Effect: Cyclosporine's blood levels may be reduced during concurrent therapy. Rifampin may decreased gemfibrozil blood levels.

Drug Uptake
Onset of action: May require several days
Absorption: Well absorbed
Half-life, elimination: 1.4 hours
Time to peak: 1-2 hours

Pregnancy Risk Factor C
Generic Available Yes

Gemtuzumab Ozogamicin (gem TUZ yu mab oh zog a MY sin)

U.S. Brand Names Mylotarg™
Canadian Brand Names Mylotarg™
Pharmacologic Category Antineoplastic Agent, Monoclonal Antibody
Use Treatment of acute myeloid leukemia (CD33 positive) in first relapse in patients who are ≥60 years of age and who are not considered candidates for cytotoxic chemotherapy.
Local Anesthetic/Vasoconstrictor Precautions No information available to require special precautions
Effects on Dental Treatment High incidence (25%) of stomatitis/mucositis reported in patients >60 years of age
Mechanism of Action Antibody to CD33 antigen, which is expressed on leukemic blasts in 80% of patients with acute myeloid leukemia (AML), as well as normal myeloid cells. Binding results in internalization of the antibody-antigen complex. Following internalization, the calicheamicin derivative is released inside the myeloid cell. The calicheamicin derivative binds to DNA resulting in double strand breaks and cell death. Pluripotent stem cells and nonhematopoietic cells are not affected.
Other Adverse Effects Percentages established in adults >60 years of age.

>10%:

- Cardiovascular: Peripheral edema (21%), hypertension (20%), hypotension (16%)
- Central nervous system: Chills (66%), fever (80%), headache (26%), pain (25%), dizziness (11%), insomnia (18%)
- Dermatologic: Rash (23%), petechiae (21%), ecchymosis (15%)
- Endocrine & metabolic: Hypokalemia (30%)
- Gastrointestinal: Nausea (64%), vomiting (55%), diarrhea (38%), anorexia (31%), abdominal pain (29%), constipation (28%), stomatitis/mucositis (25%), abdominal distention (11%), dyspepsia (11%)
- Hematologic: Neutropenia (98%; median recovery 40.5 days), thrombocytopenia (99%; median recovery 39 days); anemia (47%), bleeding (15%), lymphopenia
- Hepatic: Hyperbilirubinemia (23%) increased LDH (18%), increased transaminases (9% to 17%)
- Local: Local reaction (25%)
- Neuromuscular & skeletal: Weakness (45%), back pain (18%)
- Respiratory: Dyspnea (36%), epistaxis (29%; severe 3%), cough (19%), pharyngitis (14%)
- Miscellaneous: Infection (28%), sepsis (24%), neutropenic fever (20%)

1% to 10%:

- Cardiovascular: Tachycardia (10%)
- Central nervous system: Depression (10%), cerebral hemorrhage (2%), intracranial hemorrhage (2%)
- Endocrine & metabolic: Hypomagnesemia (4%), hyperglycemia (2%)
- Genitourinary: Hematuria (10%; severe 1%), vaginal hemorrhage (7%)
- Hematologic: Hemorrhage (8%), disseminated intravascular coagulation (DIC) (2%)
- Hepatic: Elevated PT
- Neuromuscular & skeletal: Arthralgia (10%)
- Respiratory: Rhinitis (10%), hypoxia (6%), pneumonia (10%)

Drug Uptake Half-life, elimination:
Total calicheamicin: 45 hours (initial dose); 60 hours on repeat dosing
Unconjugated calicheamicin: 100 hours (no change noted in repeat dosing)
Pregnancy Risk Factor D
Generic Available No

Gemzar® *see* Gemcitabine *on page 551*
Genaced [OTC] *see* Acetaminophen, Aspirin, and Caffeine *on page 33*
Genac® Tablet [OTC] *see* Triprolidine and Pseudoephedrine *on page 1213*
Genahist® *see* DiphenhydrAMINE *on page 398*
Genapap® [OTC] *see* Acetaminophen *on page 26*
Genapap® Children [OTC] *see* Acetaminophen *on page 26*
Genapap® Extra Strength [OTC] *see* Acetaminophen *on page 26*
Genapap® Infant [OTC] *see* Acetaminophen *on page 26*
Genaphed® [OTC] *see* Pseudoephedrine *on page 1022*
Genasoft® Plus [OTC] *see* Docusate and Casanthranol *on page 407*
Genaspor® [OTC] *see* Tolnaftate *on page 1181*
Genatuss® [OTC] *see* Guaifenesin *on page 568*
Genatuss DM® [OTC] *see* Guaifenesin and Dextromethorphan *on page 569*
Gencalc® 600 [OTC] *see* Calcium Carbonate *on page 201*
Genebs® [OTC] *see* Acetaminophen *on page 26*
Genebs® Extra Strength [OTC] *see* Acetaminophen *on page 26*

Genesec® [OTC] *see* Acetaminophen and Phenyltoloxamine *on page 30*
Geneye® [OTC] *see* Tetrahydrozoline *on page 1150*
Gengraf™ *see* CycloSPORINE *on page 337*
Gen-K® *see* Potassium Chloride *on page 977*
Genoptic® *see* Gentamicin *on page 554*
Genoptic® S.O.P. *see* Gentamicin *on page 554*
Genotropin® *see* Human Growth Hormone *on page 589*
Genotropin Miniquick® *see* Human Growth Hormone *on page 589*
Genpril® [OTC] *see* Ibuprofen *on page 621*
Gentacidin® *see* Gentamicin *on page 554*
Gentak® *see* Gentamicin *on page 554*

Gentamicin (jen ta MYE sin)

Related Information
Cardiovascular Diseases *on page 1308*

U.S. Brand Names Garamycin®; Genoptic®; Genoptic® S.O.P.; Gentacidin®; Gentak®; G-myticin®

Canadian Brand Names Alcomicin®; Diogent®; Garamycin®; Garatec; Scheinpharm Gentamicin

Mexican Brand Names Garalen; Garamicina®; Genemicin®; Genenicina®; Genkova®; Genrex; Gentabac®; Gentacin®; Genta Grin®; Gentarim; Gentazaf®; Ikatin®; Nozolon; Quilagen; Servigenta; Tondex®; Yectamicina

Pharmacologic Category Antibiotic, Aminoglycoside; Antibiotic, Ophthalmic; Antibiotic, Topical

Synonyms Gentamicin Sulfate

Use Treatment of susceptible bacterial infections, normally gram-negative organisms including *Pseudomonas, Proteus, Serratia*, and gram-positive *Staphylococcus*; treatment of bone infections, respiratory tract infections, skin and soft tissue infections, as well as abdominal and urinary tract infections, endocarditis, and septicemia; used topically in treatment of superficial infections of the skin or ophthalmic infections caused by susceptible bacteria

Local Anesthetic/Vasoconstrictor Precautions No information available to require special precautions

Effects on Dental Treatment Increased salivation has been reported.

Dosage Individualization is critical because of the low therapeutic index

Use of ideal body weight (IBW) for determining the mg/kg/dose appears to be more accurate than dosing on the basis of total body weight (TBW).

In morbid obesity, dosage requirement may best be estimated using a dosing weight of IBW + 0.4 (TBW - IBW)

Initial and periodic peak and trough plasma drug levels should be determined, particularly in critically ill patients with serious infections or in disease states known to significantly alter aminoglycoside pharmacokinetics (eg, cystic fibrosis, burns, or major surgery)

Newborns: Intrathecal: 1 mg every day
Infants >3 months: Intrathecal: 1-2 mg/day
Infants and Children <5 years: I.M., I.V.: 2.5 mg/kg/dose every 8 hours*
- Cystic fibrosis: 2.5 mg/kg/dose every 6 hours

Children >5 years: I.M., I.V.: 1.5-2.5 mg/kg/dose every 8 hours*
- Prevention of bacterial endocarditis: Dental, oral, upper respiratory procedures, GI/GU procedures: 2 mg/kg with ampicillin (50 mg/kg) 30 minutes prior to procedure

*Some patients may require larger or more frequent doses (eg, every 6 hours) if serum levels document the need (ie, cystic fibrosis or febrile granulocytopenic patients)

Adults: I.M., I.V.:
- Severe life-threatening infections: 2-2.5 mg/kg/dose
- Urinary tract infections: 1.5 mg/kg/dose
- Synergy (for gram-positive infections): 1 mg/kg/dose
- Prevention of bacterial endocarditis:
  - Dental, oral, or upper respiratory procedures: 1.5 mg/kg not to exceed 80 mg with ampicillin (1-2 g) 30 minutes prior to procedure
  - GI/GU surgery: 1.5 mg/kg not to exceed 80 mg with ampicillin 2 g 30 minutes prior to procedure

Some clinicians suggest a daily dose of 4-7 mg/kg for all patients with normal renal function. This dose is at least as efficacious with similar, if not less, toxicity than conventional dosing.

Children and Adults:
- Intrathecal: 4-8 mg/day
- Ophthalmic:
  - Ointment: Instill 1/2" (1.25 cm) 2-3 times/day to every 3-4 hours
  - Solution: Instill 1-2 drops every 2-4 hours, up to 2 drops every hour for severe infections
- Topical: Apply 3-4 times/day to affected area

Dosing interval in renal impairment:
Cl_{cr} ≥60 mL/minute: Administer every 8 hours
Cl_{cr} 40-60 mL/minute: Administer every 12 hours
Cl_{cr} 20-40 mL/minute: Administer every 24 hours
Cl_{cr} <20 mL/minute: Loading dose, then monitor levels
Hemodialysis: Dialyzable; removal by hemodialysis: 30% removal of aminoglycosides occurs during 4 hours of HD; administer dose after dialysis and follow levels
Removal by continuous ambulatory peritoneal dialysis (CAPD):
Administration via CAPD fluid:
Gram-negative infection: 4-8 mg/L (4-8 mcg/mL) of CAPD fluid
Gram-positive infection (ie, synergy): 3-4 mg/L (3-4 mcg/mL) of CAPD fluid
Administration via I.V., I.M. route during CAPD: Dose as for Cl_{cr}<10 mL/minute and follow levels
Removal via continuous arteriovenous or venovenous hemofiltration: Dose as for Cl_{cr} 10-40 mL/minute and follow levels
Dosing adjustment/comments in hepatic disease: Monitor plasma concentrations

Mechanism of Action Interferes with bacterial protein synthesis by binding to 30S and 50S ribosomal subunits resulting in a defective bacterial cell membrane

Other Adverse Effects
>10%:
Central nervous system: Neurotoxicity (vertigo, ataxia)
Neuromuscular & skeletal: Gait instability
Otic: Ototoxicity (auditory), ototoxicity (vestibular)
Renal: Nephrotoxicity, decreased creatinine clearance
1% to 10%:
Cardiovascular: Edema
Dermatologic: Skin itching, reddening of skin, rash
<1%: Drowsiness, headache, pseudomotor cerebri, photosensitivity, allergic reaction, erythema, anorexia, nausea, vomiting, weight loss, increased salivation, enterocolitis, granulocytopenia, agranulocytosis, thrombocytopenia, elevated LFTs, burning, stinging, tremors, muscle cramps, weakness, dyspnea

Contraindications Hypersensitivity to gentamicin, other aminoglycosides, or any component of their formulation

Warnings/Precautions Not intended for long-term therapy due to toxic hazards associated with extended administration; pre-existing renal insufficiency, vestibular or cochlear impairment, myasthenia gravis, hypocalcemia, conditions which depress neuromuscular transmission

Parenteral aminoglycosides have been associated with significant nephrotoxicity or ototoxicity; the ototoxicity may be directly proportional to the amount of drug given and the duration of treatment; tinnitus or vertigo are indications of vestibular injury and impending hearing loss; renal damage is usually reversible

Drug Interactions Increased Toxicity: Aminoglycosides may potentiate the effects of neuromuscular-blocking agents. Penicillins, cephalosporins, amphotericin B, loop diuretics may increase nephrotoxic potential.

Drug Uptake
Absorption: Oral: None
Half-life, elimination:
Infants: <1 week old: 3-11.5 hours; 1 week to 6 months old: 3-3.5 hours
Adults: 1.5-3 hours; End-stage renal disease: 36-70 hours
Time to peak: I.M.: 30-90 minutes; I.V.: 30 minutes after 30-minute infusion

Pregnancy Risk Factor C

Breast-feeding Considerations No data reported; however, gentamicin not absorbed orally and other aminoglycosides may be taken while breast-feeding.

Dosage Forms CRM (Garamycin®, G-myticin®): 0.1% (15 g). **INF** [in D_5W]: 60 mg, 80 mg, 100 mg. **INF** [in NS]: 40 mg, 60 mg, 80 mg, 90 mg, 100 mg, 120 mg. **INJ:** 40 mg/mL (1 mL, 1.5 mL, 2 mL, 20 mL). **INJ, intrathecal** [preservative free] (Garamycin®): 2 mg/mL (2 mL). **INJ, pediatric:** 10 mg/mL (2 mL). **OINT, ophthalmic:** 0.3% [3 mg/g] (3.5 g); (Garamycin®, Genoptic® S.O.P., Gentacidin®, Gentak®): 0.3% [3 mg/g] (3.5 g). **OINT, topical** (Garamycin®, G-myticin®): 0.1% (15 g). **SOLN, ophthalmic:** 0.3% (5 mL, 15 mL); (Garamycin®, Genoptic®, Gentacidin®, Gentak®): 0.3% (1 mL, 5 mL, 15 mL)

Generic Available Yes

GenTeal™ [OTC] *see* Hydroxypropyl Methylcellulose *on page 615*

Gentian Violet (JEN shun VYE oh let)

Pharmacologic Category Antibiotic, Topical; Antifungal Agent, Topical

Synonyms Crystal Violet; Methylrosaniline Chloride

Use Treatment of cutaneous or mucocutaneous infections caused by *Candida albicans* and other superficial skin infections - antibacterial and antifungal dye

Local Anesthetic/Vasoconstrictor Precautions No information available to require special precautions

Effects on Dental Treatment No effects or complications reported

(Continued)

Gentian Violet *(Continued)*

Dosage Children and Adults: Topical: Apply 0.5% to 2% locally with cotton to lesion 2-3 times/day for 3 days, do not swallow and avoid contact with eyes

Mechanism of Action Topical antiseptic/germicide effective against some vegetative gram-positive bacteria, particularly *Staphylococcus* sp, and some yeast; it is much less effective against gram-negative bacteria and is ineffective against acid-fast bacteria

Other Adverse Effects Frequency not defined:

- Dermatologic: Vesicle formation
- Gastrointestinal: Esophagitis, ulceration of mucous membranes
- Local: Burning, irritation
- Respiratory: Laryngitis, laryngeal obstruction, tracheitis
- Miscellaneous: Sensitivity reactions

Pregnancy Risk Factor C

Generic Available Yes

Gentran® *see* Dextran *on page 369*

Geocillin® *see* Carbenicillin *on page 219*

Germinal® *see* Ergoloid Mesylates *on page 447*

Gevrabon® [OTC] *see* Vitamin B Complex *on page 1244*

Gingi-Aid® Gingival Retraction Cord *see* Aluminum Chloride *on page 61*

Gingi-Aid® Solution *see* Aluminum Chloride *on page 61*

Glatiramer Acetate (gla TIR a mer AS e tate)

U.S. Brand Names Copaxone®

Canadian Brand Names Copaxone®

Pharmacologic Category Biological, Miscellaneous

Synonyms Copolymer-1

Use Treatment of relapsing-remitting type multiple sclerosis; studies indicate that it reduces the frequency of attacks and the severity of disability; appears to be most effective for patients with minimal disability

Local Anesthetic/Vasoconstrictor Precautions No information available to require special precautions

Effects on Dental Treatment No effects or complications reported

Dosage Adults: S.C.: 20 mg daily

Mechanism of Action Glatiramer is a mixture of random polymers of four amino acids; L-alanine, L-glutamic acid, L-lysine and L-tyrosine, the resulting mixture is antigenically similar to myelin basic protein, which is an important component of the myelin sheath of nerves; glatiramer is thought to suppress T-lymphocytes specific for a myelin antigen, it is also proposed that glatiramer interferes with the antigen-presenting function of certain immune cells opposing pathogenic T-cell function

Other Adverse Effects Reported in >2% of patients in placebo-controlled trials:

>10%:

- Cardiovascular: Chest pain (21%)
- Central nervous system: Pain (28%), vasodilation (27%), anxiety (23%), palpitations (17%)
- Dermatologic: Pruritus (18%), rash (18%), diaphoresis (15%)
- Gastrointestinal: Nausea (22%), diarrhea (12%)
- Local: Injection site reactions: Pain (73%), erythema (66%), inflammation (49%), pruritus (40%), mass (27%), induration (13%), welt (11%)
- Neuromuscular & skeletal: Weakness (41%), arthralgia (24%), hypertonia (22%), back pain (16%)
- Respiratory: Dyspnea (19%), rhinitis (14%)
- Miscellaneous: Infection (50%), flu-like syndrome (19%), lymphadenopathy (12%)

1% to 10%:

- Cardiovascular: Peripheral edema (7%), facial edema (6%), edema (3%), tachycardia (5%), hypertension (1%)
- Central nervous system: Fever (8%), vertigo (6%), migraine (5%), syncope (5%), agitation (4%), chills (4%), confusion (2%), nervousness (2%), speech disorder (2%), abnormal dreams (1%), emotional lability (1%), stupor (1%)
- Dermatologic: Bruising (8%), erythema (4%), urticaria (4%), skin nodule (2%), eczema, herpes zoster, pustular rash, skin atrophy
- Endocrine & metabolic: Dysmenorrhea (6%), amenorrhea (1%), menorrhagia (1%), vaginal hemorrhage (1%)
- Gastrointestinal: Anorexia (8%), vomiting (6%), gastrointestinal disorder (5%), gastroenteritis (3%), weight gain (3%), oral moniliasis (1%), ulcerative stomatitis (1%), salivary gland enlargement
- Genitourinary: Urinary urgency (10%), vaginal moniliasis (8%), hematuria (1%), impotence (1%)
- Local: Injection site reactions: Hemorrhage (5%), urticaria (5%), edema (1%), atrophy (1%), abscess (1%), hypersensitivity (1%)
- Neuromuscular & skeletal: Tremor (7%), foot drop (3%)

Ocular: Eye disorder (4%), nystagmus (2%), visual field defect (1%)
Otic: Ear pain (7%)
Respiratory: Bronchitis (9%), laryngismus (5%)
Miscellaneous: Neck pain (8%), bacterial infection (5%), herpes simplex (4%), cyst (2%)

Contraindications Previous hypersensitivity to any component of the copolymer formulation

Pregnancy Risk Factor B

Generic Available No

Glaucon® *see* Epinephrine *on page 438*
Gliadel® *see* Carmustine *on page 225*

Glimepiride (GLYE me pye ride)

Related Information

Endocrine Disorders and Pregnancy *on page 1331*

U.S. Brand Names Amaryl®

Canadian Brand Names Amaryl®

Mexican Brand Names Amaryl®

Pharmacologic Category Antidiabetic Agent, Sulfonylurea

Use

Management of noninsulin-dependent diabetes mellitus (type 2) as an adjunct to diet and exercise to lower blood glucose

Use in combination with insulin to lower blood glucose in patients whose hyperglycemia cannot be controlled by diet and exercise in conjunction with an oral hypoglycemic agent

Local Anesthetic/Vasoconstrictor Precautions No information available to require special precautions

Effects on Dental Treatment Glimepiride-dependent diabetics (noninsulin dependent, type 2) should be appointed for dental treatment in morning in order to minimize chance of stress-induced hypoglycemia

Dosage Oral (allow several days between dose titrations):

Adults: Initial: 1-2 mg once daily, administered with breakfast or the first main meal; usual maintenance dose: 1-4 mg once daily; after a dose of 2 mg once daily, increase in increments of 2 mg at 1- to 2-week intervals based upon the patient's blood glucose response to a maximum of 8 mg once daily

Elderly: Initial: 1 mg/day

Combination with insulin therapy (fasting glucose level for instituting combination therapy is in the range of >150 mg/dL in plasma or serum depending on the patient): initial recommended dose: 8 mg once daily with the first main meal

After starting with low-dose insulin, upward adjustments of insulin can be done ~ weekly as guided by frequent measurements of fasting blood glucose. Once stable, combination-therapy patients should monitor their capillary blood glucose on an ongoing basis, preferably daily.

Mechanism of Action Stimulates insulin release from the pancreatic beta cells; reduces glucose output from the liver; insulin sensitivity is increased at peripheral target sites

Other Adverse Effects 1% to 10%:

Central nervous system: Headache, dizziness
Gastrointestinal: Nausea
Other reactions reported with sulfonylureas: Porphyria, vasculitis

Contraindications Hypersensitivity to glimepiride, other sulfonamides, or any component of their formulation; diabetic ketoacidosis (with or without coma)

Warnings/Precautions All sulfonylurea drugs are capable of producing severe hypoglycemia. Hypoglycemia is more likely to occur when caloric intake is deficient, after severe or prolonged exercise, when alcohol is ingested, or when >1 glucose-lowering drug is used.

Chemical similarities are present among sulfonamides, sulfonylureas, carbonic anhydrase inhibitors, thiazides, and loop diuretics (except ethacrynic acid). Use in patients with sulfonamide allergy is specifically contraindicated in product labeling, however a risk of cross-reaction exists in patients with allergy to any of these compounds; avoid use when previous reaction has been severe.

Product labeling states oral hypoglycemic drugs may be associated with an increased cardiovascular mortality as compared to treatment with diet alone or diet plus insulin. Data to support this association are limited, and several studies, including a large prospective trial (UKPDS) have not supported an association.

Drug Interactions CYP2C9 enzyme substrate

Increased Effect/Toxicity: Anticoagulants, androgens, fluconazole, miconazole, salicylates, gemfibrozil, sulfonamides, tricyclic antidepressants, probenecid, MAO inhibitors, beta-blockers, methyldopa, digitalis glycosides, urinary acidifiers may increase the hypoglycemic effects of glimepiride.

Decreased Effect: There may be a decreased effect of glimepiride with corticosteroids, cholestyramine, estrogens, oral contraceptives, phenytoin, rifampin, thiazide and other diuretics, phenothiazines, NSAIDs, thyroid products, nicotinic acid,

(Continued)

Glimepiride *(Continued)*

isoniazid, sympathomimetics, urinary alkalinizers, and charcoal. **Note:** However, data from pooled data did **not** demonstrate drug interactions with calcium channel blockers, estrogens, NSAIDs, HMG-CoA reductase inhibitors, sulfonamides, or thyroid hormone.

Drug Uptake

Onset of action: Peak effect: Blood glucose reductions: 2-3 hours
Absorption: 100%; delayed when given with food
Duration: 24 hours
Half-life, elimination: 5-9 hours
Time to peak: Within 2-3 hours

Pregnancy Risk Factor C

Generic Available No

GlipiZIDE (GLIP i zide)

Related Information

Endocrine Disorders and Pregnancy *on page 1331*

U.S. Brand Names Glucotrol®; Glucotrol® XL

Mexican Brand Names Glupitel®; Minodiab

Pharmacologic Category Antidiabetic Agent, Sulfonylurea

Synonyms Glydiazinamide

Use Management of type 2 diabetes mellitus (noninsulin dependent, NIDDM)

Local Anesthetic/Vasoconstrictor Precautions No information available to require special precautions

Effects on Dental Treatment Glipizide-dependent diabetics (noninsulin dependent, type 2) should be appointed for dental treatment in morning in order to minimize chance of stress-induced hypoglycemia.

Dosage Oral (allow several days between dose titrations): Give ~30 minutes before a meal to obtain the greatest reduction in postprandial hyperglycemia

Adults: Initial: 5 mg/day; adjust dosage at 2.5-5 mg daily increments as determined by blood glucose response at intervals of several days. Maximum recommended once-daily dose: 15 mg; maximum recommended total daily dose: 40 mg; extended release (Glucotrol® XL) maximum recommended dose: 20 mg.

Elderly: Initial: 2.5 mg/day; increase by 2.5-5 mg/day at 1- to 2-week intervals

Dosing adjustment/comments in renal impairment: Cl_{cr} <10 mL/minute: Some investigators recommend not using

Dosing adjustment in hepatic impairment: Initial dosage should be 2.5 mg/day

Mechanism of Action Stimulates insulin release from the pancreatic beta cells; reduces glucose output from the liver; insulin sensitivity is increased at peripheral target sites

Other Adverse Effects Frequency not defined:

Cardiovascular: Edema
Central nervous system: Headache
Dermatologic: Rash, urticaria, photosensitivity
Endocrine & metabolic: Hypoglycemia, hyponatremia, SIADH (rare)
Gastrointestinal: Anorexia, nausea, vomiting, diarrhea, epigastric fullness, constipation, heartburn
Hematologic: Blood dyscrasias, aplastic anemia, hemolytic anemia, bone marrow suppression, thrombocytopenia, agranulocytosis
Hepatic: Cholestatic jaundice, hepatic porphyria
Renal: Diuretic effect (minor)
Miscellaneous: Disulfiram-like reaction

Warnings/Precautions Use with caution in patients with severe hepatic disease; a useful agent since few drug to drug interactions and not dependent upon renal elimination of active drug.

Chemical similarities are present among sulfonamides, sulfonylureas, carbonic anhydrase inhibitors, thiazides, and loop diuretics (except ethacrynic acid). Use in patients with sulfonamide allergy is specifically contraindicated in product labeling, however a risk of cross-reaction exists in patients with allergy to any of these compounds; avoid use when previous reaction has been severe.

Product labeling states oral hypoglycemic drugs may be associated with an increased cardiovascular mortality as compared to treatment with diet alone or diet plus insulin. Data to support this association are limited, and several studies, including a large prospective trial (UKPDS) have not supported an association.

Drug Interactions

Increased Effect/Toxicity: Increased effects/hypoglycemic effects of glipizide with H_2 antagonists, anticoagulants, androgens, cimetidine, fluconazole, salicylates, gemfibrozil, sulfonamides, tricyclic antidepressants, probenecid, MAO inhibitors, methyldopa, digitalis glycosides, and urinary acidifiers.

Decreased Effect: Decreased effect of glipizide with beta-blockers, cholestyramine, hydantoins, rifampin, thiazide diuretics, urinary alkalinizers, and charcoal.

Drug Uptake

Onset of action: Peak effect: Blood glucose reductions: 1.5-2 hours

Absorption: Delayed when given with food
Duration: 12-24 hours
Half-life, elimination: 2-4 hours
Time to peak: Maximum blood glucose reductions within 1.5-2 hours

Pregnancy Risk Factor C

Generic Available Yes

GlucaGen® *see* Glucagon *on page 559*

Glucagon (GLOO ka gon)

U.S. Brand Names GlucaGen®

Pharmacologic Category Antidote; Diagnostic Agent

Use Hypoglycemia; diagnostic aid in the radiologic examination of GI tract when a hypotonic state is needed; used with some success as a cardiac stimulant in management of severe cases of beta-adrenergic blocking agent overdosage

Local Anesthetic/Vasoconstrictor Precautions No information available to require special precautions

Effects on Dental Treatment No effects or complications reported

Dosage

Hypoglycemia or insulin shock therapy: I.M., I.V., S.C.:
- Children: 0.025-0.1 mg/kg/dose, not to exceed 1 mg/dose, repeated in 20 minutes as needed
- Adults: 0.5-1 mg, may repeat in 20 minutes as needed

If patient fails to respond to glucagon, I.V. dextrose must be given

Diagnostic aid: Adults: I.M., I.V.: 0.25-2 mg 10 minutes prior to procedure

Mechanism of Action Stimulates adenylate cyclase to produce increased cyclic AMP, which promotes hepatic glycogenolysis and gluconeogenesis, causing a raise in blood glucose levels

Other Adverse Effects 1% to 10%:
Cardiovascular: Hypotension
Dermatologic: Urticaria
Gastrointestinal: Nausea, vomiting
Respiratory: Respiratory distress

Drug Interactions Glucagon and warfarin - hypoprothrombinemic effects may be increased, possibly with bleeding.

Drug Uptake
Onset of action: Peak effect: Blood glucose levels: Parenteral: 5-20 minutes
Duration: 60-90 minutes
Half-life, elimination, plasma: 3-10 minutes

Pregnancy Risk Factor B

Generic Available No

Comments 1 unit = 1 mg

Glucophage® *see* Metformin *on page 777*
Glucophage® XR *see* Metformin *on page 777*

Glucose (GLOO kose, IN stant)

Related Information
Dental Office Emergencies *on page 1418*

U.S. Brand Names B-D Glucose® [OTC]; Glutose® [OTC]; Insta-Glucose® [OTC]

Pharmacologic Category Antihypoglycemic Agent

Use Management of hypoglycemia

Local Anesthetic/Vasoconstrictor Precautions No information available to require special precautions

Effects on Dental Treatment No effects or complications reported

Dosage Adults: Oral: 10-20 g

Other Adverse Effects 1% to 10%:
Cardiovascular: Syncope
Gastrointestinal: Nausea, vomiting, diarrhea

Pregnancy Risk Factor A

Generic Available Yes

Comments 4 calories/g

Glucose Polymers (GLOO kose POL i merz)

U.S. Brand Names Moducal® [OTC]; Polycose® [OTC]; Sumacal® [OTC]

Pharmacologic Category Dietary Supplement

Use Supplies calories for those persons not able to meet the caloric requirement with usual food intake

Local Anesthetic/Vasoconstrictor Precautions No information available to require special precautions

Effects on Dental Treatment No effects or complications reported

Dosage Adults: Oral: Add to foods or beverages or mix in water

Generic Available No

Glucotrol® *see* GlipiZIDE *on page 558*

Glucotrol® XL *see* GlipiZIDE *on page 558*
Glucovance™ *see* Glyburide and Metformin *on page 561*
Glu-K® [OTC] *see* Potassium Gluconate *on page 979*

Glutamic Acid (gloo TAM ik AS id)

U.S. Brand Names Feracid®

Pharmacologic Category Gastrointestinal Agent, Miscellaneous

Synonyms Glutamic Acid Hydrochloride

Use Treatment of hypochlorhydria and achlorhydria

Local Anesthetic/Vasoconstrictor Precautions No information available to require special precautions

Effects on Dental Treatment No effects or complications reported

Dosage Adults: Oral:

Tablet/powder: 500-1000 mg/day before meals or food

Capsule: 1-3 capsules 3 times/day before meals

Other Adverse Effects Systemic acidosis may occur with massive overdosage

Pregnancy Risk Factor C

Generic Available Yes

Glutose® [OTC] *see* Glucose *on page 559*
Glyate® [OTC] *see* Guaifenesin *on page 568*

GlyBURIDE (GLYE byoor ide)

Related Information

Endocrine Disorders and Pregnancy *on page 1331*

U.S. Brand Names Diaβeta®; Glynase™ PresTab™; Micronase®

Canadian Brand Names Albert® Glyburide; Apo®-Glyburide; Diaβeta®; Euglucon®; Gen-Glybe; Novo-Glyburide; Nu-Glyburide; PMS-Glyburide

Mexican Brand Names Daonil; Euglucon®; Glibenil; Glucal; Glucoven®; Nadib®; Norboral

Pharmacologic Category Antidiabetic Agent, Sulfonylurea

Synonyms Glibenclamide; Glybenclamide; Glybenzcyclamide

Use Management of noninsulin-dependent diabetes mellitus (type 2)

Unlabeled/Investigational: Alternative to insulin in women for the treatment of gestational diabetes (11-33 weeks gestation)

Local Anesthetic/Vasoconstrictor Precautions No information available to require special precautions

Effects on Dental Treatment Glyburide-dependent diabetics (noninsulin dependent, type 2) should be appointed for dental treatment in morning in order to minimize chance of stress-induced hypoglycemia.

Dosage Oral:

Adults: 1.25-5 mg to start then increase at weekly intervals to 1.25-20 mg maintenance dose/day divided in 1-2 doses

Elderly: Initial: 1.25-2.5 mg/day, increase by 1.25-2.5 mg/day every 1-3 weeks

PresTab™: Initial: 0.75-3 mg/day, increase by 1.5 mg/day in weekly intervals, maximum: 12 mg/day

Mechanism of Action Stimulates insulin release from the pancreatic beta cells; reduces glucose output from the liver; insulin sensitivity is increased at peripheral target sites

Other Adverse Effects Frequency not defined:

Dermatologic: Pruritus, rash, urticaria, photosensitivity reaction

Endocrine & metabolic: Hypoglycemia, hyponatremia (SIADH reported with other sulfonylureas)

Gastrointestinal: Nausea, epigastric fullness, heartburn, constipation, diarrhea, anorexia

Genitourinary: Nocturia

Hematologic: Leukopenia, thrombocytopenia, hemolytic anemia, aplastic anemia, bone marrow suppression, agranulocytosis

Hepatic: Cholestatic jaundice, hepatitis

Neuromuscular & skeletal: Arthralgia, paresthesia

Ocular: Blurred vision

Renal: Diuretic effect (minor)

Warnings/Precautions Elderly: Rapid and prolonged hypoglycemia (>12 hours) despite hypertonic glucose injections have been reported; age and hepatic and renal impairment are independent risk factors for hypoglycemia; dosage titration should be made at weekly intervals. Use with caution in patients with renal and hepatic impairment, malnourished or debilitated conditions, or adrenal or pituitary insufficiency.

Chemical similarities are present among sulfonamides, sulfonylureas, carbonic anhydrase inhibitors, thiazides, and loop diuretics (except ethacrynic acid). Use in patients with sulfonamide allergy is specifically contraindicated in product labeling, however a risk of cross-reaction exists in patients with allergy to any of these compounds; avoid use when previous reaction has been severe.

Product labeling states oral hypoglycemic drugs may be associated with an increased cardiovascular mortality as compared to treatment with diet alone or diet plus insulin. Data to support this association are limited, and several studies, including a large prospective trial (UKPDS) have not supported an association.

Drug Interactions CYP3A3/4 enzyme substrate

Possible interactions between glyburide and coumarin derivatives have been reported that may either potentiate or weaken the effects of coumarin derivatives

Increased Effect: Possible interaction between glyburide and fluoroquinolone antibiotics has been reported resulting in a potentiation of hypoglycemic action of glyburide

Increased Toxicity:

Since this agent is highly protein bound, the toxic potential is increased when given concomitantly with other highly protein bound drugs (ie, phenylbutazone, oral anticoagulants, hydantoins, salicylates, NSAIDs, beta-blockers, sulfonamides) - increase hypoglycemic effect

Ethanol increases disulfiram reactions

Phenylbutazone can increase hypoglycemic effects

Certain drugs tend to produce hyperglycemia and may lead to loss of control (ie, thiazides and other diuretics, corticosteroids, phenothiazines, thyroid products, estrogens, oral contraceptives, phenytoin, nicotinic acid, sympathomimetics, calcium channel blocking drugs, and isoniazid)

Decreased Effect: Thiazides may decrease effectiveness of glyburide

Drug Uptake

Onset of action: Serum insulin levels begin to increase 15-60 minutes after a single dose

Duration: ≤24 hours

Half-life, elimination: 5-16 hours (may increase with renal or hepatic insufficiency)

Time to peak: Adults: 2-4 hours

Pregnancy Risk Factor C

Generic Available Yes

Glyburide and Metformin (GLYE byoor ide & met FOR min)

U.S. Brand Names Glucovance™

Pharmacologic Category Antidiabetic Agent, Biguanide; Antidiabetic Agent, Sulfonylurea

Synonyms Glyburide and Metformin Hydrochloride

Use Initial therapy for management of type 2 (noninsulin-dependent) diabetes mellitus when hyperglycemia cannot be managed with diet and exercise alone. Second-line therapy for management of type 2 (noninsulin-dependent) diabetes mellitus when hyperglycemia cannot be managed with a sulfonylurea or metformin along with diet and exercise.

Local Anesthetic/Vasoconstrictor Precautions No information available to require special precautions

Effects on Dental Treatment Glyburide-dependent diabetics (noninsulin dependent, type 2) should be appointed for dental treatment in morning in order to minimize chance of stress-induced hypoglycemia. Metformin-dependent diabetics (noninsulin dependent, type 2) should be appointed for dental treatment in morning in order to minimize chance of stress-induced hypoglycemia.

Dosage Adults: Oral: Dose should be individualized based on effectiveness and tolerance; titrate to minimum effective dose needed to achieve blood glucose control; **do not exceed maximum recommended doses**

Initial therapy: Glucovance™ 1.25 mg/250 mg once daily with a meal; patients with Hb A_{1c} >9% or fasting plasma glucose (FPG) >200 mg/dL may start with Glucovance™ 1.25 mg/250 mg twice daily with meals

Dosage increases may be made every 2 weeks, in increments of Glucovance™ 1.25 mg/250 mg, until a dose of glyburide 10 mg/metformin 2000 mg per day has been reached

Due to increased risk of hypoglycemia, do not start with Glucovance™ 5 mg/500 mg.

Second-line therapy: Patients previously treated with a sulfonylurea or metformin alone: Starting dose: Glucovance™ 2.5 mg/500 mg or Glucovance™ 5 mg/500 mg twice daily with the morning and evening meals; doses may be increased in increments no larger than glyburide 5 mg/metformin 500 mg, up to a maximum dose of glyburide 20 mg/metformin 2000 mg.

When switching patients previously on a sulfonylurea and metformin together, do not exceed the daily dose of glyburide (or glyburide equivalent) or metformin.

Mechanism of Action The combination of glyburide and metformin is used to improve glycemic control in patients with type 2 diabetes mellitus by using two different, but complementary, mechanisms of action:

Glyburide: Stimulates insulin release from the pancreatic beta cells; reduces glucose output from the liver; insulin sensitivity is increased at peripheral target sites

Metformin: Decreases hepatic glucose production, decreasing intestinal absorption of glucose and improves insulin sensitivity (increases peripheral glucose uptake and utilization)

(Continued)

Glyburide and Metformin *(Continued)*

Other Adverse Effects (Also refer to Glyburide *on page 560* and Metformin *on page 777*)

>10%:

Endocrine & metabolic: Hypoglycemia (11% to 38%, effects higher when increased doses were used as initial therapy)

Gastrointestinal: Diarrhea (17%)

Respiratory: Upper respiratory infection (17%)

1% to 10%:

Central nervous system: Headache (9%), dizziness (6%)

Gastrointestinal: Nausea (8%), vomiting (8%), abdominal pain (7%) (combined GI effects increased to 38% in patients taking high doses as initial therapy)

Warnings/Precautions Age, hepatic and renal impairment are independent risk factors for hypoglycemia. Use with caution in patients with hepatic impairment, malnourished or debilitated conditions, or adrenal or pituitary insufficiency. Use caution in patients with renal impairment. Metformin is substantially excreted by the kidney. The risk of accumulation and lactic acidosis increases with the degree of impairment in renal function. Alcohol will potentiate this effect. Patients with renal function below the limit of normal for their age should not receive metformin. In elderly patients, renal function should be monitored regularly. Use of concomitant medications that may affect renal function (ie, affect tubular secretion) may affect metformin disposition. Suspend treatment for surgical procedures which restrict the intake of food and fluids; do not restart treatment until oral intake and renal function are normal.

Chemical similarities are present among sulfonamides, sulfonylureas, carbonic anhydrase inhibitors, thiazides, and loop diuretics (except ethacrynic acid). Use in patients with sulfonamide allergy is specifically contraindicated in product labeling, however a risk of cross-reaction exists in patients with allergy to any of these compounds; avoid use when previous reaction has been severe.

Drug Interactions See Metformin *on page 777* and Glyburide *on page 560*

Drug Uptake

Glucovance™:

Time to peak: 2.75 hours when taken with food

Metformin: This component of Glucovance™ is bioequivalent to metformin coadministration with glyburide.

See Glyburide *on page 560* and Metformin *on page 777*

Pregnancy Risk Factor B (manufacturer); C (expert analysis)

Generic Available No

Comments

Glyburide: Symptoms of overdose include severe hypoglycemia, seizures, cerebral damage, tingling of lips and tongue, nausea, yawning, confusion, agitation, tachycardia, sweating, convulsions, stupor, and coma. Intoxications with sulfonylureas can cause hypoglycemia and are best managed with glucose administration (orally for milder hypoglycemia or by injection in more severe forms).

Metformin: Lactic acidosis may occur. Hemodialysis may be used in suspected cases of overdose.

Glycerin (GLIS er in)

U.S. Brand Names Fleet® Babylax® [OTC]; Ophthalgan®; Osmoglyn®; Sani-Supp® [OTC]

Mexican Brand Names Senosiain®

Pharmacologic Category Laxative; Ophthalmic Agent, Miscellaneous

Synonyms Glycerol

Use Constipation; reduction of intraocular pressure; reduction of corneal edema; glycerin has been administered orally to reduce intracranial pressure

Local Anesthetic/Vasoconstrictor Precautions No information available to require special precautions

Effects on Dental Treatment No effects or complications reported

Dosage

Constipation: Rectal:

Children <6 years: 1 infant suppository 1-2 times/day as needed or 2-5 mL as an enema

Children >6 years and Adults: 1 adult suppository 1-2 times/day as needed or 5-15 mL as an enema

Children and Adults:

Reduction of intraocular pressure: Oral: 1-1.8 g/kg 1-1½ hours preoperatively; additional doses may be administered at 5-hour intervals

Reduction of intracranial pressure: Oral: 1.5 g/kg/day divided every 4 hours; 1 g/kg/dose every 6 hours has also been used

Reduction of corneal edema: Ophthalmic solution: Instill 1-2 drops in eye(s) prior to examination OR for lubricant effect, instill 1-2 drops in eye(s) every 3-4 hours

Mechanism of Action Osmotic dehydrating agent which increases osmotic pressure; draws fluid into colon and thus stimulates evacuation

Other Adverse Effects Frequency not defined:

Cardiovascular: Arrhythmias

Central nervous system: Headache, confusion, dizziness, hyperosmolar nonketotic coma

Endocrine: Polydipsia, hyperglycemia, dehydration

Gastrointestinal: Nausea, vomiting, tenesmus, rectal irritation, cramping pain, diarrhea, xerostomia

Drug Uptake

Onset of action:

Decrease in intraocular pressure: Oral: 10-30 minutes

Reduction of intracranial pressure: Oral: 10-60 minutes

Constipation: Suppository: 15-30 minutes

Peak effect:

Decrease in intraocular pressure: Oral: 60-90 minutes

Reduction of intracranial pressure: Oral: 60-90 minutes

Absorption: Oral: Well absorbed; Rectal: Poor

Duration:

Decrease in intraocular pressure: Oral: 4-8 hours

Reduction of intracranial pressure: Oral: ~2-3 hours

Half-life, elimination: 30-45 minutes

Pregnancy Risk Factor C

Generic Available Yes

Glycerin, Lanolin, and Peanut Oil

(GLIS er in, LAN oh lin, & PEE nut oyl)

U.S. Brand Names Massé® Breast Cream [OTC]

Pharmacologic Category Topical Skin Product

Use Nipple care of pregnant and nursing women

Local Anesthetic/Vasoconstrictor Precautions No information available to require special precautions

Effects on Dental Treatment No effects or complications reported

Dosage Apply as often as needed

Generic Available No

Glycerol-T® *see* Theophylline and Guaifenesin *on page 1155*
Glycofed® *see* Guaifenesin and Pseudoephedrine *on page 570*

Glycopyrrolate (glye koe PYE roe late)

U.S. Brand Names Robinul®; Robinul® Forte

Pharmacologic Category Anticholinergic Agent

Synonyms Glycopyrronium Bromide

Use Inhibit salivation and excessive secretions of the respiratory tract preoperatively; reversal of neuromuscular blockade; control of upper airway secretions; adjunct in treatment of peptic ulcer

Local Anesthetic/Vasoconstrictor Precautions No information available to require special precautions

Effects on Dental Treatment >10%: Significant xerostomia; disappears with discontinuation

Dosage

Children:

Control of secretions:

Oral: 40-100 mcg/kg/dose 3-4 times/day

I.M., I.V.: 4-10 mcg/kg/dose every 3-4 hours; maximum: 0.2 mg/dose or 0.8 mg/24 hours

Intraoperative: I.V.: 4 mcg/kg not to exceed 0.1 mg; repeat at 2- to 3-minute intervals as needed

Preoperative: I.M.:

<2 years: 4.4-8.8 mcg/kg 30-60 minutes before procedure

>2 years: 4.4 mcg/kg 30-60 minutes before procedure

Children and Adults: Reverse neuromuscular blockade: I.V.: 0.2 mg for each 1 mg of neostigmine or 5 mg of pyridostigmine administered or 5-15 mcg/kg glycopyrrolate with 25-70 mcg/kg of neostigmine or 0.1-0.3 mg/kg of pyridostigmine (agents usually administered simultaneously, but glycopyrrolate may be administered first if bradycardia is present)

Adults:

Intraoperative: I.V.: 0.1 mg repeated as needed at 2- to 3-minute intervals

Preoperative: I.M.: 4.4 mcg/kg 30-60 minutes before procedure

Peptic ulcer:

Oral: 1-2 mg 2-3 times/day

I.M., I.V.: 0.1-0.2 mg 3-4 times/day

Mechanism of Action Blocks the action of acetylcholine at parasympathetic sites in smooth muscle, secretory glands, and the CNS

Other Adverse Effects

>10%:

Dermatologic: Dry skin

(Continued)

Glycopyrrolate *(Continued)*

Gastrointestinal: Constipation, dry throat, xerostomia
Local: Irritation at injection site
Respiratory: Dry nose
Miscellaneous: Diaphoresis (decreased)

1% to 10%:

Dermatologic: Increased sensitivity to light
Endocrine & metabolic: Decreased flow of breast milk
Gastrointestinal: Dysphagia

Drug Interactions

Increased Effect/Toxicity: Increased toxicity with amantadine and cyclopropane. Effects of other anticholinergic agents may be increased by glycopyrrolate.

Decreased Effect: Decreased effect of levodopa.

Drug Uptake

Onset of action: Oral: ≤50 minutes; I.M.: 20-40 minutes; I.V.: 10-15 minutes
Peak effect: Oral: ~1 hour

Absorption: Oral: Poor and erratic

Duration: Vagal effect: 2-3 hours; Inhibition of salivation: Up to 7 hours; Anticholinergic: Oral: 8-12 hours

Half-life, elimination: 20-40 minutes

Pregnancy Risk Factor B

Generic Available Yes

Glycotuss® [OTC] *see* Guaifenesin *on page 568*
Glycotuss-dM® [OTC] *see* Guaifenesin and Dextromethorphan *on page 569*
Glynase™ PresTab™ *see* GlyBURIDE *on page 560*
Gly-Oxide® Oral [OTC] *see* Carbamide Peroxide *on page 218*
Glyset™ *see* Miglitol *on page 814*
Glytuss® [OTC] *see* Guaifenesin *on page 568*
G-myticin® *see* Gentamicin *on page 554*

Gold Sodium Thiomalate (gold SOW dee um thye oh MAL ate)

U.S. Brand Names Aurolate®

Canadian Brand Names Myochrysine®

Pharmacologic Category Gold Compound

Use Treatment of progressive rheumatoid arthritis

Local Anesthetic/Vasoconstrictor Precautions No information available to require special precautions

Effects on Dental Treatment No effects or complications reported

Dosage I.M.:

Children: Initial: Test dose of 10 mg is recommended, followed by 1 mg/kg/week for 20 weeks; maintenance: 1 mg/kg/dose at 2- to 4-week intervals thereafter for as long as therapy is clinically beneficial and toxicity does not develop. Administration for 2-4 months is usually required before clinical improvement is observed.

Adults: 10 mg first week; 25 mg second week; then 25-50 mg/week until 1 g cumulative dose has been given; if improvement occurs without adverse reactions, give 25-50 mg every 2-3 weeks for 2-20 weeks, then every 3-4 weeks indefinitely

Mechanism of Action Unknown, may decrease prostaglandin synthesis or may alter cellular mechanisms by inhibiting sulfhydryl systems

Other Adverse Effects

>10%:

Dermatologic: Itching, rash
Gastrointestinal: Stomatitis, gingivitis, glossitis
Ocular: Conjunctivitis

1% to 10%:

Dermatologic: Urticaria, alopecia
Hematologic: Eosinophilia, leukopenia, thrombocytopenia
Renal: Proteinuria, hematuria

Drug Interactions Penicillamine and acetylcysteine may decrease effect of gold sodium thiomalate.

Drug Uptake

Onset of action: Delayed; may require up to 3 months
Half-life, elimination: 5 days (may increase with multiple doses)
Time to peak: 4-6 hours

Pregnancy Risk Factor C

Generic Available No

Comments Approximately 50% gold

GoLYTELY® *see* Polyethylene Glycol-Electrolyte Solution *on page 970*
Gonak™ [OTC] *see* Hydroxypropyl Methylcellulose *on page 615*
Gonal-F® *see* Follitropins *on page 531*
Goniosol® [OTC] *see* Hydroxypropyl Methylcellulose *on page 615*

Goody's® Extra Strength Headache Powder [OTC] *see* Acetaminophen, Aspirin, and Caffeine *on page 33*

Goody's PM® Powder *see* Acetaminophen and Diphenhydramine *on page 30*

Gordofilm® [OTC] *see* Salicylic Acid *on page 1072*

Gormel® Creme [OTC] *see* Urea *on page 1221*

Goserelin (GOE se rel in)

U.S. Brand Names Zoladex® Implant

Canadian Brand Names Zoladex®; Zoladex® LA

Mexican Brand Names Prozoladex; Zoladex®

Pharmacologic Category Antineoplastic Agent, Miscellaneous; Gonadotropin Releasing Hormone Analog; Luteinizing Hormone-Releasing Hormone Analog

Synonyms Goserelin Acetate

Use Prostate carcinoma: Palliative treatment of advanced carcinoma of the prostate. An alternative treatment of prostatic cancer when orchiectomy or estrogen administration are either not indicated or unacceptable to the patient. Combination with flutamide for the management of locally confined stage T2b-T4 (stage B2-C) carcinoma of the prostate.

3.6 mg implant **only**:

Unlabeled/Investigational Use:

Endometriosis: Management of endometriosis, including pain relief and reduction of endometriotic lesions for the duration of therapy

Advanced breast cancer: Palliative treatment of advanced breast cancer in pre- and perimenopausal women. Estrogen and progesterone receptor values may help to predict whether goserelin therapy is likely to be beneficial.

Note: The 10.8 mg implant is not indicated in women as the data are insufficient to support reliable suppression of serum estradiol

Local Anesthetic/Vasoconstrictor Precautions No information available to require special precautions

Effects on Dental Treatment No effects or complications reported

Dosage

Adults: S.C.: 3.6 mg injected into upper abdomen every 28 days; do not try to aspirate with the goserelin syringe, if the needle is in a large vessel, blood will immediately appear in syringe chamber

Prostate carcinoma: Intended for long-term administration

Endometriosis: Recommended duration is 6 months; retreatment is not recommended since safety data is not available

Mechanism of Action LHRH synthetic analog of luteinizing hormone-releasing hormone also known as gonadotropin-releasing hormone (GnRH) incorporated into a biodegradable depot material which allows for continuous slow release over 28 days; mechanism of action is similar to leuprolide

Other Adverse Effects Hormone replacement therapy may decrease vasomotor symptoms and loss of bone mineral density. Adverse reaction profile varies with gender and therapeutic use.

>10%:

Central nervous system: Headache (11%)

Endocrine & metabolic: Hot flashes (53% to 62% of men, 100% of women), sexual dysfunction (15% to 21%), decreased libido, impotence, impaired erection (16% to 18%), tumor flare, bone pain (23% of women, 1% to 10% of men), vaginal dryness (10% to 14%)

1% to 10%:

Cardiovascular: Anginal pain, arrhythmias, hypertension, thromboembolic events, CHF, myocardial infarction (1% to 5%), edema

Central nervous system: Lethargy (5% to 8%), anxiety, depression, dizziness, insomnia

Dermatologic: Urticaria, maculopapular rashes (10%)

Endocrine & metabolic: Gynecomastia, breast swelling (3% to 5%), bone loss, diaphoresis

Gastrointestinal: Abdominal pain, taste disturbances, diarrhea, nausea, vomiting (5%), anorexia

Changes in BP (usually transient) have been associated with goserelin use. Osteoporosis, decreased bone mineral density, and fracture have been reported rarely in men treated with goserelin.

Drug Uptake

Absorption: Oral: Inactive; S.C.: Rapid and can be detected in the serum in 10 minutes

Half-life, elimination: Bolus S.C. dose: 5 hours; Impaired renal function: 12 hours

Time to peak: S.C.: 12-15 days

Pregnancy Risk Factor X

Generic Available No

Granisetron (gra NI se tron)

U.S. Brand Names Kytril®

Canadian Brand Names Kytril®

(Continued)

Granisetron *(Continued)*

Mexican Brand Names Kytril®

Pharmacologic Category Selective 5-HT_3 Receptor Antagonist

Use Prophylaxis and treatment of chemotherapy-related emesis; may be prescribed for patients who are refractory to or have severe adverse reactions to standard antiemetic therapy. Prophylaxis of nausea and vomiting associated with radiation therapy, including total body irradiation and fractionated abdominal radiation. Granisetron may be prescribed for young patients (ie, <45 years of age who are more likely to develop extrapyramidal reactions to high-dose metoclopramide) who are to receive highly emetogenic chemotherapeutic agents (see Comments); granisetron should not be prescribed for chemotherapeutic agents with a low emetogenic potential (eg, bleomycin, busulfan, cyclophosphamide <1000 mg, etoposide, 5-fluorouracil, vinblastine, vincristine)

Unlabeled/Investigational: Prophylaxis and treatment of postoperative nausea and vomiting

Local Anesthetic/Vasoconstrictor Precautions No information available to require special precautions

Effects on Dental Treatment No effects or complications reported

Dosage Refer to individual protocols or/and institutional guidelines. A number of different dosing schedules, for varying emetic potentials, have been reported.

Oral: 2 mg once daily or 1 mg every 12 hours on days of chemotherapy

- Prophylaxis of radiation therapy-associated emesis: 2 mg once daily 1 hour before radiation therapy
- Postoperative nausea and vomiting: 40 mcg/kg

I.V.:

- Postoperative nausea and vomiting: 40 mcg/kg
  - Prophylaxis associated with cancer chemotherapy:
    - Within U.S.: 10 mcg/kg/dose (or 1 mg/dose): for some drugs (eg, carboplatin, cyclophosphamide) with a later onset of emetic action, 10 mcg/kg every 12 hours may be necessary.
    - Outside U.S.: 40 mcg/kg/dose (or 3 mg/dose); maximum: 9 mg/24 hours
  - Breakthrough: Repeat the dose 2-3 times within the first 24 hours as necessary (suggested by anecdotal information; **not** based on controlled trials, or generally recommended).

Note: Granisetron should only be given on the day(s) of chemotherapy

Dosing interval in renal impairment: No dosage adjustment required.

Dosing interval in hepatic impairment: Kinetic studies in patients with hepatic impairment showed that total clearance was ~ halved, however, standard doses were very well tolerated

Mechanism of Action Selective 5-HT_3 receptor antagonist, blocking serotonin, both peripherally on vagal nerve terminals and centrally in the chemoreceptor trigger zone

Other Adverse Effects

>10%:

- Central nervous system: Headache (10% to 21%)
- Gastrointestinal: Constipation (3% to 18%)

1% to 10%:

- Cardiovascular: Hypertension (1%)
- Central nervous system: Dizziness, insomnia, anxiety, somnolence, fever
- Gastrointestinal: Abdominal pain, diarrhea (1% to 9%), dyspepsia
- Hepatic: Elevated liver enzymes (5% to 6%)
- Neuromuscular & skeletal: Weakness (5% to 18%)

Drug Interactions CYP3A3/4 enzyme substrate

Drug Uptake

Onset of antiemetic effect: 1-3 minutes

Duration: ≤24 hours maximum

Half-life, elimination: 3-4 hours; Cancer: 10-12 hours

Pregnancy Risk Factor B

Generic Available No

Comments

Agents with high emetogenic potential (>90%) (dose/m^2):

- Amifostine
- Azacitidine
- Carmustine ≥200 mg/m^2
- Cisplatin ≥50 mg/m^2
- Cyclophosphamide ≥1 g/m^2
- Cytarabine ≥1500 mg/m^2
- Dacarbazine ≥500 mg/m^2
- Dactinomycin
- Doxorubicin ≥60 mg/m^2
- Lomustine ≥60 mg/m^2
- Mechlorethamine
- Melphalan ≥100 mg/m^2
- Streptozocin

Thiotepa ≥100 mg/m²

or two agents classified as having high or moderately high emetogenic potential as listed:

Agents with moderately high emetogenic potential (60% to 90%) (dose/m²):
- Carboplatin 200-400 mg/m²
- Carmustine <200 mg/m²
- Cisplatin <50 mg/m²
- Cyclophosphamide 600-999 mg/m²
- Dacarbazine <500 mg/m²
- Doxorubicin 21-59 mg/m²
- Hexamethyl melamine
- Ifosfamide ≥5000 mg/m²
- Lomustine <60 mg/m²
- Methotrexate ≥250 mg/m²
- Pentostatin
- Procarbazine

Granulex *see* Trypsin, Balsam Peru, and Castor Oil *on page 1218*
Grifulvin® V *see* Griseofulvin *on page 567*

Griseofulvin (gri see oh FUL vin)

U.S. Brand Names Fulvicin® P/G; Fulvicin-U/F®; Grifulvin® V; Gris-PEG®

Canadian Brand Names Fulvicin® U/F

Mexican Brand Names Fulvina® P/G; Grisovin®; Grisovin-FP

Pharmacologic Category Antifungal Agent, Oral

Synonyms Griseofulvin Microsize; Griseofulvin Ultramicrosize

Use Treatment of susceptible tinea infections of the skin, hair, and nails

Local Anesthetic/Vasoconstrictor Precautions No information available to require special precautions

Effects on Dental Treatment May cause soreness or irritation of mouth or tongue

Dosage Oral:

Children >2 years:
- Microsize: 10-15 mg/kg/day in single or divided doses
- Ultramicrosize: 5.5-7.3 mg/kg/day in single or divided doses

Adults:
- Microsize: 500-1000 mg/day in single or divided doses
- Ultramicrosize: 330-375 mg/day in single or divided doses; doses up to 750 mg/day have been used for infections more difficult to eradicate such as tinea unguium and tinea pedis

Duration of therapy depends on the site of infection:
- Tinea corporis: 2-4 weeks
- Tinea capitis: 4-6 weeks or longer
- Tinea pedis: 4-8 weeks
- Tinea unguium: 4-6 months

Mechanism of Action Inhibits fungal cell mitosis at metaphase; binds to human keratin making it resistant to fungal invasion

Other Adverse Effects Frequency not defined:
- Central nervous system: Headache, fatigue, dizziness, insomnia, mental confusion
- Dermatologic: Rash (most common), urticaria (most common), photosensitivity, angioneurotic edema (rare)
- Gastrointestinal: Nausea, vomiting, epigastric distress, diarrhea, GI bleeding
- Genitourinary: Menstrual irregularities (rare)
- Hematologic: Leukopenia
- Neuromuscular & skeletal: Paresthesia (rare)
- Renal: Hepatotoxicity, proteinuria, nephrosis
- Miscellaneous: Oral thrush, drug-induced lupus-like syndrome (rare)

Drug Interactions CYP1A2 enzyme inducer

Decreased effect:
- Barbiturates may decrease levels of griseofulvin
- Decreased warfarin, cyclosporine, and salicylate activity with griseofulvin
- Griseofulvin decreases oral contraceptive effectiveness

Increased toxicity: With ethanol, may cause tachycardia and flushing

Drug Uptake

Absorption: Ultramicrosize griseofulvin absorption is almost complete; absorption of microsize griseofulvin is variable (25% to 70% of an oral dose); absorption is enhanced by ingestion of a fatty meal

Half-life, elimination: 9-22 hours

Pregnancy Risk Factor C

Generic Available Yes: Ultramicrosized product

Gris-PEG® *see* Griseofulvin *on page 567*
Guaifed® [OTC] *see* Guaifenesin and Pseudoephedrine *on page 570*
Guaifed-PD® *see* Guaifenesin and Pseudoephedrine *on page 570*

Guaifenesin (gwye FEN e sin)

Related Information

Guaifenesin and Phenylephrine *on page 569*
Guaifenesin, Pseudoephedrine, and Dextromethorphan *on page 571*

U.S. Brand Names Anti-Tuss® Expectorant [OTC]; Breonesin® [OTC]; Diabetic Tussin® EX [OTC]; Duratuss-G®; Fenesin™; Gee Gee® [OTC]; Genatuss® [OTC]; Glyate® [OTC]; Glycotuss® [OTC]; Glytuss® [OTC]; Guaifenex® LA; Guiatuss® [OTC]; Humibid® L.A.; Humibid® Sprinkle; Hytuss® [OTC]; Hytuss-2X® [OTC]; Liquibid®; Monafed®; Muco-Fen-LA®; Mytussin® [OTC]; Naldecon® Senior EX [OTC]; Organidin® NR; Pneumomist®; Respa-GF®; Robitussin® [OTC]; Scot-Tussin® [OTC]; Siltussin® [OTC]; Sinumist®-SR Capsulets®; Touro Ex®; Tusibron® [OTC]; Uni-tussin® [OTC]

Canadian Brand Names Balminil Expectorant; Benylin® E Extra Strength; Koffex Expectorant; Robitussin®

Mexican Brand Names Formula E; Tukol®

Pharmacologic Category Expectorant

Synonyms GG; Glycerol Guaiacolate

Use Temporary control of cough due to minor throat and bronchial irritation

Local Anesthetic/Vasoconstrictor Precautions No information available to require special precautions

Effects on Dental Treatment No effects or complications reported

Dosage Oral:

Children:
- <2 years: 12 mg/kg/day in 6 divided doses
- 2-5 years: 50-100 mg every 4 hours, not to exceed 600 mg/day
- 6-11 years: 100-200 mg every 4 hours, not to exceed 1.2 g/day

Children >12 years and Adults: 200-400 mg every 4 hours to a maximum of 2.4 g/day

Mechanism of Action Thought to act as an expectorant by irritating the gastric mucosa and stimulating respiratory tract secretions, thereby increasing respiratory fluid volumes and decreasing phlegm viscosity

Other Adverse Effects 1% to 10%:

Central nervous system: Drowsiness, headache
Dermatologic: Rash
Gastrointestinal: Nausea, vomiting, stomach pain

Drug Interactions May increase toxicity/effect of disulfiram, MAO inhibitors, metronidazole, and procarbazine

Drug Uptake

Absorption: Well absorbed
Half-life, elimination: ~1 hour

Pregnancy Risk Factor C

Generic Available Yes

Guaifenesin and Codeine (gwye FEN e sin & KOE deen)

U.S. Brand Names Brontex® Liquid; Brontex® Tablet; Cheracol®; Guaituss AC®; Guiatussin® With Codeine; Mytussin® AC; Robafen® AC; Robitussin® A-C; Tussi-Organidin® NR

Pharmacologic Category Antitussive; Cough Preparation; Expectorant

Synonyms Codeine and Guaifenesin

Use Temporary control of cough due to minor throat and bronchial irritation

Local Anesthetic/Vasoconstrictor Precautions No information available to require special precautions

Effects on Dental Treatment No effects or complications reported

Restrictions C-V

Dosage Oral:

Children:
- 2-6 years: 1-1.5 mg/kg codeine/day divided into 4 doses administered every 4-6 hours (maximum: 30 mg/24 hours)
- 6-12 years: 5 mL every 4 hours, not to exceed 30 mL/24 hours

Children >12 years and Adults: 5-10 mL every 4-8 hours not to exceed 60 mL/24 hours

Mechanism of Action

Guaifenesin is thought to act as an expectorant by irritating the gastric mucosa and stimulating respiratory tract secretions, thereby increasing respiratory fluid volumes and decreasing phlegm viscosity

Codeine is an antitussive that controls cough by depressing the medullary cough center

Other Adverse Effects

Based on **guaifenesin** component:
Central nervous system: Drowsiness, headache
Dermatologic: Rash
Gastrointestinal: Nausea, vomiting, stomach pain

Based on **codeine** component:

>10%:

Central nervous system: Drowsiness

Gastrointestinal: Constipation

1% to 10%:

Cardiovascular: Tachycardia or bradycardia, hypotension

Central nervous system: Dizziness, lightheadedness, false feeling of well being, malaise, headache, restlessness, paradoxical CNS stimulation, confusion

Dermatologic: Rash, urticaria

Gastrointestinal: Xerostomia, anorexia, nausea, vomiting,

Genitourinary: Decreased urination, ureteral spasm

Hepatic: Increased LFTs

Local: Burning at injection site

Neuromuscular & skeletal: Weakness

Ocular: Blurred vision

Respiratory: Dyspnea

Miscellaneous: Histamine release

Drug Interactions See Guaifenesin *on page 568* and Codeine *on page 317*

Drug Uptake See Guaifenesin *on page 568* and Codeine *on page 317*

Pregnancy Risk Factor C

Generic Available Yes

Guaifenesin and Dextromethorphan

(gwye FEN e sin & deks troe meth OR fan)

U.S. Brand Names Benylin® Expectorant [OTC]; Cheracol® D [OTC]; Clear Tussin® 30; Diabetic Tussin® DM [OTC]; Extra Action Cough Syrup [OTC]; Fenesin™ DM; Genatuss DM® [OTC]; Glycotuss-dM® [OTC]; Guaifenex® DM; GuiaCough® [OTC]; Guiatuss-DM® [OTC]; Halotussin® DM [OTC]; Humibid® DM [OTC]; Iobid DM®; Kolephrin® GG/DM [OTC]; Monafed® DM; Muco-Fen-DM®; Mytussin® DM [OTC]; Naldecon® Senior DX [OTC]; Phanatuss® Cough Syrup [OTC]; Phenadex® Senior [OTC]; Respa®-DM; Rhinosyn-DMX® [OTC]; Robafen DM® [OTC]; Robitussin®-DM [OTC]; Safe Tussin® 30 [OTC]; Scot-Tussin® Senior Clear [OTC]; Siltussin DM® [OTC]; Synacol® CF [OTC]; Syracol-CF® [OTC]; Tolu-Sed® DM [OTC]; Tusibron-DM® [OTC]; Tuss-DM® [OTC]; Tussi-Organidin® DM NR; Uni-tussin® DM [OTC]; Vicks® 44E [OTC]; Vicks® Pediatric Formula 44E [OTC]

Canadian Brand Names Balminil DM E; Benylin® DM-E; Koffex DM-Expectorant; Robitussin® DM

Pharmacologic Category Antitussive; Cough Preparation; Expectorant

Synonyms Dextromethorphan and Guaifenesin

Use Temporary control of cough due to minor throat and bronchial irritation

Local Anesthetic/Vasoconstrictor Precautions No information available to require special precautions

Effects on Dental Treatment No effects or complications reported

Dosage Oral:

Children: Dextromethorphan: 1-2 mg/kg/24 hours divided 3-4 times/day

Children >12 years and Adults: 5 mL every 4 hours or 10 mL every 6-8 hours not to exceed 40 mL/24 hours

Mechanism of Action

Guaifenesin is thought to act as an expectorant by irritating the gastric mucosa and stimulating respiratory tract secretions, thereby increasing respiratory fluid volumes and decreasing phlegm viscosity

Dextromethorphan is a chemical relative of morphine lacking narcotic properties except in overdose; controls cough by depressing the medullary cough center

Other Adverse Effects 1% to 10%:

Central nervous system: Drowsiness, headache

Dermatologic: Rash

Gastrointestinal: Nausea, vomiting

Warnings/Precautions Research on chicken embryos exposed to concentrations of dextromethorphan relative to those typically taken by humans has shown to cause birth defects and fetal death; more study is needed, but it is suggested that pregnant women should be advised not to use dextromethorphan-containing medications

Drug Interactions See Guaifenesin *on page 568* and Dextromethorphan *on page 372*

Drug Uptake

Onset of action: Oral: Antitussive: 15-30 minutes

See Guaifenesin *on page 568* and Dextromethorphan *on page 372*

Pregnancy Risk Factor C

Generic Available Yes

Guaifenesin and Phenylephrine (gwye FEN e sin & fen il EF rin)

U.S. Brand Names Deconsal® Sprinkle®; Endal®; Sinupan®

Pharmacologic Category Decongestant; Expectorant

Synonyms Phenylephrine and Guaifenesin

(Continued)

Guaifenesin and Phenylephrine *(Continued)*

Use Symptomatic relief of those respiratory conditions where tenacious mucous plugs and congestion complicate the problem such as sinusitis, pharyngitis, bronchitis, asthma, and as an adjunctive therapy in serous otitis media

Local Anesthetic/Vasoconstrictor Precautions Use with caution since phenylephrine is a sympathomimetic amine which could interact with epinephrine to cause a pressor response

Effects on Dental Treatment

Guaifenesin: No effects or complications reported

Phenylephrine: Up to 10% of patients could experience tachycardia, palpitations, and xerostomia; use vasoconstrictor with caution

Dosage Oral: Adults: 1 or 2 every 12 hours

Mechanism of Action See Guaifenesin *on page 568* and Phenylephrine *on page 950*

Other Adverse Effects See Guaifenesin *on page 568* and Phenylephrine *on page 950*

Drug Interactions See Guaifenesin *on page 568* and Phenylephrine *on page 950*

Drug Uptake See Guaifenesin *on page 568* and Phenylephrine *on page 950*

Generic Available No

Guaifenesin and Pseudoephedrine

(gwye FEN e sin & soo doe e FED rin)

U.S. Brand Names Congess® Jr; Congess® Sr; Congestac®; Deconsal® II; Defen-LA®; Duratuss™; Entex® PSE; Eudal®-SR; Fedahist® Expectorant [OTC]; Glycofed®; Guaifed® [OTC]; Guaifed-PD®; Guaifenex® PSE; GuaiMAX-D®; Guaitab®; Guaivent®; Guai-Vent/PSE®; Histalet® X; Maxifed®; Maxifed-G®; Nasabid™; Respa-1st®; Respaire®-60 SR; Respaire®-120 SR; Robitussin-PE® [OTC]; Robitussin® Severe Congestion Liqui-Gels® [OTC]; Ru-Tuss® DE; Rymed®; Sinufed® Timecelles®; Touro LA®; V-Dec-m®; Versacaps®; Zephrex®; Zephrex LA®

Canadian Brand Names Novahistex® Expectorant with Decongestant

Pharmacologic Category Decongestant; Expectorant

Synonyms Pseudoephedrine and Guaifenesin

Use Enhance the output of respiratory tract fluid and reduce mucosal congestion and edema in the nasal passage

Local Anesthetic/Vasoconstrictor Precautions Use with caution since pseudoephedrine is a sympathomimetic amine which could interact with epinephrine to cause a pressor response

Effects on Dental Treatment

Guaifenesin: No effects or complications reported

Pseudoephedrine: Up to 10% of patients could experience tachycardia, palpitations, and xerostomia; use vasoconstrictor with caution

Dosage Oral:

Children:

- 2-6 years: 2.5 mL every 4 hours not to exceed 15 mL/24 hours
- 6-12 years: 5 mL every 4 hours not to exceed 30 mL/24 hours

Children >12 years and Adults: 10 mL every 4 hours not to exceed 60 mL/24 hours

Drug Interactions See Guaifenesin *on page 568* and Pseudoephedrine *on page 1022*

Drug Uptake See Guaifenesin *on page 568* and Pseudoephedrine *on page 1022*

Pregnancy Risk Factor C

Generic Available Yes

Guaifenesin, Pseudoephedrine, and Codeine

(gwye FEN e sin, soo doe e FED rin, & KOE deen)

U.S. Brand Names Codafed® Expectorant; Cycofed® Pediatric; Decohistine® Expectorant; Deproist® Expectorant With Codeine; Dihistine® Expectorant; Guiatuss DAC®; Guiatussin® DAC; Halotussin® DAC; Isoclor® Expectorant; Mytussin® DAC; Nucofed®; Nucofed® Pediatric Expectorant; Nucotuss®; Phenhist® Expectorant; Robitussin®-DAC; Ryna-CX®; Tussar® SF Syrup

Canadian Brand Names Benylin® 3.3 mg-D-E; Calmylin with Codeine

Pharmacologic Category Antitussive/Decongestant/Expectorant

Synonyms Codeine, Guaifenesin, and Pseudoephedrine; Pseudoephedrine, Guaifenesin, and Codeine

Use Temporarily relieves nasal congestion and controls cough due to minor throat and bronchial irritation; helps loosen phlegm and thin bronchial secretions to make coughs more productive

Local Anesthetic/Vasoconstrictor Precautions Use with caution since pseudoephedrine is a sympathomimetic amine which could interact with epinephrine to cause a pressor response

Effects on Dental Treatment

Codeine: <1%: Xerostomia

Guaifenesin: No effects or complications reported

Pseudoephedrine: Up to 10% of patients could experience tachycardia, palpitations, and xerostomia; use vasoconstrictor with caution

Restrictions C-III; C-V

Dosage Oral:

Children 6-12 years: 5 mL every 4 hours, not to exceed 40 mL/24 hours

Children >12 years and Adults: 10 mL every 4 hours, not to exceed 40 mL/24 hours

Drug Interactions See Guaifenesin *on page 568*, Pseudoephedrine *on page 1022* and Codeine *on page 317*

Drug Uptake See Guaifenesin *on page 568*, Pseudoephedrine *on page 1022* and Codeine *on page 317*

Pregnancy Risk Factor C

Generic Available Yes

Guaifenesin, Pseudoephedrine, and Dextromethorphan

(gwye FEN e sin, soo doe e FED rin, & deks troe meth OR fan)

U.S. Brand Names Anatuss® DM [OTC]; Dimacol® Caplets [OTC]; Maxifed® DM; Rhinosyn-X® Liquid [OTC]; Ru-Tuss® Expectorant [OTC]; Sudafed® Cold & Cough Liquid Caps [OTC]

Canadian Brand Names Balminil DM + Decongestant + Expectorant; Benylin® DM-D-E; Koffex DM + Decongestant + Expectorant; Novahistex® DM Decongestant Expectorant; Novahistine® DM Decongestant Expectorant; Robitussin® Cough & Cold®

Pharmacologic Category Antitussive/Decongestant/Expectorant

Synonyms Dextromethorphan, Guaifenesin, and Pseudoephedrine; Pseudoephedrine, Dextromethorphan, and Guaifenesin

Use Temporarily relieves nasal congestion and controls cough due to minor throat and bronchial irritation; helps loosen phlegm and thin bronchial secretions to make coughs more productive

Local Anesthetic/Vasoconstrictor Precautions Use with caution since pseudoephedrine is a sympathomimetic amine which could interact with epinephrine to cause a pressor response

Effects on Dental Treatment

Guaifenesin: No effects or complications reported

Pseudoephedrine: Up to 10% of patients could experience tachycardia, palpitations, and xerostomia; use vasoconstrictor with caution

Dextromethorphan: No effects or complications reported

Dosage Adults: Oral: 2 capsules (caplets) or 10 mL every 4 hours

Mechanism of Action See Guaifenesin *on page 568*, Pseudoephedrine *on page 1022*, and Dextromethorphan *on page 372*

Other Adverse Effects See Guaifenesin *on page 568*, Pseudoephedrine *on page 1022*, and Dextromethorphan *on page 372*

Warnings/Precautions Research on chicken embryos exposed to concentrations of dextromethorphan relative to those typically taken by humans has shown to cause birth defects and fetal death; more study is needed, but it is suggested that pregnant women should be advised not to use dextromethorphan-containing medications

Drug Interactions See Guaifenesin *on page 568*, Pseudoephedrine *on page 1022* and Dextromethorphan *on page 372*

Drug Uptake See Guaifenesin *on page 568*, Pseudoephedrine *on page 1022* and Dextromethorphan *on page 372*

Generic Available Yes

Guaifenex® DM *see* Guaifenesin and Dextromethorphan *on page 569*

Guaifenex® LA *see* Guaifenesin *on page 568*

Guaifenex® PSE *see* Guaifenesin and Pseudoephedrine *on page 570*

GuaiMAX-D® *see* Guaifenesin and Pseudoephedrine *on page 570*

Guaitab® *see* Guaifenesin and Pseudoephedrine *on page 570*

Guaituss AC® *see* Guaifenesin and Codeine *on page 568*

Guaivent® *see* Guaifenesin and Pseudoephedrine *on page 570*

Guai-Vent/PSE® *see* Guaifenesin and Pseudoephedrine *on page 570*

Guanabenz (GWAHN a benz)

Related Information

Cardiovascular Diseases *on page 1308*

U.S. Brand Names Wytensin®

Canadian Brand Names Wytensin®

Pharmacologic Category $Alpha_2$-Adrenergic Agonist

Synonyms Guanabenz Acetate

Use Management of hypertension

Local Anesthetic/Vasoconstrictor Precautions No information available to require special precautions

Effects on Dental Treatment >10%: Significant xerostomia; normal salivation occurs with discontinuation

(Continued)

Guanabenz *(Continued)*

Dosage Adults: Oral: Initial: 4 mg twice daily, increase in increments of 4-8 mg/day every 1-2 weeks to a maximum of 32 mg twice daily

Mechanism of Action Stimulates $alpha_2$-adrenoreceptors in the brain stem, thus activating an inhibitory neuron, resulting in reduced sympathetic outflow, producing a decrease in vasomotor tone and heart rate

Other Adverse Effects Higher rates with larger doses

>5% (at doses of 16 mg/day):
- Cardiovascular: Orthostasis
- Central nervous system: Drowsiness or sedation (39%), dizziness (12% to 17%), headache (5%)
- Gastrointestinal: Xerostomia (28% to 38%)
- Neuromuscular & skeletal: Weakness (~10%)

≤3% (may be similar to placebo):
- Cardiovascular: Arrhythmias, palpitations, chest pain, edema
- Central nervous system: Anxiety, ataxia, depression, sleep disturbances
- Dermatologic: Rash, pruritus
- Endocrine & metabolic: Disturbances of sexual function, gynecomastia, decreased sexual function
- Gastrointestinal: Diarrhea, vomiting, constipation, nausea
- Genitourinary: Polyuria
- Neuromuscular & skeletal: Myalgia
- Ocular: Blurring of vision
- Respiratory: Nasal congestion, dyspnea
- Miscellaneous: Taste disorders

Drug Interactions

Increased Effect/Toxicity: Nitroprusside and guanabenz have additive hypotensive effects. Noncardioselective beta-blockers (nadolol, propranolol, timolol) may exacerbate rebound hypertension when guanabenz is withdrawn. The beta-blocker should be withdrawn first. The gradual withdrawal of guanabenz or a cardioselective beta-blocker could be substituted.

Decreased Effect: TCAs decrease the hypotensive effect of guanabenz. Hypoglycemic agents: Hypoglycemic symptoms may be reduced. Educate patient about decreased signs and symptoms of hypoglycemia or avoid use in patients with frequent episodes of hypoglycemia.

Drug Uptake

Onset of action: Antihypertensive: ~1 hour
Absorption: ~75%
Half-life, elimination: 7-10 hours

Pregnancy Risk Factor C

Generic Available Yes

Guanadrel (GWAHN a drel)

Related Information

Cardiovascular Diseases *on page 1308*

U.S. Brand Names Hylorel®

Canadian Brand Names Hylorel®

Pharmacologic Category False Neurotransmitter

Synonyms Guanadrel Sulfate

Use Considered a second line agent in the treatment of hypertension, usually with a diuretic

Local Anesthetic/Vasoconstrictor Precautions

Manufacturer's information states that guanadrel may block vasopressor activity of epinephrine. This has not been observed during use of epinephrine as a vasoconstrictor in local anesthesia.

Effects on Dental Treatment No effects or complications reported

Dosage Oral: Initial:

Adults: 10 mg/day (5 mg twice daily); adjust dosage until BP is controlled, usual dosage: 20-75 mg/day, given twice daily

Elderly: 5 mg once daily

Mechanism of Action Acts as a false neurotransmitter that blocks the adrenergic actions of norepinephrine; it displaces norepinephrine from its presynaptic storage granules and thus exposes it to degradation; it thereby produces a reduction in total peripheral resistance and, therefore, BP

Other Adverse Effects

>10%:
- Cardiovascular: Palpitations (30%), chest pain (28%), peripheral edema (29%)
- Central nervous system: Fatigue (64%), headache (58%), faintness (47% to 49%), drowsiness (45%), confusion (15%)
- Gastrointestinal: Increased bowel movements (31%), gas pain (24% to 32%), constipation (21%), anorexia (19%), weight gain/loss (42% to 44%)
- Genitourinary: Nocturia (48%), polyuria (34%), ejaculation disturbances (18%)
- Neuromuscular & skeletal: Paresthesia (25%), aching limbs (43%), leg cramps (20% to 26%)

Ocular: Visual disturbances (29%)
Respiratory: Dyspnea at rest (18%), coughing (27%)
1% to 10%:
Cardiovascular: Orthostatic hypotension
Central nervous system: Psychological problems (4%), depression (2%), sleep disorders (2%)
Gastrointestinal: Glossitis (8%), nausea/vomiting (4%), xerostomia (2%)
Genitourinary: Impotence (5%)
Renal: Hematuria (2%)

Drug Interactions

Increased Effect/Toxicity: Increased toxicity of direct-acting amines (epinephrine, norepinephrine) by guanadrel; the hypotensive effect of guanadrel may be potentiated. Increased effect of beta-blockers, vasodilators. Norepinephrine/phenylephrine have exaggerated pressor response; monitor BP closely. MAO inhibitors may cause severe hypertension; give at least 1 week apart.

Decreased Effect: TCAs decrease hypotensive effect of guanadrel. Phenothiazines may inhibit the antihypertensive response to guanadrel; consider an alternative antihypertensive with different mechanism of action. Amphetamines, related sympathomimetics, and methylphenidate decrease the antihypertensive response to guanadrel; consider an alternative antihypertensive with different mechanism of action. Reassess the need for amphetamine, related sympathomimetic, or methylphenidate; consider alternatives. Ephedrine may inhibit the antihypertensive response to guanadrel; consider an alternative antihypertensive with different mechanism of action. Reassess the need for ephedrine.

Drug Uptake

Onset of action: Peak effect: 4-6 hours
Absorption: Oral: Rapid
Duration: 4-14 hours
Half-life, elimination: Biphasic: Initial: 1-4 hours; Terminal: 5-45 hours
Time to peak: 1.5-2 hours

Pregnancy Risk Factor B

Generic Available No

Guanethidine (gwahn ETH i deen)

Related Information

Cardiovascular Diseases *on page 1308*

U.S. Brand Names Ismelin®

Pharmacologic Category False Neurotransmitter

Synonyms Guanethidine Monosulfate

Use Treatment of moderate to severe hypertension

Local Anesthetic/Vasoconstrictor Precautions Manufacturer's information states that haloperidol may block vasopressor activity of epinephrine. This has not been observed during use of epinephrine as a vasoconstrictor in local anesthesia.

Effects on Dental Treatment No effects or complications reported

Dosage Oral:

Children: Initial: 0.2 mg/kg/day, increase by 0.2 mg/kg/day at 7- to 10-day intervals to a maximum of 3 mg/kg/day
Adults:
Ambulatory patients: Initial: 10 mg/day, increase at 5- to 7-day intervals to a maximum of 25-50 mg/day
Hospitalized patients: Initial: 25-50 mg/day, increase by 25-50 mg/day or every other day to desired therapeutic response
Elderly: Initial: 5 mg once daily

Mechanism of Action Acts as a false neurotransmitter that blocks the adrenergic actions of norepinephrine; it displaces norepinephrine from its presynaptic storage granules and thus exposes it to degradation; it thereby produces a reduction in total peripheral resistance and, therefore, BP

Other Adverse Effects Frequency not defined:

Cardiovascular: Palpitations, bradycardia, chest pain, peripheral edema, orthostatic hypotension
Central nervous system: Fatigue, headache, faintness, drowsiness, confusion, psychological problems, depression, sleep disorders, syncope, dizziness
Gastrointestinal: Increased bowel movements, gas pain, constipation, anorexia, weight gain/loss, glossitis, nausea, vomiting, xerostomia
Genitourinary: Nocturia, polyuria, impotence, ejaculation disturbances
Neuromuscular & skeletal: Paresthesia, aching limbs, leg cramps, backache, arthralgia
Ocular: Visual disturbances
Renal: Hematuria
Respiratory: Dyspnea, coughing

Drug Interactions

Increased Effect/Toxicity: Norepinephrine/phenylephrine may have exaggerated pressor response; monitor BP closely. Minoxidil may cause severe orthostatic hypotension; avoid concurrent use. Enflurane may cause hypotension; avoid concurrent use.

(Continued)

Guanethidine *(Continued)*

Decreased Effect: TCAs and phenothiazines may inhibit the antihypertensive response to guanethidine consider an alternative antihypertensive with different mechanism of action. Amphetamines, related sympathomimetics, and methylphenidate decrease the antihypertensive response to guanethidine; consider an alternative antihypertensive with different mechanism of action. Reassess the need for amphetamine, related sympathomimetic, or methylphenidate; consider alternatives. Ephedrine may inhibit the antihypertensive response to guanethidine; consider an alternative antihypertensive with different mechanism of action. Reassess the need for ephedrine. Oral contraceptives may decrease hypotensive effect; avoid concurrent use.

Drug Uptake

Onset of action: 0.5-2 hours; Peak effect: Antihypertensive: 6-8 hours
Absorption: Irregular (3% to 55%)
Duration: 24-48 hours
Half-life, elimination: 5-10 days

Pregnancy Risk Factor C

Generic Available No

Guanfacine (GWAHN fa seen)

Related Information

Cardiovascular Diseases *on page 1308*

U.S. Brand Names Tenex®

Canadian Brand Names Tenex®

Pharmacologic Category $Alpha_2$-Adrenergic Agonist

Synonyms Guanfacine Hydrochloride

Use Management of hypertension

Local Anesthetic/Vasoconstrictor Precautions No information available to require special precautions

Effects on Dental Treatment >10%: Xerostomia

Dosage Adults: Oral: 1 mg usually at bedtime, may increase if needed at 3- to 4-week intervals to a maximum of 3 mg/day; 1 mg/day is most common dose

Mechanism of Action Stimulates $alpha_2$-adrenoreceptors in the brain stem, thus activating an inhibitory neuron, resulting in reduced sympathetic outflow, producing a decrease in vasomotor tone and heart rate

Other Adverse Effects

>10%:
- Central nervous system: Somnolence (~10%), fatigue (12%)
- Gastrointestinal: Xerostomia (47%), constipation (16%)

1% to 10%:
- Cardiovascular; Hypotension, orthostasis
- Central nervous system: Headache (4%), insomnia (4%), dizziness (6%)
- Endocrine & metabolic: Decreased sexual ability
- Gastrointestinal: Nausea, vomiting
- Ocular: Conjunctivitis **Note:** Mania and aggressive behavior have been reported in pediatric patients with ADHD who received guanfacine.

Drug Interactions

Increased Effect/Toxicity: Nitroprusside and guanfacine have additive hypotensive effects. Noncardioselective beta-blockers (nadolol, propranolol, timolol) may exacerbate rebound hypertension when guanfacine is withdrawn. The beta-blocker should be withdrawn first. The gradual withdrawal of guanfacine or a cardioselective beta-blocker could be substituted.

Decreased Effect: TCAs decrease the hypotensive effect of guanfacine.

Hypoglycemic agents: Hypoglycemic symptoms may be decreased. Educate patient about decreased signs and symptoms of hypoglycemia or avoid use in patients with frequent episodes of hypoglycemia.

Drug Uptake

Onset of action: Peak effect: 8-11 hours
Duration: 24 hours following a single dose
Half-life, elimination: 17 hours
Time to peak: 1-4 hours

Pregnancy Risk Factor B

Generic Available No

GuiaCough® [OTC] *see* Guaifenesin and Dextromethorphan *on page 569*
Guiatuss® [OTC] *see* Guaifenesin *on page 568*
Guiatuss DAC® *see* Guaifenesin, Pseudoephedrine, and Codeine *on page 570*
Guiatuss-DM® [OTC] *see* Guaifenesin and Dextromethorphan *on page 569*
Guiatussin® DAC *see* Guaifenesin, Pseudoephedrine, and Codeine *on page 570*
Guiatussin® With Codeine *see* Guaifenesin and Codeine *on page 568*
G-well® *see* Lindane *on page 714*
Gynazole-1™ *see* Butoconazole *on page 195*
Gynecort® [OTC] *see* Hydrocortisone *on page 608*

Gyne-Lotrimin® [OTC] *see* Clotrimazole *on page 312*
Gyne-Lotrimin® 3 [OTC] *see* Clotrimazole *on page 312*
Gynix® [OTC] *see* Clotrimazole *on page 312*
Gynodiol™ *see* Estradiol *on page 457*
Gynol II® [OTC] *see* Nonoxynol 9 *on page 874*
Habitrol™ Patch *see* Nicotine *on page 863*

Haemophilus b Conjugate Vaccine

(he MOF fi lus bee KON joo gate vak SEEN)

U.S. Brand Names ActHIB®; HibTITER®; PedvaxHIB®

Canadian Brand Names ActHIB®; PedvaxHIB®

Pharmacologic Category Vaccine

Synonyms Diphtheria CRM_{197} Protein Conjugate; Diphtheria Toxoid Conjugate; *Haemophilus* b Oligosaccharide Conjugate Vaccine; *Haemophilus* b Polysaccharide Vaccine; HbCV; Hib Polysaccharide Conjugate; PRP-D

Use Routine immunization of children 2 months to 5 years of age against invasive disease caused by *H. influenzae*

Unimmunized children ≥5 years of age with a chronic illness known to be associated with increased risk of *Haemophilus influenzae* type b disease, specifically, persons with anatomic or functional asplenia or sickle cell anemia or those who have undergone splenectomy, should receive Hib vaccine.

Haemophilus b conjugate vaccines are not indicated for prevention of bronchitis or other infections due to *H. influenzae* in adults; adults with specific dysfunction or certain complement deficiencies who are at especially high risk of *H. influenzae* type b infection (HIV-infected adults); patients with Hodgkin's disease (vaccinated at least 2 weeks before the initiation of chemotherapy or 3 months after the end of chemotherapy)

Local Anesthetic/Vasoconstrictor Precautions No information available to require special precautions

Effects on Dental Treatment No effects or complications reported

Dosage Children: I.M.: 0.5 mL as a single dose should be administered according to one of the "brand-specific" schedules; do not inject I.V. See table.

Vaccination Schedule for *Haemophilus* b Conjugate Vaccines

Age at 1st Dose	HibTITER®		PedvaxHIB®		ProHIBiT®	
	Primary Series	Booster	Primary Series	Booster	Primary Series	Booster
2-6 months*	3 doses 2 months apart	15 months**	2 doses 2 months apart	12 months**	—	—
7-11 months	2 doses 2 months apart	15 months**	2 doses 2 months apart	15 months**	—	—
12-14 months	1 dose	15 months**	1 dose	15 months**	—	—
15-60 months	1 dose	—	1 dose	—	1 dose	—

*It is not currently recommended that the various *Haemophilus* b conjugate vaccines be interchanged (ie, the same brand should be used throughout the entire vaccination series). If the health care provider does not know which vaccine was previously used, it is prudent that an infant, 2-6 months of age, be given a primary series of three doses.

**At least 2 months after previous dose.

Mechanism of Action Stimulates production of anticapsular antibodies and provides active immunity to *Haemophilus influenzae*; Hib conjugate vaccines use covalent binding of capsular polysaccharide of *Haemophilus influenzae* type b to diphtheria CRM 197 (HibTITER®) to produce an antigen which is postulated to convert a T-independent antigen into a T-dependent antigen to result in enhanced antibody response and on immunologic memory

Other Adverse Effects When administered during the same visit that DTP vaccine is given, the rates of systemic reactions do not differ from those observed only when DTP vaccine is administered. **All serious adverse reactions must be reported to the U.S. Department of Health and Human Services (DHHS) Vaccine Adverse Event Reporting System (VAERS) 1-800-822-7967.**

25%:

- Cardiovascular: Edema
- Dermatologic: Local erythema
- Local: Increased risk of *Haemophilus* b infections in the week after vaccination
- Miscellaneous: Warmth

>10%: Acute febrile reactions

1% to 10%:

- Central nervous system: Fever (up to 102.2°F), irritability, lethargy
- Gastrointestinal: Anorexia, diarrhea
- Local: Irritation at injection site

(Continued)

Haemophilus b Conjugate Vaccine *(Continued)*

Drug Interactions Decreased effect with immunosuppressive agents; immunoglobulins within 1 month may decrease antibody production.

Drug Uptake The seroconversion following one dose of Hib vaccine for children 18 months or 24 months of age or older is 75% to 90% respectively.

Onset of action: Serum antibody response: 1-2 weeks

Duration: Immunity: 1.5 years

Pregnancy Risk Factor C

Generic Available No

Comments Federal law requires that the date of administration, the vaccine manufacturer, lot number of vaccine, and the administering person's name, title and address be entered into the patient's permanent medical record

Halazepam (hal AZ e pam)

U.S. Brand Names Paxipam®

Canadian Brand Names Paxipam®

Pharmacologic Category Benzodiazepine

Use Management of anxiety disorders; short-term relief of the symptoms of anxiety

Unlabeled/Investigational: Hostility; ethanol withdrawal

Local Anesthetic/Vasoconstrictor Precautions No information available to require special precautions

Effects on Dental Treatment >10%: Significant xerostomia; normal salivary flow resumes with discontinuation

Restrictions C-IV

Dosage Oral:

Adults: 20-40 mg 3-4 times/day; optimal dosage usually ranges from 80-160 mg/day. If side effects occur with the starting dose, lower the dose.

Elderly ≥70 years or debilitated patients: 20 mg 1-2 times/day and adjust dose accordingly

Mechanism of Action Binds to stereospecific benzodiazepine receptors on the postsynaptic GABA neuron at several sites within the CNS, including the limbic system, reticular formation. Enhancement of the inhibitory effect of GABA on neuronal excitability results by increased neuronal membrane permeability to chloride ions. This shift in chloride ions results in hyperpolarization (a less excitable state) and stabilization.

Other Adverse Effects

>10%: Central nervous system: Drowsiness

1% to 10%:

- Cardiovascular: Tachycardia, hypotension, bradycardia
- Central nervous system: Confusion, headache, apathy, euphoria, disorientation
- Dermatologic: Dermatitis, rash
- Gastrointestinal: Increased salivation, xerostomia, nausea, sense of seasickness, constipation
- Ocular: Blurred vision

Drug Interactions CYP3A3/4 enzyme substrate

Increased Effect/Toxicity: Serum levels and/or toxicity of halazepam may be increased by cimetidine, ciprofloxacin, clarithromycin, clozapine, CNS depressants, diltiazem, disulfiram, digoxin, erythromycin, fluconazole, fluoxetine, fluvoxamine, isoniazid, itraconazole, ketoconazole, labetalol, levodopa, loxapine, metoprolol, metronidazole, miconazole, nefazodone, omeprazole, phenytoin, rifabutin, rifampin, troleandomycin, valproic acid, and verapamil.

Decreased Effect: Carbamazepine, rifampin, rifabutin may enhance the metabolism of halazepam and decrease its therapeutic effect. Theophylline may antagonize effects of benzodiazepines.

Drug Uptake

Half-life, elimination: Parent drug: 14 hours; Active metabolite (desmethyldiazepam): 50-100 hours

Time to peak: 1-3 hours

Pregnancy Risk Factor D

Generic Available No

Comments Halazepam offers no significant advantage over other benzodiazepines

Halcinonide (hal SIN oh nide)

U.S. Brand Names Halog®; Halog®-E

Canadian Brand Names Halog®

Mexican Brand Names Dermalog®

Pharmacologic Category Corticosteroid, Topical

Use Inflammation of corticosteroid-responsive dermatoses [high potency topical corticosteroid]

Local Anesthetic/Vasoconstrictor Precautions No information available to require special precautions

Effects on Dental Treatment No effects or complications reported

Dosage Children and Adults: Topical: Apply sparingly 1-3 times/day, occlusive dressing may be used for severe or resistant dermatoses; a thin film of cream or ointment is effective; do not overuse

Therapy should be discontinued when control is achieved; if no improvement is seen, reassessment of diagnosis may be necessary.

Mechanism of Action Decreases inflammation by suppression of migration of polymorphonuclear leukocytes and reversal of increased capillary permeability

Other Adverse Effects Frequency not defined:

Dermatologic: Itching, dry skin, folliculitis, hypertrichosis, acneiform eruptions, hypopigmentation, perioral dermatitis, allergic contact dermatitis, skin maceration, skin atrophy, striae

Local: Burning, irritation, miliaria

Miscellaneous: Secondary infection

Drug Uptake Absorption: Percutaneous absorption varies by location of topical application and the use of occlusive dressings

Pregnancy Risk Factor C

Generic Available No

Halcion® *see* Triazolam *on page 1201*

Haldol® *see* Haloperidol *on page 578*

Haldol® Decanoate *see* Haloperidol *on page 578*

Haley's M-O® [OTC] *see* Magnesium Hydroxide and Mineral Oil Emulsion *on page 741*

Halfan® *see* Halofantrine *on page 577*

Halfprin® [OTC] *see* Aspirin *on page 119*

Halobetasol (hal oh BAY ta sol)

U.S. Brand Names Ultravate™

Canadian Brand Names Ultravate™

Pharmacologic Category Corticosteroid, Topical

Synonyms Halobetasol Propionate

Use Relief of inflammatory and pruritic manifestations of corticosteroid-response dermatoses [very high potency topical corticosteroid]

Local Anesthetic/Vasoconstrictor Precautions No information available to require special precautions

Effects on Dental Treatment No effects or complications reported

Dosage Children and Adults: Topical: Apply sparingly to skin twice daily, rub in gently and completely; treatment should not exceed 2 consecutive weeks and total dosage should not exceed 50 g/week

Therapy should be discontinued when control is achieved; if no improvement is seen, reassessment of diagnosis may be necessary.

Mechanism of Action Corticosteroids inhibit the initial manifestations of the inflammatory process (ie, capillary dilation and edema, fibrin deposition, and migration and diapedesis of leukocytes into the inflamed site) as well as later sequelae (angiogenesis, fibroblast proliferation)

Other Adverse Effects Frequency not defined: Topical: Burning, itching, irritation, dryness, folliculitis, hypertrichosis, acneiform eruptions, hypopigmentation, perioral dermatitis, allergic contact dermatitis, skin maceration, secondary infection, skin atrophy, striae, miliaria

Drug Uptake Absorption: Percutaneous absorption varies by location of topical application and the use of occlusive dressings; ~3% of a topically applied dose of ointment enters the circulation within 96 hours

Pregnancy Risk Factor C

Generic Available No

Halofantrine (ha loe FAN trin)

U.S. Brand Names Halfan®

Pharmacologic Category Antimalarial Agent

Synonyms Halofantrine Hydrochloride

Use Orphan drug: Treatment of mild to moderate acute malaria caused by susceptible strains of *Plasmodium falciparum* and *Plasmodium vivax*

Local Anesthetic/Vasoconstrictor Precautions No information available to require special precautions

Effects on Dental Treatment No effects or complications reported

Dosage Oral:

Children <40 kg: 8 mg/kg every 6 hours for 3 doses

Adults: 500 mg every 6 hours for 3 doses

Mechanism of Action Similar to mefloquine; destruction of asexual blood forms, possible inhibition of proton pump

Other Adverse Effects 1% to 10%:

Cardiovascular: Edema

Central nervous system: Malaise, headache (3%), dizziness (5%)

Dermatologic: Pruritus (3%)

Gastrointestinal: Nausea (3%), vomiting (4%), abdominal pain (9%), diarrhea (6%)

(Continued)

Halofantrine *(Continued)*

Hematologic: Leukocytosis
Hepatic: Elevated LFTs
Local: Tenderness
Neuromuscular & skeletal: Myalgia (1%), rigors (2%)
Respiratory: Cough
Miscellaneous: Lymphadenopathy

Drug Interactions CYP2D6 and 3A3/4 enzyme substrate

Increased toxicity (QT_c interval prolongation) with other agents that cause QT_c interval prolongation, especially mefloquine.

Drug Uptake

Absorption: Erratic and variable; serum concentration are proportional to dose up to 1000 mg; doses greater than this should be divided; may be increased 60% with high fat meals

Half-life, elimination: 23 hours; Metabolite: 82 hours; may be increased in active disease

Pregnancy Risk Factor X

Generic Available No

Halog® *see* Halcinonide *on page 576*

Halog®-E *see* Halcinonide *on page 576*

Haloperidol (ha loe PER i dole)

U.S. Brand Names Haldol®; Haldol® Decanoate

Canadian Brand Names Apo®-Haloperidol; Haldol®; Novo-Peridol; Peridol; PMS-Haloperidol LA; Rho®-Haloperidol Decanoate

Mexican Brand Names Haldol®

Pharmacologic Category Antipsychotic Agent, Butyrophenone

Synonyms Haloperidol Decanoate; Haloperidol Lactate

Use Management of schizophrenia; control of tics and vocal utterances of Tourette's disorder, and severe behavioral problems in children

Unlabeled/Investigational: Treatment of psychosis, may be used for the emergency sedation of severely agitated or delirious patients; adjunctive treatment of ethanol dependence; antiemetic

Local Anesthetic/Vasoconstrictor Precautions Manufacturer's information states that haloperidol may block vasopressor activity of epinephrine. This has not been observed during use of epinephrine as a vasoconstrictor in local anesthesia.

Effects on Dental Treatment Orthostatic hypotension and nasal congestion possible in dental patients. Since the drug is a dopamine antagonist, extrapyramidal symptoms of the TMJ are a possibility.

Dosage

Children: 3-12 years (15-40 kg): Oral:
- Initial: 0.05 mg/kg/day or 0.25-0.5 mg/day given in 2-3 divided doses; increase by 0.25-0.5 mg every 5-7 days; maximum: 0.15 mg/kg/day
- Usual maintenance:
  - Agitation or hyperkinesia: 0.01-0.03 mg/kg/day once daily
  - Nonpsychotic disorders: 0.05-0.075 mg/kg/day in 2-3 divided doses
  - Psychotic disorders: 0.05-0.15 mg/kg/day in 2-3 divided doses

Children 6-12 years: I.M. (as lactate): 1-3 mg/dose every 4-8 hours to a maximum of 0.15 mg/kg/day; change over to oral therapy as soon as able

Adults:
- Oral: 0.5-5 mg 2-3 times/day; usual maximum: 30 mg/day; some patients may require up to 100 mg/day
- I.M. (as lactate): 2-5 mg every 4-8 hours as needed
- I.M. (as decanoate): Initial: 10-15 times the daily oral dose administered at 3- to 4-week intervals

Elderly (nonpsychotic patients, dementia behavior):
- Initial: Oral: 0.25-0.5 mg 1-2 times/day; increase dose at 4- to 7-day intervals by 0.25-0.5 mg/day; increase dosing intervals (twice daily, 3 times/day, etc) as necessary to control response or side effects
- Maximum daily dose: 50 mg; gradual increases (titration) may prevent side effects or decrease their severity

Mechanism of Action Blocks postsynaptic mesolimbic dopaminergic D_1 and D_2 receptors in the brain; exhibits a strong alpha-adrenergic blocking and anticholinergic effect, depresses the release of hypothalamic and hypophyseal hormones; believed to depress the reticular activating system thus affecting basal metabolism, body temperature, wakefulness, vasomotor tone, and emesis

Other Adverse Effects Frequency not defined:

Cardiovascular: Hypotension, hypertension, tachycardia, arrhythmias, abnormal T waves with prolonged ventricular repolarization

Central nervous system: Restlessness, anxiety, extrapyramidal symptoms, dystonic reactions, pseudoparkinsonian signs and symptoms, tardive dyskinesia, neuroleptic malignant syndrome (NMS), altered central temperature regulation, akathisia, tardive dystonia, insomnia, euphoria, agitation, drowsiness, depression, lethargy, headache, confusion, vertigo, seizures

Dermatologic: Hyperpigmentation, pruritus, rash, contact dermatitis, alopecia, photosensitivity (rare)
Endocrine & metabolic: Amenorrhea, galactorrhea, gynecomastia, sexual dysfunction, lactation, breast engorgement, mastalgia, menstrual irregularities, hyperglycemia, hypoglycemia, hyponatremia
Gastrointestinal: Nausea, vomiting, anorexia, constipation, diarrhea, hypersalivation, dyspepsia, xerostomia
Genitourinary: Urinary retention, priapism
Hematologic: Cholestatic jaundice, obstructive jaundice
Ocular: Blurred vision
Respiratory: Laryngospasm, bronchospasm
Miscellaneous: Heat stroke, diaphoresis

Drug Interactions CYP1A2 (minor), CYP2D6 (minor), and CYP3A3/4 enzyme substrate; CYP2D6 enzyme inhibitor
Anticholinergics: May inhibit the therapeutic response to haloperidol and excess anticholinergic effects may occur; tardive dyskinesias have also been reported; includes benztropine and trihexyphenidyl
Antihypertensives: Concurrent use of haloperidol with an antihypertensive may produce additive hypotensive effects (particularly orthostasis)
Bromocriptine: Antipsychotics inhibit the ability of bromocriptine to lower serum prolactin concentrations
Chloroquine: Serum concentrations of haloperidol may be increased by chloroquine
CNS depressants: Sedative effects may be additive; monitor for increased effect; includes barbiturates, benzodiazepines, narcotic analgesics, ethanol and other sedative agents
Enzyme inducers: May enhance the hepatic metabolism of haloperidol, decreasing its effects; larger doses of haloperidol may be required; includes barbiturates, carbamazepine, phenytoin, rifampin, and rifabutin
Indomethacin: Haloperidol in combination with indomethacin may result in drowsiness, tiredness, and confusion; monitor for adverse effects
Inhalation anesthetics: Haloperidol in combination with certain forms of induction anesthesia may produce peripheral vasodilitation and hypotension
Levodopa: Haloperidol may inhibit the antiparkinsonian effect of levodopa; avoid this combination
Lithium: Haloperidol may produce neurotoxicity with lithium; this is a rare effect
Methyldopa: Effect of haloperidol may be altered; enhanced effects, as well as reduced efficacy have been reported
Metoclopramide: May increase extrapyramidal symptoms (EPS) or risk.
Nefazodone: Haloperidol and nefazodone may produce additive CNS toxicity, including sedation
Propranolol: Serum concentrations of haloperidol may be increased
Quinidine: May increase haloperidol concentrations; monitor for EPS and/or QT_c prolongation
SSRIs: Fluoxetine, fluvoxamine, and paroxetine may inhibit the metabolism of haloperidol resulting in EPS; monitor for EPS
Sulfadoxine-pyrimethamine: May increase fluphenazine concentrations
Tricyclic antidepressants: Concurrent use may produce increased toxicity or altered therapeutic response
Trazodone: Haloperidol and trazodone may produce additive hypotensive effects

Drug Uptake
Onset of sedative effect: I.V.: ≤1 hour
Duration: Decanoate: ~3 weeks
Half-life, elimination: 20 hours
Time to peak: 20 minutes

Pregnancy Risk Factor C

Generic Available Yes

Halotestin® *see* Fluoxymesterone *on page 519*
Halotussin® DAC *see* Guaifenesin, Pseudoephedrine, and Codeine *on page 570*
Halotussin® DM [OTC] *see* Guaifenesin and Dextromethorphan *on page 569*
Haltran® [OTC] *see* Ibuprofen *on page 621*
Havrix® *see* Hepatitis A Vaccine *on page 583*
Hayfebrol® [OTC] *see* Chlorpheniramine and Pseudoephedrine *on page 270*
HDA® Toothache [OTC] *see* Benzocaine *on page 151*
Head & Shoulders® [OTC] *see* Pyrithione Zinc *on page 1029*
Healon® *see* Sodium Hyaluronate *on page 1097*
Healon® GV *see* Sodium Hyaluronate *on page 1097*
Hectorol® *see* Doxercalciferol *on page 416*
Helidac® *see* Bismuth, Metronidazole, and Tetracycline *on page 167*
Helistat® *see* Microfibrillar Collagen Hemostat *on page 808*
Helixate® FS *see* Antihemophilic Factor (Recombinant) *on page 106*
Hemabate™ *see* Carboprost Tromethamine *on page 223*

Hemin (HEE min)

U.S. Brand Names Panhematin®

Pharmacologic Category Blood Modifiers

Use Orphan drug: Treatment of recurrent attacks of acute intermittent porphyria (AIP) only after an appropriate period of alternate therapy has been tried

Local Anesthetic/Vasoconstrictor Precautions No information available to require special precautions

Effects on Dental Treatment No effects or complications reported

Dosage I.V.: 1-4 mg/kg/day administered over 10-15 minutes for 3-14 days; may be repeated no earlier than every 12 hours; not to exceed 6 mg/kg in any 24-hour period

Other Adverse Effects 1% to 10%:

Central nervous system: Mild pyrexia

Hematologic: Leukocytosis

Local: Phlebitis

Drug Interactions

Anticoagulants: May increase anticoagulant effects; avoid concurrent use

Estrogens, barbiturates, corticosteroids: Increase the effects of delta-aminolevulinic acid synthesis; hemin works oppositely to inhibit this enzyme; avoid concurrent use

Generic Available No

Hemocyte® [OTC] *see* Ferrous Fumarate *on page 497*

Hemodent® Gingival Retraction Cord *see* Aluminum Chloride *on page 61*

Hemofil® M *see* Antihemophilic Factor (Human) *on page 104*

Hemonyne® *see* Factor IX Complex (Human) *on page 484*

Hemotene® *see* Microfibrillar Collagen Hemostat *on page 808*

Hemril-HC® Uniserts® *see* Hydrocortisone *on page 608*

Heparin (HEP a rin)

U.S. Brand Names Hep-Lock®

Canadian Brand Names Hepalean®; Hepalean® Leo; Hepalean®-LOK

Mexican Brand Names Dixaparine; Helberina; Inhepar; Proparin®

Pharmacologic Category Anticoagulant

Synonyms Heparin Calcium; Heparin Lock Flush; Heparin Sodium

Use Prophylaxis and treatment of thromboembolic disorders

Local Anesthetic/Vasoconstrictor Precautions No information available to require special precautions

Effects on Dental Treatment Heparin, being a potent antithrombin agent, has caused bleeding from the gums.

Dosage Line flushing: When using daily flushes of heparin to maintain patency of single and double lumen central catheters, 10 units/mL is commonly used for younger infants (eg, <10 kg) while 100 units/mL is used for older infants, children, and adults. Capped PVC catheters and peripheral heparin locks require flushing more frequently (eg, every 6-8 hours). Volume of heparin flush is usually similar to volume of catheter (or slightly greater). Additional flushes should be given when

Standard Heparin Solution
(25,000 units/500 mL D_5W)

To Administer a Dose of:	Set Infusion Rate at:
400 units/hour	8 mL/hour
500 units/hour	10 mL/hour
600 units/hour	12 mL/hour
700 units/hour	14 mL/hour
800 units/hour	16 mL/hour
900 units/hour	18 mL/hour
1000 units/hour	20 mL/hour
1100 units/hour	22 mL/hour
1200 units/hour	24 mL/hour
1300 units/hour	26 mL/hour
1400 units/hour	28 mL/hour
1500 units/hour	30 mL/hour
1600 units/hour	32 mL/hour
1700 units/hour	34 mL/hour
1800 units/hour	36 mL/hour
1900 units/hour	38 mL/hour
2000 units/hour	40 mL/hour

stagnant blood is observed in catheter, after catheter is used for drug or blood administration, and after blood withdrawal from catheter.

Addition of heparin (0.5-1 unit/mL) to peripheral and central TPN has been shown to increase duration of line patency. The final concentration of heparin used for TPN solutions may need to be decreased to 0.5 units/mL in small infants receiving larger amounts of volume in order to avoid approaching therapeutic amounts. Arterial lines are heparinized with a final concentration of 1 unit/mL.

Children:

Intermittent I.V.: Initial: 50-100 units/kg, then 50-100 units/kg every 4 hours

I.V. infusion: Initial: 50 units/kg, then 15-25 units/kg/hour; increase dose by 2-4 units/kg/hour every 6-8 hours as required

Adults:

Prophylaxis (low-dose heparin): S.C.: 5000 units every 8-12 hours

Intermittent I.V.: Initial: 10,000 units, then 50-70 units/kg (5000-10,000 units) every 4-6 hours

I.V. infusion: 50 units/kg to start, then 15-25 units/kg/hour as continuous infusion; increase dose by 5 units/kg/hour every 4 hours as required according to PTT results, usual range: 10-30 units/hour

Weight-based protocol: 80 units/kg I.V. push followed by continuous infusion of 18 units/kg/hour. See table on previous page.

Dosing adjustments in the elderly: Patients >60 years of age may have higher serum concentration and clinical response (longer aPTTs) as compared to younger patients receiving similar dosages; lower dosages may be required

Mechanism of Action Potentiates the action of antithrombin III and thereby inactivates thrombin (as well as activated coagulation factors IX, X, XI, XII, and plasmin) and prevents the conversion of fibrinogen to fibrin; heparin also stimulates release of lipoprotein lipase (lipoprotein lipase hydrolyzes triglycerides to glycerol and free fatty acids)

Other Adverse Effects Frequency not defined:

Cardiovascular: Chest pain, vasospasm (possibly related to thrombosis), hemorrhagic shock

Central nervous system: Fever, headache, chills

Dermatologic: Unexplained bruising, urticaria, alopecia, dysesthesia pedis, purpura, eczema, cutaneous necrosis (following deep S.C. injection), erythematous plaques (case reports)

Endocrine & metabolic: Hyperkalemia (supression of aldosterone), rebound hyperlipidemia on discontinuation

Gastrointestinal: Nausea, vomiting, constipation, hematemesis

Genitourinary: Frequent or persistent erection

Hematologic: Hemorrhage, blood in urine, bleeding from gums, epistaxis, adrenal hemorrhage, ovarian hemorrhage, retroperitoneal hemorrhage, thrombocytopenia (see note)

Hepatic: Elevated liver enzymes (AST/ALT) Local: Irritation, ulceration, cutaneous necrosis have been rarely reported with deep S.C. injections, I.M. injection (not recommended) is associated with a high incidence of these effects

Neuromuscular & skeletal: Peripheral neuropathy, osteoporosis (chronic therapy effect)

Ocular: Conjunctivitis (allergic reaction)

Respiratory: Hemoptysis, pulmonary hemorrhage, asthma, rhinitis, bronchospasm (case reports)

Miscellaneous: Allergic reactions, anaphylactoid reactions

Note: Thrombocytopenia has been reported to occur at an incidence between 0% and 30%. It is often of no clinical significance. However, immunologically mediated heparin-induced thrombocytopenia has been estimated to occur in 1% to 2% of patients, and is marked by a progressive fall in platelet counts and, in some cases, thromboembolic complications (skin necrosis, pulmonary embolism, gangrene of the extremities, stroke or myocardial infarction); daily platelet counts for 5-7 days at initiation of therapy may help detect the onset of this complication.

Drug Interactions

Increased Effect/Toxicity: The risk of hemorrhage associated with heparin may be increased by oral anticoagulants (warfarin), thrombolytics, dextran, and drugs which affect platelet function (eg, aspirin, NSAIDs, dipyridamole, ticlopidine, clopidogrel, IIb/IIIa antagonists). However, heparin is often used in conjunction with thrombolytic therapy or during the initiation of warfarin therapy to assure anticoagulation and to protect against possible transient hypercoagulability. Cephalosporins which contain the MTT side chain and parenteral penicillins (may inhibit platelet aggregation) may increase the risk of hemorrhage. Other drugs reported to increase heparin's anticoagulant effect include antihistamines, tetracycline, quinine, nicotine, and cardiac glycosides (digoxin).

Decreased Effect: Nitroglycerin (I.V.) may decrease heparin's anticoagulant effect. This interaction has not been validated in some studies, and may only occur at high nitroglycerin dosages.

Drug Uptake

Onset of anticoagulant effect: I.V.: Immediate; S.C.: 20-30 minutes

(Continued)

Heparin *(Continued)*

Absorption: Oral, rectal, I.M.: Erratic at best from all these routes of administration; S.C. absorption is also erratic, but considered acceptable for prophylactic use

Half-life, elimination: Mean: 1.5 hours; Range: 1-2 hours; affected by obesity, renal and hepatic function, malignancy, presence of pulmonary embolism, and infections

Pregnancy Risk Factor C

Generic Available Yes

Comments Heparin does not possess fibrinolytic activity and, therefore, cannot lyse established thrombi; discontinue heparin if hemorrhage occurs; severe hemorrhage or overdosage may require protamine; monitor platelet counts, signs of bleeding, PTT.

When using daily flushes of heparin to maintain patency of single and double lumen central catheters, 10 units/mL is commonly used for younger infants (eg, <10 kg) while 100 units/mL is used for older infants and children (eg, ≥10 kg). Capped PVC catheters and peripheral heparin locks require flushing more frequently (eg, every 6-8 hours). Volume of heparin flush is usually similar to volume of catheter (or slightly greater) or may be standardized according to specific hospital's policy (eg, 2-5 mL/flush). Dose of heparin flush used should not approach therapeutic per kg dose. Additional flushes should be given when stagnant blood is observed in catheter, after catheter is used for drug or blood administration, and after blood withdrawal from catheter.

Heparin 1 unit/mL (final concentration) may be added to TPN solutions, both central and peripheral. (Addition of heparin to peripheral TPN has been shown to increase duration of line patency.) The final concentration of heparin used for TPN solutions may need to be decreased to 0.5 units/mL in small infants receiving larger amounts of volume in order to avoid approaching therapeutic amounts.

Arterial lines are heparinized with a final concentration of 1 unit/mL.

Hepatitis A Inactivated and Hepatitis B (Recombinant) Vaccine

(hep a TYE tis aye in ak ti VAY ted & hep a TYE tis bee ree KOM be nant vak SEEN)

Related Information

Systemic Viral Diseases *on page 1354*

U.S. Brand Names Twinrix®

Canadian Brand Names Twinrix™

Pharmacologic Category Vaccine

Synonyms Engerix-B® and Havrix®; Havrix® and Engerix-B®; Hepatitis B (Recombinant) and Hepatitis A Inactivated Vaccine

Use Active immunization against disease caused by hepatitis A virus and hepatitis B virus (all known subtypes) in populations desiring protection against or at high risk of exposure to these viruses.

Populations include travelers to areas of intermediate/high endemicity for **both** HAV and HBV; those at increased risk of HBV infection due to behavioral or occupational factors; patients with chronic liver disease; laboratory workers who handle live HAV and HBV; healthcare workers, police, and other personnel who render medical assistance; workers who come in contact with sewage; employees of day care centers and correctional facilities; patients/staff of hemodialysis units; male homosexuals; patients frequently receiving blood products; military personnel; users of injectable illicit drugs; close household contacts of patients with hepatitis A and hepatitis B infection.

Local Anesthetic/Vasoconstrictor Precautions No information available to require special precautions

Effects on Dental Treatment No effects or complications reported

Dosage I.M.: Adults: Primary immunization: Three doses (1 mL each) given on a 0-, 1-, and 6-month schedule

Mechanism of Action

Hepatitis A vaccine (Havrix®), an inactivated virus vaccine, offers active immunization against hepatitis A virus infection at an effective immune response rate in up to 99% of subjects.

Recombinant hepatitis B vaccine (Engerix-B®) is a noninfectious subunit viral vaccine. The vaccine is derived from hepatitis B surface antigen (HB_sAg) produced through recombinant DNA techniques from yeast cells. The portion of the hepatitis B gene which codes for HB_sAg is cloned into yeast which is then cultured to produce hepatitis B vaccine.

In immunocompetent people, Twinrix® provides active immunization against hepatitis A virus infection (at an effective immune response rate >99% of subjects) and against hepatitis B virus infection (at an effective immune response rate of 93% to 97%) 30 days after completion of the 3-dose series. This is comparable to using hepatitis A vaccine (Havrix®) and hepatitis B vaccine (Engerix-B®) concomitantly.

Other Adverse Effects

All serious adverse reactions must be reported to the U.S. Department of Health and Human Services (DHHS) Vaccine Adverse Event Reporting System (VAERS) 1-800-822-7967.

Incidence of adverse effects of the combination product were similar to those occurring after administration of hepatitis A vaccine and hepatitis B vaccine alone. (Incidence reported is not versus placebo.)

>10%:

Central nervous system: Headache (13% to 22%), fatigue (11% to 14%)
Local: Injection site reaction: Soreness (37% to 41%), redness (9% to 11%)

1% to 10%:

Central nervous system: Fever (2% to 3%)
Gastrointestinal: Diarrhea (4% to 6%), nausea (2% to 4%), vomiting (≤1%)
Local: Injection site reaction: Swelling (4% to 6%), induration
Respiratory: Upper respiratory tract infection
Miscellaneous: Flu-like syndrome

Drug Interactions Immunosuppressant agents: May decrease immune response to vaccine

Drug Uptake

Onset of action: Seroconversion for antibodies against HAV and HBV were detected one month after completion of the 3-dose series.

Duration: Patients remained seropositive for at least 4 years during the clinical studies.

Pregnancy Risk Factor C

Generic Available No

Hepatitis A Vaccine (hep a TYE tis aye vak SEEN)

Related Information

Systemic Viral Diseases *on page 1354*

U.S. Brand Names Havrix®; VAQTA®

Canadian Brand Names Avaxim®; Epaxal Berna®; Havrix™; VAQTA®

Pharmacologic Category Vaccine

Use For populations desiring protection against hepatitis A or for populations at high risk of exposure to hepatitis A virus (travelers to developing countries, household and sexual contacts of persons infected with hepatitis A), child day care employees, patients with chronic liver disease, illicit drug users, male homosexuals, institutional workers (eg, institutions for the mentally and physically handicapped persons, prisons, etc), and healthcare workers who may be exposed to hepatitis A virus (eg, laboratory employees); protection lasts for approximately 15 years

Local Anesthetic/Vasoconstrictor Precautions No information available to require special precautions

Effects on Dental Treatment No effects or complications reported

Dosage I.M.:

Havrix®:

Children 2-18 years: 720 ELISA units (administered as 2 injections of 360 ELISA units [0.5 mL]) 15-30 days prior to travel with a booster 6-12 months following primary immunization; the deltoid muscle should be used for I.M. injection

Adults: 1440 ELISA units(1 mL) 15-30 days prior to travel with a booster 6-12 months following primary immunization; injection should be in the deltoid

VAQTA®:

Children 2-17 years: 25 units (0.5 mL) with 25 units (0.5 mL) booster to be given 6-18 months after primary immunization

Adults: 50 units (1 mL) with 50 units (1 mL) booster to be given 6 months after primary immunization

Mechanism of Action As an inactivated virus vaccine, hepatitis A vaccine offers active immunization against hepatitis A virus infection at an effective immune response rate in up to 99% of subjects

Other Adverse Effects All serious adverse reactions must be reported to the U.S. Department of Health and Human Services (DHHS) Vaccine Adverse Event Reporting System (VAERS) 1-800-822-7967.

>10%:

Central nervous system: Headache
Local: Pain, tenderness, and warmth

1% to 10%:

Endocrine & metabolic: Pharyngitis (1%)
Gastrointestinal: Abdominal pain (1%)
Local: Cutaneous reactions at the injection site (soreness, edema, and redness)

Frequency not defined: Fatigue, fever (rare), transient LFT abnormalities

Warnings/Precautions Use caution in patients with serious active infection, cardiovascular disease, or pulmonary disorders; treatment for anaphylactic reactions should be immediately available

Drug Interactions No interference of immunogenicity was reported when mixed with hepatitis B vaccine.

(Continued)

Hepatitis A Vaccine *(Continued)*

Drug Uptake

Onset of action (protection): 3 weeks after a single dose

Duration: Neutralizing antibodies have persisted for >3 years; unconfirmed evidence indicates that antibody levels may persist for 5-10 years

Pregnancy Risk Factor C

Generic Available No

Selected Readings Centers for Disease Control, "Recommendations of the Advisory Committee on Immunization Practices (ACIP): General Recommendations on Immunization," *MMWR*, 1994, 43(RR-1):23.

Hepatitis B Immune Globulin

(hep a TYE tis bee i MYUN GLOB yoo lin)

Related Information

Occupational Exposure to Bloodborne Pathogens (Universal Precautions) *on page 1442*

Systemic Viral Diseases *on page 1354*

U.S. Brand Names BayHep B™; Nabi-HB®

Canadian Brand Names BayHep B™

Pharmacologic Category Immune Globulin

Synonyms HBIG

Use Provide prophylactic passive immunity to hepatitis B infection to those individuals exposed; newborns of mothers known to be hepatitis B surface antigen positive; hepatitis B immune globulin is not indicated for treatment of active hepatitis B infections and is ineffective in the treatment of chronic active hepatitis B infection

Local Anesthetic/Vasoconstrictor Precautions No information available to require special precautions

Effects on Dental Treatment No effects or complications reported

Dosage I.M.:

Newborns: Hepatitis B: 0.5 mL as soon after birth as possible (within 12 hours); may repeat at 3 months in order for a higher rate of prevention of the carrier state to be achieved; at this time an active vaccination program with the vaccine may begin

Adults: Postexposure prophylaxis: 0.06 mL/kg as soon as possible after exposure (ie, within 24 hours of needlestick, ocular, or mucosal exposure or within 14 days of sexual exposure); usual dose: 3-5 mL; repeat at 28-30 days after exposure

Note: HBIG may be administered at the same time (but at a different site) or up to 1 month preceding hepatitis B vaccination without impairing the active immune response

Mechanism of Action Hepatitis B immune globulin (HBIG) is a nonpyrogenic sterile solution containing 10% to 18% protein of which at least 80% is monomeric immunoglobulin G (IgG). HBIG differs from immune globulin in the amount of anti-HBs. Immune globulin is prepared from plasma that is not preselected for anti-HBs content. HBIG is prepared from plasma preselected for high titer anti-HBs. In the U.S., HBIG has an anti-HBs high titer of higher than 1:100,000 by IRA. There is no evidence that the causative agent of AIDS (HTLV-III/LAV) is transmitted by HBIG.

Other Adverse Effects Frequency not defined:

Central nervous system: Dizziness, malaise, fever, lethargy, chills

Dermatologic: Urticaria, angioedema, rash, erythema

Gastrointestinal: Vomiting, nausea

Genitourinary: Nephrotic syndrome

Local: Pain, tenderness, and muscular stiffness at injection site

Neuromuscular & skeletal: Arthralgia, myalgia

Miscellaneous: Anaphylaxis

Warnings/Precautions Have epinephrine 1:1000 available for anaphylactic reactions. As a product of human plasma, this product may potentially transmit disease; screening of donors, as well as testing and/or inactivation of certain viruses reduces this risk. Use caution in patients with thrombocytopenia or coagulation disorders (I.M. injections may be contraindicated), in patients with isolated IgA deficiency, or in patients with previous systemic hypersensitivity to human immunoglobulins. Not for I.V. administration.

Drug Interactions Interferes with immune response of live virus vaccines

Drug Uptake

Absorption: Slow

Time to peak: 1-6 days

Pregnancy Risk Factor C

Generic Available No

Hepatitis B Vaccine (hep a TYE tis bee vak SEEN)

Related Information

Systemic Viral Diseases *on page 1354*

U.S. Brand Names Engerix-B®; Recombivax HB®

Canadian Brand Names Engerix-B®; Recombivax HB®

Pharmacologic Category Vaccine

Synonyms Hepatitis B Inactivated Virus Vaccine (plasma derived); Hepatitis B Inactivated Virus Vaccine (recombinant DNA)

Use Immunization against infection caused by all known subtypes of hepatitis B virus, in individuals considered at high risk of potential exposure to hepatitis B virus or HB_sAg-positive materials. See table.

Pre-exposure Prophylaxis for Hepatitis B
Health care workers*
Special patient groups (eg, adolescents, infants born to HB_sAg–positive mothers, military personnel, etc)
Hemodialysis patients**
Recipients of certain blood products***
Lifestyle factors
Homosexual and bisexual men
Intravenous drug abusers
Heterosexually active persons with multiple sexual partners or recently acquired sexually transmitted diseases
Environmental factors
Household and sexual contacts of HBV carriers
Prison inmates
Clients and staff of institutions for the mentally handicapped
Residents, immigrants and refugees from areas with endemic HBV infection
International travelers at increased risk of acquiring HBV infection

Note: Patients with chronic renal disease should be vaccinated as early as possible, ideally before they require hemodialysis. In addition, their anti-HB_s levels should be monitored at 6-12 month intervals to assess the need for revaccination.

*The risk of hepatitis B virus (HBV) infection for health care workers varies both between hospitals and within hospitals. Hepatitis B vaccination is recommended for all health care workers with blood exposure.

**Hemodialysis patients often respond poorly to hepatitis B vaccination; higher vaccine doses or increased number of doses are required. A special formulation of one vaccine is now available for such persons (Recombivax HB®, 40 mcg/mL). The anti-Hb_s(antibody to hepatitis B surface antigen) response of such persons should be tested after they are vaccinated, and those who have not responded should be revaccinated with 1-3 additional doses

***Patients with hemophilia should be immunized subcutaneously, not intramuscularly.

Local Anesthetic/Vasoconstrictor Precautions No information available to require special precautions

Effects on Dental Treatment No effects or complications reported

Dosage I.M.:

Immunization regimen: Regimen consists of 3 doses (0, 1, and 6 months): First dose given on the elected date, second dose given 1 month later, third dose given 6 months after the first dose; see table.

Routine Immunization Regimen of Three I.M. Hepatitis B Vaccine Doses

Age	Initial		1 month		6 months	
	Recom-bivax HB® (mL)	Enger-ix-B® (mL)	Recom-bivax HB® (mL)	Enger-ix-B® (mL)	Recom-bivax HB® (mL)	Enger-ix-B® (mL)
Birth* - 10 years	0.25**	0.5	0.25**	0.5	0.25**	0.5
11-19 years	0.5	1	0.5	1	0.5	1
≥20 years	1	1	1	1	1	1
Dialysis or immu-nocompromised patients	—	2***	—	2***	—	2***

*Infants born of HB_sAg **negative** mothers.

**0.5 mL of the 5 mcg/0.5 mL (adolescent/high-risk infant) product or 0.5 mL of the 25 mcg/0.5 mL pediatric formulation

***Two 1 mL doses given at different sites.

Alternative dosing schedule for **Recombivax HB®:** Children 11-15 years (10 mcg/mL adult formulation): First dose of 1 mL given on the elected date, second dose given 4-6 months later

Alternative dosing schedules for **Engerix-B®:**

Children ≤10 years (10 mcg/0.5 mL formulation): High-risk children: 0.5 mL at 0, 1, 2, and 12 months; lower-risk children ages 5-10 who are candidates for an extended administration schedule may receive an alternative regimen of 0.5 mL at 0, 12, and 24 months. If booster dose is needed, revaccinate with 0.5 mL.

Adolescents 11-19 years (20 mcg/mL formulation): 1 mL at 0, 1, and 6 months. High-risk adolescents: 1 mL at 0, 1, 2, and 12 months; lower-risk adolescents 11-16 years who are candidates for an extended administration schedule may receive an alternative regimen of 0.5 mL (using the 10 mcg/0.5 mL)

(Continued)

Hepatitis B Vaccine *(Continued)*

formulation at 0, 12, and 24 months. If booster dose is needed, revaccinate with 20 mcg.

Adults ≥20 years: High-risk adults (20 mcg/mL formulation): 1 mL at 0, 1, 2, and 12 months. If booster dose is needed, revaccinate with 1 mL.

Postexposure prophylaxis: See table.

Postexposure Prophylaxis
Recommended Dosage for Infants Born to HB_sAg-Positive Mothers

Treatment	Birth	Within 7 days	1 month	6 months
Engerix-B® (pediatric product dose 10 mcg/0.5 mL)	*	0.5 mL*	0.5 mL	0.5 mL
Recombivax HB® (high-risk infant product dose 5 mcg/0.5 mL)	*	0.25 mL*†	0.25 mL†	0.25 mL†
Hepatitis B immune globulin	0.5 mL	—	—	—

Note: An alternate regimen is administration of the vaccine at birth, within 7 days of birth, and 1, 2, and 12 months later.

Dialysis regimen: Use Recombivax HB® formulation (40 mcg/mL); initial: 40 mcg/mL, then at 1 and 6 months; revaccination: if anti-HB_s <10 mIU/mL ≥1-2 months after 3rd dose

*The first dose may be given at birth at the same time as HBIG, but give in the opposite anterolateral thigh. This may better ensure vaccine absorption.

†Or 0.5 mL of the pediatric product (0.25 mcg/0.5 mL)

Mechanism of Action Recombinant hepatitis B vaccine is a noninfectious subunit viral vaccine. The vaccine is derived from hepatitis B surface antigen (HB_sAg) produced through recombinant DNA techniques from yeast cells. The portion of the hepatitis B gene which codes for HB_sAg is cloned into yeast which is then cultured to produce hepatitis B vaccine.

Other Adverse Effects

All serious adverse reactions must be reported to the U.S. Department of Health and Human Services (DHHS) Vaccine Adverse Event Reporting System (VAERS) 1-800-822-7967.

The most common adverse effects reported with both products included injection site reactions (>10%). Frequency not defined:

Cardiovascular: Hypotension

Central nervous system: Agitation, chills, dizziness, fatigue, fever (≥37.5°C/100°F), flushing, headache, insomnia, irritability, lightheadedness, malaise, vertigo

Dermatologic: Angioedema, petechiae, pruritus, rash, urticaria

Gastrointestinal: Abdominal pain, appetite decreased, cramps, diarrhea, dyspepsia, nausea, vomiting

Genitourinary: Dysuria

Local: Injection site reactions: Ecchymosis, erythema, induration, pain, nodule formation, soreness, swelling, tenderness, warmth

Neuromuscular & skeletal: Achiness, arthralgia, back pain, myalgia, neck pain, neck stiffness, paresthesia, shoulder pain, weakness

Otic: Earache

Respiratory: Cough, pharyngitis, rhinitis, upper respiratory tract infection

Miscellaneous: Lymphadenopathy, diaphoresis

Drug Interactions

DTaP: Vaccines may be administered together (using separate sites and syringes).

Haemophilus b conjugate vaccine (PedvaxHIB®): Vaccines may be administered together (using separate sites and syringes).

Immunosuppressant medications: The effect of the vaccine may be decreased; consider deferring vaccination for 3 months after immunosuppressant therapy is discontinued.

MMR: Vaccines may be administered together (using separate sites and syringes).

OPV: Vaccines may be administered together.

Drug Uptake Following all 3 doses of hepatitis B vaccine, immunity will last approximately 5-7 years.

Pregnancy Risk Factor C

Generic Available No

Selected Readings

Centers for Disease Control, "Recommendations of the Advisory Committee on Immunization Practices (ACIP): General Recommendations on Immunization," *MMWR*, 1994, 43(RR-1):23.

Gardner P and Schaffner W, "Immunization of Adults," *N Engl J Med*, 1993, 328(17):1252-8.

Hep-Lock® *see* Heparin *on page 580*

Herceptin® *see* Trastuzumab *on page 1192*

Hespan® *see* Hetastarch *on page 587*

Hetastarch (HET a starch)

U.S. Brand Names Hespan®; Hextend®

Mexican Brand Names HAES-steril®

Pharmacologic Category Plasma Volume Expander, Colloid

Synonyms HES; Hydroxyethyl Starch

Use Blood volume expander used in treatment of shock or impending shock when blood or blood products are not available; does not have oxygen-carrying capacity and is not a substitute for blood or plasma; an adjunct in leukapheresis to enhance the yield of granulocytes by centrifugal means

Unlabeled/Investigational: Has also been used as an adjunct in leukapheresis (Hextend® contraindicated for this use per manufacturer), as a priming fluid in pump oxygenators during cardiopulmonary bypass, and as a plasma volume expander during cardiopulmonary bypass.

Local Anesthetic/Vasoconstrictor Precautions No information available to require special precautions

Effects on Dental Treatment No effects or complications reported

Dosage I.V. infusion (requires an infusion pump):

Children: Safety and efficacy have not been established

Shock:

Adults: 500-1000 mL (up to 1500 mL/day) or 20 mL/kg/day (up to 1500 mL/day); larger volumes (15,000 mL/24 hours) have been used safely in small numbers of patients

Leukapheresis: 250-700 mL hetastarch

Dosing adjustment in renal impairment: Cl_{cr} <10 mL/minute: Initial dose is the same but subsequent doses should be reduced by 20% to 50% of normal

Mechanism of Action Produces plasma volume expansion by virtue of its highly colloidal starch structure, similar to albumin

Other Adverse Effects Frequency not defined:

Cardiovascular: Circulatory overload, heart failure, peripheral edema

Central nervous system: Chills, fever, headache

Dermatologic: Itching, pruritus

Endocrine & metabolic: Increased amylase levels, parotid gland enlargement, elevated indirect bilirubin

Gastrointestinal: Vomiting

Hematologic: Bleeding, decreased factor VIII:C plasma levels, decreased plasma aggregation, decreased von Willebrand factor, dilutional coagulopathy; prolongation of PT, PTT, clotting time, and bleeding time; thrombocytopenia

Neuromuscular & skeletal: Myalgia

Miscellaneous: Anaphylactoid reactions, hypersensitivity

Drug Uptake

Onset of action: Volume expansion: I.V.: ~30 minutes

Duration: 24-36 hours

Pregnancy Risk Factor C

Generic Available No

Comments Does not have oxygen-carrying capacity and is not a substitute for blood or plasma; large volumes may interfere with platelet function and prolong PT and PTT times; safety and efficacy in children have not been established; hetastarch is a synthetic polymer derived from a waxy starch composed of amylopectin; average molecular weight = 450,000

Hexachlorophene (heks a KLOR oh feen)

U.S. Brand Names pHisoHex®

Canadian Brand Names pHisoHex®

Pharmacologic Category Antibiotic, Topical

Use Surgical scrub and as a bacteriostatic skin cleanser; control an outbreak of gram-positive infection when other procedures have been unsuccessful

Local Anesthetic/Vasoconstrictor Precautions No information available to require special precautions

Effects on Dental Treatment No effects or complications reported

Dosage Children and Adults: Topical: Apply 5 mL cleanser and water to area to be cleansed; lather and rinse thoroughly under running water

Mechanism of Action Bacteriostatic polychlorinated biphenyl which inhibits membrane-bound enzymes and disrupts the cell membrane

Other Adverse Effects Frequency not defined:

Central nervous system: CNS injury, seizures, irritability

Dermatologic: Photosensitivity, dermatitis, redness, dry skin

Drug Uptake

Absorption: Percutaneously through inflamed, excoriated, and intact skin

Half-life, elimination: Infants: 6.1-44.2 hours

Pregnancy Risk Factor C

Generic Available No

Hexadrol® *see* Dexamethasone *on page 363*

Hexadrol® Phosphate *see* Dexamethasone *on page 363*

Hexalen® *see* Altretamine *on page 60*

Hextend® *see* Hetastarch *on page 587*

Hexylresorcinol (heks il re ZOR si nole)

U.S. Brand Names Sucrets® Sore Throat [OTC]

Pharmacologic Category Local Anesthetic

Use Minor antiseptic and local anesthetic for sore throat

Local Anesthetic/Vasoconstrictor Precautions No information available to require special precautions

Effects on Dental Treatment No effects or complications reported

Dosage May be used as needed, allow to dissolve slowly in mouth

Generic Available Yes

Hibiclens® [OTC] *see* Chlorhexidine Gluconate *on page 263*

Hibistat® [OTC] *see* Chlorhexidine Gluconate *on page 263*

HibTITER® *see Haemophilus* b Conjugate Vaccine *on page 575*

Hi-Cor® 1.0 *see* Hydrocortisone *on page 608*

Hi-Cor® 2.5 *see* Hydrocortisone *on page 608*

Hiprex® *see* Methenamine *on page 781*

Histafed® [OTC] *see* Triprolidine and Pseudoephedrine *on page 1213*

Histalet® [OTC] *see* Chlorpheniramine and Pseudoephedrine *on page 270*

Histalet® X *see* Guaifenesin and Pseudoephedrine *on page 570*

Histatab® Plus [OTC] *see* Chlorpheniramine and Phenylephrine *on page 269*

Hista-Tabs® [OTC] *see* Triprolidine and Pseudoephedrine *on page 1213*

Histolyn-CYL® *see* Histoplasmin *on page 588*

Histoplasmin (his toe PLAZ min)

U.S. Brand Names Histolyn-CYL®

Pharmacologic Category Diagnostic Agent

Synonyms Histoplasmosis Skin Test Antigen

Use Diagnosing histoplasmosis; to assess cell-mediated immunity

Local Anesthetic/Vasoconstrictor Precautions No information available to require special precautions

Effects on Dental Treatment No effects or complications reported

Dosage Adults: Intradermally: 0.1 mL of 1:100 dilution into volar surface of forearm; induration of ≥5 mm in diameter indicates a positive reaction

Other Adverse Effects Frequency not defined:

- Cardiovascular: Angioedema
- Dermatologic: Pruritus, urticaria
- Local: Ulceration or necrosis may occur at test site
- Respiratory: Dyspnea
- Miscellaneous: Diaphoresis

Pregnancy Risk Factor C

Generic Available No

Histor-D® *see* Chlorpheniramine and Phenylephrine *on page 269*

Histrelin (his TREL in)

U.S. Brand Names Supprelin™

Pharmacologic Category Gonadotropin Releasing Hormone Analog; Luteinizing Hormone-Releasing Hormone Analog

Use Treatment of estrogen-associated gynecological disorders (eg, acute intermittent porphyria, endometriosis, leiomyomata uteri, premenstrual syndrome)

Orphan drug: Treatment of central precocious puberty

Local Anesthetic/Vasoconstrictor Precautions No information available to require special precautions

Effects on Dental Treatment No effects or complications reported

Dosage

- Central idiopathic precocious puberty: S.C.: Usual dose is 10 mcg/kg/day given as a single daily dose at the same time each day
- Acute intermittent porphyria in women: S.C.: 5 mcg/day
- Endometriosis: S.C.: 100 mcg/day
- Leiomyomata uteri: S.C.: 20-50 mcg/day or 4 mcg/kg/day

Mechanism of Action Histrelin is a synthetic long-acting gonadotropin-releasing hormone analog; with daily administration, it desensitizes the pituitary to endogenous gonadotropin-releasing hormone (ie, suppresses gonadotropin release by causing down regulation of the pituitary); this results in a decrease in gonadal sex steroid production which stops the secondary sexual development

Other Adverse Effects

>10%:

- Cardiovascular: Vasodilation
- Central nervous system: Headache
- Gastrointestinal: Abdominal pain
- Genitourinary: Vaginal bleeding, vaginal dryness

Local: Skin reaction at injection site

1% to 10%:

Central nervous system: Mood swings, headache, pain

Dermatologic: Rashes, urticaria

Endocrine & metabolic: Breast tenderness, hot flashes

Gastrointestinal: Nausea, vomiting

Genitourinary: Increased urinary calcium excretion

Neuromuscular & skeletal: Joint stiffness

Drug Uptake

Precocious puberty: Onset of hormonal responses: ≤3 months

Acute intermittent porphyria associated with menses: Amelioration of symptoms: 1-2 months

Treatment of endometriosis or leiomyomata uteri: Onset of responses: 3-6 months

Pregnancy Risk Factor X

Generic Available No

Histrodrix® *see* Dexbrompheniramine and Pseudoephedrine *on page 365*

Hi-Vegi-Lip® [OTC] *see* Pancreatin *on page 913*

Hivid® *see* Zalcitabine *on page 1254*

HMS Liquifilm® *see* Medrysone *on page 753*

Hold® DM [OTC] *see* Dextromethorphan *on page 372*

Homatropine (hoe MA troe peen)

U.S. Brand Names Isopto® Homatropine

Pharmacologic Category Anticholinergic Agent, Ophthalmic; Ophthalmic Agent, Mydriatic

Synonyms Homatropine Hydrobromide

Use Producing cycloplegia and mydriasis for refraction; treatment of acute inflammatory conditions of the uveal tract

Local Anesthetic/Vasoconstrictor Precautions No information available to require special precautions

Effects on Dental Treatment No effects or complications reported

Dosage

Children:

Mydriasis and cycloplegia for refraction: Instill 1 drop of 2% solution immediately before the procedure; repeat at 10-minute intervals as needed

Uveitis: Instill 1 drop of 2% solution 2-3 times/day

Adults:

Mydriasis and cycloplegia for refraction: Instill 1-2 drops of 2% solution or 1 drop of 5% solution before the procedure; repeat at 5- to 10-minute intervals as needed

Uveitis: Instill 1-2 drops of 2% or 5% 2-3 times/day up to every 3-4 hours as needed

Mechanism of Action Blocks response of iris sphincter muscle and the accommodative muscle of the ciliary body to cholinergic stimulation resulting in dilation and loss of accommodation

Other Adverse Effects

>10%: Ocular: Blurred vision, photophobia

1% to 10%:

Local: Stinging, local irritation

Ocular: Increased intraocular pressure

Respiratory: Congestion

Drug Uptake

Mydriasis:

Peak effect: 10-30 minutes

Duration: 6 hours to 4 days

Cycloplegia:

Peak effect: 30-90 minutes

Duration: 10-48 hours

Pregnancy Risk Factor C

Generic Available Yes

H.P. Acthar® Gel *see* Corticotropin *on page 327*

Humalog® *see* Insulin Preparations *on page 639*

Humalog® Mix 75/25™ *see* Insulin Preparations *on page 639*

Human Growth Hormone (HYU man grothe HOR mone)

U.S. Brand Names Genotropin®; Genotropin Miniquick®; Humatrope®; Norditropin®; Norditropin® Cartridges; Nutropin®; Nutropin AQ ®; Nutropin Depot®; Protropin®; Saizen®; Serostim®

Canadian Brand Names Humatrope®; Nutropin® AQ; Nutropine®; Protropine®; Saizen®; Serostim®

Pharmacologic Category Growth Hormone

Synonyms Growth Hormone; Somatrem; Somatropin

(Continued)

Human Growth Hormone *(Continued)*

Use

Children:

Long-term treatment of growth failure due to lack of adequate endogenous growth hormone secretion (Genotropin®, Humatrope®, Norditropin®, Nutropin®, Nutropin AQ®, Nutropin® Depot™, Protropin®, Saizen®)

Long-term treatment of short stature associated with Turner syndrome (Humatrope®, Nutropin®, Nutropin AQ®)

Treatment of Prader-Willi syndrome (Genotropin®)

Treatment of growth failure associated with chronic renal insufficiency (CRI) up until the time of renal transplantation (Nutropin®, Nutropin AQ®)

Long-term treatment of growth failure in children born small for gestational age who fail to manifest catch-up growth by 2 years of age (Genotropin®)

Adults:

AIDS wasting or cachexia with concomitant antiviral therapy (Serostim®)

Replacement of endogenous growth hormone in patients with adult growth hormone deficiency who meet both of the following criteria (Genotropin®, Humatrope®, Nutropin®, Nutropin AQ®):

Biochemical diagnosis of adult growth hormone deficiency by means of a subnormal response to a standard growth hormone stimulation test (peak growth hormone ≤5 μg/L)

and

Adult-onset: Patients who have adult growth hormone deficiency whether alone or with multiple hormone deficiencies (hypopituitarism) as a result of pituitary disease, hypothalamic disease, surgery, radiation therapy, or trauma

or

Childhood-onset: Patients who were growth hormone deficient during childhood, confirmed as an adult before replacement therapy is initiated

Unlabeled/Investigational: Congestive heart failure

Local Anesthetic/Vasoconstrictor Precautions No information available to require special precautions

Effects on Dental Treatment No effects or complications reported

Dosage

Children (individualize dose):

Growth hormone deficiency:

Somatrem: Protropin®: I.M., S.C.: Weekly dosage: 0.3 mg/kg divided into daily doses

Somatropin:

Genotropin®: S.C.: Weekly dosage: 0.16-0.24 mg/kg divided into 6-7 doses

Humatrope®: I.M., S.C.: Weekly dosage: 0.18 mg/kg; maximum replacement dose: 0.3 mg/kg/week; dosing should be divided into equal doses given 3 times/week on alternating days, 6 times/week, or daily

Norditropin®: S.C.: Weekly dosage: 0.024-0.034 mg/kg administered in the evening, divided into doses 6-7 times/week; cartridge and vial formulations are bioequivalent; cartridge formulation does not need to be reconstituted prior to use; cartridges must be administered using the corresponding color-coded NordiPen® injection pen

Nutropin® Depot™: S.C.:

Once-monthly injection: 1.5 mg/kg administered on the same day of each month; patients >15 kg will require more than 1 injection per dose

Twice-monthly injection: 0.75 mg/kg administered twice each month on the same days of each month (eg, days 1 and 15 of each month); patients >30 kg will require more than 1 injection per dose

Nutropin®, Nutropin® AQ: S.C.: Weekly dosage: 0.3 mg/kg divided into daily doses; pubertal patients: ≤0.7 mg/kg/week divided daily

Saizen®: I.M., S.C.: Weekly dosage: 0.06 mg/kg administered 3 times/week

Note: Therapy should be discontinued when patient has reached satisfactory adult height, when epiphyses have fused, or when the patient ceases to respond. Growth of 5 cm/year or more is expected, if growth rate does not exceed 2.5 cm in a 6-month period, double the dose for the next 6 months; if there is still no satisfactory response, discontinue therapy

Chronic renal insufficiency (CRI): Nutropin®, Nutropin® AQ: S.C.: Weekly dosage: 0.35 mg/kg divided into daily injections; continue until the time of renal transplantation

Dosage recommendations in patients treated for CRI who require dialysis:

Hemodialysis: Administer dose at night prior to bedtime or at least 3-4 hours after hemodialysis to prevent hematoma formation from heparin

CCPD: Administer dose in the morning following dialysis

CAPD: Administer dose in the evening at the time of overnight exchange

Turner syndrome: Humatrope®, Nutropin®, Nutropin® AQ: S.C.: Weekly dosage: ≤0.375 mg/kg divided into equal doses 3-7 times per week

Prader-Willi syndrome: Genotropin®: S.C.: Weekly dosage: 0.24 mg/kg divided into 6-7 doses

Small for gestational age: Genotropin®: S.C.: Weekly dosage: 0.48 mg/kg divided into 6-7 doses

Adults:

Growth hormone deficiency: To minimize adverse events in older or overweight patients, reduced dosages may be necessary. During therapy, dosage should be decreased if required by the occurrence of side effects or excessive IGF-I levels.

Somatropin:

Nutropin®, Nutropin® AQ: S.C.: ≤0.006 mg/kg/day; dose may be increased according to individual requirements, up to a maximum of 0.025 mg/kg/day in patients <35 years of age, or up to a maximum of 0.0125 mg/kg/day in patients ≥35 years of age

Humatrope®: S.C.: ≤0.006 mg/kg/day; dose may be increased according to individual requirements, up to a maximum of 0.0125 mg/kg/day

Genotropin®: S.C.: Weekly dosage: ≤0.04 mg/kg divided into 6-7 doses; dose may be increased at 4- to 8-week intervals according to individual requirements, to a maximum of 0.08 mg/kg/week

AIDS wasting or cachexia:

Serostim®: S.C.: Dose should be given once daily at bedtime; patients who continue to lose weight after 2 weeks should be re-evaluated for opportunistic infections or other clinical events; rotate injection sites to avoid lipodystrophy

Daily dose based on body weight:

<35 kg: 0.1 mg/kg
35-45 kg: 4 mg
45-55 kg: 5 mg
>55 kg: 6 mg

Dosage adjustment in renal impairment Reports indicate patients with chronic renal failure tend to have decreased clearance; specific dosing suggestions not available

Dosage adjustment in hepatic impairment: Clearance may be reduced in patients with severe hepatic dysfunction; specific dosing suggestions not available

Elderly: Patients ≥65 years of age may be more sensitive to the action of growth hormone and more prone to adverse effects; in general, dosing should be cautious, beginning at low end of dosing range

Mechanism of Action Somatrem and somatropin are purified polypeptide hormones of recombinant DNA origin; somatrem contains the identical sequence of amino acids found in human growth hormone while somatropin's amino acid sequence is identical plus an additional amino acid, methionine; human growth hormone stimulates growth of linear bone, skeletal muscle, and organs; stimulates erythropoietin which increases red blood cell mass; exerts both insulin-like and diabetogenic effects

Other Adverse Effects Frequency not defined:

Growth hormone deficiency: Antigrowth hormone antibodies, carpal tunnel syndrome (rare), fluid balance disturbances, glucosuria, gynocomastia (rare), headache, hematuria, hyperglycemia (mild), hypoglycemia, hypothyroidism, leukemia, lipoatrophy, muscle pain, increased growth of pre-existing nevi (rare), pain/ local reactions at the injection site, pancreatitis (rare), peripheral edema, exacerbation of psoriasis, seizures

Prader-Willi syndrome: Aggressiveness, arthralgia, edema, hair loss, headache, benign intracranial hypertension, myalgia

Turner syndrome: Humatrope®: Surgical procedures (45%), otitis media (43%), ear disorders (18%), hypothyroidism (13%), increased nevi (11%), peripheral edema (7%)

Adult growth hormone replacement: Increased ALT, increased AST, arthralgia, back pain, carpal tunnel syndrome, diabetes mellitus, fatigue, flu-like syndrome, generalized edema, gastritis, gynocomastia (rare), headache, hypoesthesia, joint disorder, myalgia, increased growth of pre-existing nevi, pain, pancreatitis (rare), paresthesia, peripheral edema, pharyngitis, rhinitis, stiffness in extremities, weakness

AIDS wasting or cachexia (limited): Serostim®: Musculoskeletal discomfort (54%), increased tissue turgor (27%), diarrhea (26%), neuropathy (26%), nausea (26%), fatigue (17%), albuminuria (15%), increased diaphoresis (14%), anorexia (12%), anemia (12%), increased AST (12%), insomnia (11%), tachycardia (11%), hyperglycemia (10%), increased ALT (10%)

Small for gestational age: Mild, transient hyperglycemia; benign intracranial hypertension (rare); central precocious puberty; jaw prominence (rare); aggravation of pre-existing scoliosis (rare); injection site reactions; progression of pigmented nevi

Drug Interactions Limited data suggest somatropin may increase clearance of medications metabolized via CYP2B6, 2C, and 3A3/4.

Decreased Effect: Glucocorticoid therapy may inhibit growth-promoting effects. Growth hormone may induce insulin resistance in patients with diabetes mellitus; monitor glucose and adjust insulin dose as necessary.

Drug Uptake Somatrem and somatropin have equivalent pharmacokinetic properties.

Absorption: I.M., S.C.: Well absorbed

Duration: Maintains supraphysiologic levels for 18-20 hours

(Continued)

Human Growth Hormone *(Continued)*

Half-life, elimination: Dependent on formulation and route of administration

Pregnancy Risk Factor B/C (depending upon manufacturer)

Generic Available No

Humate-P® *see* Antihemophilic Factor (Human) *on page 104*
Humatin® *see* Paromomycin *on page 918*
Humatrope® *see* Human Growth Hormone *on page 589*
Humegon™ *see* Menotropins *on page 759*
Humibid® DM [OTC] *see* Guaifenesin and Dextromethorphan *on page 569*
Humibid® L.A. *see* Guaifenesin *on page 568*
Humibid® Sprinkle *see* Guaifenesin *on page 568*
Humorsol® *see* Demecarium *on page 356*
Humulin® *see* Insulin Preparations *on page 639*
Humulin® 50/50 *see* Insulin Preparations *on page 639*
Humulin® 70/30 *see* Insulin Preparations *on page 639*
Humulin® L *see* Insulin Preparations *on page 639*
Humulin® N *see* Insulin Preparations *on page 639*
Humulin® R *see* Insulin Preparations *on page 639*
Humulin® R (Concentrated) U-500 *see* Insulin Preparations *on page 639*
Hurricaine® *see* Benzocaine *on page 151*
Hyalgan® *see* Sodium Hyaluronate *on page 1097*

Hyaluronidase (hye al yoor ON i dase)

U.S. Brand Names Wydase®

Canadian Brand Names Wydase®

Pharmacologic Category Antidote

Use Increase the dispersion and absorption of other drugs; increase rate of absorption of parenteral fluids administered by hypodermoclysis; management of I.V. extravasations

Local Anesthetic/Vasoconstrictor Precautions No information available to require special precautions

Effects on Dental Treatment No effects or complications reported

Dosage

Children:

Management of I.V. extravasation: Reconstitute the 150 unit vial of lyophilized powder with 1 mL normal saline; take 0.1 mL of this solution and dilute with 0.9 mL normal saline to yield 15 units/mL; using a 25- or 26-gauge needle, five 0.2 mL injections are made subcutaneously or intradermally into the extravasation site at the leading edge, changing the needle after each injection

Hypodermoclysis:

S.C.: 1 mL (150 units) is added to 1000 mL of infusion fluid and 0.5 mL (75 units) in injected into each clysis site at the initiation of the infusion

I.V.: 15 units is added to each 100 mL of I.V. fluid to be administered

Adults: Absorption and dispersion of drugs: 150 units are added to the vehicle containing the drug

Mechanism of Action Modifies the permeability of connective tissue through hydrolysis of hyaluronic acid, one of the chief ingredients of tissue cement which offers resistance to diffusion of liquids through tissues

Other Adverse Effects Urticaria (rare), anaphylactic-like reactions (rare)

Case report: Cardiac fibrillation

Drug Interactions Decreased Effect: Salicylates, cortisone, ACTH, estrogens, antihistamines

Drug Uptake

Onset of action: Extravasation: S.C., intradermal: Immediate

Duration: 24-48 hours

Pregnancy Risk Factor C

Generic Available No

Comments The USP hyaluronidase unit is equivalent to the turbidity-reducing (TR) unit and the International Unit; each unit is defined as being the activity contained in 100 mcg of the International Standard Preparation

Hyate:C® *see* Antihemophilic Factor (Porcine) *on page 105*
Hybolin™ Decanoate *see* Nandrolone *on page 846*
Hybolin™ Improved Injection *see* Nandrolone *on page 846*
Hycamtin™ *see* Topotecan *on page 1183*
HycoClear Tuss® *see* Hydrocodone and Guaifenesin *on page 603*
Hycodan® *see* Hydrocodone and Homatropine *on page 604*
Hycomine® Compound *see* Hydrocodone, Chlorpheniramine, Phenylephrine, Acetaminophen and Caffeine *on page 607*
Hycort® *see* Hydrocortisone *on page 608*
Hycotuss® Expectorant Liquid *see* Hydrocodone and Guaifenesin *on page 603*

Hydergine® *see* Ergoloid Mesylates *on page 447*
Hydergine® LC *see* Ergoloid Mesylates *on page 447*

HydrALAZINE (hye DRAL a zeen)

Related Information
Cardiovascular Diseases *on page 1308*

U.S. Brand Names Apresoline®

Canadian Brand Names Apo®-Hydralazine; Apresoline®; Novo-Hylazin; Nu-Hydral

Mexican Brand Names Apresolina

Pharmacologic Category Vasodilator

Synonyms Hydralazine Hydrochloride

Use Management of moderate to severe hypertension, CHF, hypertension secondary to pre-eclampsia/eclampsia; also used in treatment of primary pulmonary hypertension

Local Anesthetic/Vasoconstrictor Precautions No information available to require special precautions

Effects on Dental Treatment No effects or complications reported

Dosage

Children:
- Oral: Initial: 0.75-1 mg/kg/day in 2-4 divided doses; increase over 3-4 weeks to maximum of 7.5 mg/kg/day in 2-4 divided doses; maximum daily dose: 200 mg/day
- I.M., I.V.: 0.1-0.2 mg/kg/dose (not to exceed 20 mg) every 4-6 hours as needed, up to 1.7-3.5 mg/kg/day in 4-6 divided doses

Adults:
- Oral: Hypertension:
  - Initial dose: 10 mg 4 times/day for first 2-4 days; increase to 25 mg 4 times/day for the balance of the first week
  - Increase by 10-25 mg/dose gradually to 50 mg 4 times/day; 300 mg/day may be required for some patients
- Oral: Congestive heart failure:
  - Initial dose: 10-25 mg 3-4 times/day
  - Adjustment: Dosage must be adjusted based on individual response
  - Target dose: 75 mg 4 times/day in combination with isosorbide dinitrate (40 mg 4 times/day)
  - Range: Typically 200-600 mg daily in 2-4 divided doses; dosages as high as 3 g/day have been used in some patients for symptomatic and hemodynamic improvement. Hydralazine 75 mg 4 times/day combined with isosorbide dinitrate 40 mg 4 times/day were shown in clinical trials to provide a mortality benefit in the treatment of CHF. Higher doses may be used for symptomatic and hemodynamic improvement following optimization of standard therapy.
- I.M., I.V.:
  - Hypertension: Initial: 10-20 mg/dose every 4-6 hours as needed, may increase to 40 mg/dose; change to oral therapy as soon as possible.
  - Pre-eclampsia/eclampsia: 5 mg/dose then 5-10 mg every 20-30 minutes as needed.

Elderly: Oral: Initial: 10 mg 2-3 times/day; increase by 10-25 mg/day every 2-5 days.

Dosing interval in renal impairment:
- Cl_{cr} 10-50 mL/minute: Administer every 8 hours.
- Cl_{cr} <10 mL/minute: Administer every 8-16 hours in fast acetylators and every 12-24 hours in slow acetylators.

Hemodialysis/peritoneal dialysis: Supplemental dose is not necessary.

Mechanism of Action Direct vasodilation of arterioles (with little effect on veins) with decreased systemic resistance

Other Adverse Effects Frequency not defined:
- Cardiovascular: Tachycardia, angina pectoris, orthostatic hypotension (rare), dizziness (rare), paradoxical hypertension, peripheral edema, vascular collapse (rare), flushing
- Central nervous system: Increased intracranial pressure (I.V., in patient with pre-existing increased intracranial pressure), fever (rare), chills (rare), anxiety*, disorientation*, depression*, coma*
- Dermatologic: Rash (rare), urticaria (rash), pruritus (rash)
- Gastrointestinal: Anorexia, nausea, vomiting, diarrhea, constipation, adynamic ileus
- Genitourinary: Difficulty in micturition, impotence
- Hematologic: Hemolytic anemia (rare), eosinophilia (rare), decreased hemoglobin concentration (rare), reduced erythrocyte count (rare), leukopenia (rare), agranulocytosis (rare), thrombocytopenia (rare)
- Neuromuscular & skeletal: Rheumatoid arthritis, muscle cramps, weakness, tremors, peripheral neuritis (rare)
- Ocular: Lacrimation, conjunctivitis
- Respiratory: Nasal congestion, dyspnea
- Miscellaneous: Drug-induced lupus-like syndrome (dose-related; fever, arthralgia, splenomegaly, lymphadenopathy, asthenia, myalgia, malaise, pleuritic chest

(Continued)

HydrALAZINE *(Continued)*

pain, edema, positive ANA, positive LE cells, maculopapular facial rash, positive direct Coombs' test, pericarditis, pericardial tamponade), diaphoresis

*Seen in uremic patients and severe hypertension where rapidly escalating doses may have caused hypotension leading to these effects.

Drug Interactions

Increased Effect/Toxicity: Hydralazine may increase levels of beta-blockers (metoprolol, propranolol). Some beta-blockers (acebutolol, atenolol, and nadolol) are unlikely to be affected due to limited hepatic metabolism. Concurrent use of hydralazine with MAO inhibitors may cause a significant decrease in BP. Propranolol may increase hydralazine serum concentration.

Decreased Effect: NSAIDs (eg, indomethacin) may decrease the hemodynamic effects of hydralazine.

Drug Uptake

Onset of action: Oral: 20-30 minutes; I.V.: 5-20 minutes

Duration: Oral: 2-4 hours; I.V.: 2-6 hours

Half-life, elimination: 2-8 hours; End-stage renal disease: 7-16 hours

Pregnancy Risk Factor C

Generic Available Yes

Hydralazine and Hydrochlorothiazide

(hye DRAL a zeen & hye droe klor oh THYE a zide)

U.S. Brand Names Hydra-Zide®

Pharmacologic Category Antihypertensive Agent Combination

Synonyms Apresazide® [DSC]; Hydrochlorothiazide and Hydralazine

Use Management of moderate to severe hypertension and treatment of CHF

Local Anesthetic/Vasoconstrictor Precautions No information available to require special precautions

Effects on Dental Treatment No effects or complications reported

Dosage Adults: Oral: 1 capsule twice daily

Other Adverse Effects

Based on **hydralazine** component: Frequency not defined:

Cardiovascular: Tachycardia, angina pectoris, orthostatic hypotension (rare), dizziness (rare), paradoxical hypertension, peripheral edema, vascular collapse (rare), flushing

Central nervous system: Increased intracranial pressure (I.V., in patient with pre-existing increased intracranial pressure), fever (rare), chills (rare), anxiety*, disorientation*, depression*, coma*

Dermatologic: Rash (rare), urticaria (rash), pruritus (rash)

Gastrointestinal: Anorexia, nausea, vomiting, diarrhea, constipation, adynamic ileus

Genitourinary: Difficulty in micturition, impotence

Hematologic: Hemolytic anemia (rare), eosinophilia (rare), decreased hemoglobin concentration (rare), reduced erythrocyte count (rare), leukopenia (rare), agranulocytosis (rare), thrombocytopenia (rare)

Neuromuscular & skeletal: Rheumatoid arthritis, muscle cramps, weakness, tremors, peripheral neuritis (rare)

Ocular: Lacrimation, conjunctivitis

Respiratory: Nasal congestion, dyspnea

Miscellaneous: Drug-induced lupus-like syndrome (dose-related; fever, arthralgia, splenomegaly, lymphadenopathy, asthenia, myalgia, malaise, pleuritic chest pain, edema, positive ANA, positive LE cells, maculopapular facial rash, positive direct Coombs' test, pericarditis, pericardial tamponade), diaphoresis

*Seen in uremic patients and severe hypertension where rapidly escalating doses may have caused hypotension leading to these effects.

Based on **hydrochlorothiazide** component: 1% to 10%:

Cardiovascular: Orthostatic hypotension, hypotension

Endocrine & metabolic: Hypokalemia

Dermatologic: Photosensitivity

Gastrointestinal: Anorexia, epigastric distress

Drug Interactions See Hydralazine *on page 593* and Hydrochlorothiazide *on page 595*

Drug Uptake See Hydralazine *on page 593* and Hydrochlorothiazide *on page 595*

Pregnancy Risk Factor C

Generic Available Yes

Hydralazine, Hydrochlorothiazide, and Reserpine

(hye DRAL a zeen, hye droe klor oh THYE a zide, & re SER peen)

U.S. Brand Names Hydrap-ES®; Ser-Ap-Es®

Pharmacologic Category Antihypertensive Agent Combination

Synonyms Hydrochlorothiazide, Hydralazine, and Reserpine; Reserpine, Hydralazine, and Hydrochlorothiazide

Use Hypertensive disorders

Local Anesthetic/Vasoconstrictor Precautions No information available to require special precautions

Effects on Dental Treatment No effects or complications reported

Dosage Adults: Oral: 1-2 tablets 3 times/day

Other Adverse Effects

Based on **hydralazine** component: Frequency not defined:

Cardiovascular: Tachycardia, angina pectoris, orthostatic hypotension (rare), dizziness (rare), paradoxical hypertension, peripheral edema, vascular collapse (rare), flushing

Central nervous system: Increased intracranial pressure (I.V., in patient with pre-existing increased intracranial pressure), fever (rare), chills (rare), anxiety*, disorientation*, depression*, coma*

Dermatologic: Rash (rare), urticaria (rash), pruritus (rash)

Gastrointestinal: Anorexia, nausea, vomiting, diarrhea, constipation, adynamic ileus

Genitourinary: Difficulty in micturition, impotence

Hematologic: Hemolytic anemia (rare), eosinophilia (rare), decreased hemoglobin concentration (rare), reduced erythrocyte count (rare), leukopenia (rare), agranulocytosis (rare), thrombocytopenia (rare)

Neuromuscular & skeletal: Rheumatoid arthritis, muscle cramps, weakness, tremors, peripheral neuritis (rare)

Ocular: Lacrimation, conjunctivitis

Respiratory: Nasal congestion, dyspnea

Miscellaneous: Drug-induced lupus-like syndrome (dose-related; fever, arthralgia, splenomegaly, lymphadenopathy, asthenia, myalgia, malaise, pleuritic chest pain, edema, positive ANA, positive LE cells, maculopapular facial rash, positive direct Coombs' test, pericarditis, pericardial tamponade), diaphoresis

*Seen in uremic patients and severe hypertension where rapidly escalating doses may have caused hypotension leading to these effects.

Based on **hydrochlorothiazide** component: 1% to 10%:

Cardiovascular: Orthostatic hypotension, hypotension

Dermatologic: Photosensitivity

Endocrine & metabolic: Hypokalemia

Gastrointestinal: Anorexia, epigastric distress

Based on **reserpine** component:

Cardiovascular: Peripheral edema, arrhythmias, bradycardia, chest pain, PVC, hypotension

Central nervous system: Dizziness, headache, nightmares, nervousness, drowsiness, fatigue, mental depression, parkinsonism, dull sensorium, syncope, paradoxical anxiety

Dermatologic: Rash, pruritus, flushing of skin

Gastrointestinal: Anorexia, diarrhea, xerostomia, nausea, vomiting, increased salivation, weight gain, increased gastric acid secretion

Genitourinary: Impotence, decreased libido

Hematologic: Thrombocytopenia purpura

Ocular: Blurred vision

Respiratory: Nasal congestion, dyspnea, epistaxis

Drug Interactions See Hydralazine *on page 593*, Hydrochlorothiazide *on page 595* and Reserpine *on page 1046*

Drug Uptake See Hydralazine *on page 593*, Hydrochlorothiazide *on page 595* and Reserpine *on page 1046*

Pregnancy Risk Factor C

Generic Available Yes

Hydrap-ES® *see* Hydralazine, Hydrochlorothiazide, and Reserpine *on page 594*

Hydrate® *see* DimenhyDRINATE *on page 396*

Hydra-Zide® *see* Hydralazine and Hydrochlorothiazide *on page 594*

Hydrea® *see* Hydroxyurea *on page 615*

Hydrocet® *see* Hydrocodone and Acetaminophen *on page 598*

Hydrochlorothiazide (hye droe klor oh THYE a zide)

Related Information

Cardiovascular Diseases *on page 1308*

Moexipril and Hydrochlorothiazide *on page 824*

U.S. Brand Names Aquazide®; Esidrix®; Ezide®; Hydrocot®; HydroDIURIL®; Microzide™; Oretic®

Canadian Brand Names Apo®-Hydro; HydroDIURIL®

Mexican Brand Names Diclotride®

Pharmacologic Category Diuretic, Thiazide

Synonyms HCTZ

Use Management of mild to moderate hypertension; treatment of edema in CHF and nephrotic syndrome

(Continued)

Hydrochlorothiazide *(Continued)*

Unlabeled/Investigational: Treatment of lithium-induced diabetes insipidus

Local Anesthetic/Vasoconstrictor Precautions No information available to require special precautions

Effects on Dental Treatment No effects or complications reported

Dosage Oral (effect of drug may be decreased when used every day):

Children:

<6 months: 2-3 mg/kg/day in 2 divided doses

>6 months: 2 mg/kg/day in 2 divided doses

Adults: 25-100 mg/day in 1-2 doses

Maximum: 200 mg/day

Elderly: 12.5-25 mg once daily

Minimal increase in response and more electrolyte disturbances are seen with doses >50 mg/day

Mechanism of Action Inhibits sodium reabsorption in the distal tubules causing increased excretion of sodium and water as well as potassium and hydrogen ions

Other Adverse Effects 1% to 10%:

Cardiovascular: Orthostatic hypotension, hypotension

Dermatologic: Photosensitivity

Endocrine & metabolic: Hypokalemia

Gastrointestinal: Anorexia, epigastric distress

Warnings/Precautions Avoid in severe renal disease (ineffective). Electrolyte disturbances (hypokalemia, hypochloremic alkalosis, hyponatremia) can occur. Use with caution in severe hepatic dysfunction; hepatic encephalopathy can be caused by electrolyte disturbances. Gout can be precipitated in certain patients with a history of gout, a familial predisposition to gout, or chronic renal failure. Cautious use in diabetics; may see a change in glucose control. Hypersensitivity reactions can occur. Can cause SLE exacerbation or activation. Use with caution in patients with moderate or high cholesterol concentrations. Photosensitization may occur. Correct hypokalemia before initiating therapy.

Chemical similarities are present among sulfonamides, sulfonylureas, carbonic anhydrase inhibitors, thiazides, and loop diuretics (except ethacrynic acid). Use in patients with sulfonamide allergy is specifically contraindicated in product labeling, however a risk of cross-reaction exists in patients with allergy to any of these compounds; avoid use when previous reaction has been severe.

Drug Interactions

Increased Effect/Toxicity: Increased effect of hydrochlorothiazide with furosemide and other loop diuretics. Increased hypotension and/or renal adverse effects of ACE inhibitors may result in aggressively diuresed patients. Beta-blockers increase hyperglycemic effects of thiazides in type 2 diabetes mellitus. Cyclosporine and thiazides can increase the risk of gout or renal toxicity. Digoxin toxicity can be exacerbated if a thiazide induces hypokalemia or hypomagnesemia. Lithium toxicity can occur with thiazides due to reduced renal excretion of lithium. Thiazides may prolong the duration of action with neuromuscular blocking agents.

Decreased Effect: Effects of oral hypoglycemics may be decreased. Decreased absorption of hydrochlorothiazide with cholestyramine and colestipol. NSAIDs can decrease the efficacy of thiazides, reducing the diuretic and antihypertensive effects.

Drug Uptake

Onset of diuretic action: Oral: ≤2 hours; Peak effect: 4-6 hours

Absorption: ~50% to 80%

Duration: 6-12 hours

Half-life, elimination: 5.6-14.8 hours

Time to peak: 1-2.5 hours

Pregnancy Risk Factor B (manufacturer); D (expert analysis)

Generic Available Yes

Hydrochlorothiazide and Spironolactone

(hye droe klor oh THYE a zide & speer on oh LAK tone)

Related Information

Cardiovascular Diseases *on page 1308*

U.S. Brand Names Aldactazide®

Canadian Brand Names Aldactazide 25®; Aldactazide 50®; Novo-Spirozine

Pharmacologic Category Antihypertensive Agent Combination

Synonyms Spironolactone and Hydrochlorothiazide

Use Management of mild to moderate hypertension; treatment of edema in CHF and nephrotic syndrome, and cirrhosis of the liver accompanied by edema and/or ascites

Local Anesthetic/Vasoconstrictor Precautions No information available to require special precautions

Effects on Dental Treatment No effects or complications reported

Dosage Oral:
Children: 1.66-3.3 mg/kg/day (of spironolactone) in 2-4 divided doses
Adults: 1-8 tablets in 1-2 divided doses

Other Adverse Effects
Based on **hydrochlorothiazide** component:
1% to 10%:
Cardiovascular: Orthostatic hypotension, hypotension
Dermatologic: Photosensitivity
Endocrine & metabolic: Hypokalemia
Gastrointestinal: Anorexia, epigastric distress
Based on **spironolactone** component:
Incidence of adverse events is not always reported. (Mean daily dose 26 mg)
Cardiovascular: Edema (2%, placebo 2%)
Central nervous system: Disorders (23%, placebo 21%) which may include drowsiness, lethargy, headache, mental confusion, drug fever, ataxia, fatigue
Dermatologic: Maculopapular, erythematous cutaneous eruptions, urticaria, hirsutism, eosinophilia
Endocrine & metabolic: Gynecomastia (men 9%; placebo 1%), breast pain (men 2%; placebo 0.1%), serious hyperkalemia (2%, placebo 1%), hyponatremia, dehydration, hyperchloremic metabolic acidosis in decompensated hepatic cirrhosis, inability to achieve or maintain an erection, irregular menses, amenorrhea, postmenopausal bleeding
Gastrointestinal: Disorders (29%, placebo 29%) which may include anorexia, nausea, cramping, diarrhea, gastric bleeding, ulceration, gastritis, vomiting
Genitourinary: Disorders (12%, placebo 11%)
Hematologic: Agranulocytosis
Hepatic: Cholestatic/hepatocellular toxicity
Renal: Increased BUN concentration
Respiratory: Disorders (32%, placebo 34%)
Miscellaneous: Deepening of the voice, anaphylactic reaction, breast cancer

Contraindications Hypersensitivity to hydrochlorothiazide, spironolactone, or any component of their formulation; anuria; hyperkalemia; renal or hepatic failure

Drug Interactions See Hydrochlorothiazide *on page 595* and Spironolactone *on page 1106*

Drug Uptake See Hydrochlorothiazide *on page 595* and Spironolactone *on page 1106*

Pregnancy Risk Factor C

Generic Available Yes

Hydrochlorothiazide and Triamterene

(hye droe klor oh THYE a zide & trye AM ter een)

Related Information
Cardiovascular Diseases *on page 1308*

U.S. Brand Names Dyazide®; Maxzide®; Maxzide®-25

Canadian Brand Names Apo®-Triazide; Dyazide®; Novo-Triamzide; Nu-Triazide

Pharmacologic Category Antihypertensive Agent Combination; Diuretic, Potassium Sparing; Diuretic, Thiazide

Synonyms Triamterene and Hydrochlorothiazide

Use Management of mild to moderate hypertension; treatment of edema in CHF and nephrotic syndrome

Local Anesthetic/Vasoconstrictor Precautions No information available to require special precautions

Effects on Dental Treatment No effects or complications reported

Dosage Oral: Adults:
Triamterene/hydrochlorothiazide 37.5 mg/25 mg: 1-2 tablets/capsules once daily
Triamterene/hydrochlorothiazide 75 mg/50 mg: 1 tablet daily

Mechanism of Action Competes with aldosterone for receptor sites in the distal renal tubules, increasing sodium, chloride, and water excretion while conserving potassium and hydrogen ions; may block the effect of aldosterone on arteriolar smooth muscle as well

Inhibits sodium reabsorption in the distal tubules causing increased excretion of sodium and water as well as potassium and hydrogen ions

Other Adverse Effects Frequency not defined:
Central nervous system: Dizziness, fatigue
Dermatologic: Purpura, cracked corners of mouth
Endocrine & metabolic: Electrolyte disturbances
Gastrointestinal: Bright orange tongue, burning of tongue,loss of appetite, nausea, vomiting, stomach cramps, diarrhea, upset stomach
Hematologic: Aplastic anemia, agranulocytosis, hemolytic anemia, leukopenia, thrombocytopenia, megaloblastic anemia
Neuromuscular & skeletal: Muscle cramps
Ocular: Xanthopsia, transient blurred vision
Respiratory: Allergic pneumonitis, pulmonary edema, respiratory distress
(Continued)

Hydrochlorothiazide and Triamterene *(Continued)*

Based on **hydrochlorothiazide** component: 1% to 10%:
Cardiovascular: Orthostatic hypotension, hypotension
Dermatologic: Photosensitivity
Endocrine & metabolic: Hypokalemia
Gastrointestinal: Anorexia, epigastric distress

Based on **triamterene** component: 1% to 10%:
Cardiovascular: Hypotension, edema, CHF, bradycardia
Central nervous system: Dizziness, headache, fatigue
Gastrointestinal: Constipation, nausea
Respiratory: Dyspnea

Warnings/Precautions Hydrochlorothiazide: Avoid in severe renal disease (ineffective). Electrolyte disturbances (hypokalemia, hypochloremic alkalosis, hyponatremia) can occur. Use with caution in severe hepatic dysfunction; hepatic encephalopathy can be caused by electrolyte disturbances. Gout can be precipitate in certain patients with a history of gout, a familial predisposition to gout, or chronic renal failure. Cautious use in diabetics; may see a change in glucose control. Hypersensitivity reactions can occur. Can cause SLE exacerbation or activation. Use with caution in patients with moderate or high cholesterol concentrations. Photosensitization may occur. Correct hypokalemia before initiating therapy. Chemical similarities are present among sulfonamides, sulfonylureas, carbonic anhydrase inhibitors, thiazides, and loop diuretics (except ethacrynic acid). In patients with allergy to one of these compounds, a risk of cross-reaction exists; avoid use when previous reaction has been severe.

Triamterene: Avoid potassium supplements, potassium-containing salt substitutes, a diet rich in potassium, or other drugs that can cause hyperkalemia. Monitor for fluid and electrolyte imbalances. Diuretic therapy should be carefully used in severe hepatic dysfunction; electrolyte and fluid shifts can cause or exacerbate encephalopathy. Use cautiously in patients with history of kidney stones and diabetes. Can cause photosensitivity.

Drug Interactions See Hydrochlorothiazide *on page 595* and Triamterene *on page 1200*

Drug Uptake See Hydrochlorothiazide *on page 595* and Triamterene *on page 1200*

Pregnancy Risk Factor C (per manufacturer)

Generic Available Yes

Hydrocil® [OTC] *see* Psyllium *on page 1025*
Hydro Cobex® *see* Hydroxocobalamin *on page 612*

Hydrocodone and Acetaminophen

(hye droe KOE done & a seet a MIN oh fen)

Related Information

Acetaminophen *on page 26*
Dental Drug Interactions: Update on Drug Combinations Requiring Special Considerations *on page 1434*
Oral Pain *on page 1360*

U.S. Brand Names Anexsia®; Anodynos-DHC®; Bancap HC®; Co-Gesic®; DHC®; Dolacet®; DuoCet™; Hydrocet®; Hydrogesic®; Hy-Phen®; Lorcet® 10/650; Lorcet®-HD; Lorcet® Plus; Lortab®; Margesic® H; Medipain 5®; Norco®; Stagesic®; T-Gesic®; Vicodin®; Vicodin® ES; Vicodin® HP; Zydone®

Pharmacologic Category Analgesic Combination (Narcotic)

Synonyms Acetaminophen and Hydrocodone

Use

Dental: Treatment of postoperative pain
Medical: Relief of pain

Local Anesthetic/Vasoconstrictor Precautions No information available to require special precautions

Effects on Dental Treatment <1%: Xerostomia

Restrictions C-III

Dosage Oral (doses should be titrated to appropriate analgesic effect); for children ≥12 years of age and adults, the dosage of acetaminophen should be limited to ≤4 g/day (and possibly less in patients with hepatic impairment or ethanol use)

Children:
- Antitussive (hydrocodone): 0.6 mg/kg/day in 3-4 divided doses; even though dosing by hydrocodone, make sure to keep within age-specific acetaminophen doses as well
  - A single dose should not exceed 10 mg in children >12 years, 5 mg in children 2-12 years, and 1.25 mg in children <2 years of age
- Analgesic (acetaminophen): Refer to Acetaminophen monograph

Adults: Analgesic: 1-2 tablets or capsules every 4-6 hours or 5-10 mL solution every 4-6 hours as needed for pain; do not exceed 4 g/day of acetaminophen

Hydrocodone 2.5-5 mg and acetaminophen 400-500 mg; maximum: 8 tablets/capsules per day
Hydrocodone 7.5 mg and acetaminophen: 400-650 mg; maximum: 6 tablets/capsules per day
Hydrocodone 2.5 mg and acetaminophen: 167 mg/5 mL (elixir/solution); maximum: 6 Tbsp/day
Hydrocodone 7.5 mg and acetaminophen 750 mg; maximum: 5 tablets/capsules per day
Hydrocodone 10 mg and acetaminophen: 350-660 mg; maximum: 6 tablets/day per product labeling
Do not exceed 4 g/day of acetaminophen

Mechanism of Action Hydrocodone, as with other narcotic (opiate) analgesics, blocks pain perception in the cerebral cortex by binding to specific receptor molecules (opiate receptors) within the neuronal membranes of synapses. This binding results in a decreased synaptic chemical transmission throughout the CNS thus inhibiting the flow of pain sensations into the higher centers. Mu and kappa are the two subtypes of the opiate receptor which hydrocodone binds to cause analgesia.

Acetaminophen inhibits the synthesis of prostaglandins in the CNS and peripherally blocks pain impulse generation; produces antipyresis from inhibition of hypothalamic heat-regulating center.

Other Adverse Effects Frequency not defined:
Cardiovascular: Hypotension, bradycardia
Central nervous system: Lightheadedness, dizziness, sedation, drowsiness, fatigue, confusion
Gastrointestinal: Nausea, vomiting
Genitourinary: Decreased urination
Neuromuscular & skeletal: Weakness
Respiratory: Dyspnea

<1%: Hypertension, hallucinations, xerostomia, anorexia, biliary tract spasm, urinary tract spasm, diplopia, miosis, histamine release, physical and psychological dependence with prolonged use

Contraindications Hypersensitivity to hydrocodone, acetaminophen, or any component of their formulation; CNS depression; severe respiratory depression

Warnings/Precautions Use with caution in patients with hypersensitivity reactions to other phenanthrene derivative opioid agonists (morphine, codeine, levorphanol, oxycodone, oxymorphone); respiratory diseases including asthma, emphysema, COPD, or severe liver or renal insufficiency; some preparations contain sulfites which may cause allergic reactions; may be habit-forming

Drug Interactions
Increased Effect with dextroamphetamine
Increased Toxicity with CNS depressants, TCAs; effect of warfarin may be enhanced by acetaminophen
Decreased Effect with phenothiazines

Dietary/Ethanol/Herb Considerations
Ethanol: Avoid use or limit to <3 drinks/day; may increase acetaminophen toxicity and cause CNS depression.
Food: Rate of absorption of acetaminophen may be decreased when administered with food high in carbohydrates.
Herb/Nutraceutical: Avoid kava, SAMe, St John's wort, and valerian; may increase risk of excessive sedation.

Drug Uptake
See Acetaminophen *on page 26*
Duration: 3-6 hours
Half-life, elimination: 3.8 hours
Hydrocodone:
Onset of action: Narcotic analgesic: 10-20 minutes
Duration: 4-8 hours
Half-life, elimination: 3.3-4.4 hours

Pregnancy Risk Factor C

Breast-feeding Considerations Acetaminophen: May be taken while breast-feeding.

Dosage Forms CAP (Bancap HC®, Dolacet®, Hydrocet®, Hydrogesic®, Lorcet®-HD, Margesic® H, Medipain 5®, Norcet®, Stagesic®, T-Gesic®, Zydone®): Hydrocodone 5 mg and acetaminophen 500 mg. **ELIX** (Lortab®): Hydrocodone 2.5 mg and acetaminophen 167 mg per 5 mL (480 mL). **SOLN, oral** (Lortab®): Hydrocodone 2.5 mg and acetaminophen 167 mg per 5 mL (480 mL). **TAB:** Hydrocodone 5 mg and acetaminophen 400 mg; hydrocodone 5 mg and acetaminophen 500 mg; hydrocodone 7.5 mg and acetaminophen 400 mg; hydrocodone 7.5 mg and acetaminophen 750 mg; hydrocodone 7.5 mg and acetaminophen 500 mg; hydrocodone 7.5 mg and acetaminophen 650 mg; hydrocodone 10 mg and acetaminophen 400 mg; hydrocodone 10 mg and acetaminophen 650 mg; (Anexsia® 5/500, Anodynos-DHC®, Co-Gesic®, DuoCet™, DHC®; Hy-Phen®, Lorcet®-HD, Lortab® 5/500, Vicodin®): Hydrocodone 5 mg and acetaminophen 500 mg; (Anexsia® 7.5/650, Lorcet® Plus): Hydrocodone 7.5 mg and acetaminophen 650 mg; (Lorcet® 10/650):
(Continued)

Hydrocodone and Acetaminophen *(Continued)*

Hydrocodone 10 mg and acetaminophen 650 mg; (Lortab® 2.5/500): Hydrocodone 2.5 mg and acetaminophen 500 mg; (Lortab® 7.5/500): Hydrocodone 7.5 mg and acetaminophen 500 mg; (Lortab® 10/500): Hydrocodone 10 mg and acetaminophen 500 mg; (Norco®): Hydrocodone 10 mg and acetaminophen 325 mg; (Vicodin® ES): Hydrocodone 7.5 mg and acetaminophen 750 mg; (Vicodin® HP): Hydrocodone 10 mg and acetaminophen 660 mg; (Zydone®): Hydrocodone 5 mg and acetaminophen 400 mg, hydrocodone 7.5 mg and acetaminophen 400 mg, hydrocodone 10 mg and acetaminophen 400 mg

Generic Available Yes

Comments Neither hydrocodone nor acetaminophen elicit anti-inflammatory effects. Because of addiction liability of opiate analgesics, the use of hydrocodone should be limited to 2-3 days postoperatively for treatment of dental pain. Nausea is the most common adverse effect seen after use in dental patients; sedation and constipation are second. Nausea elicited by narcotic analgesics is centrally mediated and the presence or absence of food will not affect the degree nor incidence of nausea.

Acetaminophen:

A study by Hylek, et al, suggested that the combination of acetaminophen with warfarin (Coumadin®) may cause enhanced anticoagulation. The following recommendations have been made by Hylek, et al, and supported by an editorial in *JAMA* by Bell.

Dose and duration of acetaminophen should be as low as possible, individualized and monitored

The study by Hylek reported the following:

For patients who reported taking the equivalent of at least 4 regular strength (325 mg) tablets for longer than a week, the odds of having an INR >6.0 were increased 10-fold above those not taking acetaminophen. Risk decreased with lower intakes of acetaminophen reaching a background level of risk at a dose of 6 or fewer 325 mg tablets per week.

Selected Readings

Bell WR, "Acetaminophen and Warfarin: Undesirable Synergy," *JAMA*, 1998, 279(9):702-3.
Botting RM, "Mechanism of Action of Acetaminophen: Is There a Cyclooxygenase 3?," *Clin Infect Dis*, 2000, Suppl 5:S202-10.
Dart RC, Kuffner EK, and Rumack BH, "Treatment of Pain or Fever with Paracetamol (Acetaminophen) in the Alcoholic Patient: A Systematic Review," *Am J Ther*, 2000, 7(2):123-34.
Dionne RA, "New Approaches to Preventing and Treating Postoperative Pain," *J Am Dent Assoc*, 1992, 123(6):26-34.
Gobetti JP, "Controlling Dental Pain," *J Am Dent Assoc*, 1992, 123(6):47-52.
Grant JA and Weiler JM, "A Report of a Rare Immediate Reaction After Ingestion of Acetaminophen," *Ann Allergy Asthma Immunol*, 2001, 87(3):227-9.
Hylek EM, Heiman H, Skates SJ, et al, "Acetaminophen and Other Risk factors for excessive warfarin anticoagulation, " *JAMA*, 1998, 279(9):657-62.
Kwan D, Bartle WR, and Walker SE, "The Effects of Acetaminophen on Pharmacokinetics and Pharmacodynamics of Warfarin," *J Clin Pharmacol*, 1999, 39(1):68-75.
McClain CJ, Price S, Barve S, et al, "Acetaminophen Hepatotoxicity: An Update," *Curr Gastroenterol Rep*, 1999, 1(1):42-9.
Shek KL, Chan LN, and Nutescu E, "Warfarin-Acetaminophen Drug Interaction Revisited," *Pharmacotherapy*, 1999, 19(10):1153-8.
Tanaka E, Yamazaki K, and Misawa S, "Update: The Clinical Importance of Acetaminophen Hepatotoxicity in Nonalcoholic and Alcoholic Subjects," *J Clin Pharm Ther*, 2000, 25(5):325-32.
Wynn RL, "Narcotic Analgesics for Dental Pain: Available Products, Strengths, and Formulations," *Gen Dent*, 2001, 49(2):126-8, 130, 132 passim.

Hydrocodone and Aspirin (hye droe KOE done & AS pir in)

Related Information

Dental Drug Interactions: Update on Drug Combinations Requiring Special Considerations *on page 1434*

U.S. Brand Names Lortab® ASA

Pharmacologic Category Analgesic Combination (Narcotic)

Synonyms Aspirin and Hydrocodone

Use Relief of moderate to moderately severe pain

Local Anesthetic/Vasoconstrictor Precautions No information available to require special precautions

Effects on Dental Treatment

<1%: Xerostomia

Use with caution in patients with platelet and bleeding disorders, renal dysfunction, erosive gastritis, or peptic ulcer disease, previous nonreaction does not guarantee future safe taking of medication; use with caution in impaired hepatic function. Do not use aspirin in children <16 years of age for chickenpox or flu symptoms due to the association with Reye's syndrome Avoid aspirin, if possible, for 1 week prior to surgery due to possibility of postoperative bleeding.

Elderly are a high-risk population for adverse effects from nonsteroidal anti-inflammatory agents. As much as 60% of elderly with GI complications to NSAIDs can develop peptic ulceration and/or hemorrhage asymptomatically. Also, concomitant disease and drug use contribute to the risk for GI adverse effects. Use lowest effective dose for shortest period possible. Consider renal function decline with age. Use with caution in patients with history of asthma.

Restrictions C-III

Dosage Oral:

Children: Not recommended in pediatric dental patients

Adults: 1-2 tablets every 4-6 hours as needed for pain

Mechanism of Action Hydrocodone, as with other narcotic (opiate) analgesics, blocks pain perception in the cerebral cortex by binding to specific receptor molecules (opiate receptors) within the neuronal membranes of synapsis. This binding results in a decreased synaptic chemical transmission throughout the CNS thus inhibiting the flow of pain sensations into the higher centers. Mu and kappa are the two subtypes of the opiate receptor which hydrocodone binds to cause analgesia; suppresses cough in medullary center; produces generalized CNS depression

Aspirin inhibits prostaglandin synthesis by decreasing the activity of the enzyme, cyclo-oxygenase, which results in decreased formation of prostaglandin precursors, acts on the hypothalamic heat-regulating center to reduce fever, blocks thromboxane synthetase action which prevents formation of the platelet-aggregating substance thromboxane A_2

Other Adverse Effects

>10%:

- Cardiovascular: Hypotension
- Central nervous system: Lightheadedness, dizziness, sedation, drowsiness, fatigue
- Gastrointestinal: Nausea, heartburn, stomach pains, dyspepsia, epigastric discomfort
- Neuromuscular & skeletal: Weakness

1% to 10%:

- Cardiovascular: Bradycardia
- Central nervous system: Confusion
- Dermatologic: Rash
- Gastrointestinal: Vomiting, gastrointestinal ulceration
- Genitourinary: Decreased urination
- Hematologic: Hemolytic anemia
- Respiratory: Dyspnea
- Miscellaneous: Anaphylactic shock

<1%: Hypertension, hallucinations, insomnia, nervousness, jitters, xerostomia, anorexia, biliary tract spasm, urinary tract spasm, occult bleeding, prolongated bleeding time, leukopenia, thrombocytopenia, iron-deficiency anemia, hepatotoxicity, diplopia, miosis, impaired renal function, bronchospasm, histamine release, physical and psychological dependence with prolonged use

Contraindications

Based on **hydrocodone** component: Hypersensitivity to hydrocodone or any component of the formulation

Based on **aspirin** component: Hypersensitivity to salicylates, other NSAIDs, or any component of their formulation; asthma; rhinitis; nasal polyps; inherited or acquired bleeding disorders (including factor VII and factor IX deficiency); pregnancy (in 3rd trimester especially); children (<16 years) for viral infections (chickenpox or flu symptoms), with or without fever (due to a potential association with Reye's syndrome)

Warnings/Precautions Use with caution in patients with impaired renal function, erosive gastritis, or peptic ulcer disease; children and teenagers should not use for chickenpox or flu symptoms before a physician is consulted about Reye's syndrome; tolerance or drug dependence may result from extended use

Based on **hydrocodone** component: Use with caution in patients with hypersensitivity reactions to other phenanthrene-derivative opioid agonists (morphine, codeine, hydromorphone, levorphanol, oxycodone, oxymorphone); should be used with caution in elderly or debilitated patients, and those with severe impairment of hepatic or renal function, prostatic hyperplasia, or urethral stricture. Also use caution in patients with head injury, increased intracranial pressure, acute abdomen, or impaired thyroid function. Hydrocodone suppresses the cough reflex; caution should be exercised when this agent is used postoperatively and in patients with pulmonary diseases (including asthma, emphysema, COPD)

Based on **aspirin** component: Use with caution in patients with platelet and bleeding disorders, renal dysfunction, dehydration, erosive gastritis, or peptic ulcer disease. Heavy ethanol use (>3 drinks/day) can increase bleeding risks. Avoid use in severe renal failure or in severe hepatic failure. Discontinue use if tinnitus or impaired hearing occurs. Caution in mild-moderate renal failure (only at high dosages). Patients with sensitivity to tartrazine dyes, nasal polyps and asthma may have an increased risk of salicylate sensitivity. Surgical patients should avoid ASA if possible, for 1-2 weeks prior to surgery, to reduce the risk of excessive bleeding.

Drug Interactions

Based on **hydrocodone** component:

Increased Toxicity: CNS depressants, monoamine oxidase inhibitors, general anesthetics, and tricyclic antidepressants may potentiate the effects of opiate agonists; dextroamphetamine may enhance the analgesic effect of opiate agonists

(Continued)

Hydrocodone and Aspirin *(Continued)*

Decreased Effect: Phenothiazines may antagonize the analgesic effect of opiate agonists

Based on **aspirin** component:

ACE inhibitors: The effects of ACE inhibitors may be blunted by aspirin administration, particularly at higher dosages.

Buspirone increases aspirin's free % *in vitro*.

Carbonic anhydrase inhibitors and corticosteroids have been associated with alteration in salicylate serum concentration.

Heparin and low molecular weight heparins: Concurrent use may increase the risk of bleeding

Methotrexate serum concentration may be increased; consider discontinuing aspirin 2-3 days before high-dose methotrexate treatment or avoid concurrent use.

NSAIDs may increase the risk of GI adverse effects and bleeding. Serum concentrations of some NSAIDs may be decreased by aspirin.

Platelet inhibitors (IIb/IIIa antagonists): Risk of bleeding may be increased.

Probenecid effects may be antagonized by aspirin.

Sulfonylureas: The effects of older sulfonylurea agents (tolazamide, tolbutamide) may be potentiated due to displacement from plasma proteins. This effect does not appear to be clinically significant for newer sulfonylurea agents (glyburide, glipizide, glimepiride).

Valproic acid may be displaced from its binding sites which can result in toxicity.

Verapamil may potentiate the prolongation of bleeding time associated with aspirin.

Warfarin and oral anticoagulants may increase the risk of bleeding.

Dietary/Ethanol/Herb Considerations

Ethanol: Avoid use; may increase gastric mucosal irritation and CNS depression. Based on **hydrocodone** component, watch for sedation.

Food may decrease the rate but not the extent of oral absorption. Based on **aspirin** component, administer with food or milk to reduce GI upset. Avoid garlic, ginger, and green tea.

Herb/Nutraceutical: Avoid cat's claw, dong quai, evening primrose, feverfew, garlic, ginger, ginkgo biloba, ginseng, green tea, horse chestnut, and red clover due to additional antiplatelet activity. Avoid gotu kola, kava, SAMe, St John's wort, and valerian; may increase CNS depression.

Drug Uptake

See Aspirin *on page 119*

Duration: 3-6 hours

Half-life, elimination: 3.8 hours

Hydrocodone:

Onset of action: Narcotic analgesic: 10-20 minutes

Duration: 4-8 hours

Half-life, elimination: 3.3-4.4 hours

Pregnancy Risk Factor D

Breast-feeding Considerations Aspirin: Cautious use due to potential adverse effects in nursing infants.

Dosage Forms TAB: Hydrocodone 5 mg and aspirin 500 mg

Generic Available Yes

Comments Because of addiction liability of opiate analgesics, the use of hydrocodone should be limited to 2-3 days postoperatively for treatment of dental pain; nausea is the most common adverse effect seen after use in dental patients; sedation and constipation are second; aspirin component affects bleeding times and could influence time of wound healing

Selected Readings

Dionne RA, "New Approaches to Preventing and Treating Postoperative Pain," *J Am Dent Assoc*, 1992, 123(6):26-34.

Gobetti JP, "Controlling Dental Pain," *J Am Dent Assoc*, 1992, 123(6):47-52.

Wynn RL, "Narcotic Analgesics for Dental Pain: Available Products, Strengths, and Formulations," *Gen Dent*, 2001, 49(2):126-8, 130, 132 passim.

Hydrocodone and Chlorpheniramine

(hye droe KOE done & klor fen IR a meen)

U.S. Brand Names Tussionex®

Pharmacologic Category Antihistamine/Antitussive

Synonyms Chlorpheniramine and Hydrocodone

Use Symptomatic relief of cough

Local Anesthetic/Vasoconstrictor Precautions No information available to require special precautions

Effects on Dental Treatment Prolonged use will cause significant xerostomia.

Restrictions C-III

Dosage Oral:

Children 6-12 years: 2.5 mL every 12 hours; do not exceed 5 mL/24 hours

Adults: 5 mL every 12 hours; do not exceed 10 mL/24 hours

Mechanism of Action

Based on **hydrocodone** component: Binds to opiate receptors in the CNS, altering the perception of and response to pain; suppresses cough in medullary center; produces generalized CNS depression

Based on **chlorpheniramine** component: Competes with histamine for H_1-receptor sites on effector cells in the GI tract, blood vessels, and respiratory tract

Warnings/Precautions Based on **hydrocodone** component: Use with caution in patients with hypersensitivity reactions to other phenanthrene derivative opioid agonists (morphine, codeine, hydromorphone, levorphanol, oxycodone, oxymorphone); should be used with caution in elderly or debilitated patients, and those with severe impairment of hepatic or renal function, prostatic hyperplasia, or urethral stricture. Also use caution in patients with head injury, increased intracranial pressure, acute abdomen, or impaired thyroid function. Hydrocodone suppresses the cough reflex; caution should be exercised when this agent is used postoperatively and in patients with pulmonary diseases (including asthma, emphysema, COPD); tolerance or drug dependence may result from extended use

Drug Interactions Increased Effect/Toxicity:

Based on **hydrocodone** component: Increased toxicity: CNS depressants, monoamine oxidase inhibitors, general anesthetics, and tricyclic antidepressants may potentiate the effects of opiate agonists; dextroamphetamine may enhance the analgesic effect of opiate agonists

Based on **chlorpheniramine** component: CYP2D6 enzyme substrate; Increased toxicity (CNS depression): CNS depressants, MAO inhibitors, tricyclic antidepressants, phenothiazines

Decreased Effect: Based on **hydrocodone** component: Decreased effect: Phenothiazines may antagonize the analgesic effect of opiate agonists

Drug Uptake

See Chlorpheniramine *on page 268*

Hydrocodone:

Onset of action: Narcotic analgesic: 10-20 minutes

Duration: 4-8 hours

Half-life, elimination: 3.3-4.4 hours

Pregnancy Risk Factor C

Generic Available Yes

Hydrocodone and Guaifenesin

(hye droe KOE done & gwye FEN e sin)

U.S. Brand Names Codiclear® DH; HycoClear Tuss®; Hycotuss® Expectorant Liquid; Kwelcof®; Vicodin Tuss™

Pharmacologic Category Antitussive/Expectorant

Synonyms Guaifenesin and Hydrocodone

Use Symptomatic relief of nonproductive coughs associated with upper and lower respiratory tract congestion

Local Anesthetic/Vasoconstrictor Precautions No information available to require special precautions

Effects on Dental Treatment No effects or complications reported

Restrictions C-III

Dosage Oral:

Children:

<2 years: 0.3 mg/kg/day (hydrocodone) in 4 divided doses

2-12 years: 2.5 mL every 4 hours, after meals and at bedtime

>12 years: 5 mL every 4 hours, after meals and at bedtime

Adults: 5 mL every 4 hours, after meals and at bedtime, not to exceed 30 mL in a 24-hour period

Mechanism of Action

Based on **hydrocodone** component: Binds to opiate receptors in the CNS, altering the perception of and response to pain; suppresses cough in medullary center; produces generalized CNS depression

Based on **guaifenesin** component: Thought to act as an expectorant by irritating the gastric mucosa and stimulating respiratory tract secretions, thereby increasing respiratory fluid volumes and decreasing phlegm viscosity

Other Adverse Effects Frequency not defined:

Cardiovascular: Hypertension, postural hypotension, palpitations

Central nervous system: Drowsiness, sedation, mental clouding, mental and physical impairment, anxiety, fear, dysphoria, dizziness, psychotic dependence, mood changes

Gastrointestinal: Nausea, vomiting, constipation with prolonged use

Genitourinary: Ureteral spasm, urinary retention

Ocular: Blurred vision

Respiratory: Respiratory depression (dose related)

Drug Interactions

Increased Effect/Toxicity:

Based on **hydrocodone** component: CNS depressants, monoamine oxidase inhibitors, general anesthetics, and tricyclic antidepressants may potentiate the

(Continued)

Hydrocodone and Guaifenesin *(Continued)*

effects of opiate agonists; dextroamphetamine may enhance the analgesic effect of opiate agonists

Based on **guaifenesin** component: Disulfiram, MAO inhibitors, metronidazole, procarbazine

Decreased Effect:

Based on **hydrocodone** component: Phenothiazines may antagonize the analgesic effect of opiate agonists

Based on **guaifenesin** component: Disulfiram, MAO inhibitors, metronidazole, procarbazine

Drug Uptake

See Guaifenesin *on page 568*

Hydrocodone:

Onset of action: Narcotic analgesic: 10-20 minutes

Duration: 4-8 hours

Half-life, elimination: 3.3-4.4 hours

Pregnancy Risk Factor C

Generic Available Yes

Hydrocodone and Homatropine

(hye droe KOE done & hoe MA troe peen)

U.S. Brand Names Hycodan®; Hydromet®; Hydropane®; Hydrotropine®; Tussigon®

Pharmacologic Category Antitussive

Synonyms Homatropine and Hydrocodone

Use Symptomatic relief of cough

Local Anesthetic/Vasoconstrictor Precautions No information available to require special precautions

Effects on Dental Treatment Xerostomia

Restrictions C-III

Dosage Oral (based on hydrocodone component):

Children: 0.6 mg/kg/day in 3-4 divided doses; do not administer more frequently than every 4 hours

A single dose should not exceed 1.25 mg in children <2 years of age, 5 mg in children 2-12 years, and 10 mg in children >12 years

Adults: 5-10 mg every 4-6 hours, a single dose should not exceed 15 mg; do not administer more frequently than every 4 hours

Mechanism of Action

Based on **hydrocodone** component: Binds to opiate receptors in the CNS, altering the perception of and response to pain; suppresses cough in medullary center; produces generalized CNS depression

Based on **homatropine** component: Blocks response of iris sphincter muscle and the accommodative muscle of the ciliary body to cholinergic stimulation resulting in dilation and loss of accommodation

Other Adverse Effects Frequency not defined:

Cardiovascular: Bradycardia, tachycardia, hypotension, hypertension

Central nervous system: Lightheadedness, dizziness, sedation, drowsiness, fatigue, confusion, hallucinations

Gastrointestinal: Nausea, vomiting, xerostomia, anorexia, impaired GI motility

Genitourinary: Decreased urination, urinary tract spasm

Hepatic: Biliary tract spasm

Neuromuscular & skeletal: Weakness

Ocular: Diplopia, miosis, mydriasis, blurred vision

Respiratory: Dyspnea

Miscellaneous: Histamine release, physical and psychological dependence with prolonged use

Drug Interactions

Increased Effect/Toxicity:

Based on **hydrocodone** component: Increased toxicity: CNS depressants, monoamine oxidase inhibitors, general anesthetics, and tricyclic antidepressants may potentiate the effects of opiate agonists; dextroamphetamine may enhance the analgesic effect of opiate agonists

Based on **homatropine** component:

Phenothiazine and TCAs may increase anticholinergic effects when used concurrently.

Sympathomimetic amines may cause tachyarrhythmias; avoid concurrent use

Decreased Effect: Based on **hydrocodone** component: Decreased effect: Phenothiazines may antagonize the analgesic effect of opiate agonists

Drug Uptake Duration: Hydrocodone: 4-6 hours

Pregnancy Risk Factor C

Generic Available Yes

Hydrocodone and Ibuprofen

(hye droe KOE done & eye byoo PROE fen)

Related Information

Oral Pain *on page 1360*

U.S. Brand Names Vicoprofen®

Canadian Brand Names Vicoprofen®

Pharmacologic Category Analgesic, Narcotic

Synonyms Ibuprofen and Hydrocodone

Use Relief of moderate to moderately severe pain

Local Anesthetic/Vasoconstrictor Precautions No information available to require special precautions

Effects on Dental Treatment Use with caution in patients taking anticoagulants due to ibuprofen component.

Restrictions C-III

Dosage Adults: Oral: 1-2 tablets every 4-6 hours as needed for pain

Mechanism of Action Hydrocodone, as with other narcotic (opiate) analgesics, blocks pain perception in the cerebral cortex by binding to specific receptor molecules (opiate receptors) within the neuronal membranes of synapsis. This binding results in a decreased synaptic chemical transmission throughout the CNS thus inhibiting the flow of pain sensations into the higher centers. Mu and kappa are the two subtypes of the opiate receptor to which hydrocodone binds to cause analgesia.

Based on **ibuprofen** component: Inhibits prostaglandin synthesis by decreasing the activity of the enzyme, cyclo-oxygenase, which results in decreased formation of prostaglandin precursors (see Ibuprofen *on page 621*)

Other Adverse Effects

>10%:

- Central nervous system: Headache (27%), dizziness (14%), sedation (22%)
- Dermatologic: Rash, urticaria
- Gastrointestinal: Constipation (22%), nausea (21%), dyspepsia (12%)

1% to 10%:

- Cardiovascular: Bradycardia, palpitations (<3%), vasodilation (<3%), edema (3% to 9%)
- Central nervous system: Headache, nervousness, confusion, fever (<3%), pain (3% to 9%), anxiety (3% to 9%), thought abnormalities
- Dermatologic: Itching (3% to 9%)
- Endocrine & metabolic: Fluid retention
- Gastrointestinal: Vomiting (3% to 9%), anorexia, diarrhea (3% to 9%), xerostomia (3% to 9%), flatulence (3% to 9%), gastritis (<3%), melena (<3%), mouth ulcers (<3%)
- Genitourinary: Polyuria (<3%)
- Neuromuscular & skeletal: Weakness (3% to 9%)
- Otic: Tinnitus
- Respiratory: Dyspnea, hiccups, pharyngitis, rhinitis
- Miscellaneous: Flu syndrome (<3%), infection (3% to 9%)

<1%: Congestive heart failure, arrhythmias, tachycardia, hypertension, hallucinations, mental depression, insomnia, aseptic meningitis, urticaria, erythema multiforme, toxic epidermal necrolysis, Stevens-Johnson syndrome, polydipsia, hot flashes, biliary tract spasm, cystitis, urinary tract spasm, neutropenia, anemia, agranulocytosis, inhibition of platelet aggregation, hemolytic anemia, bone marrow suppression, leukopenia, thrombocytopenia, hepatitis, peripheral neuropathy, vision changes, blurred vision, conjunctivitis, dry eyes, toxic amblyopia, diplopia, miosis, decreased hearing, acute renal failure, polyuria, allergic rhinitis, epistaxis, histamine release, physical and psychological dependence with prolonged use

Contraindications Hypersensitivity to hydrocodone, ibuprofen, aspirin, other NSAIDs, or any component of their formulation; pregnancy (3rd trimester)

Warnings/Precautions As with any opioid analgesic agent, this agent should be used with caution in elderly or debilitated patients, and those with severe impairment of hepatic or renal function, hypothyroidism, Addison's disease, prostatic hypertrophy, or urethral stricture. The usual precautions should be observed and the possibility of respiratory depression should be kept in mind. Patients with head injury, increased intracranial pressure, acute abdomen, active peptic ulcer disease, history of upper GI disease, impaired thyroid function, asthma, hypertension, edema, heart failure, and any bleeding disorder should use this agent cautiously. Hydrocodone suppresses the cough reflex; as with opioids, caution should be exercised when this agent is used postoperatively and in patients with pulmonary disease.

Drug Interactions

Based on **hydrocodone** component:

- Increased Toxicity (potential): Aspirin, other CNS depressants, alcohol, MAO inhibitors, ACE inhibitors, tricyclic antidepressants, lithium, anticoagulants, anticholinergics, methotrexate
- Decreased Effect: May decrease efficacy of ACE inhibitors and diuretics

(Continued)

Hydrocodone and Ibuprofen *(Continued)*

Based on **ibuprofen** component: CYP2C8 and 2C9 enzyme substrate

ACE-inhibitors: Antihypertensive effects may be decreased by concurrent therapy with NSAIDs; monitor BP.

Angiotensin II antagonists: Antihypertensive effects may be decreased by concurrent therapy with NSAIDs; monitor BP.

Anticoagulants (warfarin, heparin, LMWHs) in combination with NSAIDs can cause increased risk of bleeding.

Other antiplatelet drugs (ticlopidine, clopidogrel, aspirin, abciximab, dipyridamole, eptifibatide, tirofiban) can cause an increased risk of bleeding.

Loop diuretics efficacy (diuretic and antihypertensive effect) is reduced. Indomethacin reduces this efficacy, however, it may be anticipated with any NSAID.

Cholestyramine and colestipol reduce the bioavailability of diclofenac; separate administration times.

Cyclosporine: NSAIDs may increase serum creatinine, potassium, BP, and cyclosporine levels; monitor cyclosporine levels and renal function carefully.

Lithium levels can be increased; avoid concurrent use if possible or monitor lithium levels and adjust dose. Sulindac may have the least effect. When NSAID is stopped, lithium will need adjustment again.

Verapamil plasma concentration is decreased by diclofenac; avoid concurrent use.

Gentamicin and amikacin serum concentration are increased by indomethacin in premature infants. Results may apply to other aminoglycosides and NSAIDs.

Hydralazine's antihypertensive effect is decreased; avoid concurrent use.

Warfarin's INRs may be increased by piroxicam. Other NSAIDs may have the same effect depending on dose and duration. Monitor INR closely. Use the lowest dose of NSAIDs possible and for the briefest duration.

Corticosteroids may increase the risk of GI ulceration; avoid concurrent use.

Thiazides antihypertensive effects are decreased; avoid concurrent use.

Vancomycin's serum concentration is increased by indomethacin in neonates.

Dietary/Ethanol/Herb Considerations

Ethanol: Based on **hydrocodone** component, avoid use; may increase CNS depression (watch for sedation)

Food may decrease ibuprofen peak serum concentration. Avoid garlic, ginger, and green tea.

Herb/Nutraceutical: Avoid cat's claw, dong quai, evening primrose, feverfew, garlic, ginger, ginkgo biloba, ginseng, green tea, horse chestnut, and red clover due to additional antiplatelet activity.

Drug Uptake

See Ibuprofen *on page 621*

Hydrocodone:

Onset of action: Narcotic analgesic: 10-20 minutes

Duration: 4-8 hours

Half-life, elimination: 3.3-4.4 hours

Time to peak: Ibuprofen: 1.8 hours; Hydrocodone: 1.7 hours

Pregnancy Risk Factor C/D (3rd trimester)

Dosage Forms TAB: Hydrocodone 7.5 mg and ibuprofen 200 mg

Generic Available No

Comments The combination of 15 mg hydrocodone bitartrate with 400 mg ibuprofen was compared to 400 mg ibuprofen alone and placebo for the ability to diminish postoperative pain (pain after cesarean section or gynecologic surgery, 120 patients). Analgesia was measured during a 6-hour period after dosing based on onset of relief, hourly and summary variables, and duration of effect. A significantly greater proportion of patients treated with the hydrocodone/ibuprofen combination reported onset of relief compared with ibuprofen or placebo. Time to onset of relief did not differ among treatments. Hydrocodone with ibuprofen and ibuprofen alone were significantly more effective than placebo for all measures. The combination of hydrocodone with ibuprofen was significantly superior to ibuprofen for all hourly analgesic evaluations, weighted sum of pain intensity differences, total pain relief, and global rating of study medications. This report demonstrated an analgesic superiority of 15 mg hydrocodone bitartrate combined with 400 mg ibuprofen compared to 400 mg ibuprofen alone.

Selected Readings

Dionne R, "To Tame the Pain?" *Compend Contin Educ Dent*, 1998, 19(4):426-8, 430-1.

Hargreaves KM, "Management of Pain in Endodontic Patients," *Tex Dent J*, 1997, 114(10):27-31.

Sunshine A, Olson NZ, O'Neill E, et al, "Analgesic Efficacy of a Hydrocodone With Ibuprofen Combination Compared With Ibuprofen Alone for the Treatment of Acute Postoperative Pain," *J Clin Pharmacol*, 1997, 37(10):908-15.

Wynn RL, "Narcotic Analgesics for Dental Pain: Available Products, Strengths, and Formulations," *Gen Dent*, 2001, 49(2):126-8, 130, 132 passim.

Hydrocodone, Chlorpheniramine, Phenylephrine, Acetaminophen and Caffeine

(hye droe KOE done, klor fen IR a meen, fen il EF rin, a seet a MIN oh fen, & KAF een)

U.S. Brand Names Hycomine® Compound

Pharmacologic Category Antitussive/Decongestant

Synonyms Acetaminophen, Caffeine, Hydrocodone, Chlorpheniramine, and Phenylephrine; Caffeine, Hydrocodone, Chlorpheniramine, Phenylephrine, and Acetaminophen; Chlorpheniramine, Hydrocodone, Phenylephrine, Acetaminophen, and Caffeine; Phenylephrine, Hydrocodone, Chlorpheniramine, Acetaminophen, and Caffeine

Use Symptomatic relief of cough and symptoms of upper respiratory infections

Local Anesthetic/Vasoconstrictor Precautions Use with caution since phenylephrine is a sympathomimetic amine which could interact with epinephrine to cause a pressor response

Effects on Dental Treatment

Acetaminophen: No effects or complications reported

Chlorpheniramine: Prolonged use will cause significant xerostomia

Phenylephrine: Up to 10% of patients could experience tachycardia, palpitations, and xerostomia; use vasoconstrictor with caution

Restrictions C-III

Dosage Adults: Oral: 1 tablet every 4 hours, up to 4 times/day

Other Adverse Effects Frequency not defined:

Cardiovascular: Hypertension, postural hypotension, tachycardia, palpitations

Central nervous system: Sedation, drowsiness, mental clouding, lethargy, impairment of mental and physical performance, anxiety, fear, dysphoria, dizziness, psychic dependence, mood changes

Dermatologic: Rash, pruritus

Gastrointestinal: Nausea, vomiting, constipation with prolonged use

Genitourinary: Ureteral spasms, spasm of vesical sphincters and urinary retention

Ocular: Blurred vision

Respiratory: Respiratory depression

Drug Interactions See Chlorpheniramine *on page 268*, Phenylephrine *on page 950*, and Acetaminophen *on page 26*

Drug Uptake

See Chlorpheniramine *on page 268*, Phenylephrine *on page 950*, and Acetaminophen *on page 26*

Hydrocodone:

Onset of action: Narcotic analgesic: 10-20 minutes

Duration: 4-8 hours

Half-life, elimination: 3.3-4.4 hours

Pregnancy Risk Factor C

Generic Available No

Selected Readings

Barker JD Jr, de Carle DJ, and Anuras S, "Chronic Excessive Acetaminophen Use in Liver Damage," *Ann Intern Med*, 1977, 87(3):299-301.

Botting RM, "Mechanism of Action of Acetaminophen: Is There a Cyclooxygenase 3?," *Clin Infect Dis*, 2000, Suppl 5:S202-10.

Dart RC, Kuffner EK, and Rumack BH, "Treatment of Pain or Fever with Paracetamol (Acetaminophen) in the Alcoholic Patient: A Systematic Review," *Am J Ther*, 2000, 7(2):123-34.

Dionne RA, Campbell RA, Cooper SA, et al, "Suppression of Postoperative Pain by Preoperative Administration of Ibuprofen in Comparison to Placebo, Acetaminophen, and Acetaminophen Plus Codeine," *J Clin Pharmacol*, 1983, 23(1):37-43.

Grant JA and Weiler JM, "A Report of a Rare Immediate Reaction After Ingestion of Acetaminophen," *Ann Allergy Asthma Immunol*, 2001, 87(3):227-9.

Kwan D, Bartle WR, and Walker SE, "The Effects of Acetaminophen on Pharmacokinetics and Pharmacodynamics of Warfarin," *J Clin Pharmacol*, 1999, 39(1):68-75.

Licht H, Seeff LB, and Zimmerman HJ, "Apparent Potentiation of Acetaminophen Hepatotoxicity by Alcohol," *Ann Intern Med*, 1980, 92(4):511.

McClain CJ, Price S, Barve S, et al, "Acetaminophen Hepatotoxicity: An Update," *Curr Gastroenterol Rep*, 1999, 1(1):42-9.

Shek KL, Chan LN, and Nutescu E, "Warfarin-Acetaminophen Drug Interaction Revisited," *Pharmacotherapy*, 1999, 19(10):1153-8.

Tanaka E, Yamazaki K, and Misawa S, "Update: The Clinical Importance of Acetaminophen Hepatotoxicity in Nonalcoholic and Alcoholic Subjects," *J Clin Pharm Ther*, 2000, 25(5):325-32.

Hydrocodone, Phenylephrine, Pyrilamine, Phenindamine, Chlorpheniramine, and Ammonium Chloride

(hye droe KOE done, fen il EF rin, peer IL a meen, fen IN da meen, klor fen IR a meen, & a MOE nee um KLOR ide)

Pharmacologic Category Antihistamine/Decongestant/Antitussive

Use Symptomatic relief of cough and nasal congestion

Local Anesthetic/Vasoconstrictor Precautions Use with caution since phenylephrine is a sympathomimetic amine which could interact with epinephrine to cause a pressor response

(Continued)

Hydrocodone, Phenylephrine, Pyrilamine, Phenindamine, Chlorpheniramine, and Ammonium Chloride *(Continued)*

Effects on Dental Treatment

Chlorpheniramine: Prolonged use will cause significant xerostomia

Phenylephrine: Up to 10% of patients could experience tachycardia, palpitations, and xerostomia; use vasoconstrictor with caution

Dosage Adults: Oral: 10 mL every 4-6 hours, up to 40 mL/day

Drug Uptake

See Ammonium Chloride *on page 83*, Chlorpheniramine *on page 268*, and Phenylephrine *on page 950*

Hydrocodone:

Onset of action: Narcotic analgesic: 10-20 minutes

Duration: 4-8 hours

Half-life, elimination: 3.3-4.4 hours

Generic Available Yes

Hydrocodone, Pseudoephedrine, and Guaifenesin

(hye droe KOE done, soo doe e FED rin & gwye FEN e sin)

U.S. Brand Names Duratuss® HD; Hydro-Tussin® HD; K-G Tuss® HD; Su-Tuss®-HD; Tussend®

Pharmacologic Category Antitussive/Decongestant/Expectorant

Synonyms Guaifenesin, Hydrocodone, and Pseudoephedrine; Pseudoephedrine, Hydrocodone, and Guaifenesin

Use Symptomatic relief of irritating, nonproductive cough associated with respiratory conditions such as bronchitis, bronchial asthma, tracheobronchitis, and the common cold

Local Anesthetic/Vasoconstrictor Precautions Use with caution since pseudoephedrine is a sympathomimetic amine which could interact with epinephrine to cause a pressor response

Effects on Dental Treatment

Guaifenesin: No effects or complications reported

Pseudoephedrine: Up to 10% of patients could experience tachycardia, palpitations, and xerostomia; use vasoconstrictor with caution

Restrictions C-III

Dosage Adults: Oral: 5 mL every 4-6 hours

Other Adverse Effects Frequency not defined:

Cardiovascular: Arrhythmias, tachycardia, hypertension

Central nervous system: Drowsiness, fear, anxiety, tension, restlessness, pallor, insomnia, hallucinations, CNS depression

Gastrointestinal: GI upset, nausea, constipation with prolonged use

Genitourinary: Dysuria

Hepatic: Slight elevation in serum transaminase levels

Neuromuscular & skeletal: Weakness, tremor

Respiratory: Respiratory difficulty

Patients hyper-reactive to pseudoephedrine may display ephedrine-like reactions such as tachycardia, palpitations, headache, dizziness, or nausea; patient idiosyncrasy to adrenergic agents may be manifested by insomnia, dizziness, weakness, tremor, or arrhythmias.

Drug Uptake

See Acetaminophen *on page 26*, and Guaifenesin and Pseudoephedrine *on page 570*

Hydrocodone:

Onset of action: Narcotic analgesic: 10-20 minutes

Duration: 4-8 hours

Half-life, elimination: 3.3-4.4 hours

Pregnancy Risk Factor C

Generic Available Yes

Hydrocort® *see* Hydrocortisone *on page 608*

Hydrocortisone (hye droe KOR ti sone)

Related Information

Dental Office Emergencies *on page 1418*

U.S. Brand Names A-hydroCort®; Ala-Cort®; Ala-Scalp®; Anucort-HC® Suppository; Anusol® HC 1 [OTC]; Anusol® HC 2.5% [OTC]; Anusol-HC® Suppository; Cetacort®; Clocort® Maximum Strength; Cortaid® Maximum Strength [OTC]; Cortaid® With Aloe [OTC]; Cort-Dome®; Cortef®; Cortef® Feminine Itch; Cortenema®; Corticaine®; Cortifoam®; Cortizone®-5 [OTC]; Cortizone®-10 [OTC]; Delcort®; Dermacort®; DermiCort®; Dermolate® [OTC]; Dermtex® HC With Aloe; Eldecort®; Gynecort® [OTC]; Hemril-HC® Uniserts®; Hi-Cor® 1.0; Hi-Cor® 2.5; Hycort®; Hydrocort®; Hydrocortone® Acetate; Hydrocortone® Phosphate; HydroTex® [OTC]; Hytone®; LactiCare-HC®; Lanacort® [OTC]; Locoid®; Nutracort®;

Orabase® HCA; Pandel®; Penecort®; Procort® [OTC]; Proctocort™; Scalpicin®; Solu-Cortef®; S-T Cort®; Synacort®; Tegrin®-HC [OTC]; Texacort®; Westcort®

Canadian Brand Names A-Hydrocort; Aquacort®; Cortamed®; Cortate®; Cortef®; Cortenema®; Cortifoam™; Cortoderm; Emo-Cort®; Hycort™; Hyderm; Locoid®; Prevex® HC; Sarna® HC; Solu-Cortef®; Westcort®

Mexican Brand Names Aquanil HC®; Flebocorti; LactiCare-HC®; Nositrol; Nutracort®

Pharmacologic Category Corticosteroid, Rectal; Corticosteroid, Systemic; Corticosteroid, Topical

Synonyms Compound F; Cortisol; Hydrocortisone Acetate; Hydrocortisone Buteprate; Hydrocortisone Butyrate; Hydrocortisone Cypionate; Hydrocortisone Sodium Phosphate; Hydrocortisone Sodium Succinate; Hydrocortisone Valerate

Use

Dental: Treatment of a variety of oral diseases of allergic, inflammatory or autoimmune origin

Medical: Management of adrenocortical insufficiency; relief of inflammation of corticosteroid-responsive dermatoses (low and medium potency topical corticosteroid); adjunctive treatment of ulcerative colitis

Local Anesthetic/Vasoconstrictor Precautions No information available to require special precautions

Effects on Dental Treatment No effects or complications reported

Dosage Dose should be based on severity of disease and patient response

Acute adrenal insufficiency: I.M., I.V.:

- Infants and young Children: Succinate: 1-2 mg/kg/dose bolus, then 25-150 mg/day in divided doses every 6-8 hours
- Older Children: Succinate: 1-2 mg/kg bolus then 150-250 mg/day in divided doses every 6-8 hours
- Adults: Succinate: 100 mg I.V. bolus, then 300 mg/day in divided doses every 8 hours or as a continuous infusion for 48 hours; once patient is stable change to oral, 50 mg every 8 hours for 6 doses, then taper to 30-50 mg/day in divided doses

Chronic adrenal corticoid insufficiency: Adults: Oral: 20-30 mg/day

Anti-inflammatory or immunosuppressive:

- Infants and Children:
  - Oral: 2.5-10 mg/kg/day **or** 75-300 mg/m²/day every 6-8 hours
  - I.M., I.V.: Succinate: 1-5 mg/kg/day **or** 30-150 mg/m²/day divided every 12-24 hours
- Adolescents and Adults: Oral, I.M., I.V.: Succinate: 15-240 mg every 12 hours

Congenital adrenal hyperplasia: Oral: Initial: 10-20 mg/m²/day in 3 divided doses; a variety of dosing schedules have been used. **Note:** Inconsistencies have occurred with liquid formulations; tablets may provide more reliable levels. Doses must be individualized by monitoring growth, bone age, and hormonal levels. Mineralocorticoid and sodium supplementation may be required based upon electrolyte regulation and plasma renin activity.

Physiologic replacement: Children:

- Oral: 0.5-0.75 mg/kg/day **or** 20-25 mg/m²/day every 8 hours
- I.M.: Succinate: 0.25-0.35 mg/kg/day **or** 12-15 mg/m²/day once daily

Shock: I.M., I.V.: Succinate:

- Children: Initial: 50 mg/kg, then repeated in 4 hours and/or every 24 hours as needed
- Adolescents and Adults: 500 mg to 2 g every 2-6 hours

Status asthmaticus: Children and Adults: I.V.: Succinate: 1-2 mg/kg/dose every 6 hours for 24 hours, then maintenance of 0.5-1 mg/kg every 6 hours

Adults:

- Rheumatic diseases:
  - Intralesional, intra-articular, soft tissue injection: Acetate:
    - Large joints: 25 mg (up to 37.5 mg)
    - Small joints: 10-25 mg
  - Tendon sheaths: 5-12.5 mg
  - Soft tissue infiltration: 25-50 mg (up to 75 mg)
  - Bursae: 25-37.5 mg
  - Ganglia: 12.5-25 mg
- Stress dosing (surgery) in patients known to be adrenally-suppressed or on chronic systemic steroids: I.V.:
  - Minor stress (ie, inguinal herniorrhaphy): 25 mg/day for 1 day
  - Moderate stress (ie, joint replacement, cholecystectomy): 50-75 mg/day (25 mg every 8-12 hours) for 1-2 days
  - Major stress (pancreatoduodenectomy, esophagogastrectomy, cardiac surgery): 100-150 mg/day (50 mg every 8-12 hours) for 2-3 days

Dermatosis: Children >2 years and Adults: Topical: Apply to affected area 3-4 times/day (Buteprate: Apply once or twice daily). Therapy should be discontinued when control is achieved; if no improvement is seen, reassessment of diagnosis may be necessary.

Ulcerative colitis: Adults: Rectal: 10-100 mg 1-2 times/day for 2-3 weeks

(Continued)

Hydrocortisone *(Continued)*

Mechanism of Action Decreases inflammation by suppression of migration of polymorphonuclear leukocytes and reversal of increased capillary permeability

Other Adverse Effects

>10%:
- Central nervous system: Insomnia, nervousness
- Gastrointestinal: Increased appetite, indigestion

1% to 10%:
- Dermatologic: Hirsutism
- Endocrine & metabolic: Diabetes mellitus
- Neuromuscular & skeletal: Arthralgia
- Ocular: Cataracts
- Respiratory: Epistaxis

<1%: Hypertension, edema, euphoria, headache, delirium, hallucinations, seizures, mood swings, acne, dermatitis, skin atrophy, bruising, hyperpigmentation, hypokalemia, hyperglycemia, Cushing's syndrome, sodium and water retention, bone growth suppression, amenorrhea, peptic ulcer, abdominal distention, ulcerative esophagitis, pancreatitis, muscle wasting, hypersensitivity reactions, immunosuppression

Contraindications Hypersensitivity to hydrocortisone or any component of the formulation; serious infections, except septic shock or tuberculous meningitis; viral, fungal, or tubercular skin lesions

Warnings/Precautions

Use with caution in patients with hyperthyroidism, cirrhosis, nonspecific ulcerative colitis, hypertension, osteoporosis, thromboembolic tendencies, CHF, convulsive disorders, myasthenia gravis, thrombophlebitis, peptic ulcer, diabetes, glaucoma, cataracts, or tuberculosis. Use caution in hepatic impairment.

Acute adrenal insufficiency may occur with abrupt withdrawal after long-term therapy or with stress; young pediatric patients may be more susceptible to adrenal axis suppression from topical therapy

Because of the risk of adverse effects, systemic corticosteroids should be used cautiously in the elderly, in the smallest possible dose, and for the shortest possible time

Drug Interactions CYP2D6 and 3A3/4 enzyme substrate

Increased Toxicity:
- Oral anticoagulants change prothrombin time
- Potassium-depleting diuretics increase risk of hypokalemia
- Cardiac glucosides increase risk of arrhythmias or digitalis toxicity secondary to hypokalemia

Decreased Effect:
- Insulin decreases hypoglycemic effect
- Phenytoin, phenobarbital, ephedrine, and rifampin increase metabolism of hydrocortisone and decrease steroid blood level

Dietary/Ethanol/Herb Considerations

Ethanol: Avoid use; may enhance gastric mucosal irritation.

Food: Administer with food to reduce GI upset. Hydrocortisone interferes with calcium absorption; requires diet rich in pyridoxine, vitamins A, B_6, C, D, folate, calcium, phosphorus, potassium, and zinc. Limit caffeine and sodium.

Herb/Nutraceutical: Avoid cat's claw and echinacea due to immunostimulant properties. Avoid St John's wort; may decrease serum concentration.

Drug Uptake

Onset of action:
- Hydrocortisone acetate: Slow
- Hydrocortisone sodium succinate (water soluble): Rapid

Duration:
- Hydrocortisone acetate: Long
- Hydrocortisone sodium phosphate (water soluble): Short

Absorption: Rapid by all routes, except rectally

Half-life, elimination: Biologic: 8-12 hours

Pregnancy Risk Factor C

Dosage Forms **AERO, rectal, as acetate:** 10% (20 g). **AERO, topical, as base:** 0.5% (45 g, 58 g); 1% (45 mL). **CRM, as acetate:** 0.5% (15 g, 22.5 g, 30 g); 1% (15 g, 30 g, 120 g). **CRM, as base:** 0.2% (15 g, 30 g, 60 g, 120 g, 454 g); 0.5% (15 g, 30 g, 60 g, 120 g, 454 g); 1% (15 g, 20 g, 30 g, 60 g, 90 g, 120 g, 240 g, 454 g); 2.5% (15 g, 20 g, 30 g, 60 g, 120 g, 240 g, 454 g). **CRM, as buteprate:** 0.1%, 1% (15 g, 45 g). **CRM, as butyrate:** 0.1% (15 g, 45 g). **CRM, rectal, as base:** 1% (30 g); 2.5% (30 g). **CRM, as valerate:** 0.2% (15 g, 45 g, 60 g). **GEL, as base:** 0.5% (15 g, 30 g); 1% (15 g, 30 g). **INJ, as sodium phosphate:** 50 mg/mL (2 mL, 10 mL). **INJ, as sodium succinate:** 100 mg, 250 mg, 500 mg, 1000 mg. **INJ, suspension, as acetate:** 25 mg/mL (5 mL, 10 mL); 50 mg/mL (5 mL, 10 mL), **LOTION, as acetate:** 0.5%. **LOTION, as base:** 0.25% (120 mL); 0.5% (30 mL, 60 mL, 120 mL); 1% (60 mL, 118 mL, 120 mL); 2% (30 mL); 2.5% (60 mL, 120 mL). **OINT, as acetate:** 0.5% (15 g, 30 g); 1% (15 g, 21 g, 30 g). **OINT, as base:** 0.2% (15 g, 30 g); 0.5% (30 g); 1% (15 g, 20 g, 28 g, 30 g, 60 g, 120 g, 240 g, 454 g); 2.5% (20 g, 30 g). **OINT, as butyrate:** 0.1% (15 g, 45 g). **OINT, as valerate:** 0.2% (15 g, 45 g,

60 g, 120 g). **OINT, ophthalmic, as acetate:** 0.5%. **OINT, rectal, as base:** 1% (30 g). **SOLN, topical, as base:** 1% (45 mL, 75 mL, 120 mL). **SOLN, topical, as butyrate:** 0.1% (20 mL, 50 mL). **SUPP, rectal, as acetate:** 10 mg, 25 mg. **SUSP, oral, as cypionate:** 10 mg/5 mL (120 mL). **SUSP, rectal, as base:** 100 mg/60 mL (7s). **TAB, as base:** 5 mg, 10 mg, 20 mg

Generic Available Yes

Hydrocortone® Acetate *see* Hydrocortisone *on page 608*
Hydrocortone® Phosphate *see* Hydrocortisone *on page 608*
Hydrocot® *see* Hydrochlorothiazide *on page 595*
Hydro-Crysti-12® *see* Hydroxocobalamin *on page 612*
HydroDIURIL® *see* Hydrochlorothiazide *on page 595*
Hydrogesic® *see* Hydrocodone and Acetaminophen *on page 598*
Hydromet® *see* Hydrocodone and Homatropine *on page 604*

Hydromorphone (hye droe MOR fone)

U.S. Brand Names Dilaudid®; Dilaudid-5®; Dilaudid-HP®

Canadian Brand Names Dilaudid®; Dilaudid-HP®; Dilaudid-HP-Plus®; Dilaudid® Sterile Powder; Dilaudid-XP®; Hydromorph Contin®; PMS-Hydromorphone

Pharmacologic Category Analgesic, Narcotic

Synonyms Dihydromorphinone; Hydromorphone Hydrochloride

Use Management of moderate to severe pain; antitussive at lower doses

Local Anesthetic/Vasoconstrictor Precautions No information available to require special precautions

Effects on Dental Treatment 10%: Xerostomia and nausea

Restrictions C-II

Dosage Doses should be titrated to appropriate analgesic effects; when changing routes of administration, note that oral doses are less than half as effective as parenteral doses (may be only one-fifth as effective).

Pain: Older Children and Adults:
- Oral, I.M., I.V., S.C.: 1-4 mg/dose every 4-6 hours as needed; usual adult dose: 2 mg/dose
- Rectal: 3 mg every 6-8 hours

Antitussive: Oral:
- Children 6-12 years: 0.5 mg every 3-4 hours as needed
- Children >12 years and Adults: 1 mg every 3-4 hours as needed

Mechanism of Action Binds to opiate receptors in the CNS, causing inhibition of ascending pain pathways, altering the perception of and response to pain; causes cough supression by direct central action in the medulla; produces generalized CNS depression

Other Adverse Effects Frequency not defined: Antidiuretic hormone release, biliary tract spasm, miosis, urinary tract spasm, histamine release, physical and psychological dependence; increased AST, ALT

>10%:
- Cardiovascular: Palpitations, hypotension, peripheral vasodilation
- Central nervous system: Dizziness, lightheadedness, drowsiness
- Gastrointestinal: Anorexia

1% to 10%:
- Cardiovascular: Tachycardia, bradycardia, flushing of face
- Central nervous system: CNS depression, increased intracranial pressure, fatigue, headache, nervousness, restlessness
- Gastrointestinal: Nausea, vomiting, constipation, stomach cramps, xerostomia
- Genitourinary: Decreased urination, ureteral spasm
- Hepatic: Increased LFTs
- Neuromuscular & skeletal: Trembling, weakness
- Respiratory: Respiratory depression, dyspnea

Drug Interactions CNS depressants, phenothiazines, and tricyclic antidepressants may potentiate the adverse effects of hydromorphone.

Drug Uptake
- Onset of action: Analgesic: 15-30 minutes; Peak effect: 0.5-1.5 hours
- Duration: 4-5 hours
- Half-life, elimination: 1-3 hours

Pregnancy Risk Factor B/D (prolonged use or high doses at term)

Generic Available Yes

Hydromox® *see* Quinethazone *on page 1033*
Hydropane® *see* Hydrocodone and Homatropine *on page 604*
Hydrophed® *see* Theophylline, Ephedrine, and Hydroxyzine *on page 1155*

Hydroquinone (HYE droe kwin one)

U.S. Brand Names Ambi® Skin Tone [OTC]; Eldopaque® [OTC]; Eldopaque Forte®; Eldoquin® [OTC]; Eldoquin® Forte®; Esoterica® Facial [OTC]; Esoterica® Regular [OTC]; Esoterica® Sensitive Skin Formula [OTC]; Esoterica® Sunscreen [OTC]; Melanex®; Melpaque HP®; Melquin-3® [OTC]; Melquin HP®; Nuquin® Gel; Nuquin

(Continued)

Hydroquinone *(Continued)*

HP® Cream; Porcelana® [OTC]; Porcelana® Sunscreen [OTC]; Solaquin® [OTC]; Solaquin Forte®

Canadian Brand Names Eldopaque™; Eldoquin™; Neostrata® HQ; Solaquin™; Solaquin Forte™; Ultraquin™

Mexican Brand Names Crema Blanca®; Eldopaque®; Eldoquin®; Hidroquin®

Pharmacologic Category Depigmenting Agent

Synonyms Hydroquinol; Quinol

Use Gradual bleaching of hyperpigmented skin conditions

Local Anesthetic/Vasoconstrictor Precautions No information available to require special precautions

Effects on Dental Treatment No effects or complications reported

Dosage Children >12 years and Adults: Topical: Apply thin layer and rub in twice daily

Mechanism of Action Produces reversible depigmentation of the skin by suppression of melanocyte metabolic processes, in particular the inhibition of the enzymatic oxidation of tyrosine to DOPA (3,4-dihydroxyphenylalanine); sun exposure reverses this effect and will cause repigmentation.

Other Adverse Effects 1% to 10%:

Dermatologic: Dermatitis, dryness, erythema, stinging, inflammatory reaction, sensitization

Local: Irritation

Drug Uptake Onset and duration of depigmentation produced by hydroquinone varies among individuals.

Pregnancy Risk Factor C

Generic Available Yes: 3% prescription product

HydroTex® [OTC] *see* Hydrocortisone *on page 608*

Hydrotropine® *see* Hydrocodone and Homatropine *on page 604*

Hydro-Tussin™-CBX *see* Carbinoxamine and Pseudoephedrine *on page 221*

Hydro-Tussin® HD *see* Hydrocodone, Pseudoephedrine, and Guaifenesin *on page 608*

Hydroxocobalamin (hye droks oh koe BAL a min)

U.S. Brand Names Hydro Cobex®; Hydro-Crysti-12®; LA-12®

Mexican Brand Names Axofor®; Duradoce®

Pharmacologic Category Vitamin, Water Soluble

Synonyms Vitamin B_{12}

Use Treatment of pernicious anemia, vitamin B_{12} deficiency, increased B_{12} requirements due to pregnancy, thyrotoxicosis, hemorrhage, malignancy, liver or kidney disease

Unlabeled/Investigational: Neuropathies, multiple sclerosis

Local Anesthetic/Vasoconstrictor Precautions No information available to require special precautions

Effects on Dental Treatment No effects or complications reported

Dosage Vitamin B_{12} deficiency: I.M.:

Children: 1-5 mg given in single doses of 100 mcg over 2 or more weeks, followed by 30-50 mcg/month

Adults: 30 mcg/day for 5-10 days, followed by 100-200 mcg/month

Mechanism of Action Coenzyme for various metabolic functions, including fat and carbohydrate metabolism and protein synthesis, used in cell replication and hematopoiesis

Other Adverse Effects Frequency not defined:

Cardiovascular: Peripheral vascular thrombosis

Dermatologic: Itching, urticaria

Gastrointestinal: Diarrhea

Miscellaneous: Hypersensitivity reactions

Pregnancy Risk Factor A/C (dose exceeding RDA recommendation)

Generic Available Yes

Hydroxyamphetamine (hye droks ee am FET a meen)

U.S. Brand Names Paredrine®

Pharmacologic Category Adrenergic Agonist Agent, Ophthalmic

Synonyms Hydroxyamphetamine Hydrobromide

Use Produce mydriasis in diagnostic eye examination

Local Anesthetic/Vasoconstrictor Precautions No information available to require special precautions

Effects on Dental Treatment No effects or complications reported

Dosage Instill 1-2 drops into conjunctival sac

Generic Available No

Hydroxyamphetamine and Tropicamide

(hye droks ee am FET a meen & troe PIK a mide)

U.S. Brand Names Paremyd®

Pharmacologic Category Adrenergic Agonist Agent, Ophthalmic

Synonyms Tropicamide and Hydroxyamphetamine

Use Mydriasis with cycloplegia

Local Anesthetic/Vasoconstrictor Precautions No information available to require special precautions

Effects on Dental Treatment No effects or complications reported

Dosage Ophthalmic: Adults: Instill 1-2 drops into conjunctival sac(s)

Mechanism of Action Hydroxyamphetamine hydrobromide is an indirect acting sympathomimetic agent which causes the release of norepinephrine from adrenergic nerve terminals, resulting in mydriasis. Tropicamide is a parasympatholytic agent which produces mydriasis and paralysis by blocking the sphincter muscle in the iris and the ciliary muscle.

Other Adverse Effects Frequency not defined (as reported with Paremyd® or similar medications):

Cardiovascular: Hypotension, myocardial infarction, pallor, tachycardia, ventricular fibrillation

Central nervous system: Behavioral disturbances, headache, psychotic reactions

Gastrointestinal: Dry mouth, nausea, vomiting

Neuromuscular & skeletal: Muscle rigidity

Ocular: Blurred vision, intraocular pressure increased, photophobia, transient stinging

Miscellaneous: Allergic reaction, cardiorespiratory collapse, vasomotor collapse

Drug Uptake

Onset: 15 minutes

Duration: 3 hours; complete recovery usually occurs in 6-8 hours, but may take ≤24 hours

Time to peak: 60 minutes

Pregnancy Risk Factor C

Generic Available No

Hydroxychloroquine (hye droks ee KLOR oh kwin)

Related Information

Rheumatoid Arthritis and Osteoarthritis *on page 1340*

U.S. Brand Names Plaquenil®

Canadian Brand Names Plaquenil®

Pharmacologic Category Aminoquinoline (Antimalarial)

Synonyms Hydroxychloroquine Sulfate

Use Suppresses and treats acute attacks of malaria; treatment of systemic lupus erythematosus and rheumatoid arthritis

Unlabeled/Investigational: Porphyria cutanea tarda, polymorphous light eruptions

Local Anesthetic/Vasoconstrictor Precautions No information available to require special precautions

Effects on Dental Treatment No effects or complications reported

Dosage Oral:

Children:

- Chemoprophylaxis of malaria: 5 mg/kg (base) once weekly; should not exceed the recommended adult dose; begin 2 weeks before exposure; continue for 4-6 weeks after leaving endemic area
- Acute attack: 10 mg/kg (base) initial dose; followed by 5 mg/kg at 6, 24, and 48 hours
- JRA or SLE: 3-5 mg/kg/day divided 1-2 times/day to a maximum of 400 mg/day; not to exceed 7 mg/kg/day

Adults:

- Chemoprophylaxis of malaria: 2 tablets weekly on same day each week; begin 2 weeks before exposure; continue for 4-6 weeks after leaving endemic area
- Acute attack: 4 tablets first dose day 1; 2 tablets in 6 hours day 1; 2 tablets in 1 dose day 2; and 2 tablets in 1 dose on day 3
- Rheumatoid arthritis: 2-3 tablets/day to start taken with food or milk; increase dose until optimum response level is reached; usually after 4-12 weeks dose should be reduced by $1/2$ and a maintenance dose of 1-2 tablets/day given
- Lupus erythematosus: 2 tablets every day or twice daily for several weeks depending on response; 1-2 tablets/day for prolonged maintenance therapy

Mechanism of Action Interferes with digestive vacuole function within sensitive malarial parasites by increasing the pH and interfering with lysosomal degradation of hemoglobin; inhibits locomotion of neutrophils and chemotaxis of eosinophils; impairs complement-dependent antigen-antibody reactions

Other Adverse Effects Frequency not defined:

Cardiovascular: Cardiomyopathy (rare, relationship to hydroxychloroquine unclear)

Central nervous system: Irritability, nervousness, emotional changes, nightmares, psychosis, headache, dizziness, vertigo, seizures, ataxia, lassitude

(Continued)

Hydroxychloroquine *(Continued)*

Dermatologic: Bleaching of hair, alopecia, pigmentation changes (skin and mucosal; black-blue color), rash (urticarial, morbilliform, lichenoid, maculopapular, purpuric, erythema annulare centrifugum, Stevens-Johnson syndrome, acute generalized exanthematous pustulosis, and exfoliative dermatitis)

Endocrine & metabolic: Weight loss

Gastrointestinal: Anorexia, nausea, vomiting, diarrhea, abdominal cramping

Hematologic: Aplastic anemia, agranulocytosis, leukopenia, thrombocytopenia, hemolysis (in patients with glucose-6-phosphate deficiency)

Hepatic: Abnormal liver function/hepatic failure (isolated cases)

Neuromuscular & skeletal: Myopathy, palsy, or neuromyopathy leading to progressive weakness and atrophy of proximal muscle groups (may be associated with mild sensory changes, loss of deep tendon reflexes, and abnormal nerve conduction)

Ocular: Disturbance in accommodation, keratopathy, corneal changes/deposits (visual disturbances, blurred vision, photophobia - reversible on discontinuation), macular edema, atrophy, abnormal pigmentation, retinopathy (early changes reversible - may progress despite discontinuation if advanced), optic disc pallor/atrophy, attenuation of retinal arterioles, pigmentary retinopathy, scotoma, decreased visual acuity, nystagmus

Otic: Tinnitus, deafness

Miscellaneous: Exacerbation of porphyria and nonlight sensitive psoriasis

Drug Interactions

Increased Effect/Toxicity: Cimetidine increases levels of chloroquine and probably other 4-aminoquinolones.

Decreased Effect: Chloroquine and other 4-aminoquinolones absorption may be decreased due to GI binding with kaolin or magnesium trisilicate.

Drug Uptake

Onset of action: Rheumatic disease: May require 4-6 weeks to respond

Absorption: Complete

Half-life, elimination: 32-50 days

Time to peak: Rheumatic disease: Several months

Pregnancy Risk Factor C

Generic Available Yes

Hydroxyprogesterone Caproate (hye droks ee proe JES te rone)

U.S. Brand Names Hylutin®; Prodrox®

Mexican Brand Names Primolut® Depot

Pharmacologic Category Progestin

Use Treatment of amenorrhea, abnormal uterine bleeding, endometriosis, uterine carcinoma

Local Anesthetic/Vasoconstrictor Precautions No information available to require special precautions

Effects on Dental Treatment No effects or complications reported

Dosage Adults: Female: I.M.:

Amenorrhea: 375 mg; if no bleeding, begin cyclic treatment with estradiol valerate

Production of secretory endometrium and desquamation: (Medical D and C): 125-250 mg administered on day 10 of cycle; repeat every 7 days until supression is no longer desired.

Uterine carcinoma: 1 g one or more times/day (1-7 g/week) for up to 12 weeks

Mechanism of Action Natural steroid hormone that induces secretory changes in the endometrium, promotes mammary gland development, relaxes uterine smooth muscle, blocks follicular maturation and ovulation and maintains pregnancy

Other Adverse Effects Frequency not defined:

Cardiovascular: Edema

Central nervous system: Mental depression, insomnia, fever, somnolence

Dermatologic: Melasma or chloasma, allergic rash with or without pruritus, acne, hirsutism

Endocrine & metabolic: Breakthrough bleeding, spotting, changes in menstrual flow, amenorrhea

Gastrointestinal: Anorexia, nausea, weight gain/loss

Genitourinary: Changes in cervical erosion and secretions, increased breast tenderness, galactorrhea

Hepatic: Cholestatic jaundice

Local: Pain at injection site

Neuromuscular & skeletal: Weakness

Drug Interactions Rifampin may increase clearance of hydroxyprogesterone.

Drug Uptake

Duration: Concentrations measurable for 3-4 weeks after injection

Time to peak: I.M.: 3-7 days

Pregnancy Risk Factor D

Generic Available Yes

Hydroxypropyl Cellulose (hye droks ee PROE pil SEL yoo lose)

U.S. Brand Names Lacrisert®

Canadian Brand Names Lacrisert®

Pharmacologic Category Ophthalmic Agent, Miscellaneous

Use Dry eyes

Local Anesthetic/Vasoconstrictor Precautions No information available to require special precautions

Effects on Dental Treatment No effects or complications reported

Dosage Adults: Ophthalmic: Apply once daily into the inferior cul-de-sac beneath the base of tarsus, not in apposition to the cornea nor beneath the eyelid at the level of the tarsal plate

Other Adverse Effects 1% to 10%: Local: Irritation, blurred vision, edema of the eyelids

Generic Available No

Hydroxypropyl Methylcellulose

(hye droks ee PROE pil meth il SEL yoo lose)

U.S. Brand Names GenTeal™ [OTC]; Gonak™ [OTC]; Goniosol® [OTC]

Canadian Brand Names Genteal®; Isopto® Tears; Ocucoat®

Pharmacologic Category Ophthalmic Agent, Miscellaneous

Synonyms Gonioscopic Ophthalmic Solution

Use Ophthalmic surgical aid in cataract extraction and intraocular implantation; gonioscopic examinations

Local Anesthetic/Vasoconstrictor Precautions No information available to require special precautions

Effects on Dental Treatment No effects or complications reported

Dosage Introduced into anterior chamber of eye with 20-gauge or larger cannula

Other Adverse Effects 1% to 10%: Local irritation

Pregnancy Risk Factor C

Generic Available No

Hydroxyurea (hye droks ee yoor EE a)

U.S. Brand Names Droxia™; Hydrea®; Mylocel™

Canadian Brand Names Hydrea®

Mexican Brand Names Hydrea®

Pharmacologic Category Antineoplastic Agent, Antimetabolite

Synonyms Hydroxycarbamide

Use CML in chronic phase; radiosensitizing agent in the treatment of primary brain tumors, head and neck tumors, uterine cervix and nonsmall cell lung cancer, and psoriasis; treatment of hematologic conditions such as essential thrombocythemia, polycythemia vera, hypereosinophilia, and hyperleukocytosis due to acute leukemia. Has shown activity against renal cell cancer, melanoma, ovarian cancer, head and neck cancer (excluding lip cancer), and prostate cancer.

Orphan drug: Droxia™: Sickle cell anemia: Specifically for patients >18 years of age who have had at least three "painful crises" in the previous year - to reduce frequency of these crises and the need for blood transfusions

Local Anesthetic/Vasoconstrictor Precautions No information available to require special precautions

Effects on Dental Treatment No effects or complications reported

Dosage Oral (refer to individual protocols):

Adults:

HIV: 1000-1500 mg daily in a single dose or divided doses

Sickle cell anemia (moderate/severe disease): Initial: 15 mg/kg/day, increased by 5 mg/kg every 12 weeks if blood counts are in an acceptable range until the maximum tolerated dose of 35 mg/kg/day is achieved or the dose that does not produce toxic effects

Mechanism of Action Interferes with synthesis of DNA, during the S phase of cell division, without interfering with RNA synthesis; inhibits ribonucleoside diphosphate reductase preventing conversion of ribonucleotides to deoxyribonucleotides; mechanism by which hydroxyurea produces beneficial effects in sickle cell anemia is uncertain; proposed contributions include increased concentration of hemoglobin F, increased deformability of sickled cells, and reductions in neutrophils; cell-cycle specific for the S phase and may hold other cells in the G_1 phase of the cell cycle

Other Adverse Effects Frequency not defined:

Cardiovascular: Edema

Central nervous system: Drowsiness (with high doses), hallucinations, headache, dizziness, disorientation, seizures, fever, chills

Dermatologic: Erythema of the hands and face, maculopapular rash, pruritus, dry skin, dermatomyositis-like skin changes, hyperpigmentation, atrophy of skin and nails, scaling and violet papules (long-term use), nail banding, skin cancer

Endocrine & metabolic: Hyperuricemia

(Continued)

Hydroxyurea *(Continued)*

Gastrointestinal: Nausea, vomiting, stomatitis, anorexia, diarrhea, constipation, mucositis (potentiated in patients receiving radiation), pancreatitis, ulceration of buccal mucosa and GI epithelium (severe intoxication)
Emetic potential: Low (10% to 30%)
Genitourinary: Dysuria
Hematologic: Myelosuppression (primarily leukopenia); Dose-limiting toxicity, causes a rapid drop in leukocyte count (seen in 4-5 days in nonhematologic malignancy and more rapidly in leukemia); thrombocytopenia and anemia occur less often
Onset: 24-48 hours
Nadir: 10 days
Recovery: 7 days after stopping drug (reversal of WBC count occurs rapidly but the platelet count may take 7-10 days to recover)
Other hematologic effects include megaloblastic erythropoiesis, macrocytosis, hemolysis, decreased serum iron, persistent cytopenias, secondary leukemias (long-term use)
Hepatic: Elevation of hepatic enzymes, hepatotoxicity, hyperbilirubinemia (polycythemia vera)
Neuromuscular & skeletal: Weakness, peripheral neuropathy
Renal: Increased creatinine and BUN due to impairment of renal tubular function
Respiratory: Acute diffuse pulmonary infiltrates (rare), dyspnea, pulmonary fibrosis

Drug Interactions Increased Effect/Toxicity: Zidovudine, zalcitabine, didanosine may increase synergy. The potential for neurotoxicity may increase with concomitant administration with fluorouracil. Hydroxyurea modulates the metabolism and cytotoxicity of cytarabine; dose reduction is recommended. Hydroxyurea may precipitate didanosine- or stavudine-induced pancreatitis, hepatotoxicity, or neuropathy; concomitant use is not recommended.

Drug Uptake
Absorption: Readily (≥80%)
Half-life, elimination: 3-4 hours
Time to peak: ~2 hours

Pregnancy Risk Factor D

Generic Available Yes: Capsule

HydrOXYzine (hye DROKS i zeen)

Related Information
Patients Requiring Sedation *on page 1400*

U.S. Brand Names ANX®; Atarax®; Hyzine-50®; Restall®; Vistacot®; Vistaril®

Canadian Brand Names Apo®-Hydroxyzine; Atarax™; Novo-Hydroxyzin; PMS-Hydroxyzine; Vistaril®

Pharmacologic Category Antiemetic; Antihistamine

Synonyms Hydroxyzine Hydrochloride; Hydroxyzine Pamoate

Use Treatment of anxiety; preoperative sedative; antipruritic

Local Anesthetic/Vasoconstrictor Precautions No information available to require special precautions

Effects on Dental Treatment 1% to 10%: Xerostomia

Dosage
Children:
I.M.: 0.5-1.1 mg/kg/dose every 4-6 hours as needed
Oral: 0.6 mg/kg/dose every 6 hours
Adults:
Antiemetic: I.M.: 25-100 mg/dose every 4-6 hours as needed
Anxiety: Oral: 25-100 mg 4 times/day; maximum dose: 600 mg/day
Preoperative sedation:
Oral: 50-100 mg
I.M.: 25-100 mg
Management of pruritus: Oral: 25 mg 3-4 times/day
Dosing interval in hepatic impairment: Change dosing interval to every 24 hours in patients with primary biliary cirrhosis

Mechanism of Action Competes with histamine for H_1-receptor sites on effector cells in the GI tract, blood vessels, and respiratory tract. Possesses skeletal muscle relaxing, bronchodilator, antihistamine, antiemetic, and analgesic properties.

Other Adverse Effects Frequency not defined:
Central nervous system: Drowsiness, headache, fatigue, nervousness, dizziness
Gastrointestinal: Xerostomia
Neuromuscular & skeletal: Tremor, paresthesia, seizure
Ocular: Blurred vision
Respiratory: Thickening of bronchial secretions

Contraindications Hypersensitivity to hydroxyzine or any component of the formulation

Warnings/Precautions S.C., intra-arterial and I.V. administration **not** recommended since thrombosis and digital gangrene can occur; extravasation can result in sterile abscess and marked tissue induration; should be used with caution in patients with narrow-angle glaucoma, prostatic hypertrophy, and bladder neck obstruction; should also be used with caution in patients with asthma or COPD

Anticholinergic effects are not well tolerated in the elderly. Hydroxyzine may be useful as a short-term antipruritic, but it is not recommended for use as a sedative or anxiolytic in the elderly.

Drug Interactions

Amantadine, rimantadine: Central and/or peripheral anticholinergic syndrome can occur when administered with amantadine or rimantadine

Anticholinergic agents: Central and/or peripheral anticholinergic syndrome can occur when administered with narcotic analgesics, phenothiazines and other antipsychotics (especially with high anticholinergic activity), tricyclic antidepressants, quinidine and some other antiarrhythmics, and antihistamines

Antipsychotics: Hydroxyzine may antagonize the therapeutic effects of antipsychotics

CNS depressants: Sedative effects of hydroxyzine may be additive with CNS depressants; includes benzodiazepines, barbiturates, narcotic analgesics, and other sedative agents; monitor for increased effect

Dietary/Ethanol/Herb Considerations

Ethanol: Avoid use; may increase CNS depression.

Herb/Nutraceutical: Avoid gotu kola, kava, SAMe, St John's wort, and valerian; may increase CNS depression.

Drug Uptake

Onset of action: 15-30 minutes

Absorption: Oral: Rapid

Duration: 4-6 hours

Half-life, elimination: 3-7 hours

Time to peak: ~2 hours

Pregnancy Risk Factor C

Dosage Forms CAP, as pamoate: 25 mg, 50 mg, 100 mg. **INJ, as hydrochloride:** 25 mg/mL (1 mL, 2 mL, 10 mL); 50 mg/mL (1 mL, 2 mL, 10 mL). **SUSP, oral, as pamoate:** 25 mg/5 mL (120 mL, 480 mL). **SYR, as hydrochloride:** 10 mg/5 mL (120 mL, 480 mL, 4000 mL). **TAB, as hydrochloride:** 10 mg, 25 mg, 50 mg, 100 mg

Generic Available Yes

Hylorel® *see* Guanadrel *on page 572*

Hylutin® *see* Hydroxyprogesterone Caproate *on page 614*

Hyoscyamine (hye oh SYE a meen)

U.S. Brand Names Anaspaz®; A-Spas® S/L; Cystospaz®; Cystospaz-M®; ED-SPAZ®; Hyosine; Levbid®; Levsin®; Levsinex®; Levsin/SL®; NuLev™; Spacol; Spacol T/S; Symax SL; Symax SR

Canadian Brand Names Cystospaz®; Levsin®

Pharmacologic Category Anticholinergic Agent

Synonyms Hyoscyamine Sulfate; *l*-Hyoscyamine Sulfate

Use

Injection: Preoperative antimuscarinic to reduce secretions and block cardiac vagal inhibitory reflexes; to improve radiologic visibility of the kidneys; symptomatic relief of biliary and renal colic; reduce GI motility to facilitate diagnostic procedures (ie, endoscopy, hypotonic duodenography); reduce pain and hypersecretion in pancreatitis, certain cases of partial heart block associated with vagal activity; reversal of neuromuscular blockade

Oral: Adjunctive therapy for peptic ulcers, irritable bowel, neurogenic bladder/bowel; treatment of infant colic, GI tract disorders caused by spasm; to reduce rigidity, tremors, sialorrhea, and hyperhidrosis associated with parkinsonism; as a drying agent in acute rhinitis

Local Anesthetic/Vasoconstrictor Precautions No information available to require special precautions

Effects on Dental Treatment >10%: Xerostomia; normal salivary flow resumes with discontinuation

Dosage

Oral: Children: Gastrointestinal disorders: Dose as listed, based on age and weight (kg) using 0.125 mg/mL drops; repeat dose every 4 hours as needed:

Children <2 years:

3.4 kg: 4 drops; maximum: 24 drops/24 hours

5 kg: 5 drops; maximum: 30 drops/24 hours

7 kg: 6 drops; maximum: 36 drops/24 hours

10 kg: 8 drops; maximum: 48 drops/24 hours

Oral, S.L.:

Children 2-12 years: Gastrointestinal disorders: Dose as listed, based on age and weight (kg); repeat dose every 4 hours as needed:

10 kg: 0.031-0.033 mg; maximum: 0.75 mg/24 hours

20 kg: 0.0625 mg; maximum: 0.75 mg/24 hours

40 kg: 0.0938 mg; maximum: 0.75 mg/24 hours

50 kg: 0.125 mg; maximum: 0.75 mg/24 hours

(Continued)

Hyoscyamine *(Continued)*

Children >12 years and Adults: Gastrointestinal disorders: 0.125-0.25 mg every 4 hours or as needed (before meals or food); maximum: 1.5 mg/24 hours

Cystospaz®: 0.15-0.3 mg up to 4 times/day

Oral (timed release): Children >12 years and Adults: Gastrointestinal disorders: 0.375-0.75 mg every 12 hours; maximum: 1.5 mg/24 hours

I.M., I.V., S.C.: Children >12 years and Adults: Gastrointestinal disorders: 0.25-0.5 mg; may repeat as needed up to 4 times/day, at 4-hour intervals

I.V.: Children >2 year and Adults: I.V.: Preanesthesia: 5 mcg/kg given 30-60 minutes prior to induction of anesthesia or at the time preoperative narcotics or sedatives are administered

I.V.: Adults: Diagnostic procedures: 0.25-0.5 mg given 5-10 minutes prior to procedure

To reduce drug-induced bradycardia during surgery: 0.125 mg; repeat as needed

To reverse neuromuscular blockade: 0.2 mg for every 1 mg neostigmine (or the physostigmine/pyridostigmine equivalent)

Mechanism of Action Blocks the action of acetylcholine at parasympathetic sites in smooth muscle, secretory glands and the CNS; increases cardiac output, dries secretions, antagonizes histamine and serotonin

Other Adverse Effects Frequency not defined:

Cardiovascular: Palpitations, tachycardia

Central nervous system: Ataxia, dizziness, drowsiness, headache, insomnia, mental confusion/excitement, nervousness, speech disorder, weakness

Dermatologic: Urticaria

Endocrine & metabolic: Lactation suppression

Gastrointestinal: Bloating, constipation, xerostomia, loss of taste, nausea, vomiting

Genitourinary: Impotence, urinary hesitancy, urinary retention

Ocular: Blurred vision, cycloplegia, increased ocular tension, mydriasis

Miscellaneous: Allergic reactions, sweating decreased

Drug Interactions

Increased Effect/Toxicity: Increased toxicity with amantadine, antihistamines, antimuscarinics, haloperidol, phenothiazines, tricyclic antidepressants, and MAO inhibitors.

Decreased effect with antacids

Drug Uptake

Onset of action: 2-3 minutes

Absorption: Well absorbed

Duration: 4-6 hours

Half-life, elimination: 13% to 38%

Pregnancy Risk Factor C

Generic Available Yes

Hyoscyamine, Atropine, Scopolamine, and Phenobarbital

(hye oh SYE a meen, A troe peen, skoe POL a meen & fee noe BAR bi tal)

U.S. Brand Names Barbidonna®; Bellatal®; Donnatal®

Canadian Brand Names Donnatal®

Pharmacologic Category Anticholinergic Agent; Antispasmodic Agent, Gastrointestinal

Synonyms Atropine, Hyoscyamine, Scopolamine, and Phenobarbital; Phenobarbital, Hyoscyamine, Atropine, and Scopolamine; Scopolamine, Hyoscyamine, Atropine, and Phenobarbital

Use Adjunct in treatment of peptic ulcer disease, irritable bowel, spastic colitis, spastic bladder, and renal colic

Local Anesthetic/Vasoconstrictor Precautions No information available to require special precautions

Effects on Dental Treatment >10%: Xerostomia; normal salivary flow resumes with discontinuation

Dosage Oral:

Children: Donnatal® elixir: 0.1 mL/kg/dose every 4 hours; maximum dose: 5 mL **or** see table for alternative.

Weight (kg)	Dose (mL)	
	Every 4 hours	Every 6 hours
4.5	0.5	0.75
10	1	1.5
14	1.5	2
23	2.5	3.8
34	3.8	5
≥45	5	7.5

Adults: 1-2 capsules or tablets 3-4 times/day; or 1 Donnatal® Extentab® in sustained release form every 12 hours; or 5-10 mL elixir 3-4 times/day or every 8 hours

Mechanism of Action See Hyoscyamine *on page 617*, Atropine *on page 130*, Scopolamine *on page 1077*, and Phenobarbital *on page 945*

Other Adverse Effects

>10%:
- Dermatologic: Dry skin
- Gastrointestinal: Constipation, dry throat, xerostomia
- Local: Irritation at injection site
- Respiratory: Dry nose
- Miscellaneous: Diaphoresis (decreased)

1% to 10%:
- Dermatologic: Increased sensitivity to light
- Endocrine & metabolic: Decreased flow of breast milk
- Gastrointestinal: Dysphagia

Drug Interactions Increased Effect/Toxicity: May increase toxicity of CNS depressants, coumarin anticoagulants, amantadine, antihistamine, phenothiazides, antidiarrheal suspensions, corticosteroids, digitalis, griseofulvin, tetracyclines, anticonvulsants, MAO inhibitors, and tricyclic antidepressants

Drug Uptake Absorption: Well absorbed

Pregnancy Risk Factor C

Generic Available Yes

Hyoscyamine, Atropine, Scopolamine, Kaolin, and Pectin

(hye oh SYE a meen, A troe peen, skoe POL a meen, KAY oh lin & PEK tin)

Pharmacologic Category Anticholinergic Agent; Antidiarrheal

Use Antidiarrheal; also used in gastritis, enteritis, colitis, and acute GI upsets, and nausea which may accompany any of these conditions

Local Anesthetic/Vasoconstrictor Precautions No information available to require special precautions

Effects on Dental Treatment >10%: Xerostomia; normal salivary flow resumes with discontinuation

Dosage Oral:

Children:
- 10-20 lb: 2.5 mL
- 20-30 lb: 5 mL
- >30 lb: 5-10 mL

Adults:
- Diarrhea: 30 mL at once and 15-30 mL with each loose stool
- Other conditions: 15 mL every 3 hours as needed

Pregnancy Risk Factor C

Generic Available Yes

Hyoscyamine, Atropine, Scopolamine, Kaolin, Pectin, and Opium

(hye oh SYE a meen, A troe peen, skoe POL a meen, KAY oh lin, PEK tin, & OH pee um)

U.S. Brand Names Donnapectolin-PG®; Kapectolin PG®

Pharmacologic Category Anticholinergic Agent; Antidiarrheal

Use Treatment of diarrhea

Local Anesthetic/Vasoconstrictor Precautions No information available to require special precautions

Effects on Dental Treatment >10%: Xerostomia; normal salivary flow resumes with discontinuation

Restrictions C-V

Dosage

Children 6-12 years: Initial: 10 mL, then, 5-10 mL every 3 hours thereafter

Alternate children's dosing recommendations based on body weight:
- 10 lb: 2.5 mL
- 20 lb: 5 mL
- ≥ 30 lb: 5-10 mL

Do not administer >4 doses in any 24-hour period

Children >12 years and Adults: Initial: 30 mL (1 fluid oz) followed by 15 mL every 3 hours

Pregnancy Risk Factor C

Generic Available Yes

Comments Hyoscyamine is dialyzable

Hyosine *see* Hyoscyamine *on page 617*

Hyperstat® I.V. *see* Diazoxide *on page 375*

Hy-Phen® *see* Hydrocodone and Acetaminophen *on page 598*

HypoTears [OTC] *see* Artificial Tears *on page 117*

HypoTears PF [OTC] *see* Artificial Tears *on page 117*
Hyrexin-50® *see* DiphenhydrAMINE *on page 398*
Hytakerol® *see* Dihydrotachysterol *on page 394*
Hytinic® [OTC] *see* Polysaccharide-Iron Complex *on page 972*
Hytone® *see* Hydrocortisone *on page 608*
Hytrin® *see* Terazosin *on page 1140*
Hytuss® [OTC] *see* Guaifenesin *on page 568*
Hytuss-2X® [OTC] *see* Guaifenesin *on page 568*
Hyzaar® *see* Losartan and Hydrochlorothiazide *on page 732*
Hyzine-50® *see* HydrOXYzine *on page 616*
Iberet-Folic-500® *see* Ferrous Sulfate, Ascorbic Acid, Vitamin B Complex, and Folic Acid *on page 500*
Iberet®-Liquid [OTC] *see* Ferrous Sulfate, Ascorbic Acid, and Vitamin B Complex *on page 499*
Iberet®-Liquid 500 [OTC] *see* Ferrous Sulfate, Ascorbic Acid, and Vitamin B Complex *on page 499*

Ibritumomab (ib ri TYOO mo mab)

U.S. Brand Names Zevalin™

Pharmacologic Category Antineoplastic Agent, Monoclonal Antibody; Radiopharmaceutical

Synonyms Ibritumomab Tiuxetan; In-111 Zevalin; Y-90 Zevalin

Use Treatment of relapsed or refractory low-grade, follicular, or transformed B-cell non-Hodgkin's lymphoma (including rituximab-refractory follicular non-Hodgkin's lymphoma) as part of a therapeutic regimen with rituximab (Zevalin™ therapeutic regimen); **not to be used as single-agent therapy**; must be radiolabeled prior to use

Local Anesthetic/Vasoconstrictor Precautions No information available to require special precautions

Effects on Dental Treatment No effects or complications reported

Dosage I.V.: Adults: Ibritumomab is administered **only** as part of the Zevalin™ therapeutic regimen (a combined treatment regimen with rituximab). The regimen consists of two steps:

Step 1:

Rituximab infusion: 250 mg/m^2 at an initial rate of 50 mg/hour. If hypersensitivity or infusion-related events do not occur, increase infusion in increments of 50 mg/hour every 30 minutes, to a maximum of 400 mg/hour. Infusions should be temporarily slowed or interrupted if hypersensitivity or infusion-related events occur. The infusion may be resumed at one-half the previous rate upon improvement of symptoms.

In-111 ibritumomab infusion: Within 4 hours of the completion of rituximab infusion, inject 5 mCi (1.6 mg total antibody dose) over 10 minutes.

Biodistribution of In-111 ibritumomab should be assessed by imaging at 2-24 hours and at 48-72 hours postinjection. An optional third imaging may be performed 90-120 hours postinjection. If biodistribution is not acceptable, the patient should not proceed to Step 2.

Step 2 (initiated 7-9 days following Step 1):

Rituximab infusion: 250 mg/m^2 at an initial rate of 100 mg/hour (50 mg/hour if infusion-related events occurred with the first infusion). If hypersensitivity or infusion-related events do not occur, increase infusion in increments of 100 mg/hour every 30 minutes, to a maximum of 400 mg/hour, as tolerated.

Y-90 ibritumomab infusion: Within 4 hours of the completion of rituximab infusion:

Platelet count >150,000 cells/mm^3: Inject 4 mCi (14.8 MBq/kg actual body weight) over 10 minutes

Platelet count between 100,000-149,000 cells/mm^3: Inject 3 mCi (11.1 MBq/kg actual body weight) over 10 minutes

Platelet count <100,000 cells/mm^3: Do **not** administer

Maximum dose: The prescribed, measured, and administered dose of Y-90 ibritumomab must not exceed 32 mCi (1184 MBq), regardless of the patient's body weight

Mechanism of Action Ibritumomab is a monoclonal antibody directed against the CD20 antigen found on B lymphocytes (normal and malignant). Ibritumomab binding induces apoptosis in B lymphocytes *in vitro*. It is combined with the chelator tiuxetan, which acts as a specific chelation site for either Indium-111 (In-111) or Yttrium-90 (Y-90). The monoclonal antibody acts as a delivery system to direct the radioactive isotope to the targeted cells, however binding has been observed in lymphoid cells throughout the body and in lymphoid nodules in organs such as the large and small intestines. Indium-111 is a gamma-emitter used to assess biodistribution of ibritumomab, while Y-90 emits beta particles. Beta-emission induces cellular damage through the formation of free radicals (in both target cells and surrounding cells).

Other Adverse Effects Severe, potentially life-threatening allergic reactions have occurred in association with infusions. Also refer to Rituximab monograph.

>10%:
- Central nervous system: Chills (24%), fever (17%), pain (13%), headache (12%)
- Gastrointestinal: Nausea (31%), abdominal pain (16%), vomiting (12%)
- Hematologic: Thrombocytopenia (95%), neutropenia (77%), anemia (61%)
  - Myelosuppressive:
    - WBC: Severe
    - Platelets: Severe
    - Nadir: 7-9 weeks
    - Recovery: 22-35 days
- Neuromuscular & skeletal: Weakness (43%)
- Respiratory: Dyspnea (14%)
- Miscellaneous: Infection (29%)

1% to 10%:
- Cardiovascular: Peripheral edema (8%), hypotension (6%), flushing (6%), angioedema (5%)
- Central nervous system: Dizziness (10%), insomnia (5%), anxiety (4%)
- Dermatologic: Pruritus (9%), rash (8%), urticaria (4%), petechia (3%)
- Gastrointestinal: Diarrhea (9%), anorexia (8%), abdominal distension (5%), constipation (5%), dyspepsia (4%), melena (2%; life threatening in 1%), gastrointestinal hemorrhage (1%)
- Hematologic: Bruising (7%), pancytopenia (2%), secondary malignancies (2%)
- Neuromuscular & skeletal: Back pain (8%), arthralgia (7%), myalgia (7%)
- Respiratory: Cough (10%), throat irritation (10%), rhinitis (6%), bronchospasm (5%), epistaxis (3%), apnea (1%)
- Miscellaneous: Diaphoresis (4%), allergic reaction (2%; life-threatening in 1%)

Drug Interactions

Increased Effect/Toxicity: Due to the high incidence of thrombocytopenia associated with ibritumomab, the use of agents which decrease platelet function may be associated with a higher risk of bleeding (includes aspirin, NSAIDs, glycoprotein IIb/IIIa antagonists, clopidogrel and ticlopidine). In addition, the risk of bleeding may be increased with anticoagulant agents, including heparin, low molecular weight heparins, thrombolytics, and warfarin. The safety of live viral vaccines has not been established.

Decreased Effect: Response to vaccination may be impaired.

Drug Uptake

Duration: Beta cell recovery begins in ~12 weeks; generally in normal range within 9 months

Half-life, elimination: Y-90 ibritumomab: 30 hours; Indium-111 decays with a physical half-life of 67 hours; Yttrium-90 decays with a physical half-life of 64 hours

Pregnancy Risk Factor D

Generic Available No

Ibuprofen (eye byoo PROE fen)

Related Information

Dental Drug Interactions: Update on Drug Combinations Requiring Special Considerations *on page 1434*
Oral Pain *on page 1360*
Rheumatoid Arthritis and Osteoarthritis *on page 1340*
Temporomandibular Dysfunction (TMD) *on page 1397*

U.S. Brand Names Advil® [OTC]; Advil® Migraine Liqui-Gels [OTC]; Children's Advil® [OTC]; Children's Motrin® [OTC]; Genpril® [OTC]; Haltran® [OTC]; Junior Strength Motrin® [OTC]; Menadol® [OTC]; Midol® IB [OTC]; Motrin®; Motrin® IB [OTC]; Motrin® Migraine Pain [OTC]; Nuprin® [OTC]

Canadian Brand Names Advil®; Apo®-Ibuprofen; Motrin®; Motrin® (Children's); Motrin® IB; Novo-Profen®; Nu-Ibuprofen

Mexican Brand Names Advil®; Algidol®; Butacortelone; Citalgan®; Dibufen; Diprodol®; Flexafen®; Kedvil; Motrin®; Proartinal; Quadrax; Tabalon

Pharmacologic Category Nonsteroidal Anti-inflammatory Drug (NSAID)

Synonyms *p*-Isobutylhydratropic Acid

Use

Dental: Management of pain and swelling

Medical: Inflammatory diseases and rheumatoid disorders including juvenile rheumatoid arthritis, mild to moderate pain, fever, dysmenorrhea, gout, ankylosing spondylitis, acute migraine headache

Cystic fibrosis

Local Anesthetic/Vasoconstrictor Precautions No information available to require special precautions

Effects on Dental Treatment

<1%; Xerostomia

NSAID formulations are known to reversibly decrease platelet aggregation via mechanisms different than observed with aspirin. The dentist should be aware of the potential of abnormal coagulation. Caution should also be exercised in the use of NSAIDs in patients already on anticoagulant therapy with drugs such as warfarin (Coumadin®).

(Continued)

Ibuprofen *(Continued)*

Dosage Oral:

Children: Analgesic: 4-10 mg/kg/dose every 6-8 hours

Adults: 400-800 mg/dose 3-4 times/day; maximum daily dose: 3.2 (3200 mg) g/day

Mechanism of Action Inhibits prostaglandin synthesis by decreasing the activity of the enzyme, cyclo-oxygenase, which results in decreased formation of prostaglandin precursors

Other Adverse Effects

1% to 10%:

Central nervous system: Headache (1% to 3%), nervousness (<3%), fatigue (<3%)

Dermatologic: Itching (1% to 3%), rash (3% to 9%), urticaria

Endocrine & metabolic: Fluid retention

Gastrointestinal: Dyspepsia (1% to 3%), vomiting (1% to 3%), abdominal pain/cramps/distress (1% to 3%), peptic ulcer, GI bleed, GI perforation, heartburn, nausea (3% to 9%), diarrhea (1% to 3%), constipation (1% to 3%), flatulence (1% to 3%), indigestion (1% to 3%)

Otic: Tinnitus

<1%: Edema, CHF, arrhythmias, tachycardia, hypertension, confusion, hallucinations, mental depression, drowsiness, insomnia, aseptic meningitis, erythema multiforme, toxic epidermal necrolysis, Stevens-Johnson syndrome, polydipsia, hot flashes, gastritis, GI ulceration, cystitis, polyuria, neutropenia, anemia, agranulocytosis, inhibition of platelet aggregation, hemolytic anemia, bone marrow suppression, leukopenia, thrombocytopenia, hepatitis, peripheral neuropathy, vision changes, blurred vision, conjunctivitis, dry eyes, toxic amblyopia, decreased hearing, acute renal failure, allergic rhinitis, dyspnea, epistaxis

Contraindications Hypersensitivity to ibuprofen, any component of the formulation, aspirin, or other NSAIDs; patients with "aspirin triad" (bronchial asthma, aspirin intolerance, rhinitis); pregnancy (3rd trimester)

Warnings/Precautions Use with caution in patients with CHF, hypertension, dehydration, decreased renal or hepatic function, history of GI disease (bleeding or ulcers), or those receiving anticoagulants. Elderly are at a high risk for adverse effects from NSAIDs. As many as 60% of elderly can develop peptic ulceration and/or hemorrhage asymptomatically. Fatal asthmatic and anaphylactoid reactions have occurred in patients with "aspirin triad" (see Contraindications).

Use lowest effective dose for shortest period possible. Use of NSAIDs can compromise existing renal function especially when Cl_{cr} is <30 mL/minute. CNS adverse effects such as confusion, agitation, and hallucination are generally seen in overdose or high-dose situations; however, elderly may demonstrate these adverse effects at lower doses than younger adults. Do not exceed 3200 mg/day. Withhold for at least 4-6 half-lives prior to surgical or dental procedures.

Drug Interactions CYP2C8 and 2C9 enzyme substrate

ACE inhibitors: Antihypertensive effects may be decreased by concurrent therapy with NSAIDs; monitor BP.

Angiotensin II antagonists: Antihypertensive effects may be decreased by concurrent therapy with NSAIDs; monitor BP.

Anticoagulants (warfarin, heparin, LMWHs) in combination with NSAIDs can cause increased risk of bleeding.

Antiplatelet drugs (ticlopidine, clopidogrel, aspirin, abciximab, dipyridamole, eptifibatide, tirofiban) can cause an increased risk of bleeding.

Corticosteroids: May increase the risk of GI ulceration; avoid concurrent use

Cyclosporine: NSAIDs may increase serum creatinine, potassium, BP, and cyclosporine levels; monitor cyclosporine levels and renal function carefully.

Hydralazine's antihypertensive effect is decreased; avoid concurrent use

Lithium levels can be increased; avoid concurrent use if possible or monitor lithium levels and adjust dose. Sulindac may have the least effect. When NSAID is stopped, lithium will need adjustment again.

Loop diuretics efficacy (diuretic and antihypertensive effect) is reduced. Indomethacin reduces this efficacy, however, it may be anticipated with any NSAID.

Methotrexate: Severe bone marrow suppression, aplastic anemia, and GI toxicity have been reported with concomitant NSAID therapy. Avoid use during moderate or high-dose methotrexate (increased and prolonged methotrexate levels). NSAID use during low-dose treatment of rheumatoid arthritis has not been fully evaluated; extreme caution is warranted.

Warfarin's INRs may be increased by piroxicam. Other NSAIDs may have the same effect depending on dose and duration. Monitor INR closely. Use the lowest dose of NSAIDs possible and for the briefest duration. May alter the anticoagulant effects of warfarin; concurrent use with other antiplatelet agents or anticoagulants may increase risk of bleeding.

Dietary/Ethanol/Herb Considerations

Ethanol: Avoid use; may enhance gastric mucosal irritation.

Food: Administer with with food or milk to reduce GI upset. Food decreases rate of absorption but not extent; may decrease ibuprofen peak serum concentration.

Limit salicylate-containing foods (curry powder, prunes, raisins, tea, or licorice); avoid excessive amounts of vitamin C. Avoid garlic, ginger, and green tea.

Herb/Nutraceutical: Avoid cat's claw, dong quai, evening primrose, feverfew, garlic, ginger, ginkgo biloba, ginseng, green tea, horse chestnut, and red clover due to additional antiplatelet activity. Avoid kava and valerian; may enhance benzodiazepine activity.

Drug Uptake

Onset of action: Analgesic: 30-60 minutes; Anti-inflammatory: ≤7 days; Peak effect: 1-2 weeks

Absorption: Oral: Rapid (85%)

Duration: 4-6 hours

Half-life, elimination: 2-4 hours; End-stage renal disease: Unchanged

Time to peak: 1-2 hours

Pregnancy Risk Factor B/D (3rd trimester)

Breast-feeding Considerations Limited data suggests minimal excretion in breast milk.

Dosage Forms CAP: 200 mg. **CAPLET:** 200 mg. **DROPS, oral:** 40 mg/mL (15 mL). **SUSP, oral:** 100 mg/5 mL (60 mL, 120 mL, 480 mL). **TAB:** 100 mg, 200 mg, 300 mg, 400 mg, 600 mg, 800 mg. **TAB, chewable:** 50 mg, 100 mg

Generic Available Yes: Tablet

Comments Preoperative use of ibuprofen at a dose of 400-600 mg every 6 hours 24 hours before the appointment decreases postoperative edema and hastens healing time

Selected Readings

Ahmad N, Grad HA, Haas DA, et al, "The Efficacy of Nonopioid Analgesics for Postoperative Dental Pain: A Meta-Analysis," *Anesth Prog*, 1997, 44(4):119-26.

Brooks PM and Day RO, "Nonsteroidal Anti-inflammatory Drugs - Differences and Similarities," *N Engl J Med*, 1991, 324(24):1716-25.

Dionne R, "Additive Analgesia Without Opioid Side Effects," *Compend Contin Educ Dent*, 2000, 21(7):572-4, 576-7.

Dionne RA, "New Approaches to Preventing and Treating Postoperative Pain," *J Am Dent Assoc*, 1992, 123(6):26-34.

Dionne RA and Berthold CW, "Therapeutic Uses of Nonsteroidal Anti-Inflammatory Drugs in Dentistry," *Crit Rev Oral Biol Med*, 2001, 12(4):315-30.

Gobetti JP, "Controlling Dental Pain," *J Am Dent Assoc*, 1992, 123(6):47-52.

Hersh EV, Levin LM, Cooper SA, et al, "Ibuprofen Liquigel for Oral Surgery Pain," *Clin Ther*, 2000, 22(11):1306-18.

Pearlman B, Boyatzis S, Daly C, et al, "The Analgesic Efficacy of Ibuprofen in Periodontal Surgery: A Multicentre Study," *Aust Dent J*, 1997, 42(5):328-34.

Winter L Jr, Bass E, Recant B, et al, "Analgesic Activity of Ibuprofen (Motrin®) in Postoperative Oral Surgical Pain," *Oral Surg Oral Med Oral Pathol*, 1978, 45(2):159-66.

Wynn RL, "NSAIDS and Cardiovascular Effects, Celecoxib for Dental Pain, and a New Analgesic - Tramadol with Acetaminophen," *Gen Dent*, 2002, 50(3):218-222.

Nguyen AM, Graham DY, Gage T, et al, "Nonsteroidal Anti-Inflammatory Drug Use in Dentistry: Gastrointestinal Implications," *Gen Dent*, 1999, 47(6):590-6.

Ibutilide (i BYOO ti lide)

U.S. Brand Names Corvert®

Pharmacologic Category Antiarrhythmic Agent, Class III

Synonyms Ibutilide Fumarate

Use Acute termination of atrial fibrillation or flutter of recent onset; the effectiveness of ibutilide has not been determined in patients with arrhythmias of >90 days in duration

Local Anesthetic/Vasoconstrictor Precautions No information available to require special precautions

Effects on Dental Treatment No effects or complications reported

Dosage I.V.: Initial:

Adults:

<60 kg: 0.01 mg/kg over 10 minutes

≥60 kg: 1 mg over 10 minutes

If the arrhythmia does not terminate within 10 minutes after the end of the initial infusion, a second infusion of equal strength may be infused over a 10-minute period

Elderly: Dose selection should be cautious, usually starting at the lower end of the dosing range.

Mechanism of Action Exact mechanism of action is unknown; prolongs the action potential in cardiac tissue

Other Adverse Effects

1% to 10%:

Cardiovascular: Sustained polymorphic ventricular tachycardia (ie, torsade de pointes) (1.7%, often requiring cardioversion), nonsustained polymorphic ventricular tachycardia (2.7%), nonsustained monomorphic ventricular tachycardia (4.9%), ventricular extrasystoles (5.1%), nonsustained monomorphic VT (4.9%), tachycardia/supraventricular tachycardia (2.7%), hypotension (2%), bundle branch block (1.9%), AV block (1.5%), bradycardia (1.2%), QT segment prolongation, hypertension (1.2%), palpitations (1%)

Central nervous system: Headache (3.6%)

Gastrointestinal: Nausea (>1%)

(Continued)

Ibutilide *(Continued)*

Warnings/Precautions Potentially fatal arrhythmias (eg, polymorphic ventricular tachycardia) can occur with ibutilide, **usually** in association with torsade de pointes (QT prolongation). Studies indicate a 1.7% incidence of arrhythmias in treated patients. The drug should be given in a setting of continuous EKG monitoring and by personnel trained in treating arrhythmias particularly polymorphic ventricular tachycardia. Patients with chronic atrial fibrillation may not be the best candidates for ibutilide since they often revert after conversion and the risks of treatment may not be justified when compared to alternative management. Dosing adjustments in patients with renal or hepatic dysfunction since a maximum of only two 10-minute infusions are indicated and drug distribution is one of the primary mechanisms responsible for termination of the pharmacologic effect; safety and efficacy in children have not been established.

Drug Interactions Increased Effect/Toxicity: Class Ia antiarrhythmic drugs (disopyramide, quinidine, and procainamide) and other class III drugs such as amiodarone and sotalol should not be given concomitantly with ibutilide due to their potential to prolong refractoriness. Signs of digoxin toxicity may be masked when coadministered with ibutilide. Toxicity of ibutilide is potentiated by concurrent administration of other drugs which may prolong QT interval: phenothiazines, tricyclic and tetracyclic antidepressants, cisapride, sparfloxacin, gatifloxacin, moxifloxacin, erythromycin, terfenadine, and astemizole.

Drug Uptake

Onset of action: ≤90 minutes after start of infusion (1/2 of conversions to sinus rhythm occur during infusion)

Half-life, elimination: 2-12 hours; Average: 6 hours

Pregnancy Risk Factor C

Generic Available No

Idamycin® *see* Idarubicin *on page 624*

Idamycin PFS® *see* Idarubicin *on page 624*

Idarubicin (eye da ROO bi sin)

U.S. Brand Names Idamycin®; Idamycin PFS®

Canadian Brand Names Idamycin®

Mexican Brand Names Idamycin®

Pharmacologic Category Antineoplastic Agent, Anthracycline

Synonyms 4-demethoxydaunorubicin; 4-dmdr; Idarubicin Hydrochloride

Use In combination with other antineoplastic agents for treatment of acute myelogenous leukemia (AML) in adults and acute lymphocytic leukemia (ALL) in children

Local Anesthetic/Vasoconstrictor Precautions No information available to require special precautions

Effects on Dental Treatment No effects or complications reported

Mechanism of Action Similar to daunorubicin, idarubicin exhibits inhibitory effects on DNA and RNA polymerase *in vitro*, and lacks the methoxyl group at the C4 position of the aglycone. Idarubicin has an affinity for DNA similar to daunorubicin and somewhat higher efficacy in stabilizing the DNA double helix against heat denaturation. Idarubicin has been as active or more active than daunorubicin in inhibiting 3H-TdR uptake by DNA or RNA of mouse embryo fibroblasts.

Other Adverse Effects

>10%:

- Cardiovascular: Transient EKG abnormalities (supraventricular tachycardia, S-T wave changes, atrial or ventricular extrasystoles); generally asymptomatic and self-limiting. Congestive heart failure, dose-related. The relative cardiotoxicity of idarubicin compared to doxorubicin is unclear. Some investigators report no increase in cardiac toxicity at cumulative oral idarubicin doses up to 540 mg/m^2; other reports suggest a maximum cumulative I.V. dose of 150 mg/m^2.
- Central nervous system: Headache
- Dermatologic: Alopecia (25% to 30%), radiation recall, skin rash (11%), urticaria
- Gastrointestinal: Nausea, vomiting (30% to 60%); diarrhea (9% to 22%); stomatitis (11%); GI hemorrhage (30%)
- Genitourinary: Discoloration of urine (reddish)
- Hematologic: Myelosuppression, primarily leukopenia; thrombocytopenia and anemia. Effects are generally less severe with oral dosing.
  - Nadir: 10-15 days
  - Recovery: 21-28 days
- Hepatic: Elevations of bilirubin and transaminases (44%)

1% to 10%:

- Central nervous system: Seizures
- Neuromuscular & skeletal: Peripheral neuropathy

Drug Interactions Patients may experience impaired immune response to vaccines; possible infection after administration of live vaccines in patients receiving immunosuppressants.

Drug Uptake

Absorption: Oral: Rapid but erratic (20% to 30%) from GI tract

Half-life, elimination: Oral: 14-35 hours; I.V.: 12-27 hours

Time to peak: 2-4 hours; varies considerably

Pregnancy Risk Factor D

Generic Available No

Comments Discoloration of urine may persist for 48 hours

Ifex® *see* Ifosfamide *on page 625*

Ifosfamide (eye FOSS fa mide)

U.S. Brand Names Ifex®

Canadian Brand Names Ifex®

Mexican Brand Names Ifolem®; Ifoxan

Pharmacologic Category Antineoplastic Agent, Alkylating Agent

Use Treatment of lung cancer, Hodgkin's and non-Hodgkin's lymphoma, breast cancer, acute and chronic lymphocytic leukemias, ovarian cancer, sarcomas, pancreatic and gastric carcinomas

Orphan drug: Treatment of testicular cancer

Local Anesthetic/Vasoconstrictor Precautions No information available to require special precautions

Effects on Dental Treatment No effects or complications reported

Mechanism of Action Causes cross-linking of strands of DNA by binding with nucleic acids and other intracellular structures; inhibits protein synthesis and DNA synthesis; an analogue of cyclophosphamide, and like cyclophosphamide, it undergoes activation by microsomal enzymes in the liver. Ifosfamide is metabolized to active compounds, ifosfamide mustard, and acrolein

Other Adverse Effects

>10%:

- Central nervous system: Somnolence, confusion, hallucinations (12%)
- Dermatologic: Alopecia (75% to 100%)
- Endocrine & metabolic: Metabolic acidosis (31%)
- Gastrointestinal: Nausea and vomiting (58%), may be more common with higher doses or bolus infusions; constipation
- Genitourinary: Hemorrhagic cystitis (40% to 50%), patients should be vigorously hydrated (at least 2 L/day) and receive mesna
- Hematologic: Myelosuppression, leukopenia (65% to 100%), thrombocytopenia (10%) - dose-related
  - Onset: 7-14 days
  - Nadir: 21-28 days
  - Recovery: 21-28 days
- Renal: Hematuria (6% to 92%)

1% to 10%:

- Central nervous system: Hallucinations, depressive psychoses, polyneuropathy
- Dermatologic: Dermatitis, nail banding/ridging, hyperpigmentation
- Endocrine & metabolic: SIADH, sterility, elevated transaminases (3%)
- Hematologic: Anemia
- Local: Phlebitis
- Renal: Increased creatinine/BUN (6%)
- Respiratory: Nasal stuffiness

Drug Interactions CYP2B6 and 3A3/4 enzyme substrate

Increased Effect/Toxicity: Activation by microsomal enzymes may be enhanced during therapy with enzyme inducers such as phenobarbital, carbamazepine, and phenytoin.

Drug Uptake

Half-life, elimination (dose-dependent): Beta: High dose: 11-15 hours (3800-5000 mg/m^2); Lower dose: 4-7 hours (1800 mg/m^2)

Time to peak, plasma (dose-dependent): ≤1 hour

Pregnancy Risk Factor D

Generic Available No

Comments Usually used in combination with mesna, a prophylactic agent for hemorrhagic cystitis

Ilopan® *see* Dexpanthenol *on page 368*

Ilotycin® *see* Erythromycin, Topical *on page 454*

Imdur® *see* Isosorbide Mononitrate *on page 662*

Imiglucerase (imi GLOO ser ase)

U.S. Brand Names Cerezyme®

Pharmacologic Category Enzyme

Use Orphan drug: Long-term enzyme replacement therapy for patients with Type 1 Gaucher's disease

Local Anesthetic/Vasoconstrictor Precautions No information available to require special precautions

Effects on Dental Treatment No effects or complications reported

Dosage I.V.: 2.5 units/kg 3 times a week up to as much as 60 units/kg administered as frequently as once a week or as infrequently as every 4 weeks; 60 units/kg administered every 2 weeks is the most common dose

(Continued)

Imiglucerase *(Continued)*

Other Adverse Effects 1% to 10%:

Cardiovascular: Hypotension, cyanosis
Central nervous system: Headache, dizziness
Dermatologic: Rash, pruritus
Gastrointestinal: Nausea, abdominal discomfort
Genitourinary: Decreased urinary frequency
Miscellaneous: Hypersensitivity reaction (4.4%)

Pregnancy Risk Factor C

Generic Available No

Imipenem and Cilastatin (i mi PEN em & sye la STAT in)

Related Information

Animal and Human Bites Guidelines *on page 1416*

U.S. Brand Names Primaxin®

Canadian Brand Names Primaxin®

Mexican Brand Names Tienam®

Pharmacologic Category Antibiotic, Carbapenem

Synonyms Imipemide

Use Treatment of respiratory tract, urinary tract, intra-abdominal, gynecologic, bone and joint, skin structure, and polymicrobic infections as well as bacterial septicemia and endocarditis. Antibacterial activity includes resistant gram-negative bacilli (*Pseudomonas aeruginosa* and *Enterobacter* sp), gram-positive bacteria (methicillin-sensitive *Staphylococcus aureus* and *Streptococcus* sp) and anaerobes.

Note: I.M. administration is not intended for severe or life-threatening infections (eg, septicemia, endocarditis, shock)

Local Anesthetic/Vasoconstrictor Precautions No information available to require special precautions

Effects on Dental Treatment No effects or complications reported

Dosage Dosage based on **imipenem** content:

Neonates: Non-CNS infections: I.V.:
- <1 week: 25 mg/kg every 12 hours
- 1-4 weeks: 25 mg/kg every 8 hours
- 4 weeks to 3 months: 25 mg/kg every 6 hours

Children: >3 months: Non-CNS infections: I.V.: 15-25 mg/kg every 6 hours
- Maximum dosage: Susceptible infections: 2 g/day; moderately susceptible organisms: 4 g/day

Children: Cystic fibrosis: I.V.: Doses up to 90 mg/kg/day have been used

Adults:
- Mild infections:
  - I.M.: 500 mg every 12 hours; intra-abdominal infections: 750 mg every 12 hours
  - I.V.:
    - Fully-susceptible organisms: 250 mg every 6 hours (1g/day)
    - Moderately-susceptible organisms: 500 mg every 6 hours (2 g/day)
- Moderate infections:
  - I.M.: 750 mg every 12 hours
  - I.V.:
    - Fully-susceptible organisms: 500 mg every 6-8 hours (1.5-2 g/day)
    - Moderately-susceptible organisms: 500 mg every 6 hours or 1 g every 8 hours (2-3 g/day)
- Severe infections: I.V.: **Note:** I.M. administration is not intended for severe or life-threatening infections (eg, septicemia, endocarditis, shock):
  - Fully-susceptible organisms: 500 mg every 6 hours (2 g/day)
  - Moderately-susceptible organisms: 1 g every 6-8 hours (3-4 g/day)
  - Maximum daily dose should not exceed 50 mg/kg or 4 g/day, whichever is lower
- Urinary tract infection, uncomplicated: I.V.: 250 mg every 6 hours (1 g/day)
- Urinary tract infection, complicated: I.V.: 500 mg every 6 hours (2 g/day)

Dosage adjustment in renal impairment: I.V.: **Note:** Adjustments have not been established for I.M. dosing:
- Patients with a Cl_{cr} <5 mL/minute/1.73 m^2 should not receive imipenem/cilastatin unless hemodialysis is instituted within 48 hours.
- Patients weighing <30 kg with impaired renal function should not receive imipenem/cilastatin.
- Hemodialysis: Use the dosing recommendation for patients with a Cl_{cr} 6-20 mL/minute
- Peritoneal dialysis: Dose as for Cl_{cr} <10 mL/minute
- Continuous arteriovenous or venovenous hemofiltration: Dose as for Cl_{cr} 20-30 mL/minute; monitor for seizure activity; imipenem is well removed by CAVH but cilastatin is not; removes 20 mg of imipenem per liter of filtrate per day

Dosage in renal impairment is determined by daily dose required to treat the infection (see adult dosing), creatinine clearance, and body weight

Mechanism of Action Inhibits bacterial cell wall synthesis by binding to one or more of the penicillin binding proteins (PBPs); which in turn inhibits the final transpeptidation step of peptidoglycan synthesis in bacterial cell walls, thus inhibiting cell wall biosynthesis. Bacteria eventually lyse due to ongoing activity of cell wall autolytic enzymes (autolysins and murein hydrolases) while cell wall assembly is arrested. Cilastatin prevents renal metabolism of imipenem by competitive inhibition of dehydropeptidase along the brush border of the renal tubules.

Other Adverse Effects 1% to 10%:

Gastrointestinal: Nausea/diarrhea/vomiting (1% to 2%)

Local: Phlebitis (3%), pain at I.M. injection site (1.2%)

Drug Interactions Beta-lactam antibiotics and probenecid may increase potential for toxicity.

Drug Uptake

Absorption: I.M.: Imipenem: 60% to 75%; cilastatin: 95% to 100%

Half-life, elimination: 1 hour (extended with renal insufficiency):

Pregnancy Risk Factor C

Generic Available No

Imipramine (im IP ra meen)

U.S. Brand Names Tofranil®; Tofranil-PM®

Canadian Brand Names Apo®-Imipramine; Tofranil®

Mexican Brand Names Talpramin; Tofranil®; Tofranil-PM®

Pharmacologic Category Antidepressant, Tricyclic (Tertiary Amine)

Synonyms Imipramine Hydrochloride; Imipramine Pamoate

Use Treatment of various forms of depression, often in conjunction with psychotherapy; enuresis in children; analgesic for certain chronic and neuropathic pain

Unlabeled/Investigational: Enuresis in children; analgesic for certain chronic and neuropathic pain; panic disorder; attention-deficit/hyperactivity disorder (ADHD)

Local Anesthetic/Vasoconstrictor Precautions Use with caution; epinephrine, norepinephrine and levonordefrin have been shown to have an increased pressor response in combination with TCAs

Effects on Dental Treatment

>10%: Xerostomia

Long-term treatment with TCAs such as imipramine increases the risk of caries by reducing salivation and salivary buffer capacity. In a study by Rundergren, et al, pathological alterations were observed in the oral mucosa of 72% of 58 patients; 55% had new carious lesions after taking TCAs for a median of $5^1/_2$ years. Current research is investigating the use of the salivary stimulant pilocarpine to overcome the xerostomia from imipramine.

Dosage Maximum antidepressant effect may not be seen for 2 or more weeks after initiation of therapy.

Children: Oral:

Depression: 1.5 mg/kg/day with dosage increments of 1 mg/kg every 3-4 days to a maximum dose of 5 mg/kg/day in 1-4 divided doses; monitor carefully especially with doses ≥3.5 mg/kg/day

Enuresis: ≥6 years: Initial: 10-25 mg at bedtime, if inadequate response still seen after 1 week of therapy, increase by 25 mg/day; dose should not exceed 2.5 mg/kg/day or 50 mg at bedtime if 6-12 years of age or 75 mg at bedtime if ≥12 years of age

Adjunct in the treatment of cancer pain: Initial: 0.2-0.4 mg/kg at bedtime; dose may be increased by 50% every 2-3 days up to 1-3 mg/kg/dose at bedtime

Adolescents: Oral: Initial: 25-50 mg/day; increase gradually; maximum: 100 mg/day in single or divided doses

Adults:

Oral: Initial: 25 mg 3-4 times/day, increase dose gradually, total dose may be given at bedtime; maximum: 300 mg/day

I.M.: Initial: Up to 100 mg/day in divided doses; change to oral as soon as possible

Elderly: Initial: 10-25 mg at bedtime; increase by 10-25 mg every 3 days for inpatients and weekly for outpatients if tolerated; average daily dose to achieve a therapeutic concentration: 100 mg/day; range: 50-150 mg/day

Mechanism of Action Traditionally believed to increase the synaptic concentration of serotonin and/or norepinephrine in the CNS by inhibition of their reuptake by the presynaptic neuronal membrane. However, additional receptor effects have been found including desensitization of adenyl cyclase, down regulation of beta-adrenergic receptors, and down regulation of serotonin receptors.

Other Adverse Effects Frequency not defined:

Cardiovascular: Orthostatic hypotension, arrhythmias, tachycardia, hypertension, palpitations, myocardial infarction, heart block, EKG changes, CHF, stroke

Central nervous system: Dizziness, drowsiness, headache, agitation, insomnia, nightmares, hypomania, psychosis, fatigue, confusion, hallucinations, disorientation, delusions, anxiety, restlessness, seizures

Endocrine & metabolic: Gynecomastia, breast enlargement, galactorrhea, increase or decrease in libido, increase or decrease in blood sugar, SIADH

(Continued)

Imipramine *(Continued)*

Gastrointestinal: Nausea, unpleasant taste, weight gain, xerostomia, constipation, ileus, stomatitis, abdominal cramps, vomiting, anorexia, epigastric disorders, diarrhea, black tongue, weight loss

Genitourinary: Urinary retention, impotence

Neuromuscular & skeletal: Weakness, numbness, tingling, paresthesias, incoordination, ataxia, tremor, peripheral neuropathy, extrapyramidal symptoms

Ocular: Blurred vision, disturbances of accommodation, mydriasis

Otic: Tinnitus

Miscellaneous: Diaphoresis

Drug Interactions CYP1A2, 2C9, 2C19, 2D6, and 3A3/4 enzyme substrate

Increased Effect/Toxicity: Imipramine increases the effects of amphetamines, anticholinergics, other CNS depressants (sedatives, hypnotics), chlorpropamide, tolazamide, and warfarin. When used with MAO inhibitors, hyperpyrexia, hypertension, tachycardia, confusion, seizures, and **deaths have been reported** (serotonin syndrome). The SSRIs (to varying degrees), cimetidine, indinavir, methylphenidate, ritonavir, quinidine, diltiazem, and verapamil inhibit the metabolism of TCAs and clinical toxicity may result. Use of lithium with a TCA may increase the risk for neurotoxicity. Phenothiazines may increase concentration of some TCAs and TCAs may increase concentration of phenothiazines. Pressor response to I.V. epinephrine, norepinephrine, and phenylephrine may be enhanced in patients receiving TCAs (**Note:** Effect is unlikely with epinephrine or levonordefrin dosages typically administered as infiltration in combination with local anesthetics). Combined use of beta-agonists or drugs which prolong QT_c (including quinidine, procainamide, disopyramide, cisapride, sparfloxacin, gatifloxacin, moxifloxacin) with TCAs may predispose patients to cardiac arrhythmias.

Decreased Effect: Carbamazepine, phenobarbital, and rifampin may increase the metabolism of imipramine resulting in decreased effect of imipramine. Imipramine inhibits the antihypertensive response to bethanidine, clonidine, debrisoquin, guanadrel, guanethidine, guanabenz, and guanfacine. Cholestyramine and colestipol may bind TCAs and reduce their absorption; monitor for altered response.

Drug Uptake

Onset of action: Peak antidepressant effect: Usually after ≥2 weeks

Absorption: Oral: Well absorbed

Half-life, elimination: 6-18 hours

Pregnancy Risk Factor D

Generic Available Yes: Tablet

Selected Readings

Friedlander AH, Mahler ME, "Major Depressive Disorder. Psychopathology, Medical Management, and Dental Implications," *J Am Dent Assoc*, 201, 132(5):629-38.

Ganzberg S, "Psychoactive Drugs," *ADA Guide to Dental Therapeutics*, 2nd ed, Chicago, IL: ADA Publishing, a Division of ADA Business Enterprises, Inc, 2000, 376-405.

Jastak JT and Yagiela JA, "Vasoconstrictors and Local Anesthesia: A Review and Rationale for Use," *J Am Dent Assoc*, 1983, 107(4):623-30.

Mitchell JR, "Guanethidine and Related Agents. III Antagonism by Drugs Which Inhibit the Norepinephrine Pump in Man," *J Clin Invest*, 1970, 49(8):1596-604.

Rundegren J, van Dijken J, Mörnstad H, et al, "Oral Conditions in Patients Receiving Long-Term Treatment With Cyclic Antidepressant Drugs," *Swed Dent J*, 1985, 9(2):55-64.

Wynn RL, "New Antidepressant Medications," *Gen Dent*, 1997, 45(1):24-8.

Yagiela JA, "Adverse Drug Interactions in Dental Practice: Interactions Associated With Vasoconstrictors. Part V of a Series," *J Am Dent Assoc*, 1999, 130(5):701-9.

Imiquimod (i mi KWI mod)

Related Information

Oral Viral Infections *on page 1380*

Systemic Viral Diseases *on page 1354*

U.S. Brand Names Aldara™

Canadian Brand Names Aldara™

Pharmacologic Category Skin and Mucous Membrane Agent; Topical Skin Product

Use Genital and perianal warts (condyloma acuminata)

Local Anesthetic/Vasoconstrictor Precautions No information available to require special precautions

Effects on Dental Treatment No effects or complications reported

Dosage Children ≥12 years and Adults: Topical: Apply 3 times/week prior to normal sleeping hours and leave on the skin for 6-10 hours. Following treatment period, remove cream by washing the treated area with mild soap and water. Examples of 3 times/week application schedules are: Monday, Wednesday, Friday; or Tuesday, Thursday, Saturday. Continue imiquimod treatment until there is total clearance of the genital/perianal warts for ≤16 weeks. A rest period of several days may be taken if required by the patient's discomfort or severity of the local skin reaction. Treatment may resume once the reaction subsides.

Mechanism of Action Mechanism of action is unknown; however, induces cytokines, including interferon-alpha and others

Other Adverse Effects

>10%: Local, mild/moderate: Erythema (54% to 61%), itching (22% to 32%), erosion (21% to 32%), burning (9% to 26%), excoriation/flaking (18% to 25%), edema (12% to 17%), scabbing (9% to 13%)

1% to 10%:

Central nervous system: Pain (2% to 8%), headache (4% to 5%)

Local, severe: Erythema (4%), erosion (1%), edema (1%)

Local, mild/moderate: Pain, induration, ulceration (5% to 7%), vesicles (2% to 3%), soreness (<1% to 3%)

Neuromuscular & skeletal: Myalgia (1%)

Miscellaneous: Influenza-like symptoms (1% to 3%), fungal infections (2% to 11%)

Drug Uptake Absorption: Minimal

Pregnancy Risk Factor B

Generic Available No

Imitrex® *see* Sumatriptan Succinate *on page 1126*

Immune Globulin, Intramuscular

(i MYUN GLOB yoo lin, IN tra MUS kyoo ler)

Related Information

Systemic Viral Diseases *on page 1354*

U.S. Brand Names BayGam®

Canadian Brand Names Baygam™

Pharmacologic Category Immune Globulin

Synonyms Gamma Globulin; IG; IGIM; Immune Serum Globulin; ISG

Use Household and sexual contacts of persons with hepatitis A, measles, varicella, and possibly rubella; travelers to high-risk areas outside tourist routes; staff, attendees, and parents of diapered attendees in day-care center outbreaks

For travelers, IG is not an alternative to careful selection of foods and water; immune globulin can interfere with the antibody response to parenterally administered live virus vaccines. Frequent travelers should be tested for hepatitis A antibody, immune hemolytic anemia, and neutropenia (with ITP, I.V. route is usually used).

Local Anesthetic/Vasoconstrictor Precautions No information available to require special precautions

Effects on Dental Treatment No effects or complications reported

Dosage I.M.:

Hepatitis A:

Pre-exposure prophylaxis upon travel into endemic areas:

0.02 mL/kg for anticipated risk 1-3 months

0.06 mL/kg for anticipated risk >3 months

Repeat approximate dose every 4-6 months if exposure continues

Postexposure prophylaxis: 0.02 mL/kg given within 2 weeks of exposure

Measles:

Prophylaxis: 0.25 mL/kg/dose (maximum dose: 15 mL) given within 6 days of exposure followed by live attenuated measles vaccine in 3 months or at 15 months of age (whichever is later)

For patients with leukemia, lymphoma, immunodeficiency disorders, generalized malignancy, or receiving immunosuppressive therapy: 0.5 mL/kg (maximum dose: 15 mL)

Poliomyelitis: Prophylaxis: 0.3 mL/kg/dose as a single dose

Rubella: Prophylaxis: 0.55 mL/kg/dose within 72 hours of exposure

Varicella:: Prophylaxis: 0.6-1.2 mL/kg (varicella zoster immune globulin preferred) within 72 hours of exposure

IgG deficiency: 1.3 mL/kg, then 0.66 mL/kg in 3-4 weeks

Hepatitis B: Prophylaxis: 0.06 mL/kg/dose (HBIG preferred)

Mechanism of Action Provides passive immunity by increasing the antibody titer and antigen-antibody reaction potential

Other Adverse Effects Frequency not defined:

Cardiovascular: Flushing, angioedema,

Central nervous system: Chills, lethargy, fever

Dermatologic: Urticaria, erythema

Gastrointestinal: Nausea, vomiting

Local: Pain, tenderness, muscle stiffness at I.M. site

Neuromuscular & skeletal: Myalgia

Miscellaneous: Hypersensitivity reactions

Drug Interactions Increased Toxicity: Live virus, vaccines (measles, mumps, rubella); do not administer within 3 months after administration of these vaccines.

Drug Uptake

Duration: Immune effect: 3-4 weeks

Half-life, elimination: 23 days

Time to peak: I.M.: 24-48 hours

Pregnancy Risk Factor C

Generic Available No

Immune Globulin, Intravenous

(i MYUN GLOB yoo lin, IN tra VEE nus)

Related Information

Systemic Viral Diseases *on page 1354*

U.S. Brand Names Gamimune® N; Gammagard® S/D; Gammar®-P I.V.; Iveegam EN; Panglobulin®; Polygam® S/D; Sandoglobulin®; Venoglobulin®-S

Canadian Brand Names Gamimune® N; Gammagard® S/D; Iveegam Immuno®

Mexican Brand Names Citax; Intacglobin; Sandoglobulina®

Pharmacologic Category Immune Globulin

Synonyms IVIG

Use Treatment of immunodeficiency syndromes (hypogammaglobulinemia, agammaglobulinemia, IgG subclass deficiencies, severe combined immunodeficiency syndromes (SCIDS), Wiskott-Aldrich syndrome), idiopathic thrombocytopenic purpura; used in conjunction with appropriate anti-infective therapy *to prevent or modify acute bacterial or viral infections* in patients with iatrogenically-induced or disease-associated immunodepression; *chronic lymphocytic leukemia (CLL) - chronic prophylaxis autoimmune neutropenia, bone marrow transplantation patients, autoimmune hemolytic anemia or neutropenia, refractory dermatomyositis/polymyositis, autoimmune diseases* (myasthenia gravis, SLE, bullous pemphigoid, severe rheumatoid arthritis), Guillain-Barré syndrome; pediatric HIV infection to decrease frequency of serious bacterial infections; Kawasaki disease in combination with aspirin

Unlabeled/Investigational: Autoimmune diseases (myasthenia gravis, SLE, bullous pemphigoid, severe rheumatoid arthritis), Guillain-Barré syndrome; used in conjunction with appropriate anti-infective therapy to prevent or modify acute bacterial or viral infections in patients with iatrogenically-induced or disease-associated immunodepression; autoimmune hemolytic anemia or neutropenia, refractory dermatomyositis/polymyositis

Local Anesthetic/Vasoconstrictor Precautions No information available to require special precautions

Effects on Dental Treatment No effects or complications reported

Dosage Children and Adults: I.V.:

Dosages should be based on ideal body weight and not actual body weight in morbidly obese patients; approved doses and regimens may vary between brands; check manufacturer guidelines

Primary immunodeficiency disorders: 200-400 mg/kg every 4 weeks or as per monitored serum IgG concentrations

Chronic lymphocytic leukemia (CLL): 400 mg/kg/dose every 3 weeks

Idiopathic thrombocytopenic purpura (ITP): Maintenance dose:

- 400 mg/kg/day for 2-5 consecutive days; or 1000 mg/kg every other day for 3 doses, if needed or
- 1000 mg/kg/day for 2 consecutive days; or up to 2000 mg/kg/day over 2-7 consecutive days

Chronic ITP: 400-2000 mg/kg/dose as needed to maintain appropriate platelet counts

Kawasaki disease: Initiate within 10 days of disease onset: In combination with aspirin 80-100 mg/kg/day in 4 divided doses for 14 days; when fever subsides, dose aspirin at 3-5 mg/kg once daily for ≥ 6-8 weeks

- 2 g/kg for one dose only
- 400 mg/kg/day for 4 days within 10 days of onset of fever

Acquired immunodeficiency syndrome (patients must be symptomatic):

- 200-250 mg/kg/dose every 2 weeks
- 400-500 mg/kg/dose every month or every 4 weeks

Pediatric HIV: 400 mg/kg every 28 days

Autoimmune hemolytic anemia and neutropenia: 1000 mg/kg/dose for 2-3 days

Autoimmune diseases: 400 mg/kg/day for 4 days

Bone marrow transplant: 500 mg/kg beginning on days 7 and 2 pretransplant, then 500 mg/kg/week for 90 days post-transplant

Adjuvant to severe cytomegalovirus infections: 500 mg/kg/dose every other day for 7 doses

Severe systemic viral and bacterial infections: Children: 500-1000 mg/kg/week

Prevention of gastroenteritis: Infants and Children: Oral: 50 mg/kg/day divided every 6 hours

Guillain-Barré syndrome:

- 400 mg/kg/day for 4 days
- 1000 mg/kg/day for 2 days
- 2000 mg/kg/day for one day

Refractory dermatomyositis: 2 g/kg/dose every month x 3-4 doses

Refractory polymyositis: 1 g/kg/day x 2 days every month x 4 doses

Chronic inflammatory demyelinating polyneuropathy:

- 400 mg/kg/day for 5 doses once each month
- 800 mg/kg/day for 3 doses once each month
- 1000 mg/kg/day for 2 days once each month

Dosing adjustment/comments in renal impairment: Cl_{cr} <10 mL/minute: Avoid use

Mechanism of Action Replacement therapy for primary and secondary immunodeficiencies; interference with F_c receptors on the cells of the reticuloendothelial system for autoimmune cytopenias and ITP; possible role of contained antiviral-type antibodies

Other Adverse Effects Frequency not defined:

Cardiovascular: Flushing of the face, tachycardia, hypertension, hypotension, chest tightness, angioedema, lightheadedness, chest pain, myocardial infarction, CHF, pulmonary embolism

Central nervous system: Anxiety, chills, dizziness, drowsiness, fatigue, fever, headache, irritability, lethargy, malaise, aseptic meningitis syndrome

Dermatologic: Pruritus, rash, urticaria

Gastrointestinal: Abdominal cramps, nausea, vomiting

Hematologic: Autoimmune hemolytic anemia, mild hemolysis

Local: Pain or irritation at the infusion site

Neuromuscular & skeletal: Arthralgia, back or hip pain, myalgia, nuchal rigidity

Ocular: Photophobia, painful eye movements

Renal: Acute renal failure, acute tubular necrosis, anuria, BUN elevated, creatinine elevated, nephrotic syndrome, oliguria, proximal tubular nephropathy, osmotic nephrosis

Respiratory: Dyspnea, wheezing, infusion-related lung injury

Miscellaneous: Diaphoresis, hypersensitivity reactions, anaphylaxis

Drug Interactions Increased Toxicity: Live virus, vaccines (measles, mumps, rubella); do not administer within 3 months after administration of these vaccines.

Drug Uptake

Onset of action: I.V.: Provides immediate antibody levels

Duration: Immune effect: 3-4 weeks (variable)

Half-life, elimination: 21-24 days

Pregnancy Risk Factor C

Generic Available Yes

Comments Gammagard®, Polygam®, or Iveegam® have low titers of IgA and may be used in patients with IgA deficiency

Imodium® *see* Loperamide *on page 725*

Imodium® A-D [OTC] *see* Loperamide *on page 725*

Imogam® *see* Rabies Immune Globulin (Human) *on page 1038*

Imovax® Rabies Vaccine *see* Rabies Virus Vaccine *on page 1038*

Imuran® *see* Azathioprine *on page 135*

Inamrinone (eye NAM ri none)

Pharmacologic Category Phosphodiesterase Enzyme Inhibitor

Synonyms Amrinone Lactate

Use Treatment of low cardiac output states (sepsis, CHF); adjunctive therapy of pulmonary hypertension; normally prescribed for patients who have not responded well to therapy with digitalis, diuretics, and vasodilators

Local Anesthetic/Vasoconstrictor Precautions No information available to require special precautions

Effects on Dental Treatment No effects or complications reported

Dosage Dosage is based on clinical response; **Note:** Dose should not exceed 10 mg/kg/24 hours

Children and Adults: 0.75 mg/kg I.V. bolus over 2-3 minutes followed by maintenance infusion of 5-10 mcg/kg/minute; I.V. bolus may need to be repeated in 30 minutes

Mechanism of Action Inhibits myocardial cyclic adenosine monophosphate (cAMP) phosphodiesterase activity and increases cellular levels of cAMP resulting in a positive inotropic effect and increased cardiac output; also possesses systemic and pulmonary vasodilator effects resulting in pre- and afterload reduction; slightly increases atrioventricular conduction

Other Adverse Effects 1% to 10%:

Cardiovascular: Arrhythmias, hypotension (may be infusion rate-related), ventricular and supraventricular arrhythmias

Gastrointestinal: Nausea

Hematologic: Thrombocytopenia (may be dose-related)

Drug Interactions Increased Effect/Toxicity: Diuretics may cause significant hypovolemia and decrease filling pressure. Inotropic effects with digitalis are additive.

Drug Uptake

Onset of action: I.V.: 2-5 minutes

Peak effect: ~10 minutes

Duration: Dose dependent: Low dose: ~30 minutes; Higher doses: ~2 hours

Serum half-life: Adults: 3.6 hours; Adults: CHF: 5.8 hours

Pregnancy Risk Factor C

Generic Available Yes

Comments U.S. Pharmacopeia (USP) and the U.S. Adopted Name (USPNA) Council have recommended the name change of "amrinone" to "inamrinone," effective July 1, 2000. This is to eliminate confusion with similar-sounding drugs (ie, amiodarone).

Inapsine® *see* Droperidol *on page 423*

Indapamide (in DAP a mide)

Related Information

Cardiovascular Diseases *on page 1308*

U.S. Brand Names Lozol®

Canadian Brand Names Apo®-Indapamide; Gen-Indapamide; Lozide®; Lozol®; Novo-Indapamide; Nu-Indapamide; PMS-Indapamide

Pharmacologic Category Diuretic, Thiazide-Related

Use Management of mild to moderate hypertension; treatment of edema in CHF and nephrotic syndrome

Local Anesthetic/Vasoconstrictor Precautions No information available to require special precautions

Effects on Dental Treatment No effects or complications reported

Dosage Adults: Oral: 2.5-5 mg/day. **Note:** There is little therapeutic benefit to increasing the dose >5 mg/day; there is, however, an increased risk of electrolyte disturbances.

Mechanism of Action Diuretic effect is localized at the proximal segment of the distal tubule of the nephron; it does not appear to have significant effect on glomerular filtration rate nor renal blood flow; like other diuretics, it enhances sodium, chloride, and water excretion by interfering with the transport of sodium ions across the renal tubular epithelium

Other Adverse Effects 1% to 10%:

Cardiovascular: Orthostatic hypotension, palpitations (<5%), flushing

Central nervous system: Dizziness (<5%), lightheadedness (<5%), vertigo (<5%), headache (≥5%), restlessness (<5%), drowsiness (<5%), fatigue, lethargy, malaise, lassitude, anxiety, agitation, depression, nervousness (≥5%)

Dermatologic: Rash (<5%), pruritus (<5%), hives (<5%)

Endocrine & metabolic: Hyperglycemia (<5%), hyperuricemia (<5%)

Gastrointestinal: Anorexia, gastric irritation, nausea, vomiting, abdominal pain, cramping, bloating, diarrhea, constipation, xerostomia, weight loss

Genitourinary: Nocturia, frequent urination, polyuria, impotence (<5%), reduced libido (<5%), glycosuria (<5%)

Neuromuscular & skeletal: Muscle cramps, spasm, weakness (≥5%)

Ocular: Blurred vision (<5%)

Renal: Necrotizing angiitis, vasculitis, cutaneous vasculitis (<5%)

Respiratory: Rhinorrhea (<5%)

Warnings/Precautions Use with caution in severe renal disease. Electrolyte disturbances (hypokalemia, hypochloremic alkalosis, hyponatremia) can occur. Use with caution in severe hepatic dysfunction; hepatic encephalopathy can be caused by electrolyte disturbances. Gout can be precipitate in certain patients with a history of gout, a familial predisposition to gout, or chronic renal failure. Cautious use in diabetics; may see a change in glucose control. I.V. use is generally not recommended (but is available). Hypersensitivity reactions can occur. Can cause SLE exacerbation or activation. Use with caution in patients with moderate or high cholesterol concentrations. Photosensitization may occur. Correct hypokalemia before initiating therapy.

Chemical similarities are present among sulfonamides, sulfonylureas, carbonic anhydrase inhibitors, thiazides, and loop diuretics (except ethacrynic acid). Use in patients with thiazide or sulfonamide allergy is specifically contraindicated in product labeling, however a risk of cross-reaction exists in patients with allergy to any of these compounds; avoid use when previous reaction has been severe.

Drug Interactions

Increased Effect/Toxicity: The diuretic effect of indapamide is synergistic with furosemide and other loop diuretics. Increased hypotension and/or renal adverse effects of ACE inhibitors may result in aggressively diuresed patients. Cyclosporine and thiazide-type diuretics can increase the risk of gout or renal toxicity. Digoxin toxicity can be exacerbated if a diuretic induces hypokalemia or hypomagnesemia. Lithium toxicity can occur with thiazide-type diuretics due to reduced renal excretion of lithium. Thiazide-type diuretics may prolong the duration of action of neuromuscular blocking agents.

Decreased Effect: Effects of oral hypoglycemics may be decreased. Decreased absorption of indapamide with cholestyramine and colestipol. NSAIDs can decrease the efficacy of thiazide-type diuretics, reducing the diuretic and antihypertensive effects.

Drug Uptake

Onset of action: 1-2 hours

Absorption: Completely

Duration: ≤36 hours

Half-life, elimination: 14-18 hours

Time to peak: 2-2.5 hours

Pregnancy Risk Factor B (manufacturer); D (expert analysis)

Generic Available Yes

Inderal® *see* Propranolol *on page 1016*

Inderal® LA *see* Propranolol *on page 1016*

Inderide® *see* Propranolol and Hydrochlorothiazide *on page 1018*

Inderide® LA *see* Propranolol and Hydrochlorothiazide *on page 1018*

Indinavir (in DIN a veer)

Related Information

HIV Infection and AIDS *on page 1334*

U.S. Brand Names Crixivan®

Canadian Brand Names Crixivan®

Mexican Brand Names Crixivan®

Pharmacologic Category Antiretroviral Agent, Protease Inhibitor

Use Treatment of HIV infection; should always be used as part of a multidrug regimen (at least three antiretroviral agents)

Local Anesthetic/Vasoconstrictor Precautions No information available to require special precautions

Effects on Dental Treatment No effects or complications reported

Dosage

Children (investigational): 500 mg/m^2 every 8 hours (patients with smaller BSA may require lower doses of 300-400 mg/m^2 every 8 hours)

Adults: Oral: 800 mg every 8 hours

Note: Dosage adjustments for indinavir when administered in combination therapy:

Delavirdine, itraconazole, or ketoconazole: Reduce indinavir dose to 600 mg every 8 hours

Efavirenz: Increase indinavir dose to 1000 mg every 8 hours

Lopinavir and ritonavir (Kaletra™): Indinavir 600 mg twice daily

Nevirapine: Increase indinavir dose to 1000 mg every 8 hours

Rifabutin: Reduce rifabutin to ½ the standard dose plus increase indinavir to 1000 mg every 8 hours

Ritonavir: Adjustments necessary for both agents:

Ritonavir 100-200 mg twice daily plus indinavir 800 mg twice daily **or**

Ritonavir 400 mg twice daily plus indinavir 400 mg twice daily

Dosage adjustment in hepatic impairment: Mild-moderate impairment due to cirrhosis: 600 mg every 8 hours or with ketoconazole coadministration

Mechanism of Action Indinavir is a human immunodeficiency virus protease inhibitor, binding to the protease activity site and inhibiting the activity of this enzyme. HIV protease is an enzyme required for the cleavage of viral polyprotein precursors into individual functional proteins found in infectious HIV. Inhibition prevents cleavage of these polyproteins resulting in the formation of immature noninfectious viral particles.

Other Adverse Effects Protease inhibitors cause dyslipidemia which includes elevated cholesterol and triglycerides and a redistribution of body fat centrally to cause "protease paunch", buffalo hump, facial atrophy, and breast enlargement. These agents also cause hyperglycemia (exacerbation or new-onset diabetes).

10%:

Hepatic: Hyperbilirubinemia (14%)

Renal: Nephrolithiasis/urolithiasis (29%, pediatric patients)

1% to 10%:

Central nervous system: Headache (6%), insomnia (3%)

Gastrointestinal: Abdominal pain (9%), nausea (12%), diarrhea/vomiting (4% to 5%), taste perversion (3%)

Neuromuscular & skeletal: Weakness (4%), flank pain (3%)

Renal: Nephrolithiasis/urolithiasis (12%, adult patients), hematuria

Contraindications Hypersensitivity to indinavir or any component of the formulation; concurrent use of terfenadine, astemizole, cisapride, triazolam, midazolam, pimozide, or ergot alkaloids

Warnings/Precautions Use caution in patients with hepatic insufficiency; dosage reduction may be needed; nephrolithiasis may occur with use; if signs and symptoms of nephrolithiasis occur, interrupt therapy for 1-3 days; ensure adequate hydration

Drug Interactions CYP3A3/4 enzyme substrate; CYP3A3/4 enzyme inhibitor

Increased Effect/Toxicity: Levels of indinavir are increased by delavirdine, itraconazole, ketoconazole, nelfinavir, sildenafil, and ritonavir. Cisapride, terfenadine, pimozide, and astemizole should be avoided with indinavir due to life-threatening cardiotoxicity. Concurrent use of indinavir with lovastatin and simvastatin may increase the risk of myopathy or rhabdomyolysis. Cautious use of atorvastatin and cerivastatin may be possible. Benzodiazepines with indinavir may result in prolonged sedation and respiratory depression (midazolam and triazolam are contraindicated). Concurrent use of ergot alkaloids is contraindicated. Amprenavir and rifabutin concentrations are increased during concurrent therapy with indinavir. Other medications metabolized by cytochrome P450 isoenzyme 3A3/4 may be affected. Concurrent sildenafil is associated with increased risk of hypotension, visual changes, and priapism. Clarithromycin and quinidine may increase serum concentration of indinavir. Serum concentrations of

(Continued)

Indinavir *(Continued)*

these drugs may also be increased. Other CYP3A3/4 inhibitors may have similar effects.

Decreased Effect: Concurrent use of efavirenz, rifampin, and rifabutin may decrease the effectiveness of indinavir (dosage increase of indinavir is recommended); concurrent use of rifampin is not recommended; dosage decrease of rifabutin is recommended. The efficacy of protease inhibitors may be decreased when given with nevirapine. Gastric pH is lowered and absorption may be decreased when didanosine and indinavir are taken <1 hour apart. Fluconazole may decrease serum concentration of indinavir.

Drug-Herb Interactions: St John's wort (*Hypericum*) appears to induce CYP3A enzymes and has lead to 57% reductions in indinavir AUCs and 81% reductions in trough serum concentrations, which may lead to treatment failures. Grapefruit juice may decrease levels of indinavir.

Drug Uptake

Absorption: Administration with a high fat, high calorie diet resulted in a reduction in AUC and in maximum serum concentration (77% and 84% respectively). Administration with a lighter meal resulted in little or no change in these parameters.

Half-life, elimination: 1.8 ± 0.4 hour

Time to peak: 0.8 ± 0.3 hour

Pregnancy Risk Factor C

Generic Available No

Comments One study of previously untreated patients with a mean CD4-cell count of 250 cell/mm^3 found that indinavir plus zidovudine lowered serum HIV below detectable levels in 56% of 52 patients treated for 24 weeks. Other studies show similar results. Indinavir alone has suppressed serum HIV below detectable levels in 40% to 60% of patients treated up to 48 weeks.

Indocin® *see* Indomethacin *on page 634*

Indocyanine Green (in doe SYE a neen green)

U.S. Brand Names Cardio-Green®

Pharmacologic Category Diagnostic Agent

Use Determining hepatic function, cardiac output and liver blood flow and for ophthalmic angiography

Local Anesthetic/Vasoconstrictor Precautions No information available to require special precautions

Effects on Dental Treatment No effects or complications reported

Dosage

Angiography: Use 40 mg of dye in 2 mL of aqueous solvent, in some patients, half the volume (1 mL) has been found to produce angiograms of comparable resolution; immediately following the bolus dose of dye, a bolus of sodium chloride 0.9% is given; this regimen will deliver a spatially limited dye bolus of optimal concentration to the choroidal vasculature following I.V. injection

Determination of cardiac output: Dye is injected as rapidly as possible into the right atrium, right ventricle, or pulmonary artery through a cardiac catheter; the usual dose is 1.25 mg for infants, 2.5 mg for children, and 5 mg for adults; total dose should not exceed 2 mg/kg; the dye is diluted with sterile water for injection or sodium chloride 0.9% to make a final volume of 1 mL; doses are repeated periodically to obtain several dilution curves; the dye should be flushed from the catheter with sodium chloride 0.9% to prevent hemolysis

Other Adverse Effects 1% to 10%:

Central nervous system: Headache

Dermatologic: Pruritus, skin discoloration

Miscellaneous: Sweating, anaphylactoid reactions

Pregnancy Risk Factor C

Generic Available No

Indomethacin (in doe METH a sin)

Related Information

Rheumatoid Arthritis and Osteoarthritis *on page 1340*

Temporomandibular Dysfunction (TMD) *on page 1397*

U.S. Brand Names Indocin®

Canadian Brand Names Apo®-Indomethacin; Indocid®; Indocid® P.D.A.; Indocin®; Indo-Lemmon; Indotec; Novo-Methacin; Nu-Indo; Rhodacine®

Mexican Brand Names Antalgin®; Indocid®; Malival

Pharmacologic Category Nonsteroidal Anti-inflammatory Drug (NSAID)

Synonyms Indometacin; Indomethacin Sodium Trihydrate

Use Management of inflammatory diseases and rheumatoid disorders; moderate pain; acute gouty arthritis, acute bursitis/tendonitis, moderate to severe osteoarthritis, rheumatoid arthritis, ankylosing spondylitis; I.V. form used as alternative to surgery for closure of patent ductus arteriosus in neonates

Local Anesthetic/Vasoconstrictor Precautions No information available to require special precautions

Effects on Dental Treatment NSAID formulations are known to reversibly decrease platelet aggregation via mechanisms different than observed with aspirin. The dentist should be aware of the potential of abnormal coagulation. Caution should also be exercised in the use of NSAIDs in patients already on anticoagulant therapy with drugs such as warfarin (Coumadin®).

Dosage

Patent ductus arteriosus:

Neonates: I.V.: Initial: 0.2 mg/kg, followed by 2 doses depending on postnatal age (PNA):

PNA **at time of first dose** <48 hours: 0.1 mg/kg at 12- to 24-hour intervals

PNA **at time of first dose** 2-7 days: 0.2 mg/kg at 12- to 24-hour intervals

PNA **at time of first dose** >7 days: 0.25 mg/kg at 12- to 24-hour intervals

In general, may use 12-hour dosing interval if urine output >1 mL/kg/hour after prior dose; use 24-hour dosing interval if urine output is <1 mL/kg/hour but >0.6 mL/kg/hour; doses should be withheld if patient has oliguria (urine output <0.6 mL/kg/hour) or anuria

Inflammatory/rheumatoid disorders:

Oral:

Children: 1-2 mg/kg/day in 2-4 divided doses; maximum dose: 4 mg/kg/day; not to exceed 150-200 mg/day

Adults: 25-50 mg/dose 2-3 times/day; maximum dose: 200 mg/day; extended release capsule should be given on a 1-2 times/day schedule

Rectal: Adults: Persistent night pain and/or morning stiffness: 50-100 mg at bedtime (as part of total daily dose maximum of 200 mg/day)

Mechanism of Action Inhibits prostaglandin synthesis by decreasing the activity of the enzyme, cyclo-oxygenase, which results in decreased formation of prostaglandin precursors

Other Adverse Effects

>10%:

Central nervous system: Headache (11%)

Gastrointestinal: Nausea (3% to 9%), epigastric pain, abdominal pain/cramps/distress (<3%), anorexia, GI bleeding, ulcers, perforation, heartburn, indigestion

Hematologic: Inhibition of platelet aggregation

1% to 10%:

Central nervous system: Drowsiness (<3%), fatigue (<3%), vertigo (<3%), depression (<3%), malaise (<3%)

Gastrointestinal: Constipation (<3%), diarrhea (<3%), dyspepsia (3% to 9%)

Otic: Tinnitus (<3%)

Contraindications Hypersensitivity to indomethacin, any component of the formulation, aspirin, or other nonsteroidal anti-inflammatory drugs (NSAIDs); patients in whom asthma, urticaria, or rhinitis are precipitated by NSAIDs/aspirin; active GI bleeding or ulcer disease; premature neonates with necrotizing enterocolitis; impaired renal function; active bleeding; thrombocytopenia; pregnancy (3rd trimester); suppositories are contraindicated in patients with a history of proctitis or recent rectal bleeding

Warnings/Precautions Use with caution in patients with CHF, hypertension, dehydration, decreased renal or hepatic function, history of GI disease (bleeding or ulcers), or those receiving anticoagulants. Elderly are at a high risk for adverse effects from nonsteroidal anti-inflammatory agents. As many as 60% of elderly can develop peptic ulceration and/or hemorrhage asymptomatically.

Use lowest effective dose for shortest period possible. Use of NSAIDs can compromise existing renal function especially when Cl_{cr} is <30 mL/minute. Discontinue if signs/symptoms of hepatic injury occur.

CNS adverse effects such as confusion, agitation, and hallucination are generally seen in overdose or high-dose situations; but elderly may demonstrate these adverse effects at lower doses than younger adults. Use caution in patients with depression or other psychiatric disorder, epilepsy, or parkinsonism; discontinue if severe CNS adverse effects occur. Inhibits platelet aggregation. Withhold for at least 4-6 half-lives prior to surgical or dental procedures.

Drug Interactions CYP2C9 enzyme substrate

ACE inhibitors: Antihypertensive effects may be decreased by concurrent therapy with NSAIDs; monitor BP.

Angiotensin II antagonists: Antihypertensive effects may be decreased by concurrent therapy with NSAIDs; monitor BP.

Anticoagulants (warfarin, heparin, LMWHs) in combination with NSAIDs can cause increased risk of bleeding.

Other antiplatelet drugs (ticlopidine, clopidogrel, aspirin, abciximab, dipyridamole, eptifibatide, tirofiban) can cause an increased risk of bleeding.

Loop diuretics efficacy (diuretic and antihypertensive effect) is reduced. Indomethacin reduces this efficacy, however, it may be anticipated with any NSAID.

Cholestyramine and colestipol reduce the bioavailability of some NSAIDs; separate administration times.

Cyclosporine: NSAIDs may increase serum creatinine, potassium, BP, and cyclosporine levels; monitor cyclosporine levels and renal function carefully.

(Continued)

Indomethacin *(Continued)*

Gentamicin and amikacin serum concentrations are increased by indomethacin in premature infants. Results may apply to other aminoglycosides and NSAIDs.

Hydralazine's antihypertensive effect is decreased; avoid concurrent use.

Lithium levels can be increased; avoid concurrent use if possible or monitor lithium levels and adjust dose. Sulindac may have the least effect. When NSAID is stopped, lithium will need adjustment again.

Methotrexate: Severe bone marrow suppression, aplastic anemia, and GI toxicity have been reported with concomitant NSAID therapy. Avoid use during moderate or high-dose methotrexate (increased and prolonged methotrexate levels). NSAID use during low-dose treatment of rheumatoid arthritis has not been fully evaluated; extreme caution is warranted.

Thiazides antihypertensive effects are decreased; avoid concurrent use.

Warfarin's INRs may be increased by piroxicam. Other NSAIDs may have the same effect depending on dose and duration. Monitor INR closely. Use the lowest dose of NSAIDs possible and for the briefest duration.

Corticosteroids may increase the risk of GI ulceration; avoid concurrent use.

Drug Uptake

Onset of action: ~30 minutes

Absorption: Prompt and extensive

Duration: 4-6 hours

Half-life, elimination: 4.5 hours, longer in neonates

Time to peak: Oral: ~3-4 hours

Pregnancy Risk Factor B/D (3rd trimester)

Generic Available Yes

Infantaire [OTC] *see* Acetaminophen *on page 26*

Infants Tylenol® Cold [OTC] *see* Acetaminophen and Pseudoephedrine *on page 30*

Infants' Tylenol® Cold Plus Cough Concentrated Drops [OTC] *see* Acetaminophen, Dextromethorphan, and Pseudoephedrine *on page 34*

Infasurf® *see* Calfactant *on page 207*

INFeD® *see* Iron Dextran Complex *on page 655*

Inflamase® Forte *see* PrednisoLONE *on page 988*

Inflamase® Mild *see* PrednisoLONE *on page 988*

Infliximab (in FLIKS e mab)

U.S. Brand Names Remicade®

Pharmacologic Category Antirheumatic, Disease Modifying; Monoclonal Antibody

Synonyms Infliximab, Recombinant

Use

Crohn's disease: Reduce the signs and symptoms of moderate to severe disease in patients who have an inadequate response to conventional therapy; reduce the number of draining enterocutaneous fistulas in fistulizing disease

Rheumatoid arthritis: Used with methotrexate in patients who have had an inadequate response to methotrexate alone; used with methotrexate to inhibit the progression of structural damage and improve physical function in patients with moderate to severe disease

Local Anesthetic/Vasoconstrictor Precautions No information available to require special precautions

Effects on Dental Treatment ~5%: Candidiasis

Dosage I.V.: Adults:

Crohn's disease:

- Moderately- to severely-active: 5 mg/kg as a single infusion over a minimum of 2 hours
- Fistulizing: 5 mg/kg as an infusion over a minimum of 2 hours; dose repeated at 2- and 6 weeks after the initial infusion

Rheumatoid arthritis (in combination with methotrexate therapy): 3 mg/kg followed by an additional 3 mg/kg at 2- and 6 weeks after the first dose; then repeat every 8 weeks thereafter; doses have ranged from 3-10 mg/kg I.V. infusion repeated at 4-week intervals or 8-week intervals

Mechanism of Action Infliximab is a chimeric monoclonal antibody that binds to human tumor necrosis factor alpha (TNFα) receptor sites, thereby interfering with endogenous TNFα activity. Biological activities of TNFα include the induction of proinflammatory cytokines (interleukins), enhancement of leukocyte migration, activation of neutrophils and eosinophils, and the induction of acute phase reactants and tissue degrading enzymes. Animal models have shown TNFα expression causes polyarthritis, and infliximab can prevent disease as well as allow diseased joints to heal.

Other Adverse Effects Note: Although profile is similar, frequency of effects may be different in specific populations (Crohn's disease vs rheumatoid arthritis).

>10%:

Central nervous system: Headache (22% to 23%), fatigue (8% to 11%), fever (8% to 10%)

Dermatologic: Rash (6% to 12%)

Gastrointestinal: Nausea (17%), diarrhea (3% to 13%), abdominal pain (10% to 12%)

Local: Infusion reactions (19%)

Respiratory: Upper respiratory tract infection (16% to 26%), cough (5% to 13%), sinusitis (5% to 13%), pharyngitis (9% to 11%)

Miscellaneous: Development of antinuclear antibodies (34%); infections (32%); Crohn's patients with fistulizing disease: Development of new abscess (12%, 8-16 weeks after the last infusion)

2% to 10%:

Cardiovascular: Chest pain (5% to 6%, similar to placebo)

Central nervous system: Pain (8% to 9%), dizziness (8% to 10%, similar to placebo)

Dermatologic: Pruritus (5% to 6%)

Gastrointestinal: Vomiting (7% to 9%), dyspepsia (5% to 6%)

Genitourinary: Urinary tract infection (3% to 8%, similar to placebo)

Neuromuscular & skeletal: Arthralgia (5% to 6%), back pain (5% to 6%)

Respiratory: Bronchitis (6% to 7%), rhinitis (6% to 9%)

Miscellaneous: Development of antibodies to double-stranded DNA (9%)

<2%: Abscess, abdominal hernia, adult respiratory distress syndrome, ALT increased (mild, incidence increased with concomitant methotrexate therapy), anemia, anxiety, appendicitis, arrhythmia, arthritis, AST increased (mild, incidence increased with concomitant methotrexate therapy), atrioventricular block, azotemia, bacterial infection, basal cell carcinoma, biliary pain, bone fracture, bradycardia, brain infarction, breast cancer, cardiac arrest, cardiac failure, cellulitis, ceruminosis, cholecystitis, cholelithiasis, confusion, Crohn's disease, dehydration, delirium, depression, diaphragmatic hernia, dyspnea, dysuria, edema, encephalopathy, endometriosis, endophthalmitis, fungal infection, furunculosis, gastric ulcer, gastrointestinal hemorrhage, hemarthrosis, hepatitis cholestatic, herpes zoster, hydronephrosis, hypertension, hypotension, intervertebral disk herniation, inflammation, injection site inflammation, intestinal obstruction, intestinal perforation, intestinal stenosis, joint cyst, joint degeneration, kidney infarction, leukopenia, lymphangitis, lupus erythematosus syndrome, lymphoma, myalgia, myocardial ischemia, osteoarthritis, osteoporosis, peripheral ischemia, pleural effusion, pleurisy, pneumonia, pneumothorax, pulmonary edema, pulmonary embolism, pulmonary infiltration, renal calculus, renal failure, respiratory insufficiency, rheumatoid nodules, palpitation, pancreatic insufficiency, pancreatitis, peritonitis, proctalgia, pyelonephritis, rectal adenocarcinoma, sepsis, skin cancer, somnolence, splenic infarction, spondylolisthesis, spinal stenosis, splenomegaly, suicide attempt, diaphoresis increased, symphyseolysis, syncope, tachycardia, tendon disorder, tendon injury, thrombocytopenia, thrombophlebitis (deep), ulceration, upper motor neuron lesion, ureteral obstruction, weakness, weight loss, worsening rheumatoid arthritis

Drug Interactions Specific drug interaction studies have not been conducted.

Immunosuppressants: When used with infliximab, may decrease the risk of infusion related reactions, and may decrease development of anti-double-stranded DNA antibodies

Vaccines, live: Concomitant use has not been studied; currently recommended not to administer live vaccines during infliximab therapy

Drug Uptake

Onset of action: Crohn's disease: ~2 weeks

Half-life, elimination: 8-9.5 days

Pregnancy Risk Factor B (manufacturer)

Generic Available No

Influenza Virus Vaccine (in floo EN za VYE rus vak SEEN)

U.S. Brand Names Fluogen®; FluShield®; Fluvirin®; Fluzone®

Canadian Brand Names Fluviral S/F®; Fluzone®; Vaxigrip®

Pharmacologic Category Vaccine

Synonyms Influenza Virus Vaccine (inactivated whole-virus); Influenza Virus Vaccine (purified split-virus); Influenza Virus Vaccine (purified surface antigen); Influenza Virus Vaccine (split-virus)

Use Provide active immunity to influenza virus strains contained in the vaccine; for high-risk persons, previous year vaccines should not be used to prevent present year influenza

Groups at increased risk for influenza related complications:

- Persons ≥65 years of age
- Residents of nursing homes and other chronic-care facilities that house persons of any age with chronic medical conditions
- Adults and children with chronic disorders of the pulmonary or cardiovascular systems, including children with asthma

(Continued)

Influenza Virus Vaccine *(Continued)*

- Adults and children who have required regular medical follow-up or hospitalization during the preceding year because of chronic metabolic diseases (including diabetes mellitus), renal dysfunction, hemoglobinopathies, or immunosuppression (including immunosuppression caused by medications)
- Children and adolescents (6 months to 18 years of age) who are receiving long-term aspirin therapy and therefore, may be at risk for developing Reye's syndrome after influenza

Local Anesthetic/Vasoconstrictor Precautions No information available to require special precautions

Effects on Dental Treatment No effects or complications reported

Dosage I.M.:

Children:

6-35 months: 1-2 doses of 0.25 mL with ≥4 weeks between doses and the last dose administered before December

3-8 years: 1-2 doses of 0.5 mL (in anterolateral aspect of thigh) with ≥4 weeks between doses and the last dose administered before December

Children ≥9 years and Adults: 0.5 mL each year of appropriate vaccine for the year, one dose is all that is necessary; administer in late fall to allow maximum titers to develop by peak epidemic periods usually occurring in early December

Note: The split virus or purified surface antigen is recommended for children ≤12 years of age; if the child has received at least one dose of the 1978-79 or later vaccine, one dose is sufficient

Mechanism of Action Promotes immunity to influenza virus by inducing specific antibody production. Each year the formulation is standardized according to the U.S. Public Health Service. Preparations from previous seasons must not be used.

Other Adverse Effects All serious adverse reactions must be reported to the U.S. Department of Health and Human Services (DHHS) Vaccine Adverse Event Reporting System (VAERS) 1-800-822-7967.

1% to 10%:

Central nervous system: Fever, malaise

Local: Tenderness, redness, or induration at the site of injection (<33%)

Drug Interactions

Increased effect/toxicity of theophylline and warfarin possible

Decreased effect with immunosuppressive agents; some manufacturers and clinicians recommend that the flu vaccine not be administered with the DTP for the potential for increased febrile reactions (specifically whole-cell pertussis), and that one should wait at least 3 days. ACIP recommends that children at high risk for influenza may get the vaccine concomitantly with DTP.

Pregnancy Risk Factor C

Generic Available No

Selected Readings Centers for Disease Control, "Recommendations of the Advisory Committee on Immunization Practices (ACIP): General Recommendations on Immunization," *MMWR*, 1994, 43(RR-1):23.

Infumorph® *see* Morphine Sulfate *on page 829*

Innohep® *see* Tinzaparin *on page 1171*

INOmax® *see* Nitric Oxide *on page 869*

Insect Sting Kit (IN sekt sting kit)

U.S. Brand Names Ana-Kit®

Pharmacologic Category Antidote

Use Anaphylaxis emergency treatment of insect bites or stings by the sensitive patient that may occur within minutes of insect sting or exposure to an allergic substance

Local Anesthetic/Vasoconstrictor Precautions No information available to require special precautions

Effects on Dental Treatment No effects or complications reported

Dosage Children and Adults:

Epinephrine:

<2 years: 0.05-0.1 mL

2-6 years: 0.15 mL

6-12 years: 0.2 mL

>12 years : 0.3 mL

Chlorpheniramine:

<6 years: 1 tablet

6-12 years: 2 tablets

>12 years: 4 tablets

Generic Available No

Comments Not intended for I.V. use (I.M. or S.C. only)

Insta-Glucose® [OTC] *see* Glucose *on page 559*

Insulin Preparations (IN su lin prep a RAY shuns)

Related Information

Endocrine Disorders and Pregnancy *on page 1331*

U.S. Brand Names Humalog®; Humalog® Mix 75/25™; Humulin®; Humulin® 50/50; Humulin® 70/30; Humulin® L; Humulin® N; Humulin® R; Humulin® R (Concentrated) U-500; Lantus®; Lente® Iletin® II; Novolin® 70/30; Novolin® L; Novolin® N; Novolin® R; NovoLog®; NPH Iletin® II; Regular Iletin® II; Velosulin® BR (Buffered)

Canadian Brand Names Humalog®; Humalog® Mix25™; Humulin®; Iletin® II Pork; Novolin® ge

Mexican Brand Names Humulin 20/80®; Humulin® 30/70®; Humulin L®; Humulin N®; Humulin R®; Novolin 30/70®; Novolin L®; Novolin N®; Novolin R®

Pharmacologic Category Antidiabetic Agent, Insulin; Antidote

Use Treatment of insulin-dependent diabetes mellitus, also noninsulin-dependent diabetes mellitus unresponsive to treatment with diet and/or oral hypoglycemics; to assure proper utilization of glucose and reduce glucosuria in nondiabetic patients receiving parenteral nutrition whose glucosuria cannot be adequately controlled with infusion rate adjustments or those who require assistance in achieving optimal caloric intakes; hyperkalemia (use with glucose to shift potassium into cells to lower serum potassium levels)

Local Anesthetic/Vasoconstrictor Precautions No information available to require special precautions

Effects on Dental Treatment Type 1 diabetics (insulin-dependent) should be appointed for dental treatment in the morning in order to minimize chance of stress-induced hypoglycemia.

Dosage Dose requires continuous medical supervision; may administer I.V. (regular), I.M., S.C.

Diabetes mellitus: The number and size of daily doses, time of administration, and diet and exercise require continuous medical supervision. In addition, specific formulations may require distinct administration procedures.

- Lispro should be given within 15 minutes before or immediately after a meal
- Aspart should be given immediately before a meal (within 5-10 minutes of the start of a meal)
- Human regular insulin should be given within 30-60 minutes before a meal.
- Intermediate-acting insulins may be administered 1-2 times/day.
- Long-acting insulins may be administered once daily.
- Insulin glargine (Lantus®) should be administered subcutaneously once daily at bedtime. Maintenance doses should be administered subcutaneously and sites should be rotated to prevent lipodystrophy.
- Children and Adults: 0.5-1 unit/kg/day in divided doses
- Adolescents (growth spurts): 0.8-1.2 units/kg/day in divided doses
- Adjust dose to maintain premeal and bedtime blood glucose of 80-140 mg/dL (children <5 years: 100-200 mg/dL)
- Insulin glargine (Lantus®):
  - Type 2 diabetes (patient not already on insulin): 10 units once daily, adjusted according to patient response (range in clinical study 2-100 units/day)
  - Patients already receiving insulin: In clinical studies, when changing to insulin glargine from once-daily NPH or Ultralente® insulin, the initial dose was not changed; when changing from twice-daily NPH to once-daily insulin glargine, the total daily dose was reduced by 20% and adjusted according to patient response

Hyperkalemia: Administer calcium gluconate and $NaHCO_3$ first then 50% dextrose at 0.5-1 mL/kg and insulin 1 unit for every 4-5 g dextrose given

Diabetic ketoacidosis: Children and Adults: Regular insulin: I.V. loading dose: 0.1 unit/kg, then maintenance continuous infusion: 0.1 unit/kg/hour (range: 0.05-0.2 units/kg/hour depending upon the rate of decrease of serum glucose - too rapid decrease of serum glucose may lead to cerebral edema).

- Optimum rate of decrease (serum glucose): 80-100 mg/dL/hour
- **Note:** Newly diagnosed patients with IDDM presenting in DKA and patients with blood sugars <800 mg/dL may be relatively "sensitive" to insulin and should receive loading and initial maintenance doses ~ ½ of those indicated above.

Dosing adjustment in renal impairment (regular): Insulin requirements are reduced due to changes in insulin clearance or metabolism

- Cl_{cr} 10-50 mL/minute: Administer at 75% of normal dose
- Cl_{cr} <10 mL/minute: Administer at 25% to 50% of normal dose and monitor glucose closely

Hemodialysis: Because of a large molecular weight (6000 daltons), insulin is not significantly removed by either peritoneal or hemodialysis

- Supplemental dose is not necessary

Peritoneal dialysis: Supplemental dose is not necessary

Continuous arteriovenous or venovenous hemofiltration effects: Supplemental dose is not necessary

Mechanism of Action The principal hormone required for proper glucose utilization in normal metabolic processes; it is obtained from beef or pork pancreas or a biosynthetic process converting pork insulin to human insulin; insulins are categorized into 3 groups related to promptness, duration, and intensity of action

(Continued)

Insulin Preparations *(Continued)*

Other Adverse Effects Frequency not defined:

Cardiovascular: Palpitation, tachycardia, pallor

Central nervous system: Fatigue, mental confusion, loss of consciousness, headache, hypothermia

Dermatologic: Urticaria, redness

Endocrine & metabolic: Hypoglycemia

Gastrointestinal: Hunger, nausea, numbness of mouth

Local: Itching, edema, stinging, pain or warmth at injection site; atrophy or hypertrophy of S.C. fat tissue

Neuromuscular & skeletal: Muscle weakness, paresthesia, tremors

Ocular: Transient presbyopia or blurred vision

Miscellaneous: Diaphoresis, anaphylaxis

Warnings/Precautions Safety and efficacy of NovoLog™ in children has not been established.

Drug Interactions

Increased Effect/Toxicity: Increased hypoglycemic effect of insulin with alcohol, alpha-blockers, anabolic steroids, beta-blockers (nonselective beta-blockers may delay recovery from hypoglycemic episodes and mask signs/symptoms of hypoglycemia; cardioselective beta-blocker agents may be alternatives), clofibrate, guanethidine, MAO inhibitors, pentamidine, phenylbutazone, salicylates, sulfinpyrazone, and tetracyclines. Insulin increases the risk of hypoglycemia associated with oral hypoglycemic agents (including sulfonylureas, metformin, pioglitazone, rosiglitazone, and troglitazone).

Decreased hypoglycemic effect of insulin with corticosteroids, dextrothyroxine, diltiazem, dobutamine, epinephrine, niacin, oral contraceptives, thiazide diuretics, thyroid hormone, and smoking.

Drug Uptake Onset and duration of hypoglycemic effects depend upon preparation administered. See table.

Type of Insulin	Onset (h)	Peak (h)	Duration (h)
Lispro (Humalog®)	0.25	0.5-1.5	6-8
Insulin aspart injection (NovoLog®)	0.5	1-3	3-5
Insulin, regular (Novolin® R)	0.5-1	2-3	8-12
Isophane insulin suspension (NPH) (Novolin® N)	1-1.5	4-12	24
Insulin zinc suspension (Lente®)	1-2.5	8-12	18-24
Isophane insulin suspension and regular insulin injection (Novolin® 70/30)	0.5	2-12	24
Extended insulin zinc suspension (Ultralente®)	4-8	16-18	>36
Insulin glargine (Lantus®)	—	—	24

Onset and duration: Biosynthetic NPH human insulin shows a more rapid onset and shorter duration of action than corresponding porcine insulins; human insulin and purified porcine regular insulin are similarly efficacious following S.C. administration. The duration of action of highly purified porcine insulins is shorter than that of conventional insulin equivalents. Duration depends on type of preparation and route of administration as well as patient related variables. In general, the larger the dose of insulin, the longer the duration of activity.

Absorption: Biosynthetic regular human insulin is absorbed from the S.C. injection site more rapidly than insulins of animal origin (60-90 minutes peak vs 120-150 minutes peak respectively) and lowers the initial blood glucose much faster. Human Ultralente® insulin is absorbed about twice as quickly as its bovine equivalent, and bioavailability is also improved. Human Lente® insulin preparations are also absorbed more quickly than their animal equivalents. Insulin glargine (Lantus®) is designed to form microprecipitates when injected subcutaneously. Small amounts of insulin glargine are then released over a 24-hour period, with no pronounced peak. Insulin glargine (Lantus®) for the treatment of type 1 diabetes (insulin dependent, IDDM) and type 2 diabetes mellitus (noninsulin dependent, NIDDM) in patients who require basal (long-acting) insulin.

Pregnancy Risk Factor B; C (insulin glargine [Lantus®]; insulin aspart [NovoLog®])

Generic Available Yes

Comments Buffered insulin (Velosulin® BR) should not be mixed with any other form of insulin. Buffering agent in Velosulin® BR may alter the activity of other insulin products.

Intal® *see* Cromolyn Sodium *on page 330*

Integrilin® see Eptifibatide on page 445

Interferon Alfa-2a (in ter FEER on AL fa too aye)

Related Information

Systemic Viral Diseases *on page 1354*

U.S. Brand Names Roferon-A®

Canadian Brand Names Roferon-A®

Pharmacologic Category Interferon

Synonyms IFLrA; rIFN-A

Use

Patients >18 years of age: Hairy cell leukemia, AIDS-related Kaposi's sarcoma, chronic hepatitis C

Children and Adults: Chronic myelogenous leukemia (CML), Philadelphia chromosome positive, within 1 year of diagnosis (limited experience in children)

Unlabeled/Investigational: Adjuvant therapy for malignant melanoma, AIDS-related thrombocytopenia, cutaneous ulcerations of Behçet's disease, brain tumors, metastatic ileal carcinoid tumors, cervical and colorectal cancers, genital warts, idiopathic mixed cryoglobulinemia, hemangioma, hepatitis D, hepatocellular carcinoma, idiopathic hypereosinophilic syndrome, mycosis fungoides, Sézary syndrome, low-grade non-Hodgkin's lymphoma, macular degeneration, multiple myeloma, renal cell carcinoma, basal and squamous cell skin cancer, essential thrombocythemia, cutaneous T-cell lymphoma

Local Anesthetic/Vasoconstrictor Precautions No information available to require special precautions

Effects on Dental Treatment >10%: Significant xerostomia and metallic taste

Dosage

Adults:

Hepatitis C: S.C., I.M.: 3 million units 3 times/week for 12 months

Mechanism of Action Alpha interferons are a family of proteins, produced by nucleated cells, that have antiviral, antiproliferative, and immune-regulating activity. There are 16 known subtypes of alpha interferons. Interferons interact with cells through high affinity cell surface receptors. Following activation, multiple effects can be detected including induction of gene transcription. Inhibits cellular growth, alters the state of cellular differentiation, interferes with oncogene expression, alters cell surface antigen expression, increases phagocytic activity of macrophages, and augments cytotoxicity of lymphocytes for target cells

Other Adverse Effects Note: A flu-like syndrome (fever, chills, tachycardia, malaise, myalgia, arthralgia, headache) occurs within 1-2 hours of administration; may last up to 24 hours and may be dose-limiting (symptoms in up to 92% of patients). For the listing below, the percentage of incidence noted generally corresponds to highest reported ranges. Incidence depends upon dosage and indication.

>10%:

Cardiovascular: Chest pain (4% to 11%), edema (11%), hypertension (11%)

Central nervous system: Psychiatric disturbances (including depression and suicidal behavior/ideation; reported incidence highly variable, generally >15%), fatigue (90%), headache (52%), dizziness (21%), irritability (15%), insomnia (14%), somnolence, lethargy, confusion, mental impairment, and motor weakness (most frequently seen at high doses [>100 million units], usually reverses within a few days); vertigo (19%); mental status changes (12%)

Dermatologic: Rash (usually maculopapular) on the trunk and extremities (7% to 18%), alopecia (19% to 22%), pruritus (13%), dry skin

Endocrine & metabolic: Hypocalcemia (10% to 51%), hyperglycemia (33% to 39%), elevation of transaminase levels (25% to 30%), elevation of alkaline phosphatase (48%)

Gastrointestinal: Loss of taste, anorexia (30% to 70%), nausea (28% to 53%), vomiting (10% to 30%, usually mild), diarrhea (22% to 34%, may be severe), taste change (13%), dry throat, xerostomia, abdominal cramps, abdominal pain

Hematologic (often due to underlying disease): Myelosuppression; neutropenia (32% to 70%); thrombocytopenia (22% to 70%); anemia (24% to 65%, may be dose-limiting, usually seen only during the first 6 months of therapy)

Onset: 7-10 days

Nadir: 14 days, may be delayed 20-40 days in hairy cell leukemia

Recovery: 21 days

Hepatic: Elevation of AST (SGOT) (77% to 80%), LDH (47%), bilirubin (31%)

Local: Injection site reaction (29%)

Neuromuscular & skeletal: Weakness (may be severe at doses >20,000,000 units/day); arthralgia and myalgia (5% to 73%, usually during the first 72 hours of treatment); rigors

Renal: Proteinuria (15% to 25%)

Respiratory: Cough (27%), irritation of oropharynx (14%)

Miscellaneous: Flu-like syndrome (up to 92% of patients), loss of taste, diaphoresis (15%)

1% to 10%:

Cardiovascular: Hypotension (6%), supraventricular tachyarrhythmias, palpitations (<3%), acute myocardial infarction (<1% to 1%)

(Continued)

Interferon Alfa-2a *(Continued)*

Central nervous system: Confusion (10%), delirium
Dermatologic: Erythema (diffuse), urticaria
Endocrine & metabolic: Hyperphosphatemia (2%)
Gastrointestinal: Stomatitis, pancreatitis (<5%), flatulence, liver pain
Genitourinary: Impotence (6%), menstrual irregularities
Neuromuscular & skeletal: Leg cramps; peripheral neuropathy, paresthesias (7%), and numbness (4%) are more common in patients previously treated with vinca alkaloids or receiving concurrent vinblastine
Ocular: Conjunctivitis (4%)
Respiratory: Dyspnea (7.5%), epistaxis (4%), rhinitis (3%)
Miscellaneous: Antibody production to interferon (10%)

Drug Interactions Inhibits metabolism by cytochrome P450 (isoenzyme profiles not defined)

Increased Effect/Toxicity: Cimetidine may augment the antitumor effects of interferon in melanoma. Theophylline clearance has been reported to be decreased in hepatitis patients receiving interferon. Vinblastine enhances interferon toxicity in several patients; increased incidence of paresthesia has also been noted. Interferons may increase the adverse/toxic effects of ACE inhibitors, specifically the development of granulocytopenia. Agranulocytosis has been reported with concurrent use of clozapine (case report). Interferons may increase the anticoagulant effects of warfarin, and interferons may increase serum concentration of zidovudine.

Decreased Effect: Prednisone may decrease the therapeutic effects of interferon alpha. A decreased response to erythropoietin has been reported (case reports) in patients receiving interferons. Interferon alpha may decrease the serum concentration of melphalan (may or may not decrease toxicity of melphalan).

Drug Uptake

Absorption: Filtered and absorbed at the renal tubule
Half-life, elimination: I.V.: 3.7-8.5 hours (mean ~5 hours)
Time to peak: I.M., S.C.: ~6-8 hours

Pregnancy Risk Factor C

Generic Available No

Interferon Alfa-2b (in ter FEER on AL fa too bee)

Related Information

Systemic Viral Diseases *on page 1354*

U.S. Brand Names Intron® A

Canadian Brand Names Intron® A

Pharmacologic Category Interferon

Synonyms INF-alpha 2; α-2-interferon; rLFN-α2

Use

Patients >1 year of age: Chronic hepatitis B

Patients >18 years of age: Condyloma acuminata, chronic hepatitis C, hairy cell leukemia, malignant melanoma, AIDS-related Kaposi's sarcoma, follicular non-Hodgkin's lymphoma

Unlabeled/Investigational: AIDS-related thrombocytopenia, cutaneous ulcerations of Behçet's disease, carcinoid syndrome, cervical cancer, lymphomatoid granulomatosis, genital herpes, hepatitis D, chronic myelogenous leukemia (CML), non-Hodgkin's lymphomas (other than follicular lymphoma, see approved use), polycythemia vera, medullary thyroid carcinoma, multiple myeloma, renal cell carcinoma, basal and squamous cell skin cancers, essential thrombocytopenia, thrombocytopenic purpura

Local Anesthetic/Vasoconstrictor Precautions No information available to require special precautions

Effects on Dental Treatment >10%: Xerostomia and metallic taste

Dosage

Children 1-17 years: Chronic hepatitis B: S.C.: 3 million units/m² 3 times/week for 1 week; then 6 million units/m² 3 times/week; maximum: 10 million units 3 times/week; total duration of therapy 16-24 weeks

Adults:

Chronic hepatitis B: I.M., S.C.: 5 million units/day or 10 million units 3 times/week for 16 weeks

Chronic hepatitis C: I.M., S.C.: 3 million units 3 times/week for 16 weeks. In patients with normalization of ALT at 16 weeks, continue treatment for 18-24 months; consider discontinuation if normalization does not occur at 16 weeks. **Note:** May be used in combination therapy with ribavirin in previously untreated patients or in patients who relapse following alpha interferon therapy; refer to Interferon Alfa-2b and Ribavirin Combination Pack monograph.

Condyloma acuminata: Intralesionally: 1 million units/lesion (maximum: 5 lesions/treatment) 3 times/week (on alternate days) for 3 weeks. Use 1 million unit per 0.1 mL concentration.

Mechanism of Action Alpha interferons are a family of proteins, produced by nucleated cells, that have antiviral, antiproliferative, and immune-regulating activity.

There are 16 known subtypes of alpha interferons. Interferons interact with cells through high affinity cell surface receptors. Following activation, multiple effects can be detected including induction of gene transcription. Inhibits cellular growth, alters the state of cellular differentiation, interferes with oncogene expression, alters cell surface antigen expression, increases phagocytic activity of macrophages, and augments cytotoxicity of lymphocytes for target cells

Other Adverse Effects Note: In a majority of patients, a flu-like syndrome (fever, chills, tachycardia, malaise, myalgia, headache), occurs within 1-2 hours of administration; may last up to 24 hours and may be dose-limiting.

>10%:

- Cardiovascular: Chest pain (2% to 28%)
- Central nervous system: Fatigue (8% to 96%), headache (21% to 62%), fever (34% to 94%), depression (4% to 40%), somnolence (1% to 33%), irritability (1% to 22%), paresthesia (1% to 21%, more common in patients previously treated with vinca alkaloids or receiving concurrent vinblastine), dizziness (7% to 23%), confusion (1% to 12%), malaise (3% to 14%), pain (3% to 15%), insomnia (1% to 12%), impaired concentration (1% to 14%, usually reverses within a few days), amnesia (1% to 14%), chills (45% to 54%),
- Dermatologic: Alopecia (8% to 38%), rash (usually maculopapular) on the trunk and extremities (1% to 25%), pruritus (3% to 11%), dry skin (1% to 10%)
- Endocrine & metabolic: Hypocalcemia (10% to 51%), hyperglycemia (33% to 39%), amenorrhea (up to 12% in lymphoma)
- Gastrointestinal: Anorexia (1% to 69%), nausea (19% to 66%), vomiting (2% to 32%, usually mild), diarrhea (2% to 45%, may be severe), taste change (2% to 24%), xerostomia (1% to 28%), abdominal pain (2% to 23%), gingivitis (2% to 14%), constipation (1% to 14%)
- Hematologic: Myelosuppression; neutropenia (30% to 66%); thrombocytopenia (5% to 15%); anemia (15% to 32%, may be dose-limiting, usually seen only during the first 6 months of therapy)
  - Onset: 7-10 days
  - Nadir: 14 days, may be delayed 20-40 days in hairy cell leukemia
  - Recovery: 21 days
- Hepatic: Increased transaminases (increased SGOT in up to 63%), elevation of alkaline phosphatase (48%), right upper quadrant pain (15% in hepatitis C)
- Local: Injection site reaction (1% to 20%)
- Neuromuscular & skeletal: Weakness (5% to 63%) may be severe at doses >20,000,000 units/day; mild arthralgia and myalgia (5% to 75% - usually during the first 72 hours of treatment), rigors (2% to 42%), back pain (1% to 19%), musculoskeletal pain (1% to 21%), paresthesia (1% to 21%)
- Renal: Urinary tract infection (up to 5% in hepatitis C)
- Respiratory: Dyspnea (1% to 34%), cough (1% to 31%), pharyngitis (1% to 31%),
- Miscellaneous: Loss of smell, flu-like symptoms (5% to 79%), diaphoresis (2% to 21%)

5% to 10%:

- Cardiovascular: Hypertension (9% in hepatitis C)
- Central nervous system: Anxiety (1% to 9%), nervousness (1% to 3%), vertigo (up to 8% in lymphoma)
- Dermatologic: Dermatitis (1% to 8%)
- Endocrine & metabolic: Decreased libido (1% to 5%)
- Gastrointestinal: Loose stools (1% to 21%), dyspepsia (2% to 8%)
- Neuromuscular & skeletal: Hypoesthesia (1% to 10%)
- Respiratory: Nasal congestion (1% to 10%)

<5% (Limited to important or life-threatening):

- Cardiovascular: Angina, arrhythmia, atrial fibrillation, bradycardia, tachycardia, vasculitis, CHF, cardiomegaly, cardiomyopathy, hypotension, Raynaud's phenomenon, thrombosis, pulmonary embolism, myocardial infarction
- Central nervous system: Abnormal coordination, aggravated depression, aphasia, ataxia, Bell's palsy, coma, seizures, dysphonia, extrapyramidal disorder, flushing, hallucinations, manic reaction, migraine, neuropathy, paranoia, psychosis, stroke, suicidal ideation, suicide attempt, syncope, tremor
- Dermatologic: Diffuse erythema, eczema, epidermal necrolysis, hirsutism, psoriasis, urticaria
- Endocrine & metabolic: Diabetes mellitus, hyperthyroidism, hypothyroidism, hypertriglyceridemia, hyperglycemia, goiter, pancreatitis
- Gastrointestinal: Ascites, colitis, esophagitis, gastritis, gastrointestinal hemorrhage, gingival hyperplasia, mucositis, rectal hemorrhage, stomatitis, taste loss
- Genitourinary: Cystitis, incontinence, dysuria
- Hematologic: Anemia, granulocytopenia, leukopenia, hemolytic anemia, thrombocytopenic purpura
- Hepatic: Hyperbilirubinemia, jaundice, hepatic encephalopathy (rare), hepatic failure (rare), hepatotoxic reaction
- Neuromuscular & skeletal: Arthritis, leg cramps, polyarteritis nodosa, tendonitis, rheumatoid arthritis, spondylitis, lupus erythematosus
- Ocular: Abnormal vision, nystagmus
- Renal: Proteinuria, hematuria, increased BUN, nephrotic syndrome, renal failure

(Continued)

Interferon Alfa-2b *(Continued)*

Respiratory: Asthma, bronchospasm, hemoptysis, hypoventilation, pulmonary fibrosis, pleural effusion, pneumonitis, respiratory insufficiency

Miscellaneous: Acute hypersensitivity reactions, allergic reactions

Drug Interactions Inhibits metabolism by cytochrome P450 (isoenzyme profiles not defined)

Increased Effect/Toxicity: Cimetidine may augment the antitumor effects of interferon in melanoma. Theophylline clearance has been reported to be decreased in hepatitis patients receiving interferon. Vinblastine enhances interferon toxicity in several patients; increased incidence of paresthesia has also been noted. Interferons may increase the adverse/toxic effects of ACE inhibitors, specifically the development of granulocytopenia. Agranulocytosis has been reported with concurrent use of clozapine (case report). Interferons may increase the anticoagulant effects of warfarin, and interferons may increase serum concentration of zidovudine.

Drug Uptake

Half-life, elimination: I.M., I.V.: 2 hours; S.C.: 3 hours

Time to peak: I.M., S.C.: ~3-12 hours

Pregnancy Risk Factor C

Generic Available No

Interferon Alfa-2b and Ribavirin Combination Pack

(in ter FEER on AL fa too bee & rye ba VYE rin com bi NAY shun pak)

U.S. Brand Names Rebetron™

Canadian Brand Names Rebetron™

Pharmacologic Category Antiviral Agent; Interferon

Synonyms Ribavirin and Interferon Alfa-2b Combination Pack

Use The combination therapy of oral ribavirin with interferon alfa-2b, recombinant (Intron® A) injection is indicated for the treatment of chronic hepatitis C in patients with compensated liver disease who have relapsed after alpha interferon therapy.

Local Anesthetic/Vasoconstrictor Precautions No information available to require special precautions

Effects on Dental Treatment >10%: Xerostomia and metallic taste

Dosage

Children: Chronic hepatitis C: **Note:** Safety and efficacy have not been established; dosing based on pharmacokinetic profile: Recommended dosage of combination therapy (Intron® A with Rebetrol®):

- Intron® A: S.C.:
  - 25-61 kg: 3 million int. units/m² 3 times/week
  - >61 kg: Refer to adult dosing
- Rebetrol® capsule: Oral:
  - 25-36 kg: 400 mg/day (200 mg twice daily)
  - 37-49 kg: 600 mg/day (200 mg in morning and 400 mg in evening)
  - 50-61 kg: 800 mg/day (400 mg twice daily)
  - >61 kg: Refer to adult dosing

Adults: Chronic hepatitis C: Recommended dosage of combination therapy:

- Intron® A: S.C.: 3 million int. units 3 times/week **and**
- Rebetrol® capsule: Oral: Range: 1000-1200 mg in a divided daily (morning and evening) dose for 24 weeks
  - ≤75 kg (165 pounds): 1000 mg/day (two 200 mg capsules in the morning and three 200 mg capsules in the evening)
  - >75 kg: 1200 mg/day (three 200 mg capsules in the morning and three 200 mg capsules in the evening)

Mechanism of Action

Interferon Alfa-2b: Alpha interferons are a family of proteins, produced by nucleated cells, that have antiviral, antiproliferative, and immune-regulating activity. There are 16 known subtypes of alpha interferons. Interferons interact with cells through high affinity cell surface receptors. Following activation, multiple effects can be detected including induction of gene transcription. Inhibits cellular growth, alters the state of cellular differentiation, interferes with oncogene expression, alters cell surface antigen expression, increases phagocytic activity of macrophages, and augments cytotoxicity of lymphocytes for target cells

Ribavirin: Inhibits replication of RNA and DNA viruses; inhibits influenza virus RNA polymerase activity and inhibits the initiation and elongation of RNA fragments resulting in inhibition of viral protein synthesis

Other Adverse Effects Note: Adverse reactions listed are specific to combination regimen in previously untreated hepatitis patients. See individual monographs for additional adverse reactions reported with each agent during therapy for other diseases.

>10%

Central nervous system: Fatigue (68%), headache (63%), insomnia (39%), fever (37%), depression (32%), irritability (23%), dizziness (17%), impaired concentration (11%)

Dermatologic: Alopecia (28%), pruritus (21%), rash (20%)

Gastrointestinal: Nausea (38%), anorexia (27%), dyspepsia (14%), vomiting (11%)
Hematologic: Leukopenia, neutropenia (usually recovers within 4 weeks of treatment discontinuation), anemia
Hepatic: Hyperbilirubinemia (27% - only 0.9% >3.0 mg/dL)
Local: Injection site inflammation (13%)
Neuromuscular & skeletal: Myalgia (61%), rigors (40%), arthralgia (30%), musculoskeletal pain (20%)
Respiratory: Dyspnea (19%)
Miscellaneous: Flu-like syndrome (14%)

1% to 10%:
Cardiovascular: Chest pain (5%)
Central nervous system: Emotional lability (7%), nervousness (4%)
Endocrine & metabolic: Thyroid abnormalities (hyper- or hypothyroidism), increased serum uric acid, hyperglycemia
Gastrointestinal; taste perversion (7%)
Hematologic: Hemolytic anemia (10%), thrombocytopenia, anemia
Local: Injection site reaction (7%)
Neuromuscular & skeletal: Weakness (9%)
Respiratory: Sinusitis (9%)

Contraindications Hypersensitivity to interferon alfa-2b, ribavirin, or any component of the formulation; autoimmune hepatitis; males with a pregnant female partner; pregnancy

Warnings/Precautions

Interferon alfa-2b: Use with caution in patients with a history of seizures, brain metastases, multiple sclerosis, cardiac disease (ischemic or thromboembolic), arrhythmias, myelosuppression, hepatic impairment, or renal dysfunction (Cl_{cr} <50 mL/minute). Use caution in patients with a history of pulmonary disease, coagulopathy, thyroid disease, hypertension, or diabetes mellitus (particularly if prone to DKA). Caution in patients receiving drugs that may cause lactic acidosis (eg, nucleoside analogues). May cause severe psychiatric adverse events (psychosis, mania, depression, suicidal behavior/ideation) in patients with and without previous psychiatric symptoms, avoid use in severe psychiatric disorders or in patients with a history of depression; careful neuropsychiatric monitoring is required during therapy. Avoid use in patient with autoimmune disorders; worsening of psoriasis and/or development of autoimmune disorders has been associated with alpha interferons. Higher doses in elderly patients, or diseases other than hairy cell leukemia, may result in increased CNS toxicity. Treatment should be discontinued in patients who develop severe pulmonary symptoms with chest x-ray changes, autoimmune disorders, worsening of hepatic function, psychiatric symptoms (including depression and/or suicidal thoughts/behaviors), ischemic and/or infectious disorders. Ophthalmologic disorders (including retinal hemorrhages, cotton wool spots and retinal artery or vein obstruction) have occurred in patients receiving alpha interferons. Hypertriglyceridemia has been reported (discontinue if severe).

Safety and efficacy in children <18 years of age have not been established. Do not treat patients with visceral AIDS-related Kaposi's sarcoma associated with rapidly-progressing or life-threatening disease. A transient increase in SGOT (>2x baseline) is common in patients treated with interferon alfa-2b for chronic hepatitis. Therapy generally may continue, however functional indicators (albumin, prothrombin time, bilirubin) should be monitored at 2-week intervals. **Due to differences in dosage, patients should not change brands of interferons.**

Intron® A may cause bone marrow suppression, including very rarely, aplastic anemia. Hemolytic anemia (hemoglobin <10 g/dL) was observed in 10% of treated patients in clinical trials; anemia occurred within 1-2 weeks of initiation of therapy.

Ribavirin: Oral: Anemia has been observed in patients receiving the interferon/ribavirin combination. Severe psychiatric events have also occurred including depression and suicidal behavior during combination therapy; avoid use in patients with a psychiatric history. Hemolytic anemia is a significant toxicity; usually occurring within 1-2 weeks. Assess cardiac disease before initiation. Anemia may worsen underlying cardiac disease; use caution. If any deterioration in cardiovascular status occurs, discontinue therapy. Negative pregnancy test is required before initiation and monthly thereafter. Avoid pregnancy in female patients and female partners of patients during therapy by using two effective forms of contraception; continue contraceptive measures for at least 6 months after completion of therapy. If patient or female partner becomes pregnant during treatment, she should be counseled about potential risks of exposure. Discontinue therapy in suspected/confirmed pancreatitis. Use caution in elderly patients; higher frequency of anemia; take renal function into consideration before initiating. Safety and efficacy have not been established in organ transplant patients, decompensated liver disease, concurrent hepatitis B virus or HIV exposure, or pediatric patients. Use caution in patients receiving concurrent medications which may cause lactic acidosis (ie, nucleoside analogues).

(Continued)

Interferon Alfa-2b and Ribavirin Combination Pack *(Continued)*

Drug Interactions

Increased Effect/Toxicity: Interferon alpha: Cimetidine may augment the antitumor effects of interferon in melanoma. Theophylline clearance has been reported to be decreased in hepatitis patients receiving interferon. Vinblastine enhances interferon toxicity in several patients; increased incidence of paresthesia has also been noted. Interferons may increase the adverse/toxic effects of ACE inhibitors, specifically the development of granulocytopenia. Agranulocytosis has been reported with concurrent use of clozapine (case report). Interferons may increase the anticoagulant effects of warfarin, and interferons may increase serum concentration of zidovudine.

Decreased Effect: Interferon alpha: Prednisone may decrease the therapeutic effects of interferon alpha. A decreased response to erythropoietin has been reported (case reports) in patients receiving interferons. Interferon alpha may decrease the serum concentration of melphalan (may or may not decrease toxicity of melphalan). Ribavirin decreases the effect of zidovudine.

Drug Uptake See Interferon Alfa-2b *on page 642* and Ribavirin *on page 1048*

Pregnancy Risk Factor X

Generic Available No

Interferon Alfa-n3 (in ter FEER on AL fa en three)

Related Information

Systemic Viral Diseases *on page 1354*

U.S. Brand Names Alferon® N

Canadian Brand Names Alferon® N

Pharmacologic Category Interferon

Use Patients ≥18 years of age: Intralesional treatment of refractory or recurring genital or venereal warts (condylomata acuminata)

Local Anesthetic/Vasoconstrictor Precautions No information available to require special precautions

Effects on Dental Treatment >10%: Xerostomia and metallic taste

Dosage Adults: Inject 250,000 units (0.05 mL) in each wart twice weekly for a maximum of 8 weeks; therapy should not be repeated for at least 3 months after the initial 8-week course of therapy

Mechanism of Action Interferons interact with cells through high affinity cell surface receptors. Following activation, multiple effects can be detected including induction of gene transcription. Inhibits cellular growth, alters the state of cellular differentiation, interferes with oncogene expression, alters cell surface antigen expression, increases phagocytic activity of macrophages, and augments cytotoxicity of lymphocytes for target cells

Other Adverse Effects Note: Adverse reaction incidence noted below is specific to intralesional administration in patients with condylomata acuminata. Flu-like reactions, consisting of headache, fever, and/or myalgia, was reported in 30% of patients, and abated with repeated dosing.

>10%:

- Central nervous system: Fever (40%), headache (31%), chills (14%), fatigue (14%)
- Hematologic: Decreased WBC (11%)
- Neuromuscular & skeletal: Myalgia (45%)
- Miscellaneous: Flu-like syndrome (30%)

1% to 10%:

- Central nervous system: Malaise (9%), dizziness (9%), depression (2%), insomnia (2%), thirst (1%)
- Dermatologic: Pruritus (2%)
- Gastrointestinal: Nausea (45), vomiting (3%), dyspepsia (3%), diarrhea (2%), tongue hyperesthesia (1%), taste disturbance (1%)
- Genitourinary: Groin lymph node swelling (1%)
- Neuromuscular & skeletal: Arthralgia (5%), back pain (4%), cramps (1%), paresthesia (1%)
- Ocular: Visual disturbance (1%)
- Respiratory: Rhinitis (2%), pharyngitis (1%), nosebleed (1%)
- Miscellaneous: Increased diaphoresis (2%), vasovagal reaction (2%)

Drug Interactions

Increased Effect/Toxicity: Interferons may increase the adverse/toxic effects of ACE inhibitors, specifically the development of granulocytopenia. Risk: Monitor A case report of agranulocytosis has been reported with concurrent use of clozapine. Case reports of decreased hematopoietic effect with erythropoietin. Interferon alpha may decrease the P450 isoenzyme metabolism of theophylline. Interferons may increase the anticoagulant effects of warfarin. Interferons may decrease the metabolism of zidovudine.

Decreased Effect: Interferon alpha may decrease the serum concentration of melphalan; this may or may not decrease the potential toxicity of melphalan. Prednisone may decrease the therapeutic effects of Interferon alpha.

Pregnancy Risk Factor C

Generic Available No

Interferon Beta-1a (in ter FEER on BAY ta won aye)

U.S. Brand Names Avonex®; Rebif®

Canadian Brand Names Avonex®; Rebif®

Mexican Brand Names Rebif®

Pharmacologic Category Interferon

Synonyms rIFN beta-1a

Use Treatment of relapsing forms of multiple sclerosis (MS); to slow the accumulation of physical disability and decrease the frequency of clinical exacerbations

Local Anesthetic/Vasoconstrictor Precautions No information available to require special precautions

Effects on Dental Treatment No effects or complications reported

Dosage Adults >18 years: I.M.: 30 mcg once weekly

Mechanism of Action Interferon beta differs from naturally occurring human protein by a single amino acid substitution and the lack of carbohydrate side chains; alters the expression and response to surface antigens and can enhance immune cell activities. Properties of interferon beta that modify biologic responses are mediated by cell surface receptor interactions; mechanism in the treatment of MS is unknown.

Other Adverse Effects Note: Flu-like symptoms (including headache, fever, myalgia, and weakness) are the most common adverse reaction (up to 61%) and may diminish with repeated dosing. Frequencies noted here indicate the highest reported frequency for either product, either from placebo-controlled trials or comparative studies (some effects reported for only one product).

In a comparative study, the adverse effect profiles of Avonex® and Rebif® were noted to be similar; with the exception of three adverse events noted to occur more frequently in the Rebif® group: Transaminase elevations, local reactions, and reductions in white blood cell counts.

>10%:

- Central nervous system: Headache (30% to 70%), fever (23% to 28%), chills (21%), sleep disturbance (19%), dizziness (15%), depression (11% to 13%), insomnia (10% to 13%)
- Gastrointestinal: Nausea (33%), abdominal pain (9% to 22%) diarrhea (16%), dyspepsia (11%)
- Hematologic: Leukopenia (up to 36% in Rebif® patients), lymphadenopathy (12%)
- Hepatic: Transaminases increased (up to 27% with Rebif®; hepatic dysfunction noted in <10%)
- Local: Injection site disorders: A comparative trial noted events in 80% with Rebif® versus 24% with Avonex® (includes inflammation, pain, bruising, or site reaction)
- Neuromuscular & skeletal: Myalgia (25% to 34%), back pain (23% to 25%), skeletal pain (15%), weakness (21%)
- Ocular: Visual abnormalities (13%)
- Respiratory: Upper respiratory tract infection (31%), sinusitis (18%), rhinitis (15% to 17%)
- Miscellaneous; Flu-like symptoms (61%), infection (11%)

1% to 10%:

- Cardiovascular: Chest pain (8%), syncope (4%), vasodilation (4%)
- Central nervous system: Somnolence (5%), suicidal tendency (4%), malaise (5%), seizure (5%), ataxia (5%)
- Dermatologic: Urticaria (5%), alopecia (4%), rash (7%)
- Endocrine & metabolic: Thyroid abnormalities (up to 6% with Rebif®)
- Gastrointestinal: Abdominal pain (9%), anorexia (7%), xerostomia (5%)
- Genitourinary: Vaginitis (4%), ovarian cyst (3%), urinary frequency (7%), incontinence (4%)
- Hematologic: Thrombocytopenia (8%), anemia (8%), eosinophilia (5%)
- Hepatic: Hepatic function abnormalities (9%), hyperbilirubinemia (3%)
- Neuromuscular & skeletal: Arthralgia (9%), muscle spasm (7%), rigors (13%)
- Ocular: Dry eyes (3%)
- Otic: Otitis media (6%), hearing decreased (3%)
- Respiratory: Dyspnea (6%)
- Miscellaneous: Herpesvirus infection (3%), hypersensitivity reaction (3%)

Warnings/Precautions Interferon beta-1a should be used with caution in patients with a history of depression, seizures, or cardiac disease; because its use has not been evaluated during lactation, its use in breast-feeding mothers may not be safe and should be warned against

Drug Interactions Inhibits metabolism by cytochrome P450 (isoenzyme profiles not defined)

(Continued)

Interferon Beta-1a *(Continued)*

Increased Effect/Toxicity: Theophylline clearance has been reported to be decreased in hepatitis patients receiving interferon. Vinblastine enhances interferon toxicity in several patients; increased incidence of paresthesia has also been noted. Interferons may increase the adverse/toxic effects of ACE inhibitors, specifically the development of granulocytopenia. Agranulocytosis has been reported with concurrent use of clozapine (case report). Interferons may increase the anticoagulant effects of warfarin, and interferons may increase serum concentration of zidovudine.

Decreased Effect: A decreased response to erythropoietin has been reported (case reports) in patients receiving interferons. Interferon alpha may decrease the serum concentration of melphalan (may or may not decrease toxicity of melphalan).

Drug Uptake Limited data due to small doses used

Half-life, elimination: Avonex®: 10 hours; Rebif®: 69 hours

Time to peak: Avonex® (I.M.): 3-15 hours; Rebif® (S.C.): 14 hours

Pregnancy Risk Factor C

Generic Available No

Interferon Beta-1b (in ter FEER on BAY ta won bee)

U.S. Brand Names Betaseron®

Canadian Brand Names Betaseron®

Mexican Brand Names Betaferon®

Pharmacologic Category Interferon

Synonyms rIFN beta-1b

Use Reduces the frequency of clinical exacerbations in ambulatory patients with relapsing-remitting multiple sclerosis (MS)

Local Anesthetic/Vasoconstrictor Precautions No information available to require special precautions

Effects on Dental Treatment No effects or complications reported

Dosage S.C.:

Children <18 years: Not recommended

Adults >18 years: 0.25 mg (8 million units) every other day

Mechanism of Action Interferon beta-1b differs from naturally occurring human protein by a single amino acid substitution and the lack of carbohydrate side chains; alters the expression and response to surface antigens and can enhance immune cell activities. Properties of interferon beta-1b that modify biologic responses are mediated by cell surface receptor interactions; mechanism in the treatment of MS is unknown.

Other Adverse Effects Note: Flu-like symptoms (including at least two of the following - headache, fever, chills, malaise, diaphoresis, and myalgias) are reported in the majority of patients (76%).

>10%:

- Central nervous system: Headache (84%), fever (59%), pain (52%), chills (46%), dizziness (35%), malaise (15%), anxiety (15%), migraine (12%)
- Endocrine & metabolic: Dysmenorrhea (18%), menstrual disorder (17%), metrorrhagia (15%), hypoglycemia (15%)
- Gastrointestinal: Diarrhea (35%), abdominal pain (32%), constipation (24%), vomiting (21%)
- Hematologic: Lymphopenia (82%), neutropenia (18%), leukopenia (16%), lymphadenopathy (14%)
- Hepatic: SGPT increased >5x baseline (19%), SGOT increased >5x baseline (4%)
- Local: injection site reaction (85%)
- Neuromuscular & skeletal: Weakness (49%), myalgia (44%). Hypertonia (26%), myasthenia (13%)
- Ocular: Conjunctivitis (12%)
- Respiratory: Sinusitis (36%)
- Miscellaneous: Flu-like symptoms (76%), increased diaphoresis (23%)

1% to 10%:

- Cardiovascular: edema (8%), palpitation (8%), hypertension (7%), tachycardia (6%), peripheral vascular disorder (5%), hemorrhage (3%)
- Central nervous system: Nervousness (8%), somnolence (6%), confusion (4%), speech disorder (3%), seizure (2%), suicide attempt (2%), hyperkinesias (2%), amnesia (2%)
- Dermatologic: Alopecia (4%)
- Endocrine & metabolic: Breast pain (7%), menorrhagia (6%), fibrocystic breast (3%), breast neoplasm (2%), goiter (2%)
- Genitourinary: Pelvic pain (6%), cystitis (8%), urinary urgency (4%), weight gain (4%), weight loss (4%)
- Hepatic: Bilirubin increased >2.5x baseline (6%), SGOT increased >5x baseline (4%)
- Local: Injection site necrosis (5%)
- Ocular: Abnormal vision (7%)

Renal: Proteinuria (5%)
Respiratory: Dyspnea (8%), laryngitis (6%)

Drug Interactions

Increased Effect/Toxicity: Interferons may increase the adverse/toxic effects of ACE inhibitors, specifically the development of granulocytopenia; monitor. A case report of agranulocytosis has been reported with concurrent use of clozapine. Case reports of decreased hematopoietic effect with erythropoietin. Interferon alpha may decrease the P450 isoenzyme metabolism of theophylline. Interferons may increase the anticoagulant effects of warfarin. Interferons may decrease the metabolism of zidovudine.

Decreased Effect: Prednisone may decrease the therapeutic effects of Interferon alpha.

Drug Uptake Limited data due to small doses used
Half-life, elimination: 8 minutes to 4.3 hours
Time to peak: 1-8 hours

Pregnancy Risk Factor C

Generic Available No

Interferon Gamma-1b (in ter FEER on GAM ah won bee)

U.S. Brand Names Actimmune®

Canadian Brand Names Actimmune®

Pharmacologic Category Interferon

Use Reduce frequency and severity of serious infections associated with chronic granulomatous disease; delay time to disease progression in patients with severe, malignant osteopetrosis

Local Anesthetic/Vasoconstrictor Precautions No information available to require special precautions

Effects on Dental Treatment No effects or complications reported

Dosage If severe reactions occur, modify dose (50% reduction) or therapy should be discontinued until adverse reactions abate.

Chronic granulomatous disease: Children >1 year and Adults: S.C.:
BSA ≤0.5 m^2: 1.5 mcg/kg/dose 3 times/week
BSA >0.5 m^2: 50 mcg/m^2 (1.5 million int. units/m^2) 3 times/week

Severe, malignant osteopetrosis: Children >1 year: S.C.:
BSA ≤0.5 m^2: 1.5 mcg/kg/dose 3 times/week
BSA >0.5 m^2: 50 mcg/m^2 (1.5 million int. units/m^2) 3 times/week

Other Adverse Effects Based on 50 mcg/m^2 dose administered 3 times weekly for chronic granulomatous disease

>10%:
Central nervous system: Fever (52%), headache (33%), chills (14%), fatigue (14%)
Dermatologic: Rash (17%)
Gastrointestinal: Diarrhea (14%), vomiting (13%)
Local: Injection site erythema or tenderness (14%)

1% to 10%:
Central nervous system: Depression (3%)
Gastrointestinal: Nausea (10%), abdominal pain (8%)
Neuromuscular & skeletal: Myalgia (6%), arthralgia (2%), back pain (2%)

Drug Interactions Increased Effect/Toxicity: Interferon gamma-1b may increase hepatic enzymes or enhance myelosuppression when taken with other myelosuppressive agents. May decrease cytochrome P450 concentrations leading to increased serum concentration of drugs metabolized by this pathway.

Drug Uptake
Absorption: I.M., S.C.: Slowly
Half-life, elimination: I.V.: 38 minutes; I.M., S.C.: 3-6 hours
Time to peak, plasma: I.M.: 4 hours (1.5 ng/mL); S.C.: 7 hours (0.6 ng/mL)

Pregnancy Risk Factor C

Generic Available No

Comments More heat- and acid-labile than alfa interferons

Intralipid® *see* Fat Emulsion *on page 487*
Intron® A *see* Interferon Alfa-2b *on page 642*
Invanz™ *see* Ertapenem *on page 449*
Inversine® *see* Mecamylamine *on page 749*
Invirase® *see* Saquinavir *on page 1075*
Iobid DM® *see* Guaifenesin and Dextromethorphan *on page 569*
Iodex® [OTC] *see* Povidone-Iodine *on page 982*
Iodex-p® [OTC] *see* Povidone-Iodine *on page 982*

Iodine (EYE oh dyne)

Pharmacologic Category Mineral

Use Used topically as an antiseptic in the management of minor, superficial skin wounds and has been used to disinfect the skin preoperatively

(Continued)

Iodine *(Continued)*

Local Anesthetic/Vasoconstrictor Precautions No information available to require special precautions

Effects on Dental Treatment No effects or complications reported

Dosage Apply topically as necessary to affected areas of skin

Other Adverse Effects Frequency not defined:
- Central nervous system: Fever, headache
- Dermatologic: Skin rash, angioedema, urticaria, acne
- Endocrine & metabolic: Hypothyroidism
- Gastrointestinal: Metallic taste, diarrhea
- Hematologic: Eosinophilia, hemorrhage (mucosal)
- Neuromuscular & skeletal: Arthralgia
- Ocular: Swelling of eyelids
- Respiratory: Pulmonary edema
- Miscellaneous: Lymph node enlargement

Pregnancy Risk Factor D

Generic Available Yes

Comments Sodium thiosulfate inactivates iodine and is an effective chemical antidote for codeine poisoning; solutions of sodium thiosulfate may be used to remove iodine stains from skin and clothing

Iodopen® *see* Trace Metals *on page 1186*

Iodoquinol (eye oh doe KWIN ole)

U.S. Brand Names Yodoxin®

Canadian Brand Names Diodoquin®

Pharmacologic Category Amebicide

Synonyms Diiodohydroxyquin

Use Treatment of acute and chronic intestinal amebiasis; asymptomatic cyst passers; *Blastocystis hominis* infections; ineffective for amebic hepatitis or hepatic abscess

Local Anesthetic/Vasoconstrictor Precautions No information available to require special precautions

Effects on Dental Treatment No effects or complications reported

Dosage Oral:
- Children: 30-40 mg/kg/day (maximum: 650 mg/dose) in 3 divided doses for 20 days; not to exceed 1.95 g/day
- Adults: 650 mg 3 times/day after meals for 20 days; not to exceed 2 g/day

Mechanism of Action Contact amebicide that works in the lumen of the intestine by an unknown mechanism

Other Adverse Effects Frequency not defined:
- Central nervous system: Fever, chills, agitation, retrograde amnesia, headache
- Dermatologic: Rash, urticaria, pruritus
- Endocrine & metabolic: Thyroid gland enlargement
- Gastrointestinal: Diarrhea, nausea, vomiting, stomach pain, abdominal cramps
- Neuromuscular & skeletal: Peripheral neuropathy, weakness
- Ocular: Optic neuritis, optic atrophy, visual impairment
- Miscellaneous: Itching of rectal area

Drug Uptake Absorption: Oral: Poor and irregular

Pregnancy Risk Factor C

Generic Available No

Iodoquinol and Hydrocortisone

(eye oh doe KWIN ole & hye droe KOR ti sone)

U.S. Brand Names Vytone®

Pharmacologic Category Antifungal Agent, Topical; Corticosteroid, Topical

Synonyms Hydrocortisone and Iodoquinol

Use Treatment of eczema; infectious dermatitis; chronic eczematoid otitis externa; mycotic dermatoses

Local Anesthetic/Vasoconstrictor Precautions No information available to require special precautions

Effects on Dental Treatment No effects or complications reported

Dosage Apply 3-4 times/day

Therapy should be discontinued when control is achieved; if no improvement is seen, reassessment of diagnosis may be necessary.

Other Adverse Effects

Based on **iodoquinol** component: Frequency not defined:
- Central nervous system: Fever, chills, agitation, retrograde amnesia, headache
- Dermatologic: Rash, urticaria, pruritus
- Endocrine & metabolic: Thyroid gland enlargement
- Gastrointestinal: Diarrhea, nausea, vomiting, stomach pain, abdominal cramps
- Neuromuscular & skeletal: Peripheral neuropathy, weakness
- Ocular: Optic neuritis, optic atrophy, visual impairment
- Miscellaneous: Itching of rectal area

Based on **hydrocortisone** component:

>10%:

Central nervous system: Insomnia, nervousness

Gastrointestinal: Increased appetite, indigestion

1% to 10%:

Dermatologic: Hirsutism

Endocrine & metabolic: Diabetes mellitus

Neuromuscular & skeletal: Arthralgia

Ocular: Cataracts

Respiratory: Epistaxis

Drug Interactions See Iodoquinol *on page 650* and Hydrocortisone *on page 608*

Drug Uptake See Iodoquinol *on page 650* and Hydrocortisone *on page 608*

Pregnancy Risk Factor C

Generic Available No

Ionamin® *see* Phentermine *on page 948*

Iopidine® *see* Apraclonidine *on page 108*

Iosopan® Plus *see* Magaldrate and Simethicone *on page 739*

Ipecac Syrup (IP e kak SIR up)

Pharmacologic Category Antidote

Use Treatment of acute oral drug overdosage and certain poisonings

Local Anesthetic/Vasoconstrictor Precautions No information available to require special precautions

Effects on Dental Treatment No effects or complications reported

Dosage Oral:

Children:

6-12 months: 5-10 mL followed by 10-20 mL/kg of water; repeat dose one time if vomiting does not occur within 20 minutes

1-12 years: 15 mL followed by 10-20 mL/kg of water; repeat dose one time if vomiting does not occur within 20 minutes

If emesis does not occur within 30 minutes after second dose, ipecac must be removed from stomach by gastric lavage

Adults: 15-30 mL followed by 200-300 mL of water; repeat dose one time if vomiting does not occur within 20 minutes

Mechanism of Action Irritates the gastric mucosa and stimulates the medullary chemoreceptor trigger zone to induce vomiting

Other Adverse Effects Frequency not defined:

Cardiovascular: Cardiotoxicity

Central nervous system: Lethargy

Gastrointestinal: Protracted vomiting, diarrhea

Neuromuscular & skeletal: Myopathy

Drug Interactions

Increased Effect/Toxicity: Phenothiazines (chlorpromazine has been associated with serious dystonic reactions).

Decreased effect with activated charcoal.

Drug Uptake

Onset of action: 15-30 minutes

Absorption: Significant amounts, mainly when it does not produce emesis

Duration: 20-25 minutes; ≤1 hour

Pregnancy Risk Factor C

Generic Available Yes

I-Pentolate® *see* Cyclopentolate *on page 334*

IPOL™ *see* Poliovirus Vaccine, Inactivated *on page 969*

Ipratropium (i pra TROE pee um)

Related Information

Ipratropium and Albuterol *on page 652*

Respiratory Diseases *on page 1328*

U.S. Brand Names Atrovent®

Canadian Brand Names Alti-Ipratropium; Apo®-Ipravent; Atrovent®; Gen-Ipratropium; Novo-Ipramide; Novo-Ipramide; Nu-Ipratropium; PMS-Ipratropium

Mexican Brand Names Atrovent®

Pharmacologic Category Anticholinergic Agent

Synonyms Ipratropium Bromide

Use Anticholinergic bronchodilator used in bronchospasm associated with asthma, COPD, bronchitis, and emphysema; symptomatic relief of rhinorrhea associated with the common cold and allergic and nonallergic rhinitis

Local Anesthetic/Vasoconstrictor Precautions No information available to require special precautions

Effects on Dental Treatment >10%: Xerostomia

(Continued)

Ipratropium *(Continued)*

Dosage

Nebulization:

Infants and Children ≤12 years: 125-250 mcg 3 times/day

Children >12 years and Adults: 500 mcg (one unit-dose vial) 3-4 times/day with doses 6-8 hours apart

Metered dose inhaler:

Children 3-12 years: 1-2 inhalations 3 times/day, up to 6 inhalations/24 hours

Children >12 years and Adults: 2 inhalations 4 times/day, up to 12 inhalations/24 hours

Nasal spray:

Symptomatic relief of rhinorrhea associated with the common cold (safety and efficacy of use beyond 4 days in patients with the common cold have not been established):

Children 5-11 years: 0.06%: 2 sprays in each nostril 3 times/day

Children ≥5 years and Adults: 0.06%: 2 sprays in each nostril 3-4 times/day

Symptomatic relief of rhinorrhea associated with allergic/nonallergic rhinitis: Children ≥6 years and Adults: 0.03%: 2 sprays in each nostril 2-3 times/day

Mechanism of Action Blocks the action of acetylcholine at parasympathetic sites in bronchial smooth muscle causing bronchodilation

Other Adverse Effects Note: Poorly absorbed from the lung, so systemic effects are rare.

Inhalation aerosol and inhalation solution:

<10%: Respiratory: Upper respiratory infection (13%), bronchitis (15%)

1% to 10%:

Cardiovascular: Palpitations (2%)

Central nervous system: Nervousness (3%), dizziness (2%), fatigue, headache (6%), pain (4%)

Dermatologic: Rash (1%)

Gastrointestinal: Nausea, xerostomia, stomach upset, dry mucous membranes

Respiratory: Nasal congestion, dyspnea (10%), increased sputum (1%), bronchospasm (2%), pharyngitis (3%), rhinitis (2%), sinusitis (5%)

Miscellaneous: Influenza-like symptoms

Nasal spray: Epistaxis (8%), nasal dryness (5%), nausea (2%)

Drug Interactions Increased Effect/Toxicity: Increased therapeutic effect with albuterol. Increased toxicity with anticholinergics or drugs with anticholinergic properties and dronabinol.

Drug Uptake

Onset of action: Bronchodilation: 1-3 minutes; Peak effect: 1.5-2 hours

Absorption: Not readily absorbed into the systemic circulation from the surface of the lung or from the GI tract; negligible

Duration: 4-6 hours

Pregnancy Risk Factor B

Generic Available Yes

Ipratropium and Albuterol (i pra TROE pee um & al BYOO ter ole)

U.S. Brand Names Combivent®; DuoNeb™

Canadian Brand Names Combivent®

Pharmacologic Category Bronchodilator

Synonyms Albuterol and Ipratropium

Use Treatment of chronic obstructive pulmonary disease (COPD) in those patients that are currently on a regular bronchodilator who continue to have bronchospasms and require a second bronchodilator

Local Anesthetic/Vasoconstrictor Precautions No information available to require special precautions

Effects on Dental Treatment >10%: Xerostomia

Dosage

Inhalation: 2 inhalations 4 times/day (maximum: 12 inhalations/24 hours)

Inhalation via nebulization: Initial: 3 mL every 6 hours (maximum: 3 mL every 4 hours)

Mechanism of Action See Ipratropium *on page 651* and Albuterol *on page 45*

Other Adverse Effects

Based on **ipratropium** component: **Note:** Ipratropium is poorly absorbed from the lung, so systemic effects are rare.

Inhalation aerosol and inhalation solution:

<10%: Respiratory: Upper respiratory infection (13%), bronchitis (15%)

1% to 10%:

Cardiovascular: Palpitations (2%)

Central nervous system: Nervousness (3%), dizziness (2%), fatigue, headache (6%), pain (4%)

Dermatologic: Rash (1%)

Gastrointestinal: Nausea, xerostomia, stomach upset, dry mucous membranes

Respiratory: Nasal congestion, dyspnea (10%), increased sputum (1%), bronchospasm (2%), pharyngitis (3%), rhinitis (2%), sinusitis (5%)
Miscellaneous: Influenza-like symptoms

Based on **albuterol** component:
>10%:
Cardiovascular: Tachycardia, palpitations, pounding heartbeat
Gastrointestinal: GI upset, nausea
1% to 10%:
Cardiovascular: Flushing of face, hypertension or hypotension
Central nervous system: Nervousness, CNS stimulation, hyperactivity, insomnia, dizziness, lightheadedness, drowsiness, headache
Gastrointestinal: Xerostomia, heartburn, vomiting, unusual taste
Genitourinary: Dysuria
Neuromuscular & skeletal: Muscle cramping, tremor, weakness
Respiratory: Coughing
Miscellaneous: Diaphoresis (increased)

Drug Interactions See Ipratropium *on page 651* and Albuterol *on page 45*
Drug Uptake See Ipratropium *on page 651* and Albuterol *on page 45*
Pregnancy Risk Factor C
Generic Available No

Irbesartan (ir be SAR tan)

U.S. Brand Names Avapro®
Canadian Brand Names Avapro™
Mexican Brand Names Aprovel; Avapro®
Pharmacologic Category Angiotensin II Receptor Blocker
Use Treatment of hypertension alone or in combination with other antihypertensives
Local Anesthetic/Vasoconstrictor Precautions No information available to require special precautions
Effects on Dental Treatment No effects or complications reported
Dosage Oral:
Children:
<6 years: Safety and efficacy have not been established.
≥6-12 years: Initial: 75 mg once daily; may be titrated to a maximum of 150 mg once daily
Children ≥13 years and Adults: 150 mg once daily; patients may be titrated to 300 mg once daily

Mechanism of Action Irbesartan is an angiotensin receptor antagonist. Angiotensin II acts as a vasoconstrictor. In addition to causing direct vasoconstriction, angiotensin II also stimulates the release of aldosterone. Once aldosterone is released, sodium as well as water are reabsorbed. The end result is an elevation in BP. Irbesartan binds to the AT1 angiotensin II receptor. This binding prevents angiotensin II from binding to the receptor thereby blocking the vasoconstriction and the aldosterone secreting effects of angiotensin II.

Other Adverse Effects
1% to 10%:
Central nervous system: Fatigue (4%)
Gastrointestinal: Diarrhea (3%), dyspepsia (2%)
Respiratory: Upper respiratory infection (9%), cough (2.8% versus 2.7% in placebo)
>1% but frequency ≤ placebo: Abdominal pain, anxiety, nervousness, chest pain, dizziness, edema, headache, influenza, musculoskeletal pain, pharyngitis, nausea, vomiting, rash, rhinitis, sinus abnormality, tachycardia, urinary tract infection, dizziness, syncope, vertigo

Drug Interactions CYP2C9 enzyme substrate
Increased Effect/Toxicity: Blood levels of irbesartan may be increased by inhibitors of cytochrome P450 isoenzyme 2C9 (eg, sulfaphenazole, tolbutamide, nifedipine). Potassium salts/supplements, co-trimoxazole (high dose), ACE inhibitors, and potassium-sparing diuretics (amiloride, spironolactone, triamterene) may increase the risk of hyperkalemia.

Drug Uptake
Onset of action: Peak effect: 1-2 hours
Duration: >24 hours
Half-life, elimination: Terminal: 11-15 hours
Time to peak: 1.5-2 hours

Pregnancy Risk Factor C/D (2nd and 3rd trimesters)
Generic Available No

Irbesartan and Hydrochlorothiazide
(ir be SAR tan & hye droe klor oh THYE a zide)

U.S. Brand Names Avalide®
Canadian Brand Names Avalide®
Pharmacologic Category Antihypertensive Agent Combination
Synonyms Avapro® HCT; Hydrochlorothiazide and Irbesartan
(Continued)

Irbesartan and Hydrochlorothiazide *(Continued)*

Use Combination therapy for the management of hypertension

Local Anesthetic/Vasoconstrictor Precautions No information available to require special precautions

Effects on Dental Treatment No effects or complications reported

Dosage Dose must be individualized. A patient who is not controlled with either agent alone may be switched to the combination product. Mean effect increases with the dose of each component. The lowest dosage available is irbesartan 150 mg/hydrochlorothiazide 12.5 mg. Dose increases should be made not more frequently than every 2-4 weeks.

Mechanism of Action Irbesartan is an angiotensin receptor antagonist. Angiotensin II acts as a vasoconstrictor. In addition to causing direct vasoconstriction, angiotensin II also stimulates the release of aldosterone. Once aldosterone is released, sodium as well as water are reabsorbed. The end result is an elevation in BP. Irbesartan binds to the AT1 angiotensin II receptor. This binding prevents angiotensin II from binding to the receptor thereby blocking the vasoconstriction and the aldosterone secreting effects of angiotensin II.

Hydrochlorothiazide inhibits sodium reabsorption in the distal tubules causing increased excretion of sodium and water as well as potassium and hydrogen ions

Other Adverse Effects

Based on **irbesartan** component:

- Central nervous system: Fatigue (4%)
- Gastrointestinal: Diarrhea (3%), dyspepsia (2%)
- Respiratory: Upper respiratory infection (9%), cough (2.8% versus 2.7% in placebo)
- >1% but frequency ≤ placebo: Abdominal pain, anxiety, nervousness, chest pain, dizziness, edema, headache, influenza, musculoskeletal pain, pharyngitis, nausea, vomiting, rash, rhinitis, sinus abnormality, tachycardia, urinary tract infection, dizziness, syncope, vertigo

Based on **hydrochlorothiazide** component:

1% to 10%:

- Cardiovascular: Orthostatic hypotension, hypotension
- Dermatologic: Photosensitivity
- Endocrine & metabolic: Hypokalemia
- Gastrointestinal: Anorexia, epigastric distress

Drug Interactions

Based on **irbesartan** component: CYP2C9 enzyme substrate

- Inhibitors of CYP2C9 may increase blood levels.
- Lithium: Risk of toxicity may be increased by irbesartan; monitor lithium levels.
- NSAIDs: May decrease angiotensin II antagonist efficacy; effect has been seen with losartan, but may occur with other medications in this class; monitor BP
- Potassium-sparing diuretics (amiloride, potassium, spironolactone, triamterene): Increased risk of hyperkalemia.
- Potassium supplements may increase the risk of hyperkalemia.
- Trimethoprim (high dose) may increase the risk of hyperkalemia.

Based on **hydrochlorothiazide** component:

- ACE inhibitors: Increased hypotension if aggressively diuresed with a thiazide diuretic.
- Beta-blockers increase hyperglycemic effects in type 2 diabetes mellitus (noninsulin dependent, NIDDM)
- Cyclosporine and thiazides can increase the risk of gout or renal toxicity; avoid concurrent use.
- Digoxin toxicity can be exacerbated if a thiazide induces hypokalemia or hypomagnesemia.
- Lithium toxicity can occur by reducing renal excretion of lithium; monitor lithium concentration and adjust as needed.
- Neuromuscular blocking agents can prolong blockade; monitor serum potassium and neuromuscular status.
- NSAIDs can decrease the efficacy of thiazides reducing the diuretic and antihypertensive effects.

Pregnancy Risk Factor C/D (2nd and 3rd trimesters)

Generic Available No

Ircon® [OTC] *see* Ferrous Fumarate *on page 497*

Irinotecan (eye rye no TEE kan)

U.S. Brand Names Camptosar®

Canadian Brand Names Camptosar®

Mexican Brand Names Camptosar®

Pharmacologic Category Antineoplastic Agent, Natural Source (Plant) Derivative

Synonyms Camptothecin-11; CPT-11

Use A component of first-line therapy in combination with 5-fluorouracil and leucovorin for the treatment of metastatic carcinoma of the colon or rectum; treatment of metastatic carcinoma of the colon or rectum which has recurred or progressed following fluorouracil-based therapy

Unlabeled/Investigational: Lung cancer (small cell and nonsmall cell), cervical cancer, gastric cancer, pancreatic cancer, leukemia, lymphoma, breast cancer

Local Anesthetic/Vasoconstrictor Precautions No information available to require special precautions

Effects on Dental Treatment No effects or complications reported

Mechanism of Action Irinotecan and its active metabolite (SN-38) bind reversibly to topoisomerase I and stabilize the cleavable complex so that religation of the cleaved DNA strand cannot occur. This results in the accumulation of cleavable complexes and single-strand DNA breaks. This interaction results in double-stranded DNA breaks and cell death consistent with S-phase cell cycle specificity.

Other Adverse Effects

>10%:

Cardiovascular: Vasodilation

Central nervous system: Insomnia, dizziness, fever (45.4%)

Dermatologic: Alopecia (60.5%), rash

Gastrointestinal: Irinotecan therapy may induce two different forms of diarrhea. Onset, symptoms, proposed mechanisms and treatment are different. Overall, 56.9% of patients treated experience abdominal pain and/or cramping during therapy. Anorexia, constipation, flatulence, stomatitis, and dyspepsia have also been reported.

Diarrhea: Dose-limiting toxicity with weekly dosing regimen

Early diarrhea (50.7% incidence, grade 3/4 8%) usually occurs during or within 24 hours of administration. May be accompanied by symptoms of cramping, vomiting, flushing, and diaphoresis. It is thought to be mediated by cholinergic effects which can be successfully managed with atropine (refer to Warnings/Precautions).

Late diarrhea (87.8% incidence) usually occurs >24 hours after treatment. National Cancer Institute (NCI) grade 3 or 4 diarrhea (31%) occurs in 30.6% of patients. Late diarrhea generally occurs with a median of 11 days after therapy and lasts ~ 3 days. Patients experiencing grade 3 or 4 diarrhea were noted to have symptoms a total of 7 days. Correlated with irinotecan or SN-38 levels in plasma and bile. Due to the duration, dehydration and electrolyte imbalances are significant clinical concerns. Loperamide therapy is recommended. The incidence of grade 3 or 4 late diarrhea is significantly higher in patients ≥65 years of age; close monitoring and prompt initiation of high-dose loperamide therapy is prudent (refer to Warnings/Precautions).

Emetic potential: Moderately high (86.2% incidence, however, only 12.5% grade 3 or 4 vomiting)

Hematologic: Myelosuppressive: Dose-limiting toxicity with 3 week dosing regimen

Grade 1-4 neutropenia occurred in 53.9% of patients. Patients who had previously received pelvic or abdominal radiation therapy were noted to have a significantly increased incidence of grade 3 or 4 neutropenia. White blood cell count nadir is 15 days after administration and is more frequent than thrombocytopenia. Recovery is usually within 24-28 days and cumulative toxicity has not been observed.

WBC: Mild to severe

Platelets: Mild

Onset: 10 days

Nadir: 14-16 days

Recovery: 21-28 days

Neuromuscular & skeletal: Weakness (75.7%)

Respiratory: Dyspnea (22%), coughing, rhinitis, decreased DLCO (in a few patients)

Miscellaneous: Diaphoresis

1% to 10%: **Irritant chemotherapy**; thrombophlebitis has been reported

Drug Interactions Increased Effect/Toxicity: Hold diuretics during dosing due to potential risk of dehydration secondary to vomiting and/or diarrhea induced by irinotecan. Prophylactic dexamethasone as an antiemetic may enhance lymphocytopenia. Prochlorperazine may increase incidence of akathisia. Adverse reactions such as myelosuppression and diarrhea would be expected to be exacerbated by other antineoplastic agents.

Drug Uptake

Half-life, elimination: Parent drug: Alpha: 0.2 hours, beta: 2.5 hours, gamma: 14.2 hours; SN-38: 3-23.9 hours

Time to peak: SN-38: 30-minute infusion: ~1 hour

Pregnancy Risk Factor D

Generic Available No

Iron Dextran Complex (EYE ern DEKS tran KOM pleks)

U.S. Brand Names Dexferrum®; INFeD®

Canadian Brand Names Dexiron™; Infufer®

(Continued)

Iron Dextran Complex *(Continued)*

Mexican Brand Names Driken

Pharmacologic Category Iron Salt

Use Treatment of microcytic, hypochromic anemia resulting from iron deficiency when oral iron administration is infeasible or ineffective

Local Anesthetic/Vasoconstrictor Precautions No information available to require special precautions

Effects on Dental Treatment No effects or complications reported

Dosage I.M. (Z-track method should be used for I.M. injection); I.V.:

A 0.5 mL test dose (0.25 mL in infants) should be given prior to starting iron dextran therapy; total dose should be divided into a daily schedule for I.M., total dose may be given as a single continuous infusion

Iron deficiency anemia: Dose (mL) = 0.0476 x LBW (kg) x (normal hemoglobin - observed hemoglobin) + (1 mL/5 kg of LBW to maximum of 14 mL for iron stores)
LBW = Lean Body Weight

Iron replacement therapy for blood loss: Replacement iron (mg) = blood loss (mL) x hematocrit

Maximum daily dose (can administer total dose at one time I.V.):
- Infants <5 kg: 25 mg iron (0.5 mL)
- Children:
  - 5-10 kg: 50 mg iron (1 mL)
  - 10-50 kg: 100 mg iron (2 mL)
- Adults >50 kg: 100 mg iron (2 mL)

Mechanism of Action The released iron, from the plasma, eventually replenishes the depleted iron stores in the bone marrow where it is incorporated into hemoglobin

Other Adverse Effects

>10%:
- Cardiovascular: Flushing
- Central nervous system: Dizziness, fever, headache, pain
- Gastrointestinal: Nausea, vomiting, metallic taste
- Local: Staining of skin at the site of I.M. injection
- Miscellaneous: Diaphoresis

1% to 10%:
- Cardiovascular: Hypotension (1% to 2%)
- Dermatologic: Urticaria (1% to 2%), phlebitis (1% to 2%)
- Gastrointestinal: Diarrhea
- Genitourinary: Discoloration of urine

Note: Diaphoresis, urticaria, arthralgia, fever, chills, dizziness, headache, and nausea may be delayed 24-48 hours after I.V. administration or 3-4 days after I.M. administration.

Anaphylactoid reactions: Respiratory difficulties and cardiovascular collapse have been reported and occur most frequently within the first several minutes of administration.

Drug Interactions Decreased effect with chloramphenicol

Drug Uptake Absorption:

I.M.: 50% to 90% is promptly absorbed, the balance is slowly absorbed over month

I.V.: Uptake of iron by the reticuloendothelial system appears to be constant at about 10-20 mg/hour

Pregnancy Risk Factor C

Generic Available Yes

Comments 2 mL of undiluted iron dextran is the maximum recommended daily dose; epinephrine should be immediately available in the event of acute hypersensitivity reaction

Iron Sucrose (EYE ern SOO krose)

U.S. Brand Names Venofer®

Pharmacologic Category Iron Salt

Use Treatment of iron-deficiency anemia in patients undergoing chronic hemodialysis who are receiving supplemental erythropoietin therapy

Local Anesthetic/Vasoconstrictor Precautions No information available to require special precautions

Effects on Dental Treatment No effects or complications reported

Dosage Doses expressed in mg of **elemental** iron: Iron-deficiency anemia: I.V.: 100 mg (5 mL of iron sucrose injection) administered 1-3 times/week during dialysis, to a total dose of 1000 mg (10 doses); administer ≤3 times/week; may continue to administer at lowest dose necessary to maintain target hemoglobin, hematocrit, and iron storage parameters

Test dose: Product labeling does not indicate need for a test dose in product-naive patients; test doses were administered in some clinical trials as 50 mg (2.5 mL) in 50 mL 0.9% NaCl administered over 3-10 minutes

Mechanism of Action Iron sucrose is dissociated by the reticuloendothelial system into iron and sucrose. The released iron increases serum iron concentrations and is incorporated into hemoglobin.

Other Adverse Effects Fatal and life-threatening anaphylactoid reactions (characterized by anaphylactic shock, loss of consciousness, collapse, hypotension, dyspnea, or convulsion) have been reported; hypotension may be related to total dose or rate of administration.

>5%:

Cardiovascular: Hypotension (36%)
Central nervous system: Headache
Gastrointestinal: Nausea, vomiting, diarrhea
Neuromuscular & skeletal: Leg cramps (23%)

1% to 5%:

Cardiovascular: Chest pain, hypertension, hypervolemia
Central nervous system: Fever, malaise, dizziness
Dermatologic: Pruritus
Gastrointestinal: Abdominal pain
Hepatic: Elevated enzymes
Local: Application site reaction
Neuromuscular & skeletal: Musculoskeletal pain, weakness
Respiratory: Dyspnea, pneumonia, cough

Warnings/Precautions

Fatal and potentially fatal hypersensitivity reactions (characterized by anaphylactic shock, loss of consciousness, collapse, hypotension, dyspnea, and convulsion) have been reported. Facilities for cardiopulmonary resuscitation must be available during administration. Hypotension has been reported frequently in patients receiving I.V. iron, may be related to total dose or rate of administration (avoid rapid I.V. injection), follow recommended guidelines. Withhold iron in the presence of tissue iron overload, periodic monitoring of hemoglobin, hematocrit, serum ferritin, and transferrin saturation is recommended. Safety and efficacy in children have not been established.

Drug Interactions Decreased Effect: Chloramphenicol may diminish the therapeutic effects of iron sucrose injection. Iron sucrose injection may reduce the absorption of oral iron preparations.

Drug Uptake Half-life, elimination: Adults: 6 hours

Pregnancy Risk Factor B

Ismelin® *see* Guanethidine *on page 573*
Ismo® *see* Isosorbide Mononitrate *on page 662*
Ismotic® *see* Isosorbide *on page 661*
Isocaine® HCl *see* Mepivacaine *on page 764*

Isocarboxazid (eye soe kar BOKS a zid)

U.S. Brand Names Marplan®

Pharmacologic Category Antidepressant, Monoamine Oxidase Inhibitor

Use Symptomatic treatment of atypical, nonendogenous or neurotic depression

Local Anesthetic/Vasoconstrictor Precautions Attempts should be made to avoid use of vasoconstrictor due to possibility of hypertensive episodes with monoamine oxidase inhibitors

Effects on Dental Treatment

>10%: Orthostatic hypotension

Avoid use as an analgesic due to toxic reactions with MAO inhibitors.

Dosage Adults: Oral: 10 mg 3 times/day; reduce to 10-20 mg/day in divided doses when condition improves

Mechanism of Action Thought to act by increasing endogenous concentrations of epinephrine, norepinephrine, dopamine, and serotonin through inhibition of the enzyme (monoamine oxidase) responsible for the breakdown of these neurotransmitters

Other Adverse Effects

>10%:

Cardiovascular: Orthostatic hypotension
Central nervous system: Drowsiness
Endocrine & metabolic: Decreased sexual ability
Neuromuscular & skeletal: Weakness, trembling
Ocular: Blurred vision

1% to 10%:

Cardiovascular: Tachycardia, peripheral edema
Central nervous system: Nervousness, chills
Dermatologic: Xerostomia
Gastrointestinal: Diarrhea, anorexia, constipation

Drug Interactions

Increased Effect/Toxicity: In general, the combined use with TCAs, venlafaxine, trazodone, dexfenfluramine, sibutramine, lithium, meperidine, fenfluramine, dextromethorphan, and SSRIs should be avoided due to the potential for severe adverse reactions (serotonin syndrome, death). MAO inhibitors (including isocarboxazid) may inhibit the metabolism of barbiturates and prolong their effect. Isocarboxazid in combination with amphetamines, other stimulants (methylphenidate), levodopa, metaraminol, reserpine, and decongestants (pseudoephedrine)

(Continued)

Isocarboxazid *(Continued)*

may result in severe hypertensive reactions. Isocarboxazid may increase the pressor response of norepinephrine and may prolong neuromuscular blockade produced by succinylcholine. Tramadol may increase the risk of seizures and serotonin syndrome in patients receiving an MAO inhibitor. Isocarboxazid may produce additive hypoglycemic effect in patients receiving hypoglycemic agents and may produce delirium in patients receiving disulfiram.

Decreased Effect: MAO inhibitors may inhibit the antihypertensive response to guanadrel or guanethidine.

Pregnancy Risk Factor C

Generic Available No

Isoclor® Expectorant *see* Guaifenesin, Pseudoephedrine, and Codeine *on page 570*

Isoetharine (eye soe ETH a reen)

Related Information

Respiratory Diseases *on page 1328*

U.S. Brand Names Arm-a-Med® Isoetharine; Beta-2®; Bronkometer®; Bronkosol®; Dey-Lute® Isoetharine

Canadian Brand Names Beta-2®; Bronkometer®; Bronkosol®

Pharmacologic Category Adrenergic Agonist Agent; Sympathomimetic

Synonyms Isoetharine Hydrochloride; Isoetharine Mesylate

Use Bronchodilator in bronchial asthma and for reversible bronchospasm occurring with bronchitis and emphysema

Local Anesthetic/Vasoconstrictor Precautions Isoetharine is selective for beta-adrenergic receptors and not alpha receptors; therefore, there is no precaution in the use of vasoconstrictor

Effects on Dental Treatment 1% to 10%: Xerostomia

Dosage Treatments are usually not repeated more often than every 4 hours, except in severe cases

Nebulizer: Children: 0.01 mL/kg; minimum dose 0.1 mL; maximum dose: 0.5 mL diluted in 2-3 mL normal saline

Inhalation: Oral: Adults: 1-2 inhalations every 4 hours as needed

Mechanism of Action Relaxes bronchial smooth muscle by action on beta$_2$-receptors with very little effect on heart rate

Other Adverse Effects Frequency not defined:

Cardiovascular: Tachycardia, hypertension, pounding heartbeat

Central nervous system: Dizziness, lightheadedness, headache, nervousness, insomnia

Gastrointestinal: Xerostomia, nausea, vomiting

Neuromuscular & skeletal: Trembling, weakness

Respiratory: Paradoxical bronchospasm

Drug Interactions

Increased Effect/Toxicity: Increased toxicity with other sympathomimetics (eg, epinephrine).

Decreased effect with beta-blockers.

Drug Uptake

Onset of action: Peak effect: Inhalation: 5-15 minutes

Duration: 1-4 hours

Pregnancy Risk Factor C

Generic Available Yes

Isoflurophate (eye soe FLURE oh fate)

U.S. Brand Names Floropryl®

Pharmacologic Category Acetylcholinesterase Inhibitor; Ophthalmic Agent, Antiglaucoma; Ophthalmic Agent, Miotic

Synonyms DFP; Diisopropyl Fluorophosphate; Dyflos; Fluostigmin

Use Treatment of primary open-angle glaucoma and conditions that obstruct aqueous outflow; treatment of accommodative convergent strabismus

Local Anesthetic/Vasoconstrictor Precautions No information available to require special precautions

Effects on Dental Treatment No effects or complications reported

Dosage Adults: Ophthalmic:

Glaucoma: Instill 0.25" strip in eye every 8-72 hours

Strabismus: Instill 0.25" strip to each eye every night for 2 weeks then reduce to 0.25" every other night to once weekly for 2 months

Mechanism of Action Cholinesterase inhibitor that causes contraction of the iris and ciliary muscles producing miosis, reduced intraocular pressure, and increased aqueous humor outflow

Other Adverse Effects 1% to 10%: Ocular: Stinging, burning eyes, myopia, visual blurring

Drug Interactions Succinylcholine, systemic anticholinesterases, carbamate or organic phosphate insecticides, may decrease cholinesterase levels.

Drug Uptake
Onset of action: Miosis: 5-10 minutes
Peak effect: IOP reduction: 24 hours
Duration: Miosis: ≤4 weeks; IOP reduction: 1 week
Pregnancy Risk Factor X
Generic Available No

Isoniazid (eye soe NYE a zid)

Related Information
Nonviral Infectious Diseases *on page 1342*
U.S. Brand Names Nydrazid®
Canadian Brand Names Isotamine®; PMS-Isoniazid
Pharmacologic Category Antitubercular Agent
Synonyms INH; Isonicotinic Acid Hydrazide
Use Treatment of susceptible tuberculosis infections and prophylactically to those individuals exposed to tuberculosis
Local Anesthetic/Vasoconstrictor Precautions No information available to require special precautions
Effects on Dental Treatment No effects or complications reported
Dosage Recommendations often change due to resistant strains and newly developed information; consult *MMWR* for current CDC recommendations: **Oral** (injectable is available for patients who are unable to either take or absorb oral therapy):
A four-drug regimen (isoniazid, rifampin, pyrazinamide, and either streptomycin or ethambutol) is preferred for the initial, empiric treatment of TB. When the drug susceptibility results are available, the regimen should be altered as appropriate.
Infants and Children:
Prophylaxis: 10 mg/kg/day in 1-2 divided doses (maximum: 300 mg/day) 6 months in patients who do not have HIV infection and 12 months in patients who have HIV infection
Treatment:
Daily therapy: 10-20 mg/kg/day in 1-2 divided doses (maximum: 300 mg/day)
Directly observed therapy (DOT): Twice weekly therapy: 20-40 mg/kg (maximum: 900 mg/day); 3 times/week therapy: 20-40 mg/kg (maximum: 900 mg)
Adults:
Prophylaxis: 300 mg/day for 6 months in patients who do not have HIV infection and 12 months in patients who have HIV infection
Treatment:
Daily therapy: 5 mg/kg/day given daily (usual dose: 300 mg/day); 10 mg/kg/day in 1-2 divided doses in patients with disseminated disease
Directly observed therapy (DOT): Twice weekly therapy: 15 mg/kg (maximum: 900 mg); 3 times/week therapy: 15 mg/kg (maximum: 900 mg)
Note: Concomitant administration of 6-50 mg/day pyridoxine is recommended in malnourished patients or those prone to neuropathy (eg, alcoholics, diabetics)
Hemodialysis: Dialyzable (50% to 100%)
Administer dose postdialysis
Peritoneal dialysis effects: Dose for Cl_{cr} <10 mL/minute
Continuous arteriovenous or venovenous hemofiltration: Dose for Cl_{cr} <10 mL/minute
Dosing adjustment in hepatic impairment: Dose should be reduced in severe hepatic disease
Mechanism of Action Unknown, but may include the inhibition of myocolic acid synthesis resulting in disruption of the bacterial cell wall
Other Adverse Effects
>10%:
Gastrointestinal: Loss of appetite, nausea, vomiting, stomach pain
Hepatic: Mild increased LFTs (10% to 20%)
Neuromuscular & skeletal: Weakness, peripheral neuropathy (dose-related incidence, 10% to 20% incidence with 10 mg/kg/day)
1% to 10%:
Central nervous system: Dizziness, slurred speech, lethargy
Hepatic: Progressive liver damage (increases with age; 2.3% in patients >50 years)
Neuromuscular & skeletal: Hyper-reflexia
Drug Interactions CYP2E1 enzyme substrate; CYP2E1 enzyme inducer; and CYP1A2, 2C, 2C9, 2C18, 2C19, and 3A3/4 enzyme inhibitor
Increased Effect/Toxicity: Increased toxicity/levels of oral anticoagulants, carbamazepines, cycloserine, hydantoins, and hepatically metabolized benzodiazepines; reaction with disulfiram; enflurane with isoniazid may result in renal failure especially in rapid acetylators
Increased hepatic toxicity with ethanol or with rifampin and isoniazid
Decreased effect/levels of isoniazid with aluminum salts.
Drug Uptake
Absorption: Rapid and complete; rate can be slowed with food
(Continued)

Isoniazid *(Continued)*

Half-life, elimination: Fast acetylators: 30-100 minutes; Slow acetylators: 2-5 hours; may be prolonged with impaired hepatic function or severe renal impairment

Time to peak: 1-2 hours

Pregnancy Risk Factor C

Generic Available Yes

Isoproterenol (eye soe proe TER e nole)

Related Information

Cardiovascular Diseases *on page 1308*

U.S. Brand Names Isuprel®

Canadian Brand Names Isuprel®

Pharmacologic Category $Beta_1/Beta_2$ Agonist

Synonyms Isoprenaline Hydrochloride; Isoproterenol Hydrochloride; Isoproterenol Sulfate

Use Treatment of reversible airway obstruction as in asthma or COPD; used parenterally in ventricular arrhythmias due to A-V nodal block; hemodynamically compromised bradyarrhythmias or atropine-resistant bradyarrhythmias; temporary use in third degree A-V block until pacemaker insertion; low cardiac output; vasoconstrictive shock states

Unlabeled/Investigational: Temporizing measure before transvenous pacing for torsade de pointes; diagnostic aid (vasovagal syncope)

Local Anesthetic/Vasoconstrictor Precautions Isoproterenol is selective for beta-adrenergic receptors and not alpha receptors; therefore, there is no precaution in the use of vasoconstrictor such as epinephrine

Effects on Dental Treatment >10%: Xerostomia

Dosage

Children:

Bronchodilation: Inhalation: Metered dose inhaler: 1-2 metered doses up to 5 times/day

Bronchodilation (using 1:200 inhalation solution) 0.01 mL/kg/dose every 4 hours as needed (maximum: 0.05 mL/dose) diluted with NS to 2 mL

Sublingual: 5-10 mg every 3-4 hours, not to exceed 30 mg/day

Cardiac arrhythmias: I.V.: Start 0.1 mcg/kg/minute (usual effective dose 0.2-2 mcg/kg/minute)

Adults:

Bronchodilation: Inhalation: Metered dose inhaler: 1-2 metered doses 4-6 times/day

Bronchodilation: 1-2 inhalations of a 0.25% solution, ≤2 inhalations at any one time (1-5 minutes between inhalations); no more than 6 inhalations in any hour during a 24-hour period; maintenance therapy: 1-2 inhalations 4-6 times/day. Alternatively: 0.5% solution via hand bulb nebulizer is 5-15 deep inhalations repeated once in 5-10 minutes if necessary; treatments may be repeated up to 5 times/day.

Sublingual: 10-20 mg every 3-4 hours; not to exceed 60 mg/day

Cardiac arrhythmias: I.V.: 5 mcg/minute initially, titrate to patient response (2-20 mcg/minute)

Shock: I.V.: 0.5-5 mcg/minute; adjust according to response

Mechanism of Action Stimulates $beta_1$- and $beta_2$-receptors resulting in relaxation of bronchial, GI, and uterine smooth muscle, increased heart rate and contractility, vasodilation of peripheral vasculature

Other Adverse Effects

>10%:

Central nervous system: Insomnia, restlessness

Gastrointestinal: Dry throat, xerostomia, discoloration of saliva (pinkish-red) [inhalation and sublingual dosage forms]

1% to 10%:

Cardiovascular: Flushing of the face or skin, ventricular arrhythmias, tachycardia, profound hypotension, hypertension, pounding heartbeat

Central nervous system: Nervousness, anxiety, dizziness, headache, lightheadedness

Gastrointestinal: Vomiting, nausea

Neuromuscular & skeletal: Trembling, tremor, weakness

Respiratory: Coughing

Miscellaneous: Sweating

Parenteral (cardiovascular use):

>10%:

Central nervous system: Headache

Gastrointestinal: Nausea, vomiting

1% to 10%:

Cardiovascular: Premature ventricular beats, bradycardia, hypertension, hypotension, chest pain, palpitations, tachycardia, ventricular arrhythmias, myocardial infarction size increased

Central nervous system: Headache, nervousness or restlessness

Respiratory: Dyspnea

Drug Interactions Increased Effect/Toxicity: Sympathomimetic agents may cause headaches and elevate BP. General anesthetics may cause arrhythmias.

Drug Uptake

Onset of action: Bronchodilation: Oral, I.V.: Immediate

Duration: Oral inhalation: 1 hour; S.C.: ≤2 hours; I.V.: 10-15 minutes

Half-life, elimination: 2.5-5 minutes

Time to peak: Oral: 1-2 hours

Pregnancy Risk Factor C

Generic Available Yes

Isoptin® *see* Verapamil *on page 1236*

Isoptin® SR *see* Verapamil *on page 1236*

Isopto® Atropine *see* Atropine *on page 130*

Isopto® Carbachol *see* Carbachol *on page 215*

Isopto® Carpine *see* Pilocarpine *on page 955*

Isopto® Carpine *see* Pilocarpine (Dental) *on page 956*

Isopto® Cetapred® *see* Sulfacetamide Sodium and Prednisolone *on page 1116*

Isopto® Homatropine *see* Homatropine *on page 589*

Isopto® Hyoscine *see* Scopolamine *on page 1077*

Isopto® Tears [OTC] *see* Artificial Tears *on page 117*

Isordil® *see* Isosorbide Dinitrate *on page 661*

Isosorbide (eye soe SOR bide)

U.S. Brand Names Ismotic®

Pharmacologic Category Diuretic, Osmotic; Ophthalmic Agent, Antiglaucoma; Ophthalmic Agent, Osmotic

Synonyms OZIZ

Use Short-term emergency treatment of acute angle-closure glaucoma and short-term reduction of intraocular pressure prior to and following intraocular surgery; may be used to interrupt an acute glaucoma attack; preferred agent when need to avoid nausea and vomiting

Local Anesthetic/Vasoconstrictor Precautions No information available to require special precautions

Effects on Dental Treatment No effects or complications reported

Dosage Adults: Oral: Initial: 1.5 g/kg with a usual range of 1-3 g/kg 2-4 times/day as needed

Mechanism of Action Elevates osmolarity of glomerular filtrate to hinder the tubular resorption of water and increase excretion of sodium and chloride to result in diuresis; creates an osmotic gradient between plasma and ocular fluids

Other Adverse Effects Frequency not defined:

Central nervous system: Headache, confusion, disorientation, syncope, lethargy, vertigo, dizziness, lightheadedness, irritability

Dermatologic: Rash

Endocrine & metabolic: Hypernatremia, hyperosmolarity

Gastrointestinal: Vomiting, nausea, abdominal/gastric discomfort (infrequently), anorexia,

Miscellaneous: Hiccups, thirst

Drug Uptake

Onset of action: 10-30 minutes

Duration: 5-6 hours

Half-life, elimination: 5-9.5 hours

Time to peak: 1-1.5 hours

Pregnancy Risk Factor B

Generic Available No

Isosorbide Dinitrate (eye soe SOR bide dye NYE trate)

Related Information

Cardiovascular Diseases *on page 1308*

U.S. Brand Names Dilatrate®-SR; Isordil®; Sorbitrate®

Canadian Brand Names Apo®-ISDN; Cedocard®-SR; Isordil®

Mexican Brand Names Isoket; Isorbid

Pharmacologic Category Vasodilator

Synonyms ISD; ISDN

Use Prevention and treatment of angina pectoris; for CHF; to relieve pain, dysphagia, and spasm in esophageal spasm with GE reflux

Local Anesthetic/Vasoconstrictor Precautions No information available to require special precautions

Effects on Dental Treatment No effects or complications reported

Dosage Adults (elderly should be given lowest recommended daily doses initially and titrate upward):

Oral: Angina: 5-40 mg 4 times/day or 40 mg every 8-12 hours in sustained released dosage form

(Continued)

Isosorbide Dinitrate *(Continued)*

Oral: Congestive heart failure:
Initial dose: 10 mg 3 times/day
Target dose: 40 mg 3 times/day
Maximum dose: 80 mg 3 times/day
Sublingual: 2.5-10 mg every 4-6 hours
Chew: 5-10 mg every 2-3 hours
Tolerance to nitrate effects develops with chronic exposure
Dose escalation does not overcome this effect. Tolerance can only be overcome by short periods of nitrate absence from the body. Short periods (10-12 hours) or nitrate withdrawal help minimize tolerance.

Mechanism of Action Stimulation of intracellular cyclic-GMP results in vascular smooth muscle relaxation of both arterial and venous vasculature. Increased venous pooling decreases left ventricular pressure (preload) and arterial dilatation decreases arterial resistance (afterload). Therefore, this reduces cardiac oxygen demand by decreasing left ventricular pressure and systemic vascular resistance by dilating arteries. Additionally, coronary artery dilation improves collateral flow to ischemic regions; esophageal smooth muscle is relaxed via the same mechanism.

Other Adverse Effects Frequency not defined:
Cardiovascular: Hypotension (infrequent), postural hypotension, crescendo angina (uncommon), rebound hypertension (uncommon), pallor, cardiovascular collapse, tachycardia, shock, flushing, peripheral edema
Central nervous system: Headache (most common), lightheadedness (related to BP changes), syncope (uncommon), dizziness, restlessness
Gastrointestinal: Nausea, vomiting, bowel incontinence, xerostomia
Genitourinary: Urinary incontinence
Hematologic: Methemoglobinemia (rare, overdose)
Neuromuscular & skeletal: Weakness
Ocular: Blurred vision
Miscellaneous: Cold sweat
The incidence of hypotension and adverse cardiovascular events may be increased when used in combination with sildenafil (Viagra®).

Drug Interactions
Increased Effect/Toxicity: Combinations of sildenafil and nitrates has been associated with severe hypotensive reactions and death. Nitrate-induced hypotension may be exacerbated by calcium channel blockers. Nitrates and aspirin may increase serum nitrate concentrations and therapeutic effect. Nitrates and dihydroergotamine may lead to elevated BP or decrease antianginal effects.
Decreased Effect: Nitrates may decrease the effect of heparin.

Drug Uptake
Onset of action: Sublingual tablet: 2-10 minutes; Chewable tablet: 3 minutes; Oral tablet: 45-60 minutes; Sustained release tablet: 30 minutes
Duration: Sublingual tablet: 1-2 hours; Chewable tablet: 0.5-2 hours; Oral tablet: 4-6 hours; Sustained release tablet: 6-12 hours;
Half-life, elimination: Parent drug: 1-4 hours; Metabolite (5-mononitrate): 4 hours

Pregnancy Risk Factor C
Generic Available Yes

Isosorbide Mononitrate (eye soe SOR bide mon oh NYE trate)

Related Information
Cardiovascular Diseases *on page 1308*

U.S. Brand Names Imdur®; Ismo®; Monoket®
Canadian Brand Names Imdur®; ISMO®
Mexican Brand Names Elantan; Imdur®; Mono Mack
Pharmacologic Category Vasodilator
Synonyms ISMN
Use Long-acting metabolite of the vasodilator isosorbide dinitrate used for the prophylactic treatment of angina pectoris
Local Anesthetic/Vasoconstrictor Precautions No information available to require special precautions
Effects on Dental Treatment No effects or complications reported
Dosage Adults and Geriatrics (start with lowest recommended dose): Oral:
Regular tablet: 5-10 mg twice daily with the two doses given 7 hours apart (eg, 8 AM and 3 PM) to decrease tolerance development; then titrate to 10 mg twice daily in first 2-3 days.
Extended release tablet: Initial: 30-60 mg given in morning as a single dose; titrate upward as needed, giving at least 3 days between increases; maximum daily single dose: 240 mg
Tolerance to nitrate effects develops with chronic exposure. Dose escalation does not overcome this effect. Tolerance can only be overcome by short periods of nitrate absence from the body. Short periods (10-12 hours) of nitrate withdrawal help minimize tolerance. Recommended dosage regimens incorporate this interval. General recommendations are to take the last dose of short-acting

agents no later than 7 PM; administer 2 times/day rather than 4 times/day. Administer sustained release tablet once daily in the morning.

Mechanism of Action Prevailing mechanism of action for nitroglycerin (and other nitrates) is systemic venodilation, decreasing preload as measured by pulmonary capillary wedge pressure and left ventricular end diastolic volume and pressure; the average reduction in LVEDV is 25% at rest, with a corresponding increase in ejection fractions of 50% to 60%. This effect improves congestive symptoms in heart failure and improves the myocardial perfusion gradient in patients with coronary artery disease.

Other Adverse Effects

>10%: Central nervous system: Headache (19% to 38%)

1% to 10%:

Central nervous system: Dizziness (3% to 5%)

Gastrointestinal: Nausea/vomiting (2% to 4%)

The incidence of hypotension and adverse cardiovascular events may be increased when used in combination with sildenafil (Viagra®).

Drug Interactions

Increased Effect/Toxicity: Combinations of sildenafil and nitrates has been associated with severe hypotensive reactions and death. Nitrate-induced hypotension may be exacerbated by calcium channel blockers. Nitrates and aspirin may increase serum nitrate concentrations and therapeutic effect. Nitrates and dihydroergotamine may lead to elevated BP or decrease antianginal effects. Do not administer sildenafil within 24 hours of a nitrate preparation.

Decreased Effect: Nitrates may decrease the effect of heparin.

Drug Uptake

Onset of action: 30-60 minutes

Absorption: Nearly complete and low intersubject variability in its pharmacokinetic parameters and plasma concentrations

Half-life, elimination: Mononitrate: ~4 hours

Pregnancy Risk Factor C

Generic Available Yes

Isotretinoin (eye soe TRET i noyn)

U.S. Brand Names Accutane®

Canadian Brand Names Accutane®; Isotrex®

Mexican Brand Names Isotrex®; Roaccutan®

Pharmacologic Category Retinoic Acid Derivative

Synonyms 13-*cis*-Retinoic Acid

Use Treatment of severe recalcitrant nodular acne unresponsive to conventional therapy

Unlabeled/Investigational: Treatment of children with metastatic neuroblastoma or leukemia that does not respond to conventional therapy

Local Anesthetic/Vasoconstrictor Precautions No information available to require special precautions

Effects on Dental Treatment >10%: Xerostomia

Restrictions Prescriptions for Accutane® may not be dispensed unless they are affixed with a yellow self-adhesive Accutane® qualification sticker filled out by the prescriber. Telephone, fax, or computer-generated prescriptions are no longer valid. Prescriptions may not be written for more than a 1-month supply and must be dispensed with a patient education guide every month. In addition, prescriptions for females must be filled within 7 days of the date noted on the yellow sticker; prescriptions filled after 7 days of the noted date are considered to be expired and cannot be honored. Pharmacists may call the manufacturer to confirm the prescriber's authority to write for this medication, however, this is not mandatory.

Prescribers will be provided with Accutane® qualification stickers after they have read the details of the S.M.A.R.T. program and have signed and mailed to the manufacturer their agreement to participate. A half-day continuing education program is also available. Audits of pharmacies will be conducted to monitor program compliance.

Dosage Oral:

Children: Maintenance therapy for neuroblastoma (investigational): 100-250 mg/m²/day in 2 divided doses

Children and Adults: Severe recalcitrant nodular acne: 0.5-2 mg/kg/day in 2 divided doses (dosages as low as 0.05 mg/kg/day have been reported to be beneficial) for 15-20 weeks or until the total cyst count decreases by 70%, whichever is sooner. A second course of therapy may be initiated after a period of ≥2 months off therapy.

Dosing adjustment in hepatic impairment: Dose reductions empirically are recommended in hepatitis disease

Mechanism of Action Reduces sebaceous gland size and reduces sebum production; regulates cell proliferation and differentiation

Other Adverse Effects Frequency not defined:

Cardiovascular: Palpitation, tachycardia, vascular thrombotic disease, stroke, chest pain, syncope, flushing

(Continued)

Isotretinoin *(Continued)*

Central nervous system: Edema, fatigue, pseudotumor cerebri, dizziness, drowsiness, headache, insomnia, lethargy, malaise, nervousness, paresthesias, seizures, stroke, suicidal ideation, suicide attempts, suicide, depression, psychosis, emotional instability

Dermatologic: Cutaneous allergic reactions, purpura, acne fulminans, alopecia, bruising, cheilitis, xerostomia, dry nose, dry skin, epistaxis, eruptive xanthomas, fragility of skin, hair abnormalities, hirsutism, hyperpigmentation, hypopigmentation, peeling of palms, peeling of soles, photoallergic reactions, photosensitizing reactions, pruritus, rash, dystrophy, paronychia, facial erythema, seborrhea, eczema, increased sunburn susceptibility, diaphoresis, urticaria, abnormal wound healing

Endocrine & metabolic: Increased triglycerides (25%), elevated blood glucose, increased HDL, increased cholesterol, abnormal menses

Gastrointestinal: Weight loss, inflammatory bowel disease, regional ileitis, pancreatitis, bleeding and inflammation of the gums, colitis, nausea, nonspecific gastrointestinal symptoms

Genitourinary: Nonspecific urogenital findings

Hematologic: Anemia, thrombocytopenia, neutropenia, agranulocytosis, pyogenic granuloma

Hepatic: Hepatitis

Neuromuscular & skeletal: Skeletal hyperostosis, calcification of tendons and ligaments, premature epiphyseal closure, arthralgia, CPK elevations, arthritis, tendonitis, bone abnormalities, weakness

Ocular: Corneal opacities, decreased night vision, cataracts, color vision disorder, conjunctivitis, dry eyes, eyelid inflammation, keratitis, optic neuritis, photophobia, visual disturbances

Otic: Hearing impairment, tinnitus

Renal: Vasculitis, glomerulonephritis,

Respiratory: Bronchospasms, respiratory infection, voice alteration, Wegener's granulomatosis

Miscellaneous: Allergic reactions, anaphylactic reactions, lymphadenopathy, infection, disseminated herpes simplex

Drug Interactions

Increased Effect/Toxicity: Cases of pseudotumor cerebri have been reported with concurrent use of tetracycline; avoid combination.

Decreased Effect: Isotretinoin may increase clearance of carbamazepine resulting in reduced carbamazepine levels. Microdosed progesterone preparations ("minipills") may not be an adequate form of contraception.

Drug Uptake

Absorption: Biphasic

Half-life, elimination: Terminal: Parent drug: 21 hours; Metabolite: 21-24 hours

Time to peak: 3-5 hours

Pregnancy Risk Factor X

Generic Available No

Comments On October 31, 2001, the FDA and Roche Laboratories announced an addition to the existing Pregnancy Prevention Program (PPP) currently in place to prevent pregnancy during Accutane® use. The new program, S.M.A.R.T. (System to Manage Accutane® Related Teratogenicity), was developed due to increased use of Accutane® in women. Reports have indicated that although many warnings and guidelines to prevent pregnancy are currently in place, pregnancies are still reported with Accutane® use. The S.M.A.R.T. program requires enrollment by the prescribing physician, two negative pregnancy tests and signed consent by female patients, and additional restrictions for pharmacy dispensing. Details and notice of the program were distributed to physicians, pharmacists, and all State Boards of Pharmacy. In addition, a half-day continuing education program for physicians is available. Audits of pharmacies are planned to monitor program compliance (see Restrictions). The FDA notice is viewable at http://www.fda.gov/bbs/topics/ANSWERS/2001/ANSO1113.html (last accessed November 15, 2001).

Isovue® *see* Radiological/Contrast Media (Nonionic) *on page 1039*

Isoxsuprine (eye SOKS syoo preen)

U.S. Brand Names Vasodilan®

Pharmacologic Category Vasodilator

Synonyms Isoxsuprine Hydrochloride

Use Treatment of peripheral vascular diseases, such as arteriosclerosis obliterans and Raynaud's disease

Local Anesthetic/Vasoconstrictor Precautions No information available to require special precautions

Effects on Dental Treatment No effects or complications reported

Dosage Adults: 10-20 mg 3-4 times/day; start with lower dose in elderly due to potential hypotension

Mechanism of Action In studies on normal human subjects, isoxsuprine increases muscle blood flow, but skin blood flow is usually unaffected. Rather than increasing muscle blood flow by beta-receptor stimulation, isoxsuprine probably has a direct action on vascular smooth muscle. The generally accepted mechanism of action of isoxsuprine on the uterus is beta-adrenergic stimulation. Isoxsuprine was shown to inhibit prostaglandin synthetase at high serum concentration, with low concentrations there was an increase in the P-G synthesis.

Other Adverse Effects Frequency not defined:

Cardiovascular: Hypotension, tachycardia, chest pain
Central nervous system: Dizziness
Dermatologic: Rash
Gastrointestinal: Nausea, vomiting
Neuromuscular & skeletal: Weakness

Drug Interactions May enhance effects of other vasodilators/hypotensive agents; use with caution in elderly

Drug Uptake

Absorption: Nearly complete
Half-life, elimination, mean: 1.25 hours
Time to peak: Oral, I.M.: ≤1 hour

Pregnancy Risk Factor C

Generic Available Yes

Isradipine (iz RA di peen)

Related Information

Calcium Channel Blockers and Gingival Hyperplasia *on page 1432*
Cardiovascular Diseases *on page 1308*

U.S. Brand Names DynaCirc®; DynaCirc® CR

Canadian Brand Names DynaCirc®

Mexican Brand Names DynaCirc®

Pharmacologic Category Calcium Channel Blocker

Use Treatment of hypertension, CHF, migraine prophylaxis

Local Anesthetic/Vasoconstrictor Precautions No information available to require special precautions

Effects on Dental Treatment Other drugs of this class can cause gingival hyperplasia (ie, nifedipine) but there have been no reports for isradipine.

Dosage Adults: 2.5 mg twice daily; antihypertensive response seen in 2-3 hours; maximal response in 2-4 weeks; increase dose at 2- to 4-week intervals at 2.5-5 mg increments; usual dose range: 5-20 mg/day. **Note**: Most patients show no improvement with doses >10 mg/day except adverse reaction rate increases; therefore, maximal dose in elderly should be 10 mg/day.

Mechanism of Action Inhibits calcium ion from entering the "slow channels" or select voltage-sensitive areas of vascular smooth muscle and myocardium during depolarization, producing a relaxation of coronary vascular smooth muscle and coronary vasodilation; increases myocardial oxygen delivery in patients with vasospastic angina

Other Adverse Effects

>10%: Central nervous system: Headache (dose-related 2% to 22%)

1% to 10%:

- Cardiovascular: Edema (dose-related 1% to 9%), palpitations (dose-related 1% to 5%), flushing (dose-related 1% to 5%), tachycardia (1% to 3%), chest pain (2% to 3%)
- Central nervous system: Dizziness (2% to 8%), fatigue (dose-related 1% to 9%), flushing (9%)
- Dermatologic: Rash (1.5% to 2%)
- Gastrointestinal: Nausea (1% to 5%), abdominal discomfort (≤3%), vomiting (≤1%), diarrhea (≤3%)
- Renal: Urinary frequency (1% to 3%)
- Respiratory: Dyspnea (1% to 3%)

Drug Interactions CYP3A3/4 enzyme substrate

Increased Effect/Toxicity: Isradipine may increase cardiovascular adverse effects of beta-blockers. Isradipine may minimally increase cyclosporine levels. Azole antifungals (and potentially other inhibitors of CYP3A3/4) may increase levels of isradipine; avoid this combination.

Decreased Effect: NSAIDs (diclofenac) may decrease the antihypertensive response of isradipine. Isradipine may cause a decrease in lovastatin effect. Rifampin may reduce blood levels and effects of isradipine due to enzyme induction (other enzyme inducers may share this effect).

Drug Uptake

Absorption: Oral: 90% to 95%
Duration: 8-16 hours
Half-life, elimination: 8 hours
Time to peak: 1-1.5 hours

Pregnancy Risk Factor C

Generic Available No

(Continued)

Isradipine *(Continued)*

Selected Readings Westbrook P, Bednarczyk EM, Carlson M, et al, "Regression of Nifedipine-Induced Gingival Hyperplasia Following Switch to a Same Class Calcium Channel Blocker, Isradipine," *J Periodontol*, 1997, 68(7):645-50.

Isuprel® *see* Isoproterenol *on page 660*

Itch-X® [OTC] *see* Pramoxine *on page 984*

Itraconazole (i tra KOE na zole)

Related Information

Oral Fungal Infections *on page 1377*

U.S. Brand Names Sporanox®

Canadian Brand Names Sporanox®

Mexican Brand Names Carexan; Isox; Itranax; Sporanox®

Pharmacologic Category Antifungal Agent, Oral

Use

Dental: Treatment of susceptible fungal infections in immunocompromised and immunocompetent patients including blastomycosis and histoplasmosis; also has activity against *Aspergillus, Candida, Coccidioides, Cryptococcus, Sporothrix*, and chromomycosis

Medical: Treatment of susceptible fungal infections in immunocompromised and immunocompetent patients including blastomycosis and histoplasmosis; indicated for aspergillosis, and onychomycosis of the toenail; treatment of onychomycosis of the fingernail without concomitant toenail infection via a pulse-type dosing regimen; has activity against *Aspergillus, Candida, Coccidioides, Cryptococcus, Sporothrix*, tinea unguium

Useful in superficial mycoses including dermatophytoses (eg, tinea capitis), pityriasis versicolor, sebopsoriasis, vaginal and chronic mucocutaneous candidiases; systemic mycoses including candidiasis, meningeal and disseminated cryptococcal infections, paracoccidioidomycosis, coccidioidomycoses; miscellaneous mycoses such as sporotrichosis, chromomycosis, leishmaniasis, fungal keratitis, alternariosis, zygomycosis

Intravenous solution is indicated in the treatment of blastomycosis, histoplasmosis (nonmeningeal), and aspergillosis (in patients intolerant or refractory to amphotericin B therapy)

Local Anesthetic/Vasoconstrictor Precautions No information available to require special precautions

Effects on Dental Treatment No effects or complications reported

Dosage Note: **Capsule:** Absorption is best if taken with food, therefore, it is best to administer itraconazole after meals. **Solution:** Should be taken on an empty stomach. Absorption of both products is significantly increased when taken with a cola beverage.

Children: Efficacy and safety have not been established; a small number of patients 3-16 years of age have been treated with 100 mg/day for systemic fungal infections with no serious adverse effects reported

Adults:

Oral:

Blastomycosis/histoplasmosis: 200 mg once daily, if no obvious improvement or there is evidence of progressive fungal disease, increase the dose in 100 mg increments to a maximum of 400 mg/day; doses >200 mg/day are given in 2 divided doses; length of therapy varies from 1 day to >6 months depending on the condition and mycological response

Aspergillosis: 200-400 mg/day

Onychomycosis: 200 mg once daily for 12 consecutive weeks

Life-threatening infections: Loading dose: 200 mg 3 times/day (600 mg/day) should be given for the first 3 days of therapy

Oropharyngeal and esophageal candidiasis: Oral solution: 100-200 mg once daily

I.V.: 200 mg twice daily for 4 doses, followed by 200 mg daily

Dosing adjustment in renal impairment: Injection is not recommended in patients with Cl_{cr} <30 mL/minute

Dosing adjustment in hepatic impairment: May be necessary, but specific guidelines are not available. Risk-to-benefit evaluation should be undertaken in patients who develop liver function abnormalities during treatment.

Mechanism of Action Inhibits fungal cytochrome P450-dependent enzymes (cytochrome P450 3A4 and cytochrome P450 2C); this blocks the synthesis of ergosterol which is the vital component in the fungal cell membrane. Triazoles contain three nitrogen atoms in the five-membered azole ring; the triazole ring increases tissue penetration, prolongs half-life, and enhances efficacy while decreasing toxicity compared with the imidazoles.

Other Adverse Effects Listed incidences are for higher doses appropriate for systemic fungal infections.

>10%: Gastrointestinal: Nausea (11%)

1% to 10%:
- Cardiovascular: Edema (4%), hypertension (3%)
- Central nervous system: Headache (4%), fatigue (2% to 3%), malaise (1%), fever (3%), dizziness (2%)
- Dermatologic: Rash (9%), pruritus (3%)
- Endocrine & metabolic: Decreased libido (1%), hypertriglyceridemia, hypokalemia (2%)
- Gastrointestinal: Abdominal pain (2%), anorexia (1%), vomiting (5%), diarrhea (3%)
- Hepatic: Abnormal LFTs (3%), hepatitis
- Renal: Albuminuria (1%)

<1%: Adrenal suppression, constipation, gastritis, gynecomastia, impotence, somnolence, tinnitus

Postmarketing and/or case reports: Allergic reactions (urticaria, angioedema), alopecia, anaphylaxis, arrhythmia, CHF, hepatic failure, menstrual disorders, neuropathy, neutropenia, Stevens-Johnson syndrome

Contraindications Hypersensitivity itraconazole, other azoles, or any component of their formulation; concurrent administration with astemizole, cisapride, dofetilide, lovastatin, midazolam, pimozide, quinidine, or simvastatin; treatment of onychomycosis in patients with evidence of left ventricular dysfunction, CHF, or a history of CHF

Warnings/Precautions Rare cases of serious cardiovascular adverse events, including death, ventricular tachycardia and torsade de pointes have been observed due to increased terfenadine and cisapride concentrations induced by itraconazole. Patients who develop abnormal LFTs during itraconazole therapy should be monitored and therapy discontinued if symptoms of liver disease develop. Itraconazole injection is not recommended in patients with Cl_{cr} <30 mL/minute. Discontinue if signs or symptoms of CHF occur during treatment.

Drug Interactions CYP3A3/4 enzyme substrate, CYP3A3/4 inhibitor
- Benzodiazepines: Alprazolam, diazepam, temazepam, triazolam, and midazolam serum concentration may be increased; consider a benzodiazepine not metabolized by CYP3A3/4 (such as lorazepam) or another antifungal that is metabolized by CYP3A3/4
- Buspirone: Serum concentrations may be increased; monitor for sedation
- Busulfan: Serum concentrations may be increased; avoid concurrent use
- Calcium channel blockers: Serum concentrations may be increased (applies to those agents metabolized by CYP3A3/4, including felodipine, nifedipine, and verapamil); consider another agent instead of a calcium channel blocker, another antifungal, or reduce the dose of the calcium channel blocker; monitor BP
- Cisapride and terfenadine: serum concentration is increased which may lead to malignant arrhythmias; concurrent use is contraindicated
- Didanosine: May decrease absorption of itraconazole (due to buffering capacity of oral solution); applies only to oral solution formulation of didanosine
- Docetaxel: Serum concentrations may be increased; avoid concurrent use
- Dofetilide: Serum levels/toxicity may be increased; concurrent use is contraindicated.
- Enzyme inducers: Rifampin decreases itraconazole's serum concentration to levels which are no longer effective; avoid concurrent use. Other inducers (barbiturates, carbamazepine, rifabutin) may share this effect.
- Erythromycin (and clarithromycin): May increase serum concentration of itraconazole.
- H_2 blockers: May decrease itraconazole absorption. Itraconazole depends on gastric acidity for absorption. Avoid concurrent use.
- HMG-CoA reductase inhibitors (except pravastatin and fluvastatin): Serum concentrations may be increased. The risk of myopathy/rhabdomyolysis may be increased. Switch to pravastatin/fluvastatin or monitor for development of myopathy.
- Immunosuppressants: Cyclosporine, sirolimus, and tacrolimus: Serum concentrations may be increased; monitor serum concentration and renal function
- Methylprednisolone: Serum concentrations may be increased; monitor
- Nevirapine: May decrease serum concentration of itraconazole; monitor
- Oral contraceptives: Efficacy may be reduced by itraconazole (limited data); use barrier birth control method during concurrent use
- Phenytoin: Serum concentrations may be increased; monitor phenytoin levels and adjust dose as needed.
- Pimozide: Serum levels/toxicity may be increased; concurrent use is contraindicated.
- Protease inhibitors: May increase serum concentration of itraconazole. Includes amprenavir, indinavir, nelfinavir, ritonavir, and saquinavir; monitor
- Proton pump inhibitors: May decrease itraconazole absorption. Itraconazole depends on gastric acidity for absorption. Avoid concurrent use (includes omeprazole, lansoprazole).
- Quinidine: Serum levels may be increased. Concurrent use is contraindicated.
- Trimetrexate: Serum concentrations may be increased; monitor
- Warfarin: Anticoagulant effects may be increased; monitor INR and adjust warfarin's dose as needed

(Continued)

Itraconazole *(Continued)*

Vinca alkaloids: Serum concentrations may be increased; avoid concurrent use
Zolpidem: Serum levels may be increased; monitor

Dietary/Ethanol/Herb Considerations

Ethanol: Avoid use; disulfiram-like reaction may occur.

Food: Administer capsules with food; gastric acidity required for absorption. Administer solution on an empty stomach, if possible; time to peak concentration prolonged by food. Avoid grapefruit products. Absorption of both products is increased when administered with a cola beverage.

Herb/Nutraceutical: Avoid St John's wort; may decrease serum concentration.

Drug Uptake

Absorption: Requires gastric acidity; capsule better absorbed with food, solution better absorbed on empty stomach; hypochlorhydria has been reported in HIV-infected patients; therefore, oral absorption in these patients may be decreased

Half-life, elimination: Oral: After single 200 mg dose: 21 ± 5 hours; 64 hours at steady-state; I.V.: steady-state: 35 hours; steady-state concentrations are achieved in 13 days with multiple administration of itraconazole 100-400 mg/day.

Pregnancy Risk Factor C

Breast-feeding Considerations Not recommended

Dosage Forms CAP: 100 mg. **KIT, injection:** 10 mg/mL - 25 mL ampul, one 50 mL (100 mL capacity) bag 0.9% sodium chloride, one filtered infusion set. **SOLN, oral:** 100 mg/10 mL (150 mL)

Generic Available No

Iveegam EN *see* Immune Globulin, Intravenous *on page 630*

Ivermectin (eye ver MEK tin)

U.S. Brand Names Stromectol®

Pharmacologic Category Antibiotic, Miscellaneous

Use Treatment of the following infections: Strongyloidiasis of the intestinal tract due the nematode parasite *Strongyloides stercoralis.* Onchocerciasis due to the nematode parasite *Onchocerca volvulus.* **Note:** Ivermectin is ineffective against adult *Onchocerca volvulus* parasites because they reside in subcutaneous nodules which are infrequently palpable. Surgical excision of these nodules may be considered in the management of patients with onchocerciasis.

Local Anesthetic/Vasoconstrictor Precautions No information available to require special precautions

Effects on Dental Treatment No effects or complications reported

Dosage Oral:

Children ≥5 years: 150 mcg/kg as a single dose; treatment for onchocerciasis may need to be repeated every 3-12 months until the adult worms die

Adults:

Strongyloidiasis: 200 mcg/kg as a single dose; follow-up stool examinations

Onchocerciasis: 150 mcg/kg as a single dose; retreatment may be required every 3-12 months until the adult worms die

Mechanism of Action Ivermectin is a semisynthetic antihelminthic agent; it binds selectively and with strong affinity to glutamate-gated chloride ion channels which occur in invertebrate nerve and muscle cells. This leads to increased permeability of cell membranes to chloride ions then hyperpolarization of the nerve or muscle cell, and death of the parasite.

Other Adverse Effects Frequency not defined:

Cardiovascular: Hypotension, mild EKG changes, peripheral and facial edema, transient tachycardia

Central nervous system: Dizziness, headache, hyperthermia, insomnia, somnolence, vertigo

Dermatologic: Pruritus, rash, urticaria

Gastrointestinal: Abdominal pain, diarrhea, nausea, vomiting

Hematologic: Eosinophilia, leukopenia

Hepatic: Increased ALT/AST

Neuromuscular & skeletal: Limbitis, myalgia, tremor, weakness

Ocular: Blurred vision, mild conjunctivitis, punctate opacity

Mazzotti reaction (with onchocerciasis): Edema, fever, lymphadenopathy, ocular damage, pruritus, rash

Drug Uptake

Onset of action: Peak effect: 3-6 months

Absorption: Well absorbed

Half-life, elimination: 16-35 hours

Pregnancy Risk Factor C

Generic Available No

IvyBlock® [OTC] *see* Bentoquatam *on page 150*

Japanese Encephalitis Virus Vaccine, Inactivated

(jap a NEESE en sef a LYE tis VYE rus vak SEEN, in ak ti VAY ted)

U.S. Brand Names JE-VAX®

Canadian Brand Names JE-VAX®

Pharmacologic Category Vaccine

Use Active immunization against Japanese encephalitis for persons 1 year of age and older who plan to spend 1 month or more in endemic areas in Asia, especially persons traveling during the transmission season or visiting rural areas; consider vaccination for shorter trips to epidemic areas or extensive outdoor activities in rural endemic areas; elderly (>55 years of age) individuals should be considered for vaccination, since they have increased risk of developing symptomatic illness after infection; those planning travel to or residence in endemic areas should consult the Travel Advisory Service (Central Campus) for specific advice

Local Anesthetic/Vasoconstrictor Precautions No information available to require special precautions

Effects on Dental Treatment No effects or complications reported

Dosage US recommended primary immunization schedule:

Children >3 years and Adults: S.C.: Three 1 mL doses given on days 0, 7, and 30. Give third dose on day 14 when time does not permit waiting; 2 doses a week apart produce immunity in about 80% of vaccines; the longest regimen yields highest titers after 6 months

Children 1-3 years: S.C.: Three 0.5 mL doses given on days 0, 7, and 30; abbreviated schedules should be used only when necessary due to time constraints

Booster dose: Give after 2 years, or according to current recommendation

Note: Travel should not commence for at least 10 days after the last dose of vaccine, to allow adequate antibody formation and recognition of any delayed adverse reaction

Advise concurrent use of other means to reduce the risk of mosquito exposure when possible, including bed nets, insect repellents, protective clothing, avoidance of travel in endemic areas, and avoidance of outdoor activity during twilight and evening periods

Other Adverse Effects

Report allergic or unusual adverse reactions to the Vaccine Adverse Event Reporting System (VAERS) 1-800-822-7967.

Frequency not defined: Tenderness, redness, and swelling at injection site; systemic side effects include fever, headache, malaise, rash, chills, dizziness, myalgia, nausea, vomiting, abdominal pain, urticaria, itching with or without accompanying rash, and hypotension; rarely, anaphylactic reaction, encephalitis, encephalopathy, seizure, peripheral neuropathy, erythema multiforme, erythema nodosum, angioedema, dyspnea, joint swelling

Drug Interactions Simultaneous administration of DTP vaccine and Japanese encephalitis vaccine does not compromise the immunogenicity of either vaccine; data on administration with other vaccines, chloroquine, or mefloquine are lacking.

Pregnancy Risk Factor C

Generic Available No

Comments Japanese encephalitis vaccine is currently available only from the Centers for Disease Control. Contact Centers for Disease Control at (404) 639-6370 (Mon-Fri) or (404) 639-2888 (nights, weekends, or holidays).

Jenest™-28 *see* Combination Hormonal Contraceptives *on page 323*

JE-VAX® *see* Japanese Encephalitis Virus Vaccine, Inactivated *on page 669*

Junior Strength Motrin® [OTC] *see* Ibuprofen *on page 621*

K+ 10® *see* Potassium Chloride *on page 977*

Kadian® *see* Morphine Sulfate *on page 829*

Kala® [OTC] *see* *Lactobacillus acidophilus* and *Lactobacillus bulgaricus* *on page 682*

Kaletra™ *see* Lopinavir and Ritonavir *on page 725*

Kanamycin

(kan a MYE sin)

Related Information

Nonviral Infectious Diseases *on page 1342*

U.S. Brand Names Kantrex®

Canadian Brand Names Kantrex®

Mexican Brand Names Koptin®; Randikan

Pharmacologic Category Antibiotic, Aminoglycoside

Synonyms Kanamycin Sulfate

Use

Oral: Preoperative bowel preparation in the prophylaxis of infections and adjunctive treatment of hepatic coma (oral kanamycin is not indicated in the treatment of systemic infections); treatment of susceptible bacterial infection including gram-negative aerobes, gram-positive *Bacillus* as well as some mycobacteria

Parenteral: Rarely used in antibiotic irrigations during surgery

(Continued)

Kanamycin *(Continued)*

Local Anesthetic/Vasoconstrictor Precautions No information available to require special precautions

Effects on Dental Treatment No effects or complications reported

Dosage

Children: Infections: I.M., I.V.: 15 mg/kg/day in divided doses every 8-12 hours

Adults:

- Infections: I.M., I.V.: 5-7.5 mg/kg/dose in divided doses every 8-12 hours (<15 mg/kg/day)
- Preoperative intestinal antisepsis: Oral: 1 g every 4-6 hours for 36-72 hours
- Hepatic coma: Oral: 8-12 g/day in divided doses
- Intraperitoneal: After contamination in surgery: 500 mg diluted in 20 mL distilled water; other irrigations: 0.25% solutions
- Aerosol: 250 mg 2-4 times/day (250 mg diluted with 3 mL of NS and nebulized)

Dosing adjustment/interval in renal impairment:

- Cl_{cr} 50-80 mL/minute: Administer 60% to 90% of dose or administer every 8-12 hours
- Cl_{cr} 10-50 mL/minute: Administer 30% to 70% of dose or administer every 12 hours
- Cl_{cr} <10 mL/minute: Administer 20% to 30% of dose or administer every 24-48 hours

Hemodialysis: Dialyzable (50% to 100%)

Mechanism of Action Interferes with protein synthesis in bacterial cell by binding to ribosomal subunit

Other Adverse Effects Frequency not defined: Edema, neurotoxicity, drowsiness, headache, pseudomotor cerebri, skin itching, redness, rash, photosensitivity, erythema, nausea, vomiting, diarrhea (most common with oral form), malabsorption syndrome with prolonged and high-dose therapy of hepatic coma; anorexia, weight loss, increased salivation, enterocolitis, granulocytopenia, agranulocytosis, thrombocytopenia, burning, stinging, weakness, tremors, muscle cramps, ototoxicity (auditory), ototoxicity (vestibular), nephrotoxicity, dyspnea

Drug Interactions

Increased Effect/Toxicity: Penicillins, cephalosporins, amphotericin B, diuretics may increase nephrotoxicity; polypeptide antibiotics may increase risk of respiratory paralysis and renal dysfunction. Neuromuscular-blocking agents with kanamycin may increase neuromuscular blockade. A small increase in warfarin's effect may occur due to decreased absorption of vitamin K.

Decreased Effect: Methotrexate with kanamycin (oral) may be less well absorbed as may digoxin (minor) and vitamin A.

Drug Uptake

Absorption: Oral: None

Half-life, elimination: 2-4 hours; Anuria: 80 hours; End-stage renal disease: 40-96 hours

Time to peak: I.M.: 1-2 hours

Pregnancy Risk Factor D

Generic Available Yes

Kantrex® *see* Kanamycin *on page 669*

Kaochlor® *see* Potassium Chloride *on page 977*

Kaochlor® SF *see* Potassium Chloride *on page 977*

Kaodene® NN [OTC] *see* Kaolin and Pectin *on page 670*

Kaolin and Pectin (KAY oh lin & PEK tin)

U.S. Brand Names Kaodene® NN [OTC]; Kao-Spen® [OTC]; Kapectolin® [OTC]

Pharmacologic Category Antidiarrheal

Synonyms Pectin and Kaolin

Use Treatment of uncomplicated diarrhea

Local Anesthetic/Vasoconstrictor Precautions No information available to require special precautions

Effects on Dental Treatment No effects or complications reported

Dosage Oral:

Children:

- <6 years: Do not use
- 6-12 years: 30-60 mL after each loose stool

Adults: 60-120 mL after each loose stool

Other Adverse Effects 1% to 10%: Gastrointestinal: Constipation, fecal impaction

Drug Interactions May decrease absorption of many drugs, including chloroquine, atenolol, metoprolol, propranolol, diflunisal, isoniazid, penicillamine, clindamycin, digoxin (give kaolin/pectin 2 hours before or 4 hours after medication).

Pregnancy Risk Factor C

Generic Available Yes

Kaolin and Pectin With Opium

(KAY oh lin & PEK tin with OH pee um)

U.S. Brand Names Parepectolin®

Canadian Brand Names Donnagel®-PG Suspension

Pharmacologic Category Antidiarrheal

Synonyms Pectin With Opium and Kaolin

Use Symptomatic relief of diarrhea

Local Anesthetic/Vasoconstrictor Precautions No information available to require special precautions

Effects on Dental Treatment No effects or complications reported

Restrictions C-V

Dosage Oral:

Children:

3-6 years: 7.5 mL with each loose bowel movement, not to exceed 30 mL in 12 hours

6-12 years: 5-10 mL with each loose bowel movement, not to exceed 40 mL in 12 hours

Children >12 years and Adults: 15-30 mL with each loose bowel movement, not to exceed 120 mL in 12 hours

Other Adverse Effects Frequency not defined:

Central nervous system: Drowsiness

Gastrointestinal: Constipation, fecal impaction

Pregnancy Risk Factor C

Generic Available Yes

Kaon® *see* Potassium Gluconate *on page 979*

Kaon-Cl® *see* Potassium Chloride *on page 977*

Kaon-Cl-10® *see* Potassium Chloride *on page 977*

Kaopectate® Advanced Formula [OTC] *see* Attapulgite *on page 132*

Kaopectate® II [OTC] *see* Loperamide *on page 725*

Kaopectate® Maximum Strength Caplets [OTC] *see* Attapulgite *on page 132*

Kao-Spen® [OTC] *see* Kaolin and Pectin *on page 670*

Kapectolin® [OTC] *see* Kaolin and Pectin *on page 670*

Kapectolin PG® *see* Hyoscyamine, Atropine, Scopolamine, Kaolin, Pectin, and Opium *on page 619*

Karidium® *see* Fluoride *on page 514*

Karigel® *see* Fluoride *on page 514*

Karigel®-N *see* Fluoride *on page 514*

Kariva™ *see* Combination Hormonal Contraceptives *on page 323*

Kay Ciel® *see* Potassium Chloride *on page 977*

K+ Care® *see* Potassium Chloride *on page 977*

K+ Care® ET *see* Potassium Bicarbonate *on page 976*

K-Dur® 10 *see* Potassium Chloride *on page 977*

K-Dur® 20 *see* Potassium Chloride *on page 977*

Keflex® *see* Cephalexin *on page 251*

Keftab® *see* Cephalexin *on page 251*

Kefurox® *see* Cefuroxime *on page 246*

Kefzol® *see* Cefazolin *on page 234*

Kemadrin® *see* Procyclidine *on page 1002*

Kenacort® *see* Triamcinolone *on page 1197*

Kenaject-40® *see* Triamcinolone *on page 1197*

Kenalog® *see* Triamcinolone *on page 1197*

Kenalog-10® *see* Triamcinolone *on page 1197*

Kenalog-40® *see* Triamcinolone *on page 1197*

Kenalog® H *see* Triamcinolone *on page 1197*

Kenalog® in Orabase® *see* Triamcinolone *on page 1197*

Kenalog® in Orabase® *see* Triamcinolone Acetonide Dental Paste *on page 1199*

Kenonel® *see* Triamcinolone *on page 1197*

Keppra® *see* Levetiracetam *on page 695*

Keralyt® Gel [OTC] *see* Salicylic Acid and Propylene Glycol *on page 1072*

Kerlone® *see* Betaxolol *on page 161*

Kestrone® *see* Estrone *on page 468*

Ketalar® *see* Ketamine *on page 671*

Ketamine (KEET a meen)

U.S. Brand Names Ketalar®

Canadian Brand Names Ketalar®

Mexican Brand Names Ketalin®

Pharmacologic Category General Anesthetic

Synonyms Ketamine Hydrochloride

(Continued)

Ketamine *(Continued)*

Use Induction and maintenance of general anesthesia, especially when cardiovascular depression must be avoided (ie, hypotension, hypovolemia, cardiomyopathy, constrictive pericarditis); sedation; analgesia

Local Anesthetic/Vasoconstrictor Precautions No information available to require special precautions

Effects on Dental Treatment No effects or complications reported

Restrictions C-III

Dosage Used in combination with anticholinergic agents to ↓ hypersalivation

Children: Initial induction:

- Oral: 6-10 mg/kg for 1 dose (mixed in 0.2-0.3 mL/kg of cola or other beverage) given 30 minutes before the procedure
- I.M.: 3-7 mg/kg
- I.V.: Range: 0.5-2 mg/kg, use smaller doses (0.5-1 mg/kg) for sedation for minor procedures; usual induction dosage: 1-2 mg/kg
- Continuous I.V. infusion: Sedation: 5-20 mcg/kg/minute

Adults: Initial induction:

- I.M.: 3-8 mg/kg
- I.V.: Range: 1-4.5 mg/kg; usual induction dosage: 1-2 mg/kg

Children and Adults: Maintenance: Supplemental doses of $1/2$ to the full induction dose; repeat as needed

Mechanism of Action Produces a cataleptic-like state in which the patient is dissociated from the surrounding environment by direct action on the cortex and limbic system. Releases endogenous catecholamines (epinephrine, norepinephrine) which maintain BP and heart rate. Reduces polysynaptic spinal reflexes.

Other Adverse Effects

>10%:

- Cardiovascular: Hypertension, increased cardiac output, paradoxical direct myocardial depression, tachycardia
- Central nervous system: Increased intracranial pressure, visual hallucinations, vivid dreams
- Neuromuscular & skeletal: Tonic-clonic movements, tremors
- Miscellaneous: Emergence reactions, vocalization

1% to 10%:

- Cardiovascular: Bradycardia, hypotension
- Dermatologic: Pain at injection site, skin rash
- Gastrointestinal: Anorexia, nausea, vomiting
- Ocular: Diplopia, nystagmus
- Respiratory: Respiratory depression

Drug Interactions CYP2D6 and CYP3A enzyme substrate

Increased Effect/Toxicity: Barbiturates, narcotics, hydroxyzine increase prolonged recovery; nondepolarizing neuromuscular blockers may increase effects. Muscle relaxants, thyroid hormones may increase BP and heart rate. Halothane may decrease BP.

Drug Uptake

Onset of sedative effect:

- I.V.: General anesthesia: 1-2 minutes; Sedation: 1-2 minutes
- I.M.: General anesthesia: 3-8 minutes
- Oral: Sedation: 15-30 minutes

Duration: I.V.: 5-15 minutes; I.M.: 12-25 minutes

Half-life: 11-17 minutes; Elimination: 2.5-3.1 hours

Pregnancy Risk Factor D

Generic Available Yes

Ketoconazole (kee toe KOE na zole)

Related Information

Dental Drug Interactions: Update on Drug Combinations Requiring Special Considerations *on page 1434*
Oral Fungal Infections *on page 1377*
Respiratory Diseases *on page 1328*

U.S. Brand Names Nizoral®; Nizoral® A-D [OTC]

Canadian Brand Names Apo®-Ketoconazole; Nizoral®; Novo-Ketoconazole

Mexican Brand Names Akorazol; Conazol; Cremosan®; Fungoral®; Konaderm®; Mycodib®; Nizoral®; Onofin-K®; Termizol®; Tiniazol

Pharmacologic Category Antifungal Agent, Oral; Antifungal Agent, Topical

Use Treatment of susceptible fungal infections, including candidiasis, oral thrush, blastomycosis, histoplasmosis, paracoccidioidomycosis, coccidioidomycosis, chromomycosis, candiduria, chronic mucocutaneous candidiasis, as well as certain recalcitrant cutaneous dermatophytoses; used topically for treatment of tinea corporis, tinea cruris, tinea versicolor, and cutaneous candidiasis, seborrheic dermatitis

Local Anesthetic/Vasoconstrictor Precautions No information available to require special precautions

Effects on Dental Treatment No effects or complications reported

Dosage

Oral:

Children ≥2 years: 3.3-6.6 mg/kg/day as a single dose for 1-2 weeks for candidiasis, for at least 4 weeks in recalcitrant dermatophyte infections, and for up to 6 months for other systemic mycoses

Adults: 200-400 mg/day as a single daily dose for durations as stated above

Shampoo: Apply twice weekly for 4 weeks with at least 3 days between each shampoo

Topical: Rub gently into the affected area once daily to twice daily

Dosing adjustment in hepatic impairment: Dose reductions should be considered in patients with severe liver disease

Hemodialysis: Not dialyzable (0% to 5%)

Mechanism of Action Alters the permeability of the cell wall; inhibits biosynthesis of triglycerides and phospholipids by fungi; inhibits several fungal enzymes that results in a build-up of toxic concentrations of hydrogen peroxide

Other Adverse Effects

Oral:

1% to 10%:

Dermatologic: Pruritus (2%)

Gastrointestinal: Nausea/vomiting (3% to 10%), abdominal pain (1%)

<1%: Headache, dizziness, somnolence, fever, chills, bulging fontanelles, depression, gynecomastia, diarrhea, impotence, thrombocytopenia, leukopenia, hemolytic anemia, hepatotoxicity, photophobia

Cream: Severe irritation, pruritus, stinging (~5%)

Shampoo: Increases in normal hair loss, irritation (<1%), abnormal hair texture, scalp pustules, mild dryness of skin, itching, oiliness/dryness of hair

Contraindications Hypersensitivity to ketoconazole or any component of the formulation; CNS fungal infections (due to poor CNS penetration); coadministration with terfenadine, astemizole, or cisapride due to risk of potentially fatal cardiac arrhythmias

Warnings/Precautions Rare cases of serious cardiovascular adverse event, including death, ventricular tachycardia and torsade de pointes have been observed due to increased terfenadine concentrations induced by ketoconazole. Use with caution in patients with impaired hepatic function; has been associated with hepatotoxicity, including some fatalities; perform periodic LFTs; high doses of ketoconazole may depress adrenocortical function.

Drug Interactions CYP3A3/4 enzyme substrate; CYP1A2, 2C, 2C9, 2C18, 2C19, 3A3/4, and 3A5-7 enzyme inhibitor

Benzodiazepines: Alprazolam, diazepam, temazepam, triazolam, and midazolam serum concentration may be increased; consider a benzodiazepine not metabolized by CYP3A3/4 (such as lorazepam) or another antifungal that is metabolized by CYP3A3/4. Concurrent use is contraindicated.

Buspirone: Serum concentrations may be increased; monitor for sedation

Busulfan: Serum concentrations may be increased; avoid concurrent use

Calcium channel blockers: Serum concentrations may be increased (applies to those agents metabolized by CYP3A3/4, including felodipine, nifedipine, and verapamil); consider another agent instead of a calcium channel blocker, another antifungal, or reduce the dose of the calcium channel blocker; monitor BP

Cisapride and terfenadine: Serum concentration is increased which may lead to malignant arrhythmias; concurrent use is contraindicated

Didanosine: May decrease absorption of ketoconazole (due to buffering capacity of oral solution); applies only to oral solution formulation of didanosine

Docetaxel: Serum concentrations may be increased; avoid concurrent use

Enzyme inducers: Rifampin decreases ketoconazole's serum concentration to levels which are no longer effective; avoid concurrent use. Other inducers (barbiturates, carbamazepine, rifabutin) may share this effect.

Erythromycin (and clarithromycin): May increase serum concentration of ketoconazole.

H_2 blockers: May decrease ketoconazole absorption. Ketoconazole depends on gastric acidity for absorption. Avoid concurrent use.

HMG-CoA reductase inhibitors (except pravastatin and fluvastatin): Serum concentrations may be increased. The risk of myopathy/rhabdomyolysis may be increased. Switch to pravastatin/fluvastatin or monitor for development of myopathy.

Immunosuppressants: Cyclosporine, sirolimus, and tacrolimus: Serum concentrations may be increased; monitor serum concentration and renal function

Methylprednisolone: Serum concentrations may be increased; monitor

Nevirapine: May decrease serum concentration of ketoconazole; monitor

Oral contraceptives: Efficacy may be reduced by ketoconazole (limited data); use barrier birth control method during concurrent use

Phenytoin: Serum concentrations may be increased; monitor phenytoin levels and adjust dose as needed

Protease inhibitors: May increase serum concentration of ketoconazole. Includes amprenavir, indinavir, nelfinavir, ritonavir, and saquinavir; monitor

(Continued)

Ketoconazole *(Continued)*

Proton-pump inhibitors: May decrease ketoconazole absorption. Ketoconazole depends on gastric acidity for absorption. Avoid concurrent use (includes omeprazole, lansoprazole).
Quinidine: Serum levels may be increased; monitor
Trimetrexate: Serum concentrations may be increased; monitor
Warfarin: Anticoagulant effects may be increased; monitor INR and adjust warfarin's dose as needed
Vinca alkaloids: Serum concentrations may be increased; avoid concurrent use
Zolpidem: Serum levels may be increased; monitor

Dietary/Ethanol/Herb Considerations
Ethanol: Avoid use; may cause disulfiram-like reaction.
Food may prolong peak serum concentration; administer with food or milk to reduce GI upset.
Herb/Nutraceutical: Avoid St John's wort; may decrease serum concentration.

Drug Uptake
Absorption: Oral: Rapid (~75%); Shampoo: None
Half-life, elimination: Biphasic: Initial: 2 hours; terminal: 8 hours
Time to peak: 1-2 hours

Pregnancy Risk Factor C

Dosage Forms CRM: 2% (15 g, 30 g, 60 g). **SHAMP:** 1% (120 mL, 207 mL); 2% (120 mL). **TAB:** 200 mg

Generic Available Yes

Ketoprofen (kee toe PROE fen)

Related Information
Oral Pain *on page 1360*
Rheumatoid Arthritis and Osteoarthritis *on page 1340*
Temporomandibular Dysfunction (TMD) *on page 1397*

U.S. Brand Names Orudis® [DSC]; Orudis® KT [OTC]; Oruvail®

Canadian Brand Names Apo®-Keto; Apo®-Keto-E; Apo®-Keto SR; Novo-Keto; Novo-Keto-EC; Nu-Ketoprofen; Nu-Ketoprofen-E; Orafen; Orudis® SR; Oruvail®; Rhodis™; Rhodis-EC™; Rhodis SR™

Mexican Brand Names Keduril®; K-Profen®; Orudis®; Profenid®

Pharmacologic Category Nonsteroidal Anti-inflammatory Drug (NSAID)

Use
Dental: Management of pain and swelling
Medical: Acute and long-term treatment of rheumatoid arthritis and osteoarthritis; primary dysmenorrhea; mild to moderate pain

Local Anesthetic/Vasoconstrictor Precautions No information available to require special precautions

Effects on Dental Treatment NSAID formulations are known to reversibly decrease platelet aggregation via mechanisms different than observed with aspirin. The dentist should be aware of the potential of abnormal coagulation. Caution should also be exercised in the use of NSAIDs in patients already on anticoagulant therapy with drugs such as warfarin (Coumadin®).

Dosage Oral:
Children 3 months to 14 years: Fever: 0.5-1 mg/kg every 6-8 hours
Children >12 years and Adults:
- Rheumatoid arthritis or osteoarthritis: 50-75 mg 3-4 times/day up to a maximum of 300 mg/day
- Mild to moderate pain: 25-50 mg every 6-8 hours up to a maximum of 300 mg/day

Mechanism of Action Inhibits prostaglandin synthesis by decreasing the activity of the enzyme, cyclo-oxygenase, which results in decreased formation of prostaglandin precursors

Other Adverse Effects
>10%:
- Central nervous system: Headache (11%)
- Gastrointestinal: Dyspepsia (11%)

1% to 10%:
- Central nervous system: Nervousness
- Dermatologic: Rash, itching
- Endocrine & metabolic: Fluid retention
- Gastrointestinal: Vomiting (>1%), diarrhea (3% to 9%), nausea (3% to 9%), constipation (3% to 9%), abdominal distress/cramping/pain (3% to 9%), flatulence (3% to 9%), anorexia (>1%), stomatitis (>1%)
- Genitourinary: Urinary tract infection (>1%)
- Otic: Tinnitus

<1%: Congestive heart failure, hypertension, arrhythmias, tachycardia, confusion, hallucinations, mental depression, drowsiness, insomnia, aseptic meningitis, urticaria, erythema multiforme, toxic epidermal necrolysis, Stevens-Johnson syndrome, angioedema, polydipsia, hot flashes, gastritis, GI ulceration, cystitis, polyuria, agranulocytosis, anemia, hemolytic anemia, bone marrow suppression, leukopenia, thrombocytopenia, hepatitis, peripheral neuropathy, toxic amblyopia,

blurred vision, conjunctivitis, dry eyes, decreased hearing, acute renal failure, allergic rhinitis, dyspnea, epistaxis

Contraindications Hypersensitivity to ketoprofen, other NSAIDs, aspirin, or any component of their formulation; pregnancy (3rd trimester)

Warnings/Precautions Use with caution in patients with CHF, hypertension, dehydration, decreased renal or hepatic function, history of GI disease (bleeding or ulcers), or those receiving anticoagulants. Elderly are at a high risk for adverse effects from nonsteroidal anti-inflammatory agents. As much as 60% of elderly can develop peptic ulceration and/or hemorrhage asymptomatically.

Use lowest effective dose for shortest period possible. Use of NSAIDs can compromise existing renal function especially when Cl_{cr} is <30 mL/minute. CNS adverse effects such as confusion, agitation, and hallucination are generally seen in overdose or high-dose situations; however, elderly may demonstrate these adverse effects at lower doses than younger adults. Withhold for at least 4-6 half-lives prior to surgical or dental procedures. Safety and efficacy in pediatric patients have not been established (per manufacturer).

Drug Interactions CYP2C and 2C9 enzyme inhibitor

ACE inhibitors: Antihypertensive effects may be decreased by concurrent therapy with NSAIDs; monitor BP

Angiotensin II antagonists: Antihypertensive effects may be decreased by concurrent therapy with NSAIDs; monitor BP

Anticoagulants (warfarin, heparin, LMWHs) in combination with NSAIDs can cause increased risk of bleeding.

Other antiplatelet drugs (ticlopidine, clopidogrel, aspirin, abciximab, dipyridamole, eptifibatide, tirofiban) can cause an increased risk of bleeding.

Loop diuretics efficacy (diuretic and antihypertensive effect) is reduced. Indomethacin reduces this efficacy, however, it may be anticipated with any NSAID.

Corticosteroids may increase the risk of GI ulceration; avoid concurrent use.

Cyclosporine: NSAIDs may increase serum creatinine, potassium, BP, and cyclosporine levels; monitor cyclosporine levels and renal function carefully

Gentamicin and amikacin serum concentrations are increased by indomethacin in premature infants. Results may apply to other aminoglycosides and NSAIDs.

Hydralazine's antihypertensive effect is decreased; avoid concurrent use

Lithium levels can be increased; avoid concurrent use if possible or monitor lithium levels and adjust dose. Sulindac may have the least effect. When NSAID is stopped, lithium will need adjustment again.

Loop diuretics efficacy (diuretic and antihypertensive effect) is reduced. Indomethacin reduces this efficacy, however, it may be anticipated with any NSAID.

Methotrexate: Severe bone marrow suppression, aplastic anemia, and GI toxicity have been reported with concomitant NSAID therapy. Avoid use during moderate or high-dose methotrexate (increased and prolonged methotrexate levels). NSAID use during low-dose treatment of rheumatoid arthritis has not been fully evaluated; extreme caution is warranted.

Thiazides antihypertensive effects are decreased; avoid concurrent use

Verapamil plasma concentration is decreased by diclofenac; avoid concurrent use

Warfarin's INRs may be increased by piroxicam. Other NSAIDs may have the same effect depending on dose and duration. Monitor INR closely. Use the lowest dose of NSAIDs possible and for the briefest duration.

Dietary/Ethanol/Herb Considerations

Ethanol: Avoid use due to GI irritation.

Food: Administer with food or milk to reduce GI upset. Although food affects the bioavailability of ketoprofen, analgesic efficacy is not significantly diminished. Food slows rate of absorption resulting in delayed and reduced peak serum concentration.

Herb/Nutraceutical: Avoid kava and valerian; may enhance benzodiazepine activity.

Drug Uptake

Onset of action: 30-60 minutes; Peak effect: 1-2 hours

Absorption: Rapid and complete

Half-life, elimination: 1-4 hours

Time to peak: 0.5-2 hours

Pregnancy Risk Factor B/D (3rd trimester)

Breast-feeding Considerations May be taken while breast-feeding

Dosage Forms **CAP** (Orudis®): 25 mg, 50 mg, 75 mg. **CAP, extended release:** (Actron®): 200 mg; (Oruvail®): 100 mg, 150 mg. **TAB** (Orudis® KT): 12.5 mg

Generic Available Yes

Selected Readings

Balevi B, "Ketorolac Versus Ibuprofen: A Simple Cost-Efficacy Comparison for Dental Use," *J Can Dent Assoc*, 1994, 60(1):31-2.

Brooks PM and Day RO, "Nonsteroidal Anti-inflammatory Drugs - Differences and Similarities," *N Engl J Med*, 1991, 324(24):1716-25.

Cooper SA, "Ketoprofen in Oral Surgery Pain: A Review," *J Clin Pharmacol*, 1988, 28(12 Suppl):S40-6.

Hersh EV, "The Efficacy and Safety of Ketoprofen in Postsurgical Dental Pain," *Compendium*, 1991, 12(4):234.

Ketorolac Tromethamine (KEE toe role ak)

Related Information

Dental Drug Interactions: Update on Drug Combinations Requiring Special Considerations *on page 1434*
Rheumatoid Arthritis and Osteoarthritis *on page 1340*
Temporomandibular Dysfunction (TMD) *on page 1397*

U.S. Brand Names Acular®; Acular® PF; Toradol®

Canadian Brand Names Acular®; Apo®-Ketorolac; Novo-Ketorolac; Toradol®; Toradol® IM

Mexican Brand Names Acularen®; Alidol; Dola; Dolac®; Dolotor®; Findol®; Supradol®

Pharmacologic Category Nonsteroidal Anti-inflammatory Drug (NSAID)

Synonyms Ketorolac

Use First parenteral NSAID for analgesia; 30 mg I.M. provides analgesia comparable to 12 mg of morphine or 100 mg of meperidine.

Oral, injection: Short-term (≤5 days) management of moderately-severe acute pain requiring analgesia at the opioid level

Ophthalmic: Temporary relief of ocular itching due to seasonal allergic conjunctivitis; postoperative inflammation following cataract extraction; reduction of ocular pain and photophobia following incisional refractive surgery

Local Anesthetic/Vasoconstrictor Precautions No information available to require special precautions

Effects on Dental Treatment NSAID formulations are known to reversibly decrease platelet aggregation via mechanisms different than observed with aspirin. The dentist should be aware of the potential of abnormal coagulation. Caution should also be exercised in the use of NSAIDs in patients already on anticoagulant therapy with drugs such as warfarin (Coumadin®).

Dosage Use in children <16 years of age is outside of product labeling.

Children 2-16 years: Dosing guidelines are not established; **do not exceed adult doses**

Single-dose treatment:

I.M., I.V.: 0.4-1 mg/kg as a single dose; **Note:** Limited information exists. Single I.V. doses of 0.5 mg/kg, 0.75 mg/kg, 0.9 mg/kg and 1 mg/kg have been studied in children 2-16 years of age for postoperative analgesia. One study (Maunuksela, 1992) used a titrating dose starting with 0.2 mg/kg up to a total of 0.5 mg/kg (median dose required: 0.4 mg/kg).

Oral: One study used 1 mg/kg as a single dose for analgesia in 30 children (mean ± SD age: 3 ± 2.5 years) undergoing bilateral myringotomy

Multiple-dose treatment: I.M., I.V., Oral: No pediatric studies exist; one report (Buck, 1994) of the clinical experience with ketorolac in 112 children, 6 months to 19 years of age (mean: 9 years), described usual I.V. maintenance doses of 0.5 mg/kg every 6 hours (mean dose: 0.52 mg/kg; range: 0.17-1 mg/kg)

Adults (pain relief usually begins within 10 minutes with parenteral forms): **Note:** The maximum combined duration of treatment (for parenteral and oral) is 5 days; do not increase dose or frequency; supplement with low dose opioids if needed for breakthrough pain. For patients <50 kg and/or ≥65 years of age, see Elderly dosing.

I.M.: 60 mg as a single dose or 30 mg every 6 hours (maximum daily dose: 120 mg)

I.V.: 30 mg as a single dose or 30 mg every 6 hours (maximum daily dose: 120 mg)

Oral: 20 mg, followed by 10 mg every 4-6 hours; do not exceed 40 mg/day; oral dosing is intended to be a continuation of I.M. or I.V. therapy only

Ophthalmic: Children ≥12 years and Adults:

Relief of ocular itching: Instill 1 drop (0.25 mg) 4 times/day for seasonal allergic conjunctivitis

Inflammation following cataract extraction: Instill 1 drop (0.25 mg) to affected eye(s) 4 times/day beginning 24 hours after surgery; continue for 2 weeks

Pain and photophobia following incisional refractive surgery: Instill 1 drop (0.25 mg) 4 times/day to affected eye for up to 3 days

Elderly >65 years: Renal insufficiency or weight <50 kg: **Note:** Ketorolac has decreased clearance and increased half-life in the elderly. In addition, the elderly have reported increased incidence of GI bleeding, ulceration, and perforation. The maximum combined duration of treatment (for parenteral and oral) is 5 days.

I.M.: 30 mg as a single dose or 15 mg every 6 hours (maximum daily dose: 60 mg)

I.V.: 15 mg as a single dose or 15 mg every 6 hours (maximum daily dose: 60 mg)

Oral: 10 mg every 4-6 hours; do not exceed 40 mg/day; oral dosing is intended to be a continuation of I.M. or I.V. therapy only

Dosage adjustment in renal impairment: Do not use in patients with advanced renal impairment. Patients with moderately-elevated serum creatinine should use half the recommended dose, not to exceed 60 mg/day I.M./I.V.

Dosage adjustment in hepatic impairment: Use with caution, may cause elevation of liver enzymes

Mechanism of Action Inhibits prostaglandin synthesis by decreasing the activity of the enzyme, cyclo-oxygenase, which results in decreased formation of prostaglandin precursors

Other Adverse Effects

>10%:

Systemic:

Central nervous system: Headache (17%)

Gastrointestinal: Gastrointestinal pain (13%), dyspepsia (12%), nausea (12%)

Ophthalmic solution: Ocular: Transient burning/stinging (Acular®: 40%; Acular® PF: 20%)

>1% to 10%:

Systemic:

Cardiovascular: Edema (4%), hypertension

Central nervous system: Dizziness (7%), drowsiness (6%)

Dermatologic: Pruritus, purpura, rash

Gastrointestinal: Diarrhea (7%), constipation, flatulence, gastrointestinal fullness, vomiting, stomatitis

Local: Injection site pain (2%)

Miscellaneous: Diaphoresis

Ophthalmic solution: Ocular: Ocular irritation, allergic reactions, superficial ocular infection, superficial keratitis, iritis, ocular inflammation

≤1%:

Systemic: Abnormal dreams, abnormal taste, abnormal thinking, abnormal vision, anemia, anorexia, appetite increased, blurred vision, cough, depression, dyspnea, eosinophilia, epistaxis, eructation, euphoria, excessive thirst, extrapyramidal symptoms, fever, gastritis, hallucinations, hearing loss, hematuria, hyperkinesis, inability to concentrate, increased urinary frequency, infections, insomnia, nervousness, oliguria, pallor, palpitation, paresthesia, polyuria, proteinuria, pulmonary edema, rectal bleeding, rhinitis, stupor, syncope, tinnitus, tremors, urinary retention, urticaria, vertigo, weakness, weight gain, xerostomia

Ophthalmic solution: Dry eyes, corneal infiltrates, corneal ulcer, blurred vision, headache

Postmarketing and/or case reports: Acute pancreatitis, acute renal failure, anaphylactoid reaction, anaphylaxis, aseptic meningitis, asthma, azotemia, bronchospasm, cholestatic jaundice, convulsions, exfoliative dermatitis, flank pain, flushing, GI hemorrhage, GI perforation, hematuria, hemolytic uremic syndrome, hepatitis, hyperkalemia, hypersensitivity reactions, hyponatremia, hypotension, laryngeal edema, leukopenia, liver failure, maculopapular rash, melena, myalgia, nephritis, peptic ulceration, psychosis, Stevens-Johnson syndrome, thrombocytopenia, tongue edema, toxic epidermal necrolysis, urticaria, wound hemorrhage (postoperative)

Contraindications Hypersensitivity to ketorolac, aspirin, other NSAIDs, or any component of their formulation; history of nasal polyps, angioedema, or bronchospastic reactions to other NSAIDs; active or history of peptic ulcer disease; recent or history of GI bleeding or perforation; advanced renal disease or risk of renal failure, labor and delivery; nursing mothers; prophylaxis before major surgery; suspected or confirmed cerebrovascular bleeding; hemorrhagic diathesis; concurrent ASA or other NSAIDs; epidural or intrathecal administration, concomitant probenecid; pregnancy (3rd trimester)

Warnings/Precautions Systemic: Treatment should be started with I.V./I.M. administration then changed to oral only as a continuation of treatment. Total therapy is not to exceed 5 days. Should not be used for minor or chronic pain. Hypersensitivity reactions have occurred flowing the first dose of ketorolac injection, including patients without prior exposure to ketorolac, aspirin, or other NSAIDs. Use extra caution and reduce dosages in the elderly because it is cleared renally somewhat slower, and the elderly are also more sensitive to the renal effects of NSAIDs and have a greater risk of GI perforation and bleeding; use with caution in patients with CHF, hypertension, decreased renal or hepatic function, or those receiving anticoagulants. May prolong bleeding time; do not use when hemostasis is critical. Patients should be euvolemic prior to treatment. Low doses of narcotics may be needed for breakthrough pain. Withhold for at least 4-6 half-lives prior to surgical or dental procedures.

Ophthalmic: May increase bleeding time associated with ocular surgery. Use with caution in patients with known bleeding tendencies or those receiving anticoagulants. Do not administer while wearing soft contact lenses. Safety and efficacy in pediatric patients <12 years of age have not been established.

Drug Interactions

ACE inhibitors: Antihypertensive effects may be decreased by concurrent therapy with NSAIDs; monitor BP.

Angiotensin II antagonists: Antihypertensive effects may be decreased by concurrent therapy with NSAIDs; monitor BP.

Anticoagulants: Increased risk of bleeding complications with concomitant use; monitor closely.

(Continued)

Ketorolac Tromethamine *(Continued)*

Antiepileptic drugs (carbamazepine, phenytoin): Sporadic cases of seizures have been reported with concomitant use.

Diuretics: May see decreased effect of diuretics.

Lithium: May increase lithium levels; monitor.

Methotrexate: Severe bone marrow suppression, aplastic anemia, and GI toxicity have been reported with concomitant NSAID therapy. Avoid use during moderate or high-dose methotrexate (increased and prolonged methotrexate levels). NSAID use during low-dose treatment of rheumatoid arthritis has not been fully evaluated; extreme caution is warranted.

Nondepolarizing muscle relaxants: Concomitant use has resulted in apnea.

NSAIDs, salicylates: Concomitant use increases NSAID-induced adverse effects; contraindicated.

Probenecid: Probenecid significantly decreases ketorolac clearance, increases ketorolac plasma levels, and doubles the half-life of ketorolac; concomitant use is contraindicated.

Psychoactive drugs (alprazolam, fluoxetine, thiothixene): Hallucinations have been reported with concomitant use.

ACE inhibitors: Antihypertensive effects may be decreased by concurrent therapy with NSAIDs; monitor BP.

Angiotensin II antagonists: Antihypertensive effects may be decreased by concurrent therapy with NSAIDs; monitor BP.

Anticoagulants: Increased risk of bleeding complications with concomitant use; monitor closely.

Antiepileptic drugs (carbamazepine, phenytoin): Sporadic cases of seizures have been reported with concomitant use.

Diuretics: May see decreased effect of diuretics.

Lithium: May increase lithium levels; monitor.

Methotrexate: May increase methotrexate toxicity, effect seen with other NSAIDs; monitor.

Nondepolarizing muscle relaxants: Concomitant use has resulted in apnea.

NSAIDs, salicylates: Concomitant use increases NSAID-induced adverse effects; contraindicated.

Probenecid: Probenecid significantly decreases ketorolac clearance, increases ketorolac plasma concentrations, and doubles the half-life of ketorolac; concomitant use is contraindicated.

Psychoactive drugs (alprazolam, fluoxetine, thiothixene): Hallucinations have been reported with concomitant use.

Dietary/Ethanol/Herb Considerations

Ethanol: Avoid use; may enhance gastric mucosal irritation.

Food: Administer with food or milk to reduce GI upset. Food decreases rate of absorption but extent remains the same. Oral: High-fat meals may delay time to peak (by ~1 hour) and decrease peak concentrations. Avoid garlic, ginger, and green tea.

Herb/Nutraceutical: Avoid cat's claw, dong quai, evening primrose, feverfew, garlic, ginger, ginkgo biloba, ginseng, green tea, horse chestnut, and red clover due to additional antiplatelet activity. Avoid kava and valerian; may enhance benzodiazepine activity.

Drug Uptake

Onset of action: I.M.: 10 minutes; Peak effect: Analgesic: 2-3 hours

Absorption: Oral: Well absorbed

Duration: 6-8 hours

Half-life, elimination: 2-8 hours; increased 30% to 50% in elderly

Time to peak: I.M.: 30-60 minutes

Pregnancy Risk Factor C/D (3rd trimester); ophthalmic: C

Dosage Forms INJ: 15 mg/mL (1 mL); 30 mg/mL (1 mL, 2 mL). **SOLN, ophthalmic:** (Acular®): 0.5% (3 mL, 5 mL, 10 mL); (Acular® PF) [preservative free]: 0.5% (0.4 mL). **TAB:** 10 mg

Generic Available Yes

Comments According to the manufacturer, ketorolac has been used inappropriately by physicians in the past. The drug had been prescribed to NSAID-sensitive patients, patients with GI bleeding, and for long-term use; a warning has been issued regarding increased incidence and severity of GI complications with increasing doses and duration of use. Labeling now includes the statement that ketorolac inhibits platelet function and is indicated for up to 5 days use only.

Selected Readings

Ahmad N, Grad HA, Haas DA, et al, "The Efficacy of Nonopioid Analgesics for Postoperative Dental Pain: A Meta-analysis," *Anesth Prog*, 1997, 44(4):119-26.

Balevi B, "Ketorolac Versus Ibuprofen: A Simple Cost-Efficacy Comparison for Dental Use," *J Can Dent Assoc*, 1994, 60(1):31-2.

Forbes JA, Butterworth GA, Burchfield WH, et al, "Evaluation of Ketorolac, Aspirin, and an Acetaminophen-Codeine Combination in Postoperative Oral Surgery Pain," *Pharmacotherapy*, 1990, 10(6 Pt 2): 77S-93S.

Forbes JA, Kehm CJ, Grodin CD, et al, "Evaluation of Ketorolac, Ibuprofen, Acetaminophen, and an Acetaminophen-Codeine Combination in Postoperative Oral Surgery Pain," *Pharmacotherapy*, 1990, 10(6 Pt 2):94S-105S.

Fricke JR Jr, Angelocci D, Fox K, et al, "Comparison of the Efficacy and Safety of Ketorolac and Meperidine in the Relief of Dental Pain," *J Clin Pharmacol*, 1992, 32(4):376-84.

Fricke J, Halladay SC, Bynum L, et al, "Pain Relief After Dental Impaction Surgery Using Ketorolac, Hydrocodone Plus Acetaminophen, or Placebo," *Clin Ther*, 1993, 15(3):500-9.

Pendeville PE, Van Boven MJ, Contreras V, et al, "Ketorolac Tromethamine for Postoperative Analgesia in Oral Surgery," *Acta Anaesthesiol Belg*, 1995, 46(1):25-30.

Swift JQ, Roszkowski MT, Alton T, "Effect of Intra-articular Versus Systemic Anti-inflammatory Drugs in a Rabbit Model of Temporomandibular Joint Inflammation," *J Oral Maxillofac Surg*, 1998, 56(11):1288-95 (discussion 1295-6).

Walton GM, Rood JP, Snowdon AT, et al, "Ketorolac and Diclofenac for Postoperative Pain Relief Following Oral Surgery," *Br J Oral Maxillofac Surg*, 1993, 31(3):158-60.

Wynn RL, "Ketorolac (Toradol®) for Dental Pain," *Gen Dent*, 1992, 40(6):476-9.

Ketotifen (kee toe TYE fen)

U.S. Brand Names Zaditor™

Canadian Brand Names Apo®-Ketotifen; Novo-Ketotifen; Zaditen®; Zaditor™

Mexican Brand Names Kasmal®; Ventisol®; Zaditen®

Pharmacologic Category Antihistamine, H_1 Blocker, Ophthalmic

Synonyms Ketotifen Fumarate

Use Temporary prevention of eye itching due to allergic conjunctivitis

Local Anesthetic/Vasoconstrictor Precautions No information available to require special precautions

Effects on Dental Treatment No effects or complications reported

Dosage Children ≥3 years and Adults: Ophthalmic: Instill 1 drop into the affected eye(s) twice daily, every 8-12 hours

Mechanism of Action Relatively selective, noncompetitive H_1-receptor antagonist and mast cell stabilizer, inhibiting the release of mediators from cells involved in hypersensitivity reactions

Other Adverse Effects 1% to 10%:

Ocular: Allergic reactions, burning or stinging, conjunctivitis, discharge, dry eyes, eye pain, eyelid disorder, itching, keratitis, lacrimation disorder, mydriasis, photophobia, rash

Respiratory: Pharyngitis

Miscellaneous: Flu syndrome

Contraindications Hypersensitivity to ketotifen or any component (the preservative is benzalkonium chloride) of the formulation

Warnings/Precautions For topical ophthalmic use only; not to treat contact lens-related irritation. Soft contact lens wearers should wait at least 10 minutes after instillation before putting in lenses in and should not wear contact lenses if eyes are red. Do not contaminate dropper tip or solution when placing drops in eyes. Safety and efficacy not established in patients <3 years of age.

Drug Uptake

Absorption: Minimal systemic

Onset of action: Minutes

Duration: 8-12 hours

Pregnancy Risk Factor C

Generic Available No

Keygesic-10® *see* Magnesium Salicylate *on page 742*

Key-Pred® *see* PrednisoLONE *on page 988*

Key-Pred-SP® *see* PrednisoLONE *on page 988*

K-G® *see* Potassium Gluconate *on page 979*

K-G Tuss® HD *see* Hydrocodone, Pseudoephedrine, and Guaifenesin *on page 608*

Kineret™ *see* Anakinra *on page 100*

Kinevac® *see* Sincalide *on page 1090*

Klaron® *see* Sulfacetamide Sodium *on page 1115*

K-Lease® *see* Potassium Chloride *on page 977*

Klerist-D® [OTC] *see* Chlorpheniramine and Pseudoephedrine *on page 270*

Klonopin™ *see* Clonazepam *on page 307*

K-Lor™ *see* Potassium Chloride *on page 977*

Klor-Con® *see* Potassium Chloride *on page 977*

Klor-Con® 8 *see* Potassium Chloride *on page 977*

Klor-Con® 10 *see* Potassium Chloride *on page 977*

Klor-Con®/25 *see* Potassium Chloride *on page 977*

Klor-Con®/EF *see* Potassium Bicarbonate and Potassium Citrate, Effervescent *on page 976*

Klorvess® *see* Potassium Chloride *on page 977*

Klorvess® Effervescent *see* Potassium Bicarbonate and Potassium Chloride, Effervescent *on page 976*

Klotrix® *see* Potassium Chloride *on page 977*

K-Lyte® *see* Potassium Bicarbonate and Potassium Citrate, Effervescent *on page 976*

K-Lyte/Cl® *see* Potassium Bicarbonate and Potassium Chloride, Effervescent *on page 976*

K-Norm® *see* Potassium Chloride *on page 977*

Koāte®-DVI *see* Antihemophilic Factor (Human) *on page 104*
Kogenate® FS *see* Antihemophilic Factor (Recombinant) *on page 106*
Kolephrin® GG/DM [OTC] *see* Guaifenesin and Dextromethorphan *on page 569*
Kolyum® *see* Potassium Chloride and Potassium Gluconate *on page 978*
Kondon's Nasal® [OTC] *see* Ephedrine *on page 437*
Konsyl® [OTC] *see* Psyllium *on page 1025*
Konsyl-D® [OTC] *see* Psyllium *on page 1025*
Konȳne® 80 *see* Factor IX Complex (Human) *on page 484*
Koromex® [OTC] *see* Nonoxynol 9 *on page 874*
K-Pek® [OTC] *see* Attapulgite *on page 132*
K-Phos® MF *see* Potassium Phosphate and Sodium Phosphate *on page 982*
K-Phos® Neutral *see* Potassium Phosphate and Sodium Phosphate *on page 982*
K-Phos® No. 2 *see* Potassium Phosphate and Sodium Phosphate *on page 982*
K-Phos® Original *see* Potassium Acid Phosphate *on page 975*
Kristalose™ *see* Lactulose *on page 682*
K-Tab® *see* Potassium Chloride *on page 977*
Kutrase® *see* Pancreatin *on page 913*
Ku-Zyme® *see* Pancreatin *on page 913*
Ku-Zyme® HP *see* Pancrelipase *on page 914*
Kwelcof® *see* Hydrocodone and Guaifenesin *on page 603*
Kytril® *see* Granisetron *on page 565*
LA-12® *see* Hydroxocobalamin *on page 612*

Labetalol (la BET a lole)

Related Information

Cardiovascular Diseases *on page 1308*

U.S. Brand Names Normodyne®; Trandate®

Canadian Brand Names Normodyne®; Trandate®

Mexican Brand Names Midotens

Pharmacologic Category Beta Blocker With Alpha-Blocking Activity

Synonyms Ibidomide Hydrochloride; Labetalol Hydrochloride

Use Treatment of mild to severe hypertension; I.V. for hypertensive emergencies

Local Anesthetic/Vasoconstrictor Precautions Use with caution; epinephrine has interacted with nonselective beta-blockers to result in initial hypertensive episode followed by bradycardia

Effects on Dental Treatment Noncardioselective beta-blockers (ie, propranolol, nadolol) enhance the pressor response to epinephrine, resulting in hypertension and bradycardia. Many nonsteroidal anti-inflammatory drugs such as ibuprofen and indomethacin can reduce the hypotensive effect of beta-blockers after 3 or more weeks of therapy with the NSAID. Short-term NSAID use (ie, 3 days) requires no special precautions in patients taking beta-blockers.

Dosage Due to limited documentation of its use, labetalol should be initiated cautiously in pediatric patients with careful dosage adjustment and BP monitoring

Children:

- Oral: Limited information regarding labetalol use in pediatric patients is currently available in literature. Some centers recommend initial oral doses of 4 mg/kg/day in 2 divided doses. Reported oral doses have started at 3 mg/kg/day and 20 mg/kg/day and have increased up to 40 mg/kg/day.
- I.V., intermittent bolus doses of 0.3-1 mg/kg/dose have been reported
- For treatment of pediatric hypertensive emergencies, initial continuous infusions of 0.4-1 mg/kg/hour with a maximum of 3 mg/kg/hour have been used; administration requires the use of an infusion pump

Adults:

- Oral: Initial: 100 mg twice daily, may increase as needed every 2-3 days by 100 mg until desired response is obtained; usual dose: 200-400 mg twice daily; not to exceed 2.4 g/day
- I.V.: 20 mg or 1-2 mg/kg whichever is lower, IVP over 2 minutes, may give 40-80 mg at 10-minute intervals, up to 300 mg total dose
- I.V. infusion: Initial: 2 mg/minute; titrate to response up to 300 mg total dose; administration requires the use of an infusion pump
- **I.V. infusion** (500 mg/250 mL D_5W) rates:
  - 1 mg/minute: 30 mL/hour
  - 2 mg/minute: 60 mL/hour
  - 3 mg/minute: 90 mL/hour
  - 4 mg/minute: 120 mL/hour
  - 5 mg/minute: 150 mL/hour
  - 6 mg/minute: 180 mL/hour

Mechanism of Action Blocks alpha-, $beta_1$-, and $beta_2$-adrenergic receptor sites; elevated renins are reduced

Other Adverse Effects

>10%:

Central nervous system: Dizziness (1% to 16%)

Gastrointestinal: Nausea (0% to 19%)

1% to 10%:

Cardiovascular: Edema (0% to 2%), hypotension (1% to 5%); with IV use, hypotension may occur in up to 58%

Central nervous system: Fatigue (1% to 10%), paresthesia (1% to 5%), headache (2%), vertigo (2%), weakness (1%)

Dermatologic: Rash (1%), scalp tingling (1% to 5%)

Gastrointestinal: Vomiting (<1% to 3%), dyspepsia (1% to 4%)

Genitourinary: Ejaculatory failure (0% to 5%), impotence (1% to 4%)

Hepatic: Increased transaminases (4%)

Respiratory: Nasal congestion (1% to 6%), dyspnea (2%)

Miscellaneous: Taste disorder (1%), abnormal vision (1%)

Other adverse reactions noted with beta-adrenergic blocking agents include mental depression, catatonia, disorientation, short-term memory loss, emotional lability, clouded sensorium, intensification of pre-existing AV block, laryngospasm, respiratory distress, agranulocytosis, thrombocytopenic purpura, nonthrombocytopenic purpura, mesenteric artery thrombosis, and ischemic colitis.

Drug Interactions CYP2D6 enzyme substrate; CYP2D6 enzyme inhibitor

Increased Effect/Toxicity: Inhibitors of CYP2D6 including quinidine, paroxetine, and propafenone are likely to increase blood levels of labetalol. Cimetidine increases the bioavailability of labetalol. Labetalol has additive hypotensive effects with other antihypertensive agents. Concurrent use with alpha-blockers (prazosin, terazosin) and beta-blockers increases the risk of orthostasis. Concurrent use with diltiazem, verapamil, or digoxin may increase the risk of bradycardia with beta-blocking agents. Halothane, enflurane, isoflurane, and potentially other inhalation anesthetics may cause synergistic hypotension. Beta-blockers may affect the action or levels of disopyramide, nondepolarizing muscle relaxants, and theophylline although the effects are difficult to predict.

Decreased Effect: Decreased effect of beta-blockers with aluminum salts, barbiturates, calcium salts, cholestyramine, colestipol, NSAIDs, penicillins (ampicillin), rifampin, salicylates, and sulfinpyrazone due to decreased bioavailability and plasma concentrations. Beta-blockers may decrease the effect of sulfonylureas.

Drug Uptake

Onset of action: Oral: 20 minutes to 2 hours; I.V.: 2-5 minutes

Duration: Oral: 8-24 hours (dose-dependent); I.V.: 2-4 hours

Half-life, elimination: Normal renal function: 2.5-8 hours

Time to peak: Oral: 1-4 hours; I.V.: 5-15 minutes

Pregnancy Risk Factor C (manufacturer); D (2nd and 3rd trimesters - expert analysis)

Generic Available Yes

Lac-Hydrin® *see* Lactic Acid With Ammonium Hydroxide *on page 682*

Lacrisert® *see* Hydroxypropyl Cellulose *on page 615*

Lactaid® [OTC] *see* Lactase *on page 681*

Lactase (LAK tase)

U.S. Brand Names Dairy Ease® [OTC]; Lactaid® [OTC]; Lactrase® [OTC]

Canadian Brand Names Dairyaid®

Pharmacologic Category Enzyme

Use Help digest lactose in milk for patients with lactose intolerance

Local Anesthetic/Vasoconstrictor Precautions No information available to require special precautions

Effects on Dental Treatment No effects or complications reported

Dosage

Capsule: 1-2 capsules taken with milk or meal; pretreat milk with 1-2 capsules/quart of milk

Liquid: 5-15 drops/quart of milk

Tablet: 1-3 tablets with meals

Generic Available No

Lactic Acid and Sodium-PCA

(LAK tik AS id & SOW dee um-pee see aye)

U.S. Brand Names LactiCare® [OTC]

Pharmacologic Category Topical Skin Product

Synonyms Sodium-PCA and Lactic Acid

Use Lubricate and moisturize the skin counteracting dryness and itching

Local Anesthetic/Vasoconstrictor Precautions No information available to require special precautions

Effects on Dental Treatment No effects or complications reported

Dosage Apply as needed

Generic Available No

Lactic Acid With Ammonium Hydroxide

(LAK tik AS id with a MOE nee um hye DROKS ide)

U.S. Brand Names Lac-Hydrin®

Pharmacologic Category Topical Skin Product

Synonyms Ammonium Lactate

Use Treatment of moderate to severe xerosis and ichthyosis vulgaris

Local Anesthetic/Vasoconstrictor Precautions No information available to require special precautions

Effects on Dental Treatment No effects or complications reported

Dosage Children ≥2 years and Adults: Topical: Apply twice daily to affected area; rub in well

Mechanism of Action Exact mechanism of action unknown; lactic acid is a normal component in blood and tissues. When applied topically to the skin, acts as a humectant.

Other Adverse Effects

>10%: Dermatologic: Rash, including erythema and irritation (2% to 15%); burning/stinging (2% to 15%)

1% to 10%: Dermatologic: Itching (5%), dry skin (2%)

Drug Uptake Absorption: 6%

Pregnancy Risk Factor B

Generic Available No

LactiCare® [OTC] *see* Lactic Acid and Sodium-PCA *on page 681*

LactiCare-HC® *see* Hydrocortisone *on page 608*

Lactinex® [OTC] *see Lactobacillus acidophilus* and *Lactobacillus bulgaricus on page 682*

Lactobacillus acidophilus and *Lactobacillus bulgaricus*

(lak toe ba SIL us)

Related Information

Oral Nonviral Soft Tissue Ulcerations or Erosions *on page 1384*

U.S. Brand Names Bacid® [OTC]; Kala® [OTC]; Lactinex® [OTC]; MoreDophilus® [OTC]; Pro-Bionate® [OTC]; Probiotica® [OTC]; Superdophilus® [OTC]

Canadian Brand Names Bacid®; Fermalac

Mexican Brand Names Lacteol® Fort; Sinuberase®

Pharmacologic Category Antidiarrheal; Gastrointestinal Agent, Miscellaneous

Synonyms *Lactobacillus acidophilus*

Use Treatment of uncomplicated diarrhea particularly that caused by antibiotic therapy; re-establish normal physiologic and bacterial flora of the intestinal tract

Local Anesthetic/Vasoconstrictor Precautions No information available to require special precautions

Effects on Dental Treatment No effects or complications reported

Dosage Children >3 years and Adults: Oral:

Capsules: 2 capsules 2-4 times/day

Granules: 1 packet added to or taken with cereal, food, milk, fruit juice, or water, 3-4 times/day

Powder: 1 teaspoonful daily with liquid

Tablet, chewable: 4 tablets 3-4 times/day; may follow each dose with a small amount of milk, fruit juice, or water

Mechanism of Action Creates an environment unfavorable to potentially pathogenic fungi or bacteria through the production of lactic acid, and favors establishment of an aciduric flora, thereby suppressing the growth of pathogenic microorganisms; helps re-establish normal intestinal flora

Other Adverse Effects 1% to 10%: Gastrointestinal: Intestinal flatus

Pregnancy Risk Factor Not available

Generic Available No

Lactrase® [OTC] *see* Lactase *on page 681*

Lactulose (LAK tyoo lose)

U.S. Brand Names Cholac®; Chronulac®; Constilac®; Constulose®; Duphalac®; Enulose®; Evalose®; Kristalose™

Canadian Brand Names Acilac; Laxilose; PMS-Lactulose

Mexican Brand Names Lactulax®; Regulact®

Pharmacologic Category Ammonium Detoxicant; Laxative, Miscellaneous

Use Adjunct in the prevention and treatment of portal-systemic encephalopathy (PSE); treatment of chronic constipation

Local Anesthetic/Vasoconstrictor Precautions No information available to require special precautions

Effects on Dental Treatment No effects or complications reported

Dosage Diarrhea may indicate overdosage and responds to dose reduction

Prevention of portal systemic encephalopathy (PSE): Oral: Older Children: Daily dose of 40-90 mL divided 3-4 times/day; if initial dose causes diarrhea, then reduce it immediately; adjust dosage to produce 2-3 stools/day

Constipation: Oral: Children: 5 g/day (7.5 mL) after breakfast

Adults:

Acute PSE:

Oral: 20-30 g (30-45 mL) every 1-2 hours to induce rapid laxation; adjust dosage daily to produce 2-3 soft stools; doses of 30-45 mL may be given hourly to cause rapid laxation, then reduce to recommended dose; usual daily dose: 60-100 g or 20-30 g (30-45 mL), 3-4 times/day

Rectal administration: 200 g (300 mL) diluted with 700 mL of H_2O or NS; administer rectally via rectal balloon catheter and retain 30-60 minutes every 4-6 hours

Constipation: Oral: 15-30 mL/day increased to 60 mL/day if necessary

Mechanism of Action The bacterial degradation of lactulose resulting in an acidic pH inhibits the diffusion of NH_3 into the blood by causing the conversion of NH_3 to NH_4+; also enhances the diffusion of NH_3 from the blood into the gut where conversion to NH_4+ occurs; produces an osmotic effect in the colon with resultant distention promoting peristalsis

Other Adverse Effects

>10%: Gastrointestinal: Flatulence, diarrhea (excessive dose)

1% to 10%: Gastrointestinal: Abdominal discomfort, nausea, vomiting, cramping

Drug Interactions Decreased Effect: Oral neomycin, laxatives, antacids

Drug Uptake Absorption: Oral: Not appreciable; this is desirable since the intended site of action is within the colon

Pregnancy Risk Factor B

Generic Available Yes

Lamictal® *see* Lamotrigine *on page 684*

Lamisil® Cream *see* Terbinafine, Topical *on page 1141*

Lamisil® Oral *see* Terbinafine, Oral *on page 1141*

Lamivudine (la MI vyoo deen)

Related Information

HIV Infection and AIDS *on page 1334*

Zidovudine and Lamivudine *on page 1258*

U.S. Brand Names Epivir®; Epivir-HBV®

Canadian Brand Names Heptovir®; 3TC®

Pharmacologic Category Antiretroviral Agent, Reverse Transcriptase Inhibitor (Nucleoside)

Synonyms 3TC

Use Treatment of HIV infection when antiretroviral therapy is warranted; should always be used as part of a multidrug regimen (at least three antiretroviral agents); indicated for the treatment of chronic hepatitis B associated with evidence of hepatitis B viral replication and active liver inflammation

Unlabeled/Investigational: Prevention of HIV following needlesticks (with or without protease inhibitor)

Local Anesthetic/Vasoconstrictor Precautions No information available to require special precautions

Effects on Dental Treatment No effects or complications reported

Dosage The formulation and dosage of Epivir-HBV® are not appropriate for patients infected with both HBV and HIV. Use with at least two other antiretroviral agents when treating HIV.

Oral:

Children 3 months to 16 years: HIV: 4 mg/kg twice daily (maximum: 150 mg twice daily)

Children 2-17 years: Treatment of hepatitis B: 3 mg/kg once daily (maximum: 100 mg/day)

Adolescents and Adults: Prevention of HIV following needlesticks: 150 mg twice daily (with zidovudine with or without a protease inhibitor, depending on risk)

Adults:

HIV: 150 mg twice daily; <50 kg: 2 mg/kg twice daily

Treatment of hepatitis B: 100 mg/day

Dosing interval in renal impairment in patients >16 years for HIV:

Cl_{cr} 30-49 mL/minute: Administer 150 mg once daily

Cl_{cr} 15-29 mL/minute: Administer 150 mg first dose, then 100 mg once daily

Cl_{cr} 5-14 mL/minute: Administer 150 mg first dose, then 50 mg once daily

Cl_{cr} <5 mL/minute: Administer 50 mg first dose, then 25 mg once daily

Dosing interval in renal impairment in adult patients with hepatitis B:

Cl_{cr} 30-49: Administer 100 mg first dose then 50 mg once daily

Cl_{cr} 15-29: Administer 100 mg first dose then 25 mg once daily

Cl_{cr} 5-14: Administer 35 mg first dose then 15 mg once daily

Cl_{cr} <5: Administer 35 mg first dose then 10 mg once daily

Dialysis: No data available

Mechanism of Action After lamivudine is triphosphorylated, the principle mode of action is inhibition of HIV reverse transcription via viral DNA chain termination;

(Continued)

Lamivudine *(Continued)*

inhibits RNA- and DNA-dependent DNA polymerase activities of reverse transcriptase. The monophosphate form of lamivudine is incorporated into the viral DNA by hepatitis B virus polymerase, resulting in DNA chain termination.

Other Adverse Effects (As reported in adults treated for HIV infection)

>10%:

Central nervous system: Headache, fatigue

Gastrointestinal: Nausea, diarrhea, vomiting, pancreatitis (range: 0.5% to 18%; higher percentage in pediatric patients)

Neuromuscular & skeletal: Peripheral neuropathy, paresthesia, musculoskeletal pain

1% to 10%:

Central nervous system: Dizziness, depression, fever, chills, insomnia

Dermatologic: Rash

Gastrointestinal: Anorexia, abdominal pain, heartburn, elevated amylase

Hematologic: Neutropenia

Hepatic: Elevated AST, ALT

Neuromuscular & skeletal: Myalgia, arthralgia

Respiratory: Nasal signs and symptoms, cough

Drug Interactions

Increased Effect/Toxicity: Zidovudine concentrations increase significantly (~39%) with lamivudine coadministration. Trimethoprim/sulfamethoxazole increases lamivudine's blood levels. Concomitant use of ribavirin and nucleoside analogues may increase the risk of developing lactic acidosis (including adefovir, didanosine, lamivudine, stavudine, zalcitabine, zidovudine).

Decreased Effect: Zalcitabine and lamivudine may inhibit the intracellular phosphorylation of each other; concomitant use should be avoided.

Drug Uptake

Absorption: Oral: Rapid

Half-life, elimination: Children: 2 hours; Adults: 5-7 hours

Pregnancy Risk Factor C

Generic Available No

Lamotrigine (la MOE tri jeen)

U.S. Brand Names Lamictal®

Canadian Brand Names Lamictal®

Mexican Brand Names Lamictal®

Pharmacologic Category Anticonvulsant, Miscellaneous

Synonyms BW-430C; LTG

Use Adjunctive therapy in the treatment of partial seizures in adults with epilepsy (safety and effectiveness in children <16 years of age have not been established); conversion to monotherapy in adults with partial seizures who are receiving treatment with a single enzyme-inducing antiepileptic drug

Orphan drug: Adjunctive therapy in the generalized seizures of Lennox-Gastaut syndrome in pediatrics and adults

Unlabeled/Investigational: Bipolar disorder

Local Anesthetic/Vasoconstrictor Precautions No information available to require special precautions

Effects on Dental Treatment No effects or complications reported

Dosage Oral:

Children <6.7 kg: Not recommended

Children 2-12 years: Lennox-Gastaut (adjunctive): **Note:** Children 2-6 years will likely require maintenance doses at the higher end of recommended range; only whole tablets should be used for dosing, rounded down to the nearest whole tablet

Patients receiving AED regimens containing valproic acid:

Weeks 1 and 2: 0.15 mg/kg/day in 1-2 divided doses; round dose down to the nearest whole tablet. For patients >6.7 kg and <14 kg, dosing should be 2 mg every other day.

Weeks 3 and 4: 0.3 mg/kg/day in 1-2 divided doses; round dose down to the nearest whole tablet; may use combinations of 2 mg and 5 mg tablets. For patients >6.7 kg and <14 kg, dosing should be 2 mg/day.

Maintenance dose: Titrate dose to effect; after week 4, increase dose every 1-2 weeks by a calculated increment; calculate increment as 0.3 mg/kg/day rounded down to the nearest whole tablet; add this amount to the previously administered daily dose; usual maintenance: 1-5 mg/kg/day in 1-2 divided doses; maximum: 200 mg/day given in 1-2 divided doses

Patients receiving enzyme-inducing AED regimens without valproic acid:

Weeks 1 and 2: 0.6 mg/kg/day in 2 divided doses; round dose down to the nearest whole tablet

Weeks 3 and 4: 1.2 mg/kg/day in 2 divided doses; round dose down to the nearest whole tablet

Maintenance dose: Titrate dose to effect; after week 4, increase dose every 1-2 weeks by a calculated increment; calculate increment as 1.2 mg/kg/day rounded down to the nearest whole tablet; add this amount to the previously administered daily dose; usual maintenance: 5-15 mg/kg/day in 2 divided doses; maximum: 400 mg/day

Children >12 years: Lennox-Gastaut (adjunctive): See adult dosing

Children ≥16 years: Treatment of partial seizures (adjunctive) or conversion from single enzyme-inducing AED regimen to monotherapy: See adult dosing

Adults:

Lennox-Gastaut (adjunctive) or treatment of partial seizures (adjunctive):

Patients receiving AED regimens containing valproic acid:

Initial dose: 25 mg every other day for 2 weeks, then 25 mg every day for 2 weeks

Maintenance dose: 100-400 mg/day in 1-2 divided doses (usual range 100-200 mg/day). Dose may be increased by 25-50 mg every day for 1-2 weeks in order to achieve maintenance dose.

Patients receiving enzyme-inducing AED regimens without valproic acid:

Initial dose: 50 mg/day for 2 weeks, then 100 mg in 2 doses for 2 weeks; thereafter, daily dose can be increased by 100 mg every 1-2 weeks to be given in 2 divided doses

Usual maintenance dose: 300-500 mg/day in 2 divided doses; doses as high as 700 mg/day have been reported

Partial seizures (monotherapy) conversion from single enzyme-inducing AED regimen: Initial dose: 50 mg/day for 2 weeks, then 100 mg in 2 doses for 2 weeks; thereafter, daily dose should be increased by 100 mg every 1-2 weeks to be given in 2 divided doses until reaching a dose of 500 mg/day. Concomitant enzyme inducing AED should then be withdrawn by 20% decrements each week over a 4-week period. Patients should be monitored for rash.

Bipolar disorder (unlabeled use): 25 mg/day for 2 weeks, followed by 50 mg/day for 2 weeks, followed by 100 mg/day for 1 week; thereafter, daily dosage may be increased by 100 mg/week, up to a maximum of 500 mg/day as clinically indicated

Dosage adjustment in renal impairment: Decreased dosage may be effective in patients with significant renal impairment; use with caution

Mechanism of Action A triazine derivative which inhibits release of glutamate (an excitatory amino acid) and inhibits voltage-sensitive sodium channels, which stabilizes neuronal membranes. Lamotrigine has weak inhibitory effect on the 5-HT_3 receptor; *in vitro* inhibits dihydrofolate reductase.

Other Adverse Effects

>10%:

Central nervous system: Headache (29%), dizziness (7% to 38%), ataxia (7% to 22%), somnolence

Gastrointestinal: Nausea (7% to 19%)

Ocular: Diplopia (28%), blurred vision (16%)

Respiratory: Rhinitis (7% to 14%)

1% to 10%:

Central nervous system: Depression (4%), anxiety (4%), irritability, emotional lability, confusion, speech disorder, difficulty concentrating, malaise, seizure (3% to 4%), incoordination, insomnia (5% to 6%)

Dermatologic: Hypersensitivity rash (10%), pruritus (3%)

Gastrointestinal: Abdominal pain, vomiting (9%), diarrhea (6%), dyspepsia (5% to 7%), constipation (4%), anorexia (2%)

Genitourinary: Vaginitis (4%), dysmenorrhea (7%)

Neuromuscular & skeletal: Tremor (6%), arthralgia, joint pain

Ocular: Nystagmus (2%)

Miscellaneous: Flu syndrome (7%), fever (2% to 6%)

Warnings/Precautions Use caution in writing and/or interpreting prescriptions/orders; medication dispensing errors have occurred with similar-sounding medications (Lamisil®, Ludiomil®, lamivudine, labetalol, and Lomotil®).

Drug Interactions Effects on CYP not characterized, may act as inducer.

Increased Effect/Toxicity: Lamotrigine may increase the epoxide metabolite of carbamazepine resulting in toxicity. Valproic acid increases blood levels of lamotrigine. Toxicity has been reported following addition of sertraline (limited documentation).

Decreased Effect: Acetaminophen, carbamazepine, phenytoin, phenobarbital may decrease concentrations of lamotrigine. Lamotrigine enhances the metabolism of valproic acid.

Drug Uptake

Half-life, elimination: 24 hours; Concomitant valproic acid therapy: 59 hours; Concomitant phenytoin or carbamazepine therapy: 15 hours

Time to peak: 1-4 hours

Pregnancy Risk Factor C

Generic Available No

Lamprene® *see* Clofazimine *on page 304*

Lanacane® [OTC] *see* Benzocaine *on page 151*

Lanacort® [OTC] *see* Hydrocortisone *on page 608*

Lanaphilic® [OTC] *see* Urea *on page 1221*

Lanolin, Cetyl Alcohol, Glycerin, and Petrolatum

(LAN oh lin, SEE til AL koe hol, GLIS er in, pe troe LAY tum, & MIN er al oyl)

U.S. Brand Names Lubriderm® [OTC]; Lubriderm® Fragrance Free [OTC]

Pharmacologic Category Topical Skin Product

Synonyms Mineral Oil, Petrolatum, Lanolin, Cetyl Alcohol, and Glycerin

Use Treatment of dry skin

Local Anesthetic/Vasoconstrictor Precautions No information available to require special precautions

Effects on Dental Treatment No effects or complications reported

Dosage Topical: Apply to skin as necessary

Other Adverse Effects 1% to 10%: Local irritation

Pregnancy Risk Factor C

Generic Available Yes

Lanoxicaps® *see* Digoxin *on page 389*

Lanoxin® *see* Digoxin *on page 389*

Lansoprazole (lan SOE pra zole)

Related Information

Gastrointestinal Disorders *on page 1326*

U.S. Brand Names Prevacid®

Canadian Brand Names Prevacid®

Mexican Brand Names Ilsatec®; Ogastro®; Ulpax®

Pharmacologic Category Proton Pump Inhibitor

Use Short-term treatment of active duodenal ulcers; maintenance treatment of healed duodenal ulcers; as part of a multidrug regimen for *H. pylori* eradication to reduce the risk of duodenal ulcer recurrence; short-term treatment of active benign gastric ulcer; treatment of NSAID-associated gastric ulcer; to reduce the risk of NSAID-associated gastric ulcer in patients with a history of gastric ulcer who require an NSAID; short-term treatment of symptomatic GERD; short-term treatment for all grades of erosive esophagitis; to maintain healing of erosive esophagitis; long-term treatment of pathological hypersecretory conditions, including Zollinger-Ellison syndrome

Local Anesthetic/Vasoconstrictor Precautions No information available to require special precautions

Effects on Dental Treatment No effects or complications reported

Dosage Oral:

Adults:

Duodenal ulcer: Short-term treatment: 15 mg once daily for 4 weeks; maintenance therapy: 15 mg once daily

Gastric ulcer: Short-term treatment: 30 mg once daily for up to 8 weeks

NSAID-associated gastric ulcer (healing): 30 mg once daily for 8 weeks; controlled studies did not extend past 8 weeks of therapy

NSAID-associated gastric ulcer (to reduce risk): Oral: 15 mg once daily for up to 12 weeks; controlled studies did not extend past 12 weeks of therapy

Symptomatic GERD: Short-term treatment: 15 mg once daily for up to 8 weeks

Erosive esophagitis: Short-term treatment: 30 mg once daily for up to 8 weeks; continued treatment for an additional 8 weeks may be considered for recurrence or for patients that do not heal after the first 8 weeks of therapy; maintenance therapy: 15 mg once daily

Hypersecretory conditions: Initial: 60 mg once daily; adjust dose based upon patient response and to reduce acid secretion to <10 mEq/hour (5 mEq/hour in patients with prior gastric surgery); doses of 90 mg twice daily have been used; administer doses >120 mg/day in divided doses

Helicobacter pylori eradication: Currently accepted recommendations (may differ from product labeling): Dose varies with regimen: 30 mg once daily or 60 mg/day in 2 divided doses; requires combination therapy with antibiotics

Elderly: No dosage adjustment is needed in elderly patients with normal hepatic function

Dosing adjustment in hepatic impairment: Dose reduction is necessary for severe hepatic impairment

Mechanism of Action A proton pump inhibitor which decreases acid secretion in gastric parietal cells

Other Adverse Effects 1% to 10%: Gastrointestinal: Abdominal pain (2%), diarrhea (4%, more likely at doses of 60 mg/day), constipation (1%), nausea (1%)

Drug Interactions CYP2C19 enzyme substrate, CYP3A3/4 enzyme substrate (minor)

Ampicillin esters: Decreased absorption of ampicillin possible due to decreased acid levels produced by lansoprazole.

Antifungal agents (Itraconazole, ketoconazole): Decreased absorption of antifungal agent possible due to decreased acid levels produced by lansoprazole.

Digoxin: Decreased absorption of digoxin possible due to decreased acid levels produced by lansoprazole.

Iron salts: Decreased absorption of iron possible due to decreased acid levels produced by lansoprazole.

Sucralfate: Sucralfate delays the absorption and reduces the bioavailability of lansoprazole; lansoprazole should be taken ≥30 minutes prior to sucralfate to avoid this interaction.

Theophylline: Clearance of theophylline increased by ~10%; monitor theophylline levels when lansoprazole therapy is started and stopped.

Drug Uptake

Absorption: Rapid

Duration: >24 hours

Half-life, elimination: 1.5 hours; Elderly: 2.9 hours; Cirrhosis: 7 hours

Time to peak, plasma: 1.7 hours

Pregnancy Risk Factor B

Generic Available No

Lantus® *see* Insulin Preparations *on page 639*

Lariam® *see* Mefloquine *on page 755*

Larodopa® *see* Levodopa *on page 699*

Lasix® *see* Furosemide *on page 544*

Latanoprost (la TAN oh prost)

U.S. Brand Names Xalatan®

Canadian Brand Names Xalatan™

Mexican Brand Names Xalatan®

Pharmacologic Category Ophthalmic Agent, Antiglaucoma; Prostaglandin, Ophthalmic

Use Reduction of elevated intraocular pressure in patients with open-angle glaucoma and ocular hypertension who are intolerant of the other IOP lowering medications or insufficiently responsive (failed to achieve target IOP determined after multiple measurements over time) to another IOP lowering medication

Local Anesthetic/Vasoconstrictor Precautions No information available to require special precautions

Effects on Dental Treatment No effects or complications reported

Dosage Ophthalmic: Recommended dosage is one drop (1.5 g) in the affected eye(s) once daily in the evening. Dosage should not exceed once daily.

Mechanism of Action Latanoprost is a prostaglandin F_2-alpha analog believed to reduce intraocular pressure by increasing the outflow of the aqueous humor

Other Adverse Effects

>10%: Ocular: Blurred vision, burning and stinging, conjunctival hyperemia, foreign body sensation, itching, increased pigmentation of the iris, and punctate epithelial keratopathy

1% to 10%:

Cardiovascular: Chest pain, angina pectoris

Dermatologic: Rash, allergic skin reaction

Neuromuscular & skeletal: Myalgia, arthralgia, back pain

Ocular: Dry eye, excessive tearing, eye pain, lid crusting, lid edema, lid erythema, lid discomfort/pain, photophobia

Respiratory: Upper respiratory tract infection, cold, flu

Drug Interactions *In vitro* studies have shown that precipitation occurs when eye drops containing thimerosal are mixed with latanoprost. If such drugs are used, administer with an interval of at least 5 minutes between applications

Drug Uptake

Onset of action: 3-4 hours; Peak effect: Maximum: 8-12 hours

Absorption: Through the cornea where the isopropyl ester prodrug is hydrolyzed by esterases to the biologically active acid

Half-life, elimination: 17 minutes

Time to peak: Topical: 2 hours, in the aqueous humor

Pregnancy Risk Factor C

Generic Available No

Lederplex® [OTC] *see* Vitamin B Complex *on page 1244*

Leflunomide (le FLU no mide)

Related Information

Rheumatoid Arthritis and Osteoarthritis *on page 1340*

U.S. Brand Names Arava™

Canadian Brand Names Arava™

Pharmacologic Category Antirheumatic, Disease Modifying

Use Treatment of active rheumatoid arthritis to reduce signs and symptoms and to retard structural damage as evidenced by x-ray erosions and joint space narrowing

Local Anesthetic/Vasoconstrictor Precautions No information available to require special precautions

Effects on Dental Treatment 1% to 10%: Stomatitis (3%), gingivitis, candidiasis (oral), enlarged salivary gland, tooth disorder, xerostomia, taste disturbance

(Continued)

Leflunomide *(Continued)*

Dosage

Adults: Oral: Initial: 100 mg/day for 3 days, followed by 20 mg/day; dosage may be decreased to 10 mg/day in patients who have difficulty tolerating the 20 mg dose. Due to the long half-life of the active metabolite, plasma levels may require a prolonged period to decline after dosage reduction.

Dosing adjustment in renal impairment: No specific dosage adjustment is recommended. There is no clinical experience in the use of leflunomide in patients with renal impairment. The free fraction of MI is doubled in dialysis patients. Patients should be monitored closely for adverse effects requiring dosage adjustment.

Dosing adjustment in hepatic impairment: No specific dosage adjustment is recommended. Since the liver is involved in metabolic activation and subsequent metabolism/elimination of leflunomide, patients with hepatic impairment should be monitored closely for adverse effects requiring dosage adjustment.

Guidelines for dosage adjustment or discontinuation based on the severity and persistence of ALT elevation secondary to leflunomide have been developed. For ALT elevations >2 times the upper limit of normal, dosage reduction to 10 mg/day may allow continued administration (consider increased monitoring frequency - ie, weekly). Cholestyramine 8 g 3 times/day for 1-3 days may be administered to decrease plasma levels. If elevations >2 times but ≤3 times the upper limit of normal persist, liver biopsy is recommended. If elevations >3 times the upper limit of normal persist despite cholestyramine administration and dosage reduction, leflunomide should be discontinued and drug elimination should be enhanced with additional cholestyramine as indicated.

Elderly: Although hepatic function may decline with age, no specific dosage adjustment is recommended. Patients should be monitored closely for adverse effects which may require dosage adjustment.

Mechanism of Action Inhibits pyrimidine synthesis, resulting in antiproliferative and anti-inflammatory effects

Other Adverse Effects

>10%:

Gastrointestinal: Diarrhea (17%)

Respiratory: Respiratory tract infection (15%)

1% to 10%:

Cardiovascular: Hypertension (10%), chest pain (2%), palpitation, tachycardia, vasculitis, vasodilation, varicose vein, edema (peripheral)

Central nervous system: Headache (7%), dizziness (4%), pain (2%), fever, malaise, migraine, anxiety, depression, insomnia, sleep disorder

Dermatologic: Alopecia (10%), rash (10%), pruritus (4%), dry skin (2%), eczema (2%), acne, dermatitis, hair discoloration, hematoma, herpes infection, nail disorder, subcutaneous nodule, skin disorder/discoloration, skin ulcer, bruising

Endocrine & metabolic: Hypokalemia (1%), diabetes mellitus, hyperglycemia, hyperlipidemia, hyperthyroidism, menstrual disorder

Gastrointestinal: Nausea (9%), abdominal pain (5%), dyspepsia (5%), weight loss (4%), anorexia (3%), gastroenteritis (3%), stomatitis (3%), vomiting (3%), cholelithiasis, colitis, constipation, esophagitis, flatulence, gastritis, gingivitis, melena, candidiasis (oral), enlarged salivary gland, tooth disorder, xerostomia, taste disturbance

Genitourinary: Urinary tract infection (5%), albuminuria, cystitis, dysuria, hematuria, vaginal candidiasis, prostate disorder, urinary frequency

Hematologic: Anemia

Hepatic: Abnormal LFTs (5%)

Neuromuscular & skeletal: Back pain (5%), joint disorder (4%), weakness (3%), tenosynovitis (3%), synovitis (2%), arthralgia (1%), paresthesia (2%), muscle cramps (1%), neck pain, pelvic pain, increased CPK, arthrosis, bursitis, myalgia, bone necrosis, bone pain, tendon rupture, neuralgia, neuritis

Ocular: Blurred vision, cataract, conjunctivitis, eye disorder

Respiratory: Bronchitis (7%), cough (3%), pharyngitis (3%), pneumonia (2%), rhinitis (2%), sinusitis (2%), asthma, dyspnea, epistaxis, lung disorder

Miscellaneous: Infection (4%), accidental injury (5%), allergic reactions (2%), diaphoresis

Drug Interactions CYP2C9 enzyme inhibitor (*in vitro* only)

Increased Effect/Toxicity: Theoretically, concomitant use of drugs metabolized by this enzyme, including many NSAIDs, may result in increased serum concentration and possible toxic effects. Coadministration with methotrexate increases the risk of hepatotoxicity. Leflunomide may also enhance the hepatotoxicity of other drugs. Tolbutamide free fraction may be increased. Rifampin may increase serum concentration of leflunomide. Leflunomide has uricosuric activity and may enhance activity of other uricosuric agents.

Decreased Effect: Administration of cholestyramine and activated charcoal enhance the elimination of leflunomide's active metabolite.

Drug Uptake

Half-life, elimination, mean: 14-15 days; enterohepatic recycling appears to contribute to the long half-life of this agent, since activated charcoal and cholestyramine substantially reduce plasma half-life

Time to peak: 6-12 hours

Pregnancy Risk Factor X

Generic Available No

Legatrin PM® [OTC] *see* Acetaminophen and Diphenhydramine *on page 30*

Lente® Iletin® II *see* Insulin Preparations *on page 639*

Lepirudin (leh puh ROO din)

Related Information

Cardiovascular Diseases *on page 1308*

U.S. Brand Names Refludan®

Canadian Brand Names Refludan®

Pharmacologic Category Anticoagulant, Thrombin Inhibitor

Synonyms Lepirudin (rDNA); Recombinant Hirudin

Use Indicated for anticoagulation in patient with heparin-induced thrombocytopenia (HIT) and associated thromboembolic disease in order to prevent further thromboembolic complications

Unlabeled/Investigational: Prevention or reduction of ischemic complications associated with unstable angina

Local Anesthetic/Vasoconstrictor Precautions No information available to require special precautions

Effects on Dental Treatment Mouth bleeding and tongue edema reported

Dosage Adults: Maximum dose: Do not exceed 0.21 mg/kg/hour unless an evaluation of coagulation abnormalities limiting response has been completed. **Dosing is weight-based, however patients weighing >110 kg should not receive doses greater than the recommended dose for a patient weighing 110 kg (44 mg bolus and initial maximal infusion rate of 16.5 mg/hour).**

Heparin-induced thrombocytopenia: Bolus dose: 0.4 mg/kg IVP (over 15-20 seconds), followed by continuous infusion at 0.15 mg/kg/hour; bolus and infusion must be reduced in renal insufficiency

Concomitant use with thrombolytic therapy: Bolus dose: 0.2 mg/kg IVP (over 15-20 seconds), followed by continuous infusion at 0.1 mg/kg/hour

Dosing adjustments during infusions: Monitor first aPTT 4 hours after the start of the infusion. Subsequent determinations of aPTT should be obtained at least once daily during treatment. More frequent monitoring is recommended in renally impaired patients. Any aPTT ratio measurement out of range (1.5-2.5) should be confirmed prior to adjusting dose, unless a clinical need for immediate reaction exists. If the aPTT is below target range, increase infusion by 20%. If the aPTT is in excess of the target range, decrease infusion rate by 50%. A repeat aPTT should be obtained 4 hours after any dosing change.

Use in patients scheduled for switch to oral anticoagulants: Reduce lepirudin dose gradually to reach aPTT ratio just above 1.5 before starting warfarin therapy; as soon as INR reaches 2.0, lepirudin therapy should be discontinued.

Dosing adjustment in renal impairment: All patients with a creatinine clearance of <60 mL/minute or a serum creatinine of >1.5 mg/dL should receive a reduction in lepirudin dosage; there is only limited information on the therapeutic use of lepirudin in HIT patients with significant renal impairment; the following dosage recommendations are mainly based on single-dose studies in a small number of patients with renal impairment.

Initial: Bolus dose: 0.2 mg/kg IVP (over 15-20 seconds), followed by adjusted infusion based on renal function; refer to the following infusion rate adjustments based on creatinine clearance (mL/minute) and serum creatinine (mg/dL): See table.

Lepirudin Infusion Rates in Patients With Renal Impairment

Creatinine Clearance (mL/minute)	Serum Creatinine (mg/dL)	Adjusted Infusion Rate	
		% of Standard Initial Infusion Rate	mg/kg/hour
45-60	1.6-2.0	50%	0.075
30-44	2.1-3.0	30%	0.045
15-29	3.1-6.0	15%	0.0225
<15	>6.0	Avoid or STOP infusion	

Acute renal failure or hemodialysis: Infusion is to be avoided or stopped. Following the bolus dose, additional bolus doses of 0.1 mg/kg may be administered every other day (only if aPTT falls below lower therapeutic limit).

(Continued)

Lepirudin *(Continued)*

Mechanism of Action Lepirudin is a highly specific direct thrombin inhibitor. Each molecule is capable of binding one molecule of thrombin and inhibiting its thrombogenic activity. Lepirudin is a recombinant hirudin derived from yeast cells.

Other Adverse Effects As with all anticoagulants, bleeding is the most common adverse event associated with lepirudin. Hemorrhage may occur at virtually any site. Risk is dependent on multiple variables.

HIT patients:

>10%: Hematologic: Anemia (12%), bleeding from puncture sites (11%), hematoma (11%)

1% to 10%:

Cardiovascular: Heart failure (3%), pericardial effusion (1%), ventricular fibrillation (1%)
Central nervous system: Fever (7%)
Dermatologic: Eczema (3%), maculopapular rash (4%)
Gastrointestinal: GI bleeding/rectal bleeding (5%)
Genitourinary: Vaginal bleeding (2%)
Hepatic: Increased transaminases (6%)
Renal: Hematuria (4%)
Respiratory: Epistaxis (4%)

Non-HIT populations (including those receiving thrombolytics and/or contrast media):

1% to 10%: Respiratory: Bronchospasm/stridor/dyspnea/cough

Drug Interactions Increased Effect/Toxicity: Thrombolytics may enhance anticoagulant properties of lepirudin on aPTT and can increase the risk of bleeding complications. Bleeding risk may also be increased by oral anticoagulants (warfarin) and platelet function inhibitors (nonsteroidal anti-inflammatory drugs, dipyridamole, ticlopidine, clopidogrel, IIb/IIIa antagonists, and aspirin).

Drug Uptake Half-life, elimination: Initial: ~10 minutes: Terminal: Healthy volunteers: 1.3 hours; Marked renal insufficiency (Cl_{cr} <15 mL/minute and on hemodialysis: ≤2 days)

Pregnancy Risk Factor B

Generic Available No

Lescol® *see* Fluvastatin *on page 527*
Lescol® XL *see* Fluvastatin *on page 527*
Lessina™ *see* Combination Hormonal Contraceptives *on page 323*

Letrozole (LET roe zole)

U.S. Brand Names Femara®

Canadian Brand Names Femara®

Pharmacologic Category Antineoplastic Agent, Aromatase Inhibitor

Use First-line treatment of hormone receptor positive or hormone receptor unknown, locally advanced, or metastatic breast cancer in postmenopausal women; treatment of advanced breast cancer in postmenopausal women with disease progression following antiestrogen therapy

Local Anesthetic/Vasoconstrictor Precautions No information available to require special precautions

Effects on Dental Treatment No effects or complications reported

Mechanism of Action Nonsteroidal, competitive inhibitor of the aromatase enzyme system which binds to the heme group of aromatase, a cytochrome P450 enzyme which catalyzes conversion of androgens to estrogens (specifically, androstenedione to estrone and testosterone to estradiol). This leads to inhibition of the enzyme and a significant reduction in plasma estrogen levels. Does not affect synthesis of adrenal or thyroid hormones, aldosterone, or androgens.

Other Adverse Effects

>10% :

Cardiovascular: Hot flushes (5% to 18%)
Central nervous system: Headache (8% to 12%), fatigue (6% to 11%)
Gastrointestinal: Nausea (13% to 15%)
Neuromuscular & skeletal: Musculoskeletal pain, bone pain (20%), back pain (17%), arthralgia (8% to 14%),
Respiratory: Dyspnea (7% to 14%), cough (5% to 11%)

2% to 10%:

Cardiovascular: Chest pain (3% to 8%), peripheral edema (5%), hypertension (5% to 7%)
Central nervous system: Pain (5%), insomnia (6%), dizziness (3% to 5%), somnolence (2% to 3%), depression (<5%), anxiety (<5%), vertigo (<5%)
Dermatologic: Rash (5%), alopecia (<5% to 5%), pruritus (1%)
Endocrine & metabolic: Breast pain (5%), hypercholesterolemia (3%)
Gastrointestinal: Vomiting (7%), constipation (6% to 9%), diarrhea (5% to 7%), abdominal pain (4% to 6%), anorexia (4%), dyspepsia (3% to 4%), weight loss (6%), weight gain (2%)
Neuromuscular & skeletal: Weakness (4% to 5%)

Miscellaneous: Flu (5% to 6%)

<2% Angina, cardiac ischemia, coronary artery disease, hemiparesis, hemorrhagic stroke, increased bilirubin, increased transaminases, lymphopenia, myocardial infarction, portal vein thrombosis, pulmonary embolism, thrombocytopenia, thrombophlebitis, thrombotic stroke, transient ischemic attack, vaginal bleeding, venous thrombosis

Drug Interactions CYP3A3/4 and 2A6 enzyme substrate; CYP2A6 and 2C19 enzyme inhibitor

Increased Effect/Toxicity: Inhibitors of this enzyme may, in theory, increase letrozole blood levels. Letrozole inhibits cytochrome P450 isoenzyme 2A6 and 2C19 *in vitro* and may increase blood levels of drugs metabolized by these enzymes. Specific drug interaction studies have not been reported.

Drug Uptake

Absorption: Well, nearly 100%; not affected by food

Half-life, elimination: Terminal: 2 days

Time to steady state, plasma: 2-6 weeks

Pregnancy Risk Factor D

Generic Available No

Leucovorin (loo koe VOR in)

U.S. Brand Names Wellcovorin®

Mexican Brand Names Dalisol; Flynoken A; Medsavorin

Pharmacologic Category Antidote; Vitamin, Water Soluble

Synonyms Calcium Leucovorin; Citrovorum Factor; Folinic Acid; 5-Formyl Tetrahydrofolate; Leucovorin Calcium

Use Antidote for folic acid antagonists; treatment of folate deficient megaloblastic anemias of infancy, sprue, pregnancy; nutritional deficiency when oral folate therapy is not possible; in combination with fluorouracil in the treatment of malignancy

Local Anesthetic/Vasoconstrictor Precautions No information available to require special precautions

Effects on Dental Treatment No effects or complications reported

Dosage Children and Adults:

Treatment of folic acid antagonist overdosage (eg, pyrimethamine or trimethoprim): Oral: 2-15 mg/day for 3 days or until blood counts are normal or 5 mg every 3 days; doses of 6 mg/day are needed for patients with platelet counts <100,000/ mm^3

Folate-deficient megaloblastic anemia: I.M.: 1 mg/day

Megaloblastic anemia secondary to congenital deficiency of dihydrofolate reductase: I.M.: 3-6 mg/day

Rescue dose (rescue therapy should start within 24 hours of MTX therapy): I.V.: 10 mg/m^2 to start, then 10 mg/m^2 every 6 hours orally for 72 hours until serum MTX concentration is $<10^{-8}$ molar; if serum creatinine 24 hours after methotrexate is elevated 50% or more above the pre-MTX serum creatinine **or** the serum MTX concentration is $>5 \times 10^{-6}$ molar (see graph), increase dose to 100 mg/m^2/dose every 3 hours until serum methotrexate level is $<1 \times 10^{-8}$ molar

Unlabeled/Investigational: Post I.T. methotrexate: Oral, I.V.: 12 mg/m^2 as a single dose; post high-dose methotrexate: 100-1000 mg/m^2/dose until the serum methotrexate level is less than 1×10^{-7} molar. See figure.

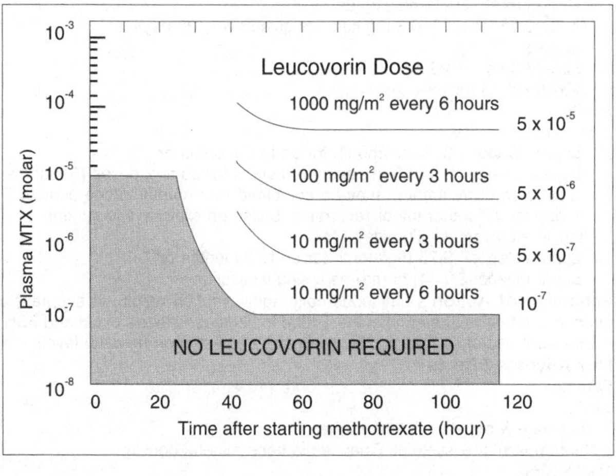

(Continued)

Leucovorin *(Continued)*

The drug should be given parenterally instead of orally in patients with GI toxicity, nausea, vomiting, and when individual doses are >25 mg

Mechanism of Action A reduced form of folic acid, but does not require a reduction reaction by an enzyme for activation, allows for purine and thymidine synthesis, a necessity for normal erythropoiesis; leucovorin supplies the necessary cofactor blocked by MTX, enters the cells via the same active transport system as MTX

Other Adverse Effects Frequency not defined:
Dermatologic: Rash, pruritus, erythema, urticaria,
Hematologic: Thrombocytosis
Respiratory: Wheezing
Miscellaneous: Anaphylactoid reactions

Drug Interactions
Increased Effect/Toxicity: Increased toxicity of fluorouracil
Decreased Effect: May decrease efficacy of co-trimoxazole against *Pneumocystis carinii* pneumonitis

Drug Uptake
Onset of action: Oral: ~30 minutes; I.V.: ~5 minutes
Absorption: Oral, I.M.: Rapid and well
Half-life, elimination: Leucovorin: 15 minutes; 5MTHF: 33-35 minutes

Pregnancy Risk Factor C

Generic Available Yes

Comments Drug should be given parenterally instead of orally in patients with GI toxicity, nausea, vomiting, and when individual doses are >25 mg

Leukeran® *see* Chlorambucil *on page 261*
Leukine™ *see* Sargramostim *on page 1075*

Leuprolide Acetate (loo PROE lide)

U.S. Brand Names Eligard™; Lupron®; Lupron Depot®; Lupron Depot-Ped®; Viadur™

Canadian Brand Names Lupron®; Lupron® Depot®; Viadur™

Mexican Brand Names Lucrin; Lucrin Depot

Pharmacologic Category Antineoplastic Agent, Miscellaneous; Luteinizing Hormone-Releasing Hormone Analog

Synonyms Leuprolide; Leuprorelin; Leuprorelin Acetate

Use Palliative treatment of advanced prostate carcinoma (alternative when orchiectomy or estrogen administration are not indicated or are unacceptable to the patient); combination therapy with flutamide for treating metastatic prostatic carcinoma; treatment of endometriosis as initial treatment and/or treatment of recurrent symptoms; central precocious puberty (may be used an agent to treat precocious puberty because of its effect in lowering levels of LH and FSH, testosterone, and estrogen).

Unlabeled/Investigational: Treatment of breast, ovarian, and endometrial cancer; leiomyoma uteri; infertility; prostatic hyperplasia

Local Anesthetic/Vasoconstrictor Precautions No information available to require special precautions

Effects on Dental Treatment No effects or complications reported

Dosage Requires parenteral administration
Children: Precocious puberty:
S.C. (Lupron®): 20-45 mcg/kg/day
I.M. (Lupron Depot®): 0.3 mg/kg/dose given every 28 days
≤25 kg: 7.5 mg
>25-37.5 kg: 11.25 mg
>37.5 kg: 15 mg
Adults:
Endometriosis: I.M.:
Lupron Depot®: 3.75 mg/month for up to 6 months **or**
Lupron Depot-3®: 11.25 mg every 3 months for up to 2 doses (6 months total duration of treatment); may be combined with norethindrone acetate 5 mg/day for initial therapy or recurrence based on clinician's judgment
Uterine leiomyomata (fibroids): I.M.:
Lupron Depot®: 3.75 mg/month for up to 3 months **or**
Lupron Depot-3®: 11.25 mg as a single injection

Mechanism of Action Continuous daily administration results in suppression of ovarian and testicular steroidogenesis due to decreased levels of LH and FSH with subsequent decrease in testosterone (male) and estrogen (female) levels

Other Adverse Effects
Female:
>10%:
Endocrine & metabolic: Amenorrhea
Neuromuscular & skeletal: Changes in bone mineral density
1% to 10%:
Endocrine & metabolic: Libido decreased, breast tenderness

Miscellaneous: Deepening of voice

Male/Female:

>10%: Cardiovascular: Hot flashes

1% to 10%:

Cardiovascular: Arrhythmias, palpitations, edema
Central nervous system: Dizziness, headache, insomnia, paresthesias
Gastrointestinal: Weight gain, nausea, vomiting
Ocular: Blurred vision
Miscellaneous: Pain at injection site

Male:

1% to 10%:

Cardiovascular: Chest pain
Endocrine & metabolic: Gynecomastia, impotence or decreased libido
Gastrointestinal: Constipation, anorexia
Genitourinary: Testicle size decreased

Drug Uptake

Onset of action: Serum testosterone levels: Increase within 3 days
Duration: Levels decrease after 2-4 weeks with continued therapy
Half-life, elimination: 3-4.25 hours

Pregnancy Risk Factor X

Generic Available Yes

Comments Has the advantage of not increasing risk of atherosclerotic vascular disease, causing swelling of breasts, fluid retention, and thromboembolism as compared to estrogen therapy

Leustatin™ *see* Cladribine *on page 295*

Levalbuterol (leve al BYOO ter ole)

U.S. Brand Names Xopenex®

Canadian Brand Names Xopenex®

Pharmacologic Category $Beta_2$ Agonist

Synonyms R-albuterol

Use Treatment or prevention of bronchospasm in adults and adolescents ≥6 years of age with reversible obstructive airway disease

Local Anesthetic/Vasoconstrictor Precautions No information available to require special precautions

Effects on Dental Treatment No effects or complications reported

Dosage

Children 6-11 years: 0.31 mg 3 times/day via nebulization (maximum dose: 0.63 mg 3 times/day)

Children >12 years and Adults: Inhalation: 0.63 mg 3 times/day at intervals of 6-8 hours, via nebulization. Dosage may be increased to 1.25 mg 3 times/day with close monitoring for adverse effects. Most patients gain optimal benefit from regular use

Elderly: Only a small number of patients have been studied. Although greater sensitivity of some elderly patients cannot be ruled out, no overall differences in safety or effectiveness were observed. An initial dose of 0.63 mg should be used in all patients >65 years of age.

Mechanism of Action Relaxes bronchial smooth muscle by action on $beta_2$ receptors with little effect on heart rate.

Other Adverse Effects Events reported include those ≥2% with incidence higher than placebo in patients ≥12 years of age.

>10%:

Endocrine & metabolic: Increased serum glucose, decreased serum potassium
Respiratory: Viral infection (7% to 12%), rhinitis (3% to 11%)

>2% to 10%:

Central nervous system: Nervousness (3% to 10%), tremor (≤7%), anxiety (≤3%), dizziness (1% to 3%), migraine (≤3%), pain (1% to 3%)
Cardiovascular: Tachycardia (~3%)
Gastrointestinal: Dyspepsia (1% to 3%)
Neuromuscular & skeletal: Leg cramps (≤3%)
Respiratory: Cough (1% to 4%), nasal edema (1% to 3%), sinusitis (1% to 4%)
Miscellaneous: Flu-like syndrome (1% to 4%), accidental injury (≤3%)

<2%: Abnormal EKG, anxiety, asthma exacerbation, chest pain, chills, diaphoresis, diarrhea, dyspepsia, gastroenteritis, hypertension, hypesthesia (hand), hypotension, insomnia, itching eyes, lymphadenopathy, myalgia, nausea, oropharyngeal dryness, paresthesia, syncope, vomiting, wheezing; immediate hypersensitivity reactions have occurred (including angioedema, oropharyngeal edema, urticaria, rash, and anaphylaxis)

Contraindications Hypersensitivity to levalbuterol or any component of the formulation

Warnings/Precautions May provoke paradoxical bronchospasm (similar to other bronchodilators). Immediate hypersensitivity reactions have occurred, including angioedema, oropharyngeal edema, urticaria, rash, and anaphylaxis. Use with caution in patients with cardiovascular disease, including coronary artery disease,
(Continued)

Levalbuterol *(Continued)*

hypertension and a history of arrhythmias (may increase heart rate, BP or other symptoms, including EKG changes). Do not use doses higher than recommended - fatalities have been associated with excessive use of other sympathomimetics. The need to use bronchodilators more frequently than usual should prompt an evaluation of the need for additional anti-inflammatory medication. Additional anti-inflammatory medication (such as corticosteroids) may be required to control asthma. Use with caution in diabetic patients and in patients with hypokalemia. Use with caution during labor and delivery. Safety and efficacy in patients <6 years of age have not been established.

Drug Interactions

Increased Effect/Toxicity: May add to effects of medications which deplete potassium (eg, loop or thiazide diuretics). Cardiac effects of levalbuterol may be potentiated in patients receiving MAO inhibitors, tricyclic antidepressants, sympathomimetics (eg, amphetamine, dobutamine), or inhaled anesthetics (eg, enflurane).

Decreased Effect: Beta-blockers (particularly nonselective agents) block the effect of levalbuterol. Digoxin levels may be decreased.

Drug Uptake

Onset of action: 10-17 minutes (measured as a 15% increase in FEV_1)
Peak effect: 1.5 hours
Absorption: A portion of inhaled dose is absorbed to systemic circulation
Duration: 5-8 hours; Average: 5-6 hours
Half-life, elimination: 3.3-4 hours
Time to peak: 0.2 hours

Pregnancy Risk Factor C

Generic Available No

Levamisole (lee VAM i sole)

U.S. Brand Names Ergamisol®

Canadian Brand Names Ergamisol®; Novo-Levamisole

Mexican Brand Names Decaris

Pharmacologic Category Immune Modulator

Synonyms Levamisole Hydrochloride

Use Adjuvant treatment with fluorouracil in Dukes stage C colon cancer

Local Anesthetic/Vasoconstrictor Precautions No information available to require special precautions

Effects on Dental Treatment No effects or complications reported

Dosage Adults: Oral: Initial: 50 mg every 8 hours for 3 days, then 50 mg every 8 hours for 3 days every 2 weeks (fluorouracil is always given concomitantly)

Mechanism of Action Clinically, combined therapy with levamisole and 5-fluorouracil has been effective in treating colon cancer patients. Due to the broad range of pharmacologic activities of levamisole, it has been suggested that the drug may act as a biochemical modulator (of fluorouracil, for example, in colon cancer), an effect entirely independent of immune modulation. Further studies are needed to evaluate the mechanisms of action of the drug in cancer patients.

Other Adverse Effects

>10%: Gastrointestinal: Nausea, diarrhea

1% to 10%:

- Cardiovascular: Edema
- Central nervous system: Fatigue, fever, dizziness, headache, somnolence, depression, nervousness, insomnia
- Dermatologic: Dermatitis, alopecia
- Gastrointestinal: Stomatitis, vomiting, anorexia, abdominal pain, constipation, taste perversion
- Hematologic: Leukopenia
- Neuromuscular & skeletal: Rigors, arthralgia, myalgia, paresthesia
- Miscellaneous: Infection

Drug Interactions Increased Effect/Toxicity: Increased toxicity/serum concentration of phenytoin

Drug Uptake

Absorption: Well absorbed
Half-life, elimination: 2-6 hours
Time to peak: 1-2 hours

Pregnancy Risk Factor C

Generic Available No

Comments Should not be used at dose exceeding the recommended dose or frequency due to increasing adverse reactions

Levaquin® *see* Levofloxacin *on page 701*
Levatol® *see* Penbutolol *on page 925*
Levbid® *see* Hyoscyamine *on page 617*

Levetiracetam (lev e tir AS e tam)

U.S. Brand Names Keppra®

Canadian Brand Names Keppra®

Pharmacologic Category Anticonvulsant, Miscellaneous

Use Adjunctive therapy in the treatment of partial onset seizures in adults

Local Anesthetic/Vasoconstrictor Precautions No information available to require special precautions

Effects on Dental Treatment No effects or complications reported

Dosage Adults: Oral: Initial: 500 mg twice daily; additional dosing adjustments should be made at 2 week intervals. The maximum daily dose is 3000 mg/day.

Mechanism of Action Precise mechanism has not been defined. Does not appear to bind receptors or increase second messengers currently known to be involved in inhibitory or excitatory neurotransmission. Anticonvulsant activity is related to protection from secondary generalization from focal seizure activity. May selectively prevent hypersynchronization of epileptiform activity, inhibiting propagation of seizure activity.

Other Adverse Effects

>10%:

- Central nervous system: Somnolence (15% vs 8% with placebo)
- Neuromuscular & skeletal: Weakness (15% vs 9% with placebo)

<10%:

- Central nervous system: Psychotic symptoms (1%), amnesia (2% vs 1% with placebo), ataxia (3% vs 1% with placebo), depression (4% vs 2% with placebo), dizziness (9% vs 4% with placebo), emotional lability (2%), nervousness (4% vs 2% with placebo), vertigo (3% vs 1% with placebo)
- Hematologic: Decreased erythrocyte counts (3%), decreased leukocytes (2% to 3%)
- Neuromuscular & skeletal: Ataxia and other coordination difficulties (3% vs 2% with placebo), pain (7% vs 6% with placebo)
- Ocular: Diplopia (2% vs 1% with placebo)

Contraindications Hypersensitivity to levetiracetam or any component of the formulation

Warnings/Precautions May cause neuropsychiatric adverse events, including somnolence, fatigue, incoordination and behavioral abnormalities (most frequently within the first 4 weeks). Behavioral changes may include psychosis. **Risk of suicide may be increased.** Antiepileptic drugs should be withdrawn gradually to minimize the potential to increase seizure frequency. Use with caution in patients with hematologic disorders. Use caution in renal impairment (dosage reduction required). Safety and efficacy in pediatric patients has not been established.

Drug Interactions No interaction was observed in pharmacokinetic trials with other anticonvulsants, including phenytoin, carbamazepine, valproic acid, phenobarbital, lamotrigine, gabapentin, and primidone.

Drug Uptake

- Onset of action: Peak effect: 1 hour
- Absorption: Rapid and complete
- Half-life, elimination: 6-8 hours
- Dialyzable: ~50% of pooled levetiracetam removed during standard 4-hour hemodialysis

Pregnancy Risk Factor C

Generic Available No

Levlen® *see* Combination Hormonal Contraceptives *on page 323*

Levlite™ *see* Combination Hormonal Contraceptives *on page 323*

Levobetaxolol (lee voe be TAX oh lol)

U.S. Brand Names Betaxon®

Canadian Brand Names Betaxon®

Pharmacologic Category Beta Blocker, Beta$_1$ Selective; Ophthalmic Agent, Antiglaucoma

Use Lowers intraocular pressure in patients with chronic open-angle glaucoma or ocular hypertension

Local Anesthetic/Vasoconstrictor Precautions No information available to require special precautions

Effects on Dental Treatment No effects or complications reported

Dosage Adults: Ophthalmic: Instill 1 drop in affected eye(s) twice daily

Mechanism of Action Levobetaxolol is a cardioselective, beta$_1$-adrenergic receptor antagonist. It is the more active enantiomer of betaxolol. Reduces intraocular pressure by reducing the production of aqueous humor.

Other Adverse Effects

>10%: Ocular: Transient discomfort (11%)

2% to 10%: Ocular: Transient blurred vision (2%)

<2%:

- Cardiovascular: Bradycardia, heart block, hypertension, hypotension, tachycardia
- Central nervous system: Anxiety, dizziness, vertigo, headache

(Continued)

Levobetaxolol *(Continued)*

Dermatologic: Alopecia, dermatitis, psoriasis
Endocrine & metabolic: Diabetes, hyperthyroidism, gout, hypercholesterolemia, hyperlipidemia
Gastrointestinal: Constipation, dyspepsia, taste perversion
Genitourinary: Cystitis
Neuromuscular & skeletal: Hypertonia, arthritis, tendonitis
Ocular: Cataracts, vitreous disorders
Otic: Ear pain, otitis media, tinnitus
Respiratory: Bronchitis, dyspnea, pharyngitis, pneumonia, rhinitis, sinusitis
Miscellaneous: Breast abscess, infection

Drug Interactions Concurrent use of systemic beta-blockers, catecholamine-depleting agents (reserpine), antipsychotic agents may increase hypotension.

Drug Uptake
Onset of action: 30 minutes; Peak effect: 2 hours
Duration: 12 hours
Half-life, elimination: 20 hours

Pregnancy Risk Factor C

Generic Available No

Levobunolol (lee voe BYOO noe lole)

U.S. Brand Names AKBeta®; Betagan® Liquifilm®

Canadian Brand Names Betagan®; Novo-Levobunolol; Optho-Bunolol®; PMS-Levobunolol

Mexican Brand Names Betagan®

Pharmacologic Category Beta Blocker, Nonselective; Ophthalmic Agent, Antiglaucoma

Synonyms *l*-Bunolol Hydrochloride; Levobunolol Hydrochloride

Use To lower intraocular pressure in chronic open-angle glaucoma or ocular hypertension

Local Anesthetic/Vasoconstrictor Precautions No information available to require special precautions

Effects on Dental Treatment No effects or complications reported

Dosage Adults: Instill 1 drop in the affected eye(s) 1-2 times/day

Mechanism of Action A nonselective beta-adrenergic blocking agent that lowers intraocular pressure by reducing aqueous humor production and possibly increases the outflow of aqueous humor

Other Adverse Effects
>10%: Ocular: Stinging/burning eyes
1% to 10%:
Cardiovascular: Bradycardia, arrhythmia, hypotension
Central nervous system: Dizziness, headache
Dermatologic: Alopecia, erythema
Local: Stinging, burning
Ocular: Blepharoconjunctivitis, conjunctivitis
Respiratory: Bronchospasm

Drug Interactions Increased Effect/Toxicity: Toxic effects may be increased with systemic beta-adrenergic blocking agents, ophthalmic epinephrine (increased BP/loss of IOP effect), quinidine (sinus bradycardia), and verapamil (bradycardia and asystole have been reported).

Drug Uptake
Onset of action: ~1 hour; Peak effect: 2-6 hours
Duration: 1-7 days

Pregnancy Risk Factor C

Generic Available Yes

Levobupivacaine (LEE voe byoo PIV a kane)

Related Information
Oral Pain *on page 1360*

U.S. Brand Names Chirocaine®

Canadian Brand Names Chirocaine®

Pharmacologic Category Local Anesthetic

Use Production of local or regional anesthesia for surgery and obstetrics, and for postoperative pain management

Local Anesthetic/Vasoconstrictor Precautions No information available to require special precautions

Effects on Dental Treatment No effects or complications reported

Dosage Adults: **Note:** Rapid injection of a large volume of local anesthetic solution should be avoided. Fractional (incremental) doses are recommended.
Guidelines (individual response varies): See table on following page.
Maximum dosage: Epidural doses up to 375 mg have been administered incrementally to patients during a surgical procedure.
Intraoperative block and postoperative pain: 695 mg in 24 hours

Postoperative epidural infusion over 24 hours: 570 mg
Single-fractionated injection for brachial plexus block: 300 mg

	Concentration	Volume	Dose	Motor Block
Surgical Anesthesia				
Epidural for surgery	0.5%-0.75%	10-20 mL	50-150 mg	Moderate to complete
Epidural for C-section	0.5%	20-30 mL	100-150 mg	Moderate to complete
Peripheral nerve	0.25%-0.5%	0.4 mL/kg (30 mL)	1-2 mg/kg (75-150 mg)	Moderate to complete
Ophthalmic	0.75%	5-15 mL	37.5-112.5 mg	Moderate to complete
Local infiltration	0.25%	60 mL	150 mg	N/A
Pain Management				
Labor analgesia (epidural bolus)	0.25%	10-20 mL	25-50 mg	Minimal to moderate
Postoperative pain (epidural infusion)	0.125%*-0.25%	4-10 mL/hour	5-25 mg/hour	Minimal to moderate

* 0.125%: Adjunct therapy with fentanyl or clonidine

Mechanism of Action Levobupivacaine is the S-enantiomer of bupivacaine. It blocks both the initiation and transmission of nerve impulses by decreasing the neuronal membrane's permeability to sodium ions, which results in inhibition of depolarization with resultant blockade of conduction. Local anesthetics reversibly prevent generation and conduction of electrical impulses in neurons by decreasing the transient increase in permeability to sodium. The differential sensitivity generally depends on the size of the fiber; small fibers are more sensitive than larger fibers and require a longer period for recovery. Sensory pain fibers are usually blocked first, followed by fibers that transmit sensations of temperature, touch, and deep pressure. High concentrations block sympathetic somatic sensory and somatic motor fibers. The spread of anesthesia depends upon the distribution of the solution. This is primarily dependent on the site of administration and volume of drug injected.

Other Adverse Effects

>10%:

Cardiovascular: Hypotension (20% to 31%)
Central nervous system: Pain (postoperative) (7% to 18%), fever (7% to 17%)
Gastrointestinal: Nausea (12% to 21%), vomiting (8% to 14%)
Hematologic: Anemia (10% to 12%)

1% to 10%:

Cardiovascular: Abnormal EKG (3%), bradycardia (2%), tachycardia (2%), hypertension (1%)
Central nervous system: Pain (4% to 8%), headache (5% to 7%), dizziness (5% to 6%), hypoesthesia (3%), somnolence (1%), anxiety (1%), hypothermia (2%)
Dermatologic: Pruritus (4% to 9%), purpura (1%)
Endocrine & metabolic: Breast pain - female (1%)
Gastrointestinal: Constipation (3% to 7%), enlarged abdomen (3%), flatulence (2%), abdominal pain (2%), dyspepsia (2%), diarrhea (1%)
Genitourinary: Urinary incontinence (1%), urine flow decreased (1%), urinary tract infection (1%)
Hematologic: Leukocytosis (1%)
Local: Anesthesia (1%)
Neuromuscular & skeletal: Back pain (6%), rigors (3%), paresthesia (2%)
Ocular: Diplopia (3%)
Renal: Albuminuria (3%), hematuria (2%)
Respiratory: Cough (1%)
Miscellaneous: Fetal distress (5% to 10%), delayed delivery (6%), hemorrhage in pregnancy (2%), uterine abnormality (2%), increased wound drainage (1%)

Contraindications Hypersensitivity to levobupivacaine, bupivacaine, any local anesthetic of the amide type, or any component of their formulation

Warnings/Precautions Unintended I.V. injection may result in cardiac arrest. Use caution when the higher concentration formulations of levobupivacaine are used. Volumes of the high concentration are more likely to produce cardiac toxicity. The 0.75% solution should not be used in obstetrical patients. Use with caution in patients with hypotension, hypovolemia, heart block, hepatic or cardiac impairment.

Local anesthetics should be administered by clinicians familiar with the use of local anesthetic agents and performance of anesthetic procedures, as well as the management of drug-related toxicity and other acute emergencies. Resuscitative equipment and medications should be readily available. Not for use in I.V. regional anesthesia (Bier block) or to produce obstetrical paracervical block anesthesia. Use with caution in patients receiving other local anesthetics or structurally related agents.

Drug Interactions CYP1A2 and 3A3/4 enzyme substrate

Although not specifically studied, inhibitors of CYP3A3/4 and CYP1A2 may increase levels/toxicity of levobupivacaine.

(Continued)

Levobupivacaine *(Continued)*

Drug Uptake

Onset of action: Epidural: 10-14 minutes
Absorption: Dependent on route of administration and dose
Duration (dose-dependent): 1-8 hours
Half-life, elimination: 1.3 hours
Time to peak: Epidural: 30 minutes

Pregnancy Risk Factor B

Generic Available No

Levocabastine (LEE voe kab as teen)

U.S. Brand Names Livostin®

Canadian Brand Names Livostin®

Mexican Brand Names Livostin®

Pharmacologic Category Antihistamine, H_1 Blocker, Ophthalmic

Synonyms Levocabastine Hydrochloride

Use Treatment of allergic conjunctivitis

Local Anesthetic/Vasoconstrictor Precautions No information available to require special precautions

Effects on Dental Treatment No effects or complications reported

Dosage Children >12 years and Adults: Instill 1 drop in affected eye(s) 4 times/day for up to 2 weeks

Mechanism of Action Potent, selective histamine H_1-receptor antagonist for topical ophthalmic use

Other Adverse Effects

>10%: Local: Transient burning, stinging, discomfort
1% to 10%:
- Central nervous system: Headache, somnolence, fatigue
- Dermatologic: Rash
- Gastrointestinal: Xerostomia
- Ocular: Blurred vision, eye pain, somnolence, red eyes, eyelid edema
- Respiratory: Dyspnea

Drug Uptake Absorption: Topical: Systemically

Pregnancy Risk Factor C

Generic Available No

Levocarnitine (lee voe KAR ni teen)

U.S. Brand Names Carnitor®; Vitacarn®

Canadian Brand Names Carnitor®

Mexican Brand Names Cardispan®

Pharmacologic Category Dietary Supplement

Synonyms L-Carnitine

Use Orphan drug:

I.V.: Acute and chronic treatment of patients with an inborn error of metabolism which results in secondary carnitine deficiency; prevention and treatment of carnitine deficiency in patients with end-stage renal disease who are undergoing hemodialysis.

Oral: Primary systemic carnitine deficiency; acute and chronic treatment of patients with an inborn error of metabolism which results in secondary carnitine deficiency

Local Anesthetic/Vasoconstrictor Precautions No information available to require special precautions

Effects on Dental Treatment No effects or complications reported

Dosage

Oral:
- Children: 50-100 mg/kg/day divided 2-3 times/day, maximum: 3 g/day; dosage must be individualized based upon patient response; higher dosages have been used
- Adults: 990 mg (oral tablets) 2-3 times/day or 1-3 g/day (oral solution)

I.V.: Children and Adults: 50 mg/kg as a loading dose, followed (in severe cases) by 50 mg/kg/day infusion; maintenance: 50 mg/kg/day given every 4-6 hours, increase as needed to a maximum of 300 mg/kg/day

Mechanism of Action Carnitine is a naturally occurring metabolic compound which functions as a carrier molecule for long-chain fatty acids within the mitochondria, facilitating energy production. Carnitine deficiency is associated with accumulation of excess acyl CoA esters and disruption of intermediary metabolism. Carnitine supplementation increases carnitine plasma concentrations. The effects on specific metabolic alterations have not been evaluated. ESRD patients on maintenance HD may have low plasma carnitine levels because of reduced intake of meat and dairy products, reduced renal synthesis, and dialytic losses. Certain clinical conditions (malaise, muscle weakness, cardiomyopathy and arrhythmias) in HD patients may be related to carnitine deficiency.

Other Adverse Effects Frequencies noted with I.V. therapy (hemodialysis patients):

Cardiovascular: Hypertension (18% to 21%), peripheral edema (3% to 6%)
Central nervous system: Dizziness (10% to 18%), fever (5% to 12%), paresthesia (3% to 12%), depression (5% to 6%)
Endocrine & metabolic: Hypercalcemia (6% to 15%)
Gastrointestinal: Diarrhea (9% to 35%), abdominal pain (5% to 21%), vomiting (9% to 21%), nausea (5% to 12%)
Neuromuscular & skeletal: Weakness (9% to 12%)
Miscellaneous: Allergic reaction (2% to 6%)

Drug Interactions Valproic acid, sodium benzoate

Drug Uptake
Half-life, elimination: 17.4 hours
Time to peak: Tablet/solution: 3.3 hours

Pregnancy Risk Factor B

Generic Available Yes

Comments Tolerance may be improved by mixing the product with liquids or food and spacing doses evenly throughout the day with meals

Levodopa (lee voe DOE pa)

U.S. Brand Names Dopar®; Larodopa®

Canadian Brand Names Dopar®; Larodopa®

Pharmacologic Category Anti-Parkinson's Agent, Dopamine Agonist

Synonyms *L*-3-Hydroxytyrosine; *L*-Dopa

Use Treatment of Parkinson's disease
Unlabeled/Investigational: Diagnostic agent for growth hormone deficiency

Local Anesthetic/Vasoconstrictor Precautions No information available to require special precautions

Effects on Dental Treatment Dopaminergic therapy in Parkinson's disease (ie, treatment with levodopa) is associated with orthostatic hypotension. Patients medicated with levodopa should be carefully assisted from the chair and observed for signs of orthostatic hypotension.

Dosage Oral:
Children (administer as a single dose to evaluate growth hormone deficiency [unlabeled use]):
0.5 g/m^2 **or**
<30 lb: 125 mg
30-70 lb: 250 mg
>70 lb: 500 mg
Adults: Parkinson's disease: 500-1000 mg/day in divided doses every 6-12 hours; increase by 100-750 mg/day every 3-7 days until response or total dose of 8000 mg is reached
A significant therapeutic response may not be obtained for 6 months

Mechanism of Action Increases dopamine levels in the brain, then stimulates dopaminergic receptors in the basal ganglia to improve the balance between cholinergic and dopaminergic activity

Other Adverse Effects Frequency not defined:
Cardiovascular: Orthostatic hypotension, arrhythmias, chest pain, hypertension, syncope, palpitations, phlebitis
Central nervous system: Dizziness, anxiety, confusion, nightmares, headache, hallucinations, on-off phenomenon, decreased mental acuity, memory impairment, disorientation, delusions, euphoria, agitation, somnolence, insomnia, gait abnormalities, nervousness, ataxia, EPS, falling, psychosis
Gastrointestinal: Anorexia, nausea, vomiting, constipation, GI bleeding, duodenal ulcer, diarrhea, dyspepsia, taste alterations, sialorrhea, heartburn
Genitourinary: Discoloration of urine, urinary frequency
Hematologic: Hemolytic anemia, agranulocytosis, thrombocytopenia, leukopenia, decreased hemoglobin and hematocrit, abnormalities in AST and ALT, LDH, bilirubin, BUN, Coombs' test
Neuromuscular & skeletal: Choreiform and involuntary movements, paresthesia, bone pain, shoulder pain, muscle cramps, weakness
Ocular: Blepharospasm
Renal: Difficult urination
Respiratory: Dyspnea, cough
Miscellaneous: Hiccups, discoloration of sweat

Drug Interactions
Increased Effect/Toxicity: Concurrent use of levodopa with nonselective MAO inhibitors may result in hypertensive reactions via an increased storage and release of dopamine, norepinephrine, or both. Use with carbidopa to minimize reactions if combination is necessary; otherwise avoid combination.
Decreased Effect: Antipsychotics, benzodiazepines, L-methionine, phenytoin, pyridoxine, spiramycin, and tacrine may inhibit the antiparkinsonian effects of levodopa; monitor for reduced effect. Antipsychotics may inhibit the antiparkinsonian effects of levodopa via dopamine receptor blockade. Use antipsychotics with low dopamine blockade (clozapine, olanzapine, quetiapine). High-protein diets may inhibit levodopa's efficacy; avoid high protein foods. Iron binds levodopa and reduces its bioavailability; separate doses of iron and levodopa.
(Continued)

Levodopa *(Continued)*

Drug Uptake

Absorption: May be decreased if given with a high protein meal
Duration: Variable, usually 6-12 hours
Half-life, elimination: 1.2-2.3 hours
Time to peak: Oral: 1-2 hours

Pregnancy Risk Factor C

Generic Available No

Levodopa and Carbidopa (lee voe DOE pa & kar bi DOE pa)

U.S. Brand Names Sinemet®; Sinemet® CR

Canadian Brand Names Apo®-Levocarb; Endo®-Levodopa/Carbidopa; Nu-Levocarb; Sinemet®; Sinemet® CR

Mexican Brand Names Racovel

Pharmacologic Category Anti-Parkinson's Agent, Dopamine Agonist

Synonyms Carbidopa and Levodopa

Use Treatment of parkinsonian syndrome; 50-100 mg/day of carbidopa is needed to block the peripheral conversion of levodopa to dopamine. "On-off" can be managed by giving smaller, more frequent doses of Sinemet® or adding a dopamine agonist or selegiline; when adding a new agent, doses of Sinemet® should usually be decreased.

Unlabeled/Investigational: Restless leg syndrome

Local Anesthetic/Vasoconstrictor Precautions No information available to require special precautions

Effects on Dental Treatment Dopaminergic therapy in Parkinson's disease (ie, treatment with levodopa and carbidopa combination) is associated with orthostatic hypotension. Patients medicated with this drug combination should be carefully assisted from the chair and observed for signs of orthostatic hypotension.

Dosage Oral:

Adults: Initial: Carbidopa 25 mg/levodopa 100 mg 2-4 times/day, increase as necessary to a maximum of carbidopa 200 mg/levodopa 2000 mg per day
Restless leg syndrome (unlabeled use): Carbidopa 25 mg/levodopa 100 mg given 30-60 minutes before bedtime; may repeat dose once
Elderly: Initial: Carbidopa 25 mg/levodopa 100 mg twice daily, increase as necessary

Conversion from Sinemet® to Sinemet® CR (50/200): (Sinemet® [total daily dose of levodopa] / Sinemet® CR)
300-400 mg / 1 tablet twice daily
500-600 mg / 1½ tablets twice daily or one 3 times/day
700-800 mg / 4 tablets in 3 or more divided doses
900-1000 mg / 5 tablets in 3 or more divided doses
Intervals between doses of Sinemet® CR should be 4-8 hours while awake

Mechanism of Action Parkinson's symptoms are due to a lack of striatal dopamine; levodopa circulates in the plasma to the blood-brain-barrier (BBB), where it crosses, to be converted by striatal enzymes to dopamine; carbidopa inhibits the peripheral plasma breakdown of levodopa by inhibiting its decarboxylation, and thereby increases available levodopa at the BBB

Other Adverse Effects Frequency not defined:

Cardiovascular: Orthostatic hypotension, arrhythmias, chest pain, hypertension, syncope, palpitations, phlebitis
Central nervous system: Dizziness, anxiety, confusion, nightmares, headache, hallucinations, on-off phenomenon, decreased mental acuity, memory impairment, disorientation, delusions, euphoria, agitation, somnolence, insomnia, gait abnormalities, nervousness, ataxia, EPS, falling, psychosis, peripheral neuropathy, seizures (causal relationship not established)
Dermatologic: Rash, alopecia, malignant melanoma, hypersensitivity (angioedema, urticaria, pruritus, bullous lesions, Henoch-Schönlein purpura)
Endocrine & metabolic: Increased libido
Gastrointestinal: Anorexia, nausea, vomiting, constipation, GI bleeding, duodenal ulcer, diarrhea, dyspepsia, taste alterations, sialorrhea, heartburn
Genitourinary: Discoloration of urine, urinary frequency
Hematologic: Hemolytic anemia, agranulocytosis, thrombocytopenia, leukopenia; decreased hemoglobin and hematocrit; abnormalities in AST and ALT, LDH, bilirubin, BUN, Coombs' test
Neuromuscular & skeletal: Choreiform and involuntary movements, paresthesia, bone pain, shoulder pain, muscle cramps, weakness
Ocular: Blepharospasm, oculogyric crises (may be associated with acute dystonic reactions)
Renal: Difficult urination
Respiratory: Dyspnea, cough
Miscellaneous: Hiccups, discoloration of sweat, diaphoresis (increased)

Drug Interactions

Increased Effect/Toxicity: Concurrent use of levodopa with nonselective MAO inhibitors may result in hypertensive reactions via an increased storage and release of dopamine, norepinephrine, or both. Use with carbidopa to minimize reactions if combination is necessary; otherwise avoid combination.

Decreased Effect: Antipsychotics, benzodiazepines, L-methionine, phenytoin, pyridoxine, spiramycin, and tacrine may inhibit the antiparkinsonian effects of levodopa; monitor for reduced effect. Antipsychotics may inhibit the antiparkinsonian effects of levodopa via dopamine receptor blockade. Use antipsychotics with low dopamine blockade (clozapine, olanzapine, quetiapine). High-protein diets may inhibit levodopa's efficacy; avoid high protein foods. Iron binds levodopa and reduces its bioavailability; separate doses of iron and levodopa.

Drug Uptake

Carbidopa:

Absorption: Oral: 40% to 70%

Duration: Variable, 6-12 hours; longer with sustained release forms

Half-life, elimination: 1-2 hours

Levodopa:

Absorption: May be decreased if given with a high protein meal

Duration: Variable, 6-12 hours; longer with sustained release forms

Half-life, elimination: 1.2-2.3 hours

Pregnancy Risk Factor C

Generic Available Yes

Levo-Dromoran® *see* Levorphanol *on page 704*

Levofloxacin (lee voe FLOKS a sin)

U.S. Brand Names Levaquin®; Quixin™ Ophthalmic

Canadian Brand Names Levaquin®

Mexican Brand Names Elequine; Tavanic

Pharmacologic Category Antibiotic, Quinolone

Use

Systemic:

Acute bacterial exacerbation of chronic bronchitis and community-acquired pneumonia due to *S. aureus*, *S. pneumoniae* (including penicillin-resistant strains), *H. influenzae*, *H. parainfluenzae*, or *M. catarrhalis*, *C. pneumoniae*, *L. pneumophila*, or *M. pneumoniae*

Acute maxillary sinusitis due to *S. pneumoniae*, *H. influenzae*, or *M. catarrhalis*

Acute pyelonephritis caused by *E. coli*

Skin or skin structure infections:

Complicated, due to methcillin-susceptible *S. aureus*, *Enterococcus fecalis*, *S. pyogenes*, or *Proteus mirabilis*

Uncomplicated, due to *S. aureus* or *S. pyogenes*

Urinary tract infections:

Complicated, due to gram-negative bacteria (*E. coli*, *Enterobacter cloacae*, *Klebsiella pneumoniae*, *Proteus mirabilis*, *Enterococcus fecalis*, or *Pseudomonas aeruginosa*)

Uncomplicated, due to *E. coli*, *K. pneumoniae*, or *S. saprophyticus*

Ophthalmic: Bacterial conjunctivitis due to *S. aureus* (methicillin-susceptible strains), *S. epidermidis* (methicillin-susceptible strains), *S. pneumoniae*, *Streptococcus* (groups C/F), *Streptococcus* (group G), Viridans group streptococci, *Corynebacterium* spp, *H. influenzae*, *Acinetobacter lwoffii*, or *Serratia marcescens*

Local Anesthetic/Vasoconstrictor Precautions No information available to require special precautions

Effects on Dental Treatment No effects or complications reported

Dosage

Adults: Oral, I.V. (infuse I.V. solution over 60 minutes):

Acute bacterial exacerbation of chronic bronchitis: 500 mg every 24 hours for at least 7 days

Community-acquired pneumonia: 500 mg every 24 hours for 7-14 days

Acute maxillary sinusitis: 500 mg every 24 hours for 10-14 days

Uncomplicated skin infections: 500 mg every 24 hours for 7-10 days

Complicated skin infections: 750 mg every 24 hours for 7-14 days

Uncomplicated urinary tract infections: 250 mg once daily for 3 days

Complicated urinary tract infections, including acute pyelonephritis: 250 mg every 24 hours for 10 days

Children ≥1 year and Adults: Ophthalmic:

Treatment day 1 and day 2: Instill 1-2 drops into affected eye(s) every 2 hours while awake, up to 8 times/day

Treatment day 3 through day 7: Instill 1-2 drops into affected eye(s) every 4 hours while awake, up to 4 times/day

Dosing adjustment in renal impairment:

Chronic bronchitis, acute maxillary sinusitis, uncomplicated skin infection, community-acquired pneumonia:

Cl_{cr} 20-49 mL/minute: Administer 250 mg every 24 hours (initial: 500 mg)

Cl_{cr} 10-19 mL/minute: Administer 250 mg every 48 hours (initial: 500 mg)

Complicated UTI, acute pyelonephritis:

Cl_{cr} 20-49 mL/minute: No dosage adjustment required required

Cl_{cr} 10-19 mL/minute: Administer 250 mg every 48 hours

(Continued)

Levofloxacin *(Continued)*

Uncomplicated UTI: No dosage adjustment required

Complicated skin infection

Cl_{cr} 20-49 mL/minute: Administer 750 mg every 48 hours mg

Cl_{cr} 10-19 mL/minute: Administer 500 mg every 48 hours (initial: 750 mg)

Hemodialysis/CAPD: 250 mg every 48 hours (initial: 500 mg for most infections; initial: 750 mg for complicated skin/soft tissue infections followed by 500 mg every 48 hours)

Mechanism of Action As the S (-) enantiomer of the fluoroquinolone, ofloxacin, levofloxacin, inhibits DNA-gyrase in susceptible organisms thereby inhibits relaxation of supercoiled DNA and promotes breakage of DNA strands. DNA gyrase (topoisomerase II), is an essential bacterial enzyme that maintains the superhelical structure of DNA and is required for DNA replication and transcription, DNA repair, recombination, and transposition.

Other Adverse Effects 1% to 10%:

Central nervous system: Dizziness, fever, headache, insomnia

Gastrointestinal: Nausea, vomiting, diarrhea, constipation

Ocular (with ophthalmic solution use): Decreased vision (transient), foreign body sensation, transient ocular burning, ocular pain or discomfort, photophobia

Respiratory: Pharyngitis

Contraindications Hypersensitivity to levofloxacin, other quinolones, or any component of their formulation

Warnings/Precautions

Systemic: Not recommended in children <18 years of age; CNS stimulation may occur (tremor, restlessness, confusion, and very rarely hallucinations or seizures); use with caution in patients with known or suspected CNS disorders or renal dysfunction; use caution to avoid possible photosensitivity reactions during and for several days following fluoroquinolone therapy

Rare cases of torsade de pointes have been reported in patients receiving levofloxacin. Use caution in patients with bradycardia, hypokalemia, hypomagnesemia, or in those receiving concurrent therapy with Class Ia or Class III antiarrhythmics.

Severe hypersensitivity reactions, including anaphylaxis, have occurred with quinolone therapy. If an allergic reaction occurs (itching, urticaria, dyspnea or facial edema, loss of consciousness, tingling, cardiovascular collapse), discontinue drug immediately. Prolonged use may result in superinfection; pseudomembranous colitis may occur and should be considered in all patients who present with diarrhea. Tendon inflammation and/or rupture has been reported; discontinue at first sign of tendon inflammation or pain. Quinolones may exacerbate myasthenia gravis, use with caution (rare, potentially life-threatening weakness of respiratory muscles may occur).

Ophthalmic solution: For topical use only. Do not inject subconjunctivally or introduce into anterior chamber of the eye. Contact lenses should not be worn during treatment for bacterial conjunctivitis. Safety and efficacy in children <1 year of age have not been established.

Drug Interactions CYP1A2 enzyme inhibitor (minor)

Increased Effect/Toxicity: Quinolones may cause increased levels of azlocillin, cyclosporine, and caffeine/theophylline (effect of levofloxacin on theophylline metabolism appears limited). Azlocillin, cimetidine, loop diuretics (furosemide, torsemide), and probenecid increase quinolone levels (decreased renal secretion). An increased incidence of seizures may occur with foscarnet or NSAIDs. The hypoprothrombinemic effect of warfarin is enhanced by some quinolone antibiotics. Levofloxacin does not alter warfarin levels, but may alter the GI flora. Monitor INR closely during therapy.

Decreased Effect: Metal cations (magnesium, aluminum, iron, and zinc) bind quinolones in the GI tract and inhibit absorption (by up to 98%). Due to electrolyte content, antacids, electrolyte supplements, sucralfate, quinapril, and some didanosine formulations should be avoided. Levofloxacin should be administered 4 hours before or 8 hours (a minimum of 2 hours before and 2 hours after) after these agents. Antineoplastic agents may decrease the absorption of quinolones.

Drug Uptake

Absorption: Well absorbed

Half-life, elimination: 6 hours

Time to peak: 1 hour

Pregnancy Risk Factor C

Generic Available No

Levomethadyl Acetate Hydrochloride

(lee voe METH a dil AS e tate hye droe KLOR ide)

U.S. Brand Names ORLAAM®

Pharmacologic Category Analgesic, Narcotic

Use Management of opiate dependence; should be reserved for use in treatment of opiate-addicted patients who fail to show an acceptable response to other adequate treatments for addiction

Local Anesthetic/Vasoconstrictor Precautions No information available to require special precautions

Effects on Dental Treatment No effects or complications reported

Restrictions C-II; must be dispensed in a designated clinic setting only

Dosage Adults: Oral: 20-40 mg at 48- or 72-hour intervals, with ranges of 10 mg to as high as 140 mg 3 times/week; adjust dose in increments of 5-10 mg (too rapid induction may lead to overdose); always dilute before administration and mix with diluent prior to dispensing

Mechanism of Action A synthetic opioid agonist with actions similar to morphine; principal actions are analgesia and sedation. Its clinical effects in the treatment of opiate abuse occur through two mechanisms: 1) cross-sensitivity for opiates of the morphine type, suppressing symptoms of withdrawal in opiate-dependent persons; 2) with chronic oral administration, can produce sufficient tolerance to block the subjective high of usual doses of parenterally administered opiates

Other Adverse Effects

>10%:

Central nervous system: Malaise

Miscellaneous: Flu syndrome

1% to 10%:

Central nervous system: CNS depression, sedation, chills, abnormal dreams, anxiety, euphoria, headache, insomnia, nervousness, hypesthesia

Endocrine & metabolic: Hot flashes (males 2:1)

Gastrointestinal: Abdominal pain, constipation, diarrhea, xerostomia, nausea, vomiting

Genitourinary: Urinary tract spasm, difficult ejaculation, impotence, decreased sex drive

Neuromuscular & skeletal: Arthralgia, back pain, weakness

Ocular: Miosis, blurred vision

Contraindications Hypersensitivity of levomethadyl or any component of the formulation; known or suspected QT_c prolongation (males: 430 milliseconds, females: 450 milliseconds); concurrent use of any drug known to have the potential to cause abnormal heart rhythm, including class I and III antiarrhythmics, MAO inhibitors; hypokalemia, hypomagnesemia; bradycardia (<50 bpm); significant cardiac disease

Drug Interactions CYP3A3/4 enzyme substrate

Increased Effect/Toxicity: CNS depressants, including sedatives, tranquilizers, propoxyphene, antidepressants, and benzodiazepines may result in serious overdose when used with levomethadyl. Enzyme inducers (carbamazepine, phenobarbital, rifampin, phenytoin) may enhance the metabolism of levomethadyl leading to an increase in levomethadyl peak effect (however duration of action is shortened). Enzyme inhibitors such as erythromycin, cimetidine, and ketoconazole may increase the risk of arrhythmia (including torsade de pointes) or may increase the duration of action of levomethadyl. Concurrent use of QT_c-prolonging agents is contraindicated (includes class I and III antiarrhythmics, cisapride, erythromycin, select quinolones, mesoridazine, thioridazine, zonisamide). Concurrent use of MAO inhibitors is contraindicated (per manufacturer), or drugs with MAO-blocking activity (linezolid). Safety of selegiline (selective MAO type B inhibitor) not established.

Decreased Effect: Levomethadyl used in combination with naloxone, naltrexone, pentazocine, nalbuphine, butorphanol, and buprenorphine may result in withdrawal symptoms. The effect of meperidine may be decreased by levomethadyl. Enzyme inducers (carbamazepine, phenobarbital, rifampin, phenytoin) may shorten levomethadyl's duration of action. Enzyme inhibitors, such as erythromycin, cimetidine, and ketoconazole may slow the onset, lower the activity levomethadyl (may also increase duration of action).

Pregnancy Risk Factor C

Generic Available No

Levonorgestrel (LEE voe nor jes trel)

Related Information

Endocrine Disorders and Pregnancy *on page 1331*

U.S. Brand Names Mirena®; Norplant® Implant; Plan B™

Canadian Brand Names Norplant® Implant; Plan B™

Mexican Brand Names Microlut®

Pharmacologic Category Contraceptive

Synonyms LNg 20

Use Prevention of pregnancy

Local Anesthetic/Vasoconstrictor Precautions No information available to require special precautions

Effects on Dental Treatment Progestins may predispose the patient to gingival bleeding.

Dosage Adults:

Long-term prevention of pregnancy:

Subdermal capsules: Total administration doses (implanted): 216 mg in 6 capsules which should be implanted during the first 7 days of onset of menses

(Continued)

Levonorgestrel *(Continued)*

subdermally in the upper arm; each Norplant® silastic capsule releases 80 mcg of levonorgestrel/day for 6-18 months, following which a rate of release of 25-30 mcg/day is maintained for ≤5 years; capsules should be removed by end of 5th year

Intrauterine system: To be inserted into uterine cavity; should be inserted within 7 days of onset of menstruation or immediately after first trimester abortion; releases 20 mcg levonorgestrel/day over 5 years. May be removed and replaced with a new unit at anytime during menstrual cycle; do not leave any one system in place for >5 years

Emergency contraception: Oral tablet: One 0.75 mg tablet as soon as possible within 72 hours of unprotected sexual intercourse; a second 0.75 mg tablet should be taken 12 hours after the first dose; may be used at any time during menstrual cycle

Dosage adjustment in renal/hepatic impairment: Safety and efficacy have not been established

Elderly: Not intended for use in postmenopausal women

Mechanism of Action Pregnancy may be prevented through several mechanisms: Thickening of cervical mucus, which inhibits sperm passage through the uterus and sperm survival; inhibition of ovulation, from a negative feedback mechanism on the hypothalamus, leading to reduced secretion of follicle stimulating hormone (FSH) and luteinizing hormone (LH); inhibition of implantation. Levonorgestrel is not effective once the implantation process has begun.

Other Adverse Effects

Intrauterine system:

>5%:
- Cardiovascular: Hypertension
- Central nervous system: Headache, depression, nervousness
- Dermatologic: Acne
- Endocrine & metabolic: Breast pain, dysmenorrhea, decreased libido, abnormal Pap smear, amenorrhea (20% at 1 year), enlarged follicles (12%)
- Gastrointestinal: Abdominal pain, nausea, weight gain
- Genitourinary: Leukorrhea, vaginitis
- Neuromuscular & skeletal: Back pain
- Respiratory: Upper respiratory tract infection, sinusitis

<3% and postmarketing reports: Alopecia, anemia, cervicitis, dyspareunia, eczema, failed insertion, migraine, sepsis, vomiting

Oral tablets:

>10%:
- Central nervous system: Fatigue (17%), headache (17%), dizziness (11%)
- Endocrine & metabolic: Heavier menstrual bleeding (14%), lighter menstrual bleeding (12%), breast tenderness (11%)
- Gastrointestinal: Nausea (23%), abdominal pain (18%),

1% to 10%: Gastrointestinal: Vomiting (6%), diarrhea (5%)

Subdermal capsules:

>10%: Endocrine & metabolic: Increased/prolonged bleeding (28%), spotting (17%)

1% to 10%:
- Endocrine & metabolic: Breast discharge (≥5%), menstrual irregularities
- Gastrointestinal: Abdominal discomfort (≥5%)
- Genitourinary: Cervicitis (≥5%), leukorrhea (≥5%), vaginitis (≥5%)
- Local: Pain/itching at implant site (4%, usually transient)
- Neuromuscular & skeletal: Musculoskeletal pain (≥5%)
- Miscellaneous: Removal difficulties (6%); these may include multiple incisions, remaining capsule fragments, pain, multiple visits, deep placement, lengthy procedure

Drug Interactions CYP3A3/4 enzyme substrate

Enzyme inducers may increase the metabolism of levonorgestrel resulting in decreased effect; includes carbamazepine, phenobarbital, phenytoin, and rifampin; additional contraceptive measures may be needed with use of enzyme inducers or following their withdrawal.

Drug Uptake

Absorption: Rapid and complete

Duration: Subdermal capsules, intrauterine system: ≤5 years

Half-life, elimination: Oral tablet: ~24 hours

Pregnancy Risk Factor X

Generic Available No

Levophed® *see* Norepinephrine *on page 875*

Levora® *see* Combination Hormonal Contraceptives *on page 323*

Levorphanol (lee VOR fa nole)

U.S. Brand Names Levo-Dromoran®

Pharmacologic Category Analgesic, Narcotic

Synonyms Levorphanol Tartrate; Levorphan Tartrate

Use Relief of moderate to severe pain; also used parenterally for preoperative sedation and an adjunct to nitrous oxide/oxygen anesthesia; 2 mg levorphanol produces analgesia comparable to that produced by 10 mg of morphine

Local Anesthetic/Vasoconstrictor Precautions No information available to require special precautions

Effects on Dental Treatment ~10%: Xerostomia; disappears with discontinuation

Restrictions C-II

Dosage Adults:

Oral: 2 mg every 6-24 hours as needed

S.C.: 2 mg, up to 3 mg if necessary, every 6-8 hours

Mechanism of Action Levorphanol tartrate is a synthetic opioid agonist that is classified as a morphinan derivative. Opioids interact with stereospecific opioid receptors in various parts of the CNS and other tissues. Analgesic potency parallels the affinity for these binding sites. These drugs do not alter the threshold or responsiveness to pain, but the perception of pain.

Other Adverse Effects Frequency not defined:

Cardiovascular: Palpitations, hypotension, bradycardia, peripheral vasodilation, cardiac arrest, shock, tachycardia

Central nervous system: CNS depression, fatigue, drowsiness, dizziness, nervousness, headache, restlessness, anorexia, malaise, confusion, coma, convulsion, insomnia, amnesia, mental depression, hallucinations, paradoxical CNS stimulation, intracranial pressure (increased),

Dermatologic: Pruritus, urticaria, rash

Endocrine & metabolic: Antidiuretic hormone release

Gastrointestinal: Nausea, vomiting, dyspepsia, stomach cramps, xerostomia, constipation, abdominal pain, xerostomia, biliary tract spasm, paralytic ileus

Genitourinary: Decreased urination, urinary tract spasm, urinary retention

Local: Pain at injection site

Neuromuscular & skeletal: Weakness

Ocular: Miosis, diplopia

Respiratory: Respiratory depression, apnea, hypoventilation, cyanosis

Miscellaneous: Histamine release, physical and psychological dependence

Drug Interactions CNS depression is enhanced with coadministration of other CNS depressants.

Drug Uptake

Onset of action: Oral: 10-60 minutes

Duration: 4-8 hours

Pregnancy Risk Factor B/D (prolonged use or high doses at term)

Generic Available No

Levo-T™ *see* Levothyroxine *on page 705*

Levothroid® *see* Levothyroxine *on page 705*

Levothyroxine (lee voe thye ROKS een)

Related Information

Endocrine Disorders and Pregnancy *on page 1331*

U.S. Brand Names Levo-T™; Levothroid®; Levoxyl®; Novothyrox; Synthroid®; Unithroid™

Canadian Brand Names Eltroxin®; Synthroid®

Mexican Brand Names Eutirox; Tiroidine

Pharmacologic Category Thyroid Product

Synonyms Levothyroxine Sodium; *L*-Thyroxine Sodium; T_4

Use Replacement or supplemental therapy in hypothyroidism; some clinicians suggest levothyroxine is the drug of choice for replacement therapy

Local Anesthetic/Vasoconstrictor Precautions No precautions with vasoconstrictor are necessary if patient is well controlled with levothyroxine

Effects on Dental Treatment No effects or complications reported

Dosage

Children:

Oral:

0-6 months: 8-10 mcg/kg/day **or** 25-50 mcg/day

6-12 months: 6-8 mcg/kg/day **or** 50-75 mcg/day

1-5 years: 5-6 mcg/kg/day **or** 75-100 mcg/day

6-12 years: 4-5 mcg/kg/day **or** 100-150 mcg/day

>12 years: 2-3 mcg/kg/day **or** ≥150 mcg/day

I.M., I.V.: 50% to 75% of the oral dose

Adults:

Oral: 12.5-50 mcg/day to start, then increase by 25-50 mcg/day at intervals of 2-4 weeks; average adult dose: 100-200 mcg/day

I.M., I.V.: 50% of the oral dose

Myxedema coma or stupor: I.V.: 200-500 mcg one time, then 100-300 mcg the next day if necessary

Thyroid suppression therapy: Oral: 2-6 mcg/kg/day for 7-10 days

Mechanism of Action Exact mechanism of action is unknown; however, it is believed the thyroid hormone exerts its many metabolic effects through control of

(Continued)

Levothyroxine *(Continued)*

DNA transcription and protein synthesis; involved in normal metabolism, growth, and development; promotes gluconeogenesis, increases utilization and mobilization of glycogen stores, and stimulates protein synthesis, increases basal metabolic rate

Other Adverse Effects Frequency not defined:

Cardiovascular: Palpitations, cardiac arrhythmias, tachycardia, chest pain
Central nervous system: Nervousness, headache, insomnia, fever, ataxia
Dermatologic: Alopecia
Endocrine & metabolic: Changes in menstrual cycle, weight loss, increased appetite
Gastrointestinal: Diarrhea, abdominal cramps, constipation, vomiting
Neuromuscular & skeletal: Myalgia, hand tremors, tremor
Respiratory: Dyspnea
Miscellaneous: Diaphoresis, allergic skin reactions (rare)

Drug Interactions CYP enzyme substrate (T_3 and T_4); thyroid hormone may alter metabolic activity of cytochrome P450 enzymes

Increased Effect/Toxicity: Levothyroxine may potentiate the hypoprothrombinemic effect of warfarin (and other oral anticoagulants). Effect of warfarin may be dramatically increased when levothyroxine is added. However, the addition of warfarin in a patient previously receiving a stable dose of levothyroxine does not require a significantly different dosing strategy. Tricyclic antidepressants (TCAs) coadministered with levothyroxine may increase potential for toxicity of both drugs. Excessive thyroid replacement in patients receiving growth hormone may lead to accelerated epiphyseal closure; inadequate replacement interferes with growth response. Coadministration with ketamine may lead to hypertension and tachycardia.

Decreased Effect: Aluminum- and magnesium-containing antacids, iron preparations, sucralfate, cholestyramine, colestipol, and Kayexalate® may decrease levothyroxine absorption (separate administration by 8 hours). Enzyme inducers (phenytoin, phenobarbital, carbamazepine, and rifampin/rifabutin) may decrease levothyroxine levels. Levothyroxine may decrease effect of oral sulfonylureas. Dosage of levothyroxine may need to be increased when SSRIs are added. Serum levels of digoxin and theophylline may be altered by thyroid function.

Drug Uptake

Onset of action: Therapeutic: Oral: 3-5 days; I.V. 6-8 hours
 Peak effect: I.V.: ~24 hours
Absorption: Oral: Erratic
Half-life, elimination: Euthyroid: 6-7 days; Hypothyroid: 9-10 days; Hyperthyroid: 3-4 days
Time to peak: 2-4 hours

Pregnancy Risk Factor A

Generic Available Yes

Levoxyl® *see* Levothyroxine *on page 705*
Levsin® *see* Hyoscyamine *on page 617*
Levsinex® *see* Hyoscyamine *on page 617*
Levsin/SL® *see* Hyoscyamine *on page 617*
Levulan® Kerastick™ *see* Aminolevulinic Acid *on page 70*
Lexxel™ *see* Enalapril and Felodipine *on page 433*
Librax® *see* Clidinium and Chlordiazepoxide *on page 299*
Librium® *see* Chlordiazepoxide *on page 262*
Lida-Mantle HC® *see* Lidocaine and Hydrocortisone *on page 710*
Lidex® *see* Fluocinonide *on page 513*
Lidex-E® *see* Fluocinonide *on page 513*

Lidocaine (LYE doe kane)

Related Information

Cardiovascular Diseases *on page 1308*
Management of Patients Undergoing Cancer Therapy *on page 1402*
Oral Pain *on page 1360*
Oral Viral Infections *on page 1380*

U.S. Brand Names Anestacon®; Dermaflex® Gel; ELA-Max® [OTC]; Lidoderm®; LidoPen® Auto-Injector; Solarcaine® Aloe Extra Burn Relief [OTC]; Xylocaine®; Zilactin-L® [OTC]

Canadian Brand Names Lidodan™; Lidoderm®; Xylocaine®; Xylocard®; Zilactin®

Mexican Brand Names Pisacaina; Uvega®; Xylocaina

Pharmacologic Category Analgesic, Topical; Antiarrhythmic Agent, Class Ib; Local Anesthetic

Synonyms Lidocaine Hydrochloride; Lignocaine Hydrochloride

Use Local anesthetic and acute treatment of ventricular arrhythmias from myocardial infarction, cardiac manipulation, digitalis intoxication; drug of choice for ventricular ectopy, ventricular tachycardia (VT), ventricular fibrillation (VF); for pulseless VT or VF preferably administer **after** defibrillation and epinephrine; control of premature ventricular contractions, wide-complex paroxysmal supraventricular tachycardia (PSVT); control of hemodynamically compromising PVCs; hemodynamically stable VT

ELA-Max® is a topical local anesthetic for use in laser, cosmetic, and outpatient surgeries; minor burns, cuts, and abrasions of the skin

Orphan drug: Lidoderm® Patch: Relief of allodynia (painful hypersensitivity) and chronic pain in postherpetic neuralgia

Local Anesthetic/Vasoconstrictor Precautions No information available to require special precautions

Effects on Dental Treatment No effects or complications reported

Dosage

Topical: Apply to affected area as needed; maximum: 3 mg/kg/dose; do not repeat within 2 hours.

ELA-Max® cream; Apply 1/4 inch thick layer to intact skin. Leave on until adequate anesthetic effect is obtained. Remove cream and cleanse area before beginning procedure.

Injectable local anesthetic: Varies with procedure, degree of anesthesia needed, vascularity of tissue, duration of anesthesia required, and physical condition of patient; maximum: 4.5 mg/kg/dose; do not repeat within 2 hours.

Patch: Postherpetic neuralgia: Apply patch to most painful area. Up to 3 patches may be applied in a single application. Patch may remain in place for up to 12 hours in any 24-hour period.

Antiarrhythmic:

I.V.: 1-1.5 mg/kg bolus over 2-3 minutes; may repeat doses of 0.5-0.75 mg/kg in 5-10 minutes up to a total of 3 mg/kg; continuous infusion: 1-4 mg/minute

I.V. (2 g/250 mL D_5W) infusion rates (infusion pump should be used for I.V. infusion administration):

1 mg/minute: 7.5 mL/hour
2 mg/minute: 15 mL/hour
3 mg/minute: 22.5 mL/hour
4 mg/minute: 30 mL/hour

Ventricular fibrillation (after defibrillation and epinephrine): Initial: 1-1.5 mg/kg. Repeat 0.5-0.75 mg/kg bolus may be given 3-5 minutes after initial dose. Total dose should not exceed 200-300 mg during a 1-hour period or 3 mg/kg total dose. Follow with continuous infusion after return of perfusion.

Endotracheal: 2-2.5 times the I.V. dose (2-4 mg/kg diluted with NS to a total volume of 10 mL)

Decrease dose in patients with CHF, shock, or hepatic disease.

Dosage adjustment in renal impairment: Not dialyzable (0% to 5%) by hemo- or peritoneal dialysis; supplemental dose is not necessary.

Dosage adjustment in hepatic impairment: Reduce dose in acute hepatitis and decompensated cirrhosis by 50%.

Mechanism of Action Class IB antiarrhythmic; local anesthetics bind selectively to the intracellular surface of sodium channels to block influx of sodium into the axon. As a result, depolarization necessary for action potential propagation and subsequent nerve function is prevented. The block at the sodium channel is reversible. Local anesthetics reversibly prevent generation and conduction of electrical impulses in neurons by decreasing the transient increase in permeability to sodium. The differential sensitivity generally depends on the size of the fiber; small fibers are more sensitive than larger fibers and require a longer period for recovery. Sensory pain fibers are usually blocked first, followed by fibers that transmit sensations of temperature, touch, and deep pressure. High concentrations block sympathetic somatic sensory and somatic motor fibers. The spread of anesthesia depends upon the distribution of the solution. This is primarily dependent on the site of administration and volume of drug injected. When drug diffuses away from the axon, sodium channel function is restored and nerve propagation returns.

Other Adverse Effects Effects vary with route of administration. Many effects are dose-related.

Frequency not defined:

Cardiovascular: Bradycardia, hypotension, heart block, arrhythmias, cardiovascular collapse, sinus node supression, increase defibrillator threshold, vascular insufficiency (periarticular injections), arterial spasms

Central nervous system: Drowsiness after administration is usually a sign of a high blood level. Other effects may include lightheadedness, dizziness, tinnitus, blurred vision, vomiting, twitching, tremors, lethargy, coma, agitation, slurred speech, seizures, anxiety, euphoria, hallucinations, paresthesia, psychosis.

Dermatologic: Itching, rash, edema of the skin, contact dermatitis

Gastrointestinal: Nausea, vomiting, taste disorder

Local: Thrombophlebitis

Neuromuscular & skeletal: Transient radicular pain (subarachnoid administration; 0-1.9%)

Ocular: Blurred vision, diplopia

Respiratory: Dyspnea, respiratory depression or arrest, bronchospasm

Miscellaneous: Allergic reactions, urticaria, edema, anaphylactoid reaction

(Continued)

Lidocaine *(Continued)*

Following spinal anesthesia positional headache (3%), shivering (2%) nausea, peripheral nerve symptoms, respiratory inadequacy and double vision (<1%), hypotension, cauda equina syndrome

Case reports: ARDS (inhalation), severe back pain, methemoglobinemia, asystole

Contraindications Hypersensitivity to lidocaine, other local anesthetics of the amide type, or any component of their formulation; Adam-Stokes syndrome; severe degrees of SA, AV, or intraventricular heart block (except in patients with a functioning artificial pacemaker)

Warnings/Precautions

Intravenous: Constant EKG monitoring is necessary during I.V. administration. Use cautiously in hepatic impairment, any degree of heart block, Wolff-Parkinson-White syndrome, CHF, marked hypoxia, severe respiratory depression, hypovolemia, history of malignant hyperthermia, or shock. Increased ventricular rate may be seen when administered to a patient with atrial fibrillation. Correct any underlying causes of ventricular arrhythmias. Monitor closely for signs and symptoms of CNS toxicity. The elderly may be prone to increased CNS and cardiovascular side effects. Reduce dose in hepatic dysfunction and CHF.

Injectable anesthetic: Follow appropriate administration techniques so as not to administer any intravascularly. Solutions containing antimicrobial preservatives should not be used for epidural or spinal anesthesia. Some solutions contain a bisulfite; avoid in patients who are allergic to bisulfite. Resuscitative equipment, medicine and oxygen should be available in case of emergency. Use products containing epinephrine cautiously in patients with significant vascular disease, compromised blood flow, or during or following general anesthesia (increased risk of arrhythmias). Adjust the dose for the elderly, pediatric, acutely ill, and debilitated patients.

Topical: ELA-Max® cream: Do not leave on large body areas for >2 hours. Observe young children closely to prevent accidental ingestion. Not for use ophthalmic use or for use on mucous membranes.

Drug Interactions CYP1A2, 2B6, and 3A3/4 enzyme substrate; CYP1A2 enzyme inhibitor

Cimetidine increases lidocaine blood levels; monitor levels or use an alternative H_2 antagonist.

Drugs which inhibit CYP3A3/4 may increase lidocaine blood levels.

Protease inhibitors like amprenavir and ritonavir may increase lidocaine blood levels.

Propranolol increases lidocaine blood levels.

Dietary/Ethanol/Herb Considerations

Food: Do not eat or drink for 1 hour following oral administration. Avoid grapefruit products; may increase serum concentration/toxicity.

Herb/Nutraceutical: Avoid St John's wort; may decrease serum concentration. Ginger has positive inotropic effects and theoretically could affect antiarrhythmic activity.

Drug Uptake

Onset of action (single bolus dose): 45-90 seconds

Duration: 10-20 minutes

Initial: 7-30 minutes

Terminal:

Infants, premature: 3.2 hours

Adults: 1.5-2 hours

Half-life, elimination: Biphasic: Increased with CHF, liver disease, shock, severe renal disease; Initial: 7-30 minutes; Terminal: Infants, premature: 3.2 hours, Adults: 1.5-2 hours

Pregnancy Risk Factor B (manufacturer); C (expert analysis)

Breast-feeding Considerations May be taken while breast-feeding

Dosage Forms CRM: 2% (56 g); 4% (5 g, 30 g). **GEL:** 0.5% (15 mL); 2.5% (15 mL). **INJ:** 0.5% [5 mg/mL] (50 mL); 1% [10 mg/mL] (2 mL, 5 mL, 10 mL, 20 mL, 30 mL, 50 mL); 1.5% [15 mg/mL] (20 mL); 2% [20 mg/mL] (2 mL, 5 mL, 10 mL, 20 mL, 30 mL, 50 mL); 4% [40 mg/mL] (5 mL); 10% [100 mg/mL] (10 mL); 20% [200 mg/mL] (10 mL, 20 mL). **INJ:** 10% [100 mg/mL] (3 mL). **INJ, I.V. admixture** [preservative free]: 4% [40 mg/mL] (5 mL, 25 mL, 50 mL); 10% [100 mg/mL] (10 mL); 20% [200 mg/mL] (5 mL, 10 mL). **INJ, I.V. direct:** 1% [10 mg/mL] (5 mL, 20 mL, 30 mL, 50 mL); 2% [20 mg/mL] (5 mL, 10 mL, 20 mL, 30 mL, 50 mL). **INJ, infusion** [in D_5W]: 0.2% [2 mg/mL] (500 mL); 0.4% [4 mg/mL] (250 mL, 500 mL, 1000 mL); 0.8% [8 mg/mL] (250 mL, 500 mL). **JELLY:** 2%. **LIQ, topical:** 2.5% (7.5 mL). **LIQ, viscous:** 2% (20 mL, 100 mL). **OINT:** 2.5% [OTC], 5% (35 g). **PATCH, transdermal:** 5%. **SOLN, topical:** 2% (15 mL, 240 mL); 4% (50 mL)

Generic Available Yes

Comments Lidocaine without epinephrine is not marketed as a dental 1.8 mL carpule and as such is not used as a dental local anesthetic

Lidocaine and Epinephrine (LYE doe kane & ep i NEF rin)

Related Information

Oral Pain *on page 1360*

U.S. Brand Names Xylocaine® With Epinephrine

Canadian Brand Names Xylocaine® With Epinephrine

Mexican Brand Names Pisacaina; Uvega; Xylocaina

Pharmacologic Category Local Anesthetic

Synonyms Epinephrine and Lidocaine

Use Dental: Amide-type anesthetic used for local infiltration anesthesia; injection near nerve trunks to produce nerve block

Local Anesthetic/Vasoconstrictor Precautions No information available to require special precautions

Effects on Dental Treatment No effects or complications reported

Dosage

Children <10 years: Dental anesthesia, infiltration, or conduction block: 20-30 mg (1-1.5 mL) of lidocaine hydrochloride as a 2% solution with epinephrine 1:100,000; maximum: 4-5 mg of lidocaine hydrochloride/kg of body weight or 100-150 mg as a single dose

Children >10 years and Adults: Dental anesthesia, infiltration, or conduction block: Do not exceed 6.6 mg/kg body weight or 300 mg of lidocaine hydrochloride and 3 mcg (0.003 mg) of epinephrine/kg of body weight or 0.2 mg epinephrine per dental appointment. The effective anesthetic dose varies with procedure, intensity of anesthesia needed, duration of anesthesia required, and physical condition of the patient. Always use the lowest effective dose along with careful aspiration. The following numbers of dental carpules (1.8 mL) provide the indicated amounts of lidocaine hydrochloride 2% and epinephrine 1:100,000. See table.

# of Cartridges (1.8 mL)	Lidocaine (2%) (mg)	Epinephrine 1:100,000 (mg)
1	36	0.018
2	72	0.036
3	108	0.054
4	144	0.072
5	180	0.090
6	216	0.108
7	252	0.126
8	288	0.144
9	324	0.162
10	360	0.180

For most routine dental procedures, lidocaine hydrochloride 2% with epinephrine 1:100,000 is preferred. When a more pronounced hemostasis is required, a 1:50,000 epinephrine concentration should be used. The following numbers of dental carpules (1.8 mL) provide the indicated amounts of lidocaine hydrochloride 2% and epinephrine 1:50,000. See table.

# of Cartridges (1.8 mL)	Lidocaine (2%) (mg)	Epinephrine 1:50,000 (mg)
1	36	0.036
2	72	0.072
3	108	0.108
4	144	0.144
5	180	0.180
6	216	0.216

Note: Doses of lidocaine hydrochloride and epinephrine cited from USP Dispensing Information (USP DI) 17th ed, The United States Pharmacopeial Convention, Inc, Rockville, MD, 1997, 138-9.

Mechanism of Action Local anesthetics bind selectively to the intracellular surface of sodium channels to block influx of sodium into the axon. As a result, depolarization necessary for action potential propagation and subsequent nerve function is prevented. The block at the sodium channel is reversible. Local anesthetics reversibly prevent generation and conduction of electrical impulses in neurons by decreasing the transient increase in permeability to sodium. The differential sensitivity generally depends on the size of the fiber; small fibers are more sensitive than larger fibers and require a longer period for recovery. Sensory pain fibers are usually blocked first, followed by fibers that transmit sensations of temperature, touch, and deep pressure. High concentrations block sympathetic somatic sensory and somatic motor fibers. The spread of anesthesia depends upon the distribution of the solution. This is primarily dependent on the site of administration and volume

(Continued)

Lidocaine and Epinephrine *(Continued)*

of drug injected. When drug diffuses away from the axon, sodium channel function is restored and nerve propagation returns.

Epinephrine prolongs the duration of the anesthetic actions of lidocaine by causing vasoconstriction (alpha adrenergic receptor agonist) of the vasculature surrounding the nerve axons. This prevents the diffusion of lidocaine away from the nerves resulting in a longer retention in the axon.

Other Adverse Effects Degree of adverse effects in the central nervous system and cardiovascular system are directly related to the blood levels of lidocaine. The effects below are more likely to occur after systemic administration rather than infiltration.

Cardiovascular: Myocardial effects include a decrease in contraction force as well as a decrease in electrical excitability and myocardial conduction rate resulting in bradycardia and reduction in cardiac output.

Central nervous system: High blood levels result in anxiety, restlessness, disorientation, confusion, dizziness, tremors and seizures. This is followed by depression of CNS resulting in somnolence, unconsciousness and possible respiratory arrest. In some cases, symptoms of CNS stimulation may be absent and the primary CNS effects are somnolence and unconsciousness.

Gastrointestinal: Nausea and vomiting may occur

Hypersensitivity reactions: Extremely rare, but may be manifest as dermatologic reactions and edema at injection site. Asthmatic syndromes have occurred. Patients may exhibit hypersensitivity to bisulfites contained in local anesthetic solution to prevent oxidation of epinephrine. In general, patients reacting to bisulfites have a history of asthma and their airways are hyper-reactive to asthmatic syndrome.

Psychogenic reactions: It is common to misinterpret psychogenic responses to local anesthetic injection as an allergic reaction. Intraoral injections are perceived by many patients as a stressful procedure in dentistry. Common symptoms to this stress are diaphoresis, palpitations, hyperventilation, generalized pallor and a fainting feeling

Contraindications Hypersensitivity to lidocaine, epinephrine, local anesthetics of the amide type, or any component of their formulation; myasthenia gravis; shock; cardiac conduction disease

See Epinephrine (Dental) *on page 438* and Lidocaine *on page 706*

Warnings/Precautions Aspirate the syringe after tissue penetration and before injection to minimize chance of direct vascular injection; do not use solutions in distal portions of the body (digits, nose, ears, penis). Use with caution in endocrine, heart, hepatic, or thyroid disease.

Drug Interactions Epinephrine (and other direct alpha-agonists): Pressor response to I.V. epinephrine, norepinephrine, and phenylephrine may be enhanced in patients receiving TCAs (**Note:** Effect is unlikely with epinephrine or levonordefrin dosages typically administered as infiltration in combination with local anesthetics)

Drug Uptake

Onset of action: Infiltration <2 minutes; nerve block 2-4 minutes; Peak effect: ~5 minutes

Duration:

Infiltration: Soft tissue anesthesia ~2.5 hours; pulp anesthesia <60 minutes

Nerve block: Soft tissue anesthesia ~3.25 hours; pulp anesthesia ≥90 minutes

See Lidocaine *on page 706* and Epinephrine *on page 438*

Pregnancy Risk Factor B

Breast-feeding Considerations Usual infiltration doses of lidocaine with epinephrine given to nursing mothers has not been shown to affect the health of the nursing infant.

Dosage Forms INJ:

Epinephrine 1:200,000: Lidocaine 0.5% [5 mg/mL] (50 mL); 1% [10 mg/mL] (30 mL); 1.5% [15 mg/mL] (5 mL, 10 mL, 30 mL); 2% [20 mg/mL] (20 mL)

Epinephrine 1:100,000: Lidocaine 1% [10 mg/mL] (20 mL, 50 mL); 2% [20 mg/mL] (1.8 mL, 20 mL, 30 mL, 50 mL)

Epinephrine 1:50,000: Lidocaine 2% [20 mg/mL] (1.8 mL)

Generic Available Yes

Selected Readings

Ayoub ST and Coleman AE, "A Review of Local Anesthetics," *Gen Dent*, 1992, 40(4):285-7, 289-90.

Jastak JT and Yagiela JA, "Vasoconstrictors and Local Anesthesia: A Review and Rationale for Use," *J Am Dent Assoc*, 1983, 107(4):623-30.

MacKenzie TA and Young ER, "Local Anesthetic Update," *Anesth Prog*, 1993, 40(2):29-34.

Wynn RL, "Epinephrine Interactions With Beta-Blockers," *Gen Dent*, 1994, 42(1):16, 18.

Wynn RL, "Recent Research on Mechanisms of Local Anesthetics," *Gen Dent*, 1995, 43(4):316-8.

Yagiela JA, "Local Anesthetics," *Anesth Prog*, 1991, 38(4-5):128-41.

Lidocaine and Hydrocortisone

(LYE doe kane & hye droe KOR ti sone)

U.S. Brand Names Lida-Mantle HC®

Pharmacologic Category Anesthetic/Corticosteroid

Synonyms Hydrocortisone and Lidocaine

Use Topical anti-inflammatory and anesthetic for skin disorders

Local Anesthetic/Vasoconstrictor Precautions No information available to require special precautions

Effects on Dental Treatment No effects or complications reported

Dosage Topical: Apply 2-4 times/day

Therapy should be discontinued when control is achieved; if no improvement is seen, reassessment of diagnosis may be necessary.

Drug Uptake See Lidocaine *on page 706* and Hydrocortisone *on page 608*

Pregnancy Risk Factor B (lidocaine); C (hydrocortisone)

Generic Available No

Lidocaine and Prilocaine (LYE doe kane & PRIL oh kane)

U.S. Brand Names EMLA®

Canadian Brand Names EMLA®

Pharmacologic Category Local Anesthetic

Synonyms Prilocaine and Lidocaine

Use

Dental: Amide-type topical anesthetic for use on normal intact skin to provide local analgesia for minor procedures such as I.V. cannulation or venipuncture

Medical: Has also been used for painful procedures such as lumbar puncture and skin graft harvesting; topical anesthetic for local anesthesia on normal skin; topical anesthetic for superficial minor surgery of genital mucous membranes; adjunct for local infiltration anesthesia in genital mucous membranes

Local Anesthetic/Vasoconstrictor Precautions No information available to require special precautions

Effects on Dental Treatment No effects or complications reported

Dosage Although the incidence of systemic adverse effects with EMLA® is very low, caution should be exercised, particularly when applying over large areas and leaving on for >2 hours

Children (intact skin): EMLA® should **not** be used in neonates with a gestation age <37 weeks nor in infants <12 months of age who are receiving treatment with methemoglobin-inducing agents

Dosing is based on child's age and weight:

Age 0-3 months or <5 kg: Apply a maximum of 1 g over no more than 10 cm^2 of skin; leave on for no longer than 1 hour

Age 3 months to 12 months and >5 kg: Apply no more than a maximum 2 g total over no more than 20 cm^2 of skin; leave on for no longer than 4 hours

Age 1-6 years and >10 kg: Apply no more than a maximum of 10 g total over no more than 100 cm^2 of skin; leave on for no longer than 4 hours.

Age 7-12 years and >20 kg: Apply no more than a maximum 20 g total over no more than 200 cm^2 of skin; leave on for no longer than 4 hours.

Note: If a patient greater than 3 months old does not meet the minimum weight requirement, the maximum total dose should be restricted to the corresponding maximum based on patient weight.

Adults (intact skin):

EMLA® cream and EMLA® anesthetic disc: A thick layer of EMLA® cream is applied to intact skin and covered with an occlusive dressing, or alternatively, an EMLA® anesthetic disc is applied to intact skin

Minor dermal procedures (eg, I.V. cannulation or venipuncture): Apply 2.5 g of cream (1/2 of the 5 g tube) over 20-25 cm of skin surface area, or 1 anesthetic disc (1 g over 10 cm^2) for at least 1 hour. **Note:** In clinical trials, 2 sites were usually prepared in case there was a technical problem with cannulation or venipuncture at the first site.

Major dermal procedures (eg, more painful dermatological procedures involving a larger skin area such as split thickness skin graft harvesting): Apply 2 g of cream per 10 cm^2 of skin and allow to remain in contact with the skin for at least 2 hours.

Adult male genital skin (eg, pretreatment prior to local anesthetic infiltration): Apply a thick layer of cream (1 g/10 cm^2) to the skin surface for 15 minutes. Local anesthetic infiltration should be performed immediately after removal of EMLA® cream.

Note: Dermal analgesia can be expected to increase for up to 3 hours under occlusive dressing and persist for 1-2 hours after removal of the cream

Adult females: Genital mucous membranes: Minor procedures (eg, removal of condylomata acuminata, pretreatment for local anesthetic infiltration): Apply 5-10 g (thick layer) of cream for 5-10 minutes

Mechanism of Action Local anesthetics bind selectively to the intracellular surface of sodium channels to block influx of sodium into the axon. As a result, depolarization necessary for action potential propagation and subsequent nerve function is prevented. The block at the sodium channel is reversible. When drug diffuses away from the axon, sodium channel function is restored and nerve propagation returns.

Other Adverse Effects Frequency not defined:

Cardiovascular: Hypotension, angioedema

Central nervous system: Shock

(Continued)

Lidocaine and Prilocaine *(Continued)*

Dermatologic: Hyperpigmentation, erythema, itching, rash, burning, urticaria
Genitourinary: Blistering of foreskin (rare)
Local: Burning, stinging, edema
Respiratory: Bronchospasm
Miscellaneous: Alteration in temperature sensation, hypersensitivity reactions

Contraindications Hypersensitivity to lidocaine, prilocaine, other amide type anesthetic agents (dibucaine, mepivacaine, bupivacaine, etidocaine), or any component of their formulation; application on mucous membranes or broken or inflamed skin; infants <1 month of age if gestational age is <37 weeks; infants <12 months of age receiving therapy with methemoglobin-inducing agents; children with congenital or idiopathic methemoglobinemia; children receiving medications associated with drug-induced methemoglobinemia [ie, acetaminophen (overdosage), benzocaine, chloroquine, dapsone, nitrofurantoin, nitroglycerin, nitroprusside, phenazopyridine, phenelzine, phenobarbital, phenytoin, quinine, sulfonamides]

Warnings/Precautions EMLA® should not be used in patients with congenital or idiopathic methemoglobinemia and in infants <12 months of age who are receiving treatment with methemoglobin-inducing agents. Very young patients or patients with glucose-6-phosphate deficiencies are more susceptible to methemoglobinemia. Patients taking drugs associated with drug-induced methemoglobinemia (sulfonamides, acetaminophen, acetanilide, aniline dyes, benzocaine, chloroquine, dapsone, naphthalene, nitrates/nitrites, nitrofurantoin, nitroglycerin, nitroprusside, pamoquine, para-aminosalicylic acid, phenacetin, phenobarbital, phenytoin, primaquine, quinine) are at greater risk for developing methemoglobinemia. Reports of significant methemoglobinemia have occurred in infants and children following excessive applications of EMLA® cream. These cases involved the use of large doses, larger than recommended areas of application, infants <3 months of age who did not have fully mature enzyme systems. Treatment with I.V. methylene blue may be effective if required.

Neonates and infants up to 3 months of age should be monitored for Met-Hb levels before, during, and after application of EMLA®, provided the test results can be obtained quickly.

Use with caution in patients who may be more sensitive to the systemic effects of lidocaine and prilocaine, including acutely ill, debilitated, or elderly patients.

Use with caution in patients with severe hepatic disease, because their inability to metabolize local anesthetics normally puts them at greater risk of developing toxic plasma concentrations of lidocaine and prilocaine.

Drug Interactions Increased Toxicity:

Class I antiarrhythmic drugs (tocainide, mexiletine): Effects are additive and potentially synergistic
Drugs known to induce methemoglobinemia

Drug Uptake

EMLA®:

Onset of dermal analgesic effect: 1 hour; Peak effect: 2-3 hours
Absorption: Related to duration of application and area over which it is applied
- 3-hour application: 3.6% lidocaine and 6.1% prilocaine were absorbed
- 24-hour application: 16.2% lidocaine and 33.5% prilocaine were absorbed

Duration: 1-2 hours after removal
Half-life, elimination:
- Lidocaine: 65-150 minutes (increases with cardiac or hepatic dysfunction)
- Prilocaine: 10-150 minutes (increases with hepatic or renal dysfunction)

See Lidocaine *on page 706* and Prilocaine *on page 992*

Pregnancy Risk Factor B

Breast-feeding Considerations Usual infiltration doses of lidocaine and prilocaine given to nursing mothers has not been shown to affect the health of the nursing infant.

Dosage Forms CRM: Lidocaine 2.5% and prilocaine 2.5% [2 Tegaderm® dressings] (5 g, 30 g). **DISC, anesthetic:** 1 g (25 mg lidocaine and 25 mg prilocaine in each 10 square centimeter disc)

Generic Available No

Selected Readings

Broadman LM, Soliman IE, Hannallah RS, et al, "Analgesic Efficacy of Eutectic Mixture of Local Anesthetics (EMLA®) vs Intradermal Infiltration Prior to Venous Cannulation in Children," *Am J Anaesth*, 1987, 34:S56.

Halperin DL, Koren G, Attias D, et al, "Topical Skin Anesthesia for Venous Subcutaneous Drug Reservoir and Lumbar Puncture in Children," *Pediatrics*, 1989, 84(2):281-4.

Robieux I, Kumar R, Radhakrishnan S, et al, "Assessing Pain and Analgesia With a Lidocaine-Prilocaine Emulsion in Infants and Toddlers During Venipuncture," *J Pediatr*, 1991, 118(6):971-3.

Taddio A, Shennan AT, Stevens B, et al, "Safety of Lidocaine-Prilocaine Cream in the Treatment of Preterm Neonates," *J Pediatr*, 1995, 127(6):1002-5.

Vickers ER, Mazbani N, Gerzina TM, et al, "Pharmacokinetics of EMLA Cream 5% Application to Oral Mucosa," *Anesth Prog*, 1997, 44:32-7.

Lidocaine Transoral (LYE doe kane trans OR al)

Related Information

Oral Pain *on page 1360*

U.S. Brand Names DentiPatch®

Pharmacologic Category Local Anesthetic, Transoral

Use Dental: Local anesthesia of the oral mucosa prior to oral injections and soft-tissue dental procedures

Local Anesthetic/Vasoconstrictor Precautions No information available to require special precautions

Effects on Dental Treatment No effects or complications reported

Dosage One patch on selected area of oral mucosa

Mechanism of Action Blocks both the initiation and conduction of nerve impulses by decreasing the neuronal membrane's permeability to sodium ions, which results in inhibition of depolarization with resultant blockade of conduction

Contraindications Hypersensitivity to lidocaine or any of component of the formulation

Drug Uptake

Onset of action: 2 minutes

Duration: ≥40 minutes based on a 15-minute application

Dosage Forms PATCH: 23 mg/2 cm^2; 46.1 mg/2 cm^2 [50s, 100s]

Generic Available No

Comments The manufacturer claims DentiPatch® is safe, with "negligible systemic absorption" of lidocaine. The agent is "clinically proven to prevent injection pain from 25-gauge needles that are inserted to the level of the bone." Data from controlled studies (235 patients) have shown no serious adverse effects with the application of lidocaine patch to the oral mucosa for 15 minutes. Peak plasma levels were 10% of those seen following local infiltration anesthesia with 1.8 mL lidocaine and 1:100,000 epinephrine. According to the manufacturer, tips for applying lidocaine patch are the following:

- Cotton roll isolation for all procedures except palatal application
- Air dry with syringe on dental unit for 30 seconds
- Apply patch to gingiva or mucosa
- Apply firm finger pressure to patch for 30 seconds

Leave patch in place during scaling and root planing procedure; remove after 15 minutes. Patch should be removed after 5-10 minutes prior to giving injection.

Selected Readings

Hersh EV, Houpt MI, Cooper SA, et al, "Analgesic Efficacy and Safety of an Intraoral Lidocaine Patch," *J Am Dent Assoc*, 1996, 127(11):1626-34.

Houpt MI, Heins P, Lamster I, et al, "An Evaluation of Intraoral Lidocaine Patches in Reducing Needle-Insertion Pain," *Compend Contin Educ Dent*, 1997, 18(4):309-10, 312-4, 316.

"The Lidocaine Patch: A New Delivery System," *Biolog Ther Dent*, 1997, 13:17-22.

Lidoderm® *see* Lidocaine *on page 706*

LidoPen® Auto-Injector *see* Lidocaine *on page 706*

Limbitrol® *see* Amitriptyline and Chlordiazepoxide *on page 76*

Limbitrol® DS *see* Amitriptyline and Chlordiazepoxide *on page 76*

Lincocin® *see* Lincomycin *on page 713*

Lincomycin (lin koe MYE sin)

U.S. Brand Names Lincocin®; Lincorex®

Canadian Brand Names Lincocin®

Mexican Brand Names Lincocin®; Princol®; Rimsalin®

Pharmacologic Category Antibiotic, Macrolide

Synonyms Lincomycin Hydrochloride

Use Treatment of susceptible bacterial infections, mainly those caused by streptococci and staphylococci resistant to other agents

Local Anesthetic/Vasoconstrictor Precautions No information available to require special precautions

Effects on Dental Treatment No effects or complications reported

Dosage

Children >1 month:

- Oral: 30-60 mg/kg/day in divided doses every 8 hours
- I.M.: 10 mg/kg every 8-12 hours
- I.V.: 10-20 mg/kg/day in divided doses every 8-12 hours

Adults:

- Oral: 500 mg every 6-8 hours
- I.M.: 600 mg every 12-24 hours
- I.V.: 600-1 g every 8-12 hours up to 8 g/day

Mechanism of Action Lincosamide antibiotic which was isolated from a strain of *Streptomyces lincolnensis*; lincomycin, like clindamycin, inhibits bacterial protein synthesis by specifically binding on the 50S subunit and affecting the process of peptide chain initiation. Other macrolide antibiotics (erythromycin) also bind to the 50S subunit. Since only one molecule of antibiotic can bind to a single ribosome, the concomitant use of erythromycin and lincomycin is not recommended.

(Continued)

Lincomycin *(Continued)*

Other Adverse Effects Frequency not defined:
Central nervous system: Vertigo
Dermatologic: Vesiculobullous dermatitis (rare)
Gastrointestinal: Nausea, vomiting, diarrhea
Hematologic: Pancytopenia (rare)
Miscellaneous: Serum sickness (rare)

Drug Interactions
Increased Effect/Toxicity: Increased activity/toxicity of neuromuscular blocking agents.
Decreased effect with erythromycin.

Drug Uptake
Absorption: Oral: ~20% to 30%
Half-life, elimination: 2-11.5 hours
Time to peak: Oral: 2-4 hours; I.M.: 1 hour

Pregnancy Risk Factor B

Generic Available Yes

Lincorex® *see* Lincomycin *on page 713*

Lindane (LIN dane)

U.S. Brand Names G-well®

Canadian Brand Names Hexit™; PMS-Lindane

Mexican Brand Names Herklin Shampoo®; Scabisan®

Pharmacologic Category Antiparasitic Agent, Topical; Pediculocide; Scabicidal Agent

Synonyms Benzene Hexachloride; Gamma Benzene Hexachloride; Hexachlorocyclohexane

Use Treatment of scabies (*Sarcoptes scabiei*), *Pediculus capitis* (head lice), and *Pediculus pubis* (crab lice); FDA recommends reserving lindane as a second-line agent or with inadequate response to other therapies

Local Anesthetic/Vasoconstrictor Precautions No information available to require special precautions

Effects on Dental Treatment No effects or complications reported

Dosage Children and Adults: Topical:
Scabies: Apply a thin layer of lotion or cream and massage it on skin from the neck to the toes (head to toe in infants). For adults, bathe and remove the drug after 8-12 hours; for children, wash off 6-8 hours after application (for infants, wash off 6 hours after application); repeat treatment in 7 days if lice or nits are still present
Pediculosis, capitis and pubis: 15-30 mL of shampoo is applied and lathered for 4-5 minutes; rinse hair thoroughly and comb with a fine tooth comb to remove nits; repeat treatment in 7 days if lice or nits are still present

Mechanism of Action Directly absorbed by parasites and ova through the exoskeleton; stimulates the nervous system resulting in seizures and death of parasitic arthropods

Drug Interactions Oil-based hair dressing may increase potential for toxicity of lindane.

Drug Uptake
Absorption: ≤13% systemically
Half-life, elimination: Children: 17-22 hours
Time to peak: Topical: Children: 6 hours

Pregnancy Risk Factor B

Generic Available Yes

Linezolid (li NE zoh lid)

U.S. Brand Names Zyvox™

Pharmacologic Category Antibiotic, Oxazolidinone

Use Treatment of vancomycin-resistant *Enterococcus faecium* (VRE) infections, nosocomial pneumonia caused by *Staphylococcus aureus* including MRSA or *Streptococcus pneumoniae* (penicillin-susceptible strains only), complicated and uncomplicated skin and skin structure infections, and community-acquired pneumonia caused by susceptible gram-positive organisms.

Local Anesthetic/Vasoconstrictor Precautions Linezolid has mild monoamine oxidase inhibitor properties. The clinician is reminded that vasoconstrictors have the potential to interact with MAOIs to result in elevation of blood pressure. Caution is suggested.

Effects on Dental Treatment ≤2%: Oral moniliasis, taste alteration, tongue discoloration

Dosage Adult:
Oral, I.V.:
VRE infections: 600 mg every 12 hours for 14-28 days
Nosocomial pneumonia, complicated skin and skin structure infections, community-acquired pneumonia including concurrent bacteremia: 600 mg every 12 hours for 10-14 days

Oral: Uncomplicated skin and skin structure infections: 400 mg every 12 hours for 10-14 days

Dosage adjustment in renal impairment: No specific adjustment recommended. The two primary metabolites may accumulate in patients with renal impairment but the clinical significance is unknown. Weigh the risk of accumulation of metabolites versus the benefit of therapy. Both linezolid and the two metabolites are eliminated by dialysis. Linezolid should be given after hemodialysis.

Mechanism of Action Inhibits bacterial protein synthesis by binding to bacterial 23S ribosomal RNA of the 50S subunit. This prevents the formation of a functional 70S initiation complex that is essential for the bacterial translation process. Linezolid is bacteriostatic against enterococci and staphylococci and bactericidal against most strains of streptococci.

Other Adverse Effects

1% to 10%:

Cardiovascular: Hypertension (1% to 3%)

Central nervous system: Headache (0.5% to 11%), insomnia (3%), dizziness (0.4% to 2%), fever (2%)

Dermatologic: Rash (2%)

Gastrointestinal: Nausea (3% to 10%), diarrhea (3% to 11%), vomiting (1% to 4%), constipation (2%), taste alteration (1% to 2%), tongue discoloration (0.2% to 1%), oral moniliasis (0.4% to 1%), pancreatitis

Genitourinary: Vaginal moniliasis (1% to 2%)

Hematologic: Thrombocytopenia (0.3% to 10%), anemia, leukopenia, neutropenia

Hepatic: Abnormal LFTs (0.4% to 1%)

Miscellaneous: Fungal infections (0.1% to 2%)

Contraindications Hypersensitivity to linezolid, other oxazolidinones, or any component of their formulation

Warnings/Precautions Linezolid has mild monoamine oxidase inhibitor properties and has the potential to have the same interactions as other MAOIs; watch for suprainfections; not for use in uncontrolled hypertension, pheochromocytoma, carcinoid syndrome, untreated hyperthyroidism

Drug Interactions Increased Effect/Toxicity: Linezolid is a reversible, nonselective inhibitor of MAO. Serotonergic agents (eg, TCAs, venlafaxine, trazodone, sibutramine, meperidine, dextromethorphan, and SSRIs) may cause a serotonin syndrome (eg, hyperpyrexia, cognitive dysfunction) when used concomitantly. Adrenergic agents (eg, phenylpropanolamine, pseudoephedrine, sympathomimetic agents, vasopressor or dopaminergic agents) may cause hypertension. Myelosuppressive medications may increase risk of myelosuppression when used concurrently with linezolid.

Drug Uptake

Absorption: Rapid and extensive

Half-life, elimination: 4-5 hours

Time to peak: 1-2 hours

Pregnancy Risk Factor C

Generic Available No

Lioresal® *see* Baclofen *on page 142*

Liothyronine (lye oh THYE roe neen)

Related Information

Endocrine Disorders and Pregnancy *on page 1331*

U.S. Brand Names Cytomel®; Triostat®

Canadian Brand Names Cytomel®

Mexican Brand Names Triyotex®

Pharmacologic Category Thyroid Product

Synonyms Liothyronine Sodium; Sodium *L*-Triiodothyronine; T_3 Sodium

Use Replacement or supplemental therapy in hypothyroidism; management of nontoxic goiter, chronic lymphocytic thyroiditis, as an adjunct in thyrotoxicosis and as a diagnostic aid; **levothyroxine is recommended for chronic therapy**; although previously thought to benefit cardiac patients with severely reduced fractions, liothyronine injection is no longer considered beneficial

Orphan drug: Triostat™: Treatment of myxedema coma/precoma

Local Anesthetic/Vasoconstrictor Precautions No precautions with vasoconstrictor are necessary if patient is well controlled with liothyronine

Effects on Dental Treatment No effects or complications reported

Dosage

Congenital hypothyroidism: Children: Oral: 5 mcg/day increase by 5 mcg every 3 days to 20 mcg/day for infants, 50 mcg/day for children 1-3 years of age, and give adult dose for children >3 years.

Hypothyroidism: Oral:

Adults: 25 mcg/day increase by 12.5-25 mcg/day every 1-2 weeks to a maximum of 100 mcg/day

Elderly: Initial: 5 mcg/day, increase by 5 mcg/day every 1-2 weeks; usual maintenance dose: 25-75 mcg/day

(Continued)

Liothyronine *(Continued)*

T_3 suppression test: Oral: 75-100 mcg/day for 7 days; use lowest dose for elderly
Myxedema coma: I.V.: 25-50 mcg
Patients with known or suspected cardiovascular disease: 10-20 mcg
Normally, at least 4 hours should be allowed between doses to adequately assess therapeutic response and ≤12 hours should elapse between doses to avoid fluctuations in hormone levels. Oral therapy should be resumed as soon as the clinical situation has been stabilized and the patient is able to take oral medication. If levothyroxine rather than liothyronine sodium is used in initiating oral therapy, the physician should bear in mind that there is a delay of several days in the onset of levothyroxine activity and that I.V. therapy should be discontinued gradually.

Mechanism of Action Primary active compound is T_3 (triiodothyronine), which may be converted from T_4 (thyroxine) and then circulates throughout the body to influence growth and maturation of various tissues; exact mechanism of action is unknown; however, it is believed the thyroid hormone exerts its many metabolic effects through control of DNA transcription and protein synthesis; involved in normal metabolism, growth, and development; promotes gluconeogenesis, increases utilization and mobilization of glycogen stores, and stimulates protein synthesis, increases basal metabolic rate

Other Adverse Effects Frequency not defined:
Cardiovascular: Palpitations, cardiac arrhythmias, tachycardia, chest pain
Central nervous system: Nervousness, headache, insomnia, fever, ataxia
Dermatologic: Alopecia
Endocrine & metabolic: Changes in menstrual cycle, weight loss, increased appetite
Gastrointestinal: Diarrhea, abdominal cramps, constipation, vomiting
Neuromuscular & skeletal: Myalgia, hand tremors, tremor
Respiratory: Dyspnea
Miscellaneous: Diaphoresis, allergic skin reactions (rare)

Drug Interactions
Aluminum- and magnesium-containing antacids, calcium carbonate, simethicone, or sucralfate: May decrease T_4 absorption; separate dose from thyroid hormones by at least 4 hours.
Antidiabetic agents (biguanides, meglitinides, sulfonylureas, thiazolidinediones, insulin): Changes in thyroid function may alter requirements of antidiabetic agent. Monitor closely at initiation of therapy, or when dose is changed or discontinued.
Cholestyramine and colestipol: Decrease T_4 absorption; separate dose from thyroid hormones by at least 4 hours.
CYP enzyme inducers: May increase the metabolism of T_3 and T_4. Inducers include barbiturates, carbamazepine, phenytoin, and rifampin/rifabutin.
Digoxin: Digoxin levels may be reduced in hyperthyroidism; therapeutic effect may be reduced. Impact of thyroid replacement should be monitored.
Iron: Decreases T_4 absorption; separate dose from thyroid hormones by at least 4 hours
Kayexalate®: Decreases T_4 absorption; separate dose from thyroid hormones by at least 4 hours
Ketamine: May cause marked hypertension and tachycardia; monitor
Ritonavir: May alter response to thyroid hormones (limited documentation/case report); monitor
Somatrem, somatropin: Excessive thyroid hormone levels lead to accelerated epiphyseal closure; inadequate replacement interferes with growth response to growth hormone. Effect of thyroid replacement not specifically evaluated; use caution.
SSRI antidepressants: May need to increase dose of thyroid hormones when SSRI is added to a previously stabilized patient.
Sympathomimetics: Effects of sympathomimetic agent or thyroid hormones may be increased. Risk of coronary insufficiency is increased in patients with coronary artery disease when these agents are used together.
Theophylline, caffeine: Decreased theophylline clearance in hypothyroid patients; monitor during thyroid replacement.
Tricyclic and tetracyclic antidepressants: Therapeutic and toxic effects of thyroid hormones and the antidepressant are increased.
Warfarin (and other oral anticoagulants): The hypoprothrombinemic response to warfarin may be altered by a change in thyroid function or replacement. Replacement may dramatically increase response to warfarin. However, initiation of warfarin in a patient stabilized on a dose of thyroid hormones does not appear to require a significantly different approach.
Note: Several medications have effects on thyroid production or conversion. The impact in thyroid replacement has not been specifically evaluated, but patient response should be monitored:
Methimazole: Decreases thyroid hormone secretion, while propylthiouracil decrease thyroid hormone secretion and decreases conversion of T_4 to T_3.
Beta-adrenergic antagonists: Decrease conversion of T_4 to T_3 (dose related, propranolol ≥160 mg/day); patients may be clinically euthyroid.

Iodide, iodine-containing radiographic contrast agents may decrease thyroid hormone secretion; may also increase thyroid hormone secretion, especially in patients with Graves' disease.

Other agents reported to impact on thyroid production/conversion include aminoglutethimide, amiodarone, chloral hydrate, diazepam, ethionamide, interferon-alpha, interleukin-2, lithium, lovastatin (case report), glucocorticoids (dose-related), 6-mercaptopurine, sulfonamides, thiazide diuretics, and tolbutamide.

In addition, a number of medications have been noted to cause transient depression in TSH secretion, which may complicate interpretation of monitoring tests for thyroid hormones, including corticosteroids, octreotide, and dopamine. Metoclopramide may increase TSH secretion.

Aluminum- and magnesium-containing antacids, calcium carbonate, simethicone, or sucralfate: May decrease T_4 absorption; separate dose from thyroid hormones by at least 4 hours.

Antidiabetic agents (biguanides, meglitinides, sulfonylureas, thiazolidinediones, insulin): Changes in thyroid function may alter requirements of antidiabetic agent. Monitor closely at initiation of therapy, or when dose is changed or discontinued.

Cholestyramine and colestipol: Decrease T_4 absorption; separate dose from thyroid hormones by at least 4 hours.

CYP enzyme inducers: May increase the metabolism of T_3 and T_4. Inducers include barbiturates, carbamazepine, phenytoin, and rifampin/rifabutin.

Digoxin: Digoxin levels may be reduced in hyperthyroidism; therapeutic effect may be reduced. Impact of thyroid replacement should be monitored.

Iron: Decreases T_4 absorption; separate dose from thyroid hormones by at least 4 hours

Kayexalate®: Decreases T_4 absorption; separate dose from thyroid hormones by at least 4 hours

Ketamine: May cause marked hypertension and tachycardia; monitor

Ritonavir: May alter response to thyroid hormones (limited documentation/case report); monitor

Somatrem, somatropin: Excessive thyroid hormone levels lead to accelerated epiphyseal closure; inadequate replacement interferes with growth response to growth hormone. Effect of thyroid replacement not specifically evaluated; use caution.

SSRI antidepressants: May need to increase dose of thyroid hormones when SSRI is added to a previously stabilized patient.

Sympathomimetics: Effects of sympathomimetic agent or thyroid hormones may be increased. Risk of coronary insufficiency is increased in patients with coronary artery disease when these agents are used together.

Theophylline, caffeine: Decreased theophylline clearance in hypothyroid patients; monitor during thyroid replacement.

Tricyclic and tetracyclic antidepressants: Therapeutic and toxic effects of thyroid hormones and the antidepressant are increased.

Warfarin (and other oral anticoagulants): The hypoprothrombinemic response to warfarin may be altered by a change in thyroid function or replacement. Replacement may dramatically increase response to warfarin. However, initiation of warfarin in a patient stabilized on a dose of thyroid hormones does not appear to require a significantly different approach.

Note: Several medications have effects on thyroid production or conversion. The impact in thyroid replacement has not been specifically evaluated, but patient response should be monitored:

Methimazole: Decreases thyroid hormone secretion, while propylthiouracil decrease thyroid hormone secretion and decreases conversion of T_4 to T_3.

Beta-adrenergic antagonists: Decrease conversion of T_4 to T_3 (dose related, propranolol ≥160 mg/day); patients may be clinically euthyroid.

Iodide, iodine-containing radiographic contrast agents may decrease thyroid hormone secretion; may also increase thyroid hormone secretion, especially in patients with Graves' disease.

Other agents reported to impact on thyroid production/conversion include aminoglutethimide, amiodarone, chloral hydrate, diazepam, ethionamide, interferon-alpha, interleukin-2, lithium, lovastatin (case report), glucocorticoids (dose-related), 6-mercaptopurine, sulfonamides, thiazide diuretics, and tolbutamide.

In addition, a number of medications have been noted to cause transient depression in TSH secretion, which may complicate interpretation of monitoring tests for thyroid hormones, including corticosteroids, octreotide, and dopamine. Metoclopramide may increase TSH secretion.

Drug Uptake

Onset of action: 24-72 hours

Absorption: Oral: Well absorbed (~85% to 90%)

Duration: ≤72 hours

Half-life, elimination: 16-49 hours

Pregnancy Risk Factor A

Generic Available Yes

Liotrix (LYE oh triks)

Related Information

Endocrine Disorders and Pregnancy *on page 1331*

U.S. Brand Names Thyrolar®

Canadian Brand Names Thyrolar®

Pharmacologic Category Thyroid Product

Synonyms T_3/T_4 Liotrix

Use Replacement or supplemental therapy in hypothyroidism (uniform mixture of $T_4:T_3$ in 4:1 ratio by weight); little advantage to this product exists and cost is not justified

Local Anesthetic/Vasoconstrictor Precautions No precautions with vasoconstrictor are necessary if patient is well controlled with liotrix

Effects on Dental Treatment No effects or complications reported

Dosage Oral:

Congenital hypothyroidism:

Children (dose of T_4 or levothyroxine/day):

- 0-6 months: 8-10 mcg/kg or 25-50 mcg/day
- 6-12 months: 6-8 mcg/kg or 50-75 mcg/day
- 1-5 years: 5-6 mcg/kg or 75-100 mcg/day
- 6-12 years: 4-5 mcg/kg or 100-150 mcg/day
- >12 years: 2-3 mcg/kg or >150 mcg/day

Hypothyroidism (dose of thyroid equivalent):

Adults: 30 mg/day, increasing by 15 mg/day at 2- to 3-week intervals to a maximum of 180 mg/day (usual maintenance dose: 60-120 mg/day)

Elderly: Initial: 15 mg, adjust dose at 2- to 4-week intervals by increments of 15 mg

Mechanism of Action The primary active compound is T_3 (triiodothyronine), which may be converted from T_4 (thyroxine) and then circulates throughout the body to influence growth and maturation of various tissues. Liotrix is uniform mixture of synthetic T_4 and T_3 in 4:1 ratio; exact mechanism of action is unknown; however, it is believed the thyroid hormone exerts its many metabolic effects through control of DNA transcription and protein synthesis; involved in normal metabolism, growth, and development; promotes gluconeogenesis, increases utilization and mobilization of glycogen stores and stimulates protein synthesis, increases basal metabolic rate

Other Adverse Effects Frequency not defined:

Cardiovascular: Palpitations, cardiac arrhythmias, tachycardia, chest pain

Central nervous system: Nervousness, headache, insomnia, fever, ataxia

Dermatologic: Alopecia

Endocrine & metabolic: Changes in menstrual cycle, weight loss, increased appetite

Gastrointestinal: Diarrhea, abdominal cramps, constipation, vomiting

Neuromuscular & skeletal: Myalgia, hand tremors, tremor

Respiratory: Dyspnea

Miscellaneous: Diaphoresis, allergic skin reactions (rare)

Drug Interactions

Aluminum- and magnesium-containing antacids, calcium carbonate, simethicone, or sucralfate: May decrease T_4 absorption; separate dose from thyroid hormones by at least 4 hours.

Antidiabetic agents (biguanides, meglitinides, sulfonylureas, thiazolidinediones, insulin): Changes in thyroid function may alter requirements of antidiabetic agent. Monitor closely at initiation of therapy, or when dose is changed or discontinued.

Cholestyramine and colestipol: Decrease T_4 absorption; separate dose from thyroid hormones by at least 4 hours.

CYP enzyme inducers: May increase the metabolism of T_3 and T_4. Inducers include barbiturates, carbamazepine, phenytoin, and rifampin/rifabutin.

Digoxin: Digoxin levels may be reduced in hyperthyroidism; therapeutic effect may be reduced. Impact of thyroid replacement should be monitored.

Iron: Decreases T_4 absorption; separate dose from thyroid hormones by at least 4 hours

Kayexalate®: Decreases T_4 absorption; separate dose from thyroid hormones by at least 4 hours

Ketamine: May cause marked hypertension and tachycardia; monitor

Ritonavir: May alter response to thyroid hormones (limited documentation/case report); monitor

Somatrem, somatropin: Excessive thyroid hormone levels lead to accelerated epiphyseal closure; inadequate replacement interferes with growth response to growth hormone. Effect of thyroid replacement not specifically evaluated; use caution.

SSRI antidepressants: May need to increase dose of thyroid hormones when SSRI is added to a previously stabilized patient.

Sympathomimetics: Effects of sympathomimetic agent or thyroid hormones may be increased. Risk of coronary insufficiency is increased in patients with coronary artery disease when these agents are used together.

Theophylline, caffeine: Decreased theophylline clearance in hypothyroid patients; monitor during thyroid replacement.

Tricyclic and tetracyclic antidepressants: Therapeutic and toxic effects of thyroid hormones and the antidepressant are increased.

Warfarin (and other oral anticoagulants): The hypoprothrombinemic response to warfarin may be altered by a change in thyroid function or replacement. Replacement may dramatically increase response to warfarin. However, initiation of warfarin in a patient stabilized on a dose of thyroid hormones does not appear to require a significantly different approach.

Note: Several medications have effects on thyroid production or conversion. The impact in thyroid replacement has not been specifically evaluated, but patient response should be monitored:

Methimazole: Decreases thyroid hormone secretion, while propylthiouracil decrease thyroid hormone secretion and decreases conversion of T_4 to T_3.

Beta-adrenergic antagonists: Decrease conversion of T_4 to T_3 (dose related, propranolol ≥160 mg/day); patients may be clinically euthyroid.

Iodide, iodine-containing radiographic contrast agents may decrease thyroid hormone secretion; may also increase thyroid hormone secretion, especially in patients with Graves' disease.

Other agents reported to impact on thyroid production/conversion include aminoglutethimide, amiodarone, chloral hydrate, diazepam, ethionamide, interferon-alpha, interleukin-2, lithium, lovastatin (case report), glucocorticoids (dose-related), 6-mercaptopurine, sulfonamides, thiazide diuretics, and tolbutamide.

In addition, a number of medications have been noted to cause transient depression in TSH secretion, which may complicate interpretation of monitoring tests for thyroid hormones, including corticosteroids, octreotide, and dopamine. Metoclopramide may increase TSH secretion.

Drug Uptake

Absorption: 50% to 95%

Half-life, elimination: 6-7 days

Time to peak: 12-48 hours

Pregnancy Risk Factor A

Generic Available No

Lipitor® *see* Atorvastatin *on page 126*
Liposyn® *see* Fat Emulsion *on page 487*
Lipovite® [OTC] *see* Vitamin B Complex *on page 1244*
Lipram® *see* Pancrelipase *on page 914*
Lipram® 4500 *see* Pancrelipase *on page 914*
Lipram-CR® *see* Pancrelipase *on page 914*
Lipram-PN® *see* Pancrelipase *on page 914*
Lipram-UL® *see* Pancrelipase *on page 914*
Liquibid® *see* Guaifenesin *on page 568*
Liqui-Char® [OTC] *see* Charcoal *on page 258*
Liquid Pred® *see* PredniSONE *on page 990*
Liqui-E® *see* Tocophersolan *on page 1177*
Liquifilm® Tears [OTC] *see* Artificial Tears *on page 117*
Liquiprin® for Children [OTC] *see* Acetaminophen *on page 26*

Lisinopril (lyse IN oh pril)

Related Information

Cardiovascular Diseases *on page 1308*

U.S. Brand Names Prinivil®; Zestril®

Canadian Brand Names Apo®-Lisinopril; Prinivil®; Zestril®

Mexican Brand Names Prinivil®; Zestril®

Pharmacologic Category Angiotensin-Converting Enzyme (ACE) Inhibitor

Use Treatment of hypertension, either alone or in combination with other antihypertensive agents; adjunctive therapy in treatment of CHF (afterload reduction); treatment of hemodynamically stable patients within 24 hours of acute myocardial infarction, to improve survival; treatment of acute myocardial infarction within 24 hours in hemodynamically stable patients to improve survival; treatment of left ventricular dysfunction after myocardial infarction

Local Anesthetic/Vasoconstrictor Precautions No information available to require special precautions

Effects on Dental Treatment No effects or complications reported

Dosage

Hypertension:

Adults: Initial: 10 mg/day; increase doses 5-10 mg/day at 1- to 2-week intervals; maximum daily dose: 40 mg

Elderly: Initial: 2.5-5 mg/day; increase doses 2.5-5 mg/day at 1- to 2-week intervals; maximum daily dose: 40 mg

Patients taking diuretics should have them discontinued 2-3 days prior to initiating lisinopril if possible. Restart diuretic after BP is stable if needed. If diuretic

(Continued)

Lisinopril *(Continued)*

cannot be discontinued prior to therapy, begin with 5 mg with close supervision until stable BP. In patients with hyponatremia (<130 mEq/L), start dose at 2.5 mg/day,

Congestive heart failure: Adults: Oral: Initial: 5 mg; then increase by no more than 10 mg increments at intervals no less than 2 weeks to a maximum daily dose of 40 mg. Usual maintenance: 5-40 mg/day as a single dose. Patients should start/continue standard therapy, including diuretics, beta-blockers, and digoxin, as indicated.

Acute myocardial infarction (within 24 hours in hemodynamically stable patients): Oral: 5 mg immediately, then 5 mg at 24 hours, 10 mg at 48 hours, and 10 mg every day thereafter for 6 weeks. Patients should continue to receive standard treatments such as thrombolytics, aspirin, and beta-blockers.

Dosing adjustment in renal impairment:

Cl_{cr} 10-50 mL/minute: Administer 50% to 75% of normal dose.

Cl_{cr} <10 mL/minute: Administer 25% to 50% of normal dose.

Hemodialysis: Dialyzable (50%)

Mechanism of Action Competitive inhibitor of angiotensin-converting enzyme (ACE); prevents conversion of angiotensin I to angiotensin II, a potent vasoconstrictor; results in lower levels of angiotensin II which causes an increase in plasma renin activity and a reduction in aldosterone secretion; a CNS mechanism may also be involved in hypotensive effect as angiotensin II increases adrenergic outflow from CNS; vasoactive kallikreins may be decreased in conversion to active hormones by ACE inhibitors, thus reducing BP

Other Adverse Effects Note: Frequency ranges include data from hypertension and heart failure trials. Higher rates of adverse reactions have generally been noted in patients with CHF. However, the frequency of adverse effects associated with placebo is also increased in this population.

1% to 10%:

Cardiovascular: Orthostatic effects (1%), hypotension (1% to 4%)

Central nervous system: Headache (4% to 6%), dizziness (5% to 12%), fatigue (3%), weakness (1%)

Dermatologic: Rash (1% to 2%)

Endocrine & metabolic: Hyperkalemia (2% to 5%)

Gastrointestinal: Diarrhea (3% to 4%), nausea (2%), vomiting (1%), abdominal pain (2%)

Genitourinary: Impotence (1%)

Hematologic: Decreased hemoglobin (small)

Neuromuscular & skeletal: Chest pain (3%)

Renal: Increased serum creatinine (often transient), increased BUN (2%); deterioration in renal function (in patients with bilateral renal artery stenosis or hypovolemia)

Respiratory: Cough (4% to 9%), upper respiratory infection (2% to 2%)

Drug Interactions

Increased Effect/Toxicity: Potassium supplements, co-trimoxazole (high dose), angiotensin II receptor antagonists (candesartan, losartan, irbesartan, etc), or potassium-sparing diuretics (amiloride, spironolactone, triamterene) may result in elevated serum potassium levels when combined with lisinopril. ACE inhibitor effects may be increased by phenothiazines or probenecid (increases levels of captopril). ACE inhibitors may increase serum concentration/effects of digoxin, lithium, and sulfonlyureas. Diuretics have additive hypotensive effects with ACE inhibitors, and hypovolemia increases the potential for adverse renal effects of ACE inhibitors. In patients with compromised renal function, coadministration with nonsteroidal anti-inflammatory drugs may result in further deterioration of renal function. Allopurinol and ACE inhibitors may cause a higher risk of hypersensitivity reaction when taken concurrently.

Decreased Effect: Aspirin (high dose) may reduce the therapeutic effects of ACE inhibitors; at low dosages this does not appear to be significant. Rifampin may decrease the effect of ACE inhibitors. Antacids may decrease the bioavailability of ACE inhibitors (may be more likely to occur with captopril); separate administration times by 1-2 hours. NSAIDs, specifically indomethacin, may reduce the hypotensive effects of ACE inhibitors. More likely to occur in low renin or volume dependent hypertensive patients.

Drug Uptake

Onset of action: 1 hour; Peak effect: Hypotensive: Oral: ~6 hours

Absorption: Well absorbed; unaffected by food

Duration: 24 hours

Half-life, elimination: 11-12 hours

Pregnancy Risk Factor C/D (2nd and 3rd trimesters)

Generic Available No

Lisinopril and Hydrochlorothiazide

(lyse IN oh pril & hye droe klor oh THYE a zide)

Related Information

Cardiovascular Diseases *on page 1308*

U.S. Brand Names Prinzide®; Zestoretic®

Canadian Brand Names Prinzide®; Zestoretic®

Pharmacologic Category Antihypertensive Agent Combination

Synonyms Hydrochlorothiazide and Lisinopril

Use Treatment of hypertension

Local Anesthetic/Vasoconstrictor Precautions No information available to require special precautions

Effects on Dental Treatment No effects or complications reported

Dosage Adults: Oral: Dosage is individualized; see each component for appropriate dosing suggestions; doses >80 mg/day lisinopril or >50 mg/day hydrochlorothiazide are not recommended.

Other Adverse Effects

Based on **lisinopril** component: **Note:** Frequency ranges include data from hypertension and heart failure trials. Higher rates of adverse reactions have generally been noted in patients with CHF. However, the frequency of adverse effects associated with placebo is also increased in this population.

1% to 10%:

- Cardiovascular: Orthostatic effects (1%), hypotension (1% to 4%)
- Central nervous system: Headache (4% to 6%), dizziness (5% to 12%), fatigue (3%), weakness (1%)
- Dermatologic: Rash (1% to 2%)
- Endocrine & metabolic: Hyperkalemia (2% to 5%)
- Gastrointestinal: Diarrhea (3% to 4%), nausea (2.%), vomiting (1%), abdominal pain (2%)
- Genitourinary: Impotence (1%)
- Hematologic: Decreased hemoglobin (small)
- Neuromuscular & skeletal: Chest pain (3%)
- Renal: Increased serum creatinine (often transient), increased BUN (2%); deterioration in renal function (in patients with bilateral renal artery stenosis or hypovolemia)
- Respiratory: Cough (4% to 9%), upper respiratory infection (2% to 2%)

Based on **hydrochlorothiazide** component:

1% to 10%:

- Cardiovascular: Orthostatic hypotension, hypotension
- Dermatologic: Photosensitivity
- Endocrine & metabolic: Hypokalemia
- Gastrointestinal: Anorexia, epigastric distress

Drug Interactions

Based on **lisinopril** component:

- Allopurinol: Case reports (rare) indicate a possible increased risk of hypersensitivity reactions when combined with lisinopril.
- Alpha$_1$ blockers: Hypotensive effect increased.
- Aspirin: The effects of ACE inhibitors may be blunted by aspirin administration, particularly at higher dosages (see Cardiovascular Considerations) and/or increase adverse renal effects.
- Diuretics: Hypovolemia due to diuretics may precipitate acute hypotensive events or acute renal failure.
- Insulin: Risk of hypoglycemia may be increased.
- Lithium: Risk of lithium toxicity may be increased; monitor lithium levels, especially the first 4 weeks of therapy.
- Mercaptopurine: Risk of neutropenia may be increased.
- NSAIDs: May attenuate hypertensive efficacy; effect has been seen with captopril and may occur with other ACE inhibitors; monitor BP. May increase adverse renal effects.
- Potassium-sparing diuretics (amiloride, spironolactone, triamterene): Increased risk of hyperkalemia.
- Potassium supplements may increase the risk of hyperkalemia.
- Trimethoprim (high dose) may increase the risk of hyperkalemia.

Based on **hydrochlorothiazide** component:

- ACE inhibitors: Increased hypotension if aggressively diuresed with a thiazide diuretic.
- Beta-blockers increase hyperglycemic effects in type 2 diabetes mellitus (noninsulin dependent, NIDDM)
- Cyclosporine and thiazides can increase the risk of gout or renal toxicity; avoid concurrent use.
- Digoxin toxicity can be exacerbated if a thiazide induces hypokalemia or hypomagnesemia.
- Lithium toxicity can occur by reducing renal excretion of lithium; monitor lithium concentration and adjust as needed.

(Continued)

Lisinopril and Hydrochlorothiazide *(Continued)*

Neuromuscular blocking agents can prolong blockade; monitor serum potassium and neuromuscular status.

NSAIDs can decrease the efficacy of thiazides reducing the diuretic and antihypertensive effects.

Drug Uptake See Lisinopril *on page 719* and Hydrochlorothiazide *on page 595*

Pregnancy Risk Factor C/D (2nd and 3rd trimesters)

Generic Available No

Lithium (LITH ee um)

Related Information

Dental Drug Interactions: Update on Drug Combinations Requiring Special Considerations *on page 1434*

U.S. Brand Names Eskalith®; Eskalith CR®; Lithobid®

Canadian Brand Names Carbolith™; Duralith®; Lithane™; PMS-Lithium Carbonate; PMS-Lithium Citrate

Mexican Brand Names Carbolit®; Litheum®

Pharmacologic Category Lithium

Synonyms Lithium Carbonate; Lithium Citrate

Use Management of bipolar disorders

Unlabeled/Investigational: Potential augmenting agent for antidepressants; aggression, post-traumatic stress disorder, conduct disorder in children

Local Anesthetic/Vasoconstrictor Precautions No information available to require special precautions

Effects on Dental Treatment Avoid NSAIDs if analgesics are required since lithium toxicity has been reported with concomitant administration; acetaminophen products (ie, singly or with narcotics) are recommended.

Dosage Oral: Monitor serum concentration and clinical response (efficacy and toxicity) to determine proper dose

Children 6-12 years:

- Bipolar disorder: 15-60 mg/kg/day in 3-4 divided doses; dose not to exceed usual adult dosage
- Conduct disorder (unlabeled use): 15-30 mg/kg/day in 3-4 divided doses; dose not to exceed usual adult dosage

Adults: Bipolar disorder: 900-2400 mg/day in 3-4 divided doses or 900-1800 mg/day (sustained release) in 2 divided doses

Elderly: Bipolar disorder: Initial dose: 300 mg once or twice daily; increase weekly in increments of 300 mg/day, monitoring levels; rarely need >900-1200 mg/day

Dosing adjustment in renal impairment:

- Cl_{cr} 10-50 mL/minute: Administer 50% to 75% of normal dose
- Cl_{cr} <10 mL/minute: Administer 25% to 50% of normal dose

Hemodialysis: Dialyzable (50% to 100%)

Mechanism of Action Alters cation transport across cell membrane in nerve and muscle cells and influences reuptake of serotonin and/or norepinephrine; second messenger systems involving the phosphatidylinositol cycle are inhibited; postsynaptic D2 receptor supersensitivity is inhibited

Other Adverse Effects Frequency not defined:

Cardiovascular: Cardiac arrhythmias, hypotension, sinus node dysfunction, flattened or inverted T waves (reversible), edema

Central nervous system: Dizziness, vertigo, slurred speech, blackout spells, seizures, sedation, restlessness, confusion, psychomotor retardation, stupor, coma, dystonia, fatigue, lethargy, headache, pseudotumor cerebri

Dermatologic: Dry or thinning of hair, folliculitis, alopecia, exacerbation of psoriasis, rash

Endocrine & metabolic: Euthyroid goiter and/or hypothyroidism, hyperthyroidism, hyperglycemia, diabetes insipidus

Gastrointestinal: Polydipsia, anorexia, nausea, vomiting, diarrhea, xerostomia, metallic taste, weight gain

Genitourinary: Incontinence, polyuria, glycosuria, oliguria, albuminuria

Hematologic: Leukocytosis

Neuromuscular & skeletal: Tremor, muscle hyperirritability, ataxia, choreoathetoid movements, hyperactive deep tendon reflexes

Ocular: Nystagmus, blurred vision

Miscellaneous: Discoloration of fingers and toes

Drug Interactions

Increased Effect/Toxicity: Concurrent use of lithium with carbamazepine, diltiazem, SSRIs (fluoxetine, fluvoxamine), haloperidol, methyldopa, metronidazole (rare), phenothiazines, phenytoin, TCAs, and verapamil may increase the risk for neurotoxicity. Lithium concentrations/toxicity may be increased by diuretics, NSAIDs (sulindac and aspirin may be exceptions), ACE inhibitors, angiotensin receptor antagonists (losartan), or tetracyclines. Lithium and MAO inhibitors should generally be avoided due to use reports of fatal malignant hyperpyrexia; risk with selective MAO type B inhibitors (selegiline) appears to be lower. Potassium iodide may enhance the hypothyroid effects of lithium. Combined use of lithium with tricyclic antidepressants or sibutramine may increase the risk of serotonin syndrome; this combination is best avoided. Lithium may potentiate effect of neuromuscular blockers.

Decreased Effect: Combined use of lithium and chlorpromazine may lower serum concentration of both drugs. Sodium bicarbonate and high sodium intake may reduce serum lithium concentrations via enhanced excretion. Lithium may blunt the pressor response to sympathomimetics (epinephrine, norepinephrine).

Drug Uptake

Half-life, elimination: 18-24 hours; can increase to >36 hours in renal impairment or elderly

Time to peak (nonsustained release product): Oral: ~0.5-2 hours

Pregnancy Risk Factor D

Generic Available Yes

Lithobid® *see* Lithium *on page 722*
Lithostat® *see* Acetohydroxamic Acid *on page 38*
Livostin® *see* Levocabastine *on page 698*
LMD® *see* Dextran *on page 369*
LoCHOLEST® *see* Cholestyramine Resin *on page 279*
LoCHOLEST® Light *see* Cholestyramine Resin *on page 279*
Locoid® *see* Hydrocortisone *on page 608*
Lodine® *see* Etodolac *on page 479*
Lodine® XL *see* Etodolac *on page 479*
Lodosyn® *see* Carbidopa *on page 220*

Lodoxamide Tromethamine (loe DOKS a mide)

U.S. Brand Names Alomide®

Canadian Brand Names Alomide®

Pharmacologic Category Mast Cell Stabilizer

Use Treatment of vernal keratoconjunctivitis, vernal conjunctivitis, and vernal keratitis

Local Anesthetic/Vasoconstrictor Precautions No information available to require special precautions

Effects on Dental Treatment No effects or complications reported

Dosage Children >2 years and Adults: Instill 1-2 drops in eye(s) 4 times/day for up to 3 months

Mechanism of Action Mast cell stabilizer that inhibits the *in vivo* type I immediate hypersensitivity reaction to increase cutaneous vascular permeability associated with IgE and antigen-mediated reactions

Other Adverse Effects

>10%: Local: Transient burning, stinging, discomfort

1% to 10%:

- Central nervous system: Headache
- Ocular: Blurred vision, corneal erosion/ulcer, eye pain, corneal abrasion, blepharitis

Drug Uptake Absorption: Topical: Negligible

Pregnancy Risk Factor B

Generic Available No

Loestrin® *see* Combination Hormonal Contraceptives *on page 323*
Loestrin® Fe *see* Combination Hormonal Contraceptives *on page 323*

Lomefloxacin (loe me FLOKS a sin)

U.S. Brand Names Maxaquin®

Mexican Brand Names Lomacin®; Maxaquin®

Pharmacologic Category Antibiotic, Quinolone

Synonyms Lomefloxacin Hydrochloride

Use Lower respiratory infections, acute bacterial exacerbation of chronic bronchitis, and urinary tract infections caused by *E. coli, K. pneumoniae, P. mirabilis, P. aeruginosa*; also has gram-positive activity including *S. pneumoniae* and some staphylococci; surgical prophylaxis (transrectal prostate biopsy or transurethral procedures)

Unlabeled/Investigational: Skin infections, sexually-transmitted diseases

Local Anesthetic/Vasoconstrictor Precautions No information available to require special precautions

Effects on Dental Treatment No effects or complications reported

Dosage Adults:

Lower respiratory and urinary tract infections (UTI): 400 mg once daily for 10-14 days

Urinary tract infection (UTI) due to susceptible organisms:

Females:

- Uncomplicated cystitis caused by *Escherichia coli*: 400 mg once daily for 3 successive days
- Uncomplicated cystitis caused by *Klebsiella pneumoniae, Proteus mirabilis*, or *Staphylococcus saprophyticus*: 400 mg once daily for 10 successive days

(Continued)

Lomefloxacin *(Continued)*

Complicated UTI caused by *Escherichia coli, Klebsiella pneumoniae, Proteus mirabilis,* or *Pseudomonas aeruginosa*: 400 mg once daily for 14 successive days

Surgical prophylaxis: 400 mg 2-6 hours before surgery

Uncomplicated gonorrhea: 400 mg as a single dose

Elderly: No dosage adjustment is needed for elderly patients with normal renal function

Dosing adjustment in renal impairment:

Cl_{cr} 11-39 mL/minute: Loading dose: 400 mg, then 200 mg every day

Hemodialysis: Same as above

Mechanism of Action Inhibits DNA-gyrase in susceptible organisms thereby inhibits relaxation of supercoiled DNA and promotes breakage of DNA strands. DNA gyrase (topoisomerase II), is an essential bacterial enzyme that maintains the superhelical structure of DNA and is required for DNA replication and transcription, DNA repair, recombination, and transposition.

Other Adverse Effects 1% to 10%:

Central nervous system: Headache (3%), dizziness (2%)

Dermatologic: Photosensitivity (2%)

Gastrointestinal: Nausea (4%)

Drug Interactions CYP1A2 enzyme inhibitor (minor)

Increased Effect/Toxicity: Quinolones can cause elevated levels of caffeine, warfarin, cyclosporine, and theophylline. Azlocillin, imipenem, cimetidine, loop diuretics, and probenecid may increase lomefloxacin serum concentration. Increased CNS stimulation may occur with caffeine, theophylline, NSAIDs. Foscarnet has been associated with seizures in patients receiving quinolones.

Decreased Effect: Decreased absorption with antacids containing aluminum, magnesium, and/or calcium (by up to 98% if given at the same time). Antineoplastic agents may decrease quinolone absorption.

Drug Uptake

Absorption: Well absorbed

Half-life, elimination: 5-7.5 hours

Pregnancy Risk Factor C

Generic Available No

Lomocot® *see* Diphenoxylate and Atropine *on page 400*

Lomotil® *see* Diphenoxylate and Atropine *on page 400*

Lomustine (loe MUS teen)

U.S. Brand Names CeeNU®

Canadian Brand Names CeeNU®

Mexican Brand Names CeeNU®

Pharmacologic Category Antineoplastic Agent, Alkylating Agent

Synonyms CCNU

Use Treatment of brain tumors, Hodgkin's and non-Hodgkin's lymphomas, melanoma, renal carcinoma, lung cancer, colon cancer

Local Anesthetic/Vasoconstrictor Precautions No information available to require special precautions

Effects on Dental Treatment No effects or complications reported

Mechanism of Action Inhibits DNA and RNA synthesis via carbamylation of DNA polymerase, alkylation of DNA, and alteration of RNA, proteins, and enzymes

Other Adverse Effects

>10%:

Gastrointestinal: Nausea and vomiting, usually within 3-6 hours after oral administration. Administration of the dose at bedtime, with an antiemetic, significantly reduces both the incidence and severity of nausea.

Hematologic: Myelosuppression, common, dose-limiting, may be cumulative and irreversible

Onset: 10-14 days

Nadir: Leukopenia: 6 weeks

Thrombocytopenia: 4 weeks

Recovery: 6-8 weeks

1% to 10%:

Dermatologic: Rash

Gastrointestinal: Anorexia, stomatitis, diarrhea

Genitourinary: Progressive azotemia, renal failure, decrease in kidney size

Hematologic: Anemia

Hepatic: Elevated liver enzymes, transient, reversible

Drug Interactions CYP2D6 enzyme inhibitor

Increased Effect/Toxicity: Increased toxicity with cimetidine, reported to cause bone marrow depression or to potentiate the myelosuppressive effects of lomustine.

Decreased effect with phenobarbital, resulting in reduced efficacy of both drugs.

Drug Uptake

Absorption: Complete; appears in plasma ~3 minutes after administration

Duration: Marrow recovery: ≤6 weeks
Half-life, elimination: Parent drug: 16-72 hours; Active metabolite: Terminal: 1.3-2 days
Time to peak: Active metabolite: ~3 hours

Pregnancy Risk Factor D
Generic Available No

Loniten® *see* Minoxidil *on page 818*
Lonox® *see* Diphenoxylate and Atropine *on page 400*
Lo/Ovral® *see* Combination Hormonal Contraceptives *on page 323*

Loperamide (loe PER a mide)

U.S. Brand Names Diar-Aid® [OTC]; Imodium®; Imodium® A-D [OTC]; Kaopectate® II [OTC]; Pepto® Diarrhea Control [OTC]
Canadian Brand Names Apo®-Loperamide; Diarr-Eze; Imodium®; Loperacap; Novo-Loperamide; PMS-Loperamine; Rho®-Loperamine; Riva-Loperamine
Mexican Brand Names Acanol; Cryoperacid®; Pramidal; Raxedin; Top-Dal®
Pharmacologic Category Antidiarrheal
Synonyms Loperamide Hydrochloride
Use Treatment of acute diarrhea and chronic diarrhea associated with inflammatory bowel disease; chronic functional diarrhea (idiopathic), chronic diarrhea caused by bowel resection or organic lesions; to decrease the volume of ileostomy discharge
Unlabeled/Investigational: Treatment of traveler's diarrhea in combination with trimethoprim-sulfamethoxazole (co-trimoxazole) (3 days therapy)
Local Anesthetic/Vasoconstrictor Precautions No information available to require special precautions
Effects on Dental Treatment No effects or complications reported
Dosage Oral:
Children:
Acute diarrhea: Initial doses (in first 24 hours):
2-6 years: 1 mg 3 times/day
6-8 years: 2 mg twice daily
8-12 years: 2 mg 3 times/day
Maintenance: After initial dosing, 0.1 mg/kg doses after each loose stool, but not exceeding initial dosage
Chronic diarrhea: 0.08-0.24 mg/kg/day divided 2-3 times/day, maximum: 2 mg/dose
Adults:
Acute diarrhea: Initial: 4 mg (2 capsules), followed by 2 mg after each loose stool, up to 16 mg/day (8 capsules)
Chronic diarrhea: Initial: Follow acute diarrhea; maintenance dose should be slowly titrated downward to minimum required to control symptoms (typically, 4-8 mg/day in divided doses)
Traveler's diarrhea: Treat for no more than 2 days
6-8 years: 1 mg after first loose stool followed by 1 mg after each subsequent stool; maximum dose: 4 mg/day
9-11 years: 2 mg after first loose stool followed by 1 mg after each subsequent stool; maximum dose: 6 mg/day
12 years to Adults: 4 mg after first loose stool followed by 2 mg after each subsequent stool; maximum dose: 8 mg/day

Mechanism of Action Acts directly on intestinal muscles to inhibit peristalsis and prolongs transit time enhancing fluid and electrolyte movement through intestinal mucosa; reduces fecal volume, increases viscosity, and diminishes fluid and electrolyte loss; demonstrates antisecretory activity; exhibits peripheral action
Other Adverse Effects Frequency not defined:
Cardiovascular: Shock
Central nervous system: Dizziness, drowsiness, fatigue, sedation
Dermatologic: Rash, toxic epidermal necrolysis
Gastrointestinal: Abdominal cramping, abdominal distention, constipation, xerostomia, nausea, paralytic ileus, vomiting
Miscellaneous: Anaphylaxis
Drug Interactions May potentiate the adverse effects of CNS depressants, phenothiazines, tricyclic antidepressants
Drug Uptake
Onset of action: Oral: 0.5-1 hour
Absorption: Oral: <40%; levels in breast milk expected to be very low
Half-life, elimination: 7-14 hours
Pregnancy Risk Factor B
Generic Available Yes

Lopid® *see* Gemfibrozil *on page 552*

Lopinavir and Ritonavir (loe PIN a veer & rit ON uh veer)

U.S. Brand Names Kaletra™
Pharmacologic Category Antiretroviral Agent, Protease Inhibitor
(Continued)

Lopinavir and Ritonavir *(Continued)*

Synonyms Lopinavir

Use For use in combination with other antiretroviral agents in the treatment of HIV infection

Local Anesthetic/Vasoconstrictor Precautions No information available to require special precautions

Effects on Dental Treatment No effects or complications reported

Dosage Oral (take with food):

Children 6 months to 12 years: Dosage based on weight, presented based on mg of lopinavir (maximum dose: Lopinavir 400 mg/ritonavir 100 mg)

7-<15 kg: 12 mg/kg twice daily

15-40 kg: 10 mg/kg twice daily

>40 kg: Refer to adult dosing

Children >12 years and Adults: Lopinavir 400 mg/ritonavir 100 mg twice daily

Dosage adjustment when taken with efavirenz or nevirapine:

Children 6 months to 12 years:

7-<15 kg: 13 mg/kg twice daily

15-50 kg: 11 mg/kg twice daily

>50 kg: Refer to adult dosing

Children >12 years and Adults: Lopinavir 533 mg/ritonavir 133 mg twice daily

Elderly: Initial studies did not include enough elderly patients to determine effects based on age. Use with caution due to possible decreased hepatic, renal, and cardiac function.

Dosage adjustment in hepatic impairment: Plasma levels may be increased

Mechanism of Action A coformulation of lopinavir and ritonavir. The lopinavir component is the active inhibitor of HIV protease. Lopinavir inhibits HIV protease and renders the enzyme incapable of processing polyprotein precursor which leads to production of noninfectious immature HIV particles. The ritonavir component inhibits the CYP3A metabolism of lopinavir, allowing increased plasma concentrations of lopinavir.

Other Adverse Effects Protease inhibitors cause dyslipidemia which includes elevated cholesterol and triglycerides and a redistribution of body fat centrally to cause "protease paunch," buffalo hump, facial atrophy, and breast enlargement. These agents also cause hyperglycemia.

>10%:

Endocrine & metabolic: Hypercholesterolemia (9% to 28%), triglycerides increased (9% to 28%)

Gastrointestinal: Diarrhea (16% to 24%), nausea (3% to 15%)

Hepatic: GGT increased (4% to 25%)

2% to 10%:

Central nervous system: Headache (2% to 7%), pain (0% to 2%), insomnia (1% to 2%)

Dermatologic: Rash (1% to 4%)

Endocrine & metabolic: Hyperglycemia (1% to 4%), hyperuricemia (up to 4%), sodium decreased (3% children), organic phosphorus decreased (up to 2%), amylase increased (2% to 10%)

Gastrointestinal: Abnormal stools (up to 6%), abdominal pain (2% to 4%), vomiting (2% to 5%), dyspepsia (0.5% to 2%)

Hematologic: Platelets decreased (4% children), neutrophils decreased (1% to 3%)

Hepatic: AST increased (2% to 9%), ALT increased (4% to 8%), bilirubin increased (children 3%)

Neuromuscular & skeletal: Weakness (4% to 7%)

<2%:

Cardiovascular: Chest pain, deep vein thrombosis, edema, facial edema, hypertension, palpitation, peripheral edema, vasculitis

Central nervous system: Abnormal dreams, abnormal thinking, agitation, amnesia, anxiety, ataxia, chills, confusion, depression, dizziness, emotional lability, encephalopathy, facial paralysis, fever, malaise, migraine, nervousness, neuropathy, paresthesia, peripheral neuritis, somnolence, tremor

Dermatologic: Acne, alopecia, benign neoplasm, dry skin, exfoliative dermatitis, furunculosis, maculopapular rash, nail disorder, pruritus, skin discoloration

Endocrine & metabolic: Cushing's syndrome, dehydration, diabetes mellitus, glucose intolerance, gynecomastia, hypogonadism (male), hypothyroidism, lactic acidosis, libido decreased, weight gain

Gastrointestinal: Anorexia, constipation, xerostomia, dyspepsia, dysphagia, enterocolitis, eructation, esophagitis, fecal incontinence, flatulence, gastritis, gastroenteritis, gastrointestinal disorder, hemorrhagic colitis, increased appetite, pancreatitis, sialadenitis, stomatitis, taste perversion, ulcerative stomatitis, weight loss

Genitourinary: Abnormal ejaculation

Hematologic: Anemia, leukopenia, lymphadenopathy

Hepatic: Cholecystitis, hepatic dysfunction

Local: Thrombophlebitis

Neuromuscular & skeletal: Arthralgia, arthrosis, back pain, dyskinesia, hypertonia, myalgia

Ocular: Abnormal vision, eye disorder

Otic: Otitis media, tinnitus

Renal: Kidney calculus, urine abnormality

Respiratory: Bronchitis, dyspnea, lung edema, rhinitis, sinusitis

Miscellaneous: Avitaminosis, diaphoresis, flu-like syndrome, obesity, viral infection

Contraindications Hypersensitivity to lopinavir, ritonavir, or any component of their formulation; administration with medications highly dependent upon CYP3A or CYP2D6 for clearance for which increased levels are associated with serious and/or life-threatening events

Ritonavir is contraindicated with amiodarone, bepridil, flecainide, propafenone, quinidine, astemizole, terfenadine, dihydroergotamine, ergotamine, midazolam, triazolam, cisapride, pimozide.

Warnings/Precautions Cases of pancreatitis, some fatal, have been associated with lopinavir/ritonavir; use caution in patients with a history of pancreatitis. Patients with signs or symptoms of pancreatitis should be evaluated and therapy suspended as clinically appropriate. Diabetes mellitus and exacerbation of diabetes mellitus have been reported in patients taking protease inhibitors. Use caution in patients with hepatic impairment; patients with hepatitis or elevations in transaminases prior to the start of therapy may be at increased risk for further increases in transaminases. Large increases in total cholesterol and triglycerides have been reported; screening should be done prior to therapy and periodically throughout treatment. Hemophilia type A and type B have been reported with protease inhibitor use. Redistribution or accumulation of body fat has been observed in patients using antiretroviral therapy. The potential for cross-resistance with other protease inhibitors is currently under study. Safety and efficacy in children <6 months of age are not yet established.

Drug Interactions CYP2D6 enzyme inhibitors

Increased Effect/Toxicity:

Contraindicated drugs: Life-threatening arrhythmias may result from concurrent use of flecainide or propafenone. Concurrent use is contraindicated. Concurrent use of cisapride, pimozide, astemizole, terfenadine is also contraindicated. Some benzodiazepines (midazolam and triazolam) are contraindicated, due to the potential for increased response/respiratory depression. Concurrent use of ergot alkaloids is contraindicated, due to potential toxicity.

Serum levels of other antiarrhythmics, including amiodarone, bepridil, lidocaine (systemic), and quinidine may be increased with concurrent use. Serum levels of calcium channel blockers (including felodipine, nicardipine, and nifedipine), clarithromycin, immunosuppressants (cyclosporin, tacrolimus, sirolimus), HMG-CoA reductase inhibitors (lovastatin and simvastatin are not recommended, atorvastatin and cerivastatin should be used at lowest possible dose), itraconazole, ketoconazole, methadone, and rifabutin (decreased dose recommended) may be increased. Serum levels of protease inhibitors may be altered during concurrent therapy. Ritonavir may increase serum concentration of amprenavir, indinavir, or saquinavir. Serum levels of sildenafil may be substantially increased (use caution at decreased dose of sildenafil, maximum of 25 mg in 48 hours). Warfarin serum concentration may also be increased.

Delavirdine increases levels of lopinavir; dosing recommendations are not yet established.

Lopinavir/ritonavir solution contains alcohol, concurrent use with disulfiram or metronidazole should be avoided. May cause Antabuse®-like reaction.

Decreased Effect: Carbamazepine, dexamethasone, phenobarbital, phenytoin, and rifampin may decrease levels of lopinavir. Non-nucleoside reverse transcriptase inhibitors: Efavirenz, nevirapine may decrease levels of lopinavir. To avoid incompatibility with didanosine, administer didanosine 1 hour before or 2 hours after lopinavir/ritonavir. Decreased levels of ethinyl estradiol may result from concurrent use. Lopinavir/ritonavir may decrease levels of abacavir, atovaquone, or zidovudine.

Drug Uptake See Ritonavir *on page 1059*

Lopinavir: Half-life, elimination: Lopinavir: 5-6 hours

Pregnancy Risk Factor C

Generic Available No

Comments Oral solution contains 42.4% alcohol.

Lopressor® *see* Metoprolol *on page 803*

Loprox® *see* Ciclopirox *on page 283*

Lorabid™ *see* Loracarbef *on page 727*

Loracarbef (lor a KAR bef)

U.S. Brand Names Lorabid™

Canadian Brand Names Lorabid™

Mexican Brand Names Carbac; Lorabid®

Pharmacologic Category Antibiotic, Carbacephem

(Continued)

Loracarbef *(Continued)*

Use Infections caused by susceptible organisms involving the respiratory tract, acute otitis media, sinusitis, skin and skin structure, bone and joint, and urinary tract and gynecologic

Local Anesthetic/Vasoconstrictor Precautions No information available to require special precautions

Effects on Dental Treatment No effects or complications reported

Dosage Oral:

Children:

Acute otitis media: 15 mg/kg twice daily for 10 days

Pharyngitis: 7.5-15 mg/kg twice daily for 10 days

Adults: Women:

Uncomplicated urinary tract infections: 200 mg once daily for 7 days

Skin and soft tissue: 200-400 mg every 12-24 hours

Uncomplicated pyelonephritis: 400 mg every 12 hours for 14 days

Mechanism of Action Inhibits bacterial cell wall synthesis by binding to one or more of the penicillin binding proteins (PBPs); inhibits the final transpeptidation step of peptidoglycan synthesis in bacterial cell walls, thus inhibiting cell wall biosynthesis. It is thought that beta-lactam antibiotics inactivate transpeptidase via acylation of the enzyme with cleavage of the CO-N bond of the beta-lactam ring. Upon exposure to beta-lactam antibiotics, bacteria eventually lyse due to ongoing activity of cell wall autolytic enzymes (autolysins and murein hydrolases) while cell wall assembly is arrested.

Other Adverse Effects ≥1%:

Central nervous system: Headache (1% to 3%), somnolence (<2%)

Dermatologic: Rash (1% to 3%)

Gastrointestinal: Diarrhea (4% to 6%), nausea (2%), vomiting (1% to 3%), anorexia (<2%), abdominal pain (1%)

Genitourinary: Vaginitis (1%)

Respiratory: Rhinitis (2% to 6%)

Drug Interactions Loracarbef serum concentration are increased with coadministered probenecid.

Drug Uptake

Absorption: Oral: Rapid

Half-life, elimination: ~1 hour

Time to peak: Oral: ~1 hour

Pregnancy Risk Factor B

Generic Available No

Loratadine (lor AT a deen)

U.S. Brand Names Claritin®; Claritin® RediTabs®

Canadian Brand Names Claritin®

Mexican Brand Names Clarityne®; Lertamine; Lowadina; Sensibit

Pharmacologic Category Antihistamine, Nonsedating

Use Relief of nasal and non-nasal symptoms of seasonal allergic rhinitis; treatment of chronic idiopathic urticaria

Local Anesthetic/Vasoconstrictor Precautions No information available to require special precautions

Effects on Dental Treatment >10%: Xerostomia; normal salivary flow resumes with discontinuation

Dosage Oral: Seasonal allergic rhinitis, chronic idiopathic urticaria:

Children 2-5 years: 5 mg once daily

Children ≥6 years and Adults: 10 mg once daily

Dosage adjustment in renal impairment: Cl_{cr} ≤30 mL/minute:

Children 2-5 years: 5 mg every other day

Children ≥6 years and Adults: 10 mg every other day

Dosage adjustment in hepatic impairment: Elimination half-life increases with severity of disease

Children 2-5 years: 5 mg every other day

Children ≥6 years and Adults: 10 mg every other day

Elderly: Peak plasma concentrations are increased; elimination half-life is slightly increased; specific dosing adjustments are not available

Mechanism of Action Long-acting tricyclic antihistamine with selective peripheral histamine H_1 receptor antagonistic properties

Other Adverse Effects

Adults:

Central nervous system: Headache (12%), somnolence (8%), fatigue (4%)

Gastrointestinal: Xerostomia (3%)

Children:

Central nervous system: Nervousness (4% ages 6-12 years), fatigue (3% ages 6-12 years, 2% to 3% ages 2-5 years), malaise (2% ages 6-12 years)

Dermatologic: Rash (2% to 3% ages 2-5 years)

Gastrointestinal: Abdominal pain (2% ages 6-12 years), stomatitis (2% to 3% ages 2-5 years)

Neuromuscular & skeletal: Hyperkinesia (3% ages 6-12 years)
Ocular: Conjunctivitis (2% ages 6-12 years)
Respiratory: Wheezing (4% ages 6-12 years), dysphonia (2% ages 6-12 years), upper respiratory infection (2% ages 6-12 years), epistaxis (2% to 3% ages 2-5 years), pharyngitis (2% to 3% ages 2-5 years), flu-like symptoms (2% to 3% ages 2-5 years)
Miscellaneous: Viral infection (2% to 3% ages 2-5 years)

Adults and Children: <2%: Agitation, altered lacrimation, altered micturition, altered salivation, altered taste, amnesia, angioneurotic edema, anorexia, anxiety, appetite increased, arthralgia, back pain, blepharospasm, blurred vision, breast pain, bronchitis, bronchospasm, chest pain, confusion, constipation, coughing, depression, dermatitis, diaphoresis increased, diarrhea, dizziness, dry hair, dry skin, dysmenorrhea, dyspepsia, dysphonia, dyspnea, earache, eye pain, flatulence, flushing, gastritis, hemoptysis, hiccup, hypertension, hypertonia, hypoesthesia, hypotension, impaired concentration, impotence, insomnia, irritability, laryngitis, leg cramps, libido decreased, loose stools, malaise, menorrhagia, migraine, myalgia, nasal dryness, nausea, palpitations, paresthesia, paroniria, photosensitivity, pruritus, purpura, rigors, sinusitis, sneezing, supraventricular tachyarrhythmia, syncope, tachycardia, thirst, tinnitus, tremor, urinary discoloration, urinary incontinence, urinary retention, urticaria, vaginitis, vertigo, vomiting, weakness, weight gain

Drug Interactions CYP2D6 and 3A3/4 enzyme substrate

Increased Effect/Toxicity: Increased plasma concentrations of loratadine and its active metabolite with ketoconazole and erythromycin, however no change in QT_c interval was seen. Increased toxicity with procarbazine, other antihistamines, alcohol. Protease inhibitors (amprenavir, ritonavir, nelfinavir) may increase the serum concentration of loratadine.

Drug Uptake

Onset of action: 1-3 hours; Peak effect: 8-12 hours
Absorption: Rapid
Duration: >24 hours
Half-life, elimination: 12-15 hours

Pregnancy Risk Factor B

Generic Available No

Loratadine and Pseudoephedrine

(lor AT a deen & soo doe e FED rin)

Related Information

Oral Bacterial Infections *on page 1367*

U.S. Brand Names Claritin-D® 12-Hour; Claritin-D® 24-Hour

Canadian Brand Names Chlor-Tripolon ND®; Claritin® Extra

Pharmacologic Category Antihistamine/Decongestant Combination

Synonyms Pseudoephedrine and Loratadine

Use Temporary relief of symptoms of seasonal and perennial allergic rhinitis, and vasomotor rhinitis, including nasal obstruction

Local Anesthetic/Vasoconstrictor Precautions Use with caution since pseudoephedrine is a sympathomimetic amine which could interact with epinephrine to cause a pressor response

Effects on Dental Treatment ≤10%: Tachycardia, palpitations (use vasoconstrictor with caution); >10%: Xerostomia; disappears with discontinuation

Dosage Adults: Oral: 1 tablet every 12 hours

Other Adverse Effects 1% to 10%:

Central nervous system: Headache, fatigue (3%), dizziness (4%), slight to moderate drowsiness (6%), nervousness (3%), insomnia (5%)
Gastrointestinal: Weight gain, nausea (3%), diarrhea, abdominal pain, xerostomia, xerostomia (8%), anorexia (2%)
Genitourinary: Dysuria, dysmenorrhea (2%)
Neuromuscular & skeletal: Arthralgia, weakness
Respiratory: Pharyngitis (5%), thickening of bronchial secretions, cough
Miscellaneous: Diaphoresis

Drug Interactions See Loratadine *on page 728* and Pseudoephedrine *on page 1022*

Drug Uptake See Loratadine *on page 728* and Pseudoephedrine *on page 1022*

Pregnancy Risk Factor B

Generic Available No

Lorazepam (lor A ze pam)

Related Information

Patients Requiring Sedation *on page 1400*
Temporomandibular Dysfunction (TMD) *on page 1397*

U.S. Brand Names Ativan®

Canadian Brand Names Apo®-Lorazepam; Ativan®; Novo-Lorazepam®; Nu-Loraz; Riva-Lorazepam

Mexican Brand Names Ativan®; Sinestron®

(Continued)

Lorazepam *(Continued)*

Pharmacologic Category Benzodiazepine

Use

I.V.: Status epilepticus, preanesthesia for desired amnesia, antiemetic adjunct

Oral: Management of anxiety disorders or short-term relief of the symptoms of anxiety or anxiety associated with depressive symptoms

Unlabeled/Investigational: Ethanol detoxification; insomnia; psychogenic catatonia; partial complex seizures

Local Anesthetic/Vasoconstrictor Precautions No information available to require special precautions

Effects on Dental Treatment >10%: Xerostomia; normal salivary flow resumes with discontinuation

Restrictions C-IV

Dosage

Antiemetic:

Children 2-15 years: I.V.: 0.05 mg/kg (up to 2 mg/dose) prior to chemotherapy

Adults: Oral, I.V.: 0.5-2 mg every 4-6 hours as needed

Anxiety and sedation:

Infants and Children: Oral, I.M., I.V.: Usual: 0.05 mg/kg/dose (range: 0.02-0.09 mg/kg) every 4-8 hours

I.V.: May use smaller doses (eg, 0.01-0.03 mg/kg) and repeat every 20 minutes, as needed to titrate to effect

Adults: Oral: 1-10 mg/day in 2-3 divided doses; usual dose: 2-6 mg/day in divided doses

Elderly: 0.5-4 mg/day; initial dose not to exceed 2 mg

Insomnia: Adults: Oral: 2-4 mg at bedtime

Preoperative: Adults:

I.M.: 0.05 mg/kg administered 2 hours before surgery (maximum: 4 mg/dose)

I.V.: 0.044 mg/kg 15-20 minutes before surgery (usual maximum: 2 mg/dose)

Operative amnesia: Adults: I.V.: Up to 0.05 mg/kg (maximum: 4 mg/dose)

Sedation (preprocedure): Infants and Children:

Oral, I.M., I.V.: Usual: 0.05 mg/kg (range: 0.02-0.09 mg/kg);

I.V.: May use smaller doses (eg, 0.01-0.03 mg/kg) and repeat every 20 minutes, as needed to titrate to effect

Status epilepticus: I.V.:

Infants and Children: 0.1 mg/kg slow I.V. over 2-5 minutes; do not exceed 4 mg/single dose; may repeat second dose of 0.05 mg/kg slow I.V. in 10-15 minutes if needed

Adolescents: 0.07 mg/kg slow I.V. over 2-5 minutes; maximum: 4 mg/dose; may repeat in 10-15 minutes

Adults: 4 mg/dose slow I.V. over 2-5 minutes; may repeat in 10-15 minutes; usual maximum dose: 8 mg

Rapid tranquilization of agitated patient (administer every 30-60 minutes):

Oral: 1-2 mg

I.M.: 0.5-1 mg

Average total dose for tranquilization: Oral, I.M.: 4-8 mg

Mechanism of Action Binds to stereospecific benzodiazepine receptors on the postsynaptic GABA neuron at several sites within the CNS, including the limbic system, reticular formation. Enhancement of the inhibitory effect of GABA on neuronal excitability results by increased neuronal membrane permeability to chloride ions. This shift in chloride ions results in hyperpolarization (a less excitable state) and stabilization.

Other Adverse Effects

>10%:

Central nervous system: Sedation

Respiratory: Respiratory depression

1% to 10%:

Cardiovascular: Hypotension

Central nervous system: Confusion, dizziness, akathisia, unsteadiness, headache, depression, disorientation, amnesia

Dermatologic: Dermatitis, rash

Gastrointestinal: Weight gain/loss, nausea, changes in appetite

Neuromuscular & skeletal: Weakness

Respiratory: Nasal congestion, hyperventilation, apnea

Contraindications Hypersensitivity to lorazepam or any component of the formulation (cross-sensitivity with other benzodiazepines may exist); acute narrow-angle glaucoma; sleep apnea (parenteral); intra-arterial injection of parenteral formulation; severe respiratory insufficiency (except during mechanical ventilation); pregnancy

Warnings/Precautions Use with caution in elderly or debilitated patients, patients with hepatic disease (including alcoholics) or renal impairment. Use with caution in patients with respiratory disease or impaired gag reflex. Initial doses in elderly or debilitated patients should not exceed 2 mg. Prolonged lorazepam use may have a possible relationship to GI disease, including esophageal dilation.

The parenteral formulation of lorazepam contains polyethylene glycol and propylene glycol. Each agent has been associated with specific toxicities when administered in prolonged infusions at high dosages. Also contains benzyl alcohol - avoid rapid injection in neonates or prolonged infusions. Intra-arterial injection or extravasation should be avoided. Concurrent administration with scopolamine results in an increased risk of hallucinations, sedation, and irrational behavior.

Causes CNS depression (dose-related) resulting in sedation, dizziness, confusion, or ataxia which may impair physical and mental capabilities. Patients must be cautioned about performing tasks which require mental alertness (ie, operating machinery or driving). Use with caution in patients receiving other CNS depressants or psychoactive agents. Effects with other sedative drugs or ethanol may be potentiated. Benzodiazepines have been associated with falls and traumatic injury and should be used with extreme caution in patients who are at risk of these events (especially the elderly).

Lorazepam may cause anterograde amnesia. Paradoxical reactions, including hyperactive or aggressive behavior have been reported with benzodiazepines, particularly in adolescent/pediatric or psychiatric patients. Does not have analgesic, antidepressant, or antipsychotic properties.

Use caution in patients with depression, particularly if suicidal risk may be present. Use with caution in patients with a history of drug dependence. Benzodiazepines have been associated with dependence and acute withdrawal symptoms on discontinuation or reduction in dose. Acute withdrawal, including seizures, may be precipitated after administration of flumazenil to patients receiving long-term benzodiazepine therapy.

As a hypnotic agent, should be used only after evaluation of potential causes of sleep disturbance. Failure of sleep disturbance to resolve after 7-10 days may indicate psychiatric or medical illness. A worsening of insomnia or the emergence of new abnormalities of thought or behavior may represent unrecognized psychiatric or medical illness and requires immediate and careful evaluation.

Drug Interactions CYP3A3/4 enzyme substrate

CNS depressants: Sedative effects and/or respiratory depression may be additive with CNS depressants; includes ethanol, barbiturates, narcotic analgesics, and other sedative agents; monitor for increased effect

CYP3A3/4 inhibitors: Serum level and/or toxicity of some benzodiazepines may be increased; inhibitors include amiodarone, cimetidine, clarithromycin, erythromycin, delavirdine, diltiazem, dirithromycin, disulfiram, fluoxetine, fluvoxamine, grapefruit juice, indinavir, itraconazole, ketoconazole, metronidazole, nefazodone, nevirapine, propoxyphene, quinupristin-dalfopristin, ritonavir, saquinavir, verapamil, zafirlukast, zileuton; monitor for altered benzodiazepine response

Enzyme inducers: Metabolism of some benzodiazepines may be increased, decreasing their therapeutic effect; consider using an alternative sedative/hypnotic agent; potential inducers include phenobarbital, phenytoin, carbamazepine, rifampin, and rifabutin

Levodopa: Lorazepam may decrease the antiparkinsonian efficacy of levodopa (limited documentation); monitor

Loxapine: There are rare reports of significant respiratory depression, stupor, and/or hypotension with concomitant use of loxapine and lorazepam; use caution if concomitant administration of loxapine and CNS drugs is required

Oral contraceptives: May decrease the clearance of some benzodiazepines (those which undergo oxidative metabolism); monitor for increased benzodiazepine effect

Scopolamine: May increase the incidence of sedation, hallucinations, and irrational behavior; reported only with parenteral lorazepam

Theophylline: May partially antagonize some of the effects of benzodiazepines; monitor for decreased response; may require higher doses for sedation

Drug Uptake

Onset of action: Hypnosis: I.M.: 20-30 minutes; Sedation, anticonvulsant: I.V.: 5 minutes; oral: 0.5-1 hour

Absorption: Oral, I.M.: Prompt

Duration: 6-8 hours

Half-life, elimination: Neonates: 40.2 hours; Older children: 10.5 hours; Adults: 12.9 hours; Elderly: 15.9 hours; End-stage renal disease: 32-70 hours

Pregnancy Risk Factor D

Generic Available Yes

Lorcet® 10/650 *see* Hydrocodone and Acetaminophen *on page 598*

Lorcet®-HD *see* Hydrocodone and Acetaminophen *on page 598*

Lorcet® Plus *see* Hydrocodone and Acetaminophen *on page 598*

Loroxide® [OTC] *see* Benzoyl Peroxide *on page 153*

Lortab® *see* Hydrocodone and Acetaminophen *on page 598*

Lortab® ASA *see* Hydrocodone and Aspirin *on page 600*

Losartan (loe SAR tan)

Related Information

Cardiovascular Diseases *on page 1308*

U.S. Brand Names Cozaar®

Canadian Brand Names Cozaar®

Mexican Brand Names Cozaar®

Pharmacologic Category Angiotensin II Receptor Blocker

Synonyms DuP 753; Losartan Potassium; MK594

Use Treatment of hypertension with or without concurrent use of thiazide diuretics

Local Anesthetic/Vasoconstrictor Precautions No information available to require special precautions

Effects on Dental Treatment No effects or complications reported

Dosage Oral: The usual starting dose is 50 mg once daily; can be administered once or twice daily with total daily doses ranging from 25 mg to 100 mg

Usual initial doses in patients receiving diuretics or those with intravascular volume depletion: 25 mg

Patients not receiving diuretics: 50 mg

Mechanism of Action As a selective and competitive, nonpeptide angiotensin II receptor antagonist, losartan blocks the vasoconstrictor and aldosterone-secreting effects of angiotensin II; losartan interacts reversibly at the AT1 and AT2 receptors of many tissues and has slow dissociation kinetics; its affinity for the AT1 receptor is 1000 times greater than the AT2 receptor. Angiotensin II receptor antagonists may induce a more complete inhibition of the renin-angiotensin system than ACE inhibitors, they do not affect the response to bradykinin, and are less likely to be associated with nonrenin-angiotensin effects (eg, cough and angioedema). Losartan increases urinary flow rate and in addition to being natriuretic and kaliuretic, increases excretion of chloride, magnesium, uric acid, calcium, and phosphate.

Other Adverse Effects

1% to 10%:

Central nervous system: Dizziness (4%), insomnia (1%)

Cardiovascular: First dose hypotension (dose-related; <1% with 50 mg, 2% with 100 mg)

Gastrointestinal: Diarrhea (2%), dyspepsia (1%), abdominal pain (2%), nausea (2%)

Neuromuscular & skeletal: Back pain (2%), muscle cramps (1%), myalgia (1%), leg pain (1%)

Respiratory: Upper respiratory infection (8%), cough (3.4% versus 3.3% in placebo), nasal congestion (2%), sinus disorder (1%), sinusitis (1%)

>1% but frequency ≤ placebo: Asthenia, fatigue, edema, abdominal pain, chest pain, nausea, headache, pharyngitis

Drug Interactions CYP2C9 and 3A3/4 enzyme substrate

Increased Effect/Toxicity: Potassium salts/supplements, co-trimoxazole (high dose), ACE inhibitors, and potassium-sparing diuretics (amiloride, spironolactone, triamterene) may increase the risk of hyperkalemia. Cimetidine may increase the absorption of losartan by 18% (clinical effect is unknown). Blood levels of losartan may be increased by inhibitors of cytochrome P450 isoenzymes 2C9 (amiodarone, fluoxetine, isoniazid, ritonavir, sulfonamides) and 3A4 (diltiazem, erythromycin, verapamil, ketoconazole, itraconazole). Potassium salts/supplements, co-trimoxazole (high dose), ACE inhibitors, and potassium-sparing diuretics (amiloride, spironolactone, triamterene) may increase the risk of hyperkalemia.

Decreased Effect: Phenobarbital caused a reduction of losartan in serum by 20%, clinical effect is unknown. Other enzyme inducers may affect serum concentration of losartan.

Drug Uptake

Onset of action: 6 hours

Half-life, elimination: Losartan: 1.5-2 hours; E-3174: 6-9 hours

Time to peak: Losartan: 1 hour; E-3174: 3-4 hours

Pregnancy Risk Factor C/D (2nd and 3rd trimesters)

Generic Available No

Comments Cozaar® may be administered with other antihypertensive agents

Losartan and Hydrochlorothiazide

(loe SAR tan & hye droe klor oh THYE a zide)

U.S. Brand Names Hyzaar®

Canadian Brand Names Hyzaar®; Hyzaar® DS

Pharmacologic Category Antihypertensive Agent Combination

Synonyms Hydrochlorothiazide and Losartan

Use Treatment of hypertension

Local Anesthetic/Vasoconstrictor Precautions No information available to require special precautions

Effects on Dental Treatment No effects or complications reported

Dosage Adults: Oral: 1 tablet daily

Other Adverse Effects

Based on **losartan** component:

1% to 10%:

Central nervous system: Dizziness (4%), insomnia (1%)

Cardiovascular: First dose hypotension (dose-related; <1% with 50 mg, 2% with 100 mg)

Gastrointestinal: Diarrhea (2%), dyspepsia (1%), abdominal pain (2%), Nausea (2%)

Neuromuscular & skeletal: Back pain (2%), muscle cramps (1%), myalgia (1%), leg pain (1%)

Respiratory: Upper respiratory infection (8%), cough (3% versus 3% in placebo), nasal congestion (2%), sinus disorder (1%), sinusitis (1%)

>1% but frequency ≤ placebo: Asthenia, fatigue, edema, abdominal pain, chest pain, nausea, headache, pharyngitis

Based on **hydrochlorothiazide** component:

1% to 10%:

Cardiovascular: Orthostatic hypotension, hypotension

Dermatologic: Photosensitivity

Endocrine & metabolic: Hypokalemia

Gastrointestinal: Anorexia, epigastric distress

Drug Interactions See Losartan *on page 732* and Hydrochlorothiazide *on page 595*

Drug Uptake See Losartan *on page 732* and Hydrochlorothiazide *on page 595*

Pregnancy Risk Factor C/D (2nd and 3rd trimesters)

Generic Available No

Lotemax™ *see* Loteprednol *on page 733*

Lotensin® *see* Benazepril *on page 149*

Lotensin® HCT *see* Benazepril and Hydrochlorothiazide *on page 150*

Loteprednol (loe te PRED nol)

U.S. Brand Names Alrex™; Lotemax™

Canadian Brand Names Alrex™; Lotemax™

Pharmacologic Category Corticosteroid, Ophthalmic

Synonyms Loteprednol Etabonate

Use

0.2% suspension (Alrex™): Temporary relief of signs and symptoms of seasonal allergic conjunctivitis

0.5% suspension (Lotemax™): Inflammatory conditions (treatment of steroid-responsive inflammatory conditions of the palpebral and bulbar conjunctiva, cornea, and anterior segment of the globe such as allergic conjunctivitis, acne rosacea, superficial punctate keratitis, herpes zoster keratitis, iritis, cyclitis, selected infective conjunctivitis, when the inherent hazard of steroid use is accepted to obtain an advisable diminution in edema and inflammation) and treatment of postoperative inflammation following ocular surgery

Local Anesthetic/Vasoconstrictor Precautions No information available to require special precautions

Effects on Dental Treatment No effects or complications reported

Dosage Adults: Ophthalmic:

0.2% suspension (Alrex™): Instill 1 drop into affected eye(s) 4 times/day

0.5% suspension (Lotemax®):

Inflammatory conditions: Apply 1-2 drops into the conjunctival sac of the affected eye(s) 4 times/day. During the initial treatment within the first week, the dosing may be increased up to 1 drop every hour. Advise patients not to discontinue therapy prematurely. If signs and symptoms fail to improve after 2 days, re-evaluate the patient.

Postoperative inflammation: Apply 1-2 drops into the conjunctival sac of the operated eye(s) 4 times/day beginning 24 hours after surgery and continuing throughout the first 2 weeks of the postoperative period

Mechanism of Action Corticosteroids inhibit the inflammatory response including edema, capillary dilation, leukocyte migration, and scar formation. Loteprednol is highly lipid soluble and penetrates cells readily to induce the production of lipocortins. These proteins modulate the activity of prostaglandins and leukotrienes.

Other Adverse Effects

>10%:

Central nervous system: Headache

Respiratory: Rhinitis, pharyngitis

1% to 10%: Ocular: Abnormal vision/blurring, burning on instillation, chemosis, dry eyes, itching, injection, conjunctivitis/irritation, corneal abnormalities, eyelid erythema, papillae uveitis

Pregnancy Risk Factor C

Generic Available No

Lotrel® *see* Amlodipine and Benazepril *on page 82*

Lotrimin® *see* Clotrimazole *on page 312*

Lotrimin® AF [OTC] *see* Clotrimazole *on page 312*
Lotrimin® AF Powder/Spray [OTC] *see* Miconazole *on page 807*
Lotrimin® Ultra™ [OTC] *see* Butenafine *on page 195*
Lotrisone® *see* Betamethasone and Clotrimazole *on page 160*
Lotronex® *see* Alosetron *on page 55*

Lovastatin (LOE va sta tin)

Related Information
Cardiovascular Diseases *on page 1308*

U.S. Brand Names Altocor™; Mevacor®

Canadian Brand Names Apo®-Lovastatin; Mevacor®

Mexican Brand Names Mevacor®

Pharmacologic Category Antilipemic Agent, HMG-CoA Reductase Inhibitor

Synonyms Mevinolin; Monacolin K

Use
Adjunct to dietary therapy to decrease elevated serum total and LDL cholesterol concentrations in primary hypercholesterolemia
Primary prevention of coronary artery disease (patients without symptomatic disease with average to moderately elevated total and LDL cholesterol and below average HDL cholesterol)
Adjunct to dietary therapy in adolescent patients (10-17 years of age, females >1 year postmenarche) with heterozygous familial hypercholesterolemia having LDL >189 mg/dL, **or** LDL >160 mg/dL with positive family history of premature cardiovascular disease (CVD), **or** LDL >160 mg/dL with the presence of at least two other CVD risk factors

Local Anesthetic/Vasoconstrictor Precautions No information available to require special precautions

Effects on Dental Treatment No effects or complications reported

Dosage Adults: Oral: Initial: 20 mg with evening meal, then adjust at 4-week intervals; maximum dose: 80 mg/day; before initiation of therapy, patients should be placed on a standard cholesterol-lowering diet for 3-6 months and the diet should be continued during drug therapy

Mechanism of Action Lovastatin acts by competitively inhibiting 3-hydroxyl-3-methylglutaryl-coenzyme A (HMG-CoA) reductase, the enzyme that catalyzes the rate-limiting step in cholesterol biosynthesis

Other Adverse Effects
>10%: Neuromuscular & skeletal: Increased CPK (>2x normal) (11%)
1% to 10%:
Central nervous system: Headache (2% to 3%), dizziness (0.5% to 1%)
Dermatologic: Rash (0.8% to 1%)
Gastrointestinal: Abdominal pain (2% to 3%), constipation (2% to 4%), diarrhea (2% to 3%), dyspepsia (1% to 2%), flatulence (4% to 5%), nausea (2% to 3%)
Neuromuscular & skeletal: Myalgia (2% to 3%), weakness (1% to 2%), muscle cramps (0.6% to 1%)
Ocular: Blurred vision (0.8% to 1%)

Warnings/Precautions Liver function must be monitored by periodic laboratory assessment. Rhabdomyolysis with acute renal failure has occurred. Risk is dose-related and is increased with concurrent use of lipid-lowering agents which may cause rhabdomyolysis (gemfibrozil, fibric acid derivatives, or niacin at doses ≥1 g/day) or during concurrent use with potent CYP3A3/4 inhibitors (including amiodarone, clarithromycin, cyclosporine, erythromycin, itraconazole, ketoconazole, nefazodone, grapefruit juice in large quantities, verapamil, or protease inhibitors such as indinavir, nelfinavir, or ritonavir). Weigh the risk versus benefit when combining any of these drugs with lovastatin. Temporarily discontinue in any patient experiencing an acute or serious condition predisposing to renal failure secondary to rhabdomyolysis. Use with caution in patients who consume large amounts of ethanol or have a history of liver disease. Safety and efficacy have not been evaluated in prepubertal patients, patients <10 years of age, or doses >40 mg/day in appropriately-selected adolescents.

Drug Interactions CYP3A3/4 enzyme substrate
Antacids: Plasma concentrations may be decreased when given with magnesium-aluminum hydroxide containing antacids (reported with atorvastatin and pravastatin). Clinical efficacy is not altered, no dosage adjustment is necessary
Cholestyramine reduces absorption of several HMG-CoA reductase inhibitors. Separate administration times by at least 4 hours.
Cholestyramine and colestipol (bile acid sequestrants): Cholesterol-lowering effects are additive.
Clofibrate and fenofibrate may increase the risk of myopathy and rhabdomyolysis; limit dose of lovastatin to <20 mg/day
Cyclosporine: Concurrent use may increase risk of myopathy; limit dose of lovastatin to <20 mg/day
CYP3A3/4 inhibitors (amiodarone, clarithromycin, cyclosporine, danazol, diltiazem, fluvoxamine, erythromycin, itraconazole, ketoconazole, miconazole, nefazodone,

amprenavir, indinavir, nelfinavir, ritonavir, saquinavir, troleandomycin, and verapamil) increase lovastatin blood levels; may increase the risk of lovastatin-induced myopathy and rhabdomyolysis; concurrent use is not recommended

Gemfibrozil: Increased risk of myopathy and rhabdomyolysis

Grapefruit juice may inhibit metabolism of lovastatin via CYP3A3/4; avoid high dietary intakes of grapefruit juice.

Isradipine may decrease lovastatin blood levels.

Niacin (at higher dosages ≥1 g/day) may increase risk of myopathy and rhabdomyolysis; limit dose of lovastatin to <20 mg/day

Warfarin effect (hypoprothrombinemic response) may be increased; monitor INR closely when lovastatin is initiated or discontinued.

Drug Uptake

Onset of action: LDL cholesterol reductions: 3 days

Absorption: Oral: 30%

Half-life, elimination: 1.1-1.7 hours

Time to peak: Oral: 2-4 hours

Pregnancy Risk Factor X

Generic Available Yes

Lovenox® *see* Enoxaparin *on page 434*

Low-Ogestrel® *see* Combination Hormonal Contraceptives *on page 323*

Lowsium® Plus *see* Magaldrate and Simethicone *on page 739*

Loxapine (LOKS a peen)

U.S. Brand Names Loxitane®; Loxitane® C; Loxitane® I.M.

Canadian Brand Names Apo®-Loxapine; Loxapac®; Nu-Loxapine; PMS-Loxapine

Pharmacologic Category Antipsychotic Agent, Dibenzoxazepine

Synonyms Loxapine Hydrochloride; Loxapine Succinate; Oxilapine Succinate

Use Treatment of psychoses, nausea and vomiting; Tourette's syndrome; mania; intractable hiccups (adults); behavioral problems (children)

Local Anesthetic/Vasoconstrictor Precautions Most pharmacology textbooks state that in presence of phenothiazines, systemic doses of epinephrine paradoxically decrease the blood pressure. This is the so called "epinephrine reversal" phenomenon. This has never been observed when epinephrine is given by infiltration as part of the anesthesia procedure.

Effects on Dental Treatment

>10%: Xerostomia

Significant hypotension may occur, especially when the drug is administered parenterally; orthostatic hypotension is due to alpha-receptor blockade, the elderly are at greater risk for orthostatic hypotension

Tardive dyskinesia: Prevalence rate may be 40% in elderly; development of the syndrome and the irreversible nature are proportional to duration and total cumulative dose over time. Extrapyramidal reactions are more common in elderly with up to 50% developing these reactions after 60 years of age; drug-induced **Parkinson's syndrome** occurs often; **Akathisia** is the most common extrapyramidal reaction in elderly.

Increased confusion, memory loss, psychotic behavior, and agitation frequently occur as a consequence of anticholinergic effects Antipsychotic associated sedation in nonpsychotic patients is extremely unpleasant due to feelings of depersonalization, derealization, and dysphoria

Dosage Adults:

Oral: 10 mg twice daily, increase dose until psychotic symptoms are controlled; usual dose range: 60-100 mg/day in divided doses 2-4 times/day; dosages >250 mg/day are not recommended

I.M.: 12.5-50 mg every 4-6 hours or longer as needed and change to oral therapy as soon as possible

Mechanism of Action Blocks postsynaptic mesolimbic dopaminergic receptors in the brain; exhibits a strong alpha-adrenergic blocking effect and depresses the release of hypothalamic and hypophyseal hormones; believed to depress the reticular-activating system, thus affecting basal metabolism, body temperatures, wakefulness, vasomotor tone, and emesis

Other Adverse Effects Frequency not defined:

Cardiovascular: Orthostatic hypotension, tachycardia, arrhythmias, abnormal T-waves with prolonged ventricular repolarization, hypertension, hypotension, lightheadedness, syncope

Central nervous system: Drowsiness, extrapyramidal symptoms (dystonia, akathisia, pseudoparkinsonism, tardive dyskinesia, akinesia), dizziness, faintness, ataxia, insomnia, agitation, tension, seizures, slurred speech, confusion, headache, neuroleptic malignant syndrome (NMS), altered central temperature regulation

Dermatologic: Rash, pruritus, photosensitivity, dermatitis, alopecia, seborrhea

Endocrine & metabolic: Enlargement of breasts, galactorrhea, amenorrhea, gynecomastia, menstrual irregularity

Gastrointestinal: Xerostomia, constipation, nausea, vomiting, nasal congestion, weight gain/loss, adynamic ileus, polydipsia

(Continued)

Loxapine *(Continued)*

Genitourinary: Urinary retention, sexual dysfunction
Hematologic: Agranulocytosis, leukopenia, thrombocytopenia
Neuromuscular & skeletal: Weakness
Ocular: Blurred vision

Drug Interactions

Aluminum salts: May decrease the absorption of antipsychotics; monitor
Amphetamines: Efficacy may be diminished by antipsychotics; in addition, amphetamines may increase psychotic symptoms; avoid concurrent use
Anticholinergics: May inhibit the therapeutic response to antipsychotics and excess anticholinergic effects may occur; includes benztropine, trihexyphenidyl, biperiden, and drugs with significant anticholinergic activity (TCAs, antihistamines, disopyramide)
Antihypertensives: Concurrent use of antipsychotics with an antihypertensive may produce additive hypotensive effects (particularly orthostasis)
Bromocriptine: Antipsychotics inhibit the ability of bromocriptine to lower serum prolactin concentrations
CNS depressants: Sedative effects may be additive with antipsychotics; monitor for increased effect; includes barbiturates, benzodiazepines, narcotic analgesics, ethanol, and other sedative agents
Enzyme inducers: May enhance the hepatic metabolism of antipsychotics. Larger doses may be required; includes rifampin, rifabutin, barbiturates, phenytoin, and cigarette smoking
Epinephrine: Chlorpromazine (and possibly other low potency antipsychotics) may diminish the pressor effects of epinephrine
Guanethidine and guanadrel: Antihypertensive effects may be inhibited by antipsychotics
Levodopa: Antipsychotics may inhibit the antiparkinsonian effect of levodopa; avoid this combination
Lithium: Antipsychotics may produce neurotoxicity with lithium; this is a rare effect
Metoclopramide: May increase extrapyramidal symptoms (EPS) or risk.
Phenytoin: May reduce serum levels of antipsychotics; antipsychotics may increase phenytoin serum levels
Propranolol: Serum concentrations of antipsychotics may be increased; propranolol also increases antipsychotic concentrations
QT_c-prolonging agents: Effects on QT_c interval may be additive with antipsychotics, increasing the risk of malignant arrhythmias. Includes type Ia antiarrhythmics, TCAs, and some quinolone antibiotics (sparfloxacin, moxifloxacin and gatifloxacin)
Sulfadoxine-pyrimethamine: May increase antipsychotic concentrations
Tricyclic antidepressants: Concurrent use may produce increased toxicity or altered therapeutic response
Trazodone: Antipsychotics and trazodone may produce additive hypotensive effects
Valproic acid: Serum levels may be increased by antipsychotics

Drug Uptake

Onset of action: Neuroleptic: Oral: 20-30 minutes; Peak effect: 1.5-3 hours
Duration: ~12 hours
Half-life, elimination: Biphasic: Initial: 5 hours; Terminal: 12-19 hours

Pregnancy Risk Factor C

Generic Available Yes

Loxitane® *see* Loxapine *on page 735*
Loxitane® C *see* Loxapine *on page 735*
Loxitane® I.M. *see* Loxapine *on page 735*
Lozol® *see* Indapamide *on page 632*
Lubriderm® [OTC] *see* Lanolin, Cetyl Alcohol, Glycerin, and Petrolatum *on page 686*
Lubriderm® Fragrance Free [OTC] *see* Lanolin, Cetyl Alcohol, Glycerin, and Petrolatum *on page 686*
Ludiomil® *see* Maprotiline *on page 744*
Lufyllin® *see* Dyphylline *on page 426*
Lumigan™ *see* Bimatoprost *on page 165*
Luminal® Sodium *see* Phenobarbital *on page 945*
Lumitene™ *see* Beta-Carotene *on page 158*
Lunelle™ *see* Estradiol Cypionate and Medroxyprogesterone Acetate *on page 461*
Lupron® *see* Leuprolide Acetate *on page 692*
Lupron Depot® *see* Leuprolide Acetate *on page 692*
Lupron Depot-Ped® *see* Leuprolide Acetate *on page 692*
Luride® *see* Fluoride *on page 514*
Luride® Lozi-Tab® *see* Fluoride *on page 514*
Luride®-SF Lozi-Tabs® *see* Fluoride *on page 514*
Luvox® *see* Fluvoxamine *on page 528*

Luxiq™ *see* Betamethasone *on page 159*

Lymphocyte Immune Globulin (LIM foe site i MYUN GLOB yoo lin)

U.S. Brand Names Atgam®

Canadian Brand Names Atgam®

Pharmacologic Category Immunosuppressant Agent

Synonyms Antithymocyte Globulin (Equine); Antithymocyte Immunoglobulin; ATG; Horse Antihuman Thymocyte Gamma Globulin

Use Prevention and treatment of acute allograft rejection; treatment of moderate to severe aplastic anemia in patients not considered suitable candidates for bone marrow transplantation; prevention of graft-vs-host disease following bone marrow transplantation

Local Anesthetic/Vasoconstrictor Precautions No information available to require special precautions

Effects on Dental Treatment No effects or complications reported

Dosage An intradermal skin test is recommended prior to administration of the initial dose of ATG; use 0.1 mL of a 1:1000 dilution of ATG in normal saline. A positive skin reaction consists of a wheal ≥10 mm in diameter. If a positive skin test occurs, the first infusion should be administered in a controlled environment with intensive life support immediately available. A systemic reaction precludes further administration of the drug. The absence of a reaction does **not** preclude the possibility of an immediate sensitivity reaction.

First dose: Premedicate with diphenhydramine 50 mg orally 30 minutes prior to and hydrocortisone 100 mg I.V. 15 minutes prior to infusion and acetaminophen 650 mg 2 hours after start of infusion

Children: I.V.:
- Aplastic anemia protocol: 10-20 mg/kg/day for 8-14 days; then administer every other day for 7 more doses; addition doses may be given every other day for 21 total doses in 28 days
- Renal allograft: 5-25 mg/kg/day

Adults: I.V.:
- Aplastic anemia protocol: 10-20 mg/kg/day for 8-14 days, then administer every other day for 7 more doses
- Renal allograft:
  - Rejection prophylaxis: 15 mg/kg/day for 14 days followed by 14 days of alternative day therapy at the same dose; the first dose should be administered within 24 hours before or after transplantation
  - Rejection treatment: 10-15 mg/kg/day for 14 days, then administer every other day for 10-14 days up to 21 doses in 28 days An intradermal skin test is recommended prior to administration of the initial dose of ATG; use 0.1 mL of a 1:1000 dilution of ATG in normal saline

Children: I.V.:
- Aplastic anemia protocol: 10-20 mg/kg/day for 8-14 days, then give every other day for 7 more doses
- Cardiac allograft: 10 mg/kg/day for 7 days
- Renal allograft: 5-25 mg/kg/day

Adults: I.V.:
- Aplastic anemia protocol: 10-20 mg/kg/day for 8-14 days, then give every other day for 7 more doses **or** 40 mg/kg/day for 4 days
- Rejection prevention: 15 mg/kg/day for 14 days, then give every other day for 7 more doses for a total of 21 doses in 28 days; initial dose should be administered within 24 hours before or after transplantation
- Rejection treatment: 10-15 mg/kg/day for 14 days, then give every other day for 7 more doses

Mechanism of Action May involve elimination of antigen-reactive T-lymphocytes (killer cells) in peripheral blood or alteration of T-cell function

Other Adverse Effects

>10%:
- Central nervous system: Fever, chills
- Dermatologic: Rash
- Hematologic: Leukopenia, thrombocytopenia
- Miscellaneous: Systemic infection

1% to 10%:
- Cardiovascular: Hypotension, hypertension, tachycardia, edema, chest pain
- Central nervous system: Headache, malaise, pain
- Gastrointestinal: Diarrhea, nausea, stomatitis, GI bleeding
- Local: Edema or redness at injection site, thrombophlebitis
- Neuromuscular & skeletal: Myalgia, back pain, arthralgia
- Renal: Abnormal RFTs
- Respiratory: Dyspnea
- Miscellaneous: Sensitivity reactions: Anaphylaxis may be indicated by hypotension, respiratory distress; serum sickness, viral infection

Drug Uptake Half-life, elimination, plasma: 1.5-12 days

Pregnancy Risk Factor C

Generic Available No

(Continued)

Lymphocyte Immune Globulin *(Continued)*

Comments Do not dilute with D_5W (may cause precipitation). The use of highly acidic infusion solutions is not recommended because of possible physical instability. When the dose of corticosteroids and other immunosuppressants is being reduced, some previously masked reaction to Atgam® may appear.

Lyphocin® *see* Vancomycin *on page 1231*

Lysine (el LYE seen)

U.S. Brand Names Enisyl® [OTC]

Pharmacologic Category Dietary Supplement

Synonyms L-Lysine; L-Lysine Hydrochloride

Use Improves utilization of vegetable proteins

Local Anesthetic/Vasoconstrictor Precautions No information available to require special precautions

Effects on Dental Treatment No effects or complications reported

Dosage Adults: Oral: 334-1500 mg/day

Pregnancy Risk Factor C

Generic Available Yes

Lysodren® *see* Mitotane *on page 821*

Maalox® [OTC] *see* Aluminum Hydroxide and Magnesium Hydroxide *on page 62*

Maalox® Anti-Gas [OTC] *see* Simethicone *on page 1088*

Maalox® Fast Release Liquid [OTC] *see* Aluminum Hydroxide, Magnesium Hydroxide, and Simethicone *on page 63*

Maalox® Max [OTC] *see* Aluminum Hydroxide, Magnesium Hydroxide, and Simethicone *on page 63*

Maalox® TC (Therapeutic Concentrate) [OTC] *see* Aluminum Hydroxide and Magnesium Hydroxide *on page 62*

Macrobid® *see* Nitrofurantoin *on page 870*

Macrodantin® *see* Nitrofurantoin *on page 870*

Macrodex® *see* Dextran *on page 369*

Mafenide (MA fe nide)

U.S. Brand Names Sulfamylon®

Pharmacologic Category Antibiotic, Topical

Synonyms Mafenide Acetate

Use Adjunct in the treatment of second- and third-degree burns to prevent septicemia caused by susceptible organisms such as *Pseudomonas aeruginosa*

Orphan drug: Prevention of graft loss of meshed autografts on excised burn wounds

Local Anesthetic/Vasoconstrictor Precautions No information available to require special precautions

Effects on Dental Treatment No effects or complications reported

Dosage Children and Adults: Topical: Apply once or twice daily with a sterile gloved hand; apply to a thickness of ~ 16 mm; the burned area should be covered with cream at all times

Mechanism of Action Interferes with bacterial folic acid synthesis through competitive inhibition of para-aminobenzoic acid

Other Adverse Effects Frequency not defined:

Cardiovascular: Facial edema
Central nervous system: Pain
Dermatologic: Rash, erythema
Endocrine & metabolic: Hyperchloremia, metabolic acidosis
Hematologic: Porphyria, bone marrow suppression, hemolytic anemia, bleeding
Local: Burning sensation, excoriation
Respiratory: Hyperventilation, tachypnea, dyspnea
Miscellaneous: Hypersensitivity

Drug Uptake

Absorption: Diffuses through devascularized areas and is rapidly absorbed from burned surface
Time to peak: Topical: 2-4 hours

Pregnancy Risk Factor C

Generic Available No

Magaldrate (MAG al drate)

U.S. Brand Names Riopan® [OTC]

Canadian Brand Names Riopan®

Pharmacologic Category Antacid

Synonyms Hydromagnesium Aluminate

Use Symptomatic relief of hyperacidity associated with peptic ulcer, gastritis, peptic esophagitis and hiatal hernia

Local Anesthetic/Vasoconstrictor Precautions No information available to require special precautions

Effects on Dental Treatment No effects or complications reported

Dosage Adults: Oral: 540-1080 mg between meals and at bedtime

Other Adverse Effects Frequency not defined:

Central nervous system: Encephalopathy

Endocrine & metabolic: Aluminum intoxication, hypophosphatemia, hypermagnesemia, milk-alkali syndrome

Gastrointestinal: Constipation, chalky taste, stomach cramps, fecal impaction, diarrhea, nausea, vomiting, discoloration of feces (white speckles), rebound hyperacidity

Neuromuscular & skeletal: Osteomalacia

Drug Interactions Decreased Effect: Tetracyclines, digoxin, iron salts, isoniazid or quinolones; indomethacin absorption can be decreased by the aluminum, or increased by the magnesium (appears to be insignificant).

Pregnancy Risk Factor C

Generic Available Yes

Comments Chemical entity known as hydroxy magnesium aluminate equivalent to magnesium oxide and aluminum oxide; unlike other magnesium-containing antacids, Riopan® is safe to use in renal patients

Magaldrate and Simethicone (MAG al drate & sye METH i kone)

U.S. Brand Names Iosopan® Plus; Lowsium® Plus; Riopan Plus® [OTC]; Riopan Plus® Double Strength [OTC]

Canadian Brand Names Riopan Plus®

Pharmacologic Category Antacid; Antiflatulent

Synonyms Simethicone and Magaldrate

Use Relief of hyperacidity associated with peptic ulcer, gastritis, peptic esophagitis and hiatal hernia which are accompanied by symptoms of gas

Local Anesthetic/Vasoconstrictor Precautions No information available to require special precautions

Effects on Dental Treatment No effects or complications reported

Dosage Adults: Oral: 5-10 mL between meals and at bedtime

Other Adverse Effects Frequency not defined:

Based on **magaldrate** component:

Central nervous system: Encephalopathy

Gastrointestinal: Constipation, chalky taste, stomach cramps, fecal impaction, diarrhea, nausea, vomiting, discoloration of feces (white speckles), rebound hyperacidity

Endocrine & metabolic: Hypophosphatemia, hypermagnesemia, milk-alkali syndrome

Neuromuscular & metabolic: Osteomalacia

Miscellaneous: Aluminum intoxication

Drug Interactions

Based on **magaldrate** component: Tetracyclines, digoxin, iron salts, isoniazid; indomethacin absorption can be decreased by the aluminum, or increased by the magnesium (appears to be insignificant)

Based on **simethicone** component: Hypersensitivity to simethicone

Pregnancy Risk Factor C

Generic Available Yes

Comments Chemical entity known as hydroxy magnesium aluminate equivalent to magnesium oxide and aluminum oxide; unlike other magnesium containing antacids, Riopan® is safe to use in renal patients if used cautiously

Mag Delay® *see* Magnesium Chloride *on page 739*

Mag-Gel® 600 *see* Magnesium Oxide *on page 742*

Maginex™ [OTC] *see* Magnesium L-aspartate Hydrochloride *on page 741*

Maginex™ DS [OTC] *see* Magnesium L-aspartate Hydrochloride *on page 741*

Magnesium Chloride (mag NEE zhum KLOR ide)

U.S. Brand Names Chloromag®; Mag Delay®; Mag-SR®; Slow-Mag® [OTC]

Canadian Brand Names Slow-Mag™

Pharmacologic Category Magnesium Salt

Use Correction or prevention of hypomagnesemia

Local Anesthetic/Vasoconstrictor Precautions No information available to require special precautions

Effects on Dental Treatment Magnesium products may prevent GI absorption of tetracyclines by forming a large ionized chelated molecule with the tetracyclines in the stomach. Tetracyclines should be given at least 1 hour before magnesium.

Dosage

Oral: Adults: Dietary supplement: 54-283 mg/day in divided doses

I.V. in TPN:

Children: 2-10 mEq/day

The usual recommended pediatric maintenance intake of magnesium ranges from 0.2-0.6 mEq/kg/day. The dose of magnesium may also be based on the

(Continued)

Magnesium Chloride *(Continued)*

caloric intake; on that basis, 3-10 mEq/day of magnesium are needed; maximum maintenance dose: 8-16 mEq/day

Adults: 8-24 mEq/day

Other Adverse Effects 1% to 10%:

Cardiovascular: Flushing

Central nervous system: Depressed CNS, somnolence

Gastrointestinal: Diarrhea

Neuromuscular & skeletal: Blocked peripheral neuromuscular transmission, deep tendon reflexes

Respiratory: Respiratory paralysis

Pregnancy Risk Factor D

Generic Available Yes

Magnesium Citrate (mag NEE zhum SIT rate)

Canadian Brand Names Citro-Mag®

Pharmacologic Category Laxative, Saline; Magnesium Salt

Synonyms Citrate of Magnesia

Use To evacuate bowel prior to certain surgical and diagnostic procedures

Local Anesthetic/Vasoconstrictor Precautions No information available to require special precautions

Effects on Dental Treatment Magnesium products may prevent GI absorption of tetracyclines by forming a large ionized chelated molecule with the tetracyclines in the stomach. Tetracyclines should be given at least 1 hour before magnesium.

Dosage Cathartic: Oral:

Children:

<6 years: 0.5 mL/kg up to a maximum of 200 mL repeated every 4-6 hours until stools are clear

6-12 years: 100-150 mL

Children ≥12 years and Adults: ½ to 1 full bottle (120-300 mL)

Mechanism of Action Promotes bowel evacuation by causing osmotic retention of fluid which distends the colon with increased peristaltic activity

Other Adverse Effects 1% to 10%:

Cardiovascular: Hypotension

Endocrine & metabolic: Hypermagnesemia

Gastrointestinal: Abdominal cramps, diarrhea, gas formation

Respiratory: Respiratory depression

Drug Uptake Absorption: Oral: 15% to 30%

Pregnancy Risk Factor B

Generic Available Yes

Comments Magnesium content of 5 mL: 3.85-4.71 mEq

Magnesium Gluconate (mag NEE zhum GLOO koe nate)

U.S. Brand Names Magonate® [OTC]

Pharmacologic Category Magnesium Salt

Use Dietary supplement for treatment of magnesium deficiencies

Local Anesthetic/Vasoconstrictor Precautions No information available to require special precautions

Effects on Dental Treatment Magnesium products may prevent GI absorption of tetracyclines by forming a large ionized chelated molecule with the tetracyclines in the stomach. Tetracyclines should be given at least 1 hour before magnesium.

Dosage The recommended dietary allowance (RDA) of magnesium is 4.5 mg/kg which is a total daily allowance of 350-400 mg for adult men and 280-300 mg for adult women. During pregnancy the RDA is 300 mg and during lactation the RDA is 355 mg. Average daily intakes of dietary magnesium have declined in recent years due to processing of food. The latest estimate of the average American dietary intake was 349 mg/day.

Dietary supplement: Oral:

Children: 3-6 mg/kg/day in divided doses 3-4 times/day; maximum: 400 mg/day

Adults: 27-54 mg 2-3 times/day or 100 mg 4 times/day

Mechanism of Action Magnesium is important as a cofactor in many enzymatic reactions in the body involving protein synthesis and carbohydrate metabolism, (at least 300 enzymatic reactions require magnesium). Actions on lipoprotein lipase have been found to be important in reducing serum cholesterol and on sodium/potassium ATPase in promoting polarization (ie, neuromuscular functioning).

Other Adverse Effects 1% to 10%: Gastrointestinal: Diarrhea (excessive dose)

Drug Interactions Increased Effect/Toxicity: Nondepolarizing neuromuscular blockers.

Decreased Effect: Decreased absorption of aminoquinolones, digoxin, nitrofurantoin, penicillamine, and tetracyclines may occur with magnesium salts.

Drug Uptake Absorption: Oral: 15% to 30%

Generic Available Yes

Comments Magnesium content of 500 mg: 27 mg

Magnesium Hydroxide (mag NEE zhum hye DROKS ide)

U.S. Brand Names Phillips'® Milk of Magnesia [OTC]

Pharmacologic Category Antacid; Magnesium Salt

Synonyms Magnesia Magma; Milk of Magnesia; MOM

Use Short-term treatment of occasional constipation and symptoms of hyperacidity, magnesium replacement therapy

Local Anesthetic/Vasoconstrictor Precautions No information available to require special precautions

Effects on Dental Treatment Magnesium products may prevent GI absorption of tetracyclines by forming a large ionized chelated molecule with the tetracyclines in the stomach. Tetracyclines should be given at least 1 hour before magnesium.

Dosage Oral:

Laxative:

- <2 years: 0.5 mL/kg/dose
- 2-5 years: 5-15 mL/day or in divided doses
- 6-12 years: 15-30 mL/day or in divided doses
- ≥12 years: 30-60 mL/day or in divided doses

Antacid:

- Children: 2.5-5 mL as needed up to 4 times/day
- Adults: 5-15 mL or 650 mg to 1.3 g tablets up to 4 times/day as needed

Mechanism of Action Promotes bowel evacuation by causing osmotic retention of fluid which distends the colon with increased peristaltic activity; reacts with hydrochloric acid in stomach to form magnesium chloride

Other Adverse Effects Frequency not defined:

Cardiovascular: Hypotension
Endocrine & metabolic: Hypermagnesemia
Gastrointestinal: Diarrhea, abdominal cramps
Neuromuscular & skeletal: Muscle weakness
Respiratory: Respiratory depression

Drug Interactions Absorption of tetracyclines, digoxin, iron salts, isoniazid, or quinolones may be decreased.

Drug Uptake Onset of action: Laxative: 4-8 hours

Pregnancy Risk Factor B

Generic Available Yes

Magnesium Hydroxide and Mineral Oil Emulsion

(mag NEE zhum hye DROKS ide & MIN er al oyl e MUL shun)

U.S. Brand Names Haley's M-O® [OTC]

Pharmacologic Category Laxative

Synonyms MOM/Mineral Oil Emulsion

Use Short-term treatment of occasional constipation

Local Anesthetic/Vasoconstrictor Precautions No information available to require special precautions

Effects on Dental Treatment Magnesium products may prevent GI absorption of tetracyclines by forming a large ionized chelated molecule with the tetracyclines in the stomach. Tetracyclines should be given at least 1 hour before magnesium.

Dosage Adults: Oral: 5-45 mL at bedtime

Other Adverse Effects Frequency not defined:

Cardiovascular: Hypotension
Endocrine & metabolic: Hypermagnesemia
Gastrointestinal: Diarrhea, abdominal cramps
Neuromuscular & skeletal: Muscle weakness
Respiratory: Respiratory depression

Drug Interactions Absorption of tetracyclines, digoxin, iron salts, isoniazid, or quinolones may be decreased.

Pregnancy Risk Factor B

Generic Available No

Magnesium L-aspartate Hydrochloride

(mag NEE zhum el as PAR tate hye droe KLOR ide)

U.S. Brand Names Maginex™ [OTC]; Maginex™ DS [OTC]

Pharmacologic Category Electrolyte Supplement, Oral

Synonyms MAH™

Use Dietary supplement

Local Anesthetic/Vasoconstrictor Precautions No information available to require special precautions

Effects on Dental Treatment Magnesium ions prevent GI absorption of tetracycline by forming a large, ionized, chelated molecule with the magnesium ion and tetracyclines in the stomach. Magnesium supplement should not be taken within 2-4 hours of oral tetracycline or other members of the tetracycline family.

Dosage Adults:

Recommended dietary allowance (RDA) of magnesium:

- Male: 400-420 mg

(Continued)

Magnesium L-aspartate Hydrochloride *(Continued)*

Female: 310-320 mg
During pregnancy: 360 mg
During lactation: 320 mg

Dietary supplement: Oral: Magnesium-L-aspartate 1230 mg (magnesium 122 mg) up to 3 times/day

Dosage adjustment in renal impairment: Patients with severe renal failure should not receive magnesium due to toxicity from accumulation.

Other Adverse Effects Frequency not defined: Gastrointestinal: Diarrhea, loose stools

Drug Interactions

Calcium: May increase magnesium serum concentration; use caution in patients with renal insufficiency.

Magnesium-containing antacids/laxatives: Concomitant use by lead to magnesium toxicity; use caution in patients with renal insufficiency.

Quinolone antibiotics (oral): May form nonabsorbable complexes leading to decreased antibiotic absorption; magnesium supplement should not be taken within 2-4 hours of oral quinolone.

Sodium polystyrene sulfonate: May bind with oral magnesium; concomitant use is not recommended.

Tetracycline (oral): May form nonabsorbable complexes leading to decreased antibiotic absorption; magnesium supplement should not be taken within 2-4 hours of oral tetracycline.

Magnesium Oxide (mag NEE zhum OKS ide)

U.S. Brand Names Mag-Gel® 600; Mag-Ox® 400 [OTC]; Uro-Mag® [OTC]

Pharmacologic Category Electrolyte Supplement, Oral

Use Short-term treatment of occasional constipation and symptoms of hyperacidity

Local Anesthetic/Vasoconstrictor Precautions No information available to require special precautions

Effects on Dental Treatment Magnesium products may prevent GI absorption of tetracyclines by forming a large ionized chelated molecule with the tetracyclines in the stomach. Tetracyclines should be given at least 1 hour before magnesium.

Dosage Magnesium RDA: 4.5 mg/kg, which is a total daily allowance of 350 mg for adult men and 280-300 mg for adult women. During pregnancy, the RDA is 200 mg and during lactation it is 355 mg. Average daily intakes of dietary magnesium have declined in recent years due to processing of food. The latest estimate of the average American dietary intake was 349 mg/day.

Adults: Oral:
Dietary supplement: 27-54 mEq (1-2 tablets) 2-3 times/day
Antacid: ½ to 3 tablets (0.21-1.68 g) with water or milk 4 times/day after meals and at bedtime
Laxative: 2-4 g at bedtime with full glass of water

Mechanism of Action Promotes bowel evacuation by causing osmotic retention of fluid which distends the colon with increased peristaltic activity

Other Adverse Effects

>10%: Gastrointestinal: Diarrhea

1% to 10%:
Cardiovascular: Hypotension, EKG changes
Central nervous system: Mental depression, coma
Gastrointestinal: Nausea, vomiting
Respiratory: Respiratory depression

Drug Interactions

Increased Effect/Toxicity: Nondepolarizing neuromuscular blockers

Decreased Effect: Decreased absorption of aminoquinolones, digoxin, nitrofurantoin, penicillamine, and tetracyclines may occur with magnesium salts

Drug Uptake Onset of action: Laxative: 4-8 hours

Pregnancy Risk Factor B

Generic Available Yes

Magnesium Salicylate (mag NEE zhum sa LIS i late)

Related Information

Rheumatoid Arthritis and Osteoarthritis *on page 1340*
Temporomandibular Dysfunction (TMD) *on page 1397*

U.S. Brand Names Backache Pain Relief Extra Strength; Doan's®, Original [OTC]; Extra Strength Doan's® [OTC]; Keygesic-10®; Mobidin®; Momentum® [OTC]

Mexican Brand Names Myoflex®

Pharmacologic Category Salicylate

Use Mild to moderate pain, fever, various inflammatory conditions

Local Anesthetic/Vasoconstrictor Precautions No information available to require special precautions

Effects on Dental Treatment NSAID formulations are known to reversibly decrease platelet aggregation via mechanisms different than observed with aspirin.

The dentist should be aware of the potential of abnormal coagulation. Caution should also be exercised in the use of NSAIDs in patients already on anticoagulant therapy with drugs such as warfarin (Coumadin®).

Dosage Oral: Adults: 650 mg 4 times daily or 1090 mg 3 times daily; may increase to 3.6-4.8 mg/day in 3 or 4 divided doses

Warnings/Precautions Use with caution in patients with CHF, dehydration, hypertension, decreased renal or hepatic function, history of GI disease, active GI ulceration or bleeding, or those receiving anticoagulants. Withhold for at least 4-6 half-lives prior to surgical or dental procedures.

Drug Interactions Decreased absorption of aminoquinolones, digoxin, nitrofurantoin, penicillamine, and tetracyclines may occur with magnesium salts.

Generic Available Yes

Magnesium Sulfate (mag NEE zhum SUL fate)

Pharmacologic Category Antacid; Anticonvulsant, Miscellaneous; Electrolyte Supplement, Parenteral; Laxative, Saline; Magnesium Salt

Synonyms Epsom Salts

Use Treatment and prevention of hypomagnesemia and in seizure prevention in severe pre-eclampsia or eclampsia, pediatric acute nephritis; also used as short-term treatment of constipation and torsade de pointes; treatment of cardiac arrhythmias (VT/VF) caused by hypomagnesemia

Local Anesthetic/Vasoconstrictor Precautions No information available to require special precautions

Effects on Dental Treatment Magnesium products may prevent GI absorption of tetracyclines by forming a large ionized chelated molecule with the tetracyclines in the stomach. Tetracyclines should be given at least 1 hour before magnesium.

Dosage The recommended dietary allowance (RDA) of magnesium is 4.5 mg/kg which is a total daily allowance of 350-400 mg for adult men and 280-300 mg for adult women. During pregnancy the RDA is 300 mg and during lactation the RDA is 355 mg. Average daily intakes of dietary magnesium have declined in recent years due to processing of food. The latest estimate of the average American dietary intake was 349 mg/day. Dose represented as $MgSO_4$ unless stated otherwise.

Serum magnesium is poor reflection of repletional status as the majority of magnesium is intracellular; serum concentration may be transiently normal for a few hours after a dose is given, therefore, aim for consistently high normal serum concentration in patients with normal renal function for most efficient repletion

Hypomagnesemia: Children: I.M., I.V.: 25-50 mg/kg/dose (0.2-0.4 mEq/kg/dose) every 4-6 hours for 3-4 doses, maximum single dose: 2000 mg (16 mEq), may repeat if hypomagnesemia persists (higher dosage up to 100 mg/kg/dose $MgSO_4$ I.V. has been used); maintenance: I.V.: 30-60 mg/kg/day (0.25-0.5 mEq/kg/day)

Management of seizures and hypertension:

- Children: I.M., I.V.: 20-100 mg/kg/dose every 4-6 hours as needed; in severe cases doses as high as 200 mg/kg/dose have been used
- Adults:
  - Oral: 3 g every 6 hours for 4 doses as needed
  - I.M., I.V.: 1 g every 6 hours for 4 doses; for severe hypomagnesemia: 8-12 g $MgSO_4$/day in divided doses has been used

Eclampsia, pre-eclampsia: Adults:

- I.M.: 1-4 g every 4 hours
- I.V.: Initial: 4 g, then switch to I.M. or 1-4 g/hour by continuous infusion

Maximum dose should not exceed 30-40 g/day; maximum rate of infusion: 1-2 g/hour

Maintenance electrolyte requirements:

- Daily requirements: 0.2-0.5 mEq/kg/24 hours or 3-10 mEq/1000 kcal/24 hours
- Maximum: 8-16 mEq/24 hours

Cathartic: Oral:

- Children: 0.25 g/kg every 4-6 hours given once or in divided doses
- Adults: 10-15 g in a glass of water

Mechanism of Action Promotes bowel evacuation by causing osmotic retention of fluid which distends the colon with increased peristaltic activity when taken orally; parenterally, decreases acetylcholine in motor nerve terminals and acts on myocardium by slowing rate of S-A node impulse formation and prolonging conduction time

Other Adverse Effects Hypotension and asystole may occur with rapid administration. Frequency not defined:

Serum magnesium levels >3 mg/dL:

- Central nervous system: Depressed CNS
- Gastrointestinal: Diarrhea
- Neuromuscular & skeletal: Blocked peripheral neuromuscular transmission leading to anticonvulsant effects

Serum magnesium levels >5 mg/dL:

- Cardiovascular: Flushing
- Central nervous system: Somnolence

Serum magnesium levels >12.5 mg/dL:

- Cardiovascular: Complete heart block, cardiac conduction affected
- Respiratory: Respiratory paralysis

(Continued)

Magnesium Sulfate *(Continued)*

Drug Interactions

Increased Effect: Nifedipine decreased BP and increased neuromuscular blockade.

Increased Toxicity: Aminoglycosides increased neuromuscular blockade; CNS depressants increased CNS depression; neuromuscular antagonists, betamethasone (pulmonary edema), ritodrine increased cardiotoxicity.

Drug Uptake

Onset of action: Oral: Cathartic: 1-2 hours; I.M.: 1 hour; I.V.: Immediate

Duration: I.M.: 3-4 hours; I.V.: 30 minutes

Pregnancy Risk Factor B

Generic Available Yes

Comments $MgSO_4$ 500 mg = magnesium 4.06 mEq = elemental magnesium 49.3 mg

Magonate® [OTC] *see* Magnesium Gluconate *on page 740*

Mag-Ox® 400 [OTC] *see* Magnesium Oxide *on page 742*

Mag-SR® *see* Magnesium Chloride *on page 739*

Malarone™ *see* Atovaquone and Proguanil *on page 129*

Mallamint® [OTC] *see* Calcium Carbonate *on page 201*

Mallazine® Eye Drops [OTC] *see* Tetrahydrozoline *on page 1150*

Mallisol® [OTC] *see* Povidone-Iodine *on page 982*

Malt Soup Extract (malt soop EKS trakt)

U.S. Brand Names Maltsupex® [OTC]

Pharmacologic Category Laxative

Use Short-term treatment of constipation

Local Anesthetic/Vasoconstrictor Precautions No information available to require special precautions

Effects on Dental Treatment No effects or complications reported

Dosage Oral:

Infants >1 month:

- Breast fed: 1-2 teaspoonfuls in 2-4 oz of water or fruit juice 1-2 times/day
- Bottle fed: ½ to 2 tablespoonfuls/day in formula for 3-4 days, then 1-2 teaspoonfuls/day

Children 2-11 years: 1-2 tablespoonfuls 1-2 times/day

Children ≥12 years and Adults:

- Liquid: 2 tablespoonfuls twice daily for 3-4 days, then 1-2 tablespoonfuls every evening
- Tablet: 4 tablets 4 times/day

Other Adverse Effects Frequency not defined: Gastrointestinal: Abdominal cramps, diarrhea, rectal obstruction

Generic Available No

Maltsupex® [OTC] *see* Malt Soup Extract *on page 744*

Mandol® *see* Cefamandole *on page 233*

Maolate® *see* Chlorphenesin *on page 268*

Mapap® [OTC] *see* Acetaminophen *on page 26*

Mapap® Children's [OTC] *see* Acetaminophen *on page 26*

Mapap® Extra Strength [OTC] *see* Acetaminophen *on page 26*

Mapap® Infants [OTC] *see* Acetaminophen *on page 26*

Maprotiline (ma PROE ti leen)

U.S. Brand Names Ludiomil®

Canadian Brand Names Ludiomil®; Novo-Maprotiline

Mexican Brand Names Ludiomil®

Pharmacologic Category Antidepressant, Tetracyclic

Synonyms Maprotiline Hydrochloride

Use Treatment of depression and anxiety associated with depression

Unlabeled/Investigational: Bulimia; duodenal ulcers; enuresis; urinary symptoms of multiple sclerosis; pain; panic attacks; tension headache; cocaine withdrawal

Local Anesthetic/Vasoconstrictor Precautions Use with caution; epinephrine, norepinephrine and levonordefrin have been shown to have an increased pressor response in combination with TCAs

Effects on Dental Treatment

>10%: Xerostomia

Long-term treatment with TCAs such as amoxapine increases the risk of caries by reducing salivation and salivary buffer capacity.

Dosage Oral:

Children 6-14 years: 10 mg/day, increase to a maximum daily dose of 75 mg

Adults: 75 mg/day to start, increase by 25 mg every 2 weeks up to 150-225 mg/day; given in 3 divided doses or in a single daily dose

Elderly: Initial: 25 mg at bedtime, increase by 25 mg every 3 days for inpatients and weekly for outpatients if tolerated; usual maintenance dose: 50-75 mg/day, higher doses may be necessary in nonresponders

Mechanism of Action Traditionally believed to increase the synaptic concentration of norepinephrine in the CNS by inhibition of their reuptake by the presynaptic neuronal membrane. However, additional receptor effects have been found including desensitization of adenyl cyclase, down regulation of beta-adrenergic receptors, and down regulation of serotonin receptors.

Other Adverse Effects

>10%:

Central nervous system: Drowsiness

Gastrointestinal: Xerostomia

1% to 10%:

Central nervous system: Insomnia, nervousness, anxiety, agitation, dizziness, fatigue, headache

Gastrointestinal: Constipation, nausea

Neuromuscular & skeletal: Tremor, weakness

Ocular: Blurred vision

Drug Interactions CYP1A2 and 2D6 enzyme substrate

Increased Effect/Toxicity: Maprotiline may increase the effects of amphetamines, anticholinergics, other CNS depressants (sedatives, hypnotics), carbamazepine, tolazamide, chlorpropamide, and warfarin. When used with MAO inhibitors, hyperpyrexia, hypertension, tachycardia, confusion, seizures, and **deaths have been reported** (serotonin syndrome). The SSRIs (to varying degrees), cimetidine, fenfluramine, indinavir, methylphenidate, ritonavir, quinidine, diltiazem, valproate, and verapamil inhibit the metabolism of cyclic antidepressants and clinical toxicity may result. Use of lithium with a cyclic antidepressant may increase the risk for neurotoxicity. Phenothiazines may increase concentration of some cyclic antidepressants and cyclic antidepressants may increase the concentration of phenothiazines. Pressor response to I.V. epinephrine, norepinephrine, and phenylephrine may be enhanced in patients receiving cyclic antidepressants (**Note:** Effect is unlikely with epinephrine or levonordefrin dosages typically administered as infiltration in combination with local anesthetics). Combined use of beta-agonists or drugs which prolong QT_c (including quinidine, procainamide, disopyramide, cisapride, sparfloxacin, gatifloxacin, moxifloxacin) with cyclic antidepressants may predispose patients to cardiac arrhythmias.

Decreased Effect: Carbamazepine, phenobarbital, and rifampin may increase the metabolism of maprotiline resulting in a decreased effect. Maprotiline inhibits the antihypertensive response to bethanidine, clonidine, debrisoquin, guanadrel, guanethidine, guanabenz, or guanfacine. Cholestyramine and colestipol may bind cyclic antidepressants and reduce their absorption.

Drug Uptake

Absorption: Slow

Half-life, elimination: 27-58 hours; Mean: 43 hours

Time to peak: ≤12 hours

Pregnancy Risk Factor B

Generic Available Yes

Selected Readings

Boakes AJ, Laurence DR, Teoh PC, et al, "Interactions Between Sympathomimetic Amines and Antidepressant Agents in Man," *Br Med J*, 1973, 1(849):311-5.

Jastak JT and Yagiela JA, "Vasoconstrictors and Local Anesthesia: A Review and Rationale for Use," *J Am Dent Assoc*, 1983, 107(4):623-30.

Mitchell JR, "Guanethidine and Related Agents. III Antagonism by Drugs Which Inhibit the Norepinephrine Pump in Man," *J Clin Invest*, 1970, 49(8):1596-604.

Rundegren J, van Dijken J, Mörnstad H, et al, "Oral Conditions in Patients Receiving Long-Term Treatment With Cyclic Antidepressant Drugs," *Swed Dent J*, 1985, 9(2):55-64.

Wynn RL, "New Antidepressant Medications," *Gen Dent*, 1997, 45(1):24-8.

Marax® *see* Theophylline, Ephedrine, and Hydroxyzine *on page 1155*

Marcaine® *see* Bupivacaine *on page 184*

Marcaine® Spinal *see* Bupivacaine *on page 184*

Marcaine® with Epinephrine *see* Bupivacaine and Epinephrine *on page 186*

Marcillin® *see* Ampicillin *on page 94*

Marezine® [OTC] *see* Cyclizine *on page 333*

Margesic® H *see* Hydrocodone and Acetaminophen *on page 598*

Marinol® *see* Dronabinol *on page 423*

Marplan® *see* Isocarboxazid *on page 657*

Masoprocol (ma SOE pro kole)

U.S. Brand Names Actinex®

Pharmacologic Category Topical Skin Product, Acne

Use Treatment of actinic keratosis

Local Anesthetic/Vasoconstrictor Precautions No information available to require special precautions

Effects on Dental Treatment No effects or complications reported

(Continued)

Masoprocol *(Continued)*

Dosage Adults: Topical: Wash and dry area; gently massage into affected area every morning and evening for 28 days

Mechanism of Action Antiproliferative activity against keratinocytes

Other Adverse Effects

>10%:

Dermatologic: Erythema, flaking, dryness, itching

Local: Burning

1% to 10%:

Dermatologic: Soreness, rash

Neuromuscular & skeletal: Paresthesia

Ocular: Eye irritation

Drug Uptake Absorption: Topical: <1% to 2%

Pregnancy Risk Factor B

Generic Available Yes

Massé® Breast Cream [OTC] *see* Glycerin, Lanolin, and Peanut Oil *on page 563*

Massengill® Medicated Douche w/Cepticin [OTC] *see* Povidone-Iodine *on page 982*

Matulane® *see* Procarbazine *on page 999*

Mavik® *see* Trandolapril *on page 1189*

Maxair™ *see* Pirbuterol *on page 965*

Maxair™ Autohaler™ *see* Pirbuterol *on page 965*

Maxalt® *see* Rizatriptan *on page 1063*

Maxalt-MLT™ *see* Rizatriptan *on page 1063*

Maxaquin® *see* Lomefloxacin *on page 723*

Maxidex® *see* Dexamethasone *on page 363*

Maxifed® *see* Guaifenesin and Pseudoephedrine *on page 570*

Maxifed® DM *see* Guaifenesin, Pseudoephedrine, and Dextromethorphan *on page 571*

Maxifed-G® *see* Guaifenesin and Pseudoephedrine *on page 570*

Maxiflor® *see* Diflorasone *on page 386*

Maximum Strength Nytol® [OTC] *see* DiphenhydrAMINE *on page 398*

Maxipime® *see* Cefepime *on page 236*

Maxitrol® *see* Neomycin, Polymyxin B, and Dexamethasone *on page 856*

Maxivate® *see* Betamethasone *on page 159*

Maxzide® *see* Hydrochlorothiazide and Triamterene *on page 597*

Maxzide®-25 *see* Hydrochlorothiazide and Triamterene *on page 597*

Mazanor® *see* Mazindol *on page 746*

Mazindol (MAY zin dole)

U.S. Brand Names Mazanor®; Sanorex®

Canadian Brand Names Mazanor®; Sanorex®

Mexican Brand Names Diestet®; Solucaps®

Pharmacologic Category Anorexiant

Use Short-term adjunct in exogenous obesity

Local Anesthetic/Vasoconstrictor Precautions No information available to require special precautions

Effects on Dental Treatment No effects or complications reported

Restrictions C-IV

Dosage Adults: Oral: Initial: 1 mg once daily and adjust to patient response; usual dose is 1 mg 3 times daily, 1 hour before meals, or 2 mg once daily, 1 hour before lunch; take with meals to avoid GI discomfort

Mechanism of Action An isoindole with pharmacologic activity similar to amphetamine; produces CNS stimulation in humans and animals and appears to work primarily in the limbic system

Other Adverse Effects Frequency not defined:

Cardiovascular: Palpitation, tachycardia, edema

Central nervous system: Insomnia, overstimulation, dizziness, dysphoria, drowsiness, depression, headache, restlessness

Dermatologic: Rash, clamminess

Endocrine & metabolic: Changes in libido

Gastrointestinal: Nausea, constipation, vomiting, xerostomia, unpleasant taste, diarrhea, abdominal cramps

Genitourinary: Dysuria, polyuria, impotence

Neuromuscular & skeletal: Tremor, weakness

Ocular: Blurred vision, corneal opacities

Miscellaneous: Diaphoresis (excessive)

Drug Interactions

Increased Effect/Toxicity: Mazindol enhances the pressor effect of exogenous catecholamines (norepinephrine) and potential BP increases in patients taking sympathomimetic medications.

Decreased Effect: Mazindol may decrease the hypotensive effect of guanethidine; monitor.

Pregnancy Risk Factor C

Generic Available No

3M™ Cavilon™ Skin Cleanser [OTC] *see* Benzalkonium Chloride *on page 151*

m-Cresyl Acetate (em-KREE sil AS e tate)

U.S. Brand Names Cresylate®

Pharmacologic Category Otic Agent, Anti-infective

Use Provides an acid medium; for external otitis infections caused by susceptible bacteria or fungus

Local Anesthetic/Vasoconstrictor Precautions No information available to require special precautions

Effects on Dental Treatment No effects or complications reported

Dosage Instill 2-4 drops as required

Generic Available No

MCT Oil® [OTC] *see* Medium Chain Triglycerides *on page 752*

ME-500® *see* Methionine *on page 783*

Measles and Rubella Vaccines, Combined

(MEE zels & roo BEL a vak SEENS, kom BINED)

U.S. Brand Names M-R-VAX® II

Canadian Brand Names MoRu-Viraten Berna™

Pharmacologic Category Vaccine, Live Virus

Synonyms Rubella and Measles Vaccines, Combined

Use Simultaneous immunization against measles and rubella

Note: Trivalent measles - mumps - rubella (MMR) vaccine is the preferred immunizing agent for most children and many adults. Adults born before 1957 are generally considered to be immune and need not be revaccinated.

Local Anesthetic/Vasoconstrictor Precautions No information available to require special precautions

Effects on Dental Treatment No effects or complications reported

Dosage Children at 15 months and Adults: S.C.: Inject 0.5 mL into outer aspect of upper arm; no routine booster for rubella

Mechanism of Action Promotes active immunity to measles and rubella by inducing specific antibodies including measles-specific IgG and IgM and rubella hemagglutination-inhibiting antibodies.

Other Adverse Effects All serious adverse reactions must be reported to the U.S. Department of Health and Human Services (DHHS) Vaccine Adverse Event Reporting System (VAERS) 1-800-822-7967.

>10%:

- Cardiovascular: Edema
- Central nervous system: Fever (<100°F)
- Local: Burning or stinging, induration

1% to 10%:

- Central nervous system: Fever between 100°F and 103°F usually between 5th and 12th days postvaccination
- Dermatologic: Rash (rarely generalized)

Warnings/Precautions Immunocompromised persons, history of anaphylactic reaction following receipt of neomycin

Drug Interactions Whole blood, interferon, immune globulin, radiation therapy, and immunosuppressive drugs (eg, corticosteroids) may result in insufficient response to immunization. DTP, OPV, MMR, Hib, and hepatitis B may be given concurrently; other virus vaccine administration should be separated by ≥1 month from measles.

Pregnancy Risk Factor C

Generic Available No

Comments Federal law requires that the date of administration, the vaccine manufacturer, lot number of vaccine, and the administering person's name, title and address be entered into the patient's permanent medical record

Measles, Mumps, and Rubella Vaccines, Combined

(MEE zels, mumpz & roo BEL a vak SEENS, kom BINED)

U.S. Brand Names M-M-R® II

Canadian Brand Names M-M-R® II; Priorix™

Pharmacologic Category Vaccine, Live Virus

Synonyms MMR; Mumps, Measles and Rubella Vaccines, Combined; Rubella, Measles and Mumps Vaccines, Combined

Use Measles, mumps, and rubella prophylaxis

Local Anesthetic/Vasoconstrictor Precautions No information available to require special precautions

Effects on Dental Treatment No effects or complications reported

(Continued)

Measles, Mumps, and Rubella Vaccines, Combined
(Continued)

Dosage S.C.:

Infants <12 months: If there is risk of exposure to measles, single-antigen measles vaccine should be administered at 6-11 months of age with a second dose (of MMR) at >12 months of age.

Children ≥12 months: 0.5 mL at 12 months and then repeated at 4-6 years of age. If the second dose was not received, the schedule should be completed by the 11- to 12-year old visit. Administer in outer aspect of the upper arm. Recommended age of primary immunization is 12-15 months; revaccination is recommended prior to elementary school.

Mechanism of Action As a live, attenuated vaccine, MMR vaccine offers active immunity to disease caused by the measles, mumps, and rubella viruses.

Other Adverse Effects All serious adverse reactions must be reported to the U.S. Department of Health and Human Services (DHHS) Vaccine Adverse Event Reporting System (VAERS) 1-800-822-7967.

Frequency not defined:

Cardiovascular: Syncope, vasculitis

Central nervous system: Ataxia, dizziness, febrile convulsions, fever, encephalitis, encephalopathy, Guillain-Barré syndrome, headache, irritability, malaise, measles inclusion body encephalitis, polyneuritis, polyneuropathy, seizures, subacute sclerosing panencephalitis

Dermatologic: Angioneurotic edema, erythema multiforme, purpura, rash, Stevens-Johnson syndrome, urticaria

Endocrine & metabolic: Diabetes mellitus

Gastrointestinal: Diarrhea, nausea, orchitis, pancreatitis, parotitis, sore throat, vomiting

Hematologic: Leukocytosis, thrombocytopenia

Local: Injection site reactions which include burning, induration, redness, stinging, swelling, tenderness, wheal and flare, vesiculation

Neuromuscular & skeletal: Arthralgia/arthritis (variable; highest rates in women, 12% to 26% versus children, up to 3%), myalgia, paresthesia

Ocular: Ocular palsies

Otic: Otitis media

Renal: Conjunctivitis, retinitis, optic neuritis, papillitis, retrobulbar neuritis

Respiratory: Bronchospasm, cough, pneumonitis, rhinitis

Miscellaneous: Anaphylactoid reactions, anaphylaxis, atypical measles, panniculitis, regional lymphadenopathy

Drug Interactions

Corticosteroids: In patients receiving high doses of systemic corticosteroids for ≥14 days, wait at least 1 month between discontinuing steroid therapy and administering immunization.

DTaP: Vaccines may be administered together (using separate sites and syringes).

Haemophilus b conjugate vaccine (PedvaxHIB®): Vaccines may be administered together (using separate sites and syringes).

Immune globulin, whole blood, plasma: Do not administer together; immune response may be compromised. Defer vaccine administration for ≥3 months.

Immunosuppressant medications: The effect of the vaccine may be decreased.

Live vaccines: Unless otherwise specified, MMR should be given 1 month before or 1 month after live viral vaccines.

Varicella: Vaccines may be administered together (using separate sites and syringes); if vaccines are not administered simultaneously, doses should be separated by at least 30 days.

Pregnancy Risk Factor C

Generic Available No

Comments Federal law requires that the date of administration, the vaccine manufacturer, lot number of vaccine, and the administering person's name, title and address be entered into the patient's permanent medical record

Measles Virus Vaccine, Live (MEE zels VYE rus vak SEEN, live)

U.S. Brand Names Attenuvax®

Pharmacologic Category Vaccine, Live Virus

Synonyms More Attenuated Enders Strain; Rubeola Vaccine

Use Adults born before 1957 are generally considered to be immune. All those born in or after 1957 without documentation of live vaccine on or after first birthday, physician-diagnosed measles, or laboratory evidence of immunity should be vaccinated, ideally with two doses of vaccine separated by no less than 1 month. For those previously vaccinated with one dose of measles vaccine, revaccination is recommended for students entering colleges and other institutions of higher education, for healthcare workers at the time of employment, and for international travelers who visit endemic areas.

MMR is the vaccine of choice if recipients are likely to be susceptible to rubella and/or mumps as well as to measles. Persons vaccinated between 1963 and 1967 with a killed measles vaccine, followed by live vaccine within 3 months, or with a vaccine of unknown type should be revaccinated with live measles virus vaccine.

Local Anesthetic/Vasoconstrictor Precautions No information available to require special precautions

Effects on Dental Treatment No effects or complications reported

Dosage Children >15 months and Adults: S.C.: 0.5 mL in outer aspect of the upper arm, no routine boosters

Mechanism of Action Promotes active immunity to measles virus by inducing specific measles IgG and IgM antibodies.

Other Adverse Effects All serious adverse reactions must be reported to the U.S. Department of Health and Human Services (DHHS) Vaccine Adverse Event Reporting System (VAERS) 1-800-822-7967.

>10%:

Cardiovascular: Edema

Central nervous system: Fever (<100°F)

Local: Burning or stinging, induration

1% to 10%:

Central nervous system: Fever between 100°F and 103°F usually between 5th and 12th days postvaccination

Dermatologic: Rash (rarely generalized)

Drug Interactions Whole blood, interferon immune globulin, radiation therapy, and immunosuppressive drugs (eg, corticosteroids) may result in insufficient response to immunization. DTP, OPV, MMR, Hib, and hepatitis B may be given concurrently; other virus vaccine administration should be separated by ≥1 month from measles.

Pregnancy Risk Factor X

Generic Available No

Comments Federal law requires that the date of administration, the vaccine manufacturer, lot number of vaccine, and the administering person's name, title and address be entered into the patient's permanent medical record

Mebaral® *see* Mephobarbital *on page 763*

Mebendazole (me BEN da zole)

U.S. Brand Names Vermox®

Canadian Brand Names Vermox®

Mexican Brand Names Helminzole; Mebensole; Revapol; Soltric; Vermicol; Vermidil®; Vermin®

Pharmacologic Category Anthelmintic

Use Treatment of pinworms, whipworms, roundworms, and hookworms

Local Anesthetic/Vasoconstrictor Precautions No information available to require special precautions

Effects on Dental Treatment No effects or complications reported

Dosage Children and Adults: Oral:

Pinworms: 100 mg as a single dose; may need to repeat after 2 weeks; treatment should include family members in close contact with patient

Whipworms, roundworms, hookworms: 1 tablet twice daily, morning and evening on 3 consecutive days; if patient is not cured within 3-4 weeks, a second course of treatment may be administered

Capillariasis: 200 mg twice daily for 20 days

Mechanism of Action Selectively and irreversibly blocks glucose uptake and other nutrients in susceptible adult intestine-dwelling helminths

Other Adverse Effects Frequency not defined:

Cardiovascular: Angioedema

Central nervous system: Fever, dizziness, headache, seizures

Dermatologic: Rash, itching, alopecia (with high doses)

Gastrointestinal: Abdominal pain, diarrhea, nausea, vomiting

Hematologic: Neutropenia (sore throat, unusual fatigue)

Neuromuscular & skeletal: Unusual weakness

Drug Interactions Anticonvulsants such as carbamazepine and phenytoin may increase metabolism of mebendazole

Drug Uptake

Absorption: 2% to 10%

Half-life, elimination: 1-11.5 hours

Time to peak: 2-4 hours

Pregnancy Risk Factor C

Generic Available No

Mecamylamine (mek a MIL a meen)

U.S. Brand Names Inversine®

Canadian Brand Names Inversine®

Pharmacologic Category Ganglionic Blocking Agent

Synonyms Mecamylamine Hydrochloride

Use Treatment of moderately severe to severe hypertension and in uncomplicated malignant hypertension

Unlabeled/Investigational: Tourette's syndrome

(Continued)

Mecamylamine *(Continued)*

Local Anesthetic/Vasoconstrictor Precautions No information available to require special precautions

Effects on Dental Treatment >10%: Xerostomia

Dosage Adults: Oral: 2.5 mg twice daily after meals for 2 days; increased by increments of 2.5 mg at intervals ≥2 days until desired BP response is achieved; average daily dose: 25 mg

Mechanism of Action Mecamylamine is a ganglionic blocker. This agent inhibits acetylcholine at the autonomic ganglia, causing a decrease in BP. Mecamylamine also blocks central nicotinic cholinergic receptors, which inhibits the effects of nicotine and may suppress the desire to smoke.

Other Adverse Effects Frequency not defined:

Cardiovascular: Postural hypotension
Central nervous system: Drowsiness, convulsions, confusion, mental depression
Endocrine & metabolic: Sexual ability decreased
Gastrointestinal: Xerostomia, loss of appetite, nausea, vomiting, bloating; frequent stools followed by severe constipation
Genitourinary: Dysuria
Neuromuscular & skeletal: Uncontrolled movements of hands, arms, legs, or face; trembling
Ocular: Blurred vision; enlarged pupils
Respiratory: Dyspnea

Drug Interactions Increased Effect/Toxicity: Sulfonamides and antibiotics that cause neuromuscular blockade may increase effect of mecamylamine. The action of mecamylamine may be increased by anesthesia, other antihypertensives, and alcohol.

Pregnancy Risk Factor C

Generic Available No

Meclizine (MEK li zeen)

U.S. Brand Names Antivert®; Antrizine®; Bonine® [OTC]; Dizmiss® [OTC]; Dramamine® II [OTC]; Meni-D®; Vergon® [OTC]

Canadian Brand Names Antivert®; Bonamine™; Bonine®

Pharmacologic Category Antiemetic; Antihistamine

Synonyms Meclizine Hydrochloride; Meclozine Hydrochloride

Use Prevention and treatment of symptoms of motion sickness; management of vertigo with diseases affecting the vestibular system

Local Anesthetic/Vasoconstrictor Precautions No information available to require special precautions

Effects on Dental Treatment ≤10%: Significant xerostomia; disappears with discontinuation

Dosage Children >12 years and Adults: Oral:

Motion sickness: 12.5-25 mg 1 hour before travel, repeat dose every 12-24 hours if needed; doses up to 50 mg may be needed
Vertigo: 25-100 mg/day in divided doses

Mechanism of Action Has central anticholinergic action by blocking chemoreceptor trigger zone; decreases excitability of the middle ear labyrinth and blocks conduction in the middle ear vestibular-cerebellar pathways

Other Adverse Effects

>10%:
- Central nervous system: Slight to moderate drowsiness
- Respiratory: Thickening of bronchial secretions

1% to 10%:
- Central nervous system: Headache, fatigue, nervousness, dizziness
- Gastrointestinal: Appetite increase, weight gain, nausea, diarrhea, abdominal pain, xerostomia
- Neuromuscular & skeletal: Arthralgia
- Respiratory: Pharyngitis

Drug Interactions Increased toxicity with CNS depressants, neuroleptics, and anticholinergics.

Drug Uptake

Onset of action: Oral: ≤1 hour
Duration: 8-24 hours
Half-life, elimination: 6 hours

Pregnancy Risk Factor B

Generic Available Yes

Meclocycline (me kloe SYE kleen)

Pharmacologic Category Antibiotic, Topical; Topical Skin Product, Acne

Synonyms Meclocycline Sulfosalicylate

Use Topical treatment of inflammatory acne vulgaris

Local Anesthetic/Vasoconstrictor Precautions No information available to require special precautions

Effects on Dental Treatment No effects or complications reported

Dosage Children >11 years and Adults: Topical: Apply generously to affected areas twice daily

Mechanism of Action Inhibits bacterial protein synthesis by binding with the 30S and possibly the 50S ribosomal subunit(s) of susceptible bacteria; may also cause alterations in the cytoplasmic membrane

Other Adverse Effects

>10%: Topical: Follicular staining, yellowing of the skin, burning/stinging feeling

1% to 10%: Topical: Pain, redness, skin irritation, dermatitis

Drug Uptake Absorption: Topical: Very little

Pregnancy Risk Factor B

Generic Available No

Meclofenamate (me kloe fen AM ate)

Related Information

Rheumatoid Arthritis and Osteoarthritis *on page 1340*

Temporomandibular Dysfunction (TMD) *on page 1397*

Canadian Brand Names Meclomen®

Pharmacologic Category Nonsteroidal Anti-inflammatory Drug (NSAID)

Synonyms Meclofenamate Sodium

Use Treatment of inflammatory disorders, arthritis, mild to moderate pain, dysmenorrhea

Local Anesthetic/Vasoconstrictor Precautions No information available to require special precautions

Effects on Dental Treatment NSAID formulations are known to reversibly decrease platelet aggregation via mechanisms different than observed with aspirin. The dentist should be aware of the potential of abnormal coagulation. Caution should also be exercised in the use of NSAIDs in patients already on anticoagulant therapy with drugs such as warfarin (Coumadin®). Recovery of platelet function usually occurs 1-2 days after discontinuation of NSAIDs.

Dosage Children >14 years and Adults: Oral:

Mild to moderate pain: 50 mg every 4-6 hours, not to exceed 400 mg/day

Rheumatoid arthritis/osteoarthritis: 200-400 mg/day in 3-4 equal doses

Mechanism of Action Inhibits prostaglandin synthesis by decreasing the activity of the enzyme, cyclo-oxygenase, which results in decreased formation of prostaglandin precursors

Other Adverse Effects

>10%:

- Central nervous system: Dizziness
- Dermatologic: Rash
- Gastrointestinal: Abdominal cramps, heartburn, indigestion, nausea

1% to 10%:

- Central nervous system: Headache, nervousness
- Dermatologic: Itching
- Endocrine & metabolic: Fluid retention
- Gastrointestinal: Vomiting
- Otic: Tinnitus

Warnings/Precautions Use with caution in patients with CHF, hypertension, decreased renal or hepatic function, history of GI disease (bleeding or ulcers), or those receiving anticoagulants. Elderly are at a high risk for adverse effects from nonsteroidal anti-inflammatory agents. As much as 60% of elderly can develop peptic ulceration and/or hemorrhage asymptomatically.

Use lowest effective dose for shortest period possible. Use of NSAIDs can compromise existing renal function especially when Cl_{cr} is <30 mL/minute. CNS adverse effects such as confusion, agitation, and hallucination are generally seen in overdose or high-dose situations; however, elderly may demonstrate these adverse effects at lower doses than younger adults. Withhold for at least 4-6 half-lives prior to surgical or dental procedures. May have adverse effects on fetus. Use with caution with dehydration. Use in children is not recommended.

Drug Interactions

ACE inhibitors: Antihypertensive effects may be decreased by concurrent therapy with NSAIDs; monitor BP.

Angiotensin II antagonists: Antihypertensive effects may be decreased by concurrent therapy with NSAIDs; monitor BP.

Anticoagulants (warfarin, heparin, LMWHs) in combination with NSAIDs can cause increased risk of bleeding.

Other antiplatelet drugs (ticlopidine, clopidogrel, aspirin, abciximab, dipyridamole, eptifibatide, tirofiban) can cause an increased risk of bleeding.

Corticosteroids may increase the risk of GI ulceration; avoid concurrent use.

Cyclosporine: NSAIDs may increase serum creatinine, potassium, BP, and cyclosporine levels; monitor cyclosporine levels and renal function carefully.

Gentamicin and amikacin serum concentrations are increased by indomethacin in premature infants. Results may apply to other aminoglycosides and NSAIDs.

Hydralazine's antihypertensive effect is decreased; avoid concurrent use.

(Continued)

Meclofenamate *(Continued)*

Lithium levels can be increased; avoid concurrent use if possible or monitor lithium levels and adjust dose. Sulindac may have the least effect. When NSAID is stopped, lithium will need adjustment again.

Loop diuretics efficacy (diuretic and antihypertensive effect) is reduced. Indomethacin reduces this efficacy, however, it may be anticipated with any NSAID.

Methotrexate: Severe bone marrow suppression, aplastic anemia, and GI toxicity have been reported with concomitant NSAID therapy. Avoid use during moderate or high-dose methotrexate (increased and prolonged methotrexate levels). NSAID use during low-dose treatment of rheumatoid arthritis has not been fully evaluated; extreme caution is warranted.

Thiazides antihypertensive effects are decreased; avoid concurrent use.

Verapamil plasma concentration is decreased by diclofenac; avoid concurrent use.

Warfarin's INRs may be increased by piroxicam. Other NSAIDs may have the same effect depending on dose and duration. Monitor INR closely. Use the lowest dose of NSAIDs possible and for the briefest duration.

Drug Uptake

Duration: 2-4 hours

Half-life, elimination: 2-3.3 hours

Time to peak: 0.5-1.5 hours

Pregnancy Risk Factor B/D (3rd trimester)

Generic Available Yes

Medi-Lice® [OTC] *see* Permethrin *on page 940*

Medipain 5® *see* Hydrocodone and Acetaminophen *on page 598*

Mediplast® Plaster [OTC] *see* Salicylic Acid *on page 1072*

Medi-Synal [OTC] *see* Acetaminophen and Pseudoephedrine *on page 30*

Medium Chain Triglycerides (mee DEE um chane trye GLIS er ides)

U.S. Brand Names MCT Oil® [OTC]

Canadian Brand Names MCT Oil®

Pharmacologic Category Dietary Supplement

Synonyms Triglycerides, Medium Chain

Use Dietary supplement for those who cannot digest long chain fats; malabsorption associated with disorders such as pancreatic insufficiency, bile salt deficiency, and bacterial overgrowth of the small bowel; induce ketosis as a prevention for seizures (akinetic, clonic, and petit mal)

Local Anesthetic/Vasoconstrictor Precautions No information available to require special precautions

Effects on Dental Treatment No effects or complications reported

Dosage Oral:

Infants: Initial: 0.5 mL every other feeding, then advance to every feeding, then increase in increments of 0.25-0.5 mL/feeding at intervals of 2-3 days as tolerated

Seizures: About 39 mL with each meal or 50% to 70% (800-1120 kcal) of total calories (1600 kcal) as the oil will induce ketosis necessary for seizure control

Cystic fibrosis: 3 tablespoons/day is tolerated without adverse symptoms by most children

Adults: 15 mL 3-4 times/day

Other Adverse Effects Frequency not defined:

Central nervous system: May result in **narcosis** and **coma** in cirrhotic patients due to high levels of medium chain fatty acids in the serum which then enter the cerebral spinal fluid; electroencephalogram effects include slowing of the alpha wave (can occur during infusion of fatty acids of 2-6 carbon lengths)

Endocrine & metabolic:

MCT therapy does not produce recognized metabolic side effects of any clinical importance, nor do they interfere with the metabolism of other food stuffs or with the absorption of drugs; when administered in the form of a mixed diet with carbohydrates and protein, there is no clinical evidence of **hyperketonemia**; hyperketonemia may occur in normal or diabetic subjects in the absence of carbohydrates; has been reported that MCT may increase hepatic free fatty acid synthesis and reduce ketone clearance

Fecal water, sodium and potassium excretion are decreased in patients with steatorrhea who are treated with MCT; enhanced calcium absorption has been demonstrated in patients with steatorrhea who are given MCT

Gastrointestinal: Nausea, occasional vomiting, gastritis and distention, diarrhea, and borborygmi are common adverse reactions occurring in about 10% of the patients receiving supplements or diets containing MCT; these symptoms may be related to rapid hydrolysis of MCT, high concentrations of free fatty acids in the stomach and small intestine, hyperosmolarity causing influx of large amounts of fluid, and lactose intolerance; abdominal cramps, nausea and vomiting occurred despite cautionary administration of MCT in small sips throughout meals, but subsided with continued administration

Pregnancy Risk Factor C

Generic Available No

Comments Does not provide any essential fatty acids; only saturated fats are contained; supplementation with safflower, corn oil, or other polyunsaturated vegetable oil must be given to provide the patient with the essential fatty acids. The minimum daily requirement has not been established for oral intake, but 10-15 mL of safflower oil (60% to 70% linoleic acid) appears to be satisfactory.

Contains 7.7 kcal/mL

Medralone® *see* MethylPREDNISolone *on page 797*

Medrol® *see* MethylPREDNISolone *on page 797*

MedroxyPROGESTERone Acetate

(me DROKS ee proe JES te rone)

Related Information

Endocrine Disorders and Pregnancy *on page 1331*

U.S. Brand Names Depo-Provera®; Provera®

Canadian Brand Names Alti-MPA; Depo-Provera®; Gen-Medroxy; Novo-Medrone; Provera®

Mexican Brand Names Cycrin®; Depo-Provera®; Provera®

Pharmacologic Category Contraceptive; Progestin

Synonyms Acetoxymethylprogesterone; Medroxyprogesterone; Methylacetoxyprogesterone

Use Endometrial carcinoma or renal carcinoma as well as secondary amenorrhea or abnormal uterine bleeding due to hormonal imbalance; reduction of endometrial hyperplasia in postmenopausal women receiving 0.625 mg conjugated estrogens for 12-14 consecutive days per month; Depo-Provera® injection is used for the prevention of pregnancy

Local Anesthetic/Vasoconstrictor Precautions No information available to require special precautions

Effects on Dental Treatment Progestins may predispose the patient to gingival bleeding.

Dosage

Adolescents and Adults: Oral:

- Amenorrhea: 5-10 mg/day for 5-10 days or 2.5 mg/day
- Abnormal uterine bleeding: 5-10 mg for 5-10 days starting on day 16 or 21 of cycle
- Accompanying cyclic estrogen therapy, postmenopausal: 2.5-10 mg the last 10-13 days of estrogen dosing each month

Adults: I.M.:

- Endometrial or renal carcinoma: 400-1000 mg/week
- Contraception: 150 mg every 3 months or 450 mg every 6 months

Mechanism of Action Inhibits secretion of pituitary gonadotropins, which prevents follicular maturation and ovulation, stimulates growth of mammary tissue

Other Adverse Effects Frequency not defined:

Cardiovascular: Edema, embolism, central thrombosis

Central nervous system: Mental depression, fever, insomnia, somnolence, headache (rare), dizziness

Dermatologic: Melasma or chloasma, allergic rash with or without pruritus, acne, hirsutism, angioneurotic edema

Endocrine & metabolic: Breakthrough bleeding, spotting, changes in menstrual flow, amenorrhea, increased breast tenderness, changes in cervical erosion and secretions

Gastrointestinal: Weight gain/loss, anorexia, nausea

Hepatic: Cholestatic jaundice

Local: Pain at injection site, sterile abscess, thrombophlebitis

Neuromuscular & skeletal: Weakness

Respiratory: Pulmonary embolism

Miscellaneous: Anaphylaxis

Drug Interactions Aminoglutethimide may decrease effects by increasing hepatic metabolism.

Drug Uptake

Absorption: Oral: Well absorbed; I.M.: Slow

Time to peak: Oral: 2-4 hours

Half-life, elimination: Oral: 38-46 hours; I.M.: Acetate: 50 days

Pregnancy Risk Factor X

Generic Available Yes

Medrysone (ME dri sone)

U.S. Brand Names HMS Liquifilm®

Pharmacologic Category Corticosteroid, Ophthalmic

Use Treatment of allergic conjunctivitis, vernal conjunctivitis, episcleritis, ophthalmic epinephrine sensitivity reaction

Local Anesthetic/Vasoconstrictor Precautions No information available to require special precautions

Effects on Dental Treatment No effects or complications reported

(Continued)

Medrysone *(Continued)*

Dosage Children and Adults: Ophthalmic: Instill 1 drop in conjunctival sac 2-4 times/day up to every 4 hours; may use every 1-2 hours during first 1-2 days

Mechanism of Action Decreases inflammation by suppression of migration of polymorphonuclear leukocytes and reversal of increased capillary permeability

Other Adverse Effects 1% to 10%: Ocular: Temporary mild blurred vision

Drug Uptake Absorption: Through aqueous humor

Pregnancy Risk Factor C

Generic Available No

Comments Medrysone is a synthetic corticosteroid; structurally related to progesterone; if no improvement after several days of treatment, discontinue medrysone and institute other therapy; duration of therapy: 3-4 days to several weeks dependent on type and severity of disease; taper dose to avoid disease exacerbation

Mefenamic Acid (me fe NAM ik AS id)

Related Information

Rheumatoid Arthritis and Osteoarthritis *on page 1340*
Temporomandibular Dysfunction (TMD) *on page 1397*

U.S. Brand Names Ponstel®

Canadian Brand Names Apo®-Mefenamic; Nu-Mefenamic; PMS-Mefenamic Acid; Ponstan®; Ponstel®

Mexican Brand Names Ponstan®

Pharmacologic Category Nonsteroidal Anti-inflammatory Drug (NSAID)

Use Short-term relief of mild to moderate pain including primary dysmenorrhea

Local Anesthetic/Vasoconstrictor Precautions No information available to require special precautions

Effects on Dental Treatment NSAID formulations are known to reversibly decrease platelet aggregation via mechanisms different than observed with aspirin. The dentist should be aware of the potential of abnormal coagulation. Caution should also be exercised in the use of NSAIDs in patients already on anticoagulant therapy with drugs such as warfarin (Coumadin®). Recovery of platelet function usually occurs 1-2 days after discontinuation of NSAIDs.

Dosage Children >14 years and Adults: Oral: 500 mg to start then 250 mg every 4 hours as needed; maximum therapy: 1 week

Mechanism of Action Inhibits prostaglandin synthesis by decreasing the activity of the enzyme, cyclo-oxygenase, which results in decreased formation of prostaglandin precursors

Other Adverse Effects 1% to 10%:

Central nervous system: Headache, nervousness, dizziness (3% to 9%)
Dermatologic: Itching, rash
Endocrine & metabolic: Fluid retention
Gastrointestinal: Abdominal cramps, heartburn, indigestion, nausea (1% to 10%), vomiting (1% to 10%), diarrhea (1% to 10%), constipation (1% to 10%), abdominal distress/cramping/pain (1% to 10%), dyspepsia (1% to 10%), flatulence (1% to 10%), gastric or duodenal ulcer with bleeding or perforation (1% to 10%), gastritis (1% to 10%)
Hematologic: Bleeding (1% to 10%)
Hepatic: Elevated LFTs (1% to 10%)
Otic: Tinnitus (1% to 10%)

Warnings/Precautions Use with caution in patients with CHF, hypertension, decreased renal or hepatic function, history of GI disease (bleeding or ulcers), or those receiving anticoagulants. Elderly are at a high risk for adverse effects from nonsteroidal anti-inflammatory agents. As much as 60% of elderly can develop peptic ulceration and/or hemorrhage asymptomatically.

Use lowest effective dose for shortest period possible. Use of NSAIDs can compromise existing renal function especially when Cl_{cr} is <30 mL/minute. CNS adverse effects such as confusion, agitation, and hallucination are generally seen in overdose or high-dose situations; however, elderly may demonstrate these adverse effects at lower doses than younger adults. Withhold for at least 4-6 half-lives prior to surgical or dental procedures. May have adverse effects on fetus. Use with caution with dehydration. Use in children is not recommended.

Drug Interactions

ACE inhibitors: Antihypertensive effects may be decreased by concurrent therapy with NSAIDs; monitor BP.
Angiotensin II antagonists: Antihypertensive effects may be decreased by concurrent therapy with NSAIDs; monitor BP.
Anticoagulants (warfarin, heparin, LMWHs) in combination with NSAIDs can cause increased risk of bleeding.
Other antiplatelet drugs (ticlopidine, clopidogrel, aspirin, abciximab, dipyridamole, eptifibatide, tirofiban) can cause an increased risk of bleeding.
Corticosteroids may increase the risk of GI ulceration; avoid concurrent use.

Cyclosporine: NSAIDs may increase serum creatinine, potassium, BP, and cyclosporine levels; monitor cyclosporine levels and renal function carefully.

Gentamicin and amikacin serum concentrations are increased by indomethacin in premature infants. Results may apply to other aminoglycosides and NSAIDs.

Hydralazine's antihypertensive effect is decreased; avoid concurrent use.

Lithium levels can be increased; avoid concurrent use if possible or monitor lithium levels and adjust dose. Sulindac may have the least effect. When NSAID is stopped, lithium will need adjustment again.

Loop diuretics efficacy (diuretic and antihypertensive effect) is reduced. Indomethacin reduces this efficacy, however, it may be anticipated with any NSAID.

Methotrexate: Severe bone marrow suppression, aplastic anemia, and GI toxicity have been reported with concomitant NSAID therapy. Avoid use during moderate or high-dose methotrexate (increased and prolonged methotrexate levels). NSAID use during low-dose treatment of rheumatoid arthritis has not been fully evaluated; extreme caution is warranted.

Thiazides antihypertensive effects are decreased; avoid concurrent use.

Verapamil plasma concentration is decreased by diclofenac; avoid concurrent use.

Warfarin's INRs may be increased by piroxicam. Other NSAIDs may have the same effect depending on dose and duration. Monitor INR closely. Use the lowest dose of NSAIDs possible and for the briefest duration.

Drug Uptake

Onset of action: Peak effect: 2-4 hours

Duration: ≤6 hours

Half-life, elimination: 3.5 hours

Pregnancy Risk Factor C/D (3rd trimester)

Generic Available No

Mefloquine (ME floe kwin)

U.S. Brand Names Lariam®

Canadian Brand Names Lariam®

Pharmacologic Category Antimalarial Agent

Synonyms Mefloquine Hydrochloride

Use Treatment of acute malarial infections and prevention of malaria

Local Anesthetic/Vasoconstrictor Precautions No information available to require special precautions

Effects on Dental Treatment No effects or complications reported

Dosage Oral:

Children: Malaria prophylaxis:

15-19 kg: 1/4 tablet

20-30 kg: 1/2 tablet

31-45 kg: 3/4 tablet

>45 kg: 1 tablet

Administer weekly starting 1 week before travel, continuing weekly during travel and for 4 weeks after leaving endemic area

Adults:

Treatment of mild to moderate malaria infection: 5 tablets (1250 mg) as a single dose with at least 8 oz of water

Malaria prophylaxis: 1 tablet (250 mg) weekly starting 1 week before travel, continuing weekly during travel and for 4 weeks after leaving endemic area

Mechanism of Action Mefloquine is a quinoline-methanol compound structurally similar to quinine; mefloquine's effectiveness in the treatment and prophylaxis of malaria is due to the destruction of the asexual blood forms of the malarial pathogens that affect humans, *Plasmodium falciparum*, *P. vivax*, *P. malariae*, *P. ovale*

Other Adverse Effects 1% to 10%:

Central nervous system: Difficulty concentrating, headache, insomnia, lightheadedness, vertigo

Gastrointestinal: Vomiting (3%), diarrhea, stomach pain, nausea

Ocular: Visual disturbances

Otic: Tinnitus

Drug Interactions Potentially similar to quinidine

Increased Effect/Toxicity: Increased bradycardia possible with beta-blockers; use caution with other drugs that alter cardiac conduction. Increased toxicity/levels of chloroquine, quinine, and quinidine (hold treatment until at least 12 hours after these drugs).

Decreased Effect: Mefloquine may decrease the effect of valproic acid.

Drug Uptake

Absorption: Oral: Well absorbed

Half-life, elimination: 21-22 days

Pregnancy Risk Factor C

Generic Available No

Comments To avoid relapse after initial treatment with mefloquine, patients should subsequently be treated with an 8-aminoquinolone (eg, primaquine)

Mefoxin® *see* Cefoxitin *on page 241*

Mega B® [OTC] *see* Vitamin B Complex *on page 1244*

Megace® *see* Megestrol Acetate *on page 756*

Megaton™ [OTC] *see* Vitamin B Complex *on page 1244*

Megestrol Acetate (me JES trole)

U.S. Brand Names Megace®

Canadian Brand Names Apo®-Megestrol; Lin-Megestrol; Megace®; Megace® OS; Nu-Megestrol

Pharmacologic Category Antineoplastic Agent, Miscellaneous; Progestin

Synonyms Megestrol

Use Palliative treatment of breast and endometrial carcinoma

Orphan drug: Treatment of anorexia, cachexia, or significant weight loss (≥10% baseline body weight); treatment of AIDS

Local Anesthetic/Vasoconstrictor Precautions No information available to require special precautions

Effects on Dental Treatment No effects or complications reported

Dosage Adults: Oral **(refer to individual protocols)**:

Female: Uterine bleeding: 40 mg 2-4 times/day

Male and Female: HIV-related cachexia: Initial dose: 800 mg/day; daily doses of 400 and 800 mg/day were found to be clinically effective

Mechanism of Action A synthetic progestin with antiestrogenic properties which disrupt the estrogen receptor cycle. Megace® interferes with the normal estrogen cycle and results in a lower LH titer. May also have a direct effect on the endometrium. Megestrol is an antineoplastic progestin thought to act through an antileutenizing effect mediated via the pituitary.

Other Adverse Effects Frequency not defined:

Cardiovascular: Edema, hypertension (≤8%), cardiomyopathy, palpitations

Central nervous system: Insomnia, depression (≤6%), fever (2% to 6%), headache (≤10%), pain (≤6%, similar to placebo), confusion (1% to 3%), convulsions (1% to 3%), depression (1% to 3%)

Dermatologic: Allergic rash (2% to 12%) with or without pruritus, alopecia

Endocrine & metabolic: Breakthrough bleeding and amenorrhea, spotting, changes in menstrual flow, changes in cervical erosion and secretions, increased breast tenderness, changes in vaginal bleeding pattern, edema, fluid retention, hyperglycemia (≤6%), diabetes, HPA-axis suppression, adrenal insufficiency, Cushing's syndrome

Gastrointestinal: Weight gain (not attributed to edema or fluid retention), nausea (≤5%, less than placebo), vomiting, diarrhea (8% to 15%, similar to placebo), flatulence (≤10%), constipation (1% to 3%)

Genitourinary: Impotence (4% to 14%), decreased libido (≤5%)

Hepatic: Cholestatic jaundice, hepatotoxicity, hepatomegaly (1% to 3%)

Local: Thrombophlebitis

Neuromuscular & skeletal: Carpal tunnel syndrome, weakness, paresthesia (1% to 3%)

Respiratory: Hyperpnea, dyspnea (1% to 3%), cough (1% to 3%)

Miscellaneous: Diaphoresis

Warnings/Precautions May suppress hypothalamic-pituitary-adrenal (HPA) axis during chronic administration. Consider the possibility of adrenal suppression in any patient receiving or being withdrawn from chronic therapy when signs/symptoms suggestive of hypoadrenalism are noted (during stress or in unstressed state). Laboratory evaluation and replacement/stress doses of rapid-acting glucocorticoid should be considered.

Drug Uptake

Onset of action: ≥2 months of continuous therapy

Absorption: Oral: Well absorbed

Half-life, elimination: 15-20 hours

Time to peak: Oral: 1-3 hours

Pregnancy Risk Factor X

Generic Available Yes

Melanex® *see* Hydroquinone *on page 611*

Melfiat®; Obezine® *see* Phendimetrazine *on page 943*

Mellaril® *see* Thioridazine *on page 1159*

Meloxicam (mel OX ee cam)

U.S. Brand Names MOBIC®

Canadian Brand Names MOBIC®; Mobicox®

Mexican Brand Names Masflex®; Mobicox®

Pharmacologic Category Nonsteroidal Anti-inflammatory Drug (NSAID)

Use Treatment of osteoarthritis

Local Anesthetic/Vasoconstrictor Precautions No information available to require special precautions

Effects on Dental Treatment <2%: Taste perversion, ulcerative stomatitis, xerostomia

Dosage Adult: Oral:

Initial: 7.5 mg once daily; some patients may receive additional benefit from an increased dose of 15 mg once daily; maximum dose: 15 mg/day

Dosage adjustment in renal impairment: Avoid use in significant renal impairment

Dosage adjustment in hepatic impairment: Aatients with severe hepatic impairment have not been adequately studied

Mechanism of Action Inhibits prostaglandin synthesis by decreasing the activity of the enzyme, cyclo-oxygenase, which results in decreased formation of prostaglandin precursors

Other Adverse Effects

1% to 10%:

Cardiovascular: Edema (2% to 5%)

Central nervous system: Headache and dizziness occurred in 2% to 8% of patients, but occurred less frequently than placebo in controlled trials

Dermatologic: Rash (1% to 3%)

Gastrointestinal: Diarrhea (3% to 8%), dyspepsia (5%), nausea (4%), flatulence (3%), abdominal pain (2% to 3%)

Respiratory: Upper respiratory infection (2% to 3%), pharyngitis (1% to 3%)

Miscellaneous: Flu-like symptoms (4% to 5%), falls (3%)

<2%: Allergic reaction, anaphylactic reaction, shock, fatigue, hot flashes, malaise, syncope, weight changes, angina, cardiac failure, hypertension, hypotension, myocardial infarction, vasculitis, seizures, paresthesia, tremor, vertigo, colitis, xerostomia, duodenal ulcer, gastric ulcer, gastritis, gastroesophageal reflux, gastrointestinal hemorrhage, hematemesis, intestinal perforation, melena, pancreatitis, duodenal perforation, gastric perforation, ulcerative stomatitis, arrhythmia, palpitations, tachycardia, agranulocytosis, leukopenia, purpura, thrombocytopenia, increased ALT, increased AST, hyperbilirubinemia, increased GGT, hepatitis, jaundice, hepatic failure, dehydration, abnormal dreams, anxiety, confusion, depression, nervousness, somnolence, asthma, bronchospasm, dyspnea, alopecia, angioedema, bullous eruption, erythema multiforme, photosensitivity reaction, pruritus, Stevens-Johnson syndrome, toxic epidermal necrolysis, urticaria, abnormal vision, conjunctivitis, taste perversion, tinnitus, albuminuria, increased BUN, increased creatinine, hematuria, interstitial nephritis, renal failure

Contraindications Hypersensitivity to meloxicam, aspirin, NSAIDs, or any component of their formulation

Warnings/Precautions Gastrointestinal irritation, ulceration, bleeding, and perforation may occur with NSAIDs. Serious complications may occur without prior symptoms of GI distress. Use with caution in patients with a history of GI disease (bleeding or ulcers), decreased renal function, hepatic disease, CHF, dehydration, hypertension, or asthma. Use with caution in elderly patients. Anaphylactoid reactions may occur, even with no prior exposure to meloxicam. Use in advanced renal disease is not recommended. May alter platelet function; use with caution in patients receiving anticoagulants or with hemostatic disorders. Safety and efficacy in pediatric patients have not been established. Withhold for at least 4-6 half-lives prior to surgical or dental procedures.

Drug Interactions

ACE inhibitors: Antihypertensive effects may be decreased by concurrent therapy with NSAIDs; monitor BP

Angiotensin II antagonists: Antihypertensive effects may be decreased by concurrent therapy with NSAIDs; monitor BP

Anticoagulants (warfarin, heparin, LMWHs) in combination with NSAIDs can cause increased risk of bleeding.

Antiplatelet drugs (ticlopidine, clopidogrel, aspirin, abciximab, dipyridamole, eptifibatide, tirofiban) can cause an increased risk of bleeding.

Aspirin increases serum concentrations (AUC) of meloxicam (in addition to potential for additive adverse effects); concurrent use is not recommended.

Cholestyramine (and possibly colestipol) increases the clearance of meloxicam.

Corticosteroids may increase the risk of GI ulceration; avoid concurrent use.

Cyclosporine: NSAIDs may increase serum creatinine, potassium, BP, and cyclosporine levels; monitor cyclosporine levels and renal function carefully.

Hydralazine's antihypertensive effect is decreased; avoid concurrent use.

Lithium levels can be increased; avoid concurrent use if possible or monitor lithium levels and adjust dose. When NSAID is stopped, lithium will need adjustment again.

Loop diuretic's efficacy (diuretic and antihypertensive effect) may be reduced by NSAIDs.

Methotrexate: Severe bone marrow suppression, aplastic anemia, and GI toxicity have been reported with concomitant NSAID therapy. Avoid use during moderate or high-dose methotrexate (increased and prolonged methotrexate levels). NSAID use during low-dose treatment of rheumatoid arthritis has not been fully evaluated; extreme caution is warranted.

Thiazide diuretics: Antihypertensive effects of thiazide diuretics are decreased; avoid concurrent use.

(Continued)

Meloxicam *(Continued)*

Warfarin INRs may be increased by meloxicam. Monitor INR closely, particularly during initiation or change in dose. May increase risk of bleeding. Use lowest possible dose for shortest duration possible.

Drug Uptake

Half-life, elimination: 15-20 hours

Time to peak: 5-10 hours

Pregnancy Risk Factor C/D (3rd trimester)

Generic Available No

Melpaque HP® *see* Hydroquinone *on page 611*

Melphalan (MEL fa lan)

U.S. Brand Names Alkeran®

Canadian Brand Names Alkeran®

Mexican Brand Names Alkeran®

Pharmacologic Category Antineoplastic Agent, Alkylating Agent

Synonyms L-PAM; L-Sarcolysin; Phenylalanine Mustard

Use Palliative treatment of multiple myeloma and nonresectable epithelial ovarian carcinoma; neuroblastoma, rhabdomyosarcoma, breast cancer, sarcoma; I.V. formulation: Use in patients in whom oral therapy is not appropriate

Local Anesthetic/Vasoconstrictor Precautions No information available to require special precautions

Effects on Dental Treatment No effects or complications reported

Mechanism of Action Alkylating agent which is a derivative of mechlorethamine that inhibits DNA and RNA synthesis via formation of carbonium ions; cross-links strands of DNA

Other Adverse Effects

>10%: Hematologic: Myelosuppressive: Leukopenia and thrombocytopenia are the most common effects of melphalan; irreversible bone marrow failure has been reported

WBC: Moderate

Platelets: Moderate

Onset: 7 days

Nadir: 8-10 days and 27-32 days

Recovery: 42-50 days

1% to 10%:

Cardiovascular: Vasculitis

Dermatologic: Vesiculation of skin, alopecia, pruritus, rash

Endocrine & metabolic: SIADH, sterility, amenorrhea

Gastrointestinal: Nausea and vomiting are mild; stomatitis and diarrhea are infrequent

Genitourinary: Hemorrhagic cystitis, bladder irritation

Hematologic: Anemia, agranulocytosis, hemolytic anemia

Hepatic: Transaminases increased (hepatitis, jaundice have been reported)

Respiratory: Pulmonary fibrosis, interstitial pneumonitis

Miscellaneous: Hypersensitivity, secondary malignancy

Drug Interactions

Increased Effect/Toxicity: Cyclosporine and melphalan increase the incidence of nephrotoxicity.

Decreased Effect: Cimetidine and other H_2 antagonists: The reduction in gastric pH has been reported to decrease bioavailability of melphalan by 30%.

Drug Uptake

Absorption: Oral: Variable and incomplete from the GI tract; food interferes with absorption

Half-life, elimination: Terminal: 1.5 hours

Time to peak: ~2 hours

Pregnancy Risk Factor D

Generic Available No

Melquin-3® [OTC] *see* Hydroquinone *on page 611*

Melquin HP® *see* Hydroquinone *on page 611*

Menadol® [OTC] *see* Ibuprofen *on page 621*

Menest® *see* Estrogens, Esterified *on page 467*

Meni-D® *see* Meclizine *on page 750*

Meningococcal Polysaccharide Vaccine, Groups A, C, Y, and W-135

(me NIN joe kok al pol i SAK a ride vak SEEN groops aye, see, why & dubl yoo won thur tee fyve)

U.S. Brand Names Menomune®-A/C/Y/W-135

Pharmacologic Category Vaccine

Use

Immunization of persons ≥2 years of age in epidemic or endemic areas as might be determined in a population delineated by neighborhood, school, dormitory, or other reasonable boundary. The prevalent serogroup in such a situation should match a serogroup in the vaccine. Individuals at particular high-risk include persons with terminal component complement deficiencies and those with anatomic or functional asplenia.

Travelers visiting areas of a country that are recognized as having hyperendemic or epidemic meningococcal disease

Vaccinations should be considered for household or institutional contacts of persons with meningococcal disease as an adjunct to appropriate antibiotic chemoprophylaxis as well as medical and laboratory personnel at risk of exposure to meningococcal disease

Local Anesthetic/Vasoconstrictor Precautions No information available to require special precautions

Effects on Dental Treatment No effects or complications reported

Dosage One dose S.C. (0.5 mL); the need for booster is unknown

Note: Individuals who are sensitive to thimerosal should receive single-dose pack (reconstituted with 0.78 mL vial without preservative).

Mechanism of Action Induces the formation of bactericidal antibodies to meningococcal antigens; the presence of these antibodies is strongly correlated with immunity to meningococcal disease caused by *Neisseria meningitidis* groups A, C, Y and W-135.

Other Adverse Effects

All serious adverse reactions must be reported to the U.S. Department of Health and Human Services (DHHS) Vaccine Adverse Event Reporting System (VAERS) 1-800-822-7967. Incidence of erythema, swelling, or tenderness may be higher in children

>10%: Local: Tenderness (9% to 36% as reported in adults)

1% to 10%:

- Central nervous system: Headache (2% to 5%), malaise (2%), fever (100°F to 106°F: 3%), chills (2%)
- Local: Pain at injection site (2% to 3%), erythema (1% to 4%), induration (1% to 4%)

Drug Interactions Decreased effect with administration of immunoglobulin within 1 month

Drug Uptake

Onset of action: Antibody levels: 10-14 days

Duration: Antibodies against group A and C polysaccharides decline markedly (to prevaccination levels) over the first 3 years following a single dose of vaccine, especially in children <4 years of age

Pregnancy Risk Factor C

Generic Available No

Menomune®-A/C/Y/W-135 *see* Meningococcal Polysaccharide Vaccine, Groups A, C, Y, and W-135 *on page 758*

Menotropins (men oh TROE pins)

U.S. Brand Names Humegon™; Pergonal®; Repronex®

Canadian Brand Names Pergonal®

Mexican Brand Names HMG Massone®; Humegon®

Pharmacologic Category Gonadotropin; Ovulation Stimulator

Use Sequentially with hCG to induce ovulation and pregnancy in the infertile woman with functional anovulation or in patients who have previously received pituitary suppression; used with hCG in men to stimulate spermatogenesis in those with primary hypogonadotropic hypogonadism

Local Anesthetic/Vasoconstrictor Precautions No information available to require special precautions

Effects on Dental Treatment No effects or complications reported

Dosage Adults:

Male: I.M.: Following pretreatment with hCG, 1 ampul 3 times/week and hCG 2000 units twice weekly until sperm is detected in the ejaculate (4-6 months) then may be increased to 2 ampuls of menotropins (150 units FSH/150 units LH) 3 times/week

Female: I.M.: 1 ampul/day (75 units of FSH and LH) for 9-12 days followed by 10,000 units hCG 1 day after the last dose; repeated at least twice at same level before increasing dosage to 2 ampuls (150 units FSH/150 units LH)

Repronex®: I.M., S.C.:

Infertile patients with oligo-anovulation: Initial: 150 int. units daily for the first 5 days of treatment. Adjustments should not be made more frequently than once every 2 days and should not exceed 75-150 int. units per adjustment. Maximum daily dose should not exceed 450 int. units and dosing beyond 12 days is not recommended. If patient's response to Repronex® is appropriate, hCG 5000-10,000 units should be given one day following the last dose of Repronex®.

(Continued)

Menotropins *(Continued)*

Assisted reproductive technologies: Initial (in patients who have received GnRH agonist or antagonist pituitary suppression): 225 int. units; adjustments in dose should not be made more frequently than once every 2 days and should not exceed >75-50 int. units per adjustment. The maximum daily doses of Repronex® given should not exceed 450 int. units and dosing beyond 12 days is not recommended. Once adequate follicular development is evident, hCG (5000-10,000 units) should be administered to induce final follicular maturation in preparation for oocyte retrieval.

Mechanism of Action Actions occur as a result of both follicle stimulating hormone (FSH) effects and luteinizing hormone (LH) effects; menotropins stimulate the development and maturation of the ovarian follicle (FSH), cause ovulation (LH), and stimulate the development of the corpus luteum (LH); in males it stimulates spermatogenesis (LH)

Other Adverse Effects

Male:

>10%: Endocrine & metabolic: Gynecomastia

1% to 10%: Erythrocytosis (dyspnea, dizziness, anorexia, syncope, epistaxis)

Female:

1% to 10%:

Central nervous system: Headache
Endocrine & metabolic: Breast tenderness
Gastrointestinal: Abdominal cramping, abdominal pain, diarrhea, enlarged abdomen, nausea, vomiting
Genitourinary: Ectopic pregnancy, OHSS (% is dose related), ovarian disease, vaginal hemorrhage
Local: Injection site edema/reaction
Miscellaneous: Infection, pelvic pain

Frequency not defined:

Cardiovascular: Stroke, tachycardia, thrombosis (venous or arterial)
Central nervous system: Dizziness
Dermatologic: Angioedema, urticaria
Genitourinary: Adnexal torsion, hemoperitoneum, ovarian enlargement
Neuromuscular & skeletal: Limb necrosis
Respiratory: Acute respiratory distress syndrome, atelectasis, dyspnea, embolism, laryngeal edema pulmonary infarction tachypnea
Miscellaneous: Allergic reactions, anaphylaxis, rash

Drug Interactions Clomiphene may decrease the amount of human menopausal gonadotropin (HMG) needed to induce ovulation (Gonadorelin, Factrel®); should not be used with drugs that stimulate ovulation.

Pregnancy Risk Factor X

Generic Available No

Mentax® *see* Butenafine *on page 195*

Mepenzolate Bromide (me PEN zoe late)

U.S. Brand Names Cantil®

Canadian Brand Names Cantil®

Pharmacologic Category Anticholinergic Agent; Antispasmodic Agent, Gastrointestinal

Synonyms Mepenzolate

Use Management of peptic ulcer disease; inhibit salivation and excessive secretions in respiratory tract preoperatively

Local Anesthetic/Vasoconstrictor Precautions No information available to require special precautions

Effects on Dental Treatment >10%: Xerostomia

Dosage Adults: Oral: 25-50 mg 4 times/day with meal and at bedtime

Other Adverse Effects Frequency not defined:

Cardiovascular: Palpitations, flushing
Central nervous system: Headache, nervousness, drowsiness, dizziness, confusion, fever, CNS stimulation may be produced with large doses
Dermatologic: Dry skin, urticaria
Gastrointestinal: Constipation, xerostomia, dry throat, dysphagia, nausea, vomiting
Respiratory: Dry nose
Miscellaneous: Decreased diaphoresis, hypersensitivity reactions, anaphylaxis

Pregnancy Risk Factor C

Generic Available No

Mepergan® *see* Meperidine and Promethazine *on page 762*

Meperidine (me PER i deen)

Related Information

Dental Drug Interactions: Update on Drug Combinations Requiring Special Considerations *on page 1434*
Oral Pain *on page 1360*

U.S. Brand Names Demerol®; Meperitab®

Canadian Brand Names Demerol®

Pharmacologic Category Analgesic, Narcotic

Synonyms Isonipecaine Hydrochloride; Meperidine Hydrochloride; Pethidine Hydrochloride

Use

Dental: Adjunct in preoperative I.V. conscious sedation in patients undergoing dental surgery; alternate oral narcotic in patients allergic to codeine in treatment of moderate to moderate-severe pain

Medical: Management of moderate to severe pain

Local Anesthetic/Vasoconstrictor Precautions No information available to require special precautions

Effects on Dental Treatment 1% to 10%: Xerostomia

Restrictions C-II

Dosage

Children: Oral: 25-50 mg every 4-6 hours as needed for pain

Adults:

I.V.: 50-100 mg titrated as a single dose to produce sedation

Oral: 50-100 mg every 4-6 hours as needed for pain

Mechanism of Action Binds to opiate receptors in the CNS, causing inhibition of ascending pain pathways, altering the perception of and response to pain; produces generalized CNS depression

Other Adverse Effects Frequency not defined:

Cardiovascular: Hypotension

Central nervous system: Fatigue, drowsiness, dizziness, nervousness, headache, restlessness, malaise, confusion, mental depression, hallucinations, paradoxical CNS stimulation, increased intracranial pressure, seizures (associated with metabolite accumulation)

Dermatologic: Rash, urticaria

Gastrointestinal: Nausea, vomiting, constipation, anorexia, stomach cramps, xerostomia, biliary spasm, paralytic ileus

Genitourinary: Ureteral spasms, decreased urination

Local: Pain at injection site

Neuromuscular & skeletal: Weakness

Respiratory: Dyspnea

Miscellaneous: Histamine release, physical and psychological dependence

Contraindications Hypersensitivity to meperidine or any component; use with MAO inhibitors or within the past 14 days

Warnings/Precautions Use with caution in patients with pulmonary, hepatic, renal disorders, or increased intracranial pressure; use with caution in patients with renal failure or seizure disorders or those receiving high-dose meperidine; normeperidine (an active metabolite and CNS stimulant) may accumulate and precipitate twitches, tremors, or seizures; some preparations contain sulfites which may cause allergic reaction

Enhanced analgesia has been seen in elderly patients on therapeutic doses of narcotics; duration of action may be increased in the elderly; the elderly may be particularly susceptible to the CNS depressant and constipating effects of narcotics

Drug Interactions CYP2D6 enzyme substrate

Increased Toxicity: May aggravate the adverse effects of isoniazid; MAO inhibitors, fluoxetine, and other serotonin uptake inhibitors greatly potentiate the effects of meperidine; acute opioid overdosage symptoms can be seen, including severe toxic reactions; CNS depressants, tricyclic antidepressants, phenothiazines may potentiate the effects of meperidine

Decreased Effect: Phenytoin may decrease the analgesic effects

Dietary/Ethanol/Herb Considerations

Ethanol: Avoid or limit use; may increase CNS depression.

Food: Glucose may cause hyperglycemia; monitor blood glucose concentrations.

Herb/Nutraceutical: Avoid gotu kola, kava, SAMe, St John's wort, and valerian; may increase CNS depression.

Drug Uptake

Onset of action: Analgesic: Oral, S.C., I.M.: 10-15 minutes; I.V.: ~5 minutes

Peak effect: Oral, S.C., I.M.: ~1 hour

Duration: Oral, S.C., I.M.: 2-4 hours

Half-life, elimination:

Parent drug: Terminal phase: Neonates: 23 hours; range: 12-39 hours; Adults: 2.5-4 hours; Adults with liver disease: 7-11 hours

Normeperidine (active metabolite): 15-30 hours; can accumulate with high doses or with decreased renal function

Time to peak: Oral: 90-120 minutes

Pregnancy Risk Factor B/D (prolonged use or high doses at term)

Breast-feeding Considerations Considered compatible by AAO in 1983 statement; however, not included in the 1989 statement

(Continued)

Meperidine *(Continued)*

Dosage Forms INF: 10 mg/mL (30 mL). **INJ:** 25 mg/dose (0.5 mL, 1 mL); 50 mg/dose (1 mL); 75 mg/dose (1 mL). **INJ** [multidose vial]: 50 mg/mL (30 mL); 100 mg/mL (20 mL). **SYR:** 50 mg/5 mL (500 mL). **TAB:** 50 mg, 100 mg

Generic Available Yes

Comments Meperidine is not to be used as the narcotic drug of first choice. It is recommended only to be used in codeine-allergic patients when a narcotic analgesic is indicated. Meperidine is not an anti-inflammatory agent. Meperidine, as with other narcotic analgesics, is recommended only for limited acute dosing (ie, 3 days or less); common adverse effects in the dental patient are nausea, sedation, and constipation. Meperidine has a significant addiction liability, especially when given long-term.

Meperidine and Promethazine (me PER i deen & proe METH a zeen)

U.S. Brand Names Mepergan®

Pharmacologic Category Analgesic Combination (Narcotic)

Synonyms Promethazine and Meperidine

Use Management of moderate to severe pain

Local Anesthetic/Vasoconstrictor Precautions No information available to require special precautions

Effects on Dental Treatment 1% to 10%: Xerostomia

Restrictions C-II

Dosage Adults:

Oral: 1 capsule every 4-6 hours

I.M.: Inject 1-2 mL every 3-4 hours

Other Adverse Effects Frequency not defined:

Based on **meperidine** component:

- Cardiovascular: Hypotension
- Central nervous system: Fatigue, drowsiness, dizziness, nervousness, headache, restlessness, malaise, confusion, mental depression, hallucinations, paradoxical CNS stimulation, increased intracranial pressure
- Dermatologic: Rash, urticaria
- Gastrointestinal: Nausea, vomiting, constipation, anorexia, stomach cramps, xerostomia, biliary spasm
- Genitourinary: Ureteral spasms, decreased urination, paralytic ileus
- Local: Pain at injection site
- Neuromuscular & skeletal: Weakness
- Respiratory: Dyspnea
- Miscellaneous: Histamine release, physical and psychological dependence

Based on **promethazine** component:

- Cardiovascular: Postural hypotension, tachycardia, dizziness, nonspecific QT changes
- Central nervous system: Drowsiness, dystonias, akathisia, pseudoparkinsonism, tardive dyskinesia, neuroleptic malignant syndrome, seizures
- Dermatologic: Photosensitivity, dermatitis, skin pigmentation (slate gray)
- Endocrine & metabolic: Lactation, breast engorgement, false-positive pregnancy test, amenorrhea, gynecomastia, hyper- or hypoglycemia
- Gastrointestinal: Xerostomia, constipation, nausea
- Genitourinary: Urinary retention, ejaculatory disorder, impotence
- Hematologic: Agranulocytosis, eosinophilia, leukopenia, hemolytic anemia, aplastic anemia, thrombocytopenic purpura
- Hepatic: Jaundice
- Ocular: Blurred vision, corneal and lenticular changes, epithelial keratopathy, pigmentary retinopathy

Warnings/Precautions

Based on **meperidine** component: Use with caution in patients with pulmonary, hepatic, renal disorders, or increased intracranial pressure; use with caution in patients with renal failure or seizure disorders or those receiving high-dose meperidine; normeperidine (an active metabolite and CNS stimulant) may accumulate and precipitate twitches, tremors, or seizures; some preparations contain sulfites which may cause allergic reaction; not recommended as a drug of first choice for the treatment of chronic pain in the elderly due to the accumulation of normeperidine; for acute pain, its use should be limited to 1-2 doses; tolerance or drug dependence may result from extended use

Based on **promethazine** component: May be sedating; use with caution in disorders where CNS depression is a feature. May impair physical or mental abilities; patients must be cautioned about performing tasks which require mental alertness (ie, operating machinery or driving). Effects with other sedative drugs or ethanol may be potentiated. Avoid use in Reye's syndrome. Use with caution in Parkinson's disease; hemodynamic instability; bone marrow suppression; predisposition to seizures; subcortical brain damage; and in severe cardiac, hepatic, renal, or respiratory disease. Caution in breast cancer or other prolactin-dependent tumors (may elevate prolactin levels). May alter temperature regulation or mask toxicity of other drugs due to antiemetic effects. May alter cardiac conduction (life-threatening arrhythmias have occurred with therapeutic doses of phenothiazines). May cause orthostatic hypotension; use with caution in patients at risk of hypotension or where transient hypotensive episodes would be poorly tolerated (cardiovascular disease or cerebrovascular disease).

Phenothiazines may cause anticholinergic effects (constipation, xerostomia, blurred vision, urinary retention); therefore, they should be used with caution in patients with decreased GI motility, urinary retention, BPH, xerostomia, or visual problems. Conditions which also may be exacerbated by cholinergic blockade include narrow-angle glaucoma (screening is recommended) and worsening of myasthenia gravis. May cause extrapyramidal symptoms, including pseudoparkinsonism, acute dystonic reactions, akathisia, and tardive dyskinesia. May be associated with neuroleptic malignant syndrome (NMS). Ampuls contain sodium metabisulfite.

Drug Interactions

Based on **meperidine** component: CYP2D6 enzyme substrate

Decreased effect: Phenytoin may decrease the analgesic effects

Increased toxicity: May aggravate the adverse effects of isoniazid; MAO inhibitors, fluoxetine, and other serotonin uptake inhibitors greatly potentiate the effects of meperidine; acute opioid overdosage symptoms can be seen, including severe toxic reactions; CNS depressants, tricyclic antidepressants, phenothiazines may potentiate the effects of meperidine

Based on **promethazine** component: CYP2D6 enzyme substrate

Aluminum salts: May decrease the absorption of phenothiazines; monitor

Amphetamines: Efficacy may be diminished by antipsychotics; in addition, amphetamines may increase psychotic symptoms; avoid concurrent use

Anticholinergics: May inhibit the therapeutic response to phenothiazines and excess anticholinergic effects may occur; includes benztropine, trihexyphenidyl, biperiden, and drugs with significant anticholinergic activity (TCAs, antihistamines, disopyramide)

Antihypertensives: Concurrent use of phenothiazines with an antihypertensive may produce additive hypotensive effects (particularly orthostasis)

Bromocriptine: Phenothiazines inhibit the ability of bromocriptine to lower serum prolactin concentrations

CNS depressants: Sedative effects may be additive with phenothiazines; monitor for increased effect; includes barbiturates, benzodiazepines, narcotic analgesics, ethanol, and other sedative agents

CYP2D6 inhibitors: Metabolism of phenothiazines may be decreased; increasing clinical effect or toxicity; inhibitors include amiodarone, cimetidine, delavirdine, fluoxetine, paroxetine, propafenone, quinidine, and ritonavir; monitor for increased effect/toxicity

Enzyme inducers: May enhance the hepatic metabolism of phenothiazines; larger doses may be required; includes rifampin, rifabutin, barbiturates, phenytoin, and cigarette smoking

Epinephrine: Chlorpromazine (and possibly other low potency antipsychotics) may diminish the pressor effects of epinephrine

Guanethidine and guanadrel: Antihypertensive effects may be inhibited by phenothiazines

Levodopa: Phenothiazines may inhibit the antiparkinsonian effect of levodopa; avoid this combination

Lithium: Phenothiazines may produce neurotoxicity with lithium; this is a rare effect

Phenytoin: May reduce serum levels of phenothiazines; phenothiazines may increase phenytoin serum levels

Propranolol: Serum concentrations of phenothiazines may be increased; propranolol also increases phenothiazine concentrations

Polypeptide antibiotics: Rare cases of respiratory paralysis have been reported with concurrent use of phenothiazines

QT_c-prolonging agents: Effects on QT_c interval may be additive with phenothiazines, increasing the risk of malignant arrhythmias; includes type Ia antiarrhythmics, TCAs, and some quinolone antibiotics (sparfloxacin, moxifloxacin, and gatifloxacin)

Sulfadoxine-pyrimethamine: May increase phenothiazine concentrations

Tricyclic antidepressants: Concurrent use may produce increased toxicity or altered therapeutic response

Trazodone: Phenothiazines and trazodone may produce additive hypotensive effects

Valproic acid: Serum levels may be increased by phenothiazines

Drug Uptake See Meperidine *on page 760* and Promethazine *on page 1006*

Pregnancy Risk Factor B/D (prolonged use or high doses at term)

Generic Available No

Meperitab® *see* Meperidine *on page 760*

Mephobarbital (me foe BAR bi tal)

U.S. Brand Names Mebaral®

Canadian Brand Names Mebaral®

Pharmacologic Category Barbiturate

(Continued)

Mephobarbital *(Continued)*

Synonyms Methylphenobarbital

Use Sedative; treatment of grand mal and petit mal epilepsy

Local Anesthetic/Vasoconstrictor Precautions No information available to require special precautions

Effects on Dental Treatment No effects or complications reported

Restrictions C-IV

Dosage Oral:

Epilepsy:
- Children: 6-12 mg/kg/day in 2-4 divided doses
- Adults: 200-600 mg/day in 2-4 divided doses

Sedation:
- Children:
  - <5 years: 16-32 mg 3-4 times/day
  - >5 years: 32-64 mg 3-4 times/day
- Adults: 32-100 mg 3-4 times/day

Mechanism of Action Increases seizure threshold in the motor cortex; depresses monosynaptic and polysynaptic transmission in the CNS

Other Adverse Effects

>10%: Central nervous system: Dizziness, lightheadedness, drowsiness, "hang-over" effect

1% to 10%:
- Central nervous system: Confusion, mental depression, unusual excitement, nervousness, faint feeling, headache, insomnia, nightmares
- Gastrointestinal: Constipation, nausea, vomiting

Drug Interactions CYP2C, 2C8, and 2C19 enzyme substrate

Increased Effect/Toxicity: When combined with other CNS depressants, narcotic analgesics, antidepressants, or benzodiazepines, additive respiratory and CNS depression may occur. Barbiturates may enhance the hepatotoxic potential of acetaminophen overdoses. Chloramphenicol, MAO inhibitors, valproic acid, and felbamate may inhibit barbiturate metabolism. Barbiturates may impair the absorption of griseofulvin, and may enhance the nephrotoxic effects of methoxy-flurane. Concurrent use of phenobarbital with meperidine may result in increased CNS depression.

Decreased Effect: Barbiturates are hepatic enzyme inducers, and may increase the metabolism of antipsychotics, some beta-blockers (unlikely with atenolol and nadolol), calcium channel blockers, chloramphenicol, cimetidine, corticosteroids, cyclosporine, disopyramide, doxycycline, ethosuximide, felbamate, furosemide, griseofulvin, lamotrigine, phenytoin, propafenone, quinidine, tacrolimus, TCAs, and theophylline. Barbiturates may increase the metabolism of estrogens and reduce the efficacy of oral contraceptives; an alternative method of contraception should be considered. Barbiturates inhibit the hypoprothrombinemic effects of oral anticoagulants via increased metabolism. Barbiturates may enhance the metabolism of methadone resulting in methadone withdrawal.

Drug Uptake
- Onset of action: 20-60 minutes
- Absorption: Oral: ~50%
- Duration: 6-8 hours
- Half-life, elimination: 34 hours

Pregnancy Risk Factor D

Generic Available No

Mephyton® *see* Phytonadione *on page 954*

Mepivacaine (me PIV a kane)

U.S. Brand Names Carbocaine®; Isocaine® HCl; Polocaine®

Canadian Brand Names Carbocaine®; Polocaine®

Pharmacologic Category Local Anesthetic

Synonyms Mepivacaine Hydrochloride

Use
- Dental: Local anesthesia by nerve block, infiltration in dental procedures
- Medical: Local anesthesia by nerve block; **not** for use in spinal anesthesia

Local Anesthetic/Vasoconstrictor Precautions No information available to require special precautions

Effects on Dental Treatment No effects or complications reported

Dosage Children and Adults: Injectable local anesthetic: Varies with procedure, degree of anesthesia needed, vascularity of tissue, duration of anesthesia required, and physical condition of patient

Mechanism of Action An amino amide local anesthetic similar to lidocaine; acts by preventing the generation and conduction of nerve impulses in neurons by decreasing the transient increase in permeability to sodium; differential sensitivity generally depends on the size of the fiber. Small fibers are more sensitive than larger fibers and require a longer period for recovery. Sensory pain fibers are usually blocked first, followed by fibers that transmit sensations of temperature, touch, and deep pressure. High concentrations block sympathetic somatic sensory and somatic motor fibers. The spread of anesthesia depends upon the distribution of the solution. This is primarily dependent on the site of administration and volume of drug injected.

Other Adverse Effects Degree of adverse effects in the CNS and cardiovascular system are directly related to the blood levels of mepivacaine. The effects below are more likely to occur after systemic administration rather than infiltration. Frequency not defined:

Cardiovascular: Bradycardia, cardiovascular collapse, edema, heart block, hypotension, myocardial depression, ventricular arrhythmias, angioneurotic edema

Central nervous system: High blood levels result in anxiety, restlessness, disorientation, confusion, dizziness, and seizures. This is followed by depression of CNS resulting in somnolence, unconsciousness, and possible respiratory arrest. In some cases, symptoms of CNS stimulation may be absent and the primary CNS effects are somnolence and unconsciousness.

Dermatologic: Cutaneous lesions, urticaria

Gastrointestinal: Nausea, vomiting

Local: Transient stinging or burning at injection site

Ophthalmic: Blurred vision

Otic: Tinnitus

Respiratory: Respiratory arrest

Miscellaneous: Anaphylactoid reactions

Contraindications Hypersensitivity to mepivacaine, other amide anesthetics, or any component of their formulation; allergy to sodium bisulfate

Warnings/Precautions Use with caution in patients with cardiac disease, renal disease, and hyperthyroidism; convulsions due to systemic toxicity leading to cardiac arrest have been reported presumably due to intravascular injection

Drug Uptake

Onset of action: Epidural: 7-15 minutes

Duration: 2-2.5 hours; similar onset and duration following infiltration

Half-life, elimination: 1.9 hours

Pregnancy Risk Factor C

Dosage Forms INJ: 1% [10 mg/mL] (30 mL, 50 mL); 1.5% [15 mg/mL] (30 mL); 2% [20 mg/mL] (20 mL, 50 mL); 3% [30 mg/mL] (1.8 mL)

Generic Available Yes

Selected Readings Torres MJ, Garcia JJ, del Cano Moratinos AM, et al, "Fixed Drug Eruption Induced by Mepivacaine," *J Allergy Clin Immunol*, 1995, 96(1):130-1.

Mepivacaine and Levonordefrin

(me PIV a kane & lee voe nor DEF rin)

Related Information

Oral Pain *on page 1360*

U.S. Brand Names Carbocaine® 2% with Neo-Cobefrin®

Canadian Brand Names Polocaine® 2% and Levonordefrin 1:20,000

Pharmacologic Category Local Anesthetic

Use Dental: Amide-type anesthetic used for local infiltration anesthesia; injection near nerve trunks to produce nerve block

Local Anesthetic/Vasoconstrictor Precautions No information available to require special precautions

Effects on Dental Treatment No effects or complications reported

Dosage

Children <10 years: Maximum pediatric dosage must be carefully calculated on the basis of patient's weight but should not exceed 6.6 mg/kg of body weight or 180 mg of mepivacaine hydrochloride as a 2% solution with levonordefrin 1:20,000

Children >10 years and Adults:

Dental infiltration and nerve block, single site: 36 mg (1.8 mL) of mepivacaine hydrochloride as a 2% solution with levonordefrin 1:20,000

# of Cartridges (1.8 mL)	Mepivacaine (2%) (mg)	Levonordefrin 1:20,000 (mg)
1	36	0.090
2	72	0.180
3	108	0.270
4	144	0.360
5	180	0.450
6	216	0.540
7	252	0.630
8	288	0.720
9	324	0.810
10	360	0.900

(Continued)

Mepivacaine and Levonordefrin *(Continued)*

Entire oral cavity: 180 mg (9 mL) of mepivacaine hydrochloride as a 2% solution with levonordefrin 1:20,000; up to a maximum of 6.6 mg/kg of body weight but not to exceed 400 mg of mepivacaine hydrochloride per appointment. The effective anesthetic dose varies with procedure, intensity of anesthesia needed, duration of anesthesia required, and physical condition of the patient. Always use the lowest effective dose along with careful aspiration.

The numbers of dental carpules (1.8 mL) (see table) provide the indicated amounts of mepivacaine hydrochloride 2% and levonordefrin 1:20,000.

Doses of mepivacaine hydrochloride with levonordefrin cited from USP Dispensing Information (USP DI), 17th ed, The United States Pharmacopeial Convention, Inc, Rockville, MD, 1997, 139.

Mechanism of Action Local anesthetics bind selectively to the intracellular surface of sodium channels to block influx of sodium into the axon. As a result, depolarization necessary for action potential propagation and subsequent nerve function is prevented. The block at the sodium channel is reversible. Local anesthetics reversibly prevent generation and conduction of electrical impulses in neurons by decreasing the transient increase in permeability to sodium. The differential sensitivity generally depends on the size of the fiber; small fibers are more sensitive than larger fibers and require a longer period for recovery. Sensory pain fibers are usually blocked first, followed by fibers that transmit sensations of temperature, touch, and deep pressure. High concentrations block sympathetic somatic sensory and somatic motor fibers. The spread of anesthesia depends upon the distribution of the solution. This is primarily dependent on the site of administration and volume of drug injected. When drug diffuses away from the axon, sodium channel function is restored and nerve propagation returns.

Levonordefrin prolongs the duration of the anesthetic actions of mepivacaine by causing vasoconstriction (alpha adrenergic receptor agonist) of the vasculature surrounding the nerve axons. This prevents the diffusion of mepivacaine away from the nerves resulting in a longer retention in the axon.

Other Adverse Effects Degree of adverse effects in the CNS and cardiovascular system are directly related to the blood levels of mepivacaine. The effects below are more likely to occur after systemic administration rather than infiltration.

Cardiovascular: Myocardial effects include a decrease in contraction force as well as a decrease in electrical excitability and myocardial conduction rate resulting in bradycardia and reduction in cardiac output.

Central nervous system: High blood levels result in anxiety, restlessness, disorientation, confusion, dizziness, and seizures. This is followed by depression of CNS resulting in somnolence, unconsciousness and possible respiratory arrest. In some cases, symptoms of CNS stimulation may be absent and the primary CNS effects are somnolence and unconsciousness.

Gastrointestinal: Nausea and vomiting may occur

Hypersensitivity reactions: Extremely rare, but may be manifest as dermatologic reactions and edema at injection site. Asthmatic syndromes have occurred. Patients may exhibit hypersensitivity to bisulfites contained in local anesthetic solution to prevent oxidation of levonordefrin. In general, patients reacting to bisulfites have a history of asthma and their airways are hyper-reactive to asthmatic syndrome.

Neuromuscular & skeletal: Tremors

Psychogenic reactions: It is common to misinterpret psychogenic responses to local anesthetic injection as an allergic reaction. Intraoral injections are perceived by many patients as a stressful procedure in dentistry. Common symptoms to this stress are diaphoresis, palpitations, hyperventilation, generalized pallor and a fainting feeling.

Contraindications Hypersensitivity to mepivacaine, levonordefrin, other local anesthetics of the amide-type, or any component of their formulation

Warnings/Precautions Should be avoided in patients with uncontrolled hyperthyroidism. Should be used in minimal amounts in patients with significant cardiovascular problems (because of levonordefrin component). Aspirate the syringe after tissue penetration and before injection to minimize chance of direct vascular injection.

Drug Interactions Due to levonordefrin component, use with tricyclic antidepressants or MAO inhibitors could result in increased pressor response; use with nonselective beta-blockers (ie, propranolol) could result in serious hypertension and reflex bradycardia.

Drug Uptake

Duration: Upper jaw: 1-2.5 hours; Lower jaw: 2.5-5.5 hours

Infiltration: 50 minutes

Inferior alveolar block: 60-75 minutes

Pregnancy Risk Factor C

Breast-feeding Considerations Usual infiltration doses of mepivacaine with levonordefrin given to nursing mothers has not been shown to affect the health of the nursing infant.

Dosage Forms INJ: Mepivacaine hydrochloride 2% with levonordefrin 1:20,000 (1.8 mL) [dental cartridge]

Generic Available Yes

Selected Readings

Ayoub ST and Coleman AE, "A Review of Local Anesthetics," *Gen Dent*, 1992, 40(4):285-7, 289-90.

Jastak JT and Yagiela JA, "Vasoconstrictors and Local Anesthesia: A Review and Rationale for Use," *J Am Dent Assoc*, 1983, 107(4):623-30.

MacKenzie TA and Young ER, "Local Anesthetic Update," *Anesth Prog*, 1993, 40(2):29-34.

Wynn RL, "Epinephrine Interactions With Beta-Blockers," *Gen Dent*, 1994, 42(1):16, 18.

Wynn RL, "Recent Research on Mechanisms of Local Anesthetics," *Gen Dent*, 1995, 43(4):316-8.

Yagiela JA, "Local Anesthetics," *Anesth Prog*, 1991, 38(4-5):128-41.

Mepivacaine Dental Anesthetic (me PIV a kane DEN tal)

Related Information

Oral Pain *on page 1360*

U.S. Brand Names Carbocaine® 3%

Canadian Brand Names Polocaine®

Pharmacologic Category Local Anesthetic

Use Dental: Amide-type anesthetic used for local infiltration anesthesia; injection near nerve trunks to produce nerve block

Local Anesthetic/Vasoconstrictor Precautions No information available to require special precautions

Effects on Dental Treatment No effects or complications reported

Dosage

Children <10 years: Up to 5-6 mg/kg of body weight; maximum pediatric dosage must be carefully calculated on the basis of patient's weight but must not exceed 270 mg (9 mL) of the 3% solution

Children >10 years and Adults:

Dental anesthesia, single site in upper or lower jaw: 54 mg (1.8 mL) as a 3% solution

Infiltration and nerve block of entire oral cavity: 270 mg (9 mL) as a 3% solution; up to a maximum of 6.6 mg/kg of body weight but not to exceed 300 mg per appointment. Manufacturer's maximum recommended dose is not >400 mg to normal healthy adults. The effective anesthetic dose varies with procedure, intensity of anesthesia needed, duration of anesthesia required, and physical condition of the patient. Always use the lowest effective dose along with careful aspiration.

The following number of dental carpules (1.8 mL) provide the indicated amounts of mepivacaine dental anesthetic 3%.

# of Cartridges (1.8 mL)	Mepivacaine (3%) (mg)
1	54
2	108
3	162
4	216
5	270
6	324
7	378
8	432

Adult and children doses of mepivacaine dental anesthetic cited from USP Dispensing Information (USP DI), 17th ed, The United States Pharmacopeial Convention, Inc, Rockville, MD, 1997, 138-9.

Mechanism of Action Local anesthetics bind selectively to the intracellular surface of sodium channels to block influx of sodium into the axon. As a result, depolarization necessary for action potential propagation and subsequent nerve function is prevented. The block at the sodium channel is reversible. Local anesthetics reversibly prevent generation and conduction of electrical impulses in neurons by decreasing the transient increase in permeability to sodium. The differential sensitivity generally depends on the size of the fiber; small fibers are more sensitive than larger fibers and require a longer period for recovery. Sensory pain fibers are usually blocked first, followed by fibers that transmit sensations of temperature, touch, and deep pressure. High concentrations block sympathetic somatic sensory and somatic motor fibers. The spread of anesthesia depends upon the distribution of the solution. This is primarily dependent on the site of administration and volume of drug injected. When drug diffuses away from the axon, sodium channel function is restored and nerve propagation returns.

Other Adverse Effects Degree of adverse effects in the CNS and cardiovascular system are directly related to the blood levels of local anesthetic. Frequency not defined:

Cardiovascular: Myocardial effects include a decrease in contraction force as well as a decrease in electrical excitability and myocardial conduction rate resulting in bradycardia and reduction in cardiac output

(Continued)

Mepivacaine Dental Anesthetic *(Continued)*

Central nervous system: High blood levels result in anxiety, restlessness, disorientation, confusion, dizziness, and seizures. This is followed by depression of CNS resulting in somnolence, unconsciousness and possible respiratory arrest. In some cases, symptoms of CNS stimulation may be absent and the primary CNS effects are somnolence and unconsciousness.

Gastrointestinal: Nausea and vomiting may occur

Hypersensitivity reactions: May manifest as dermatologic reactions and edema at injection site. Asthmatic syndromes have occurred.

Neuromuscular & skeletal: Tremors

Psychogenic reactions: It is common to misinterpret psychogenic responses to local anesthetic injection as an allergic reaction. Intraoral injection is perceived by many patients as a stressful procedure in dentistry. Common symptoms to this stress are diaphoresis, palpitations, hyperventilation, generalized pallor and a fainting feeling.

Contraindications Hypersensitivity to mepivacaine, other local anesthetics of the amide type, or any component of their formulation

Warnings/Precautions Aspirate the syringe after tissue penetration and before injection to minimize chance of direct vascular injection

Drug Uptake

Onset of action: 30-120 seconds in upper jaw; 1-4 minutes in lower jaw

Duration: 20 minutes in upper jaw; 40 minutes in lower jaw

Half-life, elimination: 1.9 hours

Pregnancy Risk Factor C

Breast-feeding Considerations Usual infiltration doses of mepivacaine dental anesthetic given to nursing mothers has not been shown to affect the health of the nursing infant.

Dosage Forms INJ: Mepivacaine hydrochloride 3% (1.8 mL) [dental cartridge]

Generic Available Yes

Selected Readings

Ayoub ST and Coleman AE, "A Review of Local Anesthetics," *Gen Dent*, 1992, 40(4):285-7, 289-90.

Wynn RL, "Recent Research on Mechanisms of Local Anesthetics," *Gen Dent*, 1995, 43(4):316-8.

Meprobamate (me proe BA mate)

U.S. Brand Names Equanil®; Miltown®

Canadian Brand Names Apo®-Meprobamate

Pharmacologic Category Antianxiety Agent, Miscellaneous

Use

Dental: Treatment of muscle spasm associated with acute temporomandibular joint pain; management of dental anxiety disorders

Medical: Management of anxiety disorders

Unlabeled/Investigational: Demonstrated value for muscle contraction, headache, premenstrual tension, external sphincter spasticity, muscle rigidity, opisthotonos-associated with tetanus

Local Anesthetic/Vasoconstrictor Precautions No information available to require special precautions

Effects on Dental Treatment <1%: Stomatitis

Restrictions C-IV

Dosage Oral:

Children 6-12 years: Anxiety: 100-200 mg 2-3 times/day

Adults: Anxiety: 400 mg 3-4 times/day, up to 2400 mg/day

Dosing interval in renal impairment:

Cl_{cr} 10-50 mL/minute: Administer every 9-12 hours

Cl_{cr} <10 mL/minute: Administer every 12-18 hours

Hemodialysis: Moderately dialyzable (20% to 50%)

Dosing adjustment in hepatic impairment: Probably necessary

Mechanism of Action Unclear; many effects have been ascribed to its central depressant actions; affects the thalamus and limbic system and appears to inhibit multineuronal spinal reflexes

Other Adverse Effects Frequency not defined:

Cardiovascular: Syncope, peripheral edema, palpitations, tachycardia, arrhythmia

Central nervous system: Drowsiness, ataxia, dizziness, paradoxical excitement, confusion, slurred speech, headache, euphoria, chills, vertigo, paresthesia, overstimulation

Dermatologic: Rashes, purpura, dermatitis, Stevens-Johnson syndrome, petechiae, ecchymosis

Gastrointestinal: Diarrhea, vomiting, nausea

Hematologic: Leukopenia, eosinophilia, agranulocytosis, aplastic anemia

Neuromuscular & skeletal: Weakness

Ocular: Blurred vision, impairment of accommodation

Renal: Renal failure

Respiratory: Wheezing, dyspnea, bronchospasm, angioneurotic edema

Contraindications Hypersensitivity to meprobamate, related compounds (including carisoprodol), or any component of their formulation; acute intermittent porphyria;

pre-existing CNS depression; narrow-angle glaucoma; severe uncontrolled pain; pregnancy

Warnings/Precautions Physical and psychological dependence and abuse may occur; not recommended in children <6 years of age; allergic reaction may occur in patients with history of dermatological condition (usually by fourth dose); use with caution in patients with renal or hepatic impairment, or with a history of seizures

Drug Interactions CNS depressants: Sedative effects may be additive with other CNS depressants; monitor for increased effect (includes barbiturates, benzodiazepines, narcotic analgesics, and other sedative agents).

Dietary/Ethanol/Herb Considerations

Ethanol: Avoid use; may increase CNS depression.

Herb/Nutraceutical: Avoid gotu kola, kava, SAMe, St John's wort, and valerian; may increase CNS depression.

Drug Uptake

Onset of action: Sedation: ~1 hour

Absorption: Oral: Rapid and nearly complete

Half-life, elimination: 10 hours

Pregnancy Risk Factor D

Breast-feeding Considerations Breast milk concentrations are higher than plasma; effects are unknown.

Dosage Forms TAB: 200 mg, 400 mg

Generic Available Yes

Mepron™ *see* Atovaquone *on page 128*

Mequinol and Tretinoin (ME kwi nol & TRET i noyn)

U.S. Brand Names Solagé™

Canadian Brand Names Solagé™

Pharmacologic Category Retinoic Acid Derivative; Vitamin A Derivative; Vitamin, Topical

Use Treatment of solar lentigines; the efficacy of using Solagé™ daily for >24 weeks has not been established. The local cutaneous safety of Solagé™ in non-Caucasians has not been adequately established.

Local Anesthetic/Vasoconstrictor Precautions No information available to require special precautions

Effects on Dental Treatment No effects or complications reported

Dosage Adult: Topical: Apply twice daily to solar lentigines using the applicator tip while avoiding application to the surrounding skin. Separate application by at east 8 hours or as directed by physician.

Mechanism of Action Solar lentigines are localized, pigmented, macular lesions of the skin on areas of the body chronically exposed to the sun. Mequinol is a substrate for the enzyme tyrosinase and acts as a competitive inhibitor of the formation of melanin precursors. The mechanisms of depigmentation for both drugs is unknown.

Other Adverse Effects

>10%: Dermatologic: Erythema (49%), burning, stinging or tingling (26%), desquamation (14%), pruritus (12%),

1% to 10%: Dermatologic: Skin irritation (5%), hypopigmentation (5%), halo hypopigmentation (7%), rash (3%), dry skin (3%), crusting (3%), vesicular bullae rash (2%), contact allergic reaction (1%)

Contraindications Hypersensitivity to mequinol, tretinoin, or any component of their formulation; pregnancy; women of childbearing age

Warnings/Precautions Discontinue if hypersensitivity is noted. Use extreme caution in eczematous skin conditions. Safety and efficacy have not been established in moderately or heavily pigmented skin. Not to be taken with photosensitizing drugs (eg, thiazides, tetracyclines, fluoroquinolones, phenothiazines, sulfonamides). Avoid sun (including sun lamps) or use protective clothing. Do not use in sunburned patients until they have fully recovered. Use extreme caution in patients who have significant exposure to the sun through their occupation. Use caution in patient with history or family history of vitiligo. For external use only. Weather extremes (wind, cold) may be irritating to users of Solagé™. Do not use in pediatric patients. No bathing or showering for at least 6 hours after application. Effects of chronic use (>52 weeks) are unknown.

Drug Interactions Increased Effect/Toxicity: Topical products with skin drying effects (eg, those containing alcohol, astringents, spices, or lime; medicated soaps or shampoos; permanent wave solutions; hair depilatories or waxes; and others) may increase skin irritation; avoid concurrent use. Photosensitizing drugs (eg, thiazides, tetracyclines, fluoroquinolones, phenothiazines, sulfonamides) can further increase sun sensitivity; avoid concurrent use.

Drug Uptake

Absorption: Percutaneous absorption was 4.4% of tretinoin when applied as 0.8 mL of Solagé™ to a 400 cm^2 area of the back

Time to peak: Mequinol: 2 hours

Pregnancy Risk Factor X

Generic Available No

Merbromin (mer BROE min)

U.S. Brand Names Mercurochrome®

Pharmacologic Category Topical Skin Product

Use Topical antiseptic

Local Anesthetic/Vasoconstrictor Precautions No information available to require special precautions

Effects on Dental Treatment No effects or complications reported

Dosage Apply freely, until injury has healed

Generic Available Yes

Mercaptopurine (mer kap toe PYOOR een)

U.S. Brand Names Purinethol®

Canadian Brand Names Purinethol®

Mexican Brand Names Purinethol®

Pharmacologic Category Antineoplastic Agent, Antimetabolite

Synonyms 6-Mercaptopurine; 6-MP

Use Maintenance therapy in acute lymphoblastic leukemia (ALL); other (less common) uses include chronic granulocytic leukemia, induction therapy in ALL, and treatment of non-Hodgkin's lymphomas

Local Anesthetic/Vasoconstrictor Precautions No information available to require special precautions

Effects on Dental Treatment No effects or complications reported

Restrictions Note: I.V. formulation is not commercially available in the U.S.

Mechanism of Action Purine antagonist which inhibits DNA and RNA synthesis; acts as false metabolite and is incorporated into DNA and RNA, eventually inhibiting their synthesis. 6-MP is substituted for hypoxanthine; must be metabolized to active nucleotides once inside the cell.

Other Adverse Effects

>10%:

Hematologic: Myelosuppression; leukopenia, thrombocytopenia, anemia

Onset: 7-10 days

Nadir: 14-16 days

Recovery: 21-28 days

Hepatic: Intrahepatic cholestasis and focal centralobular necrosis (40%), characterized by hyperbilirubinemia, increased alkaline phosphatase and AST, jaundice, ascites, encephalopathy; more common at doses >2.5 mg/kg/day. Usually occurs within 2 months of therapy but may occur within 1 week, or be delayed up to 8 years.

1% to 10%:

Central nervous system: Drug fever

Dermatologic: Hyperpigmentation, rash

Endocrine & metabolic: Hyperuricemia

Gastrointestinal: Nausea, vomiting, diarrhea, stomatitis, anorexia, stomach pain, mucositis

Renal: Renal toxicity

Drug Interactions

Increased Effect/Toxicity: Allopurinol can cause increased levels of 6-MP by inhibition of xanthine oxidase. Decrease dose of 6-MP by 75% when both drugs are used concomitantly. Seen only with oral 6-MP usage, not with I.V. May potentiate effect of bone marrow suppression (reduce 6-MP to 25% of dose). Doxorubicin: Synergistic liver toxicity with 6-MP in >50% of patients, which resolved with discontinuation of the 6-MP. Hepatotoxic drugs: Any agent which could potentially alter the metabolic function of the liver could produce higher drug levels and greater toxicities from either 6-MP or thioguanine (6-TG).

Decreased Effect: 6-MP inhibits the anticoagulation effect of warfarin by an unknown mechanism.

Drug Uptake

Absorption: Variable and incomplete (16% to 50%)

Half-life, elimination (age-dependent): Children: 21 minutes; Adults: 47 minutes

Time to peak: ~2 hours

Pregnancy Risk Factor D

Generic Available No

Mercuric Oxide (mer KYOOR ik OKS ide)

U.S. Brand Names Ocu-Merox®

Pharmacologic Category Antibiotic, Ophthalmic

Synonyms Yellow Mercuric Oxide

Use Treatment of irritation and minor infections of the eyelids

Local Anesthetic/Vasoconstrictor Precautions No information available to require special precautions

Effects on Dental Treatment No effects or complications reported

Dosage Apply small amount to inner surface of lower eyelid once or twice daily

Generic Available Yes

Mercurochrome® *see* Merbromin *on page 770*
Meridia® *see* Sibutramine *on page 1085*

Meropenem (mer oh PEN em)

U.S. Brand Names Merrem® I.V.

Canadian Brand Names Merrem®

Mexican Brand Names Merrem®

Pharmacologic Category Antibiotic, Carbapenem

Use Meropenem is indicated as single agent therapy for the treatment of intra-abdominal infections including complicated appendicitis and peritonitis in adults and bacterial meningitis in pediatric patients >3 months of age caused by *S. pneumoniae*, *H. influenzae*, and *N. meningitidis* (penicillin-resistant pneumococci have not been studied in clinical trials); it is better tolerated than imipenem and highly effective against a broad range of bacteria

Local Anesthetic/Vasoconstrictor Precautions No information available to require special precautions

Effects on Dental Treatment 1% to 10%: Oral moniliasis and glossitis

Dosage I.V.:

Neonates:

- Preterm: 20 mg/kg/dose every 12 hours (may be increased to 40 mg/kg/dose if treating a highly resistant organism such as *Pseudomonas aeruginosa*)
- Full-term (<3 months of age): 20 mg/kg/dose every 8 hours (may be increased to 40 mg/kg/dose if treating a highly resistant organism such as *Pseudomonas aeruginosa*)

Children >3 months (<50 kg):

- Intra-abdominal infections: 20 mg/kg every 8 hours (maximum dose: 1 g every 8 hours)
- Meningitis: 40 mg/kg every 8 hours (maximum dose: 2 g every 8 hours)

Children >50 kg:

- Intra-abdominal infections: 1 g every 8 hours
- Meningitis: 2 g every 8 hours

Adults: 1 g every 8 hours

Elderly: No differences in safety or efficacy have been reported. However, increased sensitivity may occur in some elderly patients; adjust dose based on renal function (see Warnings/Precautions)

Dosing adjustment in renal impairment: Adults:

- Cl_{cr} 26-50 mL/minute: Administer 1 g every 12 hours
- Cl_{cr} 10-25 mL/minute: Administer 500 mg every 12 hours
- Cl_{cr} <10 mL/minute: Administer 500 mg every 24 hours

Dialysis: Meropenem and its metabolites are readily dialyzable

Continuous arteriovenous or venovenous hemodiafiltration effects: Dose as Cl_{cr} 10-50 mL/minute

Mechanism of Action Inhibits bacterial cell wall synthesis by binding to several of the penicillin-binding proteins, which in turn inhibit the final transpeptidation step of peptidoglycan synthesis in bacterial cell walls, thus inhibiting cell wall biosynthesis; bacteria eventually lyse due to ongoing activity of cell wall autolytic enzymes (autolysins and murein hydrolases) while cell wall assembly is arrested

Other Adverse Effects 1% to 10%:

- Central nervous system: Headache (2%)
- Dermatologic: Rash (2% to 3%, includes diaper-area moniliasis in pediatrics), pruritus (1%)
- Gastrointestinal: Diarrhea (4% to 5%), nausea/vomiting (1% to 4%), constipation (1%), oral moniliasis (up to 2% in pediatric patients), glossitis
- Local: Inflammation at the injection site (2%), phlebitis/thrombophlebitis (1%), injection site reaction (1%)
- Respiratory: Apnea (1%)
- Miscellaneous: Sepsis (2%), septic shock (1%)

Warnings/Precautions Do not administer to patients with serious hypersensitivity reactions to beta-lactam agents. Seizures and other CNS events have been reported during treatment with meropenem; these experiences have occurred most commonly in patients with pre-existing CNS disorders, with bacterial meningitis, and/or decreased renal function; may cause pseudomembranous colitis

Drug Interactions Decreased Effect: Probenecid interferes with renal excretion of meropenem. Serum concentrations of valproic acid may be reduced during meropenem therapy (potentially to subtherapeutic levels).

Drug Uptake

Half-life, elimination:

- Normal renal function: 1-1.5 hours
- Cl_{cr} 30-80 mL/minute: 1.9-3.3 hours
- Cl_{cr} 2-30 mL/minute: 3.82-5.7 hours

Time to peak, tissue: 1 hour following infusion

Pregnancy Risk Factor B

Generic Available No

Comments 1 g of meropenem contains 90.2 mg of sodium as sodium carbonate (3.92 mEq)

(Continued)

Meropenem *(Continued)*

Selected Readings Wiseman LR, Wagstaff AJ, Brogden RN, et al, "Meropenem. A Review of Its Antibacterial Activity, Pharmacokinetic Properties, and Clinical Efficacy," *Drugs*, 1995, 50(1):73-101.

Merrem® I.V. *see* Meropenem *on page 771*

Mersol® [OTC] *see* Thimerosal *on page 1157*

Merthiolate® [OTC] *see* Thimerosal *on page 1157*

Meruvax® II *see* Rubella Virus Vaccine, Live *on page 1070*

Mesalamine (me SAL a meen)

U.S. Brand Names Asacol®; Canasa™; Pentasa®; Rowasa®

Canadian Brand Names Asacol®; Mesasal®; Novo-5 ASA; Pentasa®; Quintasa®; Rowasa®; Salofalk®

Mexican Brand Names Salofalk®

Pharmacologic Category 5-Aminosalicylic Acid Derivative

Synonyms 5-Aminosalicylic Acid; 5-ASA; Fisalamine; Mesalazine

Use

Oral: Treatment and maintenance of remission of mildly to moderately active ulcerative colitis

Rectal: Treatment of active mild to moderate distal ulcerative colitis, proctosigmoiditis, or proctitis

Local Anesthetic/Vasoconstrictor Precautions No information available to require special precautions

Effects on Dental Treatment No effects or complications reported

Dosage

Adults (usual course of therapy is 3-8 weeks):
- Oral:
  - Treatment of ulcerative colitis:
    - Capsule: 1 g 4 times/day
    - Tablet: Initial: 800 mg (2 tablets) 3 times/day for 6 weeks
  - Maintenance of remission of ulcerative colitis:
    - Capsule: 1 g 4 times/day
    - Tablet: 1.6 g/day in divided doses
- Rectal:
  - Retention enema: 60 mL (4 g) at bedtime, retained overnight, ~ 8 hours
  - Rectal suppository: Insert 1 suppository in rectum twice daily; retain suppositories for at least 1-3 hours to achieve maximum benefit
    - Canasa™: May increase to 3 times/day if inadequate response is seen after 2 weeks.
- **Note:** Some patients may require rectal and oral therapy concurrently.

Elderly: See adult dosing; use with caution

Mechanism of Action Mesalamine (5-aminosalicylic acid) is the active component of sulfasalazine; the specific mechanism of action of mesalamine is unknown; however, it is thought that it modulates local chemical mediators of the inflammatory response, especially leukotrienes; action appears topical rather than systemic

Other Adverse Effects Adverse effects vary depending upon dosage form. Effects as reported with tablets, unless otherwise noted:

>10%:
- Central nervous system: Pain (14%)
- Gastrointestinal: Abdominal pain (18%; enema: 8%)
- Genitourinary: Eructation (16%)
- Respiratory: Pharyngitis (11%)

1% to 10%:
- Cardiovascular: Chest pain (3%), peripheral edema (3%)
- Central nervous system: Chills (3%), dizziness (suppository: 3%), fever (enema: 3%; suppository: 1%), insomnia (2%), malaise (2%)
- Dermatologic: Rash (6%; suppository: 1%), pruritus (3%; enema: 1%), acne (2%; suppository: 1%)
- Gastrointestinal: Dyspepsia (6%), constipation (5%), vomiting (5%), colitis exacerbation (3%; suppository: 1%), nausea (capsule: 3%), flatulence (enema: 6%), hemorrhoids (enema: 1%), nausea and vomiting (capsule: 1%), rectal pain (enema: 1%; suppository: 2%)
- Local: Pain on insertion of enema tip (enema: 1%)
- Neuromuscular & skeletal: Back pain (7%; enema: 1%), arthralgia (5%), hypertonia (5%), myalgia (3%), arthritis (2%), leg/joint pain (enema: 2%),
- Ocular: Conjunctivitis (2%)
- Respiratory: Flu-like syndrome (3%; enema: 5%), diaphoresis (3%), cough increased (2%)

Drug Interactions Decreases digoxin bioavailability

Drug Uptake

Absorption:
- Rectal: ~15%; variable and dependent upon retention time, underlying GI disease, and colonic pH

Oral: Tablet: ~28% absorbed, capsule: ~20% to 30% absorbed
Half-life, elimination: 5-ASA: 0.5-1.5 hours; Acetyl 5-ASA: 5-10 hours
Time to peak: 4-7 hours

Pregnancy Risk Factor B

Generic Available No

Mesoridazine (mez oh RID a zeen)

U.S. Brand Names Serentil®

Canadian Brand Names Serentil®

Pharmacologic Category Antipsychotic Agent, Phenothiazine, Piperidine

Synonyms Mesoridazine Besylate

Use Management of schizophrenic patients who fail to respond adequately to treatment with other antipsychotic drugs, either because of insufficient effectiveness or the inability to achieve an effective dose due to intolerable adverse effects from these drugs

Unlabeled/Investigational: Psychosis

Local Anesthetic/Vasoconstrictor Precautions No information available to require special precautions

Effects on Dental Treatment No effects or complications reported

Dosage Concentrate may be diluted just prior to administration with distilled water, acidified tap water, orange or grape juice; do not prepare and store bulk dilutions

Adults:

Oral: 25-50 mg 3 times/day; maximum: 100-400 mg/day

I.M.: 25 mg initially, repeat in 30-60 minutes as needed; optimal dosage range: 25-200 mg/day

Mechanism of Action Blockade of postsynaptic CNS dopamine$_2$ receptors in the mesolimbic and mesocortical areas

Other Adverse Effects Frequency not defined:

Cardiovascular: Hypotension, orthostatic hypotension, tachycardia, QT prolongation (dose dependent, up to 100% of patients at higher dosages), syncope, edema

Central nervous system: Pseudoparkinsonism, akathisia, dystonias, tardive dyskinesia, dizziness, drowsiness, restlessness, ataxia, slurred speech, neuroleptic malignant syndrome (NMS), impairment of temperature regulation, lowering of seizure threshold

Dermatologic: Increased sensitivity to sun, rash, itching, angioneurotic edema, dermatitis, discoloration of skin (blue-gray)

Endocrine & metabolic: Changes in menstrual cycle, changes in libido, gynecomastia, lactation, galactorrhea

Gastrointestinal: Constipation, xerostomia, weight gain, nausea, vomiting, stomach pain

Genitourinary: Difficulty in urination, ejaculatory disturbances, impotence, enuresis, incontinence, priapism, urinary retention

Hematologic: Agranulocytosis, leukopenia, eosinophilia, thrombocytopenia, anemia, aplastic anemia

Hepatic: Cholestatic jaundice, hepatotoxicity

Neuromuscular & skeletal: Weakness, tremor, rigidity

Ocular: Pigmentary retinopathy, photophobia, blurred vision, cornea and lens changes

Respiratory: Nasal congestion

Miscellaneous: Diaphoresis (decreased), lupus-like syndrome

Contraindications Hypersensitivity to mesoridazine or any component of the formulation (cross-reactivity between phenothiazines may occur); severe CNS depression and coma; prolonged QT interval (>450 msec), including prolongation due to congenital causes; history of arrhythmias; concurrent use of medications which prolong QT_c (including type Ia and type III antiarrhythmics, cyclic antidepressants, some fluoroquinolones, cisapride); concurrent use of mesoridazine with fluvoxamine, fluoxetine, or paroxetine

Drug Interactions CYP1A2, 2D6, and 3A3/4 enzyme substrate; CYP2D6 enzyme inhibitor

Aluminum salts: May decrease the absorption of phenothiazines; monitor

Amphetamines: Efficacy may be diminished by antipsychotics; in addition, amphetamines may increase psychotic symptoms; avoid concurrent use

Anticholinergics: May inhibit the therapeutic response to phenothiazines and excess anticholinergic effects may occur; includes benztropine, trihexyphenidyl, biperiden, and drugs with significant anticholinergic activity (TCAs, antihistamines, disopyramide)

Antihypertensives: Concurrent use of phenothiazines with an antihypertensive may produce additive hypotensive effects (particularly orthostasis)

Bromocriptine: Phenothiazines inhibit the ability of bromocriptine to lower serum prolactin concentrations

Chloroquine: Serum concentrations of chlorpromazine may be increased by chloroquine

(Continued)

Mesoridazine *(Continued)*

CNS depressants: Sedative effects may be additive with phenothiazines; monitor for increased effect; includes barbiturates, benzodiazepines, narcotic analgesics, ethanol, and other sedative agents

CYP1A2 inhibitors: Metabolism of phenothiazines may be decreased; increasing clinical effect or toxicity. Inhibitors include cimetidine, ciprofloxacin, fluvoxamine, isoniazid, ritonavir, and zileuton. **Concurrent use with fluvoxamine is contraindicated.**

CYP2D6 inhibitors: Metabolism of phenothiazines may be decreased; increasing clinical effect or toxicity. Inhibitors include amiodarone, cimetidine, delavirdine, fluoxetine, paroxetine, propafenone, quinidine, and ritonavir; monitor for increased effect/toxicity. **Concurrent use with fluoxetine and paroxetine is contraindicated.**

CYP3A3/4 inhibitors: Metabolism of phenothiazines may be decreased; increasing clinical effect or toxicity; inhibitors include amiodarone, cimetidine, clarithromycin, erythromycin, delavirdine, diltiazem, dirithromycin, disulfiram, fluoxetine, fluvoxamine, grapefruit juice, indinavir, itraconazole, ketoconazole, nefazodone, nevirapine, propoxyphene, quinupristin-dalfopristin, ritonavir, saquinavir, verapamil, zafirlukast, zileuton

Enzyme inducers: May enhance the hepatic metabolism of phenothiazines; larger doses may be required. Includes rifampin, rifabutin, barbiturates, phenytoin, and cigarette smoking

Epinephrine: Chlorpromazine (and possibly other low potency antipsychotics) may diminish the pressor effects of epinephrine

Guanethidine and guanadrel: Antihypertensive effects may be inhibited by chlorpromazine

Levodopa: Chlorpromazine may inhibit the antiparkinsonian effect of levodopa; avoid this combination

Lithium: Chlorpromazine may produce neurotoxicity with lithium; this is a rare effect

Metoclopramide: May increase extrapyramidal symptoms (EPS) or risk.

Phenytoin: May reduce serum levels of phenothiazines; phenothiazines may increase phenytoin serum levels

Propranolol: Serum concentrations of phenothiazines may be increased; propranolol also increases phenothiazine concentrations; may also occur with pindolol. **These agents are contraindicated with mesoridazine.**

Polypeptide antibiotics: Rare cases of respiratory paralysis have been reported with concurrent use of phenothiazines

QT_c-prolonging agents: Effects on QT_c interval may be additive with phenothiazines, increasing the risk of malignant arrhythmias; includes type Ia antiarrhythmics, TCAs, and some quinolone antibiotics (sparfloxacin, moxifloxacin and gatifloxacin). **Concurrent use is contraindicated.**

Sulfadoxine-pyrimethamine: May increase phenothiazine concentrations

Tricyclic antidepressants: Concurrent use may produce increased toxicity or altered therapeutic response

Trazodone: Phenothiazines and trazodone may produce additive hypotensive effects

Valproic acid: Serum levels may be increased by phenothiazines

Drug Uptake

Absorption: Tablet: Erratic; Liquid: More dependable

Duration: 4-6 hours

Half-life, elimination: 24-48 hours

Time to peak: 2-4 hours; Steady-state serum: 4-7 days

Pregnancy Risk Factor C

Generic Available No

Mestranol and Norethindrone (MES tra nole & nor eth IN drone)

Related Information

Endocrine Disorders and Pregnancy *on page 1331*

U.S. Brand Names Necon® 1/50; Norinyl® 1+50; Ortho-Novum® 1/50

Canadian Brand Names Ortho-Novum® 1/50

Pharmacologic Category Contraceptive; Estrogen and Progestin Combination

Synonyms Norethindrone and Mestranol

Use Prevention of pregnancy

Unlabeled/Investigational: Treatment of hypermenorrhea, endometriosis, female hypogonadism

Local Anesthetic/Vasoconstrictor Precautions No information available to require special precautions

Effects on Dental Treatment When prescribing antibiotics, patients must be advised to use additional methods of birth control when taking hormonal contraceptives.

Dosage Oral: Adults: Female: Contraception:

Schedule 1 (Sunday starter): Dose begins on first Sunday after onset of menstruation; if the menstrual period starts on Sunday, take first tablet that very same day.

With a Sunday start, an additional method of contraception should be used until after the first 7 days of consecutive administration.

For 21-tablet package: Dosage is 1 tablet daily for 21 consecutive days, followed by 7 days off of the medication; a new course begins on the 8th day after the last tablet is taken.

For 28-tablet package: Dosage is 1 tablet daily without interruption.

Schedule 2 (Day 1 starter): Dose starts on first day of menstrual cycle taking 1 tablet daily.

For 21-tablet package: Dosage is 1 tablet daily for 21 consecutive days, followed by 7 days off of the medication; a new course begins on the 8th day after the last tablet is taken.

For 28-tablet package: Dosage is 1 tablet daily without interruption.

If all doses have been taken on schedule and one menstrual period is missed, continue dosing cycle. If two consecutive menstrual periods are missed, pregnancy test is required before new dosing cycle is started.

Missed doses **monophasic formulations** (refer to package insert for complete information):

One dose missed: Take as soon as remembered or take 2 tablets next day

Two consecutive doses missed in the first 2 weeks: Take 2 tablets as soon as remembered or 2 tablets next 2 days. **An additional method of contraception should be used for 7 days after missed dose.**

Two consecutive doses missed in week 3 or three consecutive doses missed at any time: **An additional method of contraception must be used for 7 days after a missed dose:**

Schedule 1 (Sunday starter): Continue dose of 1 tablet daily until Sunday, then discard the rest of the pack, and a new pack should be started that same day.

Schedule 2 (Day 1 starter): Current pack should be discarded, and a new pack should be started that same day.

Dosage adjustment in hepatic impairment: Contraindicated in patients with hepatic impairment

Mechanism of Action Combination oral contraceptives inhibit ovulation via a negative feedback mechanism on the hypothalamus, which alters the normal pattern of gonadotropin secretion of a follicle-stimulating hormone (FSH) and luteinizing hormone by the anterior pituitary. The follicular phase FSH and midcycle surge of gonadotropins are inhibited. In addition, combination hormonal contraceptives produce alterations in the genital tract, including changes in the cervical mucus, rendering it unfavorable for sperm penetration even if ovulation occurs. Changes in the endometrium may also occur, producing an unfavorable environment for nidation. Combination hormonal contraceptive drugs may alter the tubal transport of the ova through the fallopian tubes. Progestational agents may also alter sperm fertility.

Other Adverse Effects Frequency not defined:

Cardiovascular: Arterial thromboembolism, cerebral hemorrhage, cerebral thrombosis, edema, hypertension, mesenteric thrombosis, myocardial infarction

Central nervous system: Depression, dizziness, headache, migraine, nervousness, premenstrual syndrome, stroke

Dermatologic: Acne, erythema multiforme, erythema nodosum, hirsutism, loss of scalp hair, melasma (may persist), rash (allergic)

Endocrine & metabolic: Amenorrhea, breakthrough bleeding, breast enlargement, breast secretion, breast tenderness, carbohydrate intolerance, lactation decreased (postpartum), glucose tolerance decreased, libido changes, menstrual flow changes, sex hormone-binding globulins (SHBG) increased, spotting, temporary infertility (following discontinuation), thyroid-binding globulin increased, triglycerides increased

Gastrointestinal: Abdominal cramps, appetite changes, bloating, cholestasis, colitis, gallbladder disease, jaundice, nausea, vomiting, weight gain/loss

Genitourinary: Cervical erosion changes, cervical secretion changes, cystitis-like syndrome, vaginal candidiasis, vaginitis

Hematologic: Antithrombin III decreased, folate levels decreased, hemolytic uremic syndrome, norepinephrine induced platelet aggregability increased, porphyria, prothrombin increased; factors VII, VIII, IX, and X increased

Hepatic: Benign liver tumors, Budd-Chiari syndrome, cholestatic jaundice, hepatic adenomas

Local: Thrombophlebitis

Ocular: Cataracts, change in corneal curvature (steepening), contact lens intolerance, optic neuritis, retinal thrombosis

Renal: Impaired renal function

Respiratory: Pulmonary thromboembolism

Miscellaneous: Hemorrhagic eruption

Drug Interactions Ethinyl estradiol: CYP3A3/4 enzyme substrate; mestranol: CYP2C9 enzyme substrate

Increased Effect/Toxicity: Acetaminophen and ascorbic acid may increase plasma concentrations of estrogen component. Atorvastatin and indinavir increase plasma concentrations of combination hormonal contraceptives. Combination hormonal contraceptives increase the plasma concentrations of alprazolam, chlordiazepoxide, cyclosporine, diazepam, prednisolone, selegiline, theophylline,

(Continued)

Mestranol and Norethindrone *(Continued)*

tricyclic antidepressants. Combination hormonal contraceptives may increase (or decrease) the effects of coumarin derivatives.

Decreased Effect: Combination hormonal contraceptives may decrease plasma concentrations of acetaminophen, clofibric acid, lorazepam, morphine, oxazepam, salicylic acid, temazepam. Contraceptive effect decreased by acitretin, aminoglutethimide, amprenavir, anticonvulsants, griseofulvin, lopinavir, nelfinavir, nevirapine, penicillins (effect not consistent), rifampin, ritonavir, tetracyclines (effect not consistent) troglitazone. Combination hormonal contraceptives may decrease (or increase) the effects of coumarin derivatives.

Drug Uptake

Mestranol: Metabolism: Hepatic via demethylation to ethinyl estradiol via CYP2C9

See Norethindrone *on page 876*

See Ethinyl Estradiol *on page 474* for additional information

Pregnancy Risk Factor X

Generic Available Yes

Metadate® CD *see* Methylphenidate *on page 795*

Metadate™ ER *see* Methylphenidate *on page 795*

Metahydrin® *see* Trichlormethiazide *on page 1202*

Metamucil® [OTC] *see* Psyllium *on page 1025*

Metamucil® Smooth Texture [OTC] *see* Psyllium *on page 1025*

Metaproterenol (met a proe TER e nol)

Related Information

Respiratory Diseases *on page 1328*

U.S. Brand Names Alupent®

Pharmacologic Category $Beta_2$ Agonist

Synonyms Metaproterenol Sulfate; Orciprenaline Sulfate

Use Bronchodilator in reversible airway obstruction due to asthma or COPD; because of its delayed onset of action (1 hour) and prolonged effect (4 or more hours), this may not be the drug of choice for assessing response to a bronchodilator

Local Anesthetic/Vasoconstrictor Precautions No information available to require special precautions

Effects on Dental Treatment No effects or complications reported

Dosage

Oral:

Children:

<2 years: 0.4 mg/kg/dose given 3-4 times/day; in infants, the dose can be given every 8-12 hours

2-6 years: 1-2.6 mg/kg/day divided every 6 hours

6-9 years: 10 mg/dose 3-4 times/day

Children >9 years and Adults: 20 mg 3-4 times/day

Elderly: Initial: 10 mg 3-4 times/day, increasing as necessary up to 20 mg 3-4 times/day

Inhalation: Children >12 years and Adults: 2-3 inhalations every 3-4 hours, up to 12 inhalations in 24 hours

Nebulizer:

Children: 0.01-0.02 mL/kg of 5% solution; minimum dose: 0.1 mL; maximum dose: 0.3 mL diluted in 2-3 mL normal saline every 4-6 hours (may be given more frequently according to need)

Adolescents and Adults: 5-20 breaths of full strength 5% metaproterenol **or** 0.2 to 0.3 mL 5% metaproterenol in 2.5-3 mL normal saline until nebulized every 4-6 hours (can be given more frequently according to need)

Mechanism of Action Relaxes bronchial smooth muscle by action on $beta_2$-receptors with very little effect on heart rate

Other Adverse Effects

>10%:

Cardiovascular: Tachycardia (<17%)

Central nervous system: Nervousness (3% to 14%)

Neuromuscular & skeletal: Tremor (1% to 33%)

1% to 10%:

Cardiovascular: Palpitations (<4%)

Central nervous system: Headache (<4%), dizziness (1% to 4%), insomnia (2%)

Gastrointestinal: Nausea, vomiting, bad taste, heartburn (≥4%), xerostomia

Neuromuscular & skeletal: Trembling, muscle cramps, weakness (1%)

Respiratory: Coughing, pharyngitis (≤4%)

Miscellaneous: Diaphoresis (increased) (≤4%)

Drug Interactions

Increased Effect/Toxicity: Sympathomimetics, TCAs, MAO inhibitors taken with metaproterenol may result in toxicity.

Decreases effect of beta-blockers

Drug Uptake
Onset of action: Bronchodilation: Oral: ~15 minutes; Inhalation: ~60 seconds
Peak effect: Oral: ~1 hour
Duration: ~1-5 hours

Pregnancy Risk Factor C

Generic Available Yes (except inhaler)

Metaxalone (me TAKS a lone)

U.S. Brand Names Skelaxin®

Canadian Brand Names Skelaxin®

Pharmacologic Category Skeletal Muscle Relaxant

Use Relief of discomfort associated with acute, painful musculoskeletal conditions

Local Anesthetic/Vasoconstrictor Precautions No information available to require special precautions

Effects on Dental Treatment No effects or complications reported

Dosage Children >12 years and Adults: Oral: 800 mg 3-4 times/day

Mechanism of Action Does not have a direct effect on skeletal muscle; most of its therapeutic effect comes from actions on the CNS

Other Adverse Effects Frequency not defined:
Central nervous system: Paradoxical stimulation, headache, drowsiness, dizziness, irritability
Dermatologic: Allergic dermatitis
Gastrointestinal: Nausea, vomiting, stomach cramps
Hematologic: Leukopenia, hemolytic anemia
Hepatic: Hepatotoxicity
Miscellaneous: Anaphylaxis

Drug Interactions Additive effects with CNS depressants

Drug Uptake
Onset of action: ~1 hour
Duration: ~4-6 hours
Half-life, elimination: 2-3 hours

Pregnancy Risk Factor C

Generic Available No

Metformin (met FOR min)

Related Information
Endocrine Disorders and Pregnancy *on page 1331*

U.S. Brand Names Glucophage®; Glucophage® XR

Canadian Brand Names Apo®-Metformin; Gen-Metformin; Glucophage®; Glycon; Novo-Metformin; Nu-Metformin; Rho®-Metformin

Mexican Brand Names Dabex®; Dimefor®; Glucophage®; Glucophage® Forte

Pharmacologic Category Antidiabetic Agent, Biguanide

Synonyms Metformin Hydrochloride

Use Management of type 2 diabetes mellitus (noninsulin dependent, NIDDM) as monotherapy when hyperglycemia cannot be managed on diet alone. May be used concomitantly with a sulfonylurea or insulin to improve glycemic control.
Unlabeled/Investigational: Treatment of HIV lipodystrophy syndrome

Local Anesthetic/Vasoconstrictor Precautions No information available to require special precautions

Effects on Dental Treatment Metformin-dependent diabetics (noninsulin dependent, type 2) should be appointed for dental treatment in morning in order to minimize chance of stress-induced hypoglycemia.

Dosage Allow 1-2 weeks between dose titrations: Generally, clinically significant responses are not seen at doses <1500 mg daily; however, a lower recommended starting dose and gradual increased dosage is recommended to minimize GI symptoms
Children 10-16 years: Management of type 2 diabetes mellitus: Oral: 500 mg tablets: Initial: 500 mg twice daily (give with the morning and evening meals); dosage increases should be made in increments of 1 tablet every week, given in divided doses, up to a maximum of 2000 mg/day
Adults: ≥17 years: Management of type 2 diabetes mellitus: Oral:
500 mg tablets: Initial: 500 mg twice daily (give with the morning and evening meals); dosage increases should be made in increments of 1 tablet every week, given in divided doses, up to a maximum of 2500 mg/day. Doses of up to 2000 mg/day may be given twice daily; if a dose of 2500 mg/day is required, it may be better tolerated 3 times/day (with meals).
850 mg tablets: Initial: 850 mg once daily (give with the morning meal); dosage increases should be made in increments of 1 tablet every **other** week, given in divided doses, up to a maximum of 2550 mg/day. Usual maintenance dose: 850 mg twice daily (with the morning and evening meals). Some patients may be given 850 mg 3 times/day (with meals).
Extended release tablets: Initial: 500 mg once daily (with the evening meal); dosage may be increased by 500 mg weekly; maximum dose: 2000 mg once daily. If glycemic control is not achieved at maximum dose, may divide dose to

(Continued)

Metformin *(Continued)*

1000 mg twice daily; if doses >2000 mg/day are needed, switch to regular release tablets and titrate to maximum dose of 2550 mg/day

Elderly: The initial and maintenance dosing should be conservative, due to the potential for decreased renal function. Generally, elderly patients should not be titrated to the maximum dose of metformin. Do not use in patients ≥80 years of age unless normal renal function has been established.

Transfer from other antidiabetic agents: No transition period is generally necessary except when transferring from chlorpropamide. When transferring from chlorpropamide, care should be exercised during the first 2 weeks because of the prolonged retention of chlorpropamide in the body, leading to overlapping drug effects and possible hypoglycemia.

Concomitant metformin and oral sulfonylurea therapy: If patients have not responded to 4 weeks of the maximum dose of metformin monotherapy, consider a gradual addition of an oral sulfonylurea, even if prior primary or secondary failure to a sulfonylurea has occurred. Continue metformin at the maximum dose.

Failed sulfonylurea therapy: Patients with prior failure on glyburide may be treated by gradual addition of metformin. Initiate with glyburide 20 mg and metformin 500 mg daily. Metformin dosage may be increased by 500 mg/day at weekly intervals, up to a maximum of 2500 mg/day (dosage of glyburide maintained at 20 mg/day).

Concomitant metformin and insulin therapy: Initial: 500 mg metformin once daily, continue current insulin dose; increase by 500 mg metformin weekly until adequate glycemic control is achieved

Maximum dose: 2500 mg metformin; 2000 mg metformin extended release

Decrease insulin dose 10% to 25% when FPG <120 mg/dL; monitor and make further adjustments as needed

Dosing adjustment/comments in renal impairment: The plasma and blood half-life of metformin is prolonged and the renal clearance is decreased in proportion to the decrease in creatinine clearance. Metformin is contraindicated in the presence of renal dysfunction defined as a serum creatinine >1.5 mg/dL in males or >1.4 mg/dL in females or a creatinine clearance <60 mL/minute.

Dosing adjustment in hepatic impairment: Avoid metformin; liver disease is a risk factor for the development of lactic acidosis during metformin therapy.

Mechanism of Action Decreases hepatic glucose production, decreasing intestinal absorption of glucose and improves insulin sensitivity (increases peripheral glucose uptake and utilization)

Other Adverse Effects

>10%:

Gastrointestinal: Nausea/vomiting (6% to 25%), diarrhea (10% to 53%), flatulence (12%)

Neuromuscular & skeletal: Weakness (9%)

1% to 10%:

Cardiovascular: Chest discomfort, flushing, palpitation

Central nervous system: Headache (6%), chills, dizziness, lightheadedness

Dermatologic: Rash

Endocrine & metabolic: Hypoglycemia

Gastrointestinal: Indigestion (7%), abdominal discomfort (6%), abdominal distention, abnormal stools, constipation, dyspepsia/ heartburn, taste disorder

Neuromuscular & skeletal: Myalgia

Respiratory: Dyspnea, upper respiratory tract infection

Miscellaneous: Decreased vitamin B_{12} levels (7%), increased diaphoresis, flu-like syndrome, nail disorder

Drug Interactions

Increased Effect/Toxicity: Furosemide and cimetidine may increase metformin blood levels. Cationic drugs (eg, amiloride, digoxin, morphine, procainamide, quinidine, quinine, ranitidine, triamterene, trimethoprim, and vancomycin) which are eliminated by renal tubular secretion have the potential to increase metformin levels by competing for common renal tubular transport systems.

Decreased Effect: Drugs which tend to produce hyperglycemia (eg, diuretics, corticosteroids, phenothiazines, thyroid products, estrogens, oral contraceptives, phenytoin, nicotinic acid, sympathomimetics, calcium channel blocking drugs, isoniazid) may lead to a loss of glucose control.

Drug Uptake

Onset of action: Within days; maximum effects ≤2 weeks

Half-life, elimination, plasma: 6.2 hours

Pregnancy Risk Factor B

Generic Available Yes: Regular release only

Methadone (METH a done)

U.S. Brand Names Dolophine®; Methadose®

Canadian Brand Names Dolophine®; Metadol™; Methadose®

Pharmacologic Category Analgesic, Narcotic

Synonyms Methadone Hydrochloride

Use Management of severe pain; detoxification and maintenance treatment of narcotic addiction (if used for detoxification and maintenance treatment of narcotic addiction, it must be part of an FDA-approved program)

Local Anesthetic/Vasoconstrictor Precautions No information available to require special precautions

Effects on Dental Treatment 1% to 10%: Significant xerostomia; disappears with discontinuation

Restrictions C-II

Dosage Doses should be titrated to appropriate effects.

Children:

Analgesia:

Oral, I.M., S.C.: 0.7 mg/kg/24 hours divided every 4-6 hours as needed or 0.1-0.2 mg/kg every 4-12 hours as needed; maximum: 10 mg/dose

I.V.: 0.1 mg/kg every 4 hours initially for 2-3 doses, then every 6-12 hours as needed; maximum: 10 mg/dose

Iatrogenic narcotic dependency: Oral: General guidelines: Initial: 0.05-0.1 mg/kg/dose every 6 hours; increase by 0.05 mg/kg/dose until withdrawal symptoms are controlled; after 24-48 hours, the dosing interval can be lengthened to every 12-24 hours; to taper dose, wean by 0.05 mg/kg/day; if withdrawal symptoms recur, taper at a slower rate

Adults:

Analgesia: Oral, I.M., S.C.: 2.5-10 mg every 3-8 hours as needed, up to 5-20 mg every 6-8 hours. Higher doses may be required in patients with severe, debilitating pain or in patients who have become narcotic tolerant.

Detoxification: Oral: 15-40 mg/day

Maintenance treatment of opiate dependence: Oral: 20-120 mg/day

Dosing adjustment in renal impairment: Cl_{cr} <10 mL/minute: Administer at 50% to 75% of normal dose

Dosing adjustment/comments in hepatic disease: Avoid in severe liver disease

Important note: Methadone accumulates with repeated doses and dosage may need to be adjusted downward after 3-5 days to prevent toxic effects. Some patients may benefit from every 8- to 12-hour dosing interval (pain control).

Mechanism of Action Binds to opiate receptors in the CNS, causing inhibition of ascending pain pathways, altering the perception of and response to pain; produces generalized CNS depression

Other Adverse Effects Frequency not defined:

Cardiovascular: Bradycardia, peripheral vasodilation, cardiac arrest, syncope, faintness

Central nervous system: Euphoria, dysphoria, headache, insomnia, agitation, disorientation, drowsiness, dizziness, lightheadedness, sedation

Dermatologic: Pruritus, urticaria, rash

Endocrine & metabolic: Decreased libido

Gastrointestinal: Nausea, vomiting, constipation, anorexia, stomach cramps, xerostomia, biliary tract spasm

Genitourinary: Urinary retention or hesitancy, antidiuretic effect, impotence

Neuromuscular & skeletal: Weakness

Ocular: Miosis, visual disturbances

Respiratory: Respiratory depression, respiratory arrest

Miscellaneous: Physical and psychological dependence

Drug Interactions CYP1A2, 2D6, and 3A3/4 enzyme substrate; CYP2D6 enzyme inhibitor

Increased Effect/Toxicity: Fluconazole, itraconazole, and ketoconazole increase serum methadone concentrations via CYP3A3/4 inhibition; an increased narcotic effect may be experienced. Similar effects may be seen with ritonavir, nelfinavir, amiodarone, erythromycin, clarithromycin, diltiazem, verapamil, paroxetine, fluoxetine, and other inhibitors of CYP2D6 or CYP3A3/4.

Decreased Effect: Barbiturates, carbamazepine, nevirapine, phenytoin, primidone, rifampin and ritonavir may decrease serum methadone concentrations via enhanced hepatic metabolism; monitor for methadone withdrawal. Larger doses of methadone may be required.

Drug Uptake

Onset of action: Oral: Analgesic: 0.5-1 hour; Parenteral: 10-20 minutes; Peak effect: Parenteral: 1-2 hours

Duration: Oral: 6-8 hours; Multiple dose: 22-48 hours

Half-life, elimination: 15-29 hours (may increase with alkaline pH)

Pregnancy Risk Factor B/D (prolonged use or high doses at term)

Generic Available Yes

Methadose® *see* Methadone *on page 778*

Methamphetamine (meth am FET a meen)

U.S. Brand Names Desoxyn®; Desoxyn® Gradumet®

Canadian Brand Names Desoxyn®

Pharmacologic Category Stimulant

Synonyms Desoxyephedrine Hydrochloride; Methamphetamine Hydrochloride

(Continued)

Methamphetamine *(Continued)*

Use Treatment of attention-deficit/hyperactivity disorder (ADHD); exogenous obesity (short-term adjunct)

Unlabeled/Investigational: Narcolepsy

Local Anesthetic/Vasoconstrictor Precautions Use vasoconstriction with caution in patients taking methamphetamine. Amphetamines enhance the sympathomimetic response of epinephrine and norepinephrine leading to potential hypertension and cardiotoxicity.

Effects on Dental Treatment Up to 10% of patients taking dextroamphetamines may present with hypertension. The use of local anesthetic without vasoconstrictor is recommended in these patients.

Restrictions C-II

Dosage

Children >6 years and Adults: ADHD: 2.5-5 mg 1-2 times/day; may increase by 5 mg increments at weekly intervals until optimum response is achieved, usually 20-25 mg/day

Children >12 years and Adults: Exogenous obesity: 5 mg 30 minutes before each meal; long-acting formulation: 10-15 mg in morning; treatment duration should not exceed a few weeks

Mechanism of Action A sympathomimetic amine related to ephedrine and amphetamine with CNS stimulant activity; peripheral actions include elevation of systolic and diastolic BP and weak bronchodilator and respiratory stimulant action

Other Adverse Effects Frequency not defined:

Cardiovascular: Hypertension, tachycardia, palpitations

Central nervous system: Restlessness, headache, exacerbation of motor and phonic tics and Tourette's syndrome, dizziness, psychosis, dysphoria, overstimulation, euphoria, insomnia

Dermatologic: Rash, urticaria

Endocrine & metabolic: Change in libido

Gastrointestinal: Diarrhea, nausea, vomiting, stomach cramps, constipation, anorexia, weight loss, xerostomia, unpleasant taste

Genitourinary: Impotence

Neuromuscular & skeletal: Tremor

Miscellaneous: Suppression of growth in children, tolerance and withdrawal with prolonged use

Drug Interactions CYP2D6 enzyme substrate

Increased Effect/Toxicity: Amphetamines may precipitate hypertensive crisis or serotonin syndrome in patients receiving MAO inhibitors (selegiline >10 mg/day, isocarboxazid, phenelzine, tranylcypromine, furazolidone). Serotonin syndrome has also been associated with combinations of amphetamines and SSRIs; these combinations should be avoided. TCAs may enhance the effects of amphetamines, potentially leading to hypertensive crisis. Large doses of antacids or urinary alkalinizers increase the half-life and duration of action of amphetamines. May precipitate arrhythmias in patients receiving general anesthetics. Inhibitors of CYP2D6 may increase the effects of amphetamines (includes amiodarone, cimetidine, delavirdine, fluoxetine, paroxetine, propafenone, quinidine, and ritonavir).

Decreased Effect: Amphetamines inhibit the antihypertensive response to guanethidine and guanadrel. Urinary acidifiers decrease the half-life and duration of action of amphetamines. Enzyme inducers (barbiturates, carbamazepine, phenytoin, and rifampin) may decrease serum concentration of amphetamines.

Drug Uptake Duration: 12-24 hours

Pregnancy Risk Factor C

Generic Available Yes

Methantheline (meth AN tha leen)

U.S. Brand Names Banthine®

Canadian Brand Names Banthine®

Pharmacologic Category Anticholinergic Agent

Synonyms Methantheline Bromide; Methanthelinium Bromide

Use Adjunctive treatment of peptic ulcer, irritable bowel syndrome, pancreatitis, ureteral and urinary bladder spasm; to reduce duodenal motility during diagnostic radiologic procedures and treatment of an uninhibited neurogenic bladder

Local Anesthetic/Vasoconstrictor Precautions No information available to require special precautions

Effects on Dental Treatment >10%: Xerostomia

Dosage Oral:

Neonates: 12.5 mg twice daily then 3 times/day

Children:

- <1 year: 12.5-25 mg 4 times/day
- >1 year: 12.5-50 mg 4 times/day

Adults: 50-100 mg every 6 hours

Other Adverse Effects

>10%:

Dermatologic: Itching

Gastrointestinal: Nausea

1% to 10%:

Cardiovascular: Severe edema, hypotension

Central nervous system: Nervousness, vertigo, depression

Dermatologic: Painful blistering, burning, and peeling of skin; pruritus, freckling, hypopigmentation, rash, cheilitis, erythema

Neuromuscular & skeletal: Loss of muscle coordination

Pregnancy Risk Factor C

Generic Available No

Methazolamide (meth a ZOE la mide)

U.S. Brand Names Neptazane®

Canadian Brand Names Neptazane®

Pharmacologic Category Carbonic Anhydrase Inhibitor; Diuretic, Carbonic Anhydrase Inhibitor; Ophthalmic Agent, Antiglaucoma

Use Adjunctive treatment of open-angle or secondary glaucoma; short-term therapy of narrow-angle glaucoma when delay of surgery is desired

Local Anesthetic/Vasoconstrictor Precautions No information available to require special precautions

Effects on Dental Treatment No effects or complications reported

Dosage Adults: Oral: 50-100 mg 2-3 times/day

Mechanism of Action Noncompetitive inhibition of the enzyme carbonic anhydrase; thought that carbonic anhydrase is located at the luminal border of cells of the proximal tubule. When the enzyme is inhibited, there is an increase in urine volume and a change to an alkaline pH with a subsequent decrease in the excretion of titratable acid and ammonia.

Other Adverse Effects Frequency not defined:

Central nervous system: Malaise, fever, mental depression, drowsiness, dizziness, nervousness, headache, confusion, seizures, fatigue, trembling, unsteadiness

Dermatologic: Urticaria, pruritus, photosensitivity, rash, Stevens-Johnson syndrome

Endocrine & metabolic: Hyperchloremic metabolic acidosis, hypokalemia, hyperglycemia

Gastrointestinal: Metallic taste, anorexia, nausea, vomiting, diarrhea, constipation, weight loss, GI irritation, xerostomia, black tarry stools

Genitourinary: Polyuria, crystalluria, hematuria, polyuria, renal calculi, impotence

Hematologic: Bone marrow depression, thrombocytopenia, thrombocytopenic purpura, hemolytic anemia, leukopenia, pancytopenia, agranulocytosis

Hepatic: Hepatic insufficiency

Neuromuscular & skeletal: Weakness, ataxia, paresthesias

Miscellaneous: Hypersensitivity

Warnings/Precautions Sulfonamide-type reactions can occur. Chemical similarities are present among sulfonamides, sulfonylureas, carbonic anhydrase inhibitors, thiazides, and loop diuretics (except ethacrynic acid). In patients with allergy to one of these compounds, a risk of cross-reaction exists; avoid use when previous reaction has been severe. Use with caution in patients with respiratory acidosis and diabetes mellitus; impairment of mental alertness and/or physical coordination. Malaise and complaints of tiredness and myalgia are signs of excessive dosing and acidosis in the elderly.

Drug Interactions

Increased Effect/Toxicity: Methazolamide may induce hypokalemia which would sensitize a patient to digitalis toxicity. Hypokalemia may be compounded with concurrent diuretic use or steroids. Methazolamide may increase the potential for salicylate toxicity. Primidone absorption may be delayed.

Decreased Effect: Increased lithium excretion and altered excretion of other drugs by alkalinization of the urine, such as amphetamines, quinidine, procainamide, methenamine, phenobarbital, and salicylates.

Drug Uptake

Onset of action: Slow in comparison with acetazolamide (2-4 hours)

Absorption: Slowly

Duration: 10-18 hours

Half-life, elimination: ~14 hours

Time to peak: 6-8 hours

Pregnancy Risk Factor C

Generic Available Yes

Methenamine (meth EN a meen)

U.S. Brand Names Hiprex®; Urex®

Canadian Brand Names Dehydral®; Hiprex®; Mandelamine®; Urasal®; Urex®

Pharmacologic Category Antibiotic, Miscellaneous

Synonyms Hexamethylenetetramine; Methenamine Hippurate; Methenamine Mandelate

(Continued)

Methenamine *(Continued)*

Use Prophylaxis or suppression of recurrent urinary tract infections; urinary tract discomfort secondary to hypermotility; should not be used in treatment of infections outside of urinary tract

Local Anesthetic/Vasoconstrictor Precautions No information available to require special precautions

Effects on Dental Treatment No effects or complications reported

Dosage Oral:

Children: 6-12 years:

Hippurate: 25-50 mg/kg/day divided every 12 hours

Mandelate: 50-75 mg/kg/day divided every 6 hours

Children >12 years and Adults:

Hippurate: 1 g twice daily

Mandelate: 1 g 4 times/day after meals and at bedtime

Mechanism of Action Methenamine is hydrolyzed to formaldehyde and ammonia in acidic urine; formaldehyde has nonspecific bactericidal action

Other Adverse Effects 1% to 10%:

Dermatologic: Rash (4%)

Gastrointestinal: Nausea, dyspepsia (4%)

Genitourinary: Dysuria (4%)

Drug Interactions

Increased Effect/Toxicity: Sulfonamides may precipitate in the urine.

Decreased Effect: Sodium bicarbonate and acetazolamide will decrease effect secondary to alkalinization of urine.

Drug Uptake

Absorption: Readily

Half-life, elimination: 3-6 hours

Pregnancy Risk Factor C

Generic Available Yes

Methenamine, Sodium Biphosphate, Phenyl Salicylate, Methylene Blue, and Hyoscyamine

(meth EN a meen, SOW dee um bye FOS fate, fen nil sa LIS i late, METH i leen bloo, & hye oh SYE a meen)

U.S. Brand Names Urimax™

Pharmacologic Category Antibiotic, Miscellaneous

Synonyms Hyoscyamine, Methenamine, Sodium Biphosphate, Phenyl Salicylate, and Methylene Blue; Methylene Blue, Methenamine, Sodium Biphosphate, Phenyl Salicylate, and Hyoscyamine; Phenyl Salicylate, Methenamine, Methylene Blue, Sodium Biphosphate, and Hyoscyamine; Sodium Biphosphate, Methenamine, Methylene Blue, Phenyl Salicylate, and Hyoscyamine

Use Treatment of symptoms of irritative voiding; relief of local symptoms associated with urinary tract infections; relief of urinary tract symptoms caused by diagnostic procedures

Local Anesthetic/Vasoconstrictor Precautions No information available to require special precautions

Effects on Dental Treatment No effects or complications reported

Dosage Oral:

Children >6 years: Dosage must be individualized

Adults: One tablet 4 times daily (followed by liberal fluid intake)

Other Adverse Effects Frequency not defined:

Cardiovascular: Tachycardia, flushing

Central nervous system: Dizziness

Gastrointestinal: Xerostomia, nausea, vomiting

Genitourinary: Urinary retention (acute), micturition difficulty, discoloration of urine (blue)

Ocular: Blurred vision

Respiratory: Dyspnea, shortness of breath

Drug Interactions See Hyoscyamine *on page 617* and Methenamine *on page 781*

Pregnancy Risk Factor C

Generic Available No

Methergine® *see* Methylergonovine *on page 795*

Methimazole (meth IM a zole)

Related Information

Endocrine Disorders and Pregnancy *on page 1331*

U.S. Brand Names Tapazole®

Canadian Brand Names Tapazole®

Pharmacologic Category Antithyroid Agent

Synonyms Thiamazole

Use Palliative treatment of hyperthyroidism, return the hyperthyroid patient to a normal metabolic state prior to thyroidectomy, and to control thyrotoxic crisis that may accompany thyroidectomy. The use of antithyroid thioamides is as effective in elderly as they are in younger adults; however, the expense, potential adverse effects, and inconvenience (compliance, monitoring) make them undesirable. The use of radioiodine due to ease of administration and less concern for long-term side effects and reproduction problems (some older males) makes it a more appropriate therapy.

Local Anesthetic/Vasoconstrictor Precautions No information available to require special precautions

Effects on Dental Treatment No effects or complications reported

Dosage Oral: Administer in 3 equally divided doses at ~ 8-hour intervals

Children: Initial: 0.4 mg/kg/day in 3 divided doses; maintenance: 0.2 mg/kg/day in 3 divided doses up to 30 mg/24 hours maximum

Adults: Initial: 5 mg every 8 hours; maintenance dose: 5-15 mg/day up to 60 mg/day for severe hyperthyroidism

Adjust dosage as required to achieve and maintain serum T_3, T_4, and TSH levels in the normal range. An elevated T_3 may be the sole indicator of inadequate treatment. An elevated TSH indicates excessive antithyroid treatment.

Mechanism of Action Inhibits the synthesis of thyroid hormones by blocking the oxidation of iodine in the thyroid gland, blocking iodine's ability to combine with tyrosine to form thyroxine and triiodothyronine (T_3), does not inactivate circulating T_4 and T_3

Other Adverse Effects Frequency not defined:

Cardiovascular: Edema

Central nervous system: Headache, vertigo, drowsiness, CNS stimulation, depression

Dermatologic: Skin rash, urticaria, pruritus, erythema nodosum, skin pigmentation, exfoliative dermatitis, alopecia

Endocrine & metabolic: Goiter

Gastrointestinal: Nausea, vomiting, stomach pain, abnormal taste, constipation, weight gain, salivary gland swelling

Hematologic: Leukopenia, agranulocytosis, granulocytopenia, thrombocytopenia, aplastic anemia, hypoprothrombinemia

Hepatic: Cholestatic jaundice, jaundice, hepatitis

Neuromuscular & skeletal: Arthralgia, paresthesia

Renal: Nephrotic syndrome

Miscellaneous: SLE-like syndrome

Drug Interactions Increased Effect/Toxicity: Increased toxicity with lithium or potassium iodide. Anticoagulant effect of warfarin may be increased. Dosage of some drugs (including beta-blockers, digoxin, and theophylline) require adjustment during treatment of hyperthyroidism.

Drug Uptake

Onset of action: Antithyroid: Oral: 12-18 hours

Duration: 36-72 hours

Half-life, elimination: 4-13 hours

Pregnancy Risk Factor D

Generic Available Yes

Methionine (me THYE oh neen)

U.S. Brand Names ME-500®; Pedameth®

Pharmacologic Category Amino Acid

Use Treatment of diaper rash and control of odor, dermatitis and ulceration caused by ammoniacal urine

Local Anesthetic/Vasoconstrictor Precautions No information available to require special precautions

Effects on Dental Treatment No effects or complications reported

Dosage Oral:

Children: Control of diaper rash: 75 mg in formula or other liquid 3-4 times/day for 3-5 days

Adults:

Control of odor in incontinent adults: 200-400 mg 3-4 times/day

Dietary supplement: 500 mg/day

Generic Available Yes

Methocarbamol (meth oh KAR ba mole)

Related Information

Temporomandibular Dysfunction (TMD) *on page 1397*

U.S. Brand Names Robaxin®

Canadian Brand Names Robaxin®

Pharmacologic Category Skeletal Muscle Relaxant

Use

Dental: Treatment of muscle spasm associated with acute temporomandibular joint pain

(Continued)

Methocarbamol *(Continued)*

Medical: Treatment of muscle spasm associated with acute painful musculoskeletal conditions, supportive therapy in tetanus

Local Anesthetic/Vasoconstrictor Precautions No information available to require special precautions

Effects on Dental Treatment No effects or complications reported

Dosage Adults: Muscle spasm: Oral: 1.5 g 4 times/day for 2-3 days, then decrease to 4-4.5 g/day in 3-6 divided doses

Mechanism of Action Causes skeletal muscle relaxation by reducing the transmission of impulses from the spinal cord to skeletal muscle

Other Adverse Effects Frequency not defined:

Cardiovascular: Flushing of face, bradycardia, hypotension

Central nervous system: Drowsiness, dizziness, lightheadedness, syncope, convulsion, vertigo, headache, fever

Dermatologic: Allergic dermatitis, urticaria, pruritus, rash

Gastrointestinal: Nausea, vomiting, metallic taste

Hematologic: Leukopenia

Local: Pain at injection site, thrombophlebitis

Ocular: Nystagmus, blurred vision, diplopia, conjunctivitis

Renal: Renal impairment

Respiratory: Nasal congestion

Miscellaneous: Allergic manifestations, anaphylactic reaction

Contraindications Hypersensitivity to methocarbamol or any component of the formulation; renal impairment

Warnings/Precautions Rate of injection should not exceed 3 mL/minute; solution is hypertonic; avoid extravasation; use with caution in patients with a history of seizures

Drug Interactions Increased effect/toxicity with CNS depressants; pyridostigmine (a single case of worsening myasthenia has been reported following methocarbamol administration)

Dietary/Ethanol/Herb Considerations

Ethanol: Avoid use; may increase CNS depression.

Food: Tablets may be crushed and mixed with food or liquid.

Herb/Nutraceutical: Avoid gotu kola, kava, SAme, St John's wort, and valerian; may increase CNS depression.

Drug Uptake

Onset of action: Muscle relaxation: Oral: ~30 minutes

Absorption: Rapid

Half-life, elimination: 1-2 hours

Time to peak: ~2 hours

Pregnancy Risk Factor C

Breast-feeding Considerations May be taken while breast-feeding

Dosage Forms INJ: 100 mg/mL [in polyethylene glycol 50%] (10 mL). **TAB:** 500 mg, 750 mg

Generic Available Yes

Methocarbamol and Aspirin (meth oh KAR ba mole & AS pir in)

U.S. Brand Names Robaxisal®

Canadian Brand Names Aspirin® Backache; Methoxisal; Methoxisal-C; Robaxisal®; Robaxisal® Extra Strength

Pharmacologic Category Skeletal Muscle Relaxant

Synonyms Aspirin and Methocarbamol

Use

Dental: Treatment of muscle spasm associated with acute temporomandibular joint pain

Medical: Treatment of muscle spasm associated with acute painful musculoskeletal conditions, supportive therapy in tetanus

Local Anesthetic/Vasoconstrictor Precautions No information available to require special precautions

Dosage Children >12 years and Adults: Oral: 2 tablets 4 times/day

Mechanism of Action Causes skeletal muscle relaxation by reducing the transmission of impulses from the spinal cord to skeletal muscle

Other Adverse Effects Frequency not defined:

Based on **methocarbamol** component:

Central nervous system: Drowsiness, dizziness, lightheadedness, syncope, convulsion, vertigo, headache, fever

Cardiovascular: Flushing of face, bradycardia, hypotension

Dermatologic: Allergic dermatitis, urticaria, pruritus, rash

Gastrointestinal: Nausea, vomiting, metallic taste

Hematologic: Leukopenia

Local: Pain at injection site, thrombophlebitis

Ocular: Nystagmus, blurred vision, diplopia, conjunctivitis

Renal: Renal impairment

Respiratory: Nasal congestion

Miscellaneous: Allergic manifestations, anaphylactic reaction

Based on **aspirin** component: As with all drugs which may affect hemostasis, bleeding is associated with aspirin. Hemorrhage may occur at virtually any site. Risk is dependent on multiple variables including dosage, concurrent use of multiple agents which alter hemostasis, and patient susceptibility. Many adverse effects of aspirin are dose-related, and are rare at low dosages. Other serious reactions are idiosyncratic, related to allergy or individual sensitivity. Accurate estimation of frequencies is not possible. The reactions listed below have been reported for aspirin.

Cardiovascular: Hypotension, tachycardia, dysrhythmias, edema

Central nervous system: Fatigue, insomnia, nervousness, agitation, confusion, dizziness, headache, lethargy, cerebral edema, hyperthermia, coma

Dermatologic: Rash, angioedema, urticaria

Endocrine and metabolic: Acidosis, hyperkalemia, dehydration, hypoglycemia (children), hyperglycemia, hypernatremia (buffered forms)

Gastrointestinal: Nausea, vomiting, dyspepsia, epigastric discomfort, heartburn, stomach pains, gastrointestinal ulceration (6% to 31%), gastric erosions, gastric erythema, duodenal ulcers

Hematologic: Anemia, disseminated intravascular coagulation, prolongation of prothrombin times, coagulopathy, thrombocytopenia, hemolytic anemia, bleeding, iron-deficiency anemia

Hepatic: Hepatotoxicity, increased transaminases, hepatitis (reversible)

Neuromuscular and skeletal: Rhabdomyolysis, weakness, acetabular bone destruction (OA)

Otic: Hearing loss, tinnitus

Renal: Interstitial nephritis, papillary necrosis, proteinuria, renal impairment, renal failure (including cases caused by rhabdomyolysis), increased BUN, increased serum creatinine

Respiratory: Asthma, bronchospasm, dyspnea, laryngeal edema, hyperpnea, tachypnea, respiratory alkalosis, noncardiogenic pulmonary edema

Miscellaneous: Anaphylaxis, prolonged pregnancy and labor, stillbirths, low birth weight, peripartum bleeding, Reye's syndrome

Case reports: Colonic ulceration, esophageal stricture, esophagitis with esophageal ulcer, esophageal hematoma, oral mucosal ulcers (aspirin-containing chewing gum), coronary artery spasm, conduction defect and atrial fibrillation (toxicity), delirium, ischemic brain infarction, colitis, rectal stenosis (suppository), cholestatic jaundice, periorbital edema, rhinosinusitis

Contraindications Hypersensitivity to methocarbamol, salicylates, other NSAIDs, tartrazine dye, or any component of their formulation; asthma; bleeding disorders (factor VII or IX deficiencies); renal impairment; pregnancy (full-dose aspirin in 3rd trimester)

Warnings/Precautions Use aspirin with caution in patients with platelet and bleeding disorders, renal dysfunction, erosive gastritis, or peptic ulcer disease, previous nonreaction does not guarantee future safe taking of medication; use with caution in impaired hepatic function; do not use aspirin in children <16 years of age for chickenpox or flu symptoms due to the association with Reye's syndrome

Avoid aspirin, if possible, for 1 week prior to surgery because of the possibility of postoperative bleeding

Elderly are a high-risk population for adverse effects from nonsteroidal anti-inflammatory agents. As much as 60% of elderly with GI complications to NSAIDs can develop peptic ulceration and/or hemorrhage asymptomatically. Also, concomitant disease and drug use contribute to the risk for GI adverse effects. Use lowest effective dose for shortest period possible. Consider renal function decline with age. Use with caution in patients with history of asthma

Drug Interactions

Based on **methocarbamol** component: Increased effect/toxicity with CNS depressants; pyridostigmine (a single case of worsening myasthenia has been reported following methocarbamol administration)

Based on **aspirin** component:

ACE inhibitors: The effects of ACE inhibitors may be blunted by aspirin administration, particularly at higher dosages.

Buspirone increases aspirin's free % *in vitro*.

Carbonic anhydrase inhibitors and corticosteroids have been associated with alteration in salicylate serum concentration.

Heparin and low molecular weight heparins: Concurrent use may increase the risk of bleeding.

Methotrexate serum concentration may be increased; consider discontinuing aspirin 2-3 days before high-dose methotrexate treatment or avoid concurrent use.

NSAIDs may increase the risk of GI adverse effects and bleeding. Serum concentrations of some NSAIDs may be decreased by aspirin.

Platelet inhibitors (IIb/IIIa antagonists): Risk of bleeding may be increased.

Probenecid effects may be antagonized by aspirin.

(Continued)

Methocarbamol and Aspirin *(Continued)*

Sulfonylureas: The effects of older sulfonylurea agents (tolazamide, tolbutamide) may be potentiated due to displacement from plasma proteins. This effect does not appear to be clinically significant for newer sulfonylurea agents (glyburide, glipizide, glimepiride).
Valproic acid may be displaced from its binding sites which can result in toxicity.
Verapamil may potentiate the prolongation of bleeding time associated with aspirin.
Warfarin and oral anticoagulants may increase the risk of bleeding.

Dietary/Ethanol/Herb Considerations
Ethanol: Avoid use; may increase CNS depression and enhance gastric mucosal irritation.
Food decreases rate but not extent of oral absorption.
Herb/Nutraceutical: Avoid gotu kola, kava, SAMe, St John's wort, and valerian; may increase CNS depression.

Drug Uptake
Methocarbamol:
Absorption: Rapid
Onset of muscle relaxing effect: Oral: ≤30 minutes
Time to peak: Oral: ~2 hours
Half-life, elimination: 1-2 hours
Aspirin:
Absorption: Rapid
Time to peak: ~1-2 hours
Half-life, elimination: Parent drug: 15-20 minutes; Salicylates (dose-dependent): Low dose (300-600 mg): 3 hours; Medium dose: (1 g): 5-6 hours; High dose: 10 hours

Pregnancy Risk Factor C/D (full-dose aspirin in 3rd trimester)

Breast-feeding Considerations Use cautiously due to potential adverse effects in nursing infants.

Dosage Forms TAB: Methocarbamol 400 mg and aspirin 325 mg

Generic Available Yes

Methohexital (meth oh HEKS i tal)

U.S. Brand Names Brevital® Sodium

Canadian Brand Names Brevital®; Brietal Sodium®

Pharmacologic Category Barbiturate

Synonyms Methohexital Sodium

Use
Dental: I.V. induction and maintenance of general anesthesia for short periods
Medical: Can be used in pediatric patients >1 month of age as follows: For rectal or intramuscular induction of anesthesia prior to the use of other general anesthetic agents, as an adjunct to subpotent inhalational anesthetic agents for short surgical procedures, or for short surgical, diagnostic, or therapeutic procedures associated with minimal painful stimuli

Local Anesthetic/Vasoconstrictor Precautions No information available to require special precautions

Effects on Dental Treatment No effects or complications reported

Restrictions C-IV

Dosage Doses must be titrated to effect.
Children 3-12 years:
I.M.: Preop: 5-10 mg/kg/dose
I.V.: Induction: 1-2 mg/kg/dose
Rectal: Preop/induction: 20-35 mg/kg/dose; usual 25 mg/kg/dose; administer as 10% aqueous solution
Adults: I.V.: Induction: 50-120 mg to start; 20-40 mg every 4-7 minutes
Dosing adjustment/comments in hepatic impairment: Lower dosage and monitor closely

Mechanism of Action Ultrashort-acting I.V. barbiturate anesthetic; acts as agonist within the multisubunit $GABA_A$ receptor ion chloride-channel complex in CNS neurons; this leads to inhibition of many brain functions resulting in loss of consciousness. May also dissolve in neuronal membranes to cause stabilization and eventual loss of action potentials which also leads to inhibition of brain function.

Other Adverse Effects Frequency not defined:
Cardiovascular: Hypotension, peripheral vascular collapse,
Central nervous system: Seizures, headache
Gastrointestinal: Cramping, diarrhea, rectal bleeding, nausea, vomiting, abdominal pain
Hematologic: Hemolytic anemia, thrombophlebitis
Hepatic: Elevated transaminases
Local: Pain on I.M. injection
Neuromuscular & skeletal: Tremor, twitching, rigidity, involuntary muscle movement, radial nerve palsy
Respiratory: Apnea, respiratory depression, laryngospasm, coughing, hiccups

Contraindications Hypersensitivity to methohexital or any component of the formulation; porphyria

Warnings/Precautions Use with extreme caution in patients with liver impairment, asthma, cardiovascular instability

Drug Interactions CYP1A2, 2C, 3A3/4, and 3A5-7 inducer

Acetaminophen: Barbiturates may enhance the hepatotoxic potential of acetaminophen overdoses

Antiarrhythmics: Barbiturates may increase the metabolism of antiarrhythmics, decreasing their clinical effect; includes disopyramide, propafenone, and quinidine

Anticonvulsants: Barbiturates may increase the metabolism of anticonvulsants; includes ethosuximide, felbamate (possibly), lamotrigine, phenytoin, tiagabine, topiramate, and zonisamide; does not appear to affect gabapentin or levetiracetam

Antineoplastics: Limited evidence suggests that enzyme-inducing anticonvulsant therapy may reduce the effectiveness of some chemotherapy regimens (specifically in ALL); teniposide and methotrexate may be cleared more rapidly in these patients

Antipsychotics: Barbiturates may enhance the metabolism (decrease the efficacy) of antipsychotics; monitor for altered response; dose adjustment may be needed

Barbiturates are enzyme inducers; patients should be monitored when these drugs are started or stopped for a decreased or increased therapeutic effect respectively

Beta-blockers: Metabolism of beta-blockers may be increased and clinical effect decreased; atenolol and nadolol are unlikely to interact given their renal elimination

Calcium channel blockers: Barbiturates may enhance the metabolism of calcium channel blockers, decreasing their clinical effect

Chloramphenicol: Barbiturates may increase the metabolism of chloramphenicol and chloramphenicol may inhibit barbiturate metabolism; monitor for altered response

Cimetidine: Barbiturates may enhance the metabolism of cimetidine, decreasing its clinical effect

CNS depressants: Sedative effects and/or respiratory depression with barbiturates may be additive with other CNS depressants; monitor for increased effect; includes sedatives, antidepressants, narcotic analgesics, and benzodiazepines

Corticosteroids: Barbiturates may enhance the metabolism of corticosteroids, decreasing their clinical effect

Cyclosporine: Levels may be decreased by barbiturates; monitor

Doxycycline: Barbiturates may enhance the metabolism of doxycycline, decreasing its clinical effect; higher dosages may be required

Estrogens: Barbiturates may increase the metabolism of estrogens and reduce their efficacy

Felbamate may inhibit the metabolism of barbiturates and barbiturates may increase the metabolism of felbamate

Griseofulvin: Barbiturates may impair the absorption of griseofulvin, and griseofulvin metabolism may be increased by barbiturates, decreasing clinical effect

Guanfacine: Effect may be decreased by barbiturates

Immunosuppressants: Barbiturates may enhance the metabolism of immunosuppressants, decreasing its clinical effect; includes both cyclosporine and tacrolimus

Loop diuretics: Metabolism may be increased and clinical effects decreased; established for furosemide, effect with other loop diuretics not established

MAO inhibitors: Metabolism of barbiturates may be inhibited, increasing clinical effect or toxicity of the barbiturates

Methadone: Barbiturates may enhance the metabolism of methadone resulting in methadone withdrawal

Methoxyflurane: Barbiturates may enhance the nephrotoxic effects of methoxyflurane

Oral contraceptives: Barbiturates may enhance the metabolism of oral contraceptives, decreasing their clinical effect; an alternative method of contraception should be considered

Theophylline: Barbiturates may increase metabolism of theophylline derivatives and decrease their clinical effect

Tricyclic antidepressants: Barbiturates may increase metabolism of tricyclic antidepressants and decrease their clinical effect; sedative effects may be additive

Valproic acid: Metabolism of barbiturates may be inhibited by valproic acid; monitor for excessive sedation; a dose reduction may be needed

Warfarin: Barbiturates inhibit the hypoprothrombinemic effects of oral anticoagulants via increased metabolism; this combination should generally be avoided

Dietary/Ethanol/Herb Considerations Food: Do not administer if patient has food in stomach due to danger of vomiting during anesthesia.

Drug Uptake

Onset of action: I.V.: Immediately

Duration: Single dose: 10-20 minutes

(Continued)

Methohexital *(Continued)*

Pregnancy Risk Factor C

Dosage Forms INJ: 500 mg, 2.5 g, 5 g

Generic Available No

Selected Readings Dionne RA, Yagiela JA, Moore PA, et al, "Comparing Efficacy and Safety of Four Intravenous Sedation Regimens in Dental Outpatients," *Am Dent Assoc*, 2001, 132(6):740-51.

Methotrexate (meth oh TREKS ate)

Related Information

Rheumatoid Arthritis and Osteoarthritis *on page 1340*

U.S. Brand Names Rheumatrex®; Trexall™

Mexican Brand Names Ledertrexate; Texate®; Trixilem®

Pharmacologic Category Antineoplastic Agent, Antimetabolite

Synonyms Amethopterin; Methotrexate Sodium; MTX

Use Treatment of trophoblastic neoplasms; leukemias; psoriasis; rheumatoid arthritis (RA), including polyarticular-course juvenile rheumatoid arthritis (JRA); breast, head and neck, and lung carcinomas; osteosarcoma; sarcomas; carcinoma of gastric, esophagus, testes; lymphomas; mycosis fungoides (cutaneous T-cell lymphoma)

Local Anesthetic/Vasoconstrictor Precautions No information available to require special precautions

Effects on Dental Treatment Commonly causes ulceration stomatitis, gingivitis, and pharyngitis associated with oral discomfort

Dosage

Children:

Dermatomyositis: Oral: 15-20 mg/m²/week as a single dose once weekly or 0.3-1 mg/kg/dose once weekly

Juvenile rheumatoid arthritis: Oral, I.M.: Recommended starting dose: 10 mg/m² once weekly (at higher doses, GI side effects may be decreased with I.M. administration); 5-15 mg/m²/week as a single dose **or** as 3 divided doses given 12 hours apart

Adults:

Rheumatoid arthritis: Oral: 7.5 mg once weekly **OR** 2.5 mg every 12 hours for 3 doses/week; not to exceed 20 mg/week

Bone marrow suppression is increased at dosages >20 mg/week; absorption and GI effects may be improved with I.M. administration at higher end of dosage range

Psoriasis: Oral: 2.5-5 mg/dose every 12 hours for 3 doses given weekly **or** Oral, I.M.: 10-25 mg/dose given once weekly

Ectopic pregnancy: I.M./I.V.: 50 mg/m² single-dose without leucovorin rescue

Elderly: Rheumatoid arthritis/psoriasis: Oral: Initial: 5 mg once weekly; if nausea occurs, split dose to 2.5 mg every 12 hours for the day of administration; dose may be increased to 7.5 mg/week based on response, not to exceed 20 mg/week

Mechanism of Action Antimetabolite that inhibits DNA synthesis and cell reproduction in malignant cells; MTX enters the cell through an energy-dependent and temperature-dependent process which is mediated by an intramembrane protein. This carrier mechanism is also used by naturally occurring reduced folates, including folinic acid (leucovorin), making this a competitive process. Folates must be in the reduced form (FH_4) to be active and are activated by dihydrofolate reductase (DHFR) which is inhibited by MTX (by binding irreversibly), causing an increase in the intracellular dihydrofolate pool (the inactive cofactor) and inhibition of both purine and thymidylate synthesis (TS). At high drug concentrations (>20 μM), MTX enters the cell by a second mechanism which is not shared by reduced folates; the process may be passive diffusion or a specific, saturable process, and provides a rationale for high-dose MTX. A small fraction of MTX is converted intracellularly to polyglutamates, which leads to a prolonged inhibition of DHFR. The mechanism in the treatment of rheumatoid arthritis is unknown, but may affect immune function. In psoriasis, methotrexate is thought to target rapidly proliferating epithelial cells in the skin. Cytotoxicity is determined by both drug concentration and duration of cell exposure; extracellular drug concentrations of 1×10^{-8} M are required to inhibit thymidylate synthesis; reduced folates are able to rescue cells and reverse MTX toxicity if given within 40 hours of the MTX dose.

Other Adverse Effects

>10%:

Cardiovascular: Vasculitis

Central nervous system (with I.T. administration only):

Arachnoiditis: Acute reaction manifested as severe headache, nuchal rigidity, vomiting, and fever; may be alleviated by reducing the dose

Subacute toxicity: 10% of patients treated with 12-15 mg/m² of I.T. MTX may develop this in the second or third week of therapy; consists of motor paralysis of extremities, cranial nerve palsy, seizures, or coma. This has also been seen in pediatric cases receiving very high-dose I.V. MTX (when enough MTX can get across into the CSF).

Demyelinating encephalopathy: Seen months or years after receiving MTX; usually in association with cranial irradiation or other systemic chemotherapy
Dermatologic: Reddening of skin
Endocrine & metabolic: Hyperuricemia, defective oogenesis or spermatogenesis
Gastrointestinal: Ulcerative stomatitis, glossitis, gingivitis, nausea, vomiting, diarrhea, anorexia, intestinal perforation, mucositis (dose-dependent; appears in 3-7 days after therapy, resolving within 2 weeks)
Emetic potential:
<100 mg: Moderately low (10% to 30%)
≥100 mg or <250 mg: Moderate (30% to 60%)
≥250 mg: Moderately high (60% to 90%)
Hematologic: Leukopenia, thrombocytopenia
Renal: Renal failure, azotemia, nephropathy
Respiratory: Pharyngitis

1% to 10%:
Central nervous system: Dizziness, malaise, encephalopathy, seizures, fever, chills
Dermatologic: Alopecia, rash, photosensitivity, depigmentation or hyperpigmentation of skin
Endocrine & metabolic: Diabetes
Genitourinary: Cystitis
Hematologic: Hemorrhage
Myelosuppressive: This is the primary dose-limiting factor (along with mucositis) of MTX; occurs about 5-7 days after MTX therapy, and should resolve within 2 weeks
WBC: Mild
Platelets: Moderate
Onset: 7 days
Nadir: 10 days
Recovery: 21 days
Hepatic: Cirrhosis and portal fibrosis have been associated with chronic MTX therapy; acute elevation of liver enzymes are common after high-dose MTX, and usually resolve within 10 days.
Neuromuscular & skeletal: Arthralgia
Ocular: Blurred vision
Renal: Renal dysfunction: Manifested by an abrupt rise in serum creatinine and BUN and a fall in urine output; more common with high-dose MTX, and may be due to precipitation of the drug. The best treatment is prevention: Aggressively hydrate with 3 L/m^2/day starting 12 hours before therapy and continue for 24-36 hours; alkalinize the urine by adding 50 mEq of bicarbonate to each liter of fluid; keep urine flow over 100 mL/hour and urine pH >7.
Respiratory: Pneumonitis: Associated with fever, cough, and interstitial pulmonary infiltrates; treatment is to withhold MTX during the acute reaction; interstitial pneumonitis has been reported to occur with an incidence of 1% in patients with RA (dose 7.5-15 mg/week)

Drug Interactions Involvement with CYP isoenzymes not defined; may act as inhibitor of some isoenzymes

Increased Effect/Toxicity: Live virus vaccines → vaccinia infections; vincristine inhibits MTX efflux from the cell, leading to increased and prolonged MTX levels in the cell (the dose of VCR needed to produce this effect is not achieved clinically); organic acids (salicylates, sulfonamides, probenecid, and high doses of penicillins) compete with MTX for transport and reduce renal tubular secretion (salicylates and sulfonamides may also displace MTX from plasma proteins, increasing MTX levels); increased formation of the Ara-C nucleotide can occur when MTX precedes Ara-C, thus promoting the action of Ara-C; cyclosporine and MTX interfere with each other's renal elimination, which may result in increased toxicity; NSAIDs should not be used during moderate or high-dose methotrexate due to increased and prolonged methotrexate levels, may increase toxicity (NSAID use during treatment of rheumatoid arthritis has not been fully explored, but continuation of prior regimen has been allowed in some circumstances, with cautious monitoring); patients receiving concomitant therapy with methotrexate and other potential hepatotoxins (eg, azathioprine, retinoids, sulfasalazine) should be closely monitored for possible increased risk of hepatotoxicity.

Decreased Effect: Corticosteroids have been reported to decrease methotrexate entry into leukemia cells. Administration should be separated by 12 hours. Dexamethasone has been reported to not affect methotrexate entry. May decrease phenytoin and 5-FU activity.

Drug Uptake

Onset of action: Antirheumatic: 3-6 weeks; additional improvement may continue longer than 12 weeks
Absorption: Oral: Rapid; well absorbed at low doses (<30 mg/m^2), incomplete after large doses; I.M. injection: Complete
Half-life, elimination: High dose: 8-12 hours; Low dose: 3-10 hours
Time to peak: Oral: 1-2 hours; Parenteral: 30-60 minutes

Pregnancy Risk Factor D

(Continued)

Methotrexate *(Continued)*

Generic Available Yes

Methotrimeprazine *Not Available in U.S.*

(meth oh trye MEP ra zeen)

Canadian Brand Names Apo®-Methoprazine; Novo-Meprazine; Nozinan®

Mexican Brand Names Levocina®; Sinogan®

Pharmacologic Category Analgesic, Non-narcotic

Synonyms Levomepromazine; Methotrimeprazine Hydrochloride

Use Relief of moderate to severe pain in nonambulatory patients; for analgesia and sedation when respiratory depression is to be avoided, as in obstetrics; preanesthetic for producing sedation, somnolence and relief of apprehension and anxiety

Local Anesthetic/Vasoconstrictor Precautions No information available to require special precautions

Effects on Dental Treatment Anticholinergic side effects can cause a reduction of saliva production or secretion contributes to discomfort and dental disease (ie, caries, oral candidiasis and periodontal disease); phenothiazines can cause extrapyramidal reactions which may appear as muscle twitching or increased motor activity of the face, neck or head.

Dosage Adults: I.M.:

Sedation analgesia: 10-20 mg every 4-6 hours as needed

Preoperative medication: 2-20 mg, 45 minutes to 3 hours before surgery

Postoperative analgesia: 2.5-7.5 mg every 4-6 hours is suggested as necessary since residual effects of anesthetic may be present

Pre- and postoperative hypotension: I.M.: 5-10 mg

Mechanism of Action A phenothiazine with sites of action thought to be in the thalamus, hypothalamus, reticular and limbic systems, producing suppression of sensory impulses and resulting in sedation, an elevated pain threshold, and induction of amnesia. The analgesic effect is comparable to meperidine and morphine without the respiratory suppression; also has antihistamine, anticholinergic, and antiepinephrine effects.

Other Adverse Effects

>10%:

- Cardiovascular: Hypotension, orthostatic hypotension
- Central nervous system: Pseudoparkinsonism, akathisia, dystonias, dizziness
- Gastrointestinal: Constipation
- Neuromuscular & skeletal: Tardive dyskinesia
- Ocular: Pigmentary retinopathy
- Respiratory: Nasal congestion
- Miscellaneous: Decreased diaphoresis

1% to 10%:

- Central nervous system: Dizziness
- Dermatologic: Increased sensitivity to sun, skin rash
- Endocrine & metabolic: Changes in menstrual cycle, ejaculatory disturbances, changes in libido, pain in breasts
- Gastrointestinal: Weight gain, nausea, vomiting, stomach pain
- Genitourinary: Dysuria
- Neuromuscular & skeletal: Trembling of fingers

Drug Interactions Increased Toxicity: Additive effects with other CNS depressants

Drug Uptake

Onset of action: Peak effect: 20-40 minutes

Duration: 4 hours

Half-life, elimination: 20 hours

Time to peak: 0.5-1.5 hours

Pregnancy Risk Factor C

Generic Available No

Methoxsalen (meth OKS a len)

U.S. Brand Names 8-MOP®; Oxsoralen®; Oxsoralen-Ultra®; Uvadex®

Canadian Brand Names 8-MOP®; Oxsoralen™; Oxsoralen-Ultra™; Ultramop™; Uvadex®

Mexican Brand Names Dermox®; Meladinina®; Oxsoralen®

Pharmacologic Category Psoralen

Synonyms Methoxypsoralen; 8-Methoxypsoralen; 8-MOP

Use

Oral: Symptomatic control of severe, recalcitrant disabling psoriasis, not responsive to other therapy when the diagnosis has been supported by biopsy. Administer only in conjunction with a schedule of controlled doses of long wave ultraviolet (UV) radiation; also used with long wave ultraviolet (UV) radiation for repigmentation of idiopathic vitiligo.

Topical: Repigmenting agent in vitiligo, used in conjunction with controlled doses of UVA or sunlight

Orphan drug: Uvadex®: Palliative treatment of skin manifestations of cutaneous T-cell lymphoma

Local Anesthetic/Vasoconstrictor Precautions No information available to require special precautions

Effects on Dental Treatment No effects or complications reported

Dosage

Psoriasis: Adults: Oral: 10-70 mg 1½-2 hours before exposure to ultraviolet light, 2-3 times at least 48 hours apart; dosage is based upon patient's body weight and skin type

Vitiligo: Children >12 years and Adults:

Oral: 20 mg 2-4 hours before exposure to UVA light or sunlight; limit exposure to 15-40 minutes based on skin basic color and exposure

Topical: Apply lotion 1-2 hours before exposure to UVA light, no more than once weekly

Mechanism of Action Bonds covalently to pyrimidine bases in DNA, inhibits the synthesis of DNA, and suppresses cell division. The augmented sunburn reaction involves excitation of the methoxsalen molecule by radiation in the long-wave ultraviolet light (UVA), resulting in transference of energy to the methoxsalen molecule producing an excited state ("triplet electronic state"). The molecule, in this "triplet state", then reacts with cutaneous DNA.

Other Adverse Effects Frequency not defined:

Cardiovascular: Severe edema, hypotension

Central nervous system: Nervousness, vertigo, depression

Dermatologic: Painful blistering, burning, and peeling of skin; pruritus (10%), freckling, hypopigmentation, rash, cheilitis, erythema, itching

Gastrointestinal: Nausea (10%)

Neuromuscular & skeletal: Loss of muscle coordination

Drug Interactions Increased Effect/Toxicity: Concomitant therapy with other photosensitizing agents such as anthralin, coal tar, griseofulvin, phenothiazines, nalidixic acid, sulfanilamides, tetracyclines, and thiazide diuretics.

Drug Uptake

Absorption: Increased with food

Half-life, plasma: ~2 hours

Time to peak: Oral: 2-4 hours

Pregnancy Risk Factor C

Generic Available No

Methscopolamine (meth skoe POL a meen)

U.S. Brand Names Pamine®

Canadian Brand Names Pamine®

Pharmacologic Category Anticholinergic Agent

Synonyms Methscopolamine Bromide

Use Adjunctive therapy in the treatment of peptic ulcer

Local Anesthetic/Vasoconstrictor Precautions No information available to require special precautions

Effects on Dental Treatment

>10%: Xerostomia

Anticholinergic side effects can cause a reduction of saliva production or secretion contributes to discomfort and dental disease (ie, caries, oral candidiasis and periodontal disease).

Dosage Adults: Oral: 2.5 mg 30 minutes before meals or food and 2.5-5 mg at bedtime

Mechanism of Action A peripheral anticholinergic agent that does not cross the blood-brain barrier and provides a peripheral blockade of muscarinic receptors; reduces the volume and the total acid content of gastric secretions, inhibits salivation, and reduces GI motility

Other Adverse Effects Frequency not defined:

Cardiovascular: Palpitations

Central nervous system: Headache, flushing, nervousness, drowsiness, dizziness, confusion, fever, CNS stimulation may be produced with large doses

Dermatologic: Dry skin, urticaria

Gastrointestinal: Constipation, xerostomia, dry throat, dysphagia, nausea, vomiting

Respiratory: Dry nose

Miscellaneous: Decreased diaphoresis, hypersensitivity reactions, anaphylaxis

Pregnancy Risk Factor C

Generic Available No

Methsuximide (meth SUKS i mide)

U.S. Brand Names Celontin®

Canadian Brand Names Celontin®

Pharmacologic Category Anticonvulsant, Succinimide

Use Control of absence (petit mal) seizures that are refractory to other drugs

Unlabeled/Investigational: Adjunct in partial complex (psychomotor) seizures

Local Anesthetic/Vasoconstrictor Precautions No information available to require special precautions

Effects on Dental Treatment No effects or complications reported

(Continued)

Methsuximide *(Continued)*

Dosage Oral:

Children: Anticonvulsant: Initial: 10-15 mg/kg/day in 3-4 divided doses; increase weekly up to maximum of 30 mg/kg/day

Adults: Anticonvulsant: 300 mg/day for the first week; may increase by 300 mg/day at weekly intervals up to 1.2 g/day in 2-4 divided doses/day

Mechanism of Action Increases the seizure threshold and suppresses paroxysmal spike-and-wave pattern in absence seizures; depresses nerve transmission in the motor cortex

Other Adverse Effects Frequency not defined:

Cardiovascular: Hyperemia

Central nervous system: Ataxia, dizziness, drowsiness, headache, aggressiveness, mental depression, irritability, nervousness, insomnia, confusion, psychosis, suicidal behavior, auditory hallucinations

Dermatologic: Stevens-Johnson syndrome, rash, urticaria, pruritus

Gastrointestinal: Anorexia, nausea, vomiting, weight loss, diarrhea, epigastric and abdominal pain, constipation

Genitourinary: Proteinuria, hematuria (microscopic); cases of blood dyscrasias have been reported with succinimides

Hematologic: Leukopenia, pancytopenia, eosinophilia, monocytosis

Neuromuscular & skeletal: Cases of systemic lupus erythematosus have been reported

Ocular: Blurred vision, photophobia, peripheral edema

Drug Interactions CYP3A3/4 enzyme substrate

Increased Effect/Toxicity: Sedative effects and/or respiratory depression may be additive with CNS depressants; includes benzodiazepines, barbiturates, narcotic analgesics, and other sedative agents. Serum level and/or toxicity of succimides may be increased by inhibitors of CYP3A3/4. Methsuximide may increase phenobarbital and/or phenytoin concentration.

Decreased Effect: Metabolism of succimides may be increased by enzyme inducers, decreasing their therapeutic effect; consider using an alternative sedative/hypnotic agent; potential inducers include phenobarbital, phenytoin, carbamazepine, rifampin, and rifabutin.

Drug Uptake

Half-life, elimination: 2-4 hours

Time to peak: 1-3 hours

Pregnancy Risk Factor C

Generic Available No

Methyclothiazide (meth i kloe THYE a zide)

Related Information

Cardiovascular Diseases *on page 1308*

U.S. Brand Names Aquatensen®; Enduron®

Canadian Brand Names Aquatensen®; Enduron®

Pharmacologic Category Diuretic, Thiazide

Use Management of mild to moderate hypertension; treatment of edema in CHF and nephrotic syndrome

Local Anesthetic/Vasoconstrictor Precautions No information available to require special precautions

Effects on Dental Treatment No effects or complications reported

Dosage Oral:

Children: 0.05-0.2 mg/kg/day

Adults:

Edema: 2.5-10 mg/day

Hypertension: 2.5-5 mg/day

Mechanism of Action Inhibits sodium reabsorption in the distal tubules causing increased excretion of sodium and water, as well as, potassium and hydrogen ions

Other Adverse Effects 1% to 10%:

Cardiovascular: Orthostatic hypotension

Dermatologic: Photosensitivity

Endocrine & metabolic: Hypokalemia

Gastrointestinal: Anorexia, epigastric distress

Warnings/Precautions Chemical similarities are present among sulfonamides, sulfonylureas, carbonic anhydrase inhibitors, thiazides, and loop diuretics (except ethacrynic acid). Use in patients with thiazide or sulfonamide allergy is specifically contraindicated in product labeling, however a risk of cross-reaction exists in patients with allergy to any of these compounds; avoid use when previous reaction has been severe.

Drug Interactions

Increased Effect/Toxicity: Increased effect of methyclothiazide with furosemide and other loop diuretics. Increased hypotension and/or renal adverse effects of ACE inhibitors may result in aggressively diuresed patients. Beta-blockers increase hyperglycemic effects of thiazides in Type 2 diabetes mellitus. Cyclosporine and thiazides can increase the risk of gout or renal toxicity. Digoxin toxicity can be exacerbated if a thiazide induces hypokalemia or hypomagnesemia. Lithium toxicity can occur with thiazides due to reduced renal excretion of lithium. Thiazides may prolong the duration of action with neuromuscular blocking agents.

Decreased Effect: Effects of oral hypoglycemics may be decreased. Decreased absorption of thiazides with cholestyramine and colestipol. NSAIDs can decrease the efficacy of thiazides, reducing the diuretic and antihypertensive effects.

Drug Uptake

Onset of action: Diuresis: Oral: 2 hours; Peak effect: 6 hours

Duration: ~1 day

Pregnancy Risk Factor B

Generic Available Yes

Methyclothiazide and Deserpidine

(meth i kloe THYE a zide & de SER pi deen)

U.S. Brand Names Enduronyl®; Enduronyl® Forte

Canadian Brand Names Enduronyl®; Enduronyl® Forte

Pharmacologic Category Antihypertensive Agent Combination

Synonyms Deserpidine and Methyclothiazide

Use Management of mild to moderately severe hypertension

Local Anesthetic/Vasoconstrictor Precautions No information available to require special precautions

Effects on Dental Treatment No effects or complications reported

Dosage Oral: Individualized, normally 1-4 tablets/day

Pregnancy Risk Factor C

Generic Available No

Methylbenzethonium Chloride

(meth il ben ze THOE nee um KLOR ide)

U.S. Brand Names Diaparene® [OTC]; Puri-Clens™ [OTC]; Sween Cream® [OTC]

Pharmacologic Category Topical Skin Product

Use Diaper rash and ammonia dermatitis

Local Anesthetic/Vasoconstrictor Precautions No information available to require special precautions

Effects on Dental Treatment No effects or complications reported

Dosage Apply topically to area as needed

Generic Available No

Methylcellulose (meth il SEL yoo lose)

U.S. Brand Names Citrucel® [OTC]

Pharmacologic Category Laxative

Use Adjunct in treatment of constipation

Local Anesthetic/Vasoconstrictor Precautions No information available to require special precautions

Effects on Dental Treatment No effects or complications reported

Dosage Oral:

Children ≤12 years: Half the adult dose in 4 oz of cold water, 1-3 times/day

Children ≥12 years and Adults: 1 heaping tablespoon (19 g) in 8 oz of cold water, 1-3 times/day

Pregnancy Risk Factor C

Comments Each dose contains sodium 3 mg, potassium 105 mg, and 60 calories from sucrose

Methyldopa (meth il DOE pa)

Related Information

Cardiovascular Diseases *on page 1308*

U.S. Brand Names Aldomet®

Canadian Brand Names Aldomet®; Apo®-Methyldopa; Novo-Medopa®; Nu-Medopa

Mexican Brand Names Aldomet®

Pharmacologic Category Alpha-Adrenergic Inhibitor

Synonyms Methyldopate Hydrochloride

Use Management of moderate to severe hypertension

Local Anesthetic/Vasoconstrictor Precautions No information available to require special precautions

Effects on Dental Treatment Anticholinergic side effects can cause a reduction of saliva production or secretion; may result in discomfort and dental disease (ie, caries, oral candidiasis and periodontal disease).

Dosage

Children:

- Oral: Initial: 10 mg/kg/day in 2-4 divided doses; increase every 2 days as needed to maximum dose of 65 mg/kg/day; do not exceed 3 g/day
- I.V.: 5-10 mg/kg/dose every 6-8 hours up to a total dose of 65 mg/kg/24 hours or 3 g/24 hours

(Continued)

Methyldopa *(Continued)*

Adults:

Oral: Initial: 250 mg 2-3 times/day; increase every 2 days as needed; usual dose 1-1.5 g/day in 2-4 divided doses; maximum dose: 3 g/day

I.V.: 250-1000 mg every 6-8 hours; maximum dose: 1 g every 6 hours

Mechanism of Action Stimulation of central alpha-adrenergic receptors by a false transmitter that results in a decreased sympathetic outflow to the heart, kidneys, and peripheral vasculature

Other Adverse Effects

>10%: Cardiovascular: Peripheral edema

1% to 10%:

Central nervous system: Drug fever, mental depression, anxiety, nightmares, drowsiness, headache

Gastrointestinal: Xerostomia

Drug Interactions

Increased Effect/Toxicity: Beta-blockers, MAO inhibitors, phenothiazines, and sympathomimetics (including epinephrine) may result in hypertension (sometimes severe) when combined with methyldopa. Methyldopa may increase lithium serum concentration resulting in lithium toxicity. Levodopa may cause enhanced BP lowering; methyldopa may also potentiate the effect of levodopa. Tolbutamide, haloperidol, and anesthetics effects/toxicity are increased with methyldopa.

Decreased Effect: Iron supplements can interact and cause a significant **increase** in BP. Ferrous sulfate and ferrous gluconate decrease bioavailability. Barbiturates and TCAs may reduce response to methyldopa.

Drug Uptake

Onset of action: Peak effect: Hypotensive: Oral/parenteral: 3-6 hours

Duration: 12-24 hours

Half-life, elimination: 75-80 minutes; End-stage renal disease: 6-16 hours

Pregnancy Risk Factor B

Generic Available Yes

Methyldopa and Hydrochlorothiazide

(meth il DOE pa & hye droe klor oh THYE a zide)

U.S. Brand Names Aldoril®

Canadian Brand Names Apo®-Methazide

Pharmacologic Category Antihypertensive Agent Combination

Synonyms Hydrochlorothiazide and Methyldopa

Use Management of moderate to severe hypertension

Local Anesthetic/Vasoconstrictor Precautions No information available to require special precautions

Effects on Dental Treatment Anticholinergic side effects can cause a reduction of saliva production or secretion; may result in discomfort and dental disease (ie, caries, oral candidiasis and periodontal disease).

Dosage Oral: 1 tablet 2-3 times/day for first 48 hours, then decrease or increase at intervals of not less than 2 days until an adequate response is achieved

Other Adverse Effects

Based on **methyldopa** component:

>10%: Cardiovascular: Peripheral edema

1% to 10%:

Central nervous system: Drug fever, mental depression, anxiety, nightmares, drowsiness, headache

Gastrointestinal: Xerostomia

Based on **hydrochlorothiazide** component:

1% to 10%:

Cardiovascular: Orthostatic hypotension, hypotension

Dermatologic: Photosensitivity

Endocrine & metabolic: Hypokalemia

Gastrointestinal: Anorexia, epigastric distress

Drug Interactions

Based on **methyldopa** component:

Iron supplements can interact and cause a significant **increase** in BP.

Barbiturates and TCAs may reduce response to methyldopa.

Beta-blockers, MAO inhibitors, phenothiazines, and sympathomimetics: Hypertension, sometimes severe, may occur.

Lithium: Methyldopa may increase lithium toxicity; monitor lithium levels.

Tolbutamide, haloperidol, anesthetics, and levodopa effects/toxicity are increased with methyldopa.

Based on **hydrochlorothiazide** component:

ACE inhibitors: Increased hypotension if aggressively diuresed with a thiazide diuretic.

Beta-blockers increase hyperglycemic effects in type 2 diabetes mellitus (noninsulin dependent, NIDDM)

Cyclosporine and thiazides can increase the risk of gout or renal toxicity; avoid concurrent use.

Digoxin toxicity can be exacerbated if a thiazide induces hypokalemia or hypomagnesemia.
Lithium toxicity can occur by reducing renal excretion of lithium; monitor lithium concentration and adjust as needed.
Neuromuscular blocking agents can prolong blockade; monitor serum potassium and neuromuscular status.
NSAIDs can decrease the efficacy of thiazides reducing the diuretic and antihypertensive effects.

Drug Uptake See Methyldopa *on page 793* and Hydrochlorothiazide *on page 595*
Pregnancy Risk Factor C
Generic Available Yes

Methylergonovine (meth il er goe NOE veen)

U.S. Brand Names Methergine®
Canadian Brand Names Methergine®
Pharmacologic Category Ergot Derivative
Synonyms Methylergometrine Maleate; Methylergonovine Maleate
Use Prevention and treatment of postpartum and postabortion hemorrhage caused by uterine atony or subinvolution
Local Anesthetic/Vasoconstrictor Precautions No information available to require special precautions
Effects on Dental Treatment No effects or complications reported
Dosage Adults:
Oral: 0.2 mg 3-4 times/day for 2-7 days
I.M.: 0.2 mg after delivery of anterior shoulder, after delivery of placenta, or during puerperium; may be repeated as required at intervals of 2-4 hours
I.V.: Same dose as I.M., but should not be routinely administered I.V. because of possibility of inducing sudden hypertension and cerebrovascular accident

Mechanism of Action Similar smooth muscle actions as seen with ergotamine; however, it affects primarily uterine smooth muscles producing sustained contractions and thereby shortens the third stage of labor
Other Adverse Effects Frequency not defined:
Cardiovascular: Hypertension, temporary chest pain, palpitations
Central nervous system: Hallucinations, dizziness, seizures, headache
Endocrine & metabolic: Water intoxication
Gastrointestinal: Nausea, vomiting, diarrhea, foul taste
Local: Thrombophlebitis
Neuromuscular & skeletal: Leg cramps
Otic: Tinnitus
Renal: Hematuria
Respiratory: Dyspnea, nasal congestion
Miscellaneous: Diaphoresis

Drug Interactions Increased Effect/Toxicity: Avoid use of 5-HT_1 receptor antagonists (sumatriptan) within 24 hours (per manufacturer). Erythromycin, clarithromycin, and troleandomycin may increase levels of ergot alkaloids, resulting in toxicity (ischemia, vasospasm). Rare toxicity (peripheral vasoconstriction) has been reported with propranolol. Ritonavir, amprenavir, and nelfinavir increase blood levels of ergot alkaloids; avoid concurrent use. Concurrent use of sibutramine may cause serotonin syndrome; avoid concurrent use. Rarely, weakness and incoordination have been noted when SSRIs are used concurrently with 5-HT_1 agonists. The effects of vasoconstrictors may be increased by ergot derivatives.
Drug Uptake
Onset of oxytocic effect: Oral: 5-10 minutes; I.M.: 2-5 minutes; I.V.: Immediate
Absorption: Rapid
Duration: Oral: ~3 hours; I.M.: ~3 hours; I.V.: 45 minutes
Half-life, elimination: Biphasic: Initial: 1-5 minutes; Terminal: 0.5-2 hours
Time to peak: 0.5-3 hours

Pregnancy Risk Factor C
Generic Available No

Methylin™ *see* Methylphenidate *on page 795*
Methylin™ ER *see* Methylphenidate *on page 795*

Methylphenidate (meth il FEN i date)

U.S. Brand Names Concerta™; Metadate® CD; Metadate™ ER; Methylin™; Methylin™ ER; Ritalin®; Ritalin® LA; Ritalin-SR®
Canadian Brand Names PMS-Methylphenidate; Riphenidate; Ritalin®; Ritalin® SR
Mexican Brand Names Ritalin®
Pharmacologic Category Central Nervous System Stimulant
Synonyms Methylphenidate Hydrochloride
Use Treatment of attention-deficit/hyperactivity disorder (ADHD); symptomatic management of narcolepsy
Unlabeled/Investigational: Depression (especially elderly or medically ill)
Local Anesthetic/Vasoconstrictor Precautions No information available to require special precautions
(Continued)

Methylphenidate *(Continued)*

Effects on Dental Treatment Up to 10% of patients taking dextroamphetamines or amphetamine-like drugs may present with hypertension. The use of local anesthetic without vasoconstrictor is recommended in these patients.

Restrictions C-II

Dosage Oral (discontinue periodically to re-evaluate or if no improvement occurs within 1 month):

Children ≥6 years: ADHD: Initial: 0.3 mg/kg/dose or 2.5-5 mg/dose given before breakfast and lunch; increase by 0.1 mg/kg/dose or by 5-10 mg/day at weekly intervals; usual dose: 0.5-1 mg/kg/day; maximum dose: 2 mg/kg/day or 90 mg/day

Extended release products:

Metadate™ ER, Methylin™ ER, Ritalin® SR: Duration of action is 8 hours. May be given in place of regular tablets, once the daily dose is titrated using the regular tablets and the titrated 8-hour dosage corresponds to sustained release tablet size.

Metadate® CD: Initial: 20 mg once daily; may be adjusted in 20 mg increments at weekly intervals; maximum: 60 mg/day

Concerta™: Duration of action is 12 hours:

Children not currently taking methylphenidate:

Initial: 18 mg once daily in the morning

Adjustment: May increase to 54 mg/day; dose may be adjusted at weekly intervals

Children currently taking methylphenidate: **Note:** Dosing based on current regimen and clinical judgment; suggested dosing listed below:

Patients taking methylphenidate 5 mg 2-3 times/day or 20 mg/day sustained release formulation: Initial dose: 18 mg once every morning (maximum: 54 mg/day)

Patients taking methylphenidate 10 mg 2-3 times/day or 40 mg/day sustained release formulation: Initial dose: 36 mg once every morning (maximum: 54 mg/day)

Patients taking methylphenidate 15 mg 2-3 times/day or 60 mg/day sustained release formulation: Initial dose: 54 mg once every morning (maximum: 54 mg/day)

Adults:

Narcolepsy: 10 mg 2-3 times/day, up to 60 mg/day

Depression (unlabeled use): Initial: 2.5 mg every morning before 9 AM; dosage may be increased by 2.5-5 mg every 2-3 days as tolerated to a maximum of 20 mg/day; may be divided (ie, 7 AM and 12 noon), but should not be given after noon; do not use sustained release product

Mechanism of Action Mild CNS stimulant; blocks the reuptake mechanism of dopaminergic neurons; appears to stimulate the cerebral cortex and subcortical structures similar to amphetamines

Other Adverse Effects Frequency not defined:

Cardiovascular: Angina, cardiac arrhythmias, cerebral arteritis, cerebral occlusion, hypertension, hypotension, palpitations, pulse increase/decrease, tachycardia

Central nervous system: Depression, dizziness, drowsiness, fever, headache, insomnia, nervousness, neuroleptic malignant syndrome (NMS), Tourette's syndrome, toxic psychosis

Dermatologic: Erythema multiforme, exfoliative dermatitis, hair loss, rash, urticaria

Endocrine & metabolic: Growth retardation

Gastrointestinal: Abdominal pain, anorexia, nausea, vomiting, weight loss

Hematologic: Anemia, leukopenia, thrombocytopenic purpura

Hepatic: Abnormal LFTs, hepatic coma, transaminase elevation

Neuromuscular & skeletal: Arthralgia, dyskinesia

Ocular: Blurred vision

Renal: Necrotizing vasculitis

Respiratory: Cough increased, pharyngitis, sinusitis, upper respiratory tract infection

Miscellaneous: Hypersensitivity reactions

Contraindications Hypersensitivity to methylphenidate, any component of the formulation, or idiosyncrasy to sympathomimetic amines; marked anxiety, tension, and agitation; glaucoma; use during or within 14 days following MAO inhibitor therapy; Tourette's syndrome or tics

Warnings/Precautions Has demonstrated value as part of a comprehensive treatment program for ADHD. Safety and efficacy in children <6 years of age not established. Use with caution in patients with bipolar disorder, diabetes mellitus, cardiovascular disease, hyperthyroidism, seizure disorders, insomnia, porphyria, or hypertension. Use caution in patients with history of ethanol or drug abuse. May exacerbate symptoms of behavior and thought disorder in psychotic patients. Do not use to treat severe depression or fatigue states. Potential for drug dependency exists - avoid abrupt discontinuation in patients who have received for prolonged periods. Visual disturbances have been reported (rare). Stimulant use has been associated with growth suppression. Stimulants may unmask tics in individuals with coexisting Tourette's syndrome. Concerta™ should not be used in patients with esophageal motility disorders or pre-existing severe GI narrowing (small bowel disease, short gut syndrome, history of peritonitis, cystic fibrosis, chronic intestinal pseudo-obstruction, Meckel's diverticulum).

Drug Interactions May inhibit CYP isoenzymes (profile not defined)

Increased Effect/Toxicity: Methylphenidate may cause hypertensive effects when used in combination with MAO inhibitors or drugs with MAO-inhibiting activity (linezolid). Risk may be less with selegiline (MAO type B selective at low doses); it is best to avoid this combination. NMS has been reported in a patient receiving methylphenidate and venlafaxine. Methylphenidate may increase levels of phenytoin, phenobarbital, TCAs, and warfarin. Increased toxicity with clonidine and sibutramine.

Decreased Effect: Effectiveness of antihypertensive agents may be decreased. Carbamazepine may decrease the effect of methylphenidate.

Drug Uptake

Onset of action: Peak effect:

Immediate release tablet: Cerebral stimulation: ~2 hours

Extended release capsule (Metadate® CD): Biphasic; initial peak similar to immediate release product, followed by second rising portion (corresponding to extended release portion)

Sustained release tablet: 4-7 hours

Osmotic release tablet (Concerta™): Initial: 1-2 hours

Absorption: Readily

Duration: Immediate release tablet: 3-6 hours; Sustained release tablet: 8 hours

Half-life, elimination: 2-4 hours

Time to peak: C_{max}: 6-8 hours

Pregnancy Risk Factor C

Generic Available Yes

MethylPREDNISolone (meth il pred NIS oh lone)

Related Information

Respiratory Diseases *on page 1328*

U.S. Brand Names A-methaPred®; depMedalone®; Depoject®; Depo-Medrol®; Depopred®; Duralone®; Medralone®; Medrol®; M-Prednisol®; Solu-Medrol®

Canadian Brand Names Depo-Medrol®; Medrol®; Solu-Medrol®

Mexican Brand Names Cryosolona

Pharmacologic Category Corticosteroid, Systemic

Synonyms 6-α-Methylprednisolone; Methylprednisolone Acetate; Methylprednisolone Sodium Succinate

Use Anti-inflammatory or immunosuppressant agent in the treatment of a variety of diseases including those of hematologic, allergic, inflammatory, neoplastic, and autoimmune origin; prevention and treatment of graft-versus-host disease following allogeneic bone marrow transplantation

Unlabeled/Investigational: Treatment of fibrosing-alveolitis phase of adult respiratory distress syndrome (ARDS)

Local Anesthetic/Vasoconstrictor Precautions No information available to require special precautions

Effects on Dental Treatment No effects or complications reported

Dosage Dosing should be based on the lesser of ideal body weight or actual body weight.

Only sodium succinate may be given I.V.; methylprednisolone sodium succinate is highly soluble and has a rapid effect by I.M. and I.V. routes. Methylprednisolone acetate has a low solubility and has a sustained I.M. effect.

Children:

Anti-inflammatory or immunosuppressive: Oral, I.M., I.V. (sodium succinate): 0.5-1.7 mg/kg/day **or** 5-25 mg/m²/day in divided doses every 6-12 hours; "Pulse" therapy: 15-30 mg/kg/dose over ≥30 minutes given once daily for 3 days

Status asthmaticus: I.V. (sodium succinate): Loading dose: 2 mg/kg/dose, then 0.5-1 mg/kg/dose every 6 hours for up to 5 days

Acute spinal cord injury: I.V. (sodium succinate): 30 mg/kg over 15 minutes, followed in 45 minutes by a continuous infusion of 5.4 mg/kg/hour for 23 hours

Lupus nephritis: I.V. (sodium succinate): 30 mg/kg over ≥30 minutes every other day for 6 doses

Adults: **Only sodium succinate may be given I.V.;** methylprednisolone sodium succinate is highly soluble and has a rapid effect by I.M. and I.V. routes. Methylprednisolone acetate has a low solubility and has a sustained I.M. effect.

Acute spinal cord injury: I.V. (sodium succinate): 30 mg/kg over 15 minutes, followed in 45 minutes by a continuous infusion of 5.4 mg/kg/hour for 23 hours

Anti-inflammatory or immunosuppressive:

Oral: 2-60 mg/day in 1-4 divided doses to start, followed by gradual reduction in dosage to the lowest possible level consistent with maintaining an adequate clinical response.

I.M. (sodium succinate): 10-80 mg/day once daily

I.M. (acetate): 10-80 mg every 1-2 weeks

(Continued)

MethylPREDNISolone *(Continued)*

I.V. (sodium succinate): 10-40 mg over a period of several minutes and repeated I.V. or I.M. at intervals depending on clinical response; when high dosages are needed, give 30 mg/kg over a period ≥30 minutes and may be repeated every 4-6 hours for 48 hours.

Status asthmaticus: I.V. (sodium succinate): Loading dose: 2 mg/kg/dose, then 0.5-1 mg/kg/dose every 6 hours for up to 5 days

High-dose therapy for acute spinal cord injury: I.V. bolus: 30 mg/kg over 15 minutes, followed 45 minutes later by an infusion of 5.4 mg/kg/hour for 23 hours

Lupus nephritis: High-dose "pulse" therapy: I.V. (sodium succinate): 1 g/day for 3 days

Aplastic anemia: I.V. (sodium succinate): 1 mg/kg/day or 40 mg/day (whichever dose is higher), for 4 days. After 4 days, change to oral and continue until day 10 or until symptoms of serum sickness resolve, then rapidly reduce over ~ 2 weeks.

Pneumocystis pneumonia in AIDS patients: I.V.: 40-60 mg every 6 hours for 7-10 days

Intra-articular (acetate): Administer every 1-5 weeks.

Large joints: 20-80 mg

Small joints: 4-10 mg

Intralesional (acetate): 20-60 mg every 1-5 weeks

Mechanism of Action In a tissue-specific manner, corticosteroids regulate gene expression subsequent to binding specific intracellular receptors and translocation into the nucleus. Corticosteroids exert a wide array of physiologic effects including modulation of carbohydrate, protein, and lipid metabolism and maintenance of fluid and electrolyte homeostasis. Moreover cardiovascular, immunologic, musculoskeletal, endocrine, and neurologic physiology are influenced by corticosteroids. Decreases inflammation by suppression of migration of polymorphonuclear leukocytes and reversal of increased capillary permeability.

Other Adverse Effects Frequency not defined:

Cardiovascular: Edema, hypertension, arrhythmias

Central nervous system: Insomnia, nervousness, vertigo, seizures, psychoses, pseudotumor cerebri, headache, mood swings, delirium, hallucinations, euphoria

Dermatologic: Hirsutism, acne, skin atrophy, bruising, hyperpigmentation

Endocrine & metabolic: Diabetes mellitus, adrenal suppression, hyperlipidemia, Cushing's syndrome, pituitary-adrenal axis suppression, growth suppression, glucose intolerance, hypokalemia, alkalosis, amenorrhea, sodium and water retention, hyperglycemia

Gastrointestinal: Increased appetite, indigestion, peptic ulcer, nausea, vomiting, abdominal distention, ulcerative esophagitis, pancreatitis

Hematologic: Transient leukocytosis

Neuromuscular & skeletal: Arthralgia, muscle weakness, osteoporosis, fractures

Ocular: Cataracts, glaucoma

Miscellaneous: Infections, hypersensitivity reactions, avascular necrosis, secondary malignancy, intractable hiccups

Contraindications Hypersensitivity to methylprednisolone or any component of the formulation; viral, fungal, or tubercular skin lesions; administration of live virus vaccines; serious infections, except septic shock or tuberculous meningitis; formulations containing benzyl alcohol preservative in infants.

Warnings/Precautions Use with caution in patients with hyperthyroidism, cirrhosis, nonspecific ulcerative colitis, hypertension, osteoporosis, thromboembolic tendencies, CHF, convulsive disorders, myasthenia gravis, thrombophlebitis, peptic ulcer, diabetes. Acute adrenal insufficiency may occur with abrupt withdrawal after long-term therapy or with stress; young pediatric patients may be more susceptible to adrenal axis suppression from topical therapy. Because of the risk of adverse effects, systemic corticosteroids should be used cautiously in the elderly, in the smallest possible dose, and for the shortest possible time.

Drug Interactions CYP3A enzyme inducer

Increased Toxicity: Skin test antigens, immunizations decrease response and increase potential infections; methylprednisolone may increase circulating glucose levels and may need adjustments of insulin or oral hypoglycemics

Decreased Effect: Phenytoin, phenobarbital, rifampin increase clearance of methylprednisolone; potassium depleting diuretics enhance potassium depletion

Dietary/Ethanol/Herb Considerations

Ethanol: Avoid use; may increase gastric mucosal irritation.

Food: Administer after meals or with food or milk. Methylprednisolone interferes with calcium absorption; requires diet rich in pyridoxine, vitamin C, vitamin D, folate, calcium, phosphorus, and protein. Limit caffeine.

Herb/Nutraceutical: Avoid cat's claw and echinacea due to immunostimulant properties. Avoid St John's wort; may decrease serum concentration.

Drug Uptake Methylprednisolone sodium succinate is highly soluble and has a rapid effect by I.M. and I.V. routes. Methylprednisolone acetate has a low solubility and has a sustained I.M. effect. Time to obtain peak effect and the duration of these effects is dependent upon the route of administration.

Oral: Duration: 30-36 hours; Peak effect: 1-2 hours
I.M.: Duration: 1-4 weeks; Peak effect: 4-8 days
Intra-articular: Duration: 1-5 weeks; Peak effect: 1 week
Half-life, elimination: 3-3.5 hours; reduced in obese

Pregnancy Risk Factor C

Dosage Forms INJ, as acetate: 20 mg/mL (5 mL, 10 mL); 40 mg/mL (1 mL, 5 mL, 10 mL); 80 mg/mL (1 mL, 5 mL). **INJ, as sodium succinate:** 40 mg (1 mL, 3 mL); 125 mg (2 mL, 5 mL); 500 mg (1 mL, 4 mL, 8 mL, 20 mL); 1000 mg (1 mL, 8 mL, 50 mL); 2000 mg (30.6 mL). **TAB:** 2 mg, 4 mg, 8 mg, 16 mg, 24 mg, 32 mg. **TAB** [dose pack]: 4 mg (21s)

Generic Available Yes

MethylTESTOSTERone (meth il tes TOS te rone)

U.S. Brand Names Android®; Oreton® Methyl; Testred®; Virilon®

Pharmacologic Category Androgen

Use

Male: Hypogonadism; delayed puberty; impotence and climacteric symptoms
Female: Palliative treatment of metastatic breast cancer; postpartum breast pain and/or engorgement

Local Anesthetic/Vasoconstrictor Precautions No information available to require special precautions

Effects on Dental Treatment No effects or complications reported

Restrictions C-III

Dosage Adults (buccal absorption produces twice the androgenic activity of oral tablets):

- Male:
  - Oral: 10-40 mg/day
  - Buccal: 5-25 mg/day
- Female:
  - Breast pain/engorgement:
    - Oral: 80 mg/day for 3-5 days
    - Buccal: 40 mg/day for 3-5 days
  - Breast cancer:
    - Oral: 50-200 mg/day
    - Buccal: 25-100 mg/day

Mechanism of Action Stimulates receptors in organs and tissues to promote growth and development of male sex organs and maintains secondary sex characteristics in androgen-deficient males

Other Adverse Effects Frequency not defined:

Male: Virilism, priapism, prostatic hyperplasia, prostatic carcinoma, impotence, testicular atrophy, gynecomastia
Female: Virilism, menstrual problems (amenorrhea), breast soreness, hirsutism (increase in pubic hair growth) atrophy
Cardiovascular: Edema
Central nervous system: Headache, anxiety, depression
Dermatologic: Acne, "male pattern" baldness, seborrhea
Endocrine & metabolic: Hypercalcemia, hypercholesterolemia
Gastrointestinal: GI irritation, nausea, vomiting
Hematologic: Leukopenia, polycythemia
Hepatic: Hepatic dysfunction, hepatic necrosis, cholestatic hepatitis
Miscellaneous: Hypersensitivity reactions

Drug Interactions

Increased Effect/Toxicity: Effects of oral anticoagulants and hypoglycemic agents may be increased. Toxicity may occur with cyclosporine; avoid concurrent use.
Decreased effect of oral anticoagulants

Drug Uptake Absorption: From GI tract and oral mucosa

Pregnancy Risk Factor X

Generic Available Yes

Methysergide (meth i SER jide)

U.S. Brand Names Sansert®

Canadian Brand Names Sansert®

Pharmacologic Category Ergot Derivative

Synonyms Methysergide Maleate

Use Prophylaxis of vascular headache

Local Anesthetic/Vasoconstrictor Precautions No information available to require special precautions

Effects on Dental Treatment No effects or complications reported

Dosage Adults: Oral: 4-8 mg/day with meals; if no improvement is noted after 3 weeks, drug is unlikely to be beneficial; must not be given continuously for longer than 6 months, and a drug-free interval of 3-4 weeks must follow each 6-month course

(Continued)

Methysergide *(Continued)*

Mechanism of Action Ergotamine congener, however actions appear to differ; methysergide has minimal ergotamine-like oxytocic or vasoconstrictive properties, and has significantly greater serotonin-like properties

Other Adverse Effects Frequency not defined:

Cardiovascular: Postural hypotension, peripheral ischemia, peripheral edema, tachycardia, bradycardia, edema

Central nervous system: Insomnia, drowsiness, euphoria, dizziness, seizures, fever

Dermatologic: Rash, telangiectasia, flushing

Endocrine & metabolic: Weight gain

Gastrointestinal: Nausea, vomiting, abdominal pain, diarrhea, heartburn

Hematologic: Neutropenia, eosinophilia, thrombocytopenia

Neuromuscular & skeletal: Weakness, myalgia, arthralgia

Note: Fibrotic complications: Retroperitoneal, pleuropulmonary, cardiac (aortic root, aortic valve, mitral valve) fibrosis, and Peyronie's disease have been reported.

Drug Interactions Increased Effect/Toxicity: Serotonin agonists may produce excessive vasoconstriction; avoid concurrent use with 24 hours; includes sumatriptan, naratriptan, rizatriptan, zolmitriptan. Concurrent use of beta-blockers may cause peripheral ischemia. Erythromycin and clarithromycin may increase ergot alkaloid toxicity; avoid concurrent use. Protease inhibitors may increase ergot alkaloid toxicity; avoid concurrent use (amprenavir, ritonavir, saquinavir). Concurrent use of vasoconstrictors may produce excessive vasoconstriction and should be avoided.

Drug Uptake Half-life, elimination, plasma: ~10 hours

Pregnancy Risk Factor X

Generic Available No

Meticorten® *see* PredniSONE *on page 990*

Metimyd® *see* Sulfacetamide Sodium and Prednisolone *on page 1116*

Metipranolol (met i PRAN oh lol)

U.S. Brand Names OptiPranolol®

Canadian Brand Names OptiPranolol®

Pharmacologic Category Beta Blocker, Nonselective; Ophthalmic Agent, Antiglaucoma

Synonyms Metipranolol Hydrochloride

Use Agent for lowering intraocular pressure in patients with chronic open-angle glaucoma

Local Anesthetic/Vasoconstrictor Precautions No information available to require special precautions

Effects on Dental Treatment No effects or complications reported

Dosage Ophthalmic: Adults: Instill 1 drop in the affected eye(s) twice daily

Mechanism of Action Beta-adrenoceptor-blocking agent; lacks intrinsic sympathomimetic activity and membrane-stabilizing effects and possesses only slight local anesthetic activity; mechanism of action of metipranolol in reducing intraocular pressure appears to be via reduced production of aqueous humor. This effect may be related to a reduction in blood flow to the iris root-ciliary body. It remains unclear if the reduction in intraocular pressure observed with beta-blockers is actually secondary to beta-adrenoceptor blockade.

Other Adverse Effects

>10%: Ocular: Mild ocular stinging and discomfort, eye irritation

1% to 10%: Ocular: Blurred vision, browache

Drug Uptake

Onset of action: ≤30 minutes; Peak effect: Maximum: ~2 hours

Duration: Intraocular pressure reduction: ≤24 hours

Half-life, elimination: ~3 hours

Pregnancy Risk Factor C

Generic Available No

Metoclopramide (met oh kloe PRA mide)

Related Information

Endocrine Disorders and Pregnancy *on page 1331*

U.S. Brand Names Reglan®

Canadian Brand Names Apo®-Metoclop; Nu-Metoclopramide; Reglan®

Mexican Brand Names Carnotprim®; Clorimet®; Meclomid; Plasil; Pramotil

Pharmacologic Category Gastrointestinal Agent, Prokinetic

Use Prevention and/or treatment of nausea and vomiting associated with chemotherapy, radiation therapy, or postsurgery; symptomatic treatment of diabetic gastric stasis; gastroesophageal reflux; facilitation of intubation of the small intestine

Local Anesthetic/Vasoconstrictor Precautions No information available to require special precautions

Effects on Dental Treatment No effects or complications reported

Dosage

Children:

Gastroesophageal reflux: Oral: 0.1-0.2 mg/kg/dose up to 4 times/day; efficacy of continuing metoclopramide beyond 12 weeks in reflux has not been determined; total daily dose should not exceed 0.5 mg/kg/day

Gastrointestinal hypomotility (gastroparesis): Oral, I.M., I.V.: 0.1 mg/kg/dose up to 4 times/day, not to exceed 0.5 mg/kg/day

Antiemetic (chemotherapy-induced emesis): I.V.: 1-2 mg/kg 30 minutes before chemotherapy and every 2-4 hours

Facilitate intubation: I.V.:

<6 years: 0.1 mg/kg

6-14 years: 2.5-5 mg

Adults:

Gastroesophageal reflux: Oral: 10-15 mg/dose up to 4 times/day 30 minutes before meals or food and at bedtime; single doses of 20 mg are occasionally needed for provoking situations; efficacy of continuing metoclopramide beyond 12 weeks in reflux has not been determined

Gastrointestinal hypomotility (gastroparesis):

Oral: 10 mg 30 minutes before each meal and at bedtime for 2-8 weeks

I.V. (for severe symptoms): 10 mg over 1-2 minutes; 10 days of I.V. therapy may be necessary for best response

Antiemetic (chemotherapy-induced emesis): I.V.: 1-2 mg/kg 30 minutes before chemotherapy and every 2-4 hours to every 4-6 hours (and usually given with diphenhydramine 25-50 mg I.V./oral)

Postoperative nausea and vomiting: I.M.: 10 mg near end of surgery; 20 mg doses may be used

Facilitate intubation: I.V.: 10 mg

Elderly:

Gastroesophageal reflux: Oral: 5 mg 4 times/day (30 minutes before meals and at bedtime); increase dose to 10 mg 4 times/day if no response at lower dose

Gastrointestinal hypomotility:

Oral: Initial: 5 mg 30 minutes before meals and at bedtime for 2-8 weeks; increase if necessary to 10 mg doses

I.V.: Initiate at 5 mg over 1-2 minutes; increase to 10 mg if necessary

Postoperative nausea and vomiting: I.M.: 5 mg near end of surgery; may repeat dose if necessary

Mechanism of Action Blocks dopamine receptors in chemoreceptor trigger zone of the CNS; enhances the response to acetylcholine of tissue in upper GI tract causing enhanced motility and accelerated gastric emptying without stimulating gastric, biliary, or pancreatic secretions

Other Adverse Effects Adverse reactions are more common/severe at dosages used for prophylaxis of chemotherapy-induced emesis.

>10%:

Central nervous system: Restlessness, drowsiness, extrapyramidal symptoms (high-dose, up to 34%) - may be more severe in the elderly

Gastrointestinal: Diarrhea (may be dose-limiting)

Neuromuscular & skeletal: Weakness

1% to 10%:

Central nervous system: Insomnia, depression

Dermatologic: Rash

Endocrine & metabolic: Breast tenderness, prolactin stimulation

Gastrointestinal: Nausea, xerostomia

Warnings/Precautions Use with caution in patients with Parkinson's disease and in patients with a history of mental illness; has been associated with extrapyramidal symptoms and depression; may exacerbate seizures; neuroleptic malignant syndrome (NMS) has rarely been reported. Use lowest recommended doses initially; may cause transient increase in serum aldosterone; use caution in patients who are at risk of fluid overload (CHF, cirrhosis); dosage and/or frequency of administration should be modified in response to degree of renal impairment.

Drug Interactions CYP1A2 and 2D6 enzyme substrate

Anticholinergic agents antagonize metoclopramide's actions

Antipsychotic agents: Metoclopramide may increase extrapyramidal symptoms (EPS) or risk when used concurrently.

Opiate analgesics may increase CNS depression

Drug Uptake

Onset of action: Oral: 0.5-1 hour; I.V.: 1-3 minutes

Duration: Therapeutic: 1-2 hours, regardless of route

Half-life, elimination: 4-7 hours (may be dose-dependent)

Pregnancy Risk Factor B

Generic Available Yes

Metolazone (me TOLE a zone)

Related Information

Cardiovascular Diseases *on page 1308*

U.S. Brand Names Mykrox®; Zaroxolyn®

(Continued)

Metolazone *(Continued)*

Canadian Brand Names Mykrox®; Zaroxolyn®

Pharmacologic Category Diuretic, Thiazide-Related

Use Management of mild to moderate hypertension; treatment of edema in CHF and nephrotic syndrome, impaired renal function

Local Anesthetic/Vasoconstrictor Precautions No information available to require special precautions

Effects on Dental Treatment No effects or complications reported

Dosage Oral:

Children: 0.2-0.4 mg/kg/day divided every 12-24 hours

Adults:

Edema: 5-20 mg/dose every 24 hours

Hypertension: 2.5-5 mg/dose every 24 hours

Hypertension (Mykrox®): 0.5 mg/day; if response is not adequate, increase dose to maximum of 1 mg/day

Mechanism of Action Inhibits sodium reabsorption in the distal tubules causing increased excretion of sodium and water, as well as, potassium and hydrogen ions

Other Adverse Effects

>10%: Central nervous system: Dizziness

1% to 10%:

Cardiovascular: Orthostatic hypotension, palpitations, chest pain, cold extremities (rapidly acting), edema (rapidly acting), venous thrombosis (slow acting), syncope (slow acting)

Central nervous system: Headache, fatigue, lethargy, malaise, lassitude, anxiety, depression, nervousness, "weird" feeling (rapidly acting), chills (slow acting)

Dermatologic: Rash, pruritus, dry skin (rapidly acting)

Endocrine & metabolic: Hypokalemia, impotence, reduced libido, excessive volume depletion (slow acting), hemoconcentration (slow acting), acute gouty attach (slow acting), weakness

Gastrointestinal: Nausea, vomiting, abdominal pain, cramping, bloating, diarrhea or constipation, xerostomia

Genitourinary: Nocturia

Neuromuscular & skeletal: Muscle cramps, spasm

Ocular: Eye itching (rapidly acting)

Otic: Tinnitus (rapidly acting)

Respiratory: Cough (rapidly acting), epistaxis (rapidly acting), sinus congestion (rapidly acting), sore throat (rapidly acting),

Warnings/Precautions Electrolyte disturbances (hypokalemia, hypochloremic alkalosis, hyponatremia) can occur. Use with caution in severe hepatic dysfunction; hepatic encephalopathy can be caused by electrolyte disturbances. Gout can be precipitate in certain patients with a history of gout, a familial predisposition to gout, or chronic renal failure. Cautious use in diabetics; may see a change in glucose control. Hypersensitivity reactions can occur. Can cause SLE exacerbation or activation. Use caution in severe renal impairment. Orthostatic hypotension may occur (potentiated by alcohol, barbiturates, narcotics, other antihypertensive drugs). Mykrox® tablets are not interchangeable with Zaroxyln® tablets. Use with caution in patients with moderate or high cholesterol concentrations. Photosensitization may occur.

Chemical similarities are present among sulfonamides, sulfonylureas, carbonic anhydrase inhibitors, thiazides, and loop diuretics (except ethacrynic acid). Use in patients with thiazide or sulfonamide allergy is specifically contraindicated in product labeling, however a risk of cross-reaction exists in patients with allergy to any of these compounds; avoid use when previous reaction has been severe.

Drug Interactions

Increased Effect/Toxicity: Increased diuretic effect of metolazone with furosemide and other loop diuretics. Increased hypotension and/or renal adverse effects of ACE inhibitors may result in aggressively diuresed patients. Cyclosporine and thiazide-type diuretics can increase the risk of gout or renal toxicity. Digoxin toxicity can be exacerbated if a diuretic induces hypokalemia or hypomagnesemia. Lithium toxicity can occur with thiazide-type diuretics due to reduced renal excretion of lithium. Thiazide-type diuretics may prolong the duration of action of neuromuscular blocking agents.

Decreased Effect: Effects of oral hypoglycemics may be decreased. Decreased absorption of metolazone with cholestyramine and colestipol. NSAIDs can decrease the efficacy of thiazide-type diuretics, reducing the diuretic and antihypertensive effects.

Drug Uptake

Onset of action: Diuresis: ~60 minutes

Absorption: Oral: Incomplete

Duration: 12-24 hours

Half-life, elimination: 6-20 hours (dependent on renal function)

Pregnancy Risk Factor B (manufacturer); D (expert analysis)

Generic Available No

Metoprolol (me toe PROE lole)

Related Information

Cardiovascular Diseases *on page 1308*

U.S. Brand Names Lopressor®; Toprol-XL®

Canadian Brand Names Apo®-Metoprolol; Betaloc®; Betaloc® Durules®; Gen-Metoprolol; Lopressor®; Novo-Metoprolol; Nu-Metop; PMS-Metoprolol; Toprol-XL®

Mexican Brand Names Kenaprol; Lopresor; Proken M; Prolaken; Ritmolol®; Selectadril®; Seloken; Selopres

Pharmacologic Category Beta Blocker, $Beta_1$ Selective

Synonyms Metoprolol Tartrate

Use Treatment of hypertension and angina pectoris; prevention of myocardial infarction, atrial fibrillation, flutter, symptomatic treatment of hypertrophic subaortic stenosis; to reduce mortality/hospitalization in patients with CHF (NYHA class II or III) in patients already receiving ACE inhibitors, diuretics, and/or digoxin (sustained-release only)

Unlabeled/Investigational: Treatment of ventricular arrhythmias, atrial ectopy, migraine prophylaxis, essential tremor, aggressive behavior

Local Anesthetic/Vasoconstrictor Precautions No information available to require special precautions

Effects on Dental Treatment Noncardioselective beta-blockers (ie, propranolol, nadolol) enhance the pressor response to epinephrine, resulting in hypertension and bradycardia. This has not been reported for metoprolol, a cardioselective beta-blocker. Therefore, local anesthetic with vasoconstrictor can be safely used in patients medicated with metoprolol. Many nonsteroidal anti-inflammatory drugs such as ibuprofen and indomethacin can reduce the hypotensive effect of beta-blockers after 3 or more weeks of therapy with the NSAID. Short-term NSAID use (ie, 3 days) requires no special precautions in patients taking beta-blockers.

Dosage

Children: Oral: 1-5 mg/kg/24 hours divided twice daily; allow 3 days between dose adjustments

Adults:

Hypertension, angina, SVT, MI prophylaxis: Oral: 100-450 mg/day in 2-3 divided doses, begin with 50 mg twice daily and increase doses at weekly intervals to desired effect

Extended release: Same daily dose administered as a single dose

I.V.: Hypertension: Has been given in dosages 1.25-5 mg every 6-12 hours in patients unable to take oral medications

Congestive heart failure: Oral (extended release): Initial: 25 mg once daily (reduce to 12.5 mg once daily in NYHA class higher than class II); may double dosage every 2 weeks as tolerated, up to 200 mg/day

Myocardial infarction (acute): I.V.: 5 mg every 2 minutes for 3 doses in early treatment of myocardial infarction; thereafter give 50 mg orally every 6 hours 15 minutes after last I.V. dose and continue for 48 hours; then administer a maintenance dose of 100 mg twice daily.

Elderly: Oral: Initial: 25 mg/day; usual range: 25-300 mg/day

Hemodialysis: Administer dose posthemodialysis or administer 50 mg supplemental dose; supplemental dose is not necessary following peritoneal dialysis

Dosing adjustment/comments in hepatic disease: Reduced dose probably necessary

Mechanism of Action Selective inhibitor of $beta_1$-adrenergic receptors; competitively blocks $beta_1$-receptors, with little or no effect on $beta_2$-receptors at doses <100 mg; does not exhibit any membrane stabilizing or intrinsic sympathomimetic activity

Other Adverse Effects

>10%:

Central nervous system: Drowsiness, insomnia

Endocrine & metabolic: Decreased sexual ability

1% to 10%:

Cardiovascular: Bradycardia, palpitations, edema, CHF, reduced peripheral circulation

Central nervous system: Mental depression

Gastrointestinal: Diarrhea or constipation, nausea, vomiting, stomach discomfort

Respiratory: Bronchospasm

Miscellaneous: Cold extremities

Drug Interactions CYP2D6 enzyme substrate

Increased Effect/Toxicity: Metoprolol may increase the effects of other drugs which slow AV conduction (digoxin, verapamil, diltiazem), alpha-blockers (prazosin, terazosin), and alpha-adrenergic stimulants (epinephrine, phenylephrine). Metoprolol may mask the tachycardia from hypoglycemia caused by insulin and oral hypoglycemics. In patients receiving concurrent therapy, the risk of hypertensive crisis is increased when either clonidine or the beta-blocker is withdrawn. Reserpine has been shown to enhance the effect of beta-blockers. Beta-blockers may

(Continued)

Metoprolol *(Continued)*

increase the action or levels of disopyramide, nondepolarizing muscle relaxants, and theophylline although the effects are difficult to predict.

Decreased Effect: Decreased effect of beta-blockers with aluminum salts, barbiturates, calcium salts, cholestyramine, colestipol, NSAIDs, penicillins (ampicillin), rifampin, salicylates, and sulfinpyrazone due to decreased bioavailability and plasma concentrations. Beta-blockers may decrease the effect of sulfonylureas.

Drug Uptake

Onset of action: Peak effect: antihypertensive: Oral: 1.5-4 hours

Absorption: 95%

Duration: 10-20 hours

Half-life, elimination: 3-4 hours; End-stage renal disease: 2.5-4.5 hours

Pregnancy Risk Factor C (manufacturer); D (2nd and 3rd trimesters - expert analysis)

Generic Available Yes: Except sustained release product

Selected Readings

Foster CA and Aston SJ, "Propranolol-Epinephrine Interaction: A Potential Disaster," *Plast Reconstr Surg*, 1983, 72(1):74-8.

Wong DG, Spence JD, Lamki L, et al, "Effect of Nonsteroidal Anti-inflammatory Drugs on Control of Hypertension of Beta-Blockers and Diuretics," *Lancet*, 1986, 1(8488):997-1001.

Wynn RL, "Dental Nonsteroidal Anti-inflammatory Drugs and Prostaglandin-Based Drug Interactions, Part Two," *Gen Dent*, 1992, 40(2):104, 106, 108.

Wynn RL, "Epinephrine Interactions With Beta-Blockers," *Gen Dent*, 1994, 42(1):16, 18.

MetroCream® *see* Metronidazole *on page 804*

Metrodin® *see* Urofollitropin *on page 1222*

MetroGel® Topical *see* Metronidazole *on page 804*

MetroGel®-Vaginal *see* Metronidazole *on page 804*

Metro I.V.® *see* Metronidazole *on page 804*

MetroLotion® *see* Metronidazole *on page 804*

Metronidazole (me troe NI da zole)

Related Information

Antibiotic Prophylaxis, Preprocedural Guidelines for Dental Patients *on page 1344*

Gastrointestinal Disorders *on page 1326*

Oral Bacterial Infections *on page 1367*

Oral Nonviral Soft Tissue Ulcerations or Erosions *on page 1384*

Periodontal Diseases *on page 1375*

U.S. Brand Names Flagyl®; Flagyl ER®; MetroCream®; MetroGel® Topical; MetroGel®-Vaginal; Metro I.V.®; MetroLotion®; Noritate™; Protostat® Oral

Canadian Brand Names Apo®-Metronidazole; Flagyl®; MetroCream™; Metrogel®; Nidagel™; Noritate®; Novo-Nidazol

Mexican Brand Names Ameblin; Flagenase®; Flagyl®; Fresenizol®; MetroGel®; Milezzol; Nidrozol®; Otrozol; Selegil®; Servizol®; Vatrix-S; Vertisal

Pharmacologic Category Amebicide; Antibiotic, Topical; Antibiotic, Miscellaneous; Antiprotozoal

Synonyms Metronidazole Hydrochloride

Use

Dental: Treatment of oral soft tissue infections due to anaerobic bacteria including all anaerobic cocci, anaerobic gram-negative bacilli (*Bacteroides*), and gram-positive spore-forming bacilli (*Clostridium*). Useful as single agent or in combination with amoxicillin, Augmentin®, or ciprofloxacin in the treatment of periodontitis associated with the presence of *Actinobacillus actinomycetemcomitans*, (AA).

Medical: Treatment of susceptible anaerobic bacterial and protozoal infections in the following conditions: Amebiasis, symptomatic and asymptomatic trichomoniasis; skin and skin structure infections; CNS infections; intra-abdominal infections (as part of combination regimen); systemic anaerobic infections; treatment of antibiotic-associated pseudomembranous colitis (AAPC), bacterial vaginosis; as part of a multidrug regimen for *H. pylori* eradication to reduce the risk of duodenal ulcer recurrence; also used in Crohn's disease and hepatic encephalopathy

Orphan drug: MetroGel® Topical: Treatment of acne rosacea

Local Anesthetic/Vasoconstrictor Precautions No information available to require special precautions

Effects on Dental Treatment <1%: Xerostomia and metallic taste

Dosage

Infants and Children:

Amebiasis: Oral: 35-50 mg/kg/day in divided doses every 8 hours for 10 days

Trichomoniasis: Oral: 15-30 mg/kg/day in divided doses every 8 hours for 7 days

Anaerobic infections:

Oral: 15-35 mg/kg/day in divided doses every 8 hours

I.V.: 30 mg/kg/day in divided doses every 6 hours

Clostridium difficile (antibiotic-associated colitis): Oral: 20 mg/kg/day divided every 6 hours

Maximum dose: 2 g/day

Adults:

Amebiasis: Oral: 500-750 mg every 8 hours for 5-10 days

Trichomoniasis: Oral: 250 mg every 8 hours for 7 days or 2 g as a single dose

Anaerobic infections: Oral, I.V.: 500 mg every 6-8 hours, not to exceed 4 g/day

Antibiotic-associated pseudomembranous colitis: Oral: 250-500 mg 3-4 times/day for 10-14 days

Helicobacter pylori eradication: 250 mg with meals and at bedtime for 14 days; requires combination therapy with at least one other antibiotic and an acid-suppressing agent (proton pump inhibitor or H_2 blocker)

Vaginosis: 1 applicatorful (~37.5 mg metronidazole) intravaginally once or twice daily for 5 days; apply once in morning and evening if using twice daily, if daily, use at bedtime

Elderly: Use lower end of dosing recommendations for adults, do not administer as a single dose

Topical (acne rosacea therapy): Apply and rub a thin film twice daily, morning and evening, to entire affected areas after washing. Significant therapeutic results should be noticed within 3 weeks. Clinical studies have demonstrated continuing improvement through 9 weeks of therapy.

Dosing adjustment in renal impairment: Cl_{cr} <10 mL/minute: Administer every 12 hours

Hemodialysis: Extensively removed by hemodialysis and peritoneal dialysis (50% to 100%); administer dose posthemodialysis

Peritoneal dialysis: Dose as for Cl_{cr} <10 mL/minute

Dosing adjustment/comments in hepatic disease: Reduce dosage in severe liver disease

Mechanism of Action Reduced to a product which interacts with DNA to cause a loss of helical DNA structure and strand breakage resulting in inhibition of protein synthesis and cell death in susceptible organisms

Other Adverse Effects

Systemic:

>10%:

Central nervous system: Dizziness, headache

Gastrointestinal (12%): Nausea, diarrhea, loss of appetite, vomiting

<1%: Ataxia, seizures, disulfiram-type reaction with alcohol, pancreatitis, xerostomia, metallic taste, furry tongue, vaginal candidiasis, leukopenia, thrombophlebitis, neuropathy, hypersensitivity, change in taste sensation, dark urine

Topical:

1% to 10%:

Dermatologic: Dry skin, redness or other signs of skin irritation not present before therapy, stinging or burning of the skin

Ocular: Watering of eyes

Vaginal:

>10%: Genitourinary: *Candida* cervicitis or vaginitis

1% to 10%:

Central nervous system: Xerostomia, furry tongue, diarrhea, nausea, vomiting, anorexia

Gastrointestinal: Altered taste sensation

Genitourinary: Burning or irritation of penis of sexual partner; burning or increased frequency of urination, vulvitis, dark urine

Contraindications Hypersensitivity to metronidazole or any component of the formulation; 1st trimester of pregnancy (found to be carcinogenic in rats)

Warnings/Precautions Use with caution in patients with liver impairment due to potential accumulation, blood dyscrasias; history of seizures, CHF, or other sodium retaining states; reduce dosage in patients with severe liver impairment, CNS disease, and severe renal failure (Cl_{cr} <10 mL/minute); if *H. pylori* is not eradicated in patients being treated with metronidazole in a regimen, it should be assumed that metronidazole-resistance has occurred and it should not again be used; seizures and neuropathies have been reported especially with increased doses and chronic treatment; if this occurs, discontinue therapy

Drug Interactions CYP2C9 enzyme substrate; CYP2C9, 3A3/4, and 3A5-7 enzyme inhibitor

Cimetidine may increase metronidazole levels.

Cisapride: May inhibit metabolism of cisapride, causing potential arrhythmias; avoid concurrent use

Lithium: Metronidazole may increase lithium levels/toxicity; monitor lithium levels.

Phenytoin, phenobarbital may increase metabolism of metronidazole, potentially decreasing its effect.

Warfarin: Metronidazole increases P-T prolongation with warfarin.

Dietary/Ethanol/Herb Considerations

Ethanol: Avoid alcohol-containing drugs or food during therapy and for 72 hours following discontinuation; metronidazole inhibits ethanol's usual metabolism and may cause disulfiram-like reaction (flushing, headache, nausea, vomiting, sweating or tachycardia).

(Continued)

Metronidazole *(Continued)*

Food: Administer oral forms with food to reduce GI upset; peak antibiotic serum concentration is lowered and delayed by food, but total drug absorption is not affected.

Drug Uptake

Absorption: Oral: Well absorbed; Topical: Concentrations achieved systemically after application of 1 g topically are 10 times less than those obtained after a 250 mg oral dose

Half-life, elimination: Neonates: 25-75 hours; Others: 6-8 hours, increases with hepatic impairment; End-stage renal disease: 21 hours

Time to peak: Oral: Immediate release: 1-2 hours

Pregnancy Risk Factor B (may be contraindicated in 1st trimester)

Breast-feeding Considerations It is suggested to stop breast-feeding for 12-24 hours following single dose therapy to allow excretion of dose.

Dosage Forms CAP: 375 mg. **CRM:** 0.75% (45 g), 1% (30 g). **GEL:** 0.75% [7.5 mg/mL] (30 g). **GEL, vaginal:** 0.75% (70 g tube). **INJ:** 5 mg/mL (100 mL). **INJ, powder for reconstitution:** 500 mg. **TAB:** 250 mg, 500 mg. **TAB, extended release:** 750 mg

Generic Available Yes

Selected Readings

Eisenberg L, Suchow R, Coles RS, et al, "The Effects of Metronidazole Administration on Clinical and Microbiologic Parameters of Periodontal Disease," *Clin Prev Dent*, 1991, 13(1):28-34.

Jenkins WM, MacFarlane TW, Gilmour WH, et al, "Systemic Metronidazole in the Treatment of Periodontitis," *J Clin Periodontol*, 1989, 16(7):433-50.

Loesche WJ, Giordano JR, Hujoel P, et al, "Metronidazole in Periodontitis: Reduced Need for Surgery," *J Clin Periodontol*, 1992, 19(2):103-12.

Loesche WJ, Schmidt E, Smith BA, et al, "Effects of Metronidazole on Periodontal Treatment Needs," *J Periodontol*, 1991, 62(4):247-57.

Soder PO, Frithiof L, Wikner S, et al, "The Effect of Systemic Metronidazole After Nonsurgical Treatment in Moderate and Advanced Periodontitis in Young Adults," *J Periodontol*, 1990, 61(5):281-8.

Wynn RL, Bergman SA, Meiller TF, et al, "Antibiotics in Treating Oral-Facial Infections of Odontogenic Origin: An Update", *Gen Dent*, 2001, 49(3):238-40, 242, 244 passim.

Metyrosine (me TYE roe seen)

U.S. Brand Names Demser®

Canadian Brand Names Demser®

Pharmacologic Category Tyrosine Hydroxylase Inhibitor

Synonyms AMPT; OGMT

Use Short-term management of pheochromocytoma before surgery, long-term management when surgery is contraindicated or when malignant

Local Anesthetic/Vasoconstrictor Precautions No information available to require special precautions

Effects on Dental Treatment No effects or complications reported

Dosage Children >12 years and Adults: Oral: Initial: 250 mg 4 times/day, increased by 250-500 mg/day up to 4 g/day; maintenance: 2-3 g/day in 4 divided doses; for preoperative preparation, administer optimum effective dosage for 5-7 days

Mechanism of Action Blocks the rate-limiting step in the biosynthetic pathway of catecholamines. It is a tyrosine hydroxylase inhibitor, blocking the conversion of tyrosine to dihydroxyphenylalanine. This inhibition results in decreased levels of endogenous catecholamines. Catecholamine biosynthesis is reduced by 35% to 80% in patients treated with metyrosine 1-4 g/day.

Other Adverse Effects

>10%:
- Central nervous system: Drowsiness, extrapyramidal symptoms
- Gastrointestinal: Diarrhea

1% to 10%:
- Endocrine & metabolic: Galactorrhea, edema of the breasts
- Gastrointestinal: Nausea, vomiting, xerostomia
- Genitourinary: Impotence
- Respiratory: Nasal congestion

Contraindications Hypersensitivity to metyrosine or any component of the formulation; hypertension of unknown etiology

Warnings/Precautions Maintain fluid volume during and after surgery; use with caution in patients with impaired renal or hepatic function

Drug Interactions Phenothiazines, haloperidol may potentiate EPS.

Drug Uptake Half-life, elimination: 7.2 hours

Pregnancy Risk Factor C

Generic Available No

Mevacor® *see* Lovastatin *on page 734*

Mexiletine (MEKS i le teen)

Related Information

Cardiovascular Diseases *on page 1308*

U.S. Brand Names Mexitil®

Canadian Brand Names Mexitil®; Novo-Mexiletine

Pharmacologic Category Antiarrhythmic Agent, Class Ib

Use Management of serious ventricular arrhythmias; suppression of PVCs

Unlabeled/Investigational: Diabetic neuropathy

Local Anesthetic/Vasoconstrictor Precautions No information available to require special precautions

Effects on Dental Treatment No effects or complications reported

Dosage Adults: Oral: Initial: 200 mg every 8 hours (may load with 400 mg if necessary); adjust dose every 2-3 days; usual dose: 200-300 mg every 8 hours; maximum dose: 1.2 g/day (some patients respond to every 12-hour dosing); patients with hepatic impairment or CHF may require dose reduction; when switching from another antiarrhythmic, initiate a 200 mg dose 6-12 hours after stopping former agents, 3-6 hours after stopping procainamide

Mechanism of Action Class IB antiarrhythmic, structurally related to lidocaine, which may cause increase in systemic vascular resistance and decrease in cardiac output; no significant negative inotropic effect; inhibits inward sodium current, decreases rate of rise of phase 0, increases effective refractory period/action potential duration ratio

Other Adverse Effects

>10%:

- Central nervous system: Lightheadedness (11% to 25%), dizziness (20% to 25%), nervousness (5% to 10%), incoordination (10%)
- Gastrointestinal: GI distress (41%), nausea/vomiting (40%)
- Neuromuscular & skeletal: Trembling, unsteady gait, tremor (13%), ataxia (10% to 20%)

1% to 10%:

- Cardiovascular: Chest pain (3% to 8%), premature ventricular contractions (1% to 2%), palpitations (4% to 8%), angina (2%), proarrhythmic (10% to 15% in patients with malignant arrhythmias)
- Central nervous system: Confusion, headache, insomnia (5% to 7%), depression (2%)
- Dermatologic: Rash (4%)
- Gastrointestinal: Constipation or diarrhea (4% to 5%), xerostomia (3%), abdominal pain (1%)
- Neuromuscular & skeletal: Weakness (5%), numbness of fingers or toes (2% to 4%), paresthesias (2%), arthralgias (1%)
- Ocular: Blurred vision (5% to 7%), nystagmus (6%)
- Otic: Tinnitus (2% to 3%)
- Respiratory: Dyspnea (3%)

Drug Interactions CYP2D6 enzyme substrate; CYP1A2 enzyme inhibitor

Increased Effect/Toxicity: Mexiletine and caffeine or theophylline may result in elevated levels of theophylline and caffeine. Quinidine and urinary alkalinizers (antacids, sodium bicarbonate, acetazolamide) may increase mexiletine blood levels.

Decreased Effect: Decreased mexiletine plasma concentrations when used with phenobarbital, phenytoin, rifampin, cimetidine, or other hepatic enzyme inducers. Urinary acidifying agents may decrease mexiletine levels.

Drug Uptake

Absorption: Elderly have a slightly slower rate, but extent of absorption is the same as young adults

Half-life, elimination: Adults: 10-14 hours (average: 14.4 hours elderly, 12 hours in younger adults); increase with hepatic or heart failure

Time to peak: 2-3 hours

Pregnancy Risk Factor C

Generic Available Yes

Mexitil® *see* Mexiletine *on page 806*

Miacalcin® *see* Calcitonin *on page 199*

Micanol® *see* Anthralin *on page 102*

Micardis® *see* Telmisartan *on page 1134*

Micardis® HCT *see* Telmisartan and Hydrochlorothiazide *on page 1135*

Micatin® [OTC] *see* Miconazole *on page 807*

Miconazole (mi KON a zole)

U.S. Brand Names Aloe Vesta® 2-n-1 Antifungal [OTC]; Baza® Antifungal [OTC]; Carrington Antifungal [OTC]; Fungoid® Tincture [OTC]; Lotrimin® AF Powder/Spray [OTC]; Micatin® [OTC]; Micro-Guard® [OTC]; Mitrazol® [OTC]; Monistat® 1 Combination Pack [OTC]; Monistat® 3 [OTC]; Monistat® 7 [OTC]; Monistat-Derm®; Zeasorb®-AF [OTC]

Canadian Brand Names Micatin®; Micozole; Monazole-7; Monistat®

Mexican Brand Names Aloid; Daktarin; Dermifun; Fungiquim; Gyno-Daktarin; Gyno-Daktarin V; Lotrimin AF®; Neomicol®

Pharmacologic Category Antifungal Agent, Topical; Antifungal Agent, Vaginal

Synonyms Miconazole Nitrate

(Continued)

Miconazole *(Continued)*

Use

I.V.: Treatment of severe systemic fungal infections and fungal meningitis that are refractory to standard treatment

Topical: Treatment of vulvovaginal candidiasis and a variety of skin and mucous membrane fungal infections

Local Anesthetic/Vasoconstrictor Precautions No information available to require special precautions

Effects on Dental Treatment No effects or complications reported

Dosage Many products are available as a combination pack, with a suppository for vaginal instillation and cream to relieve external symptoms.

Topical: Children and Adults: Not for OTC use in children <2 years.

Tinea pedis and tinea corporis: Apply twice daily for 4 weeks

Tinea cruris: Apply twice daily for 2 weeks

Vaginal: Adults: Vulvovaginal candidiasis:

Cream, 2%: Insert 1 applicatorful at bedtime for 7 days

Cream, 4%: Insert 1 applicatorful at bedtime for 3 days

Suppository, 100 mg: Insert 1 suppository at bedtime for 7 days

Suppository, 200 mg: Insert 1 suppository at bedtime for 3 days

Suppository, 1200 mg: Insert 1 suppository at bedtime (a one-time dose)

Mechanism of Action Inhibits biosynthesis of ergosterol, damaging the fungal cell wall membrane, which increases permeability causing leaking of nutrients

Other Adverse Effects Frequency not defined:

Topical: Allergic contact dermatitis, burning, maceration

Vaginal: Abdominal cramps, burning, irritation, itching

Drug Interactions CYP3A3/4 enzyme substrate; CYP2C9 enzyme inhibitor, CYP3A3/4 enzyme inhibitor

Note: The majority of reported drug interactions were observed following I.V. miconazole administration. Although systemic absorption following topical and/or vaginal administration is low, potential interactions due to CYP isoenzyme inhibition may occur (rarely). This may be particularly true in situations where topical absorption may be increased (ie, inflamed tissue).

Amphotericin B: Antifungal effects of both agents may be decreased

Cisapride: Risk of cardiotoxicity may be increased due to effect on metabolism; concurrent administration is contraindicated

Phenytoin: Serum concentration may be increased by miconazole

Sulfonylureas: Hypoglycemic effects may be increased

Warfarin: An increased anticoagulant effect may occur with coadministration, including reports associated with short-term (3-day) intravaginal miconazole therapy

Drug Uptake

Absorption: Topical: Negligible

Half-life, elimination: Multiphasic: Initial: 40 minutes; Secondary: 126 minutes; Terminal: 24 hours

Pregnancy Risk Factor C

Generic Available Yes

MICRhoGAM™ *see* Rh_o(D) Immune Globulin *on page 1048*

Microfibrillar Collagen Hemostat

(mye kro FI bri lar KOL la jen HEE moe stat)

U.S. Brand Names Avitene®; Helistat®; Hemotene®

Pharmacologic Category Hemostatic Agent

Synonyms Collagen; MCH

Use Adjunct to hemostasis when control of bleeding by ligature is ineffective or impractical

Local Anesthetic/Vasoconstrictor Precautions No information available to require special precautions

Effects on Dental Treatment No effects or complications reported

Dosage Apply dry directly to source of bleeding

Mechanism of Action An absorbable topical hemostatic agent prepared from purified bovine corium collagen and shredded into fibrils; physically, microfibrillar collagen hemostat yields a large surface area. Chemically, it is collagen with hydrochloric acid noncovalently bound to some of the available amino groups in the collagen molecules. When in contact with a bleeding surface, microfibrillar collagen hemostat attracts platelets which adhere to its fibrils and undergo the release phenomenon. This triggers aggregation of the platelets into thrombi in the interstices of the fibrous mass, initiating the formation of a physiologic platelet plug.

Other Adverse Effects Frequency not defined: Miscellaneous: Adhesion formation, allergic reaction, foreign body reaction, potentiation of infection

Contraindications Hypersensitivity to any component of the formulation; closure of skin incisions; contaminated wounds

Warnings/Precautions Fragments of MCH may pass through filters of blood scavenging systems, avoid reintroduction of blood from operative sites treated with MCH; after several minutes remove excess material

Drug Uptake Absorption: By animal tissue in 3 months

Pregnancy Risk Factor C

Dosage Forms FIBROUS: 1 g. **WEB, nonwoven:** 2.5 cm x 5 cm; 5 cm x 8 cm; 8 cm x 10 cm; 35 mm x 35 mm x 1 mm; 70 mm x 70 mm x 1 mm; 70 mm x 35 mm x 1 mm

Generic Available No

Microgestin™ Fe *see* Combination Hormonal Contraceptives *on page 323*
Micro-Guard® [OTC] *see* Miconazole *on page 807*
Micro-K® 10 Extencaps® *see* Potassium Chloride *on page 977*
Micro-K® Extencaps *see* Potassium Chloride *on page 977*
Micro-K® LS *see* Potassium Chloride *on page 977*
Micronase® *see* GlyBURIDE *on page 560*
microNefrin® *see* Epinephrine, Racemic *on page 440*
Micronor® *see* Norethindrone *on page 876*
Microzide™ *see* Hydrochlorothiazide *on page 595*
Midamor® *see* Amiloride *on page 67*

Midazolam (MID aye zoe lam)

U.S. Brand Names Versed®

Canadian Brand Names Versed®

Mexican Brand Names Dormicum

Pharmacologic Category Benzodiazepine

Synonyms Midazolam Hydrochloride

Use

Dental: Sedation component in I.V. conscious sedation in oral surgery patients; syrup formulation is used for children to help alleviate anxiety before a dental procedure

Medical: In medicine, preoperative sedation and provides conscious sedation prior to diagnostic or radiographic procedures
Anxiety, status epilepticus

Local Anesthetic/Vasoconstrictor Precautions No information available to require special precautions

Effects on Dental Treatment No effects or complications reported

Restrictions C-IV

Dosage The dose of midazolam needs to be individualized based on the patient's age, underlying diseases, and concurrent medications. Decrease dose (by ~30%) if narcotics or other CNS depressants are administered concomitantly. **Personnel and equipment needed for standard respiratory resuscitation should be immediately available during midazolam administration.**

Children <6 years may require higher doses and closer monitoring than older children; calculate dose on ideal body weight

Conscious sedation for procedures or preoperative sedation:

Oral: 0.25-0.5 mg/kg as a single dose preprocedure, up to a maximum of 20 mg; administer 30-45 minutes prior to procedure. Children <6 years or less cooperative patients may require as much as 1 mg/kg as a single dose; 0.25 mg/kg may suffice for children 6-16 years of age.

Intranasal (not an approved route): 0.2 mg/kg (up to 0.4 mg/kg in some studies), to a maximum of 15 mg; may be administered 30-45 minutes prior to procedure

I.M.: 0.1-0.15 mg/kg 30-60 minutes before surgery or procedure; range 0.05-0.15 mg/kg; doses up to 0.5 mg/kg have been used in more anxious patients; maximum total dose: 10 mg

I.V.:

Infants <6 months: Limited information is available in nonintubated infants; dosing recommendations not clear; infants <6 months are at higher risk for airway obstruction and hypoventilation; titrate dose in small increments to desired effect; monitor carefully

Infants 6 months to Children 5 years: Initial: 0.05-0.1 mg/kg; titrate dose carefully; total dose of 0.6 mg/kg may be required; usual maximum total dose: 6 mg

Children 6-12 years: Initial: 0.025-0.05 mg/kg; titrate dose carefully; total doses of 0.4 mg/kg may be required; usual maximum total dose: 10 mg

Children 12-16 years: Dose as adults; usual maximum total dose: 10 mg

Conscious sedation during mechanical ventilation: Children: Loading dose: 0.05-0.2 mg/kg, followed by initial continuous infusion: 0.06-0.12 mg/kg/hour (1-2 mcg/kg/minute); titrate to the desired effect; usual range: 0.4-6 mcg/kg/minute

Status epilepticus refractory to standard therapy: Infants >2 months and Children: Loading dose: 0.15 mg/kg followed by a continuous infusion of 1 mcg/kg/minute; titrate dose upward very 5 minutes until clinical seizure activity is

(Continued)

Midazolam *(Continued)*

controlled; mean infusion rate required in 24 children was 2.3 mcg/kg/minute with a range of 1-18 mcg/kg/minute

Adults:

Preoperative sedation:

I.M.: 0.07-0.08 mg/kg 30-60 minutes prior to surgery/procedure; usual dose: 5 mg; **Note:** Reduce dose in patients with COPD, high-risk patients, patients ≥60 years of age, and patients receiving other narcotics or CNS depressants

I.V.: 0.02-0.04 mg/kg; repeat every 5 minutes as needed to desired effect or up to 0.1-0.2 mg/kg

Intranasal (not an approved route): 0.2 mg/kg (up to 0.4 mg/kg in some studies); administer 30-45 minutes prior to surgery/procedure

Conscious sedation: I.V.: Initial: 0.5-2 mg slow I.V. over at least 2 minutes; slowly titrate to effect by repeating doses every 2-3 minutes if needed; usual total dose: 2.5-5 mg; use decreased doses in elderly

Healthy Adults <60 years: Some patients respond to doses as low as 1 mg; ≤2.5 mg should be administered over a period of 2 minutes. Additional doses of midazolam may be administered after a 2-minute waiting period and evaluation of sedation after each dose increment. A total dose >5 mg is generally not needed. If narcotics or other CNS depressants are administered concomitantly, the midazolam dose should be reduced by 30%.

Anesthesia: I.V.:

Induction:

Unpremedicated patients: 0.3-0.35 mg/kg (up to 0.6 mg/kg in resistant cases)

Premedicated patients: 0.15-0.35 mg/kg

Maintenance: 0.05-0.3 mg/kg as needed, or continuous infusion 0.25-1.5 mcg/kg/minute

Sedation in mechanically-ventilated patients: I.V. continuous infusion: 100 mg in 250 mL D_5W or NS, (if patient is fluid-restricted, may concentrate up to a maximum of 0.5 mg/mL); initial dose: 0.01-0.05 mg/kg (~0.5-4 mg for a typical adult) initially and either repeated at 10-15 minute intervals until adequate sedation is achieved or continuous infusion rates of 0.02-0.1 mg/kg/hour (1-7 mg/hour) and titrate to reach desired level of sedation

Elderly: I.V.: Conscious sedation: Initial: 0.5 mg slow I.V.; give no more than 1.5 mg in a 2-minute period; if additional titration is needed, give no more than 1 mg over 2 minutes, waiting another 2 or more minutes to evaluate sedative effect; a total dose of >3.5 mg is rarely necessary

Mechanism of Action Binds to stereospecific benzodiazepine receptors on the postsynaptic GABA (gamma-aminobutyric acid) neuron at several sites within the CNS, including the limbic system, reticular formation. Enhancement of the inhibitory effect of GABA on neuronal excitability results by increased neuronal membrane permeability to chloride ions. This shift in chloride ions results in hyperpolarization (a less excitable state) and stabilization.

Other Adverse Effects As reported in adults, unless otherwise noted:

>10%: Respiratory: Decreased tidal volume and/or respiratory rate decrease, apnea (3% children)

1% to 10%:

Cardiovascular: Hypotension (3% children)

Central nervous system: Drowsiness (1%), oversedation, headache (1%), seizure-like activity (1% children)

Gastrointestinal: Nausea (3%), vomiting (3%)

Local: Pain and local reactions at injection site (4% I.M., 5% I.V.; severity less than diazepam)

Ocular: Nystagmus (1% children)

Respiratory: Cough (1%)

Miscellaneous: Physical and psychological dependence with prolonged use, hiccups (4%, 1% children), paradoxical reaction (2% children)

<1%: Acid taste, agitation, amnesia, bigeminy, bradycardia, bronchospasm, confusion, dyspnea, emergence delirium, euphoria, excessive salivation, hallucinations, hyperventilation, laryngospasm, PVC, rash, tachycardia, wheezing

Contraindications Hypersensitivity to midazolam or any component of the formulation, including benzyl alcohol (cross-sensitivity with other benzodiazepines may exist); parenteral form is not for intrathecal or epidural injection; narrow-angle glaucoma; pregnancy

Warnings/Precautions May cause severe respiratory depression, respiratory arrest, or apnea. Use with extreme caution, particularly in noncritical care settings. Appropriate resuscitative equipment and qualified personnel must be available for administration and monitoring. Initial dosing must be cautiously titrated and individualized, particularly in elderly or debilitated patients, patients with hepatic impairment (including alcoholics), or in renal impairment, particularly if other CNS depressants (including opiates) are used concurrently. Initial doses in elderly or debilitated patients should not exceed 2.5 mg. Use with caution in patients with respiratory disease or impaired gag reflex. Use during upper airway procedures may increase risk of hypoventilation. Prolonged responses have been noted following extended administration by continuous infusion (possibly due to metabolite accumulation) or in the presence of drugs which inhibit midazolam metabolism.

May cause hypotension - hemodynamic events are more common in pediatric patients or patients with hemodynamic instability. Hypotension and/or respiratory depression may occur more frequently in patients who have received narcotic analgesics. Use with caution in obese patients, chronic renal failure, and CHF. Parenteral form contains benzyl alcohol - avoid rapid injection in neonates or prolonged infusions. Does not protect against increases in heart rate or BP during intubation. Should not be used in shock, coma, or acute alcohol intoxication. Avoid intra-arterial administration or extravasation of parenteral formulation.

Causes CNS depression (dose-related) resulting in sedation, dizziness, confusion, or ataxia which may impair physical and mental capabilities. Patients must be cautioned about performing tasks which require mental alertness (ie, operating machinery or driving). A minimum of 1 day should elapse after midazolam administration before attempting these tasks. Use with caution in patients receiving other CNS depressants or psychoactive agents. Effects with other sedative drugs or ethanol may be potentiated. Benzodiazepines have been associated with falls and traumatic injury and should be used with extreme caution in patients who are at risk of these events (especially the elderly).

Midazolam causes anterograde amnesia. Paradoxical reactions, including hyperactive or aggressive behavior have been reported with benzodiazepines, particularly in adolescent/pediatric or psychiatric patients. Does not have analgesic, antidepressant, or antipsychotic properties.

Benzodiazepines have been associated with dependence and acute withdrawal symptoms on discontinuation or reduction in dose. Acute withdrawal, including seizures, may be precipitated after administration of flumazenil to patients receiving long-term benzodiazepine therapy.

Drug Interactions CYP3A3/4 enzyme substrate

CNS depressants: Sedative effects and/or respiratory depression may be additive with CNS depressants; includes barbiturates, narcotic analgesics, and other sedative agents; monitor for increased effect. **If narcotics or other CNS depressants are administered concomitantly, the midazolam dose should be reduced by 30% if <65 years of age, or by at least 50% if >65 years of age.**

Enzyme inducers: Metabolism of some benzodiazepines may be increased, decreasing their therapeutic effect; consider using an alternative sedative/hypnotic agent; potential inducers include phenobarbital, phenytoin, carbamazepine, rifampin, and rifabutin

CYP3A3/4 inhibitors: Serum level and/or toxicity of some benzodiazepines may be increased; inhibitors include amiodarone, cimetidine, clarithromycin, erythromycin, delavirdine, diltiazem, dirithromycin, disulfiram, fluoxetine, fluvoxamine, grapefruit juice, indinavir, itraconazole, ketoconazole, nefazodone, nevirapine, propoxyphene, quinupristin-dalfopristin, ritonavir, saquinavir, verapamil, zafirlukast, zileuton; monitor for altered benzodiazepine response. **Use is contraindicated with amprenavir and ritonavir.**

Levodopa: Therapeutic effects may be diminished in some patients following the addition of a benzodiazepine; limited/inconsistent data

Oral contraceptives: May decrease the clearance of some benzodiazepines (those which undergo oxidative metabolism); monitor for increased benzodiazepine effect

Theophylline: May partially antagonize some of the effects of benzodiazepines; monitor for decreased response; may require higher doses for sedation

Dietary/Ethanol/Herb Considerations

Ethanol: Avoid use; may increase CNS depression.

Food: Grapefruit products may increase serum concentration of midazolam; avoid concurrent use with oral form.

Herb/Nutraceutical: Avoid gotu kola, kava, SAMe, and valerian; may increase CNS depression. Avoid St John's wort; may decrease serum concentration and increase CNS depression. Melatonin may enhance activity of clonazepam; use cautiously.

Drug Uptake

Onset of sedative effect: Oral: 20-30 minutes; I.M.: 5-15 minutes; I.V.: 1-5 minutes; Intranasal: 8-12 minutes

Peak sedation: I.M.: 30-60 minutes; Intranasal: 10 minutes

Absorption: Oral: Rapid

Duration: I.M.: Up to 6 hours; Mean: 2 hours (increases with hepatic/renal dysfunction)

Half-life, elimination: 1-4 hours (increased with cirrhosis, congestive heart failure, obesity, and in elderly)

Pregnancy Risk Factor D

Dosage Forms INJ: 1 mg/mL (2 mL, 5 mL, 10 mL); 5 mg/mL (1 mL, 2 mL, 5 mL, 10 mL). **SYR:** 2 mg/mL (118 mL)

Generic Available No

(Continued)

Midazolam *(Continued)*

Selected Readings Dionne RA, Yagiela JA, Moore PA, et al, "Comparing Efficacy and Safety of Four Intravenous Sedation Regimens in Dental Outpatients," *Am Dent Assoc*, 2001, 132(6):740-51.

Midodrine (MI doe dreen)

U.S. Brand Names ProAmatine®

Canadian Brand Names Amatine®

Pharmacologic Category Alpha$_1$ Agonist

Synonyms Midodrine Hydrochloride

Use

Orphan drug: Treatment of symptomatic orthostatic hypotension

Unlabeled/Investigational: Management of urinary incontinence

Local Anesthetic/Vasoconstrictor Precautions No information available to require special precautions

Effects on Dental Treatment 1% to 10%: Significant xerostomia

Dosage Adults: Oral: 10 mg 3 times/day during daytime hours (every 3-4 hours) when patient is upright (maximum: 40 mg/day)

Mechanism of Action Forms an active metabolite, desglymidodrine, that is an alpha$_1$-agonist and increases arteriolar and venous tone resulting in a rise in standing, sitting, and supine systolic and diastolic BP in patients with orthostatic hypotension (see table).

Causes of Orthostatic Hypotension

Primary Autonomic Causes
Pure autonomic failure (Bradbury-Eggleston syndrome, idiopathic orthostatic hypotension)
Autonomic failure with multiple system atrophy (Shy-Drager syndrome)
Familial dysautonomia (Riley-Day syndrome)
Dopamine beta-hydroxylase deficiency
Secondary Autonomic Causes
Chronic alcoholism
Parkinson's disease
Diabetes mellitus
Porphyria
Amyloidosis
Various carcinomas
Vitamin B_1 or B_{12}deficiency
Nonautonomic Causes
Hypovolemia (such as associated with hemorrhage, burns, or hemodialysis) and dehydration
Diminished homeostatic regulation (such as associated with aging, pregnancy, fever, or prolonged best rest)
Medications (eg, antihypertensives, insulin, tricyclic antidepressants)

Other Adverse Effects

>10%:
- Dermatologic: Piloerection (13%), pruritus (12%)
- Genitourinary: Urinary urgency, retention, or polyuria, dysuria (up to 13%)
- Neuromuscular & skeletal: Paresthesia (18.3%)

1% to 10%:
- Cardiovascular: Supine hypertension (7%), facial flushing
- Central nervous system: Confusion, anxiety, dizziness, chills (5%)
- Dermatologic: Rash, dry skin (2%)
- Gastrointestinal: Xerostomia, nausea, abdominal pain
- Neuromuscular & skeletal: Pain (5%)

Warnings/Precautions Only indicated for patients for whom orthostatic hypotension significantly impairs their daily life. Use is not recommended with supine hypertension and caution should be exercised in patients with diabetes, visual problems, urinary retention (reduce initial dose) or hepatic dysfunction; monitor renal and hepatic function prior to and periodically during therapy; safety and efficacy have not been established in children; discontinue and re-evaluate therapy if signs of bradycardia occur.

Drug Interactions Increased Effect/Toxicity: Concomitant fludrocortisone results in hypernatremia or an increase in intraocular pressure and glaucoma. Bradycardia may be accentuated with concomitant administration of cardiac glycosides, psychotherapeutics, and beta-blockers. Alpha agonists may increase the pressure effects and alpha antagonists may negate the effects of midodrine.

Drug Uptake

Onset of action: ~1 hour

Absorption: Rapid
Duration: 2-3 hours
Half-life, elimination: Active drug: ~3-4 hours; Prodrug: 25 minutes
Time to peak: Active drug: 1-2 hours; Prodrug: 30 minutes

Pregnancy Risk Factor C

Generic Available No

Midol® IB [OTC] *see* Ibuprofen *on page 621*

Midrin® *see* Acetaminophen, Isometheptene, and Dichloralphenazone *on page 35*

Mifeprex® *see* Mifepristone *on page 813*

Mifepristone (mi fe PRIS tone)

U.S. Brand Names Mifeprex®

Pharmacologic Category Abortifacient; Antineoplastic Agent, Hormone Antagonist; Antiprogestin

Synonyms RU-486; RU-38486

Use Medical termination of intrauterine pregnancy, through day 49 of pregnancy. Patients may need treatment with misoprostol and possibly surgery to complete therapy

Unlabeled/Investigational: Treatment of unresectable meningioma; has been studied in the treatment of breast cancer, ovarian cancer, and adrenal cortical carcinoma

Local Anesthetic/Vasoconstrictor Precautions No information available to require special precautions

Effects on Dental Treatment No effects or complications reported

Restrictions There are currently no clinical trials with mifepristone in oncology open in the U.S.; investigators wishing to obtain the agent for use in oncology patients must apply for a patient-specific IND from the FDA. Mifepristone will be supplied only to licensed physicians who sign and return a "Prescriber's Agreement." Distribution of mifepristone will be subject to specific requirements imposed by the distributor. Mifepristone will **not** be available to the public through licensed pharmacies.

Dosage Oral:

Adults: Termination of pregnancy: Treatment consists of three office visits by the patient; the patient must read medication guide and sign patient agreement prior to treatment:

Day 1: 600 mg (three 200 mg tablets) taken as a single dose under physician supervision

Day 3: Patient must return to the healthcare provider 2 days following administration of mifepristone; if termination of pregnancy cannot be confirmed using ultrasound or clinical examination: 400 mcg (two 200 mcg tablets) of misoprostol; patient may need treatment for cramps or GI symptoms at this time

Day 14: Patient must return to the healthcare provider ~14 days after administration of mifepristone; confirm complete termination of pregnancy by ultrasound or clinical exam. Surgical termination is recommended to manage treatment failures.

Elderly: Safety and efficacy have not been established

Mechanism of Action A synthetic steroid which competitively binds to the intracellular progesterone receptor, blocking the effects of progesterone; when used for the termination of pregnancy, this leads to contraction-inducing activity in the myometrium. In the absence of progesterone, mifepristone acts as a partial progesterone agonist. Mifepristone also has weak antiglucocorticoid and antiandrogenic properties; it blocks the feedback effect of cortisol on corticotropin secretion.

Other Adverse Effects Vaginal bleeding and uterine cramping are expected to occur when this medication is used to terminate a pregnancy; 90% of women using this medication for this purpose also report adverse reactions

>10%:

Central nervous system: Headache (2% to 31%), dizziness (1% to 12%)
Gastrointestinal: Abdominal pain (cramping) (96%), nausea (43% to 61%), vomiting (18% to 26%), diarrhea (12% to 20%)
Genitourinary: Uterine cramping (83%)

1% to 10%:

Cardiovascular: Syncope (1%)
Central nervous system: Fatigue (10%), fever (4%), insomnia (3%), anxiety (2%), fainting (2%)
Gastrointestinal: Dyspepsia (3%)
Genitourinary: Uterine hemorrhage (5%), vaginitis (3%), pelvic pain (2%)
Hematologic: Decreased hemoglobin >2 g/dL (6%), anemia (2%), leukorrhea (2%)
Neuromuscular & skeletal: Back pain (9%), rigors (3%), leg pain (2%), weakness (2%)
Respiratory: Sinusitis (2%)
Miscellaneous: Viral infection (4%)

In trials for unresectable meningioma, the most common adverse effects included fatigue, hot flashes, gynecomastia or breast tenderness, hair thinning, and rash. In

(Continued)

Mifepristone *(Continued)*

premenopausal women, vaginal bleeding may be seen shortly after beginning therapy and cessation of menses is common. Thyroiditis and effects related to antiglucocorticoid activity have also been noted.

Contraindications Hypersensitivity to mifepristone, misoprostol, other prostaglandins, or any component of their formulation; chronic adrenal failure; porphyrias; hemorrhagic disorder or concurrent anticoagulant therapy; pregnancy termination >49 days; intrauterine device (IUD) in place; ectopic pregnancy or undiagnosed adnexal mass; concurrent long-term corticosteroid therapy; inadequate or lack of access to emergency medical services; inability to understand effects and/or comply with treatment

Warnings/Precautions Patient must be instructed of the treatment procedure and expected effects. A signed agreement form must be kept in the patient's file. Physicians may obtain patient agreement forms, physician enrollment forms, and medical consultation directly from Danco Laboratories at 1-877-432-7596. Adverse effects (including blood transfusions, hospitalization, ongoing pregnancy, and other major complications) must be reported in writing to the medication distributor.

To be administered only by physicians who can date pregnancy, diagnose ectopic pregnancies, provide access to surgical abortion (if needed), and can provide access to emergency care. Medication will be distributed directly to these physicians following signed agreement with the distributor. Must be administered under supervision by the qualified physician. Pregnancy is dated from day 1 of last menstrual period (presuming a 28-day cycle, ovulation occurring midcycle). Pregnancy duration can be determined using menstrual history and clinical examination. Ultrasound should be used if an ectopic pregnancy is suspected or if duration of pregnancy is uncertain.

Bleeding occurs and should be expected (average 9-16 days, may be ≥30 days). Bleeding may require blood transfusion (rare), curettage, saline infusions, and/or vasoconstrictors. Use caution in patients with severe anemia. Confirmation of pregnancy termination by clinical exam or ultrasound must be made 14 days following treatment. Manufacturer recommends surgical termination of pregnancy when medical termination fails or is not complete. Prescriber should determine in advance whether they will provide such care themselves or through other providers. Preventative measures to prevent Rhesus immunization must be taken prior to surgical abortion. Prescriber should also give the patient clear instructions on whom to call and what to do in the event of an emergency following administration of mifepristone.

Safety and efficacy have not been established for use in women with chronic cardiovascular, hypertensive, respiratory, or renal disease, diabetes mellitus, severe anemia, or heavy smokers. Women >35 years of age and smokers (>10 cigarettes/day) were excluded from clinical trials. Safety and efficacy in pediatric patients have not been established.

Drug Interactions CYP3A3/4 enzyme substrate; CYP3A3/4 enzyme inhibitor

There are no reported interactions. It might be anticipated that the effects of one or both agents would be minimized if mifepristone were administered concurrently with a progestin (exogenous). During concurrent use of CYP3A3/4 inhibitors, serum concentration and/or toxicity of mifepristone may be increased; inhibitors include amiodarone, cimetidine, clarithromycin, erythromycin, delavirdine, diltiazem, dirithromycin, disulfiram, fluoxetine, fluvoxamine, indinavir, itraconazole, ketoconazole, nefazodone, nevirapine, propoxyphene, quinupristin-dalfopristin, ritonavir, saquinavir, verapamil, zafirlukast, zileuton; monitor for altered response

Drug Uptake

Half-life, elimination: Terminal $t_{1/2}$: 18 hours following a slower phase where 50% eliminated between 12-72 hours

Time to peak: 90 minutes

Pregnancy Risk Factor X

Generic Available No

Miglitol (MIG li tol)

Related Information

Endocrine Disorders and Pregnancy *on page 1331*

U.S. Brand Names Glyset™

Canadian Brand Names Glyset™

Pharmacologic Category Antidiabetic Agent, Alpha-Glucosidase Inhibitor

Use

Noninsulin-dependent diabetes mellitus (NIDDM)

Monotherapy adjunct to diet to improve glycemic control in patients with NIDDM whose hyperglycemia cannot be managed with diet alone

Combination therapy with a sulfonylurea when diet plus either miglitol or a sulfonylurea alone do not result in adequate glycemic control. The effect of miglitol to enhance glycemic control is additive to that of sulfonylureas when used in combination.

Local Anesthetic/Vasoconstrictor Precautions No information available to require special precautions

Effects on Dental Treatment No effects or complications reported

Dosage Adults: Oral: 25 mg 3 times/day with the first bite of food at each meal; the dose may be increased to 50 mg 3 times/day after 4-8 weeks; maximum recommended dose: 100 mg 3 times/day

Mechanism of Action In contrast to sulfonylureas, miglitol does not enhance insulin secretion; the antihyperglycemic action of miglitol results from a reversible inhibition of membrane-bound intestinal alpha-glucosidases which hydrolyze oligosaccharides and disaccharides to glucose and other monosaccharides in the brush border of the small intestine; in diabetic patients, this enzyme inhibition results in delayed glucose absorption and lowering of postprandial hyperglycemia

Other Adverse Effects

>10%: Gastrointestinal: Flatulence (42%), diarrhea (29%), abdominal pain (12%)

1% to 10%: Dermatologic: Rash

Drug Interactions Decreased Effect: Miglitol may decrease the absorption and bioavailability of digoxin, propranolol, and ranitidine. Digestive enzymes (amylase, pancreatin, charcoal) may reduce the effect of miglitol and should **not** be taken concomitantly.

Drug Uptake

Absorption: Saturable at high doses: 25 mg dose: Completely absorbed; 100 mg dose: 50% to 70% absorbed

Half-life, elimination: ~2 hours

Time to peak: 2-3 hours

Pregnancy Risk Factor B

Generic Available No

Migranal® Nasal Spray *see* Dihydroergotamine *on page 393*

Migratine® *see* Acetaminophen, Isometheptene, and Dichloralphenazone *on page 35*

Miles Nervine® [OTC] *see* DiphenhydrAMINE *on page 398*

Milophene® *see* ClomiPHENE *on page 305*

Milrinone (MIL ri none)

U.S. Brand Names Primacor®

Canadian Brand Names Primacor®

Pharmacologic Category Phosphodiesterase Enzyme Inhibitor

Synonyms Milrinone Lactate

Use Short-term I.V. therapy of CHF; used for calcium antagonist intoxication

Local Anesthetic/Vasoconstrictor Precautions No information available to require special precautions

Effects on Dental Treatment No effects or complications reported

Dosage Adults: I.V.: Loading dose: 50 mcg/kg administered over 10 minutes followed by a maintenance dose titrated according to the hemodynamic and clinical response

Mechanism of Action Phosphodiesterase inhibitor resulting in vasodilation

Other Adverse Effects

1% to 10%:

- Cardiovascular: Arrhythmias, hypotension
- Central nervous system: Headache

Drug Interactions When furosemide is admixed with milrinone, a precipitate immediately forms.

Drug Uptake

Onset of action: I.V.: 5-15 minutes

Serum level: I.V.: Following a 125 mcg/kg dose, peak plasma concentrations ~1000 ng/mL were observed at 2 minutes postinjection, decreasing to <100 ng/mL in 2 hours

Drug concentration levels:

- Therapeutic:
  - Serum levels of 166 ng/mL, achieved during I.V. infusions of 0.25-1 mcg/kg/minute, were associated with sustained hemodynamic benefit in severe congestive heart failure patients over a 24-hour period
  - Maximum beneficial effects on cardiac output and pulmonary capillary wedge pressure following I.V. infusion have been associated with plasma milrinone concentrations of 150-250 ng/mL
- Toxic: Serum concentrations >250-300 ng/mL have been associated with marked reductions in mean arterial pressure and tachycardia; however, more studies are required to determine the toxic serum levels for milrinone

Half-life elimination: I.V.: 136 minutes in patients with CHF; patients with severe CHF have a more prolonged half-life, with values ranging from 1.7-2.7 hours. Patients with CHF have a reduction in the systemic clearance of milrinone, resulting in a prolonged elimination half-life. Alternatively, one study reported that 1 month of therapy with milrinone did not change the pharmacokinetic parameters for patients with CHF despite improvement in cardiac function.

Pregnancy Risk Factor C

(Continued)

Milrinone *(Continued)*

Generic Available No

Miltown® *see* Meprobamate *on page 768*
Minidyne® [OTC] *see* Povidone-Iodine *on page 982*
Minipress® *see* Prazosin *on page 986*
Minitran™ Patch *see* Nitroglycerin *on page 871*
Minizide® *see* Prazosin and Polythiazide *on page 987*
Minocin® *see* Minocycline *on page 816*

Minocycline (mi noe SYE kleen)

U.S. Brand Names Dynacin®; Minocin®; Vectrin® [DSC]

Canadian Brand Names Alti-Minocycline; Apo®-Minocycline; Gen-Minocycline; Minocin®; Novo-Minocycline; Rhoxal-Minocycline; Scheinpharm™ Minocycline

Mexican Brand Names Minocin®

Pharmacologic Category Antibiotic, Tetracycline Derivative

Synonyms Minocycline Hydrochloride

Use

Dental: Treatment of periodontitis associated with presence of *Actinobacillus actinomycetemcomitans* (AA); as adjunctive therapy in recurrent aphthous ulcers

Medical: Treatment of susceptible bacterial infections of both gram-negative and gram-positive organisms; treatment of anthrax (inhalation, cutaneous, and GI); acne, meningococcal carrier state

Local Anesthetic/Vasoconstrictor Precautions No information available to require special precautions

Effects on Dental Treatment Opportunistic "superinfection" with *Candida albicans*; tetracyclines are not recommended for use during pregnancy or in children ≤8 years of age since they have been reported to cause enamel hypoplasia and permanent teeth discoloration. The use of tetracycline's should only be used in these patients if other agents are contraindicated or alternative antimicrobials will not eradicate the organism. Long-term use associated with oral candidiasis.

Dosage

Children >8 years: Oral, I.V.: Initial: 4 mg/kg followed by 2 mg/kg/dose every 12 hours

Adults:

Infection: Oral, I.V.: 200 mg stat, 100 mg every 12 hours not to exceed 400 mg/24 hours

Acne: Oral: 50 mg 1-3 times/day

Hemodialysis: Not dialyzable (0% to 5%)

Mechanism of Action Inhibits bacterial protein synthesis by binding with the 30S and possibly the 50S ribosomal subunit(s) of susceptible bacteria; cell wall synthesis is not affected

Other Adverse Effects

>10%: Miscellaneous: Discoloration of teeth in children

1% to 10%:

Central nervous system: Lightheadedness, vertigo

Dermatologic: Photosensitivity

Gastrointestinal: Nausea, diarrhea

<1%: Pericarditis, increased intracranial pressure, bulging fontanels in infants, dermatologic effects, pruritus, exfoliative dermatitis, rash, pigmentation of nails, diabetes insipidus, vomiting, esophagitis, hepatic failure, anorexia, abdominal cramps, angioedema, paresthesia, acute renal failure, neutropenia, eosinophilia, thrombocytopenia, hemolytic anemia, thyroid dysfunction (extremely rare), hepatitis, urticaria, tinnitus, erythema multiforme, pseudotumor cerebri (blurred vision, headache), azotemia, Stevens-Johnson syndrome, superinfections, anaphylaxis

Contraindications Hypersensitivity to minocycline, other tetracyclines, or any component of their formulation; children <8 years of age; pregnancy

Warnings/Precautions Use during tooth development may cause permanent discoloration of the teeth and enamel, hypoplasia and retardation of skeletal development and bone growth with risk being the greatest for children <4 years of age and those receiving high doses. Use with caution in patients with renal or hepatic impairment and in pregnancy; dosage modification required in patients with renal impairment. Pseudotumor cerebri reported; outdated drug can cause nephropathy; photosensitivity reactions can occur.

Drug Interactions

Calcium-, magnesium-, or aluminum-containing antacids, oral contraceptives, iron, zinc, sodium bicarbonate, penicillins, cimetidine: May decrease absorption of tetracyclines

Although no clinical evidence exists, tetracyclines may bind with bismuth or calcium carbonate, an excipient in bismuth subsalicylate, during treatment for *H. pylori*.

Digoxin: Tetracyclines may rarely increase digoxin serum concentration.

Methoxyflurane anesthesia when concurrent with tetracyclines may cause fatal nephrotoxicity.

Warfarin: Hypoprothrombinemic response may be increased with tetracyclines; monitor INR closely during initiation or discontinuation.

Dietary/Ethanol/Herb Considerations Herb/Nutraceutical: Avoid dong quai and St John's wort; may cause photosensitization.

Drug Uptake

Absorption: Well absorbed

Half-life, elimination: 15 hours

Pregnancy Risk Factor D

Breast-feeding Considerations Although tetracyclines are excreted in limited amounts, the potential for staining of unerupted teeth has led some experts to recommend against breast-feeding. The AAP identified tetracyclines as "compatible" with breast-feeding.

Dosage Forms CAP: 50 mg, 75 mg, 100 mg; (Dynacin®): 50 mg, 75 mg, 100 mg; (Vectrin® [DSC]): 50 mg, 100 mg. **CAP, pellet-filled** (Minocin®): 50 mg, 100 mg. **INJ, powder for reconstitution** (Minocin®): 100 mg

Generic Available Yes

Minocycline Hydrochloride Periodontal Microspheres

(mi noe SYE kleen hye droe KLOR ide per ee oh DON tal MYE cro sferes)

U.S. Brand Names Arestin™

Pharmacologic Category Antibiotic, Tetracycline Derivative

Use Dental: Adjunct to scaling and root planing procedures for reduction of pocket depth in patients with adult periodontitis. May be used as part of a periodontal maintenance program which includes good oral hygiene, scaling, and root planing.

Local Anesthetic/Vasoconstrictor Precautions No information available to require special precautions

Effects on Dental Treatment Patients should avoid eating hard, crunchy, or sticky foods for 1 week and postpone brushing for a 12-hour period, as well as, avoid touching treated areas. Patients should avoid the use of interproximal cleaning devices for 10 days after administration of Arestin™.

Dosage Arestin™ is a variable dose product; dependent upon the size, shape, and number of pockets being treated. Administration of Arestin™ does not require local anesthesia. Professional subgingival administration is accomplished by inserting the unit-dose cartridge to the base of the periodontal pocket and then pressing the thumb ring in the handle mechanism to expel the powder while gradually withdrawing the tip from the base of the pocket. The handle mechanism should be sterilized between patients. Arestin™ does not have to be removed, it is bioresorbable, nor is an adhesive dressing required.

Mechanism of Action Broad spectrum of activity; it is bacteriostatic and exerts its antimicrobial activity by inhibiting protein synthesis.

Other Adverse Effects Frequency not defined:

Central nervous system: Headache, pain

Gastrointestinal: Dental caries, dental infection, dental pain, dyspepsia, gingivitis, mouth ulceration, mucous membrane disorder, periodontitis, stomatitis, tooth disorder

Respiratory: Pharyngitis

Miscellaneous: Flu syndrome, infection

Contraindications Known hypersensitivity to minocycline, tetracyclines, or any component of their formulation; pregnancy

Warnings/Precautions The use of the tetracycline class during tooth development (last half of pregnancy, infancy, and childhood to 8 years of age) may cause permanent discoloration of the teeth (yellow-gray brown). This adverse reaction is more common during long-term use of the drugs, but has been observed following repeated short-term courses. Enamel hypoplasia has also been reported. Tetracycline drugs, therefore, should not be used in this age group, or in pregnant or nursing women, unless the potential benefits are considered to outweigh the potential risks. Results of animal studies indicate that tetracyclines cross the placenta, are found in fetal tissues, and can have toxic effects on the developing fetus (often related to retardation of skeletal development). Evidence of embryotoxicity has also been noted in animals treated early in pregnancy. If any tetracyclines are used during pregnancy, or if the patient becomes pregnant while taking this drug, the patient should be apprised of the potential hazard to the fetus. Photosensitivity manifested by an exaggerated sunburn reaction has been observed in some individuals taking tetracyclines. Patients apt to be exposed to direct sunlight or ultraviolet light should be advised that this reaction can occur with tetracycline drugs, and treatment should be discontinued at the first evidence of skin erythema.

The use of Arestin™ in an acutely abscessed periodontal pocket has not been studied and is not recommended. While no overgrowth by opportunistic microorganisms, such as yeast, were noted during clinical studies, as with other antimicrobials, the use of Arestin™ may result in overgrowth of nonsusceptible microorganisms including fungi. The effects of treatment for >6 months have not been studied. Arestin™ should be used with caution in patients having a history of predisposition to oral candidiasis. The safety and effectiveness of Arestin™ have not been established for the treatment of periodontitis in patients with coexistent

(Continued)

Minocycline Hydrochloride Periodontal Microspheres *(Continued)*

oral candidiasis. Arestin™ has not been clinically tested in immunocompromised patients (such as those immunocompromised by diabetes, chemotherapy, radiation therapy, or infection with HIV). If superinfection is suspected, appropriate measures should be taken. Arestin™ has not been clinically tested for use in the regeneration of alveolar bone, either in preparation for or in conjunction with the placement of endosseous (dental) implants or in the treatment of failing implants.

Pregnancy Risk Factor D

Dosage Forms POWDER, dry [microspheres]: (Arestin™): 1 mg/unit-dose cartridge [12/tray]

Generic Available No

Minoxidil (mi NOKS i dil)

Related Information

Cardiovascular Diseases *on page 1308*

U.S. Brand Names Loniten®; Rogaine® Extra Strength for Men [OTC]; Rogaine® for Men [OTC]; Rogaine® for Women [OTC]

Canadian Brand Names Apo®-Gain; Minox; Rogaine®

Mexican Brand Names Regaine®

Pharmacologic Category Topical Skin Product; Vasodilator

Use Management of severe hypertension (usually in combination with a diuretic and beta-blocker); treatment of male pattern baldness (alopecia androgenetica)

Local Anesthetic/Vasoconstrictor Precautions No information available to require special precautions

Effects on Dental Treatment No effects or complications reported

Dosage

Children <12 years: Hypertension: Oral: Initial: 0.1-0.2 mg/kg once daily; maximum: 5 mg/day; increase gradually every 3 days; usual dosage: 0.25-1 mg/kg/day in 1-2 divided doses; maximum: 50 mg/day

Children >12 years and Adults:

Hypertension: Oral: Initial: 5 mg once daily, increase gradually every 3 days; usual dose: 10-40 mg/day in 1-2 divided doses; maximum: 100 mg/day

Alopecia: Topical: Apply twice daily; 4 months of therapy may be necessary for hair growth

Elderly: Initial: 2.5 mg once daily; increase gradually

Mechanism of Action Produces vasodilation by directly relaxing arteriolar smooth muscle, with little effect on veins; effects may be mediated by cyclic AMP; stimulation of hair growth is secondary to vasodilation, increased cutaneous blood flow and stimulation of resting hair follicles

Other Adverse Effects Incidence of reactions is not always reported.

Oral:

Cardiovascular: Peripheral edema (7%), sodium and water retention, CHF, tachycardia, angina pectoris, pericardial effusion with or without tamponade, pericarditis, EKG changes (T-wave changes, 60%), rebound hypertension (in children after a gradual withdrawal)

Central nervous system: Headache (rare), fatigue

Dermatologic: Hypertrichosis (common, 80%), transient pruritus, changes in pigmentation (rare), serosanguineous bullae (rare), rash (rare), Stevens-Johnson syndrome

Endocrine & metabolic: Breast tenderness (rare, <1%), gynecomastia (rare), polymenorrhea (rare)

Gastrointestinal: Weight gain, nausea (rare), vomiting

Hematologic: Intermittent claudication (rare), thrombocytopenia (rare), decreased hematocrit (hemodilution), decreased hemoglobin (hemodilution), decreased erythrocyte count (hemodilution), leukopenia (rare)

Hepatic: Increased alkaline phosphatase

Renal: Transient increase in serum BUN and creatinine

Respiratory: Pulmonary edema

Topical:

Cardiovascular: Increased left ventricular end-diastolic volume, increased cardiac output, increased left ventricular mass, dizziness, tachycardia, edema, transient chest pain, palpitation, increase or decrease in BP, increase or decrease in pulse rate (1.5%, placebo 1.6%)

Central nervous system: Headache, dizziness, weakness, taste alterations, faintness, lightheadedness (3.4%, placebo 3.5%), vertigo (1.2%, placebo 1.2%), anxiety (rare), mental depression (rare), fatigue (rare 0.4%, placebo 1%)

Dermatologic: Local irritation, dryness, erythema, allergic contact dermatitis (7.4%, placebo 5.4%), pruritus, scaling/flaking, eczema, seborrhea, papular rash, folliculitis, local erythema, flushing, exacerbation of hair loss, alopecia, hypertrichosis, increased hair growth outside the area of application (face, beard, eyebrows, ear, arm)

Endocrine & metabolic: Menstrual changes, breast symptoms (0.5%, placebo 0.5%)

Gastrointestinal: Diarrhea, nausea, vomiting (4.3%, placebo 6.6%), weight gain (1.2%, placebo 1.3%)
Genitourinary: Urinary tract infections (rare), renal calculi (rare), urethritis (rare), prostatitis (rare), epididymitis (rare), impotence (rare)
Hematologic: Lymphadenopathy, thrombocytopenia, anemia (0.3%, placebo 0.6%)
Neuromuscular & skeletal: Fractures, back pain, retrosternal chest pain of muscular origin, tendonitis (2.6%, placebo 2.2%)
Ocular: Conjunctivitis, visual disturbances, decreased visual acuity
Respiratory: Bronchitis, upper respiratory infections, sinusitis (7.2%, placebo 8.6%)

Drug Interactions Increased Effect/Toxicity: Concurrent use of guanethidine can cause severe orthostasis; avoid concurrent use - discontinue 1-3 weeks prior to initiating minoxidil. Effects of other antihypertensives may be additive with minoxidil.

Drug Uptake
Onset of action: Hypotensive: Oral: ~30 minutes
Duration: 2-5 days
Half-life, elimination: Adults: 3.5-4.2 hours
Time to peak: 2-8 hours

Pregnancy Risk Factor C

Generic Available Yes

Mintezol® *see* Thiabendazole *on page 1156*
Minute-Gel® *see* Fluoride *on page 514*
Miochol-E® *see* Acetylcholine *on page 38*
Miostat® Intraocular *see* Carbachol *on page 215*
Miradon® *see* Anisindione *on page 102*
MiraLax™ *see* Polyethylene Glycol-Electrolyte Solution *on page 970*
Mirapex® *see* Pramipexole *on page 983*
Mircette® *see* Combination Hormonal Contraceptives *on page 323*
Mirena® *see* Levonorgestrel *on page 703*

Mirtazapine (mir TAZ a peen)

U.S. Brand Names Remeron®; Remeron® SolTab™

Mexican Brand Names Remeron®

Pharmacologic Category Antidepressant, Alpha-2 Antagonist

Use Treatment of depression

Local Anesthetic/Vasoconstrictor Precautions No information available to require special precautions

Effects on Dental Treatment ≤25%: Significant xerostomia

Dosage Adults:
Treatment of depression: Oral: Initial: 15 mg nightly, titrate up to 15-45 mg/day with dose increases made no more frequently than every 1-2 weeks; there is an inverse relationship between dose and sedation
Elderly: Decreased clearance seen (40% males, 10% females); no specific dosage adjustment recommended by manufacturer
Dosage adjustment in renal impairment:
Cl_{cr} 11-39 mL/minute: 30% decreased clearance
Cl_{cr} <10 mL/minute: 50% decreased clearance
Dosage adjustment in hepatic impairment: Clearance decreased by 30%

Mechanism of Action A tetracyclic antidepressant that works by its central presynaptic $alpha_2$-adrenergic antagonist effects, which results in increased release of norepinephrine and serotonin; potent antagonist of 5HT2 and 5HT3 serotonin receptors and H1 histamine receptors and a moderate peripheral $alpha_1$-adrenergic and muscarinic antagonist; it does not inhibit the reuptake of norepinephrine or serotonin.

Other Adverse Effects
>10%:
Central nervous system: Somnolence (54%)
Endocrine & metabolic: Increased cholesterol
Gastrointestinal: Constipation (13%), xerostomia (25%), increased appetite (17%), weight gain (12%)
1% to 10%:
Cardiovascular: Hypertension, vasodilatation, peripheral edema (2%), edema (1%)
Central nervous system: Dizziness (7%), abnormal dreams (4%), abnormal thoughts (3%), confusion (2%), malaise
Endocrine & metabolic: Increased triglycerides
Gastrointestinal: Vomiting, anorexia, abdominal pain
Genitourinary: Urinary frequency (2%)
Neuromuscular & skeletal: Myalgia (2%), back pain (2%), arthralgias, tremor (2%), weakness (8%)
Respiratory: Dyspnea (1%)
Miscellaneous: Flu-like symptoms (5%), thirst
(Continued)

Mirtazapine *(Continued)*

Warnings/Precautions Use with caution in patients with cardiac conduction disturbances, history of hyperthyroid, renal, or hepatic dysfunction. Safety and efficacy in children have not been established. To avoid cholinergic crisis, do not discontinue abruptly in patients receiving high doses chronically. SolTab™ formulation contains phenylalanine.

Drug Interactions CYP1A2, 2C9, 2D6, and 3A3/4 enzyme substrate

Increased Effect/Toxicity: Increased sedative effect seen with CNS depressants, CYP inhibitors, linezolid, MAO inhibitors, selegiline, sibutramine

Decreased effect seen with clonidine, CYP inducers

Drug Uptake

Onset of action: Therapeutic: >2 weeks

Half-life, elimination: 20-40 hours; hampered with renal or hepatic dysfunction

Time to peak: 2 hours

Pregnancy Risk Factor C

Generic Available No

Misoprostol (mye soe PROST ole)

U.S. Brand Names Cytotec®

Canadian Brand Names Cytotec®

Mexican Brand Names Cytotec®

Pharmacologic Category Prostaglandin

Use Prevention of NSAID-induced gastric ulcers

Unlabeled/Investigational: Cervical ripening and labor induction, NSAID-induced nephropathy, fat malabsorption in cystic fibrosis

Local Anesthetic/Vasoconstrictor Precautions No information available to require special precautions

Effects on Dental Treatment No effects or complications reported

Dosage

Oral:

Children 8-16 years: Fat absorption in cystic fibrosis (unlabeled use): 100 mcg 4 times/day

Adults: Prevention of NSAID-induced gastric ulcers: 200 mcg 4 times/day with food; if not tolerated, may decrease dose to 100 mcg 4 times/day with food or 200 mcg twice daily with food; last dose of the day should be taken at bedtime

Intravaginal: Adult: Labor induction or cervical ripening (unlabeled use): 25 mcg; may repeat at intervals no more frequent than every 3-6 hours. Do not use in patients with previous cesarean delivery or prior major uterine surgery.

Mechanism of Action A synthetic prostaglandin E_1 analog that replaces the protective prostaglandins consumed with prostaglandin-inhibiting therapies (eg, NSAIDs)

Other Adverse Effects

>10%: Gastrointestinal: Diarrhea, abdominal pain

1% to 10%:

Central nervous system: Headache

Gastrointestinal: Constipation, flatulence, nausea, dyspepsia, vomiting

Drug Interactions Antacids may diminish absorption (not clinically significant).

Drug Uptake

Absorption: Oral: Rapid

Half-life, elimination: Metabolite: 20-40 minutes

Time to peak: Active metabolite: 15-30 minutes (fasting)

Pregnancy Risk Factor X

Generic Available No

Mithracin® *see* Plicamycin *on page 966*

Mitomycin (mye toe MYE sin)

U.S. Brand Names Mutamycin®

Canadian Brand Names Mutamycin®

Mexican Brand Names Mitocin®

Pharmacologic Category Antineoplastic Agent, Antibiotic

Synonyms Mitomycin-C; MTC

Use Therapy of disseminated adenocarcinoma of stomach or pancreas in combination with other approved chemotherapeutic agents; bladder cancer, colorectal cancer

Local Anesthetic/Vasoconstrictor Precautions No information available to require special precautions

Effects on Dental Treatment No effects or complications reported

Mechanism of Action Isolated from *Streptomyces caespitosus*; acts primarily as an alkylating agent and produces DNA cross-linking (primarily with guanine and cytosine pairs); cell-cycle nonspecific; inhibits DNA and RNA synthesis by alkylation and cross-linking the strands of DNA

Other Adverse Effects
>10%:
Cardiovascular: Congestive heart failure (3% to 15%) (doses >30 mg/m^2)
Dermatologic: Alopecia, nail banding/discoloration
Gastrointestinal: Nausea, vomiting and anorexia (14%)
Hematologic: Anemia (19% to 24%); myelosuppression, common, dose-limiting, delayed
Onset: 3 weeks
Nadir: 4-6 weeks
Recovery: 6-8 weeks
1% to 10%:
Dermatologic: Rash
Gastrointestinal: Stomatitis
Neuromuscular: Paresthesias
Respiratory: Interstitial pneumonitis, infiltrates, dyspnea, cough (7%)

Drug Interactions Increased Effect/Toxicity: *Vinca* alkaloids or doxorubicin may enhance cardiac toxicity when coadministered with mitomycin.

Drug Uptake
Absorption: Fairly well from the GI tract
Half-life, elimination: 23-78 minutes; Terminal: 50 minutes

Pregnancy Risk Factor D

Generic Available Yes

Mitotane (MYE toe tane)

U.S. Brand Names Lysodren®

Canadian Brand Names Lysodren®

Pharmacologic Category Antineoplastic Agent, Miscellaneous

Synonyms o,p'-DDD

Use Treatment of inoperable adrenal cortical carcinoma
Unlabeled/Investigational: Treatment of Cushing's syndrome

Local Anesthetic/Vasoconstrictor Precautions No information available to require special precautions

Effects on Dental Treatment No effects or complications reported

Mechanism of Action Causes adrenal cortical atrophy; drug affects mitochondria in adrenal cortical cells and decreases production of cortisol; also alters the peripheral metabolism of steroids

Other Adverse Effects The following reactions are reversible:
Central nervous system: CNS depression (32%), dizziness (15%), headache (5%), confusion (3%)
Dermatologic: Skin rash (12%)
Gastrointestinal: Anorexia (24%), nausea (39%), vomiting (37%), diarrhea (13%)
Neuromuscular & skeletal: Muscle tremor (3%), weakness (12%)

Drug Interactions
Increased Effect/Toxicity: CNS depressants taken with mitotane may enhance CNS depression.
Decreased Effect: Mitotane may enhance the clearance of barbiturates and warfarin by induction of the hepatic microsomal enzyme system resulting in a decreased effect. Coadministration of spironolactone has resulted in negation of mitotane's effect. Mitotane may increase clearance of phenytoin by microsomal enzyme stimulation.

Drug Uptake
Absorption: Oral: ~35% to 40%
Half-life, elimination: 18-159 days
Time to peak: 3-5 hours

Pregnancy Risk Factor C

Generic Available No

Mitoxantrone (mye toe ZAN trone)

U.S. Brand Names Novantrone®

Canadian Brand Names Novantrone®

Mexican Brand Names Misostol; Mitroxone®; Novantrone®

Pharmacologic Category Antineoplastic Agent, Antibiotic

Synonyms DHAD; Mitoxantrone Hydrochloride

Use Treatment of acute nonlymphocytic leukemia (ANLL) in adults in combination with other agents; very active against various leukemias, lymphoma, and breast cancer; moderately active against pediatric sarcoma; treatment of secondary (chronic) progressive, progressive relapsing, or worsening relapsing-remitting multiple sclerosis; treatment of pain related to advanced hormone-refractory prostate cancer (in combination with corticosteroids)

Local Anesthetic/Vasoconstrictor Precautions No information available to require special precautions

Effects on Dental Treatment No effects or complications reported

Mechanism of Action Analogue of the anthracyclines, but different in mechanism of action, cardiac toxicity, and potential for tissue necrosis; mitoxantrone does
(Continued)

Mitoxantrone *(Continued)*

intercalate DNA; binds to nucleic acids and inhibits DNA and RNA synthesis by template disordering and steric obstruction; replication is decreased by binding to DNA topoisomerase II (enzyme responsible for DNA helix supercoiling); active throughout entire cell cycle; does not appear to produce free radicals

Other Adverse Effects Reported with any indication; incidence varies based on treatment/dose

>10%:

Cardiovascular: Abnormal EKG, arrhythmia (3% to 18%), edema, nail bed changes

Central nervous system: Fatigue, fever, headache (6% to 13%)

Dermatologic: Alopecia (20% to 61%)

Endocrine & metabolic: Amenorrhea, menstrual disorder

Gastrointestinal: Abdominal pain, anorexia, nausea (29% to 76%), constipation, diarrhea (16% to 47%), GI bleeding, mucositis (10% to 29%), stomatitis, vomiting, weight gain/loss

Genitourinary: Abnormal urine, urinary tract infection

Hematologic: Decreased hemoglobin, leukopenia, lymphopenia, petechiae/bruising; myelosuppressive effects of chemotherapy:

WBC: Mild
Platelets: Mild
Onset: 7-10 days
Nadir: 14 days
Recovery: 21 days

Hepatic: Increased GGT

Neuromuscular & skeletal: Weakness (24%)

Respiratory: Cough, dyspnea, upper respiratory tract infection

Miscellaneous: Fungal infections, infection, sepsis

1% to 10%:

Cardiovascular: CHF, ischemia, decreased LVEF (≤5%)

Central nervous system: Chills, anxiety, depression, seizures

Dermatologic: Skin infection

Endocrine & metabolic: Hypocalcemia, hypokalemia, hyponatremia, hyperglycemia

Gastrointestinal: Dyspepsia, aphthosis

Genitourinary: Impotence, proteinuria, renal failure, sterility

Hematologic: Anemia, granulocytopenia, hemorrhage

Hepatic: Jaundice, increased SGOT, increased SGPT

Neuromuscular & skeletal: Back pain, myalgia, arthralgia

Ocular: Blurred vision, conjunctivitis

Renal: Hematuria

Respiratory: Pneumonia, rhinitis, sinusitis

Miscellaneous: Systemic infection, sweats, development of secondary leukemia (~1% to 2%)

Drug Interactions CYP2E1 enzyme inducer (weak)

Patients may experience impaired immune response to vaccines; possible infection after administration of live vaccines in patients receiving immunosuppressants.

Drug Uptake

Absorption: Oral: Poor

Half-life, elimination: Terminal: 23-215 hours (may increase with liver impairment)

Pregnancy Risk Factor D

Generic Available No

Mitrazol® [OTC] *see* Miconazole *on page 807*

Mitrolan® Chewable Tablet [OTC] *see* Calcium Polycarbophil *on page 207*

M-M-R® II *see* Measles, Mumps, and Rubella Vaccines, Combined *on page 747*

Moban® *see* Molindone *on page 825*

MOBIC® *see* Meloxicam *on page 756*

Mobidin® *see* Magnesium Salicylate *on page 742*

Modafinil (moe DAF i nil)

U.S. Brand Names Provigil®

Canadian Brand Names Alertec®; Provigil®

Pharmacologic Category Stimulant

Use Improve wakefulness in patients with excessive daytime sleepiness associated with narcolepsy

Unlabeled/Investigational: Attention-deficit/hyperactivity disorder (ADHD); treatment of fatigue in MS and other disorders

Local Anesthetic/Vasoconstrictor Precautions No information available to require special precautions

Effects on Dental Treatment Xerostomia, mouth ulceration, and gingivitis

Restrictions C-IV

Dosage

Children: ADHD (unlabeled use): 50-100 mg once daily

Adults:

ADHD (unlabeled use): 100-300 mg once daily

Narcolepsy: Initial: 200 mg as a single daily dose in the morning

Doses of 400 mg/day, given as a single dose, have been well tolerated, but there is no consistent evidence that this dose confers additional benefit

Elderly: Elimination of modafinil and its metabolites may be reduced as a consequence of aging and as a result, lower doses should be considered.

Dosing adjustment in hepatic impairment: Dose should be reduced to one-half of that recommended for patients with normal liver function

Mechanism of Action Exact mechanism unclear; does not appear to alter the release of dopamine or norepinephrine; does not appear to stimulate receptors commonly associated with sleep/wake regulation (including norepinephrine, serotonin, melatonin, GABA, dopamine, adenosine, and histamine-3 receptors); may exert its stimulant effects by decreasing GABA-mediated neurotransmission (theory not fully evaluated). Several studies also suggest that an intact central alpha-adrenergic system is required for modafinil's activity; the drug increases high-frequency alpha waves while decreasing both delta and theta wave activity, and these effects are consistent with generalized increases in mental alertness

Other Adverse Effects Limited to reports equal to or greater than placebo-related events.

<10%:

Cardiovascular: Chest pain (2%), hypertension (2%), hypotension (2%), vasodilation (1%), arrhythmia (1%), syncope (1%)

Central nervous system: Headache (50%, compared to 40% with placebo), nervousness (8%), dizziness (5%), depression (4%), anxiety (4%), cataplexy (3%), insomnia (3%), chills (2%), fever (1%), confusion (1%), amnesia (1%), emotional lability (1%), ataxia (1%)

Dermatologic: Dry skin (1%)

Endocrine & metabolic: Hyperglycemia (1%), albuminuria (1%)

Gastrointestinal: Diarrhea (8%), nausea (13%, compared to 4% with placebo), xerostomia (5%), anorexia (5%), vomiting (1%), mouth ulceration (1%), gingivitis (1%)

Genitourinary: Abnormal urine (1%), urinary retention (1%), ejaculatory disturbance (1%)

Hematologic: Eosinophilia (1%)

Hepatic: Abnormal LFTs (3%)

Neuromuscular & skeletal: Paresthesias (3%), dyskinesia (2%), neck pain (2%), hypertonia (2%), neck rigidity (1%), joint disorder (1%), tremor (1%)

Ocular: Amblyopia (2%), abnormal vision (2%)

Respiratory: Pharyngitis (6%), rhinitis (11%, compared to 8% with placebo), lung disorder (4%), dyspnea (2%), asthma (1%), epistaxis (1%)

Warnings/Precautions Caution when operating machinery or driving. Although functional impairment has not been demonstrated for modafinil, any agent affecting the CNS may alter judgment, thinking, or motor skills. Use with caution in patients with a recent history of myocardial infarction, unstable angina, hypertension, or history of psychosis. Efficacy of oral contraceptives may be reduced - use alternative contraceptive measures. Prolonged administration may lead to drug dependence.

Drug Interactions CYP3A3/4 enzyme substrate; CYP1A2, 2B6, and 3A3/4 enzyme inducer (weak); CYP2C19 enzyme inhibitor

Increased Effect/Toxicity: Modafinil may increase levels of diazepam, mephenytoin, phenytoin, propranolol, and warfarin. In populations deficient in the CYP2D6 isoenzyme, where CYP2C19 acts as a secondary metabolic pathway, concentrations of tricyclic antidepressants and selective serotonin reuptake inhibitors may be increased during coadministration.

Decreased Effect: Modafinil may decrease serum concentration of oral contraceptives, cyclosporine, and to a lesser degree, theophylline. Agents that induce CYP3A4, including phenobarbital, carbamazepine, and rifampin may result in decreased modafinil levels. There is also evidence to suggest that modafinil may induce its own metabolism.

Drug Uptake Modafinil is a racemic compound (10% *d*-isomer and 90% *l*-isomer at steady state), whose enantiomers have different pharmacokinetics.

Half-life, elimination: Effective half-life: 15 hours; time to steady-state: 2-4 days

Time to peak: 2-4 hours

Pregnancy Risk Factor C

Generic Available No

Modane® Bulk [OTC] *see* Psyllium *on page 1025*

Modane® Soft [OTC] *see* Docusate *on page 407*

Modane Tablets® [OTC] *see* Bisacodyl *on page 166*

Modicon® *see* Combination Hormonal Contraceptives *on page 323*

Moducal® [OTC] *see* Glucose Polymers *on page 559*

Moduretic® *see* Amiloride and Hydrochlorothiazide *on page 68*

Moexipril (mo EKS i pril)

Related Information

Cardiovascular Diseases *on page 1308*

Moexipril and Hydrochlorothiazide *on page 824*

U.S. Brand Names Univasc®

Pharmacologic Category Angiotensin-Converting Enzyme (ACE) Inhibitor

Synonyms Moexipril Hydrochloride

Use Treatment of hypertension, alone or in combination with thiazide diuretics; treatment of left ventricular dysfunction after myocardial infarction

Local Anesthetic/Vasoconstrictor Precautions No information available to require special precautions

Effects on Dental Treatment No effects or complications reported

Dosage Adults: Oral: Initial: 7.5 mg once daily (in patients **not** receiving diuretics), 1 hour prior to a meal **or** 3.75 mg once daily (when combined with thiazide diuretics); maintenance dose: 7.5-30 mg/day in 1 or 2 divided doses 1 hour before meals

Mechanism of Action Competitive inhibitor of angiotensin-converting enzyme (ACE); prevents conversion of angiotensin I to angiotensin II, a potent vasoconstrictor; results in lower levels of angiotensin II which causes an increase in plasma renin activity and a reduction in aldosterone secretion

Other Adverse Effects 1% to 10%:

Cardiovascular: Hypotension, peripheral edema

Central nervous system: Headache, dizziness, fatigue

Dermatologic: Rash, alopecia, flushing, rash

Endocrine & metabolic: Hyperkalemia, hyponatremia

Gastrointestinal: Diarrhea, nausea, heartburn

Genitourinary: Polyuria

Neuromuscular & skeletal: Myalgia

Renal: Reversible increases in creatinine or BUN

Respiratory: Cough, pharyngitis, upper respiratory infection, sinusitis

Drug Interactions

Increased Effect/Toxicity: Potassium supplements, co-trimoxazole (high dose), angiotensin II receptor antagonists (candesartan, losartan, irbesartan, etc), or potassium-sparing diuretics (amiloride, spironolactone, triamterene) may result in elevated serum potassium levels when combined with moexipril. ACE inhibitor effects may be increased by probenecid (increases levels of captopril). ACE inhibitors may increase serum concentration/effects of digoxin, lithium, and sulfonlyureas. Diuretics have additive hypotensive effects with ACE inhibitors, and hypovolemia increases the potential for adverse renal effects of ACE inhibitors. In patients with compromised renal function, coadministration with nonsteroidal anti-inflammatory drugs may result in further deterioration of renal function. Allopurinol and ACE inhibitors may cause a higher risk of hypersensitivity reaction when taken concurrently.

Decreased Effect: Aspirin (high dose) may reduce the therapeutic effects of ACE inhibitors; at low dosages this does not appear to be significant. Rifampin may decrease the effect of ACE inhibitors. Antacids may decrease the bioavailability of ACE inhibitors (may be more likely to occur with captopril); separate administration times by 1-2 hours. NSAIDs, specifically indomethacin, may reduce the hypotensive effects of ACE inhibitors. More likely to occur in low renin or volume dependent hypertensive patients.

Drug Uptake

Onset of action: Peak effect: 1-2 hours

Absorption: Food decreases bioavailability (AUC decreased by ~40%)

Duration: >24 hours

Half-life, elimination: Moexipril: 1 hour; Moexiprilat: 2-10 hours

Time to peak: 1.5 hours

Pregnancy Risk Factor C/D (2nd and 3rd trimesters)

Generic Available No

Moexipril and Hydrochlorothiazide

(mo EKS i pril & hye droe klor oh THYE a zide)

U.S. Brand Names Uniretic™

Canadian Brand Names Uniretic™

Pharmacologic Category Antihypertensive Agent Combination

Synonyms Hydrochlorothiazide and Moexipril

Use Combination therapy for hypertension, however, not indicated for initial treatment of hypertension; replacement therapy in patients receiving separate dosage forms (for patient convenience); when monotherapy with one component fails to achieve desired antihypertensive effect, or when dose-limiting adverse effects limit upward titration of monotherapy

Local Anesthetic/Vasoconstrictor Precautions No information available to require special precautions

Effects on Dental Treatment No effects or complications reported

Dosage Adults: Oral: 7.5-30 mg of moexipril, taken either in a single or divided dose 1 hour before meals

Mechanism of Action See Moexipril *on page 824* and Hydrochlorothiazide *on page 595*

Other Adverse Effects

Based on **moexipril** component: 1% to 10%:

Cardiovascular: Hypotension, peripheral edema
Central nervous system: Headache, dizziness, fatigue
Dermatologic: Rash, alopecia, flushing, rash
Endocrine & metabolic: Hyperkalemia
Gastrointestinal: Diarrhea, nausea, heartburn
Genitourinary: Polyuria
Neuromuscular & skeletal: Myalgia
Renal: Reversible increases in creatinine or BUN
Respiratory: Cough, pharyngitis, upper respiratory infection, sinusitis

Based on **hydrochlorothiazide** component: 1% to 10%:

Cardiovascular: Orthostatic hypotension, hypotension
Dermatologic: Photosensitivity
Endocrine & metabolic: Hypokalemia
Gastrointestinal: Anorexia, epigastric distress

Drug Interactions

Based on **moexipril** component:

Allopurinol: Potential for allergic reactions increased with moexipril.
Alpha$_1$ blockers: Hypotensive effect increased.
Aspirin: The effects of ACE inhibitors may be blunted by aspirin administration, particularly at higher dosages; may increase potential for adverse renal effects.
Diuretics: Hypovolemia due to diuretics may precipitate acute hypotensive events or acute renal failure.
Insulin: Risk of hypoglycemia may be increased.
Lithium: Risk of lithium toxicity may be increased; monitor lithium levels, especially the first 4 weeks of therapy.
Mercaptopurine: Risk of neutropenia may be increased.
NSAIDs: May attenuate hypertensive efficacy; effect has been seen with captopril and may occur with other ACE inhibitors; monitor BP. May increase potential to alter renal function.
Potassium-sparing diuretics (amiloride, potassium, spironolactone, triamterene): Increased risk of hyperkalemia.
Potassium supplements may increase the risk of hyperkalemia.
Probenecid: Blood levels of moexipril are increased (may occur with other ACE inhibitors).
Trimethoprim (high dose) may increase the risk of hyperkalemia.

Based on **hydrochlorothiazide** component:

ACE inhibitors: Increased hypotension if aggressively diuresed with a thiazide diuretic.
Beta-blockers increase hyperglycemic effects in type 2 diabetes mellitus (noninsulin dependent, NIDDM)
Cyclosporine and thiazides can increase the risk of gout or renal toxicity; avoid concurrent use.
Digoxin toxicity can be exacerbated if a thiazide induces hypokalemia or hypomagnesemia.
Lithium toxicity can occur by reducing renal excretion of lithium; monitor lithium concentration and adjust as needed.
Neuromuscular blocking agents can prolong blockade; monitor serum potassium and neuromuscular status.
NSAIDs can decrease the efficacy of thiazides reducing the diuretic and antihypertensive effects.

Drug Uptake See Moexipril *on page 824* and Hydrochlorothiazide *on page 595*

Pregnancy Risk Factor C/D (2nd and 3rd trimesters)

Generic Available No

Moi-Stir® [OTC] *see* Saliva Substitute *on page 1073*
Moisture® Eyes [OTC] *see* Artificial Tears *on page 117*
Moisture® Eyes PM [OTC] *see* Artificial Tears *on page 117*

Molindone (moe LIN done)

U.S. Brand Names Moban®

Canadian Brand Names Moban®

Pharmacologic Category Antipsychotic Agent, Dihydoindoline

Synonyms Molindone Hydrochloride

Use Management of schizophrenia

Unlabeled/Investigational: Management of psychotic disorders

Local Anesthetic/Vasoconstrictor Precautions No information available to require special precautions

Effects on Dental Treatment

>10%: Xerostomia

Anticholinergic side effects can cause a reduction of saliva production or secretion; may result in discomfort and dental disease (ie, caries, oral candidiasis and

(Continued)

Molindone *(Continued)*

periodontal disease). Molindone can cause extrapyramidal reactions which may appear as muscle twitching or increased motor activity of the face, neck or head.

Dosage Oral:

Children: Schizophrenia/psychoses:

3-5 years: 1-2.5 mg/day in 4 divided doses

5-12 years: 0.5-1 mg/kg/day in 4 divided doses

Adults: Schizophrenia/psychoses: 50-75 mg/day increase at 3- to 4-day intervals up to 225 mg/day

Elderly: Behavioral symptoms associated with dementia: Initial: 5-10 mg 1-2 times/day; increase at 4- to 7-day intervals by 5-10 mg/day; increase dosing intervals (bid, tid, etc) as necessary to control response or side effects.

Mechanism of Action Mechanism of action mimics that of chlorpromazine; however, it produces more extrapyramidal effects and less sedation than chlorpromazine

Other Adverse Effects Frequency not defined:

Cardiovascular: Orthostatic hypotension, tachycardia, arrhythmias

Central nervous system: Extrapyramidal reactions (akathisia, pseudoparkinsonism, dystonia, tardive dyskinesia), mental depression, altered central temperature regulation, sedation, drowsiness, restlessness, anxiety, hyperactivity, euphoria, seizures, neuroleptic malignant syndrome (NMS)

Dermatologic: Pruritus, rash, photosensitivity

Endocrine & metabolic: Change in menstrual periods, edema of breasts, amenorrhea, galactorrhea, gynecomastia

Gastrointestinal: Constipation, xerostomia, nausea, salivation, weight gain (minimal compared to other antipsychotics), weight loss

Genitourinary: Urinary retention, priapism

Hematologic: Leukopenia, leukocytosis

Ocular: Blurred vision, retinal pigmentation

Miscellaneous: Diaphoresis (decreased)

Drug Interactions CYP2D6 enzyme substrate

Aluminum salts: May decrease the absorption of antipsychotics; monitor

Amphetamines: Efficacy may be diminished by antipsychotics; in addition, amphetamines may increase psychotic symptoms; avoid concurrent use

Anticholinergics: May inhibit the therapeutic response to antipsychotics and excess anticholinergic effects may occur; includes benztropine, trihexyphenidyl, biperiden, and drugs with significant anticholinergic activity (TCAs, antihistamines, disopyramide)

Antihypertensives: Concurrent use of antipsychotics with an antihypertensive may produce additive hypotensive effects (particularly orthostasis)

Bromocriptine: Antipsychotics inhibit the ability of bromocriptine to lower serum prolactin concentrations

CNS depressants: Sedative effects may be additive with antipsychotics; monitor for increased effect; includes barbiturates, benzodiazepines, narcotic analgesics, ethanol and other sedative agents

CYP2D6 inhibitors: Metabolism of antipsychotics may be decreased; increasing clinical effect or toxicity; inhibitors include amiodarone, cimetidine, delavirdine, fluoxetine, paroxetine, propafenone, quinidine, and ritonavir; monitor for increased effect/toxicity

Enzyme inducers: May enhance the hepatic metabolism of antipsychotics; larger doses may be required; includes rifampin, rifabutin, barbiturates, phenytoin, and cigarette smoking

Epinephrine: Chlorpromazine (and possibly other low potency antipsychotics) may diminish the pressor effects of epinephrine

Guanethidine and guanadrel: Antihypertensive effects may be inhibited by antipsychotics Levodopa: Antipsychotics may inhibit the antiparkinsonian effect of levodopa; avoid this combination

Lithium: Antipsychotics may produce neurotoxicity with lithium; this is a rare effect

Metoclopramide: May increase extrapyramidal symptoms (EPS) or risk.

Phenytoin: May reduce serum levels of antipsychotics; antipsychotics may increase phenytoin serum levels

Propranolol: Serum concentrations of antipsychotics may be increased; propranolol also increases antipsychotic concentrations

QT_c-prolonging agents: Effects on QT_c interval may be additive with antipsychotics, increasing the risk of malignant arrhythmias; includes type Ia antiarrhythmics, TCAs, and some quinolone antibiotics (sparfloxacin, moxifloxacin, and gatifloxacin)

Sulfadoxine-pyrimethamine: May increase antipsychotics concentrations

Tricyclic antidepressants: Concurrent use may produce increased toxicity or altered therapeutic response

Trazodone: Antipsychotics and trazodone may produce additive hypotensive effects

Valproic acid: Serum levels may be increased by antipsychotics

Drug Uptake

Half-life, elimination: 1.5 hours

Time to peak: Oral: ~1.5 hours

Pregnancy Risk Factor C

Generic Available No

Mollifene® Ear Wax Removing Formula [OTC] *see* Carbamide Peroxide *on page 218*

Molypen® *see* Trace Metals *on page 1186*

Momentum® [OTC] *see* Magnesium Salicylate *on page 742*

Mometasone Furoate (moe MET a sone FYOOR oh ate)

Related Information

Respiratory Diseases *on page 1328*

U.S. Brand Names Elocon®; Nasonex®

Canadian Brand Names Elocom®; Nasonex®

Pharmacologic Category Corticosteroid, Nasal; Corticosteroid, Topical

Use Topical forms for the relief of the inflammatory and pruritic manifestations of corticosteroid-responsive dermatoses (medium potency topical corticosteroid); nasal spray used for the prophylaxis and treatment of nasal symptoms of seasonal allergic rhinitis and the treatment of nasal symptoms of perennial allergic rhinitis in adults and children 12 years of age and older

Local Anesthetic/Vasoconstrictor Precautions No information available to require special precautions

Effects on Dental Treatment No effects or complications reported

Dosage Adults: Topical: Apply sparingly to area once daily, do not use occlusive dressings

Therapy should be discontinued when control is achieved; if no improvement is seen, reassessment of diagnosis may be necessary.

Mechanism of Action May depress the formation, release, and activity of endogenous chemical mediators of inflammation (kinins, histamine, liposomal enzymes, prostaglandins). Leukocytes and macrophages may have to be present for the initiation of responses mediated by the above substances. Inhibits the margination and subsequent cell migration to the area of injury, and also reverses the dilatation and increased vessel permeability in the area resulting in decreased access of cells to the sites of injury.

Pregnancy Risk Factor C

Generic Available No

Monafed® *see* Guaifenesin *on page 568*

Monafed® DM *see* Guaifenesin and Dextromethorphan *on page 569*

Monarc® M *see* Antihemophilic Factor (Human) *on page 104*

Monistat® 1 Combination Pack [OTC] *see* Miconazole *on page 807*

Monistat® 3 [OTC] *see* Miconazole *on page 807*

Monistat® 7 [OTC] *see* Miconazole *on page 807*

Monistat-Derm® *see* Miconazole *on page 807*

Monobenzone (mon oh BEN zone)

U.S. Brand Names Benoquin®

Pharmacologic Category Topical Skin Product

Use Final depigmentation in extensive vitiligo

Local Anesthetic/Vasoconstrictor Precautions No information available to require special precautions

Effects on Dental Treatment No effects or complications reported

Dosage Adults: Topical: Apply 2-3 times daily

Other Adverse Effects 1% to 10%: Irritation, burning sensation, dermatitis

Pregnancy Risk Factor C

Generic Available No

Monocid® [DSC] *see* Cefonicid ***Not Available in U.S.*** *on page 238*

Monoclate-P® *see* Antihemophilic Factor (Human) *on page 104*

Monodox® *see* Doxycycline *on page 418*

Mono-Gesic® *see* Salsalate *on page 1074*

Monoket® *see* Isosorbide Mononitrate *on page 662*

Monopril® *see* Fosinopril *on page 539*

Monopril-HCT® *see* Fosinopril and Hydrochlorothiazide *on page 540*

Montelukast (mon te LOO kast)

Related Information

Respiratory Diseases *on page 1328*

U.S. Brand Names Singulair®

Canadian Brand Names Singulair®

Mexican Brand Names Singulair®

Pharmacologic Category Leukotriene Receptor Antagonist

Synonyms Montelukast Sodium

(Continued)

Montelukast *(Continued)*

Use Prophylaxis and chronic treatment of asthma in adults and children ≥2 years of age

Local Anesthetic/Vasoconstrictor Precautions No information available to require special precautions

Effects on Dental Treatment No effects or complications reported

Dosage Oral:

Children:

- <2 years: Safety and efficacy have not been established
- 2-5 years: Chew one 4 mg chewable tablet/day, taken in the evening
- 6 to 14 years: Chew one 5 mg chewable tablet/day, taken in the evening

Children ≥15 years and Adults: 10 mg/day, taken in the evening

Mechanism of Action Selective leukotriene receptor antagonist that inhibits the cysteinyl leukotriene receptor. Cysteinyl leukotrienes and leukotriene receptor occupation have been correlated with the pathophysiology of asthma, including airway edema, smooth muscle contraction, and altered cellular activity associated with the inflammatory process, which contribute to the signs and symptoms of asthma.

Other Adverse Effects

>10%: Central nervous system: Headache (18%)

1% to 10%:

- Central nervous system: Dizziness (2%), fatigue (2%), fever (2%)
- Dermatologic: Rash (2%)
- Gastrointestinal: Dyspepsia (2%), dental pain (2%), gastroenteritis (2%), abdominal pain (3%)
- Neuromuscular & skeletal: Weakness (2%)
- Respiratory: Cough (3%), nasal congestion (2%)
- Miscellaneous: Flu-like symptoms (4%), trauma (1%)

Drug Interactions CYP2A6, 2C9, and 3A3/4 enzyme substrate

Decreased Effect: Phenobarbital decreases montelukast area under the curve by 40%. Clinical significance is uncertain. Rifampin may increase the metabolism of montelukast similar to phenobarbital. No dosage adjustment is recommended when taking phenobarbital with montelukast.

Drug Uptake

Absorption: Rapid

Duration: >24 hours

Half-life, elimination, plasma: Mean: 2.7-5.5 hours

Time to peak: Tablet: 10 mg: 3-4 hours; 5 mg: 2-2.5 hours

Pregnancy Risk Factor B

Generic Available No

Monurol™ *see* Fosfomycin *on page 538*

8-MOP® *see* Methoxsalen *on page 790*

MoreDophilus® [OTC] *see Lactobacillus acidophilus* and *Lactobacillus bulgaricus on page 682*

Moricizine (mor I siz een)

Related Information

Cardiovascular Diseases *on page 1308*

U.S. Brand Names Ethmozine®

Canadian Brand Names Ethmozine®

Pharmacologic Category Antiarrhythmic Agent, Class I

Synonyms Moricizine Hydrochloride

Use Treatment of ventricular tachycardia and life-threatening ventricular arrhythmias

Unlabeled/Investigational: PVCs, complete and nonsustained ventricular tachycardia, atrial arrhythmias

Local Anesthetic/Vasoconstrictor Precautions No information available to require special precautions

Effects on Dental Treatment No effects or complications reported

Dosage Adults: Oral: 200-300 mg every 8 hours, adjust dosage at 150 mg/day at 3-day intervals. See table for dosage recommendations of transferring from other antiarrhythmic agents to Ethmozine®.

Moricizine

Transferred From	Start Ethmozine®
Encainide, propafenone, tocainide, or mexiletine	8-12 hours after last dose
Flecainide	12-24 hours after last dose
Procainamide	3-6 hours after last dose
Quinidine, disopyramide	6-12 hours after last dose

Mechanism of Action Class I antiarrhythmic agent; reduces the fast inward current carried by sodium ions, shortens Phase I and Phase II repolarization, resulting in decreased action potential duration and effective refractory period

Other Adverse Effects

>10%: Central nervous system: Dizziness

1% to 10%:

Cardiovascular: Proarrhythmia, palpitations, cardiac death, EKG abnormalities, CHF

Central nervous system: Headache, fatigue, insomnia

Endocrine & metabolic: Decreased libido

Gastrointestinal: Nausea, diarrhea, ileus

Ocular: Blurred vision, periorbital edema

Respiratory: Dyspnea

Drug Interactions May act an inhibitor of CYP1A2; may be a substrate for CYP isoenzymes

Increased Effect/Toxicity: Moricizine levels may be increased by cimetidine and diltiazem. Digoxin may result in additive prolongation of the PR interval when combined with moricizine (but not rate of second- and third-degree AV block). Drugs which may prolong QT interval (including cisapride, erythromycin, phenothiazines, cyclic antidepressants, and some quinolones) are contraindicated with type Ia antiarrhythmics. Moricizine has some type Ia activity, and caution should be used.

Decreased Effect: Moricizine may decrease levels of theophylline (50%) and diltiazem.

Drug Uptake Half-life, elimination: 3-4 hours; Cardiac disease: 6-13 hours

Pregnancy Risk Factor B

Generic Available No

Morphine Sulfate (MOR feen SUL fate)

Related Information

Dental Office Emergencies *on page 1418*

U.S. Brand Names Astramorph™ PF; Avinza™; Duramorph®; Infumorph®; Kadian®; MS Contin®; MSIR®; Oramorph SR®; RMS®; Roxanol®; Roxanol 100®; Roxanol®-T

Canadian Brand Names Kadian®; M-Eslon®; Morphine HP®; M.O.S.-Sulfate®; MS Contin®; MS-IR®; Oramorph SR®; Statex®

Mexican Brand Names Analfin®; Duralmor L.P.®; Graten®; Kapanol®; MST Continus

Pharmacologic Category Analgesic, Narcotic

Synonyms MS

Use Relief of moderate to severe acute and chronic pain; relief of pain of myocardial infarction; relief of dyspnea of acute left ventricular failure and pulmonary edema; preanesthetic medication

Orphan drug: Infumorph™: Used in microinfusion devices for intraspinal administration in treatment of intractable chronic pain

Local Anesthetic/Vasoconstrictor Precautions No information available to require special precautions

Effects on Dental Treatment

>10%: Xerostomia

Anticholinergic side effects can cause a reduction of saliva production or secretion contributes to discomfort and dental disease (ie, caries, oral candidiasis and periodontal disease).

Restrictions C-II

Dosage Should be titrated to appropriate effect; when changing routes of administration in chronically treated patients, please note that oral doses are ~$^1/_2$ as effective as parenteral dose.

Infants and Children:

Oral: Tablet and solution (prompt release): 0.2-0.5 mg/kg/dose every 4-6 hours as needed; tablet (controlled release): 0.3-0.6 mg/kg/dose every 12 hours

I.M., I.V., S.C.: 0.1-0.2 mg/kg/dose every 2-4 hours as needed; usual maximum: 15 mg/dose; may initiate at 0.05 mg/kg/dose

I.V., S.C. continuous infusion: Sickle cell or cancer pain: 0.025-2 mg/kg/hour; postoperative pain: 0.01-0.04 mg/kg/hour

Sedation/analgesia for procedures: I.V.: 0.05-0.1 mg/kg 5 minutes before the procedure

Adolescents >12 years: Sedation/analgesia for procedures: I.V.: 3-4 mg and repeat in 5 minutes if necessary

Adults:

Oral: Prompt release: 10-30 mg every 4 hours as needed; controlled release: 15-30 mg every 8-12 hours

I.M., I.V., S.C.: 2.5-20 mg/dose every 2-6 hours as needed; usual: 10 mg/dose every 4 hours as needed

I.V., S.C. continuous infusion: 0.8-10 mg/hour; may increase depending on pain relief/adverse effects; usual range: up to 80 mg/hour

Epidural: Initial: 5 mg in lumbar region; if inadequate pain relief within 1 hour, administer 1-2 mg, maximum dose: 10 mg/24 hours

Intrathecal ($^1/_{10}$ of epidural dose): 0.2-1 mg/dose; repeat doses **not** recommended

Rectal: 10-20 mg every 4 hours

Elderly or debilitated patients: Use with caution; may require dose reduction

(Continued)

Morphine Sulfate *(Continued)*

Dosing adjustment in renal impairment:

Cl_{cr} 10-50 mL/minute: Administer at 75% of normal dose

Cl_{cr} <10 mL/minute: Administer at 50% of normal dose

Dosing adjustment/comments in hepatic disease: Unchanged in mild liver disease; substantial extrahepatic metabolism may occur; excessive sedation may occur in cirrhosis

Mechanism of Action Binds to opiate receptors in the CNS, causing inhibition of ascending pain pathways, altering the perception of and response to pain; produces generalized CNS depression

Other Adverse Effects Note: Percentages are based on a study in 19 chronic cancer pain patients (*J Pain Symptom Manage*, 1995, 10:416-22). Chronic use of various opioids in cancer pain is accompanied by similar adverse reactions; individual patient differences are unpredictable, and percentage may differ in acute pain (surgical) treatment.

Frequency not defined:

- Cardiovascular: Flushing
- Central nervous system: CNS depression, sedation
- Endocrine & metabolic: Antidiuretic, hormone release
- Miscellaneous: Diaphoresis, physical and psychological dependence

>10%:

- Cardiovascular: Palpitations, hypotension, bradycardia
- Central nervous system: Drowsiness (48%, tolerance usually develops to drowsiness with regular dosing for 1-2 weeks); dizziness (20%); confusion
- Dermatologic: Pruritus (may be secondary to histamine release)
- Gastrointestinal: Nausea (28%, tolerance usually develops to nausea and vomiting with chronic use); vomiting (9%); constipation (40%, tolerance develops very slowly if at all); xerostomia (78%)
- Genitourinary: Urinary retention (16%)
- Local: Pain at injection site
- Neuromuscular & skeletal: Weakness
- Miscellaneous: Histamine release

1% to 10%:

- Central nervous system: Restlessness, headache, false feeling of well being
- Gastrointestinal: Anorexia, GI irritation, paralytic ileus
- Genitourinary: Decreased urination
- Neuromuscular & skeletal: Trembling
- Ocular: Vision problems
- Respiratory: Respiratory depression, dyspnea

Contraindications Hypersensitivity to morphine sulfate or any component of the formulation; increased intracranial pressure; severe respiratory depression (in absence of resuscitative equipment or ventilatory support); acute or severe asthma; known or suspected paralytic ileus (sustained release products only); sustained release products are not recommended in acute/postoperative pain; pregnancy (prolonged use or high doses at term)

Warnings/Precautions Infants <3 months of age are more susceptible to respiratory depression, use with caution and generally in reduced doses in this age group; use with caution in patients with impaired respiratory function or severe hepatic dysfunction and in patients with hypersensitivity reactions to other phenanthrene derivative opioid agonists (codeine, hydrocodone, hydromorphone, levorphanol, oxycodone, oxymorphone). May cause hypotension in patients with acute myocardial infarction. Tolerance or drug dependence may result from extended use. Extended or sustained release dosage forms should not be crushed or chewed.

Use caution in renal impairment (metabolite accumulation); use caution in GI motility disturbances (particularly with sustained release preparations), thyroid disorders (Addison's disease, myxedema, or hypothyroidism), prostatic hyperplasia, or urethral stricture.

Use caution in CNS depression, toxic psychosis, delirium tremens, or convulsive disorders. Sedation and psychomotor impairment are likely, and are additive with other CNS depressants or ethanol. MS Contin® 200 mg tablets are for use only in opioid-tolerant patients requiring >400 mg/day.

Elderly and/or debilitated may be particularly susceptible to the CNS depressant and constipating effects of narcotics. May mask diagnosis or clinical course in patients with acute abdominal conditions.

Drug Interactions CYP2D6 enzyme substrate

Increased Effect/Toxicity: CNS depressants (phenothiazines, tranquilizers, anxiolytics, sedatives, hypnotics, or alcohol), tricyclic antidepressants may potentiate the effects of morphine and other opiate agonists. Dextroamphetamine may enhance the analgesic effect of morphine and other opiate agonists. Concurrent use of MAO inhibitors and meperidine has been associated with significant adverse effects. Use caution with morphine. Some manufacturers recommend avoiding use within 14 days of MAO inhibitors.

Decreased Effect: Phenothiazines may antagonize the analgesic effect of morphine and other opiate agonists. Diuretic effects may be decreased (due to antidiuretic hormone release).

Drug Uptake

Onset of action: Oral: 1 hour; I.V.: 5-10 minutes

Duration: Pain relief (not sustained/controlled/extended release forms): 4 hours

Half-life, elimination: Adults: 2-4 hours (not sustained/controlled/extended release forms)

Pregnancy Risk Factor B/D (prolonged use or high doses at term)

Generic Available Yes

Morrhuate Sodium (MOR yoo ate SOW dee um)

U.S. Brand Names Scleromate™

Pharmacologic Category Sclerosing Agent

Use Treatment of small, uncomplicated varicose veins of the lower extremities

Local Anesthetic/Vasoconstrictor Precautions No information available to require special precautions

Effects on Dental Treatment No effects or complications reported

Dosage I.V.:

Children 1-18 years: Esophageal hemorrhage: 2, 3, or 4 mL of 5% repeated every 3-4 days until bleeding is controlled, then every 6 weeks until varices obliterated

Adults: 50-250 mg, repeated at 5- to 7-day intervals (50-100 mg for small veins, 150-250 mg for large veins)

Mechanism of Action Both varicose veins and esophageal varices are treated by the thrombotic action of morrhuate sodium. By causing inflammation of the vein's intima, a thrombus is formed. Occlusion secondary to the fibrous tissue and the thrombus results in the obliteration of the vein.

Other Adverse Effects Frequency not defined:

Cardiovascular: Thrombosis, valvular incompetency, vascular collapse

Central nervous system: Drowsiness, headache, dizziness

Dermatologic: Urticaria

Gastrointestinal: Nausea, vomiting

Local: Burning at the site of injection, severe extravasation effects

Neuromuscular & skeletal: Weakness

Respiratory: Asthma

Miscellaneous: Anaphylaxis, hypersensitivity reactions

Drug Uptake

Onset of action: ~5 minutes

Absorption: Most stays at site of injection

Pregnancy Risk Factor C

Generic Available No

Mosco® [OTC] *see* Salicylic Acid *on page 1072*

Motofen® *see* Difenoxin and Atropine *on page 386*

Motrin® *see* Ibuprofen *on page 621*

Motrin® IB [OTC] *see* Ibuprofen *on page 621*

Motrin® Migraine Pain [OTC] *see* Ibuprofen *on page 621*

Motrin® Sinus [OTC] *see* Pseudoephedrine and Ibuprofen *on page 1024*

Mouthkote® [OTC] *see* Saliva Substitute *on page 1073*

Mouthwash, Antiseptic (MOUTH wosh an tee SEP tik DEN tal)

Related Information

Dentin Hypersensitivity, High Caries Index, and Xerostomia *on page 1388*

Oral Bacterial Infections *on page 1367*

Oral Nonviral Soft Tissue Ulcerations or Erosions *on page 1384*

Oral Rinse Products *on page 1462*

Periodontal Diseases *on page 1375*

Pharmacologic Category Antimicrobial Mouth Rinse; Antiplaque Agent

Use Aid in the prevention and reduction of plaque and gingivitis; bad breath

Local Anesthetic/Vasoconstrictor Precautions No information available to require special precautions

Effects on Dental Treatment No effects or complications reported

Dosage Rinse full strength for 30 seconds with 20 mL (2/3 fluid ounce or 4 teaspoonfuls) morning and night

Contraindications Hypersensitivity to any components

Comments Active ingredients:

Listerine® Antiseptic: Thymol 0.064%, eucalyptus 0.092%, methyl salicylate 0.060%, menthol 0.042%, alcohol 26.9%, water, benzoic acid, poloxamer 407, sodium benzoate, caramel

Fresh Burst Listerine® Antiseptic: Thymol 0.064%, eucalyptus 0.092%, methyl salicylate 0.060%, menthol 0.042%, alcohol 26.9%, water, benzoic acid, poloxamer 407, sodium benzoate, flavoring, sodium, saccharin, sodium citrate, citric acid, D&C yellow #10, FD&C green #3

(Continued)

Mouthwash, Antiseptic *(Continued)*

Cool Mint Listerine® Antiseptic: Thymol 0.064%, eucalyptus 0.092%, methyl salicylate 0.060%, menthol 0.042%, alcohol 26.9%, water, benzoic acid, poloxamer 407, sodium benzoate, flavoring, sodium, saccharin, sodium citrate, citric acid, FD&C green #3

The following information is endorsed on the label of the Listerine® products by the Council on Scientific Affairs, American Dental Association: "Listerine® Antiseptic has been shown to help prevent and reduce supragingival plaque accumulation and gingivitis when used in a conscientiously applied program of oral hygiene and regular professional care. Its effect on periodontitis has not been determined."

Moxifloxacin (mox i FLOKS a sin)

Related Information

Oral Bacterial Infections *on page 1367*
Respiratory Diseases *on page 1328*

U.S. Brand Names ABC Pack™ (Avelox®); Avelox®

Canadian Brand Names Avelox®

Pharmacologic Category Antibiotic, Quinolone

Synonyms Moxifloxacin Hydrochloride

Use Treatment of mild to moderate community-acquired pneumonia, acute bacterial exacerbation of chronic bronchitis, acute bacterial sinusitis, uncomplicated skin infections

Special cardiovascular considerations: Moxifloxacin causes a dose-dependent QT prolongation; coadministration with other drugs that prolong the QT interval or induce bradycardia (eg, beta blockers, amiodarone) should be avoided. Use in patients with cardiovascular disease should be carefully considered, especially in those with conduction abnormalities.

Local Anesthetic/Vasoconstrictor Precautions No information available to require special precautions

Effects on Dental Treatment No effects or complications reported

Dosage Adults: Oral, I.V.:

Acute bacterial sinusitis: 400 mg every 24 hours for 10 days

Chronic bronchitis, acute bacterial exacerbation: 400 mg every 24 hours for 5 days

Note: Avelox® ABC Pack™ (Avelox® Bronchitis Course) contains five tablets of 400 mg each.

Community-acquired pneumonia: 400 mg every 24 hours for 7-14 days

Uncomplicated skin infections: 400 mg every 24 hours for 7 days

Dosage adjustment in hepatic impairment: No dosage adjustment is required in mild to moderate hepatic insufficiency (Child-Pugh Classes A and B). Not recommended in patients with severe hepatic insufficiency.

Mechanism of Action DNA gyrase inhibitor which also inhibits topoisomerase IV; DNA gyrase (topoisomerase II) is an essential bacterial enzyme that maintains the superhelical structure of DNA. DNA gyrase is required for DNA replication and transcription, DNA repair, recombination, and transposition; inhibition is bactericidal.

Other Adverse Effects

3% to 10%:

- Central nervous system: Dizziness (3%)
- Gastrointestinal: Nausea (7%), diarrhea (6%)

0.1 to 3%:

- Cardiovascular: Chest pain, hypertension, palpitation, peripheral edema, QT prolongation, tachycardia
- Central nervous system: Anxiety, chills, confusion, headache, insomnia, nervousness, pain, somnolence, tremor, vertigo
- Dermatologic: Dry skin, pruritus, rash
- Endocrine & metabolic: Serum chloride increased (≥2%), serum ionized calcium increased (≥2%), serum glucose decreased (≥2%)
- Gastrointestinal: Abdominal pain, amylase increased, amylase decreased (≥2%), anorexia, constipation, xerostomia, dyspepsia, flatulence, glossitis, lactic dehydrogenase increased, stomatitis, taste perversion, vomiting
- Hematologic: Eosinophilia, leukopenia, prothrombin time decreased, thrombocythemia, thrombocytopenia
  - Increased serum levels of the following (≥2%): MCH, neutrophils, PT ratio, WBC
  - Decreased serum levels of the following (≥2%): Basophils, eosinophils, hemoglobin, PT ratio, RBC, neutrophils
- Hepatic: Bilirubin decreased (≥2%), cholestatic jaundice, GGTP increased, liver function test abnormal
- Local: Injection site reaction
- Neuromuscular & skeletal: Arthralgia, back pain, leg pain, myalgia, paresthesia, malaise, weakness
- Renal: Serum albumin increased (≥2%)
- Respiratory: Dyspnea, pharyngitis, pneumonia, rhinitis, sinusitis, PO_2 increased (≥2%)

Miscellaneous: Allergic reaction, infection, moniliasis, diaphoresis

Contraindications Hypersensitivity to moxifloxacin, other quinolone antibiotics, or any component of their formulation; known prolongation of QT interval; uncorrected hypokalemia; concurrent administration of other medications known to prolong the QT interval (including Class Ia and Class III antiarrhythmics, cisapride, erythromycin, antipsychotics, and tricyclic antidepressants)

Warnings/Precautions Use with caution in patients with significant bradycardia or acute myocardial ischemia. Moxifloxacin causes a dose-dependent QT prolongation. Coadministration of moxifloxacin with other drugs that also prolong the QT interval or induce bradycardia (eg, beta-blockers, amiodarone) should be avoided. Careful consideration should be given in the use of moxifloxacin in patients with cardiovascular disease, particularly in those with conduction abnormalities. Use with caution in individuals at risk of seizures (CNS disorders or concurrent therapy with medications which may lower seizure threshold). Discontinue in patients who experience significant CNS adverse effects (dizziness, hallucinations, suicidal ideation or actions). Not recommended in patients with moderate to severe hepatic insufficiency. Use with caution in diabetes; glucose regulation may be altered. Tendon inflammation and/or rupture has been reported with quinolone antibiotics. Risk may be increased with concurrent corticosteroids, particularly in the elderly. Discontinue at first signs or symptoms of tendon pain.

Severe hypersensitivity reactions, including anaphylaxis, have occurred with quinolone therapy. If an allergic reaction occurs (itching, urticaria, dyspnea or facial edema, loss of consciousness, tingling, cardiovascular collapse) discontinue drug immediately. Prolonged use may result in superinfection; pseudomembranous colitis may occur and should be considered in all patients who present with diarrhea. Quinolones may exacerbate myasthenia gravis, use with caution (rare, potentially life-threatening weakness of respiratory muscles may occur).

Drug Interactions

Increased Effect/Toxicity: Drugs which prolong QT interval (including Class Ia and Class III antiarrhythmics, erythromycin, cisapride, antipsychotics, and cyclic antidepressants) are contraindicated with moxifloxacin. Azlocillin, cimetidine, and probenecid increase quinolone levels. An increased incidence of seizures may occur with foscarnet or NSAIDs. Serum levels of some quinolones are increased by loop diuretic administration. Digoxin levels may be increased in some patients by quinolones. The hypoprothrombinemic effect of warfarin is enhanced by some quinolone antibiotics. No significant effect has been demonstrated for moxifloxacin, however, monitoring of the INR during concurrent therapy is recommended by the manufacturer.

Decreased Effect: Metal cations (magnesium, aluminum, iron, and zinc) bind quinolones in the GI tract and inhibit absorption (by up to 98%). Antacids, electrolyte supplements, multivitamins, sucralfate, quinapril, and some didanosine formulations should be avoided. Moxifloxacin should be administered 4 hours before or 8 hours (a minimum of 2 hours before and 2 hours after) after these agents. Antineoplastic agents may decrease the absorption of quinolones.

Drug Uptake

Absorption: Well absorbed; not affected by high fat meal or yogurt

Half-life, elimination: Oral: 12 hours; I.V.: 15 hours

Pregnancy Risk Factor C

Generic Available No

Moxilin® *see* Amoxicillin *on page 86*

M-Prednisol® *see* MethylPREDNISolone *on page 797*

M-R-VAX® II *see* Measles and Rubella Vaccines, Combined *on page 747*

MS Contin® *see* Morphine Sulfate *on page 829*

MSIR® *see* Morphine Sulfate *on page 829*

M.T.E.-4® *see* Trace Metals *on page 1186*

M.T.E.-5® *see* Trace Metals *on page 1186*

M.T.E.-6® *see* Trace Metals *on page 1186*

Muco-Fen-DM® *see* Guaifenesin and Dextromethorphan *on page 569*

Muco-Fen-LA® *see* Guaifenesin *on page 568*

Mucomyst® *see* Acetylcysteine *on page 38*

Mucoplex® [OTC] *see* Vitamin B Complex *on page 1244*

Mucosil™ *see* Acetylcysteine *on page 38*

MulTE-PAK-4® *see* Trace Metals *on page 1186*

MulTE-PAK-5® *see* Trace Metals *on page 1186*

Multitest CMI® *see* Skin Test Antigens, Multiple *on page 1092*

Mumpsvax® *see* Mumps Virus Vaccine, Live, Attenuated *on page 833*

Mumps Virus Vaccine, Live, Attenuated

(mumpz VYE rus vak SEEN, live, a ten YOO ate ed)

U.S. Brand Names Mumpsvax®

Canadian Brand Names Mumpsvax®

Pharmacologic Category Vaccine

(Continued)

Mumps Virus Vaccine, Live, Attenuated *(Continued)*

Use Mumps prophylaxis by promoting active immunity

Note: Trivalent measles-mumps-rubella (MMR) vaccine is the preferred agent for most children and many adults; persons born prior to 1957 are generally considered immune and need not be vaccinated

Local Anesthetic/Vasoconstrictor Precautions No information available to require special precautions

Effects on Dental Treatment No effects or complications reported

Dosage Children ≥15 months and Adults: 0.5 mL S.C. in outer aspect of the upper arm, no booster

Mechanism of Action Promotes active immunity to mumps virus by inducing specific antibodies

Other Adverse Effects All serious adverse reactions must be reported to the U.S. Department of Health and Human Services (DHHS) Vaccine Adverse Event Reporting System (VAERS) 1-800-822-7967.

>10%: Local: Burning or stinging at injection site

1% to 10%:

Central nervous system: Fever (≤100°F)

Dermatologic: Rash

Endocrine & metabolic: Parotitis

Drug Interactions Whole blood, interferon immune globulin, radiation therapy, and immunosuppressive drugs (eg, corticosteroids) may result in insufficient response to immunization; may temporarily depress tuberculin skin test sensitivity and reduce the seroconversion. DTP, OPV, MMR, Hib, and hepatitis B may be given concurrently; other virus vaccine administration should be separated by ≥1 month.

Pregnancy Risk Factor X

Generic Available No

Comments Federal law requires that the date of administration, the vaccine manufacturer, lot number of vaccine, and the administering person's name, title and address be entered into the patient's permanent medical record

Mupirocin (myoo PEER oh sin)

U.S. Brand Names Bactroban®; Bactroban® Nasal

Canadian Brand Names Bactroban®

Mexican Brand Names Bactroban®; Mupiban

Pharmacologic Category Antibiotic, Topical

Synonyms Mupirocin Calcium; Pseudomonic Acid A

Use Topical treatment of impetigo due to *Staphylococcus aureus*, beta-hemolytic *Streptococcus* and *S. pyogenes*; intranasally for the eradication of nasal colonization with methicillin-resistant *Staphylococcus aureus* in adult patients and health-care workers during institutional outbreaks; eradication of nasal colonization with methicillin-resistant *Staphylococcus aureus* in adult patients and health care workers; use as part of a comprehensive infection control program to reduce the risk of infection among patients at high risk of methicillin-resistant *S. aureus* infection during institutional outbreaks of infections with this pathogen

Local Anesthetic/Vasoconstrictor Precautions No information available to require special precautions

Effects on Dental Treatment No effects or complications reported

Dosage Children and Adults: Topical: Apply small amount to affected area 2-5 times/day for 5-14 days

Mechanism of Action Binds to bacterial isoleucyl transfer-RNA synthetase resulting in the inhibition of protein and RNA synthesis

Other Adverse Effects Frequency not defined:

Central nervous system: Dizziness, headache

Dermatologic: Pruritus, rash, erythema, dry skin, cellulitis, dermatitis

Gastrointestinal: Nausea, taste perversion

Local: Burning, stinging, tenderness, edema, pain

Respiratory: Rhinitis, upper respiratory tract infection, pharyngitis, cough

Drug Uptake

Absorption: Topical: Penetrates the outer layers of skin; systemic absorption minimal through intact skin

Half-life, elimination: 17-36 minutes

Pregnancy Risk Factor B

Generic Available No

Murine® Ear Drops [OTC] *see* Carbamide Peroxide *on page 218*

Murine® Plus Ophthalmic [OTC] *see* Tetrahydrozoline *on page 1150*

Murine® Tears [OTC] *see* Artificial Tears *on page 117*

Muro 128® [OTC] *see* Sodium Chloride *on page 1094*

Murocel® [OTC] *see* Artificial Tears *on page 117*

Murocoll-2® *see* Phenylephrine and Scopolamine *on page 951*

Muromonab-CD3 (myoo roe MOE nab see dee three)

U.S. Brand Names Orthoclone OKT® 3

Canadian Brand Names Orthoclone OKT® 3

Mexican Brand Names Orthoclone OKT3

Pharmacologic Category Immunosuppressant Agent

Synonyms Monoclonal Antibody; OKT3

Use Treatment of acute allograft rejection in renal transplant patients; effective in reversing acute hepatic, kidney, pancreas, cardiac, and bone marrow transplant rejection episodes resistant to conventional treatment. Acute graft-versus-host disease following bone marrow transplantation resistant to conventional treatment.

Local Anesthetic/Vasoconstrictor Precautions No information available to require special precautions

Effects on Dental Treatment No effects or complications reported

Dosage I.V. (refer to individual protocols):

Children <30 kg: 2.5 mg/day once daily for 7-14 days

Children >30 kg: 5 mg/day once daily for 7-14 days

OR

Children <12 years: 0.1 mg/kg/day once daily for 10-14 days

Children ≥12 years and Adults: 5 mg/day once daily for 10-14 days

Hemodialysis: Molecular size of OKT3 is 150,000 daltons; not dialyzed by most standard dialyzers; however, may be dialyzed by high flux dialysis; OKT3 will be removed by plasmapheresis; administer following dialysis treatments

Peritoneal dialysis: Significant drug removal is unlikely based on physiochemical characteristics

Mechanism of Action Reverses graft rejection by binding to T cells and interfering with their function by binding T-cell receptor-associated CD3 glycoprotein

Other Adverse Effects

>10%:

"First-dose" (cytokine release) effects: Onset: 1-3 hours after the dose; duration: 12-16 hours. Severity is mild to life-threatening. Signs and symptoms include fever, chilling, dyspnea, wheezing, chest pain, chest tightness, nausea, vomiting, and diarrhea. Hypervolemic pulmonary edema, nephrotoxicity, meningitis, and encephalopathy are possible. Reactions tend to decrease with repeated doses.

Cardiovascular: Tachycardia (including ventricular)

Central nervous system: Dizziness, faintness

Gastrointestinal: Diarrhea, nausea, vomiting

Hematologic: Transient lymphopenia

Neuromuscular & skeletal: Trembling

Respiratory: Dyspnea

1% to 10%:

Central nervous system: Headache

Neuromuscular & skeletal: Stiff neck

Ocular: Photophobia

Respiratory: Pulmonary edema

Drug Interactions

Increased Effect/Toxicity: Recommend decreasing dose of prednisone to 0.5 mg/kg, azathioprine to 0.5 mg/kg (approximate 50% decrease in dose), and discontinuing cyclosporine while patient is receiving OKT3.

Decreased Effect: Decreased effect with immunosuppressive drugs

Drug Uptake

Absorption: I.V.: Immediate

Duration: 7 days after discontinuation

Time to steady-state: Trough level: 3-14 days; pretreatment levels restored within 7 days after discontinuation

Pregnancy Risk Factor C

Generic Available No

Comments Recommend decreasing dose of prednisone to 0.5 mg/kg, azathioprine to 0.5 mg/kg (approximate 50% decrease in dose), and discontinuing cyclosporine while patient is receiving OKT3

Muse® Pellet *see* Alprostadil *on page 58*
Mutamycin® *see* Mitomycin *on page 820*
Myambutol® *see* Ethambutol *on page 472*
Mycelex® *see* Clotrimazole *on page 312*
Mycelex®-3 [OTC] *see* Butoconazole *on page 195*
Mycelex®-3 *see* Clotrimazole *on page 312*
Mycelex®-7 [OTC] *see* Clotrimazole *on page 312*
Mycelex® Twin Pack [OTC] *see* Clotrimazole *on page 312*
Mycifradin® Sulfate *see* Neomycin *on page 854*
Mycinettes® [OTC] *see* Benzocaine *on page 151*
Mycitracin® [OTC] *see* Bacitracin, Neomycin, and Polymyxin B *on page 141*
Mycobutin® *see* Rifabutin *on page 1050*

Mycogen II *see* Nystatin and Triamcinolone *on page 881*
Mycolog®-II *see* Nystatin and Triamcinolone *on page 881*

Mycophenolate (mye koe FEN oh late)

U.S. Brand Names CellCept®

Canadian Brand Names CellCept®

Pharmacologic Category Immunosuppressant Agent

Synonyms Mycophenolate Mofetil

Use Prophylaxis of organ rejection concomitantly with cyclosporine and corticosteroids in patients receiving allogenic renal, cardiac, or hepatic transplants. Intravenous formulation is an alternative dosage form to oral capsules, suspension, and tablets.

Unlabeled/Investigational: Treatment of rejection in liver transplant patients unable to tolerate tacrolimus or cyclosporine due to neurotoxicity; mild rejection in heart transplant patients; treatment of moderate-severe psoriasis

Local Anesthetic/Vasoconstrictor Precautions No information available to require special precautions

Effects on Dental Treatment No effects or complications reported

Dosage

Children: Renal transplant: Oral:
- Suspension: 600 mg/m²/dose twice daily; maximum dose: 1 g twice daily
- Alternatively, may use solid dosage forms according to BSA as follows:
  - BSA 1.25-1.5 m²: 750 mg capsule twice daily
  - BSA >1.5 m²: 1 g capsule or tablet twice daily

Adults: The initial dose should be given as soon as possible following transplantation; I.V. solution may be given until the oral medication can be tolerated (up to 14 days)
- Renal transplant:
  - Oral: 1 g twice daily. Although a dose of 1.5 g twice daily was used in clinical trials and shown to be effective, no efficacy advantage was established. Patients receiving 2 g/day demonstrated an overall better safety profile than patients receiving 3 g/day. Doses >2 g/day are not recommended in these patients because of the possibility for enhanced immunosuppression as well as toxicities.
  - I.V.: 1 g twice daily
- Cardiac transplantation:
  - Oral: 1.5 g twice daily
  - I.V.: 1.5 g twice daily
- Hepatic transplantation:
  - Oral: 1.5 g twice daily
  - I.V.: 1 g twice daily

Mechanism of Action Inhibition of purine synthesis of human lymphocytes and proliferation of human lymphocytes

Other Adverse Effects As reported in adults following oral dosing of mycophenolate alone in renal, cardiac, and hepatic allograft rejection studies. In general, lower doses used in renal rejection patients had less adverse effects than higher doses. Rates of adverse effects were similar for each indication, except for those unique to the specific organ involved. The type of adverse effects observed in pediatric patients was similar to those seen in adults; abdominal pain, anemia, diarrhea, fever, hypertension, infection, pharyngitis, respiratory tract infection, sepsis, and vomiting were seen in higher proportion; lymphoproliferative disorder was the only type of malignancy observed.

>10%:

Cardiovascular: Hypertension (28% to 77%), peripheral edema (27% to 64%), hypotension (18% to 32%), edema (12% to 28%), cardiovascular disorder (26%), chest pain (13% to 26%), tachycardia (20% to 22%), arrhythmia (19%), bradycardia (17%), hypervolemia (17%), pericardial effusion (16%), heart failure (12%)

Central nervous system: Pain (31% to 76%), headache (16% to 54%), fever (21% to 52%), insomnia (9% to 52%), tremor (11% to 34%), anxiety (19% to 28%), dizziness (6% to 28%), depression (16% to 17%), confusion (13% to 17%), agitation (13%), chills (11%), somnolence (11%), nervousness (10% to 11%)

Dermatologic: Rash (18% to 22%), pruritus (14%), skin disorder (12%), diaphoresis (11%), acne (10% to 12%)

Endocrine & metabolic: Hyperglycemia (9% to 47%), hypercholesterolemia (8% to 41%), hypomagnesemia (18% to 39%), hypokalemia (10% to 37%), hypocalcemia (30%), elevated LDH (23%), hyperkalemia (9% to 22%), elevated AST (17%), elevated ALT (16%), hyperuricemia (16%), hypophosphatemia (12% to 16%), acidosis (14%), hypoproteinemia (13%), hyponatremia (11%)

Gastrointestinal: Abdominal pain (25% to 62%), nausea (20% to 54%), diarrhea (31% to 51%), constipation (18% to 41%), vomiting (12% to 34%), anorexia (25%), dyspepsia (13% to 22%), abdominal enlargement (19%), weight gain (16%), flatulence (13% to 14%), oral moniliasis (10% to 12%), nausea and vomiting (10% to 11%)

Genitourinary: Urinary tract infection (13% to 37%), urinary tract disorder

Hematologic: Leukopenia (23% to 46%), anemia (26% to 43%), leukocytosis (7% to 40%), thrombocytopenia (8% to 38%), hypochromic anemia (7% to 25%), ecchymosis (17%)

Hepatic: Abnormal LFTs (25%), ascites (24%), bilirubinemia (14% to 18%), cholangitis (14%), hepatitis (13%), cholestatic jaundice (12%)

Neuromuscular & skeletal: Back pain (12% to 47%), weakness (14% to 43%), paresthesia (15% to 21%), leg cramps (17%), hypertonia (16%), myasthenia (12%), myalgia (12%)

Ocular: Amblyopia (15%)

Renal: Elevated creatinine (20% to 40%), elevated BUN (10% to 35%), abnormal kidney function (22% to 27%), oliguria (14% to 17%), hematuria (12% to 14%), kidney tubular necrosis (6% to 10%)

Respiratory: Respiratory infection (16% to 37%), dyspnea (15% to 37%), pleural effusion (17% to 34%), increased cough (13% to 31%), lung disorder (22% to 30%), sinusitis (11% to 26%), rhinitis (19%), pharyngitis (9% to 18%), pneumonia (11% to 14%), atelectasis (13%), asthma (11%), bronchitis

Miscellaneous: Infection (18% to 27%), sepsis (18% to 27%), herpes simplex (10% to 21%), accidental injury (11% to 19%), mucocutaneous *Candida* (15% to 18%), CMV viremia/syndrome (12% to 14%), hernia (12%), CMV tissue invasive disease (6% to 11%), herpes zoster cutaneous disease (6% to 11%)

1% to 10%:

Cardiovascular: I.V.: Thrombosis (4%)

Dermatologic: Nonmelanoma skin carcinomas (2% to 4%)

Endocrine & metabolic: Hypoglycemia (10%)

Hematologic: Severe neutropenia (2% to 4%), lymphoproliferative disease/lymphoma (0.4% to 1%)

Local: I.V.: Phlebitis (4%)

Miscellaneous: Abnormal healing (10%), peritonitis (10%), fatal sepsis (2% to 5%), *Aspergillus/Mucor* (<4%), *Candidia fungemia*/disseminated disease (<4%), *Candida* tissue invasive disease (<4%), *Candida* urinary tract infection (<4%), Cryptococcosis (<4%), herpes zoster visceral disease (<4%), *Pneumocystis carinii* (<4%), malignancy (0.7% to 2%)

Drug Interactions

Increased Effect/Toxicity: Acyclovir and ganciclovir levels may increase due to competition for tubular secretion of these drugs. Probenecid may increase mycophenolate levels due to inhibition of tubular secretion. High doses of salicylates may increase free fraction of mycophenolic acid. Azathioprine's bone marrow suppression may be potentiated; do not administer together.

Decreased Effect: Antacids decrease serum concentration (C_{max} and AUC); **do not administer together**. Cholestyramine resin decreases serum concentration; **do not administer together**. Avoid use of live vaccines; vaccinations may be less effective. During concurrent use of oral contraceptives, progesterone levels are not significantly affected, however, effect on estrogen component varies; an additional form of contraception should be used.

Drug Uptake

Onset of action: Peak effect: Correlation of toxicity or efficacy is still being developed, however, one study indicated that 12-hour AUCs >40 mcg/mL/hour were correlated with efficacy and decreased episodes of rejection

Absorption: Mycophenolate mofetil is hydrolyzed to mycophenolic acid (MPA) in the liver and gastrointestinal tract. The AUC values for MPA are lower in the early post-transplant period versus the later (>3 months) post-transplant period. The extent of absorption in pediatric patients is similar to that seen in adults, although there was wide variability reported.

Half-life, elimination: Oral: 17 hours; I.V.: 18 hours

Pregnancy Risk Factor C (manufacturer)

Generic Available No

Mycostatin® *see* Nystatin *on page 880*

Myco-Triacet® II *see* Nystatin and Triamcinolone *on page 881*

Mydfrin® Ophthalmic *see* Phenylephrine *on page 950*

Mydriacyl® *see* Tropicamide *on page 1217*

Mykrox® *see* Metolazone *on page 801*

Mylanta AR® [DSC] *see* Famotidine *on page 486*

Mylanta® Extra Strength Liquid [OTC] *see* Aluminum Hydroxide, Magnesium Hydroxide, and Simethicone *on page 63*

Mylanta® Gas [OTC] *see* Simethicone *on page 1088*

Mylanta® Liquid [OTC] *see* Aluminum Hydroxide, Magnesium Hydroxide, and Simethicone *on page 63*

Myleran® *see* Busulfan *on page 190*

Mylicon® [OTC] *see* Simethicone *on page 1088*

Mylocel™ *see* Hydroxyurea *on page 615*

Mylotarg™ *see* Gemtuzumab Ozogamicin *on page 553*

Myobloc® *see* Botulinum Toxin Type B *on page 175*

Myoflex® [OTC] *see* Triethanolamine Salicylate *on page 1204*

Nabumetone (na BYOO me tone)

Related Information

Rheumatoid Arthritis and Osteoarthritis *on page 1340*
Temporomandibular Dysfunction (TMD) *on page 1397*

U.S. Brand Names Relafen®

Canadian Brand Names Apo®-Nabumetone; Relafen™

Mexican Brand Names Relifex®

Pharmacologic Category Nonsteroidal Anti-inflammatory Drug (NSAID)

Use Management of osteoarthritis and rheumatoid arthritis

Unlabeled/Investigational: Sunburn, mild to moderate pain

Local Anesthetic/Vasoconstrictor Precautions No information available to require special precautions

Effects on Dental Treatment NSAID formulations are known to reversibly decrease platelet aggregation via mechanisms different than observed with aspirin. The dentist should be aware of the potential of abnormal coagulation. Caution should also be exercised in the use of NSAIDs in patients already on anticoagulant therapy with drugs such as warfarin (Coumadin®).

Dosage Adults: Oral: 1000 mg/day; an additional 500-1000 mg may be needed in some patients to obtain more symptomatic relief; may be administered once or twice daily

Mechanism of Action A nonacidic, nonsteroidal anti-inflammatory drug that is rapidly metabolized after absorption to a major active metabolite, 6-methoxy-2-naphthylacetic acid; active metabolite is felt to be primarily responsible for the therapeutic effect; it inhibits the cyclo-oxygenase enzyme indirectly responsible for production of inflammation and pain during arthritis by enhancing production of endoperoxides and prostaglandins, E_2 and I_2 (prostacyclin). Comparatively, the parent drug is a poor inhibitor of prostaglandin synthesis.

Other Adverse Effects

>10%:

- Central nervous system: Dizziness
- Dermatologic: Rash
- Gastrointestinal: Abdominal cramps, abdominal pain (12%), diarrhea (14%), dyspepsia (13%), heartburn, indigestion, nausea

1% to 10%:

- Central nervous system: Headache, nervousness
- Dermatologic: Itching
- Endocrine & metabolic: Fluid retention
- Gastrointestinal: Vomiting
- Otic: Tinnitus

Warnings/Precautions Use with caution in patients with CHF, hypertension, decreased renal or hepatic function, history of GI disease (bleeding or ulcers), or those receiving anticoagulants. Elderly are at a high risk for adverse effects from nonsteroidal anti-inflammatory agents. As much as 60% of elderly can develop peptic ulceration and/or hemorrhage asymptomatically.

Use lowest effective dose for shortest period possible. Use of NSAIDs can compromise existing renal function especially when Cl_{cr} is <30 mL/minute. CNS adverse effects such as confusion, agitation, and hallucination are generally seen in overdose or high-dose situations; however, elderly may demonstrate these adverse effects at lower doses than younger adults. Withhold for at least 4-6 half-lives prior to surgical or dental procedures.

Drug Interactions

ACE inhibitors: Antihypertensive effects may be decreased by concurrent therapy with NSAIDs; monitor BP.

Angiotensin II antagonists: Antihypertensive effects may be decreased by concurrent therapy with NSAIDs; monitor BP.

Anticoagulants (warfarin, heparin, LMWHs) in combination with NSAIDs can cause increased risk of bleeding.

Antiplatelet drugs (ticlopidine, clopidogrel, aspirin, abciximab, dipyridamole, eptifibatide, tirofiban) can cause an increased risk of bleeding.

Corticosteroids may increase the risk of GI ulceration; avoid concurrent use.

Cyclosporine: NSAIDs may increase serum creatinine, potassium, BP, and cyclosporine levels; monitor cyclosporine levels and renal function carefully.

Hydralazine's antihypertensive effect is decreased; avoid concurrent use.

Lithium levels can be increased; avoid concurrent use if possible or monitor lithium levels and adjust dose. Sulindac may have the least effect. When NSAID is stopped, lithium will need adjustment again.

Loop diuretics efficacy (diuretic and antihypertensive effect) is reduced.

Methotrexate: Severe bone marrow suppression, aplastic anemia, and GI toxicity have been reported with concomitant NSAID therapy. Avoid use during moderate or high-dose methotrexate (increased and prolonged methotrexate levels). NSAID use during low-dose treatment of rheumatoid arthritis has not been fully evaluated; extreme caution is warranted.

Thiazides antihypertensive effects are decreased; avoid concurrent use.

Warfarin's INRs may be increased by nabumetone. Monitor INR closely. Use the lowest dose of NSAIDs possible and for the briefest duration.

Drug Uptake

Onset of action: Several days

Half-life, elimination: Major metabolite: 24 hours

Time to peak: Metabolite: Oral: 3-6 hours; Synovial fluid: 4-12 hours

Pregnancy Risk Factor C/D (3rd trimester)

Generic Available No

Nadolol (nay DOE lole)

Related Information

Cardiovascular Diseases *on page 1308*

U.S. Brand Names Corgard®

Canadian Brand Names Alti-Nadolol; Apo®-Nadol; Corgard®; Novo-Nadolol

Pharmacologic Category Beta Blocker, Nonselective

Use Treatment of hypertension and angina pectoris; prevention of myocardial infarction; prophylaxis of migraine headaches

Local Anesthetic/Vasoconstrictor Precautions Use with caution; epinephrine has interacted with nonselective beta-blockers to result in initial hypertensive episode followed by bradycardia

Effects on Dental Treatment Noncardioselective beta-blockers (ie, propranolol, nadolol) may enhance the pressor response to epinephrine, resulting in hypertension and bradycardia. Many nonsteroidal anti-inflammatory drugs such as ibuprofen and indomethacin can reduce the hypotensive effect of beta-blockers after 3 or more weeks of therapy with the NSAID. Short-term NSAID use (ie, 3 days) requires no special precautions in patients taking beta-blockers.

Dosage Oral:

Adults: Initial: 40 mg/day, increase dosage gradually by 40-80 mg increments at 3- to 7-day intervals until optimum clinical response is obtained with profound slowing of heart rate; doses up to 160-240 mg/day in angina and 240-320 mg/day in hypertension may be necessary.

Elderly: Initial: 20 mg/day; increase doses by 20 mg increments at 3- to 7-day intervals; usual dosage range: 20-240 mg/day.

Dosing adjustment in renal impairment:

Cl_{cr} 31-40 mL/minute: Administer every 24-36 hours or administer 50% of normal dose.

Cl_{cr} 10-30 mL/minute: Administer every 24-48 hours or administer 50% of normal dose.

Cl_{cr} <10 mL/minute: Administer every 40-60 hours or administer 25% of normal dose.

Hemodialysis: Moderately dialyzable (20% to 50%); administer dose postdialysis or administer 40 mg supplemental dose.

Peritoneal dialysis: Supplemental dose is not necessary.

Dosing adjustment/comments in hepatic disease: Reduced dose probably necessary.

Mechanism of Action Competitively blocks response to $beta_1$- and $beta_2$-adrenergic stimulation; does not exhibit any membrane stabilizing or intrinsic sympathomimetic activity

Other Adverse Effects

>10%:

Central nervous system: Drowsiness, insomnia

Endocrine & metabolic: Decreased sexual ability

1% to 10%:

Cardiovascular: Bradycardia, palpitations, edema, CHF, reduced peripheral circulation

Central nervous system: Mental depression

Gastrointestinal: Diarrhea or constipation, nausea, vomiting, stomach discomfort

Respiratory: Bronchospasm

Miscellaneous: Cold extremities

Drug Interactions

Increased Effect/Toxicity: The heart rate lowering effects of nadolol are additive with other drugs which slow AV conduction (digoxin, verapamil, diltiazem). Concurrent use of alpha-blockers (prazosin, terazosin) with beta-blockers may increase risk of orthostasis. Nadolol may mask the tachycardia from hypoglycemia caused by insulin and oral hypoglycemics. In patients receiving concurrent

(Continued)

Nadolol *(Continued)*

therapy, the risk of hypertensive crisis is increased when either clonidine or the beta-blocker is withdrawn. Reserpine has been shown to enhance the effect of beta-blockers. Avoid using with alpha-adrenergic stimulants (phenylephrine, epinephrine, etc) which may have exaggerated hypertensive responses. Beta-blockers may affect the action or levels of disopyramide, nondepolarizing muscle relaxants, and theophylline although the effects are difficult to predict. The vasoconstrictive effects of ergot alkaloids may be enhanced.

Decreased Effect: Decreased effect of beta-blockers with aluminum salts, barbiturates, calcium salts, cholestyramine, colestipol, NSAIDs, penicillins (ampicillin), rifampin, salicylates, and sulfinpyrazone due to decreased bioavailability and plasma concentrations. Beta-blockers may decrease the effect of sulfonylureas (possibly hyperglycemia). Nonselective beta-blockers blunt the effect of beta-2 adrenergic agonists (albuterol).

Drug Uptake

Absorption: Oral: 30% to 40%

Duration: 17-24 hours

Half-life, elimination: Adults: 10-24 hours (increases with renal impairment); End-stage renal disease: 45 hours

Time to peak: 2-4 hours

Pregnancy Risk Factor C

Generic Available Yes

Selected Readings

Foster CA and Aston SJ, "Propranolol-Epinephrine Interaction: A Potential Disaster," *Plast Reconstr Surg*, 1983, 72(1):74-8.

Wong DG, Spence JD, Lamki L, et al, "Effect of Nonsteroidal Anti-inflammatory Drugs on Control of Hypertension of Beta-Blockers and Diuretics," *Lancet*, 1986, 1(8488):997-1001.

Wynn RL, "Dental Nonsteroidal Anti-inflammatory Drugs and Prostaglandin-Based Drug Interactions, Part Two," *Gen Dent*, 1992, 40(2):104, 106, 108.

Wynn RL, "Epinephrine Interactions With Beta-Blockers," *Gen Dent*, 1994, 42(1):16, 18.

Nafarelin (NAF a re lin)

U.S. Brand Names Synarel®

Canadian Brand Names Synarel®

Mexican Brand Names Synarel®

Pharmacologic Category Hormone, Posterior Pituitary; Luteinizing Hormone-Releasing Hormone Analog

Synonyms Nafarelin Acetate

Use Treatment of endometriosis, including pain and reduction of lesions; treatment of central precocious puberty (gonadotropin-dependent precocious puberty) in children of both sexes

Local Anesthetic/Vasoconstrictor Precautions No information available to require special precautions

Effects on Dental Treatment No effects or complications reported

Dosage

Endometriosis: Adults: Female: 1 spray (200 mcg) in 1 nostril each morning and the other nostril each evening starting on days 2-4 of menstrual cycle for 6 months

Central precocious puberty: Children: Male/Female: 2 sprays (400 mcg) into each nostril in the morning 2 sprays (400 mcg) into each nostril in the evening. If inadequate suppression, may increase dose to 3 sprays (600 mcg) into alternating nostrils 3 times/day.

Mechanism of Action Potent synthetic decapeptide analogue of gonadotropin-releasing hormone (GnRH; LHRH) which is approximately 200 times more potent than GnRH in terms of pituitary release of luteinizing hormone (LH) and follicle-stimulating hormone (FSH). Effects on the pituitary gland and sex hormones are dependent upon its length of administration. After acute administration, an initial stimulation of the release of LH and FSH from the pituitary is observed; an increase in androgens and estrogens subsequently follows. Continued administration of nafarelin, however, suppresses gonadotrope responsiveness to endogenous GnRH resulting in reduced secretion of LH and FSH and, secondarily, decreased ovarian and testicular steroid production.

Other Adverse Effects

>10%:

- Central nervous system: Headache, emotional lability
- Dermatologic: Acne
- Endocrine & metabolic: Hot flashes, decreased libido, decreased breast size
- Genitourinary: Vaginal dryness
- Neuromuscular & skeletal: Myalgia
- Respiratory: Nasal irritation

1% to 10%:

- Cardiovascular: Edema, chest pain
- Central nervous system: Insomnia
- Dermatologic: Urticaria, rash, pruritus, seborrhea
- Respiratory: Dyspnea

Drug Uptake

Absorption: Not absorbed from GI tract

Time to peak: 10-45 minutes

Pregnancy Risk Factor X

Generic Available No

Nafcillin (naf SIL in)

Canadian Brand Names Nallpen®; Unipen®

Pharmacologic Category Antibiotic, Penicillin

Synonyms Ethoxynaphthamido Penicillin Sodium; Nafcillin Sodium; Nallpen [DSC]; Sodium Nafcillin

Use Treatment of susceptible bacterial infections such as osteomyelitis, septicemia, endocarditis, and CNS infections due to penicillinase-producing strains of *Staphylococcus*

Local Anesthetic/Vasoconstrictor Precautions No information available to require special precautions

Effects on Dental Treatment Prolonged use of penicillins may lead to the development of oral candidiasis.

Dosage

Children: I.M., I.V.:

Mild to moderate infections: 50-100 mg/kg/day in divided doses every 6 hours

Severe infections: 100-200 mg/kg/day in divided doses every 4-6 hours

Maximum dose: 12 g/day

Adults:

I.M.: 500 mg every 4-6 hours

I.V.: 500-2000 mg every 4-6 hours

Mechanism of Action Interferes with bacterial cell wall synthesis during active multiplication, causing cell wall death and resultant bactericidal activity against susceptible bacteria

Other Adverse Effects Frequency not defined:

Central nervous system: Pain, fever

Dermatologic: Rash

Gastrointestinal: Nausea, diarrhea

Hematologic: Neutropenia

Local: Thrombophlebitis; oxacillin (less likely to cause phlebitis) is often preferred in pediatric patients

Renal: Interstitial nephritis (acute)

Miscellaneous: Hypersensitivity reactions

Drug Interactions CYP3A3/4 enzyme inducer

Increased Effect/Toxicity: Probenecid may cause an increase in nafcillin levels.

Decreased Effect: Chloramphenicol may decrease nafcillin efficacy. Oral contraceptives may have a decreased contraceptive effect when taken with nafcillin. If taken concomitantly with warfarin, nafcillin may inhibit the anticoagulant response to warfarin. This effect may persist for up to 30 days after nafcillin has been discontinued. Subtherapeutic cyclosporine levels may result when taken concomitantly with nafcillin.

Drug Uptake

Absorption: Oral: Poor and erratic

Half-life, elimination:

Neonates: <3 weeks: 2.2-5.5 hours; 4-9 weeks: 1.2-2.3 hours

Children 3 months to 14 years: 0.75-1.9 hours

Adults: 0.5-1.5 hours (dependent on hepatic function); End-stage renal disease: 1.2 hours

Time to peak: Oral: ≤2 hours; I.M.: 0.5-1 hour

Pregnancy Risk Factor B

Generic Available Yes

Naftifine (NAF ti feen)

Related Information

Oral Fungal Infections *on page 1377*

U.S. Brand Names Naftin®

Pharmacologic Category Antifungal Agent, Topical

Synonyms Naftifine Hydrochloride

Use Topical treatment of tinea cruris (jock itch), tinea corporis (ring worm), and tinea pedis (athlete's foot)

Local Anesthetic/Vasoconstrictor Precautions No information available to require special precautions

Effects on Dental Treatment No effects or complications reported

Dosage Adults: Topical: Apply cream once daily and gel twice daily (morning and evening) for up to 4 weeks

Mechanism of Action Synthetic, broad-spectrum antifungal agent in the allylamine class; appears to have both fungistatic and fungicidal activity. Exhibits antifungal activity by selectively inhibiting the enzyme squalene epoxidase in a

(Continued)

Naftifine *(Continued)*

dose-dependent manner which results in the primary sterol, ergosterol, within the fungal membrane not being synthesized.

Other Adverse Effects

>10%: Local: Burning, stinging

1% to 10%:

Dermatologic: Erythema, itching

Local: Dryness, irritation

Drug Uptake

Absorption: Systemic: Cream: 6%; Gel: ≤4%

Half-life, elimination: 2-3 days

Pregnancy Risk Factor B

Generic Available No

Naftin® *see* Naftifine *on page 841*

Nalbuphine (NAL byoo feen)

U.S. Brand Names Nubain®

Canadian Brand Names Nubain®

Mexican Brand Names Bufigen; Nalcryn®; Nubain®

Pharmacologic Category Analgesic, Narcotic

Synonyms Nalbuphine Hydrochloride

Use Relief of moderate to severe pain; preoperative analgesia, postoperative and surgical anesthesia, and obstetrical analgesia during labor and delivery

Local Anesthetic/Vasoconstrictor Precautions No information available to require special precautions

Effects on Dental Treatment Anticholinergic side effects can cause a reduction of saliva production or secretion contributes to discomfort and dental disease (ie, caries, oral candidiasis and periodontal disease).

Dosage I.M., I.V., S.C.:

Children 10 months to 14 years: Premedication: 0.2 mg/kg; maximum: 20 mg/dose

Adults: 10 mg/70 kg every 3-6 hours; maximum single dose: 20 mg; maximum daily dose: 160 mg

Mechanism of Action Binds to opiate receptors in the CNS, causing inhibition of ascending pain pathways, altering the perception of and response to pain; produces generalized CNS depression

Other Adverse Effects

>10%:

Central nervous system: Drowsiness, CNS depression, narcotic withdrawal

Miscellaneous: Histamine release

1% to 10%:

Cardiovascular: Hypotension, flushing

Central nervous system: Dizziness, headache

Dermatologic: Urticaria, rash

Gastrointestinal: Nausea, vomiting, anorexia, xerostomia

Local: Pain at injection site

Neuromuscular & skeletal: Weakness

Respiratory: Pulmonary edema

Drug Interactions Barbiturate anesthetics may increase CNS depression.

Drug Uptake

Onset of action: Peak effect: I.M.: 30 minutes; I.V.: 1-3 minutes

Half-life, elimination: 3.5-5 hours

Pregnancy Risk Factor B/D (prolonged use or high doses at term)

Generic Available Yes

Naldecon® Senior DX [OTC] *see* Guaifenesin and Dextromethorphan *on page 569*

Naldecon® Senior EX [OTC] *see* Guaifenesin *on page 568*

Nalfon® *see* Fenoprofen *on page 492*

Nalidixic Acid (nal i DIKS ik AS id)

U.S. Brand Names NegGram®

Canadian Brand Names NegGram®

Pharmacologic Category Antibiotic, Quinolone

Synonyms Nalidixinic Acid

Use Treatment of urinary tract infections

Local Anesthetic/Vasoconstrictor Precautions No information available to require special precautions

Effects on Dental Treatment No effects or complications reported

Dosage Oral:

Children 3 months to 12 years: 55 mg/kg/day divided every 6 hours; suppressive therapy is 33 mg/kg/day divided every 6 hours

Adults: 1 g 4 times/day for 2 weeks; then suppressive therapy of 500 mg 4 times/day

Mechanism of Action Inhibits DNA polymerization in late stages of chromosomal replication

Other Adverse Effects Frequency not defined:

Central nervous system: Dizziness, drowsiness, headache, increased intracranial pressure, malaise, vertigo, confusion, toxic psychosis, convulsions, fever, chills

Dermatologic: Rash, urticaria, photosensitivity reactions

Endocrine & metabolic: Metabolic acidosis

Gastrointestinal: Nausea, vomiting

Hematologic: Leukopenia, thrombocytopenia

Hepatic: Hepatotoxicity

Ocular: Visual disturbances

Miscellaneous: Quinolones have been associated with tendonitis and tendon rupture

Warnings/Precautions Use with caution in patients with impaired hepatic or renal function and prepubertal children; has been shown to cause cartilage degeneration in immature animals; may induce hemolysis in patients with G6PD deficiency; use caution in patients with seizure disorder. Tendon inflammation and/or rupture have been reported with other quinolone antibiotics. Discontinue at first sign of tendon inflammation or pain.

Severe hypersensitivity reactions, including anaphylaxis, have occurred with quinolone therapy. If an allergic reaction occurs (itching, urticaria, dyspnea, facial edema, loss of consciousness, tingling, cardiovascular collapse), discontinue drug immediately. Prolonged use may result in superinfection; pseudomembranous colitis may occur and should be considered in all patients who present with diarrhea. Quinolones may exacerbate myasthenia gravis, use with caution (rare, potentially life-threatening weakness of respiratory muscles may occur).

Drug Interactions CYP1A2 enzyme inhibitor (minor)

Increased Effect/Toxicity: Nalidixic acid increases the levels/effect of cyclosporine, caffeine, theophylline, and warfarin. The CNS-stimulating effect of some quinolones may be enhanced by NSAIDs, and foscarnet has been associated with an increased risk of seizures with some quinolones. Serum levels of some quinolones are increased by loop diuretics, probenecid, and cimetidine (and possibly other H_2 blockers) due to altered renal elimination. This effect may be more important for quinolones with high percentage of renal elimination than with nalidixic acid.

Decreased Effect: Enteral feedings may decrease plasma concentrations of nalidixic acid probably by >30% inhibition of absorption. Aluminum/magnesium products, didanosine, quinapril, and sucralfate may decrease absorption of nalidixic acid by ≥90% if administered concurrently. (Administer nalidixic acid at least 4 hours and preferably 6 hours after the dose of these agents.) Calcium, iron, zinc, and multivitamins with minerals products may decrease absorption of nalidixic acid significantly if administered concurrently. (Administer nalidixic acid 2 hours before dose or at least 2 hours after the dose of these agents). Antineoplastic agents may decrease quinolone absorption.

Drug Uptake

Half-life, elimination: 6-7 hours (increases significantly with renal impairment)

Time to peak: Oral: 1-2 hours

Pregnancy Risk Factor B

Generic Available No

Nalmefene (NAL me feen)

U.S. Brand Names Revex®

Pharmacologic Category Antidote

Synonyms Nalmefene Hydrochloride

Use Complete or partial of opioid drug effects; management of known or suspected opioid overdose

Local Anesthetic/Vasoconstrictor Precautions No information available to require special precautions

Effects on Dental Treatment No effects or complications reported

Dosage

If recurrence of respiratory depression is noted, dose may again be titrated to clinical effect using incremental doses.

Reversal of postoperative opioid depression: Blue labeled product (100 mcg/mL): Titrate to reverse the undesired effects of opioids; initial dose for nonopioid dependent patients: 0.25 mcg/kg followed by 0.25 mcg/kg incremental doses at 2- to 5-minute intervals; after a total dose >1 mcg/kg, further therapeutic response is unlikely

Management of known/suspected opioid overdose: Green labeled product (1000 mcg/mL): Initial dose: 0.5 mg/70 kg; may repeat with 1 mg/70 kg in 2-5 minutes; further increase beyond a total dose of 1.5 mg/70 kg will not likely result in improved response and may result in cardiovascular stress and precipitated withdrawal syndrome. (If opioid dependency is suspected, administer a challenge dose of 0.1 mg/70 kg; if no withdrawal symptoms are observed in 2 minutes, the recommended doses can be administered.)

(Continued)

Nalmefene *(Continued)*

Note: If I.V. access is lost or not readily obtainable, a single S.C. or I.M. dose of 1 mg may be effective in 5-15 minutes.

Dosing adjustment in renal or hepatic impairment: Not necessary with single uses, however, slow administration (over 60 seconds) of incremental doses is recommended to minimize hypertension and dizziness

Mechanism of Action As a 6-methylene analog of naltrexone, nalmefene acts as a competitive antagonist at opioid receptor sites, preventing or reversing the respiratory depression, sedation, and hypotension induced by opiates; no pharmacologic activity of its own (eg, opioid agonist activity) has been demonstrated

Other Adverse Effects

>10%: Gastrointestinal: Nausea

1% to 10%:

- Cardiovascular: Tachycardia, hypertension, hypotension, vasodilation
- Central nervous system: Fever, dizziness, headache, chills
- Gastrointestinal: Vomiting
- Miscellaneous: Postoperative pain

Warnings/Precautions May induce symptoms of acute withdrawal in opioid-dependent patients; recurrence of respiratory depression is possible if the opioid involved is long-acting; observe patients until there is no reasonable risk of recurrent respiratory depression. Safety and efficacy have not been established in children. Avoid abrupt reversal of opioid effects in patients of high cardiovascular risk or who have received potentially cardiotoxic drugs. Pulmonary edema and cardiovascular instability have been reported in association with abrupt reversal with other narcotic antagonists. Animal studies indicate nalmefene may not completely reverse buprenorphine-induced respiratory depression.

Drug Interactions Potential for increased risk of seizures may exist with use of flumazenil and nalmefene coadministration.

Drug Uptake

Onset of action: I.M., S.C.: 5-15 minutes

Half-life, elimination: 10.8 hours

Time to peak: I.M.: 2.3 hours; I.V.: <2 minutes; S.C.: 1.5 hours

Pregnancy Risk Factor B

Generic Available No

Comments Nalmefene is supplied in two concentrations 100 mcg/mL has a blue label, 1000 mcg/mL has a green label; proper steps should be used to prevent use of the incorrect dosage strength; duration of action of nalmefene is as long as most opioid analgesics; may cause acute withdrawal symptoms in individuals who have some degree of tolerance to and dependence on opioids

Naloxone (nal OKS one)

Related Information

Dental Office Emergencies *on page 1418*

U.S. Brand Names Narcan®

Canadian Brand Names Narcan®

Mexican Brand Names Narcanti®

Pharmacologic Category Antidote

Synonyms *N*-allylnoroxymorphine Hydrochloride; Naloxone Hydrochloride

Use

Dental: Reverse overdose effects of the two narcotic agents, fentanyl and meperidine, used in the technique of I.V. conscious sedation

Medical:

- Complete or partial reversal of opioid depression, including respiratory depression, induced by natural and synthetic opioids (including propoxyphene, methadone, and certain mixed agonist-antagonist analgesics, such as nalbuphine, pentazocine, and butorphanol):
- Diagnosis of suspected opioid tolerance or acute opioid overdose
- Adjunctive agent to increase BP in the management of septic shock

Local Anesthetic/Vasoconstrictor Precautions No information available to require special precautions

Effects on Dental Treatment No effects or complications reported

Dosage I.M., I.V. (preferred), intratracheal, S.C.:

Postanesthesia narcotic reversal: Infants and Children: 0.01 mg/kg; may repeat every 2-3 minutes, as needed based on response

Opiate intoxication:

Children:

- Birth (including premature infants) to 5 years or <20 kg: 0.1 mg/kg; repeat every 2-3 minutes if needed; may need to repeat doses every 20-60 minutes
- >5 years or ≥20 kg: 2 mg/dose; if no response, repeat every 2-3 minutes; may need to repeat doses every 20-60 minutes

Children and Adults: Continuous infusion: I.V.: If continuous infusion is required, calculate dosage/hour based on effective intermittent dose used and duration of adequate response seen, titrate dose 0.04-0.16 mg/kg/hour for 2-5 days in children, adult dose typically 0.25-6.25 mg/hour (short-term infusions as high as

(Continued)

2.4 mg/kg/hour have been tolerated in adults during treatment for septic shock); alternatively, continuous infusion utilizes 2/3 of the initial naloxone bolus on an hourly basis; add 10 times this dose to each liter of D_5W and infuse at a rate of 100 mL/hour; 1/2 of the initial bolus dose should be readministered 15 minutes after initiation of the continuous infusion to prevent a drop in naloxone levels; increase infusion rate as needed to assure adequate ventilation

Narcotic overdose: Adults: I.V.: 0.4-2 mg every 2-3 minutes as needed; may need to repeat doses every 20-60 minutes, if no response is observed after 10 mg, question the diagnosis. Use 0.1-0.2 mg increments in patients who are opioid dependent and in postoperative patients to avoid large cardiovascular changes.

Mechanism of Action Competes and displaces narcotics at opioid receptor sites (mu, kappa, delta, and sigma subtypes)

Other Adverse Effects Frequency not defined:

Cardiovascular: Cardiac arrest, hypertension, hypotension, tachycardia, ventricular arrhythmias

Central nervous system: Anxiety, irritability, narcotic withdrawal, restlessness, seizures

Gastrointestinal: Diarrhea, nausea, vomiting

Neuromuscular & skeletal: Tremulousness

Respiratory: Dyspnea, pulmonary edema, runny nose, sneezing

Miscellaneous: Diaphoresis

Contraindications Hypersensitivity to naloxone or any component of the formulation

Warnings/Precautions Due to an association between naloxone and acute pulmonary edema, use with caution in patients with cardiovascular disease or in patients receiving medications with potential adverse cardiovascular effects (eg, hypotension, pulmonary edema or arrhythmias). Excessive dosages should be avoided after use of opiates in surgery. Abrupt postoperative reversal may result in nausea, vomiting, sweating, tachycardia, hypertension, seizures, and other cardiovascular events (including pulmonary edema and arrhythmias). May precipitate withdrawal symptoms in patients addicted to opiates, including pain, hypertension, sweating, agitation, irritability; in neonates: shrill cry, failure to feed. Recurrence of respiratory depression is possible if the opioid involved is long-acting; observe patients until there is no reasonable risk of recurrent respiratory depression.

Drug Interactions Decreased Effect: Antagonist of all narcotic analgesics; may precipitate acute withdrawal reaction in physically dependent patients

Drug Uptake

Onset of action: Endotracheal, I.M., S.C.: 2-5 minutes; I.V.: ~2 minutes

Duration: 20-60 minutes; since shorter than that of most opioids, repeated doses are usually needed

Half-life, elimination: Neonates: 1.2-3 hours; Adults: 1-1.5 hours

Pregnancy Risk Factor B

Breast-feeding Considerations No data reported; may transfer transfer to the infant; breast-feeding not recommended

Dosage Forms INJ: 0.4 mg/mL (1 mL, 2 mL, 10 mL); 1 mg/mL (2 mL, 10 mL). **INJ, neonatal:** 0.02 mg/mL (2 mL)

Generic Available Yes

Naltrexone (nal TREKS one)

U.S. Brand Names ReVia®

Canadian Brand Names ReVia®

Pharmacologic Category Antidote

Synonyms Naltrexone Hydrochloride

Use Adjunct to the maintenance of an opioid-free state in detoxified individual

Local Anesthetic/Vasoconstrictor Precautions No information available to require special precautions

Effects on Dental Treatment No effects or complications reported

Dosage Do not give until patient is opioid-free for 7-10 days as determined by urine analysis

Adults: Oral: 25 mg; if no withdrawal signs within 1 hour give another 25 mg; maintenance regimen is flexible, variable and individualized (50 mg/day to 100-150 mg 3 times/week for 12 weeks); up to 800 mg/day has been tolerated in adults without an adverse effect

Dosing cautions in renal/hepatic impairment: Caution in patients with renal and hepatic impairment. An increase in naltrexone AUC of ~ five- and tenfold in patients with compensated or decompensated liver cirrhosis respectively, compared with normal liver function has been reported.

Mechanism of Action A cyclopropyl derivative of oxymorphone similar in structure to naloxone and nalorphine (a morphine derivative); acts as a competitive antagonist at opioid receptor sites

Other Adverse Effects

>10%:

Central nervous system: Insomnia, nervousness, headache, low energy

Gastrointestinal: Abdominal cramping, nausea, vomiting

(Continued)

Naltrexone *(Continued)*

Neuromuscular & skeletal: Arthralgia

1% to 10%:

Central nervous system: Increased energy, feeling down, irritability, dizziness, anxiety, somnolence

Dermatologic: Rash

Endocrine & metabolic: Polydipsia

Gastrointestinal: Diarrhea, constipation

Genitourinary: Delayed ejaculation, impotency

Drug Interactions

Increased Effect/Toxicity: Lethargy and somnolence reported with thioridazine

Decreased Effect: Naltrexone decreases effects of opioid-containing products.

Drug Uptake

Absorption: Oral: Almost completely

Duration: 50 mg: 24 hours; 100 mg: 48 hours; 150 mg: 72 hours

Half-life, elimination: 4 hours; 6-β-naltrexol: 13 hours

Time to peak: ~60 minutes

Pregnancy Risk Factor C

Generic Available Yes

Nandrolone (NAN droe lone)

U.S. Brand Names Deca-Durabolin®; Hybolin™ Decanoate; Hybolin™ Improved Injection

Canadian Brand Names Deca-Durabolin®; Durabolin®

Mexican Brand Names Deca-Durabolin®

Pharmacologic Category Androgen

Synonyms Nandrolone Decanoate; Nandrolone Phenpropionate

Use Control of metastatic breast cancer; management of anemia of renal insufficiency

Local Anesthetic/Vasoconstrictor Precautions No information available to require special precautions

Effects on Dental Treatment No effects or complications reported

Restrictions C-III

Dosage Deep I.M. (into gluteal muscle):

Children 2-13 years: (decanoate): 25-50 mg every 3-4 weeks

Adults:

Male:

Breast cancer (phenpropionate): 50-100 mg/week

Anemia of renal insufficiency (decanoate): 100-200 mg/week

Female: 50-100 mg/week

Breast cancer (phenpropionate): 50-100 mg/week

Anemia of renal insufficiency (decanoate): 50-100 mg/week

Mechanism of Action Promotes tissue-building processes, increases production of erythropoietin, causes protein anabolism; increases hemoglobin and red blood cell volume

Other Adverse Effects

Male:

Postpubertal:

>10%:

Dermatologic: Acne

Endocrine & metabolic: Gynecomastia

Genitourinary: Bladder irritability, priapism

1% to 10%:

Central nervous system: Insomnia, chills

Endocrine & metabolic: Decreased libido, hepatic dysfunction

Gastrointestinal: Nausea, diarrhea

Genitourinary: Prostatic hyperplasia (elderly)

Hematologic: Iron-deficiency anemia, suppression of clotting factors

Prepubertal:

>10%:

Dermatologic: Acne

Endocrine & metabolic: Virilism

1% to 10%:

Central nervous system: Chills, insomnia

Dermatologic: Hyperpigmentation

Gastrointestinal: Diarrhea, nausea

Hematologic: Iron deficiency anemia, suppression of clotting

Female:

>10%: Endocrine & metabolic: Virilism

1% to 10%:

Central nervous system: Chills, insomnia

Endocrine & metabolic: Hypercalcemia

Gastrointestinal: Nausea, diarrhea

Hematologic: Iron deficiency anemia, suppression of clotting factors

Hepatic: Hepatic dysfunction

Drug Interactions May increase the effect of oral anticoagulants, insulin, oral hypoglycemic agents, adrenal steroids, or ACTH when taken together

Drug Uptake

Onset of action: 3-6 months

Absorption: I.M.: 77%

Duration: ≤30 days

Pregnancy Risk Factor X

Generic Available Yes

Naphazoline (naf AZ oh leen)

U.S. Brand Names AK-Con®; Albalon® Liquifilm®; Allersol®; Clear Eyes® [OTC]; Clear Eyes® ACR [OTC]; Naphcon® [OTC]; Ocu-Zoline®; Privine® Nasal [OTC]; VasoClear® [OTC]; Vasocon Regular®

Canadian Brand Names Naphcon Forte®; Vasocon®

Mexican Brand Names Afazol Grin®

Pharmacologic Category $Alpha_1$ Agonist; Ophthalmic Agent, Vasoconstrictor

Synonyms Naphazoline Hydrochloride

Use Topical vasoconstrictor; temporary relief of ocular congestion, itching, and minor irritation; control of hyperemia in patients with superficial corneal vascularity; treatment of nasal congestion; adjunct to sinusitis

Local Anesthetic/Vasoconstrictor Precautions No information available to require special precautions

Effects on Dental Treatment No effects or complications reported

Dosage

Nasal:

Children:

<6 years: Intranasal: Not recommended (especially infants) due to CNS depression

6-12 years: 1 spray of 0.05% into each nostril every 6 hours if necessary; therapy should not exceed 3-5 days

Children >12 years and Adults: 0.05%, instill 1-2 drops or sprays every 6 hours if needed; therapy should not exceed 3-5 days

Ophthalmic:

Children <6 years: Not recommended for use due to CNS depression (especially in infants)

Children >6 years and Adults: Instill 1-2 drops into conjunctival sac of affected eye(s) every 3-4 hours; therapy generally should not exceed 3-4 days

Mechanism of Action Stimulates alpha-adrenergic receptors in the arterioles of the conjunctiva and the nasal mucosa to produce vasoconstriction

Other Adverse Effects Frequency not defined:

Cardiovascular: Systemic cardiovascular stimulation

Central nervous system: Dizziness, headache, nervousness

Gastrointestinal: Nausea

Local: Transient stinging, nasal mucosa irritation, dryness, rebound congestion

Ocular: Mydriasis, increased intraocular pressure, blurring of vision

Respiratory: Sneezing

Drug Interactions Increased Toxicity: Discontinue prior to use of anesthetics that sensitize the myocardium to sympathomimetics (ie, cyclopropane, halothane), MAO inhibitors, and tricyclic antidepressants; may cause hypertensive reactions

Drug Uptake

Onset of action: Decongestant: Topical: ~10 minutes

Duration: 2-6 hours

Pregnancy Risk Factor C

Generic Available Yes

Naphazoline and Antazoline (naf AZ oh leen & an TAZ oh leen)

U.S. Brand Names Vasocon-A® [OTC]

Canadian Brand Names Albalon®-A Liquifilm; Vasocon-A®

Pharmacologic Category Ophthalmic Agent, Vasoconstrictor

Synonyms Antazoline and Naphazoline

Use Topical ocular congestion, itching, and minor irritation

Local Anesthetic/Vasoconstrictor Precautions No information available to require special precautions

Effects on Dental Treatment No effects or complications reported

Dosage 1-2 drops every 3-4 hours

Other Adverse Effects Frequency not defined:

Cardiovascular: Systemic cardiovascular stimulation, hypertension

Central nervous system: Nervousness, dizziness, headache

Gastrointestinal: Nausea

Local: Transient stinging

Neuromuscular & skeletal: Weakness

Ocular: Mydriasis, increased intraocular pressure, blurring of vision

Respiratory: Nasal mucosa irritation, dryness, rebound congestion

(Continued)

Naphazoline and Antazoline *(Continued)*

Miscellaneous: Diaphoresis

Drug Interactions MAO inhibitors (exaggerated adrenergic effects may result)

Pregnancy Risk Factor C

Generic Available Yes

Comments Discontinue if patient experiences ocular pain, visual changes, ocular redness or irritation, or if condition worsens or persists for >72 hours

Naphazoline and Pheniramine (naf AZ oh leen & fen NIR a meen)

U.S. Brand Names Naphcon-A® [OTC]

Canadian Brand Names Naphcon®-A

Pharmacologic Category Ophthalmic Agent, Vasoconstrictor

Synonyms Pheniramine and Naphazoline

Use Topical ocular vasoconstrictor

Local Anesthetic/Vasoconstrictor Precautions No information available to require special precautions

Effects on Dental Treatment No effects or complications reported

Dosage 1-2 drops every 3-4 hours

Other Adverse Effects 1% to 10%:

- Ocular: Pupillary dilation, increase in intraocular pressure
- Systemic effects due to absorption:
  - Cardiovascular: Hypertension, cardiac irregularities
  - Endocrine & metabolic: Hyperglycemia

Drug Interactions MAO inhibitors (exaggerated adrenergic effects may result)

Drug Uptake See Naphazoline *on page 847*

Pregnancy Risk Factor C

Generic Available Yes

Naphcon® [OTC] *see* Naphazoline *on page 847*

Naphcon-A® [OTC] *see* Naphazoline and Pheniramine *on page 848*

Naprelan® *see* Naproxen *on page 848*

Naprosyn® *see* Naproxen *on page 848*

Naproxen (na PROKS en)

Related Information

- Dental Drug Interactions: Update on Drug Combinations Requiring Special Considerations *on page 1434*
- Oral Pain *on page 1360*
- Rheumatoid Arthritis and Osteoarthritis *on page 1340*
- Temporomandibular Dysfunction (TMD) *on page 1397*

U.S. Brand Names Aleve® [OTC]; Anaprox®; EC-Naprosyn®; Naprelan®; Naprosyn®

Canadian Brand Names Anaprox®; Anaprox® DS; Apo®-Napro-Na; Apo®-Napro-Na DS; Apo®-Naproxen; Apo®-Naproxen SR; Gen-Naproxen EC; Naprosyn®; Naxen®; Novo-Naprox; Novo-Naprox Sodium; Novo-Naprox Sodium DS; Novo-Naprox SR; Nu-Naprox; Riva-Naproxen; Synflex®; Synflex® DS

Mexican Brand Names Artron; Atiflan; Atiquim®; Dafloxen®; Faraxen; Flanax; Flexen; Flogen®; Fuxen; Naprodil®; Naxen®; Naxil; Neonaxil®; Nixal®; Novaxen®; Pactens; Pronaxil; Supradol®; Tandax®; Velsay

Pharmacologic Category Nonsteroidal Anti-inflammatory Drug (NSAID)

Synonyms Naproxen Sodium

Use

- Dental: Management of pain and swelling
- Medical: Management of inflammatory disease and rheumatoid disorders (including juvenile rheumatoid arthritis); acute gout; mild to moderate pain; dysmenorrhea; fever, migraine headache

Local Anesthetic/Vasoconstrictor Precautions No information available to require special precautions

Effects on Dental Treatment NSAID formulations are known to reversibly decrease platelet aggregation via mechanisms different than observed with aspirin. The dentist should be aware of the potential of abnormal coagulation. Caution should also be exercised in the use of NSAIDs in patients already on anticoagulant therapy with drugs such as warfarin (Coumadin®).

Dosage Oral:

- Children >2 years:
  - Fever: 2.5-10 mg/kg/dose; maximum: 10 mg/kg/day
  - Juvenile arthritis: 10 mg/kg/day in 2 divided doses
- Adults:
  - Rheumatoid arthritis, osteoarthritis, and ankylosing spondylitis: 500-1000 mg/day in 2 divided doses; may increase to 1.5 g/day of naproxen base for limited time period
  - Mild to moderate pain or dysmenorrhea: Initial: 500 mg, then 250 mg every 6-8 hours; maximum: 1250 mg/day naproxen base

Dosing adjustment in hepatic impairment: Reduce dose to 50%

Mechanism of Action Inhibits prostaglandin synthesis by decreasing the activity of the enzyme, cyclo-oxygenase, which results in decreased formation of prostaglandin precursors

Other Adverse Effects

1% to 10%:

Central nervous system: Headache (11%), nervousness, malaise (<3%), somnolence (3% to 9%)

Dermatologic: Itching, pruritus, rash, ecchymosis (3% to 9%)

Endocrine & metabolic: Fluid retention (3% to 9%)

Gastrointestinal: Abdominal discomfort, nausea (3% to 9%), heartburn, constipation (3% to 9%), GI bleeding, ulcers, perforation, indigestion, diarrhea (<3%), abdominal distress/cramps/pain (3% to 9%), dyspepsia (<3%), stomatitis (<3%), heartburn (<3%)

Hematologic: Hemolysis (3% to 9%), ecchymosis (3% to 9%)

Otic: Tinnitus (3% to 9%)

Respiratory: Dyspnea (3% to 9%)

<1%: Acute renal failure, agranulocytosis, allergic rhinitis, anemia, angioedema, arrhythmias, aseptic meningitis, blurred vision, bone marrow suppression, bronchospasm, confusion, CHF, conjunctivitis, cystitis, decreased hearing, drowsiness, dry eyes, edema epistaxis, erythema, fatigue, gastritis, GI ulceration, hallucinations, hemolytic anemia, hepatitis, hot flashes, hypertension, inhibits platelet aggregation, insomnia, leukopenia, mental depression, multiforme, peripheral neuropathy, polydipsia, polyuria, prolonged bleeding time, renal dysfunction, Stevens-Johnson syndrome, tachycardia, thrombocytopenia, toxic amblyopia, toxic epidermal necrolysis, urticaria, vomiting

Contraindications Hypersensitivity to naproxen, aspirin, other NSAIDs, or any component of their formulation; pregnancy (3rd trimester)

Warnings/Precautions Use with caution in patients with GI disease (eg, bleeding or ulcers), cardiovascular disease (eg, CHF, hypertension), dehydration, renal or hepatic impairment, and patients receiving anticoagulants; perform ophthalmologic evaluation for those who develop eye complaints during therapy (eg, blurred vision, diminished vision, changes in color vision, retinal changes); NSAIDs may mask signs/symptoms of infections; photosensitivity reported; elderly are at especially high-risk for adverse effects. Withhold for at least 4-6 half-lives prior to surgical or dental procedures.

Drug Interactions CYP2C8, 2C9, and 2C18 enzyme substrate

ACE inhibitors: Antihypertensive effects may be decreased by concurrent therapy with NSAIDs; monitor BP.

Angiotensin II antagonists: Antihypertensive effects may be decreased by concurrent therapy with NSAIDs; monitor BP.

Anticoagulants (warfarin, heparin, LMWHs) in combination with NSAIDs can cause increased risk of bleeding.

Antiplatelet drugs (ticlopidine, clopidogrel, aspirin, abciximab, dipyridamole, eptifibatide, tirofiban) can cause an increased risk of bleeding.

Corticosteroids may increase the risk of GI ulceration; avoid concurrent use.

Cyclosporine: NSAIDs may increase serum creatinine, potassium, BP, and cyclosporine levels; monitor cyclosporine levels and renal function carefully.

Hydralazine's antihypertensive effect is decreased; avoid concurrent use.

Lithium levels can be increased; avoid concurrent use if possible or monitor lithium levels and adjust dose. Sulindac may have the least effect. When NSAID is stopped, lithium will need adjustment again.

Loop diuretics efficacy (diuretic and antihypertensive effect) is reduced. Indomethacin reduces this efficacy, however, it may be anticipated with any NSAID.

Methotrexate: Severe bone marrow suppression, aplastic anemia, and GI toxicity have been reported with concomitant NSAID therapy. Avoid use during moderate or high-dose methotrexate (increased and prolonged methotrexate levels). NSAID use during low-dose treatment of rheumatoid arthritis has not been fully evaluated; extreme caution is warranted.

Thiazides antihypertensive effects are decreased; avoid concurrent use.

Warfarin's INRs may be increased by naproxen. Other NSAIDs may have the same effect depending on dose and duration. Monitor INR closely. Use the lowest dose of NSAIDs possible and for the briefest duration.

Dietary/Ethanol/Herb Considerations

Ethanol: Avoid or limit use; may enhance gastric mucosal irritation.

Food may decrease absorption. Administer with food or milk to reduce GI upset; may cause bleeding, perforation, and ulceration. Avoid garlic, ginger, and green tea.

Herb/Nutraceutical: Avoid cat's claw, dong quai, evening primrose, feverfew, garlic, ginger, ginkgo biloba, ginseng, green tea, horse chestnut, and red clover due additional antiplatelet activity. Avoid kava and valerian; may enhance benzodiazepine activity.

Drug Uptake

Onset of action: Analgesic: 1 hour; Anti-inflammatory: ~2 weeks

Peak effect: Anti-inflammatory: 2-4 weeks

Duration: Analgesic: ≤7 hours; Anti-inflammatory: ≤12 hours

(Continued)

Naproxen *(Continued)*

Absorption: Almost 100%

Half-life, elimination: Normal renal function: 12-15 hours; End-stage renal disease: Unchanged

Time to peak: 1-2 hours

Pregnancy Risk Factor B/D (3rd trimester)

Breast-feeding Considerations May be taken while breast-feeding

Dosage Forms CAPLET: 220 mg. **GELCAP:** 220 mg. **SUSP, oral:** 125 mg/5 mL (15 mL, 30 mL, 480 mL). **TAB:** 220 mg; (Anaprox®): 275 mg, 550 mg; (Naprosyn®): 250 mg, 375 mg, 500 mg. **TAB, delayed release** (EC-Naprosyn®): 375 mg, 500 mg. **TAB, extended release:** 375 mg, 500 mg, 750 mg; (Naprelan®): 375 mg, 500 mg

Generic Available Yes

Comments The sodium salt of naproxen provides better effects because of better oral absorption; the sodium salt also provides a faster onset and a longer duration of action

Selected Readings

Ahmad N, Grad HA, Haas DA, et al, "The Efficacy of Nonopioid Analgesics for Postoperative Dental Pain: A Meta-Analysis," *Anesth Prog*, 1997, 44(4):119-26.

Brooks PM and Day RO, "Nonsteroidal Anti-inflammatory Drugs - Differences and Similarities," *N Engl J Med*, 1991, 324(24):1716-25.

Dionne R, "Additive Analgesia Without Opioid Side Effects," *Compend Contin Educ Dent*, 2000, 21(7):572-4, 576-7.

Dionne RA and Berthold CW, "Therapeutic Uses of Nonsteroidal Anti-Inflammatory Drugs in Dentistry," *Crit Rev Oral Biol Med*, 2001, 12(4):315-30.

Forbes JA, Keller CK, Smith JW, et al, "Analgesic Effect of Naproxen Sodium, Codeine, a Naproxen-Codeine Combination and Aspirin on the Postoperative Pain of Oral Surgery," *Pharmacotherapy*, 1986, 6(5):211-8.

Nguyen AM, Graham DY, Gage T, et al, "Nonsteroidal Anti-Inflammatory Drug Use in Dentistry: Gastrointestinal Implications," *Gen Dent*, 1999, 47(6):590-6.

Naqua® *see* Trichlormethiazide *on page 1202*

Naratriptan (NAR a trip tan)

U.S. Brand Names Amerge®

Canadian Brand Names Amerge®

Mexican Brand Names Naramig®

Pharmacologic Category Serotonin 5-HT_{1D} Receptor Agonist

Synonyms Naratriptan Hydrochloride

Use Acute treatment of migraine with or without aura

Local Anesthetic/Vasoconstrictor Precautions No information available to require special precautions

Effects on Dental Treatment No effects or complications reported

Dosage

Adults: Oral: 1-2.5 mg at the onset of headache; it is recommended to use the lowest possible dose to minimize adverse effects. If headache returns or does not fully resolve, the dose may be repeated after 4 hours; do not exceed 5 mg in 24 hours.

Elderly: Not recommended

Mechanism of Action The therapeutic effect for migraine is due to serotonin agonist activity; potent 5HT_{-1B} and 5HT_{-1D} agonist

Other Adverse Effects 1% to 10%:

Central nervous system: Dizziness, drowsiness, malaise/fatigue

Gastrointestinal: Nausea, vomiting

Neuromuscular & skeletal: Paresthesias

Miscellaneous: Pain or pressure in throat or neck

Contraindications Hypersensitivity to naratriptan or any component of the formulation; cerebrovascular, peripheral vascular disease (ischemic bowel disease), ischemic heart disease (angina pectoris, history of myocardial infarction, or proven silent ischemia); symptoms consistent with ischemic heart disease, coronary artery vasospasm, or Prinzmetal's variant angina; uncontrolled hypertension or patients who have received within 24 hours another 5-HT agonist (rizatriptan, sumatriptan, zolmitriptan) or ergotamine-containing product; known risk factors associated with coronary artery disease; severe hepatic or renal disease (Cl_{cr} <15 mL/minute); hemiplegic or basilar migraine

Warnings/Precautions Use only if there is a clear diagnosis of migraine. Patients who are at risk of CAD but have had a satisfactory cardiovascular evaluation may receive naratriptan but with extreme caution (ie, in a physician's office where there are adequate precautions in place to protect the patient). Blood pressure may increase with the administration of naratriptan. Monitor closely, especially with the first administration of the drug. If the patient does not respond to the first dose, re-evaluate the diagnosis of migraine before trying a second dose.

Drug Interactions

Increased Effect/Toxicity: Ergot-containing drugs (dihydroergotamine or methysergide) may cause vasospastic reactions when taken with naratriptan. Avoid concomitant use with ergots; separate dose of naratriptan and ergots by at least 24 hours. Oral contraceptives taken with naratriptan reduced the clearance of naratriptan ~30% which may contribute to adverse effects. Selective serotonin reuptake inhibitors (SSRIs) (eg, fluoxetine, fluvoxamine, paroxetine, sertraline) may cause lack of coordination, hyper-reflexia, or weakness and should be avoided when taking naratriptan.

Decreased Effect: Smoking increases the clearance of naratriptan.

Drug Uptake

Onset of action: 30 minutes

Time to peak: 2-3 hours

Pregnancy Risk Factor C

Generic Available No

Narcan® *see* Naloxone *on page 844*
Nardil® *see* Phenelzine *on page 944*
Naropin® *see* Ropivacaine *on page 1068*
Nasabid™ *see* Guaifenesin and Pseudoephedrine *on page 570*
Nasacort® *see* Triamcinolone *on page 1197*
Nasacort® AQ *see* Triamcinolone *on page 1197*
NāSal™[OTC] *see* Sodium Chloride *on page 1094*
Nasalcrom® [OTC] *see* Cromolyn Sodium *on page 330*
Nasalide® *see* Flunisolide *on page 511*
Nasal Moist® [OTC] *see* Sodium Chloride *on page 1094*
Nasarel® *see* Flunisolide *on page 511*
Nascobal® *see* Cyanocobalamin *on page 331*
Nasonex® *see* Mometasone Furoate *on page 827*
Natacyn® *see* Natamycin *on page 851*

Natamycin (na ta MYE sin)

U.S. Brand Names Natacyn®

Canadian Brand Names Natacyn®

Pharmacologic Category Antifungal Agent, Ophthalmic

Synonyms Pimaricin

Use Treatment of blepharitis, conjunctivitis, and keratitis caused by susceptible fungi (*Aspergillus, Candida*), *Cephalosporium, Curvularia, Fusarium, Penicillium, Microsporum, Epidermophyton, Blastomyces dermatitidis, Coccidioides immitis, Cryptococcus neoformans, Histoplasma capsulatum, Sporothrix schenckii, Trichomonas vaginalis*

Local Anesthetic/Vasoconstrictor Precautions No information available to require special precautions

Effects on Dental Treatment No effects or complications reported

Dosage Adults: Ophthalmic: Instill 1 drop in conjunctival sac every 1-2 hours, after 3-4 days reduce to 1 drop 6-8 times/day; usual course of therapy is 2-3 weeks

Mechanism of Action Increases cell membrane permeability in susceptible fungi

Other Adverse Effects Frequency not defined: Blurred vision, photophobia, eye pain, eye irritation not present before therapy

Drug Interactions Increased Effect/Toxicity: Topical use of corticosteroids is contraindicated

Drug Uptake Absorption: Ophthalmic: Systemic, <2%

Pregnancy Risk Factor C

Generic Available No

Natrecor® *see* Nesiritide *on page 858*
Nature's Tears® [OTC] *see* Artificial Tears *on page 117*
Nature-Throid® NT *see* Thyroid *on page 1164*
Naturetin® *see* Bendroflumethiazide *on page 150*
Nausetrol® [OTC] *see* Phosphorated Carbohydrate Solution *on page 953*
Navane® *see* Thiothixene *on page 1162*
Navelbine® *see* Vinorelbine *on page 1241*
Na-Zone® [OTC] *see* Sodium Chloride *on page 1094*
Nebcin® *see* Tobramycin *on page 1175*
NebuPent™ *see* Pentamidine *on page 932*
Necon® 0.5/35 *see* Combination Hormonal Contraceptives *on page 323*
Necon® 1/35 *see* Combination Hormonal Contraceptives *on page 323*
Necon® 1/50 *see* Mestranol and Norethindrone *on page 774*
Necon® 10/11 *see* Combination Hormonal Contraceptives *on page 323*

Nedocromil Sodium (ne doe KROE mil)

Related Information

Respiratory Diseases *on page 1328*

U.S. Brand Names Alocril™; Tilade®

Canadian Brand Names Alocril™; Tilade®

Pharmacologic Category Mast Cell Stabilizer

Synonyms Nedocromil

(Continued)

Nedocromil Sodium *(Continued)*

Use Maintenance therapy in patients with mild to moderate bronchial asthma

Local Anesthetic/Vasoconstrictor Precautions No information available to require special precautions

Effects on Dental Treatment No effects or complications reported

Dosage Children >12 years and Adults: Inhalation: 2 inhalations 4 times/day; may reduce dosage to 2-3 times/day once desired clinical response to initial dose is observed

Other Adverse Effects Inhalation:

>10%: Gastrointestinal: Unpleasant taste after inhalation

1% to 10%:

Cardiovascular: Chest pain

Central nervous system: Dizziness, dysphonia, headache, fatigue

Dermatologic: Rash

Gastrointestinal: Nausea, vomiting, heartburn, diarrhea, abdominal pain, xerostomia

Hepatic: Increased ALT

Neuromuscular & skeletal: Arthritis, tremor

Respiratory: Cough, pharyngitis, rhinitis, bronchitis, upper respiratory infection, bronchospasm, increased sputum production

Drug Uptake

Duration: 2 hours

Half-life, elimination: 1.5-2 hours

Pregnancy Risk Factor B

Generic Available No

Comments Not a bronchodilator; should not be used for reversal of acute bronchospasm; no known therapeutic systemic activity when inhaled

Nefazodone (nef AY zoe done)

U.S. Brand Names Serzone®

Canadian Brand Names Serzone-5HT$_2$®

Pharmacologic Category Antidepressant, Serotonin Reuptake Inhibitor/Antagonist

Synonyms Nefazodone Hydrochloride

Use Treatment of depression

Unlabeled/Investigational: Post-traumatic stress disorder

Local Anesthetic/Vasoconstrictor Precautions No information available to require special precautions

Effects on Dental Treatment >10%: Significant xerostomia; disappears with discontinuation

Dosage Oral:

Children and Adolescents: Depression: Target dose: 300-400 mg/day (mean: 3.4 mg/kg)

Adults: Depression: 200 mg/day, administered in 2 divided doses initially, with a range of 300-600 mg/day in 2 divided doses thereafter

Mechanism of Action Inhibits neuronal reuptake of serotonin and norepinephrine; also blocks 5-HT$_2$ and alpha$_1$ receptors; has no significant affinity for alpha$_2$, beta-adrenergic, 5-HT$_{1A}$, cholinergic, dopaminergic, or benzodiazepine receptors

Other Adverse Effects

>10%:

Central nervous system: Headache, drowsiness, insomnia, agitation, dizziness

Gastrointestinal: Xerostomia, nausea, constipation

Neuromuscular & skeletal: Weakness

1% to 10%:

Cardiovascular: Bradycardia, hypotension, peripheral edema, postural hypotension, vasodilation

Central nervous system: Chills, fever, incoordination, lightheadedness, confusion, memory impairment, abnormal dreams, decreased concentration, ataxia, psychomotor retardation, tremor

Dermatologic: Pruritus, rash

Endocrine & metabolic: Breast pain, impotence, libido decreased

Gastrointestinal: Gastroenteritis, vomiting, dyspepsia, diarrhea, increased appetite, thirst, taste perversion

Genitourinary: Urinary frequency, urinary retention

Hematologic: Hematocrit decreased

Neuromuscular & skeletal: Arthralgia, hypertonia, paresthesia, neck rigidity, tremor

Ocular: Blurred vision (9%), abnormal vision (7%), eye pain, visual field defect

Otic: Tinnitus

Respiratory: Bronchitis, cough, dyspnea, pharyngitis

Miscellaneous: Flu syndrome, infection

Drug Interactions CYP3A3/4 enzyme substrate; CYP3A3/4 enzyme inhibitor

Increased Effect/Toxicity:

CYP3A3/4 substrates: Serum concentrations of drugs metabolized by CYP3A3/4 may be elevated by nefazodone; cisapride, pimozide, and triazolam are contraindicated. Nefazodone may increase the serum concentration/effects of antiarrhythmics (amiodarone, lidocaine, propafenone, quinidine), some antipsychotics (clozapine, haloperidol, mesoridazine, quetiapine, and risperidone), some benzodiazepines (triazolam is contraindicated; decrease alprazolam dose by 50%), buspirone (limit buspirone dose to <2.5 mg/day), calcium channel blockers, cyclosporine, digoxin, donepezil, HMG-CoA reductase inhibitors (lovastatin, simvastatin - increased risk of myositis), methadone, oral contraceptives, protease inhibitors (ritonavir, saquinavir), sibutramine, sildenafil, tacrolimus, tricyclic antidepressants, vinca alkaloids, and zolpidem.

CYP3A3/4 inhibitors: Serum level and/or toxicity of nefazodone may be increased; inhibitors include amiodarone, cimetidine, clarithromycin, erythromycin, delavirdine, diltiazem, dirithromycin, disulfiram, fluoxetine, fluvoxamine, indinavir, itraconazole, ketoconazole, metronidazole, nevirapine, propoxyphene, quinupristin-dalfopristin, ritonavir, saquinavir, verapamil, zafirlukast, zileuton

MAO inhibitors: Concurrent use may lead to serotonin syndrome; avoid concurrent use or use within 14 days (includes phenelzine, isocarboxazid, and linezolid). Selegiline may increase the risk of serotonin syndrome, particularly at higher doses (>10 mg/day, where selectivity for MAO type B is decreased).

Theoretically, concurrent use of buspirone, meperidine, serotonin agonists (sumatriptan, rizatriptan), SSRIs, and venlafaxine may result in serotonin syndrome.

Decreased Effect: Carbamazepine may reduce serum concentration; avoid concurrent administration

Drug Uptake

Onset of action: Therapeutic: ≤6 weeks

Half-life, elimination: Parent compound: 2-4 hours; active metabolites persist longer

Time to peak: 30 minutes; prolonged in presence of food

Pregnancy Risk Factor C

Generic Available No

NegGram® *see* Nalidixic Acid *on page 842*

Nelfinavir (nel FIN a veer)

Related Information

HIV Infection and AIDS *on page 1334*

Oral Viral Infections *on page 1380*

U.S. Brand Names Viracept®

Canadian Brand Names Viracept®

Pharmacologic Category Antiretroviral Agent, Protease Inhibitor

Use As monotherapy or preferably in combination with nucleoside analogs in the treatment of HIV infection when antiretroviral therapy is warranted

Local Anesthetic/Vasoconstrictor Precautions No information available to require special precautions

Effects on Dental Treatment <1%: Mouth ulcers

Dosage Oral:

Children 2-13 years: 20-30 mg/kg 3 times/day with a meal or light snack; if tablets are unable to be taken, use oral powder in small amount of water, milk, formula, or dietary supplements; do not use acidic food/juice or store for >6 hours

Adults: 750 mg 3 times/day with meals or 1250 mg twice daily with meals in combination with other antiretroviral therapies

Mechanism of Action Inhibits the HIV-1 protease; inhibition of the viral protease prevents cleavage of the gag-pol polyprotein resulting in the production of immature, noninfectious virus; cross-resistance with other protease inhibitors is possible although, as yet, unknown

Other Adverse Effects Protease inhibitors cause dyslipidemia which includes elevated cholesterol and triglycerides and a redistribution of body fat centrally to cause "protease paunch", buffalo hump, facial atrophy, and breast enlargement. These agents also cause hyperglycemia.

>10%: Gastrointestinal: Diarrhea (19%)

1% to 10%:

Central nervous system: Impaired concentration

Dermatologic: Rash

Gastrointestinal: Nausea, flatulence, abdominal pain

Neuromuscular & skeletal: Weakness

Warnings/Precautions Avoid use of powder in phenylketonurics since contains phenylalanine; use extreme caution when administered to patients with hepatic insufficiency since nelfinavir is metabolized in the liver and excreted predominantly in the feces; avoid use, if possible, with terfenadine, astemizole, cisapride, triazolam, or midazolam. Concurrent use with some anticonvulsants may significantly limit nelfinavir's effectiveness. Also, avoid concurrent use of amiodarone, quinidine, and ergot alkaloids. Redistribution of fate can occur with protease inhibitors.

(Continued)

Nelfinavir *(Continued)*

Drug Interactions CYP3A3/4 enzyme substrate; CYP3A3/4 enzyme inducer; CYP3A3/4 enzyme inhibitor

Increased Effect/Toxicity: Nelfinavir inhibits the metabolism of cisapride, terfenadine, astemizole, amiodarone, quinidine, lovastatin, simvastatin - should not be administered concurrently due to risk of life-threatening cardiac arrhythmias. Concentrations of atorvastatin and cerivastatin may be increased by nelfinavir. Do not administer with ergot alkaloids. Rifabutin plasma concentrations (AUC) are increased when coadministered with nelfinavir (decrease rifabutin dose by 50%). Nelfinavir increases levels of ketoconazole and indinavir. An increase in midazolam and triazolam serum concentration may occur resulting in significant oversedation when administered with nelfinavir. Indinavir and ritonavir may increase nelfinavir plasma concentrations resulting in potential increases in side effects (the safety of these combinations have not been established). Concentrations of nelfinavir may be doubled during therapy with delavirdine. Sildenafil serum concentration may be substantially increased (do not exceed single doses of 25 mg in 48 hours).

Decreased Effect: Rifampin decreases nelfinavir's blood levels (AUC decreased by ~82%); the two drugs should not be administered concurrently. Serum levels of ethinyl estradiol and norethindrone (including many oral contraceptives) may decrease significantly with administration of nelfinavir. Patients should use alternative methods of contraceptives during nelfinavir therapy. Phenobarbital, phenytoin, and carbamazepine may decrease serum concentration and consequently effectiveness of nelfinavir. Delavirdine concentrations may be decreased by up to 50% during nelfinavir treatment. Nelfinavir's effectiveness may be decreased with concomitant nevirapine use.

Drug Uptake

Absorption: Food increases plasma concentration-time curve (AUC) by two- to threefold

Half-life, elimination: 3.5-5 hours

Time to peak: 2-4 hours

Pregnancy Risk Factor B

Generic Available No

Nembutal® *see* Pentobarbital *on page 935*

Neo-Calglucon® [OTC] *see* Calcium Glubionate *on page 203*

NeoDecadron® *see* Neomycin and Dexamethasone *on page 855*

Neo-Dexameth® *see* Neomycin and Dexamethasone *on page 855*

Neo-Fradin® *see* Neomycin *on page 854*

Neoloid® [OTC] *see* Castor Oil *on page 230*

Neomycin (nee oh MYE sin)

Related Information

Neomycin and Polymyxin B *on page 855*

Neomycin, Polymyxin B, and Dexamethasone *on page 856*

Neomycin, Polymyxin B, and Prednisolone *on page 857*

U.S. Brand Names Mycifradin® Sulfate; Neo-Fradin®; Neo-Tabs®

Pharmacologic Category Ammonium Detoxicant; Antibiotic, Aminoglycoside; Antibiotic, Topical

Synonyms Neomycin Sulfate

Use Prepares GI tract for surgery; treatment of minor skin infections; treatment of diarrhea caused by *E. coli*; adjunct in the treatment of hepatic encephalopathy, as irrigant during surgery

Local Anesthetic/Vasoconstrictor Precautions No information available to require special precautions

Effects on Dental Treatment No effects or complications reported

Dosage

Children: Oral:

Preoperative intestinal antisepsis: 90 mg/kg/day divided every 4 hours for 2 days; or 25 mg/kg at 1 PM, 2 PM, and 11 PM on the day preceding surgery as an adjunct to mechanical cleansing of the intestine and in combination with erythromycin base

Hepatic coma: 50-100 mg/kg/day in divided doses every 6-8 hours or 2.5-7 g/m^2/day divided every 4-6 hours for 5-6 days not to exceed 12 g/day

Children and Adults: Topical: Apply ointment 1-4 times/day; topical solutions containing 0.1% to 1% neomycin have been used for irrigation

Adults: Oral:

Preoperative intestinal antisepsis: 1 g each hour for 4 doses then 1 g every 4 hours for 5 doses; or 1 g at 1 PM, 2 PM, and 11 PM on day preceding surgery as an adjunct to mechanical cleansing of the bowel and oral erythromycin; or 6 g/day divided every 4 hours for 2-3 days

Hepatic coma: 500-2000 mg every 6-8 hours or 4-12 g/day divided every 4-6 hours for 5-6 days

Chronic hepatic insufficiency: 4 g/day for an indefinite period

Mechanism of Action Interferes with bacterial protein synthesis by binding to 30S ribosomal subunits

Other Adverse Effects 1% to 10%:

Dermatologic: Dermatitis, rash, urticaria, erythema

Local: Burning

Ocular: Contact conjunctivitis

Drug Interactions

Increased Effect/Toxicity: Oral neomycin may potentiate the effects of oral anticoagulants. Neomycin may increase the adverse effects with other neurotoxic, ototoxic, or nephrotoxic drugs.

Decreased Effect: May decrease GI absorption of digoxin and methotrexate.

Drug Uptake

Absorption: Oral, percutaneous: Poor (3%)

Half-life, elimination: 3 hours (dependent on age and renal function)

Time to peak: Oral: 1-4 hours; I.M.: ~2 hours

Pregnancy Risk Factor C

Generic Available Yes

Neomycin and Dexamethasone

(nee oh MYE sin & deks a METH a sone)

U.S. Brand Names AK-Neo-Dex®; NeoDecadron®; Neo-Dexameth®

Pharmacologic Category Antibiotic/Corticosteroid, Ophthalmic

Synonyms Dexamethasone and Neomycin

Use Treatment of steroid responsive inflammatory conditions of the palpebral and bulbar conjunctiva, lid, cornea, and anterior segment of the globe

Local Anesthetic/Vasoconstrictor Precautions No information available to require special precautions

Effects on Dental Treatment No effects or complications reported

Dosage

Ophthalmic: Instill 1-2 drops in eye(s) every 3-4 hours

Topical: Apply thin coat 3-4 times/day until favorable response is observed, then reduce dose to one application/day

Other Adverse Effects Frequency not defined:

Local: Burning or local irritation, transient stinging,

Ocular: Epithelial punctate keratitis, increased intraocular pressure, mydriasis, ptosis, and possible corneal or scleral malacia can occur

Drug Uptake See Neomycin *on page 854* and Dexamethasone *on page 363*

Pregnancy Risk Factor C

Generic Available Yes

Neomycin and Hydrocortisone

(nee oh MYE sin & hye droe KOR ti sone)

Canadian Brand Names Neo-Cortef®

Pharmacologic Category Antibiotic/Corticosteroid, Topical

Synonyms Hydrocortisone and Neomycin

Use Treatment of susceptible topical bacterial infections with associated swelling

Local Anesthetic/Vasoconstrictor Precautions No information available to require special precautions

Effects on Dental Treatment No effects or complications reported

Dosage Topical: Apply to area in a thin film 2-4 times/day

Therapy should be discontinued when control is achieved; if no improvement is seen, reassessment of diagnosis may be necessary.

Drug Uptake See Neomycin *on page 854* and Hydrocortisone *on page 608*

Pregnancy Risk Factor C

Generic Available Yes

Neomycin and Polymyxin B (nee oh MYE sin & pol i MIKS in bee)

U.S. Brand Names Neosporin® Cream [OTC]; Neosporin® G.U. Irrigant

Canadian Brand Names Cortimyxin®; Neosporin® Irrigating Solution

Pharmacologic Category Antibiotic, Topical

Synonyms Polymyxin B and Neomycin

Use Short-term as a continuous irrigant or rinse in the urinary bladder in prevention of bacteriuria and gram-negative rod septicemia associated with the use of indwelling catheters; aid prevention of infection in minor abrasions, cuts, and burns; treatment of superficial ocular infections involving the conjunctiva or cornea

Local Anesthetic/Vasoconstrictor Precautions No information available to require special precautions

Effects on Dental Treatment No effects or complications reported

Dosage Children and Adults:

Bladder irrigation: **Not for injection**; add 1 mL irrigant to 1 liter isotonic saline solution and connect container to the inflow of lumen of 3-way catheter. Continuous irrigant or rinse in the urinary bladder for up to a maximum of 10 days with administration rate adjusted to patient's urine output; usually ≤1 L of irrigant is used per day.

(Continued)

Neomycin and Polymyxin B *(Continued)*

Topical: Apply cream 1-4 times/day to affected area

Mechanism of Action See Neomycin *on page 854* and Polymyxin B *on page 971*

Other Adverse Effects Frequency not defined:

Dermatologic: Contact dermatitis, erythema, rash, urticaria

Genitourinary: Bladder irritation

Local: Burning

Neuromuscular & skeletal: Neuromuscular blockade

Otic: Ototoxicity

Renal: Nephrotoxicity

Drug Uptake See Polymyxin B *on page 971* and Neomycin *on page 854*

Absorption: Topical: Not absorbed following application to intact skin; absorbed through denuded or abraded skin, peritoneum, wounds, or ulcers

Pregnancy Risk Factor C/D (for G.U. irrigant)

Generic Available No

Neomycin, Polymyxin B, and Dexamethasone

(nee oh MYE sin, pol i MIKS in bee, & deks a METH a sone)

U.S. Brand Names AK-Trol®; Dexacidin®; Dexasporin®; Maxitrol®

Canadian Brand Names Dioptrol®; Maxitrol®

Pharmacologic Category Antibiotic/Corticosteroid, Ophthalmic

Synonyms Dexamethasone, Neomycin, and Polymyxin B; Polymyxin B, Neomycin, and Dexamethasone

Use Steroid-responsive inflammatory ocular conditions in which a corticosteroid is indicated and where bacterial infection or a risk of bacterial infection exists

Local Anesthetic/Vasoconstrictor Precautions No information available to require special precautions

Effects on Dental Treatment No effects or complications reported

Dosage Children and Adults: Ophthalmic:

Ointment: Place a small amount (~1/2") in the affected eye 3-4 times/day or apply at bedtime as an adjunct with drops

Solution: Instill 1-2 drops into affected eye(s) every 3-4 hours; in severe disease, drops may be used hourly and tapered to discontinuation

Mechanism of Action See Neomycin *on page 854*, Polymyxin B *on page 971*, and Dexamethasone *on page 363*

Other Adverse Effects 1% to 10%:

Dermatologic: Contact dermatitis, delayed wound healing

Ocular: Cutaneous sensitization, eye pain, development of glaucoma, cataract, increased intraocular pressure, optic nerve damage

Drug Uptake See Neomycin *on page 854*, Polymyxin B *on page 971*, and Dexamethasone *on page 363*,

Pregnancy Risk Factor C

Generic Available Yes

Neomycin, Polymyxin B, and Gramicidin

(nee oh MYE sin, pol i MIKS in bee, & gram i SYE din)

U.S. Brand Names AK-Spore® Ophthalmic Solution; Neosporin® Ophthalmic Solution

Canadian Brand Names Neosporin®; Optimyxin Plus®

Mexican Brand Names Neosporin® Oftalmico

Pharmacologic Category Antibiotic, Ophthalmic

Synonyms Gramicidin, Neomycin, and Polymyxin B; Polymyxin B, Neomycin, and Gramicidin

Use Treatment of superficial ocular infection, infection prophylaxis in minor skin abrasions

Local Anesthetic/Vasoconstrictor Precautions No information available to require special precautions

Effects on Dental Treatment No effects or complications reported

Dosage Children and Adults: Ophthalmic: Instill 1-2 drops 4-6 times/day or more frequently as required for severe infections

Mechanism of Action Interferes with bacterial protein synthesis by binding to 30S ribosomal subunits; binds to phospholipids, alters permeability, and damages the bacterial cytoplasmic membrane permitting leakage of intracellular constituents

Other Adverse Effects Frequency not defined: Ocular: Transient irritation, burning, stinging, itching, inflammation, angioneurotic edema, urticaria, vesicular and maculopapular dermatitis

Drug Interactions See Neomycin *on page 854* and Polymyxin B *on page 971*

Pregnancy Risk Factor C

Generic Available Yes

Neomycin, Polymyxin B, and Hydrocortisone

(nee oh MYE sin, pol i MIKS in bee, & hye droe KOR ti sone)

U.S. Brand Names AK-Spore® H.C. Otic; AntibiOtic® Otic; Cortatrigen® Otic; Cortisporin®; Cortisporin® Ophthalmic Suspension; Octicair® Otic; Otic-Care®; Otocort®; Otosporin®; PediOtic®; UAD Otic®

Canadian Brand Names Cortimyxin®; Cortisporin®

Pharmacologic Category Antibiotic/Corticosteroid, Ophthalmic; Antibiotic/Corticosteroid, Otic; Topical Skin Product

Synonyms Hydrocortisone, Neomycin, and Polymyxin B; Polymyxin B, Neomycin, and Hydrocortisone

Use Steroid-responsive inflammatory condition for which a corticosteroid is indicated and where bacterial infection or a risk of bacterial infection exists

Local Anesthetic/Vasoconstrictor Precautions No information available to require special precautions

Effects on Dental Treatment No effects or complications reported

Dosage Duration of use should be limited to 10 days unless otherwise directed by the physician. Therapy should be discontinued when control is achieved; if no improvement is seen, reassessment of diagnosis may be necessary.

Ophthalmic: Children and Adults: Drops: Instill 1-2 drops 2-4 times/day, or more frequently as required for severe infections; in acute infections, instill 1-2 drops every 15-30 minutes gradually reducing the frequency of administration as the infection is controlled

Swimmer's ear and infections of external auditory canal: Otic:
- Children: Instill 3 drops into affected ear 3-4 times/day
- Adults: Instill 4 drops 3-4 times/day; otic suspension is the preferred otic preparation

Topical: Children and Adults: Apply a thin layer 1-4 times/day

Mechanism of Action See Neomycin *on page 854*, Polymyxin B *on page 971*, and Hydrocortisone *on page 608*

Other Adverse Effects 1% to 10%:

Dermatologic: Contact dermatitis, erythema, rash, urticaria

Local: Burning, itching, swelling, pain, stinging

Ocular: Increased intraocular pressure, glaucoma, cataracts, conjunctival erythema, transient irritation, burning, stinging, itching, inflammation, angioneurotic edema, urticaria, vesicular and maculopapular dermatitis

Otic: Ototoxicity

Miscellaneous: Hypersensitivity, sensitization to neomycin, secondary infections

Drug Uptake See Neomycin *on page 854*, Polymyxin B *on page 971* and Hydrocortisone *on page 608*

Pregnancy Risk Factor C

Generic Available Yes

Neomycin, Polymyxin B, and Prednisolone

(nee oh MYE sin, pol i MIKS in bee, & pred NIS oh lone)

U.S. Brand Names Poly-Pred®

Pharmacologic Category Antibiotic/Corticosteroid, Ophthalmic

Synonyms Polymyxin B, Neomycin, and Prednisolone; Prednisolone, Neomycin, and Polymyxin B

Use Steroid-responsive inflammatory ocular condition in which bacterial infection or a risk of bacterial ocular infection exists

Local Anesthetic/Vasoconstrictor Precautions No information available to require special precautions

Effects on Dental Treatment No effects or complications reported

Dosage Children and Adults: Ophthalmic: Instill 1-2 drops every 3-4 hours; acute infections may require every 30-minute instillation initially with frequency of administration reduced as the infection is brought under control. To treat the lids: Instill 1-2 drops every 3-4 hours, close the eye and rub the excess on the lids and lid margins.

Mechanism of Action See Neomycin *on page 854*, Polymyxin B *on page 971*, and Prednisolone *on page 988*

Other Adverse Effects 1% to 10%:

Dermatologic: Cutaneous sensitization, skin rash, delayed wound healing

Ocular: Increased intraocular pressure, glaucoma, optic nerve damage, cataracts, conjunctival sensitization, transient irritation, burning, stinging, itching, inflammation, angioneurotic edema, urticaria, vesicular and maculopapular dermatitis

Drug Uptake See Neomycin *on page 854*, Polymyxin B *on page 971*, and Prednisolone *on page 988*

Pregnancy Risk Factor C

Generic Available No

Neoral® *see* CycloSPORINE *on page 337*

Neosar® *see* Cyclophosphamide *on page 335*

Neosporin® Cream [OTC] *see* Neomycin and Polymyxin B *on page 855*

Neosporin® G.U. Irrigant *see* Neomycin and Polymyxin B *on page 855*

Neosporin® Ophthalmic Ointment *see* Bacitracin, Neomycin, and Polymyxin B *on page 141*
Neosporin® Ophthalmic Solution *see* Neomycin, Polymyxin B, and Gramicidin *on page 856*
Neosporin® Topical [OTC] *see* Bacitracin, Neomycin, and Polymyxin B *on page 141*
Neo-Synephrine® Injection *see* Phenylephrine *on page 950*
Neo-Synephrine® Nasal [OTC] *see* Phenylephrine *on page 950*
Neo-Synephrine® Ophthalmic *see* Phenylephrine *on page 950*
Neo-Tabs® *see* Neomycin *on page 854*
Neotrace-4® *see* Trace Metals *on page 1186*
NeoVadrin® [OTC] *see* Vitamins, Multiple *on page 1246*
NeoVadrin® B Complex [OTC] *see* Vitamin B Complex *on page 1244*
Nephro-Calci® [OTC] *see* Calcium Carbonate *on page 201*
Nephrocaps® *see* Vitamin B Complex With Vitamin C and Folic Acid *on page 1244*
Nephro-Fer™ [OTC] *see* Ferrous Fumarate *on page 497*
Neptazane® *see* Methazolamide *on page 781*
Nesacaine® *see* Chloroprocaine *on page 265*
Nesacaine®-MPF *see* Chloroprocaine *on page 265*

Nesiritide (ni SIR i tide)

U.S. Brand Names Natrecor®

Canadian Brand Names Powder for injection: 1.5 mg

Pharmacologic Category Natriuretic Peptide, B-type, Human; Vasodilator

Synonyms B-type Natriuretic Peptide (Human); hBNP; Natriuretic Peptide

Use Treatment of acutely decompensated CHF in patients with dyspnea at rest or with minimal activity

Local Anesthetic/Vasoconstrictor Precautions No information available to require special precautions

Effects on Dental Treatment No effects or complications reported

Dosage Should not be initiated at a dosage higher than initial recommended dose. At intervals of ≥3 hours, the dosage may be increased by 0.005 mcg/kg/minute (preceded by a bolus of 1 mcg/kg), up to a maximum of 0.03 mcg/kg/minute. Increases beyond the initial infusion rate should be limited to selected patients and accompanied by hemodynamic monitoring.

Adults: I.V.:
- Initial: 2 mcg/kg (bolus); followed by continuous infusion at 0.01 mcg/kg/minute
- Patients experiencing hypotension during the infusion: Infusion should be interrupted; may attempt to restart at a lower dose (reduce initial infusion dose by 30% and omit bolus).

Mechanism of Action Binds to guanylate cyclase receptor on vascular smooth muscle and endothelial cells, increasing intracellular cyclic GMP, resulting in smooth muscle cell relaxation. Has been shown to produce dose-dependent reductions in pulmonary capillary wedge pressure (PCWP) and systemic arterial pressure.

Other Adverse Effects Note: Frequencies cited below were recorded in VMAC trial at dosages similar to approved labeling. Higher frequencies have been observed in trials using higher dosages of nesiritide.

>10%:
- Cardiovascular: Hypotension (total: 11%; symptomatic: 4% at recommended dose, up to 17% at higher doses)
- Renal: Increased serum creatinine (28% with >0.5 mg/dL increase over baseline)

1% to 10%:
- Cardiovascular: Ventricular tachycardia (3%)*, ventricular extrasystoles (3%)*, angina (2%)*, bradycardia (1%), tachycardia, atrial fibrillation, AV node conduction abnormalities
- Central nervous system: Headache (8%)*, dizziness (3%)*, insomnia (2%), anxiety (3%), fever, confusion, paresthesia, somnolence, tremor
- Dermatologic: Pruritus, rash
- Gastrointestinal: Nausea (4%)*, abdominal pain (1%)*, vomiting (1%)*
- Hematologic: Anemia
- Local: Injection site reaction
- Neuromuscular & skeletal: Back pain (4%), leg cramps
- Ocular: Amblyopia
- Respiratory: Cough (increased), hemoptysis, apnea
- Miscellaneous: Increased diaphoresis

*Frequency less than or equal to placebo or other standard therapy

Drug Interactions Increased Effect/Toxicity: An increased frequency of symptomatic hypotension was observed with concurrent administration of ACE inhibitors. Other hypotensive agents are likely to have additive effects on hypotension. In patients receiving diuretic therapy leading to depletion of intravascular volume, the risk of hypotension and/or renal impairment may be increased. Nesiritide should be avoided in patients with low filling pressures.

Drug Uptake
Onset of action: 15 minutes (60% of 3-hour effect achieved)
Duration: >60 minutes (≤several hours) for systolic blood pressure; hemodynamic effects persist longer than half-life, elimination would predict
Half-life, elimination: Initial: 2 minutes; Terminal: 18 minutes
Time to peak: 1 hour

Pregnancy Risk Factor C

Generic Available No

Nestrex® [OTC] *see* Pyridoxine *on page 1027*
Neulasta™ *see* Pegfilgrastim *on page 922*
Neumega® *see* Oprelvekin *on page 889*
Neupogen® *see* Filgrastim *on page 502*
Neurontin® *see* Gabapentin *on page 546*
Neut® *see* Sodium Bicarbonate *on page 1093*
Neutra-Phos® *see* Potassium Phosphate and Sodium Phosphate *on page 982*
Neutra-Phos®-K *see* Potassium Phosphate *on page 981*
Neutrexin® *see* Trimetrexate Glucuronate *on page 1210*
Neutrogena® Acne Mask [OTC] *see* Benzoyl Peroxide *on page 153*
Neutrogena® On The Spot® Acne Treatment [OTC] *see* Benzoyl Peroxide *on page 153*
Neutrogena® T/Derm *see* Coal Tar *on page 315*
Neutrogena® T/Sal [OTC] *see* Coal Tar and Salicylic Acid *on page 315*

Nevirapine (ne VYE ra peen)

Related Information
HIV Infection and AIDS *on page 1334*

U.S. Brand Names Viramune®

Canadian Brand Names Viramune®

Mexican Brand Names Viramune®

Pharmacologic Category Antiretroviral Agent, Reverse Transcriptase Inhibitor (Non-nucleoside)

Use In combination therapy with nucleoside antiretroviral agents in HIV-1 infected adults previously treated for whom current therapy is deemed inadequate

Local Anesthetic/Vasoconstrictor Precautions No information available to require special precautions

Effects on Dental Treatment 1% to 10%: Ulcerative stomatitis

Dosage Adults: Oral: 200 mg once daily for 2 weeks followed by 200 mg twice daily

Mechanism of Action A non-nucleoside reverse transcriptase inhibitor specific for HIV-1; does not require intracellular phosphorylation for antiviral activity

Other Adverse Effects
>10%:
Central nervous system: Headache (11%), fever (8% to 11%)
Dermatologic: Rash (15% to 20%)
Gastrointestinal: Diarrhea (15% to 20%)
Hematologic: Neutropenia (10% to 11%)
1% to 10%:
Gastrointestinal: Ulcerative stomatitis (4%), nausea, abdominal pain (2%)
Hematologic: Anemia
Hepatic: Hepatitis, increased LFTs (2% to 4%)
Neuromuscular & skeletal: Peripheral neuropathy, paresthesia (2%), myalgia

Drug Interactions CYP3A3/4 enzyme substrate, inducer, and inhibitor
Increased Effect/Toxicity: Cimetidine, itraconazole, ketoconazole, and some macrolide antibiotics may increase nevirapine plasma concentrations. Increased toxicity when used concomitantly with protease inhibitors or oral contraceptives. Ketoconazole should NOT be coadministered. Concurrent administration of prednisone for the initial 14 days of nevirapine therapy was associated with an increased incidence and severity of rash.
Decreased Effect: Rifampin and rifabutin may decrease nevirapine concentrations due to induction of CYP3A; since nevirapine may decrease concentrations of protease inhibitors (eg, indinavir, saquinavir), they should not be administered concomitantly or doses should be increased. Nevirapine may decrease the effectiveness of oral contraceptives; suggest alternate method of birth control. Nevirapine decreases effect of ketoconazole and methadone; may decrease serum concentration of some protease inhibitors (AUC of indinavir and saquinavir may be decreased - no effect noted with ritonavir); specific dosage adjustments have not been recommended (no adjustment recommended for ritonavir).

Drug Uptake
Absorption: Rapid, >90%
Half-life, elimination: Decreases over 2- to 4-week time with chronic dosing due to autoinduction (ie, half-life, elimination = 45 hours initially and decreases to 23 hours)
Time to peak: 2-4 hours

Pregnancy Risk Factor C
(Continued)

Nevirapine *(Continued)*

Generic Available No

Nexium™ *see* Esomeprazole *on page 456*

N.G.A.® *see* Nystatin and Triamcinolone *on page 881*

Niacin (NYE a sin)

Related Information

Cardiovascular Diseases *on page 1308*

U.S. Brand Names Niacor®; Niaspan®; Nicolar® [OTC]; Nicotinex [OTC]; Slo-Niacin® [OTC]

Canadian Brand Names Niaspan®

Mexican Brand Names Hipocol®; Pepevit®

Pharmacologic Category Antilipemic Agent, Miscellaneous; Vitamin, Water Soluble

Synonyms Nicotinic Acid; Vitamin B_3

Use Adjunctive treatment of hyperlipidemias; peripheral vascular disease and circulatory disorders; treatment of pellagra; dietary supplement; use in elevating HDL in patients with dyslipidemia

Local Anesthetic/Vasoconstrictor Precautions No information available to require special precautions

Effects on Dental Treatment No effects or complications reported

Dosage

Children: Oral:

- Pellagra: 50-100 mg/dose 3 times/day
- Recommended daily allowances:
  - 0-0.5 years: 5 mg/day
  - 0.5-1 year: 6 mg/day
  - 1-3 years: 9 mg/day
  - 4-6 years: 12 mg/day
  - 7-10 years: 13 mg/day

Children and Adolescents: Recommended daily allowances:

- Male:
  - 11-14 years: 17 mg/day
  - 15-18 years: 20 mg/day
  - 19-24 years: 19 mg/day
- Female: 11-24 years: 15 mg/day

Adults: Oral:

- Recommended daily allowances:
  - Male: 25-50 years: 19 mg/day; >51 years: 15 mg/day
  - Female: 25-50 years: 15 mg/day; >51 years: 13 mg/day
- Hyperlipidemia: Usual target dose: 1.5-6 g/day in 3 divided doses with or after meals using a dosage titration schedule; extended release: 375 mg to 2 g once daily at bedtime
  - Regular release formulation (Niacor®): Initial: 250 mg once daily (with evening meal); increase frequency and/or dose every 4-7 days to desired response or first-level therapeutic dose (1.5-2 g/day in 2-3 divided doses); after 2 months, may increase at 2- to 4-week intervals to 3 g/day in 3 divided doses
  - Extended release formulation (Niaspan®): 500 mg at bedtime for 4 weeks, then 1 g at bedtime for 4 weeks; adjust dose to response and tolerance; can increase to a maximum of 2 g/day, but only at 500 mg/day at 4-week intervals
- Pellagra: 50-100 mg 3-4 times/day, maximum: 500 mg/day
- Niacin deficiency: 10-20 mg/day, maximum: 100 mg/day

Mechanism of Action Component of two coenzymes which is necessary for tissue respiration, lipid metabolism, and glycogenolysis; inhibits the synthesis of very low density lipoproteins

Other Adverse Effects 1% to 10%:

Cardiovascular: Generalized flushing

Central nervous system: Headache

Gastrointestinal: Bloating, flatulence, nausea

Hepatic: Abnormalities of hepatic function tests, jaundice

Neuromuscular & skeletal: Paresthesia in extremities

Miscellaneous: Increased sebaceous gland activity, sensation of warmth

Drug Interactions

Increased Effect/Toxicity: Niacin increase the potential for myopathy and/or rhabdomyolysis with lovastatin (and possibly other HMG-CoA reductase inhibitors). Use with adrenergic blocking agents may result in additive vasodilating effect and postural hypotension.

Decreased Effect: The effect of oral hypoglycemics may be decreased by niacin. Niacin may inhibit uricosuric effects of sulfinpyrazone and probenecid. Aspirin (or other NSAIDs) decreases niacin-induced flushing.

Drug Uptake

Half-life, elimination: 45 minutes

Time to peak: Oral: ~45 minutes

Pregnancy Risk Factor A/C (dose exceeding RDA recommendation)

Generic Available Yes

Niacinamide (nye a SIN a mide)

Pharmacologic Category Vitamin, Water Soluble

Synonyms Nicotinamide; Vitamin B_3

Use Prophylaxis and treatment of pellagra

Local Anesthetic/Vasoconstrictor Precautions No information available to require special precautions

Effects on Dental Treatment No effects or complications reported

Dosage Oral:

Children: Pellagra: 100-300 mg/day in divided doses

Adults: 50 mg 3-10 times/day

Pellagra: 300-500 mg/day

Recommended daily allowance: 13-19 mg/day

Mechanism of Action Used by the body as a source of niacin; is a component of two coenzymes which is necessary for tissue respiration, lipid metabolism, and glycogenolysis; inhibits the synthesis of very low density lipoproteins; does not have hypolipidemia or vasodilating effects

Other Adverse Effects Frequency not defined:

Cardiovascular: Tachycardia

Dermatologic: Increased sebaceous gland activity, rash

Gastrointestinal: Bloating, flatulence, nausea

Neuromuscular & skeletal: Paresthesia in extremities

Ocular: Blurred vision

Respiratory: Wheezing

Drug Interactions

Adrenergic blocking agents → additive vasodilating effect and postural hypotension.

Aspirin decreases adverse effect of flushing.

Lovastatin (and possibly other HMG-CoA reductase inhibitors): Increased

Oral hypoglycemics: Effect may be decreased by niacin.

Sulfinpyrazone and probenecid; niacin may inhibit uricosuric effects. risk of toxicity (myopathy).

Drug Uptake

Absorption: Rapid

Half-life, elimination: 45 minutes

Time to peak: 20-70 minutes

Pregnancy Risk Factor A/C (dose exceeding RDA recommendation)

Generic Available Yes

Niacin and Lovastatin (NYE a sin & LOE va sta tin)

U.S. Brand Names Advicor™

Pharmacologic Category Antilipemic Agent, HMG-CoA Reductase Inhibitor; Antilipemic Agent, Miscellaneous

Synonyms Lovastatin and Niacin

Use Treatment of primary hypercholesterolemia (heterozygous familial and nonfamilial) and mixed dyslipidemia (Fredrickson types IIa and IIb) in patients previously treated with either agent alone (patients who require further lowering of triglycerides or increase in HDL cholesterol from addition of niacin or further lowering of LDL cholesterol from addition of lovastatin). Combination product; not intended for initial treatment.

Local Anesthetic/Vasoconstrictor Precautions No information available to require special precautions

Effects on Dental Treatment No effects or complications reported

Dosage Not for use as initial therapy of dyslipidemias. Dosage forms are a fixed combination of niacin and lovastatin; may be substituted for equivalent dose of Niaspan®, however, manufacturer does not recommend direct substitution with other niacin products.

Oral: Adults: Lowest dose: Niacin 500 mg/lovastatin 20 mg; may increase by not more than 500 mg (niacin) at 4-week intervals (maximum dose: Niacin 2000 mg/lovastatin 40 mg daily); should be taken at bedtime with a low-fat snack

Mechanism of Action Acts by competitively inhibiting 3-hydroxyl-3-methylglutaryl-coenzyme A (HMG-CoA) reductase, the enzyme that catalyzes the rate-limiting step in cholesterol biosynthesis; niacin is a component of two coenzymes which is necessary for tissue respiration, lipid metabolism, and glycogenolysis; inhibits the synthesis of very low density lipoproteins

Other Adverse Effects

>10%: Cardiovascular: Flushing

1% to 10%:

Central nervous system: Headache (9%), pain (8%)

Dermatologic: Pruritus (7%), rash (5%)

Endocrine & metabolic: Hyperglycemia (4%)

Gastrointestinal: Nausea (7%), diarrhea (6%), abdominal pain (4%), dyspepsia (3%), vomiting (3%)

(Continued)

Niacin and Lovastatin *(Continued)*

Neuromuscular & skeletal: Back pain (5%), weakness (5%), myalgia (3%)
Miscellaneous: Flu-like syndrome (6%)

Other uncommon adverse reactions reported with niacin and/or lovastatin include: Alkaline phosphatase increased, alopecia, anaphylaxis, angioedema, anemia, anorexia, anxiety, arthritis, cataracts, chills, cholestatic jaundice, cirrhosis, CPK increased (>10x normal), depression, dryness of skin/mucous membranes, dyspnea, eosinophilia, erectile dysfunction, erythema multiforme, ESR increased, facial paresis, fatty liver, fever, flushing, GGT increased, gout, gynecomastia, hemolytic anemia, hepatitis, hepatic necrosis (fulminant), hepatoma, hyperbilirubinemia, hypersensitivity reaction, hypotension, impotence, impaired extraocular muscle movement, leukopenia, libido decreased, memory loss, malaise, myopathy, nail changes, nodules, ophthalmoplegia, pancreatitis, paresthesia, peptic ulcer, peripheral nerve palsy, peripheral neuropathy, photosensitivity, polymyalgia rheumatica, pruritus, psychic disturbance, positive ANA, purpura, rhabdomyolysis, rash, renal failure, skin discoloration, Stevens-Johnson syndrome, syncope, systemic lupus erythematosus-like syndrome, taste alteration, thrombocytopenia, thyroid dysfunction, toxic epidermal necrolysis, transaminases elevated, tremor, urticaria, vasculitis, vertigo, vomiting

Drug Interactions See Lovastatin *on page 734* and Niacin *on page 860*
Drug Uptake See Lovastatin *on page 734* and Niacin *on page 860*
Pregnancy Risk Factor X
Generic Available No

Niacor® *see* Niacin *on page 860*
Niaspan® *see* Niacin *on page 860*

NiCARdipine (nye KAR de peen)

Related Information
Calcium Channel Blockers and Gingival Hyperplasia *on page 1432*
Cardiovascular Diseases *on page 1308*

U.S. Brand Names Cardene®; Cardene® I.V.; Cardene® SR
Mexican Brand Names Ridene®
Pharmacologic Category Calcium Channel Blocker
Synonyms Nicardipine Hydrochloride
Use Chronic stable angina; management of essential hypertension, migraine prophylaxis
Unlabeled/Investigational: Congestive heart failure

Local Anesthetic/Vasoconstrictor Precautions No information available to require special precautions

Effects on Dental Treatment Other drugs of this class can cause gingival hyperplasia (ie, nifedipine). The first case of nicardipine-induced gingival hyperplasia has been reported in a child taking 40-50 mg daily for 20 months.

Dosage Adults:
Oral: 40 mg 3 times/day (allow 3 days between dose increases)
Sustained release: Initial: 30 mg twice daily, titrate up to 60 mg twice daily
I.V. (dilute to 0.1 mg/mL): Initial: 5 mg/hour increased by 2.5 mg/hour every 15 minutes to a maximum of 15 mg/hour

Mechanism of Action Inhibits calcium ion from entering the "slow channels" or select voltage-sensitive areas of vascular smooth muscle and myocardium during depolarization, producing a relaxation of coronary vascular smooth muscle and coronary vasodilation; increases myocardial oxygen delivery in patients with vasospastic angina

Other Adverse Effects 1% to 10%:
Cardiovascular: Flushing (6% to 10%), palpitations (3% to 4%), tachycardia (1% to 4%), peripheral edema (dose-related 7% to 8%), increased angina (dose-related 6%), hypotension (I.V. 6%), orthostasis (I.V. 1%)
Central nervous system: Headache (6% to 15%), dizziness (4% to 7%), somnolence (4% to 6%), paresthesia (1%)
Dermatologic: Rash (1%)
Gastrointestinal: Nausea (2% to 5%), xerostomia (1%)
Genitourinary: Polyuria (1%)
Local: Injection site reaction (I.V. 1%)
Neuromuscular & skeletal: Weakness (4% to 6%), myalgia (1%)
Miscellaneous: Diaphoresis

Drug Interactions CYP3A3/4 enzyme substrate; CYP2C8/9, 2C19, 2D6, 3A3/4 enzyme inhibitor
Increased Effect/Toxicity: H_2 blockers (cimetidine) may increase the bioavailability of nicardipine. Serum concentrations/toxicity of nicardipine may be increased by inhibitors of CYP3A3/4, including amprenavir, cimetidine, ciprofloxacin, clarithromycin, clozapine, diltiazem, disulfiram, digoxin, erythromycin, fluconazole, fluoxetine, fluvoxamine, isoniazid, itraconazole, ketoconazole, labetalol, levodopa, loxapine, metoprolol, metronidazole, miconazole, nefazodone, nelfinavir, omeprazole, phenytoin, propranolol, rifabutin, rifampin, ritonavir, troleandomycin, valproic acid, and verapamil. Calcium may reduce the calcium channel blocker's

effects, particularly hypotension. Cyclosporine levels (and possibly tacrolimus) may be increased by nicardipine. May increase effect of vecuronium (reduce dose 25%) and increase serum concentration of metoprolol.

Decreased Effect: Rifampin (and potentially other enzyme inducers) increase the metabolism of calcium channel blockers.

Drug Uptake

Onset of action: Oral: 1-2 hours; I.V.: 10 minutes; Hypotension: ~20 minutes

Absorption: Oral: Well absorbed, ~100%

Duration: 2-6 hours

Half-life, elimination: 2-4 hours

Time to peak: 20-120 minutes

Pregnancy Risk Factor C

Generic Available Yes

Selected Readings Pascual-Castroviejo I and Pascual Pascual SI, "Nicardipine-Induced Gingival Hyperplasia," *Neurologia*, 1997, 12(1):37-9.

NicoDerm® CQ® Patch *see* Nicotine *on page 863*

Nicolar® [OTC] *see* Niacin *on page 860*

Nicorette® DS Gum *see* Nicotine *on page 863*

Nicorette® Gum *see* Nicotine *on page 863*

Nicotine (nik oh TEEN)

Related Information

Chemical Dependency and Smoking Cessation *on page 1410*

U.S. Brand Names Habitrol™ Patch; NicoDerm® CQ® Patch; Nicorette® DS Gum; Nicorette® Gum; Nicotrol® NS; Nicotrol® Patch [OTC]; ProStep® Patch

Canadian Brand Names Habitrol®; Nicoderm®; Nicorette®; Nicorette® Plus; Nicotrol®

Mexican Brand Names Nicolan; Nicotinell TTS

Pharmacologic Category Smoking Cessation Aid

Use Treatment to aid smoking cessation for the relief of nicotine withdrawal symptoms (including nicotine craving)

Unlabeled/Investigational: Management of ulcerative colitis (transdermal)

Local Anesthetic/Vasoconstrictor Precautions No information available to require special precautions

Effects on Dental Treatment >10%: Chewing gum formulation: Salivation and mouth or throat soreness

Dosage

Gum: Chew 1 piece of gum when urge to smoke, up to 30 pieces/day; most patients require 10-12 pieces of gum/day

Transdermal patch (benefits of use beyond 3 months have not been demonstrated):

- Smoking deterrent: Patients should be advised to completely stop smoking upon initiation of therapy: Apply new patch every 24 hours to nonhairy, clean, dry skin on the upper body or upper outer arm; each patch should be applied to a different site.
  - **Note:** Adjustment may be required during initial treatment (move to higher dose if experiencing withdrawal symptoms; lower dose if side effects are experienced).
  - Habitrol®, NicoDerm CQ®:
    - Patients smoking ≥10 cigarettes/day: Begin with **step 1** (21 mg/day) for 4-6 weeks, followed by **step 2** (14 mg/day) for 2 weeks; finish with **step 3** (7 mg/day) for 2 weeks
    - Patients smoking <10 cigarettes/day: Begin with **step 2** (14 mg/day) for 6 weeks, followed by **step 3** (7 mg/day) for 2 weeks
    - Initial starting dose for patients <100 pounds, history of cardiovascular disease: 14 mg/day for 4-6 weeks, followed by 7 mg/day for 2-4 weeks
    - Patients receiving >600 mg/day of cimetidine: Decrease to the next lower patch size
  - Nicotrol®: One patch daily for 6 weeks
  - ProStep®:
    - Patients smoking >15 cigarettes/day: One 22 mg patch daily for 6 weeks
    - Patients smoking ≤15 cigarettes/day: One 11 mg patch daily for 6 weeks
- Ulcerative colitis (unlabeled use): Titrated to 22-25 mg/day

Spray: 1-2 sprays/hour; do not exceed more than 5 doses (10 sprays) per hour; each dose (2 sprays) contains 1 mg of nicotine. **Warning:** A dose of 40 mg can cause fatalities.

Mechanism of Action Potent ganglionic and CNS stimulant, the actions of which are mediated via nicotine-specific receptors; one of two naturally-occurring alkaloids which exhibit their primary effects via autonomic ganglia stimulation; the other alkaloid is lobeline which has many actions similar to those of nicotine but is less potent. Biphasic actions are observed depending upon the dose administered. The main effect of nicotine in small doses is stimulation of all autonomic ganglia; with larger doses, initial stimulation is followed by blockade of transmission. Biphasic effects are also evident in the adrenal medulla; discharge of catecholamines occurs with small doses, whereas prevention of catecholamines release is seen with

(Continued)

Nicotine *(Continued)*

higher doses as a response to splanchnic nerve stimulation. Stimulation of the CNS (CNS) is characterized by tremors and respiratory excitation. However, convulsions may occur with higher doses, along with respiratory failure secondary to both central paralysis and peripheral blockade to respiratory muscles.

Other Adverse Effects

Chewing gum:

>10%:
- Cardiovascular: Tachycardia
- Central nervous system: Headache (mild)
- Gastrointestinal: Nausea, vomiting, indigestion, excessive salivation, belching, increased appetite
- Miscellaneous: Mouth or throat soreness, jaw muscle ache, hiccups

1% to 10%:
- Central nervous system: Insomnia, dizziness, nervousness
- Endocrine & metabolic: Dysmenorrhea
- Gastrointestinal: GI distress, eructation
- Neuromuscular & skeletal: Muscle pain
- Respiratory: Hoarseness
- Miscellaneous: Hiccups

<1%: Atrial fibrillation, erythema, hypersensitivity reactions, itching

Transdermal systems:

>10%:
- Central nervous system: Insomnia, abnormal dreams
- Dermatologic: Pruritus, erythema
- Local: Application site reaction
- Respiratory: Rhinitis, cough, pharyngitis, sinusitis

1% to 10%:
- Cardiovascular: Chest pain
- Central nervous system: Dysphoria, anxiety, difficulty concentrating, dizziness, somnolence
- Dermatologic: Rash
- Gastrointestinal: Diarrhea, dyspepsia, nausea, xerostomia, constipation, anorexia, abdominal pain
- Neuromuscular & skeletal: Arthralgia, myalgia

<1%: Atrial fibrillation, hypersensitivity reactions, itching, nervousness, taste perversion, thirst, tremor

Contraindications Hypersensitivity to nicotine or any component of the formulation; patients smoking during the postmyocardial infarction period; life-threatening arrhythmias, or severe or worsening angina pectoris; active temporomandibular joint disease (gum form); pregnancy; nonsmokers

Warnings/Precautions The risk versus the benefits must be weighed for each of these groups: patients with CAD, serious cardiac arrhythmias, vasospastic disease. Use caution in patients with hyperthyroidism, pheochromocytoma, or insulin-dependent diabetes. Use with caution in oropharyngeal inflammation and in patients with history of esophagitis, peptic ulcer, coronary artery disease, vasospastic disease, angina, hypertension, hyperthyroidism, pheochromocytoma, diabetes, severe renal dysfunction, and hepatic dysfunction. The inhaler should be used with caution in patients with bronchospastic disease (other forms of nicotine replacement may be preferred). Safety and efficacy have not been established in pediatric patients. Cautious use of topical nicotine in patients with certain skin diseases. Hypersensitivity to the topical products can occur. Dental problems may be worsened by chewing the gum. Urge patients to stop smoking completely when initiating therapy.

Drug Interactions CYP2B6 and 2A6 enzyme substrate; CYP1A2 enzyme inducer
- Adenosine: Nicotine increases the hemodynamic and AV blocking effects of adenosine; monitor
- Bupropion: Monitor for treatment-emergent hypertension in patients treated with the combination of nicotine patch and bupropion
- Cimetidine; May increases nicotine concentrations; therefore, may decrease amount of gum or patches needed
- CYP1A2 substrates: May decrease serum concentration of drugs metabolized by this isoenzyme, including theophylline and tacrine

Drug Uptake
- Onset of action: Intranasal: More closely approximate the time course of plasma nicotine levels observed after cigarette smoking than other dosage forms
- Duration: Transdermal: 24 hours
- Absorption: Transdermal: Slow
- Half-life, elimination: 4 hours
- Time to peak: Transdermal: 8-9 hours

Pregnancy Risk Factor D (transdermal); X (chewing gum)

Dosage Forms GUM, chewing, as polacrilex: 2 mg/square (96 pieces/box); 4 mg/square (96 pieces/box). **LIQ, oral inhalation** (Nicotrol® Inhaler): 10 mg cartridge (42s). **PATCH, transdermal:** 15 mg/day; (Habitrol™): 7 mg/day, 14 mg/day, 21 mg/day (30 systems/box); (NicoDerm® CQ®): 7 mg/day, 14 mg/day, 21 mg/day (14 systems/box); (ProStep®): 11 mg/day, 22 mg/day (7 systems/box). **SPRAY, intranasal** (Nicotrol® NS): 0.5 mg/actuation [10 mg/mL] (10 mL)

Generic Available Yes: Transdermal patch and gum

Comments At least 10 reported studies have documented the effectiveness of nicotine patches in smoking cessation. Approximately 45% of treated patients quit smoking after 6 weeks of patch therapy. Control patients given placebo patches accounted for about a 20% success rate. At 52 weeks, approximately ½ of the 45% 6-week successful patients continued to abstain. Control placebo patients accounted for an approximate 11% success rate after 52 weeks.

Selected Readings

Christen AG and Christen JA, "The Prescription of Transdermal Nicotine Patches for Tobacco-Using Dental Patients: Current Status in Indiana," *J Indiana Dent Assoc*, 1992, 71(6):12-8.

Li Wan Po A, "Transdermal Nicotine in Smoking Cessation. A Meta-analysis," *Eur J Clin Pharmacol*, 1993, 45(6):519-28.

Stafne EE, "The Nicotine Transdermal Patch: Use in the Dental Office Tobacco Cessation Program," *Northwest Dent*, 1994, 73(3):19-22.

Transdermal Nicotine Study Group, "Transdermal Nicotine for Smoking Cessation. Six-Month Results from Two Multicenter Controlled Clinical Trials," *JAMA*, 1991, 266(22):3133-8.

Westman EC, Levin ED, and Rose JE, "The Nicotine Patch in Smoking Cessation," *Arch Intern Med*, 1993, 153(16):1917-23.

Wynn RL, "Nicotine Patches in Smoking Cessation," *AGD Impact*, 1994, 22:14.

Nicotinex [OTC] *see* Niacin *on page 860*

Nicotrol® NS *see* Nicotine *on page 863*

Nicotrol® Patch [OTC] *see* Nicotine *on page 863*

NIFEdipine (nye FED i peen)

Related Information

Calcium Channel Blockers and Gingival Hyperplasia *on page 1432*
Cardiovascular Diseases *on page 1308*

U.S. Brand Names Adalat® CC; Procardia®; Procardia XL®

Canadian Brand Names Adalat® PA; Adalat® XL®; Apo®-Nifed; Apo®-Nifed PA; Novo-Nifedin; Nu-Nifed; Procardia®

Mexican Brand Names Adalat®; Corogal; Corotrend; Nifedipres; Noviken-N

Pharmacologic Category Calcium Channel Blocker

Use Angina, hypertrophic cardiomyopathy, hypertension (sustained release only), pulmonary hypertension

Local Anesthetic/Vasoconstrictor Precautions No information available to require special precautions

Effects on Dental Treatment Nifedipine has the greatest incidence in causing gingival hyperplasia than any other calcium channel blocker. Effects from the use of nifedipine (30-100 mg/day) have appeared after 1-9 months. Discontinuance of the drug results in complete disappearance or marked regression of symptoms; symptoms will reappear upon remedication. Marked regression occurs after 1 week and complete disappearance of symptoms has occurred within 15 days. If a gingivectomy is performed and use of the drug is continued or resumed, hyperplasia usually will recur. The success of the gingivectomy usually requires that the medication be discontinued or that a switch to a noncalcium channel blocker be made. If for some reason nifedipine cannot be discontinued, hyperplasia has not recurred after gingivectomy when extensive plaque control was performed. If nifedipine is changed to another class of cardiovascular agent, the gingival hyperplasia will probably regress and disappear. A switch to another calcium channel blocker probably may result in continued hyperplasia.

Dosage Note: Doses are usually titrated upward at 7- to 14-day intervals; may increase every 3 days if clinically necessary

Children: Hypertrophic cardiomyopathy: 0.6-0.9 mg/kg/24 hours in 3-4 divided doses

Adolescents and Adults: (**Note:** When switching from immediate release to sustained release formulations, total daily dose will start the same)

- Initial: 10 mg 3 times/day as capsules or 30 mg once daily as sustained release
- Usual dose: 10-30 mg 3 times/day as capsules or 30-60 mg once daily as sustained release
- Maximum dose: 120-180 mg/day
- *Increase sustained release at 7- to 14-day intervals*

Hemodialysis: Supplemental dose is not necessary

Peritoneal dialysis effects: Supplemental dose is not necessary

Dosing adjustment in hepatic impairment: Reduce oral dose by 50% to 60% in patients with cirrhosis

Mechanism of Action Inhibits calcium ion from entering the "slow channels" or select voltage-sensitive areas of vascular smooth muscle and myocardium during depolarization, producing a relaxation of coronary vascular smooth muscle and coronary vasodilation; increases myocardial oxygen delivery in patients with vasospastic angina

Other Adverse Effects

>10%:

Cardiovascular: Flushing (10% to 25%), peripheral edema (dose-related 7% to 10%; up to 50%)

(Continued)

NIFEdipine *(Continued)*

Central nervous system: Dizziness/lightheadedness/giddiness (10% to 27%), headache (10% to 23%)
Gastrointestinal: Nausea/heartburn (10% to 11%)
Neuromuscular & skeletal: Weakness (10% to 12%)

≥1% to 10%:
Cardiovascular: Palpitations (≤2% to 7%), transient hypotension (dose-related 5%), CHF (2%)
Central nervous system: Nervousness/mood changes (≤2% to 7%), shakiness (≤2%), jitteriness (≤2%), sleep disturbances (≤2%), difficulties in balance (≤2%), fever (≤2%), chills (≤2%)
Dermatologic: Dermatitis (≤2%), pruritus (≤2%), urticaria (≤2%)
Endocrine & metabolic: Sexual difficulties (≤2%)
Gastrointestinal: Diarrhea (≤2%), constipation (≤2%), cramps (≤2%), flatulence (≤2%), gingival hyperplasia (≤10%)
Neuromuscular & skeletal: Muscle cramps/tremor (≤2% to 8%), weakness (10%), inflammation (≤2%), joint stiffness (≤2%)
Ocular: Blurred vision (≤2%)
Respiratory: Cough/wheezing (6%), nasal congestion/sore throat (≤2% to 6%), chest congestion (≤2%), dyspnea (≤2%)
Miscellaneous: Diaphoresis (≤2%)

Reported with use of sublingual short-acting nifedipine: Cerebrovascular ischemia, syncope, heart block, stroke, sinus arrest, severe hypotension, acute myocardial infarction, EKG changes, and fetal distress

Drug Interactions CYP3A3/4 and 3A5-7 enzyme substrate

Increased Effect/Toxicity: H_2 blockers may increase bioavailability and serum concentration of nifedipine. Serum concentrations/toxicity of nifedipine may be increased by inhibitors of CYP3A3/4, including amprenavir, cimetidine, ciprofloxacin, clarithromycin, clozapine, diltiazem, disulfiram, digoxin, erythromycin, fluconazole, fluoxetine, fluvoxamine, isoniazid, itraconazole, ketoconazole, labetalol, levodopa, loxapine, metoprolol, metronidazole, miconazole, nefazodone, nelfinavir, omeprazole, phenytoin, rifabutin, rifampin, ritonavir, troleandomycin, valproic acid, and verapamil. Nifedipine may increase serum concentration of digoxin, phenytoin, theophylline, and vincristine.

Decreased Effect: Phenobarbital and nifedipine may decrease nifedipine levels. Quinidine and nifedipine may decrease quinidine serum concentration. Rifampin and nifedipine may decrease nifedipine serum concentration. Calcium may reduce the hypotension from of calcium channel blockers.

Drug Uptake

Onset of action: Oral: ≤20 minutes
Half-life, elimination: Adults: 2-5 hours; Adults: Cirrhosis: 7 hours

Pregnancy Risk Factor C

Generic Available Yes: Capsule, tablet (30 mg extended release)

Selected Readings

Deen-Duggins L, Fry HR, Clay JR, et al, "Nifedipine-Associated Gingival Overgrowth: A Survey of the Literature and Report of Four Cases," *Quintessence Int*, 1996, 27(3):163-70.
Desai P and Silver JG, "Drug-Induced Gingival Enlargements," *J Can Dent Assoc*, 1998, 64(4):263-8.
Harel-Raviv M, Eckler M, Lalani K, et al, "Nifedipine-Induced Gingival Hyperplasia. A Comprehensive Review and Analysis," *Oral Surg Oral Med Oral Pathol Oral Radiol Endod*, 1995, 79(6):715-22.
Lederman D, Lumerman H, Reuben S, et al, "Gingival Hyperplasia Associated With Nifedipine Therapy," *Oral Surg Oral Med Oral Pathol*, 1984, 57(6):620-2.
Lucas RM, Howell LP, and Wall BA, "Nifedipine-Induced Gingival Hyperplasia: A Histochemical and Ultrastructural Study," *J Periodontol*, 1985, 56(4):211-5.
Nery EB, Edson RG, Lee KK, et al, "Prevalence of Nifedipine-Induced Gingival Hyperplasia," *J Periodontol*, 1995, 66(7):572-8.
Nishikawa SJ, Tada H, Hamasaki A, et al, "Nifedipine-Induced Gingival Hyperplasia: A Clinical and In Vitro Study," *J Periodontol*, 1991, 62(1):30-5.
Pilloni A, Camargo PM, Carere M, et al, "Surgical Treatment of Cyclosporine A- and Nifedipine-Induced Gingival Enlargement: Gingivectomy Versus Periodontal Flap," *J Periodontol*, 1998, 69(7):791-7.
Saito K, Mori S, Iwakura M, et al, "Immunohistochemical Localization of Transforming Growth Factor Beta, Basic Fibroblast Growth Factor and Heparin Sulphate Glycosaminoglycan in Gingival Hyperplasia Induced by Nifedipine and Phenytoin," *J Periodontal Res*, 1996, 31(8):545-5.
Silverstein LH, Koch JP, Lefkove MD, et al, "Nifedipine-Induced Gingival Enlargement Around Dental Implants: A Clinical Report," *J Oral Implantol*, 1995, 21(2):116-20.
Westbrook P, Bednarczyk EM, Carlson M, et al, "Regression of Nifedipine-Induced Gingival Hyperplasia Following Switch to a Same Class Calcium Channel Blocker, Isradipine," *J Periodontol*, 1997, 68(7):645-50.
Wynn RL, "Calcium Channel Blockers and Gingival Hyperplasia," *Gen Dent*, 1991, 39(4):240-3.
Wynn RL, "Update on Calcium Channel Blocker-Induced Gingival Hyperplasia," *Gen Dent*, 1995, 43(3):218-22.

Niferex® [OTC] *see* Polysaccharide-Iron Complex *on page 972*
Niferex®-PN *see* Vitamins, Multiple *on page 1246*
Nilandron™ *see* Nilutamide *on page 866*
Nilstat® *see* Nystatin *on page 880*

Nilutamide (ni LU ta mide)

U.S. Brand Names Nilandron™

Canadian Brand Names Anandron®

Pharmacologic Category Antineoplastic Agent, Miscellaneous

Use In combination with surgical castration in treatment of metastatic prostatic carcinoma (Stage D_2); for maximum benefit, nilutamide treatment must begin on the same day as or on the day after surgical castration

Local Anesthetic/Vasoconstrictor Precautions No information available to require special precautions

Effects on Dental Treatment No effects or complications reported

Mechanism of Action Nonsteroidal antiandrogen that inhibits androgen uptake or inhibits binding of androgen in target tissues

Other Adverse Effects

>10%:

Central nervous system: Pain, insomnia

Endocrine & metabolic: Hot flashes (60% to 80%), gynecomastia (4% to 44%); higher incidence in patients receiving the drug as a single agent

Gastrointestinal: Nausea, mild (10% to 32%); constipation, anorexia

Genitourinary: Decreased libido, impotence, sexual dysfunction (50%)

Hepatic: Transient elevation in serum transaminases (13%)

Ocular: Impaired dark adaptation (90%), usually reversible with dose reduction, may require discontinuation of the drug in 1% to 2% of patients; blurred vision

1% to 10%:

Cardiovascular: Hypertension

Central nervous system: Dizziness, drowsiness, malaise, headache, hypesthesia

Dermatologic: Disulfiram-like reaction (hot flashes, rashes) (20%); pruritus (<5%), alopecia, dry skin

Endocrine & metabolic: Flu-like syndrome, fever

Gastrointestinal: Vomiting, diarrhea, abdominal cramps

Genitourinary: Hematuria, nocturia

Hepatic: Hepatitis (1%)

Respiratory: Interstitial pneumonitis, pulmonary fibrosis (1% to 3%), usually reversible

Drug Uptake

Absorption: Well absorbed

Half-life, elimination: Variable; Mean: 50 hours (range: 23-87 hours)

Time to peak: 1-4 hours

Pregnancy Risk Factor C

Generic Available No

Nimodipine (nye MOE di peen)

Related Information

Calcium Channel Blockers and Gingival Hyperplasia *on page 1432*
Cardiovascular Diseases *on page 1308*

U.S. Brand Names Nimotop®

Canadian Brand Names Nimotop®

Mexican Brand Names Nimotop®

Pharmacologic Category Calcium Channel Blocker

Use Spasm following subarachnoid hemorrhage from ruptured intracranial aneurysms regardless of the patient's neurological condition postictus (Hunt and Hess grades I-V)

Local Anesthetic/Vasoconstrictor Precautions No information available to require special precautions

Effects on Dental Treatment Other drugs of this class can cause gingival hyperplasia (ie, nifedipine) but there have been no reports for nimodipine.

Dosage Adults: Oral: 60 mg every 4 hours for 21 days, start therapy within 96 hours after subarachnoid hemorrhage

Mechanism of Action Shares the pharmacology of other calcium channel blockers; animal studies indicate that nimodipine has a greater effect on cerebral arterials than other arterials. This increased specificity may be due to the drug's increased lipophilicity and cerebral distribution as compared to nifedipine; inhibits calcium ion from entering the "slow channels" or select voltage sensitive areas of vascular smooth muscle and myocardium during depolarization.

Other Adverse Effects 1% to 10%:

Cardiovascular: Reductions in systemic BP (1% to 8%)

Central nervous system: Headache (1% to 4%)

Dermatologic: Rash (1% to 2%)

Gastrointestinal: Diarrhea (2% to 4%), abdominal discomfort (2%)

Drug Interactions CYP3A3/4 enzyme substrate

Increased Effect/Toxicity: Calcium channel blockers and nimodipine may result in enhanced cardiovascular effects of other calcium channel blockers. Cimetidine, omeprazole, and valproic acid may increase serum nimodipine levels. The effects of antihypertensive agents may be increased by nimodipine. Azole antifungals (itraconazole, ketoconazole, fluconazole), erythromycin, protease inhibitors (amprenavir, nelfinavir, ritonavir) and other inhibitors of cytochrome P450 isoenzyme 3A4 may inhibit calcium channel blocker metabolism.

(Continued)

Nimodipine *(Continued)*

Decreased Effect: Rifampin (and potentially other enzyme inducers) increase the metabolism of calcium channel blockers.

Drug Uptake

Half-life, elimination: 3 hours (increases with renal impairment)
Time to peak: Oral: ~1 hour

Pregnancy Risk Factor C

Generic Available No

Nimotop® *see* Nimodipine *on page 867*
Nipent® *see* Pentostatin *on page 937*

Nisoldipine (NYE sole di peen)

Related Information

Cardiovascular Diseases *on page 1308*

U.S. Brand Names Sular®

Mexican Brand Names Sular®; Syscor

Pharmacologic Category Calcium Channel Blocker

Use Management of hypertension, may be used alone or in combination with other antihypertensive agents

Local Anesthetic/Vasoconstrictor Precautions No information available to require special precautions

Effects on Dental Treatment Other drugs in this class can cause gingival hyperplasia, but there have been no reports for nisoldipine.

Dosage Adults: Oral: Initial: 20 mg once daily, then increase by 10 mg/week (or longer intervals) to attain adequate control of BP; doses >60 mg once daily are not recommended. A starting dose not exceeding 10 mg/day is recommended for the elderly and those with hepatic impairment.

Mechanism of Action Impedes movement of calcium ions into vascular smooth muscle and cardiac muscle; 5-10 times as potent a vasodilator as nifedipine; not as likely to suppress cardiac contractility and slow cardiac conduction as other calcium antagonists such as verapamil and diltiazem

Other Adverse Effects

>10%:
- Cardiovascular: Peripheral edema (dose-related 7% to 29%)
- Central nervous system: Headache (22%)

1% to 10%:
- Cardiovascular: Chest pain (2%), palpitations (3%), vasodilation (4%)
- Central nervous system: Dizziness (3% to 10%)
- Dermatologic: Rash (2%)
- Gastrointestinal: Nausea (2%)
- Respiratory: Pharyngitis (5%), sinusitis (3%), dyspnea (3%), cough (5%)

Warnings/Precautions Increased angina and/or myocardial infarction in patients with coronary artery disease

Drug Interactions CYP3A3/4 enzyme substrate

Increased Effect/Toxicity: H_2 antagonists or omeprazole may cause an increase in the serum concentration of nisoldipine. Digoxin and nisoldipine may increase digoxin effect. Azole antifungals (itraconazole, ketoconazole, fluconazole), erythromycin, and other inhibitors of cytochrome P450 isoenzyme 3A4 may inhibit calcium channel blocker metabolism. Calcium may reduce the calcium channel blocker's effects, particularly hypotension.

Decreased Effect: Rifampin, phenytoin, and potentially other enzyme inducers decrease the levels of nisoldipine. Calcium may decrease the hypotension from calcium channel blockers.

Drug Uptake

Absorption: Well absorbed
Duration: >24 hours
Half-life, elimination: 7-12 hours
Time to peak: 6-12 hours

Pregnancy Risk Factor C

Generic Available No

Nitisinone (ni TIS i known)

U.S. Brand Names Orfadin®

Pharmacologic Category 4-Hydroxyphenylpyruvate Dioxygenase Inhibitor

Use Treatment of hereditary tyrosinemia type 1 (HT-1); to be used with dietary restriction of tyrosine and phenylalanine

Local Anesthetic/Vasoconstrictor Precautions No information available to require special precautions

Effects on Dental Treatment No effects or complications reported

Restrictions Distributed by Rare Disease Therapeutics, Inc (contact 615-399-0700)

Dosage Must be used in conjunction with a low protein diet restricted in tyrosine and phenylalanine.

Oral:

Infants: See dosing for Children and Adults; infants may require maximal dose once liver function has improved

Children and Adults: Initial: 1 mg/kg/day in divided doses, given in the morning and evening, 1 hour before meals; doses do not need to be divided evenly

Dose adjustment: If biochemical parameters (see Monitoring Parameters) are not normalized within in 1-month period, dose may be increased to 1.5 mg/kg/day (maximum dose: 2 mg/kg/day).

Mechanism of Action In patients with HT-1, tyrosine metabolism is interrupted due to a lack of the enzyme (fumarylacetoacetate hydrolase) needed in the last step of tyrosine degradation. Toxic metabolites of tyrosine accumulate and cause liver and kidney toxicity. Nitisinone competitively inhibits 4-hydroxyphenyl-pyruvate dioxygenase, an enzyme needed earlier in the tyrosine degradation pathway, and therefore prevents the build-up of the damaging metabolites.

Other Adverse Effects 1% to 10%:

Dermatologic: Alopecia (1%), dry skin (1%), exfoliative dermatitis (1%), maculopapular rash (1%), pruritus (1%)

Hematologic: Thrombocytopenia (3%), leukopenia (3%), porphyria (1%), epistaxis (1%)

Hepatic: Hepatic neoplasm (8%), hepatic failure (7%)

Ocular: Conjunctivitis (2%), corneal opacity (2%), keratitis, (2%), photophobia (2%), cataracts (1%), blepharitis (1%), eye pain (1%)

Drug Uptake Limited pharmacokinetic studies in children or HT-1 patients.

Half-life, elimination: Terminal: 54 hours (healthy males)

Time to peak: 3 hours

Pregnancy Risk Factor C

Generic Available No

Nitrek® Patch *see* Nitroglycerin *on page 871*

Nitric Oxide (NYE trik OKS ide)

U.S. Brand Names INOmax®

Canadian Brand Names INOmax®

Pharmacologic Category Vasodilator, Pulmonary

Use Treatment of term and near-term (>34 weeks) neonates with hypoxic respiratory failure associated with pulmonary hypertension; used concurrently with ventilatory support and other agents

Unlabeled/Investigational: Treatment of adult respiratory distress syndrome (ARDS)

Local Anesthetic/Vasoconstrictor Precautions No information available to require special precautions

Effects on Dental Treatment No effects or complications reported

Dosage Neonates (up to 14 days old): 20 ppm. Treatment should be maintained up to 14 days or until the underlying oxygen desaturation has resolved and the neonate is ready to be weaned from therapy. In the CINRGI trial, patients whose oxygenation improved had their dose reduced to 5 ppm at the end of 4 hours of treatment. Doses above 20 ppm should not be used because of the risk of methemoglobinemia and elevated NO_2.

Mechanism of Action In neonates with persistent pulmonary hypertension, nitric oxide improves oxygenation. Nitric oxide relaxes vascular smooth muscle by binding to the heme moiety of cytosolic guanylate cyclase, activating guanylate cyclase and increasing intracellular levels of cyclic guanosine 3',5'-monophosphate, which leads to vasodilation. When inhaled, pulmonary vasodilation occurs and an increase in the partial pressure of arterial oxygen results. Dilation of pulmonary vessels in well ventilated lung areas redistributes blood flow away from lung areas where ventilation/perfusion ratios are poor.

Other Adverse Effects Atelectasis occurred in 9% of patients receiving placebo and in 9% of those receiving inhaled nitric oxide.

>10%:

Cardiovascular: Hypotension (13%)

Miscellaneous: Withdrawal syndrome (12%)

1% to 10%:

Dermatologic: Cellulitis (5%)

Endocrine & metabolic: Hyperglycemia (8%)

Genitourinary: Hematuria (8%)

Respiratory: Stridor (5%)

Miscellaneous: Sepsis (7%), infection (6%)

Contraindications Hypersensitivity to nitric oxide or any component of the formulation; neonates dependent on right-to-left shunting of blood

Warnings/Precautions Abrupt discontinuation may lead to worsening oxygenation and increasing pulmonary artery pressure (PAP). Worsening oxygenation and increasing PAP may occur in patients who do not respond. Doses above 20 ppm should not be used because of the increased risk of methemoglobinemia and elevated nitrogen dioxide (NO_2) levels. Methemoglobin levels and NO_2 should be monitored.

(Continued)

Nitric Oxide *(Continued)*

Drug Interactions

No formal studies have been conducted; has been administered with tolazoline, dopamine, dobutamine, steroids, surfactant, and high-frequency ventilation.

Increased Effect/Toxicity: Concurrent use of sodium nitroprusside or nitroglycerin may result in an increased risk of developing methemoglobinemia; monitor closely if used

Drug Uptake Absorption: Systemically after inhalation

Pregnancy Risk Factor C

Generic Available No

Nitro-Bid® Ointment *see* Nitroglycerin *on page 871*

Nitrodisc® Patch *see* Nitroglycerin *on page 871*

Nitro-Dur® Patch *see* Nitroglycerin *on page 871*

Nitrofurantoin (nye troe fyoor AN toyn)

U.S. Brand Names Furadantin®; Macrobid®; Macrodantin®

Canadian Brand Names Apo®-Nitrofurantoin; MacroBID®; Macrodantin®; Novo-Furantoin

Mexican Brand Names Furadantina; Macrodantina

Pharmacologic Category Antibiotic, Miscellaneous

Use Prevention and treatment of urinary tract infections caused by susceptible gram-negative and some gram-positive organisms; *Pseudomonas*, *Serratia*, and most species of *Proteus* are generally resistant to nitrofurantoin

Local Anesthetic/Vasoconstrictor Precautions No information available to require special precautions

Effects on Dental Treatment No effects or complications reported

Dosage Oral:

Children >1 month: 5-7 mg/kg/day in divided doses every 6 hours; maximum: 400 mg/day

Chronic therapy: 1-2 mg/kg/day in divided doses every 24 hours; maximum dose: 400 mg/day

Adults: 50-100 mg/dose every 6 hours (not to exceed 400 mg/24 hours)

Prophylaxis: 50-100 mg/dose at at bedtime

Mechanism of Action Inhibits several bacterial enzyme systems including acetyl coenzyme A interfering with metabolism and possibly cell wall synthesis

Other Adverse Effects Frequency not defined:

Cardiovascular: Chest pains

Central nervous system: Chills, dizziness, drowsiness, fatigue, fever, headache

Dermatologic: Exfoliative dermatitis, itching, rash

Gastrointestinal: *C. difficile*-colitis, diarrhea, loss of appetite/vomiting/nausea (most common), sore throat, stomach upset

Hematologic: Hemolytic anemia

Hepatic: Hepatitis, increased LFTs

Neuromuscular & skeletal: Arthralgia, numbness, paresthesia, weakness

Respiratory: Cough, dyspnea, pneumonitis, pulmonary fibrosis

Miscellaneous: Hypersensitivity, lupus-like syndrome

Drug Interactions

Increased Effect/Toxicity: Probenecid decreases renal excretion of nitrofurantoin.

Decreased Effect: Antacids decrease absorption of nitrofurantoin.

Drug Uptake

Absorption: Well absorbed from GI tract; the macrocrystalline form is absorbed more slowly due to slower dissolution, but causes less GI distress

Half-life, elimination: 20-60 minutes; increases with renal impairment

Pregnancy Risk Factor B

Generic Available Yes: Macrocrystal

Nitrofurazone (nye troe FYOOR a zone)

U.S. Brand Names Furacin®

Mexican Brand Names Furacin®

Pharmacologic Category Antibiotic, Topical

Synonyms Nitrofural

Use Antibacterial agent in second and third degree burns and skin grafting

Local Anesthetic/Vasoconstrictor Precautions No information available to require special precautions

Effects on Dental Treatment No effects or complications reported

Dosage Children and Adults: Topical: Apply once daily or every few days to lesion or place on gauze

Mechanism of Action A broad antibacterial spectrum; it acts by inhibiting bacterial enzymes involved in carbohydrate metabolism; effective against a wide range of gram-negative and gram-positive organisms; bactericidal against most bacteria commonly causing surface infections including *Staphylococcus aureus*, *Streptococcus*, *Escherichia coli*, *Enterobacter cloacae*, *Clostridium perfringens*, *Aerobacter aerogenes*, and *Proteus* sp; not particularly active against most *Pseudomonas* *aeruginosa* strains and does not inhibit viruses or fungi. Topical preparations of nitrofurazone are readily soluble in blood, pus, and serum and are nonmacerating.

Drug Interactions Sutilains decrease activity of nitrofurazone.

Pregnancy Risk Factor C

Generic Available Yes

Nitrogard® Buccal *see* Nitroglycerin *on page 871*

Nitroglycerin (nye troe GLI ser in)

Related Information

Cardiovascular Diseases *on page 1308*

Dental Office Emergencies *on page 1418*

U.S. Brand Names Deponit® Patch; Minitran™ Patch; Nitrek® Patch; Nitro-Bid® Ointment; Nitrodisc® Patch; Nitro-Dur® Patch; Nitrogard® Buccal; Nitroglyn® Oral; Nitrolingual® Pumpspray; Nitrol® Ointment; Nitrong® Oral; Nitrostat® Sublingual; Transderm-Nitro® Patch; Tridil®

Canadian Brand Names Minitrans™; Nitro-Dur®; Nitrol®; Nitrong® SR; Nitrostat™; Transderm-Nitro®

Mexican Brand Names Anglix; Cardinit; Minitran®; Nitradisc; Nitroderm TTS; Nitro-Dur®

Pharmacologic Category Vasodilator

Synonyms Glyceryl Trinitrate; Nitroglycerol; NTG

Use Treatment of angina pectoris; I.V. for CHF (especially when associated with acute myocardial infarction); pulmonary hypertension; hypertensive emergencies occurring perioperatively (especially during cardiovascular surgery)

Local Anesthetic/Vasoconstrictor Precautions No information available to require special precautions

Effects on Dental Treatment No effects or complications reported

Dosage Note: Hemodynamic and antianginal tolerance often develop within 24-48 hours of continuous nitrate administration

Children: Pulmonary hypertension: Continuous infusion: Start 0.25-0.5 mcg/kg/minute and titrate by 1 mcg/kg/minute at 20- to 60-minute intervals to desired effect; usual dose: 1-3 mcg/kg/minute; maximum: 5 mcg/kg/minute

Adults:

- Buccal: Initial: 1 mg every 3-5 hours while awake (3 times/day); titrate dosage upward if angina occurs with tablet in place
- Oral: 2.5-9 mg 2-4 times/day (up to 26 mg 4 times/day)
- I.V.: 5 mcg/minute, increase by 5 mcg/minute every 3-5 minutes to 20 mcg/minute; if no response at 20 mcg/minute increase by 10 mcg/minute every 3-5 minutes, up to 200 mcg/minute
- Ointment: ½" upon rising and ½" 6 hours later; the dose may be doubled and even doubled again as needed
- Patch, transdermal: Initial: 0.2-0.4 mg/hour, titrate to doses of 0.4-0.8 mg/hour; tolerance is minimized by using a patch-on period of 12-14 hours and patch-off period of 10-12 hours
- Sublingual: 0.2-0.6 mg every 5 minutes for maximum of 3 doses in 15 minutes; may also use prophylactically 5-10 minutes prior to activities which may provoke an attack
- Translingual: 1-2 sprays into mouth under tongue every 3-5 minutes for maximum of 3 doses in 15 minutes, may also be used 5-10 minutes prior to activities which may provoke an attack prophylactically

Hemodialysis: Supplemental dose is not necessary

Peritoneal dialysis: Supplemental dose is not necessary

May need to use nitrate-free interval (10-12 hours/day) to avoid tolerance development; gradually decrease dose in patients receiving NTG for prolonged period to avoid withdrawal reaction

Elderly: In general, dose selection should be cautious, usually starting at the low end of the dosing range

Mechanism of Action Reduces cardiac oxygen demand by decreasing left ventricular pressure and systemic vascular resistance; dilates coronary arteries and improves collateral flow to ischemic regions

Other Adverse Effects

Spray or patch:

>10%: Central nervous system: Headache (patch 63%, spray 50%)

1% to 10%:

- Cardiovascular: Hypotension (patch 4%), increased angina (patch 2%)
- Central nervous system: Lightheadedness (patch 6%), syncope (patch 4%)

Topical, sublingual, I.V.: Frequency not defined:

- Cardiovascular: Hypotension (infrequent), postural hypotension, crescendo angina (uncommon), rebound hypertension (uncommon), pallor, cardiovascular collapse, tachycardia, shock, flushing, peripheral edema
- Central nervous system: Headache (most common), lightheadedness (related to BP changes), syncope (uncommon), dizziness, restlessness
- Gastrointestinal: Nausea, vomiting, bowel incontinence, xerostomia
- Genitourinary: Urinary incontinence

(Continued)

Nitroglycerin *(Continued)*

Hematologic: Methemoglobinemia (rare, overdose)
Neuromuscular & skeletal: Weakness
Ocular: Blurred vision
Miscellaneous: Cold sweat

The incidence of hypotension and adverse cardiovascular events may be increased when used in combination with sildenafil (Viagra®).

Drug Interactions

Increased Effect/Toxicity: Has been associated with severe reactions and death when sildenafil is given concurrently with nitrites.

Decreased Effect: I.V. nitroglycerin may antagonize the anticoagulant effect of heparin (possibly only at high nitroglycerin dosages); monitor closely. May need to decrease heparin dosage when nitroglycerin is discontinued. Alteplase (tissue plasminogen activator) has a lesser effect when used with I.V. nitroglycerin; avoid concurrent use. Ergot alkaloids may cause an increase in BP and decrease in antianginal effects; avoid concurrent use.

Drug Uptake

Onset of action:
Buccal tablet: 2-5 minutes
I.V. drip: Immediate
Sublingual tablet: 1-3 minutes
Sustained release: 20-45 minutes
Topical: 15-60 minutes
Transdermal: 40-60 minutes
Translingual spray: 2 minutes

Peak effect:
Buccal tablet: 4-10 minutes
I.V. drip: Immediate
Sublingual tablet: 4-8 minutes
Sustained release: 45-120 minutes
Topical: 30-120 minutes
Transdermal: 60-180 minutes
Translingual spray: 4-10 minutes

Duration:
Buccal tablet: 2 hours
I.V. drip: 3-5 minutes
Sublingual tablet: 30-60 minutes
Sustained release: 4-8 hours
Topical: 2-12 hours
Transdermal: 18-24 hours
Translingual spray: 30-60 minutes

Half-life, elimination: 1-4 minutes

Pregnancy Risk Factor C

Generic Available Yes

Nitroglyn® Oral *see* Nitroglycerin *on page 871*
Nitrolingual® Pumpspray *see* Nitroglycerin *on page 871*
Nitrol® Ointment *see* Nitroglycerin *on page 871*
Nitrong® Oral *see* Nitroglycerin *on page 871*
Nitropress® *see* Nitroprusside *on page 872*

Nitroprusside (nye troe PRUS ide)

U.S. Brand Names Nitropress®

Pharmacologic Category Vasodilator

Synonyms Nitroprusside Sodium; Sodium Nitroferricyanide; Sodium Nitroprusside

Use Management of hypertensive crises; CHF; used for controlled hypotension to reduce bleeding during surgery

Local Anesthetic/Vasoconstrictor Precautions No information available to require special precautions

Effects on Dental Treatment No effects or complications reported

Dosage I.V. (average dose: 5 mcg/kg/minute; requires infusion pump)

Children: Pulmonary hypertension: Initial: 1 mcg/kg/minute by continuous I.V. infusion; increase in increments of 1 mcg/kg/minute at intervals of 20-60 minutes; titrating to the desired response; usual dose: 3 mcg/kg/minute, rarely need >4 mcg/kg/minute; maximum: 5 mcg/kg/minute.

Adults: Initial: 0.3-0.5 mcg/kg/minute; increase in increments of 0.5 mcg/kg/minute, titrating to the desired hemodynamic effect or the appearance of headache or nausea; usual dose: 3 mcg/kg/minute; rarely need >4 mcg/kg/minute; maximum: 10 mcg/kg/minute. When >500 mcg/kg is administered by prolonged infusion of faster than 2 mcg/kg/minute, cyanide is generated faster than an unaided patient can handle.

Mechanism of Action Causes peripheral vasodilation by direct action on venous and arteriolar smooth muscle, thus reducing peripheral resistance; will increase cardiac output by decreasing afterload; reduces aortal and left ventricular impedance

Other Adverse Effects 1% to 10%:

Cardiovascular: Excessive hypotensive response, palpitations, substernal distress
Central nervous system: Disorientation, psychosis, headache, restlessness
Endocrine & metabolic: Thyroid suppression
Gastrointestinal: Nausea, vomiting
Neuromuscular & skeletal: Weakness, muscle spasm
Otic: Tinnitus
Respiratory: Hypoxia
Miscellaneous: Diaphoresis, thiocyanate toxicity

Drug Uptake

Onset of action: BP reduction <2 minutes
Duration: 1-10 minutes
Half-life, elimination: Parent drug: <10 minutes; Thiocyanate: 2.7-7 days

Pregnancy Risk Factor C

Generic Available Yes

Nitrostat® Sublingual *see* Nitroglycerin *on page 871*

Nitrous Oxide (NYE trus OKS ide)

Related Information

Patients Requiring Sedation *on page 1400*

Pharmacologic Category Dental Gases; General Anesthetic

Use

Dental: To induce sedation and analgesia in anxious dental patients

Medical: A principal adjunct to inhalation and I.V. general anesthesia in medical patients undergoing surgery; prehospital relief of pain of differing etiologies (ie, burns, fractures, back injury, abrasions, lacerations)

Local Anesthetic/Vasoconstrictor Precautions No information available to require special precautions

Effects on Dental Treatment No effects or complications reported

Dosage Adults and Children: For sedation and analgesia: Concentrations of 25% to 50% nitrous oxide with oxygen. For general anesthesia, concentrations of 40% to 70% via mask or endotracheal tube. Minimal alveolar concentration or (MAC) ED_{50} is 105%, therefore delivery in a hyperbaric chamber is necessary to use as a complete anesthetic; when administered at 70%, reduces the MAC of other anesthetics by half. Oxygen should be briefly administered during emergence from prolonged anesthesia with nitrous oxide to prevent diffusion hypoxia.

Mechanism of Action General CNS depressant action; may act similarly as inhalant general anesthetics by mildly stabilizing axonal membranes to partially inhibit action potentials leading to sedation; may partially act on opiate receptor systems to cause mild analgesia

Other Adverse Effects

Nausea and vomiting occurs postoperatively in ~15% of patients.

An increased risk of renal and hepatic diseases and peripheral neuropathy similar to that of vitamin B_{12} deficiency have been reported in dental personnel who work in areas where nitrous oxide is used.

Methionine synthase, a vitamin B_{12} dependent enzyme, is inactivated following very prolonged administration of nitrous oxide, and the subsequent interference with DNA synthesis prevents production of both leukocytes and red blood cells by bone marrow. These effects do not occur within the time frame of clinical sedation.

Female dental personnel who were exposed to unscavenged nitrous oxide for more than 5 hours/week were significantly less fertile than women who were not exposed, or who were exposed to lower levels of scavenged or unscavenged nitrous oxide. Fertility was measured by the number of menstrual cycles, without use of contraception, required to become pregnant. Women who were exposed to nitrous oxide for more than 5 hours/week were only 41% as likely as unexposed women to conceive during each monthly cycle.

Contraindications Hypersensitivity to nitrous oxide or any component of the formulation; administration without oxygen; administration after a full meal

Warnings/Precautions Prolonged use may produce bone marrow suppression and/or neurologic dysfunction. Patients with vitamin B_{12} deficiency (pernicious anemia) and those with other nutritional deficiencies (alcoholics) are at increased risk of developing neurologic disease and bone marrow suppression with exposure to nitrous oxide. May be addictive.

Drug Uptake

Onset of action: Inhalation: 2-5 minutes
Absorption: Rapidly absorbed via lungs; blood/gas partition coefficient is 0.47

Dosage Forms CYLINDER, blue

Generic Available Yes

Comments Results of a mail survey of >30,000 dentists and 30,000 chairside assistants, who were exposed to trace anesthetics in dental operatories, were

(Continued)

Nitrous Oxide *(Continued)*

published in 1980 (Cohen et al, 1980). This study suggested that long-term exposure to nitrous oxide and to nitrous oxide/halogenated anesthetics was associated with an increase in general health problems and reproductive difficulties in these dental personnel. Schuyt et al (1986) observed that 4 female dental personnel who were exposed to inhalation sedation with 35% nitrous oxide reported 6 spontaneous abortions among 7 pregnancies over 17 months.

Selected Readings

Babich S and Burakoff RP, "Occupational Hazards of Dentistry. A Review of Literature From 1990," *N Y State Dent J*, 1997, 63(8):26-31.

Baird PA, "Occupational Exposure to Nitrous Oxide - Not a Laughing Matter," *N Engl J Med*, 1992, 327(14):1026-7.

Dunning DG, McFarland K, and Safarik M, "Nitrous-Oxide Use. II. Risks, Compliance, and Exposure Levels Among Nebraska Dentists and Dental Assistants," *Gen Dent*, 1997, 45(1):82-6.

Howard WR, "Nitrous Oxide in the Dental Environment: Assessing the Risk, Reducing the Exposure," *J Am Dent Assoc*, 1997, 128(3):356-60.

Johnsen KG, "Nitrous Oxide Safety," *J Am Dent Assoc*, 1997, 128(8):1066-7.

"Nitrous Oxide in the Dental Office. ADA Council on Scientific Affairs; ADA Council on Dental Practice," *J Am Dent Assoc*, 1997, 128(3):364-5.

Petersen JK, "Nitrous Oxide Analgesia in Dental Practice," *Acta Anaesthesiol Scand*, 1994, 38(8):773-4.

Quarnstrom F, "Nitrous Oxide," *J Am Dent Assoc*, 1997, 128(6):690, 692.

Rowland AS, Baird DD, Weinberg CR, et al, "Reduced Fertility Among Women Employed as Female Dental Assistants Exposed to High Levels of Nitrous Oxide," *N Engl J Med*, 1992, 327(14):993-7.

Schuyt HC, Brakel K, Oostendorp SG, et al, "Abortions Among Dental Personnel Exposed to Nitrous Oxide," *Anaesthesia*, 1986, 41(1):82-3.

Wynn RL, "Nitrous Oxide and Fertility, Part I," *Gen Dent*, 1993, 41(2):122-3.

Wynn RL, "Nitrous Oxide and Fertility, Part II," *Gen Dent*, 1993, 41(3):212, 214.

Nix™ Creme Rinse *see* Permethrin *on page 940*

Nizatidine (ni ZA ti deen)

Related Information

Gastrointestinal Disorders *on page 1326*

U.S. Brand Names Axid®; Axid® AR [OTC]

Canadian Brand Names Apo®-Nizatidine; Axid®; Novo-Nizatidine

Mexican Brand Names Axid®

Pharmacologic Category Histamine H_2 Antagonist

Use Treatment and maintenance of duodenal ulcer; treatment of gastroesophageal reflux disease (GERD)

Unlabeled/Investigational: Part of a multidrug regimen for *H. pylori* eradication to reduce the risk of duodenal ulcer recurrence

Local Anesthetic/Vasoconstrictor Precautions No information available to require special precautions

Effects on Dental Treatment No effects or complications reported

Dosage Adults: Active duodenal ulcer: Oral:

Treatment: 300 mg at bedtime or 150 mg twice daily

Maintenance: 150 mg/day

Mechanism of Action Nizatidine is an H_2-receptor antagonist. In healthy volunteers, nizatidine has been effective in suppressing gastric acid secretion induced by pentagastrin infusion or food. Nizatidine reduces gastric acid secretion by 29.4% to 78.4%. This compares with a 60.3% reduction by cimetidine. Nizatidine 100 mg is reported to provide equivalent acid suppression as cimetidine 300 mg.

Other Adverse Effects

>10%: Central nervous system: Headache (16%)

1% to 10%:

Central nervous system: Dizziness, insomnia, somnolence, nervousness, anxiety

Dermatologic: Rash, pruritus

Gastrointestinal: Abdominal pain, constipation, diarrhea, nausea, flatulence, vomiting, heartburn, xerostomia, anorexia

Drug Interactions May decrease the absorption of itraconazole or ketoconazole

Pregnancy Risk Factor C

Generic Available No

Nizoral® *see* Ketoconazole *on page 672*

Nizoral® A-D [OTC] *see* Ketoconazole *on page 672*

Nolahist® [OTC] *see* Phenindamine *on page 945*

Nolvadex® *see* Tamoxifen *on page 1131*

Nonoxynol 9 (non OKS i nole nine)

U.S. Brand Names Because® [OTC]; Delfen® [OTC]; Emko® [OTC]; Encare® [OTC]; Gynol II® [OTC]; Koromex® [OTC]; Ramses® [OTC]; Semicid® [OTC]; Shur-Seal® [OTC]

Canadian Brand Names Advantage 24™

Pharmacologic Category Spermicide

Use Spermatocide in contraception

Local Anesthetic/Vasoconstrictor Precautions No information available to require special precautions

Effects on Dental Treatment No effects or complications reported

Dosage Insert into vagina at least 15 minutes before intercourse

Pregnancy Risk Factor C

Generic Available Yes

No Pain-HP® [OTC] *see* Capsaicin *on page 212*

Norco® *see* Hydrocodone and Acetaminophen *on page 598*

Nordette® *see* Combination Hormonal Contraceptives *on page 323*

Norditropin® *see* Human Growth Hormone *on page 589*

Norditropin® Cartridges *see* Human Growth Hormone *on page 589*

Nordryl® *see* DiphenhydrAMINE *on page 398*

Norepinephrine (nor ep i NEF rin)

U.S. Brand Names Levophed®

Canadian Brand Names Levophed®

Pharmacologic Category Alpha/Beta Agonist

Synonyms Levarterenol Bitartrate; Noradrenaline; Noradrenaline Acid Tartrate; Norepinephrine Bitartrate

Use Treatment of shock which persists after adequate fluid volume replacement; severe hypotension; cardiogenic shock

Local Anesthetic/Vasoconstrictor Precautions No information available to require special precautions

Effects on Dental Treatment No effects or complications reported

Dosage Dosage is stated in terms of norepinephrine base; I.V. formulation is norepinephrine bitartrate

Norepinephrine bitartrate 2 mg = norepinephrine base 1 mg

Continuous I.V. infusion:

Children:

Initial: 0.05-0.1 mcg/kg/minute; titrate to desired effect

Maximum dose: 1-2 mcg/kg/minute

Adults: Initiate at 4 mcg/minute and titrate to desired response; 8-12 mcg/minute is usual range

ACLS dosing range: 0.5-30 mcg/minute

Rate of infusion: 4 mg in 500 mL D_5W

2 mcg/minute = 15 mL/hour
4 mcg/minute = 30 mL/hour
6 mcg/minute = 45 mL/hour
8 mcg/minute = 60 mL/hour
10 mcg/minute = 75 mL/hour
12 mcg/minute = 90 mL/hour
14 mcg/minute = 105 mL/hour
16 mcg/minute = 120 mL/hour
18 mcg/minute = 135 mL/hour
20 mcg/minute = 150 mL/hour

Mechanism of Action Stimulates $beta_1$-adrenergic receptors and alpha-adrenergic receptors causing increased contractility and heart rate as well as vasoconstriction, thereby increasing systemic BP and coronary blood flow; clinically alpha effects (vasoconstriction) are greater than beta effects (inotropic and chronotropic effects)

Other Adverse Effects Frequency not defined:

Cardiovascular: Bradycardia, arrhythmias, peripheral (digital) ischemia

Central nervous system: Headache (transient), anxiety, nervousness or restlessness

Gastrointestinal: Nausea, vomiting

Local: Skin necrosis (with extravasation)

Respiratory: Dyspnea, respiratory difficulty

Warnings/Precautions Blood/volume depletion should be corrected, if possible, before norepinephrine therapy; extravasation may cause severe tissue necrosis, administer into a large vein. The drug should not be given to patients with peripheral or mesenteric vascular thrombosis because ischemia may be increased and the area of infarct extended; use with caution during cyclopropane and halothane anesthesia; use with caution in patients with occlusive vascular disease; some products may contain sulfites

Drug Interactions

Increased Effect/Toxicity: The effects of norepinephrine may be increased by tricyclic antidepressants, MAO inhibitors, antihistamines (diphenhydramine, tripelennamine), beta-blockers (nonselective), guanethidine, ergot alkaloids, reserpine, and methyldopa. Atropine sulfate may block the reflex bradycardia caused by norepinephrine and enhances the vasopressor response.

Decreased Effect: Alpha blockers may blunt response to norepinephrine.

Drug Uptake

Onset of action: I.V.: Very rapid-acting

Duration: Limited

Pregnancy Risk Factor C

Generic Available No

(Continued)

Norepinephrine *(Continued)*

Selected Readings Martin C, Papazian L, Perrin G, et al, "Norepinephrine or Dopamine for the Treatment of Hyperdynamic Septic Shock?" *Chest*, 1993, 103(6):1826-31.

Norethindrone (nor eth IN drone)

Related Information

Endocrine Disorders and Pregnancy *on page 1331*

U.S. Brand Names Aygestin®; Micronor®; Nor-QD®

Canadian Brand Names Micronor®; Norlutate®

Mexican Brand Names Syngestal

Pharmacologic Category Contraceptive; Progestin

Synonyms Norethindrone Acetate; Norethisterone

Use Treatment of amenorrhea; abnormal uterine bleeding; endometriosis, oral contraceptive; **higher rate of failure with progestin only contraceptives**

Local Anesthetic/Vasoconstrictor Precautions No information available to require special precautions

Effects on Dental Treatment Until we know more about the mechanism of interaction, caution is required in prescribing antibiotics to female dental patients taking progestin-only hormonal contraceptives.

Dosage Adolescents and Adults: Female: Oral:

Contraception: Progesterone only: Norethindrone 0.35 mg every day of the year starting on first day of menstruation; if one dose is missed take as soon as remembered; then next tablet at regular time; if two doses are missed, take one of the missed doses, discard the other, and take daily dose at usual time; if three doses are missed, use another form of birth control until menses appear or pregnancy is ruled out

Amenorrhea and abnormal uterine bleeding:

- Norethindrone: 5-20 mg/day on days 5-25 of menstrual cycle
- Acetate salt: 2.5-10 mg on days 5-25 of menstrual cycle

Endometriosis:

- Norethindrone: 10 mg/day for 2 weeks; increase at increments of 5 mg/day every 2 weeks until 30 mg/day; continue for 6-9 months or until breakthrough bleeding demands temporary termination
- Acetate salt: 5 mg/day for 14 days; increase at increments of 2.5 mg/day every 2 weeks up to 15 mg/day; continue for 6-9 months or until breakthrough bleeding demands temporary termination

Mechanism of Action Inhibits secretion of pituitary gonadotropin (LH) which prevents follicular maturation and ovulation

Other Adverse Effects

>10%:

- Cardiovascular: Edema
- Endocrine & metabolic: Breakthrough bleeding, spotting, changes in menstrual flow, amenorrhea
- Gastrointestinal: Anorexia
- Local: Pain at injection site
- Neuromuscular & skeletal: Weakness

1% to 10%:

- Cardiovascular: Edema
- Central nervous system: Mental depression, fever, insomnia
- Dermatologic: Melasma or chloasma, allergic rash with or without pruritus
- Endocrine & metabolic: Increased breast tenderness
- Gastrointestinal: Weight gain/loss
- Genitourinary: Changes in cervical erosion and secretions
- Hepatic: Cholestatic jaundice

Drug Interactions Rifampin (potentially other enzyme inducers) and nelfinavir decrease the pharmacologic effect of norethindrone.

Drug Uptake

Absorption: Oral, transdermal: Rapidly absorbed

Half-life, elimination: 5-14 hours

Time to peak: 1-2 hours

Pregnancy Risk Factor X

Generic Available Yes

Norflex™ *see* Orphenadrine *on page 891*

Norfloxacin (nor FLOKS a sin)

U.S. Brand Names Chibroxin®; Noroxin®

Canadian Brand Names Apo®-Norflox; Noroxin® Ophthalmic; Noroxin® Tablet; Novo-Norfloxacin; Riva-Norfloxacin

Mexican Brand Names Difoxacil®; Floxacin®; Noroxin®; Oranor

Pharmacologic Category Antibiotic, Quinolone

Use Uncomplicated urinary tract infections and cystitis caused by susceptible gram-negative and gram-positive bacteria; sexually-transmitted disease (eg, uncomplicated urethral and cervical gonorrhea) caused by *N. gonorrhoeae*; prostatitis due to *E. coli*; ophthalmic solution for conjunctivitis

Local Anesthetic/Vasoconstrictor Precautions No information available to require special precautions

Effects on Dental Treatment No effects or complications reported

Dosage

Ophthalmic: Children >1 year and Adults: Instill 1-2 drops in affected eye(s) 4 times/day for up to 7 days

Oral: Adults:

Urinary tract infections: 400 mg twice daily for 3-21 days depending on severity of infection or organism sensitivity; maximum: 800 mg/day

Prostatitis: 400 mg every 12 hours for 4 weeks

Mechanism of Action Bactericidal; inhibits DNA gyrase which is an essential bacterial enzyme that maintains the superhelical structure of DNA; required for DNA replication and transcription, DNA repair, recombination, and transposition

Other Adverse Effects

Ophthalmic:

>10%: Ocular: Burning or other discomfort of the eye, crusting or crystals in corner of eye

1% to 10%:

Gastrointestinal: Bad taste instillation

Ocular: Foreign body sensation, conjunctival hyperemia, itching of eye, corneal deposits

Systemic: 1% to 10%:

Central nervous system: Headache (3%), dizziness (2%), fatigue

Gastrointestinal: Nausea (3%)

Drug Interactions CYP1A2 and 3A3/4 enzyme inhibitor

Increased Effect/Toxicity: Quinolones cause increased levels of caffeine, warfarin, cyclosporine, and theophylline. Cimetidine and probenecid may increase norfloxacin serum concentration.

Decreased Effect: Decreased absorption with antacids containing aluminum, magnesium, and/or calcium (by up to 98% if given at the same time). Didanosine (chewable/buffered or pediatric powder) may decrease quinolone absorption.

Drug Uptake

Absorption: Oral: Rapid, ≤40%

Half-life, elimination: 4.8 hours (may be increased with reduced glomerular filtration rates, prolonged in renal impairment)

Time to peak: 1-2 hours

Pregnancy Risk Factor C

Generic Available No

Norgesic™ *see* Orphenadrine, Aspirin, and Caffeine *on page 892*

Norgesic™ Forte *see* Orphenadrine, Aspirin, and Caffeine *on page 892*

Norgestrel (nor JES trel)

Related Information

Endocrine Disorders and Pregnancy *on page 1331*

U.S. Brand Names Ovrette®

Canadian Brand Names Ovrette®

Pharmacologic Category Contraceptive

Use Prevention of pregnancy; **progestin only products have higher risk of failure in contraceptive use**

Local Anesthetic/Vasoconstrictor Precautions No information available to require special precautions

Effects on Dental Treatment Until we know more about the mechanism of interaction, caution is required in prescribing antibiotics to female dental patients taking progestin-only hormonal contraceptives.

Dosage Administer daily, starting the first day of menstruation, take 1 tablet at the same time each day, every day of the year. If 1 dose is missed, take as soon as remembered, then next tablet at regular time; if 2 doses are missed, take 1 tablet and discard the other, then take daily at usual time; if 3 doses are missed, use an additional form of birth control until menses or pregnancy is ruled out.

Mechanism of Action Inhibits secretion of pituitary gonadotropin (LH) which prevents follicular maturation and ovulation

Other Adverse Effects Frequency not defined:

Cardiovascular: Embolism, central thrombosis, edema

Central nervous system: Mental depression, fever, insomnia

Dermatologic: Melasma or chloasma, allergic rash with or without pruritus

Endocrine & metabolic: Breakthrough bleeding, spotting, changes in menstrual flow, amenorrhea, changes in cervical erosion and secretions, increased breast tenderness

Gastrointestinal: Weight gain/loss, anorexia

Hepatic: Cholestatic jaundice

Local: Thrombophlebitis

Neuromuscular & skeletal: Weakness

(Continued)

Norgestrel *(Continued)*

Drug Interactions CYP3A3/4 enzyme substrate

Increased Effect/Toxicity: Oral contraceptives may increase toxicity of acetaminophen, anticoagulants, benzodiazepines, caffeine, corticosteroids, metoprolol, theophylline, and tricyclic antidepressants.

Decreased Effect: Azole antifungals (ketoconazole, itraconazole, fluconazole), barbiturates, hydantoins (phenytoin), carbamazepine, and rifampin decrease oral contraceptive efficacy due to increased metabolism. Antibiotics (penicillins, tetracyclines, griseofulvin) may decrease efficacy of oral contraceptives.

Drug Uptake

Absorption: Oral: Well absorbed

Half-life, elimination: ~20 hours

Pregnancy Risk Factor X

Generic Available No

Norinyl® 1+35 *see* Combination Hormonal Contraceptives *on page 323*

Norinyl® 1+50 *see* Mestranol and Norethindrone *on page 774*

Noritate™ *see* Metronidazole *on page 804*

Normodyne® *see* Labetalol *on page 680*

Noroxin® *see* Norfloxacin *on page 876*

Norpace® *see* Disopyramide *on page 403*

Norpace® CR *see* Disopyramide *on page 403*

Norplant® Implant *see* Levonorgestrel *on page 703*

Norpramin® *see* Desipramine *on page 359*

Nor-QD® *see* Norethindrone *on page 876*

Nortrel™ *see* Combination Hormonal Contraceptives *on page 323*

Nortriptyline (nor TRIP ti leen)

U.S. Brand Names Aventyl®; Pamelor®

Canadian Brand Names Alti-Nortriptyline; Apo®-Nortriptyline; Aventyl®; Gen-Nortriptyline; Norventyl; Novo-Nortriptyline; Nu-Nortriptyline; PMS-Nortriptyline

Pharmacologic Category Antidepressant, Tricyclic (Secondary Amine)

Synonyms Nortriptyline Hydrochloride

Use Treatment of symptoms of depression

Unlabeled/Investigational: Chronic pain, anxiety disorders, enuresis, attention-deficit/hyperactivity disorder (ADHD)

Local Anesthetic/Vasoconstrictor Precautions Use with caution; epinephrine, norepinephrine and levonordefrin have been shown to have an increased pressor response in combination with TCAs

Effects on Dental Treatment

>10%: Xerostomia

Long-term treatment with TCAs such as nortriptyline increases the risk of caries by reducing salivation and salivary buffer capacity.

Dosage Oral:

Nocturnal enuresis:

Children:

6-7 years (20-25 kg): 10 mg/day

8-11 years (25-35 kg): 10-20 mg/day

>11 years (35-54 kg): 25-35 mg/day

Depression or ADHD (unlabeled use):

Children 6-12 years: 1-3 mg/kg/day or 10-20 mg/day in 3-4 divided doses

Adolescents: 30-100 mg/day in divided doses

Depression:

Adults: 25 mg 3-4 times/day up to 150 mg/day

Elderly (**Note:** Nortriptyline is one of the best tolerated TCAs in the elderly)

Initial: 10-25 mg at bedtime

Dosage can be increased by 25 mg every 3 days for inpatients and weekly for outpatients if tolerated

Usual maintenance dose: 75 mg as a single bedtime dose or 2 divided doses; lower or higher doses may be required to stay within the therapeutic window

Dosing adjustment in hepatic impairment: Lower doses and slower titration dependent on individualization of dosage is recommended

Mechanism of Action Traditionally believed to increase the synaptic concentration of serotonin and/or norepinephrine in the CNS by inhibiting reuptake by the presynaptic neuronal membrane; however, additional receptor effects have been found, including desensitization of adenyl cyclase and down regulation of beta-adrenergic and serotonin receptors.

Other Adverse Effects Frequency not defined:

Cardiovascular: Postural hypotension, arrhythmias, hypertension, heart block, tachycardia, palpitations, myocardial infarction

Central nervous system: Confusion, delirium, hallucinations, restlessness, insomnia, disorientation, delusions, anxiety, agitation, panic, nightmares, hypomania, exacerbation of psychosis, incoordination, ataxia, extrapyramidal symptoms, seizures

Dermatologic: Alopecia, photosensitivity, rash, petechiae, urticaria, itching

Endocrine & metabolic: Sexual dysfunction, gynecomastia, breast enlargement, galactorrhea, increase or decrease in libido, increase in blood sugar, SIADH

Gastrointestinal: Xerostomia, constipation, vomiting, anorexia, diarrhea, abdominal cramps, black tongue, nausea, unpleasant taste, weight gain/loss

Genitourinary: Urinary retention, delayed micturition, impotence, testicular edema

Hematologic: Rarely agranulocytosis, eosinophilia, purpura, thrombocytopenia

Hepatic: Increased liver enzymes, cholestatic jaundice

Neuromuscular & skeletal: Tremor, numbness, tingling, paresthesias, peripheral neuropathy

Ocular: Blurred vision, eye pain, disturbances in accommodation, mydriasis

Otic: Tinnitus

Miscellaneous: Diaphoresis (excessive), allergic reactions

Drug Interactions CYP1A2 and 2D6 enzyme substrate

Increased Effect/Toxicity: Nortriptyline increases the effects of amphetamines, anticholinergics, other CNS depressants (sedatives, hypnotics), chlorpropamide, tolazamide, and warfarin. When used with MAO inhibitors, hyperpyrexia, hypertension, tachycardia, confusion, seizures, and **deaths have been reported** (serotonin syndrome). The SSRIs (to varying degrees), cimetidine, indinavir, methylphenidate, ritonavir, quinidine, diltiazem, and verapamil inhibit the metabolism of TCAs and clinical toxicity may result. Use of lithium with a TCA may increase the risk for neurotoxicity. Phenothiazines may increase concentration of some TCAs and TCAs may increase concentration of phenothiazines. Pressor response to I.V. epinephrine, norepinephrine, and phenylephrine may be enhanced in patients receiving TCAs (**Note:** Effect is unlikely with epinephrine or levonordefrin dosages typically administered as infiltration in combination with local anesthetics). Combined use of beta-agonists or drugs which prolong QT_c (including quinidine, procainamide, disopyramide, cisapride, sparfloxacin, gatifloxacin, moxifloxacin) with TCAs may predispose patients to cardiac arrhythmias. Use with altretamine may cause orthostatic hypotension.

Decreased Effect: Carbamazepine, phenobarbital, and rifampin may increase the metabolism of nortriptyline resulting in decreased effect of nortriptyline. Nortriptyline inhibits the antihypertensive response to bethanidine, clonidine, debrisoquin, guanadrel, guanethidine, guanabenz, or guanfacine. Cholestyramine and colestipol may bind TCAs and reduce their absorption; monitor for altered response.

Drug Uptake

Onset of action: Therapeutic: 1-3 weeks

Half-life, elimination: 28-31 hours

Time to peak: Oral: 7-8.5 hours

Pregnancy Risk Factor D

Generic Available Yes

Selected Readings

Friedlander AH, Mahler ME, "Major Depressive Disorder. Psychopathology, Medical Management, and Dental Implications," *J Am Dent Assoc*, 201, 132(5):629-38.

Ganzberg S, "Psychoactive Drugs," *ADA Guide to Dental Therapeutics*, 2nd ed, Chicago, IL: ADA Publishing, a Division of ADA Business Enterprises, Inc, 2000, 376-405.

Jastak JT and Yagiela JA, "Vasoconstrictors and Local Anesthesia: A Review and Rationale for Use," *J Am Dent Assoc*, 1983, 107(4):623-30.

Mitchell JR, "Guanethidine and Related Agents. III Antagonism by Drugs Which Inhibit the Norepinephrine Pump in Man," *J Clin Invest*, 1970, 49(8):1596-604.

Rundegren J, van Dijken J, Mörnstad H, et al, "Oral Conditions in Patients Receiving Long-Term Treatment With Cyclic Antidepressant Drugs," *Swed Dent J*, 1985, 9(2):55-64.

Yagiela JA, "Adverse Drug Interactions in Dental Practice: Interactions Associated With Vasoconstrictors. Part V of a Series," *J Am Dent Assoc*, 1999, 130(5):701-9.

Norvasc® *see* Amlodipine *on page 81*

Norvir® *see* Ritonavir *on page 1059*

Norzine® *see* Thiethylperazine *on page 1157*

Nōstrilla® [OTC] *see* Oxymetazoline *on page 907*

Nostril® Nasal [OTC] *see* Phenylephrine *on page 950*

Novantrone® *see* Mitoxantrone *on page 821*

Novarel™ *see* Chorionic Gonadotropin *on page 281*

Novocain® *see* Procaine *on page 998*

Novolin® 70/30 *see* Insulin Preparations *on page 639*

Novolin® L *see* Insulin Preparations *on page 639*

Novolin® N *see* Insulin Preparations *on page 639*

Novolin® R *see* Insulin Preparations *on page 639*

NovoLog® *see* Insulin Preparations *on page 639*

Novo-Seven® *see* Factor VIIa, Recombinant *on page 484*

Novothyrox *see* Levothyroxine *on page 705*

NP-27® [OTC] *see* Tolnaftate *on page 1181*

NPH Iletin® II *see* Insulin Preparations *on page 639*

NTZ® Long Acting Nasal [OTC] *see* Oxymetazoline *on page 907*

Nubain® *see* Nalbuphine *on page 842*

Nucofed® *see* Guaifenesin, Pseudoephedrine, and Codeine *on page 570*

Nucofed® Pediatric Expectorant *see* Guaifenesin, Pseudoephedrine, and Codeine *on page 570*
Nucotuss® *see* Guaifenesin, Pseudoephedrine, and Codeine *on page 570*
Nu-Iron® [OTC] *see* Polysaccharide-Iron Complex *on page 972*
NuLev™ *see* Hyoscyamine *on page 617*
Nullo® [OTC] *see* Chlorophyll *on page 265*
NuLytely® *see* Polyethylene Glycol-Electrolyte Solution *on page 970*
Numorphan® *see* Oxymorphone *on page 908*
Nupercainal® [OTC] *see* Dibucaine *on page 376*
Nuprin® [OTC] *see* Ibuprofen *on page 621*
Nuquin® Gel *see* Hydroquinone *on page 611*
Nuquin HP® Cream *see* Hydroquinone *on page 611*
Nu-Tears® [OTC] *see* Artificial Tears *on page 117*
Nu-Tears® II [OTC] *see* Artificial Tears *on page 117*
Nutracort® *see* Hydrocortisone *on page 608*
Nutraplus® [OTC] *see* Urea *on page 1221*
Nutrilipid® *see* Fat Emulsion *on page 487*
Nutropin® *see* Human Growth Hormone *on page 589*
Nutropin AQ ® *see* Human Growth Hormone *on page 589*
Nutropin Depot® *see* Human Growth Hormone *on page 589*
NuvaRing® *see* Combination Hormonal Contraceptives *on page 323*
Nydrazid® *see* Isoniazid *on page 659*

Nylidrin (NYE li drin)

U.S. Brand Names Arlidin®

Canadian Brand Names Arlidin®

Pharmacologic Category Vasodilator, Peripheral

Use Possibly effective for increasing blood supply in treatment of peripheral disease (eg, arteriosclerosis obliterans, diabetic vascular disease, nocturnal leg cramps, Raynaud's disease, frost bite, ischemic ulcer, thrombophlebitis) and circulatory disturbances of the inner ear (eg, cochlear ischemia, macular or ampullar ischemia, etc)

Local Anesthetic/Vasoconstrictor Precautions No information available to require special precautions

Effects on Dental Treatment No effects or complications reported

Dosage Adults: Oral: 3-12 mg 3-4 times/day

Mechanism of Action A peripheral vasodilator resulting from direct relaxation of vascular smooth muscle and beta agonist action; does not appear to affect cutaneous blood flow; reportedly increases heart rate and cardiac output; cutaneous blood flow is not enhanced to any appreciable extent

Other Adverse Effects

1% to 10%:

- Central nervous system: Nervousness
- Neuromuscular & skeletal: Trembling

Pregnancy Risk Factor C

Nystatin (nye STAT in)

Related Information

Management of Patients Undergoing Cancer Therapy *on page 1402*
Oral Fungal Infections *on page 1377*

U.S. Brand Names Bio-Statin®; Mycostatin®; Nilstat®; Nystex®; Peri-Dri®

Canadian Brand Names Candistatin®; Mycostatin®; Nilstat; Nyaderm; PMS-Nystatin

Mexican Brand Names Micostatin; Nistaquim

Pharmacologic Category Antifungal Agent, Oral Nonabsorbed; Antifungal Agent, Topical; Antifungal Agent, Vaginal

Use Dental: Treatment of susceptible cutaneous, mucocutaneous, and oral cavity fungal infections normally caused by the *Candida* species

Local Anesthetic/Vasoconstrictor Precautions No information available to require special precautions

Effects on Dental Treatment No effects or complications reported

Dosage

Oral candidiasis:

- Suspension (swish and swallow orally):
  - Premature infants: 100,000 units 4 times/day
  - Infants: 200,000 units 4 times/day or 100,000 units to each side of mouth 4 times/day
  - Children and Adults: 400,000-600,000 units 4 times/day
- Troche: Children and Adults: 200,000-400,000 units 4-5 times/day
- Powder for compounding: Children and Adults: $^1/_8$ teaspoon (500,000 units) to equal ~ $^1/_2$ cup of water; give 4 times/day

Mucocutaneous infections: Children and Adults: Topical: Apply 2-3 times/day to affected areas; very moist topical lesions are treated best with powder
Intestinal infections: Adults: Oral: 500,000-1,000,000 units every 8 hours
Vaginal infections: Adults: Vaginal tablets: Insert 1 tablet/day at bedtime for 2 weeks

Mechanism of Action Binds to sterols in fungal cell membrane, changing the cell wall permeability allowing for leakage of cellular contents

Other Adverse Effects
Frequency not defined: Contact dermatitis, Stevens-Johnson syndrome
1% to 10%: Gastrointestinal: Nausea, vomiting, diarrhea, stomach pain
<1%: Hypersensitivity reactions

Contraindications Hypersensitivity to nystatin or any component of the formulation

Dietary/Ethanol/Herb Considerations Do not permit patient to eat or drink for 10 minutes after oral dosing.

Drug Uptake
Onset of action: Symptomatic relief from candidiasis: 24-72 hours
Absorption: Topical: None through mucous membranes or intact skin; Oral: Poorly absorbed

Pregnancy Risk Factor B/C (oral)

Breast-feeding Considerations Compatible (not absorbed orally)

Dosage Forms CAP: 500,000 units, 1 million units. **CRM:** 100,000 units/g (15 g, 30 g). **OINT:** 100,000 units/g (15 g, 30 g). **POWDER:** 100,000 units/g (15 g, 56.7 g). **POWDER, oral suspension:** 50 million units, 1 billion units, 2 billion units, 5 billion units. **SUSP, oral:** 100,000 units/mL (5 mL, 60 mL, 480 mL). **TAB:** 500,000 units. **TAB, vaginal:** 100,000 units (15 and 30/box). **TROCHE:** 200,000 units

Generic Available Yes

Nystatin and Triamcinolone (nye STAT in & trye am SIN oh lone)

Related Information
Oral Fungal Infections *on page 1377*

U.S. Brand Names Mycogen II; Mycolog®-II; Myco-Triacet® II; Mytrex® F; N.G.A.®; Quenalog®

Pharmacologic Category Antifungal Agent, Topical; Corticosteroid, Topical

Synonyms Triamcinolone and Nystatin

Use Treatment of cutaneous candidiasis

Local Anesthetic/Vasoconstrictor Precautions No information available to require special precautions

Effects on Dental Treatment No effects or complications reported

Dosage Children and Adults: Topical: Apply sparingly 2-4 times/day
Therapy should be discontinued when control is achieved; if no improvement is seen, reassessment of diagnosis may be necessary.

Mechanism of Action Nystatin is an antifungal agent that binds to sterols in fungal cell membrane, changing the cell wall permeability allowing for leakage of cellular contents. Triamcinolone is a synthetic corticosteroid; it decreases inflammation by suppression of migration of polymorphonuclear leukocytes and reversal of increased capillary permeability. It suppresses the immune system reducing activity and volume of the lymphatic system. It suppresses adrenal function at high doses.

Other Adverse Effects 1% to 10%:
Dermatologic: Dryness, folliculitis, hypertrichosis, acne, hypopigmentation, allergic dermatitis, maceration of the skin, skin atrophy
Local: Burning, itching, irritation
Miscellaneous: Increased incidence of secondary infection

Contraindications Hypersensitivity to nystatin, triamcinolone, or any component of their formulation

Warnings/Precautions Avoid use of occlusive dressings; limit therapy to least amount necessary for effective therapy, pediatric patients may be more susceptible to HPA axis suppression due to larger BSA to weight ratio

Drug Uptake See Nystatin *on page 880* and Triamcinolone *on page 1197*

Pregnancy Risk Factor C

Generic Available Yes

Nystex® *see* Nystatin *on page 880*
Nytol® [OTC] *see* DiphenhydrAMINE *on page 398*
Occlusal®-HP [OTC] *see* Salicylic Acid *on page 1072*
Ocean® [OTC] *see* Sodium Chloride *on page 1094*
OCL® *see* Polyethylene Glycol-Electrolyte Solution *on page 970*
Octicair® Otic *see* Neomycin, Polymyxin B, and Hydrocortisone *on page 857*

Octreotide Acetate (ok TREE oh tide)

U.S. Brand Names Sandostatin®; Sandostatin LAR®

Canadian Brand Names Sandostatin®; Sandostatin LAR®

Mexican Brand Names Sandostatina®

Pharmacologic Category Antidiarrheal; Somatostatin Analog

Synonyms Octreotide

(Continued)

Octreotide Acetate *(Continued)*

Use Control of symptoms in patients with metastatic carcinoid and vasoactive intestinal peptide-secreting tumors (VIPomas); acromegaly, insulinomas, Zollinger-Ellison syndrome, pancreatic tumors, gastrinoma, postgastrectomy dumping syndrome, bleeding esophageal varices, small bowel fistulas, AIDS-associated secretory diarrhea, chemotherapy-induced diarrhea, GVHD (graft-versus-host disease)-induced diarrhea, control of bleeding of esophageal varices; depot suspension is indicated for long-term maintenance therapy in acromegalic patients for whom medical treatment is appropriate and who have been shown to respond to and can tolerate the injection; reduction of growth hormone and IGF-1 in acromegaly, suppression of severe diarrhea and flushing associated with malignant carcinoid syndrome, and for the treatment of profuse water diarrhea associated with VIPoma (vasoactive intestinal peptide tumor).

Unlabeled/Investigational: Breast cancer, cryptosporidiosis, Cushing's syndrome, congenital hyperinsulinism

Local Anesthetic/Vasoconstrictor Precautions No information available to require special precautions

Effects on Dental Treatment No effects or complications reported

Dosage Adults: S.C.: Initial: 50 mcg 1-2 times/day and titrate dose based on patient tolerance and response

Carcinoid: 100-600 mcg/day in 2-4 divided doses

VIPomas: 200-300 mcg/day in 2-4 divided doses

Diarrhea: Initial: I.V.: 50-100 mcg every 8 hours; increase by 100 mcg/dose at 48-hour intervals; maximum dose: 500 mcg every 8 hours

Esophageal varices bleeding: I.V. bolus: 25-50 mcg followed by continuous I.V. infusion of 25-50 mcg/hour

Acromegaly: Initial: S.C.: 50 mcg 3 times/day; titrate to achieve growth hormone levels <5 ng/mL or IGF-I (somatomedin C) levels <1.9 U/mL in males and <2.2 U/mL in females; usual effective dose 100 mcg 3 times/day; range 300-1500 mcg/day

Note: Should be withdrawn yearly for a 4-week interval in patients who have received irradiation. Resume if levels increase and signs/symptoms recur.

Acromegaly, carcinoid tumors, and VIPomas (depot injection): Patients must be stabilized on subcutaneous octreotide for at least 2 weeks before switching to the long-acting depot: Upon switch: 20 mg I.M. intragluteally every 4 weeks for 2-3 months, then the dose may be modified based upon response

Dosage adjustment for acromegaly: After 3 months of depot injections the dosage may be continued or modified as follows:

GH ≤2.5 ng/mL, IGF-1 is normal, symptoms controlled: Maintain octreotide LAR® at 20 mg I.M. every 4 weeks

GH >2.5 ng/mL, IGF-1 is elevated, and/or symptoms uncontrolled: Increase octreotide LAR® to 30 mg I.M. every 4 weeks

GH ≤1 ng/mL, IGF-1 is normal, symptoms controlled: Reduce octreotide LAR® to 10 mg I.M. every 4 weeks

Dosages >40 mg are not recommended

Dosage adjustment for carcinoid tumors and VIPomas: After 2 months of depot injections the dosage may be continued or modified as follows:

Increase to 30 mg I.M. every 4 weeks if symptoms are inadequately controlled

Decrease to 10 mg I.M. every 4 weeks, for a trial period, if initially responsive to 20 mg dose

Dosage >30 mg is not recommended

Mechanism of Action Mimics natural somatostatin by inhibiting serotonin release, and the secretion of gastrin, VIP, insulin, glucagon, secretin, motilin, and pancreatic polypeptide. Decreases growth hormone and IGF-1 in acromegaly.

Other Adverse Effects

>10%:

Cardiovascular: Sinus bradycardia (19% to 25%)

Endocrine & metabolic: Hyperglycemia (15% acromegaly, 27% carcinoid)

Gastrointestinal: Diarrhea (36% to 58% acromegaly), abdominal pain (30% to 44% acromegaly), flatulence (13% to 26% acromegaly), constipation (9% to 19% acromegaly), nausea (10% to 30%)

1% to 10%:

Cardiovascular: Flushing, edema, conduction abnormalities (9% to 10%), arrhythmias (3% to 9%)

Central nervous system: Fatigue, headache, dizziness, vertigo, anorexia, depression

Endocrine & metabolic: Hypoglycemia (2% acromegaly, 4% carcinoid), hyperglycemia (1%), hypothyroidism, galactorrhea

Gastrointestinal: Nausea, vomiting, diarrhea, constipation, abdominal pain, cramping, discomfort, fat malabsorption, loose stools, flatulence, tenesmus

Hepatic: Jaundice, hepatitis, increase LFTs, cholelithiasis has occurred, presumably by altering fat absorption and decreasing the motility of the gallbladder

Local: Pain at injection site (dose-related)

Neuromuscular & skeletal: Weakness

Drug Interactions CYP2D6 (high dose) and 3A enzyme inhibitor

Increased Effect/Toxicity: Octreotide may increase the effect of insulin or sulfonylurea agents which may result in hypoglycemia.

Decreased Effect: Octreotide may lower cyclosporine serum concentration (case report of a transplant rejection due to reduction of serum cyclosporine levels). Codeine effect may be reduced.

Drug Uptake

Absorption: S.C.: Rapid

Duration: S.C.: 6-12 hours

Half-life, elimination: 60-110 minutes

Pregnancy Risk Factor B

Generic Available No

Comments Doses of 1-10 mcg/kg every 12 hours have been used in children beginning at the low end of the range and increasing by 0.3 mcg/kg/dose at 3-day intervals; suppression of growth hormone (animal data) is of concern when used as long-term therapy

Ocu-Chlor® *see* Chloramphenicol *on page 261*
OcuClear® [OTC] *see* Oxymetazoline *on page 907*
OcuCoat® [OTC] *see* Artificial Tears *on page 117*
OcuCoat® PF [OTC] *see* Artificial Tears *on page 117*
Ocufen® Ophthalmic *see* Flurbiprofen *on page 522*
Ocuflox® *see* Ofloxacin *on page 883*
Ocu-Merox® *see* Mercuric Oxide *on page 770*
Ocupress® Ophthalmic *see* Carteolol *on page 226*
Ocusert Pilo-20® [DSC] *see* Pilocarpine *on page 955*
Ocusert Pilo-20® [DSC] *see* Pilocarpine (Dental) *on page 956*
Ocusert Pilo-40® [DSC] *see* Pilocarpine *on page 955*
Ocusert Pilo-40® [DSC] *see* Pilocarpine (Dental) *on page 956*
Ocu-Sul® *see* Sulfacetamide Sodium *on page 1115*
Ocu-Zoline® *see* Naphazoline *on page 847*
Off-Ezy® Wart Remover [OTC] *see* Salicylic Acid *on page 1072*

Ofloxacin (oh FLOKS a sin)

Related Information

Nonviral Infectious Diseases *on page 1342*

U.S. Brand Names Floxin®; Ocuflox®

Canadian Brand Names Apo®-Oflox; Floxin®; Ocuflox®

Mexican Brand Names Bactocin; Floxil; Floxstat; Ocuflox®

Pharmacologic Category Antibiotic, Quinolone

Use Quinolone antibiotic for skin and skin structure, lower respiratory, and urinary tract infections and sexually-transmitted diseases; active against many gram-positive and gram-negative aerobic bacteria

Ophthalmic: Treatment of superficial ocular infections involving the conjunctiva or cornea due to strains of susceptible organisms

Otic: Otitis externa, chronic suppurative otitis media (patients >12 years of age); acute otitis media

Local Anesthetic/Vasoconstrictor Precautions No information available to require special precautions

Effects on Dental Treatment No effects or complications reported

Dosage

Children >1 year and Adults:

- Ophthalmic: Instill 1-2 drops in affected eye(s) every 2-4 hours for the first 2 days, then use 4 times/day for an additional 5 days
- Otic: 5 or 10 drops, respectively, twice daily

Adults: Oral, I.V.: 200-400 mg every 12 hours for 7-10 days for most infections or for 6 weeks for prostatitis

Mechanism of Action Inhibits DNA gyrase, an essential bacterial enzyme that maintains the superhelical structure of DNA; DNA gyrase is required for DNA replication and transcription, DNA repair, recombination, and transposition; bactericidal

Other Adverse Effects

Ophthalmic:

>10%: Ocular: Burning or other discomfort of the eye, crusting or crystals in corner of eye

1% to 10%:

- Gastrointestinal: Bad taste instillation
- Ocular: Foreign body sensation, conjunctival hyperemia, itching of eye, ocular or facial edema, redness, stinging, photophobia

Otic: Local reactions (3%), earache (1%), tinnitus, otorrhagia

Systemic:

1% to 10%:

- Cardiovascular: Chest pain (1% to 3%)

(Continued)

Ofloxacin *(Continued)*

Central nervous system: Headache (1% to 9%), insomnia (3% to 7%), dizziness (1% to 5%), fatigue (1% to 3%), somnolence (1% to 3%), sleep disorders, nervousness (1% to 3%), pyrexia (1% to 3%), pain
Dermatologic: Rash/pruritus (1% to 3%)
Gastrointestinal: Diarrhea (1% to 4%), vomiting (1% to 3%), GI distress, cramps, abdominal cramps (1% to 3%), flatulence (1% to 3%), abnormal taste (1% to 3%), xerostomia (1% to 3%), decreased appetite, nausea (3% to 10%)
Genitourinary: Vaginitis (1% to 3%), external genital pruritus in women
Local: Pain at injection site
Ocular: Superinfection (ophthalmic), photophobia, lacrimation, dry eyes, stinging, visual disturbances (1% to 3%)
Miscellaneous: Trunk pain

Drug Interactions

Increased Effect/Toxicity: Quinolones can cause increased caffeine, warfarin, cyclosporine, and theophylline levels (unlikely to occur with ofloxacin). Azlocillin, cimetidine, and probenecid may increase ofloxacin serum concentration. Foscarnet and NSAIDs have been associated with an increased risk of seizures with some quinolones. Serum levels of some quinolones are increased by loop diuretic administration. The hypoprothrombinemic effect of warfarin is enhanced by some quinolone antibiotics. Ofloxacin does not alter warfarin levels, but may alter the GI flora which may increase warfarin's effect.

Decreased Effect: Metal cations (magnesium, aluminum, iron, and zinc) bind quinolones in the GI tract and inhibit absorption (as much as 98%). Antacids, electrolyte supplements, sucralfate, quinapril, and some didanosine formulations should be avoided. Ofloxacin should be administered 4 hours before or 8 hours after these agents. Antineoplastic agents may decrease the absorption of quinolones.

Drug Uptake

Absorption: Well absorbed; taking with food causes only minor alterations
Half-life, elimination: 5-7.5 hours; prolonged in renal impairment

Pregnancy Risk Factor C

Generic Available No

Ogen® *see* Estropipate *on page 469*
Ogestrel® *see* Combination Hormonal Contraceptives *on page 323*

Olanzapine (oh LAN za peen)

U.S. Brand Names Zyprexa®; Zyprexa® Zydis®
Canadian Brand Names Zyprexa®
Mexican Brand Names Zyprexa®
Pharmacologic Category Antipsychotic Agent, Thienobenzodiazepine
Synonyms LY170053
Use Treatment of the manifestations of schizophrenia; short-term treatment of acute mania episodes associated with bipolar mania

Unlabeled/Investigational: Treatment of psychotic symptoms

Local Anesthetic/Vasoconstrictor Precautions No information available to require special precautions

Effects on Dental Treatment No effects or complications reported

Dosage Oral:

Children: Schizophrenia/bipolar disorder: Initial: 2.5 mg/day; titrate as necessary to 20 mg/day (0.12-0.29 mg/kg/day)
Adults:
Schizophrenia: Usual starting dose: 5-10 mg once daily; increase to 10 mg once daily within 5-7 days, thereafter adjust by 5-10 mg/day at 1-week intervals, up to a maximum of 20 mg/day; doses of 30-50 mg/day have been used; typical dosage range: 10-30 mg/day
Bipolar mania: Usual starting dose: 10-15 mg once daily; increase by 5 mg/day at intervals of not less than 24 hours; maximum dose: 20 mg/day
Elderly: Schizophrenia: Usual starting dose: 2.5 mg/day, increase as clinically indicated and monitor BP; typical dosage range: 2.5-10 mg/day

Mechanism of Action Olanzapine is a thienobenzodiazepine neuroleptic; thought to work by antagonizing dopamine and serotonin activities. It is a selective monoaminergic antagonist with high affinity binding to serotonin 5-HT_{2A} and 5-HT_{2C}, dopamine D_{1-4}, muscarinic M_{1-5}, histamine H_1- and alpha$_1$-adrenergic receptor sites. Olanzapine binds weakly to GABA-A, BZD, and beta-adrenergic receptors.

Other Adverse Effects

>10%: Central nervous system: Headache, somnolence, insomnia, agitation, nervousness, hostility, dizziness
1% to 10%:
Cardiovascular: Postural hypotension, tachycardia, hypotension, peripheral edema
Central nervous system: Dystonic reactions, parkinsonian events, amnesia, euphoria, stuttering, akathisia, anxiety, personality changes, fever
Dermatologic: Rash

Gastrointestinal: Xerostomia, constipation, abdominal pain, weight gain, increased appetite
Genitourinary: Premenstrual syndrome
Neuromuscular & skeletal: Arthralgia, neck rigidity, twitching, hypertonia, tremor
Ocular: Amblyopia
Respiratory: Rhinitis, cough, pharyngitis

Drug Interactions CYP1A2 enzyme substrate, CYP2C19 enzyme substrate (minor), and CYP2D6 enzyme substrate (minor)
Activated charcoal: Decreases the C_{max} and AUC of olanzapine by 60%
Antihypertensives: Increased risk of hypotension and orthostatic hypotension with antihypertensives
Clomipramine: When used in combination, clomipramine and olanzapine have been reported to be associated with the development of seizures; limited documentation (case report)
CNS depressants: Sedative effects and may be additive with CNS depressants; includes ethanol, barbiturates, narcotic analgesics, and other sedative agents; monitor for increased effect
CYP1A2 inhibitors: Serum levels may be increased and effect/toxicity increased by CYP1A2 inhibitors; examples include cimetidine, ciprofloxacin, fluvoxamine, isoniazid, and ritonavir
Enzyme inducers: May increase the metabolism of olanzapine resulting in decreased effect; includes carbamazepine, phenobarbital, phenytoin, rifampin, and cigarette smoking; monitor for decreased response
Haloperidol: A case of severe Parkinsonism following the addition of olanzapine to haloperidol therapy has been reported
Levodopa: Antipsychotics may inhibit the antiparkinsonian effect of levodopa; avoid this combination
Metoclopramide: May increase extrapyramidal symptoms (EPS) or risk.

Drug Uptake Tablets and orally-disintegrating tablets are bioequivalent
Onset of action: Therapeutic: ≥1 week
Absorption: Well and readily; unaffected by food
Half-life, elimination: 21-54 hours; ~1.5 times greater in elderly
Time to peak: ~6 hours

Pregnancy Risk Factor C

Generic Available No

Comments Olanzapine (Zyprexa®) is chemically similar to clozapine (Clozaril®), but without as many side effects. Also, olanzapine (Zyprexa®) does not produce side effects such as Parkinson's disease-like tremors which are associated with other antipsychotics such as haloperidol.

Olmesartan (ole me SAR tan)

U.S. Brand Names Benicar™

Pharmacologic Category Angiotensin II Receptor Blocker

Synonyms Olmesartan Medoxomil

Use Treatment of hypertension with or without concurrent use of other antihypertensive agents

Local Anesthetic/Vasoconstrictor Precautions No information available to require special precautions

Effects on Dental Treatment No effects or complications reported

Dosage Adults: Oral: Initial: Usual starting dose: 20 mg once daily; if initial response is inadequate, may be increased to 40 mg once daily after 2 weeks. May administer with other antihypertensive agents if BP inadequately controlled with olmesartan. Consider lower starting dose in patients with possible depletion of intravascular volume (eg, patients receiving diuretics).

Mechanism of Action As a selective and competitive, nonpeptide angiotensin II receptor antagonist, olmesartan blocks the vasoconstrictor and aldosterone-secreting effects of angiotensin II; olmesartan interacts reversibly at the AT1 and AT2 receptors of many tissues and has slow dissociation kinetics; its affinity for the AT1 receptor is 12,500 times greater than the AT2 receptor. Angiotensin II receptor antagonists may induce a more complete inhibition of the renin-angiotensin system than ACE inhibitors, they do not affect the response to bradykinin, and are less likely to be associated with nonrenin-angiotensin effects (eg, cough and angioedema). Olmesartan increases urinary flow rate and, in addition to being natriuretic and kaliuretic, increases excretion of chloride, magnesium, uric acid, calcium, and phosphate.

Other Adverse Effects 1% to 10%:
Central nervous system: Dizziness (3%), headache
Endocrine & metabolic: Hyperglycemia, hypertriglyceridemia
Gastrointestinal: Diarrhea
Neuromuscular & skeletal: Back pain, CPK increased
Renal: Hematuria
Respiratory: Bronchitis, pharyngitis, rhinitis, sinusitis, upper respiratory tract infection
Miscellaneous: Flu-like syndrome

Drug Interactions Does not affect, and is not affected by, CYP isoenzymes

(Continued)

Olmesartan *(Continued)*

Increased Effect/Toxicity: Risk of hyperkalemia may be increased with potassium-sparing diuretics, potassium supplements, and trimethoprim; may increase risk of lithium toxicity.

Decreased Effect: NSAIDs may decrease the efficacy.

Drug Uptake

Half-life, elimination: Terminal: 13 hours

Time to peak: 1-2 hours

Pregnancy Risk Factor C/D (2nd and 3rd trimesters)

Generic Available No

Olopatadine (oh LOP ah tah deen)

U.S. Brand Names Patanol®

Canadian Brand Names Patanol®

Pharmacologic Category Antihistamine; Ophthalmic Agent, Miscellaneous

Use Treatment of signs and symptoms of allergic conjunctivitis

Local Anesthetic/Vasoconstrictor Precautions No information available to require special precautions

Effects on Dental Treatment No effects or complications reported

Dosage Adults: Ophthalmic: 1 drop in affected eye(s) every 6-8 hours (2 times daily)

Other Adverse Effects

>5%: Central nervous system: Headache (7%)

<5%:

- Central nervous system: Weakness, cold syndrome
- Gastrointestinal: Taste perversion
- Ocular: Burning, stinging, dry eyes, foreign body sensation, hyperemia, keratitis, eyelid edema, itching
- Respiratory: Pharyngitis, rhinitis, sinusitis

Drug Interactions Studies evaluating drug interactions have not been conducted.

Pregnancy Risk Factor C

Generic Available No

Olsalazine (ole SAL a zeen)

U.S. Brand Names Dipentum®

Canadian Brand Names Dipentum®

Pharmacologic Category 5-Aminosalicylic Acid Derivative

Synonyms Olsalazine Sodium

Use Maintenance of remission of ulcerative colitis in patients intolerant to sulfasalazine

Local Anesthetic/Vasoconstrictor Precautions No information available to require special precautions

Effects on Dental Treatment No effects or complications reported

Dosage Adults: Oral: 1 g/day in 2 divided doses

Mechanism of Action The mechanism of action appears to be topical rather than systemic

Other Adverse Effects

>10%: Gastrointestinal: Diarrhea, cramps, abdominal pain

1% to 10%:

- Central nervous system: Headache, fatigue, depression
- Dermatologic: Rash, itching
- Gastrointestinal: Nausea, heartburn, bloating, anorexia
- Neuromuscular & skeletal: Arthralgia

Drug Interactions Olsalazine has been reported to increase the prothrombin time in patients taking warfarin.

Drug Uptake

Absorption: <3%; very little intact olsalazine is systemically absorbed

Half-life, elimination: 56 minutes or 55 hours, depending on the analysis used

Time to peak: ~1 hour

Pregnancy Risk Factor C

Generic Available No

Olux™ *see* Clobetasol *on page 303*

Omeprazole (oh ME pray zol)

Related Information

Gastrointestinal Disorders *on page 1326*

U.S. Brand Names Prilosec®

Canadian Brand Names Losec®

Mexican Brand Names Inhibitron®; Losec®; Olexin®; Osiren®; Ozoken; Prazidec; Prazolit®; Ulsen

Pharmacologic Category Proton Pump Inhibitor

Use Short-term (4-8 weeks) treatment of active duodenal ulcer disease or active benign gastric ulcer; treatment of heartburn and other symptoms associated with gastroesophageal reflux disease (GERD); short-term (4-8 weeks) treatment of endoscopically-diagnosed erosive esophagitis; maintenance healing of erosive esophagitis; long-term treatment of pathological hypersecretory conditions; as part of a multidrug regimen for *H. pylori* eradication to reduce the risk of duodenal ulcer recurrence

Unlabeled/Investigational: Healing and prevention of NSAID-induced ulcers

Local Anesthetic/Vasoconstrictor Precautions No information available to require special precautions

Effects on Dental Treatment No effects or complications reported

Dosage Adults: Oral:

Active duodenal ulcer: 20 mg/day for 4-8 weeks

GERD or severe erosive esophagitis: 20 mg/day for 4-8 weeks

Pathological hypersecretory conditions: 60 mg once daily to start; doses up to 120 mg 3 times/day have been administered; administer daily doses >80 mg in divided doses

Helicobacter pylori: 20 mg/day or 20 mg twice daily, depending on regimen

Gastric ulcers: 40 mg/day for 4-8 weeks

Mechanism of Action Suppresses gastric acid secretion by inhibiting the parietal cell H+/K+ ATP pump

Other Adverse Effects 1% to 10%:

Central nervous system: Headache (7%), dizziness (2%)

Dermatologic: Rash (2%)

Gastrointestinal: Diarrhea (3%), abdominal pain (2%), nausea (2%), vomiting (2%), constipation (1%), taste perversion (<1% to 15%)

Neuromuscular & skeletal: Weakness (1%), back pain (1%)

Respiratory: Upper respiratory infection (2%), cough (1%)

Drug Interactions CYP2C8, 2C9, 2C18, 2C19, and 3A3/4 enzyme substrate; CYP1A2 enzyme inducer; CYP2C8, 2C9, and 2C19 enzyme inhibitor, CYP3A3/4 enzyme inhibitor (weak)

Increased Toxicity: Diazepam may increase half-life; increased digoxin, increased phenytoin, increased warfarin; voriconazole may significantly increase serum levels of omeprazole (for omeprazole dosages >40 mg/day, reduce omeprazole dose by 50%); serum levels of other proton pump inhibitors may also be increased

Decreased Effect: Decreased ketoconazole; decreased itraconazole; voriconazole not affected

Drug Uptake

Onset of action: Antisecretory: ~1 hour; Peak effect: 2 hours

Duration: 72 hours

Half-life, elimination: 30-90 minutes

Pregnancy Risk Factor C

Generic Available No

Omnicef® *see* Cefdinir *on page 235*

Omnipaque® *see* Radiological/Contrast Media (Nonionic) *on page 1039*

Oncaspar® *see* Pegaspargase *on page 921*

Oncovin® *see* VinCRIStine *on page 1240*

Ondansetron (on DAN se tron)

U.S. Brand Names Zofran®; Zofran® ODT

Canadian Brand Names Zofran®; Zofran® ODT

Mexican Brand Names Zofran®

Pharmacologic Category Selective 5-HT_3 Receptor Antagonist

Synonyms Ondansetron Hydrochloride

Use Prevention of nausea and vomiting associated with moderately to highly emetogenic cancer chemotherapy; radiotherapy in patients receiving total body irradiation or fractions to the abdomen; postoperatively, when nausea and vomiting should be avoided

Unlabeled/Investigational: Treatment of early-onset alcoholism

Local Anesthetic/Vasoconstrictor Precautions No information available to require special precautions

Effects on Dental Treatment No effects or complications reported

Dosage

Children:

I.V.:

Chemotherapy-induced emesis: 4-18 years: 0.15 mg/kg/dose administered 30 minutes prior to chemotherapy, 4 and 8 hours after the first dose

Postoperative nausea and vomiting: 2-12 years:

≤40 kg: 0.1 mg/kg

>40 kg: 4 mg

Oral: Chemotherapy-induced emesis of moderately-emetogenic agents:

4-11 years: 4 mg 30 minutes before chemotherapy; repeat 4 and 8 hours after initial dose, then 4 mg every 8 hours for 1-2 days after chemotherapy completed

≥12 years: Refer to adult dosing.

(Continued)

Ondansetron *(Continued)*

Adults:

I.V.: Chemotherapy-induced emesis: Administer either three 0.15 mg/kg doses or a single 32 mg dose:

Three-dose regimen: Initial dose is given 30 minutes prior to chemotherapy with subsequent doses administered 4 and 8 hours after the first dose

Single-dose regimen: 32 mg is infused over 15 minutes beginning 30 minutes before the start of emetogenic chemotherapy

I.M., I.V.: Postoperative nausea and vomiting: 4 mg as a single dose immediately before induction of anesthesia, or shortly following procedure if vomiting occurs

Oral:

Chemotherapy-induced emesis:

Highly-emetogenic agents/single-day therapy: 24 mg given 30 minutes prior to the start of therapy

Moderately-emetogenic agents: 8 mg every 8 hours for 2 doses beginning 30 minutes before chemotherapy, then 8 mg every 12 hours for 1-2 days after chemotherapy completed

Total body irradiation: 8 mg 1-2 hours before each fraction of radiotherapy administered each day

Single high-dose fraction radiotherapy to abdomen: 8 mg 1-2 hours before irradiation, then 8 mg every 8 hours after first dose for 1-2 days after completion of radiotherapy

Daily fractionated radiotherapy to abdomen: 8 mg 1-2 hours before irradiation, then 8 mg every 8 hours after first dose for each day of radiotherapy

Postoperative nausea and vomiting: 16 mg given 1 hour prior to induction of anesthesia

Mechanism of Action Selective 5-HT_3 receptor antagonist, blocking serotonin, both peripherally on vagal nerve terminals and centrally in the chemoreceptor trigger zone

Other Adverse Effects

>10%:

Cardiovascular: Malaise/fatigue (9% to 13%)

Central nervous system: Headache (9% to 27%)

1% to 10%:

Central nervous system: Drowsiness (8%), fever (2% to 8%), dizziness (4% to 7%), anxiety (6%), cold sensation (2%)

Dermatologic: Pruritus (2% to 5%), rash (1%)

Gastrointestinal: Constipation (6% to 9%), diarrhea (3% to 7%)

Genitourinary: Gynecological disorder (7%), urinary retention (5%)

Hepatic: Increased ALT/AST (1% to 2%)

Local: Injection site reaction (4%)

Neuromuscular & skeletal: Paresthesia (2%)

Respiratory: Hypoxia (9%)

Contraindications Hypersensitivity to ondansetron, other selective 5-HT_3 antagonists, or any component of their formulation

Drug Interactions CYP1A2, 2D6, 2E1, and 3A3/4 enzyme substrate

Increased Effect/Toxicity: Increased toxicity: CYP1A2, 2D6, 2E1, and 3A3/4 enzyme inhibitors (eg, cimetidine, allopurinol, and disulfiram) may change the clearance of ondansetron; monitor

Decreased Effect: Decreased effect: CYP1A2, 2D6, 2E1, and 3A3/4 enzyme inducers (eg, barbiturates, carbamazepine, rifampin, phenytoin, and phenylbutazone) may change the clearance of ondansetron; monitor

Drug Uptake

Onset of action: ≤30 minutes

Half-life, elimination: Children <15 years: 2-3 hours, Adults: 3-6 hours

Time to peak: Oral: ~2 hours

Pregnancy Risk Factor B

Generic Available No

ONTAK® *see* Denileukin Diftitox *on page 357*

Ony-Clear [OTC] *see* Benzalkonium Chloride *on page 151*

Ony-Clear® Nail [OTC] *see* Triacetin *on page 1197*

Operand® [OTC] *see* Povidone-Iodine *on page 982*

Ophthalgan® *see* Glycerin *on page 562*

Ophthetic® *see* Proparacaine *on page 1010*

Opium Tincture (OH pee um TING chur)

Pharmacologic Category Analgesic, Narcotic; Antidiarrheal

Synonyms DTO; Opium Tincture, Deodorized

Use Treatment of diarrhea or relief of pain

Local Anesthetic/Vasoconstrictor Precautions No information available to require special precautions

Effects on Dental Treatment No effects or complications reported

Restrictions C-II

Dosage Oral:
Children:
Diarrhea: 0.005-0.01 mL/kg/dose every 3-4 hours for a maximum of 6 doses/24 hours
Analgesia: 0.01-0.02 mL/kg/dose every 3-4 hours
Adults:
Diarrhea: 0.3-1 mL/dose every 2-6 hours to maximum of 6 mL/24 hours
Analgesia: 0.6-1.5 mL/dose every 3-4 hours

Mechanism of Action Contains many narcotic alkaloids including morphine; its mechanism for gastric motility inhibition is primarily due to this morphine content; it results in a decrease in digestive secretions, an increase in GI muscle tone, and therefore a reduction in GI propulsion

Other Adverse Effects Frequency not defined:
Cardiovascular: Palpitations, hypotension, bradycardia, peripheral vasodilation,
Central nervous system: Drowsiness, dizziness, restlessness, headache, malaise, CNS depression, increased intracranial pressure, insomnia, mental depression
Gastrointestinal: Nausea, vomiting, constipation, anorexia, stomach cramps, biliary tract spasm
Genitourinary: Decreased urination, urinary tract spasm
Neuromuscular & skeletal: Weakness
Ocular: Miosis
Respiratory: Respiratory depression
Miscellaneous: Histamine release, physical and psychological dependence

Drug Interactions
Increased Effect/Toxicity: Opium tincture and CNS depressants, MAO inhibitors, tricyclic antidepressants may potentiate the effects of opiate agonists (eg, codeine, morphine, etc). Dextroamphetamine may enhance the analgesic effect of opiate agonists.
Decreased Effect: Phenothiazines may antagonize the analgesic effect of opiate agonists.

Drug Uptake
Absorption: Variable
Duration: 4-5 hours

Pregnancy Risk Factor B/D (prolonged use or high doses at term)

Generic Available No

Oprelvekin (oh PREL ve kin)

U.S. Brand Names Neumega®

Pharmacologic Category Biological Response Modulator; Human Growth Factor

Synonyms IL-11; Interleukin-11; Recombinant Human Interleukin-11; Recombinant Interleukin-11; rhIL-11; rIL-11

Use Prevention of severe thrombocytopenia and the reduction of the need for platelet transfusions following myelosuppressive chemotherapy in patients with nonmyeloid malignancies who are at high risk of severe thrombocytopenia.

Local Anesthetic/Vasoconstrictor Precautions No information available to require special precautions

Effects on Dental Treatment No effects or complications reported

Dosage S.C.:
Children: 75-100 mcg/kg once daily for 10-21 days (until postnadir platelet count ≥50,000 cells/μL)
Note: The manufacturer states that, until efficacy/toxicity parameters are established, the use of oprelvekin in pediatric patients (particularly those <12 years of age) should be restricted to use in controlled clinical trials.
Adults: 50 mcg/kg once daily for 10-21 days (until postnadir platelet count ≥50,000 cells/μL)

Mechanism of Action Stimulates multiple stages of megakaryocytopoiesis and thrombopoiesis, resulting in proliferation of megakaryocyte progenitors and megakaryocyte maturation

Other Adverse Effects
>10%:
Cardiovascular: Tachycardia (19% to 30%), palpitations (14% to 24%), atrial arrhythmias (12%), peripheral edema (60% to 75%)
Central nervous system: Headache (41%), dizziness (38%), insomnia (33%), fatigue (30%), fever (36%)
Dermatologic: Rash (25%)
Endocrine & metabolic: Fluid retention
Gastrointestinal: Nausea (50% to 77%), vomiting, anorexia
Hematologic: Anemia (100%), probably a dilutional phenomena; appears within 3 days of initiation of therapy, resolves in about 2 weeks after cessation of oprelvekin
Neuromuscular & skeletal: Arthralgia, myalgias
Ocular: Papilledema: (frequency estimated to be up to 33% in pediatric patients, 1.5% in adults)
Respiratory: Dyspnea (48%), pleural effusions (10%)
(Continued)

Oprelvekin *(Continued)*

1% to 10%:
- Cardiovascular: Syncope (6% to 13%)
- Gastrointestinal: Weight gain (5%)

Drug Uptake
Half-life, elimination: Terminal: 5-8 hours
Time to peak: 1-6 hours

Pregnancy Risk Factor C

Generic Available No

Opticrom® *see* Cromolyn Sodium *on page 330*
Opticyl® *see* Tropicamide *on page 1217*
Optigene® [OTC] *see* Tetrahydrozoline *on page 1150*
Optimine® *see* Azatadine *on page 134*
Optimoist® [OTC] *see* Saliva Substitute *on page 1073*
OptiPranolol® *see* Metipranolol *on page 800*
Optiray® *see* Radiological/Contrast Media (Nonionic) *on page 1039*
Optivar™ *see* Azelastine *on page 136*
Orabase®-B [OTC] *see* Benzocaine *on page 151*
Orabase® HCA *see* Hydrocortisone *on page 608*
Orabase® Plain [OTC] *see* Gelatin, Pectin, and Methylcellulose *on page 551*
Orabase® With Benzocaine [OTC] *see* Benzocaine, Gelatin, Pectin, and Sodium Carboxymethylcellulose *on page 153*
Oracit® *see* Sodium Citrate and Citric Acid *on page 1096*
Orajel® [OTC] *see* Benzocaine *on page 151*
Orajel® Baby [OTC] *see* Benzocaine *on page 151*
Orajel® Baby Nighttime [OTC] *see* Benzocaine *on page 151*
Orajel® Maximum Strength [OTC] *see* Benzocaine *on page 151*
Orajel® Perioseptic® [OTC] *see* Carbamide Peroxide *on page 218*
Oramorph SR® *see* Morphine Sulfate *on page 829*
Orap™ *see* Pimozide *on page 958*
Orasol® [OTC] *see* Benzocaine *on page 151*
Orasone® *see* PredniSONE *on page 990*
Orazinc® Oral [OTC] *see* Zinc Supplements *on page 1261*
Oretic® *see* Hydrochlorothiazide *on page 595*
Oreton® Methyl *see* MethylTESTOSTERone *on page 799*
Orexin® [OTC] *see* Vitamin B Complex *on page 1244*
Orfadin® *see* Nitisinone *on page 868*
Organidin® NR *see* Guaifenesin *on page 568*
Orgaran® *see* Danaparoid *on page 346*
Orimune® *see* Poliovirus Vaccine, Live, Trivalent, Oral *on page 970*
Orinase Diagnostic® *see* TOLBUTamide *on page 1178*
ORLAAM® *see* Levomethadyl Acetate Hydrochloride *on page 702*

Orlistat (OR li stat)

U.S. Brand Names Xenical®

Canadian Brand Names Xenical®

Mexican Brand Names Xenical®

Pharmacologic Category Lipase Inhibitor

Use Management of obesity, including weight loss and weight management when used in conjunction with a reduced-calorie diet; reduce the risk of weight regain after prior weight loss; indicated for obese patients with an initial body mass index (BMI) ≥30 kg/m^2 or ≥27 kg/m^2 in the presence of other risk factors

Local Anesthetic/Vasoconstrictor Precautions No information available to require special precautions

Effects on Dental Treatment No effects or complications reported

Dosage A once-daily multivitamin containing the fat-soluble vitamins (A, D, E, and K) should be administered at least 2 hours prior to orlistat.

Oral: Adults: 120 mg 3 times/day with each main meal containing fat (during or up to 1 hour after the meal); omit dose if meal is occasionally missed or contains no fat.

Mechanism of Action Orlistat is a reversible inhibitor of lipases; it exerts its therapeutic activity in the lumen of the stomach and small intestine by forming a covalent bond with the active serine residue site of gastric and pancreatic lipases; the inactivated enzymes are thus unavailable to hydrolyze dietary fat in the form of triglycerides into absorbable free fatty acids and monoglycerides; as undigested triglycerides are not absorbed, the resulting caloric deficit may have a positive effect on weight control; systemic absorption of the drug is therefore not needed for activity; at the recommended therapeutic dose of 120 mg 3 times/day, orlistat inhibits dietary fat absorption by approximately 30%

Other Adverse Effects

>10%

Central nervous system: Headache (31%)

Gastrointestinal: Oily spotting (27%), abdominal pain/discomfort (26%), flatus with discharge (24%), fatty/oily stool (20%), fecal urgency (22%), oily evacuation (12%), increased defecation (11%)

Neuromuscular & skeletal: Back pain (14%)

Respiratory: Upper respiratory infection (38%)

1% to 10%

Central nervous system: Fatigue (7%), anxiety (5%), sleep disorder (4%)

Dermatologic: Dry skin (2%)

Endocrine & metabolic: Menstrual irregularities (10%)

Gastrointestinal: Fecal incontinence (8%), nausea (8%), infectious diarrhea (5%), rectal pain/discomfort (5%), vomiting (4%)

Neuromuscular & skeletal: Arthritis (5%), myalgia (4%)

Otic: Otitis (4%)

Contraindications Hypersensitivity to orlistat or any component of the formulation; chronic malabsorption syndrome or cholestasis

Warnings/Precautions Patients should be advised to adhere to dietary guidelines; GI adverse events may increase if taken with a diet high in fat (>30% total daily calories from fat). The daily intake of fat should be distributed over three main meals. If taken with any one meal very high in fat, the possibility of GI effects increases. Patients should be counseled to take a multivitamin supplement that contains fat-soluble vitamins to ensure adequate nutrition because orlistat has been shown to reduce the absorption of some fat-soluble vitamins and beta-carotene. The supplement should be taken once daily at least 2 hours before or after the administration of orlistat (ie, bedtime). Some patients may develop increased levels of urinary oxalate following treatment; caution should be exercised when prescribing it to patients with a history of hyperoxaluria or calcium oxalate nephrolithiasis. As with any weight-loss agent, the potential exists for misuse in appropriate patient populations (eg, patients with anorexia nervosa or bulimia). Write/fill prescription carefully. Dispensing errors have been made between Xenical® (orlistat) and Xeloda® (capecitabine).

Drug Interactions Decreased Effect: Vitamin K absorption may be decreased; coadministration with cyclosporine may decrease plasma concentrations of cyclosporine.

Pregnancy Risk Factor B

Generic Available No

Ornex® [OTC] *see* Acetaminophen and Pseudoephedrine *on page 30*

Ornex® Maximum Strength [OTC] *see* Acetaminophen and Pseudoephedrine *on page 30*

Orphenadrine (or FEN a dreen)

Related Information

Temporomandibular Dysfunction (TMD) *on page 1397*

U.S. Brand Names Norflex™

Canadian Brand Names Norflex™; Rhoxal-orphendrine

Pharmacologic Category Anti-Parkinson's Agent, Anticholinergic; Skeletal Muscle Relaxant

Synonyms Orphenadrine Citrate

Use Treatment of muscle spasm associated with acute painful musculoskeletal conditions; supportive therapy in tetanus

Local Anesthetic/Vasoconstrictor Precautions No information available to require special precautions

Effects on Dental Treatment The peripheral anticholinergic effects of orphenadrine may decrease or inhibit salivary flow; normal salivation will return with cessation of drug therapy.

Dosage Adults:

Oral: 100 mg twice daily

I.M., I.V.: 60 mg every 12 hours

Mechanism of Action Indirect skeletal muscle relaxant thought to work by central atropine-like effects; has some euphorigenic and analgesic properties

Other Adverse Effects

>10%:

Central nervous system: Drowsiness, dizziness

Ocular: Blurred vision

1% to 10%:

Cardiovascular: Flushing of face, tachycardia, syncope

Dermatologic: Rash

Gastrointestinal: Nausea, vomiting, constipation

Genitourinary: Decreased urination

Neuromuscular & skeletal: Weakness

Ocular: Nystagmus, increased intraocular pressure

Respiratory: Nasal congestion

(Continued)

Orphenadrine *(Continued)*

Drug Interactions CYP2B6, 2D6, and 3A3/4 enzyme substrate; CYP2B6 enzyme inhibitor

Increased Effect/Toxicity: Orphenadrine may increase potential for anticholinergic adverse effects of anticholinergic agents; includes drugs with high anticholinergic activity (diphenhydramine, TCAs, phenothiazines). Sedative effects of may be additive in concurrent use of orphenadrine and CNS depressants (monitor). Effects of levodopa may be decreased by orphenadrine. Monitor.

Drug Uptake

Onset of effect: Peak effect: Oral: 2-4 hours

Duration: 4-6 hours

Half-life, elimination: 14-16 hours

Pregnancy Risk Factor C

Generic Available Yes

Orphenadrine, Aspirin, and Caffeine

(or FEN a dreen, AS pir in, & KAF een)

U.S. Brand Names Norgesic™; Norgesic™ Forte

Canadian Brand Names Norgesic™; Norgesic™ Forte

Pharmacologic Category Skeletal Muscle Relaxant

Synonyms Aspirin, Orphenadrine, and Caffeine; Caffeine, Orphenadrine, and Aspirin

Use Relief of discomfort associated with skeletal muscular conditions

Local Anesthetic/Vasoconstrictor Precautions No information available to require special precautions

Effects on Dental Treatment The peripheral anticholinergic effects of orphenadrine may decrease or inhibit salivary flow; normal salivation will return with cessation of drug therapy.

Dosage Oral: 1-2 tablets 3-4 times/day

Drug Uptake See Orphenadrine *on page 891* and Aspirin *on page 119*

Pregnancy Risk Factor D

Generic Available Yes

Ortho-Cept® *see* Combination Hormonal Contraceptives *on page 323*
Orthoclone OKT® 3 *see* Muromonab-CD3 *on page 835*
Ortho-Cyclen® *see* Combination Hormonal Contraceptives *on page 323*
Ortho-Est® *see* Estropipate *on page 469*
Ortho Evra™ *see* Combination Hormonal Contraceptives *on page 323*
Ortho-Novum® *see* Combination Hormonal Contraceptives *on page 323*
Ortho-Novum® 1/50 *see* Mestranol and Norethindrone *on page 774*
Ortho-Prefest® *see* Estradiol and Norgestimate *on page 460*
Ortho Tri-Cyclen® *see* Combination Hormonal Contraceptives *on page 323*
Or-Tyl® *see* Dicyclomine *on page 382*
Orudis® [DSC] *see* Ketoprofen *on page 674*
Orudis® KT [OTC] *see* Ketoprofen *on page 674*
Oruvail® *see* Ketoprofen *on page 674*
Os-Cal® 500 [OTC] *see* Calcium Carbonate *on page 201*

Oseltamivir Phosphate (o sel TAM e veer)

Related Information

Systemic Viral Diseases *on page 1354*

U.S. Brand Names Tamiflu™

Canadian Brand Names Tamiflu™

Pharmacologic Category Antiviral Agent; Neuraminidase Inhibitor

Use Treatment of uncomplicated acute illness due to influenza (A or B) infection in adults and children >1 year of age who have been symptomatic ≤2 days; prophylaxis against influenza (A or B) infection in adults and adolescents ≥13 years of age

Local Anesthetic/Vasoconstrictor Precautions No information available to require special precautions

Effects on Dental Treatment No effects or complications reported

Dosage Oral:

Treatment: Initiate treatment within 2 days of onset of symptoms; duration of treatment: 5 days:

- Children: 1-12 years:
  - ≤15 kg: 30 mg twice daily
  - >15 kg - ≤23 kg: 45 mg twice daily
  - >23 kg - ≤40 kg: 60 mg twice daily
  - >40 kg: 75 mg twice daily
- Adolescents and Adults: 75 mg twice daily

Prophylaxis: Adolescents and Adults: 75 mg once daily for at least 7 days; treatment should begin within 2 days of contact with an infected individual. During community outbreaks, dosing is 75 mg once daily. May be used for up to 6 weeks; duration of protection lasts for length of dosing period

Dosage adjustment in renal impairment:

Cl_{cr} <10 mL/minute: Has not been studied

Cl_{cr} 10-30 mL/minute:

Treatment: Reduce dose to 75 mg once daily for 5 days

Prophylaxis: 75 mg every other day

Mechanism of Action Oseltamivir, a prodrug, is hydrolyzed to the active form, oseltamivir carboxylate. It is thought to inhibit influenza virus neuraminidase, with the possibility of alteration of virus particle aggregation and release. In clinical studies of the influenza virus, 1.3% of post-treatment isolates had decreased neuraminidase susceptibility to oseltamivir carboxylate.

Other Adverse Effects

As seen with **treatment** doses: 1% to 10%:

Central nervous system: Insomnia (adults 1%), vertigo (adults 1%)

Gastrointestinal: Nausea (adults 10%), vomiting (adults 9%, children 15%), abdominal pain (children 5%)

Ocular: Conjunctivitis (children 1%)

Otic: Ear disorder (children 2%)

Respiratory: Epistaxis (children 3%)

Similar adverse effects were seen in **prophylactic** use, however, the incidence was generally less. The following reactions were seen more commonly with prophylactic use: Headache (20%), fatigue (8%), diarrhea (3%)

Contraindications Hypersensitivity to any components of the formulation

Warnings/Precautions Oseltamivir is not a substitute for the flu shot. Dosage adjustment is required for creatinine clearance between 10-30 mL/minute. Safety and efficacy in children (<1 year of age) have not been established for treatment regimens. Safety and efficacy have not been established for prophylactic use in patients <13 years of age. Also consider primary or concomitant bacterial infections. Safety and efficacy for treatment or prophylaxis in immunocompromised patients have not been established.

Drug Interactions Increased Effect/Toxicity: Cimetidine and amoxicillin have no effect on plasma concentrations. Probenecid increases oseltamivir carboxylate serum concentration by 2-fold. Dosage adjustments are not required.

Drug Uptake

Absorption: Well absorbed

Half-life, elimination: Oseltamivir carboxylate: 6-10 hours; similar in geriatrics (68-78 years)

Time to peak: C_{max}: Oseltamivir: 65 ng/mL; Oseltamivir carboxylate: 348 ng/mL

Pregnancy Risk Factor C

Dosage Forms CAP [blister pack]: 75 mg (10/pack). **POWDER, oral suspension:** 12 mg/mL (25 mL)

Generic Available No

Comments Single doses of 1000 mg have resulted in nausea and vomiting

Osmoglyn® *see* Glycerin *on page 562*

Otic-Care® *see* Neomycin, Polymyxin B, and Hydrocortisone *on page 857*

Otic Domeboro® *see* Aluminum Acetate and Acetic Acid *on page 61*

Otobiotic® *see* Polymyxin B and Hydrocortisone *on page 972*

Otocort® *see* Neomycin, Polymyxin B, and Hydrocortisone *on page 857*

Otosporin® *see* Neomycin, Polymyxin B, and Hydrocortisone *on page 857*

Otrivin® [OTC] *see* Xylometazoline *on page 1252*

Otrivin® Pediatric [OTC] *see* Xylometazoline *on page 1252*

Ovcon® *see* Combination Hormonal Contraceptives *on page 323*

Ovidrel® *see* Chorionic Gonadotropin (Recombinant) *on page 282*

Ovral® *see* Combination Hormonal Contraceptives *on page 323*

Ovrette® *see* Norgestrel *on page 877*

Oxacillin (oks a SIL in)

U.S. Brand Names Bactocill®

Canadian Brand Names Bactocill®

Pharmacologic Category Antibiotic, Penicillin

Synonyms Methylphenyl Isoxazolyl Penicillin; Oxacillin Sodium

Use Treatment of susceptible bacterial infections such as osteomyelitis, septicemia, endocarditis, and CNS infections due to penicillinase-producing strains of *Staphylococcus*

Local Anesthetic/Vasoconstrictor Precautions No information available to require special precautions

Effects on Dental Treatment Prolonged use of penicillins may lead to development of oral candidiasis.

Dosage

Neonates: I.M., I.V.:

Postnatal age <7 days:

<2000 g: 25 mg/kg/dose every 12 hours

>2000 g: 25 mg/kg/dose every 8 hours

(Continued)

Oxacillin *(Continued)*

Postnatal age >7 days:
<1200 g: 25 mg/kg/dose every 12 hours
1200-2000 g: 30 mg/kg/dose every 8 hours
>2000 g: 37.5 mg/kg/dose every 6 hours

Infants and Children:
Oral: 50-100 mg/kg/day divided every 6 hours
I.M., I.V.: 150-200 mg/kg/day in divided doses every 6 hours; maximum dose: 12 g/day

Adults:
Oral: 500-1000 mg every 4-6 hours for at least 5 days
I.M., I.V.: 250 mg to 2 g/dose every 4-6 hours

Dosing adjustment in renal impairment: Cl_{cr} <10 mL/minute: Use lower range of the usual dosage

Hemodialysis: Not dialyzable (0% to 5%)

Mechanism of Action Inhibits bacterial cell wall synthesis by binding to one or more of the penicillin binding proteins (PBPs); which in turn inhibits the final transpeptidation step of peptidoglycan synthesis in bacterial cell walls, thus inhibiting cell wall biosynthesis. Bacteria eventually lyse due to ongoing activity of cell wall autolytic enzymes (autolysins and murein hydrolases) while cell wall assembly is arrested.

Other Adverse Effects

>10%:
Central nervous system: Headache
Gastrointestinal: Nausea (mild), vomiting
Miscellaneous: Oral candidiasis, vaginal candidiasis

1% to 10%:
Dermatologic: Urticaria, exfoliative dermatitis
Miscellaneous: Allergic reactions, specifically anaphylaxis; serum sickness-like reactions

Drug Interactions

Increased Effect/Toxicity: Probenecid increases penicillin levels. Penicillins and anticoagulants may increase the effect of anticoagulants.

Decreased Effect: Efficacy of oral contraceptives may be reduced when taken with oxacillin.

Drug Uptake

Absorption: Oral: 35% to 67%
Half-life, elimination: Children 1 week to 2 years: 0.9-1.8 hours; Adults: 23-60 minutes (increases in neonates and renal impairment)
Time to peak: Oral: ~2 hours; I.M.: 30-60 minutes

Pregnancy Risk Factor B

Generic Available Yes

Oxamniquine (oks AM ni kwin)

U.S. Brand Names Vansil™

Canadian Brand Names Vansil™

Pharmacologic Category Anthelmintic

Use Treatment of all stages of *Schistosoma mansoni* infection

Local Anesthetic/Vasoconstrictor Precautions No information available to require special precautions

Effects on Dental Treatment No effects or complications reported

Dosage Oral:
Children <30 kg: 20 mg/kg in 2 divided doses of 10 mg/kg at 2- to 8-hour intervals
Adults: 12-15 mg/kg as a single dose

Mechanism of Action Not fully elucidated; causes worms to dislodge from their usual site of residence (mesenteric veins to the liver) by paralysis and contraction of musculature and subsequently phagocytized

Other Adverse Effects

>10%: Central nervous system: Dizziness, drowsiness, headache

<10%:
Central nervous system: Insomnia, malaise, hallucinations, behavior changes
Dermatologic: Rash, urticaria, pruritus
Gastrointestinal: GI effects, orange/red discoloration of urine
Hepatic: Elevated LFTs
Renal: Proteinuria

Drug Interactions May be synergistic with praziquantel

Drug Uptake

Absorption: Well absorbed
Half-life, elimination: 1-2.5 hours
Time to peak: 1-3 hours

Pregnancy Risk Factor C

Generic Available No

Comments Strains other than from the western hemisphere may require higher doses

Oxandrin® *see* Oxandrolone *on page 895*

Oxandrolone (oks AN droe lone)

U.S. Brand Names Oxandrin®

Pharmacologic Category Androgen

Use Treatment of catabolic or tissue-depleting processes

Local Anesthetic/Vasoconstrictor Precautions No information available to require special precautions

Effects on Dental Treatment No effects or complications reported

Restrictions C-III

Dosage Adults: Oral: 2.5 mg 2-4 times daily

Mechanism of Action Synthetic testosterone derivative with similar androgenic and anabolic actions

Other Adverse Effects

Male:

Postpubertal:

- >10%:
  - Dermatologic: Acne
  - Endocrine & metabolic: Gynecomastia
  - Genitourinary: Bladder irritability, priapism
- 1% to 10%:
  - Central nervous system: Insomnia, chills
  - Endocrine & metabolic: Decreased libido, hepatic dysfunction
  - Gastrointestinal: Nausea, diarrhea
  - Genitourinary: Prostatic hyperplasia (elderly)
  - Hematologic: Iron-deficiency anemia, suppression of clotting factors

Prepubertal:

- >10%:
  - Dermatologic: Acne
  - Endocrine & metabolic: Virilism
- 1% to 10%:
  - Central nervous system: Chills, insomnia,
  - Dermatologic: Hyperpigmentation
  - Gastrointestinal: Diarrhea, nausea
  - Hematologic: Iron deficiency anemia, suppression of clotting factors

Female:

- >10%: Endocrine & metabolic: Virilism
- 1% to 10%:
  - Central nervous system: Chills, insomnia
  - Endocrine & metabolic: Hypercalcemia
  - Gastrointestinal: Nausea, diarrhea
  - Hematologic: Iron deficiency anemia, suppression of clotting factors
  - Hepatic: Hepatic dysfunction

Drug Interactions Increased Effect/Toxicity: ACTH, adrenal steroids may increase risk of edema and acne. Stanozolol enhances the hypoprothrombinemic effects of oral anticoagulants, and enhances the hypoglycemic effects of insulin and sulfonylureas (oral hypoglycemics).

Drug Uptake

Onset of action: 1 month

Absorption: High

Pregnancy Risk Factor X

Generic Available No

Oxaprozin (oks a PROE zin)

Related Information

Rheumatoid Arthritis and Osteoarthritis *on page 1340*

Temporomandibular Dysfunction (TMD) *on page 1397*

U.S. Brand Names Daypro™

Canadian Brand Names Daypro™

Pharmacologic Category Nonsteroidal Anti-inflammatory Drug (NSAID)

Use Acute and long-term use in the management of signs and symptoms of osteoarthritis and rheumatoid arthritis; juvenile rheumatoid arthritis

Local Anesthetic/Vasoconstrictor Precautions No information available to require special precautions

Effects on Dental Treatment NSAID formulations are known to reversibly decrease platelet aggregation via mechanisms different than observed with aspirin. The dentist should be aware of the potential of abnormal coagulation. Caution should also be exercised in the use of NSAIDs in patients already on anticoagulant therapy with drugs such as warfarin (Coumadin®).

Dosage Oral (individualize dosage to lowest effective dose to minimize adverse effects):

Children: Juvenile rheumatoid arthritis: Maximum daily dose: 1200 mg or 26 mg/kg (whichever is lower) in divided doses

(Continued)

Oxaprozin *(Continued)*

Adults:

Osteoarthritis: 600-1200 mg once daily

Rheumatoid arthritis: 1200 mg once daily; a one-time loading dose of up to 1800 mg/day or 26 mg/kg (whichever is lower) may be given

Maximum daily dose: 1800 mg or 26 mg/kg (whichever is lower) in divided doses

Mechanism of Action Inhibits prostaglandin synthesis by decreasing the activity of the enzyme, cyclo-oxygenase, which results in decreased formation of prostaglandin precursors

Other Adverse Effects 1% to 10%:

Central nervous system: CNS inhibition, disturbance of sleep

Dermatologic: Rash

Gastrointestinal: Nausea, dyspepsia, abdominal pain, anorexia, flatulence, vomiting

Genitourinary: Dysuria or frequency

Warnings/Precautions Use with caution in patients with CHF, hypertension. GI toxicity (bleeding, ulceration, perforation); CNS effects may occur (headaches, confusion, depression); dehydration, hypersensitivity, anaphylactoid reactions (intermittent tolmetin use more often); renal function decline, acute renal insufficiency, interstitial nephritis, dysuria, cystitis, hematuria, nephrotic syndrome, hyperkalemia in acute renal insufficiency, hyponatremia, papillary necrosis, hepatic function impairment; elderly have increased risk for adverse reactions to NSAIDs. Withhold for at least 4-6 half-lives prior to surgical or dental procedures.

Drug Interactions CYP2C9 enzyme inhibitor

ACE-inhibitors: Antihypertensive effects may be decreased by concurrent therapy with NSAIDs; monitor BP. Oxaprozin may decrease serum concentration of enalapril.

Angiotensin II antagonists: Antihypertensive effects may be decreased by concurrent therapy with NSAIDs; monitor BP.

Anticoagulants (warfarin, heparin, LMWHs) in combination with NSAIDs can cause increased risk of bleeding.

Other antiplatelet drugs (ticlopidine, clopidogrel, aspirin, abciximab, dipyridamole, eptifibatide, tirofiban) can cause an increased risk of bleeding.

Corticosteroids may increase the risk of GI ulceration; avoid concurrent use.

Cyclosporine: NSAIDs may increase serum creatinine, potassium, BP, and cyclosporine levels; monitor cyclosporine levels and renal function carefully.

Hydralazine's antihypertensive effect is decreased; avoid concurrent use.

Lithium levels can be increased; avoid concurrent use if possible or monitor lithium levels and adjust dose. Sulindac may have the least effect. When NSAID is stopped, lithium will need adjustment again.

Loop diuretics efficacy (diuretic and antihypertensive effect) may be reduced.

Methotrexate: Severe bone marrow suppression, aplastic anemia, and GI toxicity have been reported with concomitant NSAID therapy. Avoid use during moderate or high-dose methotrexate (increased and prolonged methotrexate levels). NSAID use during low-dose treatment of rheumatoid arthritis has not been fully evaluated; extreme caution is warranted.

Thiazides antihypertensive effects are decreased; avoid concurrent use.

Warfarin's INRs may be increased by piroxicam. Other NSAIDs may have the same effect depending on dose and duration. Monitor INR closely. Use the lowest dose of NSAIDs possible and for the briefest duration.

Drug Uptake

Absorption: Almost completely

Half-life, elimination: 40-50 hours

Time to peak: 2-4 hours

Pregnancy Risk Factor C/D (3rd trimester)

Generic Available Yes

Oxazepam (oks A ze pam)

Related Information

Patients Requiring Sedation *on page 1400*

U.S. Brand Names Serax®

Canadian Brand Names Apo®-Oxazepam; Serax®

Pharmacologic Category Benzodiazepine

Use Treatment of anxiety; management of ethanol withdrawal

Unlabeled/Investigational: Anticonvulsant in management of simple partial seizures; hypnotic

Local Anesthetic/Vasoconstrictor Precautions No information available to require special precautions

Effects on Dental Treatment >10%: Xerostomia; disappears with discontinuation

Restrictions C-IV

Dosage Oral:

Children: Anxiety: 1 mg/kg/day has been administered

Adults:

Anxiety: 10-30 mg 3-4 times/day

Ethanol withdrawal: 15-30 mg 3-4 times/day

Hypnotic: 15-30 mg

Elderly: Oral: Anxiety: 10 mg 2-3 times/day; increase gradually as needed to a total of 30-45 mg/day. Dose titration should be slow to evaluate sensitivity.

Hemodialysis: Not dialyzable (0% to 5%)

Mechanism of Action Binds to stereospecific benzodiazepine receptors on the postsynaptic GABA neuron at several sites within the CNS, including the limbic system, reticular formation. Enhancement of the inhibitory effect of GABA on neuronal excitability results by increased neuronal membrane permeability to chloride ions. This shift in chloride ions results in hyperpolarization (a less excitable state) and stabilization.

Other Adverse Effects Frequency not defined:

Cardiovascular: Syncope (rare), edema

Central nervous system: Drowsiness, ataxia, dizziness, vertigo, memory impairment, headache, paradoxical reactions (excitement, stimulation of effect), lethargy, amnesia, euphoria

Dermatologic: Rash

Endocrine & metabolic: Decreased libido, menstrual irregularities

Genitourinary: Incontinence

Hematologic: Leukopenia, blood dyscrasias

Hepatic: Jaundice

Neuromuscular & skeletal: Dysarthria, tremor, reflex slowing

Ocular: Blurred vision, diplopia

Miscellaneous: Drug dependence

Drug Interactions

Increased Effect/Toxicity: Other CNS depressants may increase the CNS effects of oxazepam. Oxazepam may decrease the antiparkinsonian efficacy of levodopa. Flumazenil may cause seizures if administered following long-term benzodiazepine treatment.

Decreased Effect: Oral contraceptives may increase the clearance of oxazepam. Theophylline and other CNS stimulants may antagonize the sedative effects of oxazepam. Phenytoin may increase the clearance of oxazepam.

Drug Uptake

Absorption: Oral: Almost completely

Half-life, elimination: 2.8-5.7 hours

Time to peak: 2-4 hours

Pregnancy Risk Factor D

Generic Available Yes

Oxcarbazepine (ox car BAZ e peen)

U.S. Brand Names Trileptal®

Canadian Brand Names Trileptal®

Mexican Brand Names Trileptal®

Pharmacologic Category Anticonvulsant, Miscellaneous

Synonyms GP 47680

Use Monotherapy or adjunctive therapy in the treatment of partial seizures in adults with epilepsy; adjunctive therapy in the treatment of partial seizures in children ages 4-16 with epilepsy

Unlabeled/Investigational: Antimanic

Local Anesthetic/Vasoconstrictor Precautions No information available to require special precautions

Effects on Dental Treatment No effects or complications reported

Dosage Oral:

Children:

Adjunctive therapy: 8-10 mg/kg/day, not to exceed 600 mg/day, given in 2 divided daily doses. Maintenance dose should be achieved over 2 weeks, and is dependent upon patient weight, according to the following:

20-29 kg: 900 mg/day in 2 divided doses

29.1-39 kg: 1200 mg/day in 2 divided doses

>39 kg: 1800 mg/day in 2 divided doses

Adults:

Adjunctive therapy: Initial: 300 mg twice daily; dose may be increased by as much as 600 mg/day at weekly intervals; recommended daily dose: 1200 mg/day in 2 divided doses. Although daily doses >1200 mg/day demonstrated greater efficacy, most patients were unable to tolerate 2400 mg/day (due to CNS effects).

Conversion to monotherapy: Oxcarbazepine 600 mg/day in twice daily divided doses while simultaneously initiating the reduction of the dose of the concomitant antiepileptic drug. The concomitant dosage should be withdrawn over 3-6 weeks, while the maximum dose of oxcarbazepine should be reached in about 2-4 weeks. Recommended daily dose: 2400 mg/day.

Initiation of monotherapy: Oxcarbazepine should be initiated at a dose of 600 mg/day in twice daily divided doses; doses may be titrated upward by 300 mg/day every third day to a final dose of 1200 mg/day given in 2 daily divided doses

Dosing adjustment in renal impairment: Therapy should be initiated at one-half the usual starting dose (300 mg/day) and increased slowly to achieve the desired clinical response

(Continued)

Oxcarbazepine *(Continued)*

Mechanism of Action Pharmacological activity results from both oxcarbazine and its monohydroxy metabolite (MHD). Precise mechanism of anticonvulsant effect has not been defined. Oxcarbazine and MHD block voltage sensitive sodium channels, stabilizing hyperexcited neuronal membranes, inhibiting repetitive firing, and decreasing the propagation of synaptic impulses. These actions are believed to prevent the spread of seizures. Oxcarbazine and MHD also increase potassium conductance and modulate the activity of high-voltage activated calcium channels.

Other Adverse Effects As reported in adults with doses of up to 2400 mg/day (includes patients on monotherapy, adjunctive therapy, and those not previously on AEDs); incidence in children was similar.

>10%:

Central nervous system: Dizziness (22% to 49%), somnolence (20% to 36%), headache (13% to 32%, placebo 23%), ataxia (5% to 31%), fatigue (12% to 15%), vertigo (6% to 15%)

Gastrointestinal: Vomiting (7% to 36%), nausea (15% to 29%), abdominal pain (10% to 13%)

Neuromuscular & skeletal: Abnormal gait (5% to 17%), tremor (3% to 16%)

Ocular: Diplopia (14% to 40%), nystagmus (7% to 26%), abnormal vision (4% to 14%)

1% to 10%:

Cardiovascular: Hypotension (1% to 2%), leg edema (1% to 2%, placebo 1%)

Central nervous system: Nervousness (2% to 5%, placebo 1% to 2%), amnesia (4%), abnormal thinking (2% to 4%), insomnia (2% to 4%), speech disorder (1% to 3%), EEG abnormalities (2%), abnormal feelings (1% to 2%), agitation (1% to 2%, placebo 1%), confusion (1% to 2%, placebo 1%)

Dermatologic: Rash (4%), acne (1% to 2%)

Endocrine & metabolic: Hyponatremia (1% to 3%, placebo 1%)

Gastrointestinal: Diarrhea (5% to 7%), dyspepsia (5% to 6%), constipation (2% to 6%, placebo 0% to 4%), gastritis (1% to 2%, placebo 1%), weight gain (1% to 2%, placebo 1%)

Neuromuscular & skeletal: Weakness (3% to 6%, placebo 5%), back pain (4%), falling down (4%), abnormal coordination (1% to 4%, placebo 1% to 2%), dysmetria (1% to 3%), sprains/strains (2%), muscle weakness (1% to 2%)

Ocular: Abnormal accommodation (2%)

Respiratory: Upper respiratory tract infection (7%), rhinitis (2% to 5%, placebo 4%), chest infection (4%), epistaxis (4%), sinusitis (4%)

Contraindications Hypersensitivity to oxcarbazine or any component of the formulation

Warnings/Precautions Oxcarbazine has been associated with significant hyponatremia (<125 mmol/L); monitor for signs and/or symptoms of hyponatremia; usually develops in the first three months but may occur at any time during therapy. Due to a chemical similarity with carbamazepine, use caution in patients with previous hypersensitivity to this agent; cross-sensitivity occurs in 25% to 30%. Discontinue at the first sign of a hypersensitivity reaction. May cause drowsiness, dizziness, somnolence, cognitive difficulties, or difficulties with coordination. Patients should be warned to avoid operating machinery or driving until they gain experience to gauge their ability to perform these tasks. Use caution in patients receiving other sedative medications or ethanol; additive sedation may occur. May reduce the efficacy of oral contraceptives (nonhormonal contraceptive measures are recommended). Do not discontinue abruptly; withdraw gradually to reduce risk of increased seizures.

Drug Interactions CYP2C19 enzyme inhibitor; CYP3A4/5 enzyme inducer

Increased Effect/Toxicity: Serum concentrations of phenytoin and phenobarbital are increased by oxcarbazepine.

Decreased Effect: Oxcarbazine serum concentration may be reduced by carbamazepine, phenytoin, phenobarbital, valproic acid and verapamil (decreases levels of active oxcarbazepine metabolite). Oxcarbazepine reduces the serum concentration of felodipine (similar effects may be anticipated with other dihydropyridines), oral contraceptives (use alternative contraceptive measures), and verapamil.

Drug Uptake

Absorption: Completely absorbed and extensively metabolized to its pharmacologically active 10-monohydroxy metabolite (MHD); unaffected by food

Half-life, elimination: Parent Drug: 2 hours; MHD: 9 hours (19 hours with Cl_{cr} 30 mL/minute when 300 mg of oxcarbazepine is administered)

Pregnancy Risk Factor C

Generic Available No

Comments Symptoms of overdose may include CNS depression (somnolence, ataxia). Treatment is symptomatic and supportive. Experience is limited -the largest reported overdose has been 24,000 mg.

Oxiconazole (oks i KON a zole)

Related Information

Oral Fungal Infections *on page 1377*

U.S. Brand Names Oxistat®
Canadian Brand Names Oxistat®; Oxizole®
Mexican Brand Names Gyno-Myfungar®; Myfungar®; Oxistat®
Pharmacologic Category Antifungal Agent, Topical
Synonyms Oxiconazole Nitrate
Use Treatment of tinea pedis (athlete's foot), tinea cruris (jock itch), and tinea corporis (ring worm)
Local Anesthetic/Vasoconstrictor Precautions No information available to require special precautions
Effects on Dental Treatment No effects or complications reported
Dosage Children and Adults: Topical: Apply once to twice daily to affected areas for 2 weeks (tinea corporis/tinea cruris) to 1 month (tinea pedis)
Mechanism of Action Inhibition of ergosterol synthesis. Effective for treatment of tinea pedis, tinea cruris, and tinea corporis. Active against *Trichophyton rubrum, Trichophyton mentagrophytes, Trichophyton violaceum, Microsporum canis, Microsporum audouini, Microsporum gypseum, Epidermophyton floccosum, Candida albicans,* and *Malassezia furfur.*
Other Adverse Effects 1% to 10%:
Dermatologic: Itching, erythema
Local: Transient burning, local irritation, stinging, dryness
Drug Uptake Absorption: In each layer of the dermis; very little is absorbed systemically after one topical dose
Pregnancy Risk Factor B
Generic Available No

Oxipor® VHC [OTC] *see* Coal Tar *on page 315*
Oxistat® *see* Oxiconazole *on page 898*

Oxprenolol *Not Available in U.S.* (ox PREN oh lole)

Canadian Brand Names Slow-Trasicor®; Trasicor®
Pharmacologic Category Antihypertensive; Beta-adrenergic Blocker, Noncardioselective
Synonyms Oxprenolol Hydrochloride
Use Treatment of mild or moderate hypertension
Unlabeled/Investigational: Treatment of nonsevere hypertension in pregnancy (second-line agent)
Local Anesthetic/Vasoconstrictor Precautions No information available to require special precautions
Effects on Dental Treatment No effects or complications reported
Dosage Oral: Adults:
Initial: 20 mg 3 times/day (regular-release formulation); increase by 60 mg/day (in 3 divided doses) at 1-2 week intervals until adequate control is obtained
Maintenance: 120-320 mg/day; do not exceed 480 mg; may switch to slow-release formulation once-daily dosing at this time
Mechanism of Action Has a competitive ability to antagonize catecholamine-induced tachycardia at the beta-receptor sites in the heart, thus decreasing cardiac output; inhibits the vasomotor centers and renin release by the kidneys
Other Adverse Effects Frequency not defined:
Cardiovascular: Congestive heart failure, pulmonary edema, cardiac enlargement, postural hypotension, severe bradycardia, lengthening of PR interval, second- and third-degree AV block, sinus arrest, palpitations, chest pain; peripheral vascular disorders, Raynaud's phenomenon, claudication, hot flashes
Central nervous system: Vertigo, syncope, lightheadedness, headache, dizziness, anxiety, mental depression, nervousness, irritability, hallucinations, sleep disturbances, nightmares, insomnia, weakness, sedation, vivid dreams, slurred speech
Dermatological: Dry skin, rash, pruritus
Endocrine & metabolic: Decreased libido, impotence, weight gain; elevated transaminases, alkaline phosphatase, and bilirubin; hypoglycemia
Gastrointestinal: Diarrhea, constipation, flatulence, heartburn, anorexia, nausea, vomiting, abdominal pain, xerostomia
Hematological: Thrombocytopenia, leukopenia
Neuromuscular & skeletal: Paresthesia
Ocular: Keratoconjunctivitis, dry eyes, itching eyes, blurred vision
Otic: Tinnitus
Renal: Elevated BUN
Respiratory: Dyspnea, wheezing, bronchospasm, nasal congestion, status asthmaticus
Miscellaneous: Diaphoresis, exertional tiredness
Drug Interactions CYP2D6 enzyme inhibitor
Increased Effect/Toxicity:
Antiarrhythmic agents (eg, quinidine, amiodarone) may potentiate the negative inotropic and dromotropic effect of antiarrhythmic agents (quinidine, amiodarone) may be potentiated by oxprenolol.
(Continued)

Oxprenolol *Not Available in U.S.* (Continued)

I.V. calcium channel blockers with AV-blocking potential (eg, diltiazem and verapamil) may lead to severe hypotension, cardiac arrhythmias and cardiac arrest may occur.

Catecholamine-depleting drugs (reserpine, guanethidine) may produce any excessive reduction of sympathetic activity, leading to severe bradycardia and hypotension.

Ergot alkaloids may cause deterioration in peripheral blood flow, leading to peripheral ischemia.

Inhalational anesthetics may cause cardiodepressant effects in patients receiving oxprenolol.

May potentiate hypoglycemic effects of insulin and hypoglycemic agents

MAO inhibitors may produce any excessive reduction of sympathetic activity.

CNS depressants (opiate analgesics, antihistamines, ethanol, and psychoactive drugs) may potentiate CNS depressant effects of oxprenolol.

Decreased Effect:

NSAIDs (indomethacin) may decrease antihypertensive effect of oxprenolol.

Sympathomimetic agents (eg, epinephrine) may cause hypertensive reactions.

Drug Uptake

Absorption: 20% to 70%

Duration of beta-blocking effects: Immediate-release tablet: 8-12 hours; Slow-release tablet: Up to 24 hours

Half-life, elimination: 1.3-1.5 hours

Time to peak: Immediate-release tablet: 0.5-1.5 hours; Slow-release tablet: 2-4 hours

Pregnancy Risk Factor Not assigned (similar agents rated C/D)

Generic Available No

Oxsoralen® *see* Methoxsalen *on page 790*

Oxsoralen-Ultra® *see* Methoxsalen *on page 790*

Oxy 10® Balanced Medicated Face Wash [OTC] *see* Benzoyl Peroxide *on page 153*

Oxybutynin (oks i BYOO ti nin)

U.S. Brand Names Ditropan®; Ditropan® XL

Canadian Brand Names Albert® Oxybutynin; Ditropan®; Gen-Oxybutynin; Novo-Oxybutynin; Nu-Oxybutyn; PMS-Oxybutynin

Mexican Brand Names Tavor®

Pharmacologic Category Antispasmodic Agent, Urinary

Synonyms Oxybutynin Chloride

Use Antispasmodic for neurogenic bladder (urgency, frequency, urge incontinence) and uninhibited bladder

Local Anesthetic/Vasoconstrictor Precautions No information available to require special precautions

Effects on Dental Treatment

>10%: Xerostomia

Prolonged use of oxybutynin may decrease or inhibit salivary flow; normal salivation returns with cessation of drug therapy.

Dosage Oral:

Children:

1-5 years: 0.2 mg/kg/dose 2-4 times/day

>5 years: 5 mg twice daily, up to 5 mg 4 times/day maximum

Adults: 5 mg 2-3 times/day up to 5 mg 4 times/day maximum

Elderly: 2.5-5 mg twice daily; increase by 2.5 mg increments every 1-2 days

Ditropan® XL (extended release): 5 mg or 10 mg once daily

Note: Should be discontinued periodically to determine whether the patient can manage without the drug and to minimize resistance to the drug

Mechanism of Action Direct antispasmodic effect on smooth muscle, also inhibits the action of acetylcholine on smooth muscle (exhibits $^1/_5$ the anticholinergic activity of atropine, but is 4-10 times the antispasmodic activity); does not block effects at skeletal muscle or at autonomic ganglia; increases bladder capacity, decreases uninhibited contractions, and delays desire to void; therefore, decreases urgency and frequency

Other Adverse Effects

>10%:

Central nervous system: Drowsiness

Gastrointestinal: Xerostomia, constipation

Miscellaneous: Diaphoresis (decreased)

1% to 10%:

Cardiovascular: Tachycardia, palpitations

Central nervous system: Dizziness, insomnia, fever, headache

Dermatologic: Rash

Endocrine & metabolic: Decreased flow of breast milk, decreased sexual ability, hot flashes

Gastrointestinal: Nausea, vomiting

Genitourinary: Urinary hesitancy or retention
Neuromuscular & skeletal: Weakness
Ocular: Blurred vision, mydriatic effect

Drug Interactions Increased Effect/Toxicity: Additive sedation with CNS depressants. Additive anticholinergic effects with antihistamines and anticholinergic agents.

Drug Uptake
Onset of action: Oral: 0.5-1 hour; Peak effect: 3-6 hours
Absorption: Oral: Rapid and well
Duration: 6-10 hours
Half-life, elimination: 1-2.3 hours
Time to peak: ~60 minutes

Pregnancy Risk Factor B

Generic Available Yes

Oxycel® *see* Cellulose, Oxidized *on page 250*

Oxychlorosene (oks i KLOR oh seen)

U.S. Brand Names Clorpactin® WCS-90 [OTC]

Pharmacologic Category Antibiotic, Topical

Synonyms Oxychlorosene Sodium

Use Treatment of localized infections

Local Anesthetic/Vasoconstrictor Precautions No information available to require special precautions

Effects on Dental Treatment No effects or complications reported

Dosage Topical (0.1% to 0.5% solutions): Apply by irrigation, instillation, spray, soaks, or wet compresses

Generic Available No

Comments Product is available as powder which must be diluted with sterile water or isotonic saline

Oxycodone (oks i KOE done)

Related Information
Oral Pain *on page 1360*

U.S. Brand Names Endocodone™; OxyContin®; OxyIR™; Percolone®; Roxicodone™; Roxicodone™ Intensol™

Canadian Brand Names OxyContin®; Oxy.IR®; Supeudol®

Mexican Brand Names OxyContin®

Pharmacologic Category Analgesic, Narcotic

Synonyms Dihydrohydroxycodeinone; Oxycodone Hydrochloride

Use
Dental: Treatment of postoperative pain
Medical: Around-the-clock management of moderate to severe pain when an analgesic is needed for an extended period of time.
OxyContin® is not intended for use as an "as needed" analgesic or for immediately-postoperative pain management; should be used postoperatively only if the patient has received it prior to surgery or if severe, persistent pain is anticipated.

Local Anesthetic/Vasoconstrictor Precautions No information available to require special precautions

Effects on Dental Treatment 1% to 10%: Xerostomia

Restrictions C-II

Dosage Oral:
Immediate release:
Children:
6-12 years: 1.25 mg every 6 hours as needed
>12 years: 2.5 mg every 6 hours as needed
Adults: 5 mg every 6 hours as needed
Controlled release: Adults:
Opioid naive (not currently on opioid): 10 mg every 12 hours
Currently on opioid/ASA or acetaminophen or NSAID combination:
1-5 tablets: 10-20 mg every 12 hours
6-9 tablets: 20-30 mg every 12 hours
10-12 tablets: 30-40 mg every 12 hours
May continue the nonopioid as a separate drug.
Currently on opioids: Use standard conversion chart to convert daily dose to oxycodone equivalent. Divide daily dose in 2 (for every 12-hour dosing) and round down to nearest dosage form.

Dosing adjustment in hepatic impairment: Reduce dosage with severe liver disease

Mechanism of Action Blocks pain perception in the cerebral cortex by binding to specific receptor molecules (opiate receptors) within the neuronal membranes of synapses; binding results in a decreased synaptic chemical transmission throughout the CNS, thus inhibiting the flow of pain sensations into the higher
(Continued)

Oxycodone *(Continued)*

centers, altering the perception of and response to pain. Mu and kappa are the two subtypes of the opiate receptor which oxycodone binds to cause analgesia.

Other Adverse Effects Deaths due to overdose have been reported due to misuse/abuse after crushing the sustained release tablets.

>10%:

- Cardiovascular: Hypotension
- Central nervous system: Fatigue, drowsiness, dizziness
- Gastrointestinal: Nausea, vomiting
- Neuromuscular & skeletal: Weakness

1% to 10%:

- Central nervous system: Nervousness, headache, restlessness, malaise, confusion
- Gastrointestinal: Anorexia, stomach cramps, xerostomia, constipation, biliary spasm
- Genitourinary: Ureteral spasms, decreased urination
- Local: Pain at injection site
- Respiratory: Dyspnea

<1%: Mental depression, hallucinations, paradoxical CNS stimulation, increased intracranial pressure, skin rash, urticaria, paralytic ileus, histamine release, physical and psychological dependence

Contraindications Hypersensitivity to oxycodone or any component of the formulation; significant respiratory depression; hypercarbia; acute or severe bronchial asthma; OxyContin® in paralytic ileus (known or suspected); pregnancy (prolonged use or high doses at term)

Warnings/Precautions Use with caution in patients with hypersensitivity reactions to other phenanthrene derivative opioid agonists (morphine, hydrocodone, hydromorphone, levorphanol, oxycodone, oxymorphone), respiratory diseases including asthma, emphysema, or COPD. Use with caution in pancreatitis or biliary tract disease, acute alcoholism (including delirium tremens), adrenocortical insufficiency, CNS depression/coma, kyphoscoliosis (or other skeletal disorder which may alter respiratory function), hypothyroidism (including myxedema), prostatic hypertrophy, urethral stricture, and toxic psychosis.

Use with caution in the elderly, debilitated, severe hepatic or renal function. Hemodynamic effects (hypotension, orthostasis) may be exaggerated in patients with hypovolemia, concurrent vasodilating drugs, or in patients with head injury. Respiratory depressant effects and capacity to elevate CSF pressure may be exaggerated in presence of head injury, other intracranial lesion, or pre-existing intracranial pressure. Tolerance or drug dependence may result from extended use. Healthcare provider should be alert to problems of abuse, misuse, and diversion. Do **not** crush controlled-release tablets. Some preparations contain sulfites which may cause allergic reactions. OxyContin® 80 mg and 160 mg strengths are for use only in opioid-tolerant patients requiring high daily dosages >160 mg (80 mg formulation) or >320 mg (160 mg formulation).

Drug Interactions CYP2D6 enzyme substrate

Increased Toxicity: CNS depressants, MAO inhibitors, general anesthetics, and tricyclic antidepressants may potentiate the effects of opiate agonists; dextroamphetamine may enhance the analgesic effect of opiate agonists

Decreased Effect: Phenothiazines may antagonize the analgesic effect of opiate agonists

Dietary/Ethanol/Herb Considerations

Ethanol: Avoid use; may cause CNS depression.

Herb/Nutraceutical: Avoid gotu kola, kava, SAMe, St John's wort, and valerian; may increase CNS depression.

Drug Uptake

Onset of action: Pain relief: 10-15 minutes; Peak effect: 0.5-1 hour

Duration: 3-6 hours; Controlled release: ≤12 hours

Half-life, elimination: 2-3 hours

Pregnancy Risk Factor B/D (prolonged use or high doses at term)

Dosage Forms CAP, immediate release (OxyIR™): 5 mg. **CONC, oral** (Roxicodone™ Intensol™): 20 mg/mL (30 mL). **LIQ** (Roxicodone™): 5 mg/5 mL (500 mL). **TAB:** (Endocodone™, Percolone®): 5 mg; (Roxicodone™): 5 mg, 15 mg, 30 mg. **TAB, controlled release** (OxyContin®): 10 mg, 20 mg, 40 mg, 80 mg, 160 mg

Generic Available Yes

Comments Prophylactic use of a laxative should be considered; oxycodone, as with other narcotic analgesics, is recommended only for limited acute dosing (ie, 3 days or less). The most common adverse effect is nausea, followed by sedation and constipation. Oxycodone has an addictive liability, especially when given long-term.

Selected Readings Wynn RL, "Narcotic Analgesics for Dental Pain: Available Products, Strengths, and Formulations," *Gen Dent*, 2001, 49(2)126-36.

Oxycodone and Acetaminophen

(oks i KOE done & a seet a MIN oh fen)

Related Information

Acetaminophen *on page 26*

Dental Drug Interactions: Update on Drug Combinations Requiring Special Considerations *on page 1434*

Oral Pain *on page 1360*

U.S. Brand Names Endocet®; Percocet® 2.5/325; Percocet® 5/325; Percocet® 7.5/325; Percocet® 7.5/500; Percocet® 10/325; Percocet® 10/650; Roxicet®; Roxicet® 5/500; Roxilox®; Tylox®

Canadian Brand Names Endocet®; Oxycocet®; Percocet®; Percocet®-Demi

Pharmacologic Category Analgesic, Narcotic

Synonyms Acetaminophen and Oxycodone

Use

Dental: Treatment of postoperative pain

Medical: Relief of pain

Local Anesthetic/Vasoconstrictor Precautions No information available to require special precautions

Effects on Dental Treatment 1% to 10%: Xerostomia

Restrictions C-II

Dosage Oral (doses should be titrated to appropriate analgesic effects):

Children: Oxycodone: 0.05-0.15 mg/kg/dose to 5 mg/dose (maximum) every 4-6 hours as needed

Adults: 1-2 tablets every 4-6 hours as needed for pain

Maximum daily dose of acetaminophen: 4 g/day

Dosing adjustment in hepatic impairment: Reduce dose with severe liver disease

Mechanism of Action Oxycodone, as with other narcotic (opiate) analgesics, blocks pain perception in the cerebral cortex by binding to specific receptor molecules (opiate receptors) within the neuronal membranes of synapses. This binding results in a decreased synaptic chemical transmission throughout the CNS thus inhibiting the flow of pain sensations into the higher centers. Mu and kappa are the two subtypes of the opiate receptor which oxycodone binds to to cause analgesia.

Acetaminophen inhibits the synthesis of prostaglandins in the CNS and peripherally blocks pain impulse generation; produces antipyresis from inhibition of hypothalamic heat-regulating center

Other Adverse Effects Also see Acetaminophen *on page 26* and Oxycodone *on page 901*

>10%:
- Cardiovascular: Hypotension
- Central nervous system: Fatigue, drowsiness, dizziness
- Gastrointestinal: Nausea, vomiting
- Neuromuscular & skeletal: Weakness

1% to 10%:
- Central nervous system: Nervousness, headache, restlessness, malaise, confusion
- Gastrointestinal: Anorexia, stomach cramps, xerostomia, constipation, biliary spasm
- Genitourinary: Ureteral spasms, decreased urination
- Local: Pain at injection site
- Respiratory: Dyspnea

<1%: Mental depression, hallucinations, paradoxical CNS stimulation, increased intracranial pressure, rash, urticaria, paralytic ileus, blood dyscrasias (neutropenia, pancytopenia, leukopenia), hepatic necrosis with overdosage, renal injury with chronic use, physical and psychological dependence, hypersensitivity reactions (rare), histamine release

Frequency not defined:
- Central nervous system: Dizziness, dysphoria, euphoria, lightheadedness, sedation,
- Dermatologic: Allergic reaction, pruritus, skin rash,
- Gastrointestinal: Constipation, nausea, vomiting
- Respiratory: Respiratory failure

Contraindications Hypersensitivity to oxycodone, acetaminophen, or any component of their formulation; severe respiratory depression (in absence of resuscitative equipment or ventilatory support); pregnancy (if used for prolonged periods or high doses at term)

Warnings/Precautions Use with caution in patients with hypersensitivity reactions to other phenanthrene-derivative opioid agonists (morphine, codeine, hydrocodone, hydromorphone, levorphanol, oxymorphone); respiratory diseases including asthma, emphysema, COPD, or severe liver or renal insufficiency, hypothyroidism, Addison's disease, prostatic hypertrophy, or urethral stricture; some preparations contain sulfites which may cause allergic reactions; may be habit-forming

(Continued)

Oxycodone and Acetaminophen *(Continued)*

Use with caution in patients with head injury and increased intracranial pressure (respiratory depressant effects increased and may also elevate CSF pressure). May mask diagnosis or clinical course in patients with acute abdominal conditions.

Enhanced analgesia has been seen in elderly patients on therapeutic doses of narcotics; duration of action may be increased in the elderly; the elderly may be particularly susceptible to the CNS depressant and constipating effects of narcotics

Drug Interactions

See Acetaminophen *on page 26* and Oxycodone *on page 901*

Acetaminophen: CYP1A2, 2C9, 2A6, 2D6, 2E1, and 3A3/4 enzyme substrate

Oxycodone: CYP2D6 enzyme substrate

Anesthetics, general: May have additive CNS depression; consider lowering dose of one or both agents

Anticholinergics: Concomitant use may lead to paralytic ileus

CNS depressants: May have additive CNS depression; consider lowering dose of one or both agents

Phenothiazines: May have additive CNS depression with phenothiazine and other tranquilizers; consider lowering dose of one or both agents

Sedative hypnotics: May have additive CNS depression; consider lowering dose of one or both agents

Dietary/Ethanol/Herb Considerations

Ethanol: Avoid use; may increase CNS depression. Excessive intake may increase the risk of acetaminophen-induced hepatotoxicity.

Herb/Nutraceutical: Avoid gotu kola, kava, SAMe, St John's wort, and valerian; may increase CNS depression.

Drug Uptake See Acetaminophen *on page 26* and Oxycodone *on page 901*

Pregnancy Risk Factor C (D if used for prolonged periods or high doses at term)

Breast-feeding Considerations

Oxycodone: Excreted in breast milk. If occasional doses are used during breast-feeding, monitor infant for sedation, GI effects and changes in feeding pattern.

Acetaminophen: May be taken while breast-feeding

Dosage Forms CAP: (Roxilox®): Oxycodone 5 mg and acetaminophen 500 mg; (Tylox®): Oxycodone 5 mg and acetaminophen 500 mg. **CAPLET** (Roxicet® 5/500): Oxycodone 5 mg and acetaminophen 500 mg. **SOLN, oral** (Roxicet®): Oxycodone 5 mg and acetaminophen 325 mg per 5 mL (5 mL, 500 mL). **TAB:** (Endocet®, Percocet® 5/325, Roxicet®): Oxycodone 5 mg and acetaminophen 325 mg; (Percocet® 2.5/325): Oxycodone 2.5 mg and acetaminophen 325 mg; (Percocet® 7.5/325): Oxycodone 7.5 mg and acetaminophen 325 mg; (Endocet®, Percocet® 7.5/500): Oxycodone 7.5 mg and acetaminophen 500 mg; (Percocet® 10/325): Oxycodone 10 mg and acetaminophen 325 mg; (Endocet®, Percocet® 10/650): Oxycodone 10 mg and acetaminophen 650 mg

Generic Available Yes

Comments Oxycodone, as with other narcotic analgesics, is recommended only for limited acute dosing (ie, 3 days or less). The most common adverse effect is nausea, followed by sedation and constipation. Oxycodone has an addictive liability, especially when given long-term. The acetaminophen component requires use with caution in patients with alcoholic liver disease.

Acetaminophen:

A study by Hylek, et al, suggested that the combination of acetaminophen with warfarin (Coumadin®) may cause enhanced anticoagulation. The following recommendations have been made by Hylek, et al, and supported by an editorial in *JAMA* by Bell.

Dose and duration of acetaminophen should be as low as possible, individualized and monitored

The study by Hylek reported the following:

For patients who reported taking the equivalent of at least 4 regular strength (325 mg) tablets for longer than a week, the odds of having an INR >6.0 were increased 10-fold above those not taking acetaminophen. Risk decreased with lower intakes of acetaminophen reaching a background level of risk at a dose of 6 or fewer 325 mg tablets per week.

Selected Readings

Bell WR, "Acetaminophen and Warfarin: Undesirable Synergy," *JAMA*, 1998, 279(9):702-3.

Botting RM, "Mechanism of Action of Acetaminophen: Is There a Cyclooxygenase 3?," *Clin Infect Dis*, 2000, Suppl 5:S202-10.

Cooper SA, Precheur H, Rauch D, et al, "Evaluation of Oxycodone and Acetaminophen in Treatment of Postoperative Pain," *Oral Surg Oral Med Oral Pathol*, 1980, 50(6):496-501.

Dart RC, Kuffner EK, and Rumack BH, "Treatment of Pain or Fever with Paracetamol (Acetaminophen) in the Alcoholic Patient: A Systematic Review," *Am J Ther*, 2000, 7(2):123-34.

Dionne RA, "New Approaches to Preventing and Treating Postoperative Pain," *J Am Dent Assoc*, 1992, 123(6):26-34.

Gobetti JP, "Controlling Dental Pain," *J Am Dent Assoc*, 1992, 123(6):47-52.

Grant JA and Weiler JM, "A Report of a Rare Immediate Reaction After Ingestion of Acetaminophen," *Ann Allergy Asthma Immunol*, 2001, 87(3):227-9.

Hylek EM, Heiman H, Skates SJ, et al, "Acetaminophen and Other Risk Factors for Excessive Warfarin Anticoagulation 1998," *JAMA*, 1998, 279(9):702-3.

Kwan D, Bartle WR, and Walker SE, "The Effects of Acetaminophen on Pharmacokinetics and Pharmacodynamics of Warfarin," *J Clin Pharmacol*, 1999, 39(1):68-75.

McClain CJ, Price S, Barve S, et al, "Acetaminophen Hepatotoxicity: An Update," *Curr Gastroenterol Rep*, 1999, 1(1):42-9.

Shek KL, Chan LN, and Nutescu E, "Warfarin-Acetaminophen Drug Interaction Revisited," *Pharmacotherapy*, 1999, 19(10):1153-8.

Tanaka E, Yamazaki K, and Misawa S, "Update: The Clinical Importance of Acetaminophen Hepatotoxicity in Nonalcoholic and Alcoholic Subjects," *J Clin Pharm Ther*, 2000, 25(5):325-32.

Wynn RL, "Narcotic Analgesics for Dental Pain: Available Products, Strengths, and Formulations," *Gen Dent*, 2001, 49(2):126-8, 130, 132 passim.

Oxycodone and Aspirin (oks i KOE done & AS pir in)

Related Information

Dental Drug Interactions: Update on Drug Combinations Requiring Special Considerations *on page 1434*

Oral Pain *on page 1360*

U.S. Brand Names Endodan®; Percodan®; Percodan®-Demi

Canadian Brand Names Endodan®; Oxycodan®; Percodan®; Percodan®-Demi

Pharmacologic Category Analgesic, Narcotic

Synonyms Aspirin and Oxycodone

Use

Dental: Treatment of postoperative pain

Medical: Relief of pain

Local Anesthetic/Vasoconstrictor Precautions No information available to require special precautions

Effects on Dental Treatment

1% to 10%: Xerostomia

Use with caution in patients with platelet and bleeding disorders, renal dysfunction, erosive gastritis, or peptic ulcer disease, previous nonreaction does not guarantee future safe taking of medication; use with caution in impaired hepatic function; do not use aspirin in children <16 years of age for chickenpox or flu symptoms due to the association with Reye's syndrome. Avoid aspirin, if possible, for 1 week prior to surgery due to possibility of postoperative bleeding.

Elderly are a high-risk population for adverse effects from nonsteroidal anti-inflammatory agents. As much as 60% of elderly with GI complications to NSAIDs can develop peptic ulceration and/or hemorrhage asymptomatically. Also, concomitant disease and drug use contribute to the risk for GI adverse effects. Use lowest effective dose for shortest period possible. Consider renal function decline with age. Use with caution in patients with history of asthma.

Restrictions C-II

Dosage Oral (based on oxycodone combined salts):

Children: 0.05-0.15 mg/kg/dose every 4-6 hours as needed; maximum: 5 mg/dose (1 tablet Percodan® or 2 tablets Percodan®-Demi/dose)

Adults: Percodan®: 1 tablet every 6 hours as needed for pain or Percodan®-Demi: 1-2 tablets every 6 hours as needed for pain

Dosing adjustment in hepatic impairment: Reduce dose with severe liver disease

Mechanism of Action Oxycodone, as with other narcotic (opiate) analgesics, blocks pain perception in the cerebral cortex by binding to specific receptor molecules (opiate receptors) within the neuronal membranes of synapses. This binding results in a decreased synaptic chemical transmission throughout the CNS thus inhibiting the flow of pain sensations into the higher centers. Mu and kappa are the two subtypes of the opiate receptor which oxycodone binds to cause analgesia.

Aspirin inhibits prostaglandin synthesis by decreasing the activity of the enzyme, cyclo-oxygenase, which results in decreased formation of prostaglandin precursors, acts on the hypothalamic heat-regulating center to reduce fever, blocks thromboxane synthetase action which prevents formation of the platelet-aggregating substance thromboxane A_2

Other Adverse Effects

>10%:

- Cardiovascular: Hypotension
- Central nervous system: Fatigue, drowsiness, dizziness
- Gastrointestinal: Nausea, vomiting, heartburn, stomach pains, dyspepsia
- Neuromuscular & skeletal: Weakness

1% to 10%:

- Central nervous system: Nervousness, headache, restlessness, malaise, confusion
- Dermatologic: Rash
- Gastrointestinal: Anorexia, stomach cramps, xerostomia, constipation, biliary spasm, gastrointestinal ulceration
- Genitourinary: Ureteral spasms, decreased urination
- Hematologic: Hemolytic anemia
- Local: Pain at injection site
- Respiratory: Dyspnea
- Miscellaneous: Anaphylactic shock

(Continued)

Oxycodone and Aspirin *(Continued)*

<1%: Mental depression, hallucinations, paradoxical CNS stimulation, increased intracranial pressure, insomnia, jitters, rash, urticaria, paralytic ileus, occult bleeding, prolongation of bleeding time, leukopenia, thrombocytopenia, iron-deficiency anemia, hepatotoxicity, impaired renal function, bronchospasm, physical and psychological dependence, histamine release

Contraindications Hypersensitivity to oxycodone, aspirin, or any component of their formulation; severe respiratory depression; pregnancy

Warnings/Precautions Use with caution in patients with hypersensitivity to other phenanthrene derivative opioid agonists (morphine, codeine, hydrocodone, hydromorphone, oxymorphone, levorphanol); children and teenagers should not be given aspirin products if chickenpox or flu symptoms are present; aspirin use has been associated with Reye's syndrome; severe liver or renal insufficiency, pre-existing CNS and depression

Enhanced analgesia has been seen in elderly patients on therapeutic doses of narcotics; duration of action may be increased in the elderly; the elderly may be particularly susceptible to the CNS depressant and constipating effects of narcotics

Drug Interactions

Increased effect/toxicity with CNS depressants, TCAs, dextroamphetamine

Decreased effect with phenothiazines

Dietary/Ethanol/Herb Considerations

Ethanol: Avoid use; may increase CNS depression and enhance gastric mucosal irritation.

Food: May be taken with food

Herb/Nutraceutical: Avoid gotu kola, kava, SAMe, St John's wort, and valerian; may increase CNS depression.

Drug Uptake See Aspirin *on page 119* and Oxycodone *on page 901*

Pregnancy Risk Factor D

Breast-feeding Considerations Aspirin: Caution is suggested due to potential adverse effects in nursing infants.

Dosage Forms TAB: (Endodan®, Percodan®): Oxycodone 4.5 mg, oxycodone 0.38 mg, and aspirin 325 mg; (Percodan®-Demi): Oxycodone 2.25 mg, oxycodone 0.19 mg, and aspirin 325 mg

Generic Available Yes

Comments Oxycodone, as with other narcotic analgesics, is recommended only for limited acute dosing (ie, 3 days or less). The most common adverse effect is nausea, followed by sedation and constipation. Oxycodone has an addictive liability, especially when given long-term. The oxycodone with aspirin could have anticoagulant effects and could possibly affect bleeding times.

Selected Readings

Dionne RA, "New Approaches to Preventing and Treating Postoperative Pain," *J Am Dent Assoc*, 1992, 123(6):26-34.

Gobetti JP, "Controlling Dental Pain," *J Am Dent Assoc*, 1992, 123(6):47-52.

Wynn RL, "Narcotic Analgesics for Dental Pain: Available Products, Strengths, and Formulations," *Gen Dent*, 2001, 49(2):126-8, 130, 132 passim.

OxyContin® *see* Oxycodone *on page 901*

Oxygen (OKS i jen)

Related Information

Dental Office Emergencies *on page 1418*

Pharmacologic Category Dental Gases

Use

Dental: Administered as a supplement with nitrous oxide to ensure adequate ventilation during sedation; a resuscitative agent for medical emergencies in dental office

Medical: Treatment of various clinical disorders, both respiratory and nonrespiratory; relief of arterial hypoxia and secondary complications; treatment of pulmonary hypertension, polycythemia secondary to hypoxemia, chronic disease states complicated by anemia, cancer, migraine headaches, coronary artery disease, seizure disorders, sickle-cell crisis and sleep apnea

Local Anesthetic/Vasoconstrictor Precautions No information available to require special precautions

Effects on Dental Treatment No effects or complications reported

Dosage Children and Adults: Average rate of 2 L/minute

Mechanism of Action Increases oxygen in tidal volume and oxygenation of tissues at molecular level

Warnings/Precautions Oxygen-induced hypoventilation is the greatest potential hazard of oxygen therapy. In patients with severe chronic obstructive pulmonary disease (COPD), the respiratory drive results from hypoxic stimulation of the carotid chemoreceptors. If this hypoxic drive is diminished by excessive oxygen therapy, hypoventilation may occur and further carbon dioxide retention with possible cessation of ventilation could result.

Dosage Forms LIQ, system: Large reservoir holding 75-100 lb of liquid oxygen with compressed gas system consisting of high-pressure tank; tank sizes are "H" (6900 L of oxygen), "E" (622 L of oxygen) and "D" (356 L of oxygen)

Generic Available Yes

OxyIR™ *see* Oxycodone *on page 901*

Oxymetazoline (oks i met AZ oh leen)

Related Information

Oral Bacterial Infections *on page 1367*

U.S. Brand Names Afrin® Children's Nose Drops [OTC]; Afrin® Sinus [OTC]; Allerest® 12 Hour Nasal [OTC]; Chlorphed®-LA Nasal [OTC]; Dristan® Long Lasting Nasal [OTC]; Duramist® Plus [OTC]; Duration® Nasal [OTC]; Nōstrilla® [OTC]; NTZ® Long Acting Nasal [OTC]; OcuClear® [OTC]; Sinarest® 12 Hour Nasal [OTC]; Twice-A-Day® Nasal [OTC]; Visine® L.R. [OTC]; 4-Way® Long Acting Nasal [OTC]

Canadian Brand Names Dristan® Long Lasting Nasal; Drixoral® Nasal

Mexican Brand Names Afrin®; Iliadin®; Ocuclear®; Oxylin®; Visine A.D.®

Pharmacologic Category Adrenergic Agonist Agent; Vasoconstrictor

Synonyms Oxymetazoline Hydrochloride

Use

Dental: Symptomatic relief of nasal mucosal congestion

Medical:

- Adjunctive therapy of middle ear infections, associated with acute or chronic rhinitis, the common cold, sinusitis, hay fever, or other allergies
- Ophthalmic: Relief of redness of eye due to minor eye irritations

Local Anesthetic/Vasoconstrictor Precautions No information available to require special precautions

Effects on Dental Treatment No effects or complications reported

Dosage

Intranasal (therapy should not exceed 3-5 days):

- Children 2-5 years: 0.025% solution: Instill 2-3 drops in each nostril twice daily
- Children ≥6 years and Adults: 0.05% solution: Instill 2-3 drops or 2-3 sprays into each nostril twice daily

Ophthalmic: Children >6 years and Adults: 0.025% solution: Instill 1-2 drops in affected eye(s) every 6 hours as needed or as directed by healthcare provider

Mechanism of Action Stimulates alpha-adrenergic receptors in the arterioles of the nasal mucosa to produce vasoconstriction

Other Adverse Effects

>10%:

- Local: Transient burning, stinging
- Respiratory: Dryness of the nasal mucosa, sneezing

1% to 10%:

- Cardiovascular: Hypertension, palpitations
- Respiratory: Rebound congestion with prolonged use

Contraindications Hypersensitivity to oxymetazoline or any component of the formulation

Warnings/Precautions Rebound congestion may occur with extended use (>3 days); use with caution in the presence of hypertension, diabetes, hyperthyroidism, heart disease, coronary artery disease, cerebral arteriosclerosis, or long-standing bronchial asthma

Drug Interactions Increased toxicity with MAO inhibitors

Drug Uptake

Onset of action: Intranasal: 5-10 minutes

Duration: 5-6 hours

Pregnancy Risk Factor C

Dosage Forms As hydrochloride: **DROPS, intranasal:** (Afrin® Children's Nose Drops): 0.025% (20 mL); (Afrin®, NTZ® Long Acting Nasal Solution): 0.05% (15 mL, 20 mL). **SOLN, ophthalmic:** (OcuClear®, Visine® L.R.): 0.025% (15 mL, 30 mL). **SPRAY, intranasal:** (Afrin® Sinus, Allerest® 12 Hours, Chlorphed®-LA, Dristan® Long Lasting, Duration®, 4-Way® Long Acting, Genasal®, Nasal Relief®, Neo-Synephrine® 12 Hour, Nōstrilla®, NTZ® Long Acting Nasal Solution, Twice-A-Day®): 0.05% (15 mL, 30 mL)

Generic Available Yes

Oxymetholone (oks i METH oh lone)

U.S. Brand Names Anadrol®

Pharmacologic Category Anabolic Steroid

Use Anemias caused by the administration of myelotoxic drugs

Local Anesthetic/Vasoconstrictor Precautions No information available to require special precautions

Effects on Dental Treatment No effects or complications reported

Restrictions C-III

Dosage Adults: Erythropoietic effects: Oral: 1-5 mg/kg/day in one daily dose; usual effective dose: 1-2 mg/kg/day; give for a minimum trial of 3-6 months because response may be delayed

(Continued)

Oxymetholone *(Continued)*

Dosing adjustment in hepatic impairment:

Mild to moderate hepatic impairment: Oxymetholone should be used with caution in patients with liver dysfunction because of it's hepatotoxic potential

Severe hepatic impairment: Oxymetholone should **not** be used

Mechanism of Action Stimulates receptors in organs and tissues to promote growth and development of male sex organs and maintains secondary sex characteristics in androgen-deficient males

Other Adverse Effects

Male:

Postpubertal:

>10%:

Dermatologic: Acne

Endocrine & metabolic: Gynecomastia

Genitourinary: Bladder irritability, priapism

1% to 10%:

Central nervous system: Insomnia, chills

Endocrine & metabolic: Decreased libido

Gastrointestinal: Nausea, diarrhea

Genitourinary: Prostatic hyperplasia (elderly)

Hematologic: Iron-deficiency anemia, suppression of clotting factors

Hepatic: Hepatic dysfunction

Prepubertal:

>10%:

Dermatologic: Acne

Endocrine & metabolic: Virilism

1% to 10%:

Central nervous system: Chills, insomnia

Dermatologic: Hyperpigmentation

Gastrointestinal: Diarrhea, nausea

Hematologic: Iron-deficiency anemia, suppression of clotting factors

Female:

>10%: Endocrine & metabolic: Virilism

1% to 10%:

Central nervous system: Chills, insomnia

Endocrine & metabolic: Hypercalcemia

Gastrointestinal: Nausea, diarrhea

Hematologic: Iron-deficiency anemia, suppression of clotting factors

Hepatic: Hepatic dysfunction

Drug Interactions Increased Effect/Toxicity: Oxymetholone may increase prothrombin times with patients receiving warfarin leading to toxicity. Insulin effects may be enhanced leading to hypoglycemia.

Drug Uptake

Onset of action: 2-6 months

Half-life, elimination: 9 hours

Pregnancy Risk Factor X

Generic Available No

Oxymorphone (oks i MOR fone)

U.S. Brand Names Numorphan®

Canadian Brand Names Numorphan®

Pharmacologic Category Analgesic, Narcotic

Synonyms Oxymorphone Hydrochloride

Use Management of moderate to severe pain and preoperatively as a sedative and a supplement to anesthesia

Local Anesthetic/Vasoconstrictor Precautions No information available to require special precautions

Effects on Dental Treatment Anticholinergic side effects can cause a reduction of saliva production or secretion contributes to discomfort and dental disease (ie, caries, oral candidiasis and periodontal disease).

Restrictions C-II

Dosage Adults:

I.M., S.C.: 0.5 mg initially, 1-1.5 mg every 4-6 hours as needed

I.V.: 0.5 mg initially

Rectal: 5 mg every 4-6 hours

Mechanism of Action Oxymorphone hydrochloride (Numorphan®) is a potent narcotic analgesic with uses similar to those of morphine. The drug is a semisynthetic derivative of morphine (phenanthrene derivative) and is closely related to hydromorphone chemically (Dilaudid®).

Other Adverse Effects

>10%:

Cardiovascular: Hypotension

Central nervous system: Fatigue, drowsiness, dizziness

Gastrointestinal: Nausea, vomiting, constipation

Neuromuscular & skeletal: Weakness
Miscellaneous: Histamine release
1% to 10%:
Central nervous system: Nervousness, headache, restlessness, malaise, confusion
Gastrointestinal: Anorexia, stomach cramps, xerostomia, biliary spasm
Genitourinary: Decreased urination, ureteral spasms
Local: Pain at injection site
Respiratory: Dyspnea

Drug Interactions
Increased Effect/Toxicity: Increased effect/toxicity with CNS depressants (phenothiazines, tranquilizers, anxiolytics, sedatives, hypnotics, alcohol), tricyclic antidepressants, and dextroamphetamine.
Decreased Effect: Decreased effect with phenothiazines.

Drug Uptake
Onset of action: Analgesic: I.V., I.M., S.C.: 5-10 minutes; Rectal: 15-30 minutes
Duration: Analgesic: Parenteral, rectal: 3-4 hours

Pregnancy Risk Factor B/D (prolonged use or high doses at term)
Generic Available No

Oxyphencyclimine (oks i fen SYE kli meen)

U.S. Brand Names Daricon®
Pharmacologic Category Anticholinergic Agent; Antispasmodic Agent, Gastrointestinal
Synonyms Oxyphencyclimine Hydrochloride
Use Adjunctive treatment of peptic ulcer
Local Anesthetic/Vasoconstrictor Precautions No information available to require special precautions
Effects on Dental Treatment >10%: Xerostomia
Dosage Children >12 years and Adults: Oral: 10 mg twice daily or 5 mg 3 times/day
Other Adverse Effects
>10%:
Dermatologic: Dry skin
Gastrointestinal: Constipation, dry throat, xerostomia
Respiratory: Dry nose
Miscellaneous: Decreased diaphoresis
1% to 10%:
Dermatologic: Increased sensitivity to light
Gastrointestinal: Dysphagia

Drug Interactions
Increased Effect/Toxicity: Increased anticholinergic side effects by amantadine.
Decreases effects of phenothiazines, antiparkinsonian drugs, and haloperidol.

Pregnancy Risk Factor C
Generic Available No

Oxytetracycline (oks i tet ra SYE kleen)

U.S. Brand Names Terramycin® I.M.
Canadian Brand Names Terramycin®
Mexican Brand Names Oxitraklin; Terramicina
Pharmacologic Category Antibiotic, Tetracycline Derivative
Synonyms Oxytetracycline Hydrochloride
Use Treatment of susceptible bacterial infections; both gram-positive and gram-negative, as well as, *Rickettsia* and *Mycoplasma* organisms
Local Anesthetic/Vasoconstrictor Precautions No information available to require special precautions
Effects on Dental Treatment Tetracyclines are not recommended for use during pregnancy or in children ≤8 years of age since they have been reported to cause enamel hypoplasia and permanent teeth discoloration. Tetracyclines should only be used in these patients if other agents are contraindicated or alternative antimicrobials will not eradicate the organism. Long-term use associated with oral candidiasis.

Dosage
Oral:
Children >8 years: 40-50 mg/kg/day in divided doses every 6 hours (maximum: 2 g/24 hours)
Adults: 250-500 mg/dose every 6-12 hours depending on severity of the infection
I.M.:
Children >8 years: 15-25 mg/kg/day (maximum: 250 mg/dose) in divided doses every 8-12 hours
Adults: 250 mg every 24 hours or 300 mg/day divided every 8-12 hours
Syphilis: 30-40 g in divided doses over 10-15 days
Gonorrhea: 1.5 g, then 500 mg every 6 hours for total of 9 g
Uncomplicated chlamydial infections: 500 mg every 6 hours for 7 days
Severe acne: 1 g/day then decrease to 125-500 mg/day
(Continued)

Oxytetracycline *(Continued)*

Dosing interval in renal impairment:
Cl_{cr} <10 mL/minute: Administer every 24 hours or avoid use if possible

Dosing adjustment/comments in hepatic impairment: Avoid use in patients with severe liver disease

Mechanism of Action Inhibits bacterial protein synthesis by binding with the 30S and possibly the 50S ribosomal subunit(s) of susceptible bacteria, cell wall synthesis is not affected

Other Adverse Effects

>10%: Miscellaneous: Discoloration of teeth and enamel hypoplasia (infants)

1% to 10%:
- Dermatologic: Photosensitivity
- Gastrointestinal: Nausea, diarrhea

Drug Interactions

Increased Effect/Toxicity: Oral anticoagulant (warfarin) effects may be increased.

Decreased Effect: Antacids containing aluminum, calcium or magnesium, as well as iron and bismuth subsalicylate may decrease bioavailability of tetracyclines. Barbiturates, phenytoin, and carbamazepine decrease serum concentration of tetracyclines.

Drug Uptake

Absorption: Oral: Adequate (~75%); I.M.: Poor

Half-life, elimination: 8.5-9.6 hours (increases with renal impairment)

Time to peak: 2-4 hours

Pregnancy Risk Factor D

Generic Available Yes

Oxytetracycline and Hydrocortisone

(oks i tet ra SYE kleen & hye droe KOR ti sone)

U.S. Brand Names Terra-Cortril®

Pharmacologic Category Antibiotic/Corticosteroid, Ophthalmic

Synonyms Hydrocortisone and Oxytetracycline

Use Treatment of susceptible ophthalmic bacterial infections with associated swelling

Local Anesthetic/Vasoconstrictor Precautions No information available to require special precautions

Effects on Dental Treatment No effects or complications reported

Dosage Ophthalmic: Adults: Instill 1-2 drops in eye(s) every 3-4 hours

Drug Uptake See Oxytetracycline *on page 909* and Hydrocortisone *on page 608*

Pregnancy Risk Factor C

Generic Available No

Oxytetracycline and Polymyxin B

(oks i tet ra SYE kleen & pol i MIKS in bee)

U.S. Brand Names Terramycin® w/Polymyxin B Ophthalmic

Pharmacologic Category Antibiotic, Ophthalmic; Antibiotic, Otic

Synonyms Polymyxin B and Oxytetracycline

Use Treatment of superficial ocular infections involving the conjunctiva and/or cornea

Local Anesthetic/Vasoconstrictor Precautions No information available to require special precautions

Effects on Dental Treatment No effects or complications reported

Dosage Topical: Apply ½" of ointment onto the lower lid of affected eye 2-4 times/day

Drug Uptake See Oxytetracycline *on page 909* and Polymyxin B *on page 971*

Pregnancy Risk Factor D

Generic Available No

Oxytocin (oks i TOE sin)

U.S. Brand Names Pitocin®

Canadian Brand Names Pitocin®; Syntocinon®

Mexican Brand Names Oxitopisa; Syntocinon®; Xitocin

Pharmacologic Category Oxytocic Agent

Synonyms Pit

Use Induces labor at term; controls postpartum bleeding; nasal preparation used to promote milk letdown in lactating females

Local Anesthetic/Vasoconstrictor Precautions No information available to require special precautions

Effects on Dental Treatment No effects or complications reported

Dosage I.V. administration requires the use of an infusion pump

Adults:

Induction of labor: I.V.: 0.001-0.002 units/minute; increase by 0.001-0.002 units every 15-30 minutes until contraction pattern has been established; maximum dose should not exceed 20 milliunits/minute

Postpartum bleeding:

I.M.: Total dose of 10 units after delivery

I.V.: 10-40 units by I.V. infusion in 1000 mL of I.V. fluid at a rate sufficient to control uterine atony

Promotion of milk letdown: Intranasal: 1 spray or 3 drops in one or both nostrils 2-3 minutes before breast-feeding

Mechanism of Action Produces the rhythmic uterine contractions characteristic to delivery and stimulates breast milk flow during nursing

Drug Interactions Sympathomimetic pressor effects may be increased by oxytocin resulting in postpartum hypertension.

Drug Uptake

Onset of action: Uterine contractions: I.V.: ~1 minute

Duration: <30 minutes

Half-life, elimination: 1-5 minutes

Pregnancy Risk Factor X

Generic Available Yes

Oyst-Cal 500 [OTC] *see* Calcium Carbonate *on page 201*

Oystercal® 500 *see* Calcium Carbonate *on page 201*

Pacerone® *see* Amiodarone *on page 72*

Paclitaxel (PAK li taks el)

U.S. Brand Names Taxol®

Canadian Brand Names Taxol®

Mexican Brand Names Bris Taxol®; Praxel®

Pharmacologic Category Antineoplastic Agent, Natural Source (Plant) Derivative

Use Treatment of metastatic carcinoma of the ovary after failure of first-line or subsequent chemotherapy; treatment of metastatic breast cancer; in combination with cisplatin for the first-line treatment of nonsmall cell lung cancer in patients who are not candidates for potentially curative surgery and/or radiation therapy; adjuvant treatment of node-positive breast cancer administered sequentially to standard doxorubicin-containing combination therapy

Local Anesthetic/Vasoconstrictor Precautions No information available to require special precautions

Effects on Dental Treatment No effects or complications reported

Mechanism of Action Paclitaxel exerts its effects on microtubules and their protein subunits, tubulin dimers. Microtubules serve as facilitators of intracellular transport and maintain the integrity and function of cells. Paclitaxel promotes microtubule assembly by enhancing the action of tubulin dimers, stabilizing existing microtubules, and inhibiting their disassembly. Maintaining microtubule assembly inhibits mitosis and cell death. The G_2- and M-phases of the cell cycle are affected. In addition, the drug can distort mitotic spindles, resulting in the breakage of chromosomes.

Other Adverse Effects

>10%:

Allergic: Appear to be primarily nonimmunologically mediated release of histamine and other vasoactive substances; almost always seen within the first hour of an infusion (~75% occur within 10 minutes of starting the infusion); incidence is significantly reduced by premedication

Cardiovascular: Bradycardia (transient, 25%)

Hematologic: Myelosuppression, leukopenia, neutropenia (6% to 21%), thrombocytopenia

Onset: 8-11 days

Nadir: 15-21 days

Recovery: 21 days

Dermatologic: Alopecia (87%), venous erythema, tenderness, discomfort, phlebitis (2%)

Neurotoxicity: Sensory and/or autonomic neuropathy (numbness, tingling, burning pain), myopathy or myopathic effects (25% to 55%), and central nervous system toxicity. May be cumulative and dose-limiting.

Gastrointestinal: Severe, potentially dose-limiting mucositis, stomatitis (15%), most common at doses >390 mg/m^2

Hepatic: Mild increases in liver enzymes

Neuromuscular & skeletal: Arthralgia, myalgia

1% to 10%:

Cardiovascular: Myocardial infarction

Gastrointestinal: Mild nausea and vomiting (5% to 6%), diarrhea (5% to 6%)

Hematologic: Anemia

Drug Interactions CYP2C8 and 3A3/4 enzyme substrate

Increased Effect/Toxicity: In Phase I trials, myelosuppression was more profound when given after cisplatin than with alternative sequence. Pharmacokinetic data demonstrates a decrease in clearance of ~33% when administered following cisplatin. Possibility of an inhibition of metabolism in patients treated with ketoconazole. When administered as sequential infusions, observational studies indicate a potential for increased toxicity when platinum derivatives (carboplatin, cisplatin) are administered before taxane derivatives (docetaxel, paclitaxel).

(Continued)

Paclitaxel *(Continued)*

Decreased Effect: Paclitaxel metabolism is dependent on cytochrome P450 isoenzymes. Inducers of these enzymes may decrease the effect of paclitaxel.

Drug Uptake Administered by I.V. infusion; exhibits a biphasic decline in plasma concentrations

Half-life, elimination, mean: Terminal: 5.3-17.4 hours after 1- and 6-hour infusions at dosing levels of 15-275 mg/m^2

Pregnancy Risk Factor D

Generic Available No

Palgic®-D *see* Carbinoxamine and Pseudoephedrine *on page 221*

Palgic®-DS *see* Carbinoxamine and Pseudoephedrine *on page 221*

Palivizumab (pah li VIZ u mab)

U.S. Brand Names Synagis®

Pharmacologic Category Monoclonal Antibody

Use Prevention of serious lower respiratory tract disease caused by respiratory syncytial virus (RSV) in pediatric patients at high risk of RSV disease; safety and efficacy were established in infants with bronchopulmonary dysplasia (BPD) and infants with a history of prematurity ≤35 weeks gestational age

Local Anesthetic/Vasoconstrictor Precautions No information available to require special precautions

Effects on Dental Treatment No effects or complications reported

Dosage Children: I.M.: 15 mg/kg of body weight, monthly throughout RSV season (First dose administered prior to commencement of RSV season)

Mechanism of Action Exhibits neutralizing and fusion-inhibitory activity against RSV; these activities inhibit RSV replication in laboratory and clinical studies

Other Adverse Effects The incidence of adverse events was similar between the palivizumab and placebo groups.

>1%:

- Central nervous system: Nervousness
- Dermatologic: Fungal dermatitis, eczema, seborrhea, rash
- Gastrointestinal: Diarrhea, vomiting, gastroenteritis
- Hematologic: Anemia
- Hepatic: ALT increase, abnormal LFTs
- Local: Injection site reaction, erythema, induration
- Ocular: Conjunctivitis
- Otic: Otitis media
- Respiratory: Cough, wheezing, bronchiolitis, pneumonia, bronchitis, asthma, croup, dyspnea, sinusitis, apnea, upper respiratory infection, rhinitis
- Miscellaneous: Oral moniliasis, failure to thrive, viral infection, flu syndrome

Drug Uptake

Half-life, elimination: Children <24 months: 20 days; Adults: 18 days

Time to peak: 48 hours

Pregnancy Risk Factor C

Generic Available No

Selected Readings

Johnson S, Oliver C, Prince GA, et al, "Development of a Humanized Monoclonal Antibody (MEDI-493) With Potent *In Vitro* and *In Vivo* Activity Against Respiratory Syncytial Virus," *J Infect Dis*, 1997, 176(5):1215-24.

Subramanian KN, Weisman, LE, Rhodes T, et al, "Safety, Tolerance and Pharmacokinetics of a Humanized Monoclonal Antibody to Respiratory Syncytial Virus in Premature Infants With Bronchopulmonary Dysplasia. MEDI-493 Study Group," *Pediatr Infect Dis J*, 1998, 17(2):110-5.

Welliver RC, "Respiratory Syncytial Virus Immunoglobulin and Monoclonal Antibodies in the Prevention and Treatment of Respiratory Syncytial Virus Infection," *Semin Perinatol*, 1998, 22(1):87-95.

Palmer's® Skin Success Acne [OTC] *see* Benzoyl Peroxide *on page 153*

Palmitate-A® [OTC] *see* Vitamin A *on page 1243*

PALS® [OTC] *see* Chlorophyll *on page 265*

Pamelor® *see* Nortriptyline *on page 878*

Pamidronate (pa mi DROE nate)

U.S. Brand Names Aredia®

Canadian Brand Names Aredia®

Pharmacologic Category Antidote; Bisphosphonate Derivative

Synonyms Pamidronate Disodium

Use Treatment of hypercalcemia associated with malignancy; treatment of osteolytic bone lesions associated with multiple myeloma or metastatic breast cancer; moderate to severe Paget's disease of bone

Local Anesthetic/Vasoconstrictor Precautions No information available to require special precautions

Effects on Dental Treatment No effects or complications reported

Dosage Drug must be diluted properly before administration and infused slow I.V.

I.V.: Adults:

Hypercalcemia of malignancy:

Moderate cancer-related hypercalcemia (corrected serum calcium: 12-13.5 mg/dL): 60-90 mg, as a single dose, given as a slow infusion over 2-24 hours; dose should be diluted in 1000 mL 0.45% NaCl, 0.9% NaCl, or D_5W

Severe cancer-related hypercalcemia (corrected serum calcium: >13.5 mg/dL): 90 mg, as a single dose, as a slow infusion over 2-24 hours; dose should be diluted in 1000 mL 0.45% NaCl, 0.9% NaCl, or D_5W

A period of 7 days should elapse before the use of second course; repeat infusions every 2-3 weeks have been suggested, however, could be administered every 2-3 months according to the degree and of severity of hypercalcemia and/or the type of malignancy.

Note: Some investigators have suggested a lack of a dose-response relationship. Courses of pamidronate for hypercalcemia may be repeated at varying intervals, depending on the duration of normocalcemia (median 2-3 weeks), but the manufacturer recommends a minimum interval between courses of 7 days. Oral etidronate at a dose of 20 mg/kg/day has been used to maintain the calcium lowering effect following I.V. bisphosphonates, although it is of limited effectiveness.

Osteolytic bone lesions with multiple myeloma: 90 mg in 500 mL D_5W, 0.45% NaCl or 0.9% NaCl administered over 4 hours on a monthly basis

Osteolytic bone lesions with metastatic breast cancer: 90 mg in 250 mL D_5W, 0.45% NaCl or 0.9% NaCl administered over 2 hours, repeated every 3-4 weeks

Paget's disease: 30 mg in 500 mL 0.45% NaCl, 0.9% NaCl or D_5W administered over 4 hours for 3 consecutive days

Mechanism of Action A biphosphonate which inhibits bone resorption via actions on osteoclasts or on osteoclast precursors. Does not appear to produce any significant effects on renal tubular calcium handling and is poorly absorbed following oral administration (high oral doses have been reported effective); therefore, I.V. therapy is preferred.

Other Adverse Effects As reported with hypercalcemia of malignancy; percentage of adverse effect varies upon dose and duration of infusion.

>10%:

Central nervous system: Fever (18% to 26%), fatigue (12%)

Endocrine & metabolic: Hypophosphatemia (9% to 18%), hypokalemia (4% to 18%), hypomagnesemia (4% to 12%), hypocalcemia (1% to 12%)

Gastrointestinal: Nausea (0% to 18%), anorexia (1% to 12%)

Local: Infusion site reaction (0% to 18%)

1% to 10%:

Cardiovascular: Atrial fibrillation (0% to 6%), hypertension (0% to 6%), syncope (0% to 6%), tachycardia (0% to 6%), atrial flutter (0% to 1%), cardiac failure (0% to 1%)

Central nervous system: Somnolence (1% to 6%), psychosis (0% to 4%), insomnia (0% to 1%)

Endocrine & metabolic: Hypothyroidism (6%)

Gastrointestinal: Constipation (4% to 6%), stomatitis (0% to 1%)

Hematologic: Leukopenia (0% to 4%), neutropenia (0% to 1%), thrombocytopenia (0% to 1%)

Neuromuscular & skeletal: Myalgia (0% to 1%)

Renal: Uremia (0% to 4%)

Respiratory: Rales (0% to 6%), rhinitis (0% to 6%), upper respiratory tract infection (0% to 3%)

Drug Uptake

Onset of action: 24-48 hours; Peak effect: Maximum: 5-7 days

Absorption: Poor (pharmacokinetic studies lacking)

Half-life, elimination: 21-35 hours; Bone: Terminal: ~300 days

Pregnancy Risk Factor C

Generic Available Yes

Pamine® *see* Methscopolamine *on page 791*

Pan-2400™ [OTC] *see* Pancreatin *on page 913*

Pancrease® *see* Pancrelipase *on page 914*

Pancrease® MT *see* Pancrelipase *on page 914*

Pancreatin (PAN kree a tin)

U.S. Brand Names Hi-Vegi-Lip® [OTC]; Kutrase®; Ku-Zyme®; Pan-2400™ [OTC]; Pancreatin 4X [OTC]; Pancreatin 8X [OTC]; Veg-Pancreatin 4X [OTC]

Mexican Brand Names Creon®; Optifree®; Pancrease®; Selecto®

Pharmacologic Category Enzyme

Use Replacement therapy in symptomatic treatment of malabsorption syndrome caused by pancreatic insufficiency

Local Anesthetic/Vasoconstrictor Precautions No information available to require special precautions

Effects on Dental Treatment No effects or complications reported

(Continued)

Pancreatin *(Continued)*

Dosage The following dosage recommendations are only an approximation for initial dosages. The actual dosage will depend on the digestive requirements of the individual patient.

Children:

<1 year: 2000 units of lipase with meals/feedings

1-6 years: 4000-8000 units of lipase with meals and 4000 units with snacks

7-12 years: 4000-12,000 units of lipase with meals and snacks

Adults: 4000-16,000 units of lipase with meals and with snacks

Mechanism of Action An enzyme supplement, not a replacement, which contains a combination of lipase, amylase and protease. Enhances the digestion of proteins, starch and fat in the stomach and intestines.

Other Adverse Effects Frequency not defined:

Gastrointestinal: Loose stools (decrease dose)

Respiratory: Mucous membrane irritation or precipitation of asthma attack (due to inhalation of airborne powder)

Pregnancy Risk Factor C

Generic Available Yes

Comments On a weight basis, pancreatin has 1/12 the lipolytic activity of pancrelipase

Pancreatin 4X [OTC] *see* Pancreatin *on page 913*

Pancreatin 8X [OTC] *see* Pancreatin *on page 913*

Pancrecarb MS® *see* Pancrelipase *on page 914*

Pancrelipase (pan kre LI pase)

U.S. Brand Names Creon®; Ku-Zyme® HP; Lipram®; Lipram® 4500; Lipram-CR®; Lipram-PN®; Lipram-UL®; Pancrease®; Pancrease® MT; Pancrecarb MS®; Pangestyme™ CN; Pangestyme™ EC; Pangestyme™ MT; Pangestyme™ UL; Ultrase®; Ultrase® MT; Viokase®; Zymase® [DSC]

Canadian Brand Names Cotazym®; Creon® 5; Creon® 10; Creon® 20; Creon® 25; Pancrease®; Pancrease® MT; Ultrase®; Ultrase® MT; Viokase®

Pharmacologic Category Enzyme

Synonyms Lipancreatin

Use Replacement therapy in symptomatic treatment of malabsorption syndrome caused by pancreatic insufficiency

Unlabeled/Investigational: Treatment of occluded feeding tubes

Local Anesthetic/Vasoconstrictor Precautions No information available to require special precautions

Effects on Dental Treatment No effects or complications reported

Dosage Oral:

Powder: Actual dose depends on the digestive requirements of the patient

Children <1 year: Start with 1/8 teaspoonful with feedings

Adults: 0.7 g with meals

Enteric coated microspheres and microtablets: The following dosage recommendations are only an approximation for initial dosages. The actual dosage will depend on the digestive requirements of the individual patient.

Children:

<1 year: 2000 units of lipase with meals

1-6 years: 4000-8000 units of lipase with meals and 4000 units with snacks

7-12 years: 4000-12,000 units of lipase with meals and snacks

Adults: 4000-16,000 units of lipase with meals and with snacks or 1-3 tablets/capsules before or with meals and snacks; in severe deficiencies, dose may be increased to 8 tablets/capsules

Occluded feeding tubes: 1 tablet of Viokase® crushed with one 325 mg tablet of sodium bicarbonate (to activate the Viokase®) in 5 mL of water can be instilled into the nasogastric tube and clamped for 5 minutes; then, flushed with 50 mL of tap water

Mechanism of Action A natural product harvested from the hog pancreas. It contains a combination of lipase, amylase, and protease. Products are formulated to dissolve in the more basic pH of the duodenum so that they may act locally to break down fats, protein, and starch.

Other Adverse Effects Frequency not defined; may be dose related.

Central nervous system: Pain

Dermatologic: Rash

Endocrine & metabolic: Hyperuricemia

Gastrointestinal: Nausea, cramps, constipation, diarrhea, perianal irritation/inflammation (large doses), irritation of the mouth, abdominal pain, intestinal obstruction, vomiting, flatulence, melena, weight loss, fibrotic strictures, greasy stools

Ocular: Lacrimation

Renal: Hyperuricosuria

Respiratory: Sneezing, dyspnea, bronchospasm

Miscellaneous: Allergic reactions

Drug Interactions Calcium carbonate, magnesium hydroxide may decrease the effect of pancrelipase.

Drug Uptake Absorption: Not absorbed; acts locally in GI tract

Pregnancy Risk Factor B/C (product specific)

Generic Available Yes

Comments Concomitant administration of conventional pancreatin enzymes with an H_2-receptor antagonist has been used to decrease the inactivation of enzyme activity.

Pandel® *see* Hydrocortisone *on page 608*
Pangestyme™ CN *see* Pancrelipase *on page 914*
Pangestyme™ EC *see* Pancrelipase *on page 914*
Pangestyme™ MT *see* Pancrelipase *on page 914*
Pangestyme™ UL *see* Pancrelipase *on page 914*
Panglobulin® *see* Immune Globulin, Intravenous *on page 630*
Panhematin® *see* Hemin *on page 580*
PanOxyl® *see* Benzoyl Peroxide *on page 153*
PanOxyl®-AQ *see* Benzoyl Peroxide *on page 153*
PanOxyl® Bar [OTC] *see* Benzoyl Peroxide *on page 153*
Panretin® *see* Alitretinoin *on page 52*
Panscol® [OTC] *see* Salicylic Acid *on page 1072*
Panthoderm® Cream [OTC] *see* Dexpanthenol *on page 368*

Pantoprazole (pan TOE pra zole)

Related Information

Gastrointestinal Disorders *on page 1326*

U.S. Brand Names Protonix®

Canadian Brand Names Panto™ IV; Pantoloc™; Protonix®

Mexican Brand Names Pantozol®; Zurcal®

Pharmacologic Category Proton Pump Inhibitor

Use

Oral: Treatment and maintenance of healing of erosive esophagitis associated with GERD; reduction in relapse rates of daytime and nighttime heartburn symptoms in GERD; hypersecretory disorders associated with Zollinger-Ellison syndrome or other neoplastic disorders

I.V.: As an alternative to oral therapy in patients unable to continue oral pantoprazole; hypersecretory disorders associated with Zollinger-Ellison syndrome or other neoplastic disorders

Unlabeled/Investigational: Peptic ulcer disease, active ulcer bleeding with parenterally-administered pantoprazole; adjunct treatment with antibiotics for *Helicobacter pylori*

Local Anesthetic/Vasoconstrictor Precautions No information available to require special precautions

Effects on Dental Treatment No effects or complications reported

Dosage Adults:

Oral:

Erosive esophagitis associated with GERD:

Treatment: 40 mg once daily for up to 8 weeks; an additional 8 weeks may be used in patients who have not healed after an 8-week course

Maintenance of healing: 40 mg once daily

Note: Lower doses (20 mg once daily) have been used successfully in mild GERD treatment and maintenance of healing

Hypersecretory disorders (including Zollinger-Ellison): Initial: 40 mg twice daily; adjust dose based on patient needs; doses up to 240 mg/day have been administered

I.V.:

Erosive esophagitis associated with GERD: 40 mg once daily (infused over 15 minutes) for 7-10 days

Helicobacter pylori eradication (unlabeled use): Doses up to 40 mg twice daily have been used as part of combination therapy

Hypersecretory disorders: 80 mg twice daily; adjust dose based on acid output measurements; 160-240 mg/day in divided doses has been used for a limited period (up to 7 days)

Mechanism of Action Suppresses gastric acid secretion by inhibiting the parietal cell H+/K+ ATP pump

Other Adverse Effects 1% to 10%:

Cardiovascular: Chest pain (I.V. ≤6%)

Central nervous system: Pain, migraine, anxiety, dizziness, headache (I.V. >1%)

Dermatologic: Rash (I.V. 6%), pruritus (I.V. 4%)

Endocrine & metabolic: Hyperglycemia (1%), hyperlipidemia

Gastrointestinal: Diarrhea (4%), constipation, dyspepsia, gastroenteritis, nausea, rectal disorder, vomiting, abdominal pain (I.V. 12%)

Genitourinary: Urinary frequency, urinary tract infection

Hepatic: Liver function test abnormality, increased SGPT

(Continued)

Pantoprazole *(Continued)*

Local: Injection site pain (>1%)
Neuromuscular & skeletal: Weakness, back pain, neck pain, arthralgia, hypertonia
Respiratory: Bronchitis, increased cough, dyspnea, pharyngitis, rhinitis, sinusitis, upper respiratory tract infection
Miscellaneous: Flu syndrome, infection

Drug Interactions CYP2C19 and 3A3/4 enzyme substrate

Drugs (eg, itraconazole, ketoconazole, and other azole antifungals, ampicillin esters, iron salts) where absorption is determined by an acidic gastric pH, may have decreased absorption when used concurrently. Monitor for change in effectiveness.

Drug Uptake

Absorption: Well absorbed
Half-life, elimination: 1 hour
Time to peak: Oral: 2.5 hours

Pregnancy Risk Factor B

Generic Available No

Pantothenic Acid (pan toe THEN ik AS id)

Pharmacologic Category Vitamin

Synonyms Calcium Pantothenate; Vitamin B_5

Use Pantothenic acid deficiency

Local Anesthetic/Vasoconstrictor Precautions No information available to require special precautions

Effects on Dental Treatment No effects or complications reported

Dosage Adults: Oral: Recommended daily dose 4-7 mg/day

Pregnancy Risk Factor A/C (dose exceeding RDA recommendation)

Generic Available Yes

Papacon® *see* Papaverine *on page 916*

Papaverine (pa PAV er een)

U.S. Brand Names Papacon®; Para-Time S.R.®; Pavacot®

Pharmacologic Category Vasodilator

Synonyms Papaverine Hydrochloride; Pavabid® [DSC]

Use

Oral: Relief of peripheral and cerebral ischemia associated with arterial spasm; smooth muscle relaxant
Parenteral: Various vascular spasms associated with muscle spasms as in myocardial infarction, angina, peripheral and pulmonary embolism, peripheral vascular disease, angiospastic states, and visceral spasm (ureteral, biliary, and GI colic); testing for impotence

Local Anesthetic/Vasoconstrictor Precautions No information available to require special precautions

Effects on Dental Treatment No effects or complications reported

Dosage

Children: I.M., I.V.: 1.5 mg/kg 4 times/day
Adults:
Oral: 100-300 mg 3-5 times/day
Oral, sustained release: 150-300 mg every 12 hours
I.M., I.V.: 30-120 mg every 3 hours as needed; for cardiac extrasystoles, give 2 doses 10 minutes apart I.V. or I.M.

Mechanism of Action Smooth muscle spasmolytic producing a generalized smooth muscle relaxation including: vasodilatation, GI sphincter relaxation, bronchiolar muscle relaxation, and potentially a depressed myocardium (with large doses); muscle relaxation may occur due to inhibition or cyclic nucleotide phosphodiesterase, increasing cyclic AMP; muscle relaxation is unrelated to nerve innervation; papaverine increases cerebral blood flow in normal subjects; oxygen uptake is unaltered

Other Adverse Effects Frequency not defined:

Cardiovascular: Arrhythmias (with rapid I.V. use), flushing of the face, mild hypertension, tachycardias
Central nervous system: Drowsiness, headache, lethargy, sedation, vertigo
Gastrointestinal: Abdominal distress, anorexia, constipation, diarrhea, nausea
Hepatic: Chronic hepatitis, hepatic hypersensitivity
Respiratory: Apnea (with rapid I.V. use)

Drug Interactions CYP2D6 enzyme substrate

Decreased Effect: Papaverine decreases the effects of levodopa.

Drug Uptake

Onset of action: Oral: Rapid
Half-life, elimination: 0.5-1.5 hours

Pregnancy Risk Factor C

Generic Available Yes

Para-Aminosalicylate Sodium

(PAIR a-a MEE noe sa LIS i late SOW dee um)

Related Information

Nonviral Infectious Diseases *on page 1342*

Pharmacologic Category Analgesic, Non-narcotic; Salicylate

Synonyms Aminosalicylate Sodium; PAS

Use Adjunctive treatment of tuberculosis

Local Anesthetic/Vasoconstrictor Precautions No information available to require special precautions

Effects on Dental Treatment No effects or complications reported

Dosage Oral:

Children: 240-360 mg/kg/day in 3-4 divided doses

Adults: 12-15 g/day in 3-4 divided doses

Other Adverse Effects Frequency not defined:

Endocrine & metabolic: Hypokalemia

Gastrointestinal: Nausea, vomiting, diarrhea, abdominal pain

Hepatic: Hepatitis, jaundice

Miscellaneous: Allergy reactions

Pregnancy Risk Factor C

Generic Available Yes

Comments Capsules contain bentonite which may decrease absorption of concomitantly ingested drugs

Parafon Forte® DSC *see* Chlorzoxazone *on page 277*

Paraplatin® *see* Carboplatin *on page 222*

Para-Time S.R.® *see* Papaverine *on page 916*

Parcaine® *see* Proparacaine *on page 1010*

Paredrine® *see* Hydroxyamphetamine *on page 612*

Paregoric (par e GOR ik)

Pharmacologic Category Analgesic, Narcotic

Synonyms Camphorated Tincture of Opium

Use Treatment of diarrhea or relief of pain; neonatal opiate withdrawal

Local Anesthetic/Vasoconstrictor Precautions No information available to require special precautions

Effects on Dental Treatment No effects or complications reported

Restrictions C-III

Dosage Oral:

Neonatal opiate withdrawal: Instill 3-6 drops every 3-6 hours as needed, or initially 0.2 mL every 3 hours; increase dosage by ~ 0.05 mL every 3 hours until withdrawal symptoms are controlled; it is rare to exceed 0.7 mL/dose. Stabilize withdrawal symptoms for 3-5 days, then gradually decrease dosage over a 2- to 4-week period.

Children: 0.25-0.5 mL/kg 1-4 times/day

Adults: 5-10 mL 1-4 times/day

Mechanism of Action Increases smooth muscle tone in GI tract, decreases motility and peristalsis, diminishes digestive secretions

Other Adverse Effects Frequency not defined:

Cardiovascular: Hypotension, peripheral vasodilation

Central nervous system: Drowsiness, dizziness, insomnia, CNS depression, mental depression, increased intracranial pressure, restlessness, headache, malaise

Gastrointestinal: Constipation, anorexia, stomach cramps, nausea, vomiting, biliary tract spasm

Genitourinary: Ureteral spasms, decreased urination, urinary tract spasm

Hepatic: Increased LFTs

Neuromuscular & skeletal: Weakness

Ocular: Miosis

Respiratory: Respiratory depression

Miscellaneous: Physical and psychological dependence, histamine release

Drug Interactions Increased effect/toxicity with CNS depressants (eg, alcohol, narcotics, benzodiazepines, tricyclic antidepressants, MAO inhibitors, phenothiazine).

Pregnancy Risk Factor B/D (prolonged use or high doses)

Generic Available Yes

Paremyd® *see* Hydroxyamphetamine and Tropicamide *on page 613*

Parepectolin® *see* Kaolin and Pectin With Opium *on page 671*

Paricalcitol (par eh CAL ci tol)

U.S. Brand Names Zemplar™

Canadian Brand Names Zemplar™

Pharmacologic Category Vitamin D Analog

Use Prevention and treatment of secondary hyperparathyroidism associated with chronic renal failure

(Continued)

Paricalcitol *(Continued)*

Local Anesthetic/Vasoconstrictor Precautions No information available to require special precautions

Effects on Dental Treatment No effects or complications reported

Dosage Adults: I.V.: 0.04-0.1 mcg/kg (2.8-7 mcg) given as a bolus dose no more frequently than every other day at any time during dialysis; dose as high as 0.24 mcg/kg (16.8 mcg) have been administered safely

Mechanism of Action Synthetic vitamin D analog which has been shown to reduce PTH serum concentration

Other Adverse Effects The three most frequently reported events in clinical studies were nausea, vomiting, and edema, which are commonly seen in hemodialysis patients.

>10%: Gastrointestinal: Nausea (13%)

1% to 10%:

- Cardiovascular: Palpitations, peripheral edema (7%)
- Central nervous system: Chills, malaise, fever, lightheadedness (5%)
- Gastrointestinal: Vomiting (8%), GI bleeding (5%), xerostomia (3%)
- Respiratory: Pneumonia (5%)
- Miscellaneous: Flu-like symptoms, sepsis

Drug Interactions Increased Effect/Toxicity: Phosphate or vitamin D-related compounds should not be taken concurrently. Digitalis toxicity is potentiated by hypercalcemia.

Pregnancy Risk Factor C

Generic Available No

Parlodel® *see* Bromocriptine *on page 179*
Parnate® *see* Tranylcypromine *on page 1191*

Paromomycin (par oh moe MYE sin)

U.S. Brand Names Humatin®

Canadian Brand Names Humatin®

Pharmacologic Category Amebicide

Synonyms Paromomycin Sulfate

Use Treatment of acute and chronic intestinal amebiasis due to susceptible *Entamoeba histolytica* (not effective in the treatment of extraintestinal amebiasis); tapeworm infestations; adjunctive management of hepatic coma; treatment of cryptosporidial diarrhea

Local Anesthetic/Vasoconstrictor Precautions No information available to require special precautions

Effects on Dental Treatment No effects or complications reported

Dosage Oral:

Intestinal amebiasis: Children and Adults: 25-35 mg/kg/day in 3 divided doses for 5-10 days

Dientamoeba fragilis: Children and Adults: 25-30 mg/kg/day in 3 divided doses for 7 days

Cryptosporidium: Adults with AIDS: 1.5-2.25 g/day in 3-6 divided doses for 10-14 days (occasionally courses of up to 4-8 weeks may be needed)

Tapeworm (fish, dog, bovine, porcine):
- Children: 11 mg/kg every 15 minutes for 4 doses
- Adults: 1 g every 15 minutes for 4 doses

Hepatic coma: Adults: 4 g/day in 2-4 divided doses for 5-6 days

Dwarf tapeworm: Children and Adults: 45 mg/kg/dose every day for 5-7 days

Mechanism of Action Acts directly on ameba; has antibacterial activity against normal and pathogenic organisms in the GI tract; interferes with bacterial protein synthesis by binding to 30S ribosomal subunits

Other Adverse Effects 1% to 10%: Gastrointestinal: Diarrhea, abdominal cramps, nausea, vomiting, heartburn

Drug Interactions

Increased effect of oral anticoagulants, neuromuscular blockers, and polypeptide antibiotics

Decreased effect of digoxin, vitamin A, and methotrexate

Pregnancy Risk Factor C

Generic Available Yes

Paroxetine (pa ROKS e teen)

U.S. Brand Names Paxil®; Paxil® CR™

Canadian Brand Names Paxil®; Paxil® CR™

Mexican Brand Names Aropax®; Paxil®

Pharmacologic Category Antidepressant, Selective Serotonin Reuptake Inhibitor

Use Treatment of depression in adults; treatment of panic disorder with or without agoraphobia; obsessive-compulsive disorder (OCD) in adults; social anxiety disorder (social phobia); generalized anxiety disorder (GAD)

Unlabeled/Investigational: May be useful in eating disorders, impulse control disorders, self-injurious behavior, post-traumatic stress disorder; premenstrual disorders, vasomotor symptoms of menopause; treatment of depression and obsessive-compulsive disorder (OCD) in children

Local Anesthetic/Vasoconstrictor Precautions Although caution should be used in patients taking tricyclic antidepressants, no interactions have been reported with vasoconstrictor and paroxetine, a nontricyclic antidepressant which acts to increase serotonin

Effects on Dental Treatment >10%: Xerostomia; prolonged use of paroxetine may decrease or inhibit salivary flow; normal salivary flow resumes with discontinuation

Dosage Oral:

Children:

Depression (unlabeled use): Initial: 10 mg/day and adjusted upward on an individual basis to 20 mg/day

OCD (unlabeled use): Initial: 10 mg/day and titrate up as necessary to 60 mg/day

Self-Injurious behavior (unlabeled use): 20 mg/day

Adults:

Depression: Initial: 20 mg/day given once daily preferably in the morning; increase if needed by 10 mg/day increments at intervals of at least 1 week; maximum dose: 50 mg/day

GAD: Initial: 20 mg once daily preferably administered in the morning; doses of 20-50 mg/day were used in clinical trials, however, no greater benefit was seen with doses >20 mg. If dose is increased, adjust in increments of 10 mg/day at 1-week intervals.

OCD: Initial: 20 mg/day given once daily preferably in the morning; increase by 10 mg/day increments at intervals of at least 1 week; recommended dose: 40 mg/day; range: 20-60 mg/day; maximum dose: 60 mg/day

Panic disorder: Initial: 10 mg/day given once daily preferably in the morning; increase by 10 mg/day increments at intervals of at least 1 week; recommended dose: 40 mg/day; range: 10-60 mg/day; maximum dose: 60 mg/day

PTSD: Initial: 20 mg/day given once daily, preferably in the morning; if needed, dosage may by increased in increments of 10 mg/day at intervals of at least 1 week; range: 20-50 mg

Social anxiety disorder: Initial: 20 mg/day given once daily preferably in the morning; recommended dose: 20 mg/day; range: 20-60 mg/day; doses >20 mg may not have additional benefit

Elderly: Initial: 10 mg/day; increase (if needed) in increments of 10 mg/day at intervals of at least 1 week; maximum dose: 40 mg/day

Note: Upon discontinuation of paroxetine therapy, gradually taper dose (taper-phase regimen used in PTSD/GAD clinical trials involved an incremental decrease in the daily dose by 10 mg/day at weekly intervals; when 20 mg/day dose was reached, this dose was continued for 1 week before treatment was stopped).

Dosage adjustment in severe renal/hepatic impairment: Adults: Initial: 10 mg/day; increase (if needed) in increments of 10 mg/day at intervals of at least 1 week; maximum dose: 40 mg/day

Mechanism of Action A selective serotonin reuptake inhibitor, chemically unrelated to tricyclic, tetracyclic, or other antidepressants; presumably, the inhibition of serotonin reuptake from brain synapse stimulated serotonin activity in the brain

Other Adverse Effects

>10%:

Central nervous system: Headache, somnolence, dizziness, insomnia

Gastrointestinal: Nausea, xerostomia, constipation, diarrhea

Genitourinary: Ejaculatory disturbances

Neuromuscular & skeletal: Weakness

Miscellaneous: Diaphoresis

1% to 10%:

Cardiovascular: Palpitations, vasodilation, postural hypotension

Central nervous system: Nervousness, anxiety, yawning, abnormal dreams, dizziness

Dermatologic: Rash

Endocrine & metabolic: Decreased libido, delayed ejaculation

Gastrointestinal: Anorexia, flatulence, vomiting, dyspepsia, taste perversion, weight gain

Genitourinary: Urinary frequency, impotence

Neuromuscular & skeletal: Tremor, paresthesia, myopathy, myalgia

Contraindications Hypersensitivity to paroxetine or any component of the formulation; use of MAO inhibitors or within 14 days; concurrent use with thioridazine or mesoridazine

Warnings/Precautions Potential for severe reaction when used with MAO inhibitors - serotonin syndrome (eg, hyperthermia, muscular rigidity, mental status changes/agitation, autonomic instability) may occur. May precipitate a shift to mania or hypomania in patients with bipolar disease. Has a low potential to impair cognitive or motor performance - advise caution operating hazardous machinery or driving. Low potential for sedation or anticholinergic effects relative to cyclic antidepressants. Use caution in patients with depression, particularly if suicidal risk may be present. Use caution in patients with a previous seizure disorder or condition

(Continued)

Paroxetine *(Continued)*

predisposing to seizures such as brain damage, alcoholism, or concurrent therapy with other drugs which lower the seizure threshold. Use with caution in patients with hepatic or dysfunction and in elderly patients. May cause hyponatremia/SIADH. Use with caution in patients at risk of bleeding or receiving anticoagulant therapy - may cause impairment in platelet aggregation. Use with caution in patients with renal insufficiency or other concurrent illness (due to limited experience). May cause or exacerbate sexual dysfunction. Upon discontinuation of paroxetine therapy, gradually taper dose (taper-phase regimen used in PTSD/GAD clinical trials involved an incremental decrease in the daily dose by 10 mg/day at weekly intervals; when 20 mg/day dose was reached, this dose was continued for 1 week before treatment was stopped).

Drug Interactions CYP2D6 enzyme substrate (minor); CYP2D6 and 1A2 enzyme inhibitor, and CYP3A3/4 enzyme inhibitor (weak)

Increased Effect/Toxicity:

MAO inhibitors: Paroxetine should not be used with nonselective MAO inhibitors (phenelzine, isocarboxazid) or other drugs with MAO inhibition (linezolid); fatal reactions have been reported. Wait 5 weeks after stopping fluoxetine before starting a nonselective MAO inhibitor and 2 weeks after stopping an MAO inhibitor before starting paroxetine. Concurrent selegiline has been associated with mania, hypertension, or serotonin syndrome (risk may be reduced relative to nonselective MAO inhibitors).

Phenothiazines: Paroxetine may inhibit the metabolism of thioridazine or mesoridazine, resulting in increased plasma concentrations and increasing the risk of QT_c interval prolongation. This may lead to serious ventricular arrhythmias, such as torsade de pointes-type arrhythmias and sudden death. Do not use together. Wait at least 5 weeks after discontinuing paroxetine prior to starting thioridazine.

Combined used of SSRIs and amphetamines, buspirone, meperidine, nefazodone, serotonin agonists (such as sumatriptan), sibutramine, other SSRIs, sympathomimetics, ritonavir, tramadol, and venlafaxine may increase the risk of serotonin syndrome. Paroxetine may increase serum concentration/effects of benzodiazepines (alprazolam and diazepam), carbamazepine, carvedilol, clozapine, cyclosporine (and possibly tacrolimus), dextromethorphan, digoxin, haloperidol, HMG-CoA reductase inhibitors (lovastatin and simvastatin - increasing the risk of rhabdomyolysis), phenytoin, propafenone, theophylline, trazodone, tricyclic antidepressants, and valproic acid. Concurrent lithium may increase risk of nephrotoxicity. Risk of hyponatremia may increase with concurrent use of loop diuretics (bumetanide, furosemide, torsemide). Paroxetine may increase the hypoprothrombinemic response to warfarin.

Combined use of sumatriptan (and other serotonin agonists) may result in toxicity; weakness, hyper-reflexia, and incoordination have been observed with sumatriptan and SSRIs. In addition, concurrent use may theoretically increase the risk of serotonin syndrome; includes sumatriptan, naratriptan, rizatriptan, and zolmitriptan.

Decreased Effect: Cyproheptadine, a serotonin antagonist, may inhibit the effects of serotonin reuptake inhibitors (paroxetine).

Drug Uptake

Onset of action: Therapeutic: >2 weeks

Half-life, elimination: 21 hours; Steady-state: 10 days

Pregnancy Risk Factor C

Generic Available No

Comments Problems with SSRI-induced bruxism have been reported and may preclude their use; clinicians attempting to evaluate any patient with bruxism or involuntary muscle movement, who is simultaneously being treated with an SSRI drug, should be aware of the potential association.

Ventricular arrhythmias (including torsade de pointes) have been reported, as well as serotonin syndrome.

Selected Readings Gerber PE and Lynd LD, "Selective Serotonin Reuptake Inhibitor-Induced Movement Disorders," *Ann Pharmacother*, 1998, 32(6):692-8.

Patanol® *see* Olopatadine *on page 886*
Pathilon® *see* Tridihexethyl *on page 1203*
Pathocil® *see* Dicloxacillin *on page 380*
Pavacot® *see* Papaverine *on page 916*
Paxil® *see* Paroxetine *on page 918*
Paxil® CR™ *see* Paroxetine *on page 918*
Paxipam® *see* Halazepam *on page 576*
PBZ® *see* Tripelennamine *on page 1213*
PBZ-SR® *see* Tripelennamine *on page 1213*
PC-Cap® *see* Propoxyphene and Aspirin *on page 1015*
PCE® *see* Erythromycin *on page 450*
Pedameth® *see* Methionine *on page 783*

PediaCare® Decongestant Infants [OTC] *see* Pseudoephedrine *on page 1022*
Pediacof® *see* Chlorpheniramine, Phenylephrine, and Codeine *on page 271*
Pediaflor® *see* Fluoride *on page 514*
Pediamist® [OTC] *see* Sodium Chloride *on page 1094*
Pediapred® *see* PrednisoLONE *on page 988*
Pediazole® *see* Erythromycin and Sulfisoxazole *on page 453*
Pedi-Boro® [OTC] *see* Aluminum Sulfate and Calcium Acetate *on page 63*
PediOtic® *see* Neomycin, Polymyxin B, and Hydrocortisone *on page 857*
Pedi-Pro [OTC] *see* Undecylenic Acid and Derivatives *on page 1221*
Pedituss® *see* Chlorpheniramine, Phenylephrine, and Codeine *on page 271*
PedTE-PAK-4® *see* Trace Metals *on page 1186*
Pedtrace-4® *see* Trace Metals *on page 1186*
PedvaxHIB® *see* *Haemophilus* b Conjugate Vaccine *on page 575*

Pegademase Bovine (peg A de mase BOE vine)

U.S. Brand Names Adagen™

Canadian Brand Names Adagen™

Pharmacologic Category Enzyme

Use Orphan drug: Enzyme replacement therapy for adenosine deaminase (ADA) deficiency in patients with severe combined immunodeficiency disease (SCID) who can not benefit from bone marrow transplant; not a cure for SCID, unlike bone marrow transplants, injections must be used the rest of the child's life, therefore is not really an alternative

Local Anesthetic/Vasoconstrictor Precautions No information available to require special precautions

Effects on Dental Treatment No effects or complications reported

Dosage Children: I.M.: Dose given every 7 days, 10 units/kg the first dose, 15 units/kg the second dose, and 20 units/kg the third dose; maintenance dose: 20 units/kg/week is recommended depending on patient's ADA level; maximum single dose: 30 units/kg

Mechanism of Action Adenosine deaminase is an enzyme that catalyzes the deamination of both adenosine and deoxyadenosine. Hereditary lack of adenosine deaminase activity results in severe combined immunodeficiency disease, a fatal disorder of infancy characterized by profound defects of both cellular and humoral immunity. It is estimated that 25% of patients with the autosomal recessive form of severe combined immunodeficiency lack adenosine deaminase.

Drug Interactions Decreased Effect: Vidarabine

Drug Uptake

Absorption: Rapid
Half-life, elimination: 48-72 hours
Time to peak: Plasma adenosine deaminase activity: 2-3 weeks

Pregnancy Risk Factor C

Generic Available No

Peganone® *see* Ethotoin *on page 476*

Pegaspargase (peg AS par jase)

U.S. Brand Names Oncaspar®

Canadian Brand Names Oncaspar®

Pharmacologic Category Antineoplastic Agent, Miscellaneous

Synonyms PEG-L-asparaginase

Use Induction treatment of acute lymphoblastic leukemia in combination with other chemotherapeutic agents in patients who have developed hypersensitivity to native forms of asparaginase derived from *E. coli* and/or *Erwinia chrysanthemi*, treatment of lymphoma

Local Anesthetic/Vasoconstrictor Precautions No information available to require special precautions

Effects on Dental Treatment No effects or complications reported

Mechanism of Action

A modified version of the enzyme asparaginase; asparaginase used in the manufacture of pegaspargase is derived from *Escherichia coli.*

Some malignant cells (ie, lymphoblastic leukemia cells and those of lymphocyte derivation) must acquire the amino acid asparagine from surrounding fluid such as blood, whereas normal cells can synthesize their own asparagine. asparaginase is an enzyme that deaminates asparagine to aspartic acid and ammonia in the plasma and extracellular fluid and therefore deprives tumor cells of the amino acid for protein synthesis.

Other Adverse Effects In general, pegaspargase toxicities tend to be less frequent and appear somewhat later than comparable toxicities of asparaginase. Intramuscular rather than I.V. injection may decrease the incidence of coagulopathy; GI, hepatic, and renal toxicity.

>10%:

Cardiovascular: Edema

(Continued)

Pegaspargase *(Continued)*

Central nervous system: Fatigue, disorientation (10%)
Gastrointestinal: Nausea, vomiting (50% to 60%), generally mild to moderate, but may be severe and protracted in some patients; anorexia (33%); abdominal pain (38%); diarrhea (28%); increased serum lipase and amylase
Hematologic: Hypofibrinogenemia and depression of clotting factors V and VII, variable decreases in factors VII and IX, severe protein C deficiency and decrease in antithrombin III - overt bleeding is uncommon, but may be dose-limiting, or fatal in some patients
Neuromuscular & skeletal: Weakness (33%)
Miscellaneous: Acute allergic reactions, including fever, rash, urticaria, arthralgia, hypotension, angioedema, bronchospasm, anaphylaxis (10% to 30%) - dose-limiting in some patients

1% to 10%:
Cardiovascular: Hypotension, tachycardia, thrombosis
Dermatologic: Urticaria, erythema, lip edema
Endocrine & metabolic: Hyperglycemia (3%)
Gastrointestinal: Acute pancreatitis (1%)
Mild to moderate myelosuppression, leukopenia, anemia, thrombocytopenia; onset: 7 days; nadir: 14 days; recovery: 21 days

Drug Interactions
Increased Effect/Toxicity: Increased toxicity when asparaginase is administered with vincristine and prednisone; cyclophosphamide (decreased metabolism); mercaptopurine (increased hepatotoxicity); vincristine (increased neuropathy); prednisone (hyperglycemia)
Decreased Effect: Asparaginase terminates methotrexate action by inhibition of protein synthesis and prevention of cell entry into the S Phase. Aspirin, dipyridamole, heparin, warfarin, NSAIDs: Imbalances in coagulation factors have been noted with the use of pegaspargase - use with caution.

Drug Uptake
Duration: Asparaginase was measurable for at least 15 days following initial treatment with pegaspargase
Half-life, elimination: 5.73 days; unaffected by age, renal function, or hepatic function

Pregnancy Risk Factor C
Generic Available No

Pegfilgrastim (peg fil GRA stim)

U.S. Brand Names Neulasta™
Pharmacologic Category Colony Stimulating Factor
Synonyms G-CSF (PEG Conjugate); Granulocyte Colony Stimulating Factor (PEG Conjugate)
Use Decrease the incidence of infection, by stimulation of granulocyte production, in patients with nonmyeloid malignancies receiving myelosuppressive therapy associated with a significant risk of febrile neutropenia
Local Anesthetic/Vasoconstrictor Precautions No information available to require special precautions
Effects on Dental Treatment No effects or complications reported
Dosage S.C.: Adolescents >45 kg and Adults: 6 mg once per chemotherapy cycle; do not administer 14 days before and 24 hours after administration of cytotoxic chemotherapy; do not use in patients weighing <45 kg
Mechanism of Action Stimulates the production, maturation, and activation of neutrophils, increasing their migration and cytotoxicity; prolonged duration of effect relative to filgrastim and a reduced renal clearance

Other Adverse Effects
>10%
Neuromuscular & skeletal: Bone pain (medullary, 26%)
Hepatic: Increased LDH (19%)

1% to 10%
Endocrine & metabolic: Uric acid increased (8%)
Hepatic: Alkaline phosphatase increased (9%)

Drug Interactions Lithium may potentiate release of neutrophils from bone marrow.
Drug Uptake Half-life, elimination: S.C.: 15-80 hours
Pregnancy Risk Factor C
Generic Available No

Peginterferon Alfa-2b (peg in ter FEER on AL fa too bee)

Related Information
Systemic Viral Diseases *on page 1354*
U.S. Brand Names PEG-Intron™
Pharmacologic Category Interferon
Use Treatment of chronic hepatitis C (as monotherapy or in combination with ribavirin) in adult patients who have never received interferon alpha and have compensated liver disease

Local Anesthetic/Vasoconstrictor Precautions No information available to require special precautions

Effects on Dental Treatment No effects or complications reported

Restrictions Patients must have an Access Assurance ID number (obtained by calling Schering-Plough at 1-888-437-2608). Pharmacists should receive the ID number from the patient, and must obtain an order authorization number from the manufacturer prior to placing an order with their wholesaler (effective October 22, 2001). The patient's authorization number will be retained throughout therapy. This number may be inactivated if the patient fails to fill the prescription over any 60-day period, and access will no longer be assured by the manufacturer.

Dosage S.C.:

Children: Safety and efficacy have not been established

Adults: Chronic hepatitis C: Administer dose once weekly; **Note:** Usual duration is for 1 year; after 24 weeks of treatment, if serum HCV RNA is not below the limit of detection of the assay, consider discontinuation:

Monotherapy: Initial:

≤45 kg: 40 mcg
46-56 kg: 50 mcg
57-72 kg: 64 mcg
73-88 kg: 80 mcg
89-106 kg: 96 mcg
107-136 kg: 120 mcg
137-160 kg: 150 mcg

Combination therapy with ribavirin (400 mg twice daily): Initial: 1.5 mcg/kg/week

<40 kg: 50 mcg
40-50 kg: 64 mcg
51-60 kg: 80 mcg
61-75 kg: 96 mcg
76-85 kg: 120 mcg
>85 kg: 150 mcg

Elderly: May require dosage reduction based upon renal dysfunction, but no established guidelines are available.

Dosage adjustment if serious adverse event occurs: Depression (severity based upon DSM-IV criteria):

Mild depression: No dosage adjustment required; evaluate once weekly by visit/phone call. If depression remains stable, continue weekly visits. If depression improves, resume normal visit schedule.

Moderate depression: Decrease interferon dose by 50%; evaluate once weekly with an office visit at least every other week. If depression remains stable, consider psychiatric evaluation and continue with reduced dosing. If symptoms improve and remain stable for 4 weeks, resume normal visit schedule; continue reduced dosing or return to normal dose.

Severe depression: Discontinue interferon and ribavirin permanently. Obtain immediate psychiatric consultation.

Dosage adjustment in renal impairment: Monitor for signs and symptoms of toxicity and if toxicity occurs then adjust dose. Do not use patients with Cl_{cr} <50 mL/minute. Patients were excluded from the clinical trials if serum creatinine >1.5 times the upper limits of normal.

Dosage adjustment in hepatic impairment: Contraindicated in decompensated liver disease

Dosage adjustment in hematologic toxicity:

Hemoglobin:

Hemoglobin <10 g/dL: Continue current peginterferon alfa-2b dose; decrease ribavirin dose by 200 mg/day.

Hemoglobin <8.5 g/dL: Permanently discontinue peginterferon alfa-2b and ribavirin.

Hemoglobin decrease >2 g/dL in any 4-week period and stable cardiac disease: Decrease peginterferon alfa-2b dose by half; decrease ribavirin dose by 200 mg per day. Hemoglobin <12 g/dL after ribavirin dose is decreased: Permanently discontinue both peginterferon alfa-2b and ribavirin.

White blood cells:

WBC <1.5 x 10^9/L: Decrease peginterferon alfa-2b dose by half.

WBC <1.0 x 10^9/L: Permanently discontinue peginterferon alfa-2b and ribavirin.

Neutrophils:

Neutrophils <0.75 x 10^9 /L: Decrease peginterferon alfa-2b dose by half.

Neutrophils <0.5 x 10^9 /L: Permanently discontinue peginterferon alfa-2b and ribavirin.

Platelets:

Platelet count <80 x 10^9/L: Decrease peginterferon alfa-2b dose by half.

Platelet count <50 x 10^9/L: Permanently discontinue peginterferon alfa-2b and ribavirin.

Mechanism of Action Alpha interferons are a family of proteins, produced by nucleated cells, that have antiviral, antiproliferative, and immune-regulating activity. There are 16 known subtypes of alpha interferons. Interferons interact with cells through high affinity cell surface receptors. Following activation, multiple effects can

(Continued)

Peginterferon Alfa-2b *(Continued)*

be detected including induction of gene transcription. Inhibits cellular growth, alters the state of cellular differentiation, interferes with oncogene expression, alters cell surface antigen expression, increases phagocytic activity of macrophages, and augments cytotoxicity of lymphocytes for target cells.

Other Adverse Effects

>10% :

Central nervous system: Headache (56%), fatigue (52%), depression (16% to 29%), anxiety/emotional liability/irritability (28%), insomnia (23%), fever (22%), dizziness (12%), impaired concentration (5% to 12%), pain (12%)

Dermatologic: Alopecia (22%), pruritus (12%), dry skin (11%)

Gastrointestinal: Nausea (26%), anorexia (20%), diarrhea (18%), abdominal pain (15%), weight loss (11%)

Local: Injection site inflammation/reaction (47%),

Neuromuscular & skeletal: Musculoskeletal pain (56%), myalgia (38% to 42%), rigors (23% to 45%)

Respiratory: Epistaxis (14%), nasopharyngitis (11%)

Miscellaneous: Flu-like syndrome (46%), viral infection (11%)

>1% to 10%:

Cardiovascular: Flushing (6%)

Central nervous system: Malaise (8%)

Dermatologic: Rash (6%), dermatitis (7%)

Endocrine & metabolic: Hypothyroidism (5%)

Gastrointestinal: Vomiting (7%), dyspepsia (6%), taste perversion

Hematologic: Neutropenia, thrombocytopenia

Hepatic: Transient increase in transaminases (10%), hepatomegaly (6%)

Local: Injection site pain (2%)

Neuromuscular & skeletal: Hypertonia (5%)

Respiratory: Pharyngitis (10%), sinusitis (7%), cough (6%)

Miscellaneous: Diaphoresis (6%)

Drug Interactions Does not inhibit CYP1A2, 2C8/9, 2D6, 3A4 after a single dose in healthy subjects. Interferons, including alfa, have been shown to depress (to varying degrees) the CYP enzyme system.

Increased Effect/Toxicity: ACE inhibitors, clozapine, erythropoietin may increase risk of bone marrow suppression. Fluorouracil, theophylline, zidovudine concentrations may increase. Warfarin's anticoagulant effect may increase.

Decreased Effect: Melphalan concentrations may decrease. Prednisone may decrease effects of interferon alpha.

Drug Uptake

Half-life, elimination: 40 hours

Time to peak: 15-44 hours

Pregnancy Risk Factor C (manufacturer) as monotherapy; X in combination with ribavirin

Generic Available No

PEG-Intron™ *see* Peginterferon Alfa-2b *on page 922*

PemADD® *see* Pemoline *on page 925*

PemADD® CT *see* Pemoline *on page 925*

Pemirolast (pe MIR oh last)

U.S. Brand Names Alamast™

Canadian Brand Names Alamast™

Pharmacologic Category Mast Cell Stabilizer; Ophthalmic Agent, Miscellaneous

Use Prevention of itching of the eye(s) due to allergic conjunctivitis

Local Anesthetic/Vasoconstrictor Precautions No information available to require special precautions

Effects on Dental Treatment No effects or complications reported

Dosage Children >3 years and Adults: 1-2 drops instilled in affected eye(s) 4 times/day

Mechanism of Action Mast cell stabilizer that inhibits the *in vivo* type I immediate hypersensitivity reaction; in addition, inhibits chemotaxis of eosinophils into the ocular tissue and blocks their release of mediators; also reported to prevent calcium influx into mast cells following antigen stimulation

Other Adverse Effects

>10%:

Central nervous system: Headache (10% to 25%)

Respiratory: Rhinitis (10% to 25%)

Miscellaneous: Cold/flu symptoms (10% to 25%)

<5%:

Central nervous system: Fever

Endocrine & metabolic: Dysmenorrhea

Neuromuscular & skeletal: Back pain

Ocular: Burning eyes, dry eyes, foreign body sensation, ocular discomfort

Respiratory: Bronchitis, cough, sinusitis, sneezing/nasal congestion

Drug Uptake

Onset of action: A few days; Peak effect: 4 weeks

Absorption: Systemic

Half-life, elimination: 4.5 hours

Pregnancy Risk Factor C

Pemoline (PEM oh leen)

U.S. Brand Names Cylert®; PemADD®; PemADD® CT

Pharmacologic Category Stimulant

Synonyms Phenylisohydantoin; PIO

Use Treatment of attention-deficit/hyperactivity disorder (ADHD); narcolepsy

Note: Because of its association with life-threatening hepatic failure, pemoline is not considered as first-line treatment therapy for ADHD. Pemoline (Cyclert®) should not be used by patients until there has been a complete discussion of the risks and benefits, and written informed consent has been obtained.

Local Anesthetic/Vasoconstrictor Precautions Pemoline has minimal sympathomimetic effects; there are no precautions in using vasoconstrictors

Effects on Dental Treatment No effects or complications reported

Restrictions C-IV

Dosage Children ≥6 years: Oral: Initial: 37.5 mg given once daily in the morning, increase by 18.75 mg/day at weekly intervals; usual effective dose range: 56.25-75 mg/day; maximum: 112.5 mg/day; dosage range: 0.5-3 mg/kg/24 hours; significant benefit may not be evident until third or fourth week of administration

Mechanism of Action Blocks the reuptake mechanism of dopaminergic neurons, appears to act at the cerebral cortex and subcortical structures; CNS and respiratory stimulant with weak sympathomimetic effects; actions may be mediated via increase in CNS dopamine

Other Adverse Effects Frequency not defined:

Central nervous system: Insomnia, dizziness, drowsiness, mental depression, increased irritability, seizures, precipitation of Tourette's syndrome, hallucinations, headache, movement disorders

Dermatologic: Rash

Endocrine & metabolic: Suppression of growth in children

Gastrointestinal: Anorexia, weight loss, stomach pain, nausea

Hematologic: Aplastic anemia

Hepatic: Increased liver enzyme (usually reversible upon discontinuation), hepatitis, jaundice, hepatic failure

Drug Interactions

Increased Effect/Toxicity: Use caution when pemoline is used with other CNS-acting medications.

Decreased Effect: Pemoline in combination with antiepileptic medications may decrease seizure threshold.

Drug Uptake

Onset of action: Peak effect: 4 hours

Duration: 8 hours

Half-life, elimination: Children: 7-8.6 hours; Adults: 12 hours

Time to peak: Oral: 2-4 hours

Pregnancy Risk Factor B

Generic Available Yes

Penbutolol (pen BYOO toe lole)

Related Information

Cardiovascular Diseases *on page 1308*

U.S. Brand Names Levatol®

Canadian Brand Names Levatol®

Pharmacologic Category Beta Blocker With Intrinsic Sympathomimetic Activity

Synonyms Penbutolol Sulfate

Use Treatment of mild to moderate arterial hypertension

Local Anesthetic/Vasoconstrictor Precautions No information available to require special precautions

Effects on Dental Treatment No effects or complications reported

Dosage Adults: Oral: Initial: 20 mg once daily, full effect of a 20 or 40 mg dose is seen by the end of a 2-week period, doses of 40-80 mg have been tolerated but have shown little additional antihypertensive effects

Mechanism of Action Blocks both $beta_1$- and $beta_2$-receptors and has mild intrinsic sympathomimetic activity; has negative inotropic and chronotropic effects and can significantly slow A-V nodal conduction

Other Adverse Effects 1% to 10%:

Cardiovascular: Congestive heart failure, arrhythmia

Central nervous system: Mental depression, headache, dizziness, fatigue

Gastrointestinal: Nausea, diarrhea, dyspepsia

Neuromuscular & skeletal: Arthralgia

(Continued)

Penbutolol *(Continued)*

Drug Interactions

Increased Effect/Toxicity: The heart rate lowering effects of propranolol are beta-blockers are additive with other drugs which slow AV conduction (digoxin, verapamil, diltiazem). Concurrent use of beta-blockers may increase the effects of alpha-blockers (prazosin, terazosin), alpha-adrenergic stimulants (epinephrine, phenylephrine), and the vasoconstrictive effects of ergot alkaloids. Beta-blockers may mask the tachycardia from hypoglycemia caused by insulin and oral hypoglycemics. In patients receiving concurrent therapy, the risk of hypertensive crisis is increased when either clonidine or the beta-blocker is withdrawn. Beta-blockers may increase the action or levels of disopyramide, nondepolarizing muscle relaxants, and theophylline although the effects are difficult to predict. Beta-blocker effects may be enhanced by oral contraceptives, flecainide, haloperidol (hypotensive effects), H_2 antagonists (cimetidine, possibly ranitidine), hydralazine, loop diuretics, possibly MAO inhibitors, phenothiazines, propafenone, quinidine (in extensive metabolizers), ciprofloxacin, thyroid hormones (when hypothyroid patient is converted to euthyroid state). Beta-blockers may increase the effect/toxicity of flecainide, haloperidol (hypotensive effects), hydralazine, phenothiazines, acetaminophen, anticoagulants (warfarin), and benzodiazepines.

Decreased Effect: Aluminum salts, barbiturates, calcium salts, cholestyramine, colestipol, NSAIDs, penicillins (ampicillin), rifampin, salicylates, and sulfinpyrazone decrease effect of beta-blockers due to decreased bioavailability and plasma concentrations. Beta-blockers may decrease the effect of sulfonylureas. Nonselective beta-blockers blunt the response to beta-2 adrenergic agonists (albuterol).

Drug Uptake

Absorption: Well absorbed, ~100%

Half-life, elimination: 5 hours

Pregnancy Risk Factor C (manufacturer); D (2nd and 3rd trimester - expert analysis)

Generic Available No

Selected Readings

Foster CA and Aston SJ, "Propranolol-Epinephrine Interaction: A Potential Disaster," *Plast Reconstr Surg*, 1983, 72(1):74-8.

Wong DG, Spence JD, Lamki L, et al, "Effect of Nonsteroidal Anti-inflammatory Drugs on Control of Hypertension of Beta-Blockers and Diuretics," *Lancet*, 1986, 1(8488):997-1001.

Wynn RL, "Dental Nonsteroidal Anti-inflammatory Drugs and Prostaglandin-Based Drug Interactions, Part Two," *Gen Dent*, 1992, 40(2):104, 106, 108.

Wynn RL, "Epinephrine Interactions With Beta-Blockers," *Gen Dent*, 1994, 42(1):16, 18.

Penciclovir (pen SYE kloe veer)

Related Information

Oral Viral Infections *on page 1380*

Systemic Viral Diseases *on page 1354*

U.S. Brand Names Denavir™

Pharmacologic Category Antiviral Agent

Use Antiviral cream for the treatment of recurrent herpes labialis (cold sores) in adults

Local Anesthetic/Vasoconstrictor Precautions No information available to require special precautions

Effects on Dental Treatment No effects or complications reported

Dosage Apply cream at the first sign or symptom of cold sore (eg, tingling, swelling); apply every 2 hours during waking hours for 4 days

Mechanism of Action In cells infected with HSV-1 or HSV-2, viral thymidine kinase phosphorylates penciclovir to a monophosphate form which, in turn, is converted to penciclovir triphosphate by cellular kinases. Penciclovir triphosphate inhibits HSV polymerase competitively with deoxyguanosine triphosphate. Consequently, herpes viral DNA synthesis and, therefore, replication are selectively inhibited

Other Adverse Effects

>10%: Dermatologic: Mild erythema (50%)

1% to 10%: Central nervous system: Headache (5.3%)

Contraindications Hypersensitivity to penciclovir or any component of the formulation

Warnings/Precautions Should only be used on herpes labialis on the lips and face; because no data are available, application to mucous membranes is not recommended. Avoid application in or near eyes since it may cause irritation. The effect of penciclovir has not been established in immunocompromised patients.

Drug Uptake Measurable concentrations not detected in plasma or urine of healthy male volunteers following single or repeat application of the 1% cream at a dose of 180 mg penciclovir daily (~67 times the usual clinical dose)

Pregnancy Risk Factor B

Generic Available No

Penecort® *see* Hydrocortisone *on page 608*

Penicillamine (pen i SIL a meen)

U.S. Brand Names Cuprimine®; Depen®

Canadian Brand Names Cuprimine®; Depen®

Mexican Brand Names Adalken®; Sufortan®; Sufortanon®

Pharmacologic Category Chelating Agent

Synonyms D-3-Mercaptovaline; β,β-Dimethylcysteine; D-Penicillamine

Use Treatment of Wilson's disease, cystinuria, adjunct in the treatment of severe rheumatoid arthritis; lead poisoning, primary biliary cirrhosis

Local Anesthetic/Vasoconstrictor Precautions No information available to require special precautions

Effects on Dental Treatment No effects or complications reported

Dosage Oral:

Rheumatoid arthritis:

Children: Initial: 3 mg/kg/day (≤250 mg/day) for 3 months, then 6 mg/kg/day (≤500 mg/day) in divided doses twice daily for 3 months to a maximum of 10 mg/kg/day in 3-4 divided doses

Adults: 125-250 mg/day, may increase dose at 1- to 3-month intervals up to 1-1.5 g/day

Wilson's disease (doses titrated to maintain urinary copper excretion >1 mg/day):

Infants <6 months: 250 mg/dose once daily

Children <12 years: 250 mg/dose 2-3 times/day

Adults: 250 mg 4 times/day

Cystinuria:

Children: 30 mg/kg/day in 4 divided doses

Adults: 1-4 g/day in divided doses every 6 hours

Lead poisoning (continue until blood lead level is <60 μg/dL): Children and Adults: 25-35 mg/kg/d, administered in 3-4 divided doses; initiating treatment at 25% of this dose and gradually increasing to the full dose over 2-3 weeks may minimize adverse reactions

Primary biliary cirrhosis: 250 mg/day to start, increase by 250 mg every 2 weeks up to a maintenance dose of 1 g/day, usually given 250 mg 4 times/day

Arsenic poisoning: Children: 100 mg/kg/day in divided doses every 6 hours for 5 days; maximum: 1 g/day

Mechanism of Action Chelates with lead, copper, mercury and other heavy metals to form stable, soluble complexes that are excreted in urine; depresses circulating IgM rheumatoid factor, depresses T-cell but not B-cell activity; combines with cystine to form a compound which is more soluble, thus cystine calculi are prevented

Other Adverse Effects

>10%:

Dermatologic: Rash, urticaria, itching (44% to 50%)

Gastrointestinal: Hypogeusia (25% to 33%)

Neuromuscular & skeletal: Arthralgia

1% to 10%:

Cardiovascular: Edema of the face, feet, or lower legs

Central nervous system: Fever, chills

Gastrointestinal: Weight gain, sore throat

Genitourinary: Bloody or cloudy urine

Hematologic: Aplastic or hemolytic anemia, leukopenia (2%), thrombocytopenia (4%)

Miscellaneous: White spots on lips or mouth, positive ANA

Warnings/Precautions Cross-sensitivity with penicillin is possible; therefore, should be used cautiously in patients with a history of penicillin allergy. Patients on penicillamine for Wilson's disease or cystinuria should receive pyridoxine supplementation 25 mg/day; once instituted for Wilson's disease or cystinuria, continue treatment on a daily basis; interruptions of even a few days have been followed by hypersensitivity with reinstitution of therapy. Penicillamine has been associated with fatalities due to agranulocytosis, aplastic anemia, thrombocytopenia, Goodpasture's syndrome, and myasthenia gravis; patients should be warned to report promptly any symptoms suggesting toxicity; approximately 33% of patients will experience an allergic reaction; since toxicity may be dose related, it is recommended not to exceed 750 mg/day in elderly.

Drug Interactions

Increased Effect/Toxicity: Increased effect or toxicity of gold, antimalarials, immunosuppressants, and phenylbutazone (hematologic, renal toxicity).

Decreased Effect: Decreased effect of penicillamine when taken with iron and zinc salts, antacids (magnesium, calcium, aluminum), and food. Digoxin levels may be decreased when taken with penicillamine.

Drug Uptake

Absorption: Oral: 40% to 70%

Half-life, elimination: 1.7-3.2 hours

Time to peak: ~2 hours

Pregnancy Risk Factor D

Generic Available No

(Continued)

Penicillamine *(Continued)*

Selected Readings Rosa FW, "Teratogen Update. Penicillamine," *Teratology*, 1986, 33(1):127-31.

Penicillin G Benzathine (pen i SIL in jee BENZ a theen)

Related Information

Dental Drug Interactions: Update on Drug Combinations Requiring Special Considerations *on page 1434*

Nonviral Infectious Diseases *on page 1342*

U.S. Brand Names Bicillin® L-A; Permapen®

Canadian Brand Names Bicillin® L-A

Mexican Brand Names Bencelin®; Benzanil®; Benzetacil; Benzilfan

Pharmacologic Category Antibiotic, Penicillin

Synonyms Benzathine Benzylpenicillin; Benzathine Penicillin G; Benzylpenicillin Benzathine

Use Active against some gram-positive organisms, few gram-negative organisms such as *Neisseria gonorrhoeae*, and some anaerobes and spirochetes; used only for the treatment of mild to moderately severe infections caused by organisms susceptible to low concentrations of penicillin G or for prophylaxis of infections caused by these organisms; used when patient cannot be kept in a hospital environment and neurosyphilis has been ruled out

The CDC and AAP do not currently recommend the use of penicillin G benzathine in treatment of congenital syphilis or neurosyphilis due to reported treatment failures and lack of published clinical data on its efficacy

Local Anesthetic/Vasoconstrictor Precautions No information available to require special precautions

Effects on Dental Treatment No effects or complications reported

Dosage I.M.: Give undiluted injection; higher doses result in more sustained rather than higher levels. Use a penicillin G benzathine-penicillin G procaine combination to achieve early peak levels in acute infections.

Children:

- Group A streptococcal upper respiratory infection: 25,000-50,000 units/kg as a single dose; maximum: 1.2 million units
- Prophylaxis of recurrent rheumatic fever: 25,000-50,000 units/kg every 3-4 weeks; maximum: 1.2 million units/dose
- Early syphilis: 50,000 units/kg as a single injection; maximum: 2.4 million units
- Syphilis of >1-year duration: 50,000 units/kg every week for 3 doses; maximum: 2.4 million units/dose

Adults:

- Group A streptococcal upper respiratory infection: 1.2 million units as a single dose
- Prophylaxis of recurrent rheumatic fever: 1.2 million units every 3-4 weeks or 600,000 units twice monthly
- Early syphilis: 2.4 million units as a single dose in 2 injection sites
- Syphilis of more than 1-year duration: 2.4 million units in 2 injection sites once weekly for 3 doses
- Not indicated as single drug therapy for neurosyphilis, but may be given 1 time/week for 3 weeks following I.V. treatment (refer to Penicillin G monograph for dosing)

Mechanism of Action Interferes with bacterial cell wall synthesis during active multiplication, causing cell wall death and resultant bactericidal activity against susceptible bacteria

Other Adverse Effects Frequency not defined:

Central nervous system: Convulsions, confusion, drowsiness, myoclonus, fever

Dermatologic: Rash

Endocrine & metabolic: Electrolyte imbalance

Hematologic: Positive Coombs' reaction, hemolytic anemia

Local: Pain, thrombophlebitis

Renal: Acute interstitial nephritis

Miscellaneous: Anaphylaxis, hypersensitivity reactions, Jarisch-Herxheimer reaction

Warnings/Precautions Use with caution in patients with impaired renal function, seizure disorder, or history of hypersensitivity to other beta-lactams; CDC and AAP do not currently recommend the use of penicillin G benzathine to treat congenital syphilis or neurosyphilis due to reported treatment failures and lack of published clinical data on its efficacy

Drug Interactions

Increased Effect/Toxicity: Probenecid increases penicillin levels. Aminoglycosides may lead to synergistic efficacy. Heparin and parenteral penicillins may result in increased bleeding. Effects of warfarin may be increased.

Decreased Effect: Tetracyclines may decrease penicillin effectiveness. Efficacy of oral contraceptives may be reduced when taken with penicillins.

Drug Uptake

Absorption: I.M.: Slow

Duration: 1-4 weeks (dose dependent); larger doses result in more sustained levels
Time to peak (dose-dependent): 12-24 hours; usually detectable for 1-4 weeks, larger doses result in sustained levels rather than higher levels

Pregnancy Risk Factor B

Generic Available No

Penicillin G Benzathine and Procaine Combined

(pen i SIL in jee BENZ a theen & PROE kane KOM bined)

U.S. Brand Names Bicillin® C-R; Bicillin® C-R 900/300

Pharmacologic Category Antibiotic, Penicillin

Synonyms Penicillin G Procaine and Benzathine Combined

Use Active against most gram-positive organisms, mostly streptococcal and pneumococcal

Local Anesthetic/Vasoconstrictor Precautions No information available to require special precautions

Effects on Dental Treatment No effects or complications reported

Dosage I.M.:

Children:

<30 lb: 600,000 units in a single dose

30-60 lb: 900,000 units to 1.2 million units in a single dose

Children >60 lb and Adults: 2.4 million units in a single dose

Mechanism of Action Inhibits bacterial cell wall synthesis by binding to one or more of the penicillin binding proteins (PBPs); which in turn inhibits the final transpeptidation step of peptidoglycan synthesis in bacterial cell walls, thus inhibiting cell wall biosynthesis. Bacteria eventually lyse due to ongoing activity of cell wall autolytic enzymes (autolysins and murein hydrolases) while cell wall assembly is arrested.

Other Adverse Effects Frequency not defined:

Central nervous system: CNS toxicity (convulsions, confusion, drowsiness, myoclonus)

Hematologic: Positive Coombs' reaction, hemolytic anemia

Renal: Interstitial nephritis

Miscellaneous: Hypersensitivity reactions, Jarisch-Herxheimer reaction

Drug Interactions

Increased Effect/Toxicity: Probenecid increases penicillin levels. Aminoglycosides may lead to synergistic efficacy. Warfarin effects may be increased.

Decreased Effect: Tetracyclines may decrease penicillin effectiveness. Efficacy of oral contraceptives may be reduced when taken with penicillins.

Pregnancy Risk Factor B

Generic Available No

Penicillin G, Parenteral, Aqueous

(pen i SIL in jee, pa REN ter al, AYE kwee us)

Related Information

Dental Drug Interactions: Update on Drug Combinations Requiring Special Considerations *on page 1434*

Nonviral Infectious Diseases *on page 1342*

U.S. Brand Names Pfizerpen®

Canadian Brand Names Pfizerpen®

Pharmacologic Category Antibiotic, Penicillin

Synonyms Benzylpenicillin Potassium; Benzylpenicillin Sodium; Crystalline Penicillin; Penicillin G Potassium; Penicillin G Sodium

Use Active against some gram-positive organisms, generally not *Staphylococcus aureus*; some gram-negative such as *Neisseria gonorrhoeae*, and some anaerobes and spirochetes; although ceftriaxone is now the drug of choice for Lyme disease and gonorrhea

Local Anesthetic/Vasoconstrictor Precautions No information available to require special precautions

Effects on Dental Treatment No effects or complications reported

Dosage I.M., I.V.:

Children (sodium salt is preferred in children): 100,000-250,000 units/kg/day in divided doses every 4 hours; maximum: 4.8 million units/24 hours

Severe infections: Up to 400,000 units/kg/day in divided doses every 4 hours; maximum dose: 24 million units/day

Adults: 2-24 million units/day in divided doses every 4 hours

Disseminated gonococcal infections or gonococcus ophthalmia (if organism proven sensitive): 100,000 units/kg/day in 2 equal doses (4 equal doses/day for infants >1 week)

Gonococcal meningitis: 150,000 units/kg in 2 equal doses (4 doses/day for infants >1 week)

Mechanism of Action Interferes with bacterial cell wall synthesis during active multiplication, causing cell wall death and resultant bactericidal activity against susceptible bacteria

(Continued)

Penicillin G, Parenteral, Aqueous *(Continued)*

Other Adverse Effects Frequency not defined:

Central nervous system: Convulsions, confusion, drowsiness, myoclonus, fever
Dermatologic: Rash
Endocrine & metabolic: Electrolyte imbalance
Hematologic: Positive Coombs' reaction, hemolytic anemia
Local: Thrombophlebitis
Renal: Acute interstitial nephritis
Miscellaneous: Anaphylaxis, hypersensitivity reactions, Jarisch-Herxheimer reaction

Warnings/Precautions Avoid intra-arterial administration or injection into or near major peripheral nerves or blood vessels since such injections may cause severe and/or permanent neurovascular damage; use with caution in patients with renal impairment (dosage reduction required), pre-existing seizure disorders, or with a history of hypersensitivity to cephalosporins

Drug Interactions

Increased Effect/Toxicity: Probenecid increases penicillin levels. Aminoglycosides may lead to synergistic efficacy.

Decreased Effect: Tetracyclines may decrease penicillin effectiveness. Efficacy of oral contraceptives may be reduced when taken with penicillins.

Drug Uptake

Half-life, elimination:

Neonates: <6 days old: 3.2-3.4 hours; 7-13 days old: 1.2-2.2 hours; >14 days old: 0.9-1.9 hours
Children and adults: Normal renal function: 20-50 minutes
End-stage renal disease: 3.3-5.1 hours

Time to peak: I.M.: ~30 minutes; I.V. ~1 hour

Pregnancy Risk Factor B

Generic Available Yes

Penicillin G Procaine (pen i SIL in jee PROE kane)

Related Information

Dental Drug Interactions: Update on Drug Combinations Requiring Special Considerations *on page 1434*

U.S. Brand Names Wycillin®

Canadian Brand Names Pfizerpen-AS®; Wycillin®

Mexican Brand Names Penicil; Penipot; Penprocilina

Pharmacologic Category Antibiotic, Penicillin

Synonyms APPG; Aqueous Procaine Penicillin G; Procaine Benzylpenicillin; Procaine Penicillin G

Use Moderately severe infections due to *Treponema pallidum* and other penicillin G-sensitive microorganisms that are susceptible to low, but prolonged serum penicillin concentrations; anthrax due to *Bacillus anthracis* (postexposure) to reduce the incidence or progression of disease following exposure to aerolized *Bacillus anthracis*

Local Anesthetic/Vasoconstrictor Precautions No information available to require special precautions

Effects on Dental Treatment No effects or complications reported

Dosage I.M.:

Children: 25,000-50,000 units/kg/day in divided doses 1-2 times/day; not to exceed 4.8 million units/24 hours

Anthrax, inhalational (postexposure prophylaxis): 25,000 units/kg every 12 hours (maximum: 1,200,000 units every 12 hours); see "Note" in Adults dosing

Congenital syphilis: 50,000 units/kg/day for 10-14 days

Adults: 0.6-4.8 million units/day in divided doses every 12-24 hours

Anthrax:

Inhalational (postexposure prophylaxis): 1,200,000 units every 12 hours

Note: Overall treatment duration should be 60 days. Available safety data suggest continued administration of penicillin G procaine for longer than 2 weeks may incur additional risk for adverse reactions. Clinicians may consider switching to effective alternative treatment for completion of therapy beyond 2 weeks.

Cutaneous (treatment): 600,000-1,200,000 units/day; alternative therapy is recommended in severe cutaneous or other forms of anthrax infection

Endocarditis caused by susceptible viridans *Streptococcus* (when used in conjunction with an aminoglycoside): 1.2 million units every 6 hours for 2-4 weeks

Neurosyphilis: I.M.: 2-4 million units/day with 500 mg probenecid by mouth 4 times/day for 10-14 days; **penicillin G aqueous I.V. is the preferred agent**

Hemodialysis: Moderately dialyzable (20% to 50%)

Mechanism of Action Inhibits bacterial cell wall synthesis by binding to one or more of the penicillin binding proteins (PBPs); which in turn inhibits the final transpeptidation step of peptidoglycan synthesis in bacterial cell walls, thus inhibiting cell wall biosynthesis. Bacteria eventually lyse due to ongoing activity of cell wall autolytic enzymes (autolysins and murein hydrolases) while cell wall assembly is arrested.

Other Adverse Effects Frequency not defined:

Cardiovascular: Myocardial depression, vasodilation, conduction disturbances

Central nervous system: Confusion, drowsiness, myoclonus, CNS stimulation, seizures

Hematologic: Positive Coombs' reaction, hemolytic anemia, neutropenia

Local: Pain at injection site, thrombophlebitis, sterile abscess at injection site

Renal: Interstitial nephritis

Miscellaneous: Pseudoanaphylactic reactions, hypersensitivity reactions, Jarisch-Herxheimer reaction, serum sickness

Warnings/Precautions May need to modify dosage in patients with severe renal impairment, seizure disorders, or history of hypersensitivity to cephalosporins; avoid I.V., intravascular, or intra-arterial administration of penicillin G procaine since severe and/or permanent neurovascular damage may occur; use of penicillin for longer than 2 weeks may be associated with an increased risk for some adverse reactions (neutropenia, serum sickness)

Drug Interactions

Increased Effect/Toxicity: Probenecid increases penicillin levels. Aminoglycosides may lead to synergistic efficacy.

Decreased Effect: Tetracyclines may decrease penicillin effectiveness. Efficacy of oral contraceptives may be reduced when taken with penicillins.

Drug Uptake

Absorption: I.M.: Slow

Duration: Therapeutic: 15-24 hours

Time to peak: 1-4 hours

Pregnancy Risk Factor B

Generic Available Yes

Penicillin V Potassium (pen i SIL in vee poe TASS ee um)

Related Information

Antibiotic Prophylaxis, Preprocedural Guidelines for Dental Patients *on page 1344*

Dental Drug Interactions: Update on Drug Combinations Requiring Special Considerations *on page 1434*

Oral Bacterial Infections *on page 1367*

Oral Viral Infections *on page 1380*

U.S. Brand Names Suspen®; Truxcillin®; Veetids®

Canadian Brand Names Apo®-Pen VK; Nadopen-V®; Novo-Pen-VK®; Nu-Pen-VK®; PVF® K

Mexican Brand Names Anapenil; Pen-Vi-K

Pharmacologic Category Antibiotic, Penicillin

Synonyms Pen VK; Phenoxymethyl Penicillin

Use

Dental: Antibiotic of first choice in treating common orofacial infections caused by aerobic gram-positive cocci and anaerobes. These orofacial infections include cellulitis, periapical abscess, periodontal abscess, acute suppurative pulpitis, oronasal fistula, pericoronitis, osteitis, osteomyelitis, postsurgical and post-traumatic infection. It is no longer recommended for dental procedure prophylaxis.

Medical: Treatment of moderate to severe susceptible bacterial infections involving the respiratory tract, otitis media, sinusitis, skin, and urinary tract

Local Anesthetic/Vasoconstrictor Precautions No information available to require special precautions

Effects on Dental Treatment Prolonged use of penicillins may lead to development of oral candidiasis.

Dosage Oral:

Systemic infections:

- Children <12 years: 25-50 mg/kg/day in divided doses every 6-8 hours; maximum dose: 3 g/day
- Children ≥12 years and Adults: 125-500 mg every 6-8 hours

Prophylaxis of pneumococcal infections:

- Children <5 years: 125 mg twice daily
- Children ≥5 years and Adults: 250 mg twice daily

Prophylaxis of recurrent rheumatic fever:

- Children <5 years: 125 mg twice daily
- Children ≥5 years and Adults: 250 mg twice daily

Dosing interval in renal impairment: Cl_{cr} <10 mL/minute: Administer 250 mg every 6 hours

Mechanism of Action Inhibits bacterial cell wall synthesis by binding to one or more of the penicillin binding proteins (PBPs); which in turn inhibits the final transpeptidation step of peptidoglycan synthesis in bacterial cell walls, thus inhibiting cell

(Continued)

Penicillin V Potassium *(Continued)*

wall biosynthesis. Bacteria eventually lyse due to ongoing activity of cell wall autolytic enzymes (autolysins and murein hydrolases) while cell wall assembly is arrested.

Other Adverse Effects

>10%: Gastrointestinal: Mild diarrhea, vomiting, nausea, oral candidiasis

<1%: Convulsions, fever, hemolytic anemia, positive Coombs' reaction, acute interstitial nephritis, hypersensitivity reactions, anaphylaxis

Contraindications Hypersensitivity to penicillin or any component of the formulation

Warnings/Precautions Use with caution in patients with severe renal impairment (modify dosage), history of seizures, or hypersensitivity to cephalosporins

Drug Interactions

Aminoglycosides: May be synergistic against selected organisms
Oral contraceptives: Efficacy of oral contraceptives may be reduced
Probenecid, disulfiram: May increase penicillin levels
Tetracyclines: May decrease penicillin effectiveness
Warfarin: Effects of warfarin may be increased

Dietary/Ethanol/Herb Considerations Food decreases drug absorption rate and serum concentration.

Drug Uptake

Absorption: 60% to 73%
Half-life, elimination: 0.5 hours; prolonged with renal impairment
Time to peak: 0.5-1 hour

Pregnancy Risk Factor B

Dosage Forms 250 mg = 400,000 units

POWDER, oral solution: 125 mg/5 mL (80 mL, 100 mL, 150 mL, 200 mL); 250 mg/5 mL (80 mL, 100 mL, 150 mL, 200 mL). **TAB:** 250 mg, 500 mg

Generic Available Yes

Selected Readings

Wynn RL and Bergman SA, "Antibiotics and Their Use in the Treatment of Orofacial Infections, Part I," *Gen Dent*, 1994, 42(5):398, 400, 402.
Wynn RL and Bergman SA, "Antibiotics and Their Use in the Treatment of Orofacial Infections, Part II," *Gen Dent*, 1994, 42(6):498-502.
Wynn RL, Bergman SA, Meiller TF, et al, "Antibiotics in Treating Oral-Facial Infections of Odontogenic Origin: An Update", *Gen Dent*, 2001, 49(3):238-40, 242, 244 passim.

Penlac™ *see* Ciclopirox *on page 283*
Pentacarinat® *see* Pentamidine *on page 932*

Pentagastrin (pen ta GAS trin)

U.S. Brand Names Peptavlon®

Pharmacologic Category Diagnostic Agent

Use Evaluate gastric acid secretory function in pernicious anemia, gastric carcinoma; in suspected duodenal ulcer or Zollinger-Ellison tumor

Local Anesthetic/Vasoconstrictor Precautions No information available to require special precautions

Effects on Dental Treatment No effects or complications reported

Dosage Adults:

I.M., S.C.: 6 mcg/kg
I.V. infusion: 0.1-12 mcg/kg/hour in 0.9% sodium chloride

Mechanism of Action Excites the oxyntic cells of the stomach to secrete to their maximum capacity similar to the naturally occurring hormone, gastrin

Other Adverse Effects

>10%: Gastrointestinal: Abdominal pain, desire to defecate, nausea, vomiting

1% to 10%:

Cardiovascular: Flushing, tachycardia, palpitations, hypotension, faintness
Central nervous system: Dizziness, headache
Respiratory: Dyspnea

Drug Interactions

Anticonvulsants: Pemoline may decrease seizure threshold; efficacy of anticonvulsants may be decreased
CNS depressants: Effects may be additive; use caution when pemoline is used with other CNS acting medications

Drug Uptake

Absorption: I.M., S.C.: Well absorbed
Half-life, elimination: 1 minute

Pregnancy Risk Factor C

Generic Available No

Pentam-300® *see* Pentamidine *on page 932*

Pentamidine (pen TAM i deen)

U.S. Brand Names NebuPent™; Pentacarinat®; Pentam-300®

Canadian Brand Names Pentacarinat®

Mexican Brand Names Pentacarinat®

Pharmacologic Category Antibiotic, Miscellaneous

Synonyms Pentamidine Isethionate

Use Treatment and prevention of pneumonia caused by *Pneumocystis carinii*; treatment of trypanosomiasis

Local Anesthetic/Vasoconstrictor Precautions No information available to require special precautions

Effects on Dental Treatment No effects or complications reported

Dosage

Children:

Treatment: I.M., I.V. (I.V. preferred): 4 mg/kg/day once daily for 10-14 days

Prevention:

I.M., I.V.: 4 mg/kg monthly or every 2 weeks

Inhalation (aerosolized pentamidine in children ≥5 years): 300 mg/dose given every 3-4 weeks via Respirgard® II inhaler (8 mg/kg dose has also been used in children <5 years)

Treatment of trypanosomiasis: I.V.: 4 mg/kg/day once daily for 10 days

Adults:

Treatment: I.M., I.V. (I.V. preferred): 4 mg/kg/day once daily for 14 days

Prevention: Inhalation: 300 mg every 4 weeks via Respirgard® II nebulizer

Mechanism of Action Interferes with RNA/DNA, phospholipids and protein synthesis, through inhibition of oxidative phosphorylation and/or interference with incorporation of nucleotides and nucleic acids into RNA and DNA, in protozoa

Other Adverse Effects Injection (I); Aerosol (A)

>10%:

Cardiovascular: Chest pain (A - 10% to 23%)

Central nervous system: Fatigue (A - 50% to 70%); dizziness (A - 31% to 47%)

Dermatologic: Rash (31% to 47%)

Endocrine & metabolic: Hyperkalemia

Gastrointestinal: Anorexia (A - 50% to 70%), nausea (A - 10% to 23%)

Local: Local reactions at injection site

Renal: Increased creatinine (I - 23%)

Respiratory: Wheezing (A - 10% to 23%), dyspnea (A - 50% to 70%), coughing (A - 31% to 47%), pharyngitis (10% to 23%)

1% to 10%:

Cardiovascular: Hypotension (I - 4%)

Central nervous system: Confusion/hallucinations (1% to 2%), headache (A - 1% to 5%)

Dermatologic: Rash (I - 3.3%)

Endocrine & metabolic: Hypoglycemia <25 mg/dL (I - 2.4%)

Gastrointestinal: Nausea/anorexia (I - 6%), diarrhea (A - 1% to 5%), vomiting

Hematologic: Severe leukopenia (I - 2.8%), thrombocytopenia <20,000/mm^3 (I - 1.7%), anemia (A - 1% to 5%)

Hepatic: Increased LFTs (I - 8.7%)

Drug Interactions CYP2C19 enzyme substrate

May potentiate the effect of other drugs which prolong QT interval (cisapride, terfenadine, astemizole, sparfloxacin, gatifloxacin, moxifloxacin, and type Ia and type III antiarrhythmics)

Drug Uptake

Absorption: I.M.: Well absorbed; Inhalation: Limited systemic absorption

Half-life, elimination: Terminal: 6.4-9.4 hours (may increase with severe renal impairment)

Pregnancy Risk Factor C

Generic Available Yes

Pentasa® *see* Mesalamine *on page 772*

Pentaspan® *see* Pentastarch *on page 933*

Pentastarch (PEN ta starch)

U.S. Brand Names Pentaspan®

Canadian Brand Names Pentaspan®

Mexican Brand Names Pentaspan®

Pharmacologic Category Blood Modifiers

Use Orphan drug: Adjunct in leukapheresis to improve harvesting and increase yield of leukocytes by centrifugal means

Local Anesthetic/Vasoconstrictor Precautions No information available to require special precautions

Effects on Dental Treatment No effects or complications reported

Dosage 250-700 mL to which citrate anticoagulant has been added is administered by adding to the input line of the centrifugation apparatus at a ratio of 1:8-1:13 to venous whole blood

Generic Available No

Pentazocine (pen TAZ oh seen)

U.S. Brand Names Talwin®; Talwin® NX

Canadian Brand Names Talwin®

(Continued)

Pentazocine *(Continued)*

Pharmacologic Category Analgesic, Narcotic

Synonyms Pentazocine Hydrochloride; Pentazocine Lactate

Use Relief of moderate to severe pain; has also been used as a sedative prior to surgery and as a supplement to surgical anesthesia

Local Anesthetic/Vasoconstrictor Precautions No information available to require special precautions

Effects on Dental Treatment No effects or complications reported

Restrictions C-IV

Dosage

Children: I.M., S.C.:

- 5-8 years: 15 mg
- 8-14 years: 30 mg

Children >12 years and Adults: Oral: 50 mg every 3-4 hours; may increase to 100 mg/dose if needed, but should not exceed 600 mg/day

Adults:

- I.M., S.C.: 30-60 mg every 3-4 hours, not to exceed total daily dose of 360 mg
- I.V.: 30 mg every 3-4 hours

Elderly: Elderly patients may be more sensitive to the analgesic and sedating effects. The elderly may also have impaired renal function. If needed, dosing should be started at the lower end of dosing range and adjust dose for renal function.

Dosing adjustment in renal impairment:

- Cl_{cr} 10-50 mL/minute: Administer 75% of normal dose
- Cl_{cr} <10 mL/minute: Administer 50% of normal dose

Dosing adjustment in hepatic impairment: Reduce dose or avoid use in patients with liver disease

Mechanism of Action Binds to opiate receptors in the CNS, causing inhibition of ascending pain pathways, altering the perception of and response to pain; produces generalized CNS depression; partial agonist-antagonist

Other Adverse Effects Frequency not defined:

Cardiovascular: Hypotension, palpitations, peripheral vasodilation

Central nervous system: Malaise, headache, restlessness, nightmares, insomnia, CNS depression, sedation, hallucinations, confusion, disorientation, dizziness, euphoria, drowsiness

Dermatologic: Rash, pruritus

Gastrointestinal: Nausea, vomiting, xerostomia, constipation, anorexia, diarrhea, GI irritation, biliary tract spasm

Genitourinary: Urinary tract spasm

Local: Tissue damage and irritation with I.M./S.C. use

Neuromuscular & skeletal: Weakness

Ocular: Blurred vision, miosis

Respiratory: Dyspnea, respiratory depression (rare)

Miscellaneous: Histamine release, physical and psychological dependence

Drug Interactions CYP2D6 enzyme substrate

Increased Effect/Toxicity: Increased effect/toxicity with tripelennamine (can be lethal), CNS depressants (eg, phenothiazines, tranquilizers, anxiolytics, sedatives, hypnotics, alcohol).

Decreased Effect: May potentiate or reduce analgesic effect of opiate agonist (eg, morphine) depending on patients tolerance to opiates; can precipitate withdrawal in narcotic addicts.

Drug Uptake

Onset of action: Oral, I.M., S.C.: 15-30 minutes; I.V.: 2-3 minutes

Duration: Oral: 4-5 hours; Parenteral: 2-3 hours

Half-life, elimination: 2-3 hours; increases with hepatic impairment

Pregnancy Risk Factor B/D (prolonged use or high doses at term)

Generic Available Yes

Pentazocine Compound (pen TAZ oh seen kom bi NAY shuns)

U.S. Brand Names Talacen®; Talwin® Compound

Pharmacologic Category Analgesic, Narcotic

Use Relief of moderate to severe pain; has also been used as a sedative prior to surgery and as a supplement to surgical anesthesia

Local Anesthetic/Vasoconstrictor Precautions No information available to require special precautions

Effects on Dental Treatment No effects or complications reported

Dosage Adults: Oral: 2 tablets 3-4 times/day

Other Adverse Effects

>10%:

Central nervous system: Fatigue, drowsiness, false sense of well-being

Gastrointestinal: Nausea, vomiting

1% to 10%:

Cardiovascular: Tachycardia or bradycardia, hypertension or hypotension

Central nervous system: Nervousness, headache, restlessness, malaise, dizziness
Dermatologic: Rash, urticaria
Gastrointestinal: Dry mouth, biliary spasm, constipation
Genitourinary: Ureteral spasms, decreased urination
Local: Pain at injection site
Neuromuscular & skeletal: Weakness
Ocular: Blurred vision
Respiratory: Dyspnea, shortness of breath
Miscellaneous: Histamine release

Comments Abrupt discontinuation after sustained use (generally >10 days) may cause withdrawal symptoms

Pentobarbital (pen toe BAR bi tal)

U.S. Brand Names Nembutal®

Canadian Brand Names Nembutal® Sodium

Pharmacologic Category Anticonvulsant, Barbiturate; Barbiturate

Synonyms Pentobarbital Sodium

Use Sedative/hypnotic; preanesthetic; high-dose barbiturate coma for treatment of increased intracranial pressure or status epilepticus unresponsive to other therapy

Unlabeled/Investigational: Tolerance test during withdrawal of sedative hypnotics

Local Anesthetic/Vasoconstrictor Precautions No information available to require special precautions

Effects on Dental Treatment No effects or complications reported

Restrictions C-II (capsules, injection); C-III (suppositories)

Dosage

Children:
Sedative: Oral: 2-6 mg/kg/day divided in 3 doses; maximum: 100 mg/day
Hypnotic: I.M.: 2-6 mg/kg; maximum: 100 mg/dose
Sedative/hypnotic: Rectal:
2 months to 1 year (10-20 lb): 30 mg
1-4 years (20-40 lb): 30-60 mg
5-12 years (40-80 lb): 60 mg
12-14 years (80-110 lb): 60-120 mg
or
<4 years: 3-6 mg/kg/dose
>4 years: 1.5-3 mg/kg/dose
Preoperative/preprocedure sedation: ≥6 months:
Oral, I.M., rectal: 2-6 mg/kg; maximum: 100 mg/dose
I.V.: 1-3 mg/kg to a maximum of 100 mg until asleep
Conscious sedation prior to a procedure: Children 5-12 years: I.V.: 2 mg/kg 5-10 minutes before procedures, may repeat one time

Adolescents: Conscious sedation: Oral, I.V.: 100 mg prior to a procedure

Children and Adults: Barbiturate coma in head injury patients: I.V.: Loading dose: 5-10 mg/kg given slowly over 1-2 hours; monitor BP and respiratory rate; Maintenance infusion: Initial: 1 mg/kg/hour; may increase to 2-3 mg/kg/hour; maintain burst suppression on EEG

Status epilepticus: I.V.: **Note**: Intubation required; monitor hemodynamics
Children: Loading dose: 5-15 mg/kg given slowly over 1-2 hours; maintenance infusion: 0.5-5 mg/kg/hour
Adults: Loading dose: 2-15 mg/kg given slowly over 1-2 hours; maintenance infusion: 0.5-3 mg/kg/hour

Adults:
Hypnotic:
Oral: 100-200 mg at bedtime or 20 mg 3-4 times/day for daytime sedation
I.M.: 150-200 mg
I.V.: Initial: 100 mg, may repeat every 1-3 minutes up to 200-500 mg total dose
Rectal: 120-200 mg at bedtime
Preoperative sedation: I.M.: 150-200 mg
Tolerance testing (unlabeled use): 200 mg every 2 hours until signs of intoxication are exhibited at any time during the 2 hours after the dose; maximum dose: 1000 mg

Dosing adjustment in hepatic impairment: Reduce dosage in patients with severe liver dysfunction

Mechanism of Action Short-acting barbiturate with sedative, hypnotic, and anticonvulsant properties. Barbiturates depress the sensory cortex, decrease motor activity, alter cerebellar function, and produce drowsiness, sedation, and hypnosis. In high doses, barbiturates exhibit anticonvulsant activity; barbiturates produce dose-dependent respiratory depression.

Other Adverse Effects Frequency not defined:

Cardiovascular: Bradycardia, hypotension, syncope
Central nervous system: Drowsiness, lethargy, CNS excitation or depression, impaired judgment, "hangover" effect, confusion, somnolence, agitation, hyperkinesia, ataxia, nervousness, headache, insomnia, nightmares, hallucinations, anxiety, dizziness

(Continued)

Pentobarbital *(Continued)*

Dermatologic: Rash, exfoliative dermatitis, Stevens-Johnson syndrome
Gastrointestinal: Nausea, vomiting, constipation
Hematologic: Agranulocytosis, thrombocytopenia, megaloblastic anemia
Local: Pain at injection site, thrombophlebitis with I.V. use
Renal: Oliguria
Respiratory: Laryngospasm, respiratory depression, apnea (especially with rapid I.V. use), hypoventilation, apnea
Miscellaneous: Gangrene with inadvertent intra-arterial injection

Drug Interactions

Barbiturates are enzyme inducers; patients should be monitored when these drugs are started or stopped for a decreased or increased therapeutic effect respectively

Increased Effect/Toxicity: When combined with other CNS depressants, narcotic analgesics, antidepressants, or benzodiazepines, additive respiratory and CNS depression may occur. Chronic use of barbiturates may enhance the hepatotoxic potential of acetaminophen overdoses. Chloramphenicol, MAO inhibitors, valproic acid, and felbamate may inhibit barbiturate metabolism. Barbiturates may impair the absorption of griseofulvin, and may enhance the nephrotoxic effects of methoxyflurane.

Decreased Effect: Barbiturates such as pentobarbital are hepatic enzyme inducers, and (only with chronic use) may increase the metabolism of antipsychotics, some beta-blockers (unlikely with atenolol and nadolol), calcium channel blockers, chloramphenicol, cimetidine, corticosteroids, cyclosporine, disopyramide, doxycycline, ethosuximide, felbamate, furosemide, griseofulvin, lamotrigine, phenytoin, propafenone, quinidine, tacrolimus, TCAs, and theophylline. Barbiturates may increase the metabolism of estrogens and reduce the efficacy of oral contraceptives; an alternative method of contraception should be considered. Barbiturates inhibit the hypoprothrombinemic effects of oral anticoagulants via increased metabolism. Barbiturates may enhance the metabolism of methadone resulting in methadone withdrawal.

Drug Uptake

Onset of action: Oral, rectal: 15-60 minutes; I.M.: 10-15 minutes; I.V.: ~1 minute
Duration: Oral, rectal: 1-4 hours; I.V.: 15 minutes
Half-life, elimination: Terminal: Children: 25 hours; Adults: 22 hours; Range: 35-50 hours

Pregnancy Risk Factor D

Generic Available Yes

Pentosan Polysulfate Sodium

(PEN toe san pol i SUL fate SOW dee um)

U.S. Brand Names Elmiron®

Canadian Brand Names Elmiron™

Pharmacologic Category Analgesic, Urinary

Synonyms PPS

Use Orphan drug: Relief of bladder pain or discomfort due to interstitial cystitis

Local Anesthetic/Vasoconstrictor Precautions No information available to require special precautions

Effects on Dental Treatment <1%: Gum bleeding, mouth ulcers

Dosage Patients should be evaluated at 3 months and may be continued an additional 3 months if there has been no improvement and if there are no therapy-limiting side effects. **The risks and benefits of continued use beyond 6 months in patients who have not responded is not yet known.**

Adults: Oral: 100 mg 3 times/day taken with water 1 hour before or 2 hours after meals

Mechanism of Action Although pentosan polysulfate sodium is a low-molecular weight heparinoid, it is not known whether these properties play a role in its mechanism of action in treating interstitial cystitis; the drug appears to adhere to the bladder wall mucosa where it may act as a buffer to protect the tissues from irritating substances in the urine.

Other Adverse Effects 1% to 10%:

Central nervous system: Headache (3%), dizziness (1%), depression (2%)
Dermatologic: Alopecia, rash, pruritus
Gastrointestinal: Diarrhea, nausea, dyspepsia, abdominal pain
Hepatic: Liver function test abnormalities (1%)

Warnings/Precautions Pentosan polysulfate is a low-molecular weight heparin-like compound with anticoagulant and fibrinolytic effects, therefore, bleeding complications such as ecchymosis, epistaxis and gum bleeding, may occur; patients with the following diseases should be carefully evaluated before initiating therapy: aneurysm, thrombocytopenia, hemophilia, GI ulcerations, polyps, diverticula, or hepatic insufficiency; patients undergoing invasive procedures or having signs or symptoms of underlying coagulopathies or other increased risk of bleeding (eg, receiving heparin, warfarin, thrombolytics, or high dose aspirin) should be evaluated for hemorrhage; elevations in transaminases and alopecia can occur

Drug Interactions Increased Effect/Toxicity: Although there is no information about potential drug interactions, it is expected that pentosan polysulfate sodium would have at least additive anticoagulant effects when administered with anticoagulant drugs such as warfarin or heparin, and possible similar effects when administered with aspirin or thrombolytics.

Drug Uptake

Absorption: ~3%

Half-life, elimination: 4-8 hours

Pregnancy Risk Factor B

Generic Available No

Pentostatin (PEN toe stat in)

U.S. Brand Names Nipent®

Canadian Brand Names Nipent®

Pharmacologic Category Antineoplastic Agent, Antibiotic

Synonyms DCF; Deoxycoformycin; 2′-deoxycoformycin

Use Treatment of adult patients with alpha-interferon-refractory hairy cell leukemia; significant antitumor activity in various lymphoid neoplasms has been demonstrated; pentostatin also is known as 2′-deoxycoformycin; it is a purine analogue capable of inhibiting adenosine deaminase

Local Anesthetic/Vasoconstrictor Precautions No information available to require special precautions

Effects on Dental Treatment No effects or complications reported

Mechanism of Action An antimetabolite inhibiting adenosine deaminase (ADA), prevents ADA from controlling intracellular adenosine levels through the irreversible deamination of adenosine and deoxyadenosine. ADA is found to exhibit the highest activity in lymphoid tissue. Patients receiving pentostatin accumulate deoxyadenosine (dAdo) and deoxyadenosine 5′-triphosphate (dATP); accumulation of dATP results in cell death, probably through inhibiting DNA or RNA synthesis. Following a single dose, pentostatin has the ability to inhibit ADA for periods exceeding 1 week.

Other Adverse Effects

>10%:

- Central nervous system: Fever, chills, infection (57%), severe, life-threatening (35%); headache, lethargy, seizures, coma (10% to 15%), potentially dose-limiting, uncommon at doses 4 mg/m^2
- Dermatologic: Skin rashes (25% to 30%), alopecia (10%)
- Gastrointestinal: Mild to moderate nausea, vomiting (60%), controlled with non-5-HT_3 antagonist antiemetics; stomatitis, diarrhea (13%), anorexia
- Genitourinary: Acute renal failure (35%)
- Hematologic: Thrombocytopenia (50%), dose-limiting in 25% of patients; anemia (40% to 45%), neutropenia, mild to moderate, not dose-limiting (11%)
  - Nadir: 7 days
  - Recovery: 10-14 days
- Hepatic: Mild to moderate increases in transaminase levels (30%), usually transient; hepatitis (19%), usually reversible
- Respiratory: Pulmonary edema (15%), may be exacerbated by fludarabine

1% to 10%:

- Cardiovascular: Chest pain, arrhythmia, peripheral edema
- Central nervous system: Opportunistic infections (8%); anxiety, confusion, depression, dizziness, insomnia, nervousness, somnolence, myalgias, malaise
- Dermatologic: Dry skin, eczema, pruritus
- Gastrointestinal: Constipation, flatulence, weight loss
- Neuromuscular & skeletal: Paresthesia, weakness
- Ocular: Moderate to severe keratoconjunctivitis, abnormal vision, eye pain
- Otic: Ear pain
- Respiratory: Dyspnea, pneumonia, bronchitis, pharyngitis, rhinitis, epistaxis, sinusitis (3% to 7%)

Drug Interactions Increased toxicity with vidarabine, fludarabine, and allopurinol

Drug Uptake Half-life, elimination: Terminal: 5-15 hours

Pregnancy Risk Factor D

Generic Available No

Pentothal® Sodium *see* Thiopental *on page 1158*

Pentoxifylline (pen toks I fi leen)

U.S. Brand Names Trental®

Canadian Brand Names Albert® Pentoxifylline; Apo®-Pentoxifylline SR Nu-Pentoxifylline SR; Trental®

Mexican Brand Names Fixoten®; Kentadin; Peridane; Sufisal; Trental®; Vasofyl®

Pharmacologic Category Blood Viscosity Reducer Agent

Synonyms Oxpentifylline

Use Symptomatic management of peripheral vascular disease, mainly intermittent claudication

(Continued)

Pentoxifylline *(Continued)*

Unlabeled/Investigational: AIDS patients with increased TNF, CVA, cerebrovascular diseases, diabetic atherosclerosis, diabetic neuropathy, gangrene, hemodialysis shunt thrombosis, vascular impotence, cerebral malaria, septic shock, sickle cell syndromes, and vasculitis

Local Anesthetic/Vasoconstrictor Precautions No information available to require special precautions

Effects on Dental Treatment No effects or complications reported

Dosage Adults: Oral: 400 mg 3 times/day with meals; may reduce to 400 mg twice daily if GI or CNS side effects occur

Mechanism of Action Mechanism of action remains unclear; is thought to reduce blood viscosity and improve blood flow by altering the rheology of red blood cells

Other Adverse Effects 1% to 10%:

Central nervous system: Dizziness, headache

Gastrointestinal: Dyspepsia, nausea, vomiting

Drug Interactions

Increased Effect/Toxicity: Pentoxifylline levels may be increased with cimetidine and other H_2 antagonists. May increase anticoagulation with warfarin. Pentoxifylline may increase the serum concentration of theophylline.

Decreased Effect: Blood pressure changes (decreases) have been observed with the addition of pentoxifylline therapy in patients receiving antihypertensives.

Drug Uptake

Absorption: Oral: Well absorbed

Half-life, elimination: Parent drug: 24-48 minutes; Metabolites: 60-96 minutes

Time to peak: 2-4 hours

Pregnancy Risk Factor C

Generic Available Yes

Pentrax® [OTC] *see* Coal Tar *on page 315*
Pepcid® *see* Famotidine *on page 486*
Pepcid® AC [OTC] *see* Famotidine *on page 486*
Pepcid® Complete [OTC] *see* Famotidine, Calcium Carbonate, and Magnesium Hydroxide *on page 487*
Pepcid RPD™ *see* Famotidine *on page 486*
Peptavlon® *see* Pentagastrin *on page 932*
Pepto-Bismol® [OTC] *see* Bismuth *on page 167*
Pepto-Bismol® Maximum Strength [OTC] *see* Bismuth *on page 167*
Pepto® Diarrhea Control [OTC] *see* Loperamide *on page 725*
Percocet® 2.5/325 *see* Oxycodone and Acetaminophen *on page 903*
Percocet® 5/325 *see* Oxycodone and Acetaminophen *on page 903*
Percocet® 7.5/325 *see* Oxycodone and Acetaminophen *on page 903*
Percocet® 7.5/500 *see* Oxycodone and Acetaminophen *on page 903*
Percocet® 10/325 *see* Oxycodone and Acetaminophen *on page 903*
Percocet® 10/650 *see* Oxycodone and Acetaminophen *on page 903*
Percodan® *see* Oxycodone and Aspirin *on page 905*
Percodan®-Demi *see* Oxycodone and Aspirin *on page 905*
Percogesic® [OTC] *see* Acetaminophen and Phenyltoloxamine *on page 30*
Percolone® *see* Oxycodone *on page 901*
Perdiem® Plain [OTC] *see* Psyllium *on page 1025*

Pergolide Mesylate (PER go lide)

U.S. Brand Names Permax®

Canadian Brand Names Permax®

Mexican Brand Names Permax®

Pharmacologic Category Anti-Parkinson's Agent, Dopamine Agonist; Ergot Derivative

Synonyms Pergolide

Use Adjunctive treatment to levodopa/carbidopa in the management of Parkinson's disease

Unlabeled/Investigational: Tourette's disorder, chronic motor or vocal tic disorder

Local Anesthetic/Vasoconstrictor Precautions No information available to require special precautions

Effects on Dental Treatment May decrease or inhibit salivary flow; normal salivary flow resumes with discontinuation; prolonged salivary reduction could enhance development of periodontal disease, oral candidiasis and discomfort.

Dosage When adding pergolide to levodopa/carbidopa, the dose of the latter can usually and should be decreased. Patients no longer responsive to bromocriptine may benefit by being switched to pergolide. Oral:

Children and Adolescents: Tourette's disorder, chronic motor or vocal disorder (unlabeled uses): Up to 300 mcg/day

Adults: Parkinson's disease: Start with 0.05 mg/day for 2 days, then increase dosage by 0.1 or 0.15 mg/day every 3 days over next 12 days, increase dose by

0.25 mg/day every 3 days until optimal therapeutic dose is achieved, up to 5 mg/day maximum; usual dosage range: 2-3 mg/day in 3 divided doses

Mechanism of Action Pergolide is a semisynthetic ergot alkaloid similar to bromocriptine but stated to be more potent (10-1000 times) and longer-acting; it is a centrally-active dopamine agonist stimulating both D_1 and D_2 receptors. Pergolide is believed to exert its therapeutic effect by directly stimulating postsynaptic dopamine receptors in the nigrostriatal system.

Other Adverse Effects

>10%:

Central nervous system: Dizziness, somnolence, confusion, hallucinations, dystonia

Gastrointestinal: Nausea, constipation

Neuromuscular & skeletal: Dyskinesia

Respiratory: Rhinitis

1% to 10%:

Cardiovascular: Myocardial infarction, postural hypotension, syncope, arrhythmias, peripheral edema, vasodilation, palpitations, chest pain, hypertension

Central nervous system: Chills, insomnia, anxiety, psychosis, EPS, incoordination

Dermatologic: Rash

Gastrointestinal: Diarrhea, abdominal pain, xerostomia, anorexia, weight gain, dyspepsia, taste perversion

Hematologic: Anemia

Neuromuscular & skeletal: Weakness, myalgia, tremor, NMS (with rapid dose reduction), pain

Ocular: Abnormal vision, diplopia

Respiratory: Dyspnea, epistaxis

Miscellaneous: Flu syndrome, hiccups

Drug Interactions

Increased Effect/Toxicity: Use caution with other highly plasma protein bound drugs.

Decreased Effect: Dopamine antagonists (ie, antipsychotics, metoclopramide) may diminish the effects of pergolide; these combinations should generally be avoided.

Drug Uptake

Absorption: Oral: Well absorbed

Half-life, elimination: 27 hours

Pregnancy Risk Factor B

Generic Available No

Pergonal® *see* Menotropins *on page 759*

Periactin® *see* Cyproheptadine *on page 340*

Peri-Colace® [OTC] *see* Docusate and Casanthranol *on page 407*

Peridex® *see* Chlorhexidine Gluconate *on page 263*

Peri-Dri® *see* Nystatin *on page 880*

Perindopril Erbumine (per IN doe pril er BYOO meen)

U.S. Brand Names Aceon®

Canadian Brand Names Coversyl®

Mexican Brand Names Coversyl®

Pharmacologic Category Angiotensin-Converting Enzyme (ACE) Inhibitor

Use Treatment of stage I or II hypertension and CHF

Local Anesthetic/Vasoconstrictor Precautions No information available to require special precautions

Effects on Dental Treatment <1%: Taste disturbances

Dosage Adults: Oral:

Congestive heart failure: 4 mg once daily

Hypertension: Initial: 4 mg/day but may be titrated to response; usual range: 4-8 mg/day, maximum: 16 mg/day

Dosing adjustment in renal impairment:

Cl_{cr} >60 mL/minute: Administer 4 mg/day.

Cl_{cr} 30-60 mL/minute: Administer 2 mg/day.

Cl_{cr} 15-29 mL/minute: Administer 2 mg every other day.

Cl_{cr} <15 mL/minute: Administer 2 mg on the day of dialysis.

Hemodialysis: Perindopril and its metabolites are dialyzable

Dosing adjustment in geriatric patients: Due to greater bioavailability and lower renal clearance of the drug in elderly subjects, dose reduction of 50% is recommended.

Mechanism of Action Competitive inhibitor of angiotensin-converting enzyme (ACE); prevents conversion of angiotensin I to angiotensin II, a potent vasoconstrictor; results in lower levels of angiotensin II which, in turn, causes an increase in plasma renin activity and a reduction in aldosterone secretion

Other Adverse Effects

>10% Central nervous system: Headache (23%)

(Continued)

Perindopril Erbumine *(Continued)*

1% to 10%:

Cardiovascular: edema (4%), chest pain (2%)

Central nervous system: Dizziness (8%), sleep disorders (3%), depression (2%), fever (2%), weakness (8%), nervousness (1%)

Dermatologic: Rash (2%)

Endocrine & metabolic: Hyperkalemia (1%), increased triglycerides (1%)

Gastrointestinal: Nausea (2%), diarrhea (4%), vomiting (2%), dyspepsia (2%), abdominal pain (3%), flatulence (1%)

Genitourinary: Sexual dysfunction (male: 1%)

Hepatic: Increased ALT (2%)

Neuromuscular & skeletal: Back pain (6%), upper extremity pain (3%), lower extremity pain (5%), paresthesia (2%), joint pain (1%), myalgia (1%), arthritis (1%)

Renal: Proteinuria (2%)

Respiratory: Cough (incidence is higher in women, 3:1) (12%), sinusitis (5%), rhinitis (5%), pharyngitis (3%)

Otic: Tinnitus (2%)

Miscellaneous: Viral infection (3%)

Note: Some reactions occurred at an incidence >1% but ≤ placebo.

Additional adverse effects associated with with **ACE inhibitors** include agranulocytosis (especially in patients with renal impairment or collagen vascular disease), neutropenia, decreases in creatinine clearance in some elderly hypertensive patients or those with chronic renal failure, and worsening of renal function in patients with bilateral renal artery stenosis or hypovolemic patients (diuretic therapy). In addition, a syndrome which may include fever, arthralgia, interstitial nephritis, vasculitis, rash, eosinophilia and positive ANA, and elevated ESR has been reported with ACE inhibitors.

Drug Interactions

Increased Effect/Toxicity: Potassium supplements, co-trimoxazole (high dose), angiotensin II receptor antagonists (candesartan, losartan, irbesartan, etc), or potassium-sparing diuretics (amiloride, spironolactone, triamterene) may result in elevated serum potassium levels when combined with perindopril. ACE inhibitor effects may be increased by phenothiazines or probenecid (increases levels of captopril). ACE inhibitors may increase serum concentration/effects of digoxin, lithium, and sulfonlyureas. Diuretics have additive hypotensive effects with ACE inhibitors, and hypovolemia increases the potential for adverse renal effects of ACE inhibitors. In patients with compromised renal function, coadministration with nonsteroidal anti-inflammatory drugs may result in further deterioration of renal function. Allopurinol and ACE inhibitors may cause a higher risk of hypersensitivity reaction when taken concurrently.

Decreased Effect: Aspirin (high dose) may reduce the therapeutic effects of ACE inhibitors; at low dosages this does not appear to be significant. Rifampin may decrease the effect of ACE inhibitors. Antacids may decrease the bioavailability of ACE inhibitors (may be more likely to occur with captopril); separate administration times by 1-2 hours. NSAIDs, specifically indomethacin, may reduce the hypotensive effects of ACE inhibitors. More likely to occur in low renin or volume dependent hypertensive patients.

Drug Uptake

Onset of action: Peak effect: 1-2 hours

Half-life, elimination: Parent drug: 1.5-3 hours; Metabolite: Effective: 3-10 hours, Terminal: 30-120 hours

Time to peak: Chronic therapy: Perindopril: 1 hour; Perindoprilat: 3-4 hours (maximum perindoprilat serum levels are 2-3 times higher and T_{max} is shorter following chronic therapy); CHF: Perindoprilat: 6 hours

Pregnancy Risk Factor D (especially 2nd and 3rd trimesters)

Generic Available No

PerioChip® *see* Chlorhexidine Gluconate *on page 263*

PerioGard® *see* Chlorhexidine Gluconate *on page 263*

Periostat® *see* Doxycycline *on page 418*

Periostat® *see* Doxycycline Subantimicrobial *on page 422*

Permapen® *see* Penicillin G Benzathine *on page 928*

Permax® *see* Pergolide Mesylate *on page 938*

Permethrin (per METH rin)

U.S. Brand Names A200® Lice [OTC]; Acticin®; Elimite™; Medi-Lice® [OTC]; Nix™ Creme Rinse; R&C® Lice

Canadian Brand Names Kwellada-P™; Nix®

Mexican Brand Names Novo-Herklin 2000®

Pharmacologic Category Antiparasitic Agent, Topical; Scabicidal Agent

Use Single application treatment of infestation with *Pediculus humanus capitis* (head louse) and its nits or *Sarcoptes scabiei* (scabies)

Local Anesthetic/Vasoconstrictor Precautions No information available to require special precautions

Effects on Dental Treatment No effects or complications reported

Dosage Topical: Children >2 months and Adults:

Head lice: After hair has been washed with shampoo, rinsed with water, and towel dried, apply a sufficient volume of topical liquid to saturate the hair and scalp. Leave on hair for 10 minutes before rinsing off with water; remove remaining nits; may repeat in 1 week if lice or nits still present.

Scabies: Apply cream from head to toe; leave on for 8-14 hours before washing off with water; for infants, also apply on the hairline, neck, scalp, temple, and forehead; may reapply in 1 week if live mites appear

Permethrin 5% cream was shown to be safe and effective when applied to an infant <1 month of age with neonatal scabies; time of application was limited to 6 hours before rinsing with soap and water

Mechanism of Action Inhibits sodium ion influx through nerve cell membrane channels in parasites resulting in delayed repolarization and thus paralysis and death of the pest

Other Adverse Effects 1% to 10%:

Dermatologic: Pruritus, erythema, rash of the scalp

Local: Burning, stinging, tingling, numbness or scalp discomfort, edema

Drug Uptake Absorption: Topical: Minimal (<2%)

Pregnancy Risk Factor B

Generic Available Yes

Permitil® *see* Fluphenazine *on page 520*

Perphenazine (per FEN a zeen)

U.S. Brand Names Trilafon®

Canadian Brand Names Apo®-Perphenazine; Trilafon®

Mexican Brand Names Leptopsique

Pharmacologic Category Antipsychotic Agent, Phenothiazine, Piperazine

Use Treatment of severe schizophrenia; nausea and vomiting

Unlabeled/Investigational: Ethanol withdrawal; dementia in elderly; Tourette's syndrome; Huntington's chorea; spasmodic torticollis; Reye's syndrome; psychosis

Local Anesthetic/Vasoconstrictor Precautions Most pharmacology textbooks state that in presence of phenothiazines, systemic doses of epinephrine paradoxically decrease the blood pressure. This is the so called "epinephrine reversal" phenomenon. This has never been observed when epinephrine is given by infiltration as part of the anesthesia procedure.

Effects on Dental Treatment

Significant hypotension may occur, especially when the drug is administered parenterally; orthostatic hypotension is due to alpha-receptor blockade, the elderly are at greater risk for orthostatic hypotension.

Tardive dyskinesia: Prevalence rate may be 40% in elderly; development of the syndrome and the irreversible nature are proportional to duration and total cumulative dose over time. Extrapyramidal reactions are more common in elderly with up to 50% developing these reactions after 60 years of age; drug-induced **Parkinson's syndrome** occurs often; **Akathisia** is the most common extrapyramidal reaction in elderly.

Increased confusion, memory loss, psychotic behavior, and agitation frequently occur as a consequence of anticholinergic effects. Antipsychotic associated sedation in nonpsychotic patients is extremely unpleasant due to feelings of depersonalization, derealization, and dysphoria

Dosage

Children:

Schizophrenia/psychoses:

Oral:

1-6 years: 4-6 mg/day in divided doses

6-12 years: 6 mg/day in divided doses

>12 years: 4-16 mg 2-4 times/day

I.M.: 5 mg every 6 hours

Nausea/vomiting: I.M.: 5 mg every 6 hours

Adults:

Schizophrenia/psychoses:

Oral: 4-16 mg 2-4 times/day not to exceed 64 mg/day

I.M.: 5 mg every 6 hours up to 15 mg/day in ambulatory patients and 30 mg/day in hospitalized patients

Nausea/vomiting:

Oral: 8-16 mg/day in divided doses up to 24 mg/day

I.M.: 5-10 mg every 6 hours as necessary up to 15 mg/day in ambulatory patients and 30 mg/day in hospitalized patients

I.V. (severe): 1 mg at 1- to 2-minute intervals up to a total of 5 mg

(Continued)

Perphenazine *(Continued)*

Elderly: Behavioral symptoms associated with dementia: Oral: Initial: 2-4 mg 1-2 times/day; increase at 4- to 7-day intervals by 2-4 mg/day. Increase dose intervals (bid, tid, etc) as necessary to control behavior response or side effects. Maximum daily dose: 32 mg; gradual increase (titration) and bedtime administration may prevent some side effects or decrease their severity.

Hemodialysis: Not dialyzable (0% to 5%)

Dosing adjustment in hepatic impairment: Dosage reductions should be considered in patients with liver disease although no specific guidelines are available

Mechanism of Action Blocks postsynaptic mesolimbic dopaminergic receptors in the brain; exhibits a strong alpha-adrenergic blocking effect and depresses the release of hypothalamic and hypophyseal hormones

Other Adverse Effects Frequency not defined:

Cardiovascular: Hypotension, orthostatic hypotension, hypertension, tachycardia, bradycardia, dizziness, cardiac arrest

Central nervous system: Extrapyramidal symptoms (pseudoparkinsonism, akathisia, dystonias, tardive dyskinesia), dizziness, cerebral edema, seizures, headache, drowsiness, paradoxical excitement, restlessness, hyperactivity, insomnia, neuroleptic malignant syndrome (NMS), impairment of temperature regulation

Dermatologic: Increased sensitivity to sun, rash, discoloration of skin (blue-gray)

Endocrine & metabolic: Hypoglycemia, hyperglycemia, galactorrhea, lactation, breast enlargement, gynecomastia, menstrual irregularity, amenorrhea, SIADH, changes in libido

Gastrointestinal: Constipation, weight gain, vomiting, stomach pain, nausea, xerostomia, salivation, diarrhea, anorexia, ileus

Genitourinary: Difficulty in urination, ejaculatory disturbances, incontinence, polyuria, ejaculating dysfunction, priapism

Hematologic: Agranulocytosis, leukopenia, eosinophilia, hemolytic anemia, thrombocytopenic purpura, pancytopenia

Hepatic: Cholestatic jaundice, hepatotoxicity

Neuromuscular & skeletal: Tremor

Ocular: Pigmentary retinopathy, blurred vision, cornea and lens changes

Respiratory: Nasal congestion

Miscellaneous: Diaphoresis

Drug Interactions CYP2D6 enzyme substrate; CYP2D6 enzyme inhibitor

Aluminum salts: May decrease the absorption of phenothiazines; monitor

Amphetamines: Efficacy may be diminished by antipsychotics; in addition, amphetamines may increase psychotic symptoms; avoid concurrent use

Anticholinergics: May inhibit the therapeutic response to phenothiazines and excess anticholinergic effects may occur; includes benztropine, trihexyphenidyl, biperiden, and drugs with significant anticholinergic activity (TCAs, antihistamines, disopyramide)

Antihypertensives: Concurrent use of phenothiazines with an antihypertensive may produce additive hypotensive effects (particularly orthostasis)

Bromocriptine: Phenothiazines inhibit the ability of bromocriptine to lower serum prolactin concentrations

CNS depressants: Sedative effects may be additive with phenothiazines; monitor for increased effect; includes barbiturates, benzodiazepines, narcotic analgesics, ethanol, and other sedative agents

CYP2D6 inhibitors: Metabolism of phenothiazines may be decreased; increasing clinical effect or toxicity; inhibitors include amiodarone, cimetidine, delavirdine, fluoxetine, paroxetine, propafenone, quinidine, ritonavir, and sertraline; monitor for increased effect/toxicity

Enzyme inducers: May enhance the hepatic metabolism of phenothiazines; larger doses may be required; includes rifampin, rifabutin, barbiturates, phenytoin, and cigarette smoking

Epinephrine: Chlorpromazine (and possibly other low potency antipsychotics) may diminish the pressor effects of epinephrine

Guanethidine and guanadrel: Antihypertensive effects may be inhibited by phenothiazines

Levodopa: Phenothiazines may inhibit the antiparkinsonian effect of levodopa; avoid this combination

Lithium: Phenothiazines may produce neurotoxicity with lithium; this is a rare effect

Metoclopramide: May increase extrapyramidal symptoms (EPS) or risk.

Phenytoin: May reduce serum levels of phenothiazines; phenothiazines may increase phenytoin serum levels

Propranolol: Serum concentrations of phenothiazines may be increased; propranolol also increases phenothiazine concentrations

Polypeptide antibiotics: Rare cases of respiratory paralysis have been reported with concurrent use of phenothiazines

QT_c-prolonging agents: Effects on QT_c interval may be additive with phenothiazines, increasing the risk of malignant arrhythmias; includes type Ia antiarrhythmics, TCAs, and some quinolone antibiotics (sparfloxacin, moxifloxacin, and gatifloxacin)

Sulfadoxine-pyrimethamine: May increase phenothiazine concentrations
Tricyclic antidepressants: Concurrent use may produce increased toxicity or altered therapeutic response
Trazodone: Phenothiazines and trazodone may produce additive hypotensive effects
Valproic acid: Serum levels may be increased by phenothiazines

Drug Uptake
Absorption: Oral: Well absorbed
Half-life, elimination: 9 hours
Time to peak: 4-8 hours

Pregnancy Risk Factor C
Generic Available Yes

Persantine® *see* Dipyridamole *on page 401*
Pertussin® CS [OTC] *see* Dextromethorphan *on page 372*
Pertussin® ES [OTC] *see* Dextromethorphan *on page 372*
Pfizerpen® *see* Penicillin G, Parenteral, Aqueous *on page 929*
Phanatuss® Cough Syrup [OTC] *see* Guaifenesin and Dextromethorphan *on page 569*
Pharmaflur® *see* Fluoride *on page 514*
Phazyme® [OTC] *see* Simethicone *on page 1088*
Phenadex® Senior [OTC] *see* Guaifenesin and Dextromethorphan *on page 569*
Phenameth® DM *see* Promethazine and Dextromethorphan *on page 1007*
Phenaphen® With Codeine *see* Acetaminophen and Codeine *on page 28*

Phenazopyridine (fen az oh PEER i deen)

U.S. Brand Names Azo-Dine® [OTC]; Azo-Gesic® [OTC]; Azo-Standard®; Baridium®; Prodium™ [OTC]; Pyridiate®; Pyridium®; Uristat® [OTC]; Urodol® [OTC]; Urofemme® [OTC]; Urogesic®
Canadian Brand Names Phenazo™; Pyridium®
Mexican Brand Names Azo Wintomylon; Madel; Urovalidin
Pharmacologic Category Analgesic, Urinary
Synonyms Phenazopyridine Hydrochloride; Phenylazo Diamino Pyridine Hydrochloride
Use Symptomatic relief of urinary burning, itching, frequency and urgency in association with urinary tract infection or following urologic procedures
Local Anesthetic/Vasoconstrictor Precautions No information available to require special precautions
Effects on Dental Treatment No effects or complications reported
Dosage Oral:
Children: 12 mg/kg/day in 3 divided doses administered after meals for 2 days
Adults: 100-200 mg 3 times/day after meals for 2 days when used concomitantly with an antibacterial agent
Mechanism of Action An azo dye which exerts local anesthetic or analgesic action on urinary tract mucosa through an unknown mechanism
Other Adverse Effects 1% to 10%:
Central nervous system: Headache, dizziness
Gastrointestinal: Stomach cramps
Pregnancy Risk Factor B
Generic Available Yes

Phendiet® *see* Phendimetrazine *on page 943*
Phendiet®-105 *see* Phendimetrazine *on page 943*

Phendimetrazine (fen dye ME tra zeen)

U.S. Brand Names Bontril PDM®; Bontril® Slow-Release; Melfiat®; Obezine®; Phendiet®; Phendiet®-105; Prelu-2®
Canadian Brand Names Bontril®; Plegine®; Statobex®
Pharmacologic Category Anorexiant
Synonyms Phendimetrazine Tartrate
Use An appetite suppressant during the first few weeks of dieting to help establish new eating habits; its effectiveness lasts only for short periods (3-12 weeks)
Local Anesthetic/Vasoconstrictor Precautions Use vasoconstrictor with caution in patients taking phendimetrazine. Phendimetrazine can enhance the sympathomimetic response to epinephrine leading to potential hypertension and cardiotoxicity.
Effects on Dental Treatment Patients taking phendimetrazine may present with hypertension; monitor BP.
Restrictions C-III
Dosage Adults: Oral:
Regular capsule or tablet: 35 mg 2 or 3 times daily, 1 hour before meals
Sustained release: 105 mg once daily in the morning before breakfast
Other Adverse Effects Frequency not defined:
Cardiovascular: Hypertension, tachycardia, arrhythmias
(Continued)

Phendimetrazine *(Continued)*

Central nervous system: Euphoria, nervousness, insomnia, confusion, mental depression, restlessness, headache
Dermatologic: Alopecia
Endocrine & metabolic: Changes in libido
Gastrointestinal: Nausea, vomiting, constipation, diarrhea, abdominal cramps
Genitourinary: Dysuria
Hematologic: Blood dyscrasias
Neuromuscular & skeletal: Tremor, myalgia
Ocular: Blurred vision
Renal: Polyuria
Respiratory: Dyspnea
Miscellaneous: Diaphoresis (increased)

Contraindications Hypersensitivity to phendimetrazine or any component of the formulation

Warnings/Precautions Anorexigens have been reported to be associated with the occurrence of serious regurgitant cardiac valvular disease, including disease of the mitral, aortic, and/or tricuspid valves. Primary pulmonary hypertension (PPH) - a rare, frequently fatal disease of the lungs - has been found to occur with increased frequency in patients receiving anorexigens. There have been reports of PPH and valvular irregularities in users of phendimetrazine tartrate tablets. The safety and effectiveness of the combined use of phendimetrazine with other anorexigens in the treatment of obesity have not been established, and there is no approved use of these products together in the treatment of obesity. Phendimetrazine is approved only as a single agent for short-term use (ie, a few weeks).

Generic Available Yes

Phenelzine (FEN el zeen)

U.S. Brand Names Nardil®

Canadian Brand Names Nardil®

Pharmacologic Category Antidepressant, Monoamine Oxidase Inhibitor

Synonyms Phenelzine Sulfate

Use Symptomatic treatment of atypical, nonendogenous, or neurotic depression

Unlabeled/Investigational: Selective mutism

Local Anesthetic/Vasoconstrictor Precautions Attempts should be made to avoid use of vasoconstrictor due to possibility of hypertensive episodes with monoamine oxidase inhibitors

Effects on Dental Treatment

>10%: Orthostatic hypotension
Avoid use as an analgesic due to toxic reactions with MAO inhibitors.

Dosage Oral:

Children: Selective mutism (unlabeled use): 30-60 mg/day
Adults: Depression: 15 mg 3 times/day; may increase to 60-90 mg/day during early phase of treatment, then reduce to dose for maintenance therapy slowly after maximum benefit is obtained; takes 2-4 weeks for a significant response to occur
Elderly: Depression: Initial: 7.5 mg/day; increase by 7.5-15 mg/day every 3-4 days as tolerated; usual therapeutic dose: 15-60 mg/day in 3-4 divided doses

Mechanism of Action Thought to act by increasing endogenous concentrations of epinephrine, norepinephrine, dopamine and serotonin through inhibition of the enzyme (monoamine oxidase) responsible for the breakdown of these neurotransmitters

Other Adverse Effects Frequency not defined:

Cardiovascular: Orthostatic hypotension, edema
Central nervous system: Dizziness, headache, drowsiness, sleep disturbances, fatigue, hyper-reflexia, twitching, ataxia, mania
Dermatologic: Rash, pruritus
Endocrine & metabolic: Decreased sexual ability (anorgasmia, ejaculatory disturbances, impotence), hypernatremia, hypermetabolic syndrome
Gastrointestinal: Xerostomia, constipation, weight gain
Genitourinary: Urinary retention
Hematologic: Leukopenia
Hepatic: Hepatitis
Neuromuscular & skeletal: Weakness, tremor, myoclonus
Ocular: Blurred vision, glaucoma
Miscellaneous: Diaphoresis

Drug Interactions

Increased Effect/Toxicity: In general, the combined use of phenelzine with TCAs, venlafaxine, trazodone, dexfenfluramine, sibutramine, lithium, meperidine, fenfluramine, dextromethorphan, and SSRIs should be avoided due to the potential for severe adverse reactions (serotonin syndrome, death). MAO inhibitors (including phenelzine) may inhibit the metabolism of barbiturates and prolong their effect. Phenelzine in combination with amphetamines, other stimulants (methylphenidate), levodopa, metaraminol, reserpine, and decongestants (pseudoephedrine) may result in severe hypertensive reactions. Phenelzine may increase the pressor response of norepinephrine and may prolong neuromuscular blockade produced by succinylcholine. Tramadol may increase the risk of seizures and serotonin syndrome in patients receiving an MAO inhibitor. Phenelzine may produce additive hypoglycemic effect in patients receiving hypoglycemic agents and may produce delirium in patients receiving disulfiram.

Decreased Effect: Phenelzine (and other MAO inhibitors) inhibits the antihypertensive response to guanadrel or guanethidine.

Drug Uptake

Onset of action: Therapeutic: 2-4 weeks

Absorption: Oral: Well absorbed

Duration: May continue to have a therapeutic effect and interactions 2 weeks after discontinuation

Pregnancy Risk Factor C

Generic Available No

Phenergan® *see* Promethazine *on page 1006*

Phenergan® VC *see* Promethazine and Phenylephrine *on page 1008*

Phenergan® VC With Codeine *see* Promethazine, Phenylephrine, and Codeine *on page 1008*

Phenergan® With Codeine *see* Promethazine and Codeine *on page 1007*

Phenergan® With Dextromethorphan *see* Promethazine and Dextromethorphan *on page 1007*

Phenhist® Expectorant *see* Guaifenesin, Pseudoephedrine, and Codeine *on page 570*

Phenindamine (fen IN dah meen)

U.S. Brand Names Nolahist® [OTC]

Canadian Brand Names Nolahist®

Pharmacologic Category Antihistamine

Synonyms Phenindamine Tartrate

Use Treatment of perennial and seasonal allergic rhinitis and chronic urticaria

Local Anesthetic/Vasoconstrictor Precautions No information available to require special precautions

Effects on Dental Treatment No effects or complications reported

Dosage Oral:

Children <6 years: As directed by physician

Children 6 to <12 years: 12.5 mg every 4-6 hours, up to 75 mg/24 hours

Adults: 25 mg every 4-6 hours, up to 150 mg/24 hours

Generic Available No

Phenobarbital (fee noe BAR bi tal)

U.S. Brand Names Luminal® Sodium

Mexican Brand Names Alepsal

Pharmacologic Category Anticonvulsant, Barbiturate; Barbiturate

Synonyms Phenobarbital Sodium; Phenobarbitone; Phenylethylmalonylurea

Use Management of generalized tonic-clonic (grand mal) and partial seizures; sedative

Unlabeled/Investigational: Febrile seizures in children; may also be used for prevention and treatment of neonatal hyperbilirubinemia and lowering of bilirubin in chronic cholestasis; neonatal seizures; management of sedative/hypnotic withdrawal

Local Anesthetic/Vasoconstrictor Precautions No information available to require special precautions

Effects on Dental Treatment No effects or complications reported

Restrictions C-IV

Dosage

Children:

- Sedation: Oral: 2 mg/kg 3 times/day
- Hypnotic: I.M., I.V., S.C.: 3-5 mg/kg at bedtime
- Preoperative sedation: Oral, I.M., I.V.: 1-3 mg/kg 1-1.5 hours before procedure

Adults:

- Sedation: Oral, I.M.: 30-120 mg/day in 2-3 divided doses
- Hypnotic: Oral, I.M., I.V., S.C.: 100-320 mg at bedtime
- Preoperative sedation: I.M.: 100-200 mg 1-1.5 hours before procedure

Anticonvulsant: Status epilepticus: **Loading dose:** I.V.:

- Infants and Children: 10-20 mg/kg in a single or divided dose; in select patients may administer additional 5 mg/kg/dose every 15-30 minutes until seizure is controlled or a total dose of 40 mg/kg is reached
- Adults: 300-800 mg initially followed by 120-240 mg/dose at 20-minute intervals until seizures are controlled or a total dose of 1-2 g

Anticonvulsant maintenance dose: Oral, I.V.:

- Infants: 5-8 mg/kg/day in 1-2 divided doses
- Children:
  - 1-5 years: 6-8 mg/kg/day in 1-2 divided doses
  - 5-12 years: 4-6 mg/kg/day in 1-2 divided doses

(Continued)

Phenobarbital *(Continued)*

Children >12 years and Adults: 1-3 mg/kg/day in divided doses or 50-100 mg 2-3 times/day

Sedative/hypnotic withdrawal (unlabeled use): Initial daily requirement is determined by substituting phenobarbital 30 mg for every 100 mg pentobarbital used during tolerance testing; then daily requirement is decreased by 10% of initial dose

Dosing interval in renal impairment: Cl_{cr} <10 mL/minute: Administer every 12-16 hours

Hemodialysis: Moderately dialyzable (20% to 50%)

Dosing adjustment/comments in hepatic disease: Increased side effects may occur in severe liver disease; monitor plasma concentrations and adjust dose accordingly

Mechanism of Action Short-acting barbiturate with sedative, hypnotic, and anticonvulsant properties. Interferes with transmission of impulses from the thalamus to the cortex of the brain resulting in an imbalance in central inhibitory and facilitatory mechanisms. Barbiturates depress the sensory cortex, decrease motor activity, alter cerebellar function, and produce drowsiness, sedation, and hypnosis. In high doses, barbiturates exhibit anticonvulsant activity; barbiturates produce dose-dependent respiratory depression.

Other Adverse Effects Frequency not defined:

Cardiovascular: Bradycardia, hypotension, syncope

Central nervous system: Drowsiness, lethargy, CNS excitation or depression, impaired judgment, "hangover" effect, confusion, somnolence, agitation, hyperkinesia, ataxia, nervousness, headache, insomnia, nightmares, hallucinations, anxiety, dizziness

Dermatologic: Rash, exfoliative dermatitis, Stevens-Johnson syndrome

Gastrointestinal: Nausea, vomiting, constipation

Hematologic: Agranulocytosis, thrombocytopenia, megaloblastic anemia

Local: Pain at injection site, thrombophlebitis with I.V. use

Renal: Oliguria

Respiratory: Laryngospasm, respiratory depression, apnea (especially with rapid I.V. use), hypoventilation

Miscellaneous: Gangrene with inadvertent intra-arterial injection

Drug Interactions CYP1A2, 2B6, 2C, 2C8, 2C9, 2C18, 2C19, 3A3/4, and 3A5-7 enzyme inducer

Increased Effect/Toxicity: When combined with other CNS depressants, narcotic analgesics, antidepressants, or benzodiazepines, additive respiratory and CNS depression may occur. Barbiturates may enhance the hepatotoxic potential of acetaminophen overdoses. Chloramphenicol, MAO inhibitors, valproic acid, and felbamate may inhibit barbiturate metabolism. Barbiturates may impair the absorption of griseofulvin, and may enhance the nephrotoxic effects of methoxyflurane. Concurrent use of phenobarbital with meperidine may result in increased CNS depression. Concurrent use of phenobarbital with primidone may result in elevated phenobarbital serum concentration.

Decreased Effect: Barbiturates are hepatic enzyme inducers, and may increase the metabolism of antipsychotics, some beta-blockers (unlikely with atenolol and nadolol), calcium channel blockers, chloramphenicol, cimetidine, corticosteroids, cyclosporine, disopyramide, doxycycline, ethosuximide, felbamate, furosemide, griseofulvin, lamotrigine, phenytoin, propafenone, quinidine, tacrolimus, TCAs, and theophylline. Barbiturates may increase the metabolism of estrogens and reduce the efficacy of oral contraceptives; an alternative method of contraception should be considered. Barbiturates inhibit the hypoprothrombinemic effects of oral anticoagulants via increased metabolism. Barbiturates may enhance the metabolism of methadone resulting in methadone withdrawal.

Drug Uptake

Onset of action: Oral: Hypnosis: 20-60 minutes; I.V.: ~5 minutes

Peak effect: I.V.: ~30 minutes

Absorption: Oral: 70% to 90%

Duration: Oral: 6-10 hours; I.V.: 4-10 hours

Half-life, elimination: Neonates: 45-500 hours; Infants: 20-133 hours; Children: 37-73 hours; Adults: 53-140 hours

Time to peak: Oral: 1-6 hours

Pregnancy Risk Factor D

Generic Available Yes

Phenol (FEE nol)

Related Information

Mouth Pain, Cold Sore, and Canker Sore Products *on page 1458*

U.S. Brand Names Baker's P & S [OTC]; Cēpastat® [OTC]; Chloraseptic® [OTC]; Ulcerease® [OTC]

Canadian Brand Names P & S™ Liquid Phenol

Pharmacologic Category Pharmaceutical Aid

Synonyms Carbolic Acid

Use Relief of sore throat pain, mouth, gum, and throat irritations

Local Anesthetic/Vasoconstrictor Precautions No information available to require special precautions

Effects on Dental Treatment No effects or complications reported

Dosage

Allow to dissolve slowly in mouth; may be repeated every 2 hours as needed

For each neurolysis procedure: 0.5-2 mL (up to 7.5 mL may be needed)

Other Adverse Effects Frequency not defined:

In overdose situation:

Cardiovascular: Hypotension, cardiovascular collapse, tachycardia, atrial and ventricular arrhythmias, edema

Central nervous system: slurred speech, CNS depression, agitation, confusion, seizures, coma

Dermatologic: White, red, or brown skin discoloration

Gastrointestinal: Nausea, vomiting, oral burns GI ulceration, GI bleeding

Genitourinary: Urine discoloration (green)

Hematologic: Hemorrhage

Local: Irritation, burns

Renal: Nephritis

Respiratory: Bronchospasm/wheezing, coughing, dyspnea, pneumonia, pulmonary

When used for spinal neurolysis/motor point blocks:

Cardiovascular: Dysrhythmias

Central nervous system: Headache, hyperesthesia, dysesthesia

Gastrointestinal: Bowel incontinence

Genitourinary: Urinary incontinence

Local: Tissue necrosis, pain at injection site

Neuromuscular & skeletal: Motor weakness, nerve damage

Respiratory: Pleural irritation

Pregnancy Risk Factor C

Generic Available Yes

Comments Cepastat® contains 8 calories/lozenge (2 g sorbitol)

Phenoxybenzamine (fen oks ee BEN za meen)

U.S. Brand Names Dibenzyline®

Canadian Brand Names Dibenzyline®

Pharmacologic Category $Alpha_1$ Blocker

Synonyms Phenoxybenzamine Hydrochloride

Use Symptomatic management of pheochromocytoma; treatment of hypertensive crisis caused by sympathomimetic amines

Unlabeled/Investigational: Micturition problems associated with neurogenic bladder, functional outlet obstruction, and partial prostate obstruction

Local Anesthetic/Vasoconstrictor Precautions No information available to require special precautions

Effects on Dental Treatment No effects or complications reported

Dosage Oral:

Children: Initial: 0.2 mg/kg (maximum: 10 mg) once daily, increase by 0.2 mg/kg increments; usual maintenance dose: 0.4-1.2 mg/kg/day every 6-8 hours, higher doses may be necessary

Adults: Initial: 10 mg twice daily, increase by 10 mg every other day until optimum dose is achieved; usual range: 20-40 mg 2-3 times/day

Mechanism of Action Produces long-lasting noncompetitive alpha-adrenergic blockade of postganglionic synapses in exocrine glands and smooth muscle; relaxes urethra and increases opening of the bladder

Other Adverse Effects Frequency not defined:

Cardiovascular: Postural hypotension, tachycardia, syncope, shock

Central nervous system: Lethargy, headache, confusion, fatigue

Gastrointestinal: Vomiting, nausea, diarrhea, xerostomia

Genitourinary: Inhibition of ejaculation

Neuromuscular & skeletal: Weakness

Ocular: Miosis

Respiratory: Nasal congestion

Drug Interactions

Increased Effect/Toxicity: Beta-blockers may result in increased toxicity (hypotension, tachycardia).

Decreased Effect: Alpha adrenergic agonists decrease the effect of phenoxybenzamine.

Drug Uptake

Onset of action: Oral: ≤2 hours; Peak effect: 4-6 hours

Duration: ≥4 days

Half-life, elimination: 24 hours

Pregnancy Risk Factor C

Generic Available No

Phentermine (FEN ter meen)

U.S. Brand Names Adipex-P®; Ionamin®

Canadian Brand Names Ionamin®

Mexican Brand Names Ifa Reduccing "S"®

Pharmacologic Category Anorexiant

Synonyms Phentermine Hydrochloride

Use Short-term adjunct in a regimen of weight reduction based on exercise, behavioral modification, and caloric reduction in the management of exogenous obesity for patients with an initial body mass index ≥30 kg/m^2 or ≥27 kg/m^2 in the presence of other risk factors (diabetes, hypertension)

Local Anesthetic/Vasoconstrictor Precautions Use vasoconstriction with caution in patients taking phentermine. Amphetamines enhance the sympathomimetic response of epinephrine and norepinephrine leading to potential hypertension and cardiotoxicity.

Effects on Dental Treatment Up to 10% of patients may present with hypertension. The use of local anesthetic without vasoconstrictor is recommended in these patients.

Restrictions C-IV

Dosage Oral: Adults: Obesity: 8 mg 3 times/day 30 minutes before meals or food or 15-37.5 mg/day before breakfast or 10-14 hours before retiring

Mechanism of Action Phentermine is structurally similar to dextroamphetamine and is comparable to dextroamphetamine as an appetite suppressant, but is generally associated with a lower incidence and severity of CNS side effects. Phentermine, like other anorexiants, stimulates the hypothalamus to result in decreased appetite; anorexiant effects are most likely mediated via norepinephrine and dopamine metabolism. However, other CNS effects or metabolic effects may be involved.

Other Adverse Effects Frequency not defined:

Cardiovascular: Hypertension, palpitations, tachycardia, primary pulmonary hypertension and/or regurgitant cardiac valvular disease

Central nervous system: Euphoria, insomnia, overstimulation, dizziness, dysphoria, headache, restlessness, psychosis

Dermatologic: Urticaria

Endocrine & metabolic: Changes in libido, impotence

Gastrointestinal: Nausea, constipation, xerostomia, unpleasant taste, diarrhea

Hematologic: Blood dyscrasias

Neuromuscular & skeletal: Tremor

Ocular: Blurred vision

Contraindications Hypersensitivity or idiosyncrasy to sympathomimetic amines or any component of the formulation; patients with advanced arteriosclerosis, symptomatic cardiovascular disease, moderate to severe hypertension (stage II or III), hyperthyroidism, glaucoma, agitated states; patients with a history of drug abuse; use during or within 14 days following MAO inhibitor therapy; children <16 years of age (per manufacturer)

Warnings/Precautions Use with caution in patients with bipolar disorder, diabetes mellitus, cardiovascular disease, seizure disorders, insomnia, porphyria, or mild hypertension (stage I). May exacerbate symptoms of behavior and thought disorder in psychotic patients. Stimulants may unmask tics in individuals with coexisting Tourette's syndrome. Potential for drug dependency exists - avoid abrupt discontinuation in patients who have received for prolonged periods. Use in weight reduction programs only when alternative therapy has been ineffective. Stimulant use has been associated with growth suppression, and careful monitoring is recommended.

Primary pulmonary hypertension (PPH), a rare and frequently fatal pulmonary disease, has been reported to occur in patients receiving a combination of phentermine and fenfluramine or dexfenfluramine. The possibility of an association between PPH and the use of phentermine alone cannot be ruled out.

Drug Interactions

Increased Effect/Toxicity: Dosage of hypoglycemic agents may need to be adjusted when phentermine is used in a diabetic receiving a special diet. Concurrent use of MAO inhibitors and drugs with MAO activity (furazolidone, linezolid) may be associated with hypertensive episodes. Concurrent use of SSRIs may be associated with a risk of serotonin syndrome.

Decreased Effect: Phentermine may decrease the effect of antihypertensive medications The efficacy of anorexiants may be decreased by antipsychotics; in addition, amphetamines or related compounds may induce an increase in psychotic symptoms in some patients. Amphetamines (and related compounds) inhibit the antihypertensive response to guanethidine; probably also may occur with guanadrel.

Drug Uptake

Absorption: Well absorbed; resin absorbed more slowly and produces prolonged clinical effects

Duration: Resin produces more prolonged clinical effects

Half-life, elimination: 20 hours

Pregnancy Risk Factor C

Generic Available Yes

Comments Many diet physicians have prescribed fenfluramine ("fen") and phentermine ("phen"). When taken together the combination is known as "fen-phen". The diet drug dexfenfluramine (Redux®) is chemically similar to fenfluramine (Pondimin®) and was also used in combination with phentermine called "Redux-phen". While each of the three drugs alone had approval from the FDA for sale in the treatment of obesity, neither combination had an official approval. The use of the combinations in the treatment of obesity was considered an "off-label" use. Reports in medical literature have been accumulating for some years about significant side effects associated with fenfluramine and dexfenfluramine. In 1997, the manufacturers, at the urging of the FDA, agreed to voluntarily withdraw the drugs from the market. The action was based on findings from physicians who evaluated patients taking fenfluramine and dexfenfluramine with echocardiograms. The findings indicated that approximately 30% of patients had abnormal echocardiograms, even though they had no symptoms. This was a much higher than expected percentage of abnormal test results. This conclusion was based on a sample of 291 patients examined by five different physicians. Under normal conditions, fewer than 1% of patients would be expected to show signs of heart valve disease. The findings suggested that fenfluramine and dexfenfluramine were the likely cause of heart valve problems of the type that promoted FDA's earlier warnings concerning "fen-phen". The earlier warning included the following: The mitral valve and other valves in the heart are damaged by a strange white coating and allow blood to flow back, causing heart muscle damage. In several cases, valve replacement surgery has been done. As a rule, the person must, thereafter for life, be on a blood thinner to prevent clots from the mechanical valve. This type of valve damage had only been seen before in persons who were exposed to large amounts of serotonin. The fenfluramine increases the availability of serotonin.

Phentolamine (fen TOLE a meen)

U.S. Brand Names Regitine®

Canadian Brand Names Regitine®

Mexican Brand Names Z-Max®

Pharmacologic Category Alpha$_1$ Blocker

Synonyms Phentolamine Mesylate

Use Diagnosis of pheochromocytoma and treatment of hypertension associated with pheochromocytoma or other caused by excess sympathomimetic amines; as treatment of dermal necrosis after extravasation of drugs with alpha-adrenergic effects (norepinephrine, dopamine, epinephrine, dobutamine)

Local Anesthetic/Vasoconstrictor Precautions Although the alpha-adrenergic blocking effects could antagonize epinephrine, there is no information available to require special precautions

Effects on Dental Treatment No effects or complications reported

Dosage

Treatment of alpha-adrenergic drug extravasation: S.C.:

- Children: 0.1-0.2 mg/kg diluted in 10 mL 0.9% sodium chloride infiltrated into area of extravasation within 12 hours
- Adults: Infiltrate area with small amount of solution made by diluting 5-10 mg in 10 mL 0.9% sodium chloride within 12 hours of extravasation
- If dose is effective, normal skin color should return to the blanched area within 1 hour

Diagnosis of pheochromocytoma: I.M., I.V.:

- Children: 0.05-0.1 mg/kg/dose, maximum single dose: 5 mg
- Adults: 5 mg

Surgery for pheochromocytoma: Hypertension: I.M., I.V.:

- Children: 0.05-0.1 mg/kg/dose given 1-2 hours before procedure; repeat as needed every 2-4 hours until hypertension is controlled; maximum single dose: 5 mg
- Adults: 5 mg given 1-2 hours before procedure and repeated as needed every 2-4 hours

Hypertensive crisis: Adults: 5-20 mg

Mechanism of Action Competitively blocks alpha-adrenergic receptors to produce brief antagonism of circulating epinephrine and norepinephrine to reduce hypertension caused by alpha effects of these catecholamines; also has a positive inotropic and chronotropic effect on the heart

Other Adverse Effects Frequency not defined:

- Cardiovascular: Hypotension, tachycardia, arrhythmia, flushing, orthostatic hypotension
- Central nervous system: Weakness, dizziness
- Gastrointestinal: Nausea, vomiting, diarrhea
- Respiratory: Nasal congestion

Drug Interactions Decreased effect of phentolamine with epinephrine and ephedrine

Drug Uptake

Onset of action: I.M.: 15-20 minutes; I.V.: Immediate

Duration: I.M.: 30-45 minutes; I.V.: 15-30 minutes

(Continued)

Phentolamine *(Continued)*

Half-life, elimination: 19 minutes

Pregnancy Risk Factor C

Generic Available Yes

Phenylephrine (fen il EF rin)

Related Information

Guaifenesin and Phenylephrine *on page 569*

U.S. Brand Names AK-Dilate® Ophthalmic; AK-Nefrin® Ophthalmic; Alconefrin® Nasal [OTC]; Children's Nostril®; Mydfrin® Ophthalmic; Neo-Synephrine® Injection; Neo-Synephrine® Nasal [OTC]; Neo-Synephrine® Ophthalmic; Nostril® Nasal [OTC]; Prefrin™ Ophthalmic; Relief® Ophthalmic; Rhinall® Nasal [OTC]; Vicks Sinex® Nasal [OTC]

Canadian Brand Names Dionephrine®; Mydfrin®; Neo-Synephrine®

Pharmacologic Category Alpha/Beta Agonist; Ophthalmic Agent, Antiglaucoma; Ophthalmic Agent, Mydriatic

Synonyms Phenylephrine Hydrochloride

Use Treatment of hypotension, vascular failure in shock; as a vasoconstrictor in regional analgesia; symptomatic relief of nasal and nasopharyngeal mucosal congestion; as a mydriatic in ophthalmic procedures and treatment of wide-angle glaucoma; supraventricular tachycardia

Local Anesthetic/Vasoconstrictor Precautions Use with caution since phenylephrine is a sympathomimetic amine which could interact with epinephrine to cause a pressor response

Effects on Dental Treatment ≤10%: Tachycardia, palpitations, xerostomia; use vasoconstrictor with caution

Dosage

Ophthalmic procedures:

- Children and Adults: Instill 1 drop of 2.5% or 10% solution, may repeat in 10-60 minutes as needed

Nasal decongestant (therapy should not exceed 5 continuous days):

- Children:
  - 2-6 years: Instill 1 drop every 2-4 hours of 0.125% solution as needed
  - 6-12 years: Instill 1-2 sprays or instill 1-2 drops every 4 hours of 0.25% solution as needed
- Children >12 years and Adults: Instill 1-2 sprays or instill 1-2 drops every 4 hours of 0.25% to 0.5% solution as needed; 1% solution may be used in adult in cases of extreme nasal congestion; do not use nasal solutions >3 days

Hypotension/shock:

- Children:
  - I.M., S.C.: 0.1 mg/kg/dose every 1-2 hours as needed (maximum: 5 mg)
  - I.V. bolus: 5-20 mcg/kg/dose every 10-15 minutes as needed
  - I.V. infusion: 0.1-0.5 mcg/kg/minute
- Adults:
  - I.M., S.C.: 2-5 mg/dose every 1-2 hours as needed (initial dose should not exceed 5 mg)
  - I.V. bolus: 0.1-0.5 mg/dose every 10-15 minutes as needed (initial dose should not exceed 0.5 mg)
  - I.V. infusion: 10 mg in 250 mL D_5W or NS (1:25,000 dilution) (40 mcg/mL); start at 100-180 mcg/minute (2-5 mL/minute; 50-90 drops/minute) initially; when BP is stabilized, maintenance rate: 40-60 mcg/minute (20-30 drops/minute)

Paroxysmal supraventricular tachycardia: I.V.:

- Children: 5-10 mcg/kg/dose over 20-30 seconds
- Adults: 0.25-0.5 mg/dose over 20-30 seconds

Mechanism of Action Potent, direct-acting alpha-adrenergic stimulator with weak beta-adrenergic activity; causes vasoconstriction of the arterioles of the nasal mucosa and conjunctiva; activates the dilator muscle of the pupil to cause contraction; produces vasoconstriction of arterioles in the body; produces systemic arterial vasoconstriction

Other Adverse Effects Frequency not defined:

Cardiovascular: Reflex bradycardia, excitability, restlessness, arrhythmias (rare), precordial pain or discomfort, pallor, hypertension, severe peripheral and visceral vasoconstriction, decreased cardiac output

Central nervous system: Headache, anxiety, weakness, dizziness, tremor, paresthesia, restlessness

Endocrine & metabolic: Metabolic acidosis

Local: Extravasation which may lead to necrosis and sloughing of surrounding tissue, blanching of skin

Neuromuscular & skeletal: Pilomotor response, weakness

Renal: Decreased renal perfusion, reduced urine output, reduced urine output

Respiratory: Respiratory distress

Drug Interactions

Increased Effect/Toxicity: Phenylephrine, taken with sympathomimetics, may induce tachycardia or arrhythmias. If taken with MAO inhibitors or oxytocic agents, actions may be potentiated.

Decreased Effect: Alpha- and beta-adrenergic blocking agents may have a decreased effect if taken with phenylephrine.

Drug Uptake

Onset of action: I.M., S.C.: 10-15 minutes; I.V.: Immediate

Duration: I.M.: 0.5-2 hours; I.V.: 15-30 minutes; S.C.: 1 hour

Half-life, elimination: 2.5 hours (increased after long-term infusion)

Pregnancy Risk Factor C

Generic Available Yes

Phenylephrine and Scopolamine (fen il EF rin & skoe POL a meen)

U.S. Brand Names Murocoll-2®

Pharmacologic Category Anticholinergic/Adrenergic Agonist

Synonyms Scopolamine and Phenylephrine

Use Mydriasis, cycloplegia, and to break posterior synechiae in iritis

Local Anesthetic/Vasoconstrictor Precautions Use with caution since phenylephrine is a sympathomimetic amine which could interact with epinephrine to cause a pressor response

Effects on Dental Treatment This form of phenylephrine will have no effect on dental treatment when given as eye drops.

Dosage Instill 1-2 drops into eye(s); repeat in 5 minutes

Drug Uptake See Phenylephrine *on page 950* and Scopolamine *on page 1077*

Pregnancy Risk Factor C

Generic Available No

Phenylephrine and Zinc Sulfate (fen il EF rin & zingk SUL fate)

U.S. Brand Names Zincfrin® [OTC]

Canadian Brand Names Zincfrin®

Pharmacologic Category Adrenergic Agonist Agent

Synonyms Zinc Sulfate and Phenylephrine

Use Soothe, moisturize, and remove redness due to minor eye irritation

Local Anesthetic/Vasoconstrictor Precautions No information available to require special precautions

Effects on Dental Treatment No effects or complications reported

Dosage Instill 1-2 drops in eye(s) 2-4 times/day as needed

Drug Uptake See Phenylephrine *on page 950*

Generic Available Yes

Phenylgesic® [OTC] *see* Acetaminophen and Phenyltoloxamine *on page 30*

Phenytoin (FEN i toyn)

Related Information

Cardiovascular Diseases *on page 1308*

U.S. Brand Names Dilantin®

Canadian Brand Names Dilantin®

Mexican Brand Names Epamin®; Fenidantoin®; Fenitron®; Hidantoina®

Pharmacologic Category Antiarrhythmic Agent, Class Ib; Anticonvulsant, Hydantoin

Synonyms Diphenylhydantoin; DPH; Phenytoin Sodium; Phenytoin Sodium, Extended; Phenytoin Sodium, Prompt

Use Management of generalized tonic-clonic (grand mal), simple partial and complex partial seizures; prevention of seizures following head trauma/neurosurgery; ventricular arrhythmias, including those associated with digitalis intoxication, prolonged QT interval and surgical repair of congenital heart diseases in children; also used for epidermolysis bullosa

Local Anesthetic/Vasoconstrictor Precautions No information available to require special precautions

Effects on Dental Treatment Gingival hyperplasia is a common problem observed during the first 6 months of phenytoin therapy appearing as gingivitis or gum inflammation. To minimize severity and growth rate of gingival tissue begin a program of professional cleaning and patient plaque control within 10 days of starting anticonvulsant therapy.

Dosage

Status epilepticus: I.V.:

Infants and Children: Loading dose: 15-20 mg/kg in a single or divided dose; maintenance dose: Initial: 5 mg/kg/day in 2 divided doses; usual doses:

6 months to 3 years: 8-10 mg/kg/day

4-6 years: 7.5-9 mg/kg/day

7-9 years: 7-8 mg/kg/day

10-16 years: 6-7 mg/kg/day, some patients may require every 8 hours dosing

(Continued)

Phenytoin *(Continued)*

Adults: Loading dose: Manufacturer recommends 10-15 mg/kg, however 15-25 mg/kg has been used clinically; maintenance dose: 300 mg/day or 5-6 mg/kg/day in 3 divided doses or 1-2 divided doses using extended release

Anticonvulsant: Children and Adults: Oral:

Loading dose: 15-20 mg/kg; based on phenytoin serum concentrations and recent dosing history; administer oral loading dose in 3 divided doses given every 2-4 hours to decrease GI adverse effects and to ensure complete oral absorption; maintenance dose: same as I.V.

Neurosurgery (prophylactic): 100-200 mg at ~ 4-hour intervals during surgery and during the immediate postoperative period

Dosing adjustment/comments in renal impairment or hepatic disease: Safe in usual doses in mild liver disease; clearance may be substantially reduced in cirrhosis and plasma level monitoring with dose adjustment advisable. Free phenytoin levels should be monitored closely.

Mechanism of Action Stabilizes neuronal membranes and decreases seizure activity by increasing efflux or decreasing influx of sodium ions across cell membranes in the motor cortex during generation of nerve impulses; prolongs effective refractory period and suppresses ventricular pacemaker automaticity, shortens action potential in the heart

Other Adverse Effects Frequency not defined:

I.V. effects: Hypotension, bradycardia, cardiac arrhythmias, cardiovascular collapse (especially with rapid I.V. use), venous irritation and pain, thrombophlebitis

Effects not related to plasma phenytoin concentrations: Hypertrichosis, gingival hypertrophy, thickening of facial features, carbohydrate intolerance, folic acid deficiency, peripheral neuropathy, vitamin D deficiency, osteomalacia, systemic lupus erythematosus

Concentration-related effects: Nystagmus, blurred vision, diplopia, ataxia, slurred speech, dizziness, drowsiness, lethargy, coma, rash, fever, nausea, vomiting, gum tenderness, confusion, mood changes, folic acid depletion, osteomalacia, hyperglycemia

Related to elevated concentrations:

>20 mcg/mL: Far lateral nystagmus

>30 mcg/mL: 45° lateral gaze nystagmus and ataxia

>40 mcg/mL: Decreased mentation

>100 mcg/mL: Death

Cardiovascular: Hypotension, bradycardia, cardiac arrhythmias, cardiovascular collapse

Central nervous system: Psychiatric changes, slurred speech, dizziness, drowsiness, headache, insomnia

Dermatologic: Rash

Gastrointestinal: Constipation, nausea, vomiting, gingival hyperplasia, enlargement of lips

Hematologic: Leukopenia, thrombocytopenia, agranulocytosis

Hepatic: Hepatitis

Local: Thrombophlebitis

Neuromuscular & skeletal: Tremor, peripheral neuropathy, paresthesia

Ocular: Diplopia, nystagmus, blurred vision

Drug Interactions CYP2C9 and 2C19 enzyme substrate; CYP1A2, 2B6, 2C8, 2C9, 2C18, 2C19, 3A3/4, and 3A5-7 enzyme inducer

Increased Effect/Toxicity: Phenytoin serum concentration may be increased by isoniazid, chloramphenicol, ticlopidine, or fluconazole. In addition, trimethoprim, sulfamethoxazole, valproic acid, sulfamethizole, sulfaphenazole, nifedipine, omeprazole, phenylbutazone, phenobarbital, amiodarone, chloramphenicol, cimetidine, ciprofloxacin, disulfiram, enoxacin, norfloxacin, felbamate, fluconazole, fluoxetine, influenza vaccine, isoniazid, and metronidazole inhibit the metabolism of phenytoin resulting in increased serum phenytoin concentrations. Valproic acid may increase, decrease, or have no effect on phenytoin serum concentration. Phenytoin may increase the effect of dopamine (enhanced hypotension), warfarin (transiently enhanced anticoagulation), or increase the rate of conversion of primidone to phenobarbital resulting in increased phenobarbital serum concentration. Phenytoin may enhance the hepatotoxic potential of acetaminophen. Concurrent use of acetazolamide and phenytoin may result in an increased risk of osteomalacia. Concurrent use of phenytoin and lithium has resulted in lithium intoxication. Phenytoin enhances the conversion of primidone to phenobarbital resulting in elevated phenobarbital serum concentration. Valproic acid and sulfisoxazole may displace phenytoin from binding sites, transiently increasing phenytoin free levels.

Decreased Effect: The blood levels of phenytoin may be decreased by carbamazepine, rifampin, amiodarone, cisplatin, disulfiram, vinblastine, bleomycin, folic acid, phenobarbital, pyridoxine, vigabatrin, and theophylline. Sucralfate and continuous NG feedings may decrease absorption of phenytoin. Phenytoin induces hepatic enzymes, and may decrease the effect of oral contraceptives, itraconazole, mebendazole, methadone, oral midazolam, valproic acid, cyclosporine, theophylline, doxycycline, quinidine, mexiletine, disopyramide. Phenytoin also may increase the metabolism of alprazolam, amiodarone, bromfenac, carbamazepine, clozapine, cyclosporine, diazepam, disopyramide, doxycycline, felbamate, furosemide, itraconazole, lamotrigine, mebendazole, meperidine, methadone, metyrapone, mexiletine, midazolam, oral contraceptives, quetiapine, quinidine, tacrolimus, teniposide, theophylline, thyroid hormones, triazolam, and valproic acid resulting in decreased levels/effect. Phenytoin may inhibit the anti-Parkinson effect of levodopa. Long-term concurrent use of phenytoin may inhibit hypoprothrombinemic response to warfarin. Phenytoin may reduce the effectiveness of some nondepolarizing neuromuscular blocking agents.

Drug Uptake

Onset of action: I.V.: ~0.5-1 hour

Absorption: Oral: Slow

Time to peak: (form-dependent) Oral: Extended-release capsule: 4-12 hours; Immediate release preparation: 2-3 hours

Pregnancy Risk Factor D

Generic Available Yes

Selected Readings

Dooley G and Vasan N, "Dilantin® Hyperplasia: A Review of the Literature," *J N Z Soc Periodontol*, 1989, 68:19-22.

Iacopino AM, Doxey D, Cutler CW, et al, "Phenytoin and Cyclosporine A Specifically Regulate Macrophage Phenotype and Expression of Platelet-Derived Growth Factor and Interleukin-1 *In Vitro* and *In Vivo*: Possible Molecular Mechanism of Drug-Induced Gingival Hyperplasia," *J Periodontol*, 1997, 68(1):73-83.

Pihlstrom BL, "Prevention and Treatment of Dilantin®-Associated Gingival Enlargement," *Compendium*, 1990, 14:S506-10.

Saito K, Mori S, Iwakura M, et al, "Immunohistochemical Localization of Transforming Growth Factor Beta, Basic Fibroblast Growth Factor and Heparin Sulphate Glycosaminoglycan in Gingival Hyperplasia Induced by Nifedipine and Phenytoin," *J Periodontal Res*, 1996, 31(8):545-5.

Zhou LX, Pihlstrom B, Hardwick JP, et al, "Metabolism of Phenytoin by the Gingiva of Normal Humans: The Possible Role of Reactive Metabolites of Phenytoin in the Initiation of Gingival Hyperplasia," *Clin Pharmacol Ther*, 1996, 60(2):191-8.

Phicon® [OTC] *see* Pramoxine *on page 984*

Phillips'® Milk of Magnesia [OTC] *see* Magnesium Hydroxide *on page 741*

pHisoHex® *see* Hexachlorophene *on page 587*

Phos-Flur® *see* Fluoride *on page 514*

PhosLo® *see* Calcium Acetate *on page 200*

Phospholine Iodide® *see* Echothiophate Iodide *on page 427*

Phosphorated Carbohydrate Solution

(FOS for ate ed kar boe HYE drate soe LOO shun)

U.S. Brand Names Emetrol® [OTC]; Nausetrol® [OTC]

Pharmacologic Category Antiemetic

Synonyms Dextrose, Levulose and Phosphoric Acid; Levulose, Dextrose and Phosphoric Acid; Phosphoric Acid, Levulose and Dextrose

Use Relief of nausea associated with upset stomach that occurs with intestinal flu, pregnancy, food indiscretions, and emotional upsets

Local Anesthetic/Vasoconstrictor Precautions No information available to require special precautions

Effects on Dental Treatment No effects or complications reported

Dosage

Morning sickness: 15-30 mL on arising; repeat every 3 hours or when nausea threatens

Motion sickness and vomiting due to drug therapy: 5 mL doses for young children; 15 mL doses for older children and adults

Regurgitation in infants: 5 or 10 mL, 10-15 minutes before each feeding; in refractory cases: 10-15 mL, 30 minutes before each feeding

Vomiting due to psychogenic factors:

- Children: 5-10 mL; repeat dose every 15 minutes until distress subsides; do not take >1 hour
- Adults: 15-30 mL; repeat dose every 15 minutes until distress subsides; do not take for more than 1 hour

Other Adverse Effects 1% to 10%: Gastrointestinal: Abdominal pain, diarrhea

Generic Available Yes

Photofrin® *see* Porfimer *on page 974*

Physostigmine (fye zoe STIG meen)

U.S. Brand Names Antilirium®

Canadian Brand Names Eserine®; Isopto® Eserine

Pharmacologic Category Acetylcholinesterase Inhibitor; Ophthalmic Agent, Antiglaucoma

Synonyms Eserine Salicylate; Physostigmine Salicylate; Physostigmine Sulfate

Use Reverse toxic CNS effects caused by anticholinergic drugs; used as miotic in treatment of glaucoma

(Continued)

Physostigmine *(Continued)*

Local Anesthetic/Vasoconstrictor Precautions No information available to require special precautions

Effects on Dental Treatment No effects or complications reported

Dosage

Children: Anticholinergic drug overdose: Reserve for life-threatening situations only: I.V.: 0.01-0.03 mg/kg/dose, (maximum: 0.5 mg/minute); may repeat after 5-10 minutes to a maximum total dose of 2 mg or until response occurs or adverse cholinergic effects occur

Adults: Anticholinergic drug overdose:

I.M., I.V., S.C.: 0.5-2 mg to start, repeat every 20 minutes until response occurs or adverse effect occurs

Repeat 1-4 mg every 30-60 minutes as life-threatening signs (arrhythmias, seizures, deep coma) recur; maximum I.V. rate: 1 mg/minute

Ophthalmic:

Ointment: Instill a small quantity to lower fornix up to 3 times/day

Solution: Instill 1-2 drops into eye(s) up to 4 times/day

Mechanism of Action Inhibits destruction of acetylcholine by acetylcholinesterase which facilitates transmission of impulses across myoneural junction and prolongs the central and peripheral effects of acetylcholine

Other Adverse Effects Frequency not defined:

Ophthalmic:

Central nervous system: Headache, browache

Dermatologic: Burning, redness

Ocular: Lacrimation, marked miosis, blurred vision, eye pain

Miscellaneous: Diaphoresis

Systemic:

Cardiovascular: Palpitations, bradycardia

Central nervous system: Restlessness, nervousness, hallucinations, seizures

Gastrointestinal: Nausea, salivation, diarrhea, stomach pains

Genitourinary: Frequent urge to urinate

Neuromuscular & skeletal: Muscle twitching

Ocular: Lacrimation, miosis

Respiratory: Dyspnea, bronchospasm, respiratory paralysis, pulmonary edema

Miscellaneous: Diaphoresis

Drug Interactions Increased toxicity with bethanechol, methacholine. Succinylcholine may increase neuromuscular blockade with systemic administration.

Drug Uptake

Onset of action: Ophthalmic: ≤2 minutes; Parenteral: ≤5 minutes

Absorption: I.M., ophthalmic, S.C.: Readily absorbed

Duration: Ophthalmic: 12-48 hours; Parenteral: 0.5-5 hours

Half-life, elimination: 15-40 minutes

Pregnancy Risk Factor C

Generic Available Yes: Ophthalmic

Phytonadione (fye toe na DYE one)

U.S. Brand Names AquaMEPHYTON®; Mephyton®

Canadian Brand Names AquaMEPHYTON®; Konakion; Mephyton®

Mexican Brand Names Konakion®

Pharmacologic Category Vitamin, Fat Soluble

Synonyms Methylphytyl Napthoquinone; Phylloquinone; Phytomenadione; Vitamin K_1

Use Prevention and treatment of hypoprothrombinemia caused by drug-induced or anticoagulant-induced vitamin K deficiency, hemorrhagic disease of the newborn; phytonadione is more effective and is preferred to other vitamin K preparations in the presence of impending hemorrhage; oral absorption depends on the presence of bile salts

Local Anesthetic/Vasoconstrictor Precautions No information available to require special precautions

Effects on Dental Treatment No effects or complications reported

Dosage S.C. is the preferred parenteral route (per manufacturer). I.V. route should be restricted for emergency use only.

Minimum daily requirement: Not well established

Infants: 1-5 mcg/kg/day

Adults: 0.03 mcg/kg/day

Hemorrhagic disease of the newborn:

Prophylaxis: I.M.: 0.5-1 mg within 1 hour of birth

Treatment: I.M., S.C.: 1-2 mg/dose/day

Oral anticoagulant overdose:

Infants: I.M., S.C.: 1-2 mg/dose every 4-8 hours

Children and Adults: Oral, I.V.: 1-10 mg/dose depending on degree of INR elevation

Serious bleeding or major overdose: 10 mg I.V. (slow infusion); may repeat every 12 hours

Vitamin K deficiency: Due to drugs, malabsorption, or decreased synthesis of vitamin K

Infants and Children:

Oral: 2.5-5 mg/24 hours

I.M., I.V.: 1-2 mg/dose as a single dose

Adults:

Oral: 5-25 mg/24 hours

I.M., I.V.: 10 mg

Mechanism of Action Promotes liver synthesis of clotting factors (II, VII, IX, X); however, the exact mechanism as to this stimulation is unknown. Menadiol is a water soluble form of vitamin K; phytonadione has a more rapid and prolonged effect than menadione; menadiol sodium diphosphate (K_4) is half as potent as menadione (K_3).

Drug Interactions The anticoagulant effects of warfarin, dicumarol, anisindione are reversed by phytonadione; mineral oil and orlistat may decrease GI absorption of vitamin K

Drug Uptake

Onset of action: Increased coagulation factors: Oral: 6-12 hours; Parenteral: 1-2 hours; prothrombin may become normal after 12-14 hours

Absorption: Oral: From intestines in presence of bile

Pregnancy Risk Factor C

Generic Available Yes: Injection

Pilocar® *see* Pilocarpine *on page 955*

Pilocar® *see* Pilocarpine (Dental) *on page 956*

Pilocarpine (pye loe KAR peen)

Related Information

Dentin Hypersensitivity, High Caries Index, and Xerostomia *on page 1388*

Management of Patients Undergoing Cancer Therapy *on page 1402*

U.S. Brand Names Isopto® Carpine; Ocusert Pilo-20® [DSC]; Ocusert Pilo-40® [DSC]; Pilocar®; Pilopine HS®; Piloptic®; Salagen®

Canadian Brand Names Diocarpine; Isopto® Carpine; Miocarpine®; Pilopine HS®; Salagen®; Scheinpharm Pilocarpine

Mexican Brand Names Pilogrin

Pharmacologic Category Cholinergic Agonist; Ophthalmic Agent, Antiglaucoma; Ophthalmic Agent, Miotic

Synonyms Pilocarpine Hydrochloride; Pilocarpine Nitrate

Use

Ophthalmic: Management of chronic simple glaucoma, chronic and acute angle-closure glaucoma; counter effects of cycloplegics

Orphan drug: Oral: Symptomatic treatment of xerostomia caused by salivary gland hypofunction resulting from radiotherapy for cancer of the head and neck

Local Anesthetic/Vasoconstrictor Precautions No information available to require special precautions

Effects on Dental Treatment No effects or complications reported

Dosage Adults:

Ophthalmic:

Nitrate solution: Shake well before using; instill 1-2 drops 2-4 times/day

Hydrochloride solution:

Instill 1-2 drops up to 6 times/day; adjust the concentration and frequency as required to control elevated intraocular pressure

To counteract the mydriatic effects of sympathomimetic agents: Instill 1 drop of a 1% solution in the affected eye

Gel: Instill 0.5" ribbon into lower conjunctival sac once daily at bedtime

Ocular systems: Systems are labeled in terms of mean rate of release of pilocarpine over 7 days; begin with 20 mcg/hour at night and adjust based on response

Oral: 5 mg 3 times/day, titration up to 10 mg 3 times/day may be considered for patients who have not responded adequately

Mechanism of Action Directly stimulates cholinergic receptors in the eye causing miosis (by contraction of the iris sphincter), loss of accommodation (by constriction of ciliary muscle), and lowering of intraocular pressure (with decreased resistance to aqueous humor outflow)

Other Adverse Effects Note: Ocular administration results in similar systemic effects, but at lower frequency than oral.

Ophthalmic:

>10%: Ocular: Blurred vision, miosis, decrease in night vision

1% to 10%:

Central nervous system: Headache

Genitourinary: Polyuria

Local: Stinging, burning

Ocular: Ciliary spasm, retinal detachment, browache, photophobia, acute iritis, lacrimation, conjunctival and ciliary congestion early in therapy

Miscellaneous: Hypersensitivity reactions

(Continued)

Pilocarpine *(Continued)*

Systemic:

>10%: Miscellaneous: Diaphoresis

1% to 10%:

Cardiovascular: Edema, flushing, hypertension, tachycardia
Central nervous system: Muscle weakness, headache, tremors, chills
Gastrointestinal: Nausea, vomiting, heartburn, dysphagia
Genitourinary: Polyuria
Ocular: Amblyopia
Respiratory: Epistaxis, rhinitis, voice change

Drug Interactions Concurrent use with beta-blockers may cause conduction disturbances; pilocarpine may antagonize the effects of anticholinergic drugs.

Drug Uptake

Ophthalmic:
Onset of myositic effect: 10-30 minutes
Duration: 4-8 hours
Onset of IOP reduction: 1 hour
Duration: 4-12 hours

Ocusert® Pilo application:
Onset of myositic effect: 1.5-2 hours
Onset of IOP reduction: ~1.5-2 hours; miosis ~10-30 minutes
Duration: ~1 week

Oral:
Onset of action: 20 minutes
Duration: 3-5 hours
Half-life, elimination: 0.76-1.35 hours

Pregnancy Risk Factor C

Generic Available Yes: Solution

Pilocarpine and Epinephrine (pye loe KAR peen & ep i NEF rin)

U.S. Brand Names E-Pilo-x®; P_xE_x®

Canadian Brand Names E-Pilo®

Pharmacologic Category Ophthalmic Agent, Antiglaucoma; Ophthalmic Agent, Miotic

Synonyms Epinephrine and Pilocarpine

Use Treatment of glaucoma; counter effect of cycloplegics

Local Anesthetic/Vasoconstrictor Precautions No information available to require special precautions

Effects on Dental Treatment No effects or complications reported

Dosage Instill 1-2 drops up to 6 times/day

Other Adverse Effects Frequency not defined:

Cardiovascular: Tachycardia, hypertension
Central nervous system: Headache
Dermatologic: Stinging, itching
Gastrointestinal: Salivation
Hematologic: Vitreous hemorrhages
Ocular: Miosis, ciliary spasm, blurred vision, retinal detachment, lacrimation, photophobia, acute iritis
Miscellaneous: Hypersensitivity reactions

Drug Interactions Pilocarpine may antagonize the effects of anticholinergic and produce cardiac conduction abnormalities in patients receiving beta-blockers.

Drug Uptake See Pilocarpine *on page 956* and Epinephrine *on page 438*

Pregnancy Risk Factor C

Generic Available No

Pilocarpine (Dental) (pye loe KAR peen)

U.S. Brand Names Isopto® Carpine; Ocusert Pilo-20® [DSC]; Ocusert Pilo-40® [DSC]; Pilocar®; Pilopine HS®; Piloptic®; Salagen®

Canadian Brand Names Diocarpine; Isopto® Carpine; Miocarpine®; Pilopine HS®; Salagen®; Scheinpharm Pilocarpine

Mexican Brand Names Pilogrin

Pharmacologic Category Cholinergic Agonist; Ophthalmic Agent, Antiglaucoma; Ophthalmic Agent, Miotic

Use Treatment of xerostomia caused by radiation therapy in patients with head and neck cancer and from Sjögren's syndrome

Local Anesthetic/Vasoconstrictor Precautions No information available to require special precautions

Effects on Dental Treatment Salivation (therapeutic effect)

Dosage Adults: 1-2 tablets 3-4 times/day not to exceed 30 mg/day; patients should be treated for a minimum of 90 days for optimum effects

Mechanism of Action Stimulates the muscarinic-type acetylcholine receptors in the salivary glands within the parasympathetic division of the autonomic nervous system to cause an increase in serous-type saliva

Other Adverse Effects Systemic:
- >10%: Miscellaneous: Sweating
- 1% to 10%:
  - Cardiovascular: Edema, flushing, hypertension, tachycardia
  - Central nervous system: Muscle weakness, headache, tremors, chills
  - Gastrointestinal: Nausea, vomiting, heartburn, dysphagia
  - Genitourinary: Polyuria
  - Ocular: Amblyopia
  - Respiratory: Epistaxis, rhinitis, voice change

Contraindications Hypersensitivity to pilocarpine or any component of the formulation uncontrolled asthma; when miosis is undesirable (eg, narrow-angle glaucoma)

Warnings/Precautions In patients with chronic obstructive pulmonary disease, pilocarpine may stimulate the mucous cells of the respiratory tract and may increase airway resistance. Patients with cardiovascular disease may be unable to compensate for changes in heart rhythm that could be induced by pilocarpine.

Drug Interactions Increased Effect/Toxicity: Concurrent use with anticholinergics may cause antagonism of pilocarpine's cholinergic effect; medications with cholinergic actions may result in additive cholinergic effects. Beta-adrenergic receptor blocking drugs when used with pilocarpine may increase the possibility of myocardial conduction disturbances.

Drug Uptake
- Onset of action: 20 minutes after single dose
- Duration: 3-5 hours
- Half-life, elimination: 0.76 hours
- Time to peak: 1.25 hours

Pregnancy Risk Factor C

Breast-feeding Considerations May be taken while breast-feeding

Dosage Forms GEL, ophthalmic (Pilopine HS®): 4% (3.5 g). **OCULAR THERAPEUTIC SYSTEM:** (Ocusert Pilo-20® [DSC]): Releases 20 mcg/hour for 1 week (8s); (Ocusert Pilo-40® [DSC]): Releases 40 mcg/hour for 1 week (8s). **SOLN, ophthalmic** 1% (15 mL), 2% (15 mL), 4% (15 mL), 6% (15 mL); (Isopto® Carpine): 1% (15 mL); 2% (15 mL, 30 mL); 4% (15 mL, 30 mL); 6% (15 mL); 8% (15 mL); (Pilocar®): 0.5% (15 mL); 1% (1 mL, 15 mL); 2% (1 mL, 15 mL); 3% (15 mL); 4% (1 mL, 15 mL); 6% (15 mL); (Piloptic®): 0.5% (15 mL); 1% (15 mL); 2% (15 mL); 3% (15 mL); 4% (15 mL); 6% (15 mL). **TAB** (Salagen®): 5 mg

Generic Available Yes: Solution

Comments Pilocarpine may have potential as a salivary stimulant in individuals suffering from xerostomia induced by antidepressants and other medications. At the present time however, the FDA has not approved pilocarpine for use in drug-induced xerostomia. Clinical studies are needed to evaluate pilocarpine for this type of indication. In an attempt to discern the efficacy of pilocarpine as a salivary stimulant in patients suffering from Sjögren's syndrome (SS), Rhodus and Schuh studied 9 patients with SS given daily doses of pilocarpine over a 6-week period. A dose of 5 mg daily produced a significant overall increase in both whole unstimulated salivary flow and parotid stimulated salivary flow. These results support the use of pilocarpine to increase salivary flow in patients with SS.

Selected Readings

Davies AN and Singer J, "A Comparison of Artificial Saliva and Pilocarpine in Radiation-Induced Xerostomia," *J Laryngol Otol*, 1994, 108(8):663-5.

Fox PC, "Management of Dry Mouth," *Dent Clin North Am*, 1997, 41(4):863-75.

Fox PC, Atkinson JC, Macynski AA, et al, " Pilocarpine Treatment of Salivary Gland Hypofunction and Dry Mouth (Xerostomia)," *Arch Intern Med*, 1991, 151(6):1149-52.

Garg AK and Malo M, "Manifestations and Treatment of Xerostomia and Associated Oral Effects Secondary to Head and Neck Radiation Therapy," *J Am Dent Assoc*, 1997, 128(8):1128-33.

Johnson JT, Ferretti GA, Nethery WJ, et al, "Oral Pilocarpine for Postirradiation Xerostomia in Patients With Head and Neck Cancer," *N Engl J Med*, 1993, 329(6):390-5.

Nagler RM and Laufer D, "Protection Against Irradiation-Induced Damage to Salivary Glands by Adrenergic Agonist Administration," *Int J Radiat Oncol Biol Phys*, 1998, 40(2):477-81.

Nelson JD, Friedlaender M, Yeatts RP, et al, "Oral Pilocarpine for Symptomatic Relief of Keratoconjunctivitis Sicca in Patients With Sjögren's Syndrome. The MGI PHARMA Sjögren's Syndrome Study Group," *Adv Exp Med Biol*, 1998, 438:979-83.

Rhodus NL and Schuh MJ, "Effects of Pilocarpine on Salivary Flow in Patients With Sjögren's Syndrome," *Oral Surg Oral Med Oral Pathol*, 1991, 72(5):545-9.

Rieke JW, Hafermann MD, Johnson JT, et al, "Oral Pilocarpine for Radiation-Induced Xerostomia: Integrated Efficacy and Safety Results From Two Prospective Randomized Clinical Trials," *Int J Radiat Oncol Biol Phys*, 1995, 31(3):661-9.

Rousseau P, "Pilocarpine in Radiation-Induced Xerostomia," *Am J Hosp Palliat Care*, 1995, 12(2):38-9.

Schuller DE, Stevens P, Clausen KP, et al, "Treatment of Radiation Side Effects With Pilocarpine," *J Surg Oncol*, 1989, 42(4):272-6.

Singhal S, Mehta J, Rattenbury H, et al, "Oral Pilocarpine Hydrochloride for the Treatment of Refractory Xerostomia Associated With Chronic Graft-Versus-Host Disease," *Blood*, 1995, 85(4):1147-8.

Valdez IH, Wolff A, Atkinson JC, et al, "Use of Pilocarpine During Head and Neck Radiation Therapy to Reduce Xerostomia Salivary Dysfunction," *Cancer*, 1993, 71(5):1848-51.

Wiseman LR and Faulds D, "Oral Pilocarpine: A Review of Its Pharmacological Properties and Clinical Potential in Xerostomia," *Drugs*, 1995, 49(1):143-55.

Wynn RL, "Oral Pilocarpine (Salagen®) - A Recently Approved Salivary Stimulant," *Gen Dent*, 1996, 44(1):26,29-30.

Zimmerman RP, Mark RJ, Tran LM, et al, "Concomitant Pilocarpine During Head and Neck Irradiation Is Associated With Decreased Post-Treatment Xerostomia," *Int J Radiat Oncol Biol Phys*, 1997, 37(3):571-5.

Pilopine HS® *see* Pilocarpine *on page 955*
Pilopine HS® *see* Pilocarpine (Dental) *on page 956*
Piloptic® *see* Pilocarpine *on page 955*
Piloptic® *see* Pilocarpine (Dental) *on page 956*
Pima® *see* Potassium Iodide *on page 980*

Pimecrolimus (pim e KROE li mus)

U.S. Brand Names Elidel®

Pharmacologic Category Immunosuppressant Agent; Topical Skin Product

Use Short-term and intermittent long-term treatment of mild to moderate atopic dermatitis in patients not responsive to conventional therapy or when conventional therapy is not appropriate

Local Anesthetic/Vasoconstrictor Precautions No information available to require special precautions

Effects on Dental Treatment No effects or complications reported

Dosage Children ≥2 years and Adults: Topical: Apply thin layer to affected area twice daily; rub in gently and completely. **Note:** Continue as long as signs and symptoms persist; discontinue if resolution occurs; re-evaluate if symptoms persist >6 weeks.

Mechanism of Action Penetrates inflamed epidermis to inhibit T cell activation by blocking transcription of proinflammatory cytokine genes such as interleukin-2, interferon gamma (Th1-type), interleukin-4, and interleukin-10 (Th2-type). Blocks catalytic function of calcineurin. Prevents release of inflammatory cytokines and mediators from mast cells *in vitro* after stimulation by antigen/IgE.

Other Adverse Effects

>10% :

Central nervous system: Headache (7% to 25%), pyrexia (1% to 13%)

Local: Burning at application site (2% to 26%)

Respiratory: Nasopharyngitis (8% to 27%), cough (2% to 16%), upper respiratory tract infection (4% to 19%), bronchitis (0.4% to 11%)

Miscellaneous: Influenza (3% to 13%)

1% to 10%:

Dermatologic: Skin papilloma (warts) (up to 3%), molluscum contagiosum (0.7% to 2%), herpes simplex dermatitis (up to 2%)

Gastrointestinal: Diarrhea (0.6% to 8%), constipation (up to 4%)

Local: Irritation at application site (0.4% to 6%), erythema at application site (0.4% to 2%), pruritus at application site (0.6% to 6%)

Ocular: Eye infection (up to 1%)

Otic: Ear infection (0.6% to 6%), nasal congestion (0.6% to 3%)

Respiratory: Pharyngitis (0.7% to 8%), sinusitis (0.6% to 3%)

Miscellaneous: Viral infection (up to 7%), herpes simplex infections (0.4% to 4%), tonsillitis (0.4% to 6%)

Drug Interactions CYP 3A3/4 enzyme substrate (only if significantly absorbed)

Increased Effect/Toxicity: CYP3A inhibitors may increase pimecrolimus levels in patients where increased absorption expected. **Note:** Low potential for occurrence with limited application and low absorption potential.

Drug Uptake Absorption: Poor when applied to 13% to 62% body surface area for ≤1 year

Pregnancy Risk Factor C

Generic Available No

Pimozide (PI moe zide)

U.S. Brand Names Orap™

Canadian Brand Names Orap®

Pharmacologic Category Antipsychotic Agent, Diphenylbutylperidine

Use Suppression of severe motor and phonic tics in patients with Tourette's disorder who have failed to respond satisfactorily to standard treatment

Unlabeled/Investigational: Psychosis; reported use in individuals with delusions focused on physical symptoms (ie, preoccupation with parasitic infestation); Huntington's chorea

Local Anesthetic/Vasoconstrictor Precautions No information available to require special precautions

Effects on Dental Treatment >10%: Xerostomia

Dosage Oral:

Children ≤12 years: Tourette's disorder: Initial: 1-2 mg/day in divided doses; usual range: 2-4 mg/day; do not exceed 10 mg/day (0.2 mg/kg/day)

Children >12 years and Adults: Tourette's disorder: Initial: 1-2 mg/day in divided doses, then increase dosage as needed every other day; range is usually 7-16 mg/day, maximum dose: 20 mg/day or 0.3 mg/kg/day should not be exceeded.

Note: Sudden unexpected deaths have occurred in patients taking doses >10 mg. Therefore, dosages exceeding 10 mg/day are generally not recommended.

Dosing adjustment in hepatic impairment: Reduction of dose is necessary in patients with liver disease

Mechanism of Action A potent centrally-acting dopamine receptor antagonist resulting in its characteristic neuroleptic effects

Other Adverse Effects Frequency not defined:

Cardiovascular: Facial edema, tachycardia, orthostatic hypotension, chest pain, hypertension, palpitations, ventricular arrhythmias, QT prolongation

Central nervous system: Extrapyramidal symptoms (akathisia, akinesia, dystonia, pseudoparkinsonism, tardive dyskinesia), drowsiness, NMS, headache, dizziness, excitement

Dermatologic: Rash

Endocrine & metabolic: Edema of breasts, decreased libido

Gastrointestinal: Constipation, xerostomia, weight gain/loss, nausea, salivation, vomiting, anorexia

Genitourinary: Impotence

Hematologic: Blood dyscrasias

Hepatic: Jaundice

Neuromuscular & skeletal: Weakness, tremor

Ocular: Visual disturbance, decreased accommodation, blurred vision

Miscellaneous: Diaphoresis

Contraindications Hypersensitivity to pimozide or any component of the formulation; use with macrolide antibiotics such as clarithromycin, erythromycin, azithromycin, and dirithromycin; simple tics other than Tourette's, history of cardiac dysrhythmias

Warnings/Precautions Sudden, unexpected deaths have been known to occur in patients taking high doses (>10 mg) of pimozide. One possible explanation is prolongation of QT intervals predisposing the patients to arrhythmias. May alter cardiac conduction - life-threatening arrhythmias have occurred with therapeutic doses of phenothiazines. May cause hypotension, use with caution in patients with autonomic instability. Moderately sedating, use with caution in disorders where CNS depression is a feature. Use with caution in Parkinson's disease. Caution in patients with hemodynamic instability; bone marrow suppression; predisposition to seizures; subcortical brain damage; severe cardiac, hepatic, renal, or respiratory disease. Esophageal dysmotility and aspiration have been associated with antipsychotic use; use with caution in patients at risk of pneumonia (ie, Alzheimer's disease). Use caution in breast cancer or other prolactin-dependent tumors; may elevate prolactin levels. May alter temperature regulation or mask toxicity of other drugs due to antiemetic effects. May cause orthostatic hypotension - use with caution in patients at risk of this effect or those who would tolerate transient hypotensive episodes (cerebrovascular disease, cardiovascular disease, or other medications which may predispose).

May cause anticholinergic effects (confusion, agitation, constipation, xerostomia, blurred vision, urinary retention); therefore, use with caution in patients with decreased GI motility, urinary retention, BPH, xerostomia, or visual problems. Conditions which also may be exacerbated by cholinergic blockade include narrow-angle glaucoma (screening is recommended) and worsening of myasthenia gravis. Relative to neuroleptics, pimozide has a moderate potency of cholinergic blockade.

May cause extrapyramidal reactions, including pseudoparkinsonism, acute dystonic reactions, akathisia, and tardive dyskinesia (risk of these reactions is high relative to other neuroleptics). May be associated with neuroleptic malignant syndrome (NMS) or pigmentary retinopathy.

Avoid concurrent grapefruit juice, macrolide antibiotics, azole antifungal agents, protease inhibitors, nefazodone, and zileuton due to their potential inhibition of pimozide metabolism, leading to the accumulation of active compound and the increased chance of serious arrhythmias

Drug Interactions CYP3A3/4 enzyme substrate; CYP1A2 (minor)

Aluminum salts: May decrease the absorption of antipsychotics; monitor

Amphetamines: Efficacy may be diminished by antipsychotics; in addition, amphetamines may increase psychotic symptoms; avoid concurrent use

Anticholinergics: May inhibit the therapeutic response to antipsychotics and excess anticholinergic effects may occur; includes benztropine, trihexyphenidyl, biperiden, and drugs with significant anticholinergic activity (TCAs, antihistamines, disopyramide)

Antihypertensives: Concurrent use of antipsychotics with an antihypertensive may produce additive hypotensive effects (particularly orthostasis)

Bromocriptine: Antipsychotics inhibit the ability of bromocriptine to lower serum prolactin concentrations

CNS depressants: Sedative effects may be additive with antipsychotics; monitor for increased effect; includes barbiturates, benzodiazepines, narcotic analgesics, ethanol, and other sedative agents

CYP3A3/4 inhibitors: Serum level and/or toxicity of some benzodiazepines may be increased; inhibitors include amiodarone, cimetidine, clarithromycin, erythromycin, delavirdine, diltiazem, dirithromycin, disulfiram, fluoxetine, fluvoxamine, grapefruit juice, indinavir, itraconazole, ketoconazole, metronidazole, nefazodone, nevirapine, propoxyphene, quinupristin-dalfopristin, ritonavir, saquinavir, verapamil, zafirlukast, zileuton. May cause life-threatening arrhythmias; avoid these combinations.

(Continued)

Pimozide *(Continued)*

Enzyme inducers: May enhance the hepatic metabolism of antipsychotics; larger doses may be required; includes rifampin, rifabutin, barbiturates, phenytoin, and cigarette smoking

Epinephrine: Chlorpromazine (and possibly other low potency antipsychotics) may diminish the pressor effects of epinephrine

Guanethidine and guanadrel: Antihypertensive effects may be inhibited by antipsychotics

Levodopa: Antipsychotics may inhibit the antiparkinsonian effect of levodopa; avoid this combination

Lithium: Antipsychotics may produce neurotoxicity with lithium; this is a rare effect

Mesoridazine: Concurrent use with pimozide is contraindicated due to potential arrhythmias.

Metoclopramide: May increase extrapyramidal symptoms (EPS) or risk.

Phenytoin: May reduce serum levels of antipsychotics; antipsychotics may increase phenytoin serum levels

Propranolol: Serum concentrations of antipsychotics may be increased; propranolol also increases antipsychotics concentrations

QT_c-prolonging agents: Effects on QT_c interval may be additive with antipsychotics, increasing the risk of malignant arrhythmias; includes type Ia antiarrhythmics, tricyclic antidepressants, and some quinolone antibiotics (sparfloxacin, moxifloxacin, and gatifloxacin)

Sulfadoxine-pyrimethamine: May increase antipsychotics concentrations

Thioridazine: Concurrent use with pimozide is contraindicated due to potential arrhythmias.

Tricyclic antidepressants: Concurrent use may produce increased toxicity or altered therapeutic response (also see note under QT_c prolonging agents)

Trazodone: Antipsychotics and trazodone may produce additive hypotensive effects

Valproic acid: Serum levels may be increased by antipsychotics

Ziprasidone: Concurrent use with pimozide is contraindicated due to potential arrhythmias.

Drug Uptake

Absorption: Oral: 50%

Half-life, elimination: 50 hours

Time to peak: 6-8 hours

Pregnancy Risk Factor C

Generic Available No

Selected Readings "Pimozide (Orap) Contraindicated With Clarithromycin (Biaxin®) and Other Macrolide Antibiotics," *FDA Medical Bulletin*, October 1996, 26(3).

Pindolol (PIN doe lole)

Related Information

Cardiovascular Diseases *on page 1308*

U.S. Brand Names Visken®

Canadian Brand Names Apo®-Pindol; Gen-Pindolol; Novo-Pindol; Nu-Pindol; PMS-Pindolol; Visken®

Pharmacologic Category Beta Blocker With Intrinsic Sympathomimetic Activity

Use Management of hypertension

Unlabeled: Ventricular arrhythmias/tachycardia, antipsychotic-induced akathisia, situational anxiety; aggressive behavior associated with dementia; potential augmenting agent for antidepressants

Local Anesthetic/Vasoconstrictor Precautions Use with caution; epinephrine has interacted with nonselective beta-blockers to result in initial hypertensive episode followed by bradycardia

Effects on Dental Treatment Noncardioselective beta-blockers (ie, propranolol, nadolol, pindolol) enhance the pressor response to epinephrine, resulting in hypertension and bradycardia. Many nonsteroidal anti-inflammatory drugs such as ibuprofen and indomethacin can reduce the hypotensive effect of beta-blockers after 3 or more weeks of therapy with the NSAID. Short-term NSAID use (ie, 3 days) requires no special precautions in patients taking beta-blockers.

Dosage

Adults: Initial: 5 mg twice daily, increase as necessary by 10 mg/day every 3-4 weeks; maximum daily dose: 60 mg

Elderly: Initial: 5 mg once daily, increase as necessary by 5 mg/day every 3-4 weeks

Mechanism of Action Blocks both $beta_1$- and $beta_2$-receptors and has mild intrinsic sympathomimetic activity; pindolol has negative inotropic and chronotropic effects and can significantly slow AV nodal conduction. Augmentive action of antidepressants thought to be mediated via a serotonin 1A autoreceptor antagonism.

Other Adverse Effects 1% to 10%:

Cardiovascular: Chest pain (3%), edema (6%)

Central nervous system: Nightmares/vivid dreams (5%), dizziness (9%), insomnia (10%), fatigue (8%), nervousness (7%), anxiety (<2%)
Dermatologic: Rash, itching (4%)
Gastrointestinal: Nausea (5%), abdominal discomfort (4%)
Neuromuscular & skeletal: Weakness (4%), paresthesia (3%), arthralgia (7%), muscle pain (10%)
Respiratory: Dyspnea (5%)

Drug Interactions CYP2D6 enzyme substrate

Increased Effect/Toxicity: Pindolol may increase the effects of other drugs which slow AV conduction (digoxin, verapamil, diltiazem), alpha-blockers (prazosin, terazosin), and alpha-adrenergic stimulants (epinephrine, phenylephrine). Pindolol may mask the tachycardia from hypoglycemia caused by insulin and oral hypoglycemics. In patients receiving concurrent therapy, the risk of hypertensive crisis is increased when either clonidine or the beta-blocker is withdrawn. Reserpine has been shown to enhance the effect of beta-blockers. Beta-blockers may increase the action or levels of disopyramide, nondepolarizing muscle relaxants, and theophylline although the effects are difficult to predict.

Decreased Effect: Decreased levels/effect of pindolol with aluminum salts, barbiturates, calcium salts, cholestyramine, colestipol, NSAIDs, penicillins (ampicillin), rifampin, salicylates, and sulfinpyrazone due to decreased bioavailability and plasma concentrations. Beta-blockers may decrease the effect of sulfonylureas (possibly hyperglycemia). Nonselective beta-blockers blunt the effect of beta-2 adrenergic agonists (albuterol).

Drug Uptake

Absorption: Oral: Rapid, 50% to 95%
Duration: ~12 hours
Half-life, elimination: 2.5-4 hours (increases with renal insufficiency, age, and cirrhosis)
Time to peak: 1-2 hours

Pregnancy Risk Factor B

Generic Available Yes

Selected Readings

Foster CA and Aston SJ, "Propranolol-Epinephrine Interaction: A Potential Disaster," *Plast Reconstr Surg*, 1983, 72(1):74-8.
Wong DG, Spence JD, Lamki L, et al, "Effect of Nonsteroidal Anti-inflammatory Drugs on Control of Hypertension of Beta-Blockers and Diuretics," *Lancet*, 1986, 1(8488):997-1001.
Wynn RL, "Dental Nonsteroidal Anti-inflammatory Drugs and Prostaglandin-Based Drug Interactions, Part Two," *Gen Dent*, 1992, 40(2):104, 106, 108.
Wynn RL, "Epinephrine Interactions With Beta-Blockers," *Gen Dent*, 1994, 42(1):16, 18.

Pin-Rid® [OTC] *see* Pyrantel Pamoate *on page 1025*
Pin-X® [OTC] *see* Pyrantel Pamoate *on page 1025*

Pioglitazone (pye oh GLI ta zone)

U.S. Brand Names Actos®

Canadian Brand Names Actos®

Pharmacologic Category Antidiabetic Agent, Thiazolidinedione

Use

Type 2 diabetes, monotherapy: Adjunct to diet and exercise, to improve glycemic control

Type 2 diabetes, combination therapy with sulfonylurea, metformin, or insulin: When diet, exercise, and a single agent alone does not result in adequate glycemic control

Local Anesthetic/Vasoconstrictor Precautions No information available to require special precautions

Effects on Dental Treatment Pioglitazone-dependent diabetics should be appointed for dental treatment in morning in order to minimize chance of stress-induced hypoglycemia.

Dosage Adults: Oral:

Monotherapy: Initial: 15-30 mg once daily; if response is inadequate, the dosage may be increased in increments up to 45 mg once daily; maximum recommended dose: 45 mg once daily

Combination therapy:

- With sulfonylureas: Initial: 15-30 mg once daily; dose of sulfonylurea should be reduced if the patient reports hypoglycemia
- With metformin: Initial: 15-30 mg once daily; it is unlikely that the dose of metformin will need to be reduced due to hypoglycemia
- With insulin: Initial: 15-30 mg once daily; dose of insulin should be reduced by 10% to 25% if the patient reports hypoglycemia or if the plasma glucose falls to <100 mg/dL. Doses >30 mg/day have not been evaluated in combination regimens.

A 1-week washout period is recommended in patients with normal liver enzymes who are changed from troglitazone to pioglitazone therapy.

Dosage adjustment in hepatic impairment: Clearance is significantly lower in hepatic impairment. Therapy should not be initiated if the patient exhibits active liver disease or increased transaminases (>2.5 times the upper limit of normal) at baseline.

(Continued)

Pioglitazone *(Continued)*

Mechanism of Action Thiazolidinedione antidiabetic agent that lowers blood glucose by improving target cell response to insulin, without increasing pancreatic insulin secretion. It has a mechanism of action that is dependent on the presence of insulin for activity. Pioglitazone is a potent and selective agonist for peroxisome proliferator-activated receptor-gamma (PPARgamma). Activation of nuclear PPAR-gamma receptors influences the production of a number of gene products involved in glucose and lipid metabolism.

Other Adverse Effects

>10%:

- Endocrine & metabolic: Decreased serum triglycerides, increased HDL cholesterol
- Gastrointestinal: Weight gain
- Respiratory: Upper respiratory tract infection (13%)

1% to 10%:

- Cardiovascular: Edema (5%) (in combination trials with sulfonylureas or insulin, the incidence of edema was as high as 15%)
- Central nervous system: Headache (9%), fatigue (4%)
- Endocrine & metabolic: Aggravation of diabetes mellitus (5%), hypoglycemia (range 2% to 15% when used in combination with sulfonylureas or insulin)
- Hematologic; Anemia (1%)
- Neuromuscular & skeletal: Myalgia (5%)
- Respiratory: Sinusitis (6%), pharyngitis (5%)

Contraindications Hypersensitivity to pioglitazone or any component of the formulation; active liver disease (transaminases >2.5 times the upper limit of normal at baseline); patients who have experienced jaundice during troglitazone therapy

Warnings/Precautions Should not be used in diabetic ketoacidosis. Mechanism requires the presence of insulin, therefore use in type 1 diabetes is not recommended. May potentiate hypoglycemia when used in combination with sulfonylureas or insulin. Use with caution in premenopausal, anovulatory women - may result in a resumption of ovulation, increasing the risk of pregnancy. Use with caution in patients with anemia (may reduce hemoglobin and hematocrit). Use with caution in patients with heart failure or edema - may increase plasma volume and/or increase cardiac hypertrophy. In general, use should be avoided in patients with NYHA class III or IV heart failure. Use with caution in patients with elevated transaminases (AST or ALT) - see Contraindications. Idiosyncratic hepatotoxicity has been reported with another thiazolidinedione agent (troglitazone) - monitoring should include periodic determinations of liver function.

Drug Interactions CYP2C8 and CYP3A4 substrate

Increased Effect/Toxicity: Ketoconazole (*in vitro*) inhibits metabolism of pioglitazone. Other inhibitors of CYP3A4, including itraconazole, are likely to decrease pioglitazone metabolism. Patients receiving inhibitors of CYP3A4 should have their glycemic control evaluated more frequently.

Decreased Effect: Effects of oral contraceptives may be decreased, based on data from a related compound (not been specifically evaluated for pioglitazone). CYP3A3/4 inducers may decrease the therapeutic effect of pioglitazone.

Drug Uptake

Onset of action: Delayed, may require several weeks for maximum effect
Half-life, elimination: Parent drug: 3-7 hours; Total: 16-24 hours
Time to peak: ~2 hours

Pregnancy Risk Factor C

Generic Available No

Piperacillin (pi PER a sil in)

U.S. Brand Names Pipracil®

Canadian Brand Names Pipracil®

Pharmacologic Category Antibiotic, Penicillin

Synonyms Piperacillin Sodium

Use Treatment of susceptible infections such as septicemia, acute and chronic respiratory tract infections, skin and soft tissue infections, and urinary tract infections due to susceptible strains of *Pseudomonas*, *Proteus*, and *Escherichia coli* and *Enterobacter*, normally used with other antibiotics (ie, aminoglycosides); active against some streptococci and some anaerobic bacteria; febrile neutropenia (as part of combination regimen)

Local Anesthetic/Vasoconstrictor Precautions No information available to require special precautions

Effects on Dental Treatment Prolonged use of penicillins may lead to development of oral candidiasis.

Dosage

Neonates: 100 mg/kg every 12 hours

Infants and Children: I.M., I.V.: 200-300 mg/kg/day in divided doses every 4-6 hours

Higher doses have been used in cystic fibrosis: 350-500 mg/kg/day in divided doses every 4-6 hours

Adults: I.M., I.V.:
- Moderate infections (urinary tract infections): 2-3 g/dose every 6-12 hours; maximum: 2 g I.M./site
- Serious infections: 3-4 g/dose every 4-6 hours; maximum: 24 g/24 hours
- Uncomplicated gonorrhea: 2 g I.M. in a single dose accompanied by 1 g probenecid 30 minutes prior to injection

Mechanism of Action Inhibits bacterial cell wall synthesis by binding to one or more of the penicillin binding proteins (PBPs); which in turn inhibits the final transpeptidation step of peptidoglycan synthesis in bacterial cell walls, thus inhibiting cell wall biosynthesis. Bacteria eventually lyse due to ongoing activity of cell wall autolytic enzymes (autolysins and murein hydrolases) while cell wall assembly is arrested.

Other Adverse Effects Frequency not defined:
- Central nervous system: Confusion, convulsions, drowsiness, fever, Jarisch-Herxheimer reaction
- Dermatologic: Rash
- Endocrine & metabolic: Electrolyte imbalance
- Hematologic: Abnormal platelet aggregation and prolonged PT (high doses), hemolytic anemia, Coombs' reaction (positive)
- Local: Thrombophlebitis
- Neuromuscular & skeletal: Myoclonus
- Renal: Acute interstitial nephritis
- Miscellaneous: Anaphylaxis, hypersensitivity reactions

Drug Interactions
- Increased Effect/Toxicity: Probenecid may increase penicillin levels. Neuromuscular blockers may increase duration of blockade.
- Decreased Effect: Tetracyclines may decrease penicillin effectiveness. Efficacy of oral contraceptives may be reduced when taken with piperacillin. High concentrations of piperacillin may cause physical inactivation of aminoglycosides and lead to potential toxicity in patients with mild-moderate renal dysfunction.

Drug Uptake
- Absorption: I.M.: 70% to 80%
- Half-life, elimination: Dose-dependent (increases with moderately severe renal or hepatic impairment):
  - Neonates: 1-5 days old: 3.6 hours; >6 days old: 2.1-2.7 hours
  - Children: 1-6 months: 0.79 hour; 6 months to 12 years: 0.39-0.5 hour
  - Adults: 36-80 minutes
- Time to peak: I.M.: 30-50 minutes

Pregnancy Risk Factor B

Generic Available No

Piperacillin and Tazobactam Sodium

(pi PER a sil in & ta zoe BAK tam SOW dee um)

U.S. Brand Names Zosyn®

Canadian Brand Names Tacozin®

Pharmacologic Category Antibiotic, Penicillin

Synonyms Piperacillin Sodium and Tazobactam Sodium

Use

Treatment of infections of lower respiratory tract, urinary tract, skin and skin structures, gynecologic, bone and joint infections, and septicemia caused by susceptible organisms. Tazobactam expands activity of piperacillin to include beta-lactamase producing strains of *S. aureus*, *H. influenzae*, *Enterobacteriaceae*, *Pseudomonas*, *Klebsiella*, *Citrobacter*, *Serratia*, *Bacteroides*, and other gram-negative anaerobes.

Application to nosocomial infections may be limited by restricted activity against gram-negative organisms producing class I beta-lactamases and inactivity against methicillin-resistant *Staphylococcus aureus*

Local Anesthetic/Vasoconstrictor Precautions No information available to require special precautions

Effects on Dental Treatment Prolonged use of penicillins may lead to development of oral candidiasis.

Dosage
- Children <12 years: Not recommended due to lack of data
- Children >12 years and Adults:
  - Severe infections: I.V.: Piperacillin/tazobactam 4/0.5 g every 8 hours or 3/0.375 g every 6 hours
  - Moderate infections: I.M.: Piperacillin/tazobactam 2/0.25 g every 6-1 hours; treatment should be continued for ≥7-10 days depending on severity of disease

Mechanism of Action Inhibits bacterial cell wall synthesis by binding to one or more of the penicillin binding proteins (PBPs); which in turn inhibits the final transpeptidation step of peptidoglycan synthesis in bacterial cell walls, thus inhibiting cell wall biosynthesis. Bacteria eventually lyse due to ongoing activity of cell wall autolytic enzymes (autolysins and murein hydrolases) while cell wall assembly is arrested. Tazobactam inhibits many beta-lactamases, including staphylococcal penicillinase and Richmond and Sykes types II, III, IV, and V, including extended

(Continued)

Piperacillin and Tazobactam Sodium *(Continued)*

spectrum enzymes; it has only limited activity against class I beta-lactamases other than class Ic types

Other Adverse Effects

>10%: Gastrointestinal: Diarrhea (11%)

1% to 10%:

Cardiovascular: Hypertension (2%)

Central nervous system: Insomnia (7%), headache (7% to 8%), agitation (2%), fever (2%), dizziness (1%)

Dermatologic: Rash (4%), pruritus (3%)

Gastrointestinal: Constipation (7% to 8%), nausea (7%), vomiting/dyspepsia (3%)

Respiratory: Rhinitis/dyspnea (~1%)

Miscellaneous: Serum sickness-like reaction

Several laboratory abnormalities have rarely been associated with piperacillin/tazobactam including reversible eosinophilia, and neutropenia (associated most often with prolonged therapy), positive direct Coombs' test, prolonged PT and aPTT, transient elevations of LFT, increases in creatinine

Drug Interactions

Increased Effect/Toxicity: Probenecid may increase penicillin levels. Neuromuscular blockers may increase duration of blockade.

Decreased Effect: Tetracyclines may decrease penicillin effectiveness. Efficacy of oral contraceptives may be reduced when taken with piperacillin and tazobactam sodium. Aminoglycosides may cause physical inactivation of aminoglycosides in the presence of high concentrations of piperacillin and potential toxicity in patients with mild-moderate renal dysfunction.

Drug Uptake Both AUC and peak concentrations are dose proportional. Hepatic impairment does not affect kinetics.

Half-life, elimination: Piperacillin: 1 hour; Metabolite: 1-1.5 hours; Tazobactam: 0.7-0.9 hour

Pregnancy Risk Factor B

Generic Available No

Piperazine (PI per a zeen)

Canadian Brand Names Entacyl®

Mexican Brand Names Desparasil®

Pharmacologic Category Anthelmintic

Synonyms Piperazine Citrate

Use Treatment of pinworm and roundworm infections (used as an alternative to first-line agents, mebendazole, or pyrantel pamoate)

Local Anesthetic/Vasoconstrictor Precautions No information available to require special precautions

Effects on Dental Treatment No effects or complications reported

Dosage Oral:

Pinworms: Children and Adults: 65 mg/kg/day (not to exceed 2.5 g/day) as a single daily dose for 7 days; in severe infections, repeat course after a 1-week interval

Roundworms:

Children: 75 mg/kg/day as a single daily dose for 2 days; maximum: 3.5 g/day

Adults: 3.5 g/day for 2 days (in severe infections, repeat course, after a 1-week interval)

Mechanism of Action Causes muscle paralysis of the roundworm by blocking the effects of acetylcholine at the neuromuscular junction

Other Adverse Effects

>10%:

Dermatologic: Itching, rash

Gastrointestinal: Stomatitis

Ocular: Conjunctivitis

Renal: Proteinuria

1% to 10%:

Dermatologic: Urticaria, alopecia

Gastrointestinal: Glossitis

Hematologic: Eosinophilia, leukopenia, thrombocytopenia

Renal: Hematuria

Drug Interactions Decreased Effect: Pyrantel pamoate (antagonistic mode of action)

Drug Uptake

Absorption: Well absorbed

Time to peak: 1 hour

Pregnancy Risk Factor B

Generic Available Yes

Pipracil® *see* Piperacillin *on page 962*

Pirbuterol (peer BYOO ter ole)

Related Information

Respiratory Diseases *on page 1328*

U.S. Brand Names Maxair™; Maxair™ Autohaler™

Pharmacologic Category $Beta_2$ Agonist

Synonyms Pirbuterol Acetate

Use Prevention and treatment of reversible bronchospasm including asthma

Local Anesthetic/Vasoconstrictor Precautions No information available to require special precautions

Effects on Dental Treatment No effects or complications reported

Dosage Children >12 years and Adults: 2 inhalations every 4-6 hours for prevention; two inhalations at an interval of at least 1-3 minutes, followed by a third inhalation in treatment of bronchospasm, not to exceed 12 inhalations/day

Mechanism of Action Pirbuterol is a $beta_2$-adrenergic agonist with a similar structure to albuterol, specifically a pyridine ring has been substituted for the benzene ring in albuterol. The increased $beta_2$ selectivity of pirbuterol results from the substitution of a tertiary butyl group on the nitrogen of the side chain, which additionally imparts resistance of pirbuterol to degradation by monoamine oxidase and provides a lengthened duration of action in comparison to the less selective previous beta-agonist agents.

Other Adverse Effects

>10%:
- Central nervous system: Nervousness (7%)
- Neuromuscular & skeletal: Trembling (6%)

1% to 10%:
- Cardiovascular: Palpitations (2%), tachycardia (1%)
- Central nervous system: Headache (2%), dizziness (1%)
- Gastrointestinal: Nausea (2%)
- Respiratory: Cough (1%)

Drug Interactions

Increased Effect/Toxicity: Increased toxicity with other beta agonists, MAO inhibitors, tricyclic antidepressants

Decreased Effect: Decreased effect with beta-blockers

Drug Uptake

Onset of action: Peak effect: Therapeutic: Oral: 2-3 hours (6.2-9.8 mcg/L); Inhalation: 0.5-1 hour

Half-life, elimination: 2-3 hours

Pregnancy Risk Factor C

Generic Available No

Piroxicam (peer OKS i kam)

Related Information

Rheumatoid Arthritis and Osteoarthritis *on page 1340*

Temporomandibular Dysfunction (TMD) *on page 1397*

U.S. Brand Names Feldene®

Canadian Brand Names Alti-Piroxicam; Apo®-Piroxicam; Feldene™; Gen-Piroxicam; Novo-Pirocam®; Nu-Pirox; Pexicam®

Mexican Brand Names Androxicam®; Artinor®; Artyflam; Brexicam®; Citoken®; Dixonal; Dolzycam®; Facicam; Feldene®; Flogosan®; Osteral®; Oxicanol; Piroxan; Piroxen; Rogal

Pharmacologic Category Nonsteroidal Anti-inflammatory Drug (NSAID)

Use Management of inflammatory disorders; symptomatic treatment of acute and chronic rheumatoid arthritis, osteoarthritis, and ankylosing spondylitis; also used in treatment of sunburn

Local Anesthetic/Vasoconstrictor Precautions No information available to require special precautions

Effects on Dental Treatment NSAID formulations are known to reversibly decrease platelet aggregation via mechanisms different than observed with aspirin. The dentist should be aware of the potential of abnormal coagulation. Caution should also be exercised in the use of NSAIDs in patients already on anticoagulant therapy with drugs such as warfarin (Coumadin®).

Dosage Oral:

Children: 0.2-0.3 mg/kg/day once daily; maximum dose: 15 mg/day

Adults: 10-20 mg/day once daily; although associated with increase in GI adverse effects, doses >20 mg/day have been used (ie, 30-40 mg/day)

Mechanism of Action Inhibits prostaglandin synthesis, acts on the hypothalamus heat-regulating center to reduce fever, blocks prostaglandin synthetase action which prevents formation of the platelet-aggregating substance thromboxane A_2; decreases pain receptor sensitivity. Other proposed mechanisms of action for salicylate anti-inflammatory action are lysosomal stabilization, kinin and leukotriene production, alteration of chemotactic factors, and inhibition of neutrophil activation. This latter mechanism may be the most significant pharmacologic action to reduce inflammation.

(Continued)

Piroxicam *(Continued)*

Other Adverse Effects

>10%:

Central nervous system: Dizziness
Dermatologic: Rash
Gastrointestinal: Abdominal cramps, heartburn, indigestion, nausea

1% to 10%:

Central nervous system: Headache, nervousness
Dermatologic: Itching
Endocrine & metabolic: Fluid retention
Gastrointestinal: Vomiting
Otic: Tinnitus

Warnings/Precautions Use with caution in patients with impaired cardiac function, dehydration, hypertension, impaired renal function, GI disease (bleeding or ulcers) and patients receiving anticoagulants; elderly have increased risk for adverse reactions to NSAIDs. Withhold for at least 4-6 half-lives prior to surgical or dental procedures.

Drug Interactions CYP2C9 and 2C18 enzyme substrate

ACE inhibitors: Antihypertensive effects may be decreased by concurrent therapy with NSAIDs; monitor BP.

Angiotensin II antagonists: Antihypertensive effects may be decreased by concurrent therapy with NSAIDs; monitor BP.

Anticoagulants (warfarin, heparin, LMWHs) in combination with NSAIDs can cause increased risk of bleeding.

Other antiplatelet drugs (ticlopidine, clopidogrel, aspirin, abciximab, dipyridamole, eptifibatide, tirofiban) can cause an increased risk of bleeding.

Corticosteroids may increase the risk of GI ulceration; avoid concurrent use.

Cyclosporine: NSAIDs may increase serum creatinine, potassium, BP, and cyclosporine levels; monitor cyclosporine levels and renal function carefully.

Hydralazine's antihypertensive effect is decreased; avoid concurrent use.

Lithium levels can be increased; avoid concurrent use if possible or monitor lithium levels and adjust dose.

Loop diuretics efficacy (diuretic and antihypertensive effect) is reduced. Indomethacin reduces this efficacy, however, it may be anticipated with any NSAID.

Methotrexate: Severe bone marrow suppression, aplastic anemia, and GI toxicity have been reported with concomitant NSAID therapy. Avoid use during moderate or high-dose methotrexate (increased and prolonged methotrexate levels). NSAID use during low-dose treatment of rheumatoid arthritis has not been fully evaluated; extreme caution is warranted.

Thiazides antihypertensive effects are decreased; avoid concurrent use.

Warfarin's INRs may be increased by piroxicam. Other NSAIDs may have the same effect depending on dose and duration. Monitor INR closely. Use the lowest dose of NSAIDs possible and for the briefest duration.

Drug Uptake

Onset of action: Analgesic: ~1 hour; Peak effect: 3-5 hours
Half-life, elimination: 45-50 hours

Pregnancy Risk Factor B/D (3rd trimester or near term)

Generic Available Yes

Pitocin® *see* Oxytocin *on page 910*
Pitressin® *see* Vasopressin *on page 1234*
Placidyl® *see* Ethchlorvynol *on page 474*
Plan B™ *see* Levonorgestrel *on page 703*
Plaquase® *see* Collagenase *on page 322*
Plaquenil® *see* Hydroxychloroquine *on page 613*
Platinol® *see* Cisplatin *on page 292*
Platinol®-AQ *see* Cisplatin *on page 292*
Plavix® *see* Clopidogrel *on page 310*
Plendil® *see* Felodipine *on page 489*
Pletal® *see* Cilostazol *on page 285*

Plicamycin (plye kay MYE sin)

U.S. Brand Names Mithracin®

Canadian Brand Names Mithracin®

Pharmacologic Category Antidote; Antineoplastic Agent, Antibiotic

Synonyms Mithramycin

Use Malignant testicular tumors, in the treatment of hypercalcemia and hypercalciuria of malignancy not responsive to conventional treatment; Paget's disease

Local Anesthetic/Vasoconstrictor Precautions No information available to require special precautions

Effects on Dental Treatment No effects or complications reported

Dosage Dose should be diluted in 1 L of D_5W or NS and administered over 4-6 hours. Dosage should be based on the patient's body weight. If a patient has abnormal fluid retention (ie, edema, hydrothorax or ascites), the patient's ideal weight rather than actual body weight should be used to calculate the dose.

Adults: I.V.:

Paget's disease: 15 mcg/kg/day once daily for 10 days

Hypercalcemia:

25 mcg/kg single dose which may be repeated in 48 hours if no response occurs

OR 25 mcg/kg/day for 3-4 days

OR 25-50 mcg/kg/dose every other day for 3-8 doses

Dosing adjustment in renal impairment:

Cl_{cr} 10-50 mL/minute: Decrease dosage to 75% of normal dose

Cl_{cr} <10 mL/minute: Decrease dosage to 50% of normal dose

Dosing in hepatic impairment: In the treatment of hypercalcemia in patients with hepatic dysfunction: Reduce dose to 12.5 mcg/kg/day

Mechanism of Action Potent osteoclast inhibitor; may inhibit parathyroid hormone effect on osteoclasts; inhibits bone resorption; forms a complex with DNA in the presence of magnesium or other divalent cations inhibiting DNA-directed RNA synthesis

Other Adverse Effects Note: Adverse reactions appear to be dose-related and less common at the lower doses used to treat hypercalcemia.

>10%: Gastrointestinal: Anorexia, stomatitis, nausea, vomiting, diarrhea

Nausea and vomiting occur in almost 100% of patients within the first 6 hours after treatment; incidence increases with rapid injection; stomatitis has also occurred

Time course for nausea/vomiting: Onset 4-6 hours; Duration: 4-24 hours

1% to 10%:

Cardiovascular: Facial flushing

Central nervous system: Fever, headache, depression, drowsiness

Endocrine & metabolic: Hypocalcemia

Hematologic: Myelosuppressive: Mild leukopenia and thrombocytopenia

WBC: Moderate, but uncommon

Platelets: Moderate, rapid onset

Onset: 7-10 days

Nadir: 14 days

Recovery: 21 days

Clotting disorders: May also depress hepatic synthesis of clotting factors, leading to a form of coagulopathy; petechiae, prolonged PT, epistaxis, and thrombocytopenia may be seen and may require discontinuation of the drug. Epistaxis is frequently the first sign of this bleeding disorder.

Hepatic: Hepatotoxicity

Local: Pain at injection site; extravasation (ann irritant; may produce local tissue irritation or cellulitis if infiltrated; if extravasation occurs, follow hospital procedure, discontinue I.V., and apply ice for 24 hours)

Irritant chemotherapy

Renal: Azotemia, nephrotoxicity

Miscellaneous: Hemorrhagic diathesis

Drug Interactions Calcitonin, etidronate, or glucagon taken with plicamycin may result in additive hypoglycemic effects.

Drug Uptake

Onset of action: Decreasing calcium levels: ~24 hours; Peak effect: 48-72 hours

Duration: 5-15 days

Half-life, elimination, plasma: 1 hour

Pregnancy Risk Factor X

Generic Available No

Pneumococcal Conjugate Vaccine, 7-Valent

(noo moe KOK al KON ju gate vak SEEN, seven vay lent)

U.S. Brand Names Prevnar®

Pharmacologic Category Vaccine

Synonyms Diphtheria CRM_{197} Protein; PCV7; Pneumococcal 7-Valent Conjugate Vaccine

Use Immunization of infants and toddlers against *Streptococcus pneumoniae* infection caused by serotypes included in the vaccine

Advisory Committee on Immunization Practices (ACIP) guidelines also recommend PCV7 for use in:

All children ≥23 months

Children ages 24-59 months with: Sickle cell disease (including other sickle cell hemoglobinopathies, asplenia, splenic dysfunction), HIV infection, immunocompromising conditions (congenital immunodeficiencies, renal failure, nephrotic syndrome, diseases associated with immunosuppressive or radiation therapy, solid organ transplant), chronic illnesses (cardiac disease, cerebrospinal fluid leaks, diabetes mellitus, pulmonary disease excluding asthma unless on high dose corticosteroids)

(Continued)

Pneumococcal Conjugate Vaccine, 7-Valent *(Continued)*

Consider use in all children 24-59 months with priority given to:
- Children 24-35 months
- Children 24-59 months who are of Alaska native, American Indian, or African-American descent
- Children 24-59 months who attend group day care centers

Local Anesthetic/Vasoconstrictor Precautions No information available to require special precautions

Effects on Dental Treatment No effects or complications reported

Dosage I.M.:

Infants: 2-6 months: 0.5 mL at ~ 2-month intervals for 3 consecutive doses, followed by a fourth dose of 0.5 mL at 12-15 months of age; first dose may be given as young as 6 weeks of age, but is typically given at 2 months of age. In case of a moderate shortage of vaccine, defer the fourth dose until shortage is resolved; in case of a severe shortage of vaccine, defer third and fourth doses until shortage is resolved.

Previously Unvaccinated Infants and Children:

7-11 months: 0.5 mL for a total of 3 doses; 2 doses at least 4 weeks apart, followed by a third dose after the 1-year birthday (12-15 months), separated from the second dose by at least 2 months. In case of a severe shortage of vaccine, defer the third dose until shortage is resolved.

12-23 months: 0.5 mL for a total of 2 doses, separated by at least 2 months. In case of a severe shortage of vaccine, defer the second dose until shortage is resolved.

24-59 months:

Healthy Children: 0.5 mL as a single dose. In case of a severe shortage of vaccine, defer dosing until shortage is resolved.

Children with sickle cell disease, asplenia, HIV infection, chronic illness or immunocompromising conditions (not including bone marrow transplants - results pending; use PPV23 [pneumococcal polysaccharide vaccine, polyvalent] at 12- and 24-months until studies are complete): 0.5 mL for a total of 2 doses, separated by 2 months

Previously Vaccinated Children with a lapse in vaccine administration:

7-11 months: Previously received 1 or 2 doses PCV7: 0.5 mL dose at 7-11 months of age, followed by a second dose ≥2 months later at 12-15 months of age

12-23 months:

Previously received 1 dose before 12 months of age: 0.5 mL dose, followed by a second dose ≥2 months later

Previously received 2 doses before age 12 months: 0.5 mL dose ≥2 months after the most recent dose

24-59 months: Any incomplete schedule: 0.5 mL as a single dose; **Note:** Patients with chronic diseases or immunosuppressing conditions should receive 2 doses ≥2 months apart

Mechanism of Action Contains saccharides of capsular antigens of serotypes 4, 6B, 9V, 18C, 19F, and 23F, individually conjugated to CRM197 protein

Other Adverse Effects All serious adverse reactions must be reported to the U.S. Department of Health and Human Services (DHHS) Vaccine Adverse Event Reporting System (VAERS) 1-800-822-7967.

>10%:
- Central nervous system: Fever, irritability, drowsiness, restlessness
- Dermatologic: Erythema
- Gastrointestinal: Decreased appetite, vomiting, diarrhea
- Local: Induration, tenderness, nodule

1% to 10%: Dermatologic: Rash (0.5% to 1.4%)

Drug Interactions Immunosuppressants: May decrease response to active immunizations

Pregnancy Risk Factor C

Pneumomist® *see* Guaifenesin *on page 568*
Podocon-25™ *see* Podophyllum Resin *on page 969*

Podofilox (po do FIL oks)

U.S. Brand Names Condylox®

Canadian Brand Names Condyline™; Wartec®

Pharmacologic Category Keratolytic Agent; Topical Skin Product

Use Treatment of external genital warts

Local Anesthetic/Vasoconstrictor Precautions No information available to require special precautions

Effects on Dental Treatment No effects or complications reported

Dosage Adults: Apply twice daily (morning and evening) for 3 consecutive days, then withhold use for 4 consecutive days; this cycle may be repeated up to 4 times until there is no visible wart tissue

Pregnancy Risk Factor C

Generic Available Yes: Topical solution only

Podofin® *see* Podophyllum Resin *on page 969*

Podophyllum Resin (po DOF fil um REZ in)

U.S. Brand Names Podocon-25™; Podofin®

Canadian Brand Names Podofilm®

Pharmacologic Category Keratolytic Agent

Synonyms Mandrake; May Apple; Podophyllin

Use Topical treatment of benign growths including external genital and perianal warts, papillomas, fibroids; compound benzoin tincture generally is used as the medium for topical application

Local Anesthetic/Vasoconstrictor Precautions No information available to require special precautions

Effects on Dental Treatment No effects or complications reported

Dosage Topical:

Children and Adults: 10% to 25% solution in compound benzoin tincture; apply drug to dry surface, use 1 drop at a time allowing drying between drops until area is covered; total volume should be limited to <0.5 mL per treatment session

Condylomata acuminatum: 25% solution is applied daily; use a 10% solution when applied to or near mucous membranes

Verrucae: 25% solution is applied 3-5 times/day directly to the wart

Mechanism of Action Directly affects epithelial cell metabolism by arresting mitosis through binding to a protein subunit of spindle microtubules (tubulin)

Other Adverse Effects 1% to 10%:

Dermatologic: Pruritus

Gastrointestinal: Nausea, vomiting, abdominal pain, diarrhea

Pregnancy Risk Factor X

Generic Available No

Point-Two® *see* Fluoride *on page 514*

Polaramine® *see* Dexchlorpheniramine *on page 365*

Poliovirus Vaccine, Inactivated

(POE lee oh VYE rus vak SEEN, in ak ti VAY ted)

U.S. Brand Names IPOL™

Canadian Brand Names IPOL™

Pharmacologic Category Vaccine

Synonyms Enhanced-potency Inactivated Poliovirus Vaccine; IPV; Salk Vaccine

Use As the global eradication of poliomyelitis continues, the risk for importation of wild-type poliovirus into the United States decreases dramatically. To eliminate the risk for vaccine-associated paralytic poliomyelitis (VAPP), an all-IPV schedule is recommended for routine childhood vaccination in the United States. All children should receive four doses of IPV (at age 2 months, age 4 months, between ages 6-18 months, and between ages 4-6 years). Oral poliovirus vaccine (OPV), if available, may be used only for the following special circumstances:

Mass vaccination campaigns to control outbreaks of paralytic polio

Unvaccinated children who will be traveling within 4 weeks to areas where polio is endemic or epidemic

Children of parents who do not accept the recommended number of vaccine injections; these children may receive OPV only for the third or fourth dose or both. In this situation, healthcare providers should administer OPV only after discussing the risk for VAPP with parents or caregivers.

OPV supplies are expected to be very limited in the United States after inventories are depleted. ACIP reaffirms its support for the global eradication initiative and use of OPV as the vaccine of choice to eradicate polio where it is endemic.

Local Anesthetic/Vasoconstrictor Precautions No information available to require special precautions

Effects on Dental Treatment No effects or complications reported

Dosage Subcutaneous: **Enhanced-potency inactivated poliovirus vaccine (E-IPV) is preferred for primary vaccination of adults**, 2 doses S.C. 4-8 weeks apart, a third dose 6-12 months after the second. For adults with a completed primary series and for whom a booster is indicated, either OPV or E-IPV can be given. If immediate protection is needed, either OPV or E-IPV is recommended.

Other Adverse Effects

All serious adverse reactions must be reported to the U.S. Department of Health and Human Services (DHHS) Vaccine Adverse Event Reporting System (VAERS) 1-800-822-7967.

1% to 10%:

Central nervous system: Fever (>101.3°F)

Dermatologic: Rash

Local: Tenderness or pain at injection site

Drug Interactions Decreased effect with immunosuppressive agents, immune globulin, cholera vaccine; separate by 1 month if possible; may temporarily suppress tuberculin skin test sensitivity (4-6 weeks); DTP, MMR, HIB, and hepatitis B vaccines may be given concurrently if at different sites

(Continued)

Poliovirus Vaccine, Inactivated *(Continued)*

Pregnancy Risk Factor C

Generic Available No

Poliovirus Vaccine, Live, Trivalent, Oral

(POE lee oh VYE rus vak SEEN, live, try VAY lent, OR al)

U.S. Brand Names Orimune®

Pharmacologic Category Vaccine

Synonyms OPV; Sabin Vaccine; TOPV

Use Poliovirus immunization

Local Anesthetic/Vasoconstrictor Precautions No information available to require special precautions

Effects on Dental Treatment No effects or complications reported

Dosage Oral:

Infants: 0.5 mL dose at age 2 months, 4 months, and 18 months; optional dose may be given at 6 months in areas where poliomyelitis is endemic

Older Children, Adolescents, and Adults: Two 0.5 mL doses 8 weeks apart; third dose of 0.5 mL 6-12 months after second dose; a reinforcing dose of 0.5 mL should be given before entry to school, in children who received the third primary dose before their fourth birthday

Other Adverse Effects

All serious adverse reactions must be reported to the U.S. Department of Health and Human Services (DHHS) Vaccine Adverse Event Reporting System (VAERS) 1-800-822-7967.

1% to 10%:

Central nervous system: Fever (>101.3°F)

Dermatologic: Rash

Local: Tenderness or pain at injection site

Pregnancy Risk Factor C

Generic Available No

Comments

Oral vaccine: Live, attenuated vaccine

Federal law requires that the date of administration, the vaccine manufacturer, lot number of vaccine, and the administering person's name, title and address be entered into the patient's permanent medical record; live virus vaccine

Polocaine® *see* Mepivacaine *on page 764*

Polycitra® *see* Sodium Citrate and Potassium Citrate Mixture *on page 1096*

Polycitra®-K *see* Potassium Citrate and Citric Acid *on page 979*

Polycose® [OTC] *see* Glucose Polymers *on page 559*

Polydine® [OTC] *see* Povidone-Iodine *on page 982*

Polyethylene Glycol-Electrolyte Solution

(pol i ETH i leen GLY kol ee LEK troe lite soe LOO shun)

U.S. Brand Names Colyte®; GoLYTELY®; MiraLax™; NuLytely®; OCL®

Canadian Brand Names Colyte™; Klean-Prep®; Klean-Prep®; Lyteprep™; PegLyte®; Peglyte™

Pharmacologic Category Cathartic; Laxative, Bowel Evacuant

Synonyms Electrolyte Lavage Solution

Use Bowel cleansing prior to GI examination or following toxic ingestion (electrolyte containing solutions only); treatment of occasional constipation (MiraLax™)

Local Anesthetic/Vasoconstrictor Precautions No information available to require special precautions

Effects on Dental Treatment No effects or complications reported

Dosage

Oral:

Children ≥6 months: Bowel cleansing prior to GI exam (solutions with electrolytes only): 25-40 mL/kg/hour for 4-10 hours (until rectal effluent is clear). Ideally, patients should fast for ~3-4 hours prior to administration; absolutely no solid food for at least 2 hours before the solution is given. The solution may be given via nasogastric tube to patients who are unwilling or unable to drink the solution. Patients <2 years should be monitored closely.

Adults:

Bowel cleansing prior to GI exam (solutions with electrolytes only): 240 mL (8 oz) every 10 minutes, until 4 L are consumed or the rectal effluent is clear; rapid drinking of each portion is preferred to drinking small amounts continuously. Ideally, patients should fast for ~3-4 hours prior to administration; absolutely no solid food for at least 2 hours before the solution is given. The solution may be given via nasogastric tube to patients who are unwilling or unable to drink the solution.

Occasional constipation (MiraLax™): 17 g of powder (~1 heaping tablespoon) dissolved in 8 oz of water; once daily; do not use for >2 weeks.

Nasogastric tube:

Children ≥6 months: Bowel cleansing prior to GI exam (solutions with electrolytes only): 25 mL/kg/hour until rectal effluent is clear. Ideally, patients should fast for ~3-4 hours prior to administration; absolutely no solid food for at least 2 hours before the solution is given.

Adults: Bowel cleansing prior to GI exam (solutions with electrolytes only): 20-30 mL/minute (1.2-1.8 L/hour); the first bowel movement should occur ~1 hour after the start of administration. Ideally, patients should fast for ~3-4 hours prior to administration; absolutely no solid food for at least 2 hours before the solution is given.

Mechanism of Action Induces catharsis by strong electrolyte and osmotic effects

Other Adverse Effects Frequency not defined:

Dermatologic: Dermatitis, rash, urticaria

Gastrointestinal: Nausea, abdominal fullness, bloating, abdominal cramps, vomiting, anal irritation, diarrhea, flatulence

Drug Interactions Oral medications should not be administered within 1 hour of start of therapy.

Drug Uptake Onset of effect: Oral: Bowel cleansing: ~1-2 hours; Constipation: 48-96 hours

Pregnancy Risk Factor C

Generic Available No

Comments Do not add flavorings as additional ingredients before use

Polygam® S/D *see* Immune Globulin, Intravenous *on page 630*

Polymyxin B (pol i MIKS in bee)

Related Information

Neomycin and Polymyxin B *on page 855*

Neomycin, Polymyxin B, and Dexamethasone *on page 856*

Neomycin, Polymyxin B, and Prednisolone *on page 857*

Pharmacologic Category Antibiotic, Irrigation; Antibiotic, Miscellaneous

Synonyms Polymyxin B Sulfate

Use Treatment of acute infections caused by susceptible strains of *Pseudomonas aeruginosa*; used occasionally for gut decontamination; parenteral use of polymyxin B has mainly been replaced by less toxic antibiotics, reserved for life-threatening infections caused by organisms resistant to the preferred drugs (eg, pseudomonal meningitis - intrathecal administration)

Local Anesthetic/Vasoconstrictor Precautions No information available to require special precautions

Effects on Dental Treatment No effects or complications reported

Dosage Otic (in combination with other drugs): 1-2 drops, 3-4 times/day; should be used sparingly to avoid accumulation of excess debris

Infants <2 years:

I.M.: Up to 40,000 units/kg/day divided every 6 hours (not routinely recommended due to pain at injection sites)

I.V.: Up to 40,000 units/kg/day divided every 12 hours

Intrathecal: 20,000 units/day for 3-4 days, then 25,000 units every other day for at least 2 weeks after CSF cultures are negative and CSF (glucose) has returned to within normal limits

Children ≥2 years and Adults:

I.M.: 25,000-30,000 units/kg/day divided every 4-6 hours (not routinely recommended due to pain at injection sites)

I.V.: 15,000-25,000 units/kg/day divided every 12 hours

Intrathecal: 50,000 units/day for 3-4 days, then every other day for at least 2 weeks after CSF cultures are negative and CSF (glucose) has returned to within normal limits

Total daily dose should not exceed 2,000,000 units/day

Bladder irrigation (in combination with 57 mg neomycin sulfate): Continuous irrigant or rinse in the urinary bladder for up to 10 days using 20 mg (equal to 200,000 units) added to 1 L of normal saline; usually no more than 1 L of irrigant is used per day unless urine flow rate is high; administration rate is adjusted to patient's urine output

Topical irrigation or topical solution: 500,000 units/L of normal saline; topical irrigation should not exceed 2 million units/day in adults

Gut sterilization: Oral: 15,000-25,000 units/kg/day in divided doses every 6 hours

Clostridium difficile enteritis: Oral: 25,000 units every 6 hours for 10 days

Ophthalmic: A concentration of 0.1% to 0.25% is administered as 1-3 drops every hour, then increasing the interval as response indicates to 1-2 drops 4-6 times/day

Dosing adjustment/interval in renal impairment:

Cl_{cr} 20-50 mL/minute: Administer 75% to 100% of normal dose every 12 hours

Cl_{cr} 5-20 mL/minute: Administer 50% of normal dose every 12 hours

Cl_{cr} <5 mL/minute: Administer 15% of normal dose every 12 hours

Mechanism of Action Binds to phospholipids, alters permeability, and damages the bacterial cytoplasmic membrane permitting leakage of intracellular constituents

(Continued)

Polymyxin B *(Continued)*

Other Adverse Effects Frequency not defined:

Cardiovascular: Facial flushing

Central nervous system: Neurotoxicity (irritability, drowsiness, ataxia, perioral paresthesia, numbness of the extremities, and blurring of vision); dizziness, drug fever, meningeal irritation with intrathecal administration

Dermatologic: Urticarial rash

Endocrine & metabolic: Hypocalcemia, hyponatremia, hypokalemia, hypochloremia

Local: Pain at injection site

Neuromuscular & skeletal: Neuromuscular blockade, weakness

Renal: Nephrotoxicity

Respiratory: Respiratory arrest

Miscellaneous: Anaphylactoid reaction

Drug Interactions Increased/prolonged effect of neuromuscular blocking agents

Drug Uptake

Absorption: Well absorbed from the peritoneum; minimal absorption from the GI tract (except in neonates) from mucous membranes or intact skin

Half-life, elimination: 4.5-6 hours (increases with renal impairment)

Time to peak: I.M.: ~2 hours

Pregnancy Risk Factor B (per expert opinion)

Generic Available Yes

Polymyxin B and Hydrocortisone

(pol i MIKS in bee & hye droe KOR ti sone)

U.S. Brand Names Otobiotic®

Pharmacologic Category Antibiotic/Corticosteroid, Otic

Synonyms Hydrocortisone and Polymyxin B

Use Treatment of superficial bacterial infections of external ear canal

Local Anesthetic/Vasoconstrictor Precautions No information available to require special precautions

Effects on Dental Treatment No effects or complications reported

Dosage Instill 4 drops 3-4 times/day

Pregnancy Risk Factor C

Generic Available No

Poly-Pred® *see* Neomycin, Polymyxin B, and Prednisolone *on page 857*

Polysaccharide-Iron Complex (pol i SAK a ride-EYE ern KOM pleks)

U.S. Brand Names Hytinic® [OTC]; Niferex® [OTC]; Nu-Iron® [OTC]

Pharmacologic Category Iron Salt

Use Prevention and treatment of iron deficiency anemias

Local Anesthetic/Vasoconstrictor Precautions No information available to require special precautions

Effects on Dental Treatment No effects or complications reported

Dosage Oral:

Children: 3 mg/kg 3 times/day

Adults: 200 mg 3-4 times/day

Other Adverse Effects

>10%: Gastrointestinal: Stomach cramping, constipation, nausea, vomiting, dark stools, GI irritation, epigastric pain, nausea

1% to 10%:

Gastrointestinal: Heartburn, diarrhea

Genitourinary: Discolored urine

Miscellaneous: Staining of teeth

Pregnancy Risk Factor A

Generic Available Yes

Comments 100% elemental iron

Polysporin® Ophthalmic *see* Bacitracin and Polymyxin B *on page 141*
Polysporin® Topical [OTC] *see* Bacitracin and Polymyxin B *on page 141*
Polytar® [OTC] *see* Coal Tar *on page 315*

Polythiazide (pol i THYE a zide)

Related Information

Cardiovascular Diseases *on page 1308*

U.S. Brand Names Renese®

Pharmacologic Category Diuretic, Thiazide

Use Adjunctive therapy in treatment of edema and hypertension

Local Anesthetic/Vasoconstrictor Precautions No information available to require special precautions

Effects on Dental Treatment No effects or complications reported

Dosage Adults: Oral: 1-4 mg/day

Mechanism of Action The diuretic mechanism of action of the thiazides is primarily inhibition of sodium, chloride, and water reabsorption in the renal distal tubules, thereby producing diuresis with a resultant reduction in plasma volume. The antihypertensive mechanism of action of the thiazides is unknown. It is known that doses of thiazides produce greater reductions in BP than equivalent diuretic doses of loop diuretics (eg, furosemide). There has been speculation that the thiazides may have some influence on vascular tone mediated through sodium depletion, but this remains to be proven.

Other Adverse Effects 1% to 10%: Endocrine & metabolic: Hypokalemia

Warnings/Precautions Avoid in severe renal disease (ineffective). Electrolyte disturbances (hypokalemia, hypochloremic alkalosis, hyponatremia) can occur. Use with caution in severe hepatic dysfunction; hepatic encephalopathy can be caused by electrolyte disturbances. Gout can be precipitated in certain patients with a history of gout, a familial predisposition to gout, or chronic renal failure. Cautious use in diabetics; may see a change in glucose control. Hypersensitivity reactions can occur. Can cause SLE exacerbation or activation. Use with caution in patients with moderate or high cholesterol concentrations. Photosensitization may occur. Correct hypokalemia before initiating therapy.

Chemical similarities are present among sulfonamides, sulfonylureas, carbonic anhydrase inhibitors, thiazides, and loop diuretics (except ethacrynic acid). Use in patients with sulfonamide allergy is specifically contraindicated in product labeling, however a risk of cross-reaction exists in patients with allergy to any of these compounds; avoid use when previous reaction has been severe.

Drug Interactions

Increased Effect/Toxicity: Increased effect of thiazides with furosemide and other loop diuretics. Increased hypotension and/or renal adverse effects of ACE inhibitors may result in aggressively diuresed patients. Beta-blockers increase hyperglycemic effects of thiazides in type 2 diabetes mellitus. Cyclosporine and thiazides can increase the risk of gout or renal toxicity. Digoxin toxicity can be exacerbated if a thiazide induces hypokalemia or hypomagnesemia. Lithium toxicity can occur with thiazides due to reduced renal excretion of lithium. Thiazides may prolong the duration of action with neuromuscular blocking agents.

Decreased Effect: Effects of oral hypoglycemics may be decreased. Decreased absorption of hydrochlorothiazide with cholestyramine and colestipol. NSAIDs can decrease the efficacy of thiazides, reducing the diuretic and antihypertensive effects.

Drug Uptake

Onset of action: Diuresis: ~2 hours

Duration: 24-48 hours

Pregnancy Risk Factor D

Generic Available No

Polytrim® *see* Trimethoprim and Polymyxin B *on page 1210*

Ponstel® *see* Mefenamic Acid *on page 754*

Pontocaine® *see* Tetracaine *on page 1146*

Pontocaine® With Dextrose *see* Tetracaine and Dextrose *on page 1147*

Poractant Alfa (por AKT ant AL fa)

U.S. Brand Names Curosurf®

Canadian Brand Names Curosurf®

Pharmacologic Category Lung Surfactant

Use Orphan drug: Treatment and prevention of respiratory distress syndrome (RDS) in premature infants

Local Anesthetic/Vasoconstrictor Precautions No information available to require special precautions

Effects on Dental Treatment No effects or complications reported

Dosage Intratracheal use **only**: Premature infant with RDS: Initial dose is 2.5 mL/kg of birth weight. Up to 2 subsequent doses of 1.25 mL/kg birth weight can be administered at 12-hour intervals if needed in infants who continue to require mechanical ventilation and supplemental oxygen.

Mechanism of Action Endogenous pulmonary surfactant reduces surface tension at the air-liquid interface of the alveoli during ventilation and stabilizes the alveoli against collapse at resting transpulmonary pressures. A deficiency of pulmonary surfactant in preterm infants results in respiratory distress syndrome characterized by poor lung expansion, inadequate gas exchange, and atelectasis. Poractant alpha compensates for the surfactant deficiency and restores surface activity to the infant's lungs. It reduces mortality and pneumothoraces associated with RDS.

Other Adverse Effects Frequency not defined:

Cardiovascular: Bradycardia, hypotension

Gastrointestinal: Endotracheal tube blockage

Respiratory: Oxygen desaturation

Drug Uptake Information limited to animal models. No human information about pharmacokinetics exists.

Generic Available No

Porcelana® [OTC] *see* Hydroquinone *on page 611*

Porcelana® Sunscreen [OTC] *see* Hydroquinone *on page 611*

Porfimer (POR fi mer)

U.S. Brand Names Photofrin®

Canadian Brand Names Photofrin®

Pharmacologic Category Antineoplastic Agent, Miscellaneous

Synonyms CL184116; Dihematoporphyrin Ether; Porfimer Sodium

Use Orphan drug: Photodynamic therapy (PDT) with porfimer for palliation of patients with completely obstructing esophageal cancer, or of patients with partially obstructing esophageal cancer who cannot be satisfactorily treated with Nd:YAG laser therapy; completely- or partially-obstructing endobronchial nonsmall cell lung cancer; microinvasive endobronchial nonsmall cell lung cancer

Local Anesthetic/Vasoconstrictor Precautions No information available to require special precautions

Effects on Dental Treatment No effects or complications reported

Mechanism of Action Photosensitizing agent used in the photodynamic therapy (PDT) of tumors: cytotoxic and antitumor actions of porfimer are light and oxygen dependent. Cellular damage caused by porfimer PDT is a consequence of the propagation of radical reactions.

Other Adverse Effects

>10%:

- Cardiovascular: Atrial fibrillation, chest pain
- Central nervous system: Fever, pain, insomnia
- Dermatologic: Photosensitivity reaction (minor reactions may occur in up to 100%)
- Gastrointestinal: Abdominal pain, constipation, dysphagia, nausea, vomiting
- Hematologic: Anemia
- Neuromuscular & skeletal: Back pain
- Respiratory: Dyspnea, pharyngitis, pleural effusion, pneumonia, respiratory insufficiency

1% to 10%:

- Cardiovascular: Hypertension, hypotension, edema, cardiac failure, tachycardia, chest pain (substernal)
- Central nervous system: Anxiety, confusion
- Dermatologic: Increased hair growth, skin discoloration, skin wrinkles, skin nodules, increased skin fragility
- Endocrine & metabolic: Dehydration
- Gastrointestinal: Diarrhea, dyspepsia, eructation, esophageal edema, esophageal tumor bleeding, esophageal stricture, esophagitis, hematemesis, melena, weight loss, anorexia
- Genitourinary: Urinary tract infection
- Neuromuscular & skeletal: Weakness
- Respiratory: Coughing, tracheoesophageal fistula
- Miscellaneous: Moniliasis, surgical complication

Warnings/Precautions The U.S. Food and Drug Administration (FDA) currently recommends that procedures for proper handling and disposal of antineoplastic agents be considered. If the esophageal tumor is eroding into the trachea or bronchial tree, the likelihood of tracheoesophageal or bronchoesophageal fistula resulting from treatment is sufficiently high that PDT is not recommended. All patients who receive porfimer sodium will be photosensitive and must observe precautions to avoid exposure of skin and eyes to direct sunlight or bright indoor light for 30 days. The photosensitivity is due to residual drug which will be present in all parts of the skin. Exposure of the skin to ambient indoor light is, however, beneficial because the remaining drug will be inactivated gradually and safely through a photobleaching reaction. Patients should not stay in a darkened room during this period and should be encouraged to expose their skin to ambient indoor light. Ocular discomfort has been reported; for 30 days, when outdoors, patients should wear dark sunglasses which have an average white light transmittance of <4%.

Drug Interactions

Increased Effect/Toxicity: Concomitant administration of other photosensitizing agents (eg, tetracyclines, sulfonamides, phenothiazines, sulfonylureas, thiazide diuretics, griseofulvin) could increase the photosensitivity reaction.

Decreased Effect: Compounds that quench active oxygen species or scavenge radicals (eg, dimethyl sulfoxide, beta-carotene, mannitol) would be expected to decrease photodynamic therapy (PDT) activity. Allopurinol, calcium channel blockers, and some prostaglandin synthesis inhibitors could interfere with porfimer. Drugs that decrease clotting, vasoconstriction, or platelet aggregation could decrease the efficacy of PDT. Glucocorticoid hormones may decrease the efficacy of the treatment.

Drug Uptake

Half-life, elimination: 250 hours

Time to peak: ~2 hours

Pregnancy Risk Factor C

Generic Available No

Posture® [OTC] *see* Calcium Phosphate, Tribasic *on page 206*

Potasalan® *see* Potassium Chloride *on page 977*

Potassium Acetate (poe TASS ee um AS e tate)

Pharmacologic Category Electrolyte Supplement, Parenteral

Use Potassium deficiency; to avoid chloride when high concentration of potassium is needed, source of bicarbonate

Local Anesthetic/Vasoconstrictor Precautions No information available to require special precautions

Effects on Dental Treatment No effects or complications reported

Dosage I.V. doses should be incorporated into the patient's maintenance I.V. fluids, intermittent I.V. potassium administration should be reserved for severe depletion situations and requires EKG monitoring; doses listed as mEq of potassium

Treatment of hypokalemia: I.V.:
- Children: 2-5 mEq/kg/day
- Adults: 40-100 mEq/day

I.V. intermittent infusion (must be diluted prior to administration):
- Children: 0.5-1 mEq/kg/dose (maximum: 30 mEq) to infuse at 0.3-0.5 mEq/kg/hour (maximum: 1 mEq/kg/hour)
- Adults: 10-20 mEq/dose (maximum: 40 mEq/dose) to infuse over 2-3 hours (maximum: 40 mEq over 1 hour)

Mechanism of Action Potassium is the major cation of intracellular fluid and is essential for the conduction of nerve impulses in heart, brain, and skeletal muscle; contraction of cardiac, skeletal and smooth muscles; maintenance of normal renal function, acid-base balance, carbohydrate metabolism, and gastric secretion

Other Adverse Effects

>10%: Gastrointestinal: Diarrhea, nausea, stomach pain, flatulence, vomiting (oral)

1% to 10%:
- Cardiovascular: Bradycardia
- Endocrine & metabolic: Hyperkalemia
- Neuromuscular & skeletal: Weakness
- Respiratory: Dyspnea
- Local: Local tissue necrosis with extravasation

Drug Interactions Increased Effect/Toxicity: Potassium-sparing diuretics, salt substitutes, and ACE inhibitors

Drug Uptake Absorption: Well absorbed

Pregnancy Risk Factor C

Generic Available Yes

Potassium Acetate, Potassium Bicarbonate, and Potassium Citrate

(poe TASS ee um AS e tate, poe TASS ee um bye KAR bun ate, & poe TASS ee um SIT rate)

U.S. Brand Names Tri-K®

Pharmacologic Category Electrolyte Supplement, Oral

Synonyms Potassium Acetate, Potassium Citrate, and Potassium Bicarbonate; Potassium Bicarbonate, Potassium Acetate, and Potassium Citrate; Potassium Bicarbonate, Potassium Citrate, and Potassium Acetate; Potassium Citrate, Potassium Acetate, and Potassium Bicarbonate; Potassium Citrate, Potassium Bicarbonate, and Potassium Acetate

Use Treatment or prevention of hypokalemia

Local Anesthetic/Vasoconstrictor Precautions No information available to require special precautions

Effects on Dental Treatment No effects or complications reported

Dosage Oral:
- Children: 1-4 mEq/kg/24 hours in divided doses as required to maintain normal serum potassium
- Adults:
  - Prevention: 16-24 mEq/day in 2-4 divided doses
  - Treatment: 40-100 mEq/day in 2-4 divided doses

Drug Interactions Increased Effect/Toxicity: Potassium-sparing diuretics, salt substitutes, ACE inhibitors.

Pregnancy Risk Factor C

Generic Available No

Potassium Acid Phosphate (poe TASS ee um AS id FOS fate)

U.S. Brand Names K-Phos® Original

Pharmacologic Category Urinary Acidifying Agent

Use Acidifies urine and lowers urinary calcium concentration; reduces odor and rash caused by ammoniacal urine; increases the antibacterial activity of methenamine

Local Anesthetic/Vasoconstrictor Precautions No information available to require special precautions

Effects on Dental Treatment No effects or complications reported

(Continued)

Potassium Acid Phosphate *(Continued)*

Dosage Adults: Oral: 1000 mg dissolved in 6-8 oz of water 4 times/day with meals and at bedtime; for best results, soak tablets in water for 2-5 minutes, then stir and swallow

Mechanism of Action The principal intracellular cation; involved in transmission of nerve impulses, muscle contractions, enzyme activity, and glucose utilization

Other Adverse Effects

>10%: Gastrointestinal: Diarrhea, nausea, stomach pain, flatulence, vomiting

1% to 10%:

- Cardiovascular: Bradycardia
- Endocrine & metabolic: Hyperkalemia
- Local: Local tissue necrosis with extravasation
- Neuromuscular & skeletal: Weakness
- Respiratory: Dyspnea

Drug Interactions

Increased Effect/Toxicity: Potassium-sparing diuretics, salt substitutes, salicylates, and ACE inhibitors

Decreased Effect: Antacids containing magnesium, calcium or aluminum (bind phosphate and decreased its absorption)

Drug Uptake Absorption: Well absorbed

Pregnancy Risk Factor C

Generic Available No

Potassium Bicarbonate (poe TASS ee um bye KAR bun ate)

U.S. Brand Names K+ Care® ET

Pharmacologic Category Electrolyte Supplement, Oral

Use Potassium deficiency, hypokalemia

Local Anesthetic/Vasoconstrictor Precautions No information available to require special precautions

Effects on Dental Treatment No effects or complications reported

Dosage

Children: 1-4 mEq/kg/day

Adults: 25 mEq 2-4 times/day

Drug Interactions Increased Effect/Toxicity: Potassium-sparing diuretics, salt substitutes, salicylates, and ACE inhibitors

Pregnancy Risk Factor C

Generic Available No

Potassium Bicarbonate and Potassium Chloride, Effervescent

(poe TASS ee um bye KAR bun ate & poe TASS ee um KLOR ide, ef er VES ent)

U.S. Brand Names Klorvess® Effervescent; K-Lyte/Cl®

Canadian Brand Names K-Lyte/CL®

Pharmacologic Category Electrolyte Supplement, Oral

Use Treatment or prevention of hypokalemia

Local Anesthetic/Vasoconstrictor Precautions No information available to require special precautions

Effects on Dental Treatment No effects or complications reported

Dosage Oral:

Children: 1-4 mEq/kg/24 hours in divided doses as required to maintain normal serum potassium

Adults:

- Prevention: 16-24 mEq/day in 2-4 divided doses
- Treatment: 40-100 mEq/day in 2-4 divided doses

Drug Interactions Increased Effect/Toxicity: Potassium-sparing diuretics, salt substitutes, ACE inhibitors

Pregnancy Risk Factor C

Generic Available No

Potassium Bicarbonate and Potassium Citrate, Effervescent

(poe TASS ee um bye KAR bun ate & poe TASS ee um SIT rate, ef er VES ent)

U.S. Brand Names Effer-K™; Klor-Con®/EF; K-Lyte®

Canadian Brand Names K-Lyte®

Pharmacologic Category Electrolyte Supplement, Oral

Synonyms Potassium Citrate and Potassium Bicarbonate, Effervescent

Use Treatment or prevention of hypokalemia

Local Anesthetic/Vasoconstrictor Precautions No information available to require special precautions

Effects on Dental Treatment No effects or complications reported

Dosage Oral:

Children: 1-4 mEq/kg/24 hours in divided doses as required to maintain normal serum potassium

Adults:

Prevention: 16-24 mEq/day in 2-4 divided doses

Treatment: 40-100 mEq/day in 2-4 divided doses

Mechanism of Action Needed for the conduction of nerve impulses in heart, brain, and skeletal muscle; contraction of cardiac, skeletal and smooth muscles; maintenance of normal renal function

Other Adverse Effects

>10%: Gastrointestinal: Diarrhea, nausea, stomach pain, flatulence, vomiting

1% to 10%:

Cardiovascular: Bradycardia

Endocrine & metabolic: Hyperkalemia

Local: Local tissue necrosis with extravasation

Neuromuscular & skeletal: Weakness

Respiratory: Dyspnea

Drug Interactions Increased Effect/Toxicity: Potassium-sparing diuretics, salt substitutes, ACE inhibitors

Drug Uptake Absorption: Well absorbed

Pregnancy Risk Factor C

Generic Available Yes

Potassium Chloride (poe TASS ee um KLOR ide)

U.S. Brand Names Cena-K®; Gen-K®; K+ 10®; Kaochlor®; Kaochlor® SF; Kaon-Cl®; Kaon-Cl-10®; Kay Ciel®; K+ Care®; K-Dur® 10; K-Dur® 20; K-Lease®; K-Lor™; Klor-Con®; Klor-Con® 8; Klor-Con® 10; Klor-Con®/25; Klorvess®; Klotrix®; K-Norm®; K-Tab®; Micro-K® 10 Extencaps®; Micro-K® Extencaps; Micro-K® LS; Potasalan®; Rum-K®; Slow-K®; Ten-K®

Canadian Brand Names Apo®-K; K-10®; Kaochlor®; K-Dur®; K-Lor®; K-Lyte®/Cl; Micro-k Extencaps®; Roychlor®; Slow-K®

Pharmacologic Category Electrolyte Supplement, Oral; Electrolyte Supplement, Parenteral

Synonyms KCl

Use Treatment or prevention of hypokalemia

Local Anesthetic/Vasoconstrictor Precautions No information available to require special precautions

Effects on Dental Treatment No effects or complications reported

Dosage I.V. doses should be incorporated into the patient's maintenance I.V. fluids; intermittent I.V. potassium administration should be reserved for severe depletion situations in patients undergoing EKG monitoring.

Normal daily requirements: Oral, I.V.:

Children: 2-3 mEq/kg/day

Adults: 40-80 mEq/day

Prevention during diuretic therapy: Oral:

Children: 1-2 mEq/kg/day in 1-2 divided doses

Adults: 20-40 mEq/day in 1-2 divided doses

Treatment of hypokalemia: Oral, I.V.:

Neonates, Infants, and Children: 2-5 mEq/kg/day in divided doses

Adults: 40-100 mEq/day in divided doses

Treatment of hypokalemia: I.V. intermittent infusion (must be diluted prior to administration):

Neonates, Infants, and Children: 0.5-1 mEq/kg/dose (maximum dose: 30 mEq) to infuse at 0.3-0.5 mEq/kg/hour (maximum dose: 1 mEq/kg/hour)

Treatment of hypokalemia: Adults:

I.V. intermittent infusion: 10-20 mEq/hour, not to exceed 40 mEq/hour and 150 mEq/day. See table.

Potassium Dosage/Rate of Infusion Guidelines

Serum Potassium	Maximum Infusion Rate	Maximum Concentration	Maximum 24-Hour Dose
>2.5 mEq/L	10 mEq/h	40 mEq/L	200 mEq
<2.5 mEq/L	40 mEq/h	80 mEq/L	400 mEq

Potassium >2.5 mEq/L:

Oral: 60-80 mEq/day plus additional amounts if needed

I.V.: 10 mEq over 1 hour with additional doses if needed

Potassium <2.5 mEq/L:

Oral: Up to 40-60 mEq initial dose, followed by further doses based on lab values; deficits at a plasma concentration of 2 mEq/L may be as high as 400-800 mEq of potassium

(Continued)

Potassium Chloride *(Continued)*

I.V.: Up to 40 mEq over 1 hour, with doses based on frequent lab monitoring; deficits at a plasma concentration of 2 mEq/L may be as high as 400-800 mEq of potassium

Mechanism of Action Potassium is the major cation of intracellular fluid and is essential for the conduction of nerve impulses in heart, brain, and skeletal muscle; contraction of cardiac, skeletal and smooth muscles; maintenance of normal renal function, acid-base balance, carbohydrate metabolism, and gastric secretion

Other Adverse Effects

>10%: Gastrointestinal: Diarrhea, nausea, stomach pain, flatulence, vomiting (oral)

1% to 10%:

Cardiovascular: Bradycardia

Endocrine & metabolic: Hyperkalemia

Local: Local tissue necrosis with extravasation, pain at the site of injection

Neuromuscular & skeletal: Weakness

Respiratory: Dyspnea

Drug Interactions Increased Effect/Toxicity: Potassium-sparing diuretics, salt substitutes, ACE inhibitors

Drug Uptake Absorption: Well absorbed

Pregnancy Risk Factor A

Generic Available Yes

Potassium Chloride and Potassium Gluconate

(poe TASS ee um KLOR ide & poe TASS ee um GLOO coe nate)

U.S. Brand Names Kolyum®

Pharmacologic Category Electrolyte Supplement, Oral

Use Treatment or prevention of hypokalemia

Local Anesthetic/Vasoconstrictor Precautions No information available to require special precautions

Effects on Dental Treatment No effects or complications reported

Dosage Oral:

Children: 1-4 mEq/kg/24 hours in divided doses as required to maintain normal serum potassium

Adults:

Prevention: 16-24 mEq/day in 2-4 divided doses

Treatment: 40-100 mEq/day in 2-4 divided doses

Drug Interactions Increased Effect/Toxicity: Potassium-sparing diuretics, salt substitutes, ACE inhibitors

Pregnancy Risk Factor A

Generic Available No

Potassium Citrate (poe TASS ee um SIT rate)

U.S. Brand Names Urocit®-K

Canadian Brand Names K-Lyte®; Polycitra®

Pharmacologic Category Alkalinizing Agent

Use Prevention of uric acid nephrolithiasis; prevention of calcium renal stones in patients with hypocitraturia; urinary alkalinizer when sodium citrate is contraindicated

Local Anesthetic/Vasoconstrictor Precautions No information available to require special precautions

Effects on Dental Treatment No effects or complications reported

Dosage Adults: Oral: 10-20 mEq 3 times/day with meals up to 100 mEq/day

Other Adverse Effects

>10%: Gastrointestinal: Diarrhea, nausea, stomach pain, flatulence, vomiting (oral)

1% to 10%:

Cardiovascular: Bradycardia

Endocrine & metabolic: Hyperkalemia, metabolic alkalosis in patients with severe renal failure

Neuromuscular & skeletal: Weakness

Respiratory: Dyspnea

Drug Interactions Concurrent administration with potassium-containing medications, potassium-sparing diuretics, ACE inhibitors, or cardiac glycosides could lead to toxicity.

Pregnancy Risk Factor Not available

Generic Available No

Comments Parenteral K_3PO_4 contains 3 mmol of phosphorous/mL and 4.4 mEq of potassium/mL. If ordering by phosphorous content, use mmol instead of mEq since the mEq value for phosphorous varies with the pH of the solution due to valence changes of the phosphorus ion. (1 mmol of phosphorous = 31 mg)

Potassium Citrate and Citric Acid

(poe TASS ee um SIT rate & SI trik AS id)

U.S. Brand Names Polycitra®-K

Pharmacologic Category Alkalinizing Agent

Synonyms Citric Acid and Potassium Citrate

Use Treatment of metabolic acidosis; alkalinizing agent in conditions where long-term maintenance of an alkaline urine is desirable

Local Anesthetic/Vasoconstrictor Precautions No information available to require special precautions

Effects on Dental Treatment No effects or complications reported

Dosage Oral:

Mild to moderate hypocitraturia: 10 mEq 3 times/day with meals

Severe hypocitraturia: Initial: 20 mEq 3 times/day or 15 mEq 4 times/day with meals or within 30 minutes after meals; do not exceed 100 mEq/day

Other Adverse Effects

>10%: Gastrointestinal: Diarrhea, nausea, stomach pain, flatulence, vomiting (oral)

1% to 10%:

Cardiovascular: Bradycardia

Endocrine & metabolic: Hyperkalemia, metabolic alkalosis in patients with severe renal failure

Neuromuscular & skeletal: Weakness

Respiratory: Dyspnea

Drug Interactions Concurrent administration with potassium-containing medications, potassium-sparing diuretics, ACE inhibitors, or cardiac glycosides could lead to toxicity.

Pregnancy Risk Factor A

Generic Available No

Comments Potassium citrate 3.4 mmol/5 mL and citric acid 1.6 mmol/5 mL = total of 5.0 mmol/5 mL citrate content

Potassium Citrate and Potassium Gluconate

(poe TASS ee um SIT rate & poe TASS ee um GLOO coe nate)

U.S. Brand Names Twin-K®

Pharmacologic Category Electrolyte Supplement, Oral

Synonyms Potassium Gluconate and Potassium Citrate

Use Treatment or prevention of hypokalemia

Local Anesthetic/Vasoconstrictor Precautions No information available to require special precautions

Effects on Dental Treatment No effects or complications reported

Dosage Oral:

Children: 1-4 mEq/kg/24 hours in divided doses as required to maintain normal serum potassium

Adults:

Prevention: 16-24 mEq/day in 2-4 divided doses

Treatment: 40-100 mEq/day in 2-4 divided doses

Drug Interactions Concurrent administration with potassium-containing medications, potassium-sparing diuretics, ACE inhibitors, or cardiac glycosides could lead to toxicity.

Pregnancy Risk Factor C

Generic Available No

Potassium Gluconate (poe TASS ee um GLOO coe nate)

U.S. Brand Names Glu-K® [OTC]; Kaon®; K-G®

Canadian Brand Names Kaon®

Pharmacologic Category Electrolyte Supplement, Oral

Use Treatment or prevention of hypokalemia

Local Anesthetic/Vasoconstrictor Precautions No information available to require special precautions

Effects on Dental Treatment No effects or complications reported

Dosage Oral (doses listed as mEq of potassium):

Normal daily requirement:

Children: 2-3 mEq/kg/day

Adults: 40-80 mEq/day

Prevention of hypokalemia during diuretic therapy:

Children: 1-2 mEq/kg/day in 1-2 divided doses

Adults: 16-24 mEq/day in 1-2 divided doses

Treatment of hypokalemia:

Children: 2-5 mEq/kg/day in 2-4 divided doses

Adults: 40-100 mEq/day in 2-4 divided doses

Mechanism of Action Potassium is the major cation of intracellular fluid and is essential for the conduction of nerve impulses in heart, brain, and skeletal muscle; contraction of cardiac, skeletal and smooth muscles; maintenance of normal renal function, acid-base balance, carbohydrate metabolism, and gastric secretion

(Continued)

Potassium Gluconate *(Continued)*

Other Adverse Effects
>10%: Gastrointestinal: Diarrhea, nausea, stomach pain, flatulence, vomiting (oral)
1% to 10%:
Cardiovascular: Bradycardia
Endocrine & metabolic: Hyperkalemia
Neuromuscular & skeletal: Weakness
Respiratory: Dyspnea

Drug Interactions Increased Effect/Toxicity: Potassium-sparing diuretics, salt substitutes, ACE inhibitors; increased effect of digitalis

Drug Uptake Absorption: Well absorbed

Pregnancy Risk Factor A

Generic Available Yes

Potassium Iodide (poe TASS ee um EYE oh dide)

Related Information
Endocrine Disorders and Pregnancy *on page 1331*

U.S. Brand Names Pima®; SSKI®

Canadian Brand Names Thyro-Block®

Pharmacologic Category Antithyroid Agent; Expectorant

Synonyms KI; Lugol's Solution; Strong Iodine Solution

Use Expectorant for the symptomatic treatment of chronic pulmonary diseases complicated by mucous; reduce thyroid vascularity prior to thyroidectomy and management of thyrotoxic crisis; block thyroidal uptake of radioactive isotopes of iodine in a radiation emergency or other exposure to radioactive iodine

Unlabeled/Investigational: Lymphocutaneous and cutaneous sporotrichosis

Local Anesthetic/Vasoconstrictor Precautions No information available to require special precautions

Effects on Dental Treatment No effects or complications reported

Dosage Oral:
Adults: RDA: 150 mcg (iodide)
Expectorant:
Children (Pima®):
<3 years: 162 mg 3 times day
>3 years: 325 mg 3 times/day
Adults:
Pima®: 325-650 mg 3 times/day
SSKI®: 300-600 mg 3-4 times/day
Preoperative thyroidectomy: Children and Adults: 50-250 mg (1-5 drops SSKI®) 3 times/day **or** 0.1-0.3 mL (3-5 drops) of strong iodine (Lugol's solution) 3 times/day; administer for 10 days before surgery
Radiation protectant to radioactive isotopes of iodine (Pima®):
Children:
Infants up to 1 year: 65 mg once daily for 10 days; start 24 hours prior to exposure
>1 year: 130 mg once daily for 10 days; start 24 hours prior to exposure
Adults: 195 mg once daily for 10 days; start 24 hours prior to exposure
To reduce risk of thyroid cancer following nuclear accident (dosing should continue until risk of exposure has passed or other measures are implemented):
Children (see adult dose for children >68 kg):
Infants <1 month: 16 mg once daily
1 month to 3 years: 32 mg once daily
3-18 years: 65 mg once daily
Children >68 kg and Adults (including pregnant/lactating women): 130 mg once daily
Thyrotoxic crisis:
Infants <1 year: 150-250 mg (3-5 drops SSKI®) 3 times/day
Children and Adults: 300-500 mg (6-10 drops SSKI®) 3 times/day or 1 mL strong iodine (Lugol's solution) 3 times/day
Sporotrichosis (cutaneous, lymphocutaneous): Adults: Oral: Initial: 5 drops (SSKI®) 3 times/day; increase to 40-50 drops (SSKI®) 3 times/day as tolerated for 3-6 months

Mechanism of Action Reduces viscosity of mucus by increasing respiratory tract secretions; inhibits secretion of thyroid hormone, fosters colloid accumulation in thyroid follicles

Other Adverse Effects Frequency not defined:
Cardiovascular: Irregular heart beat
Central nervous system: Confusion, tiredness, fever
Dermatologic: Skin rash
Endocrine & metabolic: Goiter, salivary gland swelling/tenderness, thyroid adenoma, swelling of neck/throat, myxedema, lymph node swelling
Gastrointestinal: Diarrhea, gastrointestinal bleeding, metallic taste, nausea, stomach pain, stomach upset, vomiting
Neuromuscular & skeletal: Numbness, tingling, weakness

Miscellaneous: Chronic iodine poisoning (with prolonged treatment/high doses); iodism, hypersensitivity reactions (angioedema, cutaneous and mucosal hemorrhage, serum sickness-like symptoms)

Drug Interactions Increased Effect/Toxicity: Lithium may cause additive hypothyroid effects; ACE-inhibitors, potassium-sparing diuretics, and potassium/potassium-containing products may lead to hyperkalemia, cardiac arrhythmias, or cardiac arrest

Drug Uptake

Onset of action: 24-48 hours; Peak effect: 10-15 days after continuous therapy

Duration: ≤6 weeks

Pregnancy Risk Factor D

Generic Available Yes

Potassium Phosphate (poe TASS ee um FOS fate)

U.S. Brand Names Neutra-Phos®-K

Pharmacologic Category Electrolyte Supplement, Oral; Electrolyte Supplement, Parenteral

Synonyms Phosphate, Potassium

Use Treatment and prevention of hypophosphatemia or hypokalemia

Local Anesthetic/Vasoconstrictor Precautions No information available to require special precautions

Effects on Dental Treatment No effects or complications reported

Dosage I.V. doses should be incorporated into the patient's maintenance I.V. fluids; intermittent I.V. infusion should be reserved for severe depletion situations in patients undergoing continuous EKG monitoring. It is difficult to determine total body phosphorus deficit; the following dosages are empiric guidelines:

Normal requirements elemental phosphorus: Oral:

- 0-6 months: 240 mg
- 6-12 months: 360 mg
- 1-10 years: 800 mg
- >10 years: 1200 mg
- Pregnancy lactation: Additional 400 mg/day

Adults RDA: 800 mg

Treatment: It is difficult to provide concrete guidelines for the treatment of severe hypophosphatemia because the extent of total body deficits and response to therapy are difficult to predict. Aggressive doses of phosphate may result in a transient serum elevation followed by redistribution into intracellular compartments or bone tissue. It is recommended that repletion of severe hypophosphatemia (<1 mg/dL in adults) be done I.V. because large doses of oral phosphate may cause diarrhea and intestinal absorption may be unreliable

Pediatric I.V. phosphate repletion: Children: 0.25-0.5 mmol/kg **administer over 4-6 hours and repeat if symptomatic hypophosphatemia persists**; to assess the need for further phosphate administration, obtain serum inorganic phosphate after administration of the first dose and base further doses on serum concentration and clinical status

Adult I.V. phosphate repletion:

Initial dose: 0.08 mmol/kg if recent uncomplicated hypophosphatemia

Initial dose: 0.16 mmol/kg if prolonged hypophosphatemia with presumed total body deficits; increase dose by 25% to 50% if patient symptomatic with severe hypophosphatemia

Do not exceed 0.24 mmol/kg/day; administer over 6 hours by I.V. infusion

With orders for I.V. phosphate, there is considerable confusion associated with the use of millimoles (mmol) versus milliequivalents (mEq) to express the phosphate requirement. Because inorganic phosphate exists as monobasic and dibasic anions, with the mixture of valences dependent on pH, ordering by mEq amounts is unreliable and may lead to large dosing errors. In addition, I.V. phosphate is available in the sodium and potassium salt; therefore, the content of these cations must be considered when ordering phosphate. The most reliable method of ordering I.V. phosphate is by millimoles, then specifying the potassium or sodium salt. For example, an order for 15 mmol of phosphate as potassium phosphate in one liter of normal saline would also provide 22 mEq of potassium.

Maintenance:

I.V. solutions:

Children: 0.5-1.5 mmol/kg/24 hours I.V. or 2-3 mmol/kg/24 hours orally in divided doses

Adults: 15-30 mmol/24 hours I.V. or 50-150 mmol/24 hours orally in divided doses

Oral:

Children <4 years: 1 capsule (250 mg phosphorus/8 mmol) 4 times/day; dilute as instructed

Children >4 years and Adults: 1-2 capsules (250-500 mg phosphorus/8-16 mmol) 4 times/day; dilute as instructed

Other Adverse Effects

>10%: Gastrointestinal: Diarrhea, nausea, stomach pain, flatulence, vomiting

(Continued)

Potassium Phosphate *(Continued)*

1% to 10%:
- Cardiovascular: Bradycardia
- Endocrine & metabolic: Hyperkalemia
- Neuromuscular & skeletal: Weakness
- Respiratory: Dyspnea

Drug Interactions

Increased Effect/Toxicity: Potassium-sparing diuretics, salt substitutes, or ACE inhibitors; increased effect of digitalis

Decreased Effect: Aluminum and magnesium-containing antacids or sucralfate can act as phosphate binders

Pregnancy Risk Factor C

Generic Available Yes

Potassium Phosphate and Sodium Phosphate

(poe TASS ee um FOS fate & SOW dee um FOS fate)

U.S. Brand Names K-Phos® MF; K-Phos® Neutral; K-Phos® No. 2; Neutra-Phos®; Uro-KP-Neutral®

Pharmacologic Category Electrolyte Supplement, Oral

Synonyms Sodium Phosphate and Potassium Phosphate

Use Treatment of conditions associated with excessive renal phosphate loss or inadequate GI absorption of phosphate; to acidify the urine to lower calcium concentrations; to increase the antibacterial activity of methenamine; reduce odor and rash caused by ammonia in urine

Local Anesthetic/Vasoconstrictor Precautions No information available to require special precautions

Effects on Dental Treatment No effects or complications reported

Dosage All dosage forms to be mixed in 6-8 oz of water prior to administration

Children: 2-3 mmol phosphate/kg/24 hours given 4 times/day **or** 1 capsule 4 times/day

Adults: 1-2 capsules (250-500 mg phosphorus/8-16 mmol) 4 times/day after meals and at bedtime

Other Adverse Effects

>10%: Gastrointestinal: Diarrhea, nausea, stomach pain, flatulence, vomiting

1% to 10%:
- Cardiovascular: Bradycardia
- Endocrine & metabolic: Hyperkalemia
- Neuromuscular & skeletal: Weakness
- Respiratory: Dyspnea

Drug Interactions

Increased Effect/Toxicity: Potassium-sparing diuretics, salt substitutes, or ACE inhibitors; increased effect of digitalis

Decreased Effect: Aluminum and magnesium-containing antacids or sucralfate can act as phosphate binders

Pregnancy Risk Factor C

Generic Available Yes

Povidone-Iodine (POE vi done EYE oh dyne)

Related Information

Animal and Human Bites Guidelines *on page 1416*

Management of Patients Undergoing Cancer Therapy *on page 1402*

U.S. Brand Names ACU-dyne® [OTC]; Aerodine® [OTC]; Betadine® [OTC]; Betadine® 5% Sterile Ophthalmic Prep Solution; Betagan® [OTC]; Biodine [OTC]; Etodine® [OTC]; Iodex® [OTC]; Iodex-p® [OTC]; Mallisol® [OTC]; Massengill® Medicated Douche w/Cepticin [OTC]; Minidyne® [OTC]; Operand® [OTC]; Polydine® [OTC]; Summer's Eve® Medicated Douche [OTC]; Yeast-Gard® Medicated Douche [OTC]

Canadian Brand Names Betadine®; Proviodine

Mexican Brand Names Isodine®; Yodine®

Pharmacologic Category Antibiotic, Ophthalmic; Antibiotic, Topical; Antibiotic, Vaginal; Topical Skin Product

Use External antiseptic with broad microbicidal spectrum against bacteria, fungi, viruses, protozoa, and yeasts

Local Anesthetic/Vasoconstrictor Precautions No information available to require special precautions

Effects on Dental Treatment No effects or complications reported

Dosage

Shampoo: Apply 2 tsp to hair and scalp, lather and rinse; repeat application 2 times/week until improvement is noted, then shampoo weekly

Topical: Apply as needed for treatment and prevention of susceptible microbial infections

Mechanism of Action Povidone-iodine is known to be a powerful broad spectrum germicidal agent effective against a wide range of bacteria, viruses, fungi, protozoa, and spores.

Other Adverse Effects 1% to 10%:

Cardiovascular: Local edema

Dermatologic: Rash, pruritus

Drug Uptake Absorption: Normal individuals: Topical: Little systemic absorption; Vaginal: Rapid, serum concentrations of total iodine and inorganic iodide are increased significantly

Pregnancy Risk Factor D

Generic Available Yes

PrameGel® [OTC] *see* Pramoxine *on page 984*

Pramipexole (pra mi PEX ole)

U.S. Brand Names Mirapex®

Canadian Brand Names Mirapex®

Pharmacologic Category Anti-Parkinson's Agent, Dopamine Agonist

Use Treatment of the signs and symptoms of idiopathic Parkinson's Disease

Unlabeled/Investigational: Treatment of depression

Local Anesthetic/Vasoconstrictor Precautions No information available to require special precautions

Effects on Dental Treatment No effects or complications reported

Dosage Adults: Oral: Initial: 0.375 mg/day given in 3 divided doses, increase gradually by 0.125 mg/dose every 5-7 days; range: 1.5-4.5 mg/day

Mechanism of Action Pramipexole is a nonergot dopamine agonist with specificity for the D_2 subfamily dopamine receptor, and has also been shown to bind to D_3 and D_4 receptors. By binding to these receptors, it is thought that pramipexole can stimulate dopamine activity on the nerves of the striatum and substantia nigra.

Other Adverse Effects

>10%:

- Cardiovascular: Postural hypotension
- Central nervous system: Asthenia, dizziness, somnolence, insomnia, hallucinations, abnormal dreams
- Gastrointestinal: Nausea, constipation
- Neuromuscular & skeletal: Weakness, dyskinesia, EPS

1% to 10%:

- Cardiovascular: Edema, postural hypotension, syncope, tachycardia, chest pain
- Central nervous system: Malaise, confusion, amnesia, dystonias, akathisia, thinking abnormalities, myoclonus, hyperesthesia, gait abnormalities, hypertonia, paranoia
- Endocrine & metabolic: Decreased libido
- Gastrointestinal: Anorexia, weight loss, xerostomia
- Genitourinary: Urinary frequency (up to 6%), impotence
- Neuromuscular & skeletal: Muscle twitching, leg cramps, arthritis, bursitis
- Ocular: Vision abnormalities (3%)
- Respiratory: Dyspnea, rhinitis

Frequency not defined, dose related: Falling asleep during activities of daily living

Contraindications Hypersensitivity to pramipexole or any component of the formulation

Warnings/Precautions Caution should be taken in patients with renal insufficiency and in patients with pre-existing dyskinesias. May cause orthostatic hypotension; Parkinson's disease patients appear to have an impaired capacity to respond to a postural challenge. Use with caution in patients at risk of hypotension (such as those receiving antihypertensive drugs) or where transient hypotensive episodes would be poorly tolerated (cardiovascular disease or cerebrovascular disease). Parkinson's patients being treated with dopaminergic agonists ordinarily require careful monitoring for signs and symptoms of postural hypotension, especially during dose escalation, and should be informed of this risk. May cause hallucinations, particularly in older patients.

Although not reported for pramipexole, other dopaminergic agents have been associated with a syndrome resembling neuroleptic malignant syndrome on withdrawal or significant dosage reduction after long-term use. Dopaminergic agents from the ergot class have also been associated with fibrotic complications, such as retroperitoneum, lungs, and pleura. Pathologic retinal changes were described in some animal studies; the significance in humans has not be established.

Pramipexole has been associated with somnolence, particularly at higher dosages (>1.5 mg/day). In addition, patients have been reported to fall asleep during activities of daily living, including driving, while taking this medication. Whether these patients exhibited somnolence prior to these events is not clear. Patients should be advised of this issue and factors which may increase risk (sleep disorders, other sedating medications, or concomitant medications which increase pramipexole concentrations) and instructed to report daytime somnolence or sleepiness to the prescriber. Patients should use caution in performing activities which require alertness (driving or operating machinery), and to avoid other medications which may cause CNS depression, including ethanol.

(Continued)

Pramipexole *(Continued)*

Drug Interactions

Increased Effect/Toxicity: Cimetidine in combination with pramipexole produced a 50% increase in AUC and a 40% increase in half-life. Drugs secreted by the cationic transport system (diltiazem, triamterene, verapamil, quinidine, quinine, ranitidine) decrease the clearance of pramipexole by ~20%.

Decreased Effect: Dopamine antagonists (antipsychotics, metoclopramide) may decrease the efficiency of pramipexole.

Drug Uptake

Half-life, elimination: ~8 hours; Elderly: 12-14 hours

Time to peak: ~2 hours, 5:44-7.17 μg/mL

Pregnancy Risk Factor C

Generic Available No

Pramosone® *see* Pramoxine and Hydrocortisone *on page 984*

Pramoxine (pra MOKS een)

U.S. Brand Names Anusol® [OTC]; Fleet® Pain Relief [OTC]; Itch-X® [OTC]; Phicon® [OTC]; PrameGel® [OTC]; Prax® [OTC]; ProctoFoam® NS [OTC]; Tronolane® [OTC]; Tronothane® [OTC]

Pharmacologic Category Local Anesthetic

Synonyms Pramoxine Hydrochloride

Use Temporary relief of pain and itching associated with anogenital pruritus or irritation; dermatosis, minor burns, hemorrhoids

Local Anesthetic/Vasoconstrictor Precautions No information available to require special precautions

Effects on Dental Treatment No effects or complications reported

Dosage Adults: Topical: Apply as directed, usually every 3-4 hours to affected area (maximum adult dose: 200 mg)

Mechanism of Action Pramoxine, like other anesthetics, decreases the neuronal membrane's permeability to sodium ions; both initiation and conduction of nerve impulses are blocked, thus depolarization of the neuron is inhibited

Other Adverse Effects 1% to 10%:

Dermatologic: Angioedema

Local: Contact dermatitis, burning, stinging

Drug Uptake

Onset of action: Therapeutic: 2-5 minutes; Peak effect: 3-5 minutes

Duration: Several days

Pregnancy Risk Factor C

Generic Available Yes

Pramoxine and Hydrocortisone

(pra MOKS een & hye droe KOR ti sone)

U.S. Brand Names Analpram-HC®; Enzone®; Epifoam®; Pramosone®; ProctoFoam®-HC; Zone-A Forte®

Canadian Brand Names Pramox® HC; Proctofoam™-HC

Pharmacologic Category Anesthetic/Corticosteroid

Synonyms Hydrocortisone and Pramoxine

Use Treatment of severe anorectal or perianal swelling

Local Anesthetic/Vasoconstrictor Precautions No information available to require special precautions

Effects on Dental Treatment No effects or complications reported

Dosage Apply to affected areas 3-4 times/day

Therapy should be discontinued when control is achieved; if no improvement is seen, reassessment of diagnosis may be necessary.

Drug Uptake See Pramoxine *on page 984* and Hydrocortisone *on page 608*

Pregnancy Risk Factor C

Generic Available Yes

Prandin® *see* Repaglinide *on page 1045*

Pravachol® *see* Pravastatin *on page 984*

Pravastatin (PRA va stat in)

Related Information

Cardiovascular Diseases *on page 1308*

U.S. Brand Names Pravachol®

Canadian Brand Names Lin-Pravastatin; Pravachol®

Mexican Brand Names Pravacol®

Pharmacologic Category Antilipemic Agent, HMG-CoA Reductase Inhibitor

Synonyms Pravastatin Sodium

Use

Primary prevention of coronary events: In combination with dietary therapy in hypercholesterolemic patients without established coronary heart disease, to reduce cardiovascular morbidity (myocardial infarction, coronary revascularization procedures) and mortality.

Secondary prevention of coronary events:

In combination with dietary therapy in hypercholesterolemic patients with established coronary heart disease, to slow the progression of coronary atherosclerosis, to reduce cardiovascular morbidity (myocardial infarction, coronary vascular procedures) and to reduce mortality; to reduce the risk of stroke and transient ischemic attacks

In combination with dietary therapy in patients with a history of prior myocardial infarction or unstable angina and "normal" cholesterol concentrations (total cholesterol ~219 mg/dL, LDL-C ~150 mg/dL); pravastatin may reduce cardiovascular mortality, the risk for recurrent myocardial infarction, stroke, and TIA, and the risk for undergoing coronary revascularization procedures.

Hyperlipidemias: As an adjunct to diet to reduce elevations in total cholesterol, LDL-C, apolipoprotein B, and triglycerides (elevations of one or more components are present in Fredrickson type IIa, IIb, III, and IV hyperlipidemias).

Local Anesthetic/Vasoconstrictor Precautions No information available to require special precautions

Effects on Dental Treatment No effects of complications reported

Dosage Oral:

Adults: Initial: 40 mg once daily (10 mg in patients with renal/hepatic dysfunction or receiving immunosuppressants, such as cyclosporine); titrate dosage to response (usual range: 10-80 mg); maximum dose: 80 mg once daily (maximum dose of 20 mg once daily recommended in patients receiving immunosuppressants, such as cyclosporine)

Elderly: No specific dosage recommendations. Clearance is reduced in the elderly, resulting in an increase in AUC between 25% to 50%. However, substantial accumulation is not expected.

Dosing adjustment in renal/hepatic impairment: 10 mg/day

Mechanism of Action Pravastatin is a competitive inhibitor of 3-hydroxy-3-methylglutaryl coenzyme A (HMG-CoA) reductase, which is the rate-limiting enzyme involved in *de novo* cholesterol synthesis.

Other Adverse Effects 1% to 10%:

Cardiovascular: Chest pain (4%)

Central nervous system: Headache (2% to 6%), fatigue (4%), dizziness (1% to 3%)

Dermatologic: Rash (4%)

Gastrointestinal: Nausea/vomiting (7%), diarrhea (6%), heartburn (3%)

Hepatic: Increased transaminases (>3x normal on two occasions - 1%)

Neuromuscular & skeletal: Myalgia (2%)

Respiratory: Cough (3%)

Miscellaneous: Influenza (2%)

Additional class-related events or case reports (not necessarily reported with pravastatin therapy): Alopecia, alteration in taste, anaphylaxis, angioedema, anorexia, anxiety, arthritis, cataracts, chills, cholestatic jaundice, cirrhosis, decreased libido, depression, dermatomyositis, dryness of skin/mucous membranes, dyspnea, elevated transaminases, eosinophilia, erectile dysfunction, erythema multiforme, facial paresis, fatty liver, fever, flushing, fulminant hepatic necrosis, gynecomastia, hemolytic anemia, hepatitis, hepatoma, hyperbilirubinemia, hypersensitivity reaction, impaired extraocular muscle movement, impotence, increased alkaline, increased CPK (>10x normal), increased ESR, increased GGT, leukopenia, malaise, memory loss, myopathy, nail changes, nodules, ophthalmoplegia, pancreatitis, paresthesia, peripheral nerve palsy, peripheral neuropathy, phosphatase, photosensitivity, polymyalgia rheumatica, positive ANA, pruritus, psychic disturbance, purpura, rash, renal failure (secondary to rhabdomyolysis), rhabdomyolysis, skin discoloration, Stevens-Johnson syndrome, systemic lupus erythematosus-like syndrome, thrombocytopenia, thyroid dysfunction, toxic epidermal necrolysis, tremor, urticaria, vasculitis, vertigo

Contraindications Hypersensitivity to pravastatin or any component of the formulation; active liver disease; unexplained persistent elevations of serum transaminases; pregnancy; breast-feeding

Warnings/Precautions Liver function must be monitored by periodic laboratory assessment. Use with caution in patients who consume large amounts of ethanol or have a history of liver disease. Rhabdomyolysis with acute renal failure has occurred with other HMG-CoA reductase inhibitors. Risk is increased with concurrent use of clarithromycin, danazol, diltiazem, fluvoxamine, indinavir, nefazodone, nelfinavir, ritonavir, verapamil, troleandomycin, cyclosporine, fibric acid derivatives, erythromycin, niacin, or azole antifungals. The risk of combining any of these drugs with pravastatin is minimal. Temporarily discontinue in any patient experiencing an acute or serious condition predisposing to renal failure secondary to rhabdomyolysis. Safety and efficacy in patients <18 years of age have not been established.

Drug Interactions CYP3A3/4 (minor) enzyme substrate

Increased Effect/Toxicity: Clofibrate, fenofibrate, gemfibrozil, and niacin may increase the risk of myopathy and rhabdomyolysis. Imidazole antifungals

(Continued)

Pravastatin *(Continued)*

(itraconazole, ketoconazole), P-glycoprotein inhibitors may increase pravastatin concentrations.

Decreased Effect: Concurrent administration of cholestyramine or colestipol can decrease pravastatin absorption.

Drug Uptake

Onset of action: Several days; Peak effect: 4 weeks

Absorption: Poor

Half-life, elimination: ~2-3 hours

Time to peak: 1-1.5 hours

Pregnancy Risk Factor X

Generic Available No

Prax® [OTC] *see* Pramoxine *on page 984*

Praziquantel (pray zi KWON tel)

U.S. Brand Names Biltricide®

Canadian Brand Names Biltricide®

Mexican Brand Names Cesol®; Cisticid; Tecprazin

Pharmacologic Category Anthelmintic

Use Treatment of all stages of schistosomiasis caused by *Schistosoma* species pathogenic to humans; also active in the treatment of clonorchiasis, opisthorchiasis, cysticercosis, and many intestinal tapeworm infections and trematode

Local Anesthetic/Vasoconstrictor Precautions No information available to require special precautions

Effects on Dental Treatment No effects or complications reported

Dosage Children >4 years and Adults: Oral:

Schistosomiasis: 20 mg/kg/dose 2-3 times/day for 1 day at 4- to 6-hour intervals

Flukes: 25 mg/kg/dose every 8 hours for 1-2 days

Cysticercosis: 50 mg/kg/day divided every 8 hours for 14 days

Tapeworms: 10-20 mg/kg as a single dose (25 mg/kg for *Hymenolepis nana*)

Mechanism of Action Increases the cell permeability to calcium in schistosomes, causing strong contractions and paralysis of worm musculature leading to detachment of suckers from the blood vessel walls and to dislodgment

Other Adverse Effects 1% to 10%:

Central nervous system: Dizziness, drowsiness, headache, malaise

Gastrointestinal: Abdominal pain, loss of appetite, nausea, vomiting

Miscellaneous: Diaphoresis

Drug Interactions Hydantoins may decrease praziquantel levels causing treatment failures.

Drug Uptake

Absorption: Oral: ~80%; CSF concentration is 14% to 20% of plasma concentration

Half-life, elimination: Parent drug: 0.8-1.5 hours; Metabolites: 4.5 hours

Time to peak: 1-3 hours

Pregnancy Risk Factor B

Generic Available No

Prazosin (PRA zoe sin)

Related Information

Cardiovascular Diseases *on page 1308*

U.S. Brand Names Minipress®

Canadian Brand Names Alti-Prazosin; Apo®-Prazo; Minipress™; Novo-Prazin; Nu-Prazo

Mexican Brand Names Minipres®; Sinozzard®

Pharmacologic Category Alpha$_1$ Blocker

Synonyms Furazosin; Prazosin Hydrochloride

Use Treatment of hypertension

Unlabeled/Investigational: Benign prostatic hypertrophy; Raynaud's syndrome

Local Anesthetic/Vasoconstrictor Precautions No information available to require special precautions

Effects on Dental Treatment

≤10%: Significant xerostomia

Significant orthostatic hypotension a possibility; monitor patient when getting out of dental chair.

Dosage Oral:

Children: Initial: 5 mcg/kg/dose (to assess hypotensive effects); usual dosing interval: every 6 hours; increase dosage gradually up to maximum of 25 mcg/kg/dose every 6 hours

Adults:

Hypertension: Initial: 1 mg/dose 2-3 times/day; usual maintenance dose: 3-15 mg/day in divided doses 2-4 times/day; maximum daily dose: 20 mg

Hypertensive urgency: 10-20 mg once, may repeat in 30 minutes

Raynaud's (unlabeled use): 0.5-3 mg twice daily

Benign prostatic hyperplasia (unlabeled use): 2 mg twice daily

Mechanism of Action Competitively inhibits postsynaptic alpha-adrenergic receptors which results in vasodilation of veins and arterioles and a decrease in total peripheral resistance and BP

Other Adverse Effects

>10%: Central nervous system: Dizziness (10%)

1% to 10%:

Cardiovascular: Palpitations (5%), edema, orthostatic hypotension, syncope (1%)

Central nervous system: Headache (8%), drowsiness (8%), weakness (7%), vertigo, depression, nervousness

Dermatologic: Rash (1% to 4%)

Endocrine & metabolic: Decreased energy (7%)

Gastrointestinal: Nausea (5%), vomiting, diarrhea, constipation

Genitourinary: Urinary frequency (1% to 5%)

Ocular: Blurred vision, reddened sclera, xerostomia

Respiratory: Dyspnea, epistaxis, nasal congestion

Drug Interactions

Increased Effect/Toxicity: Prazosin's hypotensive effect may be increased with beta-blockers, diuretics, ACE inhibitors, calcium channel blockers, and other antihypertensive medications. Concurrent use with tricyclic antidepressants (TCAs) and low-potency antipsychotics may increase risk of orthostasis.

Decreased Effect: Decreased antihypertensive effect if taken with NSAIDs.

Drug Uptake

Onset of action: BP reduction: ~2 hours; Maximum decrease: 2-4 hours

Duration: 10-24 hours

Half-life, elimination: 2-4 hours (increases with CHF)

Pregnancy Risk Factor C

Generic Available Yes

Prazosin and Polythiazide (PRA zoe sin & pol i THYE a zide)

U.S. Brand Names Minizide®

Pharmacologic Category Antihypertensive Agent Combination

Synonyms Polythiazide and Prazosin

Use Management of mild to moderate hypertension

Local Anesthetic/Vasoconstrictor Precautions No information available to require special precautions

Effects on Dental Treatment

≤10%: Significant xerostomia

Significant orthostatic hypotension a possibility; monitor patient when getting out of dental chair.

Dosage Adults: Oral: 1 capsule 2-3 times/day

Other Adverse Effects

Based on **prazosin** component:

>10%: Central nervous system: Dizziness (10%)

1% to 10%:

Cardiovascular: Palpitations (5%), edema, orthostatic hypotension, syncope (1%)

Central nervous system: Headache (8%), drowsiness (8%), weakness (7%), vertigo, depression, nervousness

Dermatologic: Rash (1% to 4%)

Endocrine & metabolic: Decreased energy (7%)

Gastrointestinal: Nausea (5%), vomiting, diarrhea, constipation

Genitourinary: Urinary frequency (1% to 5%)

Ocular: Blurred vision, reddened sclera, xerostomia

Respiratory: Dyspnea, epistaxis, nasal congestion

Based on **polythiazide** component:

1% to 10%: Hypokalemia

Drug Uptake See Prazosin *on page 986* and Polythiazide *on page 972*

Pregnancy Risk Factor C

Generic Available No

Precedex™ *see* Dexmedetomidine *on page 366*

Precose® *see* Acarbose *on page 24*

Pred Forte® *see* PrednisoLONE *on page 988*

Pred-G® *see* Prednisolone and Gentamicin *on page 989*

Pred Mild® *see* PrednisoLONE *on page 988*

Prednicarbate (PRED ni kar bate)

U.S. Brand Names Dermatop®

Pharmacologic Category Corticosteroid, Topical

Use Relief of the inflammatory and pruritic manifestations of corticosteroid-responsive dermatoses (medium potency topical corticosteroid)

Local Anesthetic/Vasoconstrictor Precautions No information available to require special precautions

Effects on Dental Treatment No effects or complications reported

(Continued)

Prednicarbate *(Continued)*

Dosage Adults: Topical: Apply a thin film to affected area twice daily

Therapy should be discontinued when control is achieved; if no improvement is seen, reassessment of diagnosis may be necessary.

Mechanism of Action Topical corticosteroids have anti-inflammatory, antipruritic, vasoconstrictive, and antiproliferative actions

Other Adverse Effects

<10%:

- Dermatologic: Acne, hypopigmentation, allergic dermatitis, maceration of the skin, skin atrophy, folliculitis, hypertrichosis
- Endocrine & metabolic: HPA suppression, Cushing's syndrome, growth retardation
- Local: Burning, itching, irritation, dryness
- Miscellaneous: Secondary infection

1% to 10%: Dermatologic: Skin atrophy, shininess, thinness, mild telangiectasia

Pregnancy Risk Factor C

Generic Available No

PrednisoLONE (pred NIS oh lone)

Related Information

Neomycin, Polymyxin B, and Prednisolone *on page 857*

Respiratory Diseases *on page 1328*

U.S. Brand Names AK-Pred®; Delta-Cortef®; Econopred®; Econopred® Plus; Inflamase® Forte; Inflamase® Mild; Key-Pred®; Key-Pred-SP®; Pediapred®; Pred Forte®; Pred Mild®; Prednisol® TBA; Prelone®

Canadian Brand Names Diopred®; Hydeltra T.B.A.®; Inflamase® Forte; Inflamase® Mild; Novo-Prednisolone®; Ophtho-Tate®; Ophtho-tate®; Pediapred®; Pred Forte®; Pred Mild®

Mexican Brand Names Fisopred®; Sophipren Ofteno

Pharmacologic Category Corticosteroid, Ophthalmic; Corticosteroid, Systemic

Synonyms Deltahydrocortisone; Metacortandralone; Prednisolone Acetate; Prednisolone Acetate, Ophthalmic; Prednisolone Sodium Phosphate; Prednisolone Sodium Phosphate, Ophthalmic; Prednisolone Tebutate

Use

Dental: Treatment of a variety of oral diseases of allergic, inflammatory or autoimmune origin

Medical: Treatment of palpebral and bulbar conjunctivitis; corneal injury from chemical, radiation, thermal burns, or foreign body penetration; endocrine disorders, rheumatic disorders, collagen diseases, dermatologic diseases, allergic states, ophthalmic diseases, respiratory diseases, hematologic disorders, neoplastic diseases, edematous states, and GI diseases; useful in patients with inability to activate prednisone (liver disease)

Local Anesthetic/Vasoconstrictor Precautions No information available to require special precautions

Effects on Dental Treatment No effects or complications reported

Dosage Dose depends upon condition being treated and response of patient; dosage for infants and children should be based on severity of the disease and response of the patient rather than on strict adherence to dosage indicated by age, weight, or body surface area. Consider alternate day therapy for long-term therapy. Discontinuation of long-term therapy requires gradual withdrawal by tapering the dose.

Children:

- Acute asthma:
  - Oral: 1-2 mg/kg/day in divided doses 1-2 times/day for 3-5 days
  - I.V. (sodium phosphate salt): 2-4 mg/kg/day divided 3-4 times/day
- Anti-inflammatory or immunosuppressive dose: Oral, I.V., I.M. (sodium phosphate salt): 0.1-2 mg/kg/day in divided doses 1-4 times/day
- Nephrotic syndrome: Oral:
  - Initial (first 3 episodes): 2 mg/kg/day **or** 60 mg/m²/day (maximum: 80 mg/day) in divided doses 3-4 times/day until urine is protein free for 3 consecutive days (maximum: 28 days); followed by 1-1.5 mg/kg/dose **or** 40 mg/m²/dose given every other day for 4 weeks
  - Maintenance (long-term maintenance dose for frequent relapses): 0.5-1 mg/kg/dose given every other day for 3-6 months

Adults:

- Oral, I.V., I.M. (sodium phosphate salt): 5-60 mg/day
- Multiple sclerosis (sodium phosphate): Oral: 200 mg/day for 1 week followed by 80 mg every other day for 1 month
- Rheumatoid arthritis: Oral: Initial: 5-7.5 mg/day; adjust dose as necessary

Elderly: Use lowest effective dose

Dosing adjustment in hyperthyroidism: Prednisolone dose may need to be increased to achieve adequate therapeutic effects

Hemodialysis: Slightly dialyzable (5% to 20%); administer dose posthemodialysis

Peritoneal dialysis: Supplemental dose is not necessary

Intra-articular, intralesional, soft-tissue administration:
Tebutate salt: 4-40 mg/dose
Sodium phosphate salt: 2-30 mg/dose
Ophthalmic suspension/solution: Children and Adults: Instill 1-2 drops into conjunctival sac every hour during day, every 2 hours at night until favorable response is obtained, then use 1 drop every 4 hours

Mechanism of Action Decreases inflammation by suppression of migration of polymorphonuclear leukocytes and reversal of increased capillary permeability; suppresses the immune system by reducing activity and volume of the lymphatic system

Other Adverse Effects
>10%:
Central nervous system: Insomnia, nervousness
Gastrointestinal: Increased appetite, indigestion
1% to 10%:
Dermatologic: Hirsutism
Endocrine & metabolic: Diabetes mellitus
Neuromuscular & skeletal: Arthralgia
Ocular: Cataracts, glaucoma
Respiratory: Epistaxis
<1%: Edema, hypertension, vertigo, seizures, psychoses, pseudotumor cerebri, headache, mood swings, delirium, hallucinations, euphoria, acne, skin atrophy, bruising, hyperpigmentation, Cushing's syndrome, pituitary-adrenal axis suppression, growth suppression, glucose intolerance, hypokalemia, alkalosis, amenorrhea, sodium and water retention, hyperglycemia, peptic ulcer, nausea, vomiting, abdominal distention, ulcerative esophagitis, pancreatitis, muscle weakness, osteoporosis, fractures, muscle wasting, hypersensitivity reactions

Contraindications Hypersensitivity to prednisolone or any component of the formulation; acute superficial herpes simplex keratitis; systemic fungal infections; varicella

Warnings/Precautions Use with caution in patients with hyperthyroidism, cirrhosis, nonspecific ulcerative colitis, hypertension, osteoporosis, thromboembolic tendencies, CHF, convulsive disorders, myasthenia gravis, thrombophlebitis, peptic ulcer, diabetes; acute adrenal insufficiency may occur with abrupt withdrawal after long-term therapy or with stress; young pediatric patients may be more susceptible to adrenal axis suppression from topical therapy. Because of the risk of adverse effects, systemic corticosteroids should be used cautiously in the elderly, in the smallest possible dose, and for the shortest possible time.

Drug Interactions CYP2D6 and CYP3A enzyme substrate; inducer of cytochrome P450 enzymes
Decreased effect:
Barbiturates, phenytoin, rifampin decrease corticosteroid effectiveness
Decreases salicylates
Decreases vaccines
Decreases toxoids effectiveness

Dietary/Ethanol/Herb Considerations
Ethanol: Avoid use; may increase gastric mucosal irritation.
Food: Administer with food or milk to reduce GI upset. Prednisolone interferes with calcium absorption; increase intake of calcium, folate, phosphorus, pyridoxine, vitamin C, and vitamin D. Limit caffeine.
Herb/Nutraceutical: Avoid cat's claw and echinacea due to immunostimulant properties. Avoid St John's wort; may decrease serum concentration.

Drug Uptake
Duration: 18-36 hours
Half-life, elimination: 3.6 hours; Biological: 18-36 hours; End-stage renal disease: 3-5 hours

Pregnancy Risk Factor C

Breast-feeding Considerations May be taken while breast-feeding

Dosage Forms **INJ, solution, as sodium phosphate:** 20 mg/mL (2 mL, 5 mL, 10 mL). **INJ, suspension, as acetate:** 25 mg/mL (10 mL, 30 mL); 50 mg/mL (10 mL, 30 mL). **INJ, suspension, as tebutate:** 20 mg/mL (10 mL). **LIQ, oral, as sodium phosphate:** 5 mg/5 mL (120 mL). **SOLN, ophthalmic, as sodium phosphate:** 0.125% (5 mL, 10 mL); 1% (5 mL, 10 mL, 15 mL). **SUSP, ophthalmic, as acetate:** 0.12% (5 mL, 10 mL); 0.125% (5 mL, 10 mL, 15 mL); 1% (1 mL, 5 mL, 10 mL, 15 mL). **SYR:** 5 mg/5 mL (120 mL); 15 mg/5 mL (240 mL). **TAB:** 5 mg

Generic Available Yes

Prednisolone and Gentamicin (pred NIS oh lone & jen ta MYE sin)

U.S. Brand Names Pred-G®

Pharmacologic Category Antibiotic/Corticosteroid, Ophthalmic

Synonyms Gentamicin and Prednisolone

Use Treatment of steroid responsive inflammatory conditions and superficial ocular infections due to strains of microorganisms susceptible to gentamicin such as *Staphylococcus*, *E. coli*, *H. influenzae*, *Klebsiella*, *Neisseria*, *Pseudomonas*, *Proteus*, and *Serratia* species

(Continued)

Prednisolone and Gentamicin *(Continued)*

Local Anesthetic/Vasoconstrictor Precautions No information available to require special precautions

Effects on Dental Treatment No effects or complications reported

Dosage Children and Adults: Ophthalmic: 1 drop 2-4 times/day; during the initial 24-48 hours, the dosing frequency may be increased if necessary

Other Adverse Effects 1% to 10%:

Dermatologic: Delayed wound healing

Local: Burning, stinging

Ocular: Increased intraocular pressure, glaucoma, superficial punctate keratitis, infrequent optic nerve damage, posterior subcapsular cataract formation

Miscellaneous: Development of secondary infection, allergic sensitization

Drug Uptake See Prednisolone *on page 988* and Gentamicin *on page 554*

Pregnancy Risk Factor C

Generic Available No

Prednisol® TBA *see* PrednisoLONE *on page 988*

PredniSONE (PRED ni sone)

Related Information

Oral Nonviral Soft Tissue Ulcerations or Erosions *on page 1384*
Respiratory Diseases *on page 1328*
Rheumatoid Arthritis and Osteoarthritis *on page 1340*

U.S. Brand Names Deltasone®; Liquid Pred®; Meticorten®; Orasone®

Canadian Brand Names Apo®-Prednisone; Winpred™

Mexican Brand Names Meticorten®; Prednidib®

Pharmacologic Category Corticosteroid, Systemic

Synonyms Deltacortisone; Deltadehydrocortisone

Use

Dental: Treatment of a variety of oral diseases of allergic, inflammatory or autoimmune origin

Medical: Treatment of a variety of diseases including adrenocortical insufficiency, hypercalcemia, rheumatic and collagen disorders; dermatologic, ocular, respiratory, GI, and neoplastic diseases; organ transplantation; not available in injectable form, prednisolone must be used

Unlabeled/Investigational: Prevention of postherpetic neuralgia and relief of acute pain in the early stages

Local Anesthetic/Vasoconstrictor Precautions No information available to require special precautions

Effects on Dental Treatment No effects or complications reported

Dosage Oral: Dose depends upon condition being treated and response of patient; dosage for infants and children should be based on severity of the disease and response of the patient rather than on strict adherence to dosage indicated by age, weight, or body surface area. Consider alternate day therapy for long-term therapy. Discontinuation of long-term therapy requires gradual withdrawal by tapering the dose.

Children:

- Anti-inflammatory or immunosuppressive dose: 0.05-2 mg/kg/day divided 1-4 times/day
- Acute asthma: 1-2 mg/kg/day in divided doses 1-2 times/day for 3-5 days
  - Alternatively (for 3- to 5-day "burst"):
  - <1 year: 10 mg every 12 hours
  - 1-4 years: 20 mg every 12 hours
  - 5-13 years: 30 mg every 12 hours
  - >13 years: 40 mg every 12 hours
- Asthma long-term therapy (alternative dosing by age):
  - <1 year: 10 mg every other day
  - 1-4 years: 20 mg every other day
  - 5-13 years: 30 mg every other day
  - >13 years: 40 mg every other day
- Nephrotic syndrome:
  - Initial (first 3 episodes): 2 mg/kg/day **or** 60 mg/m^2/day (maximum: 80 mg/day) in divided doses 3-4 times/day until urine is protein free for 3 consecutive days (maximum: 28 days); followed by 1-1.5 mg/kg/dose **or** 40 mg/m^2/dose given every other day for 4 weeks
  - Maintenance dose (long-term maintenance dose for frequent relapses): 0.5-1 mg/kg/dose given every other day for 3-6 months

Children and Adults: Physiologic replacement: 4-5 mg/m^2/day

Children ≥5 years and Adults: Asthma:

- Moderate persistent: Inhaled corticosteroid (medium dose) or inhaled corticosteroid (low-medium dose) with a long-acting bronchodilator
- Severe persistent: Inhaled corticosteroid (high dose) and corticosteroid tablets or syrup long term: 2 mg/kg/day, generally not to exceed 60 mg/day

Adults:

Immunosuppression/chemotherapy adjunct: Range: 5-60 mg/day in divided doses 1-4 times/day

Allergic reaction (contact dermatitis):

Day 1: 30 mg divided as 10 mg before breakfast, 5 mg at lunch, 5 mg at dinner, 10 mg at bedtime

Day 2: 5 mg at breakfast, 5 mg at lunch, 5 mg at dinner, 10 mg at bedtime

Day 3: 5 mg 4 times/day (with meals and at bedtime)

Day 4: 5 mg 3 times/day (breakfast, lunch, bedtime)

Day 5: 5 mg 2 times/day (breakfast, bedtime)

Day 6: 5 mg before breakfast

Pneumocystis carinii pneumonia (PCP):

40 mg twice daily for 5 days **followed by**

40 mg once daily for 5 days **followed by**

20 mg once daily for 11 days or until antimicrobial regimen is completed

Thyrotoxicosis: Oral: 60 mg/day

Chemotherapy (refer to individual protocols): Oral: Range: 20 mg/day to 100 mg/m^2/day

Rheumatoid arthritis: Oral: Use lowest possible daily dose (often ≤7.5 mg/day)

Idiopathic thrombocytopenia purpura (ITP): Oral: 60 mg daily for 4-6 weeks, gradually tapered over several weeks

Systemic lupus erythematosus (SLE): Oral:

Acute: 1-2 mg/kg/day in 2-3 divided doses

Maintenance: Reduce to lowest possible dose, usually <1 mg/kg/day as single dose (morning)

Elderly: Use the lowest effective dose

Mechanism of Action Decreases inflammation by suppression of migration of polymorphonuclear leukocytes and reversal of increased capillary permeability; suppresses the immune system by reducing activity and volume of the lymphatic system; suppresses adrenal function at high doses. Antitumor effects may be related to inhibition of glucose transport, phosphorylation, or induction of cell death in immature lymphocytes. Antiemetic effects are thought to occur due to blockade of cerebral innervation of the emetic center via inhibition of prostaglandin synthesis.

Other Adverse Effects

>10%:

Central nervous system: Insomnia, nervousness

Gastrointestinal: Increased appetite, indigestion

1% to 10%:

Dermatologic: Hirsutism

Endocrine & metabolic: Diabetes mellitus, glucose intolerance, hyperglycemia

Neuromuscular & skeletal: Arthralgia

Ocular: Cataracts, glaucoma

Respiratory: Epistaxis

<1%: Edema, hypertension, vertigo, seizures, psychoses, pseudotumor cerebri, headache, mood swings, delirium, hallucinations, euphoria, acne, skin atrophy, bruising, hyperpigmentation, Cushing's syndrome, pituitary-adrenal axis suppression, growth suppression, glucose intolerance, hypokalemia, alkalosis, amenorrhea, sodium and water retention, hyperglycemia, peptic ulcer, nausea, vomiting, abdominal distention, ulcerative esophagitis, pancreatitis, muscle weakness, osteoporosis, fractures, muscle wasting, hypersensitivity reactions

Contraindications Hypersensitivity to prednisone or any component of the formulation; serious infections, except tuberculous meningitis; systemic fungal infections; varicella

Warnings/Precautions Withdraw therapy with gradual tapering of dose, may retard bone growth. Use with caution in patients with hypothyroidism, cirrhosis, hypertension, CHF, ulcerative colitis, thromboembolic disorders, and patients at increased risk for peptic ulcer disease. Corticosteroids should be used with caution in patients with diabetes, hypertension, osteoporosis, glaucoma, cataracts, or tuberculosis. Use caution in hepatic impairment. Because of the risk of adverse effects, systemic corticosteroids should be used cautiously in the elderly, in the smallest possible dose, and for the shortest possible time.

Drug Interactions CYP3A3/4 enzyme substrate

Increased Effect/Toxicity: Concurrent use of NSAIDs may increase the risk of GI ulceration.

Decreased Effect: Decreases effectiveness of salicylates, vaccines, and toxoids; barbiturates, phenytoin, and rifampin decrease corticosteroid effectiveness.

Dietary/Ethanol/Herb Considerations

Ethanol: Avoid use; may increase gastric mucosal irritation.

Food: Administer after meals or with food or milk. Prednisone interferes with calcium absorption; increase dietary intake of pyridoxine, vitamin C, vitamin D, folate, calcium, and phosphorus. Limit caffeine.

Herb/Nutraceutical: Avoid cat's claw and echinacea due to immunostimulant properties. Avoid St John's wort; may decrease serum concentration.

Drug Uptake Prednisone is inactive and must be metabolized to prednisolone which may be impaired in patients with impaired liver function.

(Continued)

PredniSONE *(Continued)*

Absorption: Rapid and nearly complete
Half-life, elimination: Normal renal function: 2.5-3.5 hours

Pregnancy Risk Factor B

Breast-feeding Considerations May be taken while breast-feeding

Dosage Forms CONC, oral: 5 mg/mL (30 mL). **SOLN, oral:** 1 mg/mL (5 mL, 120 mL, 500 mL). **SYR:** 1 mg/mL (120 mL, 240 mL). **TAB:** 1 mg, 2.5 mg, 5 mg, 10 mg, 20 mg, 50 mg

Generic Available Yes

Prefrin™ Ophthalmic *see* Phenylephrine *on page 950*
Pregnyl® *see* Chorionic Gonadotropin *on page 281*
Prelone® *see* PrednisoLONE *on page 988*
Prelu-2® *see* Phendimetrazine *on page 943*
Premarin® *see* Estrogens, Conjugated *on page 463*
Premphase® *see* Estrogens (Conjugated) and Medroxyprogesterone *on page 465*
Prempro™ *see* Estrogens (Conjugated) and Medroxyprogesterone *on page 465*
Pre-Pen® *see* Benzylpenicilloyl-polylysine *on page 156*
Prepidil® Vaginal Gel *see* Dinoprostone *on page 397*
Pretz® [OTC] *see* Sodium Chloride *on page 1094*
Pretz-D® [OTC] *see* Ephedrine *on page 437*
Prevacid® *see* Lansoprazole *on page 686*
Prevalite® *see* Cholestyramine Resin *on page 279*
PREVEN™ *see* Combination Hormonal Contraceptives *on page 323*
PreviDent® *see* Fluoride *on page 514*
PreviDent® 5000 Plus™ *see* Fluoride *on page 514*
Prevnar® *see* Pneumococcal Conjugate Vaccine, 7-Valent *on page 967*
Priftin® *see* Rifapentine *on page 1053*

Prilocaine (PRIL oh kane)

Related Information

Oral Pain *on page 1360*

U.S. Brand Names Citanest® Plain

Canadian Brand Names Citanest® Forte; Citanest® Plain

Mexican Brand Names Citanest Octapressin®

Pharmacologic Category Local Anesthetic

Use Dental: Amide-type anesthetic used for local infiltration anesthesia; injection near nerve trunks to produce nerve block

Local Anesthetic/Vasoconstrictor Precautions No information available to require special precautions

Effects on Dental Treatment No effects or complications reported

Dosage

Children <10 years: Doses >40 mg (1 mL) as a 4% solution per procedure rarely needed

Children >10 years and Adults: Dental anesthesia, infiltration, or conduction block: Initial: 40-80 mg (1-2 mL) as a 4% solution; up to a maximum of 400 mg (10 mL) as a 4% solution within a 2-hour period. Manufacturer's maximum recommended dose is ≤600 mg to normal healthy adults. The effective anesthetic dose varies with procedure, intensity of anesthesia needed, duration of anesthesia required and physical condition of the patient. Always use the lowest effective dose along with careful aspiration.

The following numbers of dental carpules (1.8 mL) provide the indicated amounts of prilocaine hydrochloride 4%. See table.

# of Cartridges (1.8 mL)	Prilocaine HCl 4% (mg)
1	72
2	144
3	216
4	288
5	360
6	432
7	504
8	576

Note: Doses of prilocaine hydrochloride cited from USP Dispensing Information (USP DI), 17th ed, The United States Pharmacopeial Convention, Inc, Rockville, MD, 1997, 139.

Mechanism of Action Local anesthetics bind selectively to the intracellular surface of sodium channels to block influx of sodium into the axon. As a result, depolarization necessary for action potential propagation and subsequent nerve function is prevented. The block at the sodium channel is reversible. Local anesthetics reversibly prevent generation and conduction of electrical impulses in neurons by decreasing the transient increase in permeability to sodium. The differential sensitivity generally depends on the size of the fiber; small fibers are more sensitive than larger fibers and require a longer period for recovery. Sensory pain fibers are usually blocked first, followed by fibers that transmit sensations of temperature, touch, and deep pressure. High concentrations block sympathetic somatic sensory and somatic motor fibers. The spread of anesthesia depends upon the distribution of the solution. This is primarily dependent on the site of administration and volume of drug injected. When drug diffuses away from the axon, sodium channel function is restored and nerve propagation returns.

Other Adverse Effects Degree of adverse effects in the CNS and cardiovascular system are directly related to the blood levels of local anesthetic. The effects below are more likely to occur after systemic administration rather than infiltration. Frequency not defined:

Cardiovascular: Myocardial effects include a decrease in contraction force as well as a decrease in electrical excitability and myocardial conduction rate resulting in bradycardia and reduction in cardiac output.

Central nervous system: High blood levels result in anxiety, restlessness, disorientation, confusion, dizziness, tremors and seizures. This is followed by depression of CNS resulting in somnolence, unconsciousness and possible respiratory arrest. Nausea and vomiting may also occur. In some cases, symptoms of CNS stimulation may be absent and the primary CNS effects are somnolence and unconsciousness.

Hypersensitivity reactions: May be manifest as dermatologic reactions and edema at injection site. Asthmatic syndromes have occurred.

Psychogenic reactions: It is common to misinterpret psychogenic responses to local anesthetic injection as an allergic reaction. Intraoral injections are perceived by many patients as a stressful procedure in dentistry. Common symptoms to this stress are diaphoresis, palpitations, hyperventilation, generalized pallor and a fainting feeling

Contraindications Hypersensitivity to prilocaine, other local anesthetics of the amide type, or any component of their formulation

Warnings/Precautions Aspirate the syringe after tissue penetration and before injection to minimize chance of direct vascular injection

Drug Uptake

Onset of action: Infiltration: ~2 minutes; Inferior alveolar nerve block: ~3 minutes

Duration: Infiltration: Complete anesthesia for procedures lasting 20 minutes; Inferior alveolar nerve block: ~2.5 hours

Half-life, elimination: 10-150 minutes; prolonged in hepatic or renal dysfunction

Pregnancy Risk Factor B

Breast-feeding Considerations Usual infiltration doses of prilocaine given to nursing mothers has not been shown to affect the health of the nursing infant.

Dosage Forms INJ: Prilocaine hydrochloride 4% (1.8 mL) [cartridge, 100/container]

Generic Available No

Selected Readings

Jastak JT and Yagiela JA, "Vasoconstrictors and Local Anesthesia: A Review and Rationale for Use," *J Am Dent Assoc*, 1983, 107(4):623-30.
MacKenzie TA and Young ER, "Local Anesthetic Update," *Anesth Prog*, 1993, 40(2):29-34.
Wynn RL, "Epinephrine Interactions With Beta-Blockers," *Gen Dent*, 1994, 42(1):16, 18.
Yagiela JA, "Local Anesthetics," *Anesth Prog*, 1991, 38(4-5):128-41.

Prilocaine With Epinephrine (PRIL oh kane with ep i NEF rin)

Related Information

Oral Pain *on page 1360*

U.S. Brand Names Citanest® Forte

Pharmacologic Category Local Anesthetic

Use Dental: Amide-type anesthetic used for local infiltration anesthesia; injection near nerve trunks to produce nerve block

Local Anesthetic/Vasoconstrictor Precautions No information available to require special precautions

Effects on Dental Treatment No effects or complications reported

Dosage

Children <10 years: Doses >40 mg (1 mL) of prilocaine hydrochloride as a 4% solution with epinephrine 1:200,000 are rarely needed

Children >10 years and Adults: Dental anesthesia, infiltration, or conduction block: Initial: 40-80 mg (1-2 mL) of prilocaine hydrochloride as a 4% solution with epinephrine 1:200,000; up to a maximum of 400 mg (10 mL) of prilocaine hydrochloride within a 2-hour period. The effective anesthetic dose varies with procedure, intensity of anesthesia needed, duration of anesthesia required, and physical condition of the patient. Always use the lowest effective dose along with careful aspiration.

The following numbers of dental carpules (1.8 mL) provide the indicated amounts of prilocaine hydrochloride 4% and epinephrine 1:200,000. See following table.

(Continued)

Prilocaine With Epinephrine *(Continued)*

# of Cartridges (1.8 mL)	Prilocaine (4%) (mg)	Epinephrine 1:200,000 (mg)
1	72	0.009
2	144	0.018
3	216	0.027
4	288	0.036
5	360	0.045
6	432	0.054
7	504	0.063
8	576	0.072

Note: Doses of prilocaine hydrochloride with epinephrine cited from USP Dispensing Information (USP DI), 17th ed, The United States Pharmacopeial Convention, Inc, Rockville, MD, 1997, 140.

Mechanism of Action Local anesthetics bind selectively to the intracellular surface of sodium channels to block influx of sodium into the axon. As a result, depolarization necessary for action potential propagation and subsequent nerve function is prevented. The block at the sodium channel is reversible. Local anesthetics reversibly prevent generation and conduction of electrical impulses in neurons by decreasing the transient increase in permeability to sodium. The differential sensitivity generally depends on the size of the fiber; small fibers are more sensitive than larger fibers and require a longer period for recovery. Sensory pain fibers are usually blocked first, followed by fibers that transmit sensations of temperature, touch, and deep pressure. High concentrations block sympathetic somatic sensory and somatic motor fibers. The spread of anesthesia depends upon the distribution of the solution. This is primarily dependent on the site of administration and volume of drug injected. When drug diffuses away from the axon, sodium channel function is restored and nerve propagation returns.

Epinephrine prolongs the duration of the anesthetic actions of prilocaine by causing vasoconstriction (alpha adrenergic receptor agonist) of the vasculature surrounding the nerve axons. This prevents the diffusion of prilocaine away from the nerves resulting in a longer retention in the axon.

Other Adverse Effects The degree of adverse effects in the CNS and cardiovascular system are directly related to the blood levels of prilocaine. The effects below are more likely to occur after systemic administration rather than infiltration.

Cardiovascular: Myocardial effects include a decrease in contraction force as well as a decrease in electrical excitability and myocardial conduction rate resulting in bradycardia and reduction in cardiac output.

Central nervous system: High blood levels result in anxiety, restlessness, disorientation, confusion, dizziness, tremors and seizures. This is followed by depression of CNS resulting in somnolence, unconsciousness and possible respiratory arrest. Nausea and vomiting may also occur. In some cases, symptoms of CNS stimulation may be absent and the primary CNS effects are somnolence and unconsciousness.

Hypersensitivity reactions: Extremely rare, but may be manifest as dermatologic reactions and edema at injection site. Asthmatic syndromes have occurred. Patients may exhibit hypersensitivity to bisulfites contained in local anesthetic solution to prevent oxidation of epinephrine. In general, patients reacting to bisulfites have a history of asthma and their airways are hyper-reactive to asthmatic syndrome.

Psychogenic reactions: It is common to misinterpret psychogenic responses to local anesthetic injection as an allergic reaction. Intraoral injections are perceived by many patients as a stressful procedure in dentistry. Common symptoms to this stress are diaphoresis, palpitations, hyperventilation, generalized pallor, and a fainting feeling.

Contraindications Hypersensitivity to prilocaine, epinephrine, other local anesthetics of the amide-type, or any component of their formulation

Warnings/Precautions Should be avoided in patients with uncontrolled hyperthyroidism. Should be used in minimal amounts in patients with significant cardiovascular problems (because of epinephrine component). Aspirate the syringe after tissue penetration and before injection to minimize chance of direct vascular injection

Drug Interactions

Beta-blockers, nonselective (ie, propranolol): Concurrent use could result in serious hypertension and reflex bradycardia

MAO inhibitors: Administration of local anesthetic solutions containing epinephrine may produce severe, prolonged hypertension

Tricyclic antidepressants: Pressor response to I.V. epinephrine, norepinephrine, and phenylephrine may be enhanced in patients receiving TCAs (**Note:** Effect is unlikely with epinephrine or levonordefrin dosages typically administered as infiltration in combination with local anesthetics)

Drug Uptake

Onset of action: Infiltration: <2 minutes; Inferior alveolar nerve block: <3 minutes

Duration: Infiltration: 2.25 hours; Inferior alveolar nerve block: 3 hours

Pregnancy Risk Factor C

Breast-feeding Considerations Usual infiltration doses of prilocaine with epinephrine given to nursing mothers has not been shown to affect the health of the nursing infant.

Dosage Forms INJ: Prilocaine hydrochloride 4% with epinephrine 1:200,000 (1.8 mL) [cartridge, 100/box]

Generic Available No

Selected Readings

Ayoub ST and Coleman AE, "A Review of Local Anesthetics," *Gen Dent*, 1992, 40(4):285-7, 289-90.

Blanton PL and Roda RS, "The Anatomy of Local Anesthesia," *J Calif Dent Assoc*, 1995, 23(4):55-65.

Jastak JT and Yagiela JA, "Vasoconstrictors and Local Anesthesia: A Review and Rationale for Use," *J Am Dent Assoc*, 1983, 107(4):623-30.

MacKenzie TA and Young ER, "Local Anesthetic Update," *Anesth Prog*, 1993, 40(2):29-34.

Wynn RL, "Epinephrine Interactions With Beta-Blockers," *Gen Dent*, 1994, 42(1):16, 18.

Yagiela JA, "Local Anesthetics," *Anesth Prog*, 1991, 38(4-5):128-41.

Yagiela JA, "Vasoconstrictor Agents for Local Anesthesia," *Anesth Prog*, 1995, 42(3-4):116-20.

Prilosec® *see* Omeprazole *on page 886*

Primacor® *see* Milrinone *on page 815*

Primaquine Phosphate (PRIM a kween)

Pharmacologic Category Aminoquinoline (Antimalarial)

Synonyms Primaquine; Prymaccone

Use Provides radical cure of *P. vivax* or *P. ovale* malaria after a clinical attack has been confirmed by blood smear or serologic titer and postexposure prophylaxis

Local Anesthetic/Vasoconstrictor Precautions No information available to require special precautions

Effects on Dental Treatment No effects or complications reported

Dosage Oral:

Children: 0.3 mg base/kg/day once daily for 14 days (not to exceed 15 mg/day) or 0.9 mg base/kg once weekly for 8 weeks not to exceed 45 mg base/week

Adults: 15 mg/day (base) once daily for 14 days or 45 mg base once weekly for 8 weeks

Mechanism of Action Eliminates the primary tissue exoerythrocytic forms of *P. falciparum*; disrupts mitochondria and binds to DNA

Other Adverse Effects

>10%:

Gastrointestinal: Abdominal pain, nausea, vomiting

Hematologic: Hemolytic anemia in G6PD deficiency

1% to 10%: Hematologic: Methemoglobinemia in NADH-methemoglobin reductase-deficient individuals

Drug Interactions CYP2D6 enzyme inhibitor

Increased toxicity/levels with quinacrine.

Drug Uptake

Absorption: Oral: Well absorbed

Half-life, elimination: 3.7-9.6 hours

Time to peak: 1-2 hours

Pregnancy Risk Factor C

Generic Available No

Primatene® Mist [OTC] *see* Epinephrine *on page 438*

Primaxin® *see* Imipenem and Cilastatin *on page 626*

Primidone (PRI mi done)

U.S. Brand Names Mysoline®

Canadian Brand Names Apo®-Primidone; Mysoline®

Mexican Brand Names Mysoline®

Pharmacologic Category Anticonvulsant, Miscellaneous; Barbiturate

Synonyms Desoxyphenobarbital; Primaclone

Use Management of grand mal, complex partial, and focal seizures

Unlabeled/Investigational: Benign familial tremor (essential tremor)

Local Anesthetic/Vasoconstrictor Precautions No information available to require special precautions

Effects on Dental Treatment No effects or complications reported

Dosage Oral:

Children <8 years: Initial: 50-125 mg/day given at bedtime; increase by 50-125 mg/day increments every 3-7 days; usual dose: 10-25 mg/kg/day in divided doses 3-4 times/day

Children ≥8 years and Adults: Initial: 125-250 mg/day at bedtime; increase by 125-250 mg/day every 3-7 days; usual dose: 750-1500 mg/day in divided doses 3-4 times/day with maximum dosage of 2 g/day

(Continued)

Primidone *(Continued)*

Dosing interval in renal impairment:

Cl_{cr} 50-80 mL/minute: Administer every 8 hours
Cl_{cr} 10-50 mL/minute: Administer every 8-12 hours
Cl_{cr} <10 mL/minute: Administer every 12-24 hours

Hemodialysis: Moderately dialyzable (20% to 50%); administer dose postdialysis or administer supplemental 30% dose

Mechanism of Action Decreases neuron excitability, raises seizure threshold similar to phenobarbital; primidone has two active metabolites, phenobarbital and phenylethylmalonamide (PEMA); PEMA may enhance the activity of phenobarbital

Other Adverse Effects Frequency not defined:

Central nervous system: Drowsiness, vertigo, ataxia, lethargy, behavior change, fatigue, hyperirritability
Dermatologic: Rash
Gastrointestinal: Nausea, vomiting, anorexia
Genitourinary: Impotence
Hematologic: Agranulocytopenia, agranulocytosis, anemia
Ocular: Diplopia, nystagmus

Drug Interactions CYP1A2, 2B6, 2C, 2C8, 3A3/4, and 3A5-7 enzyme inducer. **Note:** Primidone is metabolically converted to phenobarbital. Barbiturates are cytochrome P450 enzyme inducers. Patients should be monitored when these drugs are started or stopped for a decreased or increased therapeutic effect, respectively.

Increased Effect/Toxicity: Central nervous system depression (and possible respiratory depression) may be increased when combined with other CNS depressants, benzodiazepines, valproic acid, chloramphenicol, or antidepressants. MAO inhibitors may prolong the effect of primidone.

Decreased Effect: Primidone may induce the hepatic metabolism of many drugs due to enzyme induction, and may reduce the efficacy of beta-blockers, chloramphenicol, cimetidine, clozapine, corticosteroids, cyclosporine, disopyramide, doxycycline, ethosuximide, furosemide, griseofulvin, haloperidol, lamotrigine, methadone, nifedipine, oral contraceptives, phenothiazine, phenytoin, propafenone, quinidine, tacrolimus, TCAs, theophylline, warfarin, and verapamil.

Drug Uptake

Half-life, elimination (age-dependent): Primidone: 10-12 hours; PEMA: 16 hours; Phenobarbital: 52-118 hours
Time to peak: Oral: ~4 hours

Pregnancy Risk Factor D

Generic Available Yes: Tablet

Primsol® *see* Trimethoprim *on page 1210*
Principen® *see* Ampicillin *on page 94*
Prinivil® *see* Lisinopril *on page 719*
Prinzide® *see* Lisinopril and Hydrochlorothiazide *on page 721*
Privine® Nasal [OTC] *see* Naphazoline *on page 847*
ProAmatine® *see* Midodrine *on page 812*

Probenecid (proe BEN e sid)

Related Information

Dental Drug Interactions: Update on Drug Combinations Requiring Special Considerations *on page 1434*

Canadian Brand Names Benuryl™

Mexican Brand Names Benecid®

Pharmacologic Category Uricosuric Agent

Synonyms Benemid [DSC]

Use Prevention of gouty arthritis; hyperuricemia; prolongation of beta-lactam effect (ie, serum levels)

Local Anesthetic/Vasoconstrictor Precautions No information available to require special precautions

Effects on Dental Treatment No effects or complications reported

Dosage Oral:

Children:

<2 years: Not recommended
2-14 years: Prolong penicillin serum concentration: 25 mg/kg starting dose, then 40 mg/kg/day given 4 times/day

Adults:

Hyperuricemia with gout: 250 mg twice daily for 1 week; increase to 250-500 mg/day; may increase by 500 mg/month, if needed, to maximum of 2-3 g/day (dosages may be increased by 500 mg every 6 months if serum urate concentrations are controlled)
Prolong penicillin serum concentration: 500 mg 4 times/day
Gonorrhea: 1 g once with cefoxitin for pelvic inflammatory disease

Mechanism of Action Competitively inhibits the reabsorption of uric acid at the proximal convoluted tubule, thereby promoting its excretion and reducing serum uric acid levels; increases plasma concentrations of weak organic acids (penicillins, cephalosporins, or other beta-lactam antibiotics) by competitively inhibiting their renal tubular secretion

Other Adverse Effects Frequency not defined:

Cardiovascular: Flushing of face
Central nervous system: Headache, dizziness
Dermatologic: Rash, itching
Gastrointestinal: Anorexia, nausea, vomiting, sore gums
Genitourinary: Painful urination
Hematologic: Aplastic anemia, hemolytic anemia, leukopenia
Hepatic: Hepatic necrosis
Neuromuscular & skeletal: Gouty arthritis (acute)
Renal: Renal calculi, nephrotic syndrome, urate nephropathy
Miscellaneous: Anaphylaxis

Drug Interactions

Increased Effect/Toxicity: Increases methotrexate toxic potential. Probenecid increases the serum concentration of quinolones and beta-lactams such as penicillins and cephalosporins. Also increases levels/toxicity of acyclovir, diflunisal, ketorolac, thiopental, benzodiazepines, dapsone, fluoroquinolones, methotrexate, NSAIDs, sulfonylureas, zidovudine.

Decreased Effect: Salicylates (high-dose) may decrease uricosuria. Decreased urinary levels of nitrofurantoin may decrease efficacy.

Drug Uptake

Onset of action: Effect on penicillin levels: 2 hours
Absorption: Rapid and complete
Half-life, elimination (dose-dependent): Normal renal function: 6-12 hours
Time to peak: 2-4 hours

Pregnancy Risk Factor B

Generic Available Yes

Pro-Bionate® [OTC] *see Lactobacillus acidophilus* and *Lactobacillus bulgaricus on page 682*

Probiotica® [OTC] *see Lactobacillus acidophilus* and *Lactobacillus bulgaricus on page 682*

Procainamide (proe kane A mide)

Related Information

Cardiovascular Diseases *on page 1308*

U.S. Brand Names Procanbid®; Pronestyl®; Pronestyl-SR®

Canadian Brand Names Apo®-Procainamide; Procan® SR; Pronestyl®; Pronestyl®-SR

Pharmacologic Category Antiarrhythmic Agent, Class Ia

Synonyms PCA; Procainamide Hydrochloride; Procaine Amide Hydrochloride

Use Treatment of ventricular tachycardia, premature ventricular contractions, paroxysmal atrial tachycardia, and atrial fibrillation; prevention of recurrence of ventricular tachycardia, paroxysmal supraventricular tachycardia, atrial fibrillation or flutter

Unlabeled/Investigational: ACLS guidelines:

Intermittent/recurrent VF or pulseless VT not responsive to earlier interventions
Monomorphic VT (EF >40%, no CHF)
Polymorphic VT with normal baseline QT interval
Wide complex tachycardia of unknown type (EF >40%, no CHF, patient stable)
Refractory paroxysmal SVT
Atrial fibrillation or flutter (EF >40%, no CHF) including pre-excitation syndrome

Local Anesthetic/Vasoconstrictor Precautions No information available to require special precautions

Effects on Dental Treatment No effects or complications reported

Dosage Must be titrated to patient's response

Children:

Oral: 15-50 mg/kg/24 hours divided every 3-6 hours

I.M.: 50 mg/kg/24 hours divided into doses of 1/8 to 1/4 every 3-6 hours in divided doses until oral therapy is possible

I.V. (infusion requires use of an infusion pump):

Load: 3-6 mg/kg/dose over 5 minutes not to exceed 100 mg/dose; may repeat every 5-10 minutes to maximum of 15 mg/kg/load

Maintenance as continuous I.V. infusion: 20-80 mcg/kg/minute; maximum: 2 g/24 hours

Adults:

Oral: 250-500 mg/dose every 3-6 hours or 500 mg to 1 g every 6 hours sustained release; usual dose: 50 mg/kg/24 hours; maximum: 4 g/24 hours (**Note:** Twice daily dosing approved for Procanbid®)

I.M.: 0.5-1 g every 4-8 hours until oral therapy is possible

I.V. (infusion requires use of an infusion pump): Loading dose: 15-18 mg/kg administered as slow infusion over 25-30 minutes or 100-200 mg/dose repeated every 5 minutes as needed to a total dose of 1 g; maintenance dose: 1-4 mg/minute by continuous infusion

(Continued)

Procainamide *(Continued)*

Infusion rate: 2 g/250 mL D_5W/NS (I.V. infusion requires use of an infusion pump):
1 mg/minute: 7.5 mL/hour
2 mg/minute: 15 mL/hour
3 mg/minute: 22.5 mL/hour
4 mg/minute: 30 mL/hour
5 mg/minute: 37.5 mL/hour
6 mg/minute: 45 mL/hour

Intermittent/recurrent VF or pulseless VT:
Initial: 20-30 mg/minute (maximum: 50 mg/minute if necessary), up to a total of 17 mg/kg. ACLS guidelines: I.V.: Infuse 20 mg/minute until arrhythmia is controlled, hypotension occurs, QRS complex widens by 50% of its original width, or total of 17 mg/kg is given.
Note: Reduce to 12 mg/kg in setting of cardiac or renal dysfunction
I.V. maintenance infusion: 1-4 mg/minute; monitor levels and do not exceed 3 mg/minute for >24 hours in adults with renal failure.

Dosing interval in renal impairment:
Cl_{cr} 10-50 mL/minute: Administer every 6-12 hours.
Cl_{cr} <10 mL/minute: Administer every 8-24 hours.

Dialysis:
Procainamide: Moderately hemodialyzable (20% to 50%): 200 mg supplemental dose posthemodialysis is recommended.
N-acetylprocainamide: Not dialyzable (0% to 5%)
Procainamide/N-acetylprocainamide: Not peritoneal dialyzable (0% to 5%)
Procainamide/N-acetylprocainamide: Replace by blood level during continuous arteriovenous or venovenous hemofiltration

Dosing adjustment in hepatic impairment: Reduce dose by 50%.

Mechanism of Action Decreases myocardial excitability and conduction velocity and may depress myocardial contractility, by increasing the electrical stimulation threshold of ventricle, His-Purkinje system and through direct cardiac effects

Other Adverse Effects >1%:
Cardiovascular: Hypotension (I.V. up to 5%)
Dermatologic: Rash
Gastrointestinal: Diarrhea (3% to 4%), nausea, vomiting, taste disorder, GI complaints (3% to 4%)

Drug Interactions
Increased Effect/Toxicity: Amiodarone, cimetidine, ofloxacin (and potentially other renally eliminated quinolones), ranitidine, and trimethoprim increase procainamide and NAPA blood levels; consider reducing procainamide dosage by 25% with concurrent use. Cisapride and procainamide may increase the risk of malignant arrhythmia; concurrent use is contraindicated. Neuromuscular blocking agents: Procainamide may potentiate neuromuscular blockade.
Drugs which may prolong the QT interval include amiodarone, amitriptyline, astemizole, bepridil, cisapride, disopyramide, erythromycin, haloperidol, imipramine, pimozide, quinidine, sotalol, mesoridazine, thioridazine, and some quinolone antibiotics (sparfloxacin, gatifloxacin, moxifloxacin); concurrent use may result in additional prolongation of the QT interval.

Drug Uptake
Onset of action: I.M. 10-30 minutes
Half-life, elimination:
Procainamide: (dependent on hepatic acetylator, phenotype, cardiac and renal function): Adults: 2.5-4.7 hours; Anephric: 11 hours
NAPA: (dependent on renal function): Children: 6 hours; Adults: 6-8 hours; Anephric: 42 hours
Time to peak: Capsule: 0.75-2.5 hours; I.M.: 0.25-1 hour

Pregnancy Risk Factor C

Generic Available Yes

Procaine (PROE kane)

U.S. Brand Names Novocain®

Canadian Brand Names Novocain®

Pharmacologic Category Local Anesthetic

Synonyms Procaine Hydrochloride

Use Produces spinal anesthesia and epidural and peripheral nerve block by injection and infiltration methods

Local Anesthetic/Vasoconstrictor Precautions No information available to require special precautions

Effects on Dental Treatment This is no longer a useful anesthetic in dentistry due to high incidence of allergic reactions.

Dosage Dose varies with procedure, desired depth, and duration of anesthesia, desired muscle relaxation, vascularity of tissues, physical condition, and age of patient

Mechanism of Action Blocks both the initiation and conduction of nerve impulses by decreasing the neuronal membrane's permeability to sodium ions, which results in inhibition of depolarization with resultant blockade of conduction. Local anesthetics reversibly prevent generation and conduction of electrical impulses in neurons by decreasing the transient increase in permeability to sodium. The differential sensitivity generally depends on the size of the fiber; small fibers are more sensitive than larger fibers and require a longer period for recovery. Sensory pain fibers are usually blocked first, followed by fibers that transmit sensations of temperature, touch, and deep pressure. High concentrations block sympathetic somatic sensory and somatic motor fibers. The spread of anesthesia depends upon the distribution of the solution. This is primarily dependent on the site of administration and volume of drug injected.

Other Adverse Effects 1% to 10%: Local: Burning sensation at site of injection, tissue irritation, pain at injection site

Drug Interactions Decreased effect of sulfonamides with the PABA metabolite of procaine, chloroprocaine, and tetracaine. Decreased/increased effect of vasopressors, ergot alkaloids, and MAO inhibitors on BP when using anesthetic solutions with a vasoconstrictor.

Drug Uptake

Onset of action: Injection: 2-5 minutes

Duration: 0.5-1.5 hours (dependent upon patient, type of block, concentration, and method of anesthesia)

Half-life, elimination: 7.7 minutes

Pregnancy Risk Factor C

Generic Available Yes

Procanbid® *see* Procainamide *on page 997*

Procarbazine (proe KAR ba zeen)

U.S. Brand Names Matulane®

Canadian Brand Names Matulane®; Natulan®

Mexican Brand Names Natulan

Pharmacologic Category Antineoplastic Agent, Alkylating Agent

Synonyms Benzmethyzin; N-Methylhydrazine; Procarbazine Hydrochloride

Use Treatment of Hodgkin's disease, non-Hodgkin's lymphoma, brain tumor, bronchogenic carcinoma

Local Anesthetic/Vasoconstrictor Precautions No information available to require special precautions

Effects on Dental Treatment No effects or complications reported

Mechanism of Action Mechanism of action is not clear, methylating of nucleic acids; inhibits DNA, RNA, and protein synthesis; may damage DNA directly and suppresses mitosis; metabolic activation required by host

Other Adverse Effects Frequency not defined:

Central nervous system: Reports of neurotoxicity with procarbazine generally originate from early usage with single agent oral (continuous) or I.V. dosing; CNS depression is commonly reported to be additive with other CNS depressants

Hematologic: Myelosuppression, hemolysis in patients with G6PD deficiency

Gastrointestinal: Nausea and vomiting (60% to 90%); increasing the dose in a stepwise fashion over several days may minimize this

Genitourinary: Reproductive dysfunction >10% (in animals, hormone treatment has prevented azoospermia)

Respiratory: Pulmonary toxicity (<1%); the most commonly reported pulmonary toxicity is a hypersensitivity pneumonitis which responds to steroids and discontinuation of the drug. At least one report of persistent pulmonary fibrosis has been reported, however, a higher incidence (18%) of pulmonary toxicity (fibrosis) was reported when procarbazine was given prior to BCNU (BCNU alone does cause pulmonary fibrosis).

Miscellaneous: Second malignancies (cumulative incidence 2% to 15% reported with MOPP combination therapy)

Drug Interactions Procarbazine exhibits weak MAO inhibitor activity. Sympathomimetic amines (epinephrine and amphetamines) and antidepressants (tricyclics) should be used cautiously with procarbazine. Barbiturates, narcotics, phenothiazines, and other CNS depressants can cause somnolence, ataxia, and other symptoms of CNS depression.

Drug Uptake

Absorption: Oral: Rapid and complete

Half-life, elimination: 1 hour

Pregnancy Risk Factor D

Generic Available No

Procardia® *see* NIFEdipine *on page 865*

Procardia XL® *see* NIFEdipine *on page 865*

Prochlorperazine (proe klor PER a zeen)

U.S. Brand Names Compazine®; Compro™

Canadian Brand Names Compazine®; Nu-Prochlor; Stemetil®

(Continued)

Prochlorperazine *(Continued)*

Pharmacologic Category Antipsychotic Agent, Phenothiazine, Piperazine

Synonyms Prochlorperazine Edisylate; Prochlorperazine Maleate

Use Management of nausea and vomiting; psychosis; treatment of schizophrenia; short-term treatment of nonpsychotic anxiety

Unlabeled/Investigational: Dementia behavior

Local Anesthetic/Vasoconstrictor Precautions Most pharmacology textbooks state that in presence of phenothiazines, systemic doses of epinephrine paradoxically decrease the blood pressure. This is the so called "epinephrine reversal" phenomenon. This has never been observed when epinephrine is given by infiltration as part of the anesthesia procedure.

Effects on Dental Treatment

>10%: Xerostomia

Significant hypotension may occur especially when the drug is administered parenterally; orthostatic hypotension is due to alpha-receptor blockade, the elderly are at greater risk for orthostatic hypotension.

Tardive dyskinesia: Prevalence rate may be 40% in elderly; development of the syndrome and the irreversible nature are proportional to duration and total cumulative dose over time. Extrapyramidal reactions are more common in elderly with up to 50% developing these reactions after 60 years of age; drug-induced **Parkinson's syndrome** occurs often; **Akathisia** is the most common extrapyramidal reaction in elderly.

Increased confusion, memory loss, psychotic behavior, and agitation frequently occur as a consequence of anticholinergic effects. Antipsychotic associated sedation in nonpsychotic patients is extremely unpleasant due to feelings of depersonalization, derealization, and dysphoria.

Dosage

Antiemetic: Children:

Oral, rectal:

>10 kg: 0.4 mg/kg/24 hours in 3-4 divided doses; **or**

9-14 kg: 2.5 mg every 12-24 hours as needed; maximum: 7.5 mg/day

14-18 kg: 2.5 mg every 8-12 hours as needed; maximum: 10 mg/day

18-39 kg: 2.5 mg every 8 hours or 5 mg every 12 hours as needed; maximum: 15 mg/day

I.M.: 0.1-0.15 mg/kg/dose; usual: 0.13 mg/kg/dose; change to oral as soon as possible

I.V.: Not recommended in children <10 kg or <2 years

Antiemetic: Adults:

Oral: 5-10 mg 3-4 times/day; usual maximum: 40 mg/day

I.M.: 5-10 mg every 3-4 hours; usual maximum: 40 mg/day

I.V.: 2.5-10 mg; maximum 10 mg/dose or 40 mg/day; may repeat dose every 3-4 hours as needed

Rectal: 25 mg twice daily

Antipsychotic:

Children 2-12 years:

Oral, rectal: 2.5 mg 2-3 times/day; increase dosage as needed to maximum daily dose of 20 mg for 2-5 years and 25 mg for 6-12 years

I.M.: 0.13 mg/kg/dose; change to oral as soon as possible

Adults:

Oral: 5-10 mg 3-4 times/day; doses up to 150 mg/day may be required in some patients for treatment of severe disturbances

I.M.: 10-20 mg every 4-6 hours may be required in some patients for treatment of severe disturbances; change to oral as soon as possible

Dementia behavior (nonpsychotic): Elderly: Initial: 2.5-5 mg 1-2 times/day; increase dose at 4- to 7-day intervals by 2.5-5 mg/day; increase dosing intervals (twice daily, 3 times/day, etc) as necessary to control response or side effects; maximum daily dose should probably not exceed 75 mg in elderly; gradual increases (titration) may prevent some side effects or decrease their severity

Mechanism of Action Blocks postsynaptic mesolimbic dopaminergic D_1 and D_2 receptors in the brain, including the medullary chemoreceptor trigger zone; exhibits a strong alpha-adrenergic and anticholinergic blocking effect and depresses the release of hypothalamic and hypophyseal hormones; believed to depress the reticular activating system, thus affecting basal metabolism, body temperature, wakefulness, vasomotor tone and emesis

Other Adverse Effects Frequency not defined:

Cardiovascular: Hypotension, orthostatic hypotension, hypertension, tachycardia, bradycardia, dizziness, cardiac arrest

Central nervous system: Extrapyramidal symptoms (pseudoparkinsonism, akathisia, dystonias, tardive dyskinesia), dizziness, cerebral edema, seizures, headache, drowsiness, paradoxical excitement, restlessness, hyperactivity, insomnia, neuroleptic malignant syndrome (NMS), impairment of temperature regulation

Dermatologic: Increased sensitivity to sun, rash, discoloration of skin (blue-gray)

Endocrine & metabolic: Hypoglycemia, hyperglycemia, galactorrhea, lactation, breast enlargement, gynecomastia, menstrual irregularity, amenorrhea, SIADH, changes in libido

Gastrointestinal: Constipation, weight gain, vomiting, stomach pain, nausea, xerostomia, salivation, diarrhea, anorexia, ileus

Genitourinary: Difficulty in urination, ejaculatory disturbances, incontinence, polyuria, ejaculating dysfunction, priapism

Hematologic: Agranulocytosis, leukopenia, eosinophilia, hemolytic anemia, thrombocytopenic purpura, pancytopenia

Hepatic: Cholestatic jaundice, hepatotoxicity

Neuromuscular & skeletal: Tremor

Ocular: Pigmentary retinopathy, blurred vision, cornea and lens changes

Respiratory: Nasal congestion

Miscellaneous: Diaphoresis

Drug Interactions Possible CYP2D6 enzyme substrate

Aluminum salts: May decrease the absorption of phenothiazines; monitor

Amphetamines: Efficacy may be diminished by antipsychotics; in addition, amphetamines may increase psychotic symptoms; avoid concurrent use

Anticholinergics: May inhibit the therapeutic response to phenothiazines and excess anticholinergic effects may occur; includes benztropine, trihexyphenidyl, biperiden, and drugs with significant anticholinergic activity (TCAs, antihistamines, disopyramide)

Antihypertensives: Concurrent use of phenothiazines with an antihypertensive may produce additive hypotensive effects (particularly orthostasis)

Bromocriptine: Phenothiazines inhibit the ability of bromocriptine to lower serum prolactin concentrations

CNS depressants: Sedative effects may be additive with phenothiazines; monitor for increased effect; includes barbiturates, benzodiazepines, narcotic analgesics, ethanol and other sedative agents

CYP2D6 inhibitors: Metabolism of phenothiazines may be decreased, increasing clinical effect or toxicity; inhibitors include amiodarone, cimetidine, delavirdine, fluoxetine, paroxetine, propafenone, quinidine, and ritonavir; monitor for increased effect/toxicity

Enzyme inducers: May enhance the hepatic metabolism of phenothiazines; larger doses may be required; includes rifampin, rifabutin, barbiturates, phenytoin, and cigarette smoking

Epinephrine: Chlorpromazine (and possibly other low potency antipsychotics) may diminish the pressor effects of epinephrine

Guanethidine and guanadrel: Antihypertensive effects may be inhibited by phenothiazines

Levodopa: Phenothiazines may inhibit the antiparkinsonian effect of levodopa; avoid this combination

Lithium: Phenothiazines may produce neurotoxicity with lithium; this is a rare effect

Metoclopramide: May increase extrapyramidal symptoms (EPS) or risk.

Phenytoin: May reduce serum levels of phenothiazines; phenothiazines may increase phenytoin serum levels

Propranolol: Serum concentrations of phenothiazines may be increased; propranolol also increases phenothiazine concentrations

Polypeptide antibiotics: Rare cases of respiratory paralysis have been reported with concurrent use of phenothiazines

QT_c-prolonging agents: Effects on QT_c interval may be additive with phenothiazines, increasing the risk of malignant arrhythmias; includes type Ia antiarrhythmics, TCAs, and some quinolone antibiotics (sparfloxacin, moxifloxacin, and gatifloxacin)

Sulfadoxine-pyrimethamine: May increase phenothiazine concentrations

Tricyclic antidepressants: Concurrent use may produce increased toxicity or altered therapeutic response

Trazodone: Phenothiazines and trazodone may produce additive hypotensive effects

Valproic acid: Serum levels may be increased by phenothiazines

Drug Uptake

Onset of action: Oral: 30-40 minutes; I.M.: 10-20 minutes; Rectal: ≤1 hour

Duration: I.M., oral (extended release): 12 hours; Rectal, oral (immediate release): 3-4 hours

Half-life, elimination: 23 hours

Pregnancy Risk Factor C

Generic Available Yes: Injection and tablet

Procort® [OTC] *see* Hydrocortisone *on page 608*

Procrit® *see* Epoetin Alfa *on page 442*

Proctocort™ *see* Hydrocortisone *on page 608*

ProctoFoam®-HC *see* Pramoxine and Hydrocortisone *on page 984*

ProctoFoam® NS [OTC] *see* Pramoxine *on page 984*

Procyclidine (proe SYE kli deen)

U.S. Brand Names Kemadrin®

Canadian Brand Names Kemadrin®; Procyclid™

Pharmacologic Category Anticholinergic Agent; Anti-Parkinson's Agent, Anticholinergic

Synonyms Procyclidine Hydrochloride

Use Relieves symptoms of parkinsonian syndrome and drug-induced extrapyramidal symptoms

Local Anesthetic/Vasoconstrictor Precautions No information available to require special precautions

Effects on Dental Treatment

>10%: Xerostomia

Prolonged use of antidyskinetics may decrease or inhibit salivary flow and could contribute to development of periodontal disease, oral candidiasis or discomfort.

Dosage

Antiemetic: Children (not recommended in children <10 kg or <2 years):

Oral, rectal:

>10 kg: 0.4 mg/kg/24 hours in 3-4 divided doses; **or**

9-14 kg: 2.5 mg every 12-24 hours as needed; maximum: 7.5 mg/day

14-18 kg: 2.5 mg every 8-12 hours as needed; maximum: 10 mg/day

18-39 kg: 2.5 mg every 8 hours or 5 mg every 12 hours as needed; maximum: 15 mg/day

I.M.: 0.1-0.15 mg/kg/dose; usual: 0.13 mg/kg/dose; change to oral as soon as possible

Antiemetic: Adults:

Oral:

Tablet: 5-10 mg 3-4 times/day; usual maximum: 40 mg/day

Capsule, sustained action: 15 mg upon arising or 10 mg every 12 hours

I.M.: 5-10 mg every 3-4 hours; usual maximum: 40 mg/day

I.V.: 2.5-10 mg; maximum 10 mg/dose or 40 mg/day; may repeat dose every 3-4 hours as needed

Rectal: 25 mg twice daily

Surgical nausea/vomiting: Adults:

I.M.: 5-10 mg 1-2 hours before induction; may repeat once if necessary

I.V.: 5-10 mg 15-30 minutes before induction; may repeat once if necessary

Antipsychotic:

Children 2-12 years (not recommended in children <10 kg or <2 years):

Oral, rectal: 2.5 mg 2-3 times/day; increase dosage as needed to maximum daily dose of 20 mg for 2-5 years and 25 mg for 6-12 years

I.M.: 0.13 mg/kg/dose; change to oral as soon as possible

Adults:

Oral: 5-10 mg 3-4 times/day; doses up to 150 mg/day may be required in some patients for treatment of severe disturbances

I.M.: 10-20 mg every 4-6 hours may be required in some patients for treatment of severe disturbances; change to oral as soon as possible

Nonpsychotic anxiety: Adults: Not >20 mg/day for no longer than 12 weeks

Elderly: Behavioral symptoms associated with dementia: Initial: 2.5-5 mg 1-2 times/day; increase dose at 4- to 7-day intervals by 2.5-5 mg/day; increase dosing intervals (twice daily, 3 times/day, etc) as necessary to control response or side effects; maximum daily dose should probably not exceed 75 mg in elderly; gradual increases (titration) may prevent some side effects or decrease their severity

Hemodialysis: Not dialyzable (0% to 5%)

Mechanism of Action Thought to act by blocking excess acetylcholine at cerebral synapses; many of its effects are due to its pharmacologic similarities with atropine; it exerts an antispasmodic effect on smooth muscle, is a potent mydriatic; inhibits salivation

Other Adverse Effects Frequency not defined:

Cardiovascular: Tachycardia, palpitations

Central nervous system: Confusion, drowsiness, headache, loss of memory, fatigue, ataxia, giddiness, lightheadedness

Dermatologic: Dry skin, increased sensitivity to light, rash

Gastrointestinal: Constipation, xerostomia, dry throat, nausea, vomiting, epigastric distress

Genitourinary: Difficult urination

Neuromuscular & skeletal: Weakness

Ocular: Increased intraocular pain, blurred vision, mydriasis

Respiratory: Dry nose

Miscellaneous: Diaphoresis (decreased)

Drug Interactions

Increased Effect/Toxicity: Central and/or peripheral anticholinergic syndrome can occur when administered with amantadine, rimantadine, narcotic analgesics, phenothiazines and other antipsychotics (especially with high anticholinergic activity), tricyclic antidepressants, quinidine and some other antiarrhythmics, and antihistamines.

Decreased Effect: May increase gastric degradation of levodopa and decrease the amount of levodopa absorbed by delaying gastric emptying; the opposite may be true for digoxin. Therapeutic effects of cholinergic agents (tacrine, donepezil) and neuroleptics may be antagonized.

Drug Uptake

Onset of action: Oral: 30-40 minutes

Duration: 4-6 hours

Pregnancy Risk Factor C

Generic Available No

Prodium™ [OTC] *see* Phenazopyridine *on page 943*

Prodrox® *see* Hydroxyprogesterone Caproate *on page 614*

Profasi® *see* Chorionic Gonadotropin *on page 281*

Profilnine® SD *see* Factor IX Complex (Human) *on page 484*

Progestasert® *see* Progesterone *on page 1003*

Progesterone (proe JES ter one)

U.S. Brand Names Crinone®; Progestasert®; Prometrium®

Canadian Brand Names Crinone®; Prometrium®

Mexican Brand Names Crinone®; Crinone® V; Utrogestan

Pharmacologic Category Progestin

Synonyms Pregnenedione; Progestin

Use

I.M.: Amenorrhea; abnormal uterine bleeding due to hormonal imbalance

Intrauterine device (IUD): Contraception in women who have had at least one child, are in a stable and mutually-monogamous relationship, and have no history of pelvic inflammatory disease; amenorrhea; functional uterine bleeding

Intravaginal gel: Part of assisted reproductive technology (ART) for infertile women with progesterone deficiency; secondary amenorrhea

Oral: Prevention of endometrial hyperplasia in nonhysterectomized, postmenopausal women who are receiving conjugated estrogen tablets; secondary amenorrhea

Local Anesthetic/Vasoconstrictor Precautions No information available to require special precautions

Effects on Dental Treatment Progestins may predispose the patient to gingival bleeding.

Dosage

I.M.: Adults: Female:

- Amenorrhea: 5-10 mg/day for 6-8 consecutive days
- Functional uterine bleeding: 5-10 mg/day for 6 doses

IUD: Adults: Female: Contraception: Insert a single system into the uterine cavity; contraceptive effectiveness is retained for 1 year and system must be replaced 1 year after insertion

Oral: Adults: Female:

- Prevention of endometrial hyperplasia (in postmenopausal women with a uterus who are receiving daily conjugated estrogen tablets): 200 mg as a single daily dose every evening for 12 days sequentially per 28-day cycle
- Amenorrhea: 400 mg every evening for 10 days

Intravaginal gel: Adults: Female:

- ART in women who require progesterone supplementation: 90 mg (8% gel) once daily; if pregnancy occurs, may continue treatment for up to 10-12 weeks
- ART in women with partial or complete ovarian failure: 90 mg (8% gel) intravaginally twice daily; if pregnancy occurs, may continue up to 10-12 weeks
- Secondary amenorrhea: 45 mg (4% gel) intravaginally every other day for up to 6 doses; women who fail to respond may be increased to 90 mg (8% gel) every other day for up to 6 doses

Mechanism of Action Natural steroid hormone that induces secretory changes in the endometrium, promotes mammary gland development, relaxes uterine smooth muscle, blocks follicular maturation and ovulation, and maintains pregnancy

Other Adverse Effects Frequency not defined:

Intrauterine device:

- Cardiovascular: Bradycardia and syncope (secondary to insertion)
- Central nervous system: Pain
- Endocrine & metabolic: Amenorrhea, delayed menses, dysmenorrhea, ectopic pregnancy, endometritis, pregnancy, septic abortion, prolonged menstrual flow, spontaneous abortion, spotting
- Genitourinary: Cervical erosion, dyspareunia, leukorrhea, pelvic infection, tubal damage, tubo-ovarian abscess, vaginitis
- Hematologic: Anemia
- Local: Embedment or fragmentation of the IUD, perforation of uterus and cervix
- Neuromuscular & skeletal: Backache
- Miscellaneous: Abscess formation and erosion of adjacent area, abdominal adhesions, complete or partial IUD expulsion, congenital anomalies, cramping, cystic masses in the pelvis, death, difficult removal, fetal damage, hormonal

(Continued)

Progesterone *(Continued)*

imbalance, intestinal penetration, intestinal obstruction, local inflammatory reaction, loss of fertility, peritonitis, septicemia

Injection (I.M.):

Cardiovascular: Edema

Central nervous system: Depression, fever, insomnia, somnolence

Dermatologic: Acne, allergic rash (rare), alopecia, hirsutism, pruritus, rash, urticaria

Endocrine & metabolic: Amenorrhea, breakthrough bleeding, breast tenderness, galactorrhea, menstrual flow changes, spotting

Gastrointestinal: Nausea, weight gain, weight loss

Genitourinary: Cervical erosion changes, cervical secretion changes

Hepatic: Cholestatic jaundice

Local: Pain at the injection site

Miscellaneous: Anaphylactoid reactions

Oral capsule:

>10%:

Central nervous system: Dizziness (16%)

Endocrine & metabolic: Breast pain (11%)

5% to 10%:

Central nervous system: Headache (10%), fatigue (7%), emotional lability (6%), irritability (5%)

Gastrointestinal: Abdominal pain (10%), abdominal distention (6%)

Neuromuscular & skeletal: Musculoskeletal pain (6%)

Respiratory: Upper respiratory tract infection (5%)

Miscellaneous: Viral infection (7%)

<5%: Dry mouth, accidental injury, chest pain, fever, hypertension, confusion, somnolence, speech disorder, constipation, dyspepsia, gastroenteritis, hemorrhagic rectum, hiatus hernia, vomiting, earache, palpitation, edema, arthritis, leg cramps, hypertonia, muscle disorder, myalgia, angina pectoris, anxiety, impaired concentration, insomnia, personality disorder, leukorrhea, uterine fibroid, vaginal dryness, fungal vaginitis, vaginitis, abscess, herpes simplex, bronchitis, nasal congestion, pharyngitis, pneumonitis, sinusitis, acne, verruca, urinary tract infection, abnormal vision, lymphadenopathy

Drug Interactions CYP2C19, 3A3/4, and 3A4/5 enzyme substrate

Increased Effect/Toxicity: Ketoconazole may increase the bioavailability of progesterone. Progesterone may increase concentrations of estrogenic compounds during concurrent therapy with conjugated estrogens.

Decreased Effect: Aminoglutethimide may decrease effect by increasing hepatic metabolism.

Drug Uptake

Duration: 24 hours

Half-life, elimination: 5 minutes

Time to peak: Oral: 1.5-2.3 hours

Pregnancy Risk Factor B (Prometrium®, per manufacturer); none established for gel (Crinone®), injection (contraindicated), or intrauterine device (contraindicated)

Generic Available Yes: Injection

Comments Capsules contain peanut oil and are contraindicated in patients with allergy to peanuts. Capsules may cause some degree of fluid retention, use with caution in conditions which may be aggravated by this factor, including CHF, renal dysfunction, epilepsy, migraine, or asthma.

Proglycem® *see* Diazoxide *on page 375*

Prograf® *see* Tacrolimus *on page 1128*

ProHance® *see* Radiological/Contrast Media (Nonionic) *on page 1039*

Prolastin® *see* $Alpha_1$-Proteinase Inhibitor *on page 56*

Proleukin® *see* Aldesleukin *on page 47*

Prolixin® *see* Fluphenazine *on page 520*

Prolixin Decanoate® *see* Fluphenazine *on page 520*

Prolixin Enanthate® *see* Fluphenazine *on page 520*

Proloprim® *see* Trimethoprim *on page 1210*

Promazine (PROE ma zeen)

U.S. Brand Names Sparine®

Canadian Brand Names Sparine®

Pharmacologic Category Antipsychotic Agent, Phenothiazine, Aliphatic

Synonyms Promazine Hydrochloride

Use Management of manifestations of psychotic disorders; depressive neurosis; alcohol withdrawal; nausea and vomiting; nonpsychotic symptoms associated with dementia in elderly, Tourette's syndrome; Huntington's chorea; spasmodic torticollis and Reye's syndrome

Unlabeled/Investigational: Preoperative sedation

Local Anesthetic/Vasoconstrictor Precautions Most pharmacology textbooks state that in presence of phenothiazines, systemic doses of epinephrine paradoxically decrease the blood pressure. This is the so called "epinephrine reversal" phenomenon. This has never been observed when epinephrine is given by infiltration as part of the anesthesia procedure.

Effects on Dental Treatment

Significant hypotension may occur, especially when the drug is administered parenterally; orthostatic hypotension is due to alpha-receptor blockade, the elderly are at greater risk for orthostatic hypotension.

Tardive dyskinesia: Prevalence rate may be 40% in elderly; development of the syndrome and the irreversible nature are proportional to duration and total cumulative dose over time. Extrapyramidal reactions are more common in elderly with up to 50% developing these reactions after 60 years of age; drug-induced **Parkinson's syndrome** occurs often; **Akathisia** is the most common extrapyramidal reaction in elderly.

Increased confusion, memory loss, psychotic behavior, and agitation frequently occur as a consequence of anticholinergic effects. Antipsychotic associated sedation in nonpsychotic patients is extremely unpleasant due to feelings of depersonalization, derealization, and dysphoria

Dosage Oral, I.M.:

Children >12 years: Antipsychotic: 10-25 mg every 4-6 hours

Adults:

Psychosis: 10-200 mg every 4-6 hours not to exceed 1000 mg/day

Antiemetic: 25-50 mg every 4-6 hours as needed

Mechanism of Action Blocks postsynaptic mesolimbic dopaminergic D_1 and D_2 receptors in the brain; exhibits a strong alpha-adrenergic blocking and anticholinergic effect, depresses the release of hypothalamic and hypophyseal hormones; believed to depress the reticular activating system thus affecting basal metabolism, body temperature, wakefulness, vasomotor tone, and emesis

Other Adverse Effects Frequency not defined:

Cardiovascular: Postural hypotension, tachycardia, dizziness, nonspecific QT changes

Central nervous system: Drowsiness, dystonias, akathisia, pseudoparkinsonism, tardive dyskinesia, neuroleptic malignant syndrome, seizures

Dermatologic: Photosensitivity, dermatitis, skin pigmentation (slate gray)

Endocrine & metabolic: Lactation, breast engorgement, false-positive pregnancy test, amenorrhea, gynecomastia, hyper- or hypoglycemia

Gastrointestinal: Xerostomia, constipation, nausea

Genitourinary: Urinary retention, ejaculatory disorder, impotence

Hematologic: Agranulocytosis, eosinophilia, leukopenia, hemolytic anemia, aplastic anemia, thrombocytopenic purpura

Hepatic: Jaundice

Ocular: Blurred vision, corneal and lenticular changes, epithelial keratopathy, pigmentary retinopathy

Drug Interactions

Aluminum salts: May decrease the absorption of phenothiazines; monitor

Amphetamines: Efficacy may be diminished by antipsychotics; in addition, amphetamines may increase psychotic symptoms; avoid concurrent use

Anticholinergics: May inhibit the therapeutic response to phenothiazines and excess anticholinergic effects may occur; includes benztropine, trihexyphenidyl, biperiden, and drugs with significant anticholinergic activity (TCAs, antihistamines, disopyramide)

Antihypertensives: Concurrent use of phenothiazines with an antihypertensive may produce additive hypotensive effects (particularly orthostasis)

Bromocriptine: Phenothiazines inhibit the ability of bromocriptine to lower serum prolactin concentrations

CNS depressants: Sedative effects may be additive with phenothiazines; monitor for increased effect; includes barbiturates, benzodiazepines, narcotic analgesics, ethanol, and other sedative agents

CYP2D6 inhibitors: Metabolism of phenothiazines may be decreased; increasing clinical effect or toxicity; inhibitors include amiodarone, cimetidine, delavirdine, fluoxetine, paroxetine, propafenone, quinidine, and ritonavir; monitor for increased effect/toxicity

Enzyme inducers: May enhance the hepatic metabolism of phenothiazines; larger doses may be required; includes rifampin, rifabutin, barbiturates, phenytoin, and cigarette smoking

Epinephrine: Chlorpromazine (and possibly other low potency antipsychotics) may diminish the pressor effects of epinephrine

Guanethidine and guanadrel: Antihypertensive effects may be inhibited by phenothiazines

Levodopa: Phenothiazines may inhibit the antiparkinsonian effect of levodopa; avoid this combination

Lithium: Phenothiazines may produce neurotoxicity with lithium; this is a rare effect

Metoclopramide: May increase extrapyramidal symptoms (EPS) or risk.

(Continued)

Promazine *(Continued)*

Phenytoin: May reduce serum levels of phenothiazines; phenothiazines may increase phenytoin serum levels

Propranolol: Serum concentrations of phenothiazines may be increased; propranolol also increases phenothiazine concentrations

Polypeptide antibiotics: Rare cases of respiratory paralysis have been reported with concurrent use of phenothiazines

QT_c-prolonging agents: Effects on QT_c interval may be additive with phenothiazines, increasing the risk of malignant arrhythmias; includes type Ia antiarrhythmics, TCAs, and some quinolone antibiotics (sparfloxacin, moxifloxacin, and gatifloxacin)

Sulfadoxine-pyrimethamine: May increase phenothiazine concentrations

Tricyclic antidepressants: Concurrent use may produce increased toxicity or altered therapeutic response

Trazodone: Phenothiazines and trazodone may produce additive hypotensive effects

Valproic acid: Serum levels may be increased by phenothiazines

Drug Uptake The specific pharmacokinetics of promazine are poorly established but probably resemble those of other phenothiazines.

Absorption: Partial; great variability in plasma levels resulting from a given dose

Half-life, elimination: ≥24 hours

Pregnancy Risk Factor C

Generic Available No

Promethazine (proe METH a zeen)

U.S. Brand Names Anergan®; Phenergan®

Canadian Brand Names Phenergan®

Pharmacologic Category Antiemetic

Synonyms Promethazine Hydrochloride

Use Symptomatic treatment of various allergic conditions, antiemetic, motion sickness, and as a sedative

Local Anesthetic/Vasoconstrictor Precautions Most pharmacology textbooks state that in presence of phenothiazines, systemic doses of epinephrine paradoxically decrease the blood pressure. This is the so called "epinephrine reversal" phenomenon. This has never been observed when epinephrine is given by infiltration as part of the anesthesia procedure.

Effects on Dental Treatment

Significant hypotension may occur, especially when the drug is administered parenterally; orthostatic hypotension is due to alpha-receptor blockade, the elderly are at greater risk for orthostatic hypotension.

Tardive dyskinesia: Prevalence rate may be 40% in elderly; development of the syndrome and the irreversible nature are proportional to duration and total cumulative dose over time. Extrapyramidal reactions are more common in elderly with up to 50% developing these reactions after 60 years of age; drug-induced **Parkinson's syndrome** occurs often; **akathisia** is the most common extrapyramidal reaction in elderly.

Increased confusion, memory loss, psychotic behavior, and agitation frequently occur as a consequence of anticholinergic effects. Antipsychotic associated sedation in nonpsychotic patients is extremely unpleasant due to feelings of depersonalization, derealization, and dysphoria.

Dosage

Children:

- Antihistamine: Oral, rectal: 0.1 mg/kg/dose every 6 hours during the day and 0.5 mg/kg/dose at bedtime as needed
- Antiemetic: Oral, I.M., I.V., rectal: 0.25-1 mg/kg 4-6 times/day as needed
- Motion sickness: Oral, rectal: 0.5 mg/kg/dose 30 minutes to 1 hour before departure, then every 12 hours as needed
- Sedation: Oral, I.M., I.V., rectal: 0.5-1 mg/kg/dose every 6 hours as needed

Adults:

- Antihistamine (including allergic reactions to blood or plasma):
  - Oral, rectal: 12.5 mg 3 times/day and 25 mg at bedtime
  - I.M., I.V.: 25 mg, may repeat in 2 hours when necessary; switch to oral route as soon as feasible
- Antiemetic: Oral, I.M., I.V., rectal: 12.5-25 mg every 4 hours as needed
- Motion sickness: Oral, rectal: 25 mg 30-60 minutes before departure, then every 12 hours as needed
- Sedation: Oral, I.M., I.V., rectal: 25-50 mg/dose

Mechanism of Action Blocks postsynaptic mesolimbic dopaminergic receptors in the brain; exhibits a strong alpha-adrenergic blocking effect and depresses the release of hypothalamic and hypophyseal hormones; competes with histamine for the H_1-receptor; reduces stimuli to the brainstem reticular system

Other Adverse Effects Frequency not defined:

Cardiovascular: Postural hypotension, tachycardia, dizziness, nonspecific QT changes

Central nervous system: Drowsiness, dystonias, akathisia, pseudoparkinsonism, tardive dyskinesia, neuroleptic malignant syndrome, seizures
Dermatologic: Photosensitivity, dermatitis, skin pigmentation (slate gray)
Endocrine & metabolic: Lactation, breast engorgement, false-positive pregnancy test, amenorrhea, gynecomastia, hyper- or hypoglycemia
Gastrointestinal: Xerostomia, constipation, nausea
Genitourinary: Urinary retention, ejaculatory disorder, impotence
Hematologic: Agranulocytosis, eosinophilia, leukopenia, hemolytic anemia, aplastic anemia, thrombocytopenic purpura
Hepatic: Jaundice
Ocular: Blurred vision, corneal and lenticular changes, epithelial keratopathy, pigmentary retinopathy

Drug Interactions CYP2D6 enzyme substrate

Increased Effect/Toxicity: Chloroquine, propranolol, and sulfadoxine-pyrimethamine also may increase promethazine concentrations. Concurrent use with TCA may produce increased toxicity or altered therapeutic response. Promethazine plus lithium may rarely produce neurotoxicity. Concurrent use of promethazine and CNS depressants (narcotics) may produce additive depressant effects.

Decreased Effect: Barbiturates and carbamazepine may increase the metabolism of promethazine, lowering its serum concentration. Benztropine (and other anticholinergics) may inhibit the therapeutic response to promethazine. Promethazine may inhibit the ability of bromocriptine to lower serum prolactin concentrations. The antihypertensive effects of guanethidine and guanadrel may be inhibited by promethazine. Promethazine may inhibit the antiparkinsonian effect of levodopa. Promethazine (and possibly other low potency antipsychotics) may reverse the pressor effects of epinephrine.

Drug Uptake

Onset of action: I.V.: ≤20 minutes; I.V. injection: 3-5 minutes
Duration: 2-6 hours

Pregnancy Risk Factor C

Generic Available Yes

Promethazine and Codeine (proe METH a zeen & KOE deen)

U.S. Brand Names Phenergan® With Codeine; Prothazine-DC®

Pharmacologic Category Antihistamine/Antitussive

Synonyms Codeine and Promethazine

Use Temporary relief of coughs and upper respiratory symptoms associated with allergy or the common cold

Local Anesthetic/Vasoconstrictor Precautions No information available to require special precautions

Effects on Dental Treatment Although promethazine is a phenothiazine derivative, extrapyramidal reactions or tardive dyskinesias are not seen with the use of this drug.

Restrictions C-V

Dosage Oral (in terms of codeine):

Children: 1-1.5 mg/kg/day every 4 hours as needed; maximum: 30 mg/day **or**
- 2-6 years: 1.25-2.5 mL every 4-6 hours or 2.5-5 mg/dose every 4-6 hours as needed; maximum: 30 mg codeine/day
- 6-12 years: 2.5-5 mL every 4-6 hours as needed or 5-10 mg/dose every 4-6 hours as needed; maximum: 60 mg codeine/day

Adults: 10-20 mg/dose every 4-6 hours as needed; maximum: 120 mg codeine/day; or 5-10 mL every 4-6 hours as needed

Drug Uptake See Promethazine *on page 1006* and Codeine *on page 317*

Pregnancy Risk Factor C

Generic Available Yes

Promethazine and Dextromethorphan

(proe METH a zeen & deks troe meth OR fan)

U.S. Brand Names Phenameth® DM; Phenergan® With Dextromethorphan

Canadian Brand Names Promatussin® DM

Pharmacologic Category Antihistamine/Antitussive

Synonyms Dextromethorphan and Promethazine

Use Temporary relief of coughs and upper respiratory symptoms associated with allergy or the common cold

Local Anesthetic/Vasoconstrictor Precautions No information available to require special precautions

Effects on Dental Treatment Although promethazine is a phenothiazine derivative, extrapyramidal reactions or tardive dyskinesias are not seen with the use of this drug.

Dosage Oral:

Children:
- 2-6 years: 1.25-2.5 mL every 4-6 hours up to 10 mL in 24 hours
- 6-12 years: 2.5-5 mL every 4-6 hours up to 20 mL in 24 hours

Adults: 5 mL every 4-6 hours up to 30 mL in 24 hours

(Continued)

Promethazine and Dextromethorphan *(Continued)*

Warnings/Precautions Research on chicken embryos exposed to concentrations of dextromethorphan relative to those typically taken by humans has shown to cause birth defects and fetal death; more study is needed, but it is suggested that pregnant women should be advised not to use dextromethorphan-containing medications

Drug Uptake See Promethazine *on page 1006* and Dextromethorphan *on page 372*

Pregnancy Risk Factor C

Generic Available Yes

Promethazine and Phenylephrine

(proe METH a zeen & fen il EF rin)

U.S. Brand Names Phenergan® VC; Promethazine VC; Promethazine VC Plain; Prometh VC Plain

Pharmacologic Category Antihistamine/Decongestant Combination

Synonyms Phenylephrine and Promethazine

Use Temporary relief of upper respiratory symptoms associated with allergy or the common cold

Local Anesthetic/Vasoconstrictor Precautions

Phenylephrine: Use with caution since phenylephrine is a sympathomimetic amine which could interact with epinephrine to cause a pressor response

Promethazine: No information available to require special precautions

Effects on Dental Treatment

Phenylephrine: ≤10%: Tachycardia, palpitations, xerostomia; use vasoconstrictor with caution

Although promethazine is a phenothiazine derivative, extrapyramidal reactions or tardive dyskinesias are not seen with the use of this drug.

Dosage Oral:

Children:
- 2-6 years: 1.25 mL every 4-6 hours, not to exceed 7.5 mL in 24 hours
- 6-12 years: 2.5 mL every 4-6 hours, not to exceed 15 mL in 24 hours

Children >12 years and Adults: 5 mL every 4-6 hours, not to exceed 30 mL in 24 hours

Drug Uptake See Promethazine *on page 1006* and Phenylephrine *on page 950*

Pregnancy Risk Factor C

Generic Available Yes

Promethazine, Phenylephrine, and Codeine

(proe METH a zeen, fen il EF rin, & KOE deen)

U.S. Brand Names Phenergan® VC With Codeine; Promethist® With Codeine; Prometh® VC With Codeine

Pharmacologic Category Antihistamine/Decongestant/Antitussive

Synonyms Codeine, Promethazine, and Phenylephrine; Phenylephrine, Promethazine, and Codeine

Use Temporary relief of coughs and upper respiratory symptoms including nasal congestion

Local Anesthetic/Vasoconstrictor Precautions

Phenylephrine: Use with caution since phenylephrine is a sympathomimetic amine which could interact with epinephrine to cause a pressor response

Promethazine: No information available to require special precautions

Effects on Dental Treatment

Phenylephrine: ≤10%: Tachycardia, palpitations, xerostomia; use vasoconstrictor with caution

Although promethazine is a phenothiazine derivative, extrapyramidal reactions or tardive dyskinesias are not seen with the use of this drug.

Restrictions C-V

Dosage Oral:

Children (expressed in terms of codeine dosage): 1-1.5 mg/kg/day every 4 hours, maximum: 30 mg/day **or**
- <2 years: Not recommended
- 2 to 6 years:
  - Weight 25 lb: 1.25-2.5 mL every 4-6 hours, not to exceed 6 mL/24 hours
  - Weight 30 lb: 1.25-2.5 mL every 4-6 hours, not to exceed 7 mL/24 hours
  - Weight 35 lb: 1.25-2.5 mL every 4-6 hours, not to exceed 8 mL/24 hours
  - Weight 40 lb: 1.25-2.5 mL every 4-6 hours, not to exceed 9 mL/24 hours
- 6 to <12 years: 2.5-5 mL every 4-6 hours, not to exceed 15 mL/24 hours

Adults: 5 mL every 4-6 hours, not to exceed 30 mL/24 hours

Drug Uptake See Promethazine *on page 1006*, Phenylephrine *on page 950* and Codeine *on page 317*

Pregnancy Risk Factor C

Generic Available Yes

Promethazine VC *see* Promethazine and Phenylephrine *on page 1008*

Promethazine VC Plain *see* Promethazine and Phenylephrine *on page 1008*

Promethist® With Codeine *see* Promethazine, Phenylephrine, and Codeine *on page 1008*

Prometh VC Plain *see* Promethazine and Phenylephrine *on page 1008*

Prometh® VC With Codeine *see* Promethazine, Phenylephrine, and Codeine *on page 1008*

Prometrium® *see* Progesterone *on page 1003*

Promit® *see* Dextran 1 *on page 369*

Pronap-100® *see* Propoxyphene and Acetaminophen *on page 1013*

Pronestyl® *see* Procainamide *on page 997*

Pronestyl-SR® *see* Procainamide *on page 997*

Pronto® [OTC] *see* Pyrethrins *on page 1026*

Propafenone (proe pa FEEN one)

Related Information

Cardiovascular Diseases *on page 1308*

U.S. Brand Names Rythmol®

Canadian Brand Names Rythmol®

Mexican Brand Names Nistaken®; Norfenon®

Pharmacologic Category Antiarrhythmic Agent, Class Ic

Synonyms Propafenone Hydrochloride

Use Life-threatening ventricular arrhythmias

Unlabeled/Investigational: Supraventricular tachycardias, including those patients with Wolff-Parkinson-White syndrome

Local Anesthetic/Vasoconstrictor Precautions No information available to require special precautions

Effects on Dental Treatment >10%: Significant xerostomia; normal salivary flow resumes with discontinuation

Dosage Adults: Oral: 150 mg every 8 hours, increase at 3- to 4-day intervals up to 300 mg every 8 hours. **Note:** Patients who exhibit significant widening of QRS complex or second or third degree A-V block may need dose reduction.

Mechanism of Action Propafenone is a 1C antiarrhythmic agent which possesses local anesthetic properties, blocks the fast inward sodium current, and slows the rate of increase of the action potential. prolongs conduction and refractoriness in all areas of the myocardium, with a slightly more pronounced effect on intraventricular conduction; it prolongs effective refractory period, reduces spontaneous automaticity and exhibits some beta-blockade activity.

Other Adverse Effects

1% to 10%:

Cardiovascular: New or worsened arrhythmias (proarrhythmic effect) (2% to 10%), angina (2% to 5%), CHF (1% to 4%), ventricular tachycardia (1% to 3%), palpitations (1% to 3%), AV block (first-degree) (1% to 3%), syncope (1% to 2%), increased QRS interval (1% to 2%), chest pain (1% to 2%), PVCs (1% to 2%), bradycardia (1% to 2%), edema (0% to 1%), bundle branch block (0% to 1%), atrial fibrillation (1%), hypotension (0% to 1%), intraventricular conduction delay (0% to 1%)

Central nervous system: Dizziness (4% to 15%), fatigue (2% to 6%), headache (2% to 5%), weakness (1% to 2%), ataxia (0% to 2%), insomnia (0% to 2%), anxiety (1% to 2%), drowsiness (1%)

Dermatologic: Rash (1% to 3%)

Gastrointestinal: Nausea/vomiting (2% to 11%), unusual taste (3% to 23%), constipation (2% to 7%), dyspepsia (1% to 3%), diarrhea (1% to 3%), xerostomia (1% to 2%), anorexia (1% to 2%), abdominal pain (1% to 2%), flatulence (0% to 1%)

Neuromuscular & skeletal: Tremor (0% to 1%), arthralgia (0% to 1%)

Ocular: Blurred vision (1% to 6%)

Respiratory: Dyspnea (2% to 5%)

Miscellaneous: Diaphoresis (1%)

Drug Interactions CYP1A2, 2D6, 3A3/4 enzyme substrate; CYP2D6 enzyme inhibitor

Increased Effect/Toxicity: Amprenavir, cimetidine, metoprolol, propranolol, quinidine, and ritonavir may increase propafenone levels; concurrent use is contraindicated. Digoxin (reduce dose by 25%), cyclosporine, local anesthetics, theophylline, and warfarin blood levels are increased by propafenone.

Decreased Effect: Enzyme inducers (phenobarbital, phenytoin, rifabutin, rifampin) may decrease propafenone blood levels.

Drug Uptake

Absorption: Well absorbed

Half-life, elimination: Single dose (100-300 mg): 2-8 hours; Chronic dosing: 10-32 hours

Time to peak: 2 hours (150 mg); 3 hours (300 mg)

Pregnancy Risk Factor C

Generic Available No

Propantheline (proe PAN the leen)

Canadian Brand Names Propanthel™

Pharmacologic Category Anticholinergic Agent

Synonyms Propantheline Bromide

Use

Dental: Induce dry field (xerostomia) in oral cavity

Medical: Adjunctive treatment of peptic ulcer, irritable bowel syndrome, pancreatitis, ureteral and urinary bladder spasm; reduce duodenal motility during diagnostic radiologic procedures

Local Anesthetic/Vasoconstrictor Precautions No information available to require special precautions

Effects on Dental Treatment >10%: Significant xerostomia (therapeutic effect)

Dosage Adults: 15-30 mg as a single dose to induce xerostomia 1 hour before procedure

Mechanism of Action Competitively blocks the action of acetylcholine at postganglionic parasympathetic receptor sites

Other Adverse Effects Frequency not defined:

Dermatologic: Dry skin

Gastrointestinal: Constipation, xerostomia, dry throat, dysphagia

Respiratory: Dry nose

Miscellaneous: Diaphoresis (decreased)

Contraindications Hypersensitivity to propantheline or any component of the formulation; ulcerative colitis; toxic megacolon; obstructive disease of the GI or urinary tract; narrow-angle glaucoma

Warnings/Precautions Use with caution in patients with hyperthyroidism, hepatic, cardiac, or renal disease, hypertension, GI infections, or other endocrine diseases

Drug Interactions

Increased effect/toxicity with anticholinergics, disopyramide, narcotic analgesics, bretylium, type I antiarrhythmics, antihistamines, phenothiazines, TCAs, corticosteroids (increased IOP), CNS depressants (sedation), adenosine, amiodarone, beta-blockers, amoxapine

Decreased effect with antacids (decreased absorption); decreased effect of sustained release dosage forms (decreased absorption)

Dietary/Ethanol/Herb Considerations Food: Administer 30 minutes before meals to ensure peak effect occurs at the proper time.

Drug Uptake

Onset of action: 30-45 minutes

Duration: 4-6 hours

Half-life, elimination: 1.6 hours (average)

Pregnancy Risk Factor C

Dosage Forms **TAB:** 15 mg

Generic Available Yes

Proparacaine (proe PAR a kane)

U.S. Brand Names Alcaine®; Ophthetic®; Parcaine®

Canadian Brand Names Alcaine®; Diocaine®

Pharmacologic Category Local Anesthetic, Ophthalmic

Synonyms Proparacaine Hydrochloride; Proxymetacaine

Use Anesthesia for tonometry, gonioscopy; suture removal from cornea; removal of corneal foreign body; cataract extraction, glaucoma surgery; short operative procedure involving the cornea and conjunctiva

Local Anesthetic/Vasoconstrictor Precautions No information available to require special precautions

Effects on Dental Treatment No effects or complications reported

Dosage Children and Adults:

Ophthalmic surgery: Instill 1 drop of 0.5% solution in eye every 5-10 minutes for 5-7 doses

Tonometry, gonioscopy, suture removal: Instill 1-2 drops of 0.5% solution in eye just prior to procedure

Mechanism of Action Prevents initiation and transmission of impulse at the nerve cell membrane by decreasing ion permeability through stabilizing

Other Adverse Effects 1% to 10%: Local: Burning, stinging, redness

Drug Interactions Effects of phenylephrine and tropicamide (ophthalmics) are increased.

Drug Uptake

Onset of action: ≤20 seconds

Duration: 15-20 minutes

Pregnancy Risk Factor C

Generic Available Yes

Proparacaine and Fluorescein (proe PAR a kane & FLURE e seen)

U.S. Brand Names Fluoracaine®

Pharmacologic Category Diagnostic Agent; Local Anesthetic

Use Anesthesia for tonometry, gonioscopy; suture removal from cornea; removal of corneal foreign body; cataract extraction, glaucoma surgery

Local Anesthetic/Vasoconstrictor Precautions No information available to require special precautions

Effects on Dental Treatment No effects or complications reported

Dosage

Ophthalmic surgery: Children and Adults: Instill 1 drop in each eye every 5-10 minutes for 5-7 doses

Tonometry, gonioscopy, suture removal: Adults: Instill 1-2 drops in each eye just prior to procedure

Mechanism of Action Prevents initiation and transmission of impulse at the nerve cell membrane by decreasing ion permeability through stabilizing

Other Adverse Effects 1% to 10%: Local: Burning, stinging of eye

Drug Uptake

Onset of action: ≤20 seconds

Duration: 15-20 minutes

Pregnancy Risk Factor C

Generic Available Yes

Propecia® *see* Finasteride *on page 503*

Propine® *see* Dipivefrin *on page 401*

Proplex® T *see* Factor IX Complex (Human) *on page 484*

Propofol (PROE po fole)

U.S. Brand Names Diprivan®

Canadian Brand Names Diprivan®

Mexican Brand Names Diprivan®; Fresofol®; Recofol®

Pharmacologic Category General Anesthetic

Use Induction of anesthesia for inpatient or outpatient surgery in patients ≥3 years of age; maintenance of anesthesia for inpatient or outpatient surgery in patients >2 months of age; in adults, for the induction and maintenance of monitored anesthesia care sedation during diagnostic procedures; may be used (for patients >18 years of age who are intubated and mechanically ventilated) as an alternative to benzodiazepines for the treatment of agitation in the intensive care unit

Unlabeled/Investigational: Postoperative antiemetic; refractory delirium tremens (case reports)

Local Anesthetic/Vasoconstrictor Precautions No information available to require special precautions

Effects on Dental Treatment No effects or complications reported

Dosage Dosage must be individualized based on total body weight and titrated to the desired clinical effect; wait at least 3-5 minutes between dosage adjustments to clinically assess drug effects; smaller doses are required when used with narcotics; the following are general dosing guidelines:

General anesthesia:

Induction: I.V.:

- Children 3-16 years, ASA I or II: 2.5-3.5 mg/kg over 20-30 seconds; use a lower dose for children ASA III or IV
- Adults, ASA I or II, <55 years: 2-2.5 mg/kg (~40 mg every 10 seconds until onset of induction)
- Elderly, debilitated, hypovolemic, or ASA III or IV: 1-1.5 mg/kg (~20 mg every 10 seconds until onset of induction)
- Cardiac anesthesia: 0.5-1.5 mg/kg (~20 mg every 10 seconds until onset of induction)
- Neurosurgical patients: 1-2 mg/kg (~20 mg every 10 seconds until onset of induction)

Maintenance: I.V. infusion:

- Children 2 months to 16 years, ASA I or II: Initial: 200-300 mcg/kg/minute; decrease dose after 30 minutes if clinical signs of light anesthesia are absent; usual infusion rate: 125-150 mcg/kg/minute (range: 125-300 mcg/kg/minute; 7.5-18 mg/kg/hour); children ≤5 years may require larger infusion rates compared to older children
- Adults, ASA I or II, <55 years: Initial: 150-200 mcg/kg/minute for 10-15 minutes; decrease by 30% to 50% during first 30 minutes of maintenance; usual infusion rate: 100-200 mcg/kg/minute (6-12 mg/kg/hour)
- Elderly, debilitated, hypovolemic, ASA III or IV: 50-100 mcg/kg/minute (3-6 mg/kg/ hour)
- Cardiac anesthesia:
  - Low-dose propofol with primary opioid: 50-100 mcg/kg/minute (see manufacturer's labeling)
  - Primary propofol with secondary opioid: 100-150 mcg/kg/minute
- Neurosurgical patients: 100-200 mcg/kg/minute (6-12 mg/kg/hour)

Maintenance: I.V. intermittent bolus: Adults, ASA I or II, <55 years: 20-50 mg increments as needed

(Continued)

Propofol *(Continued)*

Monitored anesthesia care sedation:

Initiation:

Adults, ASA I or II, <55 years: Slow I.V. infusion: 100-150 mcg/kg/minute for 3-5 minutes **or** slow injection: 0.5 mg/kg over 3-5 minutes

Elderly, debilitated, neurosurgical, or ASA III or IV patients: Use similar doses to healthy adults; avoid rapid I.V. boluses

Maintenance:

Adults, ASA I or II, <55 years: I.V. infusion using variable rates (preferred over intermittent boluses): 25-75 mcg/kg/minute **or** incremental bolus doses: 10 mg or 20 mg

Elderly, debilitated, neurosurgical, or ASA III or IV patients: Use 80% of healthy adult dose; **do not** use rapid bolus doses (single or repeated)

ICU sedation in intubated mechanically-ventilated patients: Avoid rapid bolus injection; individualize dose and titrate to response

Adults: Continuous infusion: Initial: 0.3 mg/kg/hour; increase by 0.3-0.6 mg/kg/hour every 5-10 minutes until desired sedation level is achieved; usual maintenance: 0.3-3 mg/kg/hour or higher; reduce dose by 80% in elderly, debilitated, and ASA III or IV patients; reduce dose after adequate sedation established and adjust to response (ie, evaluate frequently to use minimum dose for sedation)

Mechanism of Action Propofol is a hindered phenolic compound with I.V. general anesthetic properties. The drug is unrelated to any of the currently used barbiturate, opioid, benzodiazepine, arylcyclohexylamine, or imidazole I.V. anesthetic agents.

Other Adverse Effects

>10%:

Cardiovascular: Hypotension (3% to 26% adults, 17% children)

Central nervous system: Movement (17% children)

Local: Injection site burning, stinging, or pain (adults 18%, children 10%)

Respiratory: Apnea, lasting 30-60 seconds (24% adults, 10% children); Apnea, lasting >60 seconds (12% adults, 5% children)

3% to 10%:

Cardiovascular: Hypertension (8% children)

Central nervous system: Movement (adults)

Dermatologic: Pruritus (adults), rash

Endocrine & metabolic: Hyperlipidemia

Respiratory: Respiratory acidosis during weaning

1% to 3%:

Cardiovascular: Arrhythmia, bradycardia, decreased cardiac output, tachycardia

Dermatologic: Pruritus (children)

Contraindications

Absolute contraindications: hypersensitivity to propofol or any component of the formulation; patients who are not intubated or mechanically ventilated; pregnancy or nursing; when general anesthesia or sedation is contraindicated

Relative contraindications: Pediatric intensive care unit patients (safety and efficacy not established); severe cardiac disease (ejection fraction <50%) or respiratory disease (may cause more profound adverse cardiovascular responses); history of epilepsy or seizures (risk of seizure during recovery phase); increased intracranial pressure or impaired cerebral circulation (substantial decreases in mean arterial pressure and subsequent decreases in cerebral perfusion pressure may occur); hyperlipidemia (as evidenced by increased serum triglyceride levels or serum turbidity); hypotension, hypovolemia, hemodynamically instability or abnormally low vascular tone (eg, sepsis)

Warnings/Precautions Use slower rate of induction and avoid rapid bolus administration in the elderly, debilitated, or ASA III/IV patients; transient local pain may occur during I.V. injection; perioperative myoclonia has occurred; do not administer with blood or blood products through the same I.V. catheter; not for obstetrics, including cesarean section deliveries. Abrupt discontinuation prior to weaning or daily wake up assessments should be avoided. Abrupt discontinuation can result in rapid awakening, anxiety, agitation, and resistance to mechanical ventilation. Pain should be treated with analgesic agents, propofol must be titrated separately from the analgesic agent. Several deaths associated with severe metabolic acidosis have been reported in pediatric ICU patients on long-term propofol infusion. Concurrent use of fentanyl and propofol in pediatric patients may result in bradycardia. Propofol emulsion contains soybean oil, egg phosphatide, and glycerol.

Drug Interactions

Increased Toxicity:

Neuromuscular blockers: Atracurium: Anaphylactoid reactions (including bronchospasm) have been reported in patients who have received concomitant atracurium and propofol. Vecuronium: Propofol may potentiate the neuromuscular blockade of vecuronium.

Central nervous system depressants: Additive CNS depression and respiratory depression may necessitate dosage reduction when used with anesthetics, benzodiazepines, opiates, narcotics, or phenothiazines.

Decreased Effect: Theophylline may antagonize the effect of propofol, requiring dosage increases.

Drug Uptake

Onset of action: Anesthetic: Bolus infusion (dose-dependent): 9-51 seconds (average 30 seconds)

Duration (dose- and rate-dependent): 3-10 minutes

Half-life, elimination (biphasic): Initial: 40 minutes; Terminal: 4-7 hours (1-3 days)

Pregnancy Risk Factor B

Generic Available Yes

Comments Formulated into an emulsion containing 10% w/v soybean oil, 1.2% w/v purified egg phosphatide, and 2.25% w/v glycerol; this emulsion vehicle is chemically similar to 10% Intralipid®

Injection contains EDTA as a preservative

Propoxyphene (proe POKS i feen)

U.S. Brand Names Darvon®; Darvon-N®

Canadian Brand Names Darvon-N®; 642® Tablet

Pharmacologic Category Analgesic, Narcotic

Synonyms Dextropropoxyphene; Propoxyphene Hydrochloride; Propoxyphene Napsylate

Use Management of mild to moderate pain

Local Anesthetic/Vasoconstrictor Precautions No information available to require special precautions

Effects on Dental Treatment No effects or complications reported

Restrictions C-IV

Dosage Oral:

Children: Doses for children are not well established; doses of the hydrochloride of 2-3 mg/kg/d divided every 6 hours have been used

Adults:

Hydrochloride: 65 mg every 3-4 hours as needed for pain; maximum: 390 mg/day

Napsylate: 100 mg every 4 hours as needed for pain; maximum: 600 mg/day

Mechanism of Action Weak narcotic analgesic which binds blocks pain perception in the cerebral cortex by binding to specific receptor molecules (opiate receptors) within the neuronal membranes of synapses; binding results in a decreased synaptic chemical transmission throughout the CNS thus inhibiting the flow of pain sensations into the higher centers. Mu and kappa are the two subtypes of the opiate receptor which propoxyphene binds to in order to cause analgesia.

Other Adverse Effects Frequency not defined:

Cardiovascular: Hypotension, bundle branch block

Central nervous system: Dizziness, lightheadedness, sedation, paradoxical excitement and insomnia, fatigue, drowsiness, mental depression, hallucinations, paradoxical CNS stimulation, increased intracranial pressure, nervousness, headache, restlessness, malaise, confusion

Dermatologic: Rash, urticaria

Endocrine & metabolic: May decrease glucose, urinary 17-OHCS

Gastrointestinal: Anorexia, stomach cramps, xerostomia, biliary spasm, nausea, vomiting, constipation, paralytic ileus

Genitourinary: Decreased urination, ureteral spasms

Neuromuscular & skeletal: Weakness

Hepatic: Increased liver enzymes (may increase LFTs)

Respiratory: Dyspnea

Miscellaneous: Psychologic and physical dependence with prolonged use, histamine release

Drug Interactions CYP2C9, 3A4, CYP3A5-7, and 3A7 enzyme inhibitor

Decreased effect with charcoal, cigarette smoking

Increased toxicity: CNS depressants may potentiate pharmacologic effects; propoxyphene may inhibit the metabolism and increase the serum concentrations of carbamazepine, phenobarbital, MAO inhibitors, tricyclic antidepressants, and warfarin

Drug Uptake

Onset of action: Oral: 0.5-1 hours

Duration: 4-6 hours

Half-life, elimination: Adults: Parent drug: 8-24 hours (mean: ~15 hours); Norpropoxyphene: 34 hours

Pregnancy Risk Factor C/D (prolonged use)

Generic Available Yes: Capsule

Propoxyphene and Acetaminophen

(proe POKS i feen & a seet a MIN oh fen)

U.S. Brand Names Darvocet-N® 50; Darvocet-N® 100; Pronap-100®; Wygesic®

Canadian Brand Names Darvocet-N® 50; Darvocet-N® 100

Pharmacologic Category Analgesic Combination (Narcotic)

Synonyms Propoxyphene Hydrochloride and Acetaminophen; Propoxyphene Napsylate and Acetaminophen

(Continued)

Propoxyphene and Acetaminophen *(Continued)*

Use

Dental: Management of postoperative pain

Medical: Relief of pain

Local Anesthetic/Vasoconstrictor Precautions No information available to require special precautions

Effects on Dental Treatment No effects or complications reported

Restrictions C-IV

Dosage

Children: Not recommended in pediatric dental patients

Adults:

Darvocet-N®: 1-2 tablets every 4 hours as needed; maximum: 600 mg propoxyphene napsylate/day

Darvocet-N® 100: 1 tablet every 4 hours as needed; maximum: 600 mg propoxyphene napsylate/day

Mechanism of Action Propoxyphene, a weak narcotic analgesic, blocks pain perception in the cerebral cortex by binding to specific receptor molecules (opiate receptors) within the neuronal membranes of synapses which results in a decreased synaptic chemical transmission throughout the CNS thus inhibiting the flow of pain sensations into the higher centers. Mu and kappa are the two subtypes of the opiate receptor which propoxyphene binds to cause analgesia.

Acetaminophen inhibits the synthesis of prostaglandins in the CNS and peripherally blocks pain impulse generation; produces antipyresis from inhibition of hypothalamic heat-regulating center

Other Adverse Effects Frequency not defined:

Based on **propoxyphene** component:

Cardiovascular: Hypotension

Central nervous system: Dizziness, lightheadedness, sedation, paradoxical excitement and insomnia, fatigue, drowsiness, mental depression, hallucinations, paradoxical CNS stimulation, increased intracranial pressure, nervousness, headache, restlessness, malaise, confusion

Dermatologic: Rash, urticaria

Endocrine & metabolic: May decrease glucose, urinary 17-OHCS

Gastrointestinal: Anorexia, stomach cramps, xerostomia, biliary spasm, nausea, vomiting, constipation, paralytic ileus

Genitourinary: Decreased urination, ureteral spasms

Neuromuscular & skeletal: Weakness

Hepatic: Increased liver enzymes (may increase LFTs)

Respiratory: Dyspnea

Miscellaneous: Psychologic and physical dependence with prolonged use, histamine release

Based on **acetaminophen** component: May increase chloride, bilirubin, uric acid, glucose, ammonia, alkaline phosphatase; may decrease sodium, bicarbonate, calcium

<1%: Rash, nausea, vomiting, blood dyscrasias (neutropenia, pancytopenia, leukopenia), anemia, analgesic nephropathy, nephrotoxicity with chronic overdose, hypersensitivity reactions (rare)

Contraindications Hypersensitivity to propoxyphene, acetaminophen, or any component of their formulation; G6PD deficiency

Warnings/Precautions When given in excessive doses, either alone or in combination with other CNS depressants, propoxyphene is a major cause of drug-related deaths; do not exceed recommended dosage; give with caution in patients dependent on opiates, substitution may result in acute opiate withdrawal symptoms

Drug Interactions

Increased toxicity with cimetidine, CNS depressants; increased toxicity/effect of carbamazepine, phenobarbital, TCAs, MAO inhibitors, benzodiazepines

Decreased effect with charcoal, cigarette smoking

Dietary/Ethanol/Herb Considerations Food: Administer on an empty stomach; glucose may cause hyperglycemia (monitor blood glucose concentrations).

Based on **propoxyphene** component:

Ethanol: Avoid or limit use; may increase CNS depression.

Food may decrease rate of absorption, but slightly increase bioavailability.

Based on **acetaminophen** component:

Ethanol: Excessive intake may increase the risk of acetaminophen-induced hepatotoxicity; avoid use or limit to <3 drinks/day.

Food may slightly delay absorption of extended-release preparations; rate of absorption may be decreased when given with food high in carbohydrates.

Herb/Nutraceutical: Avoid St John's wort; may decrease serum concentration.

Drug Uptake See Acetaminophen *on page 26* and Propoxyphene *on page 1013*

Pregnancy Risk Factor C

Breast-feeding Considerations Both propoxyphene and acetaminophen may be taken while breast-feeding

Dosage Forms TAB: (Darvocet-N® 50): Propoxyphene napsylate 50 mg and acetaminophen 325 mg; (Darvocet-N® 100, Pronap-100®): Propoxyphene napsylate 100 mg and acetaminophen 650 mg; (Wygesic®): Propoxyphene hydrochloride 65 mg and acetaminophen 650 mg

Generic Available Yes

Comments Propoxyphene is a narcotic analgesic and shares many properties including addiction liability. The acetaminophen component requires use with caution in patients with alcoholic liver disease.

Selected Readings

Botting RM, "Mechanism of Action of Acetaminophen: Is There a Cyclooxygenase 3?," *Clin Infect Dis*, 2000, Suppl 5:S202-10.

Dart RC, Kuffner EK, and Rumack BH, "Treatment of Pain or Fever with Paracetamol (Acetaminophen) in the Alcoholic Patient: A Systematic Review," *Am J Ther*, 2000, 7(2):123-34.

Grant JA and Weiler JM, "A Report of a Rare Immediate Reaction After Ingestion of Acetaminophen," *Ann Allergy Asthma Immunol*, 2001, 87(3):227-9.

Kwan D, Bartle WR, and Walker SE, "The Effects of Acetaminophen on Pharmacokinetics and Pharmacodynamics of Warfarin," *J Clin Pharmacol*, 1999, 39(1):68-75.

McClain CJ, Price S, Barve S, et al, "Acetaminophen Hepatotoxicity: An Update," *Curr Gastroenterol Rep*, 1999, 1(1):42-9.

Shek KL, Chan LN, and Nutescu E, "Warfarin-Acetaminophen Drug Interaction Revisited," *Pharmacotherapy*, 1999, 19(10):1153-8.

Tanaka E, Yamazaki K, and Misawa S, "Update: The Clinical Importance of Acetaminophen Hepatotoxicity in Nonalcoholic and Alcoholic Subjects," *J Clin Pharm Ther*, 2000, 25(5):325-32.

Propoxyphene and Aspirin (proe POKS i feen & AS pir in)

U.S. Brand Names Darvon® Compound-65 Pulvules®; PC-Cap®

Pharmacologic Category Analgesic Combination (Narcotic)

Synonyms Propoxyphene Hydrochloride and Aspirin; Propoxyphene Napsylate and Aspirin

Use

Dental: Management of postoperative pain

Medical: Relief of pain

Local Anesthetic/Vasoconstrictor Precautions No information available to require special precautions

Effects on Dental Treatment

Use with caution in patients with platelet and bleeding disorders, renal dysfunction, erosive gastritis, or peptic ulcer disease, previous nonreaction does not guarantee future safe taking of medication; use with caution in impaired hepatic function; do not use aspirin in children <16 years of age for chickenpox or flu symptoms due to the association with Reye's syndrome. Avoid aspirin, if possible, for 1 week prior to surgery due to possibility of postoperative bleeding.

Elderly are a high-risk population for adverse effects from nonsteroidal anti-inflammatory agents. As much as 60% of elderly with GI complications to NSAIDs can develop peptic ulceration and/or hemorrhage asymptomatically. Also, concomitant disease and drug use contribute to the risk for GI adverse effects. Use lowest effective dose for shortest period possible. Consider renal function decline with age. Use with caution in patients with history of asthma

Restrictions C-IV

Dosage Oral:

Children: Not recommended

Adults: 1-2 capsules every 4 hours as needed

Mechanism of Action Propoxyphene, a weak narcotic analgesic, block pain perception in the cerebral cortex by binding to specific receptor molecules (opiate receptors) within the neuronal membranes of synapses. This binding results in a decreased synaptic chemical transmission throughout the CNS thus inhibiting the flow of pain sensations into the higher centers. Mu and kappa are the two subtypes of the opiate receptor which propoxyphene binds to cause analgesia.

Aspirin inhibits prostaglandin synthesis by decreasing the activity of the enzyme, cyclo-oxygenase, which results in decreased formation of prostaglandin precursors, acts on the hypothalamic heat-regulating center to reduce fever, blocks thromboxane synthetase action which prevents formation of the platelet-aggregating substance thromboxane A_2

Other Adverse Effects Frequency not defined:

Based on **propoxyphene** component:

Cardiovascular: Hypotension

Central nervous system: Dizziness, lightheadedness, sedation, paradoxical excitement and insomnia, fatigue, drowsiness, mental depression, hallucinations, paradoxical CNS stimulation, increased intracranial pressure, nervousness, headache, restlessness, malaise, confusion

Dermatologic: Rash, urticaria

Endocrine & metabolic: May decrease glucose, urinary 17-OHCS

Gastrointestinal: Anorexia, stomach cramps, xerostomia, biliary spasm, nausea, vomiting, constipation, paralytic ileus

Genitourinary: Decreased urination, ureteral spasms

Neuromuscular & skeletal: Weakness

Hepatic: Increased liver enzymes (may increase LFTs)

Respiratory: Dyspnea

(Continued)

Propoxyphene and Aspirin *(Continued)*

Miscellaneous: Psychologic and physical dependence with prolonged use, histamine release

Based on **aspirin** component: As with all drugs which may affect hemostasis, bleeding is associated with aspirin. Hemorrhage may occur at virtually any site. Risk is dependent on multiple variables including dosage, concurrent use of multiple agents which alter hemostasis, and patient susceptibility. Many adverse effects of aspirin are dose-related, and are rare at low dosages. Other serious reactions are idiosyncratic, related to allergy or individual sensitivity. Accurate estimation of frequencies is not possible. The reactions listed below have been reported for aspirin. Frequency not defined:

Cardiovascular: Hypotension, tachycardia, dysrhythmias, edema

Central nervous system: Fatigue, insomnia, nervousness, agitation, confusion, dizziness, headache, lethargy, cerebral edema, hyperthermia, coma

Dermatologic: Rash, angioedema, urticaria

Endocrine and metabolic: Acidosis, hyperkalemia, dehydration, hypoglycemia (children), hyperglycemia, hypernatremia (buffered forms)

Gastrointestinal: Nausea, vomiting, dyspepsia, epigastric discomfort, heartburn, stomach pains, gastrointestinal ulceration (6% to 31%), gastric erosions, gastric erythema, duodenal ulcers

Hematologic: Anemia, disseminated intravascular coagulation, prolongation of prothrombin times, coagulopathy, thrombocytopenia, hemolytic anemia, bleeding, iron-deficiency anemia

Hepatic: Hepatotoxicity, increased transaminases, hepatitis (reversible)

Neuromuscular and skeletal: Rhabdomyolysis, weakness, acetabular bone destruction (OA)

Otic: Hearing loss, tinnitus

Renal: Interstitial nephritis, papillary necrosis, proteinuria, renal impairment, renal failure (including cases caused by rhabdomyolysis), increased BUN, increased serum creatinine

Respiratory: Asthma, bronchospasm, dyspnea, laryngeal edema, hyperpnea, tachypnea, respiratory alkalosis, noncardiogenic pulmonary edema

Miscellaneous: Anaphylaxis, prolonged pregnancy and labor, stillbirths, low birth weight, peripartum bleeding, Reye's syndrome

Case reports: Colonic ulceration, esophageal stricture, esophagitis with esophageal ulcer, esophageal hematoma, oral mucosal ulcers (aspirin-containing chewing gum), coronary artery spasm, conduction defect and atrial fibrillation (toxicity), delirium, ischemic brain infarction, colitis, rectal stenosis (suppository), cholestatic jaundice, periorbital edema, rhinosinusitis

Contraindications Hypersensitivity to propoxyphene, aspirin, or any component of their formulation

Warnings/Precautions When given in excessive doses, either alone or in combination with other CNS depressants, propoxyphene is a major cause of drug-related deaths; do not exceed recommended dosage; because of aspirin component, children and teenagers should not use for chickenpox or flu symptoms before a physician is consulted about Reye's syndrome

Drug Interactions

Increased toxicity with cimetidine, CNS depressants; increased toxicity/effect of carbamazepine, phenobarbital, TCAs, warfarin, MAO inhibitors, benzodiazepines, warfarin (bleeding); see Aspirin

Decreased effect with charcoal, cigarette smoking

Dietary/Ethanol/Herb Considerations

Ethanol: Avoid use; may increase CNS depression and enhance gastric mucosal irritation.

Herb/Nutraceutical: Avoid gotu kola, kava, SAMe, St John's wort, and valerian; may increase CNS depression.

Drug Uptake See Aspirin *on page 119* and Propoxyphene *on page 1013*

Pregnancy Risk Factor D

Breast-feeding Considerations

Propoxyphene: May be taken while breast-feeding.

Aspirin: Use cautiously due to potential adverse effects in nursing infants.

Dosage Forms CAP (Darvon® Compound-65, PC-Cap®): Propoxyphene 65 mg and aspirin 389 mg with caffeine 32.4 mg

Generic Available Yes

Comments Propoxyphene is a narcotic analgesic and shares many properties including addiction liability. The aspirin component could have anticoagulant effects and could possibly affect bleeding times.

Propranolol (proe PRAN oh lole)

Related Information

Cardiovascular Diseases *on page 1308*

Endocrine Disorders and Pregnancy *on page 1331*

U.S. Brand Names Inderal®; Inderal® LA

Canadian Brand Names Apo®-Propranolol; Inderal®; Inderal®-LA; Nu-Propranolol

Mexican Brand Names Inderalici; PMS-Propranolol®

Pharmacologic Category Antiarrhythmic Agent, Class II; Beta Blocker, Nonselective

Synonyms Propranolol Hydrochloride

Use Management of hypertension, angina pectoris, pheochromocytoma, essential tremor, tetralogy of Fallot cyanotic spells, and arrhythmias (such as atrial fibrillation and flutter, A-V nodal re-entrant tachycardias, and catecholamine-induced arrhythmias); prevention of myocardial infarction, migraine headache; symptomatic treatment of hypertrophic subaortic stenosis

Unlabeled/Investigational: Tremor due to Parkinson's disease, alcohol withdrawal, aggressive behavior, antipsychotic-induced akathisia, esophageal varices bleeding, anxiety, schizophrenia, acute panic, and gastric bleeding in portal hypertension

Local Anesthetic/Vasoconstrictor Precautions Use with caution; epinephrine has interacted with nonselective beta-blockers to result in initial hypertensive episode followed by bradycardia

Effects on Dental Treatment Noncardioselective beta-blockers (ie, propranolol, nadolol) enhance the pressor response to epinephrine, resulting in hypertension and bradycardia. Many nonsteroidal anti-inflammatory drugs such as ibuprofen and indomethacin can reduce the hypotensive effect of beta-blockers after 3 or more weeks of therapy with the NSAID. Short-term NSAID use (ie, 3 days) requires no special precautions in patients taking beta-blockers.

Dosage

Tachyarrhythmias:

Oral:

Children: Initial: 0.5-1 mg/kg/day in divided doses every 6-8 hours; titrate dosage upward every 3-7 days; usual dose: 2-4 mg/kg/day; higher doses may be needed; do not exceed 16 mg/kg/day or 60 mg/day

Adults: 10-30 mg/dose every 6-8 hours

Elderly: Initial: 10 mg twice daily; increase dosage every 3-7 days; usual dosage range: 10-320 mg given in 2 divided doses

I.V.:

Children: 0.01-0.1 mg/kg slow IVP over 10 minutes; maximum dose: 1 mg

Adults: 1 mg/dose slow IVP; repeat every 5 minutes up to a total of 5 mg

Hypertension: Oral:

Children: Initial: 0.5-1 mg/kg/day in divided doses every 6-12 hours; increase gradually every 3-7 days; maximum: 2 mg/kg/24 hours

Adults: Initial: 40 mg twice daily; increase dosage every 3-7 days; usual dose: ≤320 mg divided in 2-3 doses/day; maximum daily dose: 640 mg

Migraine headache prophylaxis: Oral:

Children: 0.6-1.5 mg/kg/day **or**

≤35 kg: 10-20 mg 3 times/day

>35 kg: 20-40 mg 3 times/day

Adults: Initial: 80 mg/day divided every 6-8 hours; increase by 20-40 mg/dose every 3-4 weeks to a maximum of 160-240 mg/day given in divided doses every 6-8 hours; if satisfactory response not achieved within 6 weeks of starting therapy, drug should be withdrawn gradually over several weeks

Tetralogy spells: Children:

Oral: 1-2 mg/kg/day every 6 hours as needed, may increase by 1 mg/kg/day to a maximum of 5 mg/kg/day, or if refractory may increase slowly to a maximum of 10-15 mg/kg/day

I.V.: 0.15-0.25 mg/kg/dose slow IVP; may repeat in 15 minutes

Thyrotoxicosis:

Adolescents and Adults: Oral: 10-40 mg/dose every 6 hours

Adults: I.V.: 1-3 mg/dose slow IVP as a single dose

Adults: Oral:

Angina: 80-320 mg/day in doses divided 2-4 times/day

Pheochromocytoma: 30-60 mg/day in divided doses

Myocardial infarction prophylaxis: 180-240 mg/day in 3-4 divided doses

Hypertrophic subaortic stenosis: 20-40 mg 3-4 times/day

Essential tremor: 40 mg twice daily initially; maintenance doses: usually 120-320 mg/day

Mechanism of Action Nonselective beta-adrenergic blocker (class II antiarrhythmic); competitively blocks response to $beta_1$- and $beta_2$-adrenergic stimulation which results in decreases in heart rate, myocardial contractility, BP, and myocardial oxygen demand

Other Adverse Effects Frequency not defined:

Cardiovascular: Bradycardia, CHF, reduced peripheral circulation, chest pain, hypotension, impaired myocardial contractility, worsening of AV conduction disturbance, cardiogenic shock, Raynaud's syndrome, mesenteric thrombosis (rare)

Central nervous system: Mental depression, lightheadedness, amnesia, emotional lability, confusion, hallucinations, dizziness, insomnia, fatigue, vivid dreams, lethargy, cold extremities, vertigo, syncope, cognitive dysfunction, psychosis, hypersomnolence

(Continued)

Propranolol *(Continued)*

Dermatologic: Rash, alopecia, exfoliative dermatitis, psoriasiform eruptions, eczematous eruptions, hyperkeratosis, nail changes, pruritus, urticaria, ulcerative lichenoid, contact dermatitis

Endocrine & metabolic: Hypoglycemia, hyperglycemia, hyperlipidemia, hyperkalemia

Gastrointestinal: Diarrhea, nausea, vomiting, stomach discomfort, constipation, anorexia

Genitourinary: Impotence, proteinuria (rare), oliguria (rare), interstitial nephritis (rare), Peyronie's disease

Hematologic: Agranulocytosis, thrombocytopenia, thrombocytopenic purpura

Neuromuscular & skeletal: Weakness, carpal tunnel syndrome (rare), paresthesias, myotonus, polyarthritis, arthropathy

Respiratory: Wheezing, pharyngitis, bronchospasm, pulmonary edema

Ocular: Hyperemia of the conjunctiva, decreased tear production, decreased visual acuity, mydriasis

Miscellaneous: Lupus-like syndrome (rare)

Drug Interactions CYP1A2, 2C18, 2C19, and 2D6 enzyme substrate

Increased Effect/Toxicity: The heart rate lowering effects of propranolol are additive with other drugs which slow AV conduction (digoxin, verapamil, diltiazem). Reserpine increases the effects of propranolol. Concurrent use of propranolol may increase the effects of alpha-blockers (prazosin, terazosin), alpha-adrenergic stimulants (epinephrine, phenylephrine), and the vasoconstrictive effects of ergot alkaloids. Propranolol may mask the tachycardia from hypoglycemia caused by insulin and oral hypoglycemics. In patients receiving concurrent therapy, the risk of hypertensive crisis is increased when either clonidine or the beta-blocker is withdrawn. Beta-blockers may increase the action or levels of disopyramide, nondepolarizing muscle relaxants, and theophylline although the effects are difficult to predict. Beta-blocker effects may be enhanced by oral contraceptives, flecainide, haloperidol (hypotensive effects), H_2 antagonists (cimetidine, possibly ranitidine), hydralazine, loop diuretics, possibly MAO inhibitors, phenothiazines, propafenone, quinidine (in extensive metabolizers), ciprofloxacin, thyroid hormones (when hypothyroid patient is converted to euthyroid state). Beta-blockers may increase the effect/toxicity of flecainide, haloperidol (hypotensive effects), hydralazine, phenothiazines, acetaminophen, anticoagulants (warfarin), and benzodiazepines.

Decreased Effect: Aluminum salts, barbiturates, calcium salts, cholestyramine, colestipol, NSAIDs, penicillins (ampicillin), rifampin, salicylates, and sulfinpyrazone decrease effect of beta-blockers due to decreased bioavailability and plasma concentrations. Beta-blockers may decrease the effect of sulfonylureas. Ascorbic acid decreases propranolol Cp_{max} and AUC and increases the T_{max} significantly resulting in a greater decrease in the reduction of heart rate, possibly due to decreased absorption and first pass metabolism (n=5). Nefazodone decreased peak plasma concentrations and AUC of propranolol and increases time to reach steady-state; monitoring of clinical response is recommended. Nonselective beta-blockers blunt the response to beta-2 adrenergic agonists (albuterol).

Drug Uptake

Onset of action: Beta-blockade: Oral: 1-2 hours

Duration: ~6 hours

Half-life, elimination: Neonates and Infants: Possible increased half-life; Children: 3.9-6.4 hours; Adults: 4-6 hours

Pregnancy Risk Factor C (manufacturer); D (2nd and 3rd trimesters - expert analysis)

Generic Available Yes

Selected Readings

Foster CA and Aston SJ, "Propranolol-Epinephrine Interaction: A Potential Disaster," *Plast Reconstr Surg*, 1983, 72(1):74-8.

Wong DG, Spence JD, Lamki L, et al, "Effect of Nonsteroidal Anti-inflammatory Drugs on Control of Hypertension of Beta-Blockers and Diuretics," *Lancet*, 1986, 1(8488):997-1001.

Wynn RL, "Dental Nonsteroidal Anti-inflammatory Drugs and Prostaglandin-Based Drug Interactions, Part Two," *Gen Dent*, 1992, 40(2):104, 106, 108.

Wynn RL, "Epinephrine Interactions With Beta-Blockers," *Gen Dent*, 1994, 42(1):16, 18.

Propranolol and Hydrochlorothiazide

(proe PRAN oh lole & hye droe klor oh THYE a zide)

U.S. Brand Names Inderide®; Inderide® LA

Canadian Brand Names Inderide®

Pharmacologic Category Antihypertensive Agent Combination

Synonyms Hydrochlorothiazide and Propranolol

Use Management of hypertension

Local Anesthetic/Vasoconstrictor Precautions Use with caution; epinephrine has interacted with nonselective beta-blockers to result in initial hypertensive episode followed by bradycardia

Effects on Dental Treatment Noncardioselective beta-blockers (ie, propranolol, nadolol) enhance the pressor response to epinephrine, resulting in hypertension and bradycardia. Many nonsteroidal anti-inflammatory drugs such as ibuprofen and indomethacin can reduce the hypotensive effect of beta-blockers after 3 or more weeks of therapy with the NSAID. Short-term NSAID use (ie, 3 days) requires no special precautions in patients taking beta-blockers.

Dosage Dose is individualized

Drug Uptake See Propranolol *on page 1016* and Hydrochlorothiazide *on page 595*

Pregnancy Risk Factor C

Generic Available Yes: Immediate release

Propulsid® *see* Cisapride *on page 291*

Propylhexedrine (proe pil HEKS e dreen)

U.S. Brand Names Benzedrex® [OTC]

Pharmacologic Category Adrenergic Agonist Agent

Use Topical nasal decongestant

Local Anesthetic/Vasoconstrictor Precautions No information available to require special precautions

Effects on Dental Treatment No effects or complications reported

Dosage Inhale through each nostril while blocking the other

Generic Available No

Comments Drug has been extracted from inhaler and injected I.V. as an amphetamine substitute

Propylthiouracil (proe pil thye oh YOOR a sil)

Related Information

Endocrine Disorders and Pregnancy *on page 1331*

Canadian Brand Names Propyl-Thyracil®

Pharmacologic Category Antithyroid Agent

Synonyms PTU

Use Palliative treatment of hyperthyroidism as an adjunct to ameliorate hyperthyroidism in preparation for surgical treatment or radioactive iodine therapy; management of thyrotoxic crisis

Local Anesthetic/Vasoconstrictor Precautions No information available to require special precautions

Effects on Dental Treatment No effects or complications reported

Dosage Oral: Administer in 3 equally divided doses at ~ 8-hour intervals. Adjust dosage to maintain T_3, T_4, and TSH levels in normal range; elevated T_3 may be sole indicator of inadequate treatment. Elevated TSH indicates excessive antithyroid treatment.

Children: Initial: 5-7 mg/kg/day in divided doses every 8 hours **or**
- 6-10 years: 50-150 mg/day
- >10 years: 150-300 mg/day
- Maintenance: $^1/_3$ to $^2/_3$ of the initial dose in divided doses every 8-12 hours. This usually begins after 2 months on an effective initial dose.

Adults: Initial: 300-450 mg/day in divided doses every 8 hours (severe hyperthyroidism may require 600-1200 mg/day); maintenance: 100-150 mg/day in divided doses every 8-12 hours

Elderly: Use lower dose recommendations; initial dose: 150-300 mg/day

Mechanism of Action Inhibits the synthesis of thyroid hormones by blocking the oxidation of iodine in the thyroid gland; blocks synthesis of thyroxine and triiodothyronine

Other Adverse Effects Frequency not defined:

Cardiovascular: Edema, cutaneous vasculitis, leukocytoclastic vasculitis, ANCA-positive vasculitis

Central nervous system: Fever, drowsiness, vertigo, headache, drug fever, dizziness, neuritis

Dermatologic: Skin rash, urticaria, pruritus, exfoliative dermatitis, alopecia, erythema nodosum

Endocrine & metabolic: Goiter, weight gain, swollen salivary glands

Gastrointestinal: Nausea, vomiting, loss of taste perception, stomach pain, constipation

Hematologic: Leukopenia, agranulocytosis, thrombocytopenia, bleeding, aplastic anemia

Hepatic: Cholestatic jaundice, hepatitis

Neuromuscular & skeletal: Arthralgia, paresthesia

Renal: Nephritis, glomerulonephritis, acute renal failure

Respiratory: Interstitial pneumonitis, alveolar hemorrhage

Miscellaneous: SLE-like syndrome

Warnings/Precautions Use with caution in patients >40 years of age because PTU may cause hypoprothrombinemia and bleeding; use with extreme caution in patients receiving other drugs known to cause agranulocytosis; may cause agranulocytosis, thyroid hyperplasia, thyroid carcinoma (usage >1 year). Discontinue in

(Continued)

Propylthiouracil *(Continued)*

the presence of agranulocytosis, aplastic anemia, ANCA-positive vasculitis, hepatitis, unexplained fever, or exfoliative dermatitis. Safety and efficacy have not been established in children <6 years of age.

Drug Interactions

Increased Effect/Toxicity: Propylthiouracil may increase the anticoagulant activity of warfarin.

Decreased Effect: Oral anticoagulant activity is increased only until metabolic effect stabilizes. Anticoagulants may be potentiated by antivitamin K effect of propylthiouracil. Correction of hyperthyroidism may alter disposition of beta-blockers, digoxin, and theophylline, necessitating a dose reduction of these agents.

Drug Uptake

Onset of action: Therapeutic: 24-36 hours

Peak effect: Remission: 4 months of continued therapy

Duration: 2-3 hours

Half-life, elimination: 1.5-5 hours; End-stage renal disease: 8.5 hours

Time to peak: Oral: ~1 hour

Pregnancy Risk Factor D

Generic Available Yes

Proscar® *see* Finasteride *on page 503*

ProSom™ *see* Estazolam *on page 456*

ProStep® Patch *see* Nicotine *on page 863*

Prostin E₂® Vaginal Suppository *see* Dinoprostone *on page 397*

Prostin VR Pediatric® *see* Alprostadil *on page 58*

Protamine Sulfate (PROE ta meen SUL fate)

Pharmacologic Category Antidote

Use Treatment of heparin overdosage; neutralize heparin during surgery or dialysis procedures

Local Anesthetic/Vasoconstrictor Precautions No information available to require special precautions

Effects on Dental Treatment No effects or complications reported

Dosage Protamine dosage is determined by the dosage of heparin; 1 mg of protamine neutralizes 90 USP units of heparin (lung) and 115 USP units of heparin (intestinal); maximum dose: 50 mg

In the situation of heparin overdosage, since blood heparin concentrations decrease rapidly **after** administration, adjust the protamine dosage depending upon the duration of time since heparin administration as follows: See table.

Time Elapsed	Dose of Protamine (mg) to Neutralize 100 units of Heparin
Immediate	1-1.5
30-60 minutes	0.5-0.75
>2 hours	0.25-0.375

If heparin administered by deep S.C. injection, use 1-1.5 mg protamine per 100 units heparin; this may be done by a portion of the dose (eg, 25-50 mg) given slowly I.V. followed by the remaining portion as a continuous infusion over 8-16 hours (the expected absorption time of the S.C. heparin dose)

Mechanism of Action Combines with strongly acidic heparin to form a stable complex (salt) neutralizing the anticoagulant activity of both drugs

Other Adverse Effects Frequency not defined:

Cardiovascular: Sudden fall in BP, bradycardia, flushing, hypotension

Central nervous system: Lassitude

Gastrointestinal: Nausea, vomiting

Hematologic: Hemorrhage

Respiratory: Dyspnea, pulmonary hypertension

Miscellaneous: Hypersensitivity reactions

Drug Uptake Onset of action: I.V.: Heparin neutralization: ~5 minutes

Pregnancy Risk Factor C

Generic Available Yes

Comments Heparin rebound associated with anticoagulation and bleeding has been reported to occur occasionally; symptoms typically occur 8-9 hours after protamine administration, but may occur as long as 18 hours later

Prothazine-DC® *see* Promethazine and Codeine *on page 1007*

Protirelin (proe TYE re lin)

U.S. Brand Names Thyrel® TRH

Canadian Brand Names Relefact® TRH

Pharmacologic Category Diagnostic Agent

Synonyms Lopremone; Thyrotropin Releasing Hormone; TRH

Use Adjunct in the diagnostic assessment of thyroid function, and an adjunct to other diagnostic procedures in assessment of patients with pituitary or hypothalamic dysfunction; also causes release of prolactin from the pituitary and is used to detect defective control of prolactin secretion.

Local Anesthetic/Vasoconstrictor Precautions No information available to require special precautions

Effects on Dental Treatment >10%: Xerostomia

Dosage I.V.:

Children <6 years: Experience limited, but doses of 7 mcg/kg have been administered

Children 6-16 years: 7 mcg/kg to a maximum dose of 500 mcg

Adults: 500 mcg (range 200-500 mcg)

Mechanism of Action Increase release of thyroid stimulating hormone from the anterior pituitary

Other Adverse Effects

>10%:

Central nervous system: Headache, lightheadedness

Dermatologic: Flushing of face

Gastrointestinal: Nausea, xerostomia

Genitourinary: Urge to urinate

1% to 10%:

Central nervous system: Anxiety

Endocrine & metabolic: Breast enlargement and leaking in lactating women

Gastrointestinal: Bad taste in mouth, abdominal discomfort

Neuromuscular & skeletal: Tingling

Miscellaneous: Diaphoresis

Drug Interactions Decreased Effect: Aspirin, levodopa, thyroid hormones, adrenocorticoid drugs

Drug Uptake

Onset of action: Peak effect: TSH: 20-30 minutes

Duration: TSH returns to baseline after ~3 hours

Half-life, elimination: Plasma (mean): 5 minutes

Pregnancy Risk Factor C

Generic Available No

Protonix® *see* Pantoprazole *on page 915*

Protopic® *see* Tacrolimus *on page 1128*

Protostat® Oral *see* Metronidazole *on page 804*

Protriptyline (proe TRIP ti leen)

U.S. Brand Names Vivactil®

Canadian Brand Names Triptil®

Pharmacologic Category Antidepressant, Tricyclic (Secondary Amine)

Synonyms Protriptyline Hydrochloride

Use Treatment of various forms of depression, often in conjunction with psychotherapy

Local Anesthetic/Vasoconstrictor Precautions No information available to require special precautions

Effects on Dental Treatment

>10%: Xerostomia

Long-term treatment with TCAs such as protriptyline increases the risk of caries by reducing salivation and salivary buffer capacity.

Dosage Oral:

Adolescents and Elderly: 15-20 mg/day

Adults: 15-60 mg in 3-4 divided doses

Mechanism of Action Increases the synaptic concentration of serotonin and/or norepinephrine in the CNS by inhibition of their reuptake by the presynaptic neuronal membrane

Other Adverse Effects Frequency not defined:

Cardiovascular: Arrhythmias, hypotension, myocardial infarction, stroke, heart block, hypertension, tachycardia, palpitations

Central nervous system: Dizziness, drowsiness, headache, confusion, delirium, hallucinations, restlessness, insomnia, nightmares, fatigue, delusions, anxiety, agitation, hypomania, exacerbation of psychosis, panic, seizures, incoordination, ataxia, EPS

Dermatologic: Alopecia, photosensitivity, rash, petechiae, urticaria, itching

Endocrine & metabolic: Breast enlargement, galactorrhea, SIADH, gynecomastia, increased or decreased libido

Gastrointestinal: Xerostomia, constipation, unpleasant taste, weight gain/loss, increased appetite, nausea, diarrhea, heartburn, vomiting, anorexia, trouble with gums, decreased lower esophageal sphincter tone may cause GE reflux

Genitourinary: Difficult urination, impotence, testicular edema

Hematologic: Agranulocytosis, leukopenia, eosinophilia, thrombocytopenia, purpura

Hepatic: Cholestatic jaundice, increased liver enzymes

(Continued)

Protriptyline *(Continued)*

Neuromuscular & skeletal: Fine muscle tremors, weakness, tremor, numbness, tingling

Ocular: Blurred vision, eye pain, increased intraocular pressure

Otic: Tinnitus

Miscellaneous: Diaphoresis (excessive), allergic reactions

Drug Interactions CYP2D6 enzyme substrate

Increased Effect/Toxicity: Protriptyline increases the effects of amphetamines, anticholinergics, other CNS depressants (sedatives, hypnotics), chlorpropamide, tolazamide, and warfarin. When used with MAO inhibitors, hyperpyrexia, hypertension, tachycardia, confusion, seizures, and **deaths have been reported** (serotonin syndrome). The SSRIs (to varying degrees), cimetidine, indinavir, methylphenidate, ritonavir, quinidine, diltiazem, and verapamil inhibit the metabolism of TCAs and clinical toxicity may result. Use of lithium with a TCA may increase the risk for neurotoxicity. Phenothiazines may increase concentration of some TCAs and TCAs may increase concentration of phenothiazines. Pressor response to I.V. epinephrine, norepinephrine, and phenylephrine may be enhanced in patients receiving TCAs (**Note:** Effect is unlikely with epinephrine or levonordefrin dosages typically administered as infiltration in combination with local anesthetics). Combined use of beta-agonists or drugs which prolong QT_c (including quinidine, procainamide, disopyramide, cisapride, sparfloxacin, gatifloxacin, moxifloxacin) with TCAs may predispose patients to cardiac arrhythmias.

Decreased Effect: Carbamazepine, phenobarbital, and rifampin may increase the metabolism of protriptyline, decreasing its effects. Protriptyline inhibits the antihypertensive response to bethanidine, clonidine, debrisoquin, guanadrel, guanethidine, guanabenz, guanfacine. Cimetidine and methylphenidate may decrease the metabolism of protriptyline. Cholestyramine and colestipol may bind TCAs and reduce their absorption.

Drug Uptake

Onset of action: Peak effect: Antidepressant effect: 2 weeks of continuous therapy

Half-life, elimination: 54-92 hours; Average: 74 hours

Time to peak: Oral: 24-30 hours

Pregnancy Risk Factor C

Generic Available Yes

Selected Readings

Friedlander AH, Mahler ME, "Major Depressive Disorder. Psychopathology, Medical Management, and Dental Implications," *J Am Dent Assoc*, 201, 132(5):629-38.

Ganzberg S, "Psychoactive Drugs," *ADA Guide to Dental Therapeutics*, 2nd ed, Chicago, IL: ADA Publishing, a Division of ADA Business Enterprises, Inc, 2000, 376-405.

Jastak JT and Yagiela JA, "Vasoconstrictors and Local Anesthesia: A Review and Rationale for Use," *J Am Dent Assoc*, 1983, 107(4):623-30.

Mitchell JR, "Guanethidine and Related Agents. III Antagonism by Drugs Which Inhibit the Norepinephrine Pump in Man," *J Clin Invest*, 1970, 49(8):1596-604.

Rundegren J, van Dijken J, Mörnstad H, et al, "Oral Conditions in Patients Receiving Long-Term Treatment With Cyclic Antidepressant Drugs," *Swed Dent J*, 1985, 9(2):55-64.

Yagiela JA, "Adverse Drug Interactions in Dental Practice: Interactions Associated With Vasoconstrictors. Part V of a Series," *J Am Dent Assoc*, 1999, 130(5):701-9.

Protropin® *see* Human Growth Hormone *on page 589*

Proventil® *see* Albuterol *on page 45*

Proventil® HFA *see* Albuterol *on page 45*

Proventil® Repetabs® *see* Albuterol *on page 45*

Provera® *see* MedroxyPROGESTERone Acetate *on page 753*

Provigil® *see* Modafinil *on page 822*

Proxigel® Oral [OTC] *see* Carbamide Peroxide *on page 218*

Prozac® *see* Fluoxetine *on page 517*

Prozac® Weekly™ *see* Fluoxetine *on page 517*

Pseudocot-T® [OTC] *see* Triprolidine and Pseudoephedrine *on page 1213*

Pseudoephedrine (soo doe e FED rin)

Related Information

Acetaminophen and Pseudoephedrine *on page 30*

Acetaminophen, Dextromethorphan, and Pseudoephedrine *on page 34*

Diphenhydramine and Pseudoephedrine *on page 400*

Guaifenesin, Pseudoephedrine, and Dextromethorphan *on page 571*

Oral Bacterial Infections *on page 1367*

U.S. Brand Names Cenafed® [OTC]; Children's Silfedrine® [OTC]; Children's Sudafed® Nasal Decongestant [OTC]; Decofed® [OTC]; Dimetapp® Decongestant Liqui-Gels® [OTC]; Efidac/24® [OTC]; Genaphed® [OTC]; PediaCare® Decongestant Infants [OTC]; Sudafed® [OTC]; Sudafed® 12 Hour [OTC]; Triaminic® AM Decongestant Formula [OTC]; Triaminic® Infant Decongestant [OTC]

Canadian Brand Names Balminil® Decongestant; Contac® Cold 12 Hour Relief Non Drowsy; Eltor®; PMS-Pseudoephedrine; Pseudofrin; Robidrine®; Sudafed® Decongestant

Mexican Brand Names Lertamine-D®; Sudafed®

Pharmacologic Category Alpha/Beta Agonist

Synonyms *d*-Isoephedrine Hydrochloride; Pseudoephedrine Hydrochloride; Pseudoephedrine Sulfate

Use Temporary symptomatic relief of nasal congestion due to common cold, upper respiratory allergies, and sinusitis; also promotes nasal or sinus drainage

Local Anesthetic/Vasoconstrictor Precautions Use with caution since pseudoephedrine is a sympathomimetic amine which could interact with epinephrine to cause a pressor response

Effects on Dental Treatment ≤10%: Tachycardia, palpitations, xerostomia; use vasoconstrictor with caution

Dosage Oral:

Children:

<2 years: 4 mg/kg/day in divided doses every 6 hours

2-5 years: 15 mg every 6 hours; maximum: 60 mg/24 hours

6-12 years: 30 mg every 6 hours; maximum: 120 mg/24 hours

Adults: 30-60 mg every 4-6 hours, sustained release: 120 mg every 12 hours; maximum: 240 mg/24 hours

Mechanism of Action Directly stimulates alpha-adrenergic receptors of respiratory mucosa causing vasoconstriction; directly stimulates beta-adrenergic receptors causing bronchial relaxation, increased heart rate and contractility

Other Adverse Effects Frequency not defined:

Cardiovascular: Tachycardia, palpitations, arrhythmias

Central nervous system: Nervousness, transient stimulation, insomnia, excitability, dizziness, drowsiness, convulsions, hallucinations, headache

Gastrointestinal: Nausea, vomiting

Genitourinary: Dysuria

Neuromuscular & skeletal: Weakness, tremor

Respiratory: Dyspnea

Miscellaneous: Diaphoresis

Drug Interactions

Increased Effect/Toxicity: MAO inhibitors may increase BP effects of pseudoephedrine. Sympathomimetic agents may increase toxicity.

Decreased Effect: Decreased effect of methyldopa, reserpine.

Drug Uptake

Onset of action: Decongestant: Oral: 15-30 minutes

Absorption: Rapid

Duration: 4-6 hours; Extended release: ≤12 hours

Half-life, elimination: 9-16 hours

Pregnancy Risk Factor C

Generic Available Yes

Pseudoephedrine and Dextromethorphan

(soo doe e FED rin & deks troe meth OR fan)

U.S. Brand Names Children's Sudafed® Cough & Cold [OTC]; Robitussin® Maximum Strength Cough & Cold [OTC]; Robitussin® Pediatric Cough & Cold [OTC]; Vicks® 44D Cough & Head Congestion [OTC]

Canadian Brand Names Balminil DM D; Benylin® DM-D; Koffex DM-D; Novahistex® DM Decongestant; Novahistine® DM Decongestant; Robitussin® Childrens Cough & Cold

Pharmacologic Category Antitussive/Decongestant

Synonyms Dextromethorphan and Pseudoephedrine

Use Temporary symptomatic relief of nasal congestion due to common cold, upper respiratory allergies, and sinusitis; also promotes nasal or sinus drainage; symptomatic relief of coughs caused by minor viral upper respiratory tract infections or inhaled irritants; most effective for a chronic nonproductive cough

Local Anesthetic/Vasoconstrictor Precautions Use with caution since pseudoephedrine is a sympathomimetic amine which could interact with epinephrine to cause a pressor response

Effects on Dental Treatment ≤10%: Tachycardia, palpitations, xerostomia; use vasoconstrictor with caution

Dosage Oral: Adults: 1 capsule or 5-10 mL every 6 hours

Other Adverse Effects Frequency not defined:

Based on **pseudoephedrine** component:

Cardiovascular: Tachycardia, palpitations, arrhythmias

Central nervous system: Nervousness, transient stimulation, insomnia, excitability, dizziness, drowsiness, convulsions, hallucinations, headache

Gastrointestinal: Nausea, vomiting

Genitourinary: Dysuria

Neuromuscular & skeletal: Weakness, tremor

Respiratory: Dyspnea

Miscellaneous: Diaphoresis

Based on **dextromethorphan** component: Abdominal discomfort, coma, constipation, dizziness, drowsiness, GI upset, nausea, respiratory depression

(Continued)

Pseudoephedrine and Dextromethorphan *(Continued)*

Warnings/Precautions Research on chicken embryos exposed to concentrations of dextromethorphan relative to those typically taken by humans has shown to cause birth defects and fetal death; more study is needed, but it is suggested that pregnant women should be advised not to use dextromethorphan-containing medications

Drug Interactions Dextromethorphan: CYP2D6, 2E1, 3A3/4 enzyme substrate

Increased Effect/Toxicity: Based on **pseudoephedrine** component: MAO inhibitors may increase BP effects of pseudoephedrine. Sympathomimetic agents may increase toxicity.

Decreased Effect: Based on **pseudoephedrine** component: Decreased effect of methyldopa, reserpine.

Drug Uptake See Pseudoephedrine *on page 1022* and Dextromethorphan *on page 372*

Generic Available Yes

Pseudoephedrine and Ibuprofen

(soo doe e FED rin & eye byoo PROE fen)

U.S. Brand Names Advil® Cold & Sinus Caplets [OTC]; Dristan® Sinus Caplets; Motrin® Sinus [OTC]

Canadian Brand Names Advil® Cold & Sinus; Dristan® Sinus

Pharmacologic Category Decongestant/Analgesic

Synonyms Ibuprofen and Pseudoephedrine

Use Temporary symptomatic relief of nasal congestion due to common cold, upper respiratory allergies, and sinusitis; also promotes nasal or sinus drainage; sinus headaches and pains

Local Anesthetic/Vasoconstrictor Precautions Use with caution since pseudoephedrine is a sympathomimetic amine which could interact with epinephrine to cause a pressor response

Effects on Dental Treatment ≤10%: Tachycardia, palpitations, xerostomia; use vasoconstrictor with caution

Dosage Oral: Adults: 1-2 caplets every 4-6 hours

Other Adverse Effects Frequency not defined:

Based on **pseudoephedrine** component:
- Cardiovascular: Tachycardia, palpitations, arrhythmias
- Central nervous system: Nervousness, transient stimulation, insomnia, excitability, dizziness, drowsiness, convulsions, hallucinations, headache
- Gastrointestinal: Nausea, vomiting
- Genitourinary: Dysuria
- Neuromuscular & skeletal: Weakness, tremor
- Respiratory: Dyspnea
- Miscellaneous: Diaphoresis

Based on **ibuprofen** component: 1% to 10%:
- Central nervous system: Headache (1% to 3%), nervousness (<3%), fatigue (<3%)
- Dermatologic: Itching (1% to 3%), rash (3% to 9%), urticaria
- Endocrine & metabolic: Fluid retention
- Gastrointestinal: Dyspepsia (1% to 3%), vomiting (1% to 3%), abdominal pain/cramps/distress (1% to 3%), peptic ulcer, GI bleed, GI perforation, heartburn, nausea (3% to 9%), diarrhea (1% to 3%), constipation (1% to 3%), flatulence (1% to 3%), indigestion (1% to 3%)
- Otic: Tinnitus

Drug Interactions Ibuprofen: CYP2C8 and 2C9 enzyme substrate

Increased Effect/Toxicity:
- Based on **pseudoephedrine** component: MAO inhibitors may increase BP effects of pseudoephedrine. Sympathomimetic agents may increase toxicity.
- Based on **ibuprofen** component: Ibuprofen may increase cyclosporine, digoxin, lithium, and methotrexate serum concentration. The renal adverse effects of ACE inhibitors may be potentiated by NSAIDs. Corticosteroids may increase the risk of GI ulceration.

Decreased Effect:
- Based on **pseudoephedrine** component: Decreased effect of methyldopa, reserpine.
- Based on **ibuprofen** component: Aspirin may decrease ibuprofen serum concentration. Ibuprofen may decrease the effect of some antihypertensive agents (including ACE inhibitors and angiotensin antagonists) and diuretics.

Drug Uptake See Pseudoephedrine *on page 1022* and Ibuprofen *on page 621*

Pregnancy Risk Factor Ibuprofen: B/D (3rd trimester)

Generic Available Yes

Pseudo-Gest Plus® [OTC] *see* Chlorpheniramine and Pseudoephedrine *on page 270*

Psor-a-set® Soap [OTC] *see* Salicylic Acid *on page 1072*

Psorcon™ *see* Diflorasone *on page 386*

Psorcon™ E *see* Diflorasone *on page 386*
psoriGel® [OTC] *see* Coal Tar *on page 315*
P & S Plus® [OTC] *see* Coal Tar and Salicylic Acid *on page 315*

Psyllium (SIL i yum)

U.S. Brand Names Fiberall® Powder [OTC]; Fiberall® Wafer [OTC]; Hydrocil® [OTC]; Konsyl® [OTC]; Konsyl-D® [OTC]; Metamucil® [OTC]; Metamucil® Smooth Texture [OTC]; Modane® Bulk [OTC]; Perdiem® Plain [OTC]; Reguloid® [OTC]; Serutan® [OTC]; Syllact® [OTC]

Canadian Brand Names Metamucil®; Novo-Mucilax

Pharmacologic Category Antidiarrheal; Laxative, Bulk-Producing

Synonyms Plantago Seed; Plantain Seed; Psyllium Hydrophilic Mucilloid

Use Treatment of chronic atonic or spastic constipation and in constipation associated with rectal disorders; management of irritable bowel syndrome

Local Anesthetic/Vasoconstrictor Precautions No information available to require special precautions

Effects on Dental Treatment No effects or complications reported

Dosage Oral (administer at least 3 hours before or after drugs):

Children 6-11 years: (Approximately ½ adult dosage) ½ to 1 rounded teaspoonful in 4 oz glass of liquid 1-3 times/day

Adults: 1-2 rounded teaspoonfuls or 1-2 packets or 1-2 wafers in 8 oz glass of liquid 1-3 times/day

Mechanism of Action Adsorbs water in the intestine to form a viscous liquid which promotes peristalsis and reduces transit time

Other Adverse Effects Frequency not defined:

Gastrointestinal: Esophageal or bowel obstruction, diarrhea, constipation, abdominal cramps

Respiratory: Bronchospasm

Miscellaneous: Anaphylaxis upon inhalation in susceptible individuals, rhinoconjunctivitis

Drug Interactions Decreased effect of warfarin, digitalis, potassium-sparing diuretics, salicylates, tetracyclines, nitrofurantoin when taken together; separate administration times to reduce potential for drug-drug interaction.

Drug Uptake

Onset of action: 12-24 hours; Peak effect: 2-3 days

Absorption: None; small amounts of grain extracts present in the preparation have been reportedly absorbed following colonic hydrolysis

Pregnancy Risk Factor B

Generic Available Yes

P.T.E.-4® *see* Trace Metals *on page 1186*
P.T.E.-5® *see* Trace Metals *on page 1186*
Pulmicort Respules™ *see* Budesonide *on page 180*
Pulmicort Turbuhaler® *see* Budesonide *on page 180*
Pulmozyme® *see* Dornase Alfa *on page 411*
Puralube® Tears [OTC] *see* Artificial Tears *on page 117*
Purge® [OTC] *see* Castor Oil *on page 230*
Puri-Clens™ [OTC] *see* Methylbenzethonium Chloride *on page 793*
Purinethol® *see* Mercaptopurine *on page 770*
P_xE_x® *see* Pilocarpine and Epinephrine *on page 956*

Pyrantel Pamoate (pi RAN tel PAM oh ate)

U.S. Brand Names Antiminth® [OTC]; Pin-Rid® [OTC]; Pin-X® [OTC]; Reese's® Pinworm Medicine [OTC]

Canadian Brand Names Combantrin™

Mexican Brand Names Combantrin®

Pharmacologic Category Anthelmintic

Use Roundworm (*Ascaris lumbricoides*), pinworm (*Enterobius vermicularis*), and hookworm (*Ancylostoma duodenale* and *Necator americanus*) infestations, and trichostrongyliasis

Local Anesthetic/Vasoconstrictor Precautions No information available to require special precautions

Effects on Dental Treatment No effects or complications reported

Dosage Children and Adults (purgation is not required prior to use): Oral:

Roundworm, pinworm, or trichostrongyliasis: 11 mg/kg administered as a single dose; maximum dose: 1 g. (**Note:** For pinworm infection, dosage should be repeated in 2 weeks and all family members should be treated).

Hookworm: 11 mg/kg administered once daily for 3 days

Mechanism of Action Causes the release of acetylcholine and inhibits cholinesterase; acts as a depolarizing neuromuscular blocker, paralyzing the helminths

Other Adverse Effects Frequency not defined:

Central nervous system: Dizziness, drowsiness, insomnia, headache

Dermatologic: Rash

(Continued)

Pyrantel Pamoate *(Continued)*

Gastrointestinal: Anorexia, nausea, vomiting, abdominal cramps, diarrhea, tenesmus
Hepatic: Elevated liver enzymes
Neuromuscular & skeletal: Weakness

Drug Interactions Decreased effect with piperazine

Drug Uptake
Absorption: Oral: Poor
Time to peak: 1-3 hours

Pregnancy Risk Factor C

Generic Available No

Comments Purgation is not required prior to use

Pyrazinamide (peer a ZIN a mide)

Related Information
Nonviral Infectious Diseases *on page 1342*

Canadian Brand Names Tebrazid™

Mexican Brand Names Braccoprial®

Pharmacologic Category Antitubercular Agent

Synonyms Pyrazinoic Acid Amide

Use Adjunctive treatment of tuberculosis in combination with other antituberculosis agents in combination with rifampin or rifabutin for prevention of tuberculosis (as an alternative to isoniazid monotherapy)

Local Anesthetic/Vasoconstrictor Precautions No information available to require special precautions

Effects on Dental Treatment No effects or complications reported

Dosage Oral (calculate dose on ideal body weight rather than total body weight):
Note: A four-drug regimen (isoniazid, rifampin, pyrazinamide, and either streptomycin or ethambutol) is preferred for the initial, empiric treatment of TB. When the drug susceptibility results are available, the regimen should be altered as appropriate.
Children and Adults:
Daily therapy: 15-30 mg/kg/day (maximum: 2 g/day)
Directly observed therapy (DOT):
Twice weekly: 50-70 mg/kg (maximum: 4 g)
Three times/week: 50-70 mg/kg (maximum: 3 g)
Prevention of tuberculosis (in combination with rifampin or rifabutin): 15-30 mg/kg/day for 2 months
Elderly: Start with a lower daily dose (15 mg/kg) and increase as tolerated
Dosing adjustment in renal impairment: Cl_{cr} <50 mL/minute: Avoid use or reduce dose to 12-20 mg/kg/day
Dosing adjustment in hepatic impairment: Reduce dose

Mechanism of Action Converted to pyrazinoic acid in susceptible strains of *Mycobacterium* which lowers the pH of the environment; exact mechanism of action has not been elucidated

Other Adverse Effects 1% to 10%:
Central nervous system: Malaise
Gastrointestinal: Nausea, vomiting, anorexia
Neuromuscular & skeletal: Arthralgia, myalgia

Drug Interactions Combination therapy with rifampin and pyrazinamide has been associated with severe and fatal hepatotoxic reactions.

Drug Uptake Bacteriostatic or bactericidal, depending on the drug's concentration at the site of infection
Absorption: Oral: Well absorbed
Half-life, elimination: 9-10 hours (increases with renal or hepatic impairment); End-stage renal disease: 9 hours
Time to peak: ≤2 hours

Pregnancy Risk Factor C

Generic Available Yes

Pyrethrins (pye RE thrins)

U.S. Brand Names A-200™ [OTC]; End Lice® [OTC]; Pronto® [OTC]; Pyrinex® Pediculicide [OTC]; Pyrinyl® [OTC]; Pyrinyl Plus® [OTC]; R & C® [OTC]; RID® [OTC]; Tisit® [OTC]; Tisit® Blue Gel [OTC]

Canadian Brand Names R & C™ II; R & C™ Shampoo/Conditioner; RID® Mousse

Pharmacologic Category Antiparasitic Agent, Topical; Pediculocide; Shampoo, Pediculocide

Use Treatment of *Pediculus humanus* infestations (head lice, body lice, pubic lice and their eggs)

Local Anesthetic/Vasoconstrictor Precautions No information available to require special precautions

Effects on Dental Treatment No effects or complications reported

Dosage Application of pyrethrins: Topical:

Apply enough solution to completely wet infested area, including hair
Allow to remain on area for 10 minutes
Wash and rinse with large amounts of warm water
Use fine-toothed comb to remove lice and eggs from hair
Shampoo hair to restore body and luster
Treatment may be repeated if necessary once in a 24-hour period
Repeat treatment in 7-10 days to kill newly hatched lice

Mechanism of Action Pyrethrins are derived from flowers that belong to the chrysanthemum family. The mechanism of action on the neuronal membranes of lice is similar to that of DDT. Piperonyl butoxide is usually added to pyrethrin to enhance the product's activity by decreasing the metabolism of pyrethrins in arthropods.

Other Adverse Effects Frequency not defined:
Dermatologic: Pruritus
Local: Burning, stinging, irritation with repeat use

Drug Uptake
Onset of action: ~30 minutes
Absorption: Minimal

Pregnancy Risk Factor C

Generic Available Yes

Pyridiate® *see* Phenazopyridine *on page 943*
Pyridium® *see* Phenazopyridine *on page 943*

Pyridoxine (peer i DOKS een)

U.S. Brand Names Aminoxin® [OTC]; Nestrex® [OTC]

Mexican Brand Names Benadon

Pharmacologic Category Vitamin

Synonyms Pyridoxine Hydrochloride; Vitamin B_6

Use Prevents and treats vitamin B_6 deficiency, pyridoxine-dependent seizures in infants, adjunct to treatment of acute toxicity from isoniazid, cycloserine, or hydralazine overdose

Local Anesthetic/Vasoconstrictor Precautions No information available to require special precautions

Effects on Dental Treatment No effects or complications reported

Dosage
Recommended daily allowance (RDA):
- Children:
  - 1-3 years: 0.9 mg
  - 4-6 years: 1.3 mg
  - 7-10 years: 1.6 mg
- Adults:
  - Male: 1.7-2.0 mg
  - Female: 1.4-1.6 mg

Dietary deficiency: Oral:
- Children: 5-25 mg/24 hours for 3 weeks, then 1.5-2.5 mg/day in multiple vitamin product
- Adults: 10-20 mg/day for 3 weeks

Drug-induced neuritis (eg, isoniazid, hydralazine, penicillamine, cycloserine): Oral:
- Children:
  - Treatment: 10-50 mg/24 hours
  - Prophylaxis: 1-2 mg/kg/24 hours
- Adults:
  - Treatment: 100-200 mg/24 hours
  - Prophylaxis: 25-100 mg/24 hours

Treatment of seizures and/or coma from acute isoniazid toxicity, a dose of pyridoxine hydrochloride equal to the amount of INH ingested can be given I.M./I.V. in divided doses together with other anticonvulsants; if the amount INH ingested is not known, administer 5 g I.V. pyridoxine

Treatment of acute hydralazine toxicity, a pyridoxine dose of 25 mg/kg in divided doses I.M./I.V. has been used

Mechanism of Action Precursor to pyridoxal, which functions in the metabolism of proteins, carbohydrates, and fats; pyridoxal also aids in the release of liver and muscle-stored glycogen and in the synthesis of GABA (within the CNS) and heme

Other Adverse Effects Frequency not defined:
Central nervous system: Headache, seizures (following very large I.V. doses), sensory neuropathy
Endocrine & metabolic: Decreased serum folic acid secretions
Gastrointestinal: Nausea
Hepatic: Increased AST
Neuromuscular & skeletal: Paresthesia
Miscellaneous: Allergic reactions

Drug Interactions Pyridoxine may decrease serum concentration of levodopa, phenobarbital, and phenytoin (patients taking levodopa without carbidopa should
(Continued)

Pyridoxine *(Continued)*

avoid supplemental vitamin B_6 >5 mg per day, which includes multivitamin preparations).

Drug Uptake

Absorption: Enteral, parenteral: Well absorbed
Half-life, elimination: 15-20 days

Pregnancy Risk Factor A/C (dose exceeding RDA recommendation)

Generic Available Yes

Pyrimethamine (peer i METH a meen)

U.S. Brand Names Daraprim®

Canadian Brand Names Daraprim®

Mexican Brand Names Daraprim®

Pharmacologic Category Antimalarial Agent

Use Prophylaxis of malaria due to susceptible strains of plasmodia; used in conjunction with quinine and sulfadiazine for the treatment of uncomplicated attacks of chloroquine-resistant *P. falciparum* malaria; used in conjunction with fast-acting schizonticide to initiate transmission control and suppression cure; synergistic combination with sulfonamide in treatment of toxoplasmosis

Local Anesthetic/Vasoconstrictor Precautions No information available to require special precautions

Effects on Dental Treatment Atrophic glossitis has been reported.

Dosage

Malaria chemoprophylaxis (for areas where chloroquine-resistant *P. falciparum* exists): Begin prophylaxis 2 weeks before entering endemic area:
- Children: 0.5 mg/kg once weekly; not to exceed 25 mg/dose

  or
- Children:
  - <4 years: 6.25 mg once weekly
  - 4-10 years: 12.5 mg once weekly
- Children >10 years and Adults: 25 mg once weekly
- Dosage should be continued for all age groups for at least 6-10 weeks after leaving endemic areas

Chloroquine-resistant *P. falciparum* malaria (when used in conjunction with quinine and sulfadiazine):
- Children:
  - <10 kg: 6.25 mg/day once daily for 3 days
  - 10-20 kg: 12.5 mg/day once daily for 3 days
  - 20-40 kg: 25 mg/day once daily for 3 days
- Adults: 25 mg twice daily for 3 days

Toxoplasmosis:
- Infants for congenital toxoplasmosis: Oral: 1 mg/kg once daily for 6 months with sulfadiazine then every other month with sulfa, alternating with spiramycin.
- Children: Loading dose: 2 mg/kg/day divided into 2 equal daily doses for 1-3 days (maximum: 100 mg/day) followed by 1 mg/kg/day divided into 2 doses for 4 weeks; maximum: 25 mg/day
  - With sulfadiazine or trisulfapyrimidines: 2 mg/kg/day divided every 12 hours for 3 days followed by 1 mg/kg/day once daily or divided twice daily for 4 weeks given with trisulfapyrimidines or sulfadiazine
- Adults: 50-75 mg/day together with 1-4 g of a sulfonamide for 1-3 weeks depending on patient's tolerance and response, then reduce dose by 50% and continue for 4-5 weeks **or** 25-50 mg/day for 3-4 weeks

Mechanism of Action Inhibits parasitic dihydrofolate reductase, resulting in inhibition of vital tetrahydrofolic acid synthesis

Other Adverse Effects Frequency not defined:

Cardiovascular: Arrhythmias (large doses)
Central nervous system: Depression, fever, insomnia, lightheadedness, malaise, seizures
Dermatologic: Abnormal skin pigmentation, dermatitis, erythema multiforme, rash, Stevens-Johnson syndrome
Gastrointestinal: Anorexia, abdominal cramps, vomiting, diarrhea, xerostomia, atrophic glossitis
Hematologic: Megaloblastic anemia, leukopenia, pancytopenia, thrombocytopenia, pulmonary eosinophilia
Miscellaneous: Anaphylaxis

Drug Interactions

Increased Effect/Toxicity: Increased effect with sulfonamides (synergy), methotrexate, and TMP/SMZ.
Decreased Effect: Pyrimethamine effectiveness is decreased by acid.

Drug Uptake

Onset of action: ~1 hour
Absorption: Oral: Well absorbed
Half-life, elimination: 80-95 hours
Time to peak: 1.5-8 hours

Pregnancy Risk Factor C
Generic Available No

Pyrinex® Pediculicide [OTC] *see* Pyrethrins *on page 1026*
Pyrinyl® [OTC] *see* Pyrethrins *on page 1026*
Pyrinyl Plus® [OTC] *see* Pyrethrins *on page 1026*

Pyrithione Zinc (peer i THYE one zingk)

U.S. Brand Names DHS Zinc® [OTC]; Head & Shoulders® [OTC]; Theraplex Z® [OTC]; Zincon® [OTC]; ZNP® Bar [OTC]
Mexican Brand Names ZNP Shampoo®
Pharmacologic Category Topical Skin Product
Use Relieves the itching, irritation and scalp flaking associated with dandruff and/or seborrheal dermatitis of the scalp
Local Anesthetic/Vasoconstrictor Precautions No information available to require special precautions
Effects on Dental Treatment No effects or complications reported
Dosage Shampoo hair twice weekly, wet hair, apply to scalp and massage vigorously, rinse and repeat
Generic Available No

Quazepam (KWAY ze pam)

U.S. Brand Names Doral®
Canadian Brand Names Doral®
Pharmacologic Category Benzodiazepine
Use Treatment of insomnia; more likely than triazolam to cause daytime sedation and fatigue; is classified as a long-acting benzodiazepine hypnotic (like flurazepam - Dalmane®), this long duration of action may prevent withdrawal symptoms when therapy is discontinued
Local Anesthetic/Vasoconstrictor Precautions No information available to require special precautions
Effects on Dental Treatment >10%: Xerostomia; disappears with discontinuation
Restrictions C-IV
Dosage Adults: Oral: Initial: 15 mg at bedtime, in some patients the dose may be reduced to 7.5 mg after a few nights
Mechanism of Action Binds to stereospecific benzodiazepine receptors on the postsynaptic GABA (gamma-aminobutyric acid) neuron at several sites within the CNS, including the limbic system, reticular formation. Enhancement of the inhibitory effect of GABA on neuronal excitability results by increased neuronal membrane permeability to chloride ions. This shift in chloride ions results in hyperpolarization (a less excitable state) and stabilization.
Other Adverse Effects Frequency not defined:

Cardiovascular: Palpitations
Central nervous system: Drowsiness, fatigue, ataxia, memory impairment, anxiety, depression, headache, confusion, nervousness, dizziness, incoordination, hypo- and hyperkinesia, agitation, euphoria, paranoid reaction, nightmares, abnormal thinking
Dermatologic: Dermatitis, pruritus, rash
Endocrine & metabolic: Decreased libido, menstrual irregularities
Gastrointestinal: Xerostomia, constipation, diarrhea, dyspepsia, anorexia, abnormal taste perception, nausea, vomiting, increased or decreased appetite, abdominal pain
Genitourinary: Impotence, incontinence
Hematologic: Blood dyscrasias
Neuromuscular & skeletal: Dysarthria, rigidity, tremor, muscle cramps, reflex slowing
Ocular: Blurred vision
Miscellaneous: Drug dependence

Drug Interactions

Increased Effect/Toxicity: Serum levels and/or toxicity of quazepam may be increased by cimetidine, ciprofloxacin, clarithromycin, clozapine, CNS depressants, diltiazem, disulfiram, digoxin, erythromycin, fluconazole, fluoxetine, fluvoxamine, isoniazid, itraconazole, ketoconazole, labetalol, levodopa, loxapine, metoprolol, metronidazole, miconazole, nefazodone, omeprazole, phenytoin, rifabutin, rifampin, troleandomycin, valproic acid, and verapamil.
Decreased Effect: Carbamazepine, rifampin, rifabutin may enhance the metabolism of quazepam and decrease its therapeutic effect.

Drug Uptake

Absorption: Oral: Rapid
Half-life, elimination: Parent drug: 25-41 hours; Active metabolite: 40-114 hours

Pregnancy Risk Factor X
Generic Available No

Quenalog® *see* Nystatin and Triamcinolone *on page 881*
Questran® *see* Cholestyramine Resin *on page 279*

Questran® Light *see* Cholestyramine Resin *on page 279*

Quetiapine (kwe TYE a peen)

U.S. Brand Names Seroquel®

Canadian Brand Names Seroquel®

Mexican Brand Names Seroquel®

Pharmacologic Category Antipsychotic Agent, Dibenzothiazepine

Synonyms Quetiapine Fumarate

Use Treatment of schizophrenia

Unlabeled/Investigational: Treatment of mania, bipolar disorder (children and adults); autism, psychosis (children)

Local Anesthetic/Vasoconstrictor Precautions No information available to require special precautions

Effects on Dental Treatment No effects or complications reported

Dosage Oral:

Children and Adolescents:

Autism (unlabeled use): 100-350 mg/day (1.6-5.2 mg/kg/day)

Psychosis and mania (unlabeled use): Initial: 25 mg twice daily; titrate as necessary to 450 mg/day

Adults: Schizophrenia/psychoses: Initial: 25 mg twice daily; increase in increments of 25-50 mg 2-3 times/day on the second and third day, if tolerated, to a target dose of 300-400 mg in 2-3 divided doses by day 4. Make further adjustments as needed at intervals of at least 2 days in adjustments of 25-50 mg twice daily. Usual maintenance range: 300-800 mg/day

Elderly: 40% lower mean oral clearance of quetiapine in adults >65 years of age; higher plasma concentrations expected and, therefore, dosage adjustment may be needed; elderly patients usually require 50-200 mg/day

Dosing comments in hepatic insufficiency: 30% lower mean oral clearance of quetiapine than normal subjects; higher plasma concentrations expected in hepatically impaired subjects; dosage adjustment may be needed

Mechanism of Action Mechanism of action of quetiapine, as with other antipsychotic drugs, is unknown. However, it has been proposed that this drug's antipsychotic activity is mediated through a combination of dopamine type 2 (D_2) and serotonin type 2 ($5HT_2$) antagonism. However, it is an antagonist at multiple neurotransmitter receptors in the brain: serotonin $5HT_{1A}$ and $5HT_2$, dopamine D_1 and D_2, histamine H_1, and adrenergic alpha$_1$- and alpha$_2$-receptors; but appears to have no appreciable affinity at cholinergic muscarinic and benzodiazepine receptors.

Antagonism at receptors other than dopamine and $5HT_2$ with similar receptor affinities may explain some of the other effects of quetiapine. The drug's antagonism of histamine H_1 receptors may explain the somnolence observed with it. The drug's antagonism of adrenergic alpha$_1$-receptors may explain the orthostatic hypotension observed with it.

Other Adverse Effects

>10%:

Central nervous system: Headache, somnolence

Gastrointestinal: Weight gain

1% to 10%:

Cardiovascular: Postural hypotension, tachycardia, palpitations

Central nervous system: Dizziness

Dermatologic: Rash

Gastrointestinal: Abdominal pain, constipation, xerostomia, dyspepsia, anorexia

Hematologic: Leukopenia

Neuromuscular & skeletal: Dysarthria, back pain, weakness

Respiratory: Rhinitis, pharyngitis, cough, dyspnea

Miscellaneous: Diaphoresis

Drug Interactions CYP3A4, 2D6 (minor); 2C9 (minor) enzyme substrate

Antihypertensives: Concurrent use with an antihypertensive may produce additive hypotensive effects (particularly orthostasis)

Cimetidine: May decrease quetiapine's clearance by 20%; increasing serum concentrations

CNS depressants: Quetiapine may enhance the sedative effects of other CNS depressants; includes antidepressants, benzodiazepines, barbiturates, ethanol, narcotic analgesics, and other sedative agents; monitor for increased effect

CYP3A3/4 inhibitors: Serum level and/or toxicity of quetiapine may be increased; inhibitors include amiodarone, cimetidine, clarithromycin, erythromycin, delavirdine, diltiazem, dirithromycin, disulfiram, fluoxetine, fluvoxamine, grapefruit juice, indinavir, itraconazole, ketoconazole, metronidazole, nefazodone, nevirapine, propoxyphene, quinupristin-dalfopristin, ritonavir, saquinavir, verapamil, zafirlukast, zileuton; monitor for altered response

Enzyme inducers: May increase the metabolism of quetiapine, reducing serum levels and effect; enzyme inducers include carbamazepine, barbiturates, and rifampin; also see note on phenytoin

Levodopa: Quetiapine may inhibit the antiparkinsonian effect of levodopa; avoid this combination

Lorazepam: Metabolism of lorazepam may be reduced by quetiapine; clearance is reduced 20% in the presence of quetiapine; monitor for increased sedative effect
Metoclopramide: May increase extrapyramidal symptoms (EPS) or risk.
Phenytoin: Metabolism/clearance of quetiapine may be increased; fivefold changes have been noted
Thioridazine: May increase clearance of quetiapine, decreasing serum concentrations; clearance may be increased by 65%

Drug Uptake
Absorption: Accumulation is predictable upon multiple dosing
Half-life, elimination: Mean: Terminal: ~6 hours
Time to peak, plasma: 1.5 hours

Pregnancy Risk Factor C

Generic Available No

Comments In healthy volunteers, administration of quetiapine with food resulted in an increase in the peak serum concentration and AUC (each by ~15%) compared to the fasting state; can be taken with or without food

Quibron® *see* Theophylline and Guaifenesin *on page 1155*
Quibron®-T *see* Theophylline *on page 1152*
Quibron®-T/SR *see* Theophylline *on page 1152*
Quinaglute® Dura-Tabs® *see* Quinidine *on page 1034*

Quinapril (KWIN a pril)

Related Information
Cardiovascular Diseases *on page 1308*

U.S. Brand Names Accupril®

Canadian Brand Names Accupril™

Mexican Brand Names Acupril

Pharmacologic Category Angiotensin-Converting Enzyme (ACE) Inhibitor

Synonyms Quinapril Hydrochloride

Use Management of hypertension; treatment of CHF
Unlabeled/Investigational: Treatment of left ventricular dysfunction after myocardial infarction

Local Anesthetic/Vasoconstrictor Precautions No information available to require special precautions

Effects on Dental Treatment No effects or complications reported

Dosage
Adults: Oral:
Hypertension: Initial: 10-20 mg once daily, adjust according to BP response at peak and trough blood levels; initial dose may be reduced to 5 mg in patients receiving diuretic therapy if the diuretic is continued (normal dosage range is 20-80 mg/day for hypertension)
Congestive heart failure or post-MI: Initial: 5 mg once daily, titrated at weekly intervals to 20-40 mg daily in 2 divided doses
Elderly: Initial: 2.5-5 mg/day; increase dosage at increments of 2.5-5 mg at 1- to 2-week intervals.
Dosing adjustment in renal impairment: Lower initial doses should be used; after initial dose (if tolerated), administer initial dose twice daily; may be increased at weekly intervals to optimal response:
Hypertension: Initial:
Cl_{cr} >60 mL/minute: Administer 10 mg/day
Cl_{cr} 30-60 mL/minute: Administer 5 mg/day
Cl_{cr} 10-30 mL/minute: Administer 2.5 mg/day
Congestive heart failure: Initial:
Cl_{cr} >30 mL/minute: Administer 5 mg/day
Cl_{cr} 10-30 mL/minute: Administer 2.5 mg/day
Dosing comments in hepatic impairment: In patients with alcoholic cirrhosis, hydrolysis of quinapril to quinaprilat is impaired; however, the subsequent elimination of quinaprilat is unaltered.

Mechanism of Action Competitive inhibitor of angiotensin-converting enzyme (ACE); prevents conversion of angiotensin I to angiotensin II, a potent vasoconstrictor; results in lower levels of angiotensin II which causes an increase in plasma renin activity and a reduction in aldosterone secretion; a CNS mechanism may also be involved in hypotensive effect as angiotensin II increases adrenergic outflow from CNS; vasoactive kallikreins may be decreased in conversion to active hormones by ACE inhibitors, thus reducing BP

Other Adverse Effects Note: Frequency ranges include data from hypertension and heart failure trials. Higher rates of adverse reactions have generally been noted in patients with CHF. However, the frequency of adverse effects associated with placebo is also increased in this population.

1% to 10%:
Cardiovascular: Hypotension (3%), chest pain (2%), first-dose hypotension (up to 3%)
Central nervous system: Dizziness (4% to 8%), headache (2% to 6%), fatigue (3%)

(Continued)

Quinapril *(Continued)*

Dermatologic: Rash (1%)
Endocrine & metabolic: Hyperkalemia (2%)
Gastrointestinal: Vomiting/nausea (1% to 2%), diarrhea (2%)
Neuromuscular & skeletal: Myalgias (2% to 5%), back pain (1%)
Renal: Increased BUN/serum creatinine (2%, transient elevations may occur with a higher frequency), worsening of renal function (in patients with bilateral renal artery stenosis or hypovolemia)
Respiratory: Upper respiratory symptoms, cough (2% to 4%; up to 13% in some studies), dyspnea (2%)

A syndrome which may include fever, myalgia, arthralgia, interstitial nephritis, vasculitis, rash, eosinophilia and positive ANA, and elevated ESR has been reported with ACE inhibitors. In addition, pancreatitis, hepatic necrosis, neutropenia, and/or agranulocytosis (particularly in patients with collagen-vascular disease or renal impairment) have been associated with many ACE inhibitors.

Drug Interactions

Increased Effect/Toxicity: Potassium supplements, co-trimoxazole (high dose), angiotensin II receptor antagonists (candesartan, losartan, irbesartan, etc), or potassium-sparing diuretics (amiloride, spironolactone, triamterene) may result in elevated serum potassium levels when combined with quinapril. ACE inhibitor effects may be increased by phenothiazines or probenecid (increases levels of captopril). ACE inhibitors may increase serum concentration/effects of digoxin, lithium, and sulfonlyureas. Diuretics have additive hypotensive effects with ACE inhibitors, and hypovolemia increases the potential for adverse renal effects of ACE inhibitors. In patients with compromised renal function, coadministration with nonsteroidal anti-inflammatory drugs may result in further deterioration of renal function. Allopurinol and ACE inhibitors may cause a higher risk of hypersensitivity reaction when taken concurrently.

Decreased Effect: Quinapril may reduce the absorption of quinolones and tetracycline antibiotics. Aspirin (high dose) may reduce the therapeutic effects of ACE inhibitors; at low dosages this does not appear to be significant. Rifampin may decrease the effect of ACE inhibitors. Antacids may decrease the bioavailability of ACE inhibitors (may be more likely to occur with captopril); separate administration times by 1-2 hours. NSAIDs, specifically indomethacin, may reduce the hypotensive effects of ACE inhibitors.

Drug Uptake

Onset of action: 1 hour
Absorption: Quinapril: ≥60%
Duration: 24 hours
Half-life, elimination: Quinapril: 0.8 hours; Quinaprilat: 2 hours; increases as Cl_{cr} decreases
Time to peak: Quinapril: 1 hour; Quinaprilat: ~2 hours

Pregnancy Risk Factor C/D (2nd and 3rd trimesters)

Generic Available No

Quinapril and Hydrochlorothiazide

(KWIN a pril & hye droe klor oh THYE a zide)

U.S. Brand Names Accuretic™

Canadian Brand Names Accuretic™

Pharmacologic Category Angiotensin-Converting Enzyme (ACE) Inhibitor; Antihypertensive; Diuretic, Thiazide

Synonyms Hydrochlorothiazide and Quinapril

Use Treatment of hypertension (not for initial therapy)

Local Anesthetic/Vasoconstrictor Precautions No information available to require special precautions

Effects on Dental Treatment No effects or complications reported

Dosage Oral:

Children: Safety and efficacy have not been established.
Adults: Initial:
Patients who have failed quinapril monotherapy:
Quinapril 10 mg/hydrochlorothiazide 12.5 mg **or**
Quinapril 20 mg/hydrochlorothiazide 12.5 mg once daily
Patients with adequate BP control on hydrochlorothiazide 25 mg/day, but significant potassium loss:
Quinapril 10 mg/hydrochlorothiazide 12.5 mg **or**
Quinapril 20 mg/hydrochlorothiazide 12.5 mg once daily
Note: Clinical trials of quinapril/hydrochlorothiazide combinations used quinapril doses of 2.5-40 mg/day and hydrochlorothiazide doses of 6.25-25 mg/day.

Dosage adjustment in renal impairment: Cl_{cr} <30 mL/minute/1.73 m² or serum creatinine ≤3 mg/dL: Use is not recommended.

Other Adverse Effects 1% to 10%:

Central nervous system: Dizziness (5%), somnolence (1%)
Neuromuscular & skeletal: Weakness (1%)
Renal: Serum creatinine increase (3%), blood urea nitrogen increase (4%)

Respiratory: Cough (3%), bronchitis (1%)

Drug Interactions See Quinapril *on page 1031* and Hydrochlorothiazide *on page 595*

Drug Uptake See Quinapril *on page 1031* and Hydrochlorothiazide *on page 595*

Pregnancy Risk Factor C (1st trimester)/D (2nd and 3rd trimesters)

Generic Available No

Quinestrol (kwin ES trole)

Related Information

Endocrine Disorders and Pregnancy *on page 1331*

Pharmacologic Category Estrogen Derivative

Use Atrophic vaginitis; hypogonadism; primary ovarian failure; vasomotor symptoms of menopause; prostatic carcinoma; osteoporosis prophylactic

Local Anesthetic/Vasoconstrictor Precautions No information available to require special precautions

Effects on Dental Treatment No effects or complications reported

Dosage Adults: Female: Oral: 100 mcg once daily for 7 days; followed by 100 mcg/week beginning 2 weeks after inception of treatment; may increase to 200 mcg/week if necessary

Mechanism of Action Increases the synthesis of DNA, RNA, and various proteins in target tissues; reduces the release of gonadotropin-releasing hormone from the hypothalamus; reduces FSH and LH release from the pituitary

Other Adverse Effects

>10%:

- Cardiovascular: Peripheral edema
- Endocrine & metabolic: Enlargement of breasts (female and male), breast tenderness
- Gastrointestinal: Nausea, anorexia, bloating

1% to 10%:

- Central nervous system: Headache
- Endocrine & metabolic: Increased libido (female), decreased libido (male)
- Gastrointestinal: Vomiting, diarrhea

Drug Interactions No significant interactions reported

Drug Uptake

Onset of action: Therapeutic: ~3 days

Duration: ≤4 months

Half-life, elimination: 120 hours

Pregnancy Risk Factor X

Generic Available No

Quinethazone (kwin ETH a zone)

Related Information

Cardiovascular Diseases *on page 1308*

U.S. Brand Names Hydromox®

Canadian Brand Names Hydromox®

Pharmacologic Category Diuretic, Thiazide

Use Adjunctive therapy in treatment of edema and hypertension

Local Anesthetic/Vasoconstrictor Precautions No information available to require special precautions

Effects on Dental Treatment No effects or complications reported

Dosage Adults: Oral: 50-100 mg once daily up to a maximum of 200 mg/day

Mechanism of Action Quinethazone is a quinazoline derivative which increases the renal excretion of sodium and chloride and an accompanying volume of water due to inhibition of the tubular mechanism of electrolyte reabsorption.

Other Adverse Effects 1% to 10%: Endocrine & metabolic: Hypokalemia

Warnings/Precautions Avoid in severe renal disease (ineffective). Electrolyte disturbances (hypokalemia, hypochloremic alkalosis, hyponatremia) can occur. Use with caution in severe hepatic dysfunction; hepatic encephalopathy can be caused by electrolyte disturbances. Gout can be precipitated in certain patients with a history of gout, a familial predisposition to gout, or chronic renal failure. Cautious use in diabetics; may see a change in glucose control. Hypersensitivity reactions can occur. Can cause SLE exacerbation or activation. Use with caution in patients with moderate or high cholesterol concentrations. Photosensitization may occur. Correct hypokalemia before initiating therapy.

Chemical similarities are present among sulfonamides, sulfonylureas, carbonic anhydrase inhibitors, thiazides, and loop diuretics (except ethacrynic acid). Use in patients with thiazide or sulfonamide allergy is specifically contraindicated in product labeling, however a risk of cross-reaction exists in patients with allergy to any of these compounds; avoid use when previous reaction has been severe.

Drug Interactions

Increased Effect/Toxicity: Increased hypotension with ACE-inhibitors if aggressively diuresed with a thiazide diuretic. Beta-blockers may increase hyperglycemic effects in type 2 diabetes mellitus (noninsulin dependent, NIDDM). Cyclosporine and thiazides can increase the risk of gout or renal toxicity; avoid concurrent use.

(Continued)

Quinethazone *(Continued)*

Digoxin toxicity can be exacerbated if a thiazide induces hypokalemia or hypomagnesemia. Lithium toxicity can occur by reducing renal excretion of lithium; monitor lithium concentration and adjust as needed. Neuromuscular blocking agents can prolong blockade; monitor serum potassium and neuromuscular status.

Decreased Effect: NSAIDs can decrease the efficacy of thiazides reducing the diuretic and antihypertensive effects.

Drug Uptake

Onset of action: 2 hours

Duration: 18-24 hours

Pregnancy Risk Factor D

Generic Available No

Quinidex® Extentabs® *see* Quinidine *on page 1034*

Quinidine (KWIN i deen)

Related Information

Cardiovascular Diseases *on page 1308*

U.S. Brand Names Cardioquin®; Quinaglute® Dura-Tabs®; Quinidex® Extentabs®

Canadian Brand Names Apo®-Quinidine; Cardioquin®; Quinidex Extentabs®

Mexican Brand Names Quini Durules®

Pharmacologic Category Antiarrhythmic Agent, Class Ia

Synonyms Quinidine Gluconate; Quinidine Polygalacturonate; Quinidine Sulfate

Use Prophylaxis after cardioversion of atrial fibrillation and/or flutter to maintain normal sinus rhythm; also used in the prevention of reoccurrence of paroxysmal supraventricular tachycardia, paroxysmal A-V junctional rhythm, paroxysmal ventricular tachycardia, paroxysmal atrial fibrillation, and atrial or ventricular premature contractions; also has activity against *Plasmodium falciparum* malaria

Local Anesthetic/Vasoconstrictor Precautions No information available to require special precautions

Effects on Dental Treatment When taken over a long period of time, the anticholinergic side effects from quinidine can cause a reduction of saliva production or secretion contributing to discomfort and dental disease (ie, caries, oral candidiasis and periodontal disease).

Dosage Dosage expressed in terms of the salt: 267 mg of quinidine gluconate = 200 mg of quinidine sulfate.

Children: Test dose for idiosyncratic reaction (sulfate, oral or gluconate, I.M.): 2 mg/kg or 60 mg/m^2

Oral (quinidine sulfate): 15-60 mg/kg/day in 4-5 divided doses or 6 mg/kg every 4-6 hours; usual 30 mg/kg/day or 900 mg/m^2/day given in 5 daily doses

I.V. **not** recommended (quinidine gluconate): 2-10 mg/kg/dose given at a rate ≤10 mg/minute every 3-6 hours as needed

Adults: Test dose: Oral, I.M.: 200 mg administered several hours before full dosage (to determine possibility of idiosyncratic reaction)

Oral (for malaria):

Sulfate: 100-600 mg/dose every 4-6 hours; begin at 200 mg/dose and titrate to desired effect (maximum daily dose: 3-4 g)

Gluconate: 324-972 mg every 8-12 hours

I.M.: 400 mg/dose every 2-6 hours; initial dose: 600 mg (gluconate)

I.V.: 200-400 mg/dose diluted and given at a rate ≤10 mg/minute; may require as much as 500-750 mg

Dosing adjustment in renal impairment: Cl_{cr} <10 mL/minute: Administer 75% of normal dose.

Hemodialysis: Slightly hemodialyzable (5% to 20%); 200 mg supplemental dose posthemodialysis is recommended.

Peritoneal dialysis: Not dialyzable (0% to 5%)

Dosing adjustment/comments in hepatic impairment: Larger loading dose may be indicated, reduce maintenance doses by 50% and monitor serum concentration closely.

Mechanism of Action Class 1A antiarrhythmic agent; depresses phase O of the action potential; decreases myocardial excitability and conduction velocity, and myocardial contractility by decreasing sodium influx during depolarization and potassium efflux in repolarization; also reduces calcium transport across cell membrane

Other Adverse Effects

Frequency not defined: Hypotension, syncope

>10%:

Cardiovascular: QT_c prolongation (modest prolongation is common, however excessive prolongation is rare and indicates toxicity)

Central nervous system: Lightheadedness (15%)

Gastrointestinal: Diarrhea (35%), upper GI distress, bitter taste, diarrhea, anorexia, nausea, vomiting, stomach cramping (22%)

1% to 10%:

Cardiovascular: Angina (6%), palpitation (7%), new or worsened arrhythmias (proarrhythmic effect)

Central nervous system: Syncope (1% to 8%), headache (7%), fatigue (7%), weakness (5%), sleep disturbance (3%), tremor (2%), nervousness (2%), incoordination (1%)

Dermatologic: Rash (5%)

Ocular: Blurred vision

Otic: Tinnitus

Respiratory: Wheezing

Note: Cinchonism, a syndrome which may include tinnitus, high-frequency hearing loss, deafness, vertigo, blurred vision, diplopia, photophobia, headache, confusion, and delirium has been associated with quinidine use. Usually associated with chronic toxicity, this syndrome has also been described after brief exposure to a moderate dose in sensitive patients. Vomiting and diarrhea may also occur as isolated reactions to therapeutic quinidine levels.

Drug Interactions CYP3A3/4 enzyme substrate; CYP2D6 (potent) and 3A3/4 (weak) enzyme inhibitor

Amiloride may cause prolonged ventricular conduction leading to arrhythmias.

Amiodarone may increase quinidine blood levels; monitor quinidine levels.

Cimetidine: Increase quinidine blood levels; closely monitor levels or use an alternative H_2 antagonist.

Cisapride and quinidine may increase risk of malignant arrhythmias; concurrent use is contraindicated.

Codeine: Analgesic efficacy may be reduced.

CYP3A3/4 inhibitors (clarithromycin, erythromycin, itraconazole, ketoconazole, troleandomycin, protease inhibitors) may increase quinidine blood levels.

Digoxin blood levels may be increased. Monitor digoxin blood levels.

Enzyme inducers (aminoglutethimide, carbamazepine, phenobarbital, phenytoin, primidone, rifabutin, rifampin) may decrease quinidine blood levels.

Metoprolol: Increased metoprolol blood levels.

Mexiletine blood levels may be increased.

Nifedipine blood levels may be increased by quinidine; nifedipine may decrease quinidine blood levels.

Drugs which prolong the QT interval include amiodarone, amitriptyline, astemizole, bepridil, disopyramide, erythromycin, haloperidol, imipramine, pimozide, procainamide, sotalol, and thioridazine. Effects may be additive; use with caution.

Propafenone blood levels may be increased.

Propranolol blood levels may be increased.

Ritonavir, nelfinavir and amprenavir may increase quinidine levels and toxicity; concurrent use is contraindicated.

Sparfloxacin, gatifloxacin, and moxifloxacin may result in additional prolongation of the QT interval; concurrent use is contraindicated.

Timolol blood levels may be increased.

Urinary alkalinizers (antacids, sodium bicarbonate, acetazolamide) increase quinidine blood levels.

Verapamil and diltiazem increase quinidine blood levels.

Warfarin effects may be increased by quinidine; monitor INR closely during addition or withdrawal of quinidine.

Drug Uptake Half-life, elimination:

Children: 2.5-6.7 hours

Adults: 6-8 hours (increases with cirrhosis, CHF, and in the elderly)

Pregnancy Risk Factor C

Generic Available Yes

Quinine (KWYE nine)

Canadian Brand Names Quinine-Odan™

Pharmacologic Category Antimalarial Agent

Synonyms Quinine Sulfate

Use Suppression or treatment of chloroquine-resistant *P. falciparum* malaria; treatment of *Babesia microti* infection; prevention and treatment of nocturnal recumbency leg muscle cramps

Local Anesthetic/Vasoconstrictor Precautions No information available to require special precautions

Effects on Dental Treatment No effects or complications reported

Dosage Oral:

Children:

Treatment of chloroquine-resistant malaria: 25 mg/kg/day in divided doses every 8 hours for 3-7 days in conjunction with another agent

Babesiosis: 25 mg/kg/day, (up to a maximum of 650 mg/dose) divided every 8 hours for 7 days

Adults:

Treatment of chloroquine-resistant malaria: 650 mg every 8 hours for 3-7 days in conjunction with another agent

(Continued)

Quinine *(Continued)*

Suppression of malaria: 325 mg twice daily and continued for 6 weeks after exposure

Babesiosis: 650 mg every 6-8 hours for 7 days

Leg cramps: 200-300 mg at bedtime

Mechanism of Action Depresses oxygen uptake and carbohydrate metabolism; intercalates into DNA, disrupting the parasite's replication and transcription; affects calcium distribution within muscle fibers and decreases the excitability of the motor end-plate region; cardiovascular effects similar to quinidine

Other Adverse Effects Frequency not defined:

Central nervous system: Severe headache

Gastrointestinal: Nausea, vomiting, diarrhea

Ocular: Blurred vision

Otic: Tinnitus

Miscellaneous: Cinchonism (risk of cinchonism is directly related to dose and duration of therapy)

Drug Interactions CYP3A3/4 enzyme substrate; CYP3A3/4 enzyme inhibitor

Increased Effect/Toxicity: Beta-blockers + quinine may increase bradycardia. Quinine may enhance warfarin anticoagulant effect. Quinine potentiates nondepolarizing and depolarizing muscle relaxants. Quinine may increase plasma concentration of digoxin. Closely monitor digoxin concentrations. Digoxin dosage may need to be reduced (by one-half) when quinine is initiated. New steady-state digoxin plasma concentrations occur in 5-7 days. Verapamil, amiodarone, alkalinizing agents, and cimetidine may increase quinine serum concentration.

Decreased Effect: Phenobarbital, phenytoin, and rifampin may decrease quinine serum concentration.

Drug Uptake

Absorption: Oral: Readily absorbed, mainly from the upper small intestine

Half-life, elimination: Children: 6-12 hours; Adults: 8-14 hours

Time to peak: 1-3 hours

Pregnancy Risk Factor X

Generic Available Yes

Quinsana Plus® [OTC] *see* Tolnaftate *on page 1181*

Quinupristin and Dalfopristin (kwi NYOO pris tin & dal FOE pris tin)

U.S. Brand Names Synercid®

Canadian Brand Names Synercid®

Pharmacologic Category Antibiotic, Streptogramin

Synonyms Pristinamycin; RP59500

Use Treatment of serious or life-threatening infections associated with vancomycin-resistant *Enterococcus faecium* bacteremia; treatment of complicated skin and skin structure infections caused by methicillin-susceptible *Staphylococcus aureus* or *Streptococcus pyogenes*

Has been studied in the treatment of a variety of infections caused by *Enterococcus faecium* (not *E. fecalis*) including vancomycin-resistant strains. May also be effective in the treatment of serious infections caused by *Staphylococcus* species including those resistant to methicillin.

Local Anesthetic/Vasoconstrictor Precautions No information available to require special precautions

Effects on Dental Treatment No effects or complications reported

Dosage I.V.:

Children (limited information): Dosages similar to adult dosing have been used in the treatment of complicated skin/soft tissue infections and infections caused by vancomycin-resistant *Enterococcus faecium*

CNS shunt infection due to vancomycin-resistant *Enterococcus faecium*: 7.5 mg/kg/dose every 8 hours; concurrent intrathecal doses of 1-2 mg/day have been administered for up to 68 days

Adults:

Vancomycin-resistant *Enterococcus faecium:* 7.5 mg/kg every 8 hours

Complicated skin and skin structure infection: 7.5 mg/kg every 12 hours

Dosage adjustment in hepatic impairment: Dosage adjustment may be necessary; no specific recommendations

Mechanism of Action Quinupristin/dalfopristin inhibits bacterial protein synthesis by binding to different sites on the 50S bacterial ribosomal subunit thereby inhibiting protein synthesis

Other Adverse Effects

>10%:

Hepatic: Hyperbilirubinemia (3% to 35%)

Local: Inflammation at infusion site (38% to 42%), local pain (40% to 44%), local edema (17% to 18%), infusion site reaction (12% to 13%)

Note: High baseline values were noted in many patients, contributing to the high incidence of this reaction in some studies.

1% to 10%:

Central nervous system: Pain (2% to 3%), headache (2%)
Dermatologic: Pruritus (2%), rash (3%)
Endocrine & metabolic: Hyperglycemia (1%)
Gastrointestinal: Nausea (3% to 5%), diarrhea (3%), vomiting (3% to 4%)
Hematologic: Anemia (3%)
Hepatic: Increased LDH (3%), increased GGT (2%)
Local: Thrombophlebitis (2%)
Neuromuscular & skeletal: Arthralgia (<1% to 8%), myalgia (<1% to 5%), Increased CPK (2%)

Warnings/Precautions Use with caution in patients with hepatic or renal dysfunction. May cause pain and phlebitis when infused through a peripheral line (not relieved by hydrocortisone or diphenhydramine). Superinfection may occur. As with many antibiotics, antibiotic-associated colitis and pseudomembranous colitis may occur. May cause arthralgias, myalgias, and hyperbilirubinemia. May inhibit the metabolism of many drugs metabolized by CYP3A4. Concurrent therapy with astemizole, terfenadine, and cisapride (which may prolong QT_c interval and lead to arrhythmias) should be avoided.

Drug Interactions CYP3A3/4 enzyme inhibitor

Increased Effect/Toxicity: Astemizole, terfenadine, and cisapride (which may prolong QT_c interval and lead to arrhythmias) should be avoided. The metabolism of midazolam, nifedipine, and terfenadine have been demonstrated to be inhibited *in vitro*. An increase in cyclosporine levels has been documented in patients receiving concomitant therapy. Other medications metabolized by CYP3A4, including protease inhibitors, non-nucleoside reverse transcriptase inhibitors, benzodiazepines, calcium channel blockers, some HMG-CoA reductase inhibitors, immunosuppressive agents, corticosteroids, carbamazepine, quinidine, lidocaine, and disopyramide are predicted to have increased plasma concentrations during concurrent dosing.

Drug Uptake Half-life, elimination: Quinupristin: 0.85 hour; Dalfopristin: 0.7 hour (mean elimination half-lives, including metabolites: 3 and 1 hours, respectively)

Pregnancy Risk Factor B

Generic Available No

Comments Symptoms of overdose may include dyspnea, emesis, tremors and ataxia. Treatment is supportive. Not removed by hemodialysis or peritoneal dialysis.

Quixin™ Ophthalmic *see* Levofloxacin *on page 701*
QVAR™ *see* Beclomethasone *on page 146*

Rabeprazole (ra BE pray zole)

U.S. Brand Names Aciphex®

Canadian Brand Names Aciphex™

Mexican Brand Names Pariet®

Pharmacologic Category Proton Pump Inhibitor

Synonyms Pariprazole

Use Short-term (4-8 weeks) treatment of erosive or ulcerative gastroesophageal reflux disease (GERD); maintenance therapy in erosive or ulcerative GERD; short-term (up to 4 weeks) treatment of duodenal ulcers; long-term treatment of pathological hypersecretory conditions, including Zollinger-Ellison syndrome

Unlabeled/Investigational: *H. pylori* eradication; symptomatic GERD; maintenance of duodenal ulcer

Local Anesthetic/Vasoconstrictor Precautions No information available to require special precautions

Effects on Dental Treatment No effects or complications reported

Dosage Adults >18 years and Elderly:

GERD: 20 mg once daily for 4-8 weeks; maintenance: 20 mg once daily
Duodenal ulcer: 20 mg/day after breakfast for 4 weeks
Hypersecretory conditions: 60 mg once daily; dose may need to be adjusted as necessary. Doses as high as 100 mg and 60 mg twice daily have been used.

Mechanism of Action Potent proton pump inhibitor; suppresses gastric acid secretion by inhibiting the parietal cell H+/K+ ATP pump

Other Adverse Effects 1% to 10%: Central nervous system: Headache

Contraindications Hypersensitivity to rabeprazole, substituted benzimidazoles, or any component of their formulation

Drug Interactions CYP3A3/4 and 2C19 (minor) enzyme substrate

Increased Effect/Toxicity: Rabeprazole (in extremely high concentrations) may increase serum concentration of digoxin and cyclosporine.

Decreased Effect: Rabeprazole may decrease bioavailability of ketoconazole or itraconazole.

Drug Uptake

Onset of action: 1 hour; Peak effect, plasma: ~2-5 hours
Absorption: Oral: Well absorbed within 1 hour
Duration: 24 hours
Half-life, elimination: 0.85-2 hours (dose-dependent)

(Continued)

Rabeprazole *(Continued)*

Time to peak: 2-5 hours

Pregnancy Risk Factor B

Generic Available No

Rabies Immune Globulin (Human)

(RAY beez i MYUN GLOB yoo lin, HYU man)

Related Information

Animal and Human Bites Guidelines *on page 1416*

U.S. Brand Names BayRab®; Imogam®

Canadian Brand Names BayRab™; Imogam® Rabies Pasteurized

Pharmacologic Category Immune Globulin

Synonyms RIG

Use Part of postexposure prophylaxis of persons with rabies exposure who lack a history or pre-exposure or postexposure prophylaxis with rabies vaccine or a recently documented neutralizing antibody response to previous rabies vaccination; although it is preferable to give RIG with the first dose of vaccine, it can be given up to 8 days after vaccination

Local Anesthetic/Vasoconstrictor Precautions No information available to require special precautions

Effects on Dental Treatment No effects or complications reported

Dosage Children and Adults: I.M.: 20 units/kg in a single dose (RIG should always be administered in conjunction with rabies vaccine (HDCV)); infiltrate 1/2 of the dose locally around the wound; administer remainder I.M. into gluteal muscle

Mechanism of Action Rabies immune globulin is a solution of globulins dried from the plasma or serum of selected adult human donors who have been immunized with rabies vaccine and have developed high titers of rabies antibody. It generally contains 10% to 18% of protein of which not less than 80% is monomeric immunoglobulin G.

Other Adverse Effects 1% to 10%:

Central nervous system: Fever (mild)

Local: Soreness at injection site

Warnings/Precautions Have epinephrine 1:1000 available for anaphylactic reactions. As a product of human plasma, this product may potentially transmit disease; screening of donors, as well as testing and/or inactivation of certain viruses reduces this risk. Use caution in patients with thrombocytopenia or coagulation disorders (I.M. injections may be contraindicated), in patients with isolated IgA deficiency, or in patients with previous systemic hypersensitivity to human immunoglobulins. Not for I.V. administration.

Drug Interactions Decreased Effect: Live virus vaccines (eg, MMR, rabies) may have delayed or diminished antibody response with immune globulin administration; should not be administered within 3 months unless antibody titers dictate as appropriate

Pregnancy Risk Factor C

Generic Available No

Rabies Virus Vaccine (RAY beez VYE rus vak SEEN)

Related Information

Animal and Human Bites Guidelines *on page 1416*

U.S. Brand Names Imovax® Rabies Vaccine

Canadian Brand Names Imovax® Rabies

Pharmacologic Category Vaccine

Synonyms HDCV; Human Diploid Cell Cultures Rabies Vaccine

Use

Pre-exposure immunization: Vaccinate persons with greater than usual risk due to occupation or avocation including veterinarians, rangers, animal handlers, certain laboratory workers, and persons living in or visiting countries for longer than 1 month where rabies is a constant threat.

Postexposure prophylaxis: If a bite from a carrier animal is unprovoked, if it is not captured and rabies is present in that species and area, administer rabies immune globulin (RIG) and the vaccine as indicated

Local Anesthetic/Vasoconstrictor Precautions No information available to require special precautions

Effects on Dental Treatment No effects or complications reported

Dosage

Pre-exposure prophylaxis: 1 mL I.M. on days 0, 7, and 21 to 28. **Note:** Prolonging the interval between doses does not interfere with immunity achieved after the concluding dose of the basic series.

Postexposure prophylaxis: All postexposure treatment should begin with immediate cleansing of the wound with soap and water

Persons not previously immunized as above: Rabies immune globulin 20 units/kg body weight, half infiltrated at bite site if possible, remainder I.M.; and 5 doses of rabies vaccine, 1 mL I.M., one each on days 0, 3, 7, 14, 28

Persons who have previously received postexposure prophylaxis with rabies vaccine, received a recommended I.M. pre-exposure series of rabies vaccine or have a previously documented rabies antibody titer considered adequate: 1 mL of either vaccine I.M. only on days 0 and 3; do not administer RIG

Booster (for occupational or other continuing risk): 1 mL I.M. every 2-5 years or based on antibody titers

Mechanism of Action Rabies vaccine is an inactivated virus vaccine which promotes immunity by inducing an active immune response. The production of specific antibodies requires about 7-10 days to develop. Rabies immune globulin or antirabies serum, equine (ARS) is given in conjunction with rabies vaccine to provide immune protection until an antibody response can occur.

Other Adverse Effects Mild systemic reactions occur at an incidence of ~8% to 10% with RVA and 20% with HDCV.

All serious adverse reactions must be reported to the U.S. Department of Health and Human Services (DHHS) Vaccine Adverse Event Reporting System (VAERS)1-800-822-7967.

Note: Serum sickness reaction is much less frequent with RVA (<1%) vs the HDCV (6%).

Frequency not defined:

- Cardiovascular: Edema
- Central nervous system: Dizziness, malaise, encephalomyelitis, transverse myelitis, fever, pain, headache, neuroparalytic reactions
- Dermatologic: Itching, erythema
- Gastrointestinal: Nausea, abdominal pain
- Local: Local discomfort, pain at injection site
- Neuromuscular & skeletal: Myalgia

Drug Interactions Decreased effect with immunosuppressive agents, corticosteroids, antimalarial drugs (ie, chloroquine); persons on these drugs should receive RIG (3 doses/1 mL each) by the I.M. route

Drug Uptake

Onset of action: I.M.: Rabies antibody: ~7-10 days; Peak effect: ~30-60 days

Duration: ≥1 year

Pregnancy Risk Factor C

Generic Available No

Radiological/Contrast Media (Nonionic)

U.S. Brand Names Amipaque®; Isovue®; Omnipaque®; Optiray®; ProHance®

Pharmacologic Category Radiopaque Agents

Synonyms Gadoteridol; Iohexol; Iopamidol; Ioversol; Metrizamide

Use Enhance visualization of structures during radiologic procedures

Local Anesthetic/Vasoconstrictor Precautions No information available to require special precautions

Effects on Dental Treatment <1%: Xerostomia, edematous and/or itching tongue, gingivitis; 1.4%: taste perversion

Generic Available Yes

Raloxifene (ral OX i feen)

Related Information

Endocrine Disorders and Pregnancy *on page 1331*

U.S. Brand Names Evista®

Canadian Brand Names Evista®

Mexican Brand Names Evista®

Pharmacologic Category Selective Estrogen Receptor Modulator (SERM)

Synonyms Keoxifene Hydrochloride; Raloxifene Hydrochloride

Use Prevention and treatment of osteoporosis in postmenopausal women

Local Anesthetic/Vasoconstrictor Precautions No information available to require special precautions

Effects on Dental Treatment No effects or complications reported

Dosage Adults: Oral: 1 tablet daily may be administered any time of the day without regard to meals

Mechanism of Action A selective estrogen receptor modulator, meaning that it affects some of the same receptors that estrogen does, but not all, and in some instances, it antagonizes or blocks estrogen; it acts like estrogen to prevent bone loss and improve lipid profiles (decreases total and LDL cholesterol but does not raise triglycerides), but it has the potential to block some estrogen effects such as those that lead to breast cancer and uterine cancer

Other Adverse Effects Note: Has been associated with increased risk of thromboembolism (DVT, PE) and superficial thrombophlebitis; risk is similar to reported risk of HRT

≥2%:

- Cardiovascular: Chest pain
- Central nervous system: Migraine, depression, insomnia, fever
- Dermatologic: Rash

(Continued)

Raloxifene *(Continued)*

Endocrine & metabolic: Hot flashes

Gastrointestinal: Nausea, dyspepsia, vomiting, flatulence, gastroenteritis, weight gain

Genitourinary: Vaginitis, urinary tract infection, cystitis, leukorrhea

Neuromuscular & skeletal: Leg cramps, arthralgia, myalgia, arthritis

Respiratory: Sinusitis, pharyngitis, cough, pneumonia, laryngitis

Miscellaneous: Infection, flu syndrome, diaphoresis

Drug Interactions

Increased Effect/Toxicity: Raloxifene has the potential to interact with highly protein-bound drugs (increase effects of either agent). Use caution with highly protein-bound drugs, warfarin, clofibrate, indomethacin, naproxen, ibuprofen, diazepam, phenytoin, or tamoxifen.

Decreased Effect: Ampicillin and cholestyramine reduce raloxifene absorption/blood levels.

Drug Uptake

Onset of action: 8 weeks

Half-life, elimination: 27.7-32.5 hours

Pregnancy Risk Factor X

Generic Available No

Comments The decrease in estrogen-related adverse effects with the selective estrogen-receptor modulators in general and raloxifene in particular should improve compliance and decrease the incidence of cardiovascular events and fractures while not increasing breast cancer

Ramipril (ra MI pril)

Related Information

Cardiovascular Diseases *on page 1308*

U.S. Brand Names Altace®

Canadian Brand Names Altace®

Mexican Brand Names Ramace; Tritace

Pharmacologic Category Angiotensin-Converting Enzyme (ACE) Inhibitor

Use Treatment of hypertension (alone or in combination with thiazide diuretics), CHF, left ventricular dysfunction after myocardial infarction; to reduce risk of heart attack, stroke, and death in patients at increased risk for these problems

Local Anesthetic/Vasoconstrictor Precautions No information available to require special precautions

Effects on Dental Treatment No effects or complications reported

Dosage Adults: Oral:

Hypertension: 2.5-5 mg once daily, maximum: 20 mg/day

Reduction in risk of MI, stroke, and death from cardiovascular causes: Initial: 2.5 mg once daily for 1 week, then 5 mg once daily for the next 3 weeks, then increase as tolerated to 10 mg once daily (may be given as divided dose)

Heart failure postmyocardial infarction: Initial: 2.5 mg twice daily titrated upward, if possible, to 5 mg twice daily.

Note: The dose of any concomitant diuretic should be reduced. If the diuretic cannot be discontinued, initiate therapy with 1.25 mg. After the initial dose, the patient should be monitored carefully until BP has stabilized.

Mechanism of Action Ramipril is an angiotensin-converting enzyme (ACE) inhibitor which prevents the formation of angiotensin II from angiotensin I and exhibits pharmacologic effects that are similar to captopril. Ramipril must undergo enzymatic saponification by esterases in the liver to its biologically active metabolite, ramiprilat. The pharmacodynamic effects of ramipril result from the high-affinity, competitive, reversible binding of ramiprilat to angiotensin-converting enzyme thus preventing the formation of the potent vasoconstrictor angiotensin II. This isomerized enzyme-inhibitor complex has a slow rate of dissociation, which results in high potency and a long duration of action; a CNS mechanism may also be involved in the hypotensive effect as angiotensin II increases adrenergic outflow from CNS; vasoactive kallikreins may be decreased in conversion to active hormones by ACE inhibitors, thus reducing BP

Other Adverse Effects Frequency ranges include data from hypertension and heart failure trials. Higher rates of adverse reactions have generally been noted in patients with CHF. However, the frequency of adverse effects associated with placebo is also increased in this population.

>10%: Respiratory: Cough (increased) (7% to 12%)

1% to 10%:

Cardiovascular: Hypotension (11%), angina (3%), postural hypotension (2%), syncope (2%)

Central nervous system: Headache (1% to 5%), dizziness (2% to 4%), fatigue (2%), vertigo (2%)

Endocrine & metabolic: Hyperkalemia (1% to 10%)

Gastrointestinal: Nausea/vomiting (1% to 2%)

Neuromuscular & skeletal: Chest pain (noncardiac) (1%)

Renal: Renal dysfunction (1%), elevation in serum creatinine (1% to 2%), increased BUN (<1% to 3%); transient elevations of creatinine and/or BUN may occur more frequently

Respiratory: Cough (estimated 1% to 10%)

Worsening of renal function may occur in patients with bilateral renal artery stenosis or in hypovolemia. In addition, a syndrome which may include fever, myalgia, arthralgia, interstitial nephritis, vasculitis, rash, eosinophilia and positive ANA, and elevated ESR has been reported with ACE inhibitors. Pancreatitis and agranulocytosis (particularly in patients with collagen vascular disease or renal impairment) have been associated with ACE inhibitors.

Drug Interactions

Increased Effect/Toxicity: Potassium supplements, co-trimoxazole (high dose), angiotensin II receptor antagonists (candesartan, losartan, irbesartan, etc), or potassium-sparing diuretics (amiloride, spironolactone, triamterene) may result in elevated serum potassium levels when combined with ramipril. ACE inhibitor effects may be increased by phenothiazines or probenecid (increases levels of captopril). ACE inhibitors may increase serum concentration/effects of digoxin, lithium, and sulfonlyureas. Diuretics have additive hypotensive effects with ACE inhibitors, and hypovolemia increases the potential for adverse renal effects of ACE inhibitors. In patients with compromised renal function, coadministration with nonsteroidal anti-inflammatory drugs may result in further deterioration of renal function. Allopurinol and ACE inhibitors may cause a higher risk of hypersensitivity reaction when taken concurrently.

Decreased Effect: Aspirin (high dose) may reduce the therapeutic effects of ACE inhibitors; at low dosages this does not appear to be significant. Rifampin may decrease the effect of ACE inhibitors. Antacids may decrease the bioavailability of ACE inhibitors (may be more likely to occur with captopril); separate administration times by 1-2 hours. NSAIDs, specifically indomethacin, may reduce the hypotensive effects of ACE inhibitors. More likely to occur in low renin or volume dependent hypertensive patients.

Drug Uptake

Onset of action: 1-2 hours

Duration: 24 hours

Absorption: Well absorbed (50% to 60%)

Half-life, elimination: Ramiprilat: Effective: 13-17 hours; Terminal: >50 hours

Time to peak: ~1 hour

Pregnancy Risk Factor C/D (2nd and 3rd trimesters)

Generic Available No

Ramses® [OTC] *see* Nonoxynol 9 *on page 874*

Ranitidine Bismuth Citrate (ra NI ti deen BIZ muth SIT rate)

Related Information

Gastrointestinal Disorders *on page 1326*

U.S. Brand Names Tritec®

Canadian Brand Names Pylorid®

Pharmacologic Category Histamine H_2 Antagonist

Synonyms GR1222311X; RBC

Use Used in combination with clarithromycin for the treatment of active duodenal ulcer associated with *H. pylori* infection; not to be used alone for the treatment of active duodenal ulcer

Local Anesthetic/Vasoconstrictor Precautions No information available to require special precautions

Effects on Dental Treatment 60% to 70%: Darkening of the tongue and/or stool; 11%: Taste disturbance

Dosage Adults: Oral: 400 mg twice daily for 3 weeks with clarithromycin plus amoxicillin **or** clarithromycin plus metronidazole **or** clarithromycin plus tetracycline

Refer to Multiple Drug Regimens for the Treatment of *H. pylori* Infection *on page 1327.*

Mechanism of Action As a complex of ranitidine and bismuth citrate, gastric acid secretion is inhibited by histamine-blocking activity at the parietal cell and the structural integrity of *H. pylori* organisms is disrupted; additionally bismuth reduces the adherence of *H. pylori* to epithelial cells of the stomach and may exert a cytoprotectant effect, inhibiting pepsin, as well. Adequate eradication of *Helicobacter pylori* is achieved with the combination of clarithromycin.

Other Adverse Effects

>10%:

Central nervous system: Headache (14%)

Gastrointestinal: Darkening of the tongue and/or stool (60% to 70%), taste disturbance (11%)

>1%:

Central nervous system: Dizziness (1% to 2%)

Gastrointestinal: Diarrhea (5%), nausea/vomiting (3%), constipation (2%), abdominal pain, gastric upset (<10%)

Miscellaneous: Flu-like symptoms (2%)

(Continued)

Ranitidine Bismuth Citrate *(Continued)*

Warnings/Precautions Use in children has not been established

Drug Interactions See Ranitidine Hydrochloride *on page 1042*

Drug Uptake

Absorption: Bismuth: Minimal systemic absorption (≤1%); Ranitidine: 50% to 60% (dose-dependent)

Half-life, elimination: Complex: 5-8 days; Bismuth: 11-28 days; Ranitidine: 3 hours

Time to peak: Bismuth: 0.25-1 hour; Ranitidine: 0.5-5 hours; Time to peak effect of complex: 1 week

Pregnancy Risk Factor C

Generic Available No

Ranitidine Hydrochloride (ra NI ti deen)

Related Information

Dental Drug Interactions: Update on Drug Combinations Requiring Special Considerations *on page 1434*

Gastrointestinal Disorders *on page 1326*

Ranitidine Bismuth Citrate *on page 1041*

U.S. Brand Names Zantac®; Zantac® 75 [OTC]

Canadian Brand Names Alti-Ranitidine; Apo®-Ranitidine; Gen-Ranidine; Novo-Ranidine; Nu-Ranit; Scheinpharm™ Ranitidine; Zantac®; Zantac 75®

Mexican Brand Names Acloral®; Alter-H2®; Alvidina; Anistal; Azanplus®; Azantac; Cauteridol®; Credaxol; Galidrin; Gastrec; Microtid; Neugal; Ranifur®; Ranisen; Raudil®; Serviradine®; Ulcedin®; Ulsaven®; Ultran®

Pharmacologic Category Histamine H_2 Antagonist

Synonyms Ranitidine

Use

Zantac®: Short-term and maintenance therapy of duodenal ulcer, gastric ulcer, gastroesophageal reflux, active benign ulcer, erosive esophagitis, and pathological hypersecretory conditions

Zantac® 75 [OTC]: Relief of heartburn, acid indigestion, and sour stomach

Unlabeled/Investigational: Recurrent postoperative ulcer, upper GI bleeding, prevention of acid-aspiration pneumonitis during surgery, and prevention of stress-induced ulcers

Local Anesthetic/Vasoconstrictor Precautions No information available to require special precautions

Effects on Dental Treatment No effects or complications reported

Dosage

Children 1 month to 16 years:

Duodenal and gastric ulcer:

Oral:

Treatment: 2-4 mg/kg/day divided twice daily; maximum treatment dose: 300 mg/day

Maintenance: 2-4 mg/kg once daily; maximum maintenance dose: 150 mg/day

I.V.: 2-4 mg/kg/day divided every 6-8 hours; maximum: 150 mg/day

GERD and erosive esophagitis:

Oral: 5-10 mg/kg/day divided twice daily; maximum: GERD: 300 mg/day, erosive esophagitis: 600 mg/day

I.V.: 2-4 mg/kg/day divided every 6-8 hours; maximum: 150 mg/day **or as an alternative**

Continuous infusion: Initial: 1 mg/kg/dose for one dose followed by infusion of 0.08-0.17 mg/kg/hour or 2-4 mg/kg/day

Children ≥12 years: Prevention of heartburn: Oral: Zantac® 75 [OTC]: 75 mg 30-60 minutes before eating food or drinking beverages which cause heartburn; maximum: 150 mg/24 hours; do not use for more than 14 days

Adults:

Duodenal ulcer: Oral: Treatment: 150 mg twice daily, or 300 mg once daily after the evening meal or at bedtime; maintenance: 150 mg once daily at bedtime

Helicobacter pylori eradication: 150 mg twice daily; requires combination therapy

Pathological hypersecretory conditions:

Oral: 150 mg twice daily; adjust dose or frequency as clinically indicated; doses of up to 6 g/day have been used

I.V.: Continuous infusion for Zollinger-Ellison: 1 mg/kg/hour; measure gastric acid output at 4 hours, if >10 mEq or if patient is symptomatic, increase dose in increments of 0.5 mg/kg/hour; doses of up to 2.5 mg/kg/hour have been used

Gastric ulcer, benign: Oral: 150 mg twice daily; maintenance: 150 mg once daily at bedtime

Erosive esophagitis: Oral: Treatment: 150 mg 4 times/day; maintenance: 150 mg twice daily

Prevention of heartburn: Oral: Zantac® 75 [OTC]: 75 mg 30-60 minutes before eating food or drinking beverages which cause heartburn; maximum: 150 mg in 24 hours; do not use for more than 14 days

Patients not able to take oral medication:
I.M.: 50 mg every 6-8 hours
I.V.: Intermittent bolus or infusion: 50 mg every 6-8 hours
Continuous I.V. infusion: 6.25 mg/hour

Elderly: Ulcer healing rates and incidence of adverse effects are similar in the elderly, when compared to younger patients; dosing adjustments not necessary based on age alone

Dosing adjustment in renal impairment: Adults: Cl_{cr} <50 mL/minute: 150 mg every 24 hours; adjust dose cautiously if needed

Hemodialysis: Adjust dosing schedule so that dose coincides with the end of hemodialysis

Dosing adjustment/comments in hepatic disease: Patients with hepatic impairment may have minor changes in ranitidine half-life, distribution, clearance, and bioavailability; dosing adjustments not necessary, monitor

Mechanism of Action Competitive inhibition of histamine at H_2-receptors of the gastric parietal cells, which inhibits gastric acid secretion, gastric volume, and hydrogen ion concentration are reduced. Does not affect pepsin secretion, pentagastrin-stimulated intrinsic factor secretion, or serum gastrin.

Other Adverse Effects Frequency not defined:

Cardiovascular: Atrioventricular block, bradycardia, premature ventricular beats, tachycardia, vasculitis

Central nervous system: Agitation, dizziness, depression, hallucinations, headache, insomnia, malaise, mental confusion, somnolence, vertigo

Dermatologic: Alopecia, erythema multiforme, rash

Endocrine & metabolic: Gynocomastia, impotence, increased prolactin levels, loss of libido

Gastrointestinal: Abdominal discomfort/pain, constipation, diarrhea, nausea, pancreatitis, vomiting

Hematologic: Acquired hemolytic anemia, agranulocytosis, aplastic anemia, granulocytopenia, leukopenia, pancytopenia, thrombocytopenia

Hepatic: Hepatic failure, hepatitis

Local: Transient pain, burning or itching at the injection site

Neuromuscular & skeletal: Arthralgia, involuntary motor disturbance, myalgia

Ocular: Blurred vision

Renal: Increased serum creatinine

Miscellaneous: Anaphylaxis, angioneurotic edema, hypersensitivity reactions

Drug Interactions CYP2D6 and 3A3/4 enzyme inhibitor

Increased Effect/Toxicity: Increases the effect/toxicity of cyclosporine (increased serum creatinine), gentamicin (neuromuscular blockade), glipizide, glyburide, midazolam (increased concentrations), metoprolol, pentoxifylline, phenytoin, quinidine, and triazolam. Optimal antimicrobial effects of ranitidine bismuth citrate occur when the drug is taken with food.

Decreased Effect: Variable effects on warfarin; antacids may decrease absorption of ranitidine; ketoconazole and itraconazole absorptions are decreased; may produce altered serum concentration of procainamide and ferrous sulfate; decreased effect of nondepolarizing muscle relaxants, cefpodoxime, cyanocobalamin (decreased absorption), diazepam, oxaprozin

Decreased toxicity of atropine

Drug Uptake

Absorption: Oral: 50%

Half-life, elimination (dependent on renal function):
Oral: Normal: 2.5-3 hours; Cl_{cr} 25-35 mL/minute: 4.8 hours
I.V.: Normal: 2-2.5 hours

Time to peak: Oral: 2-3 hours; I.M.: ≤15 minutes

Pregnancy Risk Factor B

Generic Available Yes

Rapamune® *see* Sirolimus *on page 1090*

Rauwolfia Serpentina (rah WOOL fee a ser pen TEEN ah)

Pharmacologic Category Rauwolfia Alkaloid

Synonyms Whole Root Rauwolfia

Use Mild essential hypertension; relief of agitated psychotic states

Local Anesthetic/Vasoconstrictor Precautions No information available to require special precautions

Effects on Dental Treatment No effects or complications reported

Dosage Adults: Oral: 200-400 mg/day in 2 divided doses

Other Adverse Effects Frequency not defined:

Cardiovascular: Hypotension, tachycardia, flushing

Central nervous system: Drowsiness, fatigue, CNS depression, coma, parkinsonism, hypothermia

Endocrine & metabolic: Sodium and water retention, gynecomastia, galactorrhea

Gastrointestinal: Abdominal cramps, nausea, vomiting, gastric acid secretion (increased), xerostomia, diarrhea

Ocular: Miosis, conjunctival flushing

Respiratory: Nasal congestion

(Continued)

Rauwolfia Serpentina *(Continued)*

Drug Interactions Increased Effect/Toxicity: Effects may be additive with other antihypertensives. May increase effect of CNS depressants.

Pregnancy Risk Factor C

Generic Available Yes

R & C® [OTC] *see* Pyrethrins *on page 1026*
R&C® Lice *see* Permethrin *on page 940*
Rea-Lo® [OTC] *see* Urea *on page 1221*
Rebetol® *see* Ribavirin *on page 1048*
Rebetron™ *see* Interferon Alfa-2b and Ribavirin Combination Pack *on page 644*
Rebif® *see* Interferon Beta-1a *on page 647*
Recombinate™ *see* Antihemophilic Factor (Recombinant) *on page 106*
Recombivax HB® *see* Hepatitis B Vaccine *on page 584*
Redutemp® [OTC] *see* Acetaminophen *on page 26*
Reese's® Pinworm Medicine [OTC] *see* Pyrantel Pamoate *on page 1025*
ReFacto® *see* Antihemophilic Factor (Recombinant) *on page 106*
Refludan® *see* Lepirudin *on page 689*
Refresh® [OTC] *see* Artificial Tears *on page 117*
Refresh® Plus [OTC] *see* Artificial Tears *on page 117*
Refresh® Tears [OTC] *see* Artificial Tears *on page 117*
Regitine® *see* Phentolamine *on page 949*
Reglan® *see* Metoclopramide *on page 800*
Regranex® *see* Becaplermin *on page 146*
Regular Iletin® II *see* Insulin Preparations *on page 639*
Regulax SS® [OTC] *see* Docusate *on page 407*
Reguloid® [OTC] *see* Psyllium *on page 1025*
Relafen® *see* Nabumetone *on page 838*
Relenza® *see* Zanamivir *on page 1256*
Relief® Ophthalmic *see* Phenylephrine *on page 950*
Remeron® *see* Mirtazapine *on page 819*
Remeron® SolTab™ *see* Mirtazapine *on page 819*
Remicade® *see* Infliximab *on page 636*

Remifentanil (rem i FEN ta nil)

U.S. Brand Names Ultiva™

Canadian Brand Names Ultiva®

Mexican Brand Names Ultiva®

Pharmacologic Category Analgesic, Narcotic

Synonyms GI87084B

Use Analgesic for use during general anesthesia for continued analgesia in children ≥2 years of age and adults

Local Anesthetic/Vasoconstrictor Precautions No information available to require special precautions

Effects on Dental Treatment No effects or complications reported

Restrictions C-II

Dosage I.V. continuous infusion:

Children ≥2 years: Per kg doses are the same as for adult patients
Adults:
During induction: 0.5-1 mcg/kg/minute
During maintenance:
- With nitrous oxide (66%): 0.4 mcg/kg/minute (range: 0.1-2 mcg/kg/min)
- With isoflurane: 0.25 mcg/kg/minute (range: 0.05-2 mcg/kg/min)
- With propofol: 0.25 mcg/kg/minute (range: 0.05-2 mcg/kg/min)

Continuation as an analgesic in immediate postoperative period: 0.1 mcg/kg/minute (range: 0.025-0.2 mcg/kg/min)

Elderly: Elderly patients have an increased sensitivity to effect of remifentanil, doses should be decreased by ½ and titrated

Mechanism of Action Binds with stereospecific mu-opioid receptors at many sites within the CNS, increases pain threshold, alters pain reception, inhibits ascending pain pathways

Other Adverse Effects

>10%: Gastrointestinal: Nausea, vomiting

1% to 10%:
- Cardiovascular: Hypotension, bradycardia, tachycardia, hypertension
- Central nervous system: Dizziness, headache, agitation, fever
- Dermatologic: Pruritus
- Ocular: Visual disturbances
- Respiratory: Respiratory depression, apnea, hypoxia
- Miscellaneous: Shivering, postoperative pain

Drug Interactions Additive effects with other CNS depressants

Drug Uptake
Onset of action: I.V.: 1-3 minutes
Half-life, elimination (dose-dependent): 10 minutes
Pregnancy Risk Factor C
Generic Available No

Remodulin™ *see* Treprostinil *on page 1194*
Renacidin® *see* Citric Acid Bladder Mixture *on page 295*
Renagel® *see* Sevelamer *on page 1084*
Renese® *see* Polythiazide *on page 972*
Renoquid® *see* Sulfacytine *on page 1116*
Renova® *see* Tretinoin, Topical *on page 1196*
Rentamine® [OTC] *see* Chlorpheniramine, Ephedrine, Phenylephrine, and Carbetapentane *on page 270*
ReoPro® *see* Abciximab *on page 23*

Repaglinide (re PAG li nide)

Related Information
Endocrine Disorders and Pregnancy *on page 1331*
U.S. Brand Names Prandin®
Canadian Brand Names GlucoNorm®; Prandin®
Pharmacologic Category Antidiabetic Agent, Miscellaneous
Use Management of type 2 diabetes mellitus (noninsulin dependent, NIDDM)
An adjunct to diet and exercise to lower the blood glucose in patients with type 2 diabetes mellitus whose hyperglycemia cannot be controlled satisfactorily by diet and exercise alone
In combination with metformin to lower blood glucose in patients whose hyperglycemia cannot be controlled by exercise, diet and either agent alone
Local Anesthetic/Vasoconstrictor Precautions No information available to require special precautions
Effects on Dental Treatment No effects or complications reported
Dosage Oral: Adults: 0.5-4 mg before each meal; the starting dose in oral hypoglycemic naive individuals or in those with Hb A_{1c} levels under 8% is 0.5 mg before each meal. For other patients, the starting dose is 1-2 mg before each meal. The dose can be adjusted (by prescribers) up to 4 mg before each meal. If a meal is skipped, the patient should also skip the repaglinide dose
Mechanism of Action Nonsulfonylurea hypoglycemic agent of the meglitinide class (the nonsulfonylurea moiety of glyburide) used in the management of type 2 diabetes mellitus. Stimulates insulin secretion from the beta cells of the pancreas by binding to sites on the beta cell. Prandin is minimally excreted by the kidney, which may be an advantage for patients (often elderly) who often suffer from decreased kidney function.
Other Adverse Effects
>10%:
Central nervous system: Headache (9% to 11%)
Endocrine & metabolic: Hypoglycemia (16% to 31%)
1% to 10%:
Cardiovascular: Chest pain (2% to 3%)
Gastrointestinal: Nausea (3% to 5%), heartburn (2% to 4%), vomiting (2% to 3%) constipation (2% to 3%), diarrhea (4% to 5%), tooth disorder (<1% to 2%)
Genitourinary: Urinary tract infection (2% to 3%)
Neuromuscular & skeletal: Arthralgia (3% to 6%), back pain (5% to 6%), paresthesia (2% to 3%)
Respiratory: Upper respiratory tract infection (10% to 16%), sinusitis (3% to 6%), rhinitis (3% to 7%), bronchitis (2% to 6%)
Miscellaneous: Allergy (1% to 2%)
Warnings/Precautions At higher dosages, sulfonylureas may block the ATP-sensitive potassium channels, which may correspond to an increased risk of cardiovascular events. In May, 2000, the National Diabetes Center issued a warning to avoid the use of sulfonylureas at higher dosages (repaglinide daily doses >1.5 mg).
Drug Interactions CYP2C9 and 3A3/4 enzyme substrate
CYP2C9 inducers (eg, carbamazepine, phenobarbital, phenytoin, rifampin): May increase metabolism of repaglinide.
CYP2C9 inhibitors (eg, amiodarone, isoniazid, metronidazole): May increase repaglinide concentrations.
CYP3A4 inducers (eg, barbiturates, carbamazepine, rifampin): May increase metabolism of repaglinide.
CYP3A4 inhibitors (eg, itraconazole, ketoconazole): May increase repaglinide concentrations.
HMG-CoA reductase inhibitors (eg, atorvastatin, fluvastatin, lovastatin, pravastatin, simvastatin): May increase repaglinide concentrations by decreasing metabolism.
Macrolide antibiotics (eg, clarithromycin, erythromycin, troleandomycin): May increase repaglinide concentrations by decreasing metabolism.
(Continued)

Repaglinide *(Continued)*

Oral contraceptives: Repaglinide may increase serum concentrations of contraceptives.

Estrogens (eg, estradiol, ethinyl estradiol, mestranol): May increase repaglinide concentrations.

Progestins: May increase repaglinide concentrations.

Protein-bound drugs (eg, phenylbutazone, oral anticoagulants, hydantoins, salicylates, NSAIDs, sulfonamides): Since repaglinide is highly protein bound, toxicity may occur with concurrent use of other highly protein bound drugs.

Drug Uptake

Onset of action: Single dose: Increased insulin levels: ~15-60 minutes

Absorption: Rapidly and completely

Duration: 4-6 hours

Time to peak, plasma: ~1 hour

Pregnancy Risk Factor C

Generic Available No

Comments Known as GlucoNorm® in Canada, NovoNorm™ elsewhere

Repan® *see* Butalbital, Acetaminophen, and Caffeine *on page 192*

Repronex® *see* Menotropins *on page 759*

Requip® *see* Ropinirole *on page 1067*

Rescriptor® *see* Delavirdine *on page 355*

Reserpine (re SER peen)

Related Information

Cardiovascular Diseases *on page 1308*

U.S. Brand Names Serpalan®

Pharmacologic Category Rauwolfia Alkaloid

Use Management of mild to moderate hypertension

Unlabeled/Investigational: Management of tardive dyskinesia, schizophrenia

Local Anesthetic/Vasoconstrictor Precautions No information available to require special precautions

Effects on Dental Treatment >10%: Xerostomia

Dosage When used for management of hypertension, full antihypertensive effects may take as long as 3 weeks.

Oral:

Children: Hypertension: 0.01-0.02 mg/kg/24 hours divided every 12 hours; maximum dose: 0.25 mg/day (not recommended in children)

Adults:

Hypertension: 0.1-0.25 mg/day in 1-2 doses; initial: 0.5 mg/day for 1-2 weeks; maintenance: reduce to 0.1-0.25 mg/day;

Psychiatric: Initial: 0.5 mg/day; usual range: 0.1-1 mg

Elderly: Initial: 0.05 mg once daily, increasing by 0.05 mg every week as necessary

Dosing adjustment in renal impairment: Cl_{cr} <10 mL/minute: Avoid use

Dialysis: Not removed by hemo or peritoneal dialysis; supplemental dose is not necessary

Mechanism of Action Reduces BP via depletion of sympathetic biogenic amines (norepinephrine and dopamine); this also commonly results in sedative effects

Other Adverse Effects Frequency not defined:

Cardiovascular: Peripheral edema, arrhythmias, bradycardia, chest pain, PVC, hypotension

Central nervous system: Dizziness, headache, nightmares, nervousness, drowsiness, fatigue, mental depression, parkinsonism, dull sensorium, syncope, paradoxical anxiety

Dermatologic: Rash, pruritus, flushing of skin

Gastrointestinal: Anorexia, diarrhea, xerostomia, nausea, vomiting, increased salivation, weight gain, increased gastric acid secretion

Genitourinary: Impotence, decreased libido

Hematologic: Thrombocytopenia purpura

Ocular: Blurred vision

Respiratory: Nasal congestion, dyspnea, epistaxis

Drug Interactions

Increased Effect/Toxicity: May cause hypertensive reactions in patients receiving an MAO inhibitor (use an alternative antihypertensive); may increase the effect of beta-blockers and CNS depressants; may increase the effects/toxicity of levodopa, quinidine, procainamide, and digitalis glycosides.

Decreased Effect: Tricyclic antidepressants may increase antihypertensive effect.

Drug Uptake

Onset of action: Antihypertensive: 3-6 days

Absorption: Oral: ~40%

Duration: 2-6 weeks

Half-life, elimination: 50-100 hours

Half-life elimination: 50-100 hours

Pregnancy Risk Factor C
Generic Available Yes

Respa-1st® *see* Guaifenesin and Pseudoephedrine *on page 570*
Respa®-DM *see* Guaifenesin and Dextromethorphan *on page 569*
Respa-GF® *see* Guaifenesin *on page 568*
Respaire®-60 SR *see* Guaifenesin and Pseudoephedrine *on page 570*
Respaire®-120 SR *see* Guaifenesin and Pseudoephedrine *on page 570*
Respbid® *see* Theophylline *on page 1152*
Resporal® *see* Dexbrompheniramine and Pseudoephedrine *on page 365*
Restall® *see* HydrOXYzine *on page 616*
Restoril® *see* Temazepam *on page 1136*
Retavase® *see* Reteplase *on page 1047*

Reteplase (RE ta plase)

U.S. Brand Names Retavase®
Canadian Brand Names Retavase®
Pharmacologic Category Thrombolytic Agent
Synonyms Recombinant Plasminogen Activator; r-PA
Use Management of acute myocardial infarction
Local Anesthetic/Vasoconstrictor Precautions No information available to require special precautions
Effects on Dental Treatment No effects or complications reported
Dosage Adults: 10 units I.V. over 2 minutes, followed by a second dose 30 minutes later of 10 units I.V. over 2 minutes
Withhold second dose if serious bleeding or anaphylaxis occurs
Mechanism of Action Reteplase is a nonglycosylated form of tPA produced by recombinant DNA technology using *E. coli*; it initiates local fibrinolysis by binding to fibrin in a thrombus (clot) and converts entrapped plasminogen to plasmin
Other Adverse Effects Bleeding is the most frequent adverse effect associated with reteplase. Heparin and aspirin have been administered concurrently with reteplase in clinical trials. The incidence of adverse events is a reflection of these combined therapies, and are comparable with comparison thrombolytics.

>10%: Local: Injection site bleeding (4.6% to 48.6%)
1% to 10%:
- Gastrointestinal: Bleeding (1.8% to 9.0%)
- Genitourinary: Bleeding (0.9% to 9.5%)
- Hematologic: Anemia (0.9% to 2.6%)

Other adverse effects noted are frequently associated with myocardial infarction (and therefore may or may not be attributable to Retavase®) and include arrhythmias, hypotension, cardiogenic shock, pulmonary edema, cardiac arrest, reinfarction, pericarditis, tamponade, thrombosis, and embolism.

Drug Interactions
Increased Effect/Toxicity: The risk of bleeding associated with reteplase may be increased by oral anticoagulants (warfarin), heparin, low molecular weight heparins, and drugs which affect platelet function (eg, NSAIDs, dipyridamole, ticlopidine, clopidogrel, IIb/IIIa antagonists). Concurrent use with aspirin and heparin may increase the risk of bleeding; however, aspirin and heparin were used concomitantly with reteplase in the majority of patients in clinical studies.
Decreased Effect: Aminocaproic acid (antifibrinolytic agent) may decrease effectiveness of thrombolytic agents.

Drug Uptake
Onset of action: Thrombolysis: 30-90 minutes
Half-life, elimination: 13-16 minutes

Pregnancy Risk Factor C
Generic Available No

Retin-A® *see* Tretinoin, Topical *on page 1196*
Retin-A® Micro *see* Tretinoin, Topical *on page 1196*
Retrovir® *see* Zidovudine *on page 1257*
Revex® *see* Nalmefene *on page 843*
Rēv-Eyes™ *see* Dapiprazole *on page 350*
ReVia® *see* Naltrexone *on page 845*
R-Gel® [OTC] *see* Capsaicin *on page 212*
R-Gene® *see* Arginine *on page 111*
Rheomacrodex® *see* Dextran *on page 369*
Rheumatrex® *see* Methotrexate *on page 788*
Rhinall® Nasal [OTC] *see* Phenylephrine *on page 950*
Rhinatate® *see* Chlorpheniramine, Pyrilamine, and Phenylephrine *on page 273*
Rhinocort® *see* Budesonide *on page 180*
Rhinocort® Aqua™ *see* Budesonide *on page 180*
Rhinosyn® [OTC] *see* Chlorpheniramine and Pseudoephedrine *on page 270*

Rhinosyn-DMX® [OTC] *see* Guaifenesin and Dextromethorphan *on page 569*

Rhinosyn-PD® [OTC] *see* Chlorpheniramine and Pseudoephedrine *on page 270*

Rhinosyn-X® Liquid [OTC] *see* Guaifenesin, Pseudoephedrine, and Dextromethorphan *on page 571*

Rh_o(D) Immune Globulin

(ar aych oh (dee) i MYUN GLOB yoo lin in tra MUS kue lar)

U.S. Brand Names BayRho-D®; BayRho-D® Mini-Dose; MICRhoGAM™; RhoGAM™

Pharmacologic Category Immune Globulin

Use Prevention of isoimmunization in Rh-negative individuals exposed to Rh-positive blood during delivery of an Rh-positive infant, as a result of an abortion, following amniocentesis or abdominal trauma, or following a transfusion accident; to prevent hemolytic disease of the newborn if there is a subsequent pregnancy with an Rh-positive fetus

Local Anesthetic/Vasoconstrictor Precautions No information available to require special precautions

Effects on Dental Treatment No effects or complications reported

Dosage Adults (administered I.M. to mothers **not** to infant) I.M.:

Obstetrical usage: 1 vial (300 mcg) prevents maternal sensitization if fetal packed red blood cell volume that has entered the circulation is <15 mL; if it is more, give additional vials. The number of vials = RBC volume of the calculated fetomaternal hemorrhage divided by 15 mL

Postpartum prophylaxis: 300 mcg within 72 hours of delivery

Antepartum prophylaxis: 300 mcg at ~ 26-28 weeks gestation; followed by 300 mcg within 72 hours of delivery if infant is Rh-positive

Following miscarriage, abortion, or termination of ectopic pregnancy at up to 13 weeks of gestation: 50 mcg ideally within 3 hours, but may be given up to 72 hours after; if pregnancy has been terminated at 13 or more weeks of gestation, administer 300 mcg

Mechanism of Action Suppresses the immune response and antibody formation of Rh-negative individuals to Rh-positive red blood cells

Warnings/Precautions Have epinephrine 1:1000 available for anaphylactic reactions. Use with caution in patients with IgA deficiency; do not administer to neonates. As a product of human plasma, this product may potentially transmit disease; screening of donors, as well as testing and/or inactivation of certain viruses reduces this risk. Use caution in patients with thrombocytopenia or coagulation disorders (I.M. injections may be contraindicated). Not for I.V. administration.

Drug Uptake Half-life, elimination: 23-26 days

Pregnancy Risk Factor C

Generic Available No

Comments Administered I.M. to mothers **not** to infant; will prevent hemolytic disease of newborn in subsequent pregnancy

RhoGAM™ *see* Rh_o(D) Immune Globulin *on page 1048*

Ribavirin (rye ba VYE rin)

Related Information

Systemic Viral Diseases *on page 1354*

U.S. Brand Names Rebetol®; Virazole® Aerosol

Canadian Brand Names Virazole™

Mexican Brand Names Vilona; Vilona Pediatrica; Virazide

Pharmacologic Category Antiviral Agent

Synonyms RTCA; Tribavirin

Use Inhalation: Treatment of patients with respiratory syncytial virus (RSV) infections; may also be used in other viral infections including influenza A and B and adenovirus; specially indicated for treatment of severe lower respiratory tract RSV infections in patients with an underlying compromising condition (prematurity, bronchopulmonary dysplasia and other chronic lung conditions, congenital heart disease, immunodeficiency, immunosuppression), and recent transplant recipients

Oral capsules: The combination therapy of oral ribavirin with interferon alfa-2b, recombinant (Intron® A) injection is indicated for the treatment of chronic hepatitis C in patients with compensated liver disease who have relapsed after alpha interferon therapy or were previously untreated with alpha interferons

Unlabeled/Investigational: Treatment of West Nile virus; hemorrhagic fever virus infections with renal syndrome (Lassa, Venezuelan, Korean hemorrhagic fever, Sabia, Argentian hemorrhagic fever, Bolivian hemorrhagic fever, Junin, Machupa)

Local Anesthetic/Vasoconstrictor Precautions No information available to require special precautions

Effects on Dental Treatment No effects or complications reported

Dosage

Aerosol inhalation: Infants and children: Use with Viratek® small particle aerosol generator (SPAG-2) at a concentration of 20 mg/mL (6 g reconstituted with 300 mL of sterile water without preservatives). Continuous aerosol administration: 12-18 hours/day for 3 days, up to 7 days in length

Oral:

Children: Chronic hepatitis C (in combination with interferon alfa-2b): **Note:** Safety and efficacy have not been established; dosing based on pharmacokinetic profile:

25-36 kg: 400 mg/day (200 mg twice daily)

37-49 kg: 600 mg/day (200 mg in morning and 400 mg in evening)

50-61 kg: 800 mg/day (400 mg twice daily)

>61 kg: Refer to adult dosing

Note: Also refer to Interferon Alfa-2B and Ribavirin Combination Pack monograph.

Adults:

Chronic hepatitis C (in combination with interferon alfa-2b):

≤75 kg: 400 mg in the morning, then 600 mg in the evening

>75 kg: 600 mg in the morning, then 600 mg in the evening

Note: If HCV-RNA is undetectable at 24 weeks, duration of therapy is 48 weeks. In patients who relapse following interferon therapy, duration of dual therapy is 24 weeks.

Note: Also refer to Interferon Alfa-2B and Ribavirin Combination Pack monograph.

Chronic hepatitis C (in combination with peginterferon alfa-2b): 400 mg twice daily; duration of therapy is 1 year; after 24 weeks of treatment, if serum HCV-RNA is not below the limit of detection of the assay, consider discontinuation.

Dosage adjustment in renal impairment: Cl_{cr} <50 mL/minute: Oral route is contraindicated

Dosage adjustment for toxicity: Oral:

Patient **without** cardiac history:

Hemoglobin <10 g/dL: Decrease dose to 600 mg/day

Hemoglobin <8.5 g/dL: Permanently discontinue treatment

Patient **with** cardiac history:

Hemoglobin has ≥2 g/dL decrease during any 4-week period of treatment: Decrease dose to 600 mg/day

Hemoglobin <12 g/dL after 4 weeks of reduced dose: Permanently discontinue treatment

Mechanism of Action Inhibits replication of RNA and DNA viruses; inhibits influenza virus RNA polymerase activity and inhibits the initiation and elongation of RNA fragments resulting in inhibition of viral protein synthesis

Other Adverse Effects

Inhalation:

1% to 10%:

Central nervous system: Fatigue, headache, insomnia

Gastrointestinal: Nausea, anorexia

Hematologic: Anemia

Note: Incidence of adverse effects (approximate) in healthcare workers: Headache (51%); conjunctivitis (32%); rhinitis, nausea, rash, dizziness, pharyngitis, and lacrimation (10% to 20%)

Oral (all adverse reactions are documented while receiving combination therapy with interferon alpha-2b):

>10%:

Central nervous system: Dizziness (17% to 26%), headache (63% to 66%)*, fatigue (60% to 70%)*, fever (32% to 41%)*, insomnia (26% to 39%), irritability (23% to 32%), depression (23% to 36%)*, emotional lability (7% to 12%)*, impaired concentration (10% to 14%)*

Dermatologic: Alopecia (27% to 32%), rash (20% to 28%), pruritus (13% to 21%)

Gastrointestinal: Nausea (38% to 47%), anorexia (21% to 27%), dyspepsia (14% to 16%), vomiting (9% to 12%)*

Hematologic: Decreased hemoglobin (25% to 36%), decreased WBC, absolute neutrophil count <0.5 x 10^9/L (5% to 11%), thrombocytopenia (6% to 14%), hyperbilirubinemia (24% to 34%), hemolysis

Neuromuscular & skeletal: Myalgia (61% to 64%)*, arthralgia (29% to 33%)*, musculoskeletal pain (20% to 28%), rigors (40% to 43%)

Respiratory: Dyspnea (17% to 19%), sinusitis (9% to 12%)*, nasal congestion

Miscellaneous: Flu-like syndrome (13% to 18%)*

*Similar to interferon alone

1% to 10%:

Cardiovascular: Chest pain (5% to 9%)*

Central nervous system: Nervousness (~5%)*

Gastrointestinal: Taste perversion (6% to 8%)

Hematologic: Hemolytic anemia (~10%)

Neuromuscular & skeletal: Weakness (9% to 10%)

*Similar to interferon alone

Drug Interactions Decreases effect of zidovudine

(Continued)

Ribavirin *(Continued)*

Drug Uptake

Absorption: Systemic from respiratory tract following nasal and oral inhalation; dependent upon respiratory factors and method of drug delivery; maximal absorption occurs with the use of aerosol generator via endotracheal tube; highest concentrations in respiratory tract and erythrocytes

Oral: Rapid and extensive

Half-life, elimination, plasma:

Children: 6.5-11 hours

Adults: 24 hours; Erythrocyte: 16-40 days, which can be used as a marker for intracellular metabolism

Time to peak: Inhalation: Immediate; Oral: 3 hours (multiple dose)

Pregnancy Risk Factor X

Generic Available No

Comments RSV season is usually December to April; viral shedding period for RSV is usually 3-8 days

Riboflavin (RYE boe flay vin)

Pharmacologic Category Vitamin, Water Soluble

Synonyms Lactoflavin; Vitamin B_2; Vitamin G

Use Prevention of riboflavin deficiency and treatment of ariboflavinosis

Local Anesthetic/Vasoconstrictor Precautions No information available to require special precautions

Effects on Dental Treatment No effects or complications reported

Dosage Oral:

Riboflavin deficiency:

Children: 2.5-10 mg/day in divided doses

Adults: 5-30 mg/day in divided doses

Recommended daily allowance:

Children: 0.4-1.8 mg

Adults: 1.2-1.7 mg

Mechanism of Action Component of flavoprotein enzymes that work together, which are necessary for normal tissue respiration; also needed for activation of pyridoxine and conversion of tryptophan to niacin

Other Adverse Effects Frequency not defined: Genitourinary: Discoloration of urine (yellow-orange)

Warnings/Precautions Riboflavin deficiency often occurs in the presence of other B vitamin deficiencies

Drug Interactions Decreased absorption with probenecid

Drug Uptake

Absorption: Readily via GI tract, however, food increases extent; decreased with hepatitis, cirrhosis, or biliary obstruction

Half-life, elimination: Biologic: 66-84 minutes

Pregnancy Risk Factor A/C (dose exceeding RDA recommendation)

Dosage Forms TAB: 50 mg, 100 mg

Generic Available Yes

RID® [OTC] *see* Pyrethrins *on page 1026*

Ridactate® *see* Calcium Lactate *on page 206*

Ridaura® *see* Auranofin *on page 132*

Ridifed® [OTC] *see* Triprolidine and Pseudoephedrine *on page 1213*

Rifabutin (rif a BYOO tin)

Related Information

Nonviral Infectious Diseases *on page 1342*

Systemic Viral Diseases *on page 1354*

U.S. Brand Names Mycobutin®

Canadian Brand Names Mycobutin®

Pharmacologic Category Antibiotic, Miscellaneous; Antitubercular Agent

Synonyms Ansamycin

Use Prevention of disseminated *Mycobacterium avium* complex (MAC) in patients with advanced HIV infection; also utilized in multiple drug regimens for treatment of MAC

Local Anesthetic/Vasoconstrictor Precautions No information available to require special precautions

Effects on Dental Treatment No effects or complications reported

Dosage Oral:

Children >1 year:

Treatment: Patients not receiving NNRTIs or protease inhibitors:

Initial phase (2 weeks to 2 months): 10-20 mg/kg daily (maximum: 300 mg).

Second phase: 10-20 mg/kg daily (maximum: 300 mg) or twice weekly

Prophylaxis: 5 mg/kg daily; higher dosages have been used in limited trials

Adults:
Treatment:
Patients not receiving NNRTIs or protease inhibitors:
Initial phase: 5 mg/kg daily (maximum: 300 mg)
Second phase: 5 mg/kg daily or twice weekly
Patients receiving nelfinavir, amprenavir, indinavir: Reduce dose to 150 mg/day; no change in dose if administered twice weekly
Prophylaxis: 300 mg once daily (alone or in combination with azithromycin)

Dosage adjustment in renal impairment: Cl_{cr} <30 mL/minute: Reduce dose by 50%

Mechanism of Action Inhibits DNA-dependent RNA polymerase at the beta subunit which prevents chain initiation

Other Adverse Effects

>10%:
Dermatologic: Rash (11%)
Genitourinary: Discolored urine (30%)
Hematologic: Neutropenia (25%), leukopenia (17%)

1% to 10%:
Central nervous system: Headache (3%)
Gastrointestinal: Vomiting/nausea (3%), abdominal pain (4%), diarrhea (3%), anorexia (2%), flatulence (2%), eructation (3%)
Hematologic: Anemia, thrombocytopenia (5%)
Hepatic: Increased AST/ALT (7% to 9%)
Neuromuscular & skeletal: Myalgia

Drug Interactions CYP3A3/4 enzyme inducer

Increased Effect/Toxicity: Concentrations of rifabutin are increased by indinavir (reduce rifabutin to 50% of standard dose) and ritonavir (reduce rifabutin dose to 150 mg every other day). Fluconazole increases rifabutin concentrations.

Decreased Effect: Rifabutin may decreased plasma concentrations (due to induction of liver enzymes) of verapamil, methadone, digoxin, cyclosporine, corticosteroids, oral anticoagulants, theophylline, barbiturates, chloramphenicol, itraconazole, ketoconazole, oral contraceptives, quinidine, protease inhibitors (indinavir, nelfinavir, ritonavir, saquinavir), non-nucleoside reverse transcriptase inhibitors, halothane, and clarithromycin.

Drug Uptake

Absorption: Oral: Readily absorbed (53%)
Half-life, elimination: Terminal: 45 hours; Range: 16-69 hours
Time to peak: 2-4 hours

Pregnancy Risk Factor B

Generic Available No

Rifadin® *see* Rifampin *on page 1051*

Rifamate® *see* Rifampin and Isoniazid *on page 1053*

Rifampin (RIF am pin)

Related Information

Nonviral Infectious Diseases *on page 1342*

U.S. Brand Names Rifadin®; Rimactane®

Canadian Brand Names Rifadin®; Rofact™

Mexican Brand Names Pestarin®; Rifadin®; Rimactan®

Pharmacologic Category Antibiotic, Miscellaneous; Antitubercular Agent

Synonyms Rifampicin

Use Management of active tuberculosis in combination with other agents; eliminate meningococci from asymptomatic carriers; prophylaxis of *Haemophilus influenzae* type b infection; used in combination with other anti-infectives in the treatment of staphylococcal infections; *Legionella* pneumonia

Local Anesthetic/Vasoconstrictor Precautions No information available to require special precautions

Effects on Dental Treatment No effects or complications reported

Dosage I.V. infusion dose is the same as for the oral route.

Tuberculosis therapy: Oral:

Note: A four-drug regimen (isoniazid, rifampin, pyrazinamide, and either streptomycin or ethambutol) is preferred for the initial, empiric treatment of TB. When the drug susceptibility results are available, the regimen should be altered as appropriate.

Patients with TB and without HIV infection:

OPTION 1:

Isoniazid resistance rate <4%: Administer daily isoniazid, rifampin, and pyrazinamide for 8 weeks followed by isoniazid and rifampin daily or directly observed therapy (DOT) 2-3 times/week for 16 weeks

If isoniazid resistance rate is not documented, ethambutol or streptomycin should also be administered until susceptibility to isoniazid or rifampin is demonstrated. Continue treatment for at least 6 months or 3 months beyond culture conversion.

(Continued)

Rifampin *(Continued)*

OPTION 2: Administer daily isoniazid, rifampin, pyrazinamide, and either streptomycin or ethambutol for 2 weeks followed by DOT 2 times/week administration of the same drugs for 6 weeks, and subsequently, with isoniazid and rifampin DOT 2 times/week administration for 16 weeks

OPTION 3: Administer isoniazid, rifampin, pyrazinamide, and either ethambutol or streptomycin by DOT 3 times/week for 6 months

Patients with TB and with HIV infection:

Administer any of the above OPTIONS 1, 2 or 3, however, treatment should be continued for a total of 9 months and at least 6 months beyond culture conversion

Note: Some experts recommend that the duration of therapy should be extended to 9 months for patients with disseminated disease, miliary disease, disease involving the bones or joints, or tuberculosis lymphadenitis

Children <12 years of age: Oral:

Daily therapy: 10-20 mg/kg/day in divided doses every 12-24 hours (maximum: 600 mg/day)

Directly observed therapy (DOT): Twice weekly: 10-20 mg/kg (maximum: 600 mg)

DOT: 3 times/week: 10-20 mg/kg (maximum: 600 mg)

Adults: Oral:

Daily therapy: 10 mg/kg/day (maximum: 600 mg/day)

Directly observed therapy (DOT): Twice weekly: 10 mg/kg (maximum: 600 mg)

DOT: 3 times/week: 10 mg/kg (maximum: 600 mg)

H. influenzae prophylaxis: Oral:

Children: 20 mg/kg/day every 24 hours for 4 days, not to exceed 600 mg/dose

Adults: 600 mg every 24 hours for 4 days

Meningococcal prophylaxis: Oral:

<1 month: 10 mg/kg/day in divided doses every 12 hours for 2 days

Children: 20 mg/kg/day in divided doses every 12 hours for 2 days

Adults: 600 mg every 12 hours for 2 days

Nasal carriers of *Staphylococcus aureus*: Oral:

Children: 15 mg/kg/day divided every 12 hours for 5-10 days in combination with other antibiotics

Adults: 600 mg/day for 5-10 days in combination with other antibiotics

Synergy for *Staphylococcus aureus* infections: Oral: Adults: 300-600 mg twice daily with other antibiotics

Mechanism of Action Inhibits bacterial RNA synthesis by binding to the beta subunit of DNA-dependent RNA polymerase, blocking RNA transcription

Other Adverse Effects

Frequency not defined:

Cardiovascular: Flushing, edema

Central nervous system: Headache, drowsiness, dizziness, confusion, numbness, behavioral changes, ataxia

Dermatologic: Pruritus, urticaria, pemphigoid reaction

Hematologic: Eosinophilia, leukopenia, hemolysis, hemolytic anemia, thrombocytopenia (especially with high-dose therapy)

Hepatic: Hepatitis (rare)

Neuromuscular & skeletal: Myalgia, weakness, osteomalacia

Ocular: Visual changes, exudative conjunctivitis

1% to 10%:

Dermatologic: Rash (1% to 5%)

Gastrointestinal (1% to 2%): Epigastric distress, anorexia, nausea, vomiting, diarrhea, cramps, pseudomembranous colitis, pancreatitis

Hepatic: Increased LFTs (up to 14%)

Drug Interactions CYP3A3/4 (major) enzyme substrate; CYP1A2, 2C, 2C8, 2C9, 2C18, 2C19, 2D6, 3A3/4, and 3A5-7 enzyme inducer

Increased Effect/Toxicity: Rifampin levels may be increased when given with co-trimoxazole, probenecid, or ritonavir. Rifampin given with halothane or isoniazid increases the potential for hepatotoxicity. Combination therapy with rifampin and pyrazinamide has been associated with severe and fatal hepatotoxic reactions.

Decreased Effect: Rifampin induces liver enzymes which may decrease the plasma concentration of calcium channel blockers (verapamil, diltiazem, nifedipine), methadone, digoxin, cyclosporine, corticosteroids, haloperidol, oral anticoagulants, theophylline, barbiturates, chloramphenicol, imidazole antifungals (ketoconazole), oral contraceptives, acetaminophen, benzodiazepines, hydantoins, sulfa drugs, enalapril, beta-blockers, clofibrate, dapsone, antiarrhythmics (disopyramide, mexiletine, quinidine, tocainide), doxycycline, fluoroquinolones, levothyroxine, nortriptyline, tacrolimus, zidovudine, protease inhibitors (ie, amprenavir), and non-nucleoside reverse transcriptase inhibitors.

Drug Uptake

Absorption: Oral: Well absorbed; food may delay or slightly reduce peak

Duration: ≤24 hours

Half-life, elimination: 3-4 hours; prolonged with hepatic impairment; End-stage renal disease: 1.8-11 hours

Time to peak: Oral: 2-4 hours

Pregnancy Risk Factor C

Generic Available Yes

Rifampin and Isoniazid (RIF am pin & eye soe NYE a zid)

U.S. Brand Names Rifamate®

Canadian Brand Names Rifamate®

Pharmacologic Category Antibiotic, Miscellaneous

Synonyms Isoniazid and Rifampin

Use Management of active tuberculosis; see Rifampin *on page 1051* and Isoniazid *on page 659*

Local Anesthetic/Vasoconstrictor Precautions No information available to require special precautions

Effects on Dental Treatment No effects or complications reported

Dosage Oral: 2 capsules/day

Drug Uptake See Rifampin *on page 1051* and Isoniazid *on page 659*

Pregnancy Risk Factor C

Generic Available No

Rifampin, Isoniazid, and Pyrazinamide

(RIF am pin, eye soe NYE a zid, & peer a ZIN a mide)

U.S. Brand Names Rifater®

Canadian Brand Names Rifater™

Pharmacologic Category Antibiotic, Miscellaneous

Synonyms Isoniazid, Rifampin, and Pyrazinamide; Pyrazinamide, Rifampin, and Isoniazid

Use Management of active tuberculosis

Local Anesthetic/Vasoconstrictor Precautions No information available to require special precautions

Effects on Dental Treatment No effects or complications reported

Dosage Adults: Oral: Patients weighing:

- ≤44 kg: 4 tablets
- 45-54 kg: 5 tablets
- ≥55 kg: 6 tablets

Doses should be administered in a single daily dose

Other Adverse Effects See Rifampin *on page 1051*, Isoniazid *on page 659*, and Pyrazinamide *on page 1026*

Drug Interactions Increased Effect/Toxicity: Combination therapy with rifampin and pyrazinamide has been associated with severe and fatal hepatotoxic reactions. Based on **rifampin** component: Rifampin levels may be increased when given with co-trimoxazole, probenecid, or ritonavir. Rifampin given with halothane or isoniazid increases the potential for hepatotoxicity.

Drug Uptake See Rifampin *on page 1051*, Isoniazid *on page 659*, and Pyrazinamide *on page 1026*

Pregnancy Risk Factor C

Generic Available No

Rifapentine (RIF a pen teen)

U.S. Brand Names Priftin®

Canadian Brand Names Priftin®

Pharmacologic Category Antitubercular Agent

Use Treatment of pulmonary tuberculosis (indication is based on the 6-month follow-up treatment outcome observed in controlled clinical trial). Rifapentine must always be used in conjunction with at least one other antituberculosis drug to which the isolate is susceptible; it may also be necessary to add a third agent (either streptomycin or ethambutol) until susceptibility is known.

Local Anesthetic/Vasoconstrictor Precautions No information available to require special precautions

Effects on Dental Treatment No effects or complications reported

Dosage

Children: No dosing information available

Adults: **Rifapentine should not be used alone**; initial phase should include a 3- to 4-drug regimen

Intensive phase of short-term therapy (initial 2 months): 600 mg (four 150 mg tablets) given twice weekly (at an interval not less than 72 hours); following the intensive phase, treatment should continue with rifapentine 600 mg once weekly for 4 months in combination with INH or appropriate agent for susceptible organisms

Mechanism of Action Inhibits DNA-dependent RNA polymerase in susceptible strains of *Mycobacterium tuberculosis* (but not in mammalian cells). Rifapentine is bactericidal against both intracellular and extracellular MTB organisms. Strains which are resistant to other rifamycins including rifampin are likely to be resistant to

(Continued)

Rifapentine *(Continued)*

rifapentine. Cross-resistance does not appear between rifapentine and other nonrifamycin antimycobacterial agents.

Other Adverse Effects

>10%: Endocrine & metabolic: Hyperuricemia (most likely due to pyrazinamide from initiation phase combination therapy)

1% to 10%:

Cardiovascular: Hypertension
Central nervous system: Headache, dizziness
Dermatologic: Rash, pruritus, acne
Gastrointestinal: Anorexia, nausea, vomiting, dyspepsia, diarrhea
Hematologic: Neutropenia, lymphopenia, anemia, leukopenia, thrombocytosis
Hepatic: Increased ALT/AST
Neuromuscular & skeletal: Arthralgia, pain
Renal: Pyuria, proteinuria, hematuria, urinary casts
Respiratory: Hemoptysis

Drug Interactions CYP3A3/4, 2C8, and 2C9 enzyme inducer

Increased Effect/Toxicity: Rifapentine metabolism is mediated by esterase activity, therefore, there is minimal potential for rifapentine metabolism to be affected by other drug therapy.

Decreased Effect: Rifapentine may increase the metabolism of coadministered drugs that are metabolized by these enzymes. Enzymes are induced within 4 days after the first dose and returned to baseline 14 days after discontinuation of rifapentine. The magnitude of enzyme induction is dose and frequency dependent. Rifampin has been shown to accelerate the metabolism and may reduce activity of the following drugs (therefore, rifapentine may also do the same): Phenytoin, disopyramide, mexiletine, quinidine, tocainide, chloramphenicol, clarithromycin, dapsone, doxycycline, fluoroquinolones, warfarin, fluconazole, itraconazole, ketoconazole, barbiturates, benzodiazepines, beta-blockers, diltiazem, nifedipine, verapamil, corticosteroids, cardiac glycoside preparations, clofibrate, oral or other systemic hormonal contraceptives, haloperidol, HIV protease inhibitors, sulfonylureas, cyclosporine, tacrolimus, levothyroxine, methadone, progestins, quinine, delavirdine, zidovudine, sildenafil, theophylline, amitriptyline, and nortriptyline. Rifapentine should be used with extreme caution, if at all, in patients who are also taking protease inhibitors. Patients using oral or other systemic hormonal contraceptives should be advised to change to nonhormonal methods of birth control when receiving concomitant rifapentine.

Drug Uptake

Absorption: Food increases AUC and C_{max} by 43% and 44% respectively.
Half-life, elimination: Rifapentine: 14-17 hours; 25-desacetyl rifapentine: 13 hours
Time to peak: 5-6 hours

Pregnancy Risk Factor C

Generic Available No

Rifater® *see* Rifampin, Isoniazid, and Pyrazinamide *on page 1053*
Rilutek® *see* Riluzole *on page 1054*

Riluzole (RIL yoo zole)

U.S. Brand Names Rilutek®

Mexican Brand Names Rilutek®

Pharmacologic Category Glutamate Inhibitor

Synonyms 2-Amino-6-Trifluoromethoxy-benzothiazole; RP54274

Use Orphan drug: Treatment of amyotrophic lateral sclerosis (ALS); riluzole can extend survival or time to tracheostomy

Local Anesthetic/Vasoconstrictor Precautions No information available to require special precautions

Effects on Dental Treatment No effects or complications reported

Dosage Adults: Oral: 50 mg every 12 hours; no increased benefit can be expected from higher daily doses, but adverse events are increased

Mechanism of Action Inhibitory effect on glutamate release, inactivation of voltage-dependent sodium channels; and ability to interfere with intracellular events that follow transmitter binding at excitatory amino acid receptors

Other Adverse Effects

>10%:

Gastrointestinal: Nausea (10% to 21%)
Neuromuscular & skeletal: Weakness (15% to 20%)
Respiratory: Decreased lung function (10% to 16%)

1% to 10%:

Cardiovascular: Hypertension, tachycardia, postural hypotension, edema
Central nervous system: headache, dizziness, somnolence, insomnia, malaise, depression, vertigo, agitation, tremor, circumoral paresthesia
Dermatologic: Pruritus, eczema, alopecia
Gastrointestinal: Abdominal pain, diarrhea, anorexia, dyspepsia, vomiting, stomatitis

Neuromuscular & skeletal: Arthralgia, back pain
Respiratory: Rhinitis, increased cough
Miscellaneous: Aggravation reaction

Drug Interactions CYP1A2 enzyme substrate

Increased Effect/Toxicity: Inhibitors of CYP1A2 (eg, caffeine, theophylline, amitriptyline, quinolones) could decrease the rate of riluzole elimination resulting in accumulation of riluzole.

Decreased Effect: Drugs that induce CYP1A2 (eg, cigarette smoke, charbroiled food, rifampin, omeprazole) could increase the rate of riluzole elimination.

Drug Uptake Absorption: Well absorbed (90%); decreased by a high fat meal (AUC by 20% and peak blood levels by 45%)

Pregnancy Risk Factor C

Generic Available No

Rimactane® *see* Rifampin *on page 1051*

Rimantadine (ri MAN ta deen)

Related Information

Systemic Viral Diseases *on page 1354*

U.S. Brand Names Flumadine®

Canadian Brand Names Flumadine®

Pharmacologic Category Antiviral Agent

Synonyms Rimantadine Hydrochloride

Use Prophylaxis (adults and children >1 year) and treatment (adults) of influenza A viral infection

Local Anesthetic/Vasoconstrictor Precautions No information available to require special precautions

Effects on Dental Treatment No effects or complications reported

Dosage Oral:

Prophylaxis:

Children <10 years: 5 mg/kg give once daily; maximum: 150 mg

Children >10 years and Adults: 100 mg twice daily; decrease to 100 mg/day in elderly or in patients with severe hepatic or renal impairment (Cl_{cr} ≤10 mL/minute)

Treatment: Adults: 100 mg twice daily; decrease to 100 mg/day in elderly or in patients with severe hepatic or renal impairment (Cl_{cr} ≤10 mL/minute)

Mechanism of Action Exerts its inhibitory effect on three antigenic subtypes of influenza A virus (H1N1, H2N2, H3N2) early in the viral replicative cycle, possibly inhibiting the uncoating process; it has no activity against influenza B virus and is 2- to 8-fold more active than amantadine

Other Adverse Effects 1% to 10%:

Cardiovascular: Orthostatic hypotension, edema

Central nervous system: Dizziness (2%), confusion, headache (1%), insomnia (2%), difficulty in concentrating, anxiety (1%), restlessness, irritability, hallucinations; incidence of CNS side effects may be less than that associated with amantadine

Gastrointestinal: Nausea (3%), vomiting (2%), xerostomia (2%), abdominal pain (1%), anorexia (2%)

Genitourinary: Urinary retention

Drug Interactions

Increased Effect/Toxicity: Cimetidine increases blood levels/toxicity of rimantadine.

Decreased Effect: Acetaminophen may cause a small reduction in AUC and peak concentration of rimantadine. Peak plasma and AUC concentrations of rimantadine are slightly reduced by aspirin.

Drug Uptake

Onset of action: Antiviral activity: No data exist establishing a correlation between plasma concentration and antiviral effect

Absorption: Tablet and syrup formulations are equally absorbed;

Half-life, elimination: 25.4 hours (increases in the elderly)

Time to peak: 6 hours

Pregnancy Risk Factor C

Generic Available No

Rimexolone (ri MEKS oh lone)

U.S. Brand Names Vexol®

Canadian Brand Names Vexol®

Pharmacologic Category Corticosteroid, Ophthalmic

Use Treatment of inflammation after ocular surgery and the treatment of anterior uveitis

Local Anesthetic/Vasoconstrictor Precautions No information available to require special precautions

Effects on Dental Treatment No effects or complications reported

Dosage Adults: Ophthalmic: Instill 1 drop in conjunctival sac 2-4 times/day up to every 4 hours; may use every 1-2 hours during first 1-2 days

(Continued)

Rimexolone (Continued)

Mechanism of Action Decreases inflammation by suppression of migration of polymorphonuclear leukocytes and reversal of increased capillary permeability
Other Adverse Effects 1% to 10%: Ocular: Temporary mild blurred vision
Drug Uptake Absorption: Through aqueous humor
Pregnancy Risk Factor C
Generic Available No

Riopan® [OTC] *see* Magaldrate *on page 738*
Riopan Plus® [OTC] *see* Magaldrate and Simethicone *on page 739*
Riopan Plus® Double Strength [OTC] *see* Magaldrate and Simethicone *on page 739*

Risedronate (ris ED roe nate)

U.S. Brand Names Actonel®
Canadian Brand Names Actonel®
Pharmacologic Category Bisphosphonate Derivative
Synonyms Risedronate Sodium
Use Paget's disease of the bone; treatment and prevention of glucocorticoid-induced osteoporosis; treatment and prevention of osteoporosis in postmenopausal women
Local Anesthetic/Vasoconstrictor Precautions No information available to require special precautions
Effects on Dental Treatment No effects or complications reported
Dosage Should be taken at least 30 minutes before the first food or drink of the day other than water. Oral:

Adults (patients should receive supplemental calcium and vitamin D if dietary intake is inadequate):

- Paget's disease of bone: 30 mg once daily for 2 months
  - Retreatment may be considered (following post-treatment observation of at least 2 months) if relapse occurs, or if treatment fails to normalize serum alkaline phosphatase. For retreatment, the dose and duration of therapy are the same as for initial treatment. No data are available on more than one course of retreatment.
- Osteoporosis prevention and treatment (postmenopausal or glucocorticoid-induced): 5 mg once daily; efficacy for use longer than 1 year has not been established; **alternatively,** a dose of 35 mg once weekly has been demonstrated to be effective

Dosage adjustment in elderly: Dosage adjustment is not necessary except in patients who have severe renal impairment (Cl_{cr} <30 mL/minute)

Dosage adjustment in renal impairment: Cl_{cr} <30 mL/minute: **Not** recommended for use

Mechanism of Action A bisphosphonate which inhibits bone resorption via actions on osteoclasts or on osteoclast precursors; decreases the rate of bone resorption direction, leading to an indirect decrease in bone formation.

Other Adverse Effects

Seen in patients taking 30 mg/day for Paget's disease:

- >10%:
  - Central nervous system: Headache (18%)
  - Dermatologic: Rash (11%)
  - Gastrointestinal: Diarrhea (20%), abdominal pain (11%)
  - Neuromuscular & skeletal: Arthralgia (33%)
  - Miscellaneous: Flu-like syndrome (10%)
- 1% to 10%:
  - Cardiovascular: Peripheral edema (8%)
  - Central nervous system: Chest pain (7%), dizziness (7%)
  - Gastrointestinal: Nausea (10%), constipation (7%), belching (3%), colitis (3%, placebo 3%)
  - Neuromuscular & skeletal: Weakness (5%), bone pain (5%, placebo 5%), leg cramps (3%, placebo 3%), myasthenia (3%)
  - Ocular: Amblyopia (3%, placebo 3%), dry eye (3%)
  - Otic: Tinnitus (3%, placebo 3%)
  - Respiratory: Sinusitis (5%), bronchitis (3%, placebo 5%)
  - Miscellaneous: Neoplasm (3%)

Seen in patient taking 5 mg/day for osteoporosis (events similar to those seen with placebo)

- >10%:
  - Central nervous system: Pain (14%)
  - Gastrointestinal: Abdominal pain (12%), diarrhea (11%), nausea (11%)
  - Genitourinary: Urinary tract infection (11%)
  - Neuromuscular & skeletal: Back pain (26%), arthralgia (24%)
- 1% to 10%:
  - Cardiovascular: Hypertension (10%), chest pain (5%), cardiovascular disorder (2%), angina (2%)
  - Central nervous system: Depression (7%), dizziness (6%), insomnia (5%), anxiety (4%), vertigo (3%)

Dermatologic: Rash (8%), bruising (4%), pruritus (3%), skin carcinoma (2%)
Gastrointestinal: Flatulence (5), gastritis (2%), gastrointestinal disorder (2%), rectal disorder (2%), tooth disorder (2%)
Genitourinary: Cystitis (4%)
Hematologic: Anemia (2%)
Neuromuscular & skeletal: Joint disorder (7%), myalgia (7%), neck pain (5%), asthenia (5%), bone pain (5%), bone disorder (4%), neuralgia (4%), leg cramps (4%), bursitis (3%), tendon disorder (3%), hypertonia (2%), paresthesia (2%)
Ocular: Cataract (6%), conjunctivitis (3%)
Otic: Otitis media (2%)
Respiratory: Pharyngitis (6%), rhinitis (6%), dyspnea (4%), pneumonia (3%)
Miscellaneous: Neoplasm(3%), hernia (3%)

Contraindications Hypersensitivity to bisphosphonates or any component of their formulation; hypocalcemia

Warnings/Precautions Bisphosphonates may cause upper GI disorders such as dysphagia, esophageal ulcer, and gastric ulcer. Use caution in patients with renal impairment; hypocalcemia must be corrected before therapy initiation with alendronate; ensure adequate calcium and vitamin D intake, especially for patients with Paget's disease in whom the pretreatment rate of bone turnover may be greatly elevated.

Drug Interactions Calcium supplements and antacids interfere with absorption.

Drug Uptake

Onset of action: May require weeks
Absorption: Rapid
Half-life, elimination: Terminal: 220 hours

Pregnancy Risk Factor C

Generic Available No

Risperdal® *see* Risperidone *on page 1057*

Risperidone (ris PER i done)

U.S. Brand Names Risperdal®

Canadian Brand Names Risperdal®

Mexican Brand Names Risperdal®

Pharmacologic Category Antipsychotic Agent, Benzisoxazole

Use Management of psychotic disorders (eg, schizophrenia)

Unlabeled/Investigational: Behavioral symptoms associated with dementia in elderly; treatment of bipolar disorder, mania, Tourette's disorder; treatment of pervasive developmental disorder and autism in children and adolescents

Local Anesthetic/Vasoconstrictor Precautions No information available to require special precautions

Effects on Dental Treatment ≤10%: Significant xerostomia and orthostatic hypotension; disappears with discontinuation

Dosage Oral:

Children and Adolescents:

Pervasive developmental disorder (unlabeled use): Initial: 0.25 mg twice daily; titrate up 0.25 mg/day every 5-7 days; optimal dose range: 0.75-3 mg/day
Autism (unlabeled use): Initial: 0.25 mg at bedtime; titrate to 1 mg/day (0.1 mg/kg/day)
Schizophrenia: Initial: 0.5 mg twice daily; titrate as necessary up to 2-6 mg/day
Bipolar disorder (unlabeled use): 0.5-3 mg/day
Tourette's disorder (unlabeled use): 2-4 mg/day

Adults: Recommended starting dose: 0.5-1 mg twice daily; slowly increase to the optimum range of 3-6 mg/day; may be given as a single daily dose once maintenance dose is achieved; daily dosages >10 mg does not appear to confer any additional benefit, and the incidence of extrapyramidal reactions is higher than with lower doses

Elderly: A starting dose of 0.25-1 mg in 1-2 divided doses, and titration should progress slowly. Additional monitoring of renal function and orthostatic BP may be warranted. If once-a-day dosing in the elderly or debilitated patient is considered, a twice daily regimen should be used to titrate to the target dose, and this dose should be maintained for 2-3 days prior to attempts to switch to a once-daily regimen.

Dosing adjustment in renal, hepatic impairment: Starting dose of 0.25-0.5 mg twice daily is advisable

Mechanism of Action Risperidone is a benzisoxazole derivative, mixed serotonin-dopamine antagonist; binds to 5-HT_2-receptors in the CNS and in the periphery with a very high affinity; binds to dopamine-D_2 receptors with less affinity. The binding affinity to the dopamine-D_2 receptor is 20 times lower than the 5-HT_2 affinity. The addition of serotonin antagonism to dopamine antagonism (classic neuroleptic mechanism) is thought to improve negative symptoms of psychoses and reduce the incidence of extrapyramidal side effects. Alpha$_1$, alpha$_2$ adrenergic, and histaminergic receptors are also antagonized with high affinity. Risperidone

(Continued)

Risperidone *(Continued)*

has low to moderate affinity for 5-HT_{1C}, 5-HT_{1D}, and 5-HT_{1A} receptors, weak affinity for D_1 and no affinity for muscarinics or $beta_1$ and $beta_2$ receptors

Other Adverse Effects

Frequency not defined: Gastrointestinal: Dysphagia, esophageal dysmotility

>10%: Central nervous system: Insomnia, agitation, anxiety, headache

1% to 10%:

Cardiovascular: Hypotension (especially orthostatic), tachycardia

Central nervous system: Sedation, dizziness, restlessness, extrapyramidal symptoms (dose dependent), dystonic reactions, pseudoparkinson, tardive dyskinesia, neuroleptic malignant syndrome, altered central temperature regulation

Dermatologic: Photosensitivity (rare), rash, dry skin

Endocrine & metabolic: Amenorrhea, galactorrhea, gynecomastia, sexual dysfunction

Gastrointestinal: Constipation, GI upset, xerostomia, dyspepsia, vomiting, abdominal pain, nausea, anorexia, weight gain

Genitourinary: Polyuria

Ocular: Abnormal vision

Respiratory: Rhinitis, coughing, sinusitis, pharyngitis, dyspnea

Drug Interactions CYP2D6 substrate and inhibitor (weak); CYP3A4 substrate

Antihypertensives: Risperidone may enhance the hypotensive effects of antihypertensive agents

Clozapine: Decreases clearance of risperidone, increasing its serum concentrations

CYP2D6 inhibitors: Metabolism of risperidone may be decreased; increasing clinical effect or toxicity; inhibitors include amiodarone, cimetidine, delavirdine, fluoxetine, paroxetine, propafenone, quinidine, and ritonavir; monitor for increased effect/toxicity

CYP3A3/4 inhibitors: May increase serum concentrations of risperidone; inhibitors include amiodarone, cimetidine, clarithromycin, erythromycin, delavirdine, diltiazem, dirithromycin, disulfiram, fluoxetine, fluvoxamine, grapefruit juice, indinavir, itraconazole, ketoconazole, metronidazole, nefazodone, nevirapine, propoxyphene, quinupristin-dalfopristin, ritonavir, saquinavir, verapamil, zafirlukast, zileuton; monitor for altered response

Enzyme inducers: May increase the metabolism of risperidone, reducing serum levels and effect; enzyme inducers include carbamazepine, barbiturates, phenytoin and rifampin; see note on carbamazepine

Levodopa: At high doses (>6 mg/day), risperidone may inhibit the antiparkinsonian effect of levodopa; avoid this combination when high doses are used

Metoclopramide: May increase extrapyramidal symptoms (EPS) or risk.

Valproic acid: Generalized edema has been reported as a consequence of concurrent therapy (case report)

Drug Uptake

Absorption: Oral: Rapid and well; food does not affect rate or extent

Half-life, elimination: 20 hours (risperidone and its active metabolite 9-hydroxyrisperidone)

Time to peak, plasma: Risperidone: ~1 hour; 9-hydroxyrisperidone: 3 hours in extensive metabolizers and 17 hours in poor metabolizers

Pregnancy Risk Factor C

Generic Available No

Ritalin® *see* Methylphenidate *on page 795*

Ritalin® LA *see* Methylphenidate *on page 795*

Ritalin-SR® *see* Methylphenidate *on page 795*

Ritifed® [OTC] *see* Triprolidine and Pseudoephedrine *on page 1213*

Ritodrine *No longer manufactured* (RI toe dreen)

U.S. Brand Names Yutopar®

Pharmacologic Category $Beta_2$ Agonist

Synonyms Ritodrine Hydrochloride

Use Inhibits uterine contraction in preterm labor

Local Anesthetic/Vasoconstrictor Precautions No information available to require special precautions

Effects on Dental Treatment No effects or complications reported

Dosage Adults:

I.V.: 50-100 mcg/minute; increase by 50 mcg/minute every 10 minutes; continue for 12 hours after contractions have stopped

Oral: Start 30 minutes before stopping I.V. infusion; 10 mg every 2 hours for 24 hours, then 10-20 mg every 4-6 hours up to 120 mg/day

Mechanism of Action Tocolysis due to its uterine $beta_2$-adrenergic receptor stimulating effects; this agent's $beta_2$ effects can also cause bronchial relaxation and vascular smooth muscle stimulation

Other Adverse Effects

>10%:

Cardiovascular: Increases in maternal and fetal heart rates and maternal hypertension, palpitations

Endocrine & metabolic: Temporary hyperglycemia

Gastrointestinal: Nausea, vomiting

Neuromuscular & skeletal: Tremor

1% to 10%:

Cardiovascular: Chest pain

Central nervous system: Nervousness, anxiety, restlessness

Dermatologic: Rash

Drug Interactions

Increased Effect/Toxicity: Increased effect/toxicity with meperidine, sympathomimetics, diazoxide, magnesium, betamethasone (pulmonary edema), potassium-depleting diuretics, and general anesthetics.

Decreased effect with beta-blockers

Drug Uptake

Absorption: Oral: Rapid

Half-life, elimination: 15 hours

Time to peak: 0.5-1 hour

Pregnancy Risk Factor B (contraindicated before 20th week)

Generic Available Yes

Ritonavir (rye TON a veer)

Related Information

HIV Infection and AIDS *on page 1334*

U.S. Brand Names Norvir®

Canadian Brand Names Norvir®; Norvir® SEC

Mexican Brand Names Norvir®

Pharmacologic Category Antiretroviral Agent, Protease Inhibitor

Use Treatment of HIV infection; should always be used as part of a multidrug regimen (at least 3 antiretroviral agents)

Local Anesthetic/Vasoconstrictor Precautions No information available to require special precautions

Effects on Dental Treatment No effects or complications reported

Dosage Oral:

Children ≥2 years: 250 mg/m^2 twice daily; titrate dose upward to 400 mg/m^2 twice daily (maximum: 600 mg twice daily)

Adults: 600 mg twice daily; dose escalation tends to avoid nausea that many patients experience upon initiation of full dosing. Escalate the dose as follows: 300 mg twice daily for 1 day, 400 mg twice daily for 2 days, 500 mg twice daily for 1 day, then 600 mg twice daily. Ritonavir may be better tolerated when used in combination with other antiretrovirals by initiating the drug alone and subsequently adding the second agent within 2 weeks.

Note: Dosage adjustments for ritonavir when administered in combination therapy:

Amprenavir: Adjustments necessary for each agent:

Amprenavir 1200 mg with ritonavir 200 mg once daily **or**

Amprenavir 600 mg with ritonavir 100 mg twice daily

Amprenavir plus efavirenz (3-drug regimen): Amprenavir 1200 mg twice daily plus ritonavir 200 mg twice daily plus efavirenz at standard dose

Indinavir: Adjustments necessary for both agents:

Indinavir 800 mg twice daily plus ritonavir 100-200 mg twice daily **or**

Indinavir 400 mg twice daily plus ritonavir 400 mg twice daily

Nelfinavir or saquinavir: Ritonavir 400 mg twice daily

Dosing adjustment in hepatic impairment: Caution advised with severe impairment

Mechanism of Action Ritonavir inhibits HIV protease and renders the enzyme incapable of processing of polyprotein precursor which leads to production of noninfectious immature HIV particles

Other Adverse Effects Protease inhibitors cause dyslipidemia which includes elevated cholesterol and triglycerides and a redistribution of body fat centrally to cause "protease paunch," buffalo hump, facial atrophy, and breast enlargement. These agents also cause hyperglycemia.

>10%:

Endocrine & metabolic: Increased triglycerides

Gastrointestinal: Diarrhea, nausea, vomiting, taste perversion

Hematologic: Anemia, decreased WBCs

Hepatic: Increased GGT

Neuromuscular & skeletal: Weakness

1% to 10%:

Cardiovascular: Vasodilation

Central nervous system: Fever, headache, malaise, dizziness, insomnia, somnolence, thinking abnormally

Dermatologic: Rash

(Continued)

Ritonavir *(Continued)*

Endocrine & metabolic: Hyperlipidemia, increased uric acid, increased glucose
Gastrointestinal: Abdominal pain, anorexia, constipation, dyspepsia, flatulence, local throat irritation
Hematologic: Neutropenia, eosinophilia, neutrophilia, prolonged PT, leukocytosis
Hepatic: Increased LFTs
Neuromuscular & skeletal: Increased CPK, myalgia, paresthesia
Respiratory: Pharyngitis
Miscellaneous: Diaphoresis, increased potassium, increased calcium,

Contraindications Hypersensitivity to ritonavir or any component of the formulation; concurrent amiodarone, bepridil, flecainide, propafenone, quinidine, astemizole, terfenadine, dihydroergotamine, ergotamine, midazolam, triazolam, cisapride, pimozide; breast-feeding

Warnings/Precautions Use caution in patients with hepatic insufficiency; safety and efficacy have not been established in children <16 years of age; use caution with certain analgesics (meperidine, piroxicam, propoxyphene); avoid concurrent use of St John's wort (may lead to loss of virologic response and/or resistance)

Drug Interactions CYP1A2, 2A6, 2C9, 2C19, 2E1, and 3A3/4 enzyme substrate, CYP2D6 enzyme substrate (minor); CYP1A2 enzyme inducer; CYP1A2, 2A6, 2C9, 2C19, 2D6, 2E1, and 3A3/4 enzyme inhibitor

Increased Effect/Toxicity: Concurrent use of amiodarone, astemizole, bepridil, cisapride, flecainide, pimozide, propafenone, and quinidine is contraindicated. Serum concentrations/toxicity of many benzodiazepines may be increased; midazolam and triazolam are contraindicated. Concurrent use of ergot alkaloids (dihydroergotamine, ergotamine, ergonovine, methylergonovine) with ritonavir is also contraindicated (may cause vasospasm and peripheral ischemia). HMG-CoA reductase inhibitors serum concentration may be increased by ritonavir, increasing the risk of myopathy/rhabdomyolysis; lovastatin and simvastatin are contraindicated; fluvastatin and pravastatin may be safer alternatives. Serum concentrations of meperidine's neuroexcitatory metabolite (normeperidine) are increased by ritonavir, which may increase the risk of CNS toxicity/seizures. Rifabutin and rifabutin metabolite serum concentration may be increased by ritonavir; reduce rifabutin dose to 150 mg every other day. Sildenafil serum concentration may be increased by ritonavir; when used concurrently, do not exceed a maximum sildenafil dose of 25 mg in a 48-hour period. Saquinavir's serum concentration are increased by ritonavir; the dosage of both agents should be reduced to 400 mg twice daily. Concurrent therapy with amprenavir may result in increased serum concentration: dosage adjustment is recommended. Metronidazole or disulfiram may cause Antabuse® reaction (oral solution contains 43% ethanol).

Ritonavir may also increase the serum concentration of the following drugs (dose decrease may be needed): Benzodiazepines, beta-blockers (metoprolol, timolol), bupropion, calcium channel blockers (diltiazem, nifedipine, verapamil), carbamazepine, clarithromycin, clonazepam, clorazepate, clozapine, cyclosporin, dexamethasone, disopyramide, dronabinol, ethosuximide, fluoxetine (and other SSRIs), indinavir, ketoconazole, lidocaine, methamphetamine, mexiletine, nefazodone, perphenazine, prednisone, propoxyphene, piroxicam, quinine, risperidone, tacrolimus, tramadol, thioridazine, tricyclic antidepressants (including desipramine), and zolpidem. Serum concentrations of rifabutin may be increased by ritonavir; dosage adjustment required.

Decreased Effect: The administration of didanosine (buffered formulation) should be separated from ritonavir by 2.5 hours to limit interaction with ritonavir. Concurrent use of rifampin, rifabutin, dexamethasone, and many anticonvulsants may lower serum concentration of ritonavir. Ritonavir may reduce the concentration of ethinyl estradiol which may result in loss of contraception (including combination products). Theophylline concentrations may be reduced in concurrent therapy. Levels of didanosine and zidovudine may be decreased by ritonavir, however, no dosage adjustment is necessary. In addition, ritonavir may decrease the serum concentration of the following drugs: Atovaquone, divalproex, lamotrigine, methadone, phenytoin, warfarin.

Drug Uptake

Absorption: Variable, with or without food
Half-life, elimination: 3-5 hours

Pregnancy Risk Factor B

Generic Available No

Selected Readings Ouellet D, Hsu A, Granneman GR, et al, "Pharmacokinetic Interaction Between Ritonavir and Clarithromycin," *Clin Pharmacol Ther*, 1998, 64(4):355-62.

Rituxan® *see* Rituximab *on page 1060*

Rituximab (ri TUK si mab)

U.S. Brand Names Rituxan®

Canadian Brand Names Rituxan®

Mexican Brand Names Mabthera®

Pharmacologic Category Antineoplastic Agent, Monoclonal Antibody

Synonyms C2B8

Use Treatment of patients with relapsed or refractory low-grade or follicular, CD20 positive, B-cell non-Hodgkin's lymphoma; treatment (as part of combination therapy with radiolabeled ibritumomab) of patients with relapsed or refractory low-grade, follicular, or transformed B-cell non-Hodgkin's lymphoma (including rituximab refractory follicular non-Hodgkin's lymphoma)

Local Anesthetic/Vasoconstrictor Precautions No information available to require special precautions

Effects on Dental Treatment No effects or complications reported

Mechanism of Action A monoclonal antibody directed against the CD20 antigen on B-lymphocytes; CD20 regulates cell cycle initiation; and, possibly, functions as a calcium channel. Rituximab binds to the antigen on the cell surface, activating complement-dependent cytotoxicity; and to human Fc receptors, mediating cell killing through an antibody-dependent cellular toxicity. The CD20 antigen is also expressed on >90% of B-cell non-Hodgkin's lymphomas (NHL) but is not found on hematopoietic stem cells, pro-B cells, normal plasma cells, or other normal tissues.

Other Adverse Effects

>10%:

Central nervous system: Headache, fever, chills

Gastrointestinal: Nausea

Hematologic: Leukopenia

Neuromuscular & skeletal: Asthenia

Miscellaneous: Angioedema

Immunologic: Rituximab-induced B-cell depletion occurred in 70% to 80% of patients and was associated with decreased serum immunoglobulins in a minority of patients. The incidence of infections does not appear to be increased. During the treatment period, 50 patients in the pivotal trial developed infectious events, including six grade 3 events (there were no grade 4 events. The six serious events were not associated with neutropenia).

Infusion-related: An infusion-related symptom complex consisting of fever and chills/rigors occurred in the majority of patients during the first rituximab infusion. Other frequent infusion-related symptoms included nausea, urticaria, fatigue, headache, pruritus, bronchospasm, dyspnea, sensation of tongue or throat swelling (angioedema), rhinitis, vomiting, hypotension, flushing, and pain at disease sites. These reactions generally occurred within 30 minutes to 2 hours of beginning the first infusion, and resolved with slowing or interruption of the infusion and with supportive care (I.V. saline, diphenhydramine, and acetaminophen). The incidence of infusion related events decreased from 80% during the first to ~40% with subsequent infusions. Mild to moderate hypotension requiring interruption of rituximab infusion, with or without the administration of I.V. saline, occurred in 10%. Isolated occurrences of severe reactions requiring epinephrine have been reported in patients receiving rituximab for other indicators. Angioedema was reported in 13% and was serious in one patient.

1% to 10%:

Cardiovascular: Hypotension

Central nervous system: Myalgia, dizziness

Dermatologic: Pruritus, rash, urticaria

Gastrointestinal: Vomiting, abdominal pain

Hematologic: Thrombocytopenia, neutropenia; during the treatment period (up to 30 days following the last dose), the following occurred: Severe thrombocytopenia, severe neutropenia, and severe anemia

Respiratory: Bronchospasm occurred in 8%; 25% of these patients were treated with bronchodilators; rhinitis

Miscellaneous: Throat irritation

Note: The following adverse events were reported more frequently in retreated patients: Asthenia, throat irritation, flushing, tachycardia, anorexia, leukopenia, thrombocytopenia, anemia, peripheral edema, dizziness, depression, respiratory symptoms, night sweats, pruritus

Warnings/Precautions Rituximab is associated with hypersensitivity reactions which may respond to adjustments in the infusion rate. Hypotension, bronchospasm, and angioedema have occurred as part of an infusion-related symptom complex. Interrupt rituximab infusion for severe reactions and resume at a 50% reduction in rate (eg, from 100 to 50 mg/hour) when symptoms have completely resolved. Treatment of these symptoms with diphenhydramine and acetaminophen is recommended; additional treatment with bronchodilators or I.V. saline may be indicated. In most cases, patients who have experienced nonlife-threatening reactions have been able to complete the full course of therapy. Medications for the treatment of hypersensitivity reactions (eg, epinephrine, antihistamines, corticosteroids) should be available for immediate use in the event of such a reaction during administration.

Discontinue infusions in the event of serious or life-threatening cardiac arrhythmias. Patients who develop clinically significant arrhythmias should undergo cardiac monitoring during and after subsequent infusions of rituximab. Patients with

(Continued)

Rituximab *(Continued)*

pre-existing cardiac conditions including arrhythmias and angina have had recurrences of these events during rituximab therapy; monitor these patients throughout the infusion and immediate postinfusion periods.

Drug Uptake

Absorption: I.V.: Immediate and results in a rapid and sustained depletion of circulating and tissue-based B cells

Duration: Detectable in serum 3-6 months after completion of treatment; B-cell recovery begins ~6 months following completion of treatment; median B-cell levels return to normal by 12 months following completion of treatment

Half-life elimination:

>100 mg/m^2: 4.4 days (range 1.6-10.5 days)

375 mg/m^2: 50 hours (following first dose) to 174 hours (following fourth dose)

Pregnancy Risk Factor C

Generic Available No

Rivastigmine (ri va STIG meen)

U.S. Brand Names Exelon®

Canadian Brand Names Exelon®

Mexican Brand Names Exelon®

Pharmacologic Category Acetylcholinesterase Inhibitor (Central)

Synonyms ENA 713; SDZ ENA 713

Use Treatment of mild to moderate dementia from Alzheimer's disease

Local Anesthetic/Vasoconstrictor Precautions No information available to require special precautions

Effects on Dental Treatment No effects or complications reported

Dosage Adults: Mild to moderate Alzheimer's dementia: Oral: Initial: 1.5 mg twice daily to start; if dose is tolerated for at least 2 weeks then it may be increased to 3 mg twice daily; increases to 4.5 mg twice daily and 6 mg twice daily should only be attempted after at least 2 weeks at the previous dose; maximum dose: 6 mg twice daily. If adverse events such as nausea, vomiting, abdominal pain, or loss of appetite occur, the patient should be instructed to discontinue treatment for several doses then restart at the same or next lower dosage level; antiemetics have been used to control GI symptoms. If treatment is interrupted for longer than several days, restart the treatment at the lowest dose and titrate as previously described.

Elderly: Clearance is significantly lower in patients older than 60 years of age, but dosage adjustments are not recommended. Titrate dose to individual's tolerance.

Mechanism of Action A deficiency of cortical acetylcholine is thought to account for some of the symptoms of Alzheimer's disease; rivastigmine increases acetylcholine in the CNS through reversible inhibition of its hydrolysis by cholinesterase.

Other Adverse Effects

>10%:

Central nervous system: Dizziness (21%), headache (17%)

Gastrointestinal: Nausea (47%), vomiting (31%), diarrhea (19%), anorexia (17%), abdominal pain (13%)

2% to 10%:

Cardiovascular: Syncope (3%), hypertension (3%)

Central nervous system: Fatigue (9%), insomnia (9%), confusion (8%), depression (6%), anxiety (5%), malaise (5%), somnolence (5%), hallucinations (4%), aggressiveness (3%)

Gastrointestinal: Dyspepsia (9%), constipation (5%), flatulence (4%), weight loss (3%), eructation (2%)

Genitourinary: Urinary tract infection (7%)

Neuromuscular & skeletal: Weakness (6%), tremor (4%)

Respiratory: Rhinitis (4%)

Miscellaneous: Increased diaphoresis (4%), flu-like syndrome (3%)

>2% (but frequency equal to placebo): Chest pain, peripheral edema, vertigo, back pain, arthralgia, pain, bone fracture, agitation, nervousness, delusion, paranoid reaction, upper respiratory tract infections, infection, coughing, pharyngitis, bronchitis, rash, urinary incontinence.

<2% (Limited to important or life-threatening symptoms; reactions may be at a similar frequency to placebo): Fever, edema, allergy, periorbital or facial edema, hypothermia, hypotension, postural hypotension, cardiac failure, ataxia, convulsions, apraxia, aphasia, dysphonia, hyperkinesia, hypertonia, hypokinesia, migraine, neuralgia, peripheral neuropathy, hypothyroidism, peptic ulcer, gastroesophageal reflux, GI hemorrhage, intestinal obstruction, pancreatitis, colitis, atrial fibrillation, bradycardia, AV block, bundle branch block, sick sinus syndrome, cardiac arrest, supraventricular tachycardia, tachycardia, abnormal hepatic function, cholecystitis, dehydration, arthritis, angina pectoris, myocardial infarction, epistaxis, hematoma, thrombocytopenia, purpura, delirium, emotional lability, psychosis, anemia, bronchospasm, apnea, rashes (maculopapular, eczema, bullous, exfoliative, psoriaform, erythematous), urticaria, acute renal failure,

peripheral ischemia, pulmonary embolism, thrombosis, thrombophlebitis, intracranial hemorrhage, conjunctival hemorrhage, diplopia, glaucoma, lymphadenopathy, leukocytosis.

Contraindications Hypersensitivity to rivastigmine, other carbamate derivatives, or any component of their formulation

Warnings/Precautions Significant nausea, vomiting, anorexia, and weight loss are associated with use; occurs more frequently in women and during the titration phase. If treatment is interrupted for more than several days, reinstate at the lowest daily dose. Use caution in patients with a history of peptic ulcer disease or concurrent NSAID use. Caution in patients undergoing anesthesia who will receive succinylcholine-type muscle relaxation, patients with sick sinus syndrome, bradycardia or supraventricular conduction conditions, urinary obstruction, seizure disorders, or pulmonary conditions such as asthma or COPD. There are no trials evaluating the safety and efficacy in children.

Drug Interactions

Increased Effect/Toxicity: Beta-blockers without ISA activity may increase risk of bradycardia. Calcium channel blockers (diltiazem or verapamil) may increase risk of bradycardia. Cholinergic agonists effects may be increased with rivastigmine. Cigarette use increases the clearance of rivastigmine by 23%. Depolarizing neuromuscular blocking agents effects may be increased with rivastigmine. Digoxin may increase risk of bradycardia. Cigarette use increases the clearance of rivastigmine by 23%.

Decreased Effect: Anticholinergic agents effects may be reduced with rivastigmine.

Drug Uptake

Absorption: Fasting: Rapid and complete within 1 hour

Half-life, elimination: 1.5 hours

Time to peak: 1 hour

Pregnancy Risk Factor B

Generic Available No

Rizatriptan (rye za TRIP tan)

U.S. Brand Names Maxalt®; Maxalt-MLT™

Canadian Brand Names Maxalt™; Maxalt RPD™

Mexican Brand Names Maxalt®

Pharmacologic Category Serotonin 5-HT_{1D} Receptor Agonist

Synonyms MK462

Use Acute treatment of migraine with or without aura

Local Anesthetic/Vasoconstrictor Precautions No information available to require special precautions

Effects on Dental Treatment No effects or complications reported

Dosage In patients with risk factors for coronary artery disease, following adequate evaluation to establish the absence of coronary artery disease, the initial dose should be administered in a setting where response may be evaluated (physician's office or similarly staffed setting). EKG monitoring may be considered.

Oral: 5-10 mg, repeat after 2 hours if significant relief is not attained; maximum: 30 mg in a 24-hour period (use 5 mg dose in patients receiving propranolol with a maximum of 15 mg in 24 hours)

Note: For orally-disintegrating tablets (Maxalt-MLT™): Patient should be instructed to place tablet on tongue and allow to dissolve. Dissolved tablet will be swallowed with saliva.

Mechanism of Action Selective agonist for serotonin (5-HT_{1D} receptor) in cranial arteries to cause vasoconstriction and reduce sterile inflammation associated with antidromic neuronal transmission correlating with relief of migraine

Other Adverse Effects 1% to 10%:

Cardiovascular: Systolic/diastolic BP increases (5-10 mm Hg), chest pain (5%), palpitation

Central nervous system: Dizziness, drowsiness, fatigue (13% to 30%, dose related)

Dermatologic: Skin flushing

Endocrine & metabolic: Mild increase in growth hormone, hot flashes

Gastrointestinal: Nausea, abdominal pain, xerostomia (<5%)

Respiratory: Dyspnea

Drug Interactions Increased Effect/Toxicity: Use within 24 hours of another selective 5-HT_1 antagonist or ergot-containing drug should be avoided due to possible additive vasoconstriction. Use with propranolol increased plasma concentration of rizatriptan by 70%. Rarely, concurrent use with SSRIs results in weakness and incoordination; monitor closely. MAO inhibitors and nonselective MAO inhibitors increase concentration of rizatriptan.

Drug Uptake

Onset of action: ~30 minutes

Duration: 14-16 hours

Half-life, elimination: 2-3 hours

Time to peak, serum: 1-1.5 hours

Pregnancy Risk Factor C

Generic Available No

RMS® *see* Morphine Sulfate *on page 829*
Robafen® AC *see* Guaifenesin and Codeine *on page 568*
Robafen DM® [OTC] *see* Guaifenesin and Dextromethorphan *on page 569*
Robaxin® *see* Methocarbamol *on page 783*
Robaxisal® *see* Methocarbamol and Aspirin *on page 784*
Robinul® *see* Glycopyrrolate *on page 563*
Robinul® Forte *see* Glycopyrrolate *on page 563*
Robitussin® [OTC] *see* Guaifenesin *on page 568*
Robitussin® A-C *see* Guaifenesin and Codeine *on page 568*
Robitussin® Cough Calmers [OTC] *see* Dextromethorphan *on page 372*
Robitussin®-DAC *see* Guaifenesin, Pseudoephedrine, and Codeine *on page 570*
Robitussin®-DM [OTC] *see* Guaifenesin and Dextromethorphan *on page 569*
Robitussin® Maximum Strength Cough & Cold [OTC] *see* Pseudoephedrine and Dextromethorphan *on page 1023*
Robitussin-PE® [OTC] *see* Guaifenesin and Pseudoephedrine *on page 570*
Robitussin® Pediatric [OTC] *see* Dextromethorphan *on page 372*
Robitussin® Pediatric Cough & Cold [OTC] *see* Pseudoephedrine and Dextromethorphan *on page 1023*
Robitussin® Severe Congestion Liqui-Gels® [OTC] *see* Guaifenesin and Pseudoephedrine *on page 570*
Rocaltrol® *see* Calcitriol *on page 199*
Rocephin® *see* Ceftriaxone *on page 245*

Rofecoxib (roe fe COX ib)

Related Information

Oral Pain *on page 1360*
Rheumatoid Arthritis and Osteoarthritis *on page 1340*

U.S. Brand Names Vioxx®

Canadian Brand Names Vioxx®

Pharmacologic Category Nonsteroidal Anti-inflammatory Drug (NSAID), COX-2 Selective

Use

Dental: Management of acute pain in adults

Medical: Relief of the signs and symptoms of osteoarthritis; management of acute pain in adults; treatment of primary dysmenorrhea; relief of signs and symptoms of rheumatoid arthritis in adults

Local Anesthetic/Vasoconstrictor Precautions No information available to require special precautions

Effects on Dental Treatment In models of postoperative dental pain, rofecoxib was effective against dental pain rated as moderate to severe. The analgesic efficacy of a single 50 mg dose of rofecoxib was apparently similar to 400 mg of ibuprofen or 550 mg of naproxen sodium. The onset of analgesia for postoperative dental pain with a single 50 mg dose of rofecoxib was 45 minutes.

Platelets: Bleeding time was not altered after a single dose of 500 mg or 1000 mg of rofecoxib. In addition, according to the manufacturer, multiple doses of rofecoxib 12.5 mg, 25 mg, and up to 375 mg administered daily up to 12 days, had no effect on bleeding time relative to placebo. However, according to the manufacturer, rofecoxib may increase the INR in patients receiving warfarin (see Drug Interactions).

Dosage Adult: Oral:

Osteoarthritis: 12.5 mg once daily; may be increased to a maximum of 25 mg once daily

Acute pain and management of dysmenorrhea: 50 mg once daily as needed (use for longer than 5 days has not been studied)

Rheumatoid arthritis: 25 mg once daily

Dosing comment in renal impairment: Use in advanced renal disease is not recommended

Dosing adjustment in hepatic impairment: No specific dosage adjustment is recommended (AUC may be increased by 69%)

Elderly: No specific adjustment is recommended. However, the AUC in elderly patients may be increased by 34% as compared to younger subjects. Use the lowest recommended dose.

Mechanism of Action Inhibits prostaglandin synthesis by decreasing the activity of the enzyme, cyclo-oxygenase-2 (COX-2), which results in decreased formation of prostaglandin precursors. Rofecoxib does not inhibit cyclo-oxygenase-1 (COX-1) at therapeutic concentrations.

Other Adverse Effects

2% to 10%:

Cardiovascular: Peripheral edema (3.7%), hypertension (3.5%)

Central nervous system: Headache (4.7%), dizziness (3%), weakness (2.2%)

Gastrointestinal: Diarrhea (6.5%), nausea (5.2%), heartburn (4.2%), epigastric discomfort (3.8%), dyspepsia (3.5%), abdominal pain (3.4%)

Genitourinary: Urinary tract infection (2.8%)

Neuromuscular & skeletal: Back pain (2.5%)
Respiratory: Upper respiratory infection (8.5%), bronchitis (2.0%), sinusitis (2.7%)
Miscellaneous: Flu-like syndrome (2.9%)

0.1% to 2%:

Cardiovascular: Chest pain, upper extremity edema, atrial fibrillation, bradycardia, arrhythmia, palpitation, tachycardia, venous insufficiency, fluid retention
Central nervous system: Anxiety, depression, decreased mental acuity, hypesthesia, insomnia, neuropathy, migraine, paresthesia, somnolence, vertigo, fever, pain
Dermatologic: Alopecia, atopic dermatitis, basal cell carcinoma, contact dermatitis, pruritus, rash, erythema, urticaria, dry skin
Endocrine & metabolic: Weight gain, hypercholesteremia
Gastrointestinal: Reflux, abdominal distension, abdominal tenderness, constipation, xerostomia, esophagitis, flatulence, gastritis, gastroenteritis, hematochezia, hemorrhoids, oral ulceration, dental caries, aphthous stomatitis
Genitourinary: Breast mass, cystitis, dysuria, menopausal disorder, nocturia, urinary retention, vaginitis, pelvic pain
Hematologic: Hematoma
Neuromuscular & skeletal: Muscle spasm, sciatica, arthralgia, bursitis, cartilage trauma, joint swelling, muscle cramps, muscle weakness, myalgia, tendonitis, traumatic arthropathy, fracture (wrist)
Ocular: Blurred vision, conjunctivitis
Otic: Otic pain, otitis media, tinnitus
Respiratory: Asthma, cough, dyspnea, pneumonia, respiratory infection, pulmonary congestion, rhinitis, epistaxis, laryngitis, dry throat, pharyngitis, tonsillitis, diaphragmatic hernia
Miscellaneous: Allergy, fungal infection, insect bite reaction, syncope, viral syndrome, herpes simplex, herpes zoster, increased sweating

<0.1% (Limited to severe or life-threatening symptoms): Congestive heart failure, cerebrovascular accident, deep venous thrombosis, myocardial infarction, unstable angina, transient ischemic attack, colitis, colonic neoplasm, cholecystitis, duodenal ulcer, gastrointestinal bleeding, intestinal obstruction, pancreatitis, lymphoma, breast cancer, prostatic cancer, urolithiasis, pulmonary embolism, esophageal ulcer, duodenal perforation, angioedema, aseptic meningitis, hallucinations, acute renal failure, interstitial nephritis

Contraindications Hypersensitivity to rofecoxib aspirin, other NSAIDs, or any component of their formulation; pregnancy (3rd trimester)

Warnings/Precautions Gastrointestinal irritation, ulceration, bleeding, and perforation may occur with NSAIDs (it is unclear whether rofecoxib is associated with rates of these events which are similar to nonselective NSAIDs). Use with caution in patients with a history of GI disease (bleeding or ulcers), decreased renal function, hepatic disease, CHF, hypertension, or asthma. Anaphylactoid reactions may occur, even with no prior exposure to rofecoxib.

Drug Interactions CYP2C8/9 enzyme substrate; may be a mild inducer of CYP3A4 (CYP3A3/4); may be a mild CYP1A2 inhibitor (per manufacturer)

ACE inhibitors: Antihypertensive effects may be reduced by rofecoxib.
Aspirin: Rofecoxib may be used with low-dose aspirin, however, rates of GI bleeding may be increased with coadministration.
Cimetidine increases AUC of rofecoxib by 23%.
Diuretics: Thiazide diuretics, loop diuretics: Effects may be diminished by rofecoxib.
Lithium: Serum concentrations/toxicity may be increased by rofecoxib; monitor.
Methotrexate: Severe bone marrow suppression, aplastic anemia, and GI toxicity have been reported with concomitant NSAID therapy. Selective COX-2 inhibitors appear to have a lower risk of this toxicity, however, caution is warranted.
Rifampin reduces the serum concentration of rofecoxib by ~50%.
Theophylline: Serum concentrations may be increased during therapy with rofecoxib; monitor.
Warfarin: Rofecoxib may increase the INR in patients receiving warfarin and may increase the risk of bleeding complications. However, rofecoxib does not appear to inhibit platelet aggregation.

Dietary/Ethanol/Herb Considerations

Ethanol: Avoid use; may increase gastric mucosal irritation.
Food: May be taken with food; time to peak concentrations are delayed when taken with a high-fat meal, but peak concentration and AUC are unchanged.

Drug Uptake

Onset of action: 45 minutes
Duration: Up to >24 hours
Half-life, elimination: 17 hours
Time to peak: 2-3 hours

Pregnancy Risk Factor C/D (3rd trimester)

Breast-feeding Considerations Not recommended

Dosage Forms SUSP, oral: 12.5 mg/5 mL; 25 mg/5 mL. **TAB:** 12.5 mg, 25 mg, 50 mg

Generic Available No

(Continued)

Rofecoxib *(Continued)*

Comments Recent news reports have noted an association between selective COX-2 inhibitors and increased cardiovascular risk. This was prompted by publication of a meta-analysis entitled "Risk of Cardiovascular Events Associated With Selective COX-2 Inhibitors" in the August 22, 2001, edition of the Journal of the American Medical Association (JAMA), viewable at http://jama.ama-assn.org/issues/v286n8/rfull/jsc10193.html. The researchers reanalyzed four previously published trials, assessing cardiovascular events in patients receiving either celecoxib or rofecoxib. They found an association between the use of COX-2 inhibitors and cardiovascular events (including myocardial infarction and ischemic stroke). The annualized myocardial infarction rate was found to be significantly higher in patients receiving celecoxib or rofecoxib than in the control (placebo) group from a recent meta-analysis of primary prevention trials. Although cause and effect cannot be established (these trials were originally designed to assess GI effects, not cardiovascular ones), the authors believe the available data raise a cautionary flag concerning the risk of cardiovascular events with the use of COX-2 inhibitors. The manufacturers of these agents dispute the methods and validity of the study's conclusions.

New Indications, Warnings Added to Vioxx® Labeling - April 11, 2002: The Food and Drug Administration (FDA) has approved new labeling which extends its approved indications to the symptomatic management of rheumatoid arthritis in adults and emphasizes differences in the adverse event profile as compared to nonselective NSAIDs. A reduction in GI adverse events relative to a nonselective NSAID (naproxen) is noted. Precautions concerning the use in cardiovascular disease (including ischemic disease) have also been added. The potential development of edema and hypertension with rofecoxib, particularly at high dosages (50 mg/day), is emphasized. Prescribers are reminded that rofecoxib does not possess antiplatelet activity, which may influence risk of ischemic events (as compared to nonselective NSAIDs). Data concerning ischemic cardiovascular events, including myocardial infarction, are presented but it is noted that prospective studies to evaluate cardiovascular risk have not been conducted.

Selected Readings

Bombardier C, Laine L, Reicin A, et al, "Comparison of Upper Gastrointestinal Toxicity of Rofecoxib and Naproxen in Patients With Rheumatoid Arthritis. VIGOR Study Group," *N Engl J Med*, 2000, 343(21):1520-8.

Change DJ, Fricke JR, Bird SR, et al, "Rofecoxib Versus Codeine/Acetaminophen in Postoperative Dental Pain: A Double-Blind, Randomized, Placebo- and Active Comparator-Controlled Clinical Trial," *Clin Ther*, 2001, 23(9):1446-55.

Ehrich EW, Dallob A, De Lepeleire I, et al, "Characterization of Rofecoxib as a Cyclo-oxygenase-2 Isoform Inhibitor and Demonstration of Analgesia in the Dental Pain Model," *Clin Pharmacol Ther*, 1999, 65(3):336-47.

Greenberg HE, Gottesdiener K, Huntington M, et al, "A New Cyclo-oxygenase-2 Inhibitor, Rofecoxib (Vioxx®), Did Not Alter the Antiplatelet Effects of Low-Dose Aspirin in Healthy Volunteers," *J Clin Pharmacol*, 2000, 40(12 Pt 2):1509-15.

Hawkey CJ, Jackson L, Harper SE, et al, "Review Article: The Gastrointestinal Safety Profile of Rofecoxib, a Highly Selective Inhibitor of Cyclo-oxygenase-2 in Humans," *Aliment Pharmacol Ther*, 2001, 15(1):1-9.

Malmstrom K, Daniels S, Kotey P, et al, "Comparison of Rofecoxib and Celecoxib, two Cyclooxygenase-2 Inhibitors, in Postoperative Dental Pain: A Randomized Placebo- and Active-Comparator-Controlled Clinical Trial," *Clin Ther*, 1999, 21(10):1653-63.

Moore PA and Hersh EV, "Celecoxib and Rofecoxib. The Role of COX-2 Inhibitors in Dental Practice," *J Am Dent Assoc*, 2001, 132(4):451-6.

Morrison BW, Christensen S, Yuan W, et al, "Analgesic Efficacy of the Cyclo-oxygenase-2-Specific Inhibitor Rofecoxib in Postdental Surgery Pain: A Randomized, Controlled Trial," *Clin Ther*, 1999, 21(6):943-53.

Mullican WS and Lacy JR, "Tramadol/Acetaminophen Combination Tablets and Codeine/Acetaminophen Combination Capsules for the Management of Chronic Pain: A Comparative Trial," *Clin Ther*, 2001, 23(9):1429-45.

Wynn RL, "The New COX-2 Inhibitors: Rofecoxib (Vioxx®) and Celecoxib (Celebrex™)," *Gen Dent*, 2000, 48(1):16-20.

Wynn RL, "NSAIDS and Cardiovascular Effects, Celecoxib for Dental Pain, and a New Analgesic - Tramadol with Acetaminophen," *Gen Dent*, 2002, 50(3):218-222.

Roferon-A® *see* Interferon Alfa-2a *on page 641*

Rogaine® Extra Strength for Men [OTC] *see* Minoxidil *on page 818*

Rogaine® for Men [OTC] *see* Minoxidil *on page 818*

Rogaine® for Women [OTC] *see* Minoxidil *on page 818*

Rolaids® Calcium Rich [OTC] *see* Calcium Carbonate *on page 201*

Rolatuss® Plain *see* Chlorpheniramine and Phenylephrine *on page 269*

Romazicon™ *see* Flumazenil *on page 511*

Romycin® *see* Erythromycin, Topical *on page 454*

Rondec®-DM Drops *see* Carbinoxamine, Pseudoephedrine, and Dextromethorphan *on page 221*

Rondec® Drops *see* Carbinoxamine and Pseudoephedrine *on page 221*

Rondec® Syrup *see* Brompheniramine and Pseudoephedrine *on page 180*

Rondec® Tablets *see* Carbinoxamine and Pseudoephedrine *on page 221*

Rondec-TR® *see* Carbinoxamine and Pseudoephedrine *on page 221*

Ropinirole (roe PIN i role)

U.S. Brand Names Requip®

Canadian Brand Names ReQuip™

Pharmacologic Category Anti-Parkinson's Agent, Dopamine Agonist

Synonyms Ropinirole Hydrochloride

Use Treatment of idiopathic Parkinson's disease; in patients with early Parkinson's disease who were not receiving concomitant levodopa therapy as well as in patients with advanced disease on concomitant levodopa

Local Anesthetic/Vasoconstrictor Precautions No information available to require special precautions

Effects on Dental Treatment ≤2%: Increased salivation, xerostomia

Dosage Adults: Oral: Dosage should be increased to achieve a maximum therapeutic effect, balanced against the principal side effects of nausea, dizziness, somnolence, and dyskinesia

Recommended starting dose: 0.25 mg 3 times/day; based on individual patient response, the dosage should be titrated with weekly increments

Week 1: 0.25 mg 3 times/day; total daily dose: 0.75 mg

Week 2: 0.5 mg 3 times/day; total daily dose: 1.5 mg

Week 3: 0.75 mg 3 times/day; total daily dose: 2.25 mg

Week 4: 1 mg 3 times/day; total daily dose: 3 mg

After week 4, if necessary, daily dosage may be increased by 1.5 mg/day on a weekly basis up to a dose of 9 mg/day, and then by up to 3 mg/day weekly to a total of 24 mg/day

Mechanism of Action Has a high relative *in vitro* specificity and full intrinsic activity at the D_2 and D_3 dopamine receptor subtypes, binding with higher affinity to D_3 than to D_2 or D_4 receptor subtypes; relevance of D_3 receptor binding in Parkinson's disease is unknown. Ropinirole has moderate *in vitro* affinity for opioid receptors. Ropinirole and its metabolites have negligible *in vitro* affinity for dopamine D_1, 5-HT_1, 5-HT_2, benzodiazepine, GABA, muscarinic, alpha$_1$-, alpha$_2$-, and beta-adrenoreceptors. Although precise mechanism of action of ropinirole is unknown, it is believed to be due to stimulation of postsynaptic dopamine D_2-type receptors within the caudate-putamen in the brain. Ropinirole caused decreases in systolic and diastolic BP at doses above 0.25 mg. The mechanism of ropinirole-induced postural hypotension is believed to be due to D_2-mediated blunting of the noradrenergic response to standing and subsequent decrease in peripheral vascular resistance.

Other Adverse Effects

Early Parkinson's disease (without levodopa):

>10%:

Cardiovascular: Syncope (12%)

Central nervous system: Dizziness (40%), somnolence (40%), fatigue (11%)

Gastrointestinal: Nausea (60%), vomiting (12%)

Miscellaneous: Viral infection (11%)

1% to 10%:

Cardiovascular: Dependent/leg edema (6% to 7%), orthostasis (6%), hypertension (5%), chest pain (4%), flushing (3%), palpitations (3%), peripheral ischemia (3%), hypotension (2%), tachycardia (2%),

Central nervous system: Pain (8%), confusion (5%), hallucinations (5%, dose related), hypoesthesia (4%), amnesia (3%), malaise (3%), vertigo (2%), yawning (3%)

Gastrointestinal: Constipation (>5%), dyspepsia (10%), abdominal pain (6%), xerostomia (5%), anorexia (4%), flatulence (3%)

Genitourinary: Urinary tract infection (5%), impotence (3%)

Hepatic: Elevated alkaline phosphatase (3%)

Neuromuscular & skeletal: Weakness (6%)

Ocular: Abnormal vision (6%), xerophthalmia (2%)

Respiratory: Pharyngitis (6%), rhinitis (4%), sinusitis (4%), dyspnea (3%)

Miscellaneous: Diaphoresis (increased) (6%)

Advanced Parkinson's disease (with levodopa):

>10%:

Central nervous system: Dizziness (26%), somnolence (20%), headache (17%)

Gastrointestinal: Nausea (30%)

Neuromuscular & skeletal: Dyskinesias (34%)

1% to 10%:

Cardiovascular: Syncope (3%), hypotension (2%)

Central nervous system: Hallucinations (10%, dose related), aggravated parkinsonism, confusion (9%), pain (5%), paresis (3%), amnesia (5%), anxiety (6%), abnormal dreaming (3%), insomnia

Gastrointestinal: Abdominal pain (9%), vomiting (7%), constipation (6%), diarrhea (5%), dysphagia (2%), flatulence (2%), increased salivation (2%), xerostomia, weight loss (2%)

Genitourinary: Urinary tract infections

Hematologic: Anemia (2%)

Neuromuscular & skeletal: Falls (10%), arthralgia (7%), tremor (6%), hypokinesia (5%), paresthesia (5%), arthritis (3%)

(Continued)

Ropinirole *(Continued)*

Respiratory: Upper respiratory tract infection (9%), dyspnea (3%)
Miscellaneous: Injury, increased diaphoresis (7%), viral infection, increased drug level (7%)

Other adverse effects (all phase 2/3 trials):
1% to 10%:
Central nervous system: Neuralgia (>1%)
Renal: Elevated BUN (>1%)

Drug Interactions CYP1A2 enzyme substrate

Increased Effect/Toxicity: Inhibitors of CYP1A2 inhibitors may increase serum concentration of ropinirole; inhibitors include cimetidine, ciprofloxacin, erythromycin, fluvoxamine, isoniazid, ritonavir, and zileuton. Estrogens may also reduce the metabolism of ropinirole; dosage adjustments may be needed.

Decreased Effect: Antipsychotics, enzyme inducers (barbiturates, carbamazepine, phenytoin, rifampin, rifabutin), cigarette smoking, and metoclopramide may reduce the effect or serum concentration of ropinirole.

Drug Uptake
Half-life, elimination: ~6 hours
Time to peak: ~1-2 hours; T_{max} increased by 2.5 hours when drug taken with a meal

Pregnancy Risk Factor C

Generic Available No

Ropivacaine (roe PIV a kane)

Related Information
Oral Pain *on page 1360*

U.S. Brand Names Naropin®

Canadian Brand Names Naropin®

Mexican Brand Names Naropin®

Pharmacologic Category Local Anesthetic

Synonyms Ropivacaine Hydrochloride

Use Local anesthetic (injectable) for use in surgery, postoperative pain management, and obstetrical procedures when local or regional anesthesia is needed. It can be administered via local infiltration, epidural block and epidural infusion, or intermittent bolus.

Local Anesthetic/Vasoconstrictor Precautions No information available to require special precautions

Effects on Dental Treatment No effects or complications reported

Dosage Dose varies with procedure, onset and depth of anesthesia desired, vascularity of tissues, duration of anesthesia, and condition of patient: Adults:

Surgical anesthesia:
- Lumbar epidural: 15-30 mL of 0.5% to 1% solution
- Lumbar epidural block for cesarean section:
  - 20-30 mL dose of 0.5% solution
  - 15-20 mL dose of 0.75% solution
- Thoracic epidural block: 5-15 mL dose of 0.5% to 0.75% solution
- Major nerve block:
  - 35-50 mL dose of 0.5% solution (175-250 mg)
  - 10-40 mL dose of 0.75% solution (75-300 mg)
- Field block: 1-40 mL dose of 0.5% solution (5-200 mg)

Labor pain management: Lumbar epidural: Initial: 10-20 mL 0.2% solution; continuous infusion dose: 6-14 mL/hour of 0.2% solution with incremental injections of 10-15 mL/hour of 0.2% solution

Postoperative pain management:
- Lumbar or thoracic epidural: Continuous infusion dose: 6-14 mL/hour of 0.2% solution
- Infiltration/minor nerve block:
  - 1-100 mL dose of 0.2% solution
  - 1-40 mL dose of 0.5% solution

Mechanism of Action Local anesthetics bind selectively to the intracellular surface of sodium channels to block influx of sodium into the axon. As a result, depolarization necessary for action potential propagation and subsequent nerve function is prevented. The block at the sodium channel is reversible. Local anesthetics reversibly prevent generation and conduction of electrical impulses in neurons by decreasing the transient increase in permeability to sodium. The differential sensitivity generally depends on the size of the fiber; small fibers are more sensitive than larger fibers and require a longer period for recovery. Sensory pain fibers are usually blocked first, followed by fibers that transmit sensations of temperature, touch, and deep pressure. High concentrations block sympathetic somatic sensory and somatic motor fibers. The spread of anesthesia depends upon the distribution of the solution. This is primarily dependent on the site of administration and volume of drug injected. When drug diffuses away from the axon, sodium channel function is restored and nerve propagation returns.

Other Adverse Effects

>10% (dose and route related):

Cardiovascular: Hypotension, bradycardia
Gastrointestinal: Nausea, vomiting
Neuromuscular & skeletal: Back pain
Miscellaneous: Shivering

1% to 10% (dose related):

Cardiovascular: Hypertension, tachycardia
Central nervous system: Headache, dizziness, anxiety, lightheadedness
Neuromuscular & skeletal: Hypoesthesia, paresthesia, circumoral paresthesia
Otic: Tinnitus
Respiratory: Apnea

Drug Interactions CYP2D6 enzyme substrate

Increased Effect/Toxicity: Other local anesthetics or agents structurally related to the amide-type anesthetics; increased toxicity possible (but not yet reported) with drugs that decrease cytochrome P450 1A enzyme function.

Drug Uptake

Onset of action: Anesthesia (route-dependent): 3-15 minutes
Duration (dose- and route-dependent): 3-15 hours
Half-life, elimination: Epidural: 5-7 hours; I.V.: 2.4 hours

Pregnancy Risk Factor B

Generic Available No

Comments Not available with vasoconstrictor (epinephrine) and not available in dental (1.8 mL) carpules

Rosiglitazone (roh si GLI ta zone)

U.S. Brand Names Avandia®

Canadian Brand Names Avandia®

Pharmacologic Category Antidiabetic Agent, Thiazolidinedione

Use Type 2 diabetes

Monotherapy: Improve glycemic control as an adjunct to diet and exercise

Combination therapy: In combination with metformin when diet, exercise and metformin alone or diet, exercise and rosiglitazone alone do not result in adequate glycemic control.

Local Anesthetic/Vasoconstrictor Precautions No information available to require special precautions

Effects on Dental Treatment Rosiglitazone-dependent diabetics should be appointed for dental treatment in morning in order to minimize chance of stress-induced hypoglycemia.

Dosage Adults: Oral: Initial: 4 mg/day as a single daily dose or in divided doses twice daily. If response is inadequate after 12 weeks of treatment, the dosage may be increased to 8 mg/day as a single daily dose or in divided doses twice daily.

Mechanism of Action Thiazolidinedione antidiabetic agent that lowers blood glucose by improving target cell response to insulin, without increasing pancreatic insulin secretion. It has a mechanism of action that is dependent on the presence of insulin for activity.

Other Adverse Effects Rare cases of hepatocellular injury have been reported in men in their 60s within 2-3 weeks after initiation of rosiglitazone therapy. LFTs in these patients revealed severe hepatocellular injury which responded with rapid improvement of liver function and resolution of symptoms upon discontinuation of rosiglitazone. Patients were also receiving other potentially hepatotoxic medications (*Ann Intern Med*, 2000, 132:121-4; 132:164-6).

>10%: Endocrine & metabolic: Weight gain, increase in total cholesterol, increased LDL cholesterol, increased HDL cholesterol

1% to 10%:

Cardiovascular: Edema (5%)
Central nervous system: Headache (6%), fatigue (4%)
Endocrine & metabolic: Hyperglycemia (4%), hypoglycemia (1% to 2%)
Gastrointestinal: Diarrhea (2%)
Hematologic: Anemia (2%)
Neuromuscular & skeletal: Back pain (4%)
Respiratory: Upper respiratory tract infection (10%), sinusitis (3%)
Miscellaneous: Injury (8%)

Warnings/Precautions Should not be used in diabetic ketoacidosis. Mechanism requires the presence of insulin, therefore use in type 1 diabetes is not recommended. Use with caution in premenopausal, anovulatory women; may result in resumption of ovulation, increasing the risk of pregnancy. May result in hormonal imbalance; development of menstrual irregularities should prompt reconsideration of therapy. Use with caution in patients with anemia or depressed leukocyte counts (may reduce hemoglobin, hematocrit, and/or WBC). Use with caution in patients with heart failure or edema; may increase in plasma volume and/or increase cardiac hypertrophy. In general, use should be avoided in patients with NYHA class III or IV heart failure. Use with caution in patients with elevated transaminases (AST

(Continued)

Rosiglitazone *(Continued)*

or ALT). Idiosyncratic hepatotoxicity has been reported with another thiazolidinedione agent (troglitazone). Monitoring should include periodic determinations of liver function.

Drug Interactions CYP2C8 enzyme substrate; minor metabolism by CYP2C9

When rosiglitazone was coadministered with glyburide, metformin, digoxin, warfarin, or ranitidine, no significant pharmacokinetic alterations were observed.

Drug Uptake

Onset of action: Delayed; Maximum effect: Therapeutic: ≤12 weeks

Half-life, elimination: 3.15-3.59 hours

Time to peak: 1 hour

Pregnancy Risk Factor C

Generic Available No

Rowasa® *see* Mesalamine *on page 772*

Roxanol® *see* Morphine Sulfate *on page 829*

Roxanol 100® *see* Morphine Sulfate *on page 829*

Roxanol®-T *see* Morphine Sulfate *on page 829*

Roxicet® *see* Oxycodone and Acetaminophen *on page 903*

Roxicet® 5/500 *see* Oxycodone and Acetaminophen *on page 903*

Roxicodone™ *see* Oxycodone *on page 901*

Roxicodone™ Intensol™ *see* Oxycodone *on page 901*

Roxilox® *see* Oxycodone and Acetaminophen *on page 903*

R-Tannamine® *see* Chlorpheniramine, Pyrilamine, and Phenylephrine *on page 273*

R-Tannate® *see* Chlorpheniramine, Pyrilamine, and Phenylephrine *on page 273*

Rubella Virus Vaccine, Live (rue BEL a VYE rus vak SEEN, live)

U.S. Brand Names Meruvax® II

Pharmacologic Category Vaccine

Synonyms German Measles Vaccine

Use Selective active immunization against rubella; vaccination is routinely recommended for persons from 12 months of age to puberty. All adults, both male and female, lacking documentation of live vaccine on or after first birthday, or laboratory evidence of immunity (particularly women of childbearing age and young adults who work in or congregate in hospitals, colleges, and on military bases) should be vaccinated. Susceptible travelers should be vaccinated.

Note: Trivalent measles - mumps - rubella (MMR) vaccine is the preferred immunizing agent for most children and many adults.

Local Anesthetic/Vasoconstrictor Precautions No information available to require special precautions

Effects on Dental Treatment No effects or complications reported

Dosage Children ≥12 months and Adults: S.C.: 0.5 mL in outer aspect of upper arm; children vaccinated before 12 months of age should be revaccinated. Recommended age for primary immunization is 12-15 months; revaccination with MMR-II is recommended prior to elementary school.

Mechanism of Action A live attenuated vaccine that contains the Wistar Institute RA 27/3 strain, which is adapted to and propagated in human diploid cell culture; promotes active immunity by inducing rubella hemagglutination-inhibiting antibodies; it is the only strain of rubella vaccine marketed in the U.S. Antibody titers after immunization last 6 years without significant decline; 90% of those vaccinated have protection for at least 15 years.

Other Adverse Effects All serious adverse reactions must be reported to the U.S. Department of Health and Human Services (DHHS) Vaccine Adverse Event Reporting System (VAERS) 1-800-822-7967.

Frequency not defined:

Cardiovascular: Syncope, vasculitis

Central nervous system: Dizziness, encephalitis, fever, Guillain-Barré syndrome, headache, irritability, malaise, polyneuritis, polyneuropathy

Dermatologic: Angioneurotic edema, erythema multiforme, purpura, rash, Stevens-Johnson syndrome, urticaria

Gastrointestinal: Diarrhea, nausea, sore throat, vomiting

Hematologic: Leukocytosis, thrombocytopenia

Local: Injection site reactions which include burning, induration, pain, redness, stinging, wheal and flare

Neuromuscular & skeletal: Arthralgia/arthritis (variable; highest rates in women, 12% to 26% versus children, up to 3%), myalgia, paresthesia

Ocular: Conjunctivitis, optic neuritis, papillitis, retrobulbar neuritis

Otic: Nerve deafness, otitis media

Respiratory: Bronchial spasm, cough, rhinitis

Miscellaneous: Anaphylactoid reactions, anaphylaxis, regional lymphadenopathy

Drug Interactions

Corticosteroids: In patients receiving high doses of systemic corticosteroids for ≥14 days, wait at least 1 month between discontinuing steroid therapy and administering immunization.

DTaP: Vaccines may be administered together (using separate sites and syringes).

Haemophilus b conjugate vaccine (PedvaxHIB®): Vaccines may be administered together (using separate sites and syringes).

Hepatitis B vaccine: Vaccines may be administered together (using separate sites and syringes).

Immune globulin, whole blood, plasma: Do not administer together; immune response may be compromised. Defer vaccine administration for ≥3 months.

Immunosuppressant medications: The effect of the vaccine may be decreased, increasing the risk of rubella disease in individuals who are receiving immunosuppressant drugs.

Live vaccines: Unless otherwise specified, rubella vaccine should be given 1 month before or 1 month after other live viral vaccines.

OPV: Vaccines may be administered together.

Varicella: Vaccines may be administered together (using separate sites and syringes); if vaccines are not administered simultaneously, doses should be separated by at least 30 days.

Drug Uptake

Onset of action: Antibodies to vaccine: 2-4 weeks

Duration: Protection against both clinical rubella and asymptomatic viremia is probably life-long. Vaccine-induced antibody levels have been shown to persist for at least 10 years without substantial decline. If the present pattern continues, it will provide a basis for the expectation that immunity following vaccination will be permanent. However, continued surveillance will be required to demonstrate this point.

Pregnancy Risk Factor C

Generic Available No

Comments Federal law requires that the date of administration, the vaccine manufacturer, lot number of vaccine, and the administering person's name, title and address be entered into the patient's permanent record

Rubex® *see* DOXOrubicin *on page 416*

Rum-K® *see* Potassium Chloride *on page 977*

Ru-Tuss® *see* Chlorpheniramine and Phenylephrine *on page 269*

Ru-Tuss® DE *see* Guaifenesin and Pseudoephedrine *on page 570*

Ru-Tuss® Expectorant [OTC] *see* Guaifenesin, Pseudoephedrine, and Dextromethorphan *on page 571*

Rymed® *see* Guaifenesin and Pseudoephedrine *on page 570*

Ryna® [OTC] *see* Chlorpheniramine and Pseudoephedrine *on page 270*

Ryna-C® *see* Chlorpheniramine, Pseudoephedrine, and Codeine *on page 273*

Ryna-CX® *see* Guaifenesin, Pseudoephedrine, and Codeine *on page 570*

Rynatan® Pediatric Suspension *see* Chlorpheniramine, Pyrilamine, and Phenylephrine *on page 273*

Rynatan® Tablet *see* Azatadine and Pseudoephedrine *on page 135*

Rynatuss® [OTC] *see* Chlorpheniramine, Ephedrine, Phenylephrine, and Carbetapentane *on page 270*

Rynatuss® Pediatric Suspension [OTC] *see* Chlorpheniramine, Ephedrine, Phenylephrine, and Carbetapentane *on page 270*

Rythmol® *see* Propafenone *on page 1009*

S-2® *see* Epinephrine, Racemic *on page 440*

Sacrosidase (sak RO se dase)

U.S. Brand Names Sucraid®

Canadian Brand Names Sucraid®

Pharmacologic Category Enzyme, Gastrointestinal

Use Orphan drug: Oral replacement therapy in sucrase deficiency, as seen in congenital sucrase-isomaltase deficiency (CSID)

Local Anesthetic/Vasoconstrictor Precautions No information available to require special precautions

Effects on Dental Treatment No effects or complications reported

Dosage Oral:

Infants ≥5 months and Children <15 kg: 8500 int. units (1 mL) per meal or snack

Children >15 kg and Adults: 17,000 int. units (2 mL) per meal or snack

Doses should be diluted with 2-4 oz of water, milk, or formula with each meal or snack. Approximately one-half of the dose may be taken before, and the remainder of a dose taken at the completion of each meal or snack.

Mechanism of Action A naturally occurring GI enzyme which breaks down the disaccharide sucrose to its monosaccharide components; hydrolysis is necessary to allow absorption of these nutrients.

Other Adverse Effects 1% to 10%:

Central nervous system: Insomnia, headache, nervousness

(Continued)

Sacrosidase *(Continued)*

Gastrointestinal: Abdominal pain, vomiting, nausea, diarrhea, constipation
Endocrine and metabolic: Dehydration
Respiratory: Bronchospasm
Miscellaneous: Hypersensitivity reaction

Contraindications Hypersensitivity to yeast, yeast products, or glycerin

Warnings/Precautions Hypersensitivity reactions to sacrosidase, including bronchospasm, have been reported. Administer initial doses in a setting where acute hypersensitivity reactions may be treated within a few minutes. Skin testing for hypersensitivity may be performed prior to administration to identify patients at risk.

Drug Interactions Drug interactions have not been evaluated.

Drug Uptake Absorption: Amino acids

Pregnancy Risk Factor C

Generic Available No

Comments Oral solution contains 50% glycerol

Safe Tussin® 30 [OTC] *see* Guaifenesin and Dextromethorphan *on page 569*
Saizen® *see* Human Growth Hormone *on page 589*
Sal-Acid® Plaster [OTC] *see* Salicylic Acid *on page 1072*
Salactic® Film [OTC] *see* Salicylic Acid *on page 1072*
Salagen® *see* Pilocarpine *on page 955*
Salagen® *see* Pilocarpine (Dental) *on page 956*
Salflex® *see* Salsalate *on page 1074*

Salicylic Acid (sal i SIL ik AS id)

U.S. Brand Names Compound W® [OTC]; Dr Scholl's® Disk [OTC]; Dr Scholl's® Wart Remover [OTC]; DuoFilm® [OTC]; DuoPlant® [OTC]; Freezone® [OTC]; Gordofilm® [OTC]; Mediplast® Plaster [OTC]; Mosco® [OTC]; Occlusal®-HP [OTC]; Off-Ezy® Wart Remover [OTC]; Panscol® [OTC]; Psor-a-set® Soap [OTC]; Sal-Acid® Plaster [OTC]; Salactic® Film [OTC]; Sal-Plant® [OTC]; Trans-Ver-Sal® AdultPatch [OTC]; Trans-Ver-Sal® PediaPatch [OTC]; Trans-Ver-Sal® PlantarPatch [OTC]; Wart-Off® [OTC]

Canadian Brand Names Duofilm®; Duoforte® 27; Keralyt®; Occlusal™; Occlusal™-HP; Sebcur®; Soluver®; Soluver® Plus; Trans-Plantar®; Trans-Ver-Sal®

Mexican Brand Names DuoPlant®; Ionil®; Ionil Plus®; Trans-Ver-Sal®

Pharmacologic Category Keratolytic Agent

Use Topically for its keratolytic effect in controlling seborrheic dermatitis or psoriasis of body and scalp, dandruff, and other scaling dermatoses; also used to remove warts, corns, and calluses

Local Anesthetic/Vasoconstrictor Precautions No information available to require special precautions

Effects on Dental Treatment No effects or complications reported

Dosage

Lotion, cream, gel: Apply a thin layer to affected area once or twice daily
Plaster: Cut to size that covers the corn or callus, apply and leave in place for 48 hours; do not exceed 5 applications over a 14-day period
Solution: Apply a thin layer directly to wart using brush applicator once daily as directed for 1 week or until wart is removed

Mechanism of Action Produces desquamation of hyperkeratotic epithelium via dissolution of the intercellular cement which causes the cornified tissue to swell, soften, macerate, and desquamate. Salicylic acid is keratolytic at concentrations of 3% to 6%; it becomes destructive to tissue at concentrations >6%. Concentrations of 6% to 60% are used to remove corns and warts and in the treatment of psoriasis and other hyperkeratotic disorders.

Other Adverse Effects

>10%: Local: Burning and irritation at site of exposure on normal tissue
1% to 10%:
Central nervous system: Dizziness, mental confusion, headache
Otic: Tinnitus
Respiratory: Hyperventilation

Drug Uptake

Absorption: Percutaneous; systemic toxicity unlikely with normal use
Time to peak: Within 5 hours of application with occlusion

Pregnancy Risk Factor C

Generic Available Yes

Salicylic Acid and Propylene Glycol

(sal i SIL ik AS id & PROE pi leen GLYE cole)

U.S. Brand Names Keralyt® Gel [OTC]

Canadian Brand Names Keralyt®

Pharmacologic Category Keratolytic Agent

Synonyms Propylene Glycol and Salicylic Acid

Use Removal of excessive keratin in hyperkeratotic skin disorders, including various ichthyosis, keratosis palmaris and plantaris and psoriasis; may be used to remove excessive keratin in dorsal and plantar hyperkeratotic lesions

Local Anesthetic/Vasoconstrictor Precautions No information available to require special precautions

Effects on Dental Treatment No effects or complications reported

Dosage Apply to area at night after soaking region for at least 5 minutes to hydrate area, and place under occlusion; medication is washed off in morning

Pregnancy Risk Factor C

Generic Available No

SalineX® [OTC] *see* Sodium Chloride *on page 1094*

Salivart® [OTC] *see* Saliva Substitute *on page 1073*

Saliva Substitute (sa LYE va SUB stee tute)

Related Information

Management of Patients Undergoing Cancer Therapy *on page 1402*

U.S. Brand Names Entertainer's Secret® [OTC]; Moi-Stir® [OTC]; Mouthkote® [OTC]; Optimoist® [OTC]; Salivart® [OTC]; Salix® Lozenge [OTC]

Pharmacologic Category Gastrointestinal Agent, Miscellaneous

Use Relief of xerostomia and throat in xerostomia

Local Anesthetic/Vasoconstrictor Precautions No information available to require special precautions

Effects on Dental Treatment No effects or complications reported

Dosage Use as needed

Generic Available Yes

Salix® Lozenge [OTC] *see* Saliva Substitute *on page 1073*

Salmeterol (sal ME te role)

Related Information

Respiratory Diseases *on page 1328*

U.S. Brand Names Serevent®; Serevent® Diskus®

Canadian Brand Names Serevent®

Mexican Brand Names Serevent®; Zamtirel

Pharmacologic Category $Beta_2$ Agonist

Synonyms Salmeterol Xinafoate

Use Inhalation:

Aerosol: Maintenance treatment of asthma and in prevention of bronchospasm in patients >12 years of age with reversible obstructive airway disease, including patients with symptoms of nocturnal asthma, who require regular treatment with inhaled, short-acting $beta_2$ agonists; prevention of exercise-induced bronchospasm; treatment of COPD-induced bronchospasm

Powder: Maintenance treatment of asthma and in prevention of bronchospasm in patients ≥4 years of age with reversible obstructive airway disease, including patients with symptoms of nocturnal asthma, who require regular treatment with inhaled, short-acting $beta_2$ agonists; prevention of exercise-induced bronchospasm

Local Anesthetic/Vasoconstrictor Precautions No information available to require special precautions

Effects on Dental Treatment No effects or complications reported

Dosage Do **NOT** use spacer with inhalation powder.

Asthma, maintenance and prevention:

Inhalation, aerosol: Children ≥12 years and Adults: 42 mcg (2 puffs) twice daily (12 hours apart)

Inhalation, powder (Serevent® Diskus®): Children ≥4 years and Adults: One inhalation (50 mcg) twice daily

Exercise-induced asthma, prevention:

Inhalation, aerosol: Children ≥12 years and Adults: 42 mcg (2 puffs) 30-60 minutes prior to exercise; additional doses should not be used for 12 hours

Inhalation, powder (Serevent® Diskus®): Children ≥4 years and Adults: One inhalation (50 mcg) at least 30 minutes prior to exercise; additional doses should not be used for 12 hours

COPD (maintenance treatment of associated bronchospasm):

Inhalation, aerosol: Adults: 42 micrograms (2 puffs) twice daily (morning and evening - 12 hours apart)

Mechanism of Action Relaxes bronchial smooth muscle by selective action on $beta_2$-receptors with little effect on heart rate; because salmeterol acts locally in the lung, therapeutic effect is not predicted by plasma concentrations

Other Adverse Effects

>10%:

Central nervous system: Headache

Respiratory: Pharyngitis

(Continued)

Salmeterol *(Continued)*

1% to 10%:

Cardiovascular: Tachycardia, palpitations, elevation or depression of BP, cardiac arrhythmias

Central nervous system: Nervousness, CNS stimulation, hyperactivity, insomnia, malaise, dizziness

Gastrointestinal: GI upset, diarrhea, nausea

Neuromuscular & skeletal: Tremors (may be more common in the elderly), myalgias, back pain, arthralgia

Respiratory: Upper respiratory infection, cough, bronchitis

Drug Interactions CYP3A3/4 enzyme substrate

Increased Toxicity (cardiovascular): MAO inhibitors, tricyclic antidepressants

Increased Effect: Inhaled corticosteroids: The addition of salmeterol has been demonstrated to improve response to inhaled corticosteroids (as compared to increasing steroid dosage).

Decreased Effect: Beta-adrenergic blockers (eg, propranolol)

Drug Uptake

Onset of action: 5-20 minutes (average 10 minutes); Peak effect: 2-4 hours

Duration: 12 hours

Half-life, elimination: 3-4 hours

Pregnancy Risk Factor C

Generic Available No

Sal-Plant® [OTC] *see* Salicylic Acid *on page 1072*

Salsalate (SAL sa late)

Related Information

Rheumatoid Arthritis and Osteoarthritis *on page 1340*

Temporomandibular Dysfunction (TMD) *on page 1397*

U.S. Brand Names Amigesic®; Argesic®-SA; Disalcid®; Mono-Gesic®; Salflex®

Canadian Brand Names Amigesic®; Disalcid™; Salflex®

Pharmacologic Category Salicylate

Synonyms Disalicylic Acid; Salicylsalicylic Acid

Use Treatment of minor pain or fever; arthritis

Local Anesthetic/Vasoconstrictor Precautions No information available to require special precautions

Effects on Dental Treatment NSAID formulations are known to reversibly decrease platelet aggregation via mechanisms different than observed with aspirin. The dentist should be aware of the potential of abnormal coagulation. Caution should also be exercised in the use of NSAIDs in patients already on anticoagulant therapy with drugs such as warfarin (Coumadin®).

Dosage Adults: Oral: 3 g/day in 2-3 divided doses

Mechanism of Action Inhibits prostaglandin synthesis, acts on the hypothalamus heat-regulating center to reduce fever, blocks prostaglandin synthetase action which prevents formation of the platelet-aggregating substance thromboxane A_2

Other Adverse Effects

>10%: Gastrointestinal: Nausea, heartburn, stomach pains, dyspepsia

1% to 10%:

Central nervous system: Fatigue

Dermatologic: Rash

Gastrointestinal: Gastrointestinal ulceration

Hematologic: Hemolytic anemia

Neuromuscular & skeletal: Weakness

Respiratory: Dyspnea

Miscellaneous: Anaphylactic shock

Warnings/Precautions Use with caution in patients with CHF, dehydration, hypertension, decreased renal or hepatic function, history of GI disease, active GI ulceration or bleeding, or those receiving anticoagulants. Withhold for at least 4-6 half-lives prior to surgical or dental procedures.

Drug Interactions

Increased Effect/Toxicity: Increased effect/toxicity of oral anticoagulants, hypoglycemics, and methotrexate.

Decreased Effect: Decreased effect of uricosurics and spironolactone. Decreased effect with urinary alkalinizers, antacids, and corticosteroids.

Drug Uptake

Onset of action: Therapeutic: 3-4 days of continuous dosing

Absorption: Oral: Completely from small intestine

Half-life, elimination: 7-8 hours

Pregnancy Risk Factor C/D (3rd trimester)

Generic Available Yes

Sal-Tropine™ *see* Atropine *on page 130*

Sal-Tropine™ *see* Atropine Sulfate Dental Tablets *on page 131*

Sandimmune® *see* CycloSPORINE *on page 337*

Sandoglobulin® *see* Immune Globulin, Intravenous *on page 630*

Sandostatin® *see* Octreotide Acetate *on page 881*
Sandostatin LAR® *see* Octreotide Acetate *on page 881*
Sani-Supp® [OTC] *see* Glycerin *on page 562*
Sanorex® *see* Mazindol *on page 746*
Sansert® *see* Methysergide *on page 799*
Santyl® *see* Collagenase *on page 322*

Saquinavir (sa KWIN a veer)

Related Information

HIV Infection and AIDS *on page 1334*

U.S. Brand Names Fortovase®; Invirase®

Canadian Brand Names Fortovase™; Invirase®

Mexican Brand Names Invirase®

Pharmacologic Category Antiretroviral Agent, Protease Inhibitor

Synonyms Saquinavir Mesylate

Use Treatment of advanced HIV infection, used in combination with older nucleoside analog medications

Local Anesthetic/Vasoconstrictor Precautions No information available to require special precautions

Effects on Dental Treatment No effects or complications reported

Dosage Adults: Oral: **Note:** Fortovase® and Invirase® are not bioequivalent and should not be used interchangeably; only Fortovase® should be used to initiate therapy:

Fortovase®: Six 200 mg capsules (1200 mg) 3 times/day within 2 hours after a meal in combination with a nucleoside analog

Invirase®: Three 200 mg capsules (600 mg) 3 times/day within 2 hours after a full meal in combination with a nucleoside analog

Dose of either Fortovase® or Invirase® in combination with ritonavir: 400 mg twice daily

Mechanism of Action As an inhibitor of HIV protease, saquinavir prevents the cleavage of viral polyprotein precursors which are needed to generate functional proteins in and maturation of HIV-infected cells

Other Adverse Effects Protease inhibitors cause dyslipidemia which includes elevated cholesterol and triglycerides and a redistribution of body fat centrally to cause "protease paunch", buffalo hump, facial atrophy, and breast enlargement. These agents also cause hyperglycemia.

1% to 10%:

- Dermatologic: Rash
- Endocrine & metabolic: Hyperglycemia
- Gastrointestinal: Diarrhea, abdominal discomfort, nausea, abdominal pain, buccal mucosa ulceration
- Neuromuscular & skeletal: Paresthesia, weakness, increased CPK

Drug Interactions CYP3A3/4 enzyme substrate; CYP3A3/4 enzyme inhibitor

Increased effect: Ketoconazole significantly increases plasma concentrations and AUC of saquinavir; as a known, although not potent inhibitor of the cytochrome P450 system, saquinavir may decrease the metabolism of terfenadine and astemizole, as well as cisapride and ergot derivatives (and result in rare but serious effects including cardiac arrhythmias); other drugs which may have increased adverse effects if coadministered with saquinavir include benzodiazepines (midazolam and triazolam), calcium channel blockers, clindamycin, dapsone, ergot alkaloids, and quinidine. Both clarithromycin and saquinavir levels/effects may be increased with coadministration. Delavirdine may increase concentration; ritonavir may increase AUC >17-fold; concurrent administration of nelfinavir results in increase in nelfinavir (18%) and saquinavir (mean: 392%). Saquinavir increased serum concentration of simvastatin, lovastatin, and atorvastatin; risk of myopathy/rhabdomyolysis may be increased. Use cautiously with HMG-CoA reductase inhibitors. Avoid use with simvastatin and lovastatin. Use caution with atorvastatin and cerivastatin (fluvastatin and pravastatin are not metabolized by CYP3A3/4). Sildenafil serum concentration are increased in concurrent therapy (limit sildenafil dosage to 25 mg).

Decreased Effect: Saquinavir may decrease delavirdine concentrations. Rifampin may decrease saquinavir's plasma concentrations and AUC by 40% to 80%; other enzyme inducers may induce saquinavir's metabolism (eg, phenobarbital, phenytoin, dexamethasone, carbamazepine)

Drug Uptake Absorption: Poor, increased with high fat meal; Fortovase® has improved absorption over Invirase®

Pregnancy Risk Factor B

Generic Available No

Sarafem™ *see* Fluoxetine *on page 517*

Sargramostim (sar GRAM oh stim)

U.S. Brand Names Leukine™

Canadian Brand Names Leukine™

(Continued)

Sargramostim *(Continued)*

Mexican Brand Names Leucomax®

Pharmacologic Category Colony Stimulating Factor

Synonyms GM-CSF; Granulocyte-Macrophage Colony Stimulating Factor; rGM-CSF

Use

Myeloid reconstitution:

After autologous bone marrow transplantation: Non-Hodgkin's lymphoma (NHL), acute lymphoblastic leukemia (ALL), Hodgkin's lymphoma, metastatic breast cancer

After allogeneic bone marrow transplantation

Peripheral stem cell transplantation: Metastatic breast cancer, non-Hodgkin's lymphoma, Hodgkin's lymphoma, multiple myeloma

Orphan drug:

Acute myelogenous leukemia (AML) following induction chemotherapy in older adults to shorten time to neutrophil recovery and to reduce the incidence of severe and life-threatening infections and infections resulting in death

Bone marrow transplant (allogeneic or autologous) failure or engraftment delay

Note: Safety and efficacy of GM-CSF given simultaneously with cytotoxic chemotherapy have not been established. Concurrent treatment may increase myelosuppression.

Local Anesthetic/Vasoconstrictor Precautions No information available to require special precautions

Effects on Dental Treatment No effects or complications reported

Dosage All orders should be scheduled between 8 AM and 10 AM daily

Children and Adults: I.V. infusion over ≥2 hours or S.C.

Bone marrow transplantation failure or engraftment delay: I.V.: 250 mcg/m²/day for 14 days. The dose can be repeated after 7 days off therapy if engraftment has not occurred. If engraftment still has not occurred, a third course of 500 mcg/m²/day for 14 days may be tried after another 7 days off therapy. If there is still no engraftment, it is unlikely that further dose escalation be beneficial.

Myeloid reconstitution after autologous bone marrow transplant: I.V.: 250 mcg/m²/day to begin 2-4 hours after the marrow infusion on day 0 of autologous bone marrow transplant or ≥24 hours after chemotherapy or 12 hours after last dose of radiotherapy. If significant adverse effects or "first dose" reaction is seen at this dose, discontinue the drug until toxicity resolves, then restart at a reduced dose of 125 mcg/m²/day.

Length of therapy: Bone marrow transplant patients: GM-CSF should be administered daily for up to 30 days or until the ANC has reached 1000/mm³ for 3 consecutive days following the expected chemotherapy-induced neutrophil-nadir

Cancer chemotherapy recovery: I.V.: 3-15 mcg/kg/day for 14-21 days; maximum daily dose is 15 mcg/kg/day due to dose-related adverse effects; **discontinue therapy** if the ANC count is >20,000/mm³

Excessive blood counts return to normal or baseline levels within 3-7 days following cessation of therapy

Mechanism of Action Stimulates proliferation, differentiation and functional activity of neutrophils, eosinophils, monocytes, and macrophages; see table.

Proliferation / Differentiation	G-CSF (Filgrastim)	GM-CSF (Sargramostim)
Neutrophils	Yes	Yes
Eosinophils	No	Yes
Macrophages	No	Yes
Neutrophil migration	Enhanced	Inhibited

Other Adverse Effects

>10%:

Cardiovascular: Hypotension, tachycardia, flushing, and syncope may occur with the first dose of a cycle ("first-dose effect"); peripheral edema (11%)

Central nervous system: Headache (26%)

Dermatologic: Rash, alopecia

Endocrine & metabolic: Polydypsia

Gastrointestinal: Diarrhea (52% to 89%), stomatitis, mucositis

Local: Local reactions at the injection site (~50%)

Neuromuscular & skeletal: Myalgia (18%), arthralgia (21%), bone pain

Renal: Increased serum creatinine (14%)

Respiratory: Dyspnea (28%)

1% to 10%:

Cardiovascular: Transient supraventricular arrhythmias; chest pain; capillary leak syndrome; pericardial effusion (4%)

Central nervous system: Headache

Gastrointestinal: Nausea, vomiting

Hematologic: Leukocytosis, thrombocytopenia
Neuromuscular & skeletal: Weakness
Respiratory: Cough; pleural effusion (1%)

Drug Interactions Lithium and corticosteroids may potentiate myeloproliferative effects.

Drug Uptake
Onset of action: Increase in WBC: 7-14 days
Duration: WBC returns to baseline ~1 week after discontinuation
Half-life, elimination: 2 hours
Time to peak: S.C.: 1-2 hours

Pregnancy Risk Factor C

Generic Available No

Comments Has been demonstrated to accelerate myeloid engraftment in autologous bone marrow transplant, decrease median duration of antibiotic administration, reduce the median duration of infectious episodes, and shorten the median duration of hospitalization, no difference in relapse rate or survival or disease response has been found in placebo-controlled trials. Safety and efficacy of GM-CSF given simultaneously with cytotoxic chemotherapy have not been established. Concurrent treatment may increase myelosuppression. Precaution should be exercised in the usage of GM-CSF in any malignancy with myeloid characteristics. GM-CSF can potentially act as a growth factor for any tumor type, particularly myeloid malignancies. Tumors of nonhematopoietic origin may have surface receptors for GM-CSF.

Scalpicin® *see* Hydrocortisone *on page 608*
Scleromate™ *see* Morrhuate Sodium *on page 831*
Scopace® *see* Scopolamine *on page 1077*

Scopolamine (skoe POL a meen)

U.S. Brand Names Isopto® Hyoscine; Scopace®; Transderm Scōp®

Canadian Brand Names Transderm-V®

Pharmacologic Category Anticholinergic Agent

Synonyms Hyoscine; Scopolamine Hydrobromide

Use Preoperative medication to produce amnesia and decrease salivary and respiratory secretions; to produce cycloplegia and mydriasis; treatment of iridocyclitis; prevention of motion sickness; prevention of nausea/vomiting associated with anesthesia or opiate analgesia (patch); symptomatic treatment of postencephalitic parkinsonism and paralysis agitans (oral); inhibits excessive motility and hypertonus of the GI tract in such conditions as the irritable colon syndrome, mild dysentery, diverticulitis, pylorospasm, and cardiospasm

Local Anesthetic/Vasoconstrictor Precautions No information available to require special precautions

Effects on Dental Treatment >10% of patients medicated with scopolamine patch (Transderm Scop®) will experience significant xerostomia; disappears with discontinuation

Dosage
Preoperatively:
Children: I.M., S.C.: 6 mcg/kg/dose (maximum: 0.3 mg/dose) or 0.2 mg/m^2 may be repeated every 6-8 hours **or** alternatively:
4-7 months: 0.1 mg
7 months to 3 years: 0.15 mg
3-8 years: 0.2 mg
8-12 years: 0.3 mg
Adults:
I.M., I.V., S.C.: 0.3-0.65 mg; may be repeated every 4-6 hours
Transdermal patch: Apply 2.5 cm^2 patch to hairless area behind ear the night before surgery or 1 hour prior to cesarean section (the patch should be applied no sooner than 1 hour before surgery for best results and removed 24 hours after surgery)
Motion sickness: Transdermal: Children >12 years and Adults: Apply 1 disc behind the ear at least 4 hours prior to exposure and every 3 days as needed; effective if applied as soon as 2-3 hours before anticipated need, best if 12 hours before
Ophthalmic:
Refraction:
Children: Instill 1 drop of 0.25% to eye(s) twice daily for 2 days before procedure
Adults: Instill 1-2 drops of 0.25% to eye(s) 1 hour before procedure
Iridocyclitis:
Children: Instill 1 drop of 0.25% to eye(s) up to 3 times/day
Adults: Instill 1-2 drops of 0.25% to eye(s) up to 4 times/day
Oral: Parkinsonism, spasticity, motion sickness: 0.4-0.8 mg as a range; the dosage may be cautiously increased in parkinsonism and spastic states.

Mechanism of Action Blocks the action of acetylcholine at parasympathetic sites in smooth muscle, secretory glands and the CNS; increases cardiac output, dries secretions, antagonizes histamine and serotonin
(Continued)

Scopolamine *(Continued)*

Other Adverse Effects Frequency not defined:

Ophthalmic: Note: Systemic adverse effects have been reported following ophthalmic administration.

Cardiovascular: Vascular congestion, edema
Central nervous system: Drowsiness,
Dermatologic: Eczematoid dermatitis,
Ocular: Blurred vision, photophobia, local irritation, increased intraocular pressure, follicular conjunctivitis, exudate
Respiratory: Congestion

Systemic:

Cardiovascular: Orthostatic hypotension, ventricular fibrillation, tachycardia, palpitations
Central nervous system: Confusion, drowsiness, headache, loss of memory, ataxia, fatigue
Dermatologic: Dry skin, increased sensitivity to light, rash
Endocrine & metabolic: Decreased flow of breast milk
Gastrointestinal: Constipation, xerostomia, dry throat, dysphagia, bloated feeling, nausea, vomiting
Genitourinary: Dysuria
Local: Irritation at injection site
Neuromuscular & skeletal: Weakness
Ocular: Increased intraocular pain, blurred vision
Respiratory: Dry nose, diaphoresis (decreased)

Drug Interactions

Increased Effect/Toxicity: Additive adverse effects with other anticholinergic agents.
Decreased Effect: Decreased effect of acetaminophen, levodopa, ketoconazole, digoxin, riboflavin, and potassium chloride in wax matrix preparations.

Drug Uptake

Onset of action: Oral, I.M.: 0.5-1 hour; I.V.: 10 minutes; may take 3-7 days for full recovery
Absorption: Well absorbed
Duration: Oral, I.M.: 4-6 hours; I.V.: 2 hours
Time to peak: 20-60 minutes; Transdermal: 24 hours

Pregnancy Risk Factor C

Generic Available Yes

Scot-Tussin® [OTC] *see* Guaifenesin *on page 568*
Scot-Tussin DM® Cough Chasers [OTC] *see* Dextromethorphan *on page 372*
Scot-Tussin® Senior Clear [OTC] *see* Guaifenesin and Dextromethorphan *on page 569*
SeaMist® [OTC] *see* Sodium Chloride *on page 1094*
Seba-Gel™ *see* Benzoyl Peroxide *on page 153*
Sebizon® *see* Sulfacetamide Sodium *on page 1115*

Secobarbital (see koe BAR bi tal)

U.S. Brand Names Seconal™

Pharmacologic Category Barbiturate

Synonyms Quinalbarbitone Sodium; Secobarbital Sodium

Use Short-term treatment of insomnia and as preanesthetic agent

Local Anesthetic/Vasoconstrictor Precautions No information available to require special precautions

Effects on Dental Treatment No effects or complications reported

Restrictions C-II

Dosage Hypnotic:

Children: I.M.: 3-5 mg/kg/dose; maximum: 100 mg/dose
Adults:
Oral: 100 mg at bedtime
I.M.: 100-200 mg/dose
I.V.: 50-250 mg/dose

Mechanism of Action Interferes with transmission of impulses from the thalamus to the cortex of the brain resulting in an imbalance in central inhibitory and facilitatory mechanisms. Depresses CNS activity by binding to barbiturate site at GABA-receptor complex enhancing GABA activity, depressing reticular activity system; higher doses may be gabamimetic

Other Adverse Effects Frequency not defined:

Cardiovascular: Hypotension
Central nervous system: Dizziness, lightheadedness, "hangover" effect, drowsiness, CNS depression, fever, confusion, mental depression, unusual excitement, nervousness, faint feeling, headache, insomnia, nightmares, hallucinations
Dermatologic: Exfoliative dermatitis, rash, Stevens-Johnson syndrome
Gastrointestinal: Nausea, vomiting, constipation
Hematologic: Agranulocytosis, megaloblastic anemia, thrombocytopenia, thrombophlebitis, urticaria apnea

Local: Pain at injection site
Respiratory: Respiratory depression, laryngospasm

Drug Interactions CYP2C9, 3A3/4, and 3A5-7 enzyme inducer

Increased Effect/Toxicity: Increased toxicity when combined with other CNS depressants, antidepressants, benzodiazepines, chloramphenicol, or valproic acid; respiratory and CNS depression may be additive. MAO inhibitors may prolong the effect of secobarbital. Barbiturates may enhance the hepatotoxic potential of acetaminophen (due to an increased formation of toxic metabolites). Chloramphenicol may inhibit the metabolism of barbiturates.

Decreased Effect: Barbiturates, such as secobarbital, are hepatic enzyme inducers, and may increase the metabolism of antipsychotics, some beta-blockers (unlikely with atenolol and nadolol), calcium channel blockers, chloramphenicol, cimetidine, corticosteroids, cyclosporine, disopyramide, doxycycline, ethosuximide, felbamate, furosemide, griseofulvin, lamotrigine, phenytoin, propafenone, quinidine, tacrolimus, TCAs, and theophylline. Barbiturates may increase the metabolism of estrogens and reduce the efficacy of oral contraceptives; an alternative method of contraception should be considered. Barbiturates inhibit the hypoprothrombinemic effects of oral anticoagulants via increased metabolism. Barbiturates may enhance the metabolism of methadone resulting in methadone withdrawal.

Drug Uptake

Onset of action: Hypnosis: Oral: 1-3 minutes; I.V. injection: 15-30 minutes
Absorption: Oral: Well absorbed (90%)
Duration: ~15 minutes
Half-life, elimination: 25 hours
Time to peak: 2-4 hours

Pregnancy Risk Factor D

Generic Available Yes

Seconal™ *see* Secobarbital *on page 1078*
Secran® *see* Vitamins, Multiple *on page 1246*
SecreFlo™ *see* Secretin *on page 1079*

Secretin (SEE kre tin)

U.S. Brand Names SecreFlo™

Pharmacologic Category Diagnostic Agent

Use Diagnosis of Zollinger-Ellison syndrome, chronic pancreatic dysfunction, and some hepatobiliary diseases such as obstructive jaundice resulting from cancer or stones in the biliary tract

Local Anesthetic/Vasoconstrictor Precautions No information available to require special precautions

Effects on Dental Treatment No effects or complications reported

Dosage I.V.: Adults: **Note:** A test dose of 0.2 mcg (0.1 mL) is injected to test for possible allergy. Dosing may be completed if no reaction occurs after 1 minute.

Diagnosis of pancreatic dysfunction: 0.2 mcg/kg over 1 minute
Diagnosis of gastrinoma: 0.4 mcg/kg over 1 minute

Mechanism of Action SecreFlo™ is a synthetic formulation of the porcine hormone secretin. This hormone is normally secreted by duodenal mucosa and upper jejunal mucosa which increases the volume and bicarbonate content of pancreatic juice; stimulates the flow of hepatic bile with a high bicarbonate concentration; stimulates gastrin release in patients with Zollinger-Ellison syndrome.

Other Adverse Effects 1% to 10%: Gastrointestinal: Abdominal discomfort (1%)

Drug Interactions Anticholinergics: Response to secretin stimulation may be blunted; includes drugs with high anticholinergic activity such as tricyclic antidepressants, phenothiazines, and antihistamines.

Drug Uptake Inactivated by proteolytic enzymes if administered orally.

Duration: ≥2 hours
Half-life, elimination: 27 minutes
Time to peak: Output of pancreatic secretions: ≤30 minutes

Pregnancy Risk Factor C

Generic Available No

Comments Potency of secretin is expressed in terms of clinical units

Sectral® *see* Acebutolol *on page 25*

Selegiline (seh LEDGE ah leen)

U.S. Brand Names Atapryl®; Eldepryl®; Selpak®

Canadian Brand Names Apo®-Selegiline; Eldepryl®; Gen-Selegiline; Novo-Selegiline; Nu-Selegiline

Mexican Brand Names Niar®

Pharmacologic Category Antidepressant, Monoamine Oxidase Inhibitor; Anti-Parkinson's Agent, MAO Type B Inhibitor

Synonyms Deprenyl; L-Deprenyl; Selegiline Hydrochloride

Use Adjunct in the management of parkinsonian patients in which levodopa/carbidopa therapy is deteriorating

(Continued)

Selegiline *(Continued)*

Unlabeled/Investigational: Early Parkinson's disease; attention-deficit/hyperactivity disorder (ADHD); negative symptoms of schizophrenia; extrapyramidal symptoms; depression; Alzheimer's disease (studies have shown some improvement in behavioral and cognitive performance)

Local Anesthetic/Vasoconstrictor Precautions Selegiline in doses of 10 mg a day or less does not inhibit type-A MAO. Therefore, there are no precautions with the use of vasoconstrictors.

Effects on Dental Treatment

>10%: Xerostomia

Anticholinergic side effects can cause a reduction of saliva production or secretion contributing to discomfort and dental disease (ie, caries, oral candidiasis and periodontal disease).

Dosage Oral:

Children and Adolescents: ADHD (unlabeled use): 5-15 mg/day

Adults: Parkinson's disease: 5 mg twice daily with breakfast and lunch or 10 mg in the morning

Elderly: Parkinson's disease: Initial: 5 mg in the morning, may increase to a total of 10 mg/day

Mechanism of Action Potent monoamine oxidase (MAO) type-B inhibitor; MAO-B plays a major role in the metabolism of dopamine; selegiline may also increase dopaminergic activity by interfering with dopamine reuptake at the synapse

Other Adverse Effects Frequency not defined:

Cardiovascular: Orthostatic hypotension, hypertension, arrhythmias, palpitations, angina, tachycardia, peripheral edema, bradycardia, syncope

Central nervous system: Hallucinations, dizziness, confusion, anxiety, depression, drowsiness, behavior/mood changes, dreams/nightmares, fatigue, delusions

Dermatologic: Rash, photosensitivity

Gastrointestinal: Xerostomia, nausea, vomiting, constipation, weight loss, anorexia, diarrhea, heartburn

Genitourinary: Nocturia, prostatic hyperplasia, urinary retention, sexual dysfunction

Neuromuscular & skeletal: Tremor, chorea, loss of balance, restlessness, bradykinesia

Ocular: Blepharospasm, blurred vision

Miscellaneous: Diaphoresis (increased)

Drug Interactions CYP2D6 enzyme substrate

Note: Many drug interactions involving selegiline are theoretical, primarily based on interactions with nonspecific MAO inhibitors; at doses <10 mg/day, the risk of these interactions with selegiline may be very low

Amphetamines: MAO inhibitors in combination with amphetamines may result in severe hypertensive reaction or serotonin syndrome; these combinations are best avoided

Anorexiants: Concurrent use of selegiline (high dose) in combination with CNS stimulants or anorexiants may result in serotonin syndrome; these combinations are best avoided; includes dexfenfluramine, fenfluramine, or sibutramine

Barbiturates: MAO inhibitors may inhibit the metabolism of barbiturates and prolong their effect

CNS stimulants: MAO inhibitors in combination with stimulants (methylphenidate) may result in serotonin syndrome; these combinations are best avoided

CYP2D6 inhibitors: Theoretically, inhibitors may decrease hepatic metabolism of selegiline, increasing serum concentrations; inhibitors include amiodarone, cimetidine, delavirdine, fluoxetine, paroxetine, propafenone, quinidine, and ritonavir; monitor for increased effect/toxicity

Dextromethorphan: Concurrent use of selegiline (high dose) may result in serotonin syndrome; these combinations are best avoided

Disulfiram: MAO inhibitors may produce delirium in patients receiving disulfiram; monitor

Enzyme inducers: May increase the metabolism of selegiline, reducing serum levels and effect; enzyme inducers include carbamazepine, barbiturates, phenytoin, and rifampin

Guanadrel and guanethidine: MAO inhibitors inhibit the antihypertensive response to guanadrel or guanethidine; use an alternative antihypertensive agent

Hypoglycemic agents: MAO inhibitors may produce hypoglycemia in patients with diabetes; monitor

Levodopa: MAO inhibitors in combination with levodopa may result in hypertensive reactions; monitor

Lithium: MAO inhibitors in combination with lithium have resulted in malignant hyperpyrexia; this combination is best avoided

Meperidine: Concurrent use of selegiline (high dose) may result in serotonin syndrome; these combinations are best avoided

Nefazodone: Concurrent use of selegiline (high dose) may result in serotonin syndrome; these combinations are best avoided

Norepinephrine: MAO inhibitors may increase the pressor response of norepinephrine (effect is generally small); monitor

Oral contraceptives: Increased selegiline levels have been noted with concurrent administration; monitor

Reserpine: MAO inhibitors in combination with reserpine may result in hypertensive reactions; monitor

SSRIs: Concurrent use of selegiline with an SSRI may result in mania or hypertension; it is generally best to avoid these combinations

Sympathomimetics (indirect-acting): MAO inhibitors in combination with sympathomimetics such as dopamine, metaraminol, phenylephrine, and decongestants (pseudoephedrine) may result in severe hypertensive reaction; these combinations are best avoided

Succinylcholine: MAO inhibitors may prolong the muscle relaxation produced by succinylcholine via decreased plasma pseudocholinesterase

Tramadol: May increase the risk of seizures and serotonin syndrome in patients receiving an MAO inhibitor

Trazodone: Concurrent use of selegiline (high dose) may result in serotonin syndrome; these combinations are best avoided

Tricyclic antidepressants: May cause serotonin syndrome when combined with an MAO inhibitor; avoid this combination

Tyramine: Selegiline (>10 mg/day) in combination with tyramine (cheese, ethanol) may increase the pressor response; avoid high tyramine-containing foods in patients receiving >10 mg/day of selegiline

Venlafaxine: Concurrent use of selegiline (high dose) may result in serotonin syndrome; these combinations are best avoided

Drug Uptake

Onset of action: Therapeutic: ≤1 hour

Duration: 24-72 hours

Half-life, elimination: 9 minutes

Pregnancy Risk Factor C

Generic Available Yes

Selenium Sulfide (se LEE nee um)

U.S. Brand Names Selepen®

Pharmacologic Category Mineral

Use Treatment of itching and flaking of the scalp associated with dandruff, to control scalp seborrheic dermatitis; treatment of tinea versicolor

Local Anesthetic/Vasoconstrictor Precautions No information available to require special precautions

Effects on Dental Treatment No effects or complications reported

Dosage Topical:

Dandruff, seborrhea: Massage 5-10 mL into wet scalp, leave on scalp 2-3 minutes, rinse thoroughly, and repeat application; shampoo twice weekly for 2 weeks initially, then use once every 1-4 weeks as indicated depending upon control

Tinea versicolor: Apply the 2.5% lotion to affected area and lather with small amounts of water; leave on skin for 10 minutes, then rinse thoroughly; apply every day for 7 days

Mechanism of Action May block the enzymes involved in growth of epithelial tissue; part of glutathione peroxidase which protects cell components from oxidative damage due to peroxidases produced in cellular metabolism

Other Adverse Effects Frequency not defined:

Central nervous system: Lethargy

Dermatologic: Alopecia or hair discoloration

Gastrointestinal: Vomiting following long-term use on damaged skin; abdominal pain, garlic breath

Local: Irritation

Neuromuscular & skeletal: Tremor

Miscellaneous: Diaphoresis

Drug Uptake Absorption: Topical: Not absorbed through intact skin, but through damaged skin

Pregnancy Risk Factor C

Generic Available Yes

Sele-Pak® *see* Trace Metals *on page 1186*

Selepen® *see* Selenium Sulfide *on page 1081*

Selepen® *see* Trace Metals *on page 1186*

Selpak® *see* Selegiline *on page 1079*

Semicid® [OTC] *see* Nonoxynol 9 *on page 874*

Semprex®-D *see* Acrivastine and Pseudoephedrine *on page 39*

Senexon® [OTC] *see* Senna *on page 1081*

Senna (SEN na)

U.S. Brand Names Black Draught® [OTC]; ex-lax®; ex-lax® Maximum Relief; Senexon® [OTC]; Senna-Gen® [OTC]; Senokot® [OTC]; X-Prep® [OTC]

Pharmacologic Category Laxative, Stimulant

Synonyms *C. angustifolia*; *Cassia acutifolia*; Senna Alexandria

(Continued)

Senna *(Continued)*

Use Short-term treatment of constipation; evacuate the colon for bowel or rectal examinations

Local Anesthetic/Vasoconstrictor Precautions No information available to require special precautions

Effects on Dental Treatment No effects or complications reported

Dosage Oral:

Children:

>6 years: 10-20 mg/kg/dose at bedtime; maximum daily dose: 872 mg

6-12 years, >27 kg: 1 tablet at bedtime, up to 4 tablets/day **or** $^1/_2$ teaspoonful of granules (326 mg/tsp) at bedtime (up to 2 teaspoonfuls/day)

Liquid:

2-5 years: 5-10 mL at bedtime

6-15 years: 10-15 mL at bedtime

Suppository: $^1/_2$ at bedtime

Syrup:

1 month to 1 year: 1.25-2.5 mL at bedtime up to 5 mL/day

1-5 years: 2.5-5 mL at bedtime up to 10 mL/day

5-10 years: 5-10 mL at bedtime up to 20 mL/day

Adults:

Granules (326 mg/teaspoon): 1 teaspoonful at bedtime, not to exceed 2 teaspoonfuls twice daily

Liquid: 15-30 mL with meals and at bedtime

Suppository: 1 at bedtime, may repeat once in 2 hours

Syrup: 2-3 teaspoonfuls at bedtime, not to exceed 30 mL/day

Tablet: 187 mg: 2 tablets at bedtime, not to exceed 8 tablets/day

Tablet: 374 mg: 1 at bedtime, up to 4/day; 600 mg: 2 tablets at bedtime, up to 3 tablets/day

Mechanism of Action Hydrolyzed by bacteria in the colon thus releasing active sennosides; active metabolite (aglycone) acts as a local irritant on the colon, stimulates Auerbach's plexus to produce peristalsis; contains up to 3% anthraquinone glycosides

Other Adverse Effects

1% to 10%: Gastrointestinal: Abdominal cramps, diarrhea, nausea, vomiting (from fresh plant leaves or pods)

Frequency not defined:

Cardiovascular: Palpitations

Central nervous system: Dizziness, tetany

Endocrine & metabolic: (Per Commission E) Electrolyte imbalance (from long-term use/abuse), hypokalemia

Gastrointestinal: Cachexia, melanosis coli (reversible)

Genitourinary: Discoloration of urine (red in alkaline urine, yellow-brown in acidic urine)

Hepatic: Hepatitis

Neuromuscular & skeletal: Finger clubbing (reversible)

Renal: Oliguria, proteinuria

Respiratory: Dyspnea

Contraindications Per Commission E: Abdominal pain (origin undiagnosed), acute intestinal inflammation (eg, Crohn's disease) or obstruction/perforation, colitis ulcerosa, appendicitis, children <12 years, and pregnancy

Warnings/Precautions May alter GI absorption of other herbs or drugs

Drug Interactions

Antiarrhythmics, digoxin, diuretics (potassium-depleting), laxatives, lithium, phenytoin, theophylline

Increased Effect/Toxicity: Docusate may enhance the absorption of senna. Excessive use may lead to electrolyte disturbances and potentiate the effects of various drugs with narrow therapeutic windows.

Per Commission E: Potentiation of cardiac glycosides (with long-term use) is possible due to loss in potassium.

Decreased Effect: May decrease absorption of oral medications by decreasing bowel transit time.

Per Commission E: Potassium deficiency can be increased by simultaneous application of thiazide diuretics, corticosteroids, and licorice root.

Pregnancy Risk Factor C

Generic Available Yes

Comments Some patients will experience considerable gripping

Senna-Gen® [OTC] *see* Senna *on page 1081*

Senokot® [OTC] *see* Senna *on page 1081*

Sensorcaine® *see* Bupivacaine *on page 184*

Sensorcaine®-MPF *see* Bupivacaine *on page 184*

Septocaine™ *see* Articaine Hydrochloride and Epinephrine ***U.S.*** *on page 114*

Septra® *see* Sulfamethoxazole and Trimethoprim *on page 1120*

Septra® DS *see* Sulfamethoxazole and Trimethoprim *on page 1120*

Ser-Ap-Es® *see* Hydralazine, Hydrochlorothiazide, and Reserpine *on page 594*
Serax® *see* Oxazepam *on page 896*
Serentil® *see* Mesoridazine *on page 773*
Serevent® *see* Salmeterol *on page 1073*
Serevent® Diskus® *see* Salmeterol *on page 1073*
Seromycin® Pulvules® *see* CycloSERINE *on page 336*
Serophene® *see* ClomiPHENE *on page 305*
Seroquel® *see* Quetiapine *on page 1030*
Serostim® *see* Human Growth Hormone *on page 589*
Serpalan® *see* Reserpine *on page 1046*

Sertraline (SER tra leen)

U.S. Brand Names Zoloft®

Canadian Brand Names Apo®-Sertraline; Novo-Sertraline; Zoloft™

Mexican Brand Names Altruline®

Pharmacologic Category Antidepressant, Selective Serotonin Reuptake Inhibitor

Synonyms Sertraline Hydrochloride

Use Treatment of major depression; obsessive-compulsive disorder (OCD); panic disorder; post-traumatic stress disorder (PTSD)

Unlabeled/Investigational: Eating disorders; anxiety disorders; premenstrual disorders; impulse control disorders

Local Anesthetic/Vasoconstrictor Precautions Although caution should be used in patients taking tricyclic antidepressants, no interactions have been reported with vasoconstrictor and sertraline, a nontricyclic antidepressant which acts to increase serotonin

Effects on Dental Treatment No effects or complications reported

Dosage Oral:

Children and Adolescents: Depression/OCD:
- 6-12 years: Initial: 25 mg once daily
- 13-17 years: Initial: 50 mg once daily
- **Note:** May increase by 50 mg/day increments at intervals of not less than 1 week if tolerated to 100 mg/day; additional increases may be necessary; maximum: 200 mg/day. If somnolence is noted, give at bedtime.

Adults:
- Depression/OCD: Oral: Initial: 50 mg/day (see "Note" above)
- Panic disorder/post-traumatic stress disorder (PTSD): Oral: Initial 25 mg once daily; increased after 1 week to 50 mg once daily (see "Note" above)
- Premenstrual dysphoric disorder (PMDD): 50 mg once daily; dose may be increased (by 50 mg/day) at the onset of a new menstrual cycle; may be dosed throughout the menstrual cycle or during luteal phase only
  - Maximum dose:
    - Luteal phase: 100 mg/day; If 100 mg/day dose is used during the luteal phase, a titration step of 50 mg/day for 3 days is recommended.
    - Menstrual cycle: 150 mg/day

Elderly: Depression/OCD: Start treatment with 25 mg/day in the morning and increase by 25 mg/day increments every 2-3 days if tolerated to 50-100 mg/day; additional increases may be necessary; maximum dose: 200 mg/day

Hemodialysis: Not removed by hemodialysis

Dosage comments in hepatic impairment: Sertraline is extensively metabolized by the liver; caution should be used in patients with hepatic impairment

Mechanism of Action Antidepressant with selective inhibitory effects on presynaptic serotonin (5-HT) reuptake and only very weak effects on norepinephrine and dopamine neuronal uptake

Other Adverse Effects

>10%:
- Central nervous system: Insomnia, somnolence, dizziness, headache, fatigue
- Gastrointestinal: Xerostomia, diarrhea, nausea
- Genitourinary: Ejaculatory disturbances

1% to 10%:
- Cardiovascular: Palpitations
- Central nervous system: Agitation, anxiety, nervousness
- Dermatologic: Rash
- Endocrine & metabolic: Decreased libido
- Gastrointestinal: Constipation, anorexia, dyspepsia, flatulence, vomiting, weight gain
- Genitourinary: Micturition disorders
- Neuromuscular & skeletal: Tremors, paresthesia
- Ocular: Visual difficulty, abnormal vision
- Otic: Tinnitus
- Miscellaneous: Diaphoresis (increased)

Drug Interactions CYP3A3/4 enzyme substrate, CYP2D6 enzyme substrate (minor); CYP1A2 and 2D6 enzyme inhibitor (weak); CYP2C9, 2C19, and 3A3/4 enzyme inhibitor

(Continued)

Sertraline *(Continued)*

MAO inhibitors: Sertraline should not be used with nonselective MAO inhibitors (phenelzine, isocarboxazid) or other drugs with MAO inhibition (linezolid); fatal reactions have been reported. Wait 5 weeks after stopping sertraline before starting a nonselective MAO inhibitor and 2 weeks after stopping an MAO inhibitor before starting sertraline. Concurrent selegiline has been associated with mania, hypertension, or serotonin syndrome (risk may be reduced relative to nonselective MAO inhibitors).

Combined used of SSRIs and amphetamines, buspirone, meperidine, nefazodone, serotonin agonists (such as sumatriptan), sibutramine, other SSRIs, sympathomimetics, tramadol, and venlafaxine may increase the risk of serotonin syndrome. Sertraline may increase serum concentration/effects of benzodiazepines (alprazolam and diazepam), carbamazepine, carvedilol, clozapine, cyclosporine (and possibly tacrolimus), dextromethorphan, digoxin, haloperidol, HMG-CoA reductase inhibitors (lovastatin and simvastatin - increasing the risk of rhabdomyolysis, despite sertraline's weak inhibition), phenytoin, propafenone, trazodone, tricyclic antidepressants, and valproic acid. Concurrent lithium may increase risk of nephrotoxicity. Risk of hyponatremia may increase with concurrent use of loop diuretics (bumetanide, furosemide, torsemide). Sertraline may increase the hypoprothrombinemic response to warfarin.

Combined use of sumatriptan (and other serotonin agonists) may result in toxicity; weakness, hyper-reflexia, and incoordination have been observed with sumatriptan and SSRIs. In addition, concurrent use may theoretically increase the risk of serotonin syndrome; includes sumatriptan, naratriptan, rizatriptan, and zolmitriptan.

Phenothiazines: CYP3A3/4 inhibitors (including sertraline) may inhibit the metabolism of thioridazine or mesoridazine, resulting in increased plasma concentrations and increasing the risk of QT_c interval prolongation. This may lead to serious ventricular arrhythmias, such as torsade de pointes-type arrhythmias and sudden death. Do not use together. Wait at least 5 weeks after discontinuing sertraline prior to starting thioridazine.

Drug Uptake

Onset of action: Steady-state: 7 days; Therapeutic: >2 weeks

Absorption: Slow

Half-life, elimination: Parent drug: 24 hours; Metabolites: 66 hours

Pregnancy Risk Factor C

Generic Available No

Comments Problems with SSRI-induced bruxism have been reported and may preclude their use; clinicians attempting to evaluate any patient with bruxism or involuntary muscle movement, who is simultaneously being treated with an SSRI drug, should be aware of the potential association.

Selected Readings Gerber PE and Lynd LD, "Selective Serotonin Reuptake Inhibitor-Induced Movement Disorders," *Ann Pharmacother*, 1998, 32(6):692-8.

Serutan® [OTC] *see* Psyllium *on page 1025*

Serzone® *see* Nefazodone *on page 852*

Sevelamer (se VEL a mer)

U.S. Brand Names Renagel®

Canadian Brand Names Renagel®

Pharmacologic Category Phosphate Binder

Synonyms Sevelamer Hydrochloride

Use Reduction of serum phosphorous in patients with end-stage renal disease

Local Anesthetic/Vasoconstrictor Precautions No information available to require special precautions

Effects on Dental Treatment No effects or complications reported

Dosage Adults: Oral: 2-4 capsules 3 times/day with meals; the initial dose may be based on serum phosphorous:

(Phosphorous: Initial Dose)

>6.0 mg/dL and <7.5 mg/dL: 2 capsules 3 times/day

>7.5 mg/dL and <9.0 mg/dL: 3 capsules 3 times/day

≥9.0 mg/dL: 4 capsules 3 times/day

Dosage should be adjusted based on serum phosphorous concentration, with a goal of lowering to <6.0 mg/dL; maximum daily dose studied was 30 capsules/day.

Mechanism of Action A polymeric compound which binds phosphate within the intestinal lumen, limiting absorption and decreasing serum phosphate concentrations without altering calcium, aluminum, or bicarbonate concentrations

Other Adverse Effects

>10%:

Cardiovascular: Hypotension (11%), thrombosis (10%)

Central nervous system: Headache (10%)

Endocrine & metabolic: Decreased absorption of vitamins D, E, K and folic acid

Gastrointestinal: Diarrhea (16%), dyspepsia (5% to 11%), vomiting (12%)

Neuromuscular & skeletal: Pain (13%)

Miscellaneous: Infection (15%)

1% to 10%:

Cardiovascular: Hypertension (9%)

Gastrointestinal: Nausea (7%), flatulence (4%), diarrhea (4%), constipation (2%)

Respiratory: Cough (4%)

Drug Interactions May bind to some drugs in the GI tract and decrease their absorption; when changes in absorption of oral medications may have significant clinical consequences (such as antiarrhythmic and antiseizure medications), these medications should be taken at least 1 hour before or 3 hours after a dose of sevelamer.

Pregnancy Risk Factor C

Generic Available No

Shur-Seal® [OTC] *see* Nonoxynol 9 *on page 874*

Sibutramine (si BYOO tra meen)

U.S. Brand Names Meridia®

Canadian Brand Names Meridia®

Mexican Brand Names Reductil®

Pharmacologic Category Anorexiant

Synonyms Sibutramine Hydrochloride Monohydrate

Use Management of obesity, including weight loss and maintenance of weight loss, and should be used in conjunction with a reduced calorie diet

Local Anesthetic/Vasoconstrictor Precautions No information available to require special precautions

Effects on Dental Treatment No effects or complications reported

Restrictions C-IV; recommended only for obese patients with a body mass index ≥30 kg/m² or ≥27 kg/m² in the presence of other risk factors such as hypertension, diabetes, and/or dyslipidemia

Dosage Adults ≥16 years: Initial: 10 mg once daily; after 4 weeks may titrate up to 15 mg once daily as needed and tolerated (may be used for up to 2 years, per manufacturer labeling)

Mechanism of Action Blocks the neuronal uptake of norepinephrine and, to a lesser extent, serotonin and dopamine

Other Adverse Effects

>10%

Central nervous system: Headache, insomnia

Gastrointestinal: Anorexia, xerostomia, constipation

Respiratory: Rhinitis

1% to 10%

Cardiovascular: Tachycardia, vasodilation, hypertension, palpitations, chest pain, edema

Central nervous system: Migraine, dizziness, nervousness, anxiety, depression, somnolence, CNS stimulation, emotional liability

Dermatologic: Rash

Endocrine & metabolic: Dysmenorrhea

Gastrointestinal: Increased appetite, nausea, dyspepsia, gastritis, vomiting, taste perversion, abdominal pain

Neuromuscular & skeletal: Weakness, arthralgia, back pain

Respiratory: Pharyngitis, sinusitis, cough, laryngitis

Miscellaneous: Diaphoresis, flu-like syndrome, allergic reactions, thirst

Drug Interactions CYP3A3/4 enzyme substrate

Increased Effect/Toxicity: Serotonergic agents such as buspirone, selective serotonin reuptake inhibitors (eg, citalopram, fluoxetine, fluvoxamine, paroxetine, sertraline), sumatriptan (and similar serotonin agonists), dihydroergotamine, lithium, tryptophan, some opioid/analgesics (eg, meperidine, tramadol), and venlafaxine, when combined with sibutramine may result in serotonin syndrome. Dextromethorphan, MAO inhibitors and other drugs that can raise the BP (eg decongestants, centrally-acting weight loss products, amphetamines, and amphetamine-like compounds) can increase the possibility of sibutramine-associated cardiovascular complications. Sibutramine may increase serum concentration of tricyclic antidepressants. Theoretically, inhibitors of CYP3A4 (including ketoconazole, itraconazole, erythromycin) may increase sibutramine levels.

Decreased Effect: Inducers of CYP3A4 (including phenytoin, phenobarbital, carbamazepine, and rifampin) theoretically may reduce sibutramine serum concentration.

Pregnancy Risk Factor C

Generic Available No

Comments The mechanism of action is thought to be different from the "fen" drugs. Sibutramine works to suppress the appetite by inhibiting the reuptake of norepinephrine and serotonin. Unlike dexfenfluramine and fenfluramine, it is not a serotonin releaser. Sibutramine is closer chemically to the widely used antidepressants such as fluoxetine (Prozac®). The FDA approved sibutramine over the objections of its own advisory panel, who called the drug too risky. FDA reported that the drug

(Continued)

Sibutramine *(Continued)*

causes blood pressure to increase, generally by a small amount, though in some patients the increases were higher. It is now recommended that patients taking sibutramine have their blood pressure evaluated regularly.

Selected Readings Wynn RL, "Sibutramine (Meridia) - Dental Considerations for a New Weight Control Drug," *Gen Dent*, 1998, 46(4):332-5.

Silace-C® [OTC] *see* Docusate and Casanthranol *on page 407*
Siladryl® [OTC] *see* DiphenhydrAMINE *on page 398*
Silafed® [OTC] *see* Triprolidine and Pseudoephedrine *on page 1213*
Silapap® Children's [OTC] *see* Acetaminophen *on page 26*
Silapap® Infants [OTC] *see* Acetaminophen *on page 26*

Sildenafil (sil DEN a fil)

U.S. Brand Names Viagra®

Canadian Brand Names Viagra™

Mexican Brand Names Viagra®

Pharmacologic Category Phosphodiesterase Enzyme Inhibitor

Synonyms UK 92480

Use Effective in most men with erectile dysfunction (ED), the medical term for impotence, which is associated with a broad range of physical or psychological medical conditions.

Unlabeled/Investigational: Psychotropic-induced sexual dysfunction

Local Anesthetic/Vasoconstrictor Precautions No information available to require special precautions

Effects on Dental Treatment No effects or complications reported

Dosage Adults: Oral: For most patients, the recommended dose is 50 mg taken as needed, ~ 1 hour before sexual activity. However, sildenafil may be taken anywhere from 30 minutes to 4 hours before sexual activity. Based on effectiveness and tolerance, the dose may be increased to a maximum recommended dose of 100 mg or decreased to 25 mg. The maximum recommended dosing frequency is once daily.

Dosage adjustment for patients >65 years of age, hepatic impairment (cirrhosis), severe renal impairment (creatinine clearance <30 mL/minute), or concomitant use of potent cytochrome P450 3A4 inhibitors (erythromycin, ketoconazole, itraconazole): Higher plasma concentrations have been associated which may result in increase in efficacy and adverse effects and a starting dose of 25 mg should be considered

Mechanism of Action Does not directly cause penile erections, but affects the response to sexual stimulation. The physiologic mechanism of erection of the penis involves release of nitric oxide (NO) in the corpus cavernosum during sexual stimulation. NO then activates the enzyme guanylate cyclase, which results in increased levels of cyclic guanosine monophosphate (cGMP), producing smooth muscle relaxation and inflow of blood to the corpus cavernosum. Sildenafil enhances the effect of NO by inhibiting phosphodiesterase type 5 (PDE5), which is responsible for degradation of cGMP in the corpus cavernosum; when sexual stimulation causes local release of NO, inhibition of PDE5 by sildenafil causes increased levels of cGMP in the corpus cavernosum, resulting in smooth muscle relaxation and inflow of blood to the corpus cavernosum; at recommended doses, it has no effect in the absence of sexual stimulation.

Other Adverse Effects

>10%:
- Central nervous system: Headache
  - **Note:** Dyspepsia and abnormal vision (blurred or increased sensitivity to light) occurred at an incidence of >10% with doses of 100 mg.

1% to 10%:
- Cardiovascular: Flushing
- Central nervous system: Dizziness
- Dermatologic: Rash
- Genitourinary: Urinary tract infection
- Ophthalmic: Abnormal vision (blurred or increased sensitivity to light)
- Respiratory: Nasal congestion

<2% (Limited to important of life-threatening): Shock, allergic reaction, angina pectoris, AV block, migraine, syncope, hypotension, postural hypotension, myocardial ischemia, cerebral thrombosis, cardiac arrest, heart failure, cardiomyopathy, colitis, rectal hemorrhage, edema, gout, hyperglycemia, neuralgia, vertigo, asthma, dyspnea, exfoliative dermatitis, eye hemorrhage, cataract, anorgasmia, seizures, priapism

Drug Interactions CYP3A3/4 enzyme substrate (major); CYP2C9 enzyme substrate (minor)

Increased Effect/Toxicity: Sildenafil potentiates the hypotensive effects of nitrates (amyl nitrate, isosorbide dinitrate, isosorbide mononitrate, nitroglycerin); severe reactions have occurred and concurrent use is contraindicated. Sildenafil may potentiate the effect of other antihypertensives. Serum concentrations/toxicity of sildenafil may be increased by inhibitors of CYP3A3/4, including amprenavir, cimetidine, ciprofloxacin, clarithromycin, clozapine, diltiazem, disulfiram, digoxin, erythromycin, fluconazole, fluoxetine, fluvoxamine, ritonavir, isoniazid, itraconazole, ketoconazole, labetalol, levodopa, loxapine, metoprolol, metronidazole, miconazole, nefazodone, nelfinavir, omeprazole, phenytoin, rifabutin, rifampin, ritonavir, troleandomycin, valproic acid, and verapamil. Sildenafil may potentiate bleeding in patients receiving heparin. A reduction in sildenafil's dose is recommended when used with ritonavir or indinavir (no more than 25 mg/dose; no more than 25 mg in 48 hours).

Decreased Effect: Enzyme inducers (including phenytoin, carbamazepine, phenobarbital, rifampin) may decrease the serum concentration and efficacy of sildenafil.

Drug Uptake

Onset of action: ~60 minutes

Duration: 2-4 hours

Half-life, elimination: 4 hours

Time to peak: 30-120 minutes

Pregnancy Risk Factor B

Generic Available No

Silphen® Cough [OTC] *see* DiphenhydrAMINE *on page 398*

Silphen DM® [OTC] *see* Dextromethorphan *on page 372*

Siltussin® [OTC] *see* Guaifenesin *on page 568*

Siltussin DM® [OTC] *see* Guaifenesin and Dextromethorphan *on page 569*

Silvadene® *see* Silver Sulfadiazine *on page 1088*

Silver Nitrate (SIL ver NYE trate)

Pharmacologic Category Antibiotic, Ophthalmic; Antibiotic, Topical; Cauterizing Agent, Topical; Topical Skin Product, Antibacterial

Synonyms $AgNO_3$

Use Prevention of gonococcal ophthalmia neonatorum; cauterization of wounds and sluggish ulcers, removal of granulation tissue and warts; aseptic prophylaxis of burns

Local Anesthetic/Vasoconstrictor Precautions No information available to require special precautions

Effects on Dental Treatment No effects or complications reported

Dosage Children and Adults:

Ointment: Apply in an apertured pad on affected area or lesion for ~ 5 days

Sticks: Apply to mucous membranes and other moist skin surfaces only on area to be treated 2-3 times/week for 2-3 weeks

Topical solution: Apply a cotton applicator dipped in solution on the affected area 2-3 times/week for 2-3 weeks

Mechanism of Action Free silver ions precipitate bacterial proteins by combining with chloride in tissue forming silver chloride; coagulates cellular protein to form an eschar; silver ions or salts or colloidal silver preparations can inhibit the growth of both gram-positive and gram-negative bacteria. This germicidal action is attributed to the precipitation of bacterial proteins by liberated silver ions. Silver nitrate coagulates cellular protein to form an eschar, and this mode of action is the postulated mechanism for control of benign hematuria, rhinitis, and recurrent pneumothorax.

Other Adverse Effects

>10%:

- Dermatologic: Burning and skin irritation
- Ocular: Chemical conjunctivitis

1% to 10%:

- Dermatologic: Staining of the skin
- Hematologic: Methemoglobinemia
- Ocular: Cauterization of the cornea, blindness

Drug Interactions Sulfacetamide preparations are incompatible.

Drug Uptake Absorption: Because silver ions readily combine with protein, there is minimal GI and cutaneous absorption of the 0.5% and 1% preparations

Pregnancy Risk Factor C

Generic Available Yes

Comments Applicators are **not** for ophthalmic use

Silver Protein, Mild (SIL ver PRO teen mild)

U.S. Brand Names Argyrol® S.S. 20%

Pharmacologic Category Antibiotic, Ophthalmic

Use Stain and coagulate mucus in eye surgery which is then removed by irrigation; eye infections

Local Anesthetic/Vasoconstrictor Precautions No information available to require special precautions

Effects on Dental Treatment No effects or complications reported

(Continued)

Silver Protein, Mild *(Continued)*

Dosage

Preop in eye surgery: Place 2-3 drops into eye(s), then rinse out with sterile irrigating solution

Eye infections: 1-3 drops into the affected eye(s) every 3-4 hours for several days

Pregnancy Risk Factor C

Generic Available No

Silver Sulfadiazine (SIL ver sul fa DYE a zeen)

U.S. Brand Names Silvadene®; SSD® AF; SSD® Cream; Thermazene®

Canadian Brand Names Dermazin™; Flamazine®; SSD™

Pharmacologic Category Antibiotic, Topical

Use Prevention and treatment of infection in second and third degree burns

Local Anesthetic/Vasoconstrictor Precautions No information available to require special precautions

Effects on Dental Treatment No effects or complications reported

Dosage Children and Adults: Topical: Apply once or twice daily with a sterile-gloved hand; apply to a thickness of 1/16"; burned area should be covered with cream at all times

Mechanism of Action Acts upon the bacterial cell wall and cell membrane. Bactericidal for many gram-negative and gram-positive bacteria and is effective against yeast. Active against *Pseudomonas aeruginosa, Pseudomonas maltophilia, Enterobacter* species, *Klebsiella* species, *Serratia* species, *Escherichia coli, Proteus mirabilis, Morganella morganii, Providencia rettgeri, Proteus vulgaris, Providencia* species, *Citrobacter* species, *Acinetobacter calcoaceticus, Staphylococcus aureus, Staphylococcus epidermidis, Enterococcus* species, *Candida albicans, Corynebacterium diphtheriae*, and *Clostridium perfringens*

Other Adverse Effects

Frequency not defined:

- Dermatologic: Itching, rash, erythema multiforme, discoloration of skin, photosensitivity
- Hematologic: Hemolytic anemia, leukopenia, agranulocytosis, aplastic anemia
- Hepatic: Hepatitis
- Renal: Interstitial nephritis
- Miscellaneous: Allergic reactions may be related to sulfa component

>10%: Local: Burning feeling on treated areas

Drug Interactions Topical proteolytic enzymes are inactivated by silver sulfadiazine.

Drug Uptake

Absorption: Significant percutaneous absorption of sulfadiazine can occur especially when applied to extensive burns.

Half-life, elimination: 10 hours (increases with renal insufficiency)

Time to peak: 3-11 days of continuous therapy

Pregnancy Risk Factor B

Generic Available No

Simethicone (sye METH i kone)

U.S. Brand Names Flatulex® [OTC]; Gas-X® [OTC]; Maalox® Anti-Gas [OTC]; Mylanta® Gas [OTC]; Mylicon® [OTC]; Phazyme® [OTC]

Canadian Brand Names Ovol®; Phazyme™

Pharmacologic Category Antiflatulent

Synonyms Activated Dimethicone; Activated Methylpolysiloxane

Use Relief of flatulence and functional gastric bloating, and postoperative gas pains

Local Anesthetic/Vasoconstrictor Precautions No information available to require special precautions

Effects on Dental Treatment No effects or complications reported

Dosage Oral:

Children <12 years: 40 mg 4 times/day

Children >12 years and Adults: 40-120 mg after meals and at bedtime as needed, not to exceed 500 mg/day

Mechanism of Action Decreases the surface tension of gas bubbles thereby disperses and prevents gas pockets in the GI system

Pregnancy Risk Factor C

Generic Available Yes: Tablet, drops

Simulect® *see* Basiliximab *on page 143*

Simvastatin (SIM va stat in)

Related Information

Cardiovascular Diseases *on page 1308*

U.S. Brand Names Zocor®

Canadian Brand Names Zocor®

Mexican Brand Names Zocor®

Pharmacologic Category Antilipemic Agent, HMG-CoA Reductase Inhibitor

Use Adjunct to dietary therapy to decrease elevated serum total and LDL cholesterol, apolipoprotein B (apo-B), and triglyceride levels, and to increase HDL cholesterol in patients with primary hypercholesterolemia (heterozygous, familial and nonfamilial) and mixed dyslipidemia (Fredrickson types IIa and IIb); treatment of homozygous familial hypercholesterolemia; treatment of isolated hypertriglyceridemia (Fredrickson type IV) and type III hyperlipoproteinemia

"Secondary prevention" in patients with coronary heart disease and hypercholesterolemia to reduce the risk of total mortality by reducing coronary death; reduce the risk of nonfatal myocardial infarction; reduce the risk of undergoing myocardial revascularization procedures; and reduce the risk of stroke or transient ischemic attack

Local Anesthetic/Vasoconstrictor Precautions No information available to require special precautions

Effects on Dental Treatment No effects or complications reported

Dosage Oral: Adults:

Initial: 20 mg once daily in the evening

Patients who require only a moderate reduction of LDL cholesterol may be started at 10 mg once daily

Patients who require a reduction of >45% in low-density lipoprotein (LDL) cholesterol may be started at 40 mg once daily in the evening

Maintenance: Recommended dosage range: 5-80 mg/day as a single dose in the evening; doses should be individualized according to the baseline LDL cholesterol levels, the recommended goal of therapy, and the patient's response.

Note: Adjustments: Should be made at intervals of 4 weeks or more.

Patients with homozygous familial hypercholesteremia: 40 mg in the evening or 80 mg/day in 3 divided doses of 20 mg, 20 mg, and an evening dose of 40 mg.

Patients receiving concomitant cyclosporine: Initial: 5 mg, should **not** exceed 10 mg/day.

Patients receiving concomitant fibrates or niacin: Dose should **not** exceed 10 mg/day.

Patients receiving concomitant amiodarone or verapamil: Dose should **not** exceed 20 mg/day.

Dosing adjustment/comments in renal impairment: Because simvastatin does not undergo significant renal excretion, modification of dose should not be necessary in patients with mild to moderate renal insufficiency.

Severe renal impairment: Cl_{cr} <10 mL/minute: Initial: 5 mg/day with close monitoring.

Mechanism of Action A methylated derivative of lovastatin that acts by competitively inhibiting 3-hydroxy-3-methylglutaryl-CoA reductase (HMG CoA reductase), the enzyme that catalyzes the rate-limiting step in cholesterol biosynthesis

Other Adverse Effects 1% to 10%:

Gastrointestinal: Constipation (2%), dyspepsia (1%), flatulence (2%)

Neuromuscular & skeletal: CPK elevation (>3x normal on one or more occasions - 5%)

Respiratory: Upper respiratory infection (2%)

Additional class-related events or case reports (not necessarily reported with simvastatin therapy): Myopathy, increased CPK (>10x normal), rhabdomyolysis, renal failure (secondary to rhabdomyolysis), alteration in taste, impaired extraocular muscle movement, facial paresis, tremor, headache, memory loss, vertigo, paresthesia, peripheral neuropathy, peripheral nerve palsy, anxiety, depression, psychic disturbance, hypersensitivity reaction, angioedema, anaphylaxis, systemic lupus erythematosus-like syndrome, polymyalgia rheumatica, dermatomyositis, vasculitis, purpura, thrombocytopenia, leukopenia, hemolytic anemia, positive ANA, increased ESR, eosinophilia, arthritis, urticaria, photosensitivity, fever, chills, flushing, malaise, dyspnea, rash, toxic epidermal necrolysis, erythema multiforme, Stevens-Johnson syndrome, pancreatitis, hepatitis, cholestatic jaundice, fatty liver, cirrhosis, fulminant hepatic necrosis, hepatoma, anorexia, vomiting, alopecia, pruritus, nodules, skin discoloration, dryness of skin/mucous membranes, nail changes, gynecomastia, decreased libido, erectile dysfunction/impotence, cataracts, ophthalmoplegia, elevated transaminases, increased alkaline phosphatase, increased GGT, hyperbilirubinemia, thyroid dysfunction

Warnings/Precautions Liver function must be monitored by periodic laboratory assessment. Rhabdomyolysis with acute renal failure has occurred. Risk is dose-related and is increased with concurrent use of lipid-lowering agents which may cause rhabdomyolysis (gemfibrozil, fibric acid derivatives, or niacin at doses ≥1 g/day) or during concurrent use with potent CYP3A3/4 inhibitors (including amiodarone, clarithromycin, cyclosporine, erythromycin, itraconazole, ketoconazole, nefazodone, grapefruit juice in large quantities, verapamil, or protease inhibitors such as indinavir, nelfinavir, or ritonavir). Weigh the risk versus benefit when combining any of these drugs with simvastatin. Temporarily discontinue in any patient experiencing an acute or serious condition predisposing to renal failure secondary to rhabdomyolysis.

Drug Interactions CYP3A3/4 enzyme substrate

(Continued)

Simvastatin *(Continued)*

Increased Effect/Toxicity: Risk of myopathy/rhabdomyolysis may be increased by concurrent use of lipid-lowering agents which may cause rhabdomyolysis (gemfibrozil, fibric acid derivatives, or niacin at doses ≥1 g/day), or during concurrent use of potent CYP3A3/4 inhibitors (including amiodarone, clarithromycin, cyclosporine, danazol, diltiazem, erythromycin, fluconazole, itraconazole, ketoconazole, nefazodone, verapamil or protease inhibitors such as indinavir, nelfinavir, ritonavir or saquinavir). In large quantities (ie, >1 quart/day), grapefruit juice may also increase simvastatin serum concentrations, increasing the risk of rhabdomyolysis. In general, concurrent use with CYP3A3/4 inhibitors is not recommended; manufacturer recommends limiting simvastatin dose to 20 mg/day when used with amiodarone or verapamil, and 10 mg/day when used with cyclosporine, gemfibrozil, or fibric acid derivatives. The anticoagulant effect of warfarin may be increased by simvastatin. Cholesterol-lowering effects are additive with bile-acid sequestrants (colestipol and cholestyramine).

Decreased Effect: When taken within 1 before or up to 2 hours after cholestyramine, a decrease in absorption of simvastatin can occur.

Drug Uptake

Onset of action: >3 days; Peak effect: 2 weeks

Absorption: Oral: Although 85% is absorbed following administration, <5% reaches the general circulation due to an extensive first-pass effect

Half-life, elimination: Unknown

Time to peak: 1.3-2.4 hours

Pregnancy Risk Factor X

Generic Available No

Sinarest® 12 Hour Nasal [OTC] *see* Oxymetazoline *on page 907*

Sincalide (SIN ka lide)

U.S. Brand Names Kinevac®

Pharmacologic Category Diagnostic Agent

Synonyms C8-CCK; OP-CCK

Use Postevacuation cholecystography; gallbladder bile sampling; stimulate pancreatic secretion for analysis

Local Anesthetic/Vasoconstrictor Precautions No information available to require special precautions

Effects on Dental Treatment No effects or complications reported

Dosage Adults: I.V.:

Contraction of gallbladder: 0.02 mcg/kg over 30 seconds to 1 minute, may repeat in 15 minutes a 0.04 mcg/kg dose

Pancreatic function: 0.02 mcg/kg over 30 minutes administered after secretin

Mechanism of Action Stimulates contraction of the gallbladder and simultaneous relaxation of the sphincter of Oddi, inhibits gastric emptying, and increases intestinal motility. Graded doses have been shown to produce graded decreases in small intestinal transit time, thought to be mediated by acetylcholine.

Other Adverse Effects 1% to 10%:

Cardiovascular: Flushing

Central nervous system: Dizziness

Gastrointestinal: Nausea, abdominal pain, urge to defecate

Drug Uptake

Onset of action: Contraction of the gallbladder: ~5-15 minutes

Duration: ~1 hour

Pregnancy Risk Factor B

Generic Available No

Comments Preparation of solution: To reconstitute, add 5 mL sterile water for injection to the vial; the solution may be kept at room temperature; use within 24 hours after reconstitution; delivers 1 mcg/mL

Sinemet® *see* Levodopa and Carbidopa *on page 700*

Sinemet® CR *see* Levodopa and Carbidopa *on page 700*

Sinequan® *see* Doxepin *on page 414*

Singulair® *see* Montelukast *on page 827*

Sinufed® Timecelles® *see* Guaifenesin and Pseudoephedrine *on page 570*

Sinumist®-SR Capsulets® *see* Guaifenesin *on page 568*

Sinupan® *see* Guaifenesin and Phenylephrine *on page 569*

Sinus-Relief® [OTC] *see* Acetaminophen and Pseudoephedrine *on page 30*

Sinutab® Sinus Allergy Maximum Strength [OTC] *see* Acetaminophen, Chlorpheniramine, and Pseudoephedrine *on page 33*

Sinutab® Sinus Maximum Strength Without Drowsiness [OTC] *see* Acetaminophen and Pseudoephedrine *on page 30*

Sirolimus (sir OH li mus)

U.S. Brand Names Rapamune®

Canadian Brand Names Rapamune®

Pharmacologic Category Immunosuppressant Agent

Use Prophylaxis of organ rejection in patients receiving renal transplants, in combination with cyclosporine and corticosteroids

Unlabeled/Investigational: Prophylaxis of organ rejection in solid organ transplant patients in combination with tacrolimus and corticosteroids

Local Anesthetic/Vasoconstrictor Precautions No information available to require special precautions

Effects on Dental Treatment No effects or complications reported

Dosage Oral:

Children ≥13 years or Adults <40 kg: Loading dose: 3 mg/m^2 (day 1); followed by a maintenance of 1 mg/m^2/day.

Adults ≥40 kg: Loading dose: For *de novo* transplant recipients, a loading dose of 3 times the daily maintenance dose should be administered on day 1 of dosing. Maintenance dose: 2 mg/day. Doses should be taken 4 hours after cyclosporine, and should be taken consistently either with or without food.

Mechanism of Action Inhibits T-lymphocyte activation and proliferation in response to antigenic and cytokine stimulation; mechanism differs from other immunosuppressants, it inhibits acute rejection of allografts and prolongs graft survival.

Other Adverse Effects Incidence of many adverse effects are dose related

>20%:

Cardiovascular: Hypertension (39% to 49%), peripheral edema (54% to 64%), edema (16% to 24%), chest pain (16% to 24%)

Central nervous system: Fever (23% to 34%), headache (23% to 34%), pain (24% to 33%), insomnia (13% to 22%)

Dermatologic: Acne (20% to 31%), rash (10% to 20%)

Endocrine & metabolic: Hypercholesterolemia (38% to 46%), hyperkalemia (12% to 17%), hypokalemia (11% to 21%), hypophosphatemia (15% to 23%), hyperlipidemia (38% to 57%)

Gastrointestinal: Abdominal pain (28% to 36%), nausea (25% to 36%), vomiting (19% to 25%), diarrhea (25% to 42%), constipation (28% to 38%), dyspepsia (17% to 25%), weight gain (8% to 21%)

Genitourinary: Urinary tract infection (20% to 33%)

Hematologic: Anemia (23% to 37%), leukopenia (9% to 15%), thrombocytopenia (13% to 40%)

Neuromuscular & skeletal: Arthralgia (25% to 31%), weakness (22% to 40%), back pain (16% to 26%), tremor (21% to 31%)

Renal: Increased serum creatinine (35% to 40%)

Respiratory: Dyspnea (22% to 30%), upper respiratory infection (20% to 26%), pharyngitis (16% to 21%)

3% to 20%:

Cardiovascular: Atrial fibrillation, CHF, hypervolemia, hypotension, palpitation, peripheral vascular disorder, postural hypotension, syncope, tachycardia, thrombosis, vasodilation

Central nervous system: Chills, malaise, anxiety, confusion, depression, dizziness, emotional lability, hypesthesia, hypotonia, insomnia, neuropathy, somnolence

Dermatologic: Dermatitis (fungal), hirsutism, pruritus, skin hypertrophy, dermal ulcer, ecchymosis, cellulitis

Endocrine & metabolic: Cushing's syndrome, diabetes mellitus, glycosuria, acidosis, dehydration, hypercalcemia, hyperglycemia, hyperphosphatemia, hypocalcemia, hypoglycemia, hypomagnesemia, hyponatremia

Gastrointestinal: Enlarged abdomen, anorexia, dysphagia, eructation, esophagitis, flatulence, gastritis, gastroenteritis, gingivitis, gingival hyperplasia, ileus, mouth ulceration, oral moniliasis, stomatitis, weight loss

Genitourinary: Pelvic pain, scrotal edema, testis disorder, impotence

Hematologic: Leukocytosis, polycythemia, TTP, hemolytic-uremic syndrome, hemorrhage

Hepatic: Abnormal LFTs, increased alkaline phosphatase, increased LDH, increased transaminases, ascites

Local: Thrombophlebitis

Neuromuscular & skeletal: Increased CPK, arthrosis, bone necrosis, leg cramps, myalgia, osteoporosis, tetany, hypertonia, paresthesia

Ocular: Abnormal vision, cataract, conjunctivitis

Otic: Ear pain, deafness, otitis media, tinnitus

Renal: Increased BUN, increased serum creatinine, albuminuria, bladder pain, dysuria, hematuria, hydronephrosis, kidney pain, tubular necrosis, nocturia, oliguria, pyuria, nephropathy (toxic), urinary frequency, urinary incontinence, urinary retention

Respiratory: Asthma, atelectasis, bronchitis, cough, epistaxis, hypoxia, lung edema, pleural effusion, pneumonia, rhinitis, sinusitis

Miscellaneous: Abscess, facial edema, flu-like syndrome, hernia, infection, lymphadenopathy, lymphocele, peritonitis, sepsis, diaphoresis

Contraindications Hypersensitivity to sirolimus or any component of the formulation

(Continued)

Sirolimus *(Continued)*

Warnings/Precautions Immunosuppressive agents, including sirolimus, increase the risk of infection and may be associated with the development of lymphoma. Only physicians experienced in the management of organ transplant patients should prescribe sirolimus. May increase serum lipids (cholesterol and triglycerides). Use with caution in patients with hyperlipidemia. May decrease GFR and increase serum creatinine. Use caution in patients with renal impairment, or when used concurrently with medications which may alter renal function. Has been associated with an increased risk of lymphocele. Avoid concurrent use of ketoconazole.

Sirolimus is neither approved nor recommended for use in liver transplant patients; studies indicate an association with an increase risk of hepatic artery thrombosis and graft failure in these patients.

Drug Interactions CYP3A3/4 enzyme substrate and P-glycoprotein substrate

Increased Effect/Toxicity: Cyclosporine increases sirolimus concentrations during concurrent therapy, and cyclosporine levels may be increased. Diltiazem, ketoconazole, and rifampin increase serum concentration of sirolimus. Other inhibitors of CYP3A4 (eg, calcium channel blockers, antifungal agents, macrolide antibiotics, GI prokinetic agents, HIV-protease inhibitors) are likely to increase sirolimus concentrations

Voriconazole: Sirolimus serum concentrations may be increased; concurrent use is contraindicated.

Decreased Effect: Inducers of CYP3A4 (eg, rifampin, phenobarbital, carbamazepine, rifabutin, phenytoin) are likely to decrease serum concentration of sirolimus.

Drug Uptake

Absorption: Rapid

Half-life, elimination: Mean: 62 hours

Time to peak: 1-3 hours

Pregnancy Risk Factor C

Generic Available No

Skelaxin® *see* Metaxalone *on page 777*

Skelid® *see* Tiludronate *on page 1169*

Skin Test Antigens, Multiple (skin test AN tee gens, MUL ti pul)

U.S. Brand Names Multitest CMI®

Canadian Brand Names Multitest® CMI

Pharmacologic Category Diagnostic Agent

Use Detection of nonresponsiveness to antigens by means of delayed hypersensitivity skin testing

Local Anesthetic/Vasoconstrictor Precautions No information available to require special precautions

Effects on Dental Treatment No effects or complications reported

Dosage Select only test sites that permit sufficient surface area and subcutaneous tissue to allow adequate penetration of all eight points, avoid hairy areas

Press loaded unit into the skin with sufficient pressure to puncture the skin and allow adequate penetration of all points, maintain firm contact for at least 5 seconds, during application the device should not be "rocked" back and forth and side to side without removing any of the test heads from the skin sites

If adequate pressure is applied it will be possible to observe:

1. The puncture marks of the nine tines on each of the eight test heads
2. An imprint of the circular platform surrounding each test head
3. Residual antigen and glycerin at each of the eight sites

If any of the above three criteria are not fully followed, the test results may not be reliable

Reading should be done in good light, read the test sites at both 24 and 48 hours, the largest reaction recorded from the two readings at each test site should be used; if two readings are not possible, a single 48 hour is recommended

A positive reaction from any of the seven delayed hypersensitivity skin test antigens is **induration ≥2 mm** providing there is no induration at the negative control site; the size of the induration reactions with this test may be smaller than those obtained with other intradermal procedures

Other Adverse Effects 1% to 10%: Local: Irritation

Drug Interactions Decreased Effect: Drugs or procedures that suppress immunity such as corticosteroids, chemotherapeutic agents, antilymphocyte globulin and irradiation, may possibly cause a loss of reactivity

Pregnancy Risk Factor C

Generic Available No

Comments Contains disposable plastic applicator consisting of eight sterile test heads preloaded with the following seven delayed hypersensitivity skin test antigens and glycerin negative control for percutaneous administration

Test Head No. 1 = Tetanus toxoid antigen

Test Head No. 2 = Diphtheria toxoid antigen

Test Head No. 3 = *Streptococcus* antigen

Test Head No. 4 = Tuberculin, old
Test Head No. 5 = Glycerin negative control
Test Head No. 6 = *Candida* antigen
Test Head No. 7 = *Trichophyton* antigen
Test Head No. 8 = *Proteus* antigen

Sleep-eze 3® Oral [OTC] *see* DiphenhydrAMINE *on page 398*
Sleepinal® [OTC] *see* DiphenhydrAMINE *on page 398*
Sleepwell 2-nite® [OTC] *see* DiphenhydrAMINE *on page 398*
Slo-bid™ *see* Theophylline *on page 1152*
Slo-Niacin® [OTC] *see* Niacin *on page 860*
Slo-Phyllin® *see* Theophylline *on page 1152*
Slo-Phyllin® GG *see* Theophylline and Guaifenesin *on page 1155*
Slow FE® [OTC] *see* Ferrous Sulfate *on page 498*
Slow-K® *see* Potassium Chloride *on page 977*
Slow-Mag® [OTC] *see* Magnesium Chloride *on page 739*

Sodium Ascorbate (SOW dee um a SKOR bate)

U.S. Brand Names Cenolate®
Pharmacologic Category Vitamin, Water Soluble
Use Prevention and treatment of scurvy; used to acidify urine
Local Anesthetic/Vasoconstrictor Precautions No information available to require special precautions
Effects on Dental Treatment No effects or complications reported
Dosage Oral, I.V., S.C.:
Infants:
Daily protective requirement: 30 mg
Treatment: 100-300 mg/day (75-100 mg in premature infants)
Children:
Scurvy: 100-300 mg/day in divided doses for at least 2 weeks
Urinary acidification: 500 mg every 6-8 hours
Dietary supplement: 35-45 mg/day
Adults:
Scurvy: 100-250 mg 1-2 times/day for at least 2 weeks
Urinary acidification: 4-12 g/day in divided doses
Dietary supplement: 50-60 mg/day (RDA: 60 mg)
Prevention and treatment of cold: 1-3 g/day
Other Adverse Effects 1% to 10%:
Cardiovascular: Hypotension with rapid I.V. administration
Gastrointestinal: Diarrhea
Local: Soreness at injection site
Renal: Precipitation of cystine, oxalate, or urate renal stones
Contraindications Large doses during pregnancy
Warnings/Precautions Use with caution in diabetics, patients with renal calculi, and those on sodium-restricted diets
Drug Uptake Therapeutic levels: 0.4-1.5 mg/dL
Pregnancy Risk Factor C
Dosage Forms INJ: 562.5 mg/mL [ascorbic acid 500 mg/mL] (1 mL, 2 mL)
Generic Available No

Sodium Bicarbonate (SOW dee um bye KAR bun ate)

U.S. Brand Names Neut®
Pharmacologic Category Alkalinizing Agent; Antacid; Electrolyte Supplement, Oral; Electrolyte Supplement, Parenteral
Synonyms Baking Soda; $NaHCO_3$; Sodium Acid Carbonate; Sodium Hydrogen Carbonate
Use Management of metabolic acidosis; gastric hyperacidity; as an alkalinization agent for the urine; treatment of hyperkalemia; management of overdose of certain drugs, including tricyclic antidepressants and aspirin
Local Anesthetic/Vasoconstrictor Precautions No information available to require special precautions
Effects on Dental Treatment No effects or complications reported
Dosage
Cardiac arrest:
Routine use of $NaHCO_3$ is not recommended and should be given only after adequate alveolar ventilation has been established and effective cardiac compressions are provided
Infants and Children: I.V.: 0.5-1 mEq/kg/dose repeated every 10 minutes or as indicated by arterial blood gases; rate of infusion should not exceed 10 mEq/minute; neonates and children <2 years of age should receive 4.2% (0.5 mEq/mL) solution
Adults: I.V.: Initial: 1 mEq/kg/dose one time; maintenance: 0.5 mEq/kg/dose every 10 minutes or as indicated by arterial blood gases
(Continued)

Sodium Bicarbonate *(Continued)*

Metabolic acidosis: Dosage should be based on the following formula if blood gases and pH measurements are available:

Infants and Children:

HCO_3^-(mEq) = 0.3 x weight (kg) x base deficit (mEq/L) **or**

HCO_3^-(mEq) = 0.5 x weight (kg) x [24 - serum HCO_3^- (mEq/L)]

Adults:

HCO_3^-(mEq) = 0.2 x weight (kg) x base deficit (mEq/L) **or**

HCO_3^-(mEq) = 0.5 x weight (kg) x [24 - serum HCO_3^- (mEq/L)]

If acid-base status is not available: Dose for older Children and Adults: 2-5 mEq/kg I.V. infusion over 4-8 hours; subsequent doses should be based on patient's acid-base status

Chronic renal failure: Oral: Initiate when plasma HCO_3^- <15 mEq/L

Children: 1-3 mEq/kg/day

Adults: Start with 20-36 mEq/day in divided doses, titrate to bicarbonate level of 18-20 mEq/L

Hyperkalemia: Adults: I.V.: 1 mEq/kg over 5 minutes

Renal tubular acidosis: Oral:

Distal:

Children: 2-3 mEq/kg/day

Adults: 0.5-2 mEq/kg/day in 4-5 divided doses

Proximal: Children: Initial: 5-10 mEq/kg/day; maintenance: Increase as required to maintain serum bicarbonate in the normal range

Urine alkalinization: Oral:

Children: 1-10 mEq (84-840 mg)/kg/day in divided doses every 4-6 hours; dose should be titrated to desired urinary pH

Adults: Initial: 48 mEq (4 g), then 12-24 mEq (1-2 g) every 4 hours; dose should be titrated to desired urinary pH; doses up to 16 g/day (200 mEq) in patients <60 years and 8 g (100 mEq) in patients >60 years

Antacid: Adults: Oral: 325 mg to 2 g 1-4 times/day

Mechanism of Action Dissociates to provide bicarbonate ion which neutralizes hydrogen ion concentration and raises blood and urinary pH

Other Adverse Effects Frequency not defined:

Cardiovascular: Cerebral hemorrhage, CHF (aggravated), edema

Central nervous system: Tetany

Gastrointestinal: Belching

Endocrine & metabolic: Hypernatremia, hyperosmolality, hypocalcemia, hypokalemia, increased affinity of hemoglobin for oxygen-reduced pH in myocardial tissue necrosis when extravasated, intracranial acidosis, metabolic alkalosis, milk-alkali syndrome (especially with renal dysfunction)

Gastrointestinal: Flatulence (with oral), gastric distension

Respiratory: Pulmonary edema

Warnings/Precautions Rapid administration in neonates and children <2 years of age has led to hypernatremia, decreased CSF pressure and intracranial hemorrhage. **Use of I.V. $NaHCO_3$ should be reserved for documented metabolic acidosis and for hyperkalemia-induced cardiac arrest.** Routine use in cardiac arrest is not recommended. Avoid extravasation, tissue necrosis can occur due to the hypertonicity of $NaHCO_3$. May cause sodium retention especially if renal function is impaired; not to be used in treatment of peptic ulcer; use with caution in patients with CHF, edema, cirrhosis, or renal failure. Not the antacid of choice for the elderly because of sodium content and potential for systemic alkalosis.

Drug Interactions

Increased Effect/Toxicity: Increased toxicity/levels of amphetamines, ephedrine, pseudoephedrine, flecainide, quinidine, and quinine due to urinary alkalinization.

Decreased Effect: Decreased effect/levels of lithium, chlorpropamide, and salicylates due to urinary alkalinization.

Drug Uptake

Onset of action: Oral: Rapid; I.V.: 15 minutes

Absorption: Oral: Well absorbed

Duration: Oral: 8-10 minutes; I.V.: 1-2 hours

Pregnancy Risk Factor C

Generic Available Yes

Comments

Sodium content of injection 50 mL, 8.4% = 1150 mg = 50 mEq; each 6 mg of $NaHCO_3$ contains 12 mEq sodium; 1 mEq $NaHCO_3$ = 84 mg

Each 84 mg of sodium bicarbonate provides 1 mEq of sodium and bicarbonate ions; each gram of sodium bicarbonate provides 12 mEq of sodium and bicarbonate ions

Sodium Chloride (SOW dee um KLOR ide)

U.S. Brand Names Adsorbonac® [DSC]; Altamist [OTC]; Ayr® Baby Saline [OTC]; Ayr® Saline [OTC]; Breathe Free® [OTC]; Breathe Right® Saline [OTC]; Broncho Saline®; Entsol® [OTC]; Entsol® Mist [OTC]; Entsol® Single Use [OTC]; Muro 128® [OTC]; NāSal™[OTC]; Nasal Moist® [OTC]; Na-Zone® [OTC]; Ocean® [OTC];

Pediamist® [OTC]; Pretz® [OTC]; SalineX® [OTC]; SeaMist® [OTC]; Wound Wash Saline™ [OTC]

Pharmacologic Category Electrolyte Supplement, Oral; Electrolyte Supplement, Parenteral; Lubricant, Ocular; Sodium Salt

Synonyms NaCl; Normal Saline; Salt

Use

Parenteral: Restores sodium ion in patients with restricted oral intake (especially hyponatremia states or low salt syndrome). In general, parenteral saline uses:

Bacteriostatic sodium chloride: Dilution or dissolving drugs for I.M., I.V., or S.C. injections

Concentrated sodium chloride: Additive for parenteral fluid therapy

Hypertonic sodium chloride: For severe hyponatremia and hypochloremia

Hypotonic sodium chloride: Hydrating solution

Normal saline: Restores water/sodium losses

Pharmaceutical aid/diluent for infusion of compatible drug additives

Ophthalmic: Reduces corneal edema

Oral: Restores sodium losses

Inhalation: Restores moisture to pulmonary system; loosens and thins congestion caused by colds or allergies; diluent for bronchodilator solutions that require dilution before inhalation

Intranasal: Restores moisture to nasal membranes

Irrigation: Wound cleansing, irrigation, and flushing

Local Anesthetic/Vasoconstrictor Precautions No information available to require special precautions

Effects on Dental Treatment No effects or complications reported

Dosage

Children: I.V.: Hypertonic solutions (>0.9%) should only be used for the initial treatment of acute serious symptomatic hyponatremia; maintenance: 3-4 mEq/kg/day; maximum: 100-150 mEq/day; dosage varies depending on clinical condition

Replacement: Determined by laboratory determinations mEq

Sodium deficiency (mEq/kg) = [% dehydration (L/kg)/100 x 70 (mEq/L)] + [0.6 (L/kg) x (140 - serum sodium) (mEq/L)]

Children ≥2 years and Adults:

Intranasal: 2-3 sprays in each nostril as needed

Irrigation: Spray affected area

Children and Adults:

Inhalation: Bronchodilator diluent: 1-3 sprays (1-3 mL) to dilute bronchodilator solution in nebulizer prior to administration

Ophthalmic:

Ointment: Apply once daily or more often

Solution: Instill 1-2 drops into affected eye(s) every 3-4 hours

Adults:

GU irrigant: 1-3 L/day by intermittent irrigation

Heat cramps: Oral: 0.5-1 g with full glass of water, up to 4.8 g/day

Replacement I.V.: Determined by laboratory determinations mEq

Sodium deficiency (mEq/kg) = [% dehydration (L/kg)/100 x 70 (mEq/L)] + [0.6 (L/kg) x (140 - serum sodium) (mEq/L)]

To correct acute, serious hyponatremia: mEq sodium = [desired sodium (mEq/L) - actual sodium (mEq/L)] x [0.6 x wt (kg)]; for acute correction use 125 mEq/L as the desired serum sodium; acutely correct serum sodium in 5 mEq/L/dose increments; more gradual correction in increments of 10 mEq/L/day is indicated in the asymptomatic patient

Chloride maintenance electrolyte requirement in parenteral nutrition: 2-4 mEq/kg/24 hours or 25-40 mEq/1000 kcals/24 hours; maximum: 100-150 mEq/24 hours

Sodium maintenance electrolyte requirement in parenteral nutrition: 3-4 mEq/kg/24 hours or 25-40 mEq/1000 kcals/24 hours; maximum: 100-150 mEq/24 hours.

Approximate Deficits of Water and Electrolytes in Moderately Severe Dehydration

Condition	Water (mL/kg)	Sodium (mEq/kg)
Fasting and thirsting	100-120	5-7
Diarrhea		
isonatremic	100-120	8-10
hypernatremic	100-120	2-4
hyponatremic	100-120	10-12
Pyloric stenosis	100-120	8-10
Diabetic acidosis	100-120	9-10

Note: A **negative** deficit indicates total body **excess** prior to treatment.

Adapted from Behrman RE, Kleigman RM, Nelson WE, et al, eds, *Nelson Textbook of Pediatrics*, 14th ed, WB Saunders Co, 1992.

(Continued)

Sodium Chloride *(Continued)*

Mechanism of Action Principal extracellular cation; functions in fluid and electrolyte balance, osmotic pressure control, and water distribution

Other Adverse Effects 1% to 10%:

Cardiovascular: Thrombosis, hypervolemia

Endocrine & metabolic: Hypernatremia, dilution of serum electrolytes, overhydration, hypokalemia

Local: Phlebitis

Respiratory: Pulmonary edema

Miscellaneous: Congestive conditions, extravasation

Warnings/Precautions Use with caution in patients with CHF, renal insufficiency, liver cirrhosis, hypertension, edema; sodium toxicity is almost exclusively related to how fast a sodium deficit is corrected; both rate and magnitude are extremely important

Drug Interactions Lithium serum concentration may be decreased.

Drug Uptake Absorption: Oral, I.V.: Rapid

Pregnancy Risk Factor C

Generic Available Yes

Sodium Citrate and Citric Acid

(SOW dee um SIT rate & SI trik AS id)

U.S. Brand Names Bicitra®; Oracit®

Canadian Brand Names PMS-Dicitrate™

Pharmacologic Category Alkalinizing Agent

Synonyms Modified Shohl's Solution

Use Treatment of chronic metabolic acidosis; alkalinizing agent in conditions where long-term maintenance of an alkaline urine is desirable

Local Anesthetic/Vasoconstrictor Precautions No information available to require special precautions

Effects on Dental Treatment No effects or complications reported

Dosage Oral:

Infants and Children: 2-3 mEq/kg/day in divided doses 3-4 times/day **or** 5-15 mL with water after meals and at bedtime

Adults: 15-30 mL with water after meals and at bedtime

Other Adverse Effects Frequency not defined:

Central nervous system: Tetany

Endocrine & metabolic: Metabolic alkalosis, hyperkalemia

Gastrointestinal: Diarrhea, nausea, vomiting

Warnings/Precautions Conversion to bicarbonate may be impaired in patients with hepatic failure, in shock, or who are severely ill

Drug Interactions

Increased Effect/Toxicity: Increased toxicity/levels of amphetamines, ephedrine, pseudoephedrine, flecainide, quinidine, and quinine due to urinary alkalinization.

Decreased Effect: Decreased effect/levels of lithium, chlorpropamide, and salicylates due to urinary alkalinization.

Pregnancy Risk Factor Not established

Generic Available No

Comments 1 mL of Bicitra® contains 1 mEq of sodium and the equivalent of 1 mEq of bicarbonate

Sodium Citrate and Potassium Citrate Mixture

(SOW dee um SIT rate & poe TASS ee um SIT rate MIKS chur)

U.S. Brand Names Polycitra®

Pharmacologic Category Alkalinizing Agent

Synonyms Potassium Citrate Mixture and Sodium Citrate

Use Conditions where long-term maintenance of an alkaline urine is desirable as in control and dissolution of uric acid and cystine calculi of the urinary tract

Local Anesthetic/Vasoconstrictor Precautions No information available to require special precautions

Effects on Dental Treatment No effects or complications reported

Dosage Oral:

Children: 5-15 mL diluted in water after meals and at bedtime

Adults: 15-30 mL diluted in water after meals and at bedtime

Drug Interactions

Increased Effect/Toxicity: Increased toxicity/levels of amphetamines, ephedrine, pseudoephedrine, flecainide, quinidine, and quinine due to urinary alkalinization.

Decreased Effect: Decreased effect/levels of lithium, chlorpropamide, and salicylates due to urinary alkalinization.

Pregnancy Risk Factor Not established

Generic Available Yes

Sodium Hyaluronate (SOW dee um hye al yoor ON ate)

U.S. Brand Names AMO Vitrax®; Amvisc®; Amvisc® Plus; Healon®; Healon® GV; Hyalgan®

Canadian Brand Names Biolon™; Cystistat®; Eyestil; Healon®; Healon® GV; Suplasyn®

Mexican Brand Names Biolon®; Healon®

Pharmacologic Category Ophthalmic Agent, Viscoelastic

Synonyms Hyaluronic Acid

Use Surgical aid in cataract extraction, intraocular implantation, corneal transplant, glaucoma filtration, and retinal attachment surgery

Local Anesthetic/Vasoconstrictor Precautions No information available to require special precautions

Effects on Dental Treatment No effects or complications reported

Dosage Depends upon procedure (slowly introduce a sufficient quantity into eye)

Mechanism of Action Functions as a tissue lubricant and is thought to play an important role in modulating the interactions between adjacent tissues. Sodium hyaluronate is a polysaccharide which is distributed widely in the extracellular matrix of connective tissue in man. (Vitreous and aqueous humor of the eye, synovial fluid, skin, and umbilical cord.) Sodium hyaluronate forms a viscoelastic solution in water (at physiological pH and ionic strength) which makes it suitable for aqueous and vitreous humor in ophthalmic surgery.

Other Adverse Effects 1% to 10%: Ocular: Postoperative inflammatory reactions (iritis, hypopyon), corneal edema, corneal decompensation, transient postoperative increase in IOP

Drug Uptake Absorption: Following intravitreous injection, diffusion occurs slowly

Pregnancy Risk Factor C

Generic Available No

Comments Bring drug to room temperature before instillation into eye

Sodium Hypochlorite Solution

(SOW dee um hye poe KLOR ite soe LOO shun)

U.S. Brand Names Dakin's Solution

Pharmacologic Category Disinfectant, Antibacterial, Topical

Synonyms Dakin's Solution; Modified Dakin's Solution

Use Treatment of athlete's foot (0.5%); wound irrigation (0.5%); disinfect utensils and equipment (5%)

Local Anesthetic/Vasoconstrictor Precautions No information available to require special precautions

Effects on Dental Treatment No effects or complications reported

Dosage Topical irrigation

Other Adverse Effects Frequency not defined:

Dermatologic: Irritating to skin

Hematologic: Dissolves blood clots, delays clotting

Contraindications Hypersensitivity to any component of the formulation

Warnings/Precautions For external use only; avoid eye or mucous membrane contact; do not use on open wounds

Pregnancy Risk Factor C

Generic Available No

Sodium Phenylbutyrate (SOW dee um fen il BYOO ti rate)

U.S. Brand Names Buphenyl®

Pharmacologic Category Urea Cycle Disorder (UCD) Treatment Agent

Synonyms Ammonapse

Use Orphan drug: Adjunctive therapy in the chronic management of patients with urea cycle disorder involving deficiencies of carbamoylphosphate synthetase, ornithine transcarbamylase, or argininosuccinic acid synthetase

Local Anesthetic/Vasoconstrictor Precautions No information available to require special precautions

Effects on Dental Treatment No effects or complications reported

Dosage Oral:

Powder: Patients weighing <20 kg: 450-600 mg/kg/day or 9.9-13 g/m^2/day, administered in equally divided amounts with each meal or feeding, four to six times daily; safety and efficacy of doses >20 g/day has not been established

Tablet: Children >20 kg and Adults: 450-600 mg/kg/day or 9.9-13 g/m^2/day, administered in equally divided amounts with each meal; safety and efficacy of doses >20 g/day have not been established

Mechanism of Action A prodrug that, when given orally, is rapidly converted to phenylacetate, which is in turn conjugated with glutamine to form the active compound phenylacetylglutamine; phenylacetylglutamine serves as a substitute for urea and is excreted in the urine whereby it carries with it 2 moles of nitrogen per mole of phenylacetylglutamine and can thereby assist in the clearance of nitrogenous waste in patients with urea cycle disorders.

(Continued)

Sodium Phenylbutyrate *(Continued)*

Other Adverse Effects

>10%: Endocrine & metabolic: Amenorrhea, menstrual dysfunction

1% to 10%:

Gastrointestinal: Anorexia, abnormal taste

Miscellaneous: Offensive body odor

Warnings/Precautions Since no studies have been conducted in pregnant women, sodium phenylbutyrate should be used cautiously during pregnancy; each 1 gram of drug contains 125 mg of sodium and, therefore, should be used cautiously, if at all, in patients who must maintain a low sodium intake

Pregnancy Risk Factor C

Generic Available No

Sodium Phosphates (SOW dee um FOS fates)

U.S. Brand Names Fleet® Enema [OTC]; Fleet® Phospho®-Soda [OTC]; Visicol™

Canadian Brand Names Fleet Enema®; Fleet® Phospho®-Soda Oral Laxative

Pharmacologic Category Cathartic; Electrolyte Supplement, Oral; Electrolyte Supplement, Parenteral; Laxative, Bowel Evacuant

Use

Oral, rectal: Short-term treatment of constipation and to evacuate the colon for rectal and bowel exams

I.V.: Source of phosphate in large volume I.V. fluids and parenteral nutrition; treatment and prevention of hypophosphatemia

Local Anesthetic/Vasoconstrictor Precautions No information available to require special precautions

Effects on Dental Treatment No effects or complications reported

Dosage

Oral: Normal requirements elemental phosphorus:

0-6 months: Adequate intake: 100 mg/day

6-12 months: Adequate intake: 275 mg/day

1-3 years: RDA: 460 mg

4-8 years: RDA: 500 mg

9-18 years: RDA: 1250 mg

≥19 years: RDA: 700 mg

Hypophosphatemia: It is difficult to provide concrete guidelines for the treatment of severe hypophosphatemia because the extent of total body deficits and response to therapy are difficult to predict. Aggressive doses of phosphate may result in a transient serum elevation followed by redistribution into intracellular compartments or bone tissue. Intermittent I.V. infusion should be reserved for severe depletion situations (<1 mg/dL in adults); large doses of oral phosphate may cause diarrhea and intestinal absorption may be unreliable. I.V. solutions should be infused slowly. Use caution when mixing with calcium and magnesium, precipitate may form. The following dosages are empiric guidelines. **Note:** 1 mmol phosphate = 31 mg phosphorus; 1 mg phosphorus = 0.032 mmol phosphate

Hypophosphatemia treatment: Doses listed as mmol of phosphate:

Intermittent I.V. infusion: Acute repletion or replacement:

Children:

Low dose: 0.08 mmol/kg over 6 hours; use if losses are recent and uncomplicated

Intermediate dose: 0.16-0.24 mmol/kg over 4-6 hours; use if serum phosphorus level 0.5-1 mg/dL

High dose: 0.36 mmol/kg over 6 hours; use if serum phosphorus <0.5 mg/dL

Adults: Varying dosages: 0.15-0.3 mmol/kg/dose over 12 hours; may repeat as needed to achieve desired serum concentration **or**

15 mmol/dose over 2 hours; use if serum phosphorus <2 mg/dL **or**

Low dose: 0.16 mmol/kg over 4-6 hours; use if serum phosphorus level 2.3-3 mg/dL

Intermediate dose: 0.32 mmol/kg over 4-6 hours; use if serum phosphorus level 1.6-2.2 mg/dL

High dose: 0.64 mmol/kg over 8-12 hours; use if serum phosphorus <1.5 mg/dL

Oral: Adults: 0.5-1 g elemental phosphorus 2-3 times/day may be used when serum phosphorus level is 1-2.5 mg/dL

Maintenance: Doses listed as mmol of phosphate:

Children:

Oral: 2-3 mmol/kg/day in divided doses

I.V.: 0.5-1.5 mmol/kg/day

Adults:

Oral: 50-150 mmol/day in divided doses

I.V.: 50-70 mmol/day

Laxative (Fleet®): Rectal:

Children 2-<5 years: One-half contents of one 2.25 oz pediatric enema

Children 5-12 years: Contents of one 2.25 oz pediatric enema, may repeat

Children ≥12 years and Adults: Contents of one 4.5 oz enema as a single dose, may repeat

Laxative (Fleet® Phospho®-Soda): Oral: Take on an empty stomach; dilute dose with 4 ounces cool water, then follow dose with 8 ounces water; **do not repeat dose within 24 hours**

Children 5-9 years: 5-10 mL as a single dose

Children 10-12 years: 10-20 mL as a single dose

Children ≥12 years and Adults: 20-45 mL as a single dose

Bowel cleansing prior to colonoscopy (Visicol™): Oral: Adults: A total of 40 tablets divided as follows:

Evening before colonoscopy: 3 tablets every 15 minutes for 6 doses, then 2 additional tablets in 15 minutes (total of 20 tablets)

3-5 hours prior to colonoscopy: 3 tablets every 15 minutes for 6 doses, then 2 additional tablets in 15 minutes (total of 20 tablets)

Note: Each dose should be taken with a minimum of 8 ounces of clear liquids. Do not repeat treatment within 7 days. Do not use additional agents, especially sodium phosphate products.

Dosage adjustment in renal impairment: Use with caution; ionized inorganic phosphate is excreted by the kidneys; oral solution is contraindicated in patients with kidney disease

Dosage adjustment in hepatic impairment: Not expected to be metabolized in the liver

Elderly: Use with caution due to increased risk of renal impairment.

Mechanism of Action As a laxative, exerts osmotic effect in the small intestine by drawing water into the lumen of the gut, producing distention and promoting peristalsis and evacuation of the bowel; phosphorous participates in bone deposition, calcium metabolism, utilization of B complex vitamins, and as a buffer in acid-base equilibrium

Other Adverse Effects Frequency not defined:

Cardiovascular: Edema, hypotension

Central nervous system: Dizziness, headache

Endocrine & metabolic: Hypocalcemia, hypernatremia, hyperphosphatemia, calcium phosphate precipitation

Gastrointestinal: Nausea, vomiting, diarrhea, abdominal bloating, abdominal pain, mucosal bleeding, superficial mucosal ulcerations

Renal: Acute renal failure

Drug Interactions

Increased Effect/Toxicity: Increased risk of hypoglycemia with concurrent use of bisphosphonates and sodium phosphates. Intravenous preparation: Use caution with thiazide diuretics, may lead to renal damage.

Decreased Effect: Do not give with magnesium- and aluminum-containing antacids or sucralfate which can bind with phosphate. Oral preparations: May affect absorption of other medications due to rapid intestinal peristalsis and watery diarrhea caused by agent

Drug Uptake

Onset of action: Cathartic: 3-6 hours; Rectal: 2-5 minutes

Absorption: Oral: ~1% to 20%

Pregnancy Risk Factor C

Generic Available Yes

Sodium Salicylate (SOW dee um sa LIS i late)

Pharmacologic Category Salicylate

Use Treatment of minor pain or fever; arthritis

Local Anesthetic/Vasoconstrictor Precautions No information available to require special precautions

Effects on Dental Treatment No effects or complications reported

Dosage Adults: Oral: 325-650 mg every 4 hours

Mechanism of Action Inhibits prostaglandin synthesis, acts on the hypothalamus heat-regulating center to reduce fever; decreases pain receptor sensitivity. Other proposed mechanisms of action for salicylate anti-inflammatory action are lysosomal stabilization, kinin and leukotriene production, alteration of chemotactic factors, and inhibition of neutrophil activation. This latter mechanism may be the most significant pharmacologic action to reduce inflammation.

Other Adverse Effects Frequency not defined:

Dermatologic: Rash, urticaria

Gastrointestinal: Nausea, vomiting, GI distress, GI ulcers, GI bleeding

Hematologic: Platelet inhibition

Hepatic: Hepatotoxicity

Respiratory: Bronchospasm/wheezing

Drug Interactions Decreased Effect: Ammonium chloride, vitamin C (high dose), methionine, antacids, urinary alkalinizers, carbonic anhydrase inhibitors, corticosteroids, nizatidine, alcohol, ACE inhibitors, beta-blockers, loop diuretics, methotrexate, probenecid, sulfinpyrazone, spironolactone, sulfonylureas.

(Continued)

Sodium Salicylate *(Continued)*

Drug Uptake Half-life, elimination: Aspirin (dose-dependent): 15-20 minutes; Low dose (300-600 mg): 3 hours; (1 g): 5-6 hours; High dose: 15-30 hours; Therapeutic anti-inflammatory dose: 6-12 hours

Pregnancy Risk Factor C

Generic Available Yes

Comments Sodium content of 1 g: 6.25 mEq; less effective than an equal dose of aspirin in reducing pain or fever; patients hypersensitive to aspirin may be able to tolerate

Sodium Sulamyd® *see* Sulfacetamide Sodium *on page 1115*

Sodium Tetradecyl (SOW dee um tetra DEK il)

U.S. Brand Names Sotradecol®

Canadian Brand Names Trombovar®

Pharmacologic Category Sclerosing Agent

Synonyms Sodium Tetradecyl Sulfate

Use Treatment of small, uncomplicated varicose veins of the lower extremities; endoscopic sclerotherapy in the management of bleeding esophageal varices

Local Anesthetic/Vasoconstrictor Precautions No information available to require special precautions

Effects on Dental Treatment No effects or complications reported

Dosage I.V.: Test dose: 0.5 mL given several hours prior to administration of larger dose; 0.5-2 mL in each vein, maximum: 10 mL per treatment session; 3% solution reserved for large varices

Mechanism of Action Acts by irritation of the vein intimal endothelium

Other Adverse Effects Frequency not defined:

Central nervous system: Headache

Dermatologic: Discoloration at site of injection, sloughing and tissue necrosis following extravasation, ulceration at site, urticaria

Gastrointestinal: Esophageal perforation, mucosal lesions, nausea, vomiting

Local: Pain at injection site

Respiratory: Asthma, pulmonary edema

Drug Interactions Chemically **incompatible** with heparin.

Pregnancy Risk Factor C

Generic Available No

Sodium Thiosulfate (SOW dee um thye oh SUL fate)

U.S. Brand Names Tinver®

Pharmacologic Category Antidote

Use

Parenteral: Used alone or with sodium nitrite or amyl nitrite in cyanide poisoning or arsenic poisoning; reduce the risk of nephrotoxicity associated with cisplatin therapy; local infiltration (in diluted form) of selected chemotherapy extravasation

Topical: Treatment of tinea versicolor

Local Anesthetic/Vasoconstrictor Precautions No information available to require special precautions

Effects on Dental Treatment No effects or complications reported

Dosage

Cyanide and nitroprusside antidote: I.V.:

Children <25 kg: 50 mg/kg after receiving 4.5-10 mg/kg sodium nitrite; a half dose of each may be repeated if necessary

Children >25 kg and Adults: 12.5 g after 300 mg of sodium nitrite; a half dose of each may be repeated if necessary

Variation of Sodium Nitrite and Sodium Thiosulfate Dose With Hemoglobin Concentration*

Hemoglobin (g/dL)	Initial Dose Sodium Nitrite (mg/kg)	Initial Dose Sodium Nitrite 3% (mL/kg)	Initial Dose Sodium Thiosulfate 25% (mL/kg)
7	5.8	0.19	0.95
8	6.6	0.22	1.10
9	7.5	0.25	1.25
10	8.3	0.27	1.35
11	9.1	0.30	1.50
12	10.0	0.33	1.65
13	10.8	0.36	1.80
14	11.6	0.39	1.95

Adapted from Berlin DM Jr, "The Treatment of Cyanide Poisoning in Children," *Pediatrics*, 1970, 46:793.

Cyanide poisoning: I.V.: Dose should be based on determination as with nitrite, at rate of 2.5-5 mL/minute to maximum of 50 mL. See table on previous page.

Cisplatin rescue should be given before or during cisplatin administration: I.V. infusion (in sterile water): 12 g/m^2 over 6 hours or 9 g/m^2 I.V. push followed by 1.2 g/m^2 continuous infusion for 6 hours

Arsenic poisoning: I.V.: 1 mL first day, 2 mL second day, 3 mL third day, 4 mL fourth day, 5 mL on alternate days thereafter

Children and Adults: Topical: 20% to 25% solution: Apply a thin layer to affected areas twice daily

Mechanism of Action

Cyanide toxicity: Increases the rate of detoxification of cyanide by the enzyme rhodanese by providing an extra sulfur

Cisplatin toxicity: Complexes with cisplatin to form a compound that is nontoxic to either normal or cancerous cells

Other Adverse Effects 1% to 10%:

Cardiovascular: Hypotension

Central nervous system: Coma, CNS depression secondary to thiocyanate intoxication, psychosis, confusion

Dermatologic: Contact dermatitis, local irritation

Neuromuscular & skeletal: Weakness

Otic: Tinnitus

Drug Uptake Half-life, elimination: 0.65 hour

Pregnancy Risk Factor C

Generic Available Yes

Comments White, odorless crystals or powder with a salty taste; normal body burden: 1.5 mg/kg

Solagé™ *see* Mequinol and Tretinoin *on page 769*

Solaquin® [OTC] *see* Hydroquinone *on page 611*

Solaquin Forte® *see* Hydroquinone *on page 611*

Solaraze™ *see* Diclofenac *on page 378*

Solarcaine® [OTC] *see* Benzocaine *on page 151*

Solarcaine® Aloe Extra Burn Relief [OTC] *see* Lidocaine *on page 706*

Solganal® *see* Aurothioglucose *on page 133*

Solu-Cortef® *see* Hydrocortisone *on page 608*

Solu-Medrol® *see* MethylPREDNISolone *on page 797*

Solurex® *see* Dexamethasone *on page 363*

Solurex L.A.® *see* Dexamethasone *on page 363*

Soma® *see* Carisoprodol *on page 224*

Soma® Compound *see* Carisoprodol and Aspirin *on page 224*

Soma® Compound w/Codeine *see* Carisoprodol, Aspirin, and Codeine *on page 225*

Sominex® [OTC] *see* DiphenhydrAMINE *on page 398*

Sonata® *see* Zaleplon *on page 1255*

Sorbitol (SOR bi tole)

U.S. Brand Names Arlex®

Pharmacologic Category Genitourinary Irrigant; Laxative, Miscellaneous

Use Genitourinary irrigant in transurethral prostatic resection or other transurethral resection or other transurethral surgical procedures; diuretic; humectant; sweetening agent; hyperosmotic laxative; facilitate the passage of sodium polystyrene sulfonate through the intestinal tract

Local Anesthetic/Vasoconstrictor Precautions No information available to require special precautions

Effects on Dental Treatment No effects or complications reported

Dosage Hyperosmotic laxative (as single dose, at infrequent intervals):

Children 2-11 years:

- Oral: 2 mL/kg (as 70% solution)
- Rectal enema: 30-60 mL as 25% to 30% solution

Children >12 years and Adults:

- Oral: 30-150 mL (as 70% solution)
- Rectal enema: 120 mL as 25% to 30% solution
- Adjunct to sodium polystyrene sulfonate: 15 mL as 70% solution orally until diarrhea occurs (10-20 mL/2 hours) or 20-100 mL as an oral vehicle for the sodium polystyrene sulfonate resin

When administered with charcoal:

- Oral:
  - Children: 4.3 mL/kg of 35% sorbitol with 1 g/kg of activated charcoal
  - Adults: 4.3 mL/kg of 70% sorbitol with 1 g/kg of activated charcoal every 4 hours until first stool containing charcoal is passed
- Topical: 3% to 3.3% as transurethral surgical procedure irrigation

Mechanism of Action A polyalcoholic sugar with osmotic cathartic actions

Other Adverse Effects Frequency not defined:

Cardiovascular: Edema

(Continued)

Sorbitol *(Continued)*

Endocrine & metabolic: Fluid and electrolyte losses, lactic acidosis
Gastrointestinal: Diarrhea, nausea, vomiting, abdominal discomfort, xerostomia

Contraindications Anuria

Warnings/Precautions Use with caution in patients with severe cardiopulmonary or renal impairment and in patients unable to metabolize sorbitol

Drug Uptake
Onset of action: 0.25-1 hour
Absorption: Oral, rectal: Poor

Generic Available Yes

Sorbitrate® *see* Isosorbide Dinitrate *on page 661*
Sorine™ *see* Sotalol *on page 1102*

Sotalol (SOE ta lole)

Related Information
Cardiovascular Diseases *on page 1308*

U.S. Brand Names Betapace®; Betapace AF™; Sorine™

Canadian Brand Names Alti-Sotalol; Apo®-Sotalol; Betapace AF™; Gen-Sotalol; Novo-Sotalol; Nu-Sotalol; PMS-Sotalol; Rho®-Sotalol; Sotacor®

Pharmacologic Category Antiarrhythmic Agent, Class II; Antiarrhythmic Agent, Class III; Beta Blocker, Nonselective

Synonyms Sotalol Hydrochloride

Use Treatment of documented ventricular arrhythmias (ie, sustained ventricular tachycardia), that in the judgment of the physician are life-threatening; maintenance of normal sinus rhythm in patients with symptomatic atrial fibrillation and atrial flutter who are currently in sinus rhythm. Manufacturer states substitutions should not be made for Betapace AF™ since Betapace AF™ is distributed with a patient package insert specific for atrial fibrillation/flutter.

Local Anesthetic/Vasoconstrictor Precautions Use with caution; epinephrine has interacted with nonselective beta-blockers to result in initial hypertensive episode followed by bradycardia

Effects on Dental Treatment Noncardioselective beta-blockers (ie, propranolol, nadolol) enhance the pressor response to epinephrine, resulting in hypertension and bradycardia. Many nonsteroidal anti-inflammatory drugs such as ibuprofen and indomethacin can reduce the hypotensive effect of beta-blockers after 3 or more weeks of therapy with the NSAID. Short-term NSAID use (ie, 3 days) requires no special precautions in patients taking beta-blockers.

Dosage Should be initiated and doses increased in a hospital with facilities for cardiac rhythm monitoring and assessment; proarrhythmic events can occur after initiation of therapy and with each upward dosage adjustment.

Children: Oral: The safety and efficacy of sotalol in children have not been established

Note: Dosing per manufacturer, based on pediatric pharmacokinetic data; wait at least 36 hours between dosage adjustments to allow monitoring of QT intervals

Sotalol Age Factor Nomogram for Patients ≤2 Years of Age

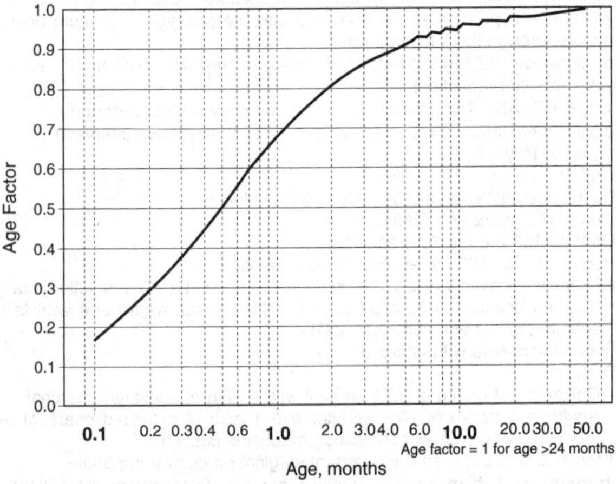

Adapted from U.S. Food and Drug Administration.
http://www.fda.gov/cder/foi/label/2001/2115s3lbl.PDF

≤2 years: Dosage should be adjusted (decreased) by plotting of the child's age on a logarithmic scale; see graph on previous page or refer to manufacturer's package labeling.

>2 years: Initial: 90 mg/m²/day in 3 divided doses; may be incrementally increased to a maximum of 180 mg/m²/day

Adults: Oral:

Ventricular arrhythmias (Betapace®, Sorine™):

Initial: 80 mg twice daily

Dose may be increased gradually to 240-320 mg/day; allow 3 days between dosing increments in order to attain steady-state plasma concentrations and to allow monitoring of QT intervals

Most patients respond to a total daily dose of 160-320 mg/day in 2-3 divided doses.

Some patients, with life-threatening refractory ventricular arrhythmias, may require doses as high as 480-640 mg/day; however, these doses should only be prescribed when the potential benefit outweighs the increased of adverse events.

Atrial fibrillation or atrial flutter (Betapace AF™): Initial: 80 mg twice daily

If the initial dose does not reduce the frequency of relapses of atrial fibrillation/flutter and is tolerated without excessive QT prolongation (not >520 msec) after 3 days, the dose may be increased to 120 mg twice daily. This may be further increased to 160 mg twice daily if response is inadequate and QT prolongation is not excessive.

Elderly: Age does not significantly alter the pharmacokinetics of sotalol, but impaired renal function in elderly patients can increase the terminal half-life, resulting in increased drug accumulation

Dosage adjustment in renal impairment:

Children: Safety and efficacy in children with renal impairment have not been established.

Adults: Impaired renal function can increase the terminal half-life, resulting in increased drug accumulation. Sotalol (Betapace AF™) is contraindicated per the manufacturer for treatment of atrial fibrillation/flutter in patients with a Cl_{cr} <40 mL/minute.

Ventricular arrhythmias (Betapace®, Sorine™):

Cl_{cr} >60 mL/minute: Administer every 12 hours
Cl_{cr} 30-60 mL/minute: Administer every 24 hours
Cl_{cr} 10-30 mL/minute: Administer every 36-48 hours
Cl_{cr} <10 mL/minute: Individualize dose

Atrial fibrillation/flutter (Betapace AF™):

Cl_{cr} >60 mL/minute: Administer every 12 hours
Cl_{cr} 40-60 mL/minute: Administer every 24 hours
Cl_{cr} <40 mL/minute: Use is contraindicated

Dialysis: Hemodialysis would be expected to reduce sotalol plasma concentrations because sotalol is not bound to plasma proteins and does not undergo extensive metabolism; administer dose postdialysis or administer supplemental 80 mg dose; peritoneal dialysis does not remove sotalol; supplemental dose is not necessary

Mechanism of Action Beta-blocker which contains both beta-adrenoreceptor-blocking (Vaughan Williams Class II) and cardiac action potential duration prolongation (Vaughan Williams Class III) properties; a racemic mixture of *d*- and *l*-sotalol; both isomers have similar Class III antiarrhythmic effects while the *l*-isomer is responsible for virtually all of the beta-blocking activity. The beta-blocking effect of sotalol is a noncardioselective [half maximal at about 80 mg/day and maximal at doses of 320-640 mg/day]. Significant beta-blockade occurs at oral doses as low as 25 mg/day.

Class II effects: Increased sinus cycle length, slowed heart rate, decreased AV nodal conduction, and increased AV nodal refractoriness

Class III effects: Prolongation of the atrial and ventricular monophasic action potentials, and effective refractory prolongation of atrial muscle, ventricular muscle, and atrioventricular accessory pathways in both the antegrade and retrograde directions (Class III effects are seen only at oral doses ≥160 mg/day).

Other Adverse Effects

>10%:

Cardiovascular: Bradycardia (16%), chest pain (16%), palpitations (14%)
Central nervous system: Fatigue (20%), dizziness (20%), lightheadedness (12%)
Neuromuscular & skeletal: Weakness (13%)
Respiratory: Dyspnea (21%)

1% to 10%:

Cardiovascular: Congestive heart failure (5%), peripheral vascular disorders (3%), edema (8%), abnormal EKG (7%), hypotension (6%), proarrhythmia (5%), syncope (5%)

Central nervous system: Mental confusion (6%), anxiety (4%), headache (8%), sleep problems (8%), depression (4%)

(Continued)

Sotalol *(Continued)*

Dermatologic: Itching/rash (5%)
Endocrine & metabolic: Decreased sexual ability (3%)
Gastrointestinal: Diarrhea (7%), nausea/vomiting (10%), stomach discomfort (3% to 6%), flatulence (2%)
Genitourinary: Impotence (2%)
Hematologic: Bleeding (2%)
Neuromuscular & skeletal: Paresthesia (4%), extremity pain (7%), back pain (3%)
Ocular: Visual problems (5%)
Respiratory: Upper respiratory problems (5% to 8%), asthma (2%)

Drug Interactions

Increased Effect/Toxicity: Increased effect/toxicity of beta-blockers with calcium blockers since there may be additive effects on AV conduction or ventricular function. Sotalol in combination with amiodarone. Other agents which prolong QT interval, including Class I antiarrhythmic agents, bepridil, cisapride (use is contraindicated), erythromycin, haloperidol, pimozide, phenothiazines, tricyclic antidepressants, specific quinolones (sparfloxacin, gatifloxacin, moxifloxacin), terfenadine, or astemizole may increase the effect of sotalol on the prolongation of QT interval. When used concurrently with clonidine, sotalol may increase the risk of rebound hypertension after or during withdrawal of either agent. Beta-blocker and catecholamine depleting agents (reserpine or guanethidine) may result in additive hypotension or bradycardia. Beta-blockers may increase the action or levels of nondepolarizing muscle relaxants, and theophylline although the effects are difficult to predict.

Decreased Effect: Decreased effect of sotalol may occur with aluminum-magnesium antacids (if taken within 2 hours), aluminum salts, barbiturates, calcium salts, cholestyramine, colestipol, NSAIDs, penicillins (ampicillin), rifampin, salicylates, and sulfinpyrazone due to decreased bioavailability and plasma concentrations. Beta-blockers may decrease the effect of sulfonylureas. Beta-agonists such as albuterol, terbutaline may have less of a therapeutic effect when administered concomitantly.

Drug Uptake

Onset of action: Rapid, 1-2 hours; Peak effect: 2.5-4 hours
Absorption: Decreased 20% to 30% by meals compared to fasting
Duration: 8-16 hours
Half-life, elimination: 12 hours (9.5 hours in children); terminal half-life decreases with age <2 years (may by ≥1 week in neonates)

Pregnancy Risk Factor B

Generic Available Yes: Betapace®

Selected Readings

Foster CA and Aston SJ, "Propranolol-Epinephrine Interaction: A Potential Disaster," *Plast Reconstr Surg*, 1983, 72(1):74-8.
Wong DG, Spence JD, Lamki L, et al, "Effect of Nonsteroidal Anti-inflammatory Drugs on Control of Hypertension of Beta-Blockers and Diuretics," *Lancet*, 1986, 1(8488):997-1001.
Wynn RL, "Dental Nonsteroidal Anti-inflammatory Drugs and Prostaglandin-Based Drug Interactions, Part Two," *Gen Dent*, 1992, 40(2):104, 106, 108.
Wynn RL, "Epinephrine Interactions With Beta-Blockers," *Gen Dent*, 1994, 42(1):16, 18.

Sotradecol® *see* Sodium Tetradecyl *on page 1100*
Soyacal® *see* Fat Emulsion *on page 487*
Spacol *see* Hyoscyamine *on page 617*
Spacol T/S *see* Hyoscyamine *on page 617*
Span-FF® *see* Ferrous Fumarate *on page 497*

Sparfloxacin (spar FLOKS a sin)

U.S. Brand Names Zagam®

Pharmacologic Category Antibiotic, Quinolone

Use Treatment of adult patients with community acquired pneumonia caused by susceptible strains of *Chlamydia pneumoniae, Haemophilus influenzae, Haemophilus parainfluenzae, Moraxella catarrhalis, Mycoplasma pneumoniae*, or *Streptococcus pneumoniae* and acute bacterial exacerbations of acute bronchitis caused by susceptible strains of *Chlamydia pneumoniae, Enterobacter cloacae, Haemophilus influenzae, Haemophilus parainfluenzae, Klebsiella pneumoniae, Moraxella catarrhalis, Staphylococcus aureus*, or *Streptococcus pneumoniae*

Local Anesthetic/Vasoconstrictor Precautions No information available to require special precautions

Effects on Dental Treatment No effects or complications reported

Dosage Adults: Oral:

Loading dose: 2 tablets (400 mg) on day 1
Maintenance: 1 tablet (200 mg) daily for 10 additional days (total 11 tablets)

Mechanism of Action Inhibits DNA-gyrase in susceptible organisms; inhibits relaxation of supercoiled DNA and promotes breakage of double-stranded DNA

Other Adverse Effects

1% to 10%:

Cardiovascular: QT_c interval prolongation (1.3%)

Central nervous system: Insomnia, dizziness, headache, agitation, sleep disorders, anxiety, delirium

Dermatologic: Photosensitivity reaction, pruritus, vasodilatation

Gastrointestinal: Diarrhea, dyspepsia, nausea, abdominal pain, vomiting, flatulence, taste perversion, xerostomia

Hematologic: Leukopenia, eosinophilia, anemia

Hepatic: Increased LFTs

Warnings/Precautions Not recommended in children <18 years of age, other quinolones have caused transient arthropathy in children; CNS stimulation may occur (tremor, restlessness, confusion, and very rarely hallucinations or seizures); use with caution in patients with known or suspected CNS disorder or renal dysfunction; prolonged use may result in superinfection; if an allergic reaction (itching, urticaria, dyspnea, pharyngeal or facial edema, loss of consciousness, tingling, cardiovascular collapse) occurs, discontinue the drug immediately; use caution to avoid possible photosensitivity reactions during and for several days following fluoroquinolone therapy; pseudomembranous colitis may occur and should be considered in patients who present with diarrhea

Drug Interactions

Increased Effect/Toxicity: Quinolones cause increased levels of caffeine, warfarin, cyclosporine, and theophylline (although one study indicates that sparfloxacin may not affect theophylline metabolism). Cimetidine, and probenecid increase quinolone levels. An increased incidence of seizures may occur with foscarnet and NSAIDs. Sparfloxacin does not appear to alter warfarin levels, but warfarin effect may be increased due possible effects on GI flora.

Decreased Effect: Decreased absorption with antacids containing aluminum, didanosine (chewable/buffered tablets or pediatric powder for oral solution), magnesium, zinc, iron and/or calcium (by up to 98% if given at the same time). Phenytoin serum concentration may be reduced by quinolones. Antineoplastic agents may also decrease serum concentration of fluoroquinolones.

Drug Uptake

Absorption: Slow and erratic; unaffected by food or milk; reduced by ~50% by concurrent administration of aluminum- and magnesium-containing antacids

Half-life, elimination: Mean terminal: 20 hours (range: 16-30 hours)

Time to peak: 3-5 hours

Pregnancy Risk Factor C

Generic Available No

Sparine® *see* Promazine *on page 1004*

Spectazole™ *see* Econazole *on page 427*

Spectinomycin (spek ti noe MYE sin)

Related Information

Nonviral Infectious Diseases *on page 1342*

U.S. Brand Names Trobicin®

Mexican Brand Names Trobicin®

Pharmacologic Category Antibiotic, Miscellaneous

Synonyms Spectinomycin Hydrochloride

Use Treatment of uncomplicated gonorrhea (ineffective against syphilis)

Local Anesthetic/Vasoconstrictor Precautions No information available to require special precautions

Effects on Dental Treatment No effects or complications reported

Dosage I.M.:

Children:

<45 kg: 40 mg/kg/dose 1 time

≥45 kg: See adult dose

Children >8 years who are allergic to PCNS/cephalosporins may be treated with oral tetracycline

Adults:

Uncomplicated urethral endocervical or rectal gonorrhea: 2 g deep I.M. or 4 g where antibiotic resistance is prevalent 1 time; 4 g (10 mL) dose should be given as two 5 mL injections, followed by doxycycline 100 mg twice daily for 7 days

Disseminated gonococcal infection: 2 g every 12 hours

Mechanism of Action A bacteriostatic antibiotic that selectively binds to the 30s subunits of ribosomes, and thereby inhibiting bacterial protein synthesis

Warnings/Precautions Since spectinomycin is ineffective in the treatment of syphilis and may mask symptoms, all patients should be tested for syphilis at the time of diagnosis and 3 months later.

Drug Uptake

Absorption: I.M.: Rapid and almost completely

Duration: ≤8 hours

Half-life, elimination: 1.7 hours

Time to peak: ≤1 hour

Pregnancy Risk Factor B

Generic Available No

Spectracef™ *see* Cefditoren *on page 235*

Spectrocin Plus® [OTC] *see* Bacitracin, Neomycin, Polymyxin B, and Lidocaine *on page 142*

Spiramycin *Not Available in U.S.* (speer a MYE sin)

Canadian Brand Names Rovamycine®

Pharmacologic Category Antibiotic, Macrolide

Use Treatment of infections of the respiratory tract, buccal cavity, skin and soft tissues due to susceptible organisms. *N. gonorrhoeae*: as an alternate choice of treatment for gonorrhea in patients allergic to the penicillins. Before treatment of gonorrhea, the possibility of concomitant infection due to *T. pallidum* should be excluded.

Unlabeled/Investigational: Treatment of *Toxoplasma gondii* to prevent transmission from mother to fetus

Local Anesthetic/Vasoconstrictor Precautions No information available to require special precautions

Effects on Dental Treatment No effects or complications reported

Dosage Oral:

Children: Dosage by body weight; usual dosage 150,000 int. units/kg; expressed as the number of 750,000 int. unit (Rovamycine® "250") capsules per day. Daily dose should be administered in 2-3 divided doses.

15 kg = 3 capsules per day
20 kg = 4 capsules per day
30 kg = 6 capsules per day

Note: In severe infections, dosage may be increased by 50%.

Adults:

Mild to moderate infections: 6,000,000 to 9,000,000 int. units (4-6 capsules of Rovamycine® "500" per day) in 2 divided doses

Severe infections: 12,000,000 to 15,000,000 int. units (8-10 capsules of Rovamycine® "500" per day) in 2 divided doses

Gonorrhea: 12,000,000 to 13,500,000 int. units (8-9 capsules of Rovamycine® "500") as a single dose

Mechanism of Action Inhibits growth of susceptible organisms; mechanism not established.

Other Adverse Effects Rare adverse reactions associated with other macrolide antibiotics include life-threatening ventricular arrhythmias, prolongation of QT_c, and neuromuscular blockade.

Frequency not defined:

Central nervous system: Paresthesia (rare)
Dermatologic: Rash, urticaria, pruritus, angioedema (rare)
Gastrointestinal: Nausea, vomiting, diarrhea, pseudomembranous colitis (rare)
Hepatic: Transaminases increased
Miscellaneous: Anaphylactic shock (rare)

Drug Interactions Decreased Effect: Reported to decrease carbidopa absorption and decrease levodopa concentrations.

Pregnancy Risk Factor Not assigned (other macrolides rated B); C per expert analysis

Generic Available No

Spironolactone (speer on oh LAK tone)

Related Information

Cardiovascular Diseases *on page 1308*

U.S. Brand Names Aldactone®

Canadian Brand Names Aldactone®; Novo-Spiroton

Mexican Brand Names Aldactone®

Pharmacologic Category Diuretic, Potassium Sparing

Use Management of edema associated with excessive aldosterone excretion; hypertension; primary hyperaldosteronism; hypokalemia; treatment of hirsutism; cirrhosis of liver accompanied by edema or ascites. The benefits of spironolactone were additive to the benefits of angiotensin-converting enzyme inhibition in patients with severe CHF (further reducing mortality by 30% over 2 years) in RALES - a large controlled clinical trial.

Local Anesthetic/Vasoconstrictor Precautions No information available to require special precautions

Effects on Dental Treatment No effects or complications reported

Dosage Administration with food increases absorption. To reduce delay in onset of effect, a loading dose of 2 or 3 times the daily dose may be administered on the first day of therapy.

Oral:

Children:

Diuretic, hypertension: 1.5-3.5 mg/kg/day in divided doses every 6-24 hours
Diagnosis of primary aldosteronism: 125-375 mg/m²/day in divided doses
Vaso-occlusive disease: 7.5 mg/kg/day in divided doses twice daily (not FDA approved)

Adults:

Edema, hypertension, hypokalemia: 25-200 mg/day in 1-2 divided doses

Diagnosis of primary aldosteronism: 100-400 mg/day in 1-2 divided doses

CHF, patients with severe heart failure already using an ACE inhibitor and a loop diuretic ± digoxin: 25 mg/day, increased or reduced depending on individual response and evidence of hyperkalemia

Elderly: Initial: 25-50 mg/day in 1-2 divided doses, increasing by 25-50 mg every 5 days as needed

Mechanism of Action Competes with aldosterone for receptor sites in the distal renal tubules, increasing sodium chloride and water excretion while conserving potassium and hydrogen ions; may block the effect of aldosterone on arteriolar smooth muscle as well

Other Adverse Effects Incidence of adverse events is not always reported. (Mean daily dose: 26 mg)

Cardiovascular: Edema (2%, placebo 2%)

Central nervous system: Disorders (23%, placebo 21%) which may include drowsiness, lethargy, headache, mental confusion, drug fever, ataxia, fatigue

Dermatologic: Maculopapular, erythematous cutaneous eruptions, urticaria, hirsutism, eosinophilia

Endocrine & metabolic: Gynecomastia (men 9%; placebo 1%), breast pain (men 2%; placebo 0.1%), serious hyperkalemia (2%, placebo 1%), hyponatremia, dehydration, hyperchloremic metabolic acidosis in decompensated hepatic cirrhosis, inability to achieve or maintain an erection, irregular menses, amenorrhea, postmenopausal bleeding

Gastrointestinal: Disorders (29%, placebo 29%) which may include anorexia, nausea, cramping, diarrhea, gastric bleeding, ulceration, gastritis, vomiting

Genitourinary: Disorders (12%, placebo 11%)

Hematologic: Agranulocytosis

Hepatic: Cholestatic/hepatocellular toxicity

Renal: Increased BUN concentration

Respiratory: Disorders (32%, placebo 34%)

Miscellaneous: Deepening of the voice, anaphylactic reaction, breast cancer

Drug Interactions

Increased Effect/Toxicity: Concurrent use of spironolactone with other potassium-sparing diuretics, potassium supplements, angiotensin-receptor antagonists, co-trimoxazole (high dose), and angiotensin-converting enzyme inhibitors can increase the risk of hyperkalemia, especially in patients with renal impairment. Cholestyramine can cause hyperchloremic acidosis in cirrhotic patients; avoid concurrent use.

Decreased Effect: The effects of digoxin (loss of positive inotropic effect) and mitotane may be reduced by spironolactone. Salicylates and NSAIDs (indomethacin) may decrease the natriuretic effect of spironolactone.

Drug Uptake

Half-life, elimination: 78-84 minutes

Time to peak: 1-3 hours (primarily as the active metabolite)

Pregnancy Risk Factor D

Generic Available Yes

Sporanox® *see* Itraconazole *on page 666*

Sportscreme® [OTC] *see* Triethanolamine Salicylate *on page 1204*

SSD® AF *see* Silver Sulfadiazine *on page 1088*

SSD® Cream *see* Silver Sulfadiazine *on page 1088*

SSKI® *see* Potassium Iodide *on page 980*

Stadol® *see* Butorphanol *on page 195*

Stadol® NS *see* Butorphanol *on page 195*

Stagesic® *see* Hydrocodone and Acetaminophen *on page 598*

Stanozolol (stan OH zoe lole)

U.S. Brand Names Winstrol®

Pharmacologic Category Anabolic Steroid

Use Prophylactic use against hereditary angioedema

Local Anesthetic/Vasoconstrictor Precautions No information available to require special precautions

Effects on Dental Treatment No effects or complications reported

Restrictions C-III

Dosage

Children: Acute attacks:

<6 years: 1 mg/day

6-12 years: 2 mg/day

Adults: Oral: Initial: 2 mg 3 times/day, may then reduce to a maintenance dose of 2 mg/day or 2 mg every other day after 1-3 months

Mechanism of Action Synthetic testosterone derivative with similar androgenic and anabolic actions

(Continued)

Stanozolol *(Continued)*

Other Adverse Effects

Male:

Postpubertal:

>10%:

Dermatologic: Acne

Endocrine & metabolic: Gynecomastia

Genitourinary: Bladder irritability, priapism

1% to 10%:

Central nervous system: Insomnia, chills

Endocrine & metabolic: Decreased libido, hepatic dysfunction

Gastrointestinal: Nausea, diarrhea

Genitourinary: Prostatic hyperplasia (elderly)

Hematologic: Iron-deficiency anemia, suppression of clotting factors

Prepubertal:

>10%:

Dermatologic: Acne

Endocrine & metabolic: Virilism

1% to 10%:

Central nervous system: Chills, insomnia, factors

Dermatologic: Hyperpigmentation

Gastrointestinal: Diarrhea, nausea

Hematologic: Iron deficiency anemia, suppression of clotting

Female:

>10%: Endocrine & metabolic: Virilism

1% to 10%:

Central nervous system: Chills, insomnia

Endocrine & metabolic: Hypercalcemia

Gastrointestinal: Nausea, diarrhea

Hematologic: Iron deficiency anemia, suppression of clotting factors

Hepatic: Hepatic dysfunction

Drug Interactions Increased Effect/Toxicity: ACTH, adrenal steroids may increase risk of edema and acne. Stanozolol enhances the hypoprothrombinemic effects of oral anticoagulants and enhances the hypoglycemic effects of insulin and sulfonylureas (oral hypoglycemics).

Pregnancy Risk Factor X

Generic Available No

Staticin® *see* Erythromycin, Topical *on page 454*

Stat Touch 2 [OTC] *see* Chlorhexidine Gluconate *on page 263*

Stavudine (STAV yoo deen)

Related Information

HIV Infection and AIDS *on page 1334*

U.S. Brand Names Zerit®

Canadian Brand Names Zerit®

Mexican Brand Names Zerit®

Pharmacologic Category Antiretroviral Agent, Reverse Transcriptase Inhibitor (Nucleoside)

Synonyms d4T

Use For the treatment of adults with advanced HIV infection who are intolerant to approved therapies with proven clinical benefit or who have experienced significant clinical or immunologic deterioration while receiving these therapies, or for whom such therapies are contraindicated

Local Anesthetic/Vasoconstrictor Precautions No information available to require special precautions

Effects on Dental Treatment No effects or complications reported

Dosage Oral:

Newborns (Birth to 13 days): 0.5 mg/kg every 12 hours

Children:

>14 days and <30 kg: 1 mg/kg every 12 hours

≥30 kg: 30 mg every 12 hours

Adults:

≥60 kg: 40 mg every 12 hours

<60 kg: 30 mg every 12 hours

Dose may be cut in half if symptoms of peripheral neuropathy occur

Dosing adjustment in renal impairment:

Cl_{cr} >50 mL/minute:

≥60 kg: 40 mg every 12 hours

<60 kg: 30 mg every 12 hours

Cl_{cr} 26-50 mL/minute:

≥60 kg: 20 mg every 12 hours

<60 kg: 15 mg every 12 hours

Hemodialysis:

≥60 kg: 20 mg every 24 hours

<60 kg: 15 mg every 24 hours

Elderly: Older patients should be closely monitored for signs and symptoms of peripheral neuropathy; dosage should be carefully adjusted to renal function.

Mechanism of Action A thymidine analog which interferes with HIV viral DNA dependent DNA polymerase resulting in inhibition of viral replication; nucleoside reverse transcriptase inhibitor

Other Adverse Effects All adverse reactions reported below were similar to comparative agent, zidovudine, except for peripheral neuropathy, which was greater for stavudine.

>10%:

Central nervous system: Headache, chills/fever, malaise, insomnia, anxiety, depression, pain

Dermatologic: Rash

Gastrointestinal: Nausea, vomiting, diarrhea, pancreatitis, abdominal pain

Neuromuscular & skeletal: Peripheral neuropathy (15% to 21%)

1% to 10%:

Hematologic: Neutropenia, thrombocytopenia

Hepatic: Increased hepatic transaminases, increased bilirubin

Neuromuscular & skeletal: Myalgia, back pain, weakness

Drug Interactions Increased Effect/Toxicity: Drugs associated with peripheral neuropathy (chloramphenicol, cisplatin, dapsone, ethionamide, gold, hydralazine, iodoquinol, isoniazid, lithium, metronidazole, nitrofurantoin, pentamidine, phenytoin, ribavirin, vincristine) may increase risk for stavudine peripheral neuropathy. Risk of neuropathy, pancreatitis, or lactic acidosis and severe hepatomegaly is increased with concurrent use of didanosine and hydroxyurea.

Drug Uptake

Half-life, elimination: 1-1.6 hours

Time to peak: 1 hour

Pregnancy Risk Factor C

Generic Available No

S-T Cort® *see* Hydrocortisone *on page 608*

Stelazine® *see* Trifluoperazine *on page 1204*

Stilphostrol® *see* Diethylstilbestrol *on page 385*

Stimate™ *see* Desmopressin Acetate *on page 361*

St. Joseph® Cough Suppressant [OTC] *see* Dextromethorphan *on page 372*

St. Joseph® Pain Reliever [OTC] *see* Aspirin *on page 119*

Stop® [OTC] *see* Fluoride *on page 514*

Streptase® *see* Streptokinase *on page 1109*

Streptokinase (strep toe KYE nase)

Related Information

Cardiovascular Diseases *on page 1308*

U.S. Brand Names Streptase®

Canadian Brand Names Kabikinase®; Streptase®

Mexican Brand Names Streptase®

Pharmacologic Category Thrombolytic Agent

Synonyms SK

Use Thrombolytic agent used in treatment of recent severe or massive deep vein thrombosis, pulmonary emboli, myocardial infarction, and occluded arteriovenous cannulas

Local Anesthetic/Vasoconstrictor Precautions No information available to require special precautions

Effects on Dental Treatment No effects or complications reported

Dosage I.V.:

Children: Safety and efficacy have not been not established. Limited studies have used 3500-4000 units/kg over 30 minutes followed by 1000-1500 units/kg/hour.

Clotted catheter: 25,000 units, clamp for 2 hours then aspirate contents and flush with normal saline.

Adults: Antibodies to streptokinase remain for at least 3-6 months after initial dose:

Administration requires the use of an infusion pump.

An intradermal skin test of 100 units has been suggested to predict allergic response to streptokinase. If a positive reaction is not seen after 15-20 minutes, a therapeutic dose may be administered.

Guidelines for acute myocardial infarction (AMI): 1.5 million units over 60 minutes

Administration:

Dilute two 750,000 unit vials of streptokinase with 5 mL dextrose 5% in water (D_5W) each, gently swirl to dissolve.

Add this dose of the 1.5 million units to 150 mL D_5W.

This should be infused over 60 minutes; an in-line filter ≥0.45 micron should be used.

(Continued)

Streptokinase *(Continued)*

Monitor for the first few hours for signs of anaphylaxis or allergic reaction. **Infusion should be slowed if lowering of 25 mm Hg in BP or terminated if asthmatic symptoms appear.**

Begin heparin 5000-10,000 unit bolus followed by 1000 units/hour ~ 3-4 hours after completion of streptokinase infusion or when PTT is <100 seconds.

Guidelines for acute pulmonary embolism (APE): 3 million unit dose over 24 hours

Administration:

Dilute four 750,000 unit vials of streptokinase with 5 mL dextrose 5% in water (D_5W) each, gently swirl to dissolve.

Add this dose of 3 million units to 250 mL D_5W, an in-line filter ≥0.45 micron should be used.

Administer 250,000 units (23 mL) over 30 minutes followed by 100,000 units/hour (9 mL/hour) for 24 hours.

Monitor for the first few hours for signs of anaphylaxis or allergic reaction. **Infusion should be slowed if BP is lowered by 25 mm Hg or if asthmatic symptoms appear.**

Begin heparin 1000 units/hour about 3-4 hours after completion of streptokinase infusion or when PTT is <100 seconds.

Monitor PT, PTT, and fibrinogen levels during therapy.

Thromboses: 250,000 units to start, then 100,000 units/hour for 24-72 hours depending on location.

Cannula occlusion: 250,000 units into cannula, clamp for 2 hours, then aspirate contents and flush with normal saline; **Not recommended; see Comments**

Mechanism of Action Activates the conversion of plasminogen to plasmin by forming a complex, exposing plasminogen-activating site, and cleaving a peptide bond that converts plasminogen to plasmin; plasmin degrades fibrin, fibrinogen and other procoagulant proteins into soluble fragments; effective both outside and within the formed thrombus/embolus

Other Adverse Effects As with all drugs which may affect hemostasis, bleeding is the major adverse effect associated with streptokinase. Hemorrhage may occur at virtually any site. Risk is dependent on multiple variables, including the dosage administered, concurrent use of multiple agents which alter hemostasis, and patient predisposition (including hypertension). Rapid lysis of coronary artery thrombi by thrombolytic agents may be associated with reperfusion-related atrial and/or ventricular arrhythmias.

>10%:

Cardiovascular: Hypotension
Local: Injection site bleeding

1% to 10%:

Central nervous system: Fever (1% to 4%)
Dermatologic: Bruising, rash, pruritus
Gastrointestinal: Gastrointestinal hemorrhage, nausea, vomiting
Genitourinary: Genitourinary hemorrhage
Hematologic: Anemia
Neuromuscular & skeletal: Muscle pain
Ocular: Eye hemorrhage, periorbital edema
Respiratory: Bronchospasm, epistaxis
Miscellaneous: Diaphoresis

Additional cardiovascular events associated with use in myocardial infarction: AV block, cardiogenic shock, heart failure, cardiac arrest, recurrent ischemia/infarction, myocardial rupture, electromechanical dissociation, pericardial effusion, pericarditis, mitral regurgitation, cardiac tamponade, thromboembolism, pulmonary edema, asystole, ventricular tachycardia

Drug Interactions

Increased Effect/Toxicity: The risk of bleeding with streptokinase is increased by oral anticoagulants (warfarin), heparin, low molecular weight heparins, and drugs which affect platelet function (eg, NSAIDs, dipyridamole, ticlopidine, clopidogrel, IIb/IIIa antagonists). Although concurrent use with aspirin and heparin may increase the risk of bleeding. Aspirin and heparin were used concomitantly with streptokinase in the majority of patients in clinical studies of MI.

Decreased Effect: Antifibrinolytic agents (aminocaproic acid) may decrease effectiveness to thrombolytic agents.

Drug Uptake

Onset of action: Activation of plasminogen occurs almost immediately
Duration: Fibrinolytic effect: Several hours; Anticoagulant effect: 12-24 hours
Half-life, elimination: 83 minutes

Pregnancy Risk Factor C

Generic Available No

Comments Avoid I.M. injections; use with caution in patients >75 years of age, patients with a history of cardiac arrhythmias, septic thrombophlebitis or occluded A-V cannula at seriously infected site, patients with a high likelihood of left heart thrombus, (eg, mitral stenosis with atrial fibrillation), major surgery within last 10 days, GI bleeding, diabetic hemorrhagic retinopathy, subacute bacterial endocarditis, cerebrovascular disease, recent trauma including cardiopulmonary resuscitation, or severe hypertension (systolic BP >180 mm Hg and/or diastolic BP >110 mm Hg); antibodies to streptokinase remain for 3-6 months after initial dose, use another thrombolytic enzyme (ie, alteplase) if thrombolytic therapy is indicated in patients with prior streptokinase therapy

Streptokinase is not indicated for restoration of patency of intravenous catheters. Serious adverse events relating to the use of streptokinase in the restoration of patency of occluded intravenous catheters have involved the use of high doses of streptokinase in small volumes (250,000 international units in 2 mL). Uses of lower doses of streptokinase in infusions over several hours, generally into partially occluded catheters, or local instillation into the catheter lumen and subsequent aspiration, have been described in the medical literature. Healthcare providers should consider the risk for potentially life-threatening reactions (eg, hypotension, hypersensitivity reactions, apnea, bleeding) associated with the use of streptokinase in the management of occluded intravenous catheters.

Streptomycin (strep toe MYE sin)

Related Information

Nonviral Infectious Diseases *on page 1342*

Pharmacologic Category Antibiotic, Aminoglycoside; Antitubercular Agent

Synonyms Streptomycin Sulfate

Use Combination therapy of active tuberculosis; used in combination with other agents for treatment of streptococcal or enterococcal endocarditis, mycobacterial infections, plague, tularemia, and brucellosis. Streptomycin is indicated for persons from endemic areas of drug-resistant *Mycobacterium tuberculosis* or who are HIV infected.

Local Anesthetic/Vasoconstrictor Precautions No information available to require special precautions

Effects on Dental Treatment No effects or complications reported

Dosage Intramuscular (may also be given I.V. piggyback):

Tuberculosis therapy: **Note:** A four-drug regimen (isoniazid, rifampin, pyrazinamide and either streptomycin or ethambutol) is preferred for the initial, empiric treatment of TB. When the drug susceptibility results are available, the regimen should be altered as appropriate.

Patients with TB and without HIV infection:

OPTION 1:

Isoniazid resistance rate <4%: Administer daily isoniazid, rifampin, and pyrazinamide for 8 weeks followed by isoniazid and rifampin daily or directly observed therapy (DOT) 2-3 times/week for 16 weeks

If isoniazid resistance rate is not documented, ethambutol or streptomycin should also be administered until susceptibility to isoniazid or rifampin is demonstrated. Continue treatment for at least 6 months or 3 months beyond culture conversion.

OPTION 2: Administer daily isoniazid, rifampin, pyrazinamide, and either streptomycin or ethambutol for 2 weeks followed by DOT 2 times/week administration of the same drugs for 6 weeks, and subsequently, with isoniazid and rifampin DOT 2 times/week administration for 16 weeks

OPTION 3: Administer isoniazid, rifampin, pyrazinamide, and either ethambutol or streptomycin by DOT 3 times/week for 6 months

Patients with TB and with HIV infection: Administer any of the above OPTIONS 1, 2 or 3, however, treatment should be continued for a total of 9 months and at least 6 months beyond culture conversion

Some experts recommend that the duration of therapy should be extended to 9 months for patients with disseminated disease, miliary disease, disease involving the bones or joints, or tuberculosis lymphadenitis

Children:

Daily therapy: 20-30 mg/kg/day (maximum: 1 g/day)

Directly observed therapy (DOT): Twice weekly: 25-30 mg/kg (maximum: 1.5 g)

DOT: 3 times/week: 25-30 mg/kg (maximum: 1 g)

Adults:

Daily therapy: 15 mg/kg/day (maximum: 1 g)

Directly observed therapy (DOT): Twice weekly: 25-30 mg/kg (maximum: 1.5 g)

DOT: 3 times/week: 25-30 mg/kg (maximum: 1 g)

Enterococcal endocarditis: 1 g every 12 hours for 2 weeks, 500 mg every 12 hours for 4 weeks in combination with penicillin

Streptococcal endocarditis: 1 g every 12 hours for 1 week, 500 mg every 12 hours for 1 week

Tularemia: 1-2 g/day in divided doses for 7-10 days or until patient is afebrile for 5-7 days

Plague: 2-4 g/day in divided doses until the patient is afebrile for at least 3 days

Elderly: 10 mg/kg/day, not to exceed 750 mg/day; dosing interval should be adjusted for renal function; some authors suggest not to give >5 days/week or give as 20-25 mg/kg/dose twice weekly

(Continued)

Streptomycin *(Continued)*

Mechanism of Action Inhibits bacterial protein synthesis by binding directly to the 30S ribosomal subunits causing faulty peptide sequence to form in the protein chain

Other Adverse Effects Frequency not defined:

Cardiovascular: Hypotension

Central nervous system: Neurotoxicity, drowsiness, headache, drug fever, paresthesia

Dermatologic: Skin rash

Gastrointestinal: Nausea, vomiting

Hematologic: Eosinophilia, anemia

Neuromuscular & skeletal: Arthralgia, weakness, tremor

Otic: Ototoxicity (auditory), ototoxicity (vestibular)

Renal: Nephrotoxicity

Respiratory: Difficulty in breathing

Drug Interactions Increased Effect/Toxicity: Increased/prolonged effect with depolarizing and nondepolarizing neuromuscular blocking agents. Concurrent use with amphotericin or loop diuretics may increase nephrotoxicity.

Drug Uptake

Absorption: I.M.: Well absorbed

Half-life, elimination: Newborns: 4-10 hours; Adults: 2-4.7 hours (increases with renal impairment)

Time to peak: ≤1 hour

Pregnancy Risk Factor D

Generic Available Yes

Streptozocin (strep toe ZOE sin)

U.S. Brand Names Zanosar®

Canadian Brand Names Zanosar®

Pharmacologic Category Antineoplastic Agent, Alkylating Agent

Use Treatment of metastatic islet cell carcinoma of the pancreas, carcinoid tumor and syndrome, Hodgkin's disease, palliative treatment of colorectal cancer

Local Anesthetic/Vasoconstrictor Precautions No information available to require special precautions

Effects on Dental Treatment No effects or complications reported

Mechanism of Action Interferes with the normal function of DNA by alkylation and cross-linking the strands of DNA, and by possible protein modification

Other Adverse Effects

>10%:

- Gastrointestinal: Nausea and vomiting in all patients usually 1-4 hours after infusion; diarrhea in 10% of patients; increased LFTs and hypoalbuminemia
  - Emetic potential: High (>90%)
  - Time course of nausea/vomiting: Onset 1-3 hours; Duration: 1-12 hours
- Renal: Renal dysfunction occurs in 65% of patients; proteinuria, decreased Cl_{cr}, increased BUN, hypophosphatemia, and renal tubular acidosis; use caution with patients on other nephrotoxic agents; nephrotoxicity (25% to 75% of patients)

1% to 10%:

- Endocrine & metabolic: Hypoglycemia: Seen in 6% of patients; may be prevented with the administration of nicotinamide
- Gastrointestinal: Diarrhea
- Hematologic: Myelosuppressive:
  - WBC: Mild
  - Platelets: Mild
  - Onset: 7 days
  - Nadir: 14 days
  - Recovery: 21 days
- Local: Pain at injection site

Drug Interactions

Increased Effect/Toxicity: Doxorubicin prolongs half-life and thus prolonged leukopenia and thrombocytopenia.

Decreased Effect: Phenytoin results in negation of streptozocin cytotoxicity.

Drug Uptake

Duration: Disappears from serum in 4 hours

Half-life, elimination: 35-40 minutes

Pregnancy Risk Factor C

Generic Available No

Stresstabs® 600 Advanced Formula [OTC] *see* Vitamins, Multiple *on page 1246*
Stromectol® *see* Ivermectin *on page 668*
Sublimaze® *see* Fentanyl *on page 493*
Sucraid® *see* Sacrosidase *on page 1071*

Sucralfate (soo KRAL fate)

Related Information

Management of Patients Undergoing Cancer Therapy *on page 1402*

U.S. Brand Names Carafate®

Canadian Brand Names Apo®-Sucralate; Novo-Sucralate; Nu-Sucralate; PMS-Sucralate; Sulcrate®; Sulcrate® Suspension Plus

Mexican Brand Names Antepsin

Pharmacologic Category Gastrointestinal Agent, Miscellaneous

Synonyms Aluminum Sucrose Sulfate, Basic

Use Short-term management of duodenal ulcers

Unlabeled/Investigational: Gastric ulcers; suspension may be used topically for treatment of stomatitis due to cancer chemotherapy and other causes of esophageal and gastric erosions; GERD, esophagitis, treatment of NSAID mucosal damage, prevention of stress ulcers, postsclerotherapy for esophageal variceal bleeding.

Local Anesthetic/Vasoconstrictor Precautions No information available to require special precautions

Effects on Dental Treatment No effects or complications reported

Dosage Oral:

Children: Dose not established, doses of 40-80 mg/kg/day divided every 6 hours have been used

Stomatitis: 2.5-5 mL (1 g/10 mL suspension), swish and spit or swish and swallow 4 times/day

Adults:

Stress ulcer prophylaxis: 1 g 4 times/day

Stress ulcer treatment: 1 g every 4 hours

Duodenal ulcer:

Treatment: 1 g 4 times/day, 1 hour before meals or food and at bedtime for 4-8 weeks, or alternatively 2 g twice daily; treatment is recommended for 4-8 weeks in adults, the elderly will require 12 weeks

Maintenance: Prophylaxis: 1 g twice daily

Stomatitis: 1 g/10 mL suspension, swish and spit or swish and swallow 4 times/day

Mechanism of Action Forms a complex by binding with positively charged proteins in exudates, forming a viscous paste-like, adhesive substance, when combined with gastric acid adheres to the damaged mucosal area. This selectively forms a protective coating that protects the lining against peptic acid, pepsin, and bile salts.

Other Adverse Effects 1% to 10%: Gastrointestinal: Constipation

Drug Interactions Decreased Effect: Sucralfate may alter the absorption of digoxin, phenytoin (hydantoins), warfarin, ketoconazole, quinidine, quinolones, tetracycline, theophylline. Because of the potential for sucralfate to alter the absorption of some drugs; separate administration (take other medications at least 2 hours before sucralfate). The potential for decreased absorption should be considered when alterations in bioavailability are believed to be critical.

Drug Uptake

Onset of action: Paste formation and ulcer adhesion: 1-2 hours

Absorption: Oral: <5%

Duration: ≤6 hours

Pregnancy Risk Factor B

Generic Available Yes

Sucrets® Cough Calmers [OTC] *see* Dextromethorphan *on page 372*

Sucrets® Sore Throat [OTC] *see* Hexylresorcinol *on page 588*

Sudafed® [OTC] *see* Pseudoephedrine *on page 1022*

Sudafed® 12 Hour [OTC] *see* Pseudoephedrine *on page 1022*

Sudafed® Cold & Allergy [OTC] *see* Chlorpheniramine and Pseudoephedrine *on page 270*

Sudafed® Cold and Sinus [OTC] *see* Acetaminophen and Pseudoephedrine *on page 30*

Sudafed® Cold & Cough Liquid Caps [OTC] *see* Guaifenesin, Pseudoephedrine, and Dextromethorphan *on page 571*

Sudafed® Severe Cold [OTC] *see* Acetaminophen, Dextromethorphan, and Pseudoephedrine *on page 34*

Sudafed® Sinus Headache [OTC] *see* Acetaminophen and Pseudoephedrine *on page 30*

Sufenta® *see* Sufentanil *on page 1113*

Sufentanil (soo FEN ta nil)

U.S. Brand Names Sufenta®

Canadian Brand Names Sufenta®

Pharmacologic Category Analgesic, Narcotic; General Anesthetic

Synonyms Sufentanil Citrate

Use Analgesic supplement in maintenance of balanced general anesthesia

(Continued)

Sufentanil *(Continued)*

Local Anesthetic/Vasoconstrictor Precautions No information available to require special precautions

Effects on Dental Treatment No effects or complications reported

Restrictions C-II

Dosage

Children 2-12 years: 10-25 mcg/kg (10-15 mcg/kg most common dose) with 100% O_2, maintenance: up to 1-2 mcg/kg total dose

Adults: Dose should be based on body weight. **Note:** In obese patients (ie, >20% above ideal body weight), use lean body weight to determine dosage.

1-2 mcg/kg with N_2O/O_2 for endotracheal intubation; maintenance: 10-25 mcg as needed

2-8 mcg/kg with N_2O/O_2 more complicated major surgical procedures; maintenance: 10-50 mcg as needed

8-30 mcg/kg with 100% O_2 and muscle relaxant produces sleep; at doses ≥8 mcg/kg maintains a deep level of anesthesia; maintenance: 10-50 mcg as needed

Mechanism of Action Binds to opioid receptors throughout the CNS. Once receptor binding occurs, effects are exerted by opening K+ channels and inhibiting Ca++ channels. These mechanisms increase pain threshold, alter pain perception, inhibit ascending pain pathways; short-acting narcotic

Other Adverse Effects

>10%:

Cardiovascular: Bradycardia, hypotension

Central nervous system: Somnolence

Gastrointestinal: Nausea, vomiting

Respiratory: Respiratory depression

1% to 10%:

Cardiovascular: Cardiac arrhythmias, orthostatic hypotension

Central nervous system: CNS depression, confusion

Gastrointestinal: Biliary spasm

Ocular: Blurred vision

Drug Interactions CYP3A3/4 enzyme substrate

Increased Effect/Toxicity: Additive effect/toxicity with CNS depressants or beta-blockers. May increase response to neuromuscular blocking agents.

Drug Uptake

Onset of action: 1-3 minutes

Duration: Dose-dependent

Pregnancy Risk Factor C

Generic Available Yes

Sular® *see* Nisoldipine *on page 868*

Sulconazole (sul KON a zole)

U.S. Brand Names Exelderm®

Canadian Brand Names Exelderm®

Pharmacologic Category Antifungal Agent, Topical

Synonyms Sulconazole Nitrate

Use Treatment of superficial fungal infections of the skin, including tinea cruris (jock itch), tinea corporis (ringworm), tinea versicolor, and possibly tinea pedis (athlete's foot - cream only)

Local Anesthetic/Vasoconstrictor Precautions No information available to require special precautions

Effects on Dental Treatment No effects or complications reported

Dosage Adults: Topical: Apply a small amount to the affected area and gently massage once or twice daily for 3 weeks (tinea cruris, tinea corporis, tinea versicolor) to 4 weeks (tinea pedis).

Mechanism of Action Substituted imidazole derivative which inhibits metabolic reactions necessary for the synthesis of ergosterol, an essential membrane component. The end result is usually fungistatic; however, sulconazole may act as a fungicide in *Candida albicans* and parapsilosis during certain growth phases.

Other Adverse Effects 1% to 10%:

Dermatologic: Itching

Local: Burning, stinging, redness

Drug Uptake Absorption: Topical: About 8.7% absorbed percutaneously

Pregnancy Risk Factor C

Generic Available No

Sulf-10® *see* Sulfacetamide Sodium *on page 1115*

Sulfabenzamide, Sulfacetamide, and Sulfathiazole

(sul fa BENZ a mide, sul fa SEE ta mide & sul fa THYE a zole)

U.S. Brand Names V.V.S.®

Pharmacologic Category Antibiotic, Vaginal

Synonyms Triple Sulfa

Use Treatment of *Haemophilus vaginalis* vaginitis

Local Anesthetic/Vasoconstrictor Precautions No information available to require special precautions

Effects on Dental Treatment No effects or complications reported

Dosage Adults:

Cream: Insert one applicatorful in vagina twice daily for 4-6 days; dosage may then be decreased to ½ to ¼ of an applicatorful twice daily

Tablet: Insert one intravaginally twice daily for 10 days

Mechanism of Action Interferes with microbial folic acid synthesis and growth via inhibition of para-aminobenzoic acid metabolism

Other Adverse Effects Frequency not defined:

Dermatologic: Pruritus, urticaria, Stevens-Johnson syndrome

Local: Local irritation

Miscellaneous: Allergic reactions

Drug Uptake Absorption: Variable and unreliable from the vagina

Pregnancy Risk Factor C (avoid if near term)

Generic Available Yes

Sulfacetamide Sodium (sul fa SEE ta mide)

U.S. Brand Names AK-Sulf®; Bleph®-10; Carmol® Scalp; Cetamide®; Klaron®; Ocu-Sul®; Sebizon®; Sodium Sulamyd®; Sulf-10®

Canadian Brand Names Cetamide™; Diosulf™; Sodium Sulamyd®

Mexican Brand Names Ceta Sulfa®

Pharmacologic Category Antibiotic, Ophthalmic; Antibiotic, Sulfonamide Derivative

Synonyms Sodium Sulfacetamide; Sulfacetamide

Use Treatment and prophylaxis of conjunctivitis due to susceptible organisms; corneal ulcers; adjunctive treatment with systemic sulfonamides for therapy of trachoma; topical application in scaling dermatosis (seborrheic); bacterial infections of the skin

Local Anesthetic/Vasoconstrictor Precautions No information available to require special precautions

Effects on Dental Treatment No effects or complications reported

Dosage

Children >2 months and Adults: Ophthalmic:

Ointment: Apply to lower conjunctival sac 1-4 times/day and at bedtime

Solution: Instill 1-3 drops several times daily up to every 2-3 hours in lower conjunctival sac during waking hours and less frequently at night

Children >12 years and Adults: Topical:

Seborrheic dermatitis: Apply at bedtime and allow to remain overnight; in severe cases, may apply twice daily

Secondary cutaneous bacterial infections: Apply 2-4 times/day until infection clears

Mechanism of Action Interferes with bacterial growth by inhibiting bacterial folic acid synthesis through competitive antagonism of PABA

Other Adverse Effects 1% to 10%: Local: Irritation, stinging, burning

Warnings/Precautions Inactivated by purulent exudates containing PABA; use with caution in severe dry eye; ointment may retard corneal epithelial healing; sulfite in some products may cause hypersensitivity reactions. Chemical similarities are present among sulfonamides, sulfonylureas, carbonic anhydrase inhibitors, thiazides, and loop diuretics (except ethacrynic acid). Use in patients with sulfonamide allergy is specifically contraindicated in product labeling, however a risk of cross-reaction exists in patients with allergy to any of these compounds; avoid use when previous reaction has been severe.

Drug Interactions Silver containing products are incompatible with sulfacetamide solutions.

Drug Uptake Half-life, elimination: 7-13 hours

Pregnancy Risk Factor C

Generic Available Yes

Sulfacetamide Sodium and Fluorometholone

(sul fa SEE ta mide SOW dee um & flure oh METH oh lone)

U.S. Brand Names FML-S®

Pharmacologic Category Antibiotic/Corticosteroid, Ophthalmic

Synonyms Fluorometholone and Sulfacetamide

Use Steroid-responsive inflammatory ocular conditions where infection is present or there is a risk of infection

Local Anesthetic/Vasoconstrictor Precautions No information available to require special precautions

Effects on Dental Treatment No effects or complications reported

Dosage Children >2 months and Adults: Ophthalmic: Instill 1-3 drops every 2-3 hours while awake

Drug Uptake See Sulfacetamide Sodium *on page 1115* and Fluorometholone *on page 515*

(Continued)

Sulfacetamide Sodium and Fluorometholone *(Continued)*

Pregnancy Risk Factor C

Generic Available No

Sulfacetamide Sodium and Phenylephrine

(sul fa SEE ta mide SOW dee um & fen il EF rin)

U.S. Brand Names Vasosulf®

Pharmacologic Category Antibiotic, Ophthalmic

Synonyms Phenylephrine and Sulfacetamide

Use Treatment of conjunctivitis, corneal ulcer, and other superficial ocular infections due to susceptible microorganisms; adjunctive in systemic sulfonamide therapy

Local Anesthetic/Vasoconstrictor Precautions No information available to require special precautions

Effects on Dental Treatment No effects or complications reported

Dosage Instill 1 or 2 drops into the lower conjunctival sac(s) every 2 or 3 hours during the day, less often at night

Drug Uptake See Sulfacetamide Sodium *on page 1115* and Phenylephrine *on page 950*

Pregnancy Risk Factor C

Generic Available No

Sulfacetamide Sodium and Prednisolone

(sul fa SEE ta mide SOW dee um & pred NIS oh lone)

U.S. Brand Names AK-Cide®; Blephamide®; Cetapred®; Isopto® Cetapred®; Metimyd®; Vasocidin®

Canadian Brand Names Blephamide®; Dioptimyd®; Vasocidin®

Pharmacologic Category Antibiotic/Corticosteroid, Ophthalmic

Synonyms Prednisolone and Sulfacetamide

Use Steroid-responsive inflammatory ocular conditions where infection is present or there is a risk of infection; ophthalmic suspension may be used as an otic preparation

Local Anesthetic/Vasoconstrictor Precautions No information available to require special precautions

Effects on Dental Treatment No effects or complications reported

Dosage Children >2 months and Adults: Ophthalmic:

Ointment: Apply to lower conjunctival sac 1-4 times/day

Solution: Instill 1-3 drops every 2-3 hours while awake

Mechanism of Action Interferes with bacterial growth by inhibiting bacterial folic acid synthesis through competitive antagonism of PABA; decreases inflammation by suppression of migration of polymorphonuclear leukocytes and reversal of increased capillary permeability; suppresses the immune system by reducing activity and volume of the lymphatic system

Other Adverse Effects 1% to 10%: Local: Burning, stinging

Drug Uptake See Sulfacetamide Sodium *on page 1115* and Prednisolone *on page 988*

Pregnancy Risk Factor C

Generic Available Yes

Sulfacytine (sul fa SYE teen)

U.S. Brand Names Renoquid®

Pharmacologic Category Antibiotic, Sulfonamide Derivative

Use Treatment of urinary tract infections

Local Anesthetic/Vasoconstrictor Precautions No information available to require special precautions

Effects on Dental Treatment No effects or complications reported

Dosage Adults: Oral: Initial: 500 mg, then 250 mg every 4 hours for 10 days

Other Adverse Effects Frequency not defined:

Central nervous system: Fever, dizziness, headache

Dermatologic: Itching, skin rash, photosensitivity, Lyell's syndrome, Stevens-Johnson syndrome

Gastrointestinal: Anorexia, nausea, vomiting, diarrhea

Hematologic: Granulocytopenia, leukopenia, thrombocytopenia, aplastic anemia, hemolytic anemia

Hepatic: Hepatitis

Warnings/Precautions Chemical similarities are present among sulfonamides, sulfonylureas, carbonic anhydrase inhibitors, thiazides, and loop diuretics (except ethacrynic acid). In patients with allergy to one of these compounds, a risk of cross-reaction exists; avoid use when previous reaction has been severe.

Pregnancy Risk Factor B/D (at term)

Generic Available No

SulfaDIAZINE (sul fa DYE a zeen)

Pharmacologic Category Antibiotic, Sulfonamide Derivative

Use Treatment of urinary tract infections and nocardiosis, rheumatic fever prophylaxis; adjunctive treatment in toxoplasmosis; uncomplicated attack of malaria

Local Anesthetic/Vasoconstrictor Precautions No information available to require special precautions

Effects on Dental Treatment No effects or complications reported

Dosage Oral:

Congenital toxoplasmosis:

Newborns and Children <2 months: 100 mg/kg/day divided every 6 hours in conjunction with pyrimethamine 1 mg/kg/day once daily and supplemental folinic acid 5 mg every 3 days for 6 months

Children >2 months: 25-50 mg/kg/dose 4 times/day

Toxoplasmosis:

Children: 120-150 mg/kg/day, maximum dose: 6 g/day; divided every 6 hours in conjunction with pyrimethamine 2 mg/kg/day divided every 12 hours for 3 days followed by 1 mg/kg/day once daily (maximum: 25 mg/day) with supplemental folinic acid

Adults: 2-8 g/day divided every 6 hours in conjunction with pyrimethamine 25 mg/day and with supplemental folinic acid

Mechanism of Action Interferes with bacterial growth by inhibiting bacterial folic acid synthesis through competitive antagonism of PABA

Other Adverse Effects Frequency not defined:

Central nervous system: Fever, dizziness, headache

Dermatologic: Lyell's syndrome, Stevens-Johnson syndrome, itching, rash, photosensitivity

Endocrine & metabolic: Thyroid function disturbance

Gastrointestinal: Anorexia, nausea, vomiting, diarrhea

Genitourinary: Crystalluria

Hematologic: Granulocytopenia, leukopenia, thrombocytopenia, aplastic anemia, hemolytic anemia

Hepatic: Hepatitis, jaundice

Renal: Hematuria, acute nephropathy, interstitial nephritis

Miscellaneous: Serum sickness-like reactions

Warnings/Precautions Use with caution in patients with impaired hepatic function or impaired renal function, G6PD deficiency; dosage modification required in patients with renal impairment; fluid intake should be maintained ≥1500 mL/day, or administer sodium bicarbonate to keep urine alkaline; more likely to cause crystalluria because it is less soluble than other sulfonamides. Chemical similarities are present among sulfonamides, sulfonylureas, carbonic anhydrase inhibitors, thiazides, and loop diuretics (except ethacrynic acid). Use in patients with sulfonamide allergy is specifically contraindicated in product labeling, however a risk of cross-reaction exists in patients with allergy to any of these compounds; avoid use when previous reaction has been severe.

Drug Interactions

Cyclosporine concentrations may be decreased; monitor levels and renal function

Hydantoin levels may be increased; monitor levels and adjust as necessary

Hypoglycemics: Increased effect of oral hypoglycemics (rare, but severe); monitor blood sugar

Methenamine: Combination may result in crystalluria; avoid use

Methotrexate-induced bone marrow suppression may be increased

NSAIDs and salicylates: May increase sulfonamide concentrations

PABA (para-aminobenzoic acid - may be found in some vitamin supplements): Interferes with the antibacterial activity of sulfonamides; avoid concurrent use

Sulfinpyrazone: May increase sulfonamide concentrations

Thiazide diuretics: May increase the incidence of thrombocytopenia purpura

Thiopental's effect may be enhanced; monitor for possible dosage reduction

Uricosuric agents: Actions of these agents are potentiated

Warfarin and other oral anticoagulants: Anticoagulant effect may be increased; decrease dose and monitor INR closely

Drug Uptake

Absorption: Oral: Well absorbed

Half-life, elimination: 10 hours

Time to peak: 3-6 hours

Pregnancy Risk Factor B/D (at term)

Generic Available Yes

Sulfadiazine, Sulfamethazine, and Sulfamerazine

(sul fa DYE a zeen sul fa METH a zeen & sul fa MER a zeen)

Pharmacologic Category Antibiotic, Sulfonamide Derivative

Synonyms Multiple Sulfonamides; Trisulfapyrimidines

Use Treatment of toxoplasmosis

Local Anesthetic/Vasoconstrictor Precautions No information available to require special precautions

(Continued)

Sulfadiazine, Sulfamethazine, and Sulfamerazine *(Continued)*

Effects on Dental Treatment No effects or complications reported

Dosage Adults: Oral: 2-4 g to start, then 2-4 g/day in 3-6 divided doses

Mechanism of Action Interferes with microbial folic acid synthesis and growth via inhibition of para-aminobenzoic acid metabolism

Warnings/Precautions Chemical similarities are present among sulfonamides, sulfonylureas, carbonic anhydrase inhibitors, thiazides, and loop diuretics (except ethacrynic acid). Use in patients with sulfonamide allergy is specifically contraindicated in product labeling, however a risk of cross-reaction exists in patients with allergy to any of these compounds; avoid use when previous reaction has been severe.

Drug Interactions

Cyclosporine concentrations may be decreased; monitor levels and renal function

Hydantoin levels may be increased; monitor levels and adjust as necessary

Hypoglycemics: Increased effect of oral hypoglycemics (rare, but severe); monitor blood sugar

Methenamine: Combination may result in crystalluria; avoid use

Methotrexate-induced bone marrow suppression may be increased

NSAIDs and salicylates: May increase sulfonamide concentrations

PABA (para-aminobenzoic acid - may be found in some vitamin supplements): Interferes with the antibacterial activity of sulfonamides; avoid concurrent use

Sulfinpyrazone: May increase sulfonamide concentrations

Thiazide diuretics: May increase the incidence of thrombocytopenia purpura

Thiopental's effect may be enhanced; monitor for possible dosage reduction

Uricosuric agents: Actions of these agents are potentiated

Warfarin and other oral anticoagulants: Anticoagulant effect may be increased; decreased dose and monitor INR closely

Pregnancy Risk Factor B/D (at term)

Generic Available No

Sulfadoxine and Pyrimethamine

(sul fa DOKS een & peer i METH a meen)

U.S. Brand Names Fansidar®

Pharmacologic Category Antimalarial Agent

Synonyms Pyrimethamine and Sulfadoxine

Use Treatment of *Plasmodium falciparum* malaria in patients in whom chloroquine resistance is suspected; malaria prophylaxis for travelers to areas where chloroquine-resistant malaria is endemic

Local Anesthetic/Vasoconstrictor Precautions No information available to require special precautions

Effects on Dental Treatment No effects or complications reported

Dosage Children and Adults: Oral:

Treatment of acute attack of malaria: A single dose of the following number of Fansidar® tablets is used in sequence with quinine or alone:

- 2-11 months: 1/4 tablet
- 1-3 years: 1/2 tablet
- 4-8 years: 1 tablet
- 9-14 years: 2 tablets
- >14 years: 2-3 tablets

Malaria prophylaxis:

The first dose of Fansidar® should be taken 1-2 days before departure to an endemic area (CDC recommends that therapy be initiated 1-2 weeks before such travel), administration should be continued during the stay and for 4-6 weeks after return. Dose = pyrimethamine 0.5 mg/kg/dose and sulfadoxine 10 mg/kg/dose up to a maximum of 25 mg pyrimethamine and 500 mg sulfadoxine/dose weekly.

- 2-11 months: 1/8 tablet weekly **or** 1/4 tablet once every 2 weeks
- 1-3 years: 1/4 tablet once weekly **or** 1/2 tablet once every 2 weeks
- 4-8 years: 1/2 tablet once weekly **or** 1 tablet once every 2 weeks
- 9-14 years: 3/4 tablet once weekly **or** 1 1/2 tablets once every 2 weeks
- >14 years: 1 tablet once weekly **or** 2 tablets once every 2 weeks

Mechanism of Action Sulfadoxine interferes with bacterial folic acid synthesis and growth via competitive inhibition of para-aminiobenzoic acid; pyrimethamine inhibits microbial dihydrofolate reductase, resulting in inhibition of tetrahydrofolic acid synthesis

Other Adverse Effects Frequency not defined:

Central nervous system: Ataxia, seizures, headache

Dermatologic: Photosensitivity, Stevens-Johnson syndrome, erythema multiforme, toxic epidermal necrolysis, rash

Endocrine & metabolic: Thyroid function dysfunction

Gastrointestinal: Atrophic glossitis, vomiting, gastritis, anorexia, glossitis

Genitourinary: Crystalluria

Hematologic: Megaloblastic anemia, leukopenia, thrombocytopenia, pancytopenia

Hepatic: Hepatic necrosis, hepatitis
Neuromuscular & skeletal: Tremors
Respiratory: Respiratory failure
Miscellaneous: Hypersensitivity

Warnings/Precautions Use with caution in patients with renal or hepatic impairment, patients with possible folate deficiency, and patients with seizure disorders, increased adverse reactions are seen in patients also receiving chloroquine; fatalities associated with sulfonamides, although rare, have occurred due to severe reactions including Stevens-Johnson syndrome, toxic epidermal necrolysis, hepatic necrosis, agranulocytosis, aplastic anemia and other blood dyscrasias; discontinue use at first sign of rash or any sign of adverse reaction; hemolysis occurs in patients with G6PD deficiency; leucovorin should be administered to reverse signs and symptoms of folic acid deficiency.

Chemical similarities are present among sulfonamides, sulfonylureas, carbonic anhydrase inhibitors, thiazides, and loop diuretics (except ethacrynic acid). Use in patients with sulfonamide allergy is specifically contraindicated in product labeling, however a risk of cross-reaction exists in patients with allergy to any of these compounds; avoid use when previous reaction has been severe.

Drug Interactions

Increased Effect/Toxicity: Hydantoin (phenytoin) levels may be increased. Effect of oral hypoglycemics (rare, but severe) may occur. Combination with methenamine may result in crystalluria; avoid use. May increase methotrexate-induced bone marrow suppression. NSAIDs and salicylates may increase sulfonamide concentrations. Effect of warfarin may be increased.

Decreased Effect: Cyclosporine concentrations may be decreased; monitor levels and renal function. PABA (para-aminobenzoic acid - may be found in some vitamin supplements): interferes with the antibacterial activity of sulfonamides; avoid concurrent use. Pyrimethamine effectiveness decreased by acid.

Drug Uptake

Absorption: Oral: Well absorbed
Half-life, elimination: Pyrimethamine: 80-95 hours; Sulfadoxine: 5-8 days
Time to peak: 2-8 hours

Pregnancy Risk Factor C/D (at term)

Generic Available No

Sulfamethoxazole (sul fa meth OKS a zole)

U.S. Brand Names Gantanol®

Pharmacologic Category Antibiotic, Sulfonamide Derivative

Use Treatment of urinary tract infections, nocardiosis, toxoplasmosis, acute otitis media, and acute exacerbations of chronic bronchitis due to susceptible organisms

Local Anesthetic/Vasoconstrictor Precautions No information available to require special precautions

Effects on Dental Treatment No effects or complications reported

Dosage Oral:

Children >2 months: 50-60 mg/kg as single dose followed by 50-60 mg/kg/day divided every 12 hours; maximum: 3 g/24 hours or 75 mg/kg/day
Adults: 2 g stat, 1 g 2-3 times/day; maximum: 3 g/24 hours

Mechanism of Action Interferes with bacterial growth by inhibiting bacterial folic acid synthesis through competitive antagonism of PABA

Other Adverse Effects Frequency not defined:

Central nervous system: Fever, dizziness, headache
Dermatologic: Itching, rash, photosensitivity, Lyell's syndrome, Stevens-Johnson syndrome
Gastrointestinal: Anorexia, nausea, vomiting, diarrhea
Hematologic: Granulocytopenia, leukopenia, thrombocytopenia, aplastic anemia, hemolytic anemia
Hepatic: Hepatitis

Warnings/Precautions Maintain adequate fluid intake to prevent crystalluria; use with caution in patients with renal or hepatic impairment, and patients with G6PD deficiency; should not be used for group A beta-hemolytic streptococcal infections. Chemical similarities are present among sulfonamides, sulfonylureas, carbonic anhydrase inhibitors, thiazides, and loop diuretics (except ethacrynic acid). Use in patients with sulfonamide allergy is specifically contraindicated in product labeling, however a risk of cross-reaction exists in patients with allergy to any of these compounds; avoid use when previous reaction has been severe.

Drug Interactions CYP2C9 enzyme inhibitor

Increased Effect/Toxicity: Increased effect of oral anticoagulants, oral hypoglycemic agents, and methotrexate.

Decreased effect with PABA or PABA metabolites of drugs (eg, procaine, proparacaine, tetracaine).

Drug Uptake

Absorption: 90%
Half-life, elimination: 9-12 hours; prolonged with renal impairment
Time to peak: 1-4 hours

(Continued)

Sulfamethoxazole *(Continued)*

Pregnancy Risk Factor B/D (at term)

Generic Available Yes

Sulfamethoxazole and Trimethoprim

(sul fa meth OKS a zole & trye METH oh prim)

Related Information

Animal and Human Bites Guidelines *on page 1416*

U.S. Brand Names Bactrim™; Bactrim™ DS; Septra®; Septra® DS; Sulfatrim®; Sulfatrim® DS

Canadian Brand Names Apo®-Sulfatrim; Novo-Trimel; Novo-Trimel D.S.; Nu-Cotrimox®; Septra®; Septra® DS; Septra® Injection

Mexican Brand Names Anitrim; Bactelan; Batrizol; Ectaprim®; Ectaprim®-F; Enterobacticel; Esteprim; Isobac; Kelfiprim; Metoxiprim; Syraprim; Tribakin; Trimesuxol; Trimetoger; Trimetox; Trimzol

Pharmacologic Category Antibiotic, Sulfonamide Derivative; Antibiotic, Miscellaneous

Synonyms Co-Trimoxazole; SMZ-TMP; TMP-SMZ; Trimethoprim and Sulfamethoxazole

Use

Oral treatment of urinary tract infections; acute otitis media in children; acute exacerbations of chronic bronchitis in adults; prophylaxis of *Pneumocystis carinii* pneumonitis (PCP)

I.V. treatment of documented PCP, empiric treatment of PCP in immune compromised patients; treatment of documented or suspected shigellosis, typhoid fever, *Nocardia asteroides* infection, or other infections caused by susceptible bacterial

Unlabeled/Investigational: Cholera and salmonella-type infections and nocardiosis; chronic prostatitis; as prophylaxis in neutropenic patients with *P. carinii* infections, in leukemics, and in patients following renal transplantation, to decrease incidence of gram-negative rod infections

Local Anesthetic/Vasoconstrictor Precautions No information available to require special precautions

Effects on Dental Treatment No effects or complications reported

Dosage Dosage recommendations are based on the trimethoprim component

Children >2 months:

Mild to moderate infections: Oral, I.V.: 8 mg TMP/kg/day in divided doses every 12 hours

Serious infection/*Pneumocystis*: I.V.: 20 mg TMP/kg/day in divided doses every 6 hours

Urinary tract infection prophylaxis: Oral: 2 mg TMP/kg/dose daily

Prophylaxis of *Pneumocystis*: Oral, I.V.: 10 mg TMP/kg/day or 150 mg TMP/m^2/day in divided doses every 12 hours for 3 days/week; dose should not exceed 320 mg trimethoprim and 1600 mg sulfamethoxazole 3 days/week

Adults:

Urinary tract infection/chronic bronchitis: Oral: 1 double strength tablet every 12 hours for 10-14 days

Sepsis: I.V.: 20 mg TMP/kg/day divided every 6 hours

Pneumocystis carinii:

Prophylaxis: Oral, I.V.: 10 mg TMP/kg/day divided every 12 hours for 3 days/week

Treatment: I.V.: 20 mg TMP/kg/day divided every 6 hours

Mechanism of Action Sulfamethoxazole interferes with bacterial folic acid synthesis and growth via inhibition of dihydrofolic acid formation from para-aminobenzoic acid; trimethoprim inhibits dihydrofolic acid reduction to tetrahydrofolate resulting in sequential inhibition of enzymes of the folic acid pathway

Other Adverse Effects The most common adverse reactions include gastrointestinal upset (nausea, vomiting, anorexia) and dermatologic reactions (rash or urticaria). Rare, life-threatening reactions have been associated with co-trimoxazole, including severe dermatologic reactions and hepatotoxic reactions. Most other reactions listed are rare, however, frequency cannot be accurately estimated.

Cardiovascular: Allergic myocarditis

Central nervous system: Confusion, depression, hallucinations, seizures, aseptic meningitis, peripheral neuritis, fever, ataxia, kernicterus in neonates

Dermatologic: Rashes, pruritus, urticaria, photosensitivity; rare reactions include erythema multiforme, Stevens-Johnson syndrome, toxic epidermal necrolysis, exfoliative dermatitis, and Henoch-Schönlein purpura

Endocrine & metabolic: Hyperkalemia (generally at high dosages), hyperglycemia

Gastrointestinal: Nausea, vomiting, anorexia, stomatitis, diarrhea, pseudomembranous colitis, pancreatitis

Hematologic: Thrombocytopenia, megaloblastic anemia, granulocytopenia, eosinophilia, pancytopenia, aplastic anemia, methemoglobinemia, hemolysis (with G6PD deficiency), agranulocytosis

Hepatic: Elevated serum transaminases, hepatotoxicity (including hepatitis, cholestasis, and hepatic necrosis), hyperbilirubinemia

Neuromuscular & skeletal: Arthralgia, myalgia, rhabdomyolysis
Renal: Interstitial nephritis, crystalluria, renal failure, nephrotoxicity (in association with cyclosporine), diuresis
Respiratory: Cough, dyspnea, pulmonary infiltrates
Miscellaneous: Serum sickness, angioedema, periarteritis nodosa (rare), systemic lupus erythematosus (rare)

Warnings/Precautions Use with caution in patients with G6PD deficiency, impaired renal or hepatic function or potential folate deficiency (malnourished, chronic anticonvulsant therapy, or elderly); maintain adequate hydration to prevent crystalluria; adjust dosage in patients with renal impairment. Injection vehicle contains benzyl alcohol and sodium metabisulfite.

Chemical similarities are present among sulfonamides, sulfonylureas, carbonic anhydrase inhibitors, thiazides, and loop diuretics (except ethacrynic acid). Use in patients with sulfonamide allergy is specifically contraindicated in product labeling, however a risk of cross-reaction exists in patients with allergy to any of these compounds; avoid use when previous reaction has been severe.

Fatalities associated with severe reactions including Stevens-Johnson syndrome, toxic epidermal necrolysis, hepatic necrosis, agranulocytosis, aplastic anemia and other blood dyscrasias; discontinue use at first sign of rash. Elderly patients appear at greater risk for more severe adverse reactions. May cause hypoglycemia, particularly in malnourished, or patients with renal or hepatic impairment. Use with caution in patients with porphyria or thyroid dysfunction. Slow acetylators may be more prone to adverse reactions. Caution in patients with allergies or asthma. May cause hyperkalemia (associated with high doses of trimethoprim). Incidence of adverse effects appears to be increased in patients with AIDS.

Drug Interactions CYP2C9 enzyme inhibitor

Increased Effect/Toxicity: Co-trimoxazole may cause an increased effect of sulfonylureas and oral anticoagulants (warfarin). Co-trimoxazole may displace highly protein-bound drugs like methotrexate, phenytoin, or cyclosporine causing increased free serum concentration, leading to increased toxicity of these agents. May also compete for renal excretion of methotrexate. Co-trimoxazole may enhance the nephrotoxicity of cyclosporine and may increase digoxin concentrations.

Decreased Effect: Co-trimoxazole causes decreased effect of cyclosporines and tricyclic antidepressants. Procaine and indomethacin may cause decreased effect of co-trimoxazole.

Drug Uptake See Sulfamethoxazole *on page 1119* and Trimethoprim *on page 1210*

Pregnancy Risk Factor C/D (at term - expert analysis)

Generic Available Yes

Sulfamylon® *see* Mafenide *on page 738*

Sulfanilamide (sul fa NIL a mide)

U.S. Brand Names AVC™

Canadian Brand Names AVC®

Pharmacologic Category Antifungal Agent, Vaginal

Use Treatment of vulvovaginitis caused by *Candida albicans*

Local Anesthetic/Vasoconstrictor Precautions No information available to require special precautions

Effects on Dental Treatment No effects or complications reported

Dosage Adults: Female: Insert one applicatorful intravaginally once or twice daily continued through 1 complete menstrual cycle or insert one suppository intravaginally once or twice daily for 30 days

Mechanism of Action Interferes with microbial folic acid synthesis and growth via inhibition of para-aminiobenzoic acid metabolism; exerts a bacteriostatic action

Other Adverse Effects 1% to 10%:

Central nervous system: Kernicterus
Dermatologic: Itching, rash, burning, irritation, exfoliative dermatitis
Gastrointestinal: Nausea, vomiting
Genitourinary: Crystalluria
Hematologic: Agranulocytosis, hemolytic anemia in patients with severe G6PD deficiency
Hepatic: Hepatic toxicity Frequency not defined:
Dermatologic: Stevens-Johnson syndrome (infrequent)
Genitourinary: Burning, increased discomfort, irritation of penis of sexual partner
Miscellaneous: Allergic reactions, systemic reactions (rare)

Pregnancy Risk Factor C (avoid use after 7th month)

Generic Available Yes

Sulfasalazine (sul fa SAL a zeen)

U.S. Brand Names Azulfidine®; Azulfidine® EN-tabs®

Canadian Brand Names Alti-Sulfasalazine; Salazopyrin®; Salazopyrin En-Tabs®; S.A.S.™

Pharmacologic Category 5-Aminosalicylic Acid Derivative

(Continued)

Sulfasalazine *(Continued)*

Synonyms Salicylazosulfapyridine

Use Management of ulcerative colitis; enteric coated tablets are also used for rheumatoid arthritis (including juvenile rheumatoid arthritis) in patients who inadequately respond to analgesics and NSAIDs

Unlabeled/Investigational: Ankylosing spondylitis, collagenous colitis, Crohn's disease, psoriasis, psoriatic arthritis, juvenile chronic arthritis

Local Anesthetic/Vasoconstrictor Precautions No information available to require special precautions

Effects on Dental Treatment No effects or complications reported

Dosage Oral:

Children ≥2 years: Ulcerative colitis: Initial: 40-60 mg/kg/day in 3-6 divided doses; maintenance dose: 20-30 mg/kg/day in 4 divided doses

Children ≥6 years: Juvenile rheumatoid arthritis: 30-50 mg/kg/day in 2 divided doses; Initial: Begin with 1/4 to 1/3 of expected maintenance dose; increase weekly; maximum: 2 g/day typically

Adults: Enteric coated tablet:

Ulcerative colitis: Initial: 1 g 3-4 times/day, 2 g/day maintenance in divided doses; may initiate therapy with 0.5-1 g/day

Rheumatoid arthritis: Initial: 0.5-1 g/day; increase weekly to maintenance dose of 2 g/day in 2 divided doses; maximum: 3 g/day (if response to 2 g/day is inadequate after 12 weeks of treatment)

Dosing interval in renal impairment:

Cl_{cr} 10-30 mL/minute: Administer twice daily

Cl_{cr} <10 mL/minute: Administer once daily

Dosing adjustment in hepatic impairment: Avoid use

Mechanism of Action Acts locally in the colon to decrease the inflammatory response and systemically interferes with secretion by inhibiting prostaglandin synthesis

Other Adverse Effects

>10%:

Central nervous system: Headache (33%)

Dermatologic: Photosensitivity

Gastrointestinal: Anorexia, nausea, vomiting, diarrhea (33%), gastric distress

Genitourinary: Reversible oligospermia (33%)

<3%:

Dermatologic: Urticaria/pruritus (<3%)

Hematologic: Hemolytic anemia (<3%), Heinz body anemia (<3%)

Contraindications Hypersensitivity to sulfasalazine, sulfa drugs, salicylates, or any component of their formulation; porphyria, GI or GU obstruction; children <2 years of age

Warnings/Precautions Use with caution in patients with renal impairment; impaired hepatic function or urinary obstruction, blood dyscrasias, severe allergies or asthma, or G6PD deficiency; may cause folate deficiency (consider providing 1 mg/day folate supplement). Chemical similarities are present among sulfonamides, sulfonylureas, carbonic anhydrase inhibitors, thiazides, and loop diuretics (except ethacrynic acid). Use in patients with sulfonamide allergy is specifically contraindicated in product labeling, however a risk of cross-reaction exists in patients with allergy to any of these compounds; avoid use when previous reaction has been severe.

Drug Interactions

Cyclosporine concentrations may be decreased; monitor levels and renal function

Digoxin's absorption may be decreased

Folic acid's absorption may be decreased

Hydantoin levels may be increased; monitor levels and adjust as necessary

Hypoglycemics: Increased effect of oral hypoglycemics (rare, but severe); monitor blood sugar

Methenamine: Combination may result in crystalluria; avoid use

Methotrexate-induced bone marrow suppression may be increased

NSAIDs and salicylates: May increase sulfonamide concentrations

PABA (para-aminobenzoic acid - may be found in some vitamin supplements): Interferes with the antibacterial activity of sulfonamides; avoid concurrent use

Sulfinpyrazone: May increase sulfonamide concentrations

Thiazide diuretics: May increase the incidence of thrombocytopenia purpura

Thiopental's effect may be enhanced; monitor for possible dosage reduction

Uricosuric agents: Actions of these agents are potentiated

Warfarin and other oral anticoagulants: Anticoagulant effect may be increased; decrease dose and monitor INR closely

Drug Uptake

Absorption: 10% to 15% as unchanged drug from small intestine

Half-life, elimination: 5.7-10 hours

Pregnancy Risk Factor B/D (at term)

Generic Available Yes

Sulfatrim® *see* Sulfamethoxazole and Trimethoprim *on page 1120*

Sulfatrim® DS *see* Sulfamethoxazole and Trimethoprim *on page 1120*

Sulfinpyrazone (sul fin PEER a zone)

U.S. Brand Names Anturane®

Canadian Brand Names Apo®-Sulfinpyrazone; Nu-Sulfinpyrazone

Pharmacologic Category Uricosuric Agent

Use Treatment of chronic gouty arthritis and intermittent gouty arthritis

Unlabeled/Investigational: To decrease the incidence of sudden death postmyocardial infarction

Local Anesthetic/Vasoconstrictor Precautions No information available to require special precautions

Effects on Dental Treatment No effects or complications reported

Dosage Adults: Oral: 100-200 mg twice daily; maximum daily dose: 800 mg

Mechanism of Action Acts by increasing the urinary excretion of uric acid, thereby decreasing blood urate levels; this effect is therapeutically useful in treating patients with acute intermittent gout, chronic tophaceous gout, and acts to promote resorption of tophi; also has antithrombic and platelet inhibitory effects

Other Adverse Effects Frequency not defined:

Cardiovascular: Flushing

Central nervous system: Dizziness, headache

Dermatologic: Dermatitis, rash

Endocrine & metabolic: Gouty arthritis

Gastrointestinal (most frequent adverse effects): Nausea, vomiting, stomach pain

Genitourinary: Polyuria

Hematologic: Anemia, leukopenia, increased bleeding time (decreased platelet aggregation)

Hepatic: Hepatic necrosis

Renal: Nephrotic syndrome, uric acid stones

Drug Interactions CYP2C and 3A3/4 enzyme inducer; CYP2C9 enzyme inhibitor

Increased Effect/Toxicity: Increased effect of oral hypoglycemics and anticoagulants. Risk of acetaminophen hepatotoxicity is increased, while therapeutic effects may be reduced.

Decreased Effect: Decreased effect/levels of theophylline, verapamil. Decreased uricosuric activity with salicylates, niacins.

Drug Uptake

Absorption: Complete and rapid

Half-life, elimination: 2.7-6 hours

Time to peak: 1.6 hours

Pregnancy Risk Factor C/D (near term - expert analysis)

Generic Available Yes

SulfiSOXAZOLE (sul fi SOKS a zole)

U.S. Brand Names Gantrisin®; Truxazole®

Canadian Brand Names Novo-Soxazole®; Sulfizole®

Pharmacologic Category Antibiotic, Sulfonamide Derivative

Synonyms Sulfisoxazole Acetyl; Sulphafurazole

Use Treatment of urinary tract infections, otitis media, *Chlamydia*; nocardiosis; treatment of acute pelvic inflammatory disease in prepubertal children; often used in combination with trimethoprim

Local Anesthetic/Vasoconstrictor Precautions No information available to require special precautions

Effects on Dental Treatment No effects or complications reported

Dosage Oral (not for use in patients <2 months of age):

Children >2 months: 75 mg/kg stat, followed by 120-150 mg/kg/day in divided doses every 4-6 hours; not to exceed 6 g/day

Pelvic inflammatory disease: 100 mg/kg/day in divided doses every 6 hours; used in combination with ceftriaxone

Chlamydia trachomatis: 100 mg/kg/day in divided doses every 6 hours

Adults: 2-4 g stat, 4-8 g/day in divided doses every 4-6 hours

Pelvic inflammatory disease: 500 mg every 6 hours for 21 days; used in combination with ceftriaxone

Chlamydia trachomatis: 500 mg every 6 hours for 10 days

Elderly: 2 g stat, then 2-8 g/day in divided doses every 6 hours

Mechanism of Action Interferes with bacterial growth by inhibiting bacterial folic acid synthesis through competitive antagonism of PABA

Other Adverse Effects Frequency not defined:

Cardiovascular: Vasculitis

Central nervous system: Fever, dizziness, headache

Dermatologic: Itching, rash, photosensitivity, Lyell's syndrome, Stevens-Johnson syndrome

Endocrine & metabolic: Thyroid function disturbance

Gastrointestinal: Anorexia, nausea, vomiting, diarrhea

Genitourinary: Crystalluria, hematuria,

(Continued)

SulfiSOXAZOLE *(Continued)*

Hematologic: Granulocytopenia, leukopenia, thrombocytopenia, aplastic anemia, hemolytic anemia
Hepatic: Jaundice, hepatitis
Renal: Interstitial nephritis
Miscellaneous: Serum sickness-like reactions

Warnings/Precautions Use with caution in patients with G6PD deficiency (hemolysis may occur), hepatic or renal impairment; dosage modification required in patients with renal impairment; risk of crystalluria should be considered in patients with impaired renal function. Chemical similarities are present among sulfonamides, sulfonylureas, carbonic anhydrase inhibitors, thiazides, and loop diuretics (except ethacrynic acid). Use in patients with sulfonamide allergy is specifically contraindicated in product labeling, however a risk of cross-reaction exists in patients with allergy to any of these compounds; avoid use when previous reaction has been severe.

Drug Interactions

Increased Effect/Toxicity: Increased effect of oral anticoagulants, methotrexate, and oral hypoglycemic agents.

Decreased effect with PABA or PABA metabolites of drugs (eg, procaine, proparacaine, tetracaine), thiopental.

Drug Uptake

Absorption: Sulfisoxazole acetyl is hydrolyzed in GI tract to sulfisoxazole which is readily absorbed
Half-life, elimination: 4-7 hours (increases with renal impairment)
Time to peak: 2-3 hours

Pregnancy Risk Factor B/D (near term)

Generic Available Yes

Sulfonated Phenolics in Aqueous Solution

(sul fo NATE ed fe NOL iks in AYE kwee us so LU shun)

U.S. Brand Names Debacterol®

Pharmacologic Category Aphthous Ulcer Treatment Agent

Use Dental: Therapeutic cauterization in the treatment of oral mucosal lesions (aphthous stomatitis, gingivitis, moderate to severe periodontitis)

Local Anesthetic/Vasoconstrictor Precautions No effects or complications reported

Effects on Dental Treatment In most patients, a stinging sensation will be felt immediately. Ulcer pain should subside almost immediately after rinsing.

Mechanism of Action Semiviscous, chemical cautery agent which provides controlled, focal debridement and sterilization of necrotic tissues; relieving pain, sealing damaged tissue, and providing local antiseptic action

Other Adverse Effects Frequency not defined: Local: Irritation upon administration

Contraindications For external use only

Warnings/Precautions Safety and effectiveness in children <12 years has not been established. prolonged Use of Debacterol® on normal tissue should be avoided; if ingested, do not induce vomiting, immediately dilute with milk or water and get medical help or contact a Poison Control Center. If eye exposure occurs, immediately remove contact lenses, irrigate eyes for at least 15 minutes with lukewarm water, and contact a physician.

Pregnancy Risk Factor C

Breast-feeding Considerations Unknown if excreted in breast milk; use with caution

Dosage Forms SOLN, top, for oral mucosa: (Debacterol®): 1 mL [22% sulfonated phenolics and 30% sulfuric acid in aqueous solution]

Generic Available No

Comments Prior to application/treatment, the ulcerated mucosal area should be thoroughly dried with a cotton-tipped applicator or similar method. After drying, dip a cotton-tipped applicator into the solution and apply directly to the ulcerated area (most patients experience a brief stinging sensation immediately) and hold the applicator in contact with the ulcer for at least 5-10 seconds. The patient should then thoroughly rinse out the mouth with water and spit out the rinse water. The stinging sensation and ulcer pain will subside almost immediately after the rinse, larger ulcers may require 1-2 minutes for relief. One application per ulcer is usually sufficient. If the ulcer pain returns shortly after rinsing, additional applications may be applied as part of the same treatment session until the ulcer remains pain-free after rinsing. It is not recommended that more than one treatment be applied to each ulcer. If excess irritation occurs during use, a rinse with sodium bicarbonate (baking soda) solution will neutralize the reaction (use 0.5 teaspoon in 120 mL water).

Note: Currently available only by direct distribution to healthcare providers from the manufacturer. Contact Northern Research Laboratories at (888)884-4675.

Selected Readings Rhodus NL and Bereuter J, "An Evaluation of a Chemical Cautery Agent and an Anti-inflammatory Ointment for the Treatment of Recurrent Aphthous Stomatitis: A Pilot Study," *Quintessence Int*, 1998, 29(12):769-73.

Sulindac (sul IN dak)

Related Information

Rheumatoid Arthritis and Osteoarthritis *on page 1340*

Temporomandibular Dysfunction (TMD) *on page 1397*

U.S. Brand Names Clinoril®

Canadian Brand Names Apo®-Sulin; Novo-Sundac; Nu-Sundac

Mexican Brand Names Clinoril®; Copal®; Kenalin®

Pharmacologic Category Nonsteroidal Anti-inflammatory Drug (NSAID)

Use Management of inflammatory disease, rheumatoid disorders; acute gouty arthritis; structurally similar to indomethacin but acts like aspirin; safest NSAID for use in mild renal impairment

Local Anesthetic/Vasoconstrictor Precautions No information available to require special precautions

Effects on Dental Treatment NSAID formulations are known to reversibly decrease platelet aggregation via mechanisms different than observed with aspirin. The dentist should be aware of the potential of abnormal coagulation. Caution should also be exercised in the use of NSAIDs in patients already on anticoagulant therapy with drugs such as warfarin (Coumadin®).

Dosage Maximum therapeutic response may not be realized for up to 3 weeks. Oral:

Children: Dose not established

Adults: 150-200 mg twice daily or 300-400 mg once daily; not to exceed 400 mg/day

Mechanism of Action Inhibits prostaglandin synthesis by decreasing the activity of the enzyme, cyclo-oxygenase, which results in decreased formation of prostaglandin precursors

Other Adverse Effects

1% to 10%:

Cardiovascular: Edema

Central nervous system: Dizziness, headache, nervousness

Dermatologic: Pruritus, rash

Gastrointestinal: GI pain, heartburn, nausea, vomiting, diarrhea, constipation, flatulence, anorexia, abdominal cramps

Otic: Tinnitus

Warnings/Precautions Use with caution in patients with peptic ulcer disease, GI bleeding, bleeding abnormalities, dehydration, impaired renal or hepatic function, CHF, hypertension, and patients receiving anticoagulants. Withhold for at least 4-6 half-lives prior to surgical or dental procedures.

Drug Interactions CYP2C9 enzyme inhibitor

ACE-inhibitors: Antihypertensive effects may be decreased by concurrent therapy with NSAIDs; monitor BP.

Angiotensin II antagonists: Antihypertensive effects may be decreased by concurrent therapy with NSAIDs; monitor BP.

Anticoagulants (warfarin, heparin, LMWHs) in combination with NSAIDs can cause increased risk of bleeding.

Other antiplatelet drugs (ticlopidine, clopidogrel, aspirin, abciximab, dipyridamole, eptifibatide, tirofiban) can cause an increased risk of bleeding.

Corticosteroids may increase the risk of GI ulceration; avoid concurrent use.

Cyclosporine: NSAIDs may increase serum creatinine, potassium, BP, and cyclosporine levels; monitor cyclosporine levels and renal function carefully.

Hydralazine's antihypertensive effect is decreased; avoid concurrent use.

Lithium levels can be increased; avoid concurrent use if possible or monitor lithium levels and adjust dose. Sulindac may have the least effect. When NSAID is stopped, lithium will need adjustment again.

Loop diuretic efficacy (diuretic and antihypertensive effect) may be reduced.

Methotrexate: Severe bone marrow suppression, aplastic anemia, and GI toxicity have been reported with concomitant NSAID therapy. Avoid use during moderate or high-dose methotrexate (increased and prolonged methotrexate levels). NSAID use during low-dose treatment of rheumatoid arthritis has not been fully evaluated; extreme caution is warranted.

Thiazides antihypertensive effects are decreased; avoid concurrent use.

Warfarin's INRs may be increased by piroxicam. Other NSAIDs may have the same effect depending on dose and duration. Monitor INR closely. Use the lowest dose of NSAIDs possible and for the briefest duration.

Drug Uptake

Onset of action: Analgesic: ~1 hour

Absorption: 90%

Duration: 12-24 hours

Half-life, elimination: Parent drug: 7 hours; Active metabolite: 18 hours

Pregnancy Risk Factor B/D (3rd trimester)

Generic Available Yes

Sumacal® [OTC] *see* Glucose Polymers *on page 559*

Sumatriptan Succinate (SOO ma trip tan SUKS i nate)

U.S. Brand Names Imitrex®

Canadian Brand Names Imitrex®

Mexican Brand Names Imigran

Pharmacologic Category Serotonin 5-HT_{1D} Receptor Agonist

Use Acute treatment of migraine with or without aura; sumatriptan injection: acute treatment of cluster headaches

Local Anesthetic/Vasoconstrictor Precautions No information available to require special precautions

Effects on Dental Treatment No effects or complications reported

Dosage Adults:

Oral: A single dose of 25 mg, 50 mg, or 100 mg (taken with fluids). If a satisfactory response has not been obtained at 2 hours, a second dose may be administered. Results from clinical trials show that initial doses of 50 mg and 100 mg are more effective than doses of 25 mg, and that 100 mg doses do not provide a greater effect than 50 mg and may have increased incidence of side effects. Although doses of up to 300 mg/day have been studied, the total daily dose should not exceed 200 mg. The safety of treating an average of >4 headaches in a 30-day period have not been established.

Intranasal: A single dose of 5 mg, 10 mg, or 20 mg administered in one nostril. A 10 mg dose may be achieved by administering a single 5 mg dose in each nostril. If headache returns, the dose may be repeated once after 2 hours, not to exceed a total daily dose of 40 mg. The safety of treating an average of >4 headaches in a 30-day period has not been established.

S.C.: 6 mg; a second injection may be administered at least 1 hour after the initial dose, but not more than 2 injections in a 24-hour period. If side effects are dose-limiting, lower doses may be used.

Mechanism of Action Selective agonist for serotonin (5HT_{-1-D} receptor) in cranial arteries to cause vasoconstriction and reduces sterile inflammation associated with antidromic neuronal transmission correlating with relief of migraine

Other Adverse Effects

>10%:

- Central nervous system: Dizziness (injection 12%), warm/hot sensation (injection 11%)
- Gastrointestinal: Bad taste (nasal spray 13% to 24%), nausea (nasal spray 11% to 13%), vomiting (nasal spray 11% to 13%)
- Local: Injection: Pain at the injection site (59%)
- Neuromuscular & skeletal: Tingling (injection 13%)

1% to 10%:

- Cardiovascular: Chest pain/tightness/heaviness/pressure (injection 2% to 3%, tablet 1% to 2%)
- Central nervous system: Burning (injection 7%), dizziness (nasal spray 1% to 2%, tablet >1%), feeling of heaviness (injection 7%), flushing (injection 7%), pressure sensation (injection 7%), feeling of tightness (injection 5%), numbness (injection 5%), drowsiness (injection 3%, tablet >1%), malaise/fatigue (tablet 2% to 3%, injection 1%), feeling strange (injection 2%), headache (injection 2%, tablet >1%), tight feeling in head (injection 2%), nonspecified pain (tablet 1% to 2%, placebo 1%), vertigo (tablet <1% to 2%, nasal spray 1% to 2%), migraine (tablet >1%), sleepiness (tablet >1%), cold sensation (injection 1%), anxiety (injection 1%)
- Gastrointestinal: Nausea (tablet >1%), vomiting (tablet >1%), hyposalivation (tablet >1%), abdominal discomfort (injection 1%), dysphagia (injection 1%)
- Neuromuscular & skeletal: Neck, throat, and jaw pain/tightness/pressure (injection 2% to 5%, tablet 2% to 3%), mouth/tongue discomfort (injection 5%), paresthesia (tablet 3% to 5%), weakness (injection 5%), myalgia (injection 2%), muscle cramps (injection 1%)
- Ocular: Vision alterations (injection 1%)
- Respiratory: Nasal disorder/discomfort (nasal spray 2% to 4%, injection 2%), throat discomfort (injection 3%, nasal spray 1% to 2%)
- Miscellaneous: Warm/cold sensation (tablet 2% to 3%, placebo 2%), nonspecified pressure/tightness/heaviness (tablet 1% to 3%, placebo 2%), diaphoresis (injection 2%)

Drug Interactions Increased Effect/Toxicity: Increased toxicity with ergot containing drugs, avoid use, wait 24 hours from last ergot containing drug (dihydroergotamine, or methysergide) before administering sumatriptan. MAO inhibitors decrease clearance of sumatriptan increasing the risk of systemic sumatriptan toxic effects. Sumatriptan may enhance CNS toxic effects when taken with selective serotonin reuptake inhibitors (SSRIs) like fluoxetine, fluvoxamine, paroxetine, or sertraline.

Drug Uptake After S.C. administration:

Onset of action: ~30 minutes

Half-life, elimination: Terminal: 115 minutes; Injection, tablet: 2.5 hours; Nasal spray: 2 hours

Time to peak: 5-20 minutes

Pregnancy Risk Factor C

Generic Available No

Summer's Eve® Medicated Douche [OTC] *see* Povidone-Iodine *on page 982*

Sumycin® *see* Tetracycline *on page 1147*

Superdophilus® [OTC] *see Lactobacillus acidophilus* and *Lactobacillus bulgaricus on page 682*

Supprelin™ *see* Histrelin *on page 588*

Suppress® [OTC] *see* Dextromethorphan *on page 372*

Suprax® *see* Cefixime *on page 237*

Surbex® [OTC] *see* Vitamin B Complex *on page 1244*

Surbex-T® Filmtabs® [OTC] *see* Vitamin B Complex With Vitamin C *on page 1244*

Surbex® With C Filmtabs® [OTC] *see* Vitamin B Complex With Vitamin C *on page 1244*

Sureprin 81™ [OTC] *see* Aspirin *on page 119*

Surfak® [OTC] *see* Docusate *on page 407*

Surgicel® *see* Cellulose, Oxidized *on page 250*

Surgicel® Absorbable Hemostat *see* Cellulose, Oxidized Regenerated *on page 250*

Surmontil® *see* Trimipramine *on page 1211*

Survanta® *see* Beractant *on page 157*

Suspen® *see* Penicillin V Potassium *on page 931*

Sus-Phrine® *see* Epinephrine *on page 438*

Sus-Phrine® (Dental) *see* Epinephrine *on page 438*

Sustiva® *see* Efavirenz *on page 429*

Su-Tuss®-HD *see* Hydrocodone, Pseudoephedrine, and Guaifenesin *on page 608*

Sween Cream® [OTC] *see* Methylbenzethonium Chloride *on page 793*

Swim-Ear® Otic [OTC] *see* Boric Acid *on page 171*

Syllact® [OTC] *see* Psyllium *on page 1025*

Symax SL *see* Hyoscyamine *on page 617*

Symax SR *see* Hyoscyamine *on page 617*

Symmetrel® *see* Amantadine *on page 64*

Synacol® CF [OTC] *see* Guaifenesin and Dextromethorphan *on page 569*

Synacort® *see* Hydrocortisone *on page 608*

Synagis® *see* Palivizumab *on page 912*

Synalar® *see* Fluocinolone *on page 512*

Synalgos®-DC *see* Dihydrocodeine Compound *on page 392*

Synarel® *see* Nafarelin *on page 840*

Synercid® *see* Quinupristin and Dalfopristin *on page 1036*

Synthroid® *see* Levothyroxine *on page 705*

Syracol-CF® [OTC] *see* Guaifenesin and Dextromethorphan *on page 569*

Tac™-3 *see* Triamcinolone *on page 1197*

Tac™-40 *see* Triamcinolone *on page 1197*

Tacrine (TAK reen)

U.S. Brand Names Cognex®

Pharmacologic Category Acetylcholinesterase Inhibitor (Central)

Synonyms Tacrine Hydrochloride; Tetrahydroaminoacrine; THA

Use Treatment of mild to moderate dementia of the Alzheimer's type

Local Anesthetic/Vasoconstrictor Precautions No information available to require special precautions

Effects on Dental Treatment No effects or complications reported

Dosage Adults: Initial: 10 mg 4 times/day; may increase by 40 mg/day adjusted every 6 weeks; maximum: 160 mg/day; best administered separate from meal times. See table.

Dose Adjustment Based Upon Transaminase Elevations

ALT	Regimen
≤3 x ULN*	Continue titration
>3 to ≤5 x ULN	Decrease dose by 40 mg/day, resume when ALT returns to normal
>5 x ULN	Stop treatment, may rechallenge upon return of ALT to normal

*ULN = upper limit of normal.

Patients with clinical jaundice confirmed by elevated total bilirubin (>3 mg/dL) should not be rechallenged with tacrine

Mechanism of Action A deficiency of cortical acetylcholine is believed to account for some of the clinical manifestations of mild to moderate dementia. Tacrine

(Continued)

Tacrine *(Continued)*

probably acts by elevating acetylcholine concentrations in the cortical areas by slowing the degradation of acetylcholine released by still intact cholinergic neurons.

Other Adverse Effects

>10%:

Central nervous system: Headache, dizziness
Gastrointestinal: Nausea, vomiting, diarrhea
Miscellaneous: Elevated transaminases

1% to 10%:

Cardiovascular: Flushing
Central nervous system: Confusion, ataxia, insomnia, somnolence, depression, anxiety, fatigue
Dermatologic: Rash
Gastrointestinal: Dyspepsia, anorexia, abdominal pain, flatulence, constipation, weight loss
Neuromuscular & skeletal: Myalgia, tremor
Respiratory: Rhinitis

Warnings/Precautions The use of tacrine has been associated with elevations in serum transaminases; serum transaminases (specifically ALT) must be monitored throughout therapy; use extreme caution in patients with current evidence of a history of abnormal LFTs; use caution in patients with bladder outlet obstruction, asthma, and sick-sinus syndrome (tacrine may cause bradycardia). Also, patients with cardiovascular disease, asthma, or peptic ulcer should use cautiously.

Drug Interactions CYP1A2 enzyme substrate; CYP1A2 inhibitor

Increased Effect/Toxicity: Tacrine in combination with other cholinergic agents (eg, ambenonium, edrophonium, neostigmine, pyridostigmine, bethanechol), will likely produce additive cholinergic effects. Tacrine in combination with beta-blockers may produce additive bradycardia. Tacrine may increase the levels/effect of succinylcholine and theophylline. in elevated plasma concentrations. Fluvoxamine, enoxacin, and cimetidine increase tacrine concentrations via enzyme inhibition (CYP1A2).

Decreased Effect: Enzyme inducers and cigarette smoking may reduce tacrine plasma concentrations via enzyme induction (CYP1A2). Tacrine may worsen Parkinson's disease and inhibit the effects of levodopa. Tacrine may antagonize the therapeutic effect of anticholinergic agents (benztropine, trihexphenidyl).

Drug Uptake

Onset of action: May require weeks
Half-life, elimination, serum: 2-4 hours; Steady-state: 24-36 hours
Time to peak, plasma: 1-2 hours

Pregnancy Risk Factor C

Generic Available No

Tacrolimus (ta KROE li mus)

U.S. Brand Names Prograf®; Protopic®

Canadian Brand Names Prograf®

Mexican Brand Names Prograf®

Pharmacologic Category Immunosuppressant Agent; Topical Skin Product

Synonyms FK506

Use

Oral/injection: Potent immunosuppressive drug used in liver or kidney transplant recipients

Topical: Moderate to severe atopic dermatitis in patients not responsive to conventional therapy or when conventional therapy is not appropriate

Unlabeled/Investigational: Potent immunosuppressive drug used in heart, lung, small bowel transplant recipients; immunosuppressive drug for peripheral stem cell/bone marrow transplantation

Local Anesthetic/Vasoconstrictor Precautions No information available to require special precautions

Effects on Dental Treatment No effects or complications reported

Dosage

Children:

Liver transplant: Patients without pre-existing renal or hepatic dysfunction have required and tolerated higher doses than adults to achieve similar blood concentrations. It is recommended that therapy be initiated at high end of the recommended adult I.V. and oral dosing ranges; dosage adjustments may be required.

Oral: Initial dose: 0.15-0.20 mg/kg/day in 2 divided doses, given every 12 hours; begin oral dose no sooner than 6 hours post-transplant; adjunctive therapy with corticosteroids is recommended; if switching from I.V. to oral, the oral dose should be started 8-12 hours after stopping the infusion

Typical whole blood trough concentrations: Months 1-12: 5-20 ng/mL

I.V.: **Note:** I.V. route should only be used in patients not able to take oral medications, anaphylaxis has been reported. Initial dose: 0.03-0.05 mg/kg/day as a continuous infusion; begin no sooner than 6 hours post-transplant;

adjunctive therapy with corticosteroids is recommended; continue only until oral medication can be tolerated

Children ≥2 years: Moderate to severe atopic dermatitis: Topical: Apply 0.03% ointment to affected area twice daily; rub in gently and completely; continue applications for 1 week after symptoms have cleared

Adults:

Kidney transplant:

Oral: Initial dose: 0.2 mg/kg/day in 2 divided doses, given every 12 hours; initial dose may be given within 24 hours of transplant, but should be delayed until renal function has recovered; African-American patients may require larger doses to maintain trough concentration

Typical whole blood trough concentrations: Months 1-3: 7- 20 ng/mL; months 4-12: 5-15 ng/mL

I.V.: **Note:** I.V. route should only be used in patients not able to take oral medications, anaphylaxis has been reported. Initial dose: 0.03-0.05 mg/kg/day as a continuous infusion; begin no sooner than 6 hours post-transplant, starting at lower end of the dosage range; adjunctive therapy with corticosteroids is recommended; continue only until oral medication can be tolerated

Liver transplant:

Oral: Initial dose: 0.1-0.15 mg/kg/day in 2 divided doses, given every 12 hours; begin oral dose no sooner than 6 hours post-transplant; adjunctive therapy with corticosteroids is recommended; if switching from I.V. to oral, the oral dose should be started 8-12 hours after stopping the infusion

Typical whole blood trough concentrations: Months 1-12: 5-20 ng/mL

I.V.: **Note:** I.V. route should only be used in patients not able to take oral medications, anaphylaxis has been reported. Initial dose: 0.03-0.05 mg/kg/day as a continuous infusion; begin no sooner than 6 hours post-transplant starting at lower end of the dosage range; adjunctive therapy with corticosteroids is recommended; continue only until oral medication can be tolerated

Prevention of graft-vs-host disease: I.V.: 0.03 mg/kg/day as continuous infusion

Moderate to severe atopic dermatitis: Topical: Apply 0.03% or 0.1% ointment to affected area twice daily; rub in gently and completely; continue applications for 1 week after symptoms have cleared

Dosing adjustment in renal impairment: Evidence suggests that lower doses should be used; patients should receive doses at the lowest value of the recommended I.V. and oral dosing ranges; further reductions in dose below these ranges may be required

Tacrolimus therapy should usually be delayed up to 48 hours or longer in patients with postoperative oliguria

Hemodialysis: Not removed by hemodialysis; supplemental dose is not necessary

Peritoneal dialysis: Significant drug removal is unlikely based on physiochemical characteristics

Dosing adjustment in hepatic impairment: Use of tacrolimus in liver transplant recipients experiencing post-transplant hepatic impairment may be associated with increased risk of developing renal insufficiency related to high whole blood levels of tacrolimus. The presence of moderate-to-severe hepatic dysfunction (serum bilirubin >2 mg/dL) appears to affect the metabolism of FK506. The half-life of the drug was prolonged and the clearance reduced after I.V. administration. The bioavailability of FK506 was also increased after oral administration. The higher plasma concentrations as determined by ELISA, in patients with severe hepatic dysfunction are probably due to the accumulation of FK506 metabolites of lower activity. These patients should be monitored closely and dosage adjustments should be considered. Some evidence indicates that lower doses could be used in these patients.

Mechanism of Action Suppressed cellular immunity (inhibits T-lymphocyte activation); possibly by binding to an intracellular protein, FKBP-12

Other Adverse Effects

Oral, I.V.:

≥15%

Cardiovascular: Chest pain, hypertension

Central nervous system: Dizziness, headache, insomnia, tremor (headache and tremor are associated with high whole blood concentrations and may respond to decreased dosage)

Dermatologic: Pruritus, rash

Endocrine & metabolic: Diabetes mellitus, hyperglycemia, hyperkalemia, hyperlipemia, hypomagnesemia, hypophosphatemia

Gastrointestinal: Abdominal pain, constipation, diarrhea, dyspepsia, nausea, vomiting

Genitourinary: Urinary tract infection

Hematologic: Anemia, leukocytosis, thrombocytopenia

Hepatic: Ascites

Neuromuscular & skeletal: Arthralgia, back pain, weakness, paresthesia

Renal: Abnormal kidney function, increased creatinine, oliguria, urinary tract infection, increased BUN

Respiratory: Atelectasis, dyspnea, increased cough

(Continued)

Tacrolimus *(Continued)*

3% to 15%:

Cardiovascular: Abnormal EKG, angina pectoris, deep thrombophlebitis, hemorrhage, hypotension, hypervolemia, generalized edema, peripheral vascular disorder, phlebitis, postural hypotension, tachycardia, thrombosis, vasodilation

Central nervous system: Abnormal dreams, abnormal thinking, agitation, amnesia, anxiety, chills, confusion, depression, emotional lability, encephalopathy, hallucinations, nervousness, psychosis, somnolence

Dermatologic: Acne, alopecia, cellulitis, exfoliative dermatitis, fungal dermatitis, hirsutism, increased diaphoresis, photosensitivity reaction, skin discoloration, skin disorder, skin ulcer

Endocrine & metabolic: Acidosis, alkalosis, Cushing's syndrome, decreased bicarbonate, decreased serum iron, diabetes mellitus, hypercalcemia, hypercholesterolemia, hyperphosphatemia, hypoproteinemia, increased alkaline phosphatase, increase LDH

Gastrointestinal: Anorexia, cramps, dysphagia, enlarged abdomen, esophagitis, flatulence, gastritis, GI perforation/hemorrhage, ileus, increased appetite, oral moniliasis, rectal disorder, stomatitis, weight gain

Genitourinary: Urinary frequency, urinary incontinence, vaginitis, cystitis, dysuria

Hematologic: Bruising, coagulation disorder, decreased prothrombin, hypochromic anemia, leukopenia, polycythemia

Hepatic: Abnormal LFTs, bilirubinemia, cholangitis, cholestatic jaundice, hepatitis, increased ALT, increased AST, increased GGT, jaundice, liver damage

Neuromuscular & skeletal: Hypertonia, incoordination, joint disorder, leg cramps, myalgia, myasthenia, myoclonus, neuropathy, osteoporosis

Ocular: Abnormal vision, amblyopia

Otic: Ear pain, otitis media, tinnitus

Renal: Albuminuria

Respiratory: Asthma, bronchitis, lung disorder, pharyngitis, pneumonia, pneumothorax, pulmonary edema, respiratory disorder, rhinitis, sinusitis, voice alteration

Miscellaneous: Abscess, abnormal healing, allergic reaction, flu-like syndrome, generalized spasm, hernia, herpes simplex, peritonitis, sepsis

Topical (as reported in children and adults, unless otherwise noted):

>10%:

Central nervous system: Headache (5% to 20%), fever (1% to 21%)

Dermatologic: Skin burning (43% to 58%), pruritus (41% to 46%), erythema (12% to 28%)

Respiratory: Increased cough (18% children)

Miscellaneous: Flu-like syndrome (23% to 28%), allergic reaction (4% to 12%)

1% to 10%:

Cardiovascular: Peripheral edema (3% to 4% adults)

Central nervous system: Hyperesthesia (3% to 7% adults), pain (1% to 2%)

Dermatologic: Skin tingling (2% to 8%), acne (4% to 7% adults), folliculitis (2% to 6%), urticaria (1% to 6%), rash (2% to 5%), pustular rash (2% to 4%), vesiculobullous rash (4% children), contact dermatitis (3% to 4%), cyst (1% to 3% adults), eczema herpeticum (1% to 2%), fungal dermatitis (1% to 2% adults), sunburn (1% to 2% adults), dry skin (1% children)

Endocrine & metabolic: Dysmenorrhea (4% women)

Gastrointestinal: Diarrhea (3% to 5%), dyspepsia (1% to 4% adults), abdominal pain (3% children), vomiting (1% adults), gastroenteritis (adults 2%), nausea (1% children)

Neuromuscular & skeletal: Myalgia (2% to 3% adults), weakness (2% to 3% adults), back pain (2% adults)

Ocular: Conjunctivitis (2% adults)

Otic: Otitis media (12% children)

Respiratory: Rhinitis (6% children), sinusitis (2% to 4% adults), bronchitis (2% adults), pneumonia (1% adults)

Miscellaneous: Ethanol intolerance (3% to 7% adults), varicella/herpes zoster (1% to 5%), lymphadenopathy (3% children)

≥1%: Alopecia, increased ALT, increased AST, anaphylactoid reaction, angina pectoris, angioedema, anorexia, anxiety, arrhythmia, arthralgia, arthritis, bilirubinemia, breast pain, cellulitis, cerebrovascular accident, cheilitis, chills, constipation, increased creatinine, dehydration, depression, dizziness, dyspnea, ear pain, ecchymosis, edema, epistaxis, exacerbation of untreated area, eye pain, furunculosis, gastritis, hernia, hyperglycemia, hypertension, hypoglycemia, hypoxia, laryngitis, leukocytosis, leukopenia, abnormal LFTs, lymphadenopathy (0.8%), malaise, migraine, neck pain, neuritis, palpitations, paresthesia, peripheral vascular disorder, photosensitivity reaction, skin discoloration, diaphoresis, taste perversion, unintended pregnancy, vaginal moniliasis, vasodilation, vertigo

Drug Interactions CYP3A3/4 enzyme substrate

Antacids: Separate administration by at least 2 hours

Anticonvulsants: Carbamazepine, phenobarbital, phenytoin: May decrease tacrolimus blood levels

Cisapride (and metoclopramide): May increase serum concentration of tacrolimus

Cyclosporine: Concomitant use is associated with synergistic immunosuppression and increased nephrotoxicity; give first dose of tacrolimus no sooner than 24 hours after last cyclosporine dose. In the presence of elevated tacrolimus or cyclosporine concentration, dosing of the other usually should be delayed longer.

CYP3A3/4 inhibitors: Serum level and/or toxicity of tacrolimus may be increased. Inhibitors include amiodarone, bromocriptine, cimetidine, clarithromycin, clotrimazole, erythromycin, danazol, delavirdine, diltiazem, dirithromycin, disulfiram, fluconazole, fluoxetine, fluvoxamine, grapefruit juice, indinavir, itraconazole, ketoconazole, methylprednisolone, metoclopramide, nefazodone, nevirapine, nicardipine, nifedipine, propoxyphene, quinupristin-dalfopristin, ritonavir, saquinavir, troleandomycin, verapamil, zafirlukast, zileuton. Although specific drug interaction studies have not been conducted with the topical product, use of tacrolimus topical ointment in patients with widespread disease should be done with caution in patients taking CYP3A3/4 inhibitors.

Ganciclovir: Also nephrotoxic, use with caution

Potassium-sparing diuretics: Tacrolimus use may lead to hyperkalemia; avoid concomitant use

Rifabutin, rifampin: May decrease tacrolimus blood levels

St John's wort: May reduce tacrolimus serum concentrations; avoid concurrent use.

Sucralfate: Separate administration by at least 2 hours

Vaccines (live): Vaccine may be less effective; avoid vaccination during treatment if possible

Voriconazole: Tacrolimus serum concentrations may be increased; monitor serum concentrations and renal function. Decrease tacrolimus dosage by 66% when initiating voriconazole.

Drug Uptake

Absorption: Better in resected patients with a closed stoma; unlike cyclosporine, clamping of the T-tube in liver transplant patients does not alter trough concentrations or AUC

Oral: Incomplete and variable; food within 15 minutes of administration decreases absorption (27%)

Topical: Serum concentrations range from undetectable to 20 ng/mL (<5 ng/mL in majority of adult patients studied)

Half-life, elimination: Variable, 21-61 hours in healthy volunteers

Time to peak: 0.5-4 hours

Pregnancy Risk Factor C

Generic Available No

Tagamet® *see* Cimetidine *on page 286*

Tagamet® HB [OTC] *see* Cimetidine *on page 286*

Talacen® *see* Pentazocine Compound *on page 934*

Talwin® *see* Pentazocine *on page 933*

Talwin® Compound *see* Pentazocine Compound *on page 934*

Talwin® NX *see* Pentazocine *on page 933*

Tambocor™ *see* Flecainide *on page 505*

Tamiflu™ *see* Oseltamivir Phosphate *on page 892*

Tamoxifen (ta MOKS i fen)

U.S. Brand Names Nolvadex®

Canadian Brand Names Apo®-Tamox; Gen-Tamoxifen; Nolvadex®; Nolvadex®-D; Novo-Tamoxifen; PMS-Tamoxifen; Tamofen®

Mexican Brand Names Bilem; Cryoxifeno; Nolvadex®; Tamoxan; Taxus®; Tecnofen®

Pharmacologic Category Antineoplastic Agent, Estrogen Receptor Antagonist

Synonyms Tamoxifen Citrate

Use Palliative or adjunctive treatment of advanced breast cancer; reduce the incidence of breast cancer in women at high risk (taking into account age, number of first-degree relatives with breast cancer, previous breast biopsies, age at first live birth, age at first menstrual period, and a history of lobular carcinoma *in situ*); reduce risk of invasive breast cancer in women with ductal carcinoma *in situ* (DCIS); metastatic male breast cancer

Unlabeled/Investigational: Treatment of mastalgia, gynecomastia, pancreatic carcinoma, and induction of ovulation. Studies have shown tamoxifen to be effective in the treatment of primary breast cancer in elderly women. Comparative studies with other antineoplastic agents in elderly women with breast cancer had more favorable survival rates with tamoxifen. Initiation of hormone therapy rather than chemotherapy is justified for elderly patients with metastatic breast cancer who are responsive.

Local Anesthetic/Vasoconstrictor Precautions No information available to require special precautions

Effects on Dental Treatment No effects or complications reported

(Continued)

Tamoxifen *(Continued)*

Dosage Oral: Adults: Induction of ovulation (unlabeled use): 5-40 mg twice daily for 4 days

Mechanism of Action Competitively binds to estrogen receptors on tumors and other tissue targets, producing a nuclear complex that decreases DNA synthesis and inhibits estrogen effects; nonsteroidal agent with potent antiestrogenic properties which compete with estrogen for binding sites in breast and other tissues; cells accumulate in the G_0 and G_1 phases; therefore, tamoxifen is cytostatic rather than cytocidal.

Other Adverse Effects

>10%:
- Cardiovascular: Flushing (64%)
- Endocrine & metabolic: Hot flashes (67%); decreased libido (29%); tumor flare (26%) (with bone pain [5%], tumor pain, erythema)
- Gastrointestinal: Mild to moderate nausea (10% to 58%), may be severe in ~3% of patients
- Genitourinary: Vaginal bleeding, discharge (18%)
- Hematologic: Thrombocytopenia (24% to 28%), leukopenia (28%)

1% to 10%:
- Cardiovascular: Arterial and venous thrombosis
- Central nervous system: Lightheadedness, depression, dizziness, headache, lassitude, mental confusion
- Dermatologic: Skin rash (5%), dry skin (7%)
- Endocrine & metabolic: Hypercalcemia, sodium and water retention, edema (8%)
- Gastrointestinal: Vomiting
- Genitourinary: Pruritus vulvae (2%), endometriosis, priapism
- Hematologic: Decreased hemoglobin/hematocrit, anemia
- Ocular: Retinopathy, including optic disk swelling, retinal hemorrhage, visual impairment, seen with high (>200 mg/day) doses

Warnings/Precautions The Food and Drug Administration (FDA) and AstraZeneca have added a black box warning to the Nolvadex (tamoxifen) product labeling, concerning its use in women taking this medication to reduce the risk of developing breast cancer. This would include women at high risk for cancer and women with ductal carcinoma in situ (DCIS).

Serious and life-threatening events (including stroke, pulmonary emboli, and uterine malignancy) have occurred at an incidence greater than placebo during use for cancer risk reduction; these events are rare, but require consideration in risk:benefit evaluation. Use with caution in patients with leukopenia, thrombocytopenia, or hyperlipidemias; ovulation may be induced; decreased visual acuity, retinopathy, corneal changes, and increased incidence of cataracts have been reported; hypercalcemia in patients with bone metastasis; hepatocellular carcinomas have been reported in some studies, relationship to treatment is unclear. Endometrial hyperplasia and polyps have occurred. Increased risk of uterine or endometrial cancer; monitor.

Drug Interactions CYP3A3/4, CYP2C9 enzyme substrate
- Allopurinol: Concurrent use may result in exacerbation of allopurinol-induced hepatotoxicity.
- Bromocriptine: May increase serum levels of tamoxifen.
- Cyclosporine: Concurrent use may result in an increase in cyclosporine serum levels.
- CYP3A3/4 inducers: May decrease serum levels of tamoxifen.
- Letrozole: Serum levels may be reduced by tamoxifen.
- Warfarin: Concomitant use is contraindicated when used for risk reduction; results in significant enhancement of the anticoagulant effects of warfarin

Drug Uptake
- Absorption: Well absorbed
- Half-life, elimination: 7 days
- Time to peak: Oral: 4-7 hours

Pregnancy Risk Factor D

Generic Available Yes

Tamsulosin (tam SOO loe sin)

U.S. Brand Names Flomax®

Canadian Brand Names Flomax®

Mexican Brand Names Secotex®

Pharmacologic Category $Alpha_1$ Blocker

Synonyms Tamsulosin Hydrochloride

Use Treatment of signs and symptoms of benign prostatic hyperplasia (BPH)

Local Anesthetic/Vasoconstrictor Precautions No information available to require special precautions

Effects on Dental Treatment No effects or complications reported

Dosage Oral: Adults: 0.4 mg once daily ~30 minutes after the same meal each day

Mechanism of Action An antagonist of $alpha_{1A}$ adrenoceptors in the prostate. Three subtypes identified: $alpha_{1A}$, $alpha_{1B}$, $alpha_{1D}$ have distribution that differs between human organs and tissue. Approximately 70% of the $alpha_1$-receptors in human prostate are of $alpha_{1A}$ subtype. The symptoms associated with benign prostatic hyperplasia (BPH) are related to bladder outlet obstruction, which is comprised of two underlying components: static and dynamic. Static is related to an increase in prostate size, partially caused by a proliferation of smooth muscle cells in the prostatic stroma. Severity of BPH symptoms and the degree of urethral obstruction do not correlate well with the size of the prostate. Dynamic is a function of an increase in smooth muscle tone in the prostate and bladder neck leading to constriction of the bladder outlet. Smooth muscle tone is mediated by the sympathetic nervous stimulation of $alpha_1$ adrenoceptors, which are abundant in the prostate, prostatic capsule, prostatic urethra, and bladder neck. Blockade of these adrenoceptors can cause smooth muscles in the bladder neck and prostate to relax, resulting in an improvement in urine flow rate and a reduction in symptoms of BPH.

Other Adverse Effects Orthostatic hypotension (by testing criteria): First-dose orthostatic hypotension at 4 hours postdose has been observed in 7% of patients following a 0.4 mg dose as compared to 3% in a placebo group. Overall, at least one positive test was observed in 16% of patients receiving 0.4 mg and 19% of patients receiving the 0.8 mg dose as compared to 11% in a placebo group. **Percentages correspond to the 0.4 mg and 0.8 mg doses, respectively.**

>10%:

Central nervous system: Headache (19% to 21%), dizziness (15% to 17%)
Genitourinary: Abnormal ejaculation (8% to 18%)
Respiratory: Rhinitis (13% to 18%)

1% to 10%:

Cardiovascular: Chest pain (~4%)
Central nervous system: Weakness (8% to 9%), somnolence (3% to 4%), insomnia (1% to 2%)
Endocrine & metabolic: Decreased libido (1% to 2%)
Gastrointestinal: Diarrhea (4% to 6%), nausea (3% to 4%), stomach discomfort (2% to 3%), bitter taste (2% to 3%)
Neuromuscular & skeletal: Back pain (7% to 8%)
Ocular: Amblyopia (0.2% to 2%)
Respiratory: Pharyngitis (6% to 5%), cough (3% to 5%), sinusitis (2% to 4%)
Miscellaneous: Infection (9% to 11%), tooth disorder (1% to 2%)

Drug Interactions Extensive metabolism via CYP isoenzymes, profile not characterized.

Increased Effect/Toxicity: Metabolized by cytochrome P450 isoenzymes. Profile of involved isoenzymes has not been established. Concurrent cimetidine therapy increased AUC of tamsulosin by 44%. Use with caution in patients receiving concurrent warfarin therapy (may increase anticoagulant effect). Do not use in combination with other alpha-blocking drugs.

Decreased Effect: Metabolism by cytochrome P450 isoenzymes may, in theory, be influenced by enzyme-inducing agents, resulting in decreased effects.

Drug Uptake

Absorption: >90%

Half-life, elimination: Healthy volunteers: 9-13 hours; Target population: 14-15 hours; Steady-state: By the fifth day of once daily dosing

Time to peak: C_{max}: Fasting: 40% to 70% increase; T_{max}: Fasting: 4-5 hours, With food: 6-7 hours

Pregnancy Risk Factor B

Generic Available No

Tanoral® *see* Chlorpheniramine, Pyrilamine, and Phenylephrine *on page 273*
Tao® *see* Troleandomycin *on page 1215*
Tapazole® *see* Methimazole *on page 782*
Targretin® *see* Bexarotene *on page 163*
Tarka® *see* Trandolapril and Verapamil *on page 1190*
Tasmar® *see* Tolcapone *on page 1179*
Tavist® *see* Clemastine *on page 299*
Tavist®-1 [OTC] *see* Clemastine *on page 299*
Taxol® *see* Paclitaxel *on page 911*
Taxotere® *see* Docetaxel *on page 406*

Tazarotene (taz AR oh teen)

U.S. Brand Names Tazorac®

Canadian Brand Names Tazorac™

Pharmacologic Category Keratolytic Agent

Use Topical treatment of facial acne vulgaris; topical treatment of stable plaque psoriasis of up to 20% body surface area involvement

Local Anesthetic/Vasoconstrictor Precautions No information available to require special precautions

Effects on Dental Treatment No effects or complications reported

(Continued)

Tazarotene *(Continued)*

Dosage Topical: **Note:** In patients experiencing excessive pruritus, burning, skin redness, or peeling, discontinue until integrity of the skin is restored, or reduce dosing to an interval the patient is able to tolerate.

Children ≥12 years and Adults:

Acne: Cream/gel 0.1%: Cleanse the face gently. After the skin is dry, apply a thin film of tazarotene (2 mg/cm^2) once daily, in the evening, to the skin where the acne lesions appear; use enough to cover the entire affected area

Psoriasis: Gel 0.05% or 0.1%: Apply once daily, in the evening, to psoriatic lesions using enough (2 mg/cm^2) to cover only the lesion with a thin film to no more than 20% of body surface area. If a bath or shower is taken prior to application, dry the skin before applying. Unaffected skin may be more susceptible to irritation, avoid application to these areas.

Children ≥18 years and Adults: Cream 0.05% or 0.1%: Apply once daily, in the evening, to psoriatic lesions using enough (2 mg/cm^2) to cover only the lesion with a thin film to no more than 20% of body surface area. If a bath or shower is taken prior to application, dry the skin before applying. Unaffected skin may be more susceptible to irritation, avoid application to these areas.

Mechanism of Action Synthetic, acetylenic retinoid which modulates differentiation and proliferation of epithelial tissue and exerts some degree of anti-inflammatory and immunological activity

Other Adverse Effects Percentage of incidence varies with formulation and/or strength:

>10%: Dermatologic: Burning/stinging, dry skin, erythema, pruritus, skin pain, worsening of psoriasis

1% to 10%: Dermatologic: Contact dermatitis, desquamation, discoloration, fissuring, hypertriglyceridemia, inflammation, localized bleeding, rash

Frequency not defined:

Dermatologic: Photosensitization

Neuromuscular & skeletal: Peripheral neuropathy

Drug Interactions Increased Effect/Toxicity: Increased toxicity may occur with sulfur, benzoyl peroxide, salicylic acid, resorcinol, or any product with strong drying effects (including alcohol-containing compounds) due to increased drying actions. May augment phototoxicity of sensitizing medications (thiazides, tetracyclines, fluoroquinolones, phenothiazines, sulfonamides).

Drug Uptake

Absorption: Minimal following cutaneous application (≤6% of dose)

Duration: Therapeutic: Psoriasis: ≤3 months after a 3-month course of topical treatment

Half-life, elimination: 18 hours

Pregnancy Risk Factor X

Generic Available No

Tazicef® *see* Ceftazidime *on page 243*

Tazidime® *see* Ceftazidime *on page 243*

Tazorac® *see* Tazarotene *on page 1133*

Teargen® [OTC] *see* Artificial Tears *on page 117*

Teargen® II [OTC] *see* Artificial Tears *on page 117*

Tearisol® [OTC] *see* Artificial Tears *on page 117*

Tears Again® [OTC] *see* Artificial Tears *on page 117*

Tears Naturale® [OTC] *see* Artificial Tears *on page 117*

Tears Naturale® Free [OTC] *see* Artificial Tears *on page 117*

Tears Naturale® II [OTC] *see* Artificial Tears *on page 117*

Tears Plus® [OTC] *see* Artificial Tears *on page 117*

Tears Renewed® [OTC] *see* Artificial Tears *on page 117*

Teczem® *see* Enalapril and Diltiazem *on page 433*

Tedral® *see* Theophylline, Ephedrine, and Phenobarbital *on page 1155*

Tegretol® *see* Carbamazepine *on page 216*

Tegretol®-XR *see* Carbamazepine *on page 216*

Tegrin® Dandruff Shampoo [OTC] *see* Coal Tar *on page 315*

Tegrin®-HC [OTC] *see* Hydrocortisone *on page 608*

Telmisartan (tel mi SAR tan)

U.S. Brand Names Micardis®

Canadian Brand Names Micardis®

Pharmacologic Category Angiotensin II Receptor Blocker

Use Treatment of hypertension; may be used alone or in combination with other antihypertensive agents

Local Anesthetic/Vasoconstrictor Precautions No information available to require special precautions

Effects on Dental Treatment No effects or complications reported

Dosage Adults: Oral: Initial: 40 mg once daily; usual maintenance dose range: 20-80 mg/day. Patients with volume depletion should be initiated on the lower dosage with close supervision.

Mechanism of Action A nonpeptide angiotensin receptor antagonist which acts as a vasoconstrictor; in addition to causing direct vasoconstriction, angiotensin II also stimulates the release of aldosterone. Once aldosterone is released, sodium as well as water are reabsorbed. The end result is an elevation in BP. Telmisartan binds to the AT1 angiotensin II receptor. This binding prevents angiotensin II from binding to the receptor thereby blocking the vasoconstriction and the aldosterone secreting effects of angiotensin II.

Other Adverse Effects May be associated with worsening of renal function in patients dependent on renin-angiotensin-aldosterone system.

1% to 10%:

- Cardiovascular: Hypertension (1%), chest pain (1%), peripheral edema (1%)
- Central nervous system: Headache (1%), dizziness (1%), pain (1%), fatigue (1%)
- Gastrointestinal: Diarrhea (3%), dyspepsia (1%), nausea (1%), abdominal pain (1%)
- Genitourinary: Urinary tract infection (1%)
- Neuromuscular & skeletal: Back pain (3%), myalgia (1%)
- Respiratory: Upper respiratory infection (7%), sinusitis (3%), pharyngitis (1%), cough (2%)
- Miscellaneous: Flu-like syndrome (1%)

Drug Interactions CYP2C19 enzyme inhibitor

Increased Effect/Toxicity: Telmisartan may increase serum digoxin concentrations. Potassium salts/supplements, co-trimoxazole (high dose), ACE inhibitors, and potassium-sparing diuretics (amiloride, spironolactone, triamterene) may increase the risk of hyperkalemia with telmisartan.

Decreased Effect: Telmisartan decreased the trough concentrations of warfarin during concurrent therapy, however INR was not changed.

Drug Uptake Orally active, not a prodrug

Onset of action: 1-2 hours

Duration: ≤24 hours

Half-life, elimination: Terminal: ~24 hours

Time to peak: 0.5-1 hour

Pregnancy Risk Factor C (1st trimester); D (2nd and 3rd trimesters)

Generic Available No

Telmisartan and Hydrochlorothiazide

(tel mi SAR tan & hye droe klor oh THYE a zide)

U.S. Brand Names Micardis® HCT

Pharmacologic Category Angiotensin II Receptor Blocker Combination; Antihypertensive Agent Combination

Synonyms HCTZ and Telmisartan; Hydrochlorothiazide and Telmisartan; Telmisartan and HCTZ

Use Treatment of hypertension; combination product should not be used for initial therapy

Local Anesthetic/Vasoconstrictor Precautions No information available to require special precautions

Effects on Dental Treatment No effects or complications reported

Dosage Adults: Oral: Replacement therapy: Combination product can be substituted for individual titrated agents. Initiation of combination therapy when monotherapy has failed to achieve desired effects:

Patients currently on telmisartan: Initial dose if BP is not currently controlled on monotherapy of 80 mg telmisartan: Telmisartan 80 mg/hydrochlorothiazide 12.5 mg once daily; may titrate up to telmisartan 160 mg/hydrochlorothiazide 25 mg if needed

Patients currently on HCTZ: Initial dose if BP is not currently controlled on monotherapy of 25 mg once daily, or is controlled and experiencing hypokalemia: Telmisartan 80 mg/hydrochlorothiazide 12.5 mg once daily; may titrate up to telmisartan 160 mg/hydrochlorothiazide 25 mg if BP remains uncontrolled after 2-4 weeks of therapy

Mechanism of Action

Telmisartan: Telmisartan is an angiotensin receptor antagonist. Angiotensin II acts as a vasoconstrictor. In addition to causing direct vasoconstriction, angiotensin II also stimulates the release of aldosterone. Once aldosterone is released, sodium as well as water are reabsorbed. The end result is an elevation in BP. Telmisartan binds to the AT1 angiotensin II receptor. This binding prevents angiotensin II from binding to the receptor thereby blocking the vasoconstriction and the aldosterone secreting effects of angiotensin II.

Hydrochlorothiazide: Inhibits sodium reabsorption in the distal tubules causing increased excretion of sodium and water as well as potassium and hydrogen ions

Other Adverse Effects The following reactions have been reported with the combination product; refer to individual product monographs for additional adverse reactions that may be expected from each agent.

(Continued)

Telmisartan and Hydrochlorothiazide *(Continued)*

2% to 10%:

Central nervous system: Dizziness (5%)

Gastrointestinal: Diarrhea (3%), nausea (2%)

Renal: Elevated BUN (3%)

Respiratory: Upper respiratory tract infection (8%), sinusitis (4%)

Miscellaneous: Flu-like syndrome (2%)

<2%: Abdominal pain, back pain, bronchitis, decreased hematocrit, decreased hemoglobin, dyspepsia, elevated bilirubin, elevated liver enzymes, elevated serum creatinine, hypokalemia, pharyngitis, postural hypotension, rash, tachycardia, vomiting

Drug Interactions

Telmisartan: CYP2C19 inhibitor (*in vitro*)

Digoxin concentrations may be increased; monitor when initiating, adjusting, or discontinuing telmisartan

Lithium: Risk of toxicity may be increased by telmisartan; monitor lithium concentrations

NSAIDs: May decrease angiotensin II antagonist efficacy; effect has been seen with losartan, but may occur with other medications in this class; monitor BP

Potassium-sparing diuretics (amiloride, potassium, spironolactone, triamterene): Increased risk of hyperkalemia

Potassium supplements: May increase the risk of hyperkalemia

Trimethoprim (high dose): May increase the risk of hyperkalemia

Warfarin serum concentrations may be slightly decreased (not associated with alteration in INR)

Hydrochlorothiazide:

ACTH: May increase hypokalemia

ACE inhibitors: Increased hypotension if aggressively diuresed with a thiazide diuretic

Antidiabetic agents: May require dosage adjustment of oral agents and insulin; monitor

Barbiturates: May potentiate orthostatic hypertension

Cholestyramine and colestipol resins: Decreased absorption of hydrochlorothiazide

Corticosteroids: May increase hypokalemia

Cyclosporine and thiazides can increase the risk of gout or renal toxicity; avoid concurrent use

Digoxin: Toxicity can be exacerbated if a thiazide induces hypokalemia or hypomagnesemia

Lithium: Toxicity can occur by reducing renal excretion of lithium; monitor lithium concentration and adjust as needed

Narcotics: May potentiate orthostatic hypertension

Neuromuscular blocking agents: Can prolong blockade; monitor serum potassium and neuromuscular status.

NSAIDs: May lead to decreased effect of thiazides; monitor

Norepinephrine: Hydrochlorothiazide may decrease response to pressor amines; monitor

Drug Uptake See Hydrochlorothiazide *on page 595* and Telmisartan *on page 1134*

Pregnancy Risk Factor C (1st trimester); D (2nd and 3rd trimesters)

Selected Readings Conlin P, Moore T, Swartz S, et al, "Effect of Indomethacin on Blood Pressure Lowering by Captopril and Losartan in Hypertensive Patients," *Hypertension*, 2000, 36(3):461-5.

Temazepam (te MAZ e pam)

U.S. Brand Names Restoril®

Canadian Brand Names Apo®-Temazepam; Gen-Temazepam; Novo-Temazepam; Nu-Temazepam; PMS-Temazepam; Restoril®

Pharmacologic Category Benzodiazepine

Use Treatment of anxiety and as an adjunct in the treatment of depression; also may be used in the management of panic attacks; transient insomnia and sleep latency

Local Anesthetic/Vasoconstrictor Precautions No information available to require special precautions

Effects on Dental Treatment >10%: Significant xerostomia; normal salivary flow resumes with discontinuation

Restrictions C-IV

Dosage Adults: Oral: 15-30 mg at bedtime; 15 mg in elderly or debilitated patients

Mechanism of Action Binds to stereospecific benzodiazepine receptors on the postsynaptic GABA neuron at several sites within the CNS, including the limbic system, reticular formation. Enhancement of the inhibitory effect of GABA on neuronal excitability results by increased neuronal membrane permeability to chloride ions. This shift in chloride ions results in hyperpolarization (a less excitable state) and stabilization; causes minimal change in REM sleep patterns

Other Adverse Effects 1% to 10%:

Central nervous system: Confusion, dizziness, drowsiness, fatigue, anxiety, headache, lethargy, hangover, euphoria, vertigo

Dermatologic: Rash

Endocrine & metabolic: Decreased libido

Gastrointestinal: Diarrhea

Neuromuscular & skeletal: Dysarthria, weakness

Otic: Blurred vision

Miscellaneous: Diaphoresis

Warnings/Precautions Safety and efficacy in children <18 years of age have not been established; do not use in pregnant women; may cause drug dependency; avoid abrupt discontinuance in patients with prolonged therapy or seizure disorders; use with caution in patients receiving other CNS depressants, in patients with hepatic dysfunction, and the elderly

Drug Interactions CYP3A3/4 enzyme substrate

Increased Effect/Toxicity: Temazepam potentiates the CNS depressant effects of narcotic analgesics, barbiturates, phenothiazines, antihistamines, MAO inhibitors, sedative-hypnotics, and cyclic antidepressants. Serum levels of temazepam may be increased by inhibitors of CYP3A3/4, including cimetidine, ciprofloxacin, clarithromycin, clozapine, diltiazem, disulfiram, digoxin, erythromycin, ethanol, fluconazole, fluoxetine, fluvoxamine, isoniazid, itraconazole, ketoconazole, labetalol, levodopa, loxapine, metoprolol, metronidazole, miconazole, nefazodone, omeprazole, phenytoin, rifabutin, rifampin, troleandomycin, valproic acid, and verapamil.

Decreased Effect: Oral contraceptives may increase the clearance of temazepam. Temazepam may decrease the antiparkinsonian efficacy of levodopa. Theophylline and other CNS stimulants may antagonize the sedative effects of temazepam. Carbamazepine, rifampin, rifabutin may enhance the metabolism of temazepam and decrease its therapeutic effect.

Drug Uptake

Half-life, elimination: 9.5-12.4 hours

Time to peak: 2-3 hours

Pregnancy Risk Factor X

Generic Available Yes

Temodar® *see* Temozolomide *on page 1137*

Temovate® *see* Clobetasol *on page 303*

Temozolomide (te mo ZOLE oh mide)

U.S. Brand Names Temodar®

Canadian Brand Names Temodal™; Tomedar®

Pharmacologic Category Antineoplastic Agent, Alkylating Agent

Use Treatment of adult patients with refractory (first relapse) anaplastic astrocytoma who have experienced disease progression on nitrosourea and procarbazine

Unlabeled/Investigational: Glioma, first relapse/advanced metastatic malignant melanoma

Local Anesthetic/Vasoconstrictor Precautions No information available to require special precautions

Effects on Dental Treatment No effects or complications reported

Mechanism of Action Temozolomide (prodrug) is hydrolyzed to MTIC (active form). The cytotoxic effects of MTIC is through alkylation of DNA (O^6, N^7 of guanine). Like DTIC, temozolomide is converted to the active alkylating metabolite MTIC. Unlike DTIC, however, this conversion is spontaneous, nonenzymatic, and occurs under physiologic conditions in all tissues to which the drug distributes.

Other Adverse Effects

>10%:

Central nervous system: Headache (41%), fatigue (34%), convulsions (23%), hemiparesis (29%), dizziness (19%), fever (11%), coordination abnormality (11%), amnesia (10%), insomnia (10%), somnolence. In the case of CNS malignancies, it is difficult to distinguish the relative contributions of temozolomide and progressive disease to CNS symptoms.

Gastrointestinal: Nausea (53%), vomiting (42%), constipation (33%), diarrhea (16%), anorexia

Hematologic: Neutropenia (grade 3-4, 14%), thrombocytopenia (grade 3-4 19%)

Neuromuscular & skeletal: Weakness (13%)

1% to 10%:

Central nervous system: Ataxia (8%), confusion (5%), anxiety (7%), depression (6%)

Dermatologic: Rash (8%), pruritus (8%)

Gastrointestinal: Dysphagia (7%), abdominal pain (9%)

Hematologic: Anemia (8%; grade 3-4, 4%)

Neuromuscular & skeletal: Paresthesia (9%), back pain (8%), myalgia (5%)

Ocular: Diplopia (5%), vision abnormality (5%)

Contraindications Hypersensitivity to temozolomide or any component of the formulation; history of hypersensitivity to Dtic®

(Continued)

Temozolomide *(Continued)*

Drug Interactions Although valproic acid reduces the clearance of temozolomide by 5%, the clinical significance of this is unknown.

Drug Uptake

Half-life, elimination: Mean: Parent compound: 1.8 hours

Time to peak: 1 hour if taken on empty stomach

Pregnancy Risk Factor D

Generic Available No

Comments Dose-limiting toxicity is hematological. In the event of an overdose, hematological evaluation is necessary. Treatment is supportive.

Tenecteplase (ten EK te plase)

U.S. Brand Names TNKase™

Pharmacologic Category Thrombolytic Agent

Use Reduce mortality associated with acute myocardial infarction

Local Anesthetic/Vasoconstrictor Precautions No information available to require special precautions

Effects on Dental Treatment No effects or complications reported

Dosage I.V.:

Adult: Recommended total dose should not exceed 50 mg and is based on patient's weight; administer as a bolus over 5 seconds

If patient's weight:

<60 kg, dose: 30 mg

≥60 to <70 kg, dose: 35 mg

≥70 to <80 kg, dose: 40 mg

≥80 to <90 kg, dose: 45 mg

≥90 kg, dose: 50 mg

All patients received 150-325 mg of aspirin as soon as possible and then daily. Intravenous heparin was initiated as soon as possible and aPTT was maintained between 50-70 seconds.

Dosage adjustment in hepatic impairment: Severe hepatic failure is a relative contraindication. Recommendations were not made for mild to moderate hepatic impairment.

Elderly: Although dosage adjustments are not recommended, the elderly have a higher incidence of morbidity and mortality with the use of tenecteplase. The 30-day mortality in the ASSENT-2 trial was 2.5% for patients <65 years, 8.5% for patients 65-74 years, and 16.2% for patients ≥75 years. The intracranial hemorrhage rate was 0.4% for patients <65, 1.6 % for patients 65-74 years, and 1.7 % for patients ≥75. The risks and benefits of use should be weighted carefully in the elderly.

Mechanism of Action Initiates fibrinolysis by binding to fibrin and converting plasminogen to plasmin.

Other Adverse Effects As with all drugs which may affect hemostasis, bleeding is the major adverse effect associated with tenecteplase. Hemorrhage may occur at virtually any site. Risk is dependent on multiple variables, including the dosage administered, concurrent use of multiple agents which alter hemostasis, and patient predisposition. Rapid lysis of coronary artery thrombi by thrombolytic agents may be associated with reperfusion-related arterial and/or ventricular arrhythmias. The incidence of stroke and bleeding increase in patients >65 years.

>10%:

Hematologic: Bleeding (22% minor: ASSENT-2 trial)

Local: Hematoma (12% minor)

1% to 10%:

Central nervous system: Stroke (2%)

Gastrointestinal: GI hemorrhage (1% major, 2% minor), epistaxis (2% minor)

Genitourinary: GU bleeding (4% minor)

Hematologic: Bleeding (5% major: ASSENT-2 trial)

Local: Bleeding at catheter puncture site (4% minor), hematoma (2% major)

Respiratory: Pharyngeal bleeding (3% minor)

Additional cardiovascular events associated with use in myocardial infarction: Cardiogenic shock, arrhythmias, AV block, pulmonary edema, heart failure, cardiac arrest, recurrent myocardial ischemia, myocardial reinfarction, myocardial rupture, cardiac tamponade, pericarditis, pericardial effusion, mitral regurgitation, thrombosis, embolism, electromechanical dissociation, hypotension, fever, nausea, vomiting

Drug Interactions

Increased Effect/Toxicity: Drugs which affect platelet function (eg, NSAIDs, dipyridamole, ticlopidine, clopidogrel, IIb/IIIa antagonists) may potentiate the risk of hemorrhage; use with caution. Heparin and aspirin: Use with aspirin and heparin may increase bleeding. However, aspirin and heparin were used concomitantly with tenecteplase in the majority of patients in clinical studies. Risk of bleeding may be increased during concurrent therapy with warfarin or oral anticoagulants.

Decreased Effect: Aminocaproic acid (antifibrinolytic agent) may decrease effectiveness.

Drug Uptake Half-life, elimination: 90-130 minutes
Pregnancy Risk Factor C
Generic Available No

Tenex® *see* Guanfacine *on page 574*

Teniposide (ten i POE side)

U.S. Brand Names Vumon
Canadian Brand Names Vumon®
Mexican Brand Names Vumon®
Pharmacologic Category Antineoplastic Agent, Miscellaneous
Synonyms EPT; VM-26
Use Treatment of Hodgkin's and non-Hodgkin's lymphomas, acute lymphocytic leukemia, bladder carcinoma and neuroblastoma
Local Anesthetic/Vasoconstrictor Precautions No information available to require special precautions
Effects on Dental Treatment No effects or complications reported
Mechanism of Action A topoisomerase II inhibitor; appears to cause DNA strand breaks by inhibition of strand-passing and DNA ligase action; does not inhibit microtubular assembly; has been shown to delay transit of cells through the S phase and arrest cells in late S or early G_2 phase
Other Adverse Effects

>10%:
- Gastrointestinal: Mucositis (75%); diarrhea, nausea, vomiting (20% to 30%); anorexia
- Hematologic: Myelosuppression, leukopenia, neutropenia (95%), thrombocytopenia (65% to 80%), anemia
  - Onset: 5-7 days
  - Nadir: 7-10 days
  - Recovery: 21-28 days

1% to 10%:
- Cardiovascular: Hypotension (2%), associated with rapid (<30 minutes) infusions
- Dermatologic: Alopecia (9%), rash (3%)
- Miscellaneous: Anaphylactoid reactions (5%) (fever, rash, hypertension, hypotension, dyspnea, bronchospasm), usually seen with rapid (<30 minutes) infusions

Drug Interactions CYP3A3/4 enzyme substrate; CYP2C19 enzyme inhibitor

Increased Effect/Toxicity: Alteration of MTX transport has been found as a slow efflux of MTX and its polyglutamated form out of the cell, leading to intercellular accumulation of MTX. Sodium salicylate, sulfamethizole, and tolbutamide displace teniposide from protein-binding sites which could cause substantial increases in free drug levels, resulting in potentiation of toxicity.

Drug Uptake Half-life, elimination: 5 hours
Pregnancy Risk Factor D
Generic Available No

Ten-K® *see* Potassium Chloride *on page 977*

Tenofovir (te NOE fo veer)

Related Information

HIV Infection and AIDS *on page 1334*

U.S. Brand Names Viread™
Pharmacologic Category Antiretroviral Agent, Reverse Transcriptase Inhibitor (Nucleotide)
Synonyms PMPA; TDF; Tenofovir Disoproxil Fumarate
Use Management of HIV infections in combination with at least two other antiretroviral agents
Local Anesthetic/Vasoconstrictor Precautions No information available to require special precautions
Effects on Dental Treatment No effects or complications reported
Dosage Oral: Adults:

HIV infection: 300 mg once daily

Note: When used concurrently with didanosine, tenofovir should be administered at least 2 hours before or 1 hour after didanosine.

Dosage adjustment in renal impairment: Avoid use in renal impairment (Cl_{cr} <60 mL/minute). No dosage guidelines available.

Mechanism of Action Tenofovir disoproxil fumarate is an analog of adensoine 5'-monophosphate; it interferes with the HIV viral RNA-dependent DNA polymerase, resulting in inhibition of viral replication. TDF is first converted intracellularly by hydrolysis to tenofovir and subsequently phosphorolated to the active tenofovir diphosphate; nucleotide reverse transcriptase inhibitor.
Other Adverse Effects Clinical trials involved addition to prior antiretroviral therapy. Frequencies listed are treatment-emergent adverse effects noted at higher frequency than in the placebo group.

>10%: Gastrointestinal: Nausea (11%)

(Continued)

Tenofovir *(Continued)*

1% to 10%:

Endocrine & metabolic: Glycosuria (3%, frequency equal to placebo); other metabolic effects (hyperglycemia, hypertriglyceridemia) noted at frequencies less than placebo

Gastrointestinal: Diarrhea (9%), vomiting (5%), flatulence (4%), abdominal pain (3%, frequency equal to placebo), anorexia (3%)

Hematologic: Neutropenia (1%, frequency equal to placebo)

Hepatic: Increased transaminases (2% to 4%)

Neuromuscular & skeletal: Weakness (8%, frequency equal to placebo)

Note: Uncommon, but significant adverse reactions reported with other reverse transcriptase inhibitors include pancreatitis, peripheral neuropathy, and myopathy. These have not been reported in clinical trials with tenofovir prior to marketing approval.

Drug Interactions CYP1A2 inhibitor (minor)

Didanosine: Serum concentrations of didanosine may be increased by tenofovir. Separate administration times (tenofovir should be given 2 hours before or 1 hour after didanosine).

Lopinavir: Serum levels of lopinavir may be decreased by tenofovir; lopinavir/ritonavir may increase serum concentrations of tenofovir.

Ritonavir: Serum concentrations of ritonavir may be decreased by tenofovir.

Note: Drugs which may compete for renal tubule secretion (including acyclovir, cidofovir, ganciclovir, valacyclovir, valganciclovir) may increase the serum concentrations of tenofovir. Drugs causing nephrotoxicity may also reduce elimination of tenofovir.

Drug Uptake Time to peak: 1 hour (fasting); 2 hours (with food)

Pregnancy Risk Factor B

Generic Available No

Tenoretic® *see* Atenolol and Chlorthalidone *on page 126*

Tenormin® *see* Atenolol *on page 125*

Tenuate® *see* Diethylpropion *on page 384*

Tenuate® Dospan® *see* Diethylpropion *on page 384*

Tequin® *see* Gatifloxacin *on page 549*

Terazol® 3 *see* Terconazole *on page 1142*

Terazol® 7 *see* Terconazole *on page 1142*

Terazosin (ter AY zoe sin)

Related Information

Cardiovascular Diseases *on page 1308*

U.S. Brand Names Hytrin®

Canadian Brand Names Alti-Terazosin; Apo®-Terazosin; Hytrin®; Novo-Terazosin; Nu-Terazosin

Mexican Brand Names Adecur®; Hytrin®

Pharmacologic Category $Alpha_1$ Blocker

Use Management of mild to moderate hypertension; alone or in combination with other agents such as diuretics or beta-blockers; benign prostate hyperplasia (BPH)

Local Anesthetic/Vasoconstrictor Precautions No information available to require special precautions

Effects on Dental Treatment ≤10%: Xerostomia

Dosage Adults: Oral:

Hypertension: Initial: 1 mg at bedtime; slowly increase dose to achieve desired BP, up to 20 mg/day; usual dose: 1-5 mg/day

Dosage reduction may be needed when adding a diuretic or other antihypertensive agent; if drug is discontinued for greater than several days, consider beginning with initial dose and retitrate as needed; dosage may be given on a twice daily regimen if response is diminished at 24 hours and hypotensive is observed at 2-4 hours following a dose

Benign prostatic hypertrophy: Initial: 1 mg at bedtime, increasing as needed; most patients require 10 mg day; if no response after 4-6 weeks of 10 mg/day, may increase to 20 mg/day

Mechanism of Action $Alpha_1$-specific blocking agent with minimal $alpha_2$ effects; this allows peripheral postsynaptic blockade, with the resultant decrease in arterial tone, while preserving the negative feedback loop which is mediated by the peripheral presynaptic $alpha_2$-receptors; terazosin relaxes the smooth muscle of the bladder neck, thus reducing bladder outlet obstruction

Other Adverse Effects Asthenia, postural hypotension, dizziness, somnolence, nasal congestion/rhinitis, and impotence were the only events noted in clinical trials to occur at a frequency significantly greater than placebo ($p < 0.05$).

>10%: Central nervous system: Dizziness, headache, muscle weakness

1% to 10%:

Cardiovascular: Edema, palpitations, chest pain, peripheral edema (3%), orthostatic hypotension (3% to 4%), tachycardia

Central nervous system: Fatigue, nervousness, drowsiness

Gastrointestinal: Dry mouth
Genitourinary: Urinary incontinence
Ocular: Blurred vision
Respiratory: Dyspnea, nasal congestion

Drug Interactions

Increased Effect/Toxicity: Terazosin's hypotensive effect is increased with beta-blockers, diuretics, ACE inhibitors, calcium channel blockers, and other antihypertensive medications.

Decreased Effect: Decreased antihypertensive response with NSAIDs. Alpha-blockers reduce the response to pressor agents (norepinephrine).

Drug Uptake

Onset of action: 1-2 hours
Absorption: Oral: Rapid
Half-life, elimination: 9.2-12 hours
Time to peak: ~1 hour

Pregnancy Risk Factor C

Generic Available Yes

Terbinafine, Oral (TER bin a feen, OR al)

U.S. Brand Names Lamisil® Oral

Pharmacologic Category Antifungal Agent

Use Treatment of onychomycosis infections of the toenail or fingernail

Local Anesthetic/Vasoconstrictor Precautions No information available to require special precautions

Effects on Dental Treatment No effects or complications reported

Dosage Adults: Oral:

Fingernail onychomycosis: 250 mg once daily for 6 weeks
Toenail onychomycosis: 250 mg once daily for 12 weeks

Mechanism of Action Synthetic allylamine derivative which inhibits squalene epoxidase, a key enzyme in sterol biosynthesis in fungi; the resulting deficiency in ergosterol within the cell wall causes fungi death

Other Adverse Effects

>10%: Central nervous system: Headache

1% to 10%:

Dermatologic: Rash, pruritus, urticaria
Gastrointestinal: Diarrhea, dyspepsia, abdominal pain, nausea, flatulence, abnormal taste
Hepatic: Elevated liver enzyme ≥2 times upper limit of normal range
Ocular: Visual disturbance

Drug Uptake

Absorption: Oral: >70%
Half-life, elimination: 200-400 hours

Terbinafine, Topical (TER bin a feen, TOP i kal)

U.S. Brand Names Lamisil® Cream

Pharmacologic Category Antifungal Agent, Topical

Use Topical antifungal for the treatment of tinea pedis (athlete's foot), tinea cruris (jock itch), and tinea corporis (ring worm)

Unlabeled/Investigational: Cutaneous candidiasis and pityriasis versicolor

Local Anesthetic/Vasoconstrictor Precautions No information available to require special precautions

Effects on Dental Treatment No effects or complications reported

Dosage Adults: Topical:

Athlete's foot: Apply to affected area twice daily for at least 1 week, not to exceed 4 weeks

Ringworm and jock itch: Apply to affected area once or twice daily for at least 1 week, not to exceed 4 weeks

Mechanism of Action Synthetic alkylamine derivative which inhibits squalene epoxidases, a key enzyme in sterol biosynthesis in fungi; the resulting deficiency in ergosterol within the cell wall causes fungi death

Other Adverse Effects 1% to 10%:

Dermatologic: Pruritus, contact dermatitis
Local: Irritation, stinging

Drug Uptake Absorption: Topical: Limited

Terbutaline (ter BYOO ta leen)

Related Information

Respiratory Diseases *on page 1328*

U.S. Brand Names Brethine®

Canadian Brand Names Bricanyl® [DSC]

Mexican Brand Names Bricanyl®; Taziken®

Pharmacologic Category $Beta_2$ Agonist

Synonyms Brethaire® [DSC]; Bricanyl® [DSC]

Use Bronchodilator in reversible airway obstruction and bronchial asthma

(Continued)

Terbutaline *(Continued)*

Unlabeled/Investigational: Tocolytic agent (management of preterm labor)

Local Anesthetic/Vasoconstrictor Precautions No information available to require special precautions

Effects on Dental Treatment No effects or complications reported

Dosage

Children <12 years:

Oral: Initial: 0.05 mg/kg/dose 3 times/day, increased gradually as required; maximum: 0.15 mg/kg/dose 3-4 times/day or a total of 5 mg/24 hours

S.C.: 0.005-0.01 mg/kg/dose to a maximum of 0.3 mg/dose every 15-20 minutes for 3 doses

Nebulization: 0.01-0.03 mg/kg/dose every 4-6 hours

Inhalation: 1-2 inhalations every 4-6 hours

Children >12 years and Adults:

Oral:

12-15 years: 2.5 mg every 6 hours 3 times/day; not to exceed 7.5 mg in 24 hours

>15 years: 5 mg/dose every 6 hours 3 times/day; if side effects occur, reduce dose to 2.5 mg every 6 hours; not to exceed 15 mg in 24 hours

S.C.: 0.25 mg/dose repeated in 15-30 minutes for one time only; a total dose of 0.5 mg should not be exceeded within a 4-hour period

Nebulization: 0.01-0.03 mg/kg/dose every 4-6 hours

Inhalation: 2 inhalations every 4-6 hours; wait 1 minute between inhalations

Mechanism of Action Relaxes bronchial smooth muscle by action on $beta_2$-receptors with less effect on heart rate

Other Adverse Effects

>10%:

Central nervous system: Nervousness, restlessness

Neuromuscular & skeletal: Trembling

1% to 10%:

Cardiovascular: Tachycardia, hypertension

Central nervous system: Dizziness, drowsiness, headache, insomnia

Gastrointestinal: Xerostomia, nausea, vomiting, bad taste in mouth

Neuromuscular & skeletal: Muscle cramps, weakness

Miscellaneous: Diaphoresis

Drug Interactions

Increased Effect/Toxicity: Increased toxicity with MAO inhibitors, tricyclic antidepressants

Decreased effect with beta-blockers

Drug Uptake

Onset of action: Oral: 30-45 minutes; S.C.: 6-15 minutes

Half-life, elimination: 11-16 hours

Pregnancy Risk Factor B

Generic Available No

Terconazole (ter KONE a zole)

U.S. Brand Names Terazol® 3; Terazol® 7

Canadian Brand Names Terazol®

Mexican Brand Names Fungistat

Pharmacologic Category Antifungal Agent, Vaginal

Synonyms Triaconazole

Use Local treatment of vulvovaginal candidiasis

Local Anesthetic/Vasoconstrictor Precautions No information available to require special precautions

Effects on Dental Treatment No effects or complications reported

Dosage Adults: Female: Insert 1 applicatorful intravaginally at bedtime for 7 consecutive days

Mechanism of Action Triazole ketal antifungal agent; involves inhibition of fungal cytochrome P450. Specifically, terconazole inhibits cytochrome P450-dependent 14-alpha-demethylase which results in accumulation of membrane disturbing 14-alpha-demethylsterols and ergosterol depletion.

Other Adverse Effects 1% to 10%:

Central nervous system; Fever, chills

Gastrointestinal: Abdominal pain

Genitourinary: Vulvar/vaginal burning, dysmenorrhea

Drug Uptake Absorption: Extent of systemic absorption after vaginal administration may be dependent on the presence of a uterus; 5% to 8% in women who had a hysterectomy versus 12% to 16% in nonhysterectomy women

Pregnancy Risk Factor C

Generic Available No

Terpin Hydrate and Codeine (TER pin HYE drate & KOE deen)

Pharmacologic Category Expectorant

Synonyms ETH and C

Use Symptomatic relief of cough

Local Anesthetic/Vasoconstrictor Precautions No information available to require special precautions

Effects on Dental Treatment No effects or complications reported

Restrictions C-V

Dosage Based on codeine content

Adults: 10-20 mg/dose every 4-6 hours as needed

Children (not recommended): 1-1.5 mg/kg/24 hours divided every 4 hours; maximum: 30 mg/24 hours

2-6 years: 1.25-2.5 mL every 4-6 hours as needed

6-12 years: 2.5-5 mL every 4-6 hours as needed

Other Adverse Effects Frequency not defined:

Central nervous system: Drowsiness

Gastrointestinal: Nausea, vomiting

Drug Uptake See Codeine monograph.

Pregnancy Risk Factor C

Generic Available Yes

Terra-Cortril® *see* Oxytetracycline and Hydrocortisone *on page 910*

Terramycin® I.M. *see* Oxytetracycline *on page 909*

Terramycin® w/Polymyxin B Ophthalmic *see* Oxytetracycline and Polymyxin B *on page 910*

Teslac® *see* Testolactone *on page 1143*

Tessalon® *see* Benzonatate *on page 153*

Testoderm® *see* Testosterone *on page 1143*

Testoderm® TTS *see* Testosterone *on page 1143*

Testoderm® with Adhesive *see* Testosterone *on page 1143*

Testolactone (tes toe LAK tone)

U.S. Brand Names Teslac®

Canadian Brand Names Teslac®

Pharmacologic Category Androgen

Use Palliative treatment of advanced disseminated breast carcinoma

Local Anesthetic/Vasoconstrictor Precautions No information available to require special precautions

Effects on Dental Treatment No effects or complications reported

Restrictions C-III

Dosage Adults: Female: Oral: 250 mg 4 times/day for at least 3 months; desired response may take as long as 3 months

Mechanism of Action A synthetic testosterone derivative without significant androgen activity; inhibits steroid aromatase activity, thereby blocking the production of estradiol and estrone from androgen precursors such as testosterone and androstenedione; enzymatic block is transient and is usually limited to a period of 3 months.

Other Adverse Effects 1% to 10%:

Cardiovascular: Edema

Central nervous system: Malaise

Dermatologic: Maculopapular rash

Endocrine & metabolic: Hypercalcemia,

Gastrointestinal: Anorexia, diarrhea, nausea, edema of the tongue

Neuromuscular & skeletal: Paresthesias, peripheral neuropathies

Drug Interactions Increases effects of oral anticoagulants

Drug Uptake Absorption: Oral: Well absorbed

Pregnancy Risk Factor C

Generic Available No

Testopel® Pellet *see* Testosterone *on page 1143*

Testosterone (tes TOS ter one)

U.S. Brand Names Androderm®; AndroGel®; Delatestryl®; Depo®-Testosterone; Testoderm®; Testoderm® TTS; Testoderm® with Adhesive; Testopel® Pellet; Testro® AQ; Testro® LA

Canadian Brand Names Andriol®; Androderm®; Androgel®; Andropository; Delatestryl®; Depotest® 100; Everone® 200; Testoderm®; Virilon® IM

Pharmacologic Category Androgen

Synonyms Aqueous Testosterone; Testosterone Cypionate; Testosterone Enanthate; Testosterone Propionate

Use Androgen replacement therapy in the treatment of delayed male puberty; inoperable breast cancer; male hypogonadism

Local Anesthetic/Vasoconstrictor Precautions No information available to require special precautions

(Continued)

Testosterone *(Continued)*

Effects on Dental Treatment No effects or complications reported

Restrictions C-III

Dosage

Children: I.M.:

Male hypogonadism:

Initiation of pubertal growth: 40-50 mg/m²/dose (cypionate or enanthate ester) monthly until the growth rate falls to prepubertal levels

Terminal growth phase: 100 mg/m²/dose (cypionate or enanthate ester) monthly until growth ceases

Maintenance virilizing dose: 100 mg/m²/dose (cypionate or enanthate ester) twice monthly

Delayed puberty: 40-50 mg/m²/dose monthly (cypionate or enanthate ester) for 6 months

Adults: Inoperable breast cancer: I.M.: 200-400 mg every 2-4 weeks

Male: Short-acting formulations: Testosterone aqueous/testosterone propionate (in oil): I.M.:

Androgen replacement therapy: 10-50 mg 2-3 times/week

Male hypogonadism: 40-50 mg/m²/dose monthly until the growth rate falls to prepubertal levels (~5 cm/year); during terminal growth phase: 100 mg/m²/dose monthly until growth ceases; maintenance virilizing dose: 100 mg/m²/dose twice monthly or 50-400 mg/dose every 2-4 weeks

Male: Long-acting formulations: Testosterone enanthate (in oil)/testosterone cypionate (in oil): I.M.:

Male hypogonadism: 50-400 mg every 2-4 weeks

Male with delayed puberty: 50-200 mg every 2-4 weeks for a limited duration

Male ≥18 years: Transdermal: Primary hypogonadism **or** hypogonadotropic hypogonadism:

Testoderm®: Apply 6 mg patch daily to scrotum (if scrotum is inadequate, use a 4 mg daily system)

Testoderm® TTS: Apply 5 mg patch daily to clean, dry area of skin on the arm, back or upper buttocks. **Do not apply Testoderm® TTS to the scrotum.**

Androderm®: Apply 2 systems nightly to clean, dry area on the back, abdomen, upper arms, or thighs for 24 hours for a total of 5 mg/day

AndroGel®: Male >18 years: 5 g (to deliver 50 mg of testosterone with 5 mg systemically absorbed) applied once daily (preferably in the morning) to clean, dry, intact skin of the shoulder and upper arms and/or abdomen. Upon opening the packet(s), the entire contents should be squeezed into the palm of the hand and immediately applied to the application site(s). Application sites should be allowed to dry for a few minutes prior to dressing. Hands should be washed with soap and water after application. **Do not apply AndroGel® to the genitals.**

Dosing adjustment/comments in hepatic disease: Reduce dose

Mechanism of Action Principal endogenous androgen responsible for promoting the growth and development of the male sex organs and maintaining secondary sex characteristics in androgen-deficient males

Other Adverse Effects Frequency not defined:

Cardiovascular: Flushing, edema

Central nervous system: Excitation, aggressive behavior, sleeplessness, anxiety, mental depression, headache

Dermatologic: Hirsutism (increase in pubic hair growth), acne

Endocrine & metabolic: Menstrual problems (amenorrhea), virilism, breast soreness, gynecomastia, hypercalcemia, hypoglycemia

Gastrointestinal: Nausea, vomiting, GI irritation

Genitourinary: Prostatic hypertrophy, prostatic carcinoma, impotence, testicular atrophy, epididymitis, priapism, bladder irritability

Hepatic: Hepatic dysfunction, cholestatic hepatitis, hepatic necrosis

Hematologic: Leukopenia, polycythemia, suppression of clotting factors

Miscellaneous: Hypersensitivity reactions

Drug Interactions CYP3A3/4 and 3A5-7 enzyme substrate

Increased Effect/Toxicity: Warfarin and testosterone: Effects of oral anticoagulants may be enhanced. Testosterone may increase levels of oxyphenbutazone. May enhance fluid retention from corticosteroids.

Drug Uptake

Absorption: Transdermal: ~10% of dose (gel) systemically

Duration: Route- and ester-dependent; I.M.: Cypionate and enanthate esters have longest duration, ≤2-4 weeks

Half-life, elimination: 10-100 minutes

Pregnancy Risk Factor X

Generic Available Yes

Testred® *see* MethylTESTOSTERone *on page 799*

Testro® AQ *see* Testosterone *on page 1143*

Testro® LA *see* Testosterone *on page 1143*

Tetanus Immune Globulin (Human)

(TET a nus i MYUN GLOB yoo lin HYU man)

Related Information

Animal and Human Bites Guidelines *on page 1416*

U.S. Brand Names BayTet™

Canadian Brand Names BayTet™

Pharmacologic Category Immune Globulin

Synonyms TIG

Use Passive immunization against tetanus; tetanus immune globulin is preferred over tetanus antitoxin for treatment of active tetanus; part of the management of an unclean, nonminor wound in a person whose history of previous receipt of tetanus toxoid is unknown or who has received less than three doses of tetanus toxoid

Local Anesthetic/Vasoconstrictor Precautions No information available to require special precautions

Effects on Dental Treatment No effects or complications reported

Dosage I.M.:

Prophylaxis of tetanus:

Children: 4 units/kg; some recommend administering 250 units to small children

Adults: 250 units

Treatment of tetanus:

Children: 500-3000 units; some should infiltrate locally around the wound

Adults: 3000-6000 units. See table.

Tetanus Prophylaxis in Wound Management

Number of Prior Tetanus Toxoid Doses	Clean, Minor Wounds		All Other Wounds	
	Td[1]	TIG[2]	Td[1]	TIG[2]
Unknown or <3	Yes	No	Yes	Yes
≥3*	No[3]	No	No[4]	No

*If only three doses of fluid tetanus toxoid have been received, a fourth dose of toxoid, preferably an adsorbed toxoid, should be given.

[1]Adult tetanus and diphtheria toxoids; use pediatric preparations (DT or DTP) if the patient is <7 years old

[2]Tetanus immune globulin

[3]Yes, if >10 years since last dose

[4]Yes, if >5 years since last dose Adapted from Report of the Committee on Infectious Diseases, American Academy of Pediatrics, Elk Grove Village, IL: American Academy of Pediatrics, 1986.

Mechanism of Action Passive immunity toward tetanus

Other Adverse Effects

>10%: Local: Pain, tenderness, erythema at injection site

1% to 10%:

Central nervous system: Fever (mild)

Dermatologic: Urticaria, angioedema

Neuromuscular & skeletal: Muscle stiffness

Miscellaneous: Anaphylaxis reaction

Warnings/Precautions Have epinephrine 1:1000 available for anaphylactic reactions. Use caution in patients with isolated immunoglobulin A deficiency or a history of systemic hypersensitivity to human immunoglobulins. As a product of human plasma, this product may potentially transmit disease; screening of donors, as well as testing and/or inactivation of certain viruses reduces this risk. Use caution in patients with thrombocytopenia or coagulation disorders (I.M. injections may be contraindicated). Not for I.V. administration.

Drug Interactions Never administer tetanus toxoid and TIG in same syringe (toxoid will be neutralized); toxoid may be given at a separate site; concomitant administration with Td may decrease its immune response, especially in individuals with low prevaccination antibody titers.

Drug Uptake Absorption: Well absorbed

Pregnancy Risk Factor C

Generic Available No

Comments Tetanus immune globulin is preferred over tetanus antitoxin for treatment of active tetanus

Tetanus Toxoid, Adsorbed (TET a nus TOKS oyd, ad SORBED)

Pharmacologic Category Toxoid

Use Selective induction of active immunity against tetanus in selected patients.

Note: Tetanus and diphtheria toxoids for adult use (Td) is the preferred immunizing agent for most adults and for children after their seventh birthday. Young children should receive trivalent DTwP or DTaP (diphtheria/tetanus/pertussis - whole cell or acellular), as part of their childhood immunization program, unless pertussis is contraindicated, then TD is warranted.

Local Anesthetic/Vasoconstrictor Precautions No information available to require special precautions

(Continued)

Tetanus Toxoid, Adsorbed *(Continued)*

Effects on Dental Treatment No effects or complications reported

Dosage Adults: I.M.:

Primary immunization: 0.5 mL; repeat 0.5 mL at 4-8 weeks after first dose and at 6-12 months after second dose

Routine booster doses are recommended only every 5-10 years

Mechanism of Action Preparations contain the toxin produced by virulent tetanus bacilli (detoxified growth products of *Clostridium tetani*). The toxin has been modified by treatment with formaldehyde so that it has lost toxicity but still retains ability to act as antigen and produce active immunity; the aluminum salt, a mineral adjuvant, delays the rate of absorption and prolongs and enhances its properties; duration ~10 years.

Other Adverse Effects

>10%: Local: Induration/redness at injection site

1% to 10%:

- Central nervous system: Chills, fever
- Local: Sterile abscess at injection site
- Miscellaneous: Allergic reaction

Drug Interactions Decreased Response: If primary immunization is started in individuals receiving an immunosuppressive agent or corticosteroids, serologic testing may be needed to ensure adequate antibody response; concurrent use of TIG and tetanus toxoid may delay the development of active immunity by several days

Drug Uptake Duration: Primary immunization: ~10 years

Pregnancy Risk Factor C

Generic Available No

Comments Routine booster doses are recommended only every 10 years

Tetanus Toxoid, Fluid (TET a nus TOKS oyd FLOO id)

Pharmacologic Category Toxoid

Synonyms Tetanus Toxoid Plain

Use Detection of delayed hypersensitivity and assessment of cell-mediated immunity; active immunization against tetanus in the rare adult or child who is allergic to the aluminum adjuvant (a product containing adsorbed tetanus toxoid is preferred)

Local Anesthetic/Vasoconstrictor Precautions No information available to require special precautions

Effects on Dental Treatment No effects or complications reported

Dosage

Anergy testing: Intradermal: 0.1 mL

Primary immunization (**Note:** Td, TD, DTaP/DTwP are recommended): Adults: Inject 3 doses of 0.5 mL I.M. or S.C. at 4- to 8-week intervals; give fourth dose 6-12 months after third dose

Booster doses: I.M., S.C.: 0.5 mL every 10 years

Mechanism of Action Preparations contain the toxin produced by virulent tetanus bacilli (detoxified growth products of *Clostridium tetani*). The toxin has been modified by treatment with formaldehyde so that is has lost toxicity but still retains ability to act as antigen and produce active immunity.

Other Adverse Effects Frequency not defined: Very hypersensitive persons may develop a local reaction at the injection site; urticaria, anaphylactic reactions, shock and death are possible.

Contraindications Hypersensitivity to tetanus toxoid or any component of the formulation

Drug Interactions Increased Effect: Cimetidine may augment delayed hypersensitivity responses to skin test antigens.

Pregnancy Risk Factor C

Generic Available No

Comments Tetanus Toxoid, Adsorbed is preferred for all basic immunizing and recall reactions because of more persistent antitoxin titer induction

Tetracaine (TET ra kane)

Related Information

Mouth Pain, Cold Sore, and Canker Sore Products *on page 1458*
Oral Nonviral Soft Tissue Ulcerations or Erosions *on page 1384*
Oral Pain *on page 1360*

U.S. Brand Names Pontocaine®

Canadian Brand Names Ametop™; Pontocaine®

Pharmacologic Category Local Anesthetic

Synonyms Amethocaine Hydrochloride; Tetracaine Hydrochloride

Use

Dental: Ester-type local anesthetic; applied topically to throat for various diagnostic procedures

Medical: Spinal anesthetic; local anesthetic applied to nose and eyes for various diagnostic and examination purposes

Local Anesthetic/Vasoconstrictor Precautions No information available to require special precautions

Effects on Dental Treatment No effects or complications reported

Dosage Children and Adults: Topical: Applied as a 1% or 2% cream to affected areas 3-4 times/day as needed

Mechanism of Action Local anesthetics bind selectively to the intracellular surface of sodium channels to block influx of sodium into the axon. As a result, depolarization necessary for action potential propagation and subsequent nerve function is prevented. The block at the sodium channel is reversible. Local anesthetics reversibly prevent generation and conduction of electrical impulses in neurons by decreasing the transient increase in permeability to sodium. The differential sensitivity generally depends on the size of the fiber; small fibers are more sensitive than larger fibers and require a longer period for recovery. Sensory pain fibers are usually blocked first, followed by fibers that transmit sensations of temperature, touch, and deep pressure. High concentrations block sympathetic somatic sensory and somatic motor fibers. The spread of anesthesia depends upon the distribution of the solution. This is primarily dependent on the site of administration and volume of drug injected. When drug diffuses away from the axon, sodium channel function is restored and nerve propagation returns.

Other Adverse Effects

1% to 10%: Dermatologic: Contact dermatitis, burning, stinging, angioedema

<1%: Tenderness, urticaria, urethritis, methemoglobinemia in infants

Contraindications Hypersensitivity to tetracaine or any component of the formulation; ophthalmic secondary bacterial infection; liver disease; CNS disease or meningitis (if used for epidural or spinal anesthesia); myasthenia gravis

Warnings/Precautions No pediatric dosage recommendations; ophthalmic preparations may delay wound healing; use with caution in patients with cardiac disease and hyperthyroidism

Drug Interactions Aminosalicylic acid, sulfonamides' effects may be antagonized.

Drug Uptake

Onset of action: Anesthetic: Ophthalmic: ~60 seconds; Topical or spinal injection: 3-8 minutes after applied to mucous membranes or when saddle block administered for spinal anesthesia

Duration: Topical: 1.5-3 hours

Pregnancy Risk Factor C

Dosage Forms **CRM:** 1% (28 g). **INJ:** 1% [10 mg/mL] (2 mL). **INJ, powder for reconstitution:** 20 mg. **INJ:** 0.2% [2 mg/mL] (2 mL); 0.3% [3 mg/mL] (5 mL). **OINT:** 0.5% [5 mg/mL] (28 g). **OINT, ophthalmic:** 0.5% [5 mg/mL] (3.75 g). **SOLN, ophthalmic:** 0.5% [5 mg/mL] (1 mL, 2 mL, 15 mL, 59 mL). **SOLN, topical:** 2% [20 mg/mL] (30 mL, 118 mL)

Generic Available Yes

Tetracaine and Dextrose (TET ra kane & DEKS trose)

Related Information

Oral Pain *on page 1360*

U.S. Brand Names Pontocaine® With Dextrose

Pharmacologic Category Local Anesthetic

Synonyms Dextrose and Tetracaine

Use Spinal anesthesia (saddle block)

Local Anesthetic/Vasoconstrictor Precautions No information available to require special precautions

Effects on Dental Treatment No effects or complications reported

Dosage Dose varies with procedure, depth of anesthesia, duration desired and physical condition of patient

Drug Uptake See Tetracaine *on page 1146*

Pregnancy Risk Factor C

Generic Available Yes

TetraCap® *see* Tetracycline *on page 1147*

Tetracycline (tet ra SYE kleen)

Related Information

Dental Drug Interactions: Update on Drug Combinations Requiring Special Considerations *on page 1434*

Gastrointestinal Disorders *on page 1326*

Oral Bacterial Infections *on page 1367*

Oral Nonviral Soft Tissue Ulcerations or Erosions *on page 1384*

Periodontal Diseases *on page 1375*

U.S. Brand Names Brodspec®; EmTet®; Sumycin®; TetraCap®; Topicycline®; Wesmycin®

Canadian Brand Names Apo®-Tetra; Novo-Tetra; Nu-Tetra

Mexican Brand Names Acromicina; Ambotetra; Quimocyclar; Terranumonyl; Tetra-Atlantis®; Zorbenal-G

Pharmacologic Category Antibiotic, Ophthalmic; Antibiotic, Tetracycline Derivative; Antibiotic, Topical

(Continued)

Tetracycline *(Continued)*

Synonyms Achromycin® [DSC]; TCN; Tetracycline Hydrochloride

Use

Dental: Treatment of periodontitis associated with presence of *Actinobacillus actinomycetemcomitans* (AA). As adjunctive therapy in recurrent aphthous ulcers

Medical: In medicine for treatment of susceptible bacterial infections of both gram-positive and gram-negative organisms; also some unusual organisms including *Mycoplasma*, *Chlamydia*, and *Rickettsia*; may also be used for acne, exacerbations of chronic bronchitis, and treatment of gonorrhea and syphilis in patients that are allergic to penicillin

Local Anesthetic/Vasoconstrictor Precautions No information available to require special precautions

Effects on Dental Treatment Opportunistic "superinfection" with *Candida albicans*; tetracyclines are not recommended for use during pregnancy or in children ≤8 years of age since they have been reported to cause enamel hypoplasia and permanent teeth discoloration. The use of tetracyclines should only be used in these patients if other agents are contraindicated or alternative antimicrobials will not eradicate the organism. Long-term use associated with oral candidiasis.

Dosage Adults: 250 mg every 6 hours until improvement (usually 10 days or more)

Mechanism of Action Inhibits bacterial protein synthesis by binding with the 30S and possibly the 50S ribosomal subunit(s) of susceptible bacteria; may also cause alterations in the cytoplasmic membrane

Other Adverse Effects

>10%: Gastrointestinal: Discoloration of teeth and enamel hypoplasia (young children)

1% to 10%:

Dermatologic: Photosensitivity

Gastrointestinal: Nausea, diarrhea

<1%: Pericarditis, increased intracranial pressure, bulging fontanels in infants, pseudotumor cerebri, pancreatitis, pruritus, pigmentation of nails, exfoliative dermatitis, diabetes insipidus syndrome, vomiting, esophagitis, anorexia, abdominal cramps, antibiotic-associated pseudomembranous colitis, staphylococcal enterocolitis, hepatotoxicity, thrombophlebitis, paresthesia, acute renal failure, azotemia, renal damage, superinfections, anaphylaxis, hypersensitivity reactions, candidal superinfection

Contraindications Hypersensitivity to tetracycline or any component of the formulation; children ≤8 years of age; pregnancy (systemic use)

Warnings/Precautions Use of tetracyclines during tooth development may cause permanent discoloration of the teeth and enamel, hypoplasia and retardation of skeletal development and bone growth with risk being the greatest for children <4 years and those receiving high doses; use with caution in patients with renal or hepatic impairment (eg, elderly) and in pregnancy; dosage modification required in patients with renal impairment since it may increase BUN as an antianabolic agent; pseudotumor cerebri has been reported with tetracycline use (usually resolves with discontinuation); outdated drug can cause nephropathy; superinfection possible; use protective measure to avoid photosensitivity

Drug Interactions Although no clinical evidence exists, may bind with bismuth or calcium carbonate, an excipient in bismuth subsalicylate, during treatment for *H. pylori*

Increased Toxicity: Methoxyflurane anesthesia when concurrent with tetracycline may cause fatal nephrotoxicity; warfarin with tetracyclines may result in increased anticoagulation; tetracyclines may rarely increase digoxin serum concentration

Decreased Effect: Calcium-, magnesium-, or aluminum-containing antacids, oral contraceptives, iron, zinc, sodium bicarbonate, penicillins, cimetidine may decrease tetracycline absorption

Dietary/Ethanol/Herb Considerations

Food: Administer on an empty stomach, 1 hour before or 2 hours after meals; food decreases absorption. Avoid dairy products and iron supplements within 3 hours of administration; tetracycline decreases absorption of magnesium, zinc, calcium, iron, and amino acids.

Herb/Nutraceutical: Avoid dong quai and St John's wort; may cause additional photosensitization.

Drug Uptake

Absorption: Oral: 75%

Half-life, elimination: Normal renal function: 8-11 hours; End-stage renal disease: 57-108 hours

Time to peak: Oral: 2-4 hours

Pregnancy Risk Factor D (systemic)/B (topical)

Breast-feeding Considerations Negligible absorption by infant; potential to stain unerupted teeth of infants

Dosage Forms CAP: 250 mg, 500 mg. **OINT:** 3% [30 mg/mL] (14.2 g, 30 g). **OINT, ophthalmic:** 1% [10 mg/mL] (3.5 g). **SOLN, topical:** 2.2 mg/mL (70 mL). **SUSP, ophthalmic:** 1% [10 mg/mL] (0.5 mL, 1 mL, 4 mL). **SUSP, oral:** 125 mg/5 mL (60 mL, 480 mL). **TAB:** 250 mg, 500 mg

Generic Available Yes

Comments *Helicobacter pylori*: Clinically effective treatment regimens: See Multiple Drug Regimens for the Treatment of *H. pylori* Infection *on page 1327*.

Selected Readings

Gordon JM and Walker CB, "Current Status of Systemic Antibiotic Usage in Destructive Periodontal Disease," *J Periodontol*, 1993, 64(8 Suppl): 760-71.

Rams TE and Slots J, "Antibiotics in Periodontal Therapy: An Update," *Compendium*, 1992, 13(12):1130, 1132, 1134.

Seymour RA and Heasman PA, "Tetracyclines in the Management of Periodontal Diseases. A Review," *J Clin Periodontol*, 1995, 22(1):22-35.

Seymour RA and Heasman PA, "Pharmacological Control of Periodontal Disease. II. Antimicrobial Agents," *J Dent*, 1995, 23(1):5-14

Tetracycline Periodontal Fibers

(tet ra SYE kleen per ee oh DON tal FYE bers)

Related Information

Dental Drug Interactions: Update on Drug Combinations Requiring Special Considerations *on page 1434*

U.S. Brand Names Actisite®

Pharmacologic Category Antibacterial, Dental

Use Dental: Treatment of adult periodontitis; as an adjunct to scaling and root planing for the reduction of pocket depth and bleeding on probing in selected patients with adult periodontitis

Local Anesthetic/Vasoconstrictor Precautions No information available to require special precautions

Effects on Dental Treatment 1% to 10%: Gingival inflammation, pain in mouth, glossitis, candidiasis, staining of tongue

Dosage Adults: Insert fiber to fill the periodontal pocket; each fiber contains 12.7 mg of tetracycline in 23 cm (9 inches) and provides continuous release of drug for 10 days; fibers are to be secured in pocket with cyanoacrylate adhesive and left in place for 10 days

Mechanism of Action Antibiotic which inhibits growth of susceptible microorganisms; binds primarily to the 30S subunits of bacterial ribosomes, and appears to prevent access of aminoacyl tRNA to the acceptor site on the mRNA-ribosome complex. The fiber releases tetracycline into the periodontal site at a rate of 2 mcg/cm/hour.

Other Adverse Effects 1% to 10%:

Dermatologic: Local erythema following removal

Miscellaneous: Discomfort from fiber placement

Contraindications Hypersensitivity to tetracyclines or any component of the formulation

Warnings/Precautions Use of tetracyclines is not recommended during pregnancy because of interference with fetal bone and dental development. Safety and efficacy in children have not been established.

Dietary/Ethanol/Herb Considerations

Food: Avoid dairy products and iron supplements within 3 hours of use; tetracycline decreases absorption of magnesium, zinc, calcium, iron, and amino acids.

Herb/Nutraceutical: Avoid dong quai and St John's wort; may cause additional photosensitization.

Drug Uptake The fiber releases tetracycline at a rate of 2 mcg/cm/hour.

Tissue fluid concentrations:

Gingival fluid: ~1590 mcg/mL of tetracycline per site over 10 days

Plasma: During fiber treatment of up to 11 teeth, the tetracycline plasma concentration was below any detectable levels (<0.1 mcg/mL)

Oral: 500 mg of tetracycline produces a peak plasma level of 3-4 mcg/mL

Saliva: ~50.7 mcg/mL of tetracycline immediately after fiber treatment of 9 teeth

Pregnancy Risk Factor C

Breast-feeding Considerations It is not known whether tetracycline from periodontal fibers is distributed into human breast milk

Dosage Forms FIBER: 23 cm (9") in length [12.7 mg of tetracycline hydrochloride per fiber]

Generic Available No

Comments A number of different facultative and obligate anaerobic bacteria have been found to be causative factors in periodontal disease. These include *Actinobacillus actinomycetemcomitans* (AA), *Fusobacterium nucleatum*, and *Porphyromonas gingivalis*. These bacteria are sensitive to tetracyclines at similar concentrations as those released from the tetracycline-impregnated fibers. Placement of tetracycline periodontal fibers into gingival pockets decreases inflammation, edema, pocket depth, and bleeding upon probing.

Selected Readings

Baer PN, "Actisite (Tetracycline Hydrochloride Periodontal Fiber): A Critique," *Periodontal Clin Investig*, 1994, 16(2):5-7.

Greenstein G, "Treating Periodontal Diseases With Tetracycline-Impregnated Fibers: Data and Controversies," *Compend Contin Educ Dent*, 1995, 16(5)448-55.

Kerry G, "Tetracycline-Loaded Fibers as Adjunctive Treatment in Periodontal Disease," *J Am Dent Assoc*, 1994, 125(9):1199-203.

(Continued)

Tetracycline Periodontal Fibers *(Continued)*

Michalowicz BS, Pihlstrom BL, Drisko CL, et al, "Evaluation of Periodontal Treatments Using Controlled-Release Tetracycline Fibers: Maintenance Response," *J Periodontol*, 1995, 66(8):708-15.
Mombelli A, Lehmann B, Tonetti M, et al, "Clinical Response to Local Delivery of Tetracycline in Relation to Overall and Local Periodontal Conditions," *J Clin Periodontol*, 1997, 24(7):470-77.
Vandekerckhove BN, Quirynen M, and van Steenberghe D, "The Use of Tetracycline-Containing Controlled-Release Fibers in the Treatment of Refractory Periodontitis," *J Periodontol*, 1997, 68(4):353-61.

Tetrahydrozoline (tet ra hye DROZ a leen)

U.S. Brand Names Collyrium Fresh® [OTC]; Eyesine® [OTC]; Geneye® [OTC]; Mallazine® Eye Drops [OTC]; Murine® Plus Ophthalmic [OTC]; Optigene® [OTC]; Tetrasine® [OTC]; Tetrasine® Extra [OTC]; Tyzine®; Visine® Extra [OTC]

Mexican Brand Names Visine®

Pharmacologic Category Adrenergic Agonist Agent; Ophthalmic Agent, Vasoconstrictor

Synonyms Tetrahydrozoline Hydrochloride; Tetryzoline

Use Symptomatic relief of nasal congestion and conjunctival congestion

Local Anesthetic/Vasoconstrictor Precautions No information available to require special precautions

Effects on Dental Treatment No effects or complications reported

Dosage

Nasal congestion: Intranasal:
- Children 2-6 years: Instill 2-3 drops of 0.05% solution every 4-6 hours as needed, no more frequent than every 3 hours
- Children >6 years and Adults: Instill 2-4 drops or 3-4 sprays of 0.1% solution every 3-4 hours as needed, no more frequent than every 3 hours

Conjunctival congestion: Ophthalmic: Adults: Instill 1-2 drops in each eye 2-4 times/day

Mechanism of Action Stimulates alpha-adrenergic receptors in the arterioles of the conjunctiva and the nasal mucosa to produce vasoconstriction

Other Adverse Effects

>10%:
- Local: Transient stinging
- Respiratory: Sneezing

1% to 10%:
- Cardiovascular: Tachycardia, palpitations, hypertension, heart rate
- Central nervous system: Headache
- Neuromuscular & skeletal: Tremor
- Ocular: Blurred vision

Drug Interactions Increased Toxicity: MAO inhibitors can cause an exaggerated adrenergic response if taken concurrently or within 21 days of discontinuing MAO inhibitor; beta-blockers can cause hypertensive episodes and increased risk of intracranial hemorrhage; anesthetics

Drug Uptake

Onset of action: Decongestant: Intranasal: 4-8 hours
Duration: Ophthalmic vasoconstriction: 2-3 hours

Pregnancy Risk Factor C

Generic Available Yes

Tetrasine® [OTC] *see* Tetrahydrozoline *on page 1150*
Tetrasine® Extra [OTC] *see* Tetrahydrozoline *on page 1150*
Teveten® *see* Eprosartan *on page 445*
Texacort® *see* Hydrocortisone *on page 608*
T/Gel® [OTC] *see* Coal Tar *on page 315*
T-Gesic® *see* Hydrocodone and Acetaminophen *on page 598*

Thalidomide (tha LI doe mide)

Related Information

HIV Infection and AIDS *on page 1334*
Oral Nonviral Soft Tissue Ulcerations or Erosions *on page 1384*

U.S. Brand Names Thalomid®

Canadian Brand Names Thalomid®

Pharmacologic Category Immunosuppressant Agent

Use Treatment and maintenance of cutaneous manifestations of erythema nodosum leprosum

Orphan drug: Treatment of Crohn's disease

Unlabeled/Investigational: Treatment or prevention of graft-versus-host reactions after bone marrow transplantation; AIDS-related aphthous stomatitis; Langerhans cell histiocytosis, Behçet's syndrome; hypnotic agent; also may be effective in rheumatoid arthritis, discoid lupus erythematosus, and erythema multiforme; useful in type 2 lepra reactions, but not type 1; renal cell carcinoma, multiple myeloma, myeloma, Waldenström's macroglobulinemia

Local Anesthetic/Vasoconstrictor Precautions No information available to require special precautions

Effects on Dental Treatment 1% to 10% of patients may experience moniliasis, tooth pain; in HIV-seropositive patients, oral moniliasis was seen in 6.3% to 11.1% of patients; aphthous stomatitis has been reported

Restrictions Approved for marketing only under a special distribution program called the "System for Thalidomide Education and Prescribing Safety" (STEPS™), approved by the FDA. Prescribing and dispensing is restricted to prescribers and pharmacists registered with the program. Prior to dispensing, an authorization number must be obtained (1-888-423-5436) from Celgene (write authorization number on prescription). No more than a 4-week supply should be dispensed. Blister packs should be dispensed intact (do not repackage capsules). Prescriptions must be filled within 7 days.

Dosage Oral:

Cutaneous ENL:

- Initiate dosing at 100-300 mg/day taken once daily at bedtime with water (at least 1 hour after evening meal)
- Patients weighing <50 kg: Initiate at lower end of the dosing range
- Severe cutaneous reaction or previously requiring high dose may be initiated at 400 mg/day; doses may be divided, but taken 1 hour after meals
- Dosing should continue until active reaction subsides (usually at least 2 weeks), then tapered in 50 mg decrements every 2-4 weeks
- Patients who flare during tapering or with a history or requiring prolonged maintenance should be maintained on the minimum dosage necessary to control the reaction. Efforts to taper should be repeated every 3-6 months, in increments of 50 mg every 2-4 weeks.

Behçet's syndrome (unlabeled use): 100-400 mg/day

Graft-vs-host reactions (unlabeled use): 100-1600 mg/day; usual initial dose: 200 mg 4 times/day for use up to 700 days

AIDS-related aphthous stomatitis (unlabeled use): 200 mg twice daily for 5 days, then 200 mg/day for up to 8 weeks

Discoid lupus erythematosus (unlabeled use): 100-400 mg/day; maintenance dose: 25-50 mg

Mechanism of Action A derivative of glutethimide; mode of action for immunosuppression is unclear; inhibition of neutrophil chemotaxis and decreased monocyte phagocytosis may occur; may cause 50% to 80% reduction of tumor necrosis factor - alpha

Other Adverse Effects

Controlled clinical trials: ENL:

>10%:

- Central nervous system: Somnolence (37.5%), headache (12.5%)
- Dermatologic: Rash (20.8%)

1% to 10%:

- Cardiovascular: Peripheral edema
- Central nervous system: Dizziness (4.2%), vertigo (8.3%), chills, malaise (8.3%)
- Dermatologic: Dermatitis (fungal) (4.2%), nail disorder (4.2%), pruritus (8.3%), rash (maculopapular) (4.2%)
- Gastrointestinal (4.2%): Constipation, diarrhea, nausea, moniliasis, tooth pain, abdominal pain
- Genitourinary: Impotence (8.2%)
- Neuromuscular & skeletal: Asthenia (8.3%), pain (8.3%), back pain (4.2%), neck pain (4.2%), neck rigidity (4.2%), tremor (4.2%)
- Respiratory (4.2%): Pharyngitis, rhinitis, sinusitis

HIV-seropositive: General: An increased viral load has been noted in patients treated with thalidomide. This is of uncertain clinical significance - see monitoring

>10%:

- Central nervous system: Somnolence (36% to 37%), dizziness (18.7% to 19.4%), fever (19.4% to 21.9%), headache (16.7% to 18.7%)
- Dermatologic: Rash (25%), maculopapular rash (16.7% to 18.7%), acne (3.1% to 11.1%)
- Gastrointestinal: AST increase (2.8% to 12.5%), diarrhea (11.1% to 18.7%), nausea (≤12.5%), oral moniliasis (6.3% to 11.1%)
- Hematologic: Leukopenia (16.7% to 25%), anemia (5.6% to 12.5%)
- Neuromuscular & skeletal: Paresthesia (5.6% to 15.6%), weakness (5.6% to 21.9%)
- Miscellaneous: Diaphoresis (≤12.5%), lymphadenopathy (5.6% to 12.5%)

1% to 10%:

- Cardiovascular: Peripheral edema (3.1% to 8.3%)
- Central nervous system: Nervousness (2.8% to 9.4%), insomnia (≤9.4%), agitation (≤9.4%), chills (≤9.4%)
- Dermatologic: Dermatitis (fungal) (5.6% to 9.4%), nail disorder (≤3.1%), pruritus (2.8% to 6.3%)
- Gastrointestinal: Anorexia (2.8% to 9.4%), constipation (2.8% to 9.4%), xerostomia (8.3% to 9.4%), flatulence (8.3% to 9.4%), multiple abnormalities LFTs (≤9.4%), abdominal pain (2.8% to 3.1%)
- Neuromuscular & skeletal: Back pain (≤5%), pain (≤3.1%)

(Continued)

Thalidomide *(Continued)*

Respiratory: Pharyngitis (6.3% to 8.3%), sinusitis (3.1% to 8.3%)
Miscellaneous: Accidental injury (≤5.6%), infection (6.3% to 8.3%)

Contraindications Hypersensitivity to thalidomide or any component of the formulation; neuropathy (peripheral); pregnancy or women in childbearing years (unless alternative therapies are inappropriate and adequate precautions are taken to avoid pregnancy); patient unable to comply with STEPS™ program; breast-feeding

Warnings/Precautions Hepatic, neurological disorders, constipation, CHF, hypertension; safety and efficacy have not been established in children <12 years of age

Drug Interactions Other medications known to cause peripheral neuropathy should be used with caution in patients receiving thalidomide; thalidomide may enhance the sedative activity of barbiturates, reserpine, and chlorpromazine.

Drug Uptake
Half-life, elimination: 8.7 hours
Time to peak, plasma: 2-6 hours

Pregnancy Risk Factor X

Generic Available No

Selected Readings Jacobson JM, Greenspan JS, Spritzler J, et al, "Thalidomide for the Treatment of Oral Aphthous Ulcers in Patients With Human Immunodeficiency Virus Infection. National Institute of Allergy and Infectious Diseases AIDS Clinical Trials Group," *N Engl J Med*, 1997, 336(21):1487-93.

Thalitone® *see* Chlorthalidone *on page 277*
Thalomid® *see* Thalidomide *on page 1150*
THAM® *see* Tromethamine *on page 1216*
Theo-24® *see* Theophylline *on page 1152*
Theochron® *see* Theophylline *on page 1152*
Theo-Dur® *see* Theophylline *on page 1152*
Theolair™ *see* Theophylline *on page 1152*

Theophylline (thee OF i lin)

Related Information

Aminophylline *on page 71*
Dental Drug Interactions: Update on Drug Combinations Requiring Special Considerations *on page 1434*
Respiratory Diseases *on page 1328*

U.S. Brand Names Aerolate III®; Aerolate JR®; Aerolate SR®; Elixophyllin®; Quibron®-T; Quibron®-T/SR; Respbid®; Slo-bid™; Slo-Phyllin®; Theo-24®; Theochron®; Theo-Dur®; Theolair™; T-Phyl®; Uni-Dur®; Uniphyl®

Canadian Brand Names Apo®-Theo LA; Novo-Theophyl SR; Quibron®-T/SR; Theochron® SR; Theo-Dur®; Theolair™; Theolair™-SR; Uniphyl®

Mexican Brand Names Slo-Bid®; Teolong®; Uni-Dur®

Pharmacologic Category Theophylline Derivative

Synonyms Theophylline Anhydrous

Use Bronchodilator in reversible airway obstruction due to asthma, chronic bronchitis, and emphysema; for neonatal apnea/bradycardia

Local Anesthetic/Vasoconstrictor Precautions No information available to require special precautions

Effects on Dental Treatment Prescribe erythromycin products with caution to patients taking theophylline products. Erythromycin will delay the normal metabolic inactivation of theophyllines leading to increased blood levels; this has resulted in nausea, vomiting, and CNS restlessness. Azithromycin does not cause these effects in combination with theophylline products.

Approximate I.V. Theophylline Dosage for Treatment of Acute Bronchospasm

Group	Dosage for next 12 hours*	Dosage after 12 hours*
Infants 6 weeks to 6 months	0.5 mg/kg/hour	—
Children 6 months to 1 year	0.6-0.7 mg/kg/hour	
Children 1-9 years	0.95 mg/kg/hour (1.2 mg/kg/hour)	0.79 mg/kg/hour (1 mg/kg/hour)
Children 9-16 years and young adult smokers	0.79 mg/kg/hour (1 mg/kg/hour)	0.63 mg/kg/hour (0.8 mg/kg/hour)
Healthy, nonsmoking adults	0.55 mg/kg/hour (0.7 mg/kg/hour)	0.39 mg/kg/hour (0.5 mg/kg/hour)
Older patients and patients with cor pulmonale	0.47 mg/kg/hour (0.6 mg/kg/hour)	0.24 mg/kg/hour (0.3 mg/kg/hour)
Patients with congestive heart failure or liver failure	0.39 mg/kg/hour (0.5 mg/kg/hour)	0.08-0.16 mg/kg/hour (0.1-0.2 mg/kg/hour)

*Equivalent hydrous aminophylline dosage indicated in parentheses

Dosage Use ideal body weight for obese patients

I.V.: Initial: Maintenance infusion rates:

Children:

6 weeks to 6 months: 0.5 mg/kg/hour

6 months to 1 year: 0.6-0.7 mg/kg/hour

Children >1 year and Adults:

Treatment of acute bronchospasm: I.V.: Loading dose (in patients not currently receiving aminophylline or theophylline): 6 mg/kg (based on aminophylline) given I.V. over 20-30 minutes; administration rate should not exceed 25 mg/minute (aminophylline). See table on previous page.

Approximate I.V. maintenance dosages are based upon continuous infusions; bolus dosing (often used in children <6 months of age) may be determined by multiplying the hourly infusion rate by 24 hours and dividing by the desired number of doses/day. See table.

Maintenance Dose for Acute Symptoms

Population Group	Oral Theophylline (mg/kg/day)	I.V. Aminophylline
Premature infant or newborn-6 weeks (for apnea/bradycardia)	4	5 mg/kg/day
6 weeks-6 months	10	12 mg/kg/day or continuous I.V. infusion*
Infants 6 months-1 year	12-18	15 mg/kg/day or continuous I.V. infusion*
Children 1-9 years	20-24	1 mg/kg/hour
Children 9-12 years, and adolescent daily smokers of cigarettes or marijuana, and otherwise healthy adult smokers <50 years	16	0.9 mg/kg/hour
Adolescents 12-16 years (nonsmokers)	13	0.7 mg/kg/hour
Otherwise healthy nonsmoking adults (including elderly patients)	10 (not to exceed 900 mg/day)	0.5 mg/kg/hour
Cardiac decompensation, cor pulmonale and/or liver dysfunction	5 (not to exceed 400 mg/day)	0.25 mg/kg/hour

*For continuous I.V. infusion divide total daily dose by 24 = mg/kg/hour.

Dosage Adjustment After Serum Theophylline Measurement

Serum Theophylline		Guidelines
Within normal limits	10-20 µg/mL	Maintain dosage if tolerated. Recheck serum theophylline concentration at 6- to 12-month intervals.*
Too high	20-25 µg/mL	Decrease doses by about 10%. Recheck serum theophylline concentration after 3 days and then at 6- to 12-month intervals.*
	25-30 µg/mL	Skip next dose and decrease subsequent doses by about 25%. Recheck serum theophylline.
	>30 µg/mL	Skip next 2 doses and decrease subsequent doses by 50%. Recheck serum theophylline.
Too low	7.5-10 µg/mL	Increase dose by about 25%.** Recheck serum theophylline concentration after 3 days and then at 6- to 12-month intervals.*
	5-7.5 µg/mL	Increase dose by about 25% to the nearest dose increment.** Recheck serum theophylline for guidance in further dosage adjustment (another increase will probably be needed, but this provides a safety check).

*Finer adjustments in dosage may be needed for some patients.

**Dividing the daily dose into 3 doses administered at 8-hour intervals may be indicated if symptoms occur repeatedly at the end of a dosing interval.

From Weinberger M and Hendeles L, "Practical Guide to Using Theophylline," *J Resp Dis*, 1981, 2:12-27.

(Continued)

Theophylline *(Continued)*

Dosage should be adjusted according to serum concentration measurements during the first 12- to 24-hour period. See table on previous page.

Oral theophylline: Initial dosage recommendation: Loading dose (to achieve a serum concentration of about 10 mcg/mL; loading doses should be given using a rapidly absorbed oral product **not** a sustained release product):

If no theophylline has been administered in the previous 24 hours: 4-6 mg/kg theophylline

If theophylline has been administered in the previous 24 hours: administer 1/2 loading dose or 2-3 mg/kg theophylline can be given in emergencies when serum concentration are not available

On the average, for every 1 mg/kg theophylline given, blood levels will rise 2 mcg/mL

Ideally, defer the loading dose if a serum theophylline concentration can be obtained rapidly. However, if this is not possible, exercise clinical judgment. If the patient is not experiencing theophylline toxicity, this is unlikely to result in dangerous adverse effects.

See table.

Oral Theophylline Dosage for Bronchial Asthma*

Age	Initial 3 Days	Second 3 Days	Steady-State Maintenance
<1 year	0.2 x (age in weeks) + 5		0.3 x (age in weeks) + 8
1-9 years	16 up to a maximum of 400 mg/24 hours	20	22
9-12 years	16 up to a maximum of 400 mg/24 hours	16 up to a maximum of 600 mg/24 hours	20 up to a maximum of 800 mg/24 hours
12-16 years	16 up to a maximum of 400 mg/24 hours	16 up to a maximum of 600 mg/24 hours	18 up to a maximum of 900 mg/24 hours
Adults	400 mg/24 hours	600 mg/24 hours	900 mg/24 hours

*Dose in mg/kg/24 hours of theophylline.

Increasing dose: The dosage may be increased in ~ 25% increments at 2- to 3-day intervals so long as the drug is tolerated or until the maximum dose is reached

Maintenance dose: In children and healthy adults, a slow-release product can be used; the total daily dose can be divided every 8-12 hours

Mechanism of Action Causes bronchodilatation, diuresis, CNS and cardiac stimulation, and gastric acid secretion by blocking phosphodiesterase which increases tissue concentrations of cyclic adenine monophosphate (cAMP) which in turn promotes catecholamine stimulation of lipolysis, glycogenolysis, and gluconeogenesis and induces release of epinephrine from adrenal medulla cells

Other Adverse Effects

Adverse reactions/theophylline serum level: (Do not necessarily occur according to serum levels; arrhythmia and seizure can occur without seeing the other adverse effects). Frequency not defined:

15-25 mcg/mL: GI upset, diarrhea, nausea/vomiting, abdominal pain, nervousness, headache, insomnia, agitation, dizziness, muscle cramp, tremor

25-35 mcg/mL: Tachycardia, occasional PVC

>35 mcg/mL: Ventricular tachycardia, frequent PVC, seizure

Uncommon at serum theophylline concentrations ≤20 mcg/mL: 1% to 10%:

Cardiovascular: Tachycardia

Central nervous system: Nervousness, restlessness

Gastrointestinal: Nausea, vomiting

Drug Interactions CYP1A2 and 3A3/4 enzyme substrate; 2E1 enzyme substrate (minor)

Increased Effect/Toxicity: Changes in diet may affect the elimination of theophylline. The following may increase serum theophylline levels: propranolol, allopurinol (>600 mg/day), erythromycin, cimetidine, troleandomycin, ciprofloxacin (other quinolone antibiotics), oral contraceptives, beta-blockers, calcium channel blockers, corticosteroids, disulfiram, ephedrine, influenza virus vaccine, interferon, macrolides, mexiletine, thiabendazole, thyroid hormones, carbamazepine, isoniazid, and loop diuretics. Other inhibitors of cytochrome P450 1A2 may increase theophylline levels.

Decreased Effect: Changes in diet may affect the elimination of theophylline. Charcoal-broiled foods may increase elimination, reducing half-life by 50%. The following factors decrease theophylline serum concentration: Smoking (cigarettes, marijuana), high protein/low carbohydrate diet, charcoal, phenytoin, phenobarbital, carbamazepine, rifampin, ritonavir, I.V. isoproterenol, aminoglutethimide, barbiturates, hydantoins, ketoconazole, sulfinpyrazone, isoniazid, loop diuretics, and sympathomimetics.

Drug Uptake

Absorption: Oral: ≤100%; depends on formulation used

Half-life, elimination: Highly variable (dependent upon age, liver and cardiac function, lung disease and smoking history)

Pregnancy Risk Factor C

Generic Available Yes

Theophylline and Guaifenesin (thee OF i lin & gwye FEN e sin)

U.S. Brand Names Bronchial®; Glycerol-T®; Quibron®; Slo-Phyllin® GG

Pharmacologic Category Theophylline Derivative

Synonyms Guaifenesin and Theophylline

Use Symptomatic treatment of bronchospasm associated with bronchial asthma, chronic bronchitis and pulmonary emphysema

Local Anesthetic/Vasoconstrictor Precautions No information available to require special precautions

Effects on Dental Treatment Prescribe erythromycin products with caution to patients taking theophylline products. Erythromycin will delay the normal metabolic inactivation of theophyllines leading to increased blood levels; this has resulted in nausea, vomiting, and CNS restlessness.

Dosage Adults: Oral: 16 mg/kg/day or 400 mg theophylline/day, in divided doses, every 6-8 hours

Drug Uptake See Theophylline *on page 1152* and Guaifenesin *on page 568*

Pregnancy Risk Factor C

Generic Available Yes

Theophylline, Ephedrine, and Hydroxyzine

(thee OF i lin, e FED rin, & hye DROKS i zeen)

U.S. Brand Names Hydrophed®; Marax®

Pharmacologic Category Theophylline Derivative

Synonyms Ephedrine, Theophylline, and Hydroxyzine; Hydroxyzine, Theophylline, and Ephedrine

Use Possibly effective for controlling bronchospastic disorders

Local Anesthetic/Vasoconstrictor Precautions Use vasoconstrictors with caution since ephedrine may enhance cardiostimulation and vasopressor effects of sympathomimetics

Effects on Dental Treatment Prescribe erythromycin products with caution to patients taking theophylline products. Erythromycin will delay the normal metabolic inactivation of theophyllines leading to increased blood levels; this has resulted in nausea, vomiting, and CNS restlessness.

Dosage

Children:

2-5 years: 1/2 tablet 2-4 times/day or 2.5 mL 3-4 times/day

>5 years: 1/2 tablet 2-4 times/day or 5 mL 3-4 times/day

Adults: 1 tablet 2-4 times/day

Drug Uptake See Theophylline *on page 1152*, Ephedrine *on page 437*, and Hydroxyzine *on page 616*

Pregnancy Risk Factor C

Generic Available Yes

Theophylline, Ephedrine, and Phenobarbital

(thee OF i lin, e FED rin, & fee noe BAR bi tal)

U.S. Brand Names Tedral®

Pharmacologic Category Theophylline Derivative

Synonyms Ephedrine, Theophylline and Phenobarbital

Use Prevention and symptomatic treatment of bronchial asthma; relief of asthmatic bronchitis and other bronchospastic disorders

Local Anesthetic/Vasoconstrictor Precautions Use vasoconstrictors with caution since ephedrine may enhance cardiostimulation and vasopressor effects of sympathomimetics

Effects on Dental Treatment Prescribe erythromycin products with caution to patients taking theophylline products. Erythromycin will delay the normal metabolic inactivation of theophyllines leading to increased blood levels; this has resulted in nausea, vomiting, and CNS restlessness.

Dosage

Children >60 lb: 1 tablet or 5 mL every 4 hours

Adults: 1-2 tablets or 10-20 mL every 4 hours

Drug Uptake See Theophylline *on page 1152*, Ephedrine *on page 437* and Phenobarbital *on page 945*

Pregnancy Risk Factor D

Generic Available Yes

Therabid® [OTC] *see* Vitamins, Multiple *on page 1246*

Thera-Combex® H-P Kapseals® [OTC] *see* Vitamin B Complex With Vitamin C *on page 1244*

TheraCys® *see* BCG Vaccine *on page 145*

Thera-Flu® Flu and Cold *see* Acetaminophen, Chlorpheniramine, and Pseudoephedrine *on page 33*

Thera-Flu® Non-Drowsy Flu, Cold and Cough [OTC] *see* Acetaminophen, Dextromethorphan, and Pseudoephedrine *on page 34*

Thera-Flur® *see* Fluoride *on page 514*

Thera-Flur-N® *see* Fluoride *on page 514*

Theragran® [OTC] *see* Vitamins, Multiple *on page 1246*

Theragran® Hematinic® *see* Vitamins, Multiple *on page 1246*

Theragran® Liquid [OTC] *see* Vitamins, Multiple *on page 1246*

Theragran-M® [OTC] *see* Vitamins, Multiple *on page 1246*

Theramycin Z® *see* Erythromycin, Topical *on page 454*

Theraplex Z® [OTC] *see* Pyrithione Zinc *on page 1029*

Thermazene® *see* Silver Sulfadiazine *on page 1088*

Thiabendazole (thye a BEN da zole)

U.S. Brand Names Mintezol®

Canadian Brand Names Mintezol®

Pharmacologic Category Anthelmintic

Synonyms Tiabendazole

Use Treatment of strongyloidiasis, cutaneous larva migrans, visceral larva migrans, dracunculiasis, trichinosis, and mixed helminthic infections

Local Anesthetic/Vasoconstrictor Precautions No information available to require special precautions

Effects on Dental Treatment No effects or complications reported

Dosage Purgation not required prior to use; drinking fruit juice aids in expulsion of worms by removing the mucous to which they are attached.

Children and Adults: Oral: 50 mg/kg/day divided every 12 hours; maximum dose: 3 g/day
- Strongyloidiasis: For 2 consecutive days
- Cutaneous larva migrans: For 2-5 consecutive days
- Visceral larva migrans: For 5-7 consecutive days
- Trichinosis: For 2-4 consecutive days
- Dracunculosis: 50-75 mg/kg/day divided every 12 hours for 3 days

Mechanism of Action Inhibits helminth-specific mitochondrial fumarate reductase

Other Adverse Effects Frequency not defined:
- Central nervous system: Seizures, hallucinations, delirium, dizziness, drowsiness, headache, chills
- Dermatologic: Rash, Stevens-Johnson syndrome, pruritus, angioedema
- Endocrine & metabolic: Hyperglycemia
- Gastrointestinal: Anorexia, diarrhea, nausea, vomiting, drying of mucous membranes, abdominal pain
- Genitourinary: Malodor of urine, hematuria, crystalluria, enuresis
- Hematologic: Leukopenia
- Hepatic: Jaundice, cholestasis, hepatic failure, hepatotoxicity
- Neuromuscular & skeletal: Numbness, incoordination
- Ocular: Visual changes, dry eyes, Sicca syndrome
- Otic: Tinnitus
- Renal: Nephrotoxicity
- Miscellaneous: Anaphylaxis, hypersensitivity reactions, lymphadenopathy

Drug Interactions Increases levels of theophylline and other xanthines

Drug Uptake
- Absorption: Rapid and well absorbed
- Half-life, elimination: 1.2 hours
- Time to peak: 1-2 hours

Pregnancy Risk Factor C

Generic Available No

Thiamilate® *see* Thiamine *on page 1156*

Thiamine (THYE a min)

U.S. Brand Names Thiamilate®

Canadian Brand Names Betaxin®

Mexican Brand Names Benerva®

Pharmacologic Category Vitamin

Synonyms Aneurine Hydrochloride; Thiamine Hydrochloride; Thiaminium Chloride Hydrochloride; Vitamin B_1

Use Treatment of thiamine deficiency including beriberi, Wernicke's encephalopathy syndrome, and peripheral neuritis associated with pellagra, alcoholic patients with altered sensorium; various genetic metabolic disorders

Local Anesthetic/Vasoconstrictor Precautions No information available to require special precautions

Effects on Dental Treatment No effects or complications reported

Dosage
Recommended daily allowance:
<6 months: 0.3 mg
6 months to 1 year: 0.4 mg
1-3 years: 0.7 mg
4-6 years: 0.9 mg
7-10 years: 1 mg
11-14 years: 1.1-1.3 mg
>14 years: 1-1.5 mg
Thiamine deficiency (beriberi):
Children: 10-25 mg/dose I.M. or I.V. daily (if critically ill), or 10-50 mg/dose orally every day for 2 weeks, then 5-10 mg/dose orally daily for 1 month
Adults: 5-30 mg/dose I.M. or I.V. 3 times/day (if critically ill); then orally 5-30 mg/day in single or divided doses 3 times/day for 1 month
Wernicke's encephalopathy: Adults: Initial: 100 mg I.V., then 50-100 mg/day I.M. or I.V. until consuming a regular, balanced diet
Dietary supplement (depends on caloric or carbohydrate content of the diet):
Children: 0.5-1 mg/day
Adults: 1-2 mg/day
Note: The above doses can be found in multivitamin preparations
Metabolic disorders: Oral: Adults: 10-20 mg/day (dosages up to 4 g/day in divided doses have been used)

Mechanism of Action An essential coenzyme in carbohydrate metabolism by combining with adenosine triphosphate to form thiamine pyrophosphate

Drug Interactions Neuromuscular blocking agents; high carbohydrate diets or I.V. dextrose solutions increase thiamine requirement

Drug Uptake Absorption: Oral: Adequate; I.M.: Rapid and complete

Pregnancy Risk Factor A/C (dose exceeding RDA recommendation)

Generic Available Yes

Thiethylperazine (thye eth il PER a zeen)

U.S. Brand Names Norzine®; Torecan®

Canadian Brand Names Torecan®

Mexican Brand Names Torecan®

Pharmacologic Category Antiemetic

Synonyms Thiethylperazine Maleate

Use Relief of nausea and vomiting
Unlabeled/Investigational: Treatment of vertigo

Local Anesthetic/Vasoconstrictor Precautions No information available to require special precautions

Effects on Dental Treatment >10%: Xerostomia

Dosage Children >12 years and Adults:
Oral, I.M., rectal: 10 mg 1-3 times/day as needed
I.V. and S.C. routes of administration are not recommended

Mechanism of Action Blocks postsynaptic mesolimbic dopaminergic receptors in the brain; exhibits a strong alpha-adrenergic blocking effect and depresses the release of hypothalamic and hypophyseal hormones; acts directly on chemoreceptor trigger zone and vomiting center

Other Adverse Effects
>10%:
Central nervous system: Drowsiness, dizziness
Gastrointestinal: Xerostomia
Respiratory: Dry nose
1% to 10%:
Cardiovascular: Tachycardia, orthostatic hypotension
Central nervous system: Confusion, convulsions, extrapyramidal symptoms, tardive dyskinesia, fever, headache
Hematologic: Agranulocytosis
Hepatic: Cholestatic jaundice
Otic: Tinnitus

Drug Interactions Increased effect with CNS depressants (eg, anesthetics, opiates, tranquilizers, alcohol), lithium, atropine, epinephrine, MAO inhibitors, TCAs

Drug Uptake
Onset of action: Antiemetic: ~30 minutes
Duration: ~4 hours

Pregnancy Risk Factor X

Generic Available No

Thimerosal (thye MER oh sal)

U.S. Brand Names Aeroaid® [OTC]; Mersol® [OTC]; Merthiolate® [OTC]

Pharmacologic Category Antibiotic, Topical

Use Organomercurial antiseptic with sustained bacteriostatic and fungistatic activity

Local Anesthetic/Vasoconstrictor Precautions No information available to require special precautions
(Continued)

Thimerosal *(Continued)*

Effects on Dental Treatment No effects or complications reported

Dosage Apply 1-3 times/day

Generic Available Yes

Thioguanine (thye oh GWAH neen)

Canadian Brand Names Lanvis®

Pharmacologic Category Antineoplastic Agent, Antimetabolite

Synonyms 2-Amino-6-Mercaptopurine; TG; 6-TG; 6-Thioguanine; Tioguanine

Use Remission induction, consolidation, and maintenance therapy of acute myelogenous (nonlymphocytic) leukemia; treatment of chronic myelogenous leukemia and granulocytic leukemia

Local Anesthetic/Vasoconstrictor Precautions No information available to require special precautions

Effects on Dental Treatment No effects or complications reported

Mechanism of Action Purine analog that is incorporated into DNA and RNA resulting in the blockage of synthesis and metabolism of purine nucleotides

Other Adverse Effects

>10%:
- Hematologic: Myelosuppressive:
  - WBC: Moderate
  - Platelets: Moderate
  - Onset: 7-10 days
  - Nadir: 14 days
  - Recovery: 21 days

1% to 10%:
- Dermatologic: Skin rash
- Endocrine & metabolic: Hyperuricemia
- Gastrointestinal: Mild nausea or vomiting, anorexia, stomatitis, diarrhea
  - Emetic potential: Low (<10%)
- Neuromuscular & skeletal: Unsteady gait

Drug Interactions Allopurinol can be used in full doses with 6-TG unlike 6-MP. Use with busulfan may cause hepatotoxicity and esophageal varices.

Drug Uptake

Absorption: Oral: 30%

Half-life, elimination: Terminal: 11 hours

Time to peak: ≤8 hours

Pregnancy Risk Factor D

Generic Available No

Thiola™ *see* Tiopronin *on page 1173*

Thiopental (thye oh PEN tal)

U.S. Brand Names Pentothal® Sodium

Canadian Brand Names Pentothal®

Mexican Brand Names Pentothal Sodico®; Sodipental®

Pharmacologic Category Anticonvulsant, Barbiturate; Barbiturate; General Anesthetic

Synonyms Thiopental Sodium

Use Induction of anesthesia; adjunct for intubation in head injury patients; control of convulsive states; treatment of elevated intracranial pressure

Local Anesthetic/Vasoconstrictor Precautions No information available to require special precautions

Effects on Dental Treatment No effects or complications reported

Restrictions C-III

Dosage

I.V.:
- Induction anesthesia:
  - Neonates: 3-4 mg/kg
  - Infants: 5-8 mg/kg
  - Children 1-12 years: 5-6 mg/kg
  - Adults: 3-5 mg/kg
- Maintenance anesthesia:
  - Children: 1 mg/kg as needed
  - Adults: 25-100 mg as needed
- Increased intracranial pressure: Children and Adults: 1.5-5 mg/kg/dose; repeat as needed to control intracranial pressure
- Seizures:
  - Children: 2-3 mg/kg/dose, repeat as needed
  - Adults: 75-250 mg/dose, repeat as needed

Rectal administration (should be NPO for no less than 3 hours prior to administration):

Suggested initial doses of thiopental rectal suspension are:

<3 months: 15 mg/kg/dose

>3 months: 25 mg/kg/dose

Note: The age of a premature infant should be adjusted to reflect the age that the infant would have been if full-term (eg, an infant, now age 4 months, who was 2 months premature should be considered to be a 2-month old infant).

Doses should be rounded downward to the nearest 50 mg increment to allow for accurate measurement of the dose

Inactive or debilitated patients and patients recently medicated with other sedatives, (eg, chloral hydrate, meperidine, chlorpromazine, and promethazine), may require smaller doses than usual

If the patient is not sedated within 15-20 minutes, a single repeat dose of thiopental can be given. The single repeat doses are:

<3 months: <7.5 mg/kg/dose

>3 months: 15 mg/kg/dose

Adults weighing >90 kg should not receive >3 g as a total dose (initial plus repeat doses)

Children weighing >34 kg should not receive >1 g as a total dose (initial plus repeat doses)

Neither adults nor children should receive more than one course of thiopental rectal suspension (initial dose plus repeat dose) per 24-hour period

Mechanism of Action Short-acting barbiturate with sedative, hypnotic, and anticonvulsant properties. Barbiturates depress the sensory cortex, decrease motor activity, alter cerebellar function, and produce drowsiness, sedation, and hypnosis. In high doses, barbiturates exhibit anticonvulsant activity; barbiturates produce dose-dependent respiratory depression.

Other Adverse Effects Frequency not defined:

Cardiovascular: Bradycardia, hypotension, syncope

Central nervous system: Drowsiness, lethargy, CNS excitation or depression, impaired judgment, "hangover" effect, confusion, somnolence, agitation, hyperkinesia, ataxia, nervousness, headache, insomnia, nightmares, hallucinations, anxiety, dizziness

Dermatologic: Rash, exfoliative dermatitis, Stevens-Johnson syndrome

Gastrointestinal: Nausea, vomiting, constipation

Hematologic: Agranulocytosis, thrombocytopenia, megaloblastic anemia

Local: Pain at injection site, thrombophlebitis with I.V. use

Renal: Oliguria

Respiratory: Laryngospasm, respiratory depression, apnea (especially with rapid I.V. use), hypoventilation, apnea

Miscellaneous: Gangrene with inadvertent intra-arterial injection

Drug Interactions Increased Effect/Toxicity: In chronic use, barbiturates are potent inducers of CYP isoenzymes resulting in multiple interactions with medication groups. When used for limited periods, thiopental is not likely to interact via this mechanism. Sedative effects and/or respiratory depression with barbiturates may be additive with other CNS depressants; includes sedatives, antidepressants, narcotic analgesics, and benzodiazepines. Felbamate may inhibit the metabolism of barbiturates and barbiturates may increase the metabolism of felbamate. Barbiturates may enhance the nephrotoxic effects of methoxyflurane

Drug Uptake

Onset of action: Anesthetic: I.V.: 30-60 seconds

Duration: 5-30 minutes

Half-life, elimination: 3-11.5 hours (decreases in children)

Pregnancy Risk Factor C

Generic Available Yes

Thioplex® *see* Thiotepa *on page 1161*

Thioridazine (thye oh RID a zeen)

U.S. Brand Names Mellaril®

Canadian Brand Names Apo®-Thioridazine; Mellaril®

Mexican Brand Names Melleril®

Pharmacologic Category Antipsychotic Agent, Phenothiazine, Piperidine

Synonyms Thioridazine Hydrochloride

Use Management of schizophrenic patients who fail to respond adequately to treatment with other antipsychotic drugs, either because of insufficient effectiveness or the inability to achieve an effective dose due to intolerable adverse effects from those medications

Unlabeled/Investigational: Psychosis

Local Anesthetic/Vasoconstrictor Precautions Most pharmacology textbooks state that in the presence of phenothiazines, systemic doses of epinephrine paradoxically decrease the blood pressure. This is the so called "epinephrine reversal" phenomenon. This has never been observed when epinephrine is given by infiltration as part of the anesthesia procedure.

Effects on Dental Treatment

Significant hypotension may occur, especially when the drug is administered parenterally; orthostatic hypotension is due to alpha-receptor blockade, the elderly are at greater risk for orthostatic hypotension.

(Continued)

Thioridazine *(Continued)*

Tardive dyskinesia; Prevalence rate may be 40% in elderly; development of the syndrome and the irreversible nature are proportional to duration and total cumulative dose over time. Extrapyramidal reactions are more common in elderly with up to 50% developing these reactions after 60 years of age; drug-induced **Parkinson's syndrome** occurs often; **Akathisia** is the most common extrapyramidal reaction in elderly.

Increased confusion, memory loss, psychotic behavior, and agitation frequently occur as a consequence of anticholinergic effects. Antipsychotic associated sedation in nonpsychotic patients is extremely unpleasant due to feelings of depersonalization, derealization, and dysphoria.

Dosage Oral:

Children >2-12 years: Range: 0.5-3 mg/kg/day in 2-3 divided doses; usual: 1 mg/kg/day; maximum: 3 mg/kg/day
- Behavior problems: Initial: 10 mg 2-3 times/day, increase gradually
- Severe psychoses: Initial: 25 mg 2-3 times/day, increase gradually

Children >12 years and Adults:
- Schizophrenia/psychoses: Initial: 50-100 mg 3 times/day with gradual increments as needed and tolerated; maximum: 800 mg/day in 2-4 divided doses; if >65 years, initial dose: 10 mg 3 times/day
- Depressive disorders/dementia: Initial: 25 mg 3 times/day; maintenance dose: 20-200 mg/day

Elderly: Behavioral symptoms associated with dementia: Initial: 10-25 mg 1-2 times/day; increase at 4- to 7-day intervals by 10-25 mg/day; increase dose intervals (qd, bid, etc) as necessary to control response or side effects. Maximum daily dose: 400 mg; gradual increases (titration) may prevent some side effects or decrease their severity.

Hemodialysis: Not dialyzable (0% to 5%)

Mechanism of Action Blocks postsynaptic mesolimbic dopaminergic receptors in the brain; exhibits a strong alpha-adrenergic blocking effect and depresses the release of hypothalamic and hypophyseal hormones

Other Adverse Effects Frequency not defined:

Cardiovascular: Hypotension, orthostatic hypotension, peripheral edema, EKG changes

Central nervous system: EPS (pseudoparkinsonism, akathisia, dystonias, tardive dyskinesia), dizziness, drowsiness, neuroleptic malignant syndrome (NMS), impairment of temperature regulation, lowering of seizures threshold, seizure

Dermatologic: Increased sensitivity to sun, rash, discoloration of skin (blue-gray)

Endocrine & metabolic: Changes in menstrual cycle, changes in libido, breast pain, galactorrhea, amenorrhea

Gastrointestinal: Constipation, weight gain, nausea, vomiting, stomach pain, xerostomia, nausea, vomiting, diarrhea

Genitourinary: Difficulty in urination, ejaculatory disturbances, urinary retention, priapism

Hematologic: Agranulocytosis, leukopenia

Hepatic: Cholestatic jaundice, hepatotoxicity

Neuromuscular & skeletal: Tremor

Ocular: Pigmentary retinopathy, blurred vision, cornea and lens changes

Respiratory: Nasal congestion

Drug Interactions CYP1A2 and 2D6 enzyme substrate; CYP2D6 enzyme inhibitor

Aluminum salts: May decrease the absorption of phenothiazines; monitor

Amphetamines: Efficacy may be diminished by antipsychotics; in addition, amphetamines may increase psychotic symptoms; avoid concurrent use

Anticholinergics: May inhibit the therapeutic response to phenothiazines and excess anticholinergic effects may occur; includes benztropine, trihexyphenidyl, biperiden, and drugs with significant anticholinergic activity (TCAs, antihistamines, disopyramide)

Antihypertensives: Concurrent use of phenothiazines with an antihypertensive may produce additive hypotensive effects (particularly orthostasis)

Beta-blockers: May increase the risk of arrhythmia; propranolol and pindolol are **contraindicated**

Bromocriptine: Phenothiazines inhibit the ability of bromocriptine to lower serum prolactin concentrations

Carvedilol: Serum concentrations may be increased, leading to hypotension and bradycardia; avoid concurrent use

CNS depressants: Sedative effects may be additive with phenothiazines; monitor for increased effect; includes barbiturates, benzodiazepines, narcotic analgesics, ethanol, and other sedative agents

CYP1A2 inhibitors: Metabolism of phenothiazines may be decreased; increasing clinical effect or toxicity. Inhibitors include cimetidine, ciprofloxacin, fluvoxamine, isoniazid, ritonavir, and zileuton. Concurrent use with fluvoxamine is contraindicated.

CYP2D6 inhibitors: Metabolism of phenothiazines may be decreased; increasing clinical effect or toxicity. Inhibitors include amiodarone, cimetidine, delavirdine, fluoxetine, paroxetine, propafenone, quinidine, and ritonavir; monitor for increased effect/toxicity. **Thioridazine is contraindicated with inhibitors of this enzyme, including fluoxetine and paroxetine.**

Enzyme inducers: May enhance the hepatic metabolism of phenothiazines; larger doses may be required; includes rifampin, rifabutin, barbiturates, phenytoin, and cigarette smoking

Epinephrine: Chlorpromazine (and possibly other low potency antipsychotics) may diminish the pressor effects of epinephrine

Guanethidine and guanadrel: Antihypertensive effects may be inhibited by phenothiazines

Levodopa: Phenothiazines may inhibit the antiparkinsonian effect of levodopa; avoid this combination

Lithium: Phenothiazines may produce neurotoxicity with lithium; this is a rare effect

Metoclopramide: May increase extrapyramidal symptoms (EPS) or risk.

Phenytoin: May reduce serum levels of phenothiazines; phenothiazines may increase phenytoin serum levels

Polypeptide antibiotics: Rare cases of respiratory paralysis have been reported with concurrent use of phenothiazines

Potassium-depleting agents: May increase the risk of serious arrhythmias with thioridazine; includes many diuretics, aminoglycosides, and amphotericin; monitor serum potassium closely

Propranolol: Serum concentrations of phenothiazines may be increased; propranolol also increases phenothiazine concentrations; may also occur with pindolol. **These agents are contraindicated with thioridazine.**

QT_c-prolonging agents: Effects on QT_c interval may be additive with phenothiazines, increasing the risk of malignant arrhythmias; includes type Ia antiarrhythmics, TCAs, and some quinolone antibiotics (sparfloxacin, moxifloxacin and gatifloxacin). **These agents are contraindicated with thioridazine.**

Sulfadoxine-pyrimethamine: May increase phenothiazine concentrations

Trazodone: Phenothiazines and trazodone may produce additive hypotensive effects

Tricyclic antidepressants: Concurrent use may produce increased toxicity or altered therapeutic response

Valproic acid: Serum levels may be increased by phenothiazines

Drug Uptake

Duration: 4-5 days

Half-life, elimination: 21-25 hours

Time to peak: ~1 hour

Pregnancy Risk Factor C

Generic Available Yes

Thiotepa (thye oh TEP a)

U.S. Brand Names Thioplex®

Pharmacologic Category Antineoplastic Agent, Alkylating Agent

Synonyms TESPA; Thiophosphoramide; Triethylenethiophosphoramide; TSPA

Use Treatment of superficial tumors of the bladder; palliative treatment of adenocarcinoma of breast or ovary; lymphomas and sarcomas; meningeal neoplasms; control pleural, pericardial or peritoneal effusions caused by metastatic tumors; high-dose regimens with autologous bone marrow transplantation

Local Anesthetic/Vasoconstrictor Precautions No information available to require special precautions

Effects on Dental Treatment No effects or complications reported

Mechanism of Action Alkylating agent that reacts with DNA phosphate groups to produce cross-linking of DNA strands leading to inhibition of DNA, RNA, and protein synthesis; mechanism of action has not been explored as thoroughly as the other alkylating agents, it is presumed that the aziridine rings open and react as nitrogen mustard; reactivity is enhanced at a lower pH

Other Adverse Effects

>10%:

Hematopoietic: Dose-limiting toxicity which is dose-related and cumulative; moderate to severe leukopenia and severe thrombocytopenia have occurred. Anemia and pancytopenia may become fatal, so careful hematologic monitoring is required; intravesical administration may cause bone marrow suppression as well.

Hematologic: Myelosuppressive:

- WBC: Moderate
- Platelets: Severe
- Onset: 7-10 days
- Nadir: 14 days
- Recovery: 28 days

Local: Pain at injection site

1% to 10%:

Central nervous system: Dizziness, fever, headache

Dermatologic: Alopecia, rash, pruritus, hyperpigmentation with high-dose therapy

Endocrine & metabolic: Hyperuricemia

Gastrointestinal: Anorexia, nausea and vomiting rarely occur

(Continued)

Thiotepa *(Continued)*

Emetic potential: Low (<10%)
Genitourinary: Hemorrhagic cystitis
Renal: Hematuria
Miscellaneous: Tightness of the throat, allergic reactions

Drug Interactions Increased Effect/Toxicity: Other alkylating agents or irradiation used concomitantly with thiotepa intensifies toxicity rather than enhancing therapeutic response. Prolonged muscular paralysis and respiratory depression may occur when neuromuscular blocking agents are administered. Succinylcholine and other neuromuscular blocking agents' action can be prolonged due to thiotepa inhibiting plasma pseudocholinesterase.

Drug Uptake

Absorption: Intracavitary instillation: Unreliable (10% to 100%) through the bladder mucosa; I.M.: Variable

Half-life, elimination: Terminal: 109 minutes (dose-dependent)

Pregnancy Risk Factor D

Generic Available Yes

Thiothixene (thye oh THIKS een)

U.S. Brand Names Navane®

Canadian Brand Names Navane®

Pharmacologic Category Antipsychotic Agent, Thioxanthene Derivative

Synonyms Tiotixene

Use Management of schizophrenia

Unlabeled/Investigational: Psychotic disorders

Local Anesthetic/Vasoconstrictor Precautions Most pharmacology textbooks state that in presence of phenothiazines, systemic doses of epinephrine paradoxically decrease the blood pressure. This is the so called "epinephrine reversal" phenomenon. This has never been observed when epinephrine is given by infiltration as part of the anesthesia procedure.

Effects on Dental Treatment

Significant hypotension may occur, especially when the drug is administered parenterally; orthostatic hypotension is due to alpha-receptor blockade, the elderly are at greater risk for orthostatic hypotension.

Tardive dyskinesia: Prevalence rate may be 40% in elderly; development of the syndrome and the irreversible nature are proportional to duration and total cumulative dose over time. Extrapyramidal reactions are more common in elderly with up to 50% developing these reactions after 60 years of age; drug-induced **Parkinson's syndrome** occurs often; **Akathisia** is the most common extrapyramidal reaction in elderly.

Increased confusion, memory loss, psychotic behavior, and agitation frequently occur as a consequence of anticholinergic effects. Antipsychotic associated sedation in nonpsychotic patients is extremely unpleasant due to feelings of depersonalization, derealization, and dysphoria.

Dosage

Children <12 years (unlabeled): Schizophrenia/psychoses: Oral: 0.25 mg/kg/24 hours in divided doses (dose not well established)

Children >12 years and Adults: Mild to moderate psychosis:

- Oral: 2 mg 3 times/day, up to 20-30 mg/day; more severe psychosis: Initial: 5 mg 2 times/day, may increase gradually, if necessary; maximum: 60 mg/day
- I.M.: 4 mg 2-4 times/day, increase dose gradually; usual: 16-20 mg/day; maximum: 30 mg/day; change to oral dose as soon as able
- Rapid tranquilization of the agitated patient (administered every 30-60 minutes):
  - Oral: 5-10 mg
  - I.M.: 10-20 mg
  - Average total dose for tranquilization: 15-30 mg

Hemodialysis: Not dialyzable (0% to 5%)

Mechanism of Action Elicits antipsychotic activity by postsynaptic blockade of CNS dopamine receptors resulting in inhibition of dopamine-mediated effects; also has alpha-adrenergic blocking activity

Other Adverse Effects Frequency not defined:

Cardiovascular: Hypotension, tachycardia, syncope, nonspecific EKG changes

Central nervous system: Extrapyramidal symptoms (pseudoparkinsonism, akathisia, dystonias, lightheadedness, tardive dyskinesia), dizziness, drowsiness, restlessness, agitation, insomnia

Dermatologic: Discoloration of skin (blue-gray), rash, pruritus, urticaria, photosensitivity

Endocrine & metabolic: Changes in menstrual cycle, changes in libido, breast pain, galactorrhea, lactation, amenorrhea, gynecomastia, hyperglycemia, hypoglycemia

Gastrointestinal: Weight gain, nausea, vomiting, stomach pain, constipation, xerostomia, increased salivation

Genitourinary: Difficulty in urination, ejaculatory disturbances, impotence

Hematologic: Leukopenia, leukocytes

Neuromuscular & skeletal: Tremors
Ocular: Pigmentary retinopathy, blurred vision
Respiratory: Nasal congestion
Miscellaneous: Diaphoresis

Drug Interactions CYP1A2 enzyme substrate

Aluminum salts: May decrease the absorption of antipsychotics; monitor
Amphetamines: Efficacy may be diminished by antipsychotics; in addition, amphetamines may increase psychotic symptoms; avoid concurrent use
Anticholinergics: May inhibit the therapeutic response to antipsychotics and excess anticholinergic effects may occur; includes benztropine, trihexyphenidyl, biperiden, and drugs with significant anticholinergic activity (TCAs, antihistamines, disopyramide)
Antihypertensives: Concurrent use of antipsychotics with an antihypertensive may produce additive hypotensive effects (particularly orthostasis)
Bromocriptine: Antipsychotics inhibit the ability of bromocriptine to lower serum prolactin concentrations
CNS depressants: Sedative effects may be additive with antipsychotics; monitor for increased effect; includes barbiturates, benzodiazepines, narcotic analgesics, ethanol, and other sedative agents
CYP1A2 inhibitors: Serum levels may be increased; inhibitors include cimetidine, ciprofloxacin, fluvoxamine, isoniazid, ritonavir, and zileuton
Enzyme inducers: May enhance the hepatic metabolism of antipsychotics; larger doses may be required; includes rifampin, rifabutin, barbiturates, phenytoin, and cigarette smoking
Epinephrine: Chlorpromazine (and possibly other low potency antipsychotics) may diminish the pressor effects of epinephrine
Guanethidine and guanadrel: Antihypertensive effects may be inhibited by antipsychotics
Levodopa: Antipsychotics may inhibit the antiparkinsonian effect of levodopa; avoid this combination
Lithium: Antipsychotics may produce neurotoxicity with lithium; this is a rare effect
Metoclopramide: May increase extrapyramidal symptoms (EPS) or risk.
Phenytoin: May reduce serum levels of antipsychotics; antipsychotics may increase phenytoin serum levels
Propranolol: Serum concentrations of antipsychotics may be increased; propranolol also increases antipsychotics concentrations
QT_c-prolonging agents: Effects on QT_c interval may be additive with antipsychotics, increasing the risk of malignant arrhythmias; includes type Ia antiarrhythmics, TCAs, and some quinolone antibiotics (sparfloxacin, moxifloxacin, and gatifloxacin)
Sulfadoxine-pyrimethamine: May increase antipsychotics concentrations
Trazodone: Antipsychotics and trazodone may produce additive hypotensive effects
Tricyclic antidepressants: Concurrent use may produce increased toxicity or altered therapeutic response
Valproic acid: Serum levels may be increased by antipsychotics

Drug Uptake Half-life, elimination: >24 hours with chronic use

Pregnancy Risk Factor C

Generic Available Yes

Thorazine® *see* ChlorproMAZINE *on page 273*
Thrombate III™ *see* Antithrombin III *on page 107*
Thrombinar® *see* Thrombin, Topical *on page 1163*

Thrombin, Topical (THROM bin, TOP i kal)

U.S. Brand Names Thrombinar®; Thrombogen®; Thrombostat®

Canadian Brand Names Thrombostat™

Pharmacologic Category Hemostatic Agent

Use Hemostasis whenever minor bleeding from capillaries and small venules is accessible

Local Anesthetic/Vasoconstrictor Precautions No information available to require special precautions

Effects on Dental Treatment No effects or complications reported

Dosage Use 1000-2000 units/mL of solution where bleeding is profuse; apply powder directly to the site of bleeding or on oozing surfaces; use 100 units/mL for bleeding from skin or mucosal surfaces

Mechanism of Action Catalyzes the conversion of fibrinogen to fibrin

Other Adverse Effects 1% to 10%:

Central nervous system: Fever
Miscellaneous: Allergic type reaction

Contraindications Hypersensitivity to thrombin or any component of the formulation

Warnings/Precautions Do not inject, for topical use only

Pregnancy Risk Factor C

(Continued)

Thrombin, Topical *(Continued)*

Dosage Forms POWDER: 1000 units, 5000 units, 10,000 units, 20,000 units, 50,000 units

Generic Available No

Comments Topical thrombin is not to be used in conjunction with oxidized cellulose.

Thrombogen® *see* Thrombin, Topical *on page 1163*

Thrombostat® *see* Thrombin, Topical *on page 1163*

Thyrel® TRH *see* Protirelin *on page 1020*

Thyrogen® *see* Thyrotropin Alpha *on page 1165*

Thyroid (THYE royd)

Related Information

Endocrine Disorders and Pregnancy *on page 1331*

U.S. Brand Names Armour® Thyroid; Nature-Throid® NT; Westhroid®

Pharmacologic Category Thyroid Product

Synonyms Desiccated Thyroid; Thyroid Extract; Thyroid USP

Use Replacement or supplemental therapy in hypothyroidism; pituitary TSH suppressants (thyroid nodules, thyroiditis, multinodular goiter, thyroid cancer), thyrotoxicosis, diagnostic suppression tests

Local Anesthetic/Vasoconstrictor Precautions No precautions with vasoconstrictor are necessary if patient is well controlled with thyroid preparations

Effects on Dental Treatment No effects or complications reported

Dosage Oral:

Children: See table.

Recommended Pediatric Dosage for Congenital Hypothyroidism

Age	Daily Dose (mg)	Daily Dose/kg (mg)
0-6 months	15-30	4.8-6
6-12 months	30-45	3.6-4.8
1-5 years	45-60	3-3.6
6-12 years	60-90	2.4-3
>12 years	>90	1.2-1.8

Adults: Initial: 15-30 mg; increase with 15 mg increments every 2-4 weeks; use 15 mg in patients with cardiovascular disease or myxedema. Maintenance dose: Usually 60-120 mg/day; monitor TSH and clinical symptoms.

Thyroid cancer: Requires larger amounts than replacement therapy

Mechanism of Action The primary active compound is T_3 (triiodothyronine), which may be converted from T_4 (thyroxine) and then circulates throughout the body to influence growth and maturation of various tissues; exact mechanism of action is unknown; however, it is believed the thyroid hormone exerts its many metabolic effects through control of DNA transcription and protein synthesis; involved in normal metabolism, growth, and development; promotes gluconeogenesis, increases utilization and mobilization of glycogen stores and stimulates protein synthesis, increases basal metabolic rate

Drug Interactions

Increased Effect/Toxicity: Thyroid may potentiate the hypoprothrombinemic effect of oral anticoagulants. Tricyclic antidepressants (TAD) coadministered with thyroid hormone may increase potential for toxicity of both drugs.

Decreased Effect: Thyroid hormones increase the therapeutic need for oral hypoglycemics or insulin. Cholestyramine can bind thyroid and reduce its absorption. Phenytoin may decrease thyroxine serum concentration. Thyroid hormone may decrease effect of oral sulfonylureas.

Drug Uptake

Absorption: T_4 is 48% to 79% absorbed; T_3 is 95% absorbed; desiccated thyroid contains thyroxine, liothyronine, and iodine (primarily bound); following absorption thyroxine is largely converted to liothyronine

Half-life, elimination: Liothyronine: 1-2 days; Thyroxine: 6-7 days

Pregnancy Risk Factor A

Generic Available Yes

Thyrolar® *see* Liotrix *on page 718*

Thyrotropin (thye roe TROE pin)

U.S. Brand Names Thytropar®

Pharmacologic Category Diagnostic Agent

Synonyms Thyroid Stimulating Hormone; Thyrotropic Hormone; TSH

Use Diagnostic aid to differentiate thyroid failure; diagnosis of decreased thyroid reserve, to differentiate between primary and secondary hypothyroidism and between primary hypothyroidism and euthyroidism in patients receiving thyroid replacement

Local Anesthetic/Vasoconstrictor Precautions No information available to require special precautions

Effects on Dental Treatment No effects or complications reported

Dosage Adults: I.M., S.C.: 10 units/day for 1-3 days; follow by a radioiodine study 24 hours past last injection, no response in thyroid failure, substantial response in pituitary failure

Mechanism of Action Stimulates formation and secretion of thyroid hormone, increases uptake of iodine by thyroid gland

Drug Uptake Half-life, elimination: 35 minutes (dependent on thyroid function)

Pregnancy Risk Factor C

Generic Available No

Thyrotropin Alpha (thye roe TROE pin AL fa)

U.S. Brand Names Thyrogen®

Pharmacologic Category Diagnostic Agent

Synonyms Human Thyroid Stimulating Hormone; TSH

Use As an adjunctive diagnostic tool for serum thyroglobulin (Tg) testing with or without radioiodine imaging in the follow-up of patients with well-differentiated thyroid cancer

Potential clinical uses:

1. Patients with an undetectable Tg on thyroid hormone suppressive therapy to exclude the diagnosis of residual or recurrent thyroid cancer
2. Patients requiring serum Tg testing and radioiodine imaging who are unwilling to undergo thyroid hormone withdrawal testing and whose treating physician believes that use of a less sensitive test is justified
3. Patients who are either unable to mount an adequate endogenous TSH response to thyroid hormone withdrawal or in whom withdrawal is medically contraindicated

Local Anesthetic/Vasoconstrictor Precautions No information available to require special precautions

Effects on Dental Treatment No effects or complications reported

Dosage Children >16 years and Adults: I.M.: 0.9 mg every 24 hours for 2 doses or every 72 hours for 3 doses. For radioiodine imaging, radioiodine administration should be given 24 hours following the final Thyrogen® injection. Scanning should be performed 48 hours after radioiodine administration (72 hours after the final injection of Thyrogen®).

Mechanism of Action An exogenous source of human TSH that offers an additional diagnostic tool in the follow-up of patients with a history of well-differentiated thyroid cancer. Binding of thyrotropin alpha to TSH receptors on normal thyroid epithelial cells or on well-differentiated thyroid cancer tissue stimulates iodine uptake and organification and synthesis and secretion of thyroglobulin, triiodothyronine, and thyroxine.

Other Adverse Effects 1% to 10%:

Central nervous system: Headache, chills, fever, dizziness
Gastrointestinal: Nausea, vomiting
Neuromuscular & skeletal: Weakness, paresthesia
Miscellaneous: Flu-like syndrome

Contraindications Hypersensitivity to thyrotropin alpha or any component of the formulation

Drug Uptake

Half-life, elimination: 25 ± 10 hours
Time to peak: Mean: 3-24 hours after injection

Pregnancy Risk Factor C

Generic Available No

Thytropar® *see* Thyrotropin *on page 1164*

Tiagabine (tye AG a bene)

U.S. Brand Names Gabitril®

Canadian Brand Names Gabitril®

Pharmacologic Category Anticonvulsant, Miscellaneous

Synonyms Tiagabine Hydrochloride

Use Adjunctive therapy in adults and children 12 years and older in the treatment of partial seizures

Unlabeled/Investigational: Bipolar disorder

Local Anesthetic/Vasoconstrictor Precautions No information available to require special precautions

Effects on Dental Treatment No effects or complications reported

Dosage Children >12 years and Adults: Oral: Starting dose: 4 mg once daily; the total daily dose may be increased in 4 mg increments beginning the second week of therapy; thereafter, the daily dose may be increased by 4-8 mg/day until clinical

(Continued)

Tiagabine *(Continued)*

response is achieved, up to a maximum of 32 mg/day; the total daily dose at higher levels should be given in divided doses 2-4 times/day

Mechanism of Action The exact mechanism by which tiagabine exerts antiseizure activity is not definitively known; however, *in vitro* experiments demonstrate that it enhances the activity of gamma aminobutyric acid (GABA), the major neuroinhibitory transmitter in the nervous system; it is thought that binding to the GABA uptake carrier inhibits the uptake of GABA into presynaptic neurons, allowing an increased amount of GABA to be available to postsynaptic neurons; based on *in vitro* studies, tiagabine does not inhibit the uptake of dopamine, norepinephrine, serotonin, glutamate or choline

Other Adverse Effects

>10%:

Central nervous system: Dizziness, somnolence
Gastrointestinal: Nausea
Neuromuscular & skeletal: Weakness

1% to 10%:

Central nervous system: Nervousness, difficulty with concentration, insomnia, ataxia, confusion, speech disorder, depression, emotional lability, abnormal gait, hostility
Dermatologic: Rash, pruritus
Gastrointestinal: Diarrhea, vomiting, increased appetite
Neuromuscular & skeletal: Tremor, paresthesia
Ocular: Nystagmus
Otic: Hearing impairment
Respiratory: Pharyngitis, cough

Contraindications Hypersensitivity to tiagabine or any component of the formulation

Warnings/Precautions Anticonvulsants should not be discontinued abruptly because of the possibility of increasing seizure frequency; clinical studies were carried out that demonstrated an increase in seizure frequency upon abrupt withdrawal; tiagabine should be withdrawn gradually to minimize the potential of increased seizure frequency, unless safety concerns require a more rapid withdrawal

Drug Interactions CYP2D6 and 3A3/4 enzyme substrate

CNS depressants: Sedative effects may be additive with other CNS depressants; monitor for increased effect; includes ethanol, sedatives, antidepressants, narcotic analgesics, other anticonvulsants, and benzodiazepines

CYP2D6 inhibitors: Serum levels and/or toxicity of tiagabine may be increased; inhibitors include amiodarone, cimetidine, delavirdine, fluoxetine, paroxetine, propafenone, quinidine, and ritonavir; monitor for increased effect/toxicity

CYP3A3/4 inhibitors: Serum level and/or toxicity of tiagabine may be increased; inhibitors include amiodarone, cimetidine, clarithromycin, erythromycin, delavirdine, diltiazem, dirithromycin, disulfiram, fluoxetine, fluvoxamine, grapefruit juice, indinavir, itraconazole, ketoconazole, nevirapine, propoxyphene, quinupristin-dalfopristin, ritonavir, saquinavir, verapamil, zafirlukast, zileuton; monitor for altered effects

Enzyme inducers: May increase the metabolism of tiagabine resulting in decreased effect. Primidone, phenobarbital, phenytoin, and carbamazepine increase tiagabine clearance by 60%

Valproate: Increased free tiagabine concentrations by 40%

Drug Uptake

Absorption: Rapid (~1 hour); prolonged with food
Half-life, elimination: 6.7 hours

Pregnancy Risk Factor C

Generic Available No

Selected Readings Patsalos PN and Sander JW, "Newer Antiepileptic Drugs: Towards an Improved Risk-Benefit Ratio," *Drug Saf*, 1994, 11(1):37-67.

Tiamate® *see* Diltiazem *on page 394*
Tiazac® *see* Diltiazem *on page 394*
Ticar® *see* Ticarcillin *on page 1166*

Ticarcillin (tye kar SIL in)

U.S. Brand Names Ticar®

Pharmacologic Category Antibiotic, Penicillin

Synonyms Ticarcillin Disodium

Use Treatment of susceptible infections such as septicemia, acute and chronic respiratory tract infections, skin and soft tissue infections, and urinary tract infections due to susceptible strains of *Pseudomonas*, *Proteus*, and *Escherichia coli* and *Enterobacter*, normally used with other antibiotics (ie, aminoglycosides)

Local Anesthetic/Vasoconstrictor Precautions No information available to require special precautions

Effects on Dental Treatment Prolonged use of penicillins may lead to development of oral candidiasis.

Dosage Generally given I.M. only for the treatment of uncomplicated urinary tract infections

Children: I.V.: Serious Infections: 200-300 mg/kg/day in divided doses every 4-6 hours; doses as high as 400 mg/kg/day divided every 4 hours have been used in acute pulmonary exacerbations of cystic fibrosis

Maximum dose: 24 g/day

Adults: I.V.: 1-4 g every 4-6 hours

Mechanism of Action Inhibits bacterial cell wall synthesis by binding to one or more of the penicillin binding proteins (PBPs); which in turn inhibits the final transpeptidation step of peptidoglycan synthesis in bacterial cell walls, thus inhibiting cell wall biosynthesis. Bacteria eventually lyse due to ongoing activity of cell wall autolytic enzymes (autolysins and murein hydrolases) while cell wall assembly is arrested.

Other Adverse Effects

>10%:

Central nervous system: Headache

Gastrointestinal: Nausea (mild), vomiting

Miscellaneous: Oral candidiasis, vaginal candidiasis

1% to 10%:

Dermatologic: Urticaria, exfoliative dermatitis

Miscellaneous: Allergic reactions, specifically anaphylaxis; serum sickness-like reactions

Frequency not defined:

Central nervous system: Confusion, convulsions, drowsiness, fever, Jarisch-Herxheimer reaction

Dermatologic: Rash

Endocrine & metabolic: Electrolyte imbalance

Gastrointestinal: *Clostridium difficile* colitis

Hematologic: Bleeding, eosinophilia, hemolytic anemia, leukopenia, neotropenia, positive Coombs' reaction, thrombocytopenia

Hepatic: Hepatotoxicity, jaundice

Local: Thrombophlebitis

Neuromuscular & skeletal: Myoclonus

Renal: Interstitial nephritis (acute)

Miscellaneous: Anaphylaxis, hypersensitivity reactions

Drug Interactions

Increased Effect/Toxicity: Probenecid may increase penicillin levels. Neuromuscular blockers may have an increased duration of action (neuromuscular blockade).

Decreased Effect: Tetracyclines may decrease penicillin effectiveness. Efficacy of oral contraceptives may be reduced when taken with ticarcillin. Aminoglycosides may cause physical inactivation of aminoglycosides in the presence of high concentrations of ticarcillin and potential toxicity in patients with mild-moderate renal dysfunction.

Drug Uptake

Absorption: I.M.: 86%

Half-life, elimination:

Neonates: <1 week old: 3.5-5.6 hours; 1-8 weeks old: 1.3-2.2 hours

Children 5-13 years: 0.9 hour

Adults: 66-72 minutes; prolonged with renal and/or hepatic impairment

Time to peak: I.M.: 30-75 minutes

Pregnancy Risk Factor B

Generic Available No

Ticarcillin and Clavulanate Potassium

(tye kar SIL in & klav yoo LAN ate poe TASS ee um)

U.S. Brand Names Timentin®

Canadian Brand Names Timentin®

Pharmacologic Category Antibiotic, Penicillin

Synonyms Ticarcillin and Clavulanic Acid

Use Treatment of infections of lower respiratory tract, urinary tract, skin and skin structures, bone and joint, and septicemia caused by susceptible organisms. Clavulanate expands activity of ticarcillin to include beta-lactamase producing strains of *S. aureus*, *H. influenzae*, *Enterobacteriaceae*, *Klebsiella*, *Citrobacter*, and *Serratia*

Local Anesthetic/Vasoconstrictor Precautions No information available to require special precautions

Effects on Dental Treatment Prolonged use of penicillins may lead to development of oral candidiasis.

Dosage I.V.:

Children: 200-300 mg of ticarcillin component/kg/day in divided doses every 4-6 hours

Adults: 3.1 g (ticarcillin 3 g plus clavulanic acid 0.1 g) every 4-6 hours; maximum: 18-24 g/day

(Continued)

Ticarcillin and Clavulanate Potassium *(Continued)*

Mechanism of Action Inhibits bacterial cell wall synthesis by binding to one or more of the penicillin binding proteins (PBPs); which in turn inhibits the final transpeptidation step of peptidoglycan synthesis in bacterial cell walls, thus inhibiting cell wall biosynthesis. Bacteria eventually lyse due to ongoing activity of cell wall autolytic enzymes (autolysins and murein hydrolases) while cell wall assembly is arrested. Clavulanic acid prevents degradation of ticarcillin by binding to the active site on beta-lactamase.

Other Adverse Effects Frequency not defined:

Central nervous system: Confusion, convulsions, drowsiness, fever, Jarisch-Herxheimer reaction

Dermatologic: Rash

Endocrine & metabolic: Electrolyte imbalance

Gastrointestinal: *Clostridium difficile* colitis

Hematologic: Bleeding, hemolytic anemia, leukopenia, neutropenia, positive Coombs' reaction, thrombocytopenia

Hepatic: Hepatotoxicity, jaundice

Local: Thrombophlebitis

Neuromuscular & skeletal: Myoclonus

Renal: Interstitial nephritis (acute)

Miscellaneous: Anaphylaxis, hypersensitivity reactions

Drug Interactions

Increased Effect/Toxicity: Probenecid may increase penicillin levels. Neuromuscular blockers may have an increased duration of action (neuromuscular blockade).

Decreased Effect: Tetracyclines may decrease penicillin effectiveness. Efficacy of oral contraceptives may be reduced when taken with ticarcillin and clavulanate potassium. Aminoglycosides may cause physical inactivation of aminoglycosides in the presence of high concentrations of ticarcillin and potential toxicity in patients with mild-moderate renal dysfunction.

Drug Uptake Half-life, elimination:

Clavulanate: 66-90 minutes

Ticarcillin: 66-72 minutes in patients with normal renal function; clavulanic acid does not affect the clearance of ticarcillin

Pregnancy Risk Factor B

Generic Available No

TICE® BCG *see* BCG Vaccine *on page 145*

Ticlid® *see* Ticlopidine *on page 1168*

Ticlopidine (tye KLOE pi deen)

Related Information

Cardiovascular Diseases *on page 1308*

U.S. Brand Names Ticlid®

Canadian Brand Names Alti-Ticlopidine; Apo®-Ticlopidine; Gen-Ticlopidine; Nu-Ticlopidine; Rhoxal-ticlopidine; Ticlid®

Mexican Brand Names Ticlid®

Pharmacologic Category Antiplatelet Agent

Synonyms Ticlopidine Hydrochloride

Use Platelet aggregation inhibitor that reduces the risk of thrombotic stroke in patients who have had a stroke or stroke precursors. **Note:** Due to its association with life-threatening hematologic disorders, ticlopidine should be reserved for patients who are intolerant to aspirin, or who have failed aspirin therapy. Adjunctive therapy (with aspirin) following successful coronary stent implantation to reduce the incidence of subacute stent thrombosis.

Unlabeled/Investigational: Protection of aortocoronary bypass grafts, diabetic microangiopathy, ischemic heart disease, prevention of postoperative DVT, reduction of graft loss following renal transplant

Local Anesthetic/Vasoconstrictor Precautions No information available to require special precautions

Effects on Dental Treatment No effects or complications reported; if a patient is to undergo elective surgery and an antiplatelet effect is not desired, ticlopidine should be discontinued at least 7 days prior to surgery.

Dosage Oral: Adults:

Stroke prevention: 250 mg twice daily with food

Coronary artery stenting (initiate after successful implantation): 250 mg twice daily with food (in combination with antiplatelet doses of aspirin) for up to 30 days

Mechanism of Action Mechanism different from other antiplatelet drugs; significantly increases bleeding time but effect may not be solely related to ticlopidine's effect on platelets; prolongation of bleeding time is further increased by aspirin in *ex vivo* experiments; although many metabolites of ticlopidine have been found, none have been shown to account for *in vivo* activity

Other Adverse Effects As with all drugs which may affect hemostasis, bleeding is associated with ticlopidine. Hemorrhage may occur at virtually any site. Risk is dependent on multiple variables, including the use of multiple agents which alter hemostasis and patient susceptibility.

>10%:

Endocrine & metabolic: Increased total cholesterol (increases of ~8% to 10% within 1 month of therapy)

Gastrointestinal: Diarrhea (13%)

1% to 10%:

Central nervous system: Dizziness (1%)

Dermatologic: Rash (5%), purpura (2%), pruritus (1%)

Gastrointestinal: Nausea (7%), dyspepsia (7%), gastrointestinal pain (4%), vomiting (2%), flatulence (2%), anorexia (1%)

Hematologic: Neutropenia (2%)

Hepatic: Abnormal liver function test (1%)

Warnings/Precautions Use with caution in patients who may have an increased risk of bleeding (such as, ulcers). Consider discontinuing 10-14 days before elective surgery. Use caution in mixing with other antiplatelet drugs. Use with caution in patients with severe liver disease or severe renal impairment (experience is limited). May cause life-threatening hematologic reactions, including neutropenia, agranulocytosis, thrombotic thrombocytopenia purpura (TTP), and aplastic anemia. Routine monitoring is required (see Monitoring Parameters). Monitor for signs and symptoms of neutropenia including WBC count. Discontinue if the absolute neutrophil count falls to <1200/mm^3 or if the platelet count falls to <80,000/mm^3.

Drug Interactions CYP3A3/4 enzyme substrate; CYP1A2 (possible), 2C19 (potent), 2D6 (weak) enzyme inhibitor

Antacids reduce absorption of ticlopidine (~18%).

Anticoagulants or other antiplatelet agents may increase the risk of bleeding; use with caution.

Carbamazepine blood levels may be increased by ticlopidine.

Cimetidine increases ticlopidine levels.

Cyclosporine blood levels may be reduced by ticlopidine.

Digoxin blood levels may be decreased by ticlopidine.

Phenytoin blood levels may be increased by ticlopidine (case reports).

Theophylline blood levels may be increased by ticlopidine.

Drug Uptake

Onset of action: ≤6 hours; Peak effect: 3-5 days; serum levels do not correlate with clinical antiplatelet activity

Half-life, elimination: 24 hours

Pregnancy Risk Factor B

Generic Available No

Tigan® *see* Trimethobenzamide *on page 1209*

Tikosyn™ *see* Dofetilide *on page 408*

Tilade® *see* Nedocromil Sodium *on page 851*

Tiludronate (tye LOO droe nate)

U.S. Brand Names Skelid®

Pharmacologic Category Bisphosphonate Derivative

Synonyms Tiludronate Disodium

Use Treatment of Paget's disease of the bone in patients who have a level of serum alkaline phosphatase (SAP) at least twice the upper limit of normal, or who are symptomatic, or who are at risk for future complications of their disease

Local Anesthetic/Vasoconstrictor Precautions No information available to require special precautions

Effects on Dental Treatment No effects or complications reported

Dosage Adults: Oral: 400 mg (2 tablets) [tiludronic acid] daily

Mechanism of Action Inhibition of normal and abnormal bone resorption. Inhibits osteoclasts through at least two mechanisms: disruption of the cytoskeletal ring structure, possibly by inhibition of protein-tyrosine-phosphatase, thus leading to the detachment of osteoclasts from the bone surface area and the inhibition of the osteoclast proton pump.

Other Adverse Effects The following events occurred >2% and at a frequency > placebo:

1% to 10%:

Cardiovascular: Chest pain (2.7%), edema (2.7%)

Central nervous system: Dizziness (4.0%), paresthesia (4.0%)

Dermatologic: Rash (2.7%), skin disorder (2.7%)

Gastrointestinal: Nausea (9.3%), diarrhea (9.3%), heartburn (5.3%), vomiting (4.0%), flatulence (2.7%)

Neuromuscular & skeletal: Arthrosis (2.7%)

Ocular: cataract (2.7%), conjunctivitis (2.7%), glaucoma (2.7%)

Respiratory: Rhinitis (5.3%), sinusitis (5.3%), coughing (2.7%), pharyngitis (2.7%)

Drug Interactions

Increased Effect/Toxicity: Administration of indomethacin increases bioavailability of tiludronate 2- to 4-fold.

(Continued)

Tiludronate *(Continued)*

Decreased Effect: Concurrent administration of calcium salts, aluminum- or magnesium-containing antacids, and aspirin markedly decrease absorption/bioavailability (by 50% to 60%) of tiludronate if given within 2 hours of a dose.

Drug Uptake

Onset of action: Delayed, may require several weeks

Time to peak, plasma: ~2 hours

Pregnancy Risk Factor C

Generic Available No

Timentin® *see* Ticarcillin and Clavulanate Potassium *on page 1167*

Timolol (TYE moe lole)

Related Information

Cardiovascular Diseases *on page 1308*

U.S. Brand Names Betimol®; Blocadren®; Timoptic®; Timoptic® OcuDose®; Timoptic-XE®

Canadian Brand Names Apo®-Timol; Apo®-Timop; Gen-Timolol; Novo-Timol; Nu-Timolol; Phoxal-timolol; PMS-Timolol; Tim-AK; Timoptic®; Timoptic-XE®

Mexican Brand Names Imot Ofteno; Shemol®; Timoptol®; Timoptol® XE

Pharmacologic Category Beta Blocker, Nonselective; Ophthalmic Agent, Antiglaucoma

Synonyms Timolol Hemihydrate; Timolol Maleate

Use Ophthalmic dosage form used in the treatment of elevated intraocular pressure such as glaucoma or ocular hypertension; orally for treatment of hypertension and angina and reduce mortality following myocardial infarction and prophylaxis of migraine

Local Anesthetic/Vasoconstrictor Precautions No information available to require special precautions

Effects on Dental Treatment No effects or complications reported

Dosage

Children and Adults: Ophthalmic: Initial: 0.25% solution, instill 1 drop twice daily; increase to 0.5% solution if response not adequate; decrease to 1 drop/day if controlled; do not exceed 1 drop twice daily of 0.5% solution

Adults: Oral:

- Hypertension: Initial: 10 mg twice daily, increase gradually every 7 days, usual dosage: 20-40 mg/day in 2 divided doses; maximum: 60 mg/day
- Prevention of myocardial infarction: 10 mg twice daily initiated within 1-4 weeks after infarction
- Migraine headache: Initial: 10 mg twice daily, increase to maximum of 30 mg/day

Mechanism of Action Blocks both $beta_1$- and $beta_2$-adrenergic receptors, reduces intraocular pressure by reducing aqueous humor production or possibly outflow; reduces BP by blocking adrenergic receptors and decreasing sympathetic outflow, produces a negative chronotropic and inotropic activity through an unknown mechanism

Other Adverse Effects

Ophthalmic:

- >10%: Ocular: Conjunctival hyperemia
- 1% to 10%: Ocular: Anisocoria, corneal punctate keratitis, keratitis, corneal staining, decreased corneal sensitivity, eye pain, vision disturbances

Systemic:

>10%:

- Central nervous system: Drowsiness, insomnia
- Endocrine & metabolic: Decreased sexual ability

1% to 10%:

- Cardiovascular: Bradycardia, palpitations, edema, CHF, reduced peripheral circulation
- Central nervous system: Mental depression
- Gastrointestinal: Diarrhea or constipation, nausea, vomiting, stomach discomfort
- Respiratory: Bronchospasm
- Miscellaneous: Cold extremities

Drug Interactions CYP2D6 enzyme substrate

Increased Effect/Toxicity: The heart rate lowering effects of timolol are additive with other drugs which slow AV conduction (digoxin, verapamil, diltiazem). Reserpine increases the effects of timolol. Concurrent use of timolol may increase the effects of alpha-blockers (prazosin, terazosin), alpha-adrenergic stimulants (epinephrine, phenylephrine), and the vasoconstrictive effects of ergot alkaloids. Timolol may mask the tachycardia from hypoglycemia caused by insulin and oral hypoglycemics. In patients receiving concurrent therapy, the risk of hypertensive crisis is increased when either clonidine or the beta-blocker is withdrawn. Beta-blockers may increase the action or levels of disopyramide, nondepolarizing muscle relaxants, and theophylline although the effects are difficult to predict.

Decreased Effect: Decreased effect of timolol with aluminum salts, barbiturates, calcium salts, cholestyramine, colestipol, NSAIDs, penicillins (ampicillin), rifampin, salicylates, and sulfinpyrazone due to decreased bioavailability and plasma concentrations. Beta-blockers may decrease the effect of sulfonylureas. Beta-blockers may affect the action or levels of ethanol, disopyramide, nondepolarizing muscle relaxants, and theophylline, although the effects are difficult to predict.

Drug Uptake

Onset of action: Hypotensive: Oral: 15-45 minutes; Peak effect: 0.5-2.5 hours

Duration: ~4 hours; Ophthalmic: Intraocular: 24 hours

Half-life, elimination: 2-2.7 hours (increases with renal impairment)

Pregnancy Risk Factor C (manufacturer); D (2nd and 3rd trimesters - expert analysis)

Generic Available No

Selected Readings

Foster CA and Aston SJ, "Propranolol-Epinephrine Interaction: A Potential Disaster," *Plast Reconstr Surg*, 1983, 72(1):74-8.

Wong DG, Spence JD, Lamki L, et al, "Effect of Nonsteroidal Anti-inflammatory Drugs on Control of Hypertension of Beta-Blockers and Diuretics," *Lancet*, 1986, 1(8488):997-1001.

Wynn RL, "Dental Nonsteroidal Anti-inflammatory Drugs and Prostaglandin-Based Drug Interactions, Part Two," *Gen Dent*, 1992, 40(2):104, 106, 108.

Wynn RL, "Epinephrine Interactions With Beta-Blockers," *Gen Dent*, 1994, 42(1):16, 18.

Timoptic® *see* Timolol *on page 1170*

Timoptic® OcuDose® *see* Timolol *on page 1170*

Timoptic-XE® *see* Timolol *on page 1170*

Tinactin® [OTC] *see* Tolnaftate *on page 1181*

Tinactin® for Jock Itch [OTC] *see* Tolnaftate *on page 1181*

TinBen® [OTC] *see* Benzoin *on page 153*

Tine Test PPD *see* Tuberculin Purified Protein Derivative *on page 1218*

Ting® [OTC] *see* Tolnaftate *on page 1181*

Tinver® *see* Sodium Thiosulfate *on page 1100*

Tinzaparin (tin ZA pa rin)

U.S. Brand Names Innohep®

Canadian Brand Names Innohep®

Pharmacologic Category Low Molecular Weight Heparin

Synonyms Tinzaparin Sodium

Use Treatment of acute symptomatic deep vein thrombosis, with or without pulmonary embolism, in conjunction with warfarin sodium

Local Anesthetic/Vasoconstrictor Precautions No information available to require special precautions

Effects on Dental Treatment

No effects or complications reported

Patients undergoing treatment with low molecular weight heparins have an increased risk of hemorrhage during surgery.

Dosage S.C.:

Adults: 175 anti-Xa int. units/kg of body weight once daily. Warfarin sodium should be started when appropriate. Administer tinzaparin for at least 6 days and until patient is adequately anticoagulated with warfarin.

Note: To calculate the volume of solution to administer per dose: Volume to be administered (mL) = patient weight (kg) x 0.00875 mL/kg (may be rounded off to the nearest 0.05 mL)

Elderly: No significant differences in safety or response were seen when used in patients ≥65 years of age. However, increased sensitivity to tinzaparin in elderly patients may be possible due to a decline in renal function.

Mechanism of Action Standard heparin consists of components with molecular weights ranging from 4000-30,000 daltons with a mean of 16,000 daltons. Heparin acts as an anticoagulant by enhancing the inhibition rate of clotting proteases by antithrombin III, impairing normal hemostasis and inhibition of factor Xa. Low molecular weight heparins have a small effect on the activated partial thromboplastin time and strongly inhibit factor Xa. The primary inhibitory activity of tinzaparin is through antithrombin. Tinzaparin is derived from porcine heparin that undergoes controlled enzymatic depolymerization. The average molecular weight of tinzaparin ranges between 5500 and 7500 daltons which is distributed as (<10%) 2000 daltons (60% to 72%) 2000-8000 daltons, and (22% to 36%) >8000 daltons. The antifactor Xa activity is approximately 100 int. units/mg.

Other Adverse Effects As with all anticoagulants, bleeding is the major adverse effect of tinzaparin. Hemorrhage may occur at virtually any site. Risk is dependent on multiple variables.

>10%:

Hepatic: Increased ALT (13%)

Local: Injection site hematoma (16%)

1% to 10%:

Cardiovascular: Angina pectoris, chest pain (2%), hypertension, hypotension, tachycardia

Central nervous system: Confusion, dizziness, fever (2%), headache (2%), insomnia, pain (2%)

(Continued)

Tinzaparin *(Continued)*

Dermatologic: Bullous eruption, pruritus, rash (1%), skin disorder

Gastrointestinal: Constipation (1%), dyspepsia, flatulence, nausea (2%), nonspecified gastrointestinal disorder, vomiting (1%)

Genitourinary: Dysuria, urinary retention, urinary tract infection (4%)

Hematologic: Anemia, hematoma, hemorrhage (2%), thrombocytopenia (1%)

Hepatic: Increased AST (9%)

Local: Deep vein thrombosis, injection site hematoma

Neuromuscular & skeletal: Back pain (2%)

Renal: Hematuria (1%)

Respiratory: Dyspnea (1%), epistaxis (2%), pneumonia, pulmonary embolism (2%), respiratory disorder

Miscellaneous: Impaired healing, infection, unclassified reactions

Additional serious adverse reactions reported in clinical trials and postmarketing experience: Abscess, acute febrile reaction, agranulocytosis, allergic purpura, allergic reaction, angioedema, anorectal bleeding, cardiac arrhythmia, cellulitis, cerebral hemorrhage, cholestatic hepatitis, coronary thrombosis, dependent edema, epidermal necrolysis, erythematous gastrointestinal hemorrhage, granulocytopenia, hemarthrosis, hematemesis, hemoptysis, intracranial hemorrhage, ischemic necrosis, melena, myocardial infarction, necrosis, neoplasm, ocular hemorrhage, pancytopenia, peripheral ischemia, priapism, purpura, retroperitoneal/intra-abdominal bleeding, severe thrombocytopenia, skin necrosis, spinal epidural hematoma, Stevens-Johnson syndrome, thromboembolism, urticaria, vaginal hemorrhage, wound hematoma

Drug Interactions Increased Effect/Toxicity: Drugs which affect platelet function (eg, aspirin, NSAIDs, dipyridamole, ticlopidine, clopidogrel, sulfinpyrazone, dextran) may potentiate the risk of hemorrhage. Thrombolytic agents increase the risk of hemorrhage. Risk of bleeding may be increased during concurrent warfarin therapy. Tinzaparin is commonly continued during the initiation of warfarin therapy to assure anticoagulation and to protect against possible transient hypercoagulability

Drug Uptake

Onset of action: 2-3 hours

Half-life, elimination: 3-4 hours

Time to peak: 4-5 hours

Pregnancy Risk Factor B

Generic Available No

Tioconazole (tye oh KONE a zole)

U.S. Brand Names 1-Day™ [OTC]; Vagistat®-1 [OTC]

Canadian Brand Names GyneCure™; Trosyd™ AF; Trosyd™ J

Pharmacologic Category Antifungal Agent, Vaginal

Use Local treatment of vulvovaginal candidiasis

Local Anesthetic/Vasoconstrictor Precautions No information available to require special precautions

Effects on Dental Treatment No effects or complications reported

Dosage Adults: Vaginal: Insert 1 applicatorful in vagina, just prior to bedtime, as a single dose

Mechanism of Action A 1-substituted imidazole derivative with a broad antifungal spectrum against a wide variety of dermatophytes and yeasts, usually at a concentration of ≤6.25 mg/L; has been demonstrated to be at least as active *in vitro* as other imidazole antifungals. *In vitro*, tioconazole has been demonstrated 2-8 times as potent as miconazole against common dermal pathogens including *Trichophyton mentagrophytes*, *T. rubrum*, *T. erinacei*, *T. tonsurans*, *Microsporum canis*, *Microsporum gypseum*, and *Candida albicans.* Both agents appear to be similarly effective against *Epidermophyton floccosum.*

Other Adverse Effects Frequency not defined:

Central nervous system: Headache

Dermatologic: Burning, desquamation

Gastrointestinal: Abdominal pain

Genitourinary: Vulvar/vaginal burning sensation, vaginal discharge, vulvar/vaginal irritation/itching, vaginal pain, vaginitis, vulvar swelling dyspareunia, dysuria nocturia

Contraindications Hypersensitivity to tioconazole or any component of the formulation

Warnings/Precautions For vaginal use only; petrolatum-based vaginal products may damage rubber or latex condoms or diaphragms; separate use by 3 days

Drug Uptake Absorption: Intravaginal: Systemic (small amounts)

Pregnancy Risk Factor C

Generic Available No

Tiopronin (tye oh PROE nin)

U.S. Brand Names Thiola™

Canadian Brand Names Thiola™

Pharmacologic Category Urinary Tract Product

Use Prevention of kidney stone (cystine) formation in patients with severe homozygous cystinuric who have urinary cystine >500 mg/day who are resistant to treatment with high fluid intake, alkali, and diet modification, or who have had adverse reactions to penicillamine

Local Anesthetic/Vasoconstrictor Precautions No information available to require special precautions

Effects on Dental Treatment No effects or complications reported

Dosage Adults: Initial dose is 800 mg/day, average dose is 1000 mg/day

Pregnancy Risk Factor C

Generic Available No

Tirofiban (tye roe FYE ban)

Related Information

Cardiovascular Diseases *on page 1308*

U.S. Brand Names Aggrastat®

Canadian Brand Names Aggrastat®

Mexican Brand Names Agrastat®

Pharmacologic Category Antiplatelet Agent, Glycoprotein IIb/IIIa Inhibitor

Synonyms MK383; Tirofiban Hydrochloride

Use In combination with heparin, indicated for the treatment of acute coronary syndrome, including patients who are to be managed medically and those undergoing PTCA or atherectomy. In this setting, it has been shown to decrease the rate of a combined endpoint of death, new myocardial infarction or refractory ischemia/ repeat cardiac procedure.

Local Anesthetic/Vasoconstrictor Precautions No information available to require special precautions

Effects on Dental Treatment No effects or complications reported

Dosage Adults: I.V.: Initial rate of 0.4 mcg/kg/minute for 30 minutes and then continued at 0.1 mcg/kg/minute; dosing should be continued through angiography and for 12-24 hours after angioplasty or atherectomy. See table.

Tirofiban Dosing
(Using 50 mcg/mL Concentration)

Patient Weight (kg)	Patients With Normal Renal Function		Patients With Renal Dysfunction	
	30-Minute Loading Infusion Rate (mL/h)	Maintenance Infusion Rate (mL/h)	30-Minute Loading Infusion Rate (mL/h)	Maintenance Infusion Rate (mL/h)
30-37	16	4	8	2
38-45	20	5	10	3
46-54	24	6	12	3
55-62	28	7	14	4
63-70	32	8	16	4
71-79	36	9	18	5
80-87	40	10	20	5
88-95	44	11	22	6
96-104	48	12	24	6
105-112	52	13	26	7
113-120	56	14	28	7
121-128	60	15	30	8
128-137	64	16	32	8
138-145	68	17	34	9
146-153	72	18	36	9

Dosing adjustment in severe renal impairment: Cl_{cr} <30 mL/minute: Reduce dose to 50% of normal rate.

Mechanism of Action A reversible antagonist of fibrinogen binding to the GP IIb/IIIa receptor, the major platelet surface receptor involved in platelet aggregation. When administered I.V., it inhibits *ex vivo* platelet aggregation in a dose- and concentration-dependent manner. When given according to the recommended regimen, >90% inhibition is attained by the end of the 30-minute infusion. Platelet aggregation inhibition is reversible following cessation of the infusion.

Other Adverse Effects Bleeding is the major drug-related adverse effect. Patients received background treatment with aspirin and heparin. Major bleeding was

(Continued)

Tirofiban *(Continued)*

reported in 1.4% to 2.2%; minor bleeding in 10.5% to 12%; transfusion was required in 4.0% to 4.3%.

>1% (nonbleeding adverse events):

Cardiovascular: Bradycardia (4%), coronary artery dissection (5%), edema (2%)
Central nervous system: Dizziness (3%), fever (>1%), headache (>1%), vasovagal reaction (2%)
Gastrointestinal: Nausea (>1%)
Genitourinary: Pelvic pain (6%)
Hematologic: Thrombocytopenia: <90,000/mm^3 (1.5%), <50,000/mm^3 (0.3%)
Neuromuscular & skeletal: Leg pain (3%)
Miscellaneous: Diaphoresis (2%)

Drug Interactions

Increased Effect/Toxicity: Use of tirofiban with aspirin and heparin is associated with an increase in bleeding over aspirin and heparin alone; however, efficacy of tirofiban is improved. Risk of bleeding is increased when used with thrombolytics, oral anticoagulants, nonsteroidal anti-inflammatory drugs, dipyridamole, ticlopidine, and clopidogrel. Avoid concomitant use of other IIb/IIIa antagonists. Cephalosporins which contain the MTT side chain may theoretically increase the risk of hemorrhage.

Decreased Effect: Levothyroxine and omeprazole decrease tirofiban levels; however, the clinical significance of this interaction remains to be demonstrated.

Drug Uptake Half-life, elimination: 2 hours

Pregnancy Risk Factor B

Generic Available No

Tisit® [OTC] *see* Pyrethrins *on page 1026*

Tisit® Blue Gel [OTC] *see* Pyrethrins *on page 1026*

Tisseel® VH Fibrin Sealant Kit *see* Fibrin Sealant Kit *on page 502*

Titralac® Plus Liquid [OTC] *see* Calcium Carbonate and Simethicone *on page 202*

Tizanidine (tye ZAN i deen)

U.S. Brand Names Zanaflex®

Canadian Brand Names Zanaflex®

Mexican Brand Names Sirdalud®

Pharmacologic Category Alpha$_2$-Adrenergic Agonist

Synonyms Sirdalud®

Use Intermittent management of increased muscle tone associated with spasticity (eg, multiple sclerosis, spinal cord injury)

Unlabeled/Investigational: Tension headaches, low back pain, and trigeminal neuralgia

Local Anesthetic/Vasoconstrictor Precautions No information available to require special precautions

Effects on Dental Treatment >10%: Significant xerostomia; disappears with discontinuation

Dosage Adults: 2-4 mg 3 times/day

Usual initial dose: 4 mg, may increase by 2-4 mg as needed for satisfactory reduction of muscle tone every 6-8 hours to a maximum of three doses in any 24-hour period

Maximum dose: 36 mg/day

Mechanism of Action An alpha$_2$-adrenergic agonist agent which decreases excitatory input to alpha motor neurons; an imidazole derivative chemically-related to clonidine, which acts as a centrally-acting muscle relaxant with alpha$_2$-adrenergic agonist properties; acts on the level of the spinal cord

Other Adverse Effects

>10%:

Cardiovascular: Hypotension
Central nervous system: Sedation, daytime drowsiness, somnolence
Gastrointestinal: Xerostomia

1% to 10%:

Cardiovascular: Bradycardia, syncope
Central nervous system: Fatigue, dizziness, anxiety, nervousness, insomnia
Dermatologic: Pruritus, skin rash
Gastrointestinal: Nausea, vomiting, dyspepsia, constipation, diarrhea
Hepatic: Elevation of liver enzymes
Neuromuscular & skeletal: Muscle weakness, tremor

Warnings/Precautions Reduce dose in patients with liver or renal disease; use with caution in patients with hypotension or cardiac disease

Drug Interactions

Increased effect: Oral contraceptives

Increased toxicity: Additive hypotensive effects may be seen with diuretics, other alpha adrenergic agonists, or antihypertensives; CNS depression with alcohol, baclofen or other CNS depressants

Drug Uptake
Duration: 3-6 hours
Half-life, elimination: 4-8 hours
Time to peak: 1-5 hours
Pregnancy Risk Factor C
Generic Available No

TNKase™ *see* Tenecteplase *on page 1138*
TOBI™ *see* Tobramycin *on page 1175*
TobraDex® *see* Tobramycin and Dexamethasone *on page 1176*

Tobramycin (toe bra MYE sin)

U.S. Brand Names AKTob®; Nebcin®; TOBI™; Tobrex®
Canadian Brand Names Nebcin®; PMS-Tobramycin; TOBI®; Tobrex®; Tomycine™
Mexican Brand Names Tobra; Tobrex®; Trazil®
Pharmacologic Category Antibiotic, Aminoglycoside; Antibiotic, Ophthalmic
Synonyms Tobramycin Sulfate
Use Treatment of documented or suspected *Pseudomonas aeruginosa* infection; infection with a nonpseudomonal enteric bacillus which is more sensitive to tobramycin than gentamicin based on susceptibility tests; empiric therapy in cystic fibrosis and immunocompromised patients; topically used in treatment of superficial ophthalmic infections caused by susceptible bacteria; inhaled version used for improving lung function and controlling *Pseudomonas aeruginosa* infections in people with cystic fibrosis (CF)
Local Anesthetic/Vasoconstrictor Precautions No information available to require special precautions
Effects on Dental Treatment No effects or complications reported
Dosage Individualization is critical because of the low therapeutic index

Use of ideal body weight (IBW) for determining the mg/kg/dose appears to be more accurate than dosing on the basis of total body weight (TBW)

In morbid obesity, dosage requirement may best be estimated using a dosing weight of IBW + 0.4 (TBW - IBW)

Initial and periodic peak and trough plasma drug levels should be determined, particularly in critically ill patients with serious infections or in disease states known to significantly alter aminoglycoside pharmacokinetics (eg, cystic fibrosis, burns, or major surgery); 2-3 serum concentration measurements should be obtained after the initial dose to measure the half-life in order to determine the frequency of subsequent doses

Once daily dosing: Higher peak serum drug concentration to MIC ratios, demonstrated aminoglycoside postantibiotic effect, decreased renal cortex drug uptake, and improved cost-time efficiency are supportive reasons for the use of once daily dosing regimens for aminoglycosides. Current research indicates these regimens to be as effective for nonlife-threatening infections, with no higher incidence of nephrotoxicity, than those requiring multiple daily doses. Doses are determined by calculating the entire day's dose via usual multiple dose calculation techniques and administering this quantity as a single dose. Doses are then adjusted to maintain mean serum concentration above the MIC(s) of the causative organism(s). (Example: 2.5-5 mg/kg as a single dose; expected Cp_{max}: 10-20 mcg/mL and Cp_{min}: <1 mcg/mL). Further research is needed for universal recommendation in all patient populations and gram-negative disease; exceptions may include those with known high clearance (eg, children, patients with cystic fibrosis, or burns who may require shorter dosage intervals) and patients with renal function impairment for whom longer than conventional dosage intervals are usually required.

Children <5 years: I.M., I.V.: 2.5 mg/kg/dose every 8 hours
Children >5 years: 1.5-2.5 mg/kg/dose every 8 hours

Note: Some patients may require larger or more frequent doses if serum concentration document the need (ie, cystic fibrosis or febrile granulocytopenic patients).

Adults: I.M., I.V.:
Severe life-threatening infections: 2-2.5 mg/kg/dose
Urinary tract infection: 1.5 mg/kg/dose
Synergy (for gram-positive infections): 1 mg/kg/dose

Children and Adults: Ophthalmic: Instill 1-2 drops of solution every 4 hours; apply ointment 2-3 times/day; for severe infections apply ointment every 3-4 hours, or solution 2 drops every 30-60 minutes initially, then reduce to less frequent intervals

Children and Adults: Inhalation: Inhaled twice daily and requires about 10-15 minutes per treatment. The TOBI™ treatment regimen consists of repeated cycles of 28-days on drug, followed by 28-days off drug.

Mechanism of Action Interferes with bacterial protein synthesis by binding to 30S and 50S ribosomal subunits resulting in a defective bacterial cell membrane
Other Adverse Effects 1% to 10%:
Neuromuscular & skeletal: Neurotoxicity (neuromuscular blockade)
Otic: Ototoxicity (auditory), ototoxicity (vestibular)
(Continued)

Tobramycin *(Continued)*

Renal: Nephrotoxicity

Drug Interactions Increased Effect/Toxicity: Increased antimicrobial effect of tobramycin with extended spectrum penicillins (synergistic). Neuromuscular blockers may have an increased duration of action (neuromuscular blockade). Amphotericin B, cephalosporins, and loop diuretics may increase the risk of nephrotoxicity.

Drug Uptake

Absorption: I.M.: Rapid and complete

Half-life, elimination:

Neonates: ≤1200 g: 11 hours; >1200 g: 2-9 hours

Adults: 2-3 hours; directly dependent upon glomerular filtration rate

Adults with impaired renal function: 5-70 hours

Time to peak: I.M.: 30-60 minutes; I.V.: ~30 minutes

Pregnancy Risk Factor C

Generic Available Yes

Tobramycin and Dexamethasone

(toe bra MYE sin & deks a METH a sone)

U.S. Brand Names TobraDex®

Canadian Brand Names Tobradex®

Pharmacologic Category Antibiotic/Corticosteroid, Ophthalmic

Synonyms Dexamethasone and Tobramycin

Use Treatment of external ocular infection caused by susceptible gram-negative bacteria and steroid responsive inflammatory conditions of the palpebral and bulbar conjunctiva, lid, cornea, and anterior segment of the globe

Local Anesthetic/Vasoconstrictor Precautions No information available to require special precautions

Effects on Dental Treatment No effects or complications reported

Dosage Children and Adults: Ophthalmic: Instill 1-2 drops of solution every 4 hours; apply ointment 2-3 times/day; for severe infections apply ointment every 3-4 hours, or solution 2 drops every 30-60 minutes initially, then reduce to less frequent intervals

Mechanism of Action See Tobramycin *on page 1175* and Dexamethasone *on page 363*

Other Adverse Effects Frequency not defined:

Dermatologic: Allergic contact dermatitis, delayed wound healing

Ocular: Lacrimation, itching, edema of eyelid, keratitis, increased intraocular pressure, glaucoma, cataract formation

Drug Interactions See Tobramycin *on page 1175* and Dexamethasone *on page 363*

Drug Uptake

Absorption: Into the aqueous humor

Time to peak: 1-2 hours in the cornea and aqueous humor

Pregnancy Risk Factor B

Generic Available No

Tobrex® *see* Tobramycin *on page 1175*

Tocainide (toe KAY nide)

Related Information

Cardiovascular Diseases *on page 1308*

U.S. Brand Names Tonocard®

Canadian Brand Names Tonocard®

Pharmacologic Category Antiarrhythmic Agent, Class Ib

Synonyms Tocainide Hydrochloride

Use Suppression and prevention of symptomatic life-threatening ventricular arrhythmias

Unlabeled/Investigational: Trigeminal neuralgia

Local Anesthetic/Vasoconstrictor Precautions No information available to require special precautions

Effects on Dental Treatment No effects or complications reported

Dosage Adults: Oral: 1200-1800 mg/day in 3 divided doses, up to 2400 mg/day

Mechanism of Action Class 1B antiarrhythmic agent; suppresses automaticity of conduction tissue, by increasing electrical stimulation threshold of ventricle, His-Purkinje system, and spontaneous depolarization of the ventricles during diastole by a direct action on the tissues; blocks both the initiation and conduction of nerve impulses by decreasing the neuronal membrane's permeability to sodium ions, which results in inhibition of depolarization with resultant blockade of conduction

Other Adverse Effects

>10%:

Central nervous system: Dizziness (8% to 15%)

Gastrointestinal: Nausea (14% to 15%)

1% to 10%:

Cardiovascular: Tachycardia (3%), bradycardia/angina/palpitations (0.5% to 1.8%), hypotension (3%)

Central nervous system: Nervousness (0.5% to 1.5%), confusion (2% to 3%), headache (4.6%), anxiety, incoordination, giddiness, vertigo

Dermatologic: Rash (0.5% to 8.4%)

Gastrointestinal: Vomiting (4.5%), diarrhea (4% to 5%), anorexia (1% to 2%), loss of taste

Neuromuscular & skeletal: Paresthesia (3.5% to 9%), tremor (dose-related: 2.9% to 8.4%), ataxia (dose-related: 2.9% to 8.4%), hot and cold sensations

Ocular: Blurred vision (~1.5%), nystagmus (1%)

Note: Rare, potentially severe hematologic reactions, have occurred (generally within the first 12 weeks of therapy). These may include agranulocytosis, bone marrow depression, aplastic anemia, hypoplastic anemia, hemolytic anemia, anemia, leukopenia, neutropenia, thrombocytopenia, and eosinophilia.

Drug Interactions

Increased Effect/Toxicity: Tocainide may increase serum concentration of caffeine and theophylline.

Decreased Effect: Decreased tocainide plasma concentrations with cimetidine, phenobarbital, phenytoin, rifampin, and other hepatic enzyme inducers.

Drug Uptake

Absorption: Oral: Extensive, 99% to 100%

Half-life, elimination: 11-14 hours; Renal/hepatic impairment: 23-27 hours

Time to peak: 30-160 minutes

Pregnancy Risk Factor C

Generic Available No

Tocophersolan (toe kof er SOE lan)

U.S. Brand Names Liqui-E®

Pharmacologic Category Vitamin, Fat Soluble

Synonyms TPGS

Use Treatment of vitamin E deficiency resulting from malabsorption due to prolonged cholestatic hepatobiliary disease

Local Anesthetic/Vasoconstrictor Precautions No information available to require special precautions

Effects on Dental Treatment No effects or complications reported

Dosage Dietary supplement: Oral: 15 mg (400 units) every day

Pregnancy Risk Factor A/C

Generic Available No

Comments Studies indicate that TPGS is absorbed better than fat soluble forms of vitamin E in patients with impaired digestion and absorption and when coadministered with cyclosporine to transplant recipients it improves cyclosporine absorption. Due to these findings, this product has a valuable role in the liver transplant patient population.

Tofranil® *see* Imipramine *on page 627*

Tofranil-PM® *see* Imipramine *on page 627*

TOLAZamide (tole AZ a mide)

Related Information

Endocrine Disorders and Pregnancy *on page 1331*

U.S. Brand Names Tolinase®

Canadian Brand Names Tolinase®

Pharmacologic Category Antidiabetic Agent, Sulfonylurea

Use Adjunct to diet for the management of mild to moderately severe, stable, noninsulin-dependent (type II) diabetes mellitus

Local Anesthetic/Vasoconstrictor Precautions No information available to require special precautions

Effects on Dental Treatment Use salicylates with caution in patients taking tolazamide due to potential increased hypoglycemia; NSAIDs such as ibuprofen and naproxen may be safely used. Tolazamide-dependent diabetics (noninsulin dependent, type 2) should be appointed for dental treatment in morning in order to minimize chance of stress-induced hypoglycemia.

Dosage Oral (doses >1000 mg/day normally do not improve diabetic control):

Adults: Initial: 100 mg/day, increase at 2- to 4-week intervals; maximum dose: 1000 mg; give as a single or twice daily dose

Conversion from insulin → tolazamide

10 units day = 100 mg/day

20-40 units/day = 250 mg/day

>40 units/day = 250 mg/day and 50% of insulin dose

Doses >500 mg/day should be given in 2 divided doses

Mechanism of Action Stimulates insulin release from the pancreatic beta cells; reduces glucose output from the liver; insulin sensitivity is increased at peripheral target sites

(Continued)

TOLAZamide *(Continued)*

Other Adverse Effects Frequency not defined:

Central nervous system: Headache, dizziness

Dermatologic: Rash, urticaria, photosensitivity

Endocrine & metabolic: Hypoglycemia, SIADH

Gastrointestinal: Anorexia, nausea, vomiting, diarrhea, constipation, heartburn, epigastric fullness

Hematologic: Aplastic anemia, hemolytic anemia, bone marrow suppression, thrombocytopenia, agranulocytosis

Hepatic: Cholestatic jaundice

Renal: Diuretic effect

Warnings/Precautions False-positive response has been reported in patients with liver disease, idiopathic hypoglycemia of infancy, severe malnutrition, acute pancreatitis, renal dysfunction. Transferring a patient from one sulfonylurea to another does not require a priming dose; doses >1000 mg/day normally do not improve diabetic control. Has not been studied in older patients; however, except for drug interactions, it appears to have a safe profile and decline in renal function does not affect its pharmacokinetics. How "tightly" an elderly patient's blood glucose should be controlled is controversial; however, a fasting blood sugar <150 mg/dL is now an acceptable end point. Such a decision should be based on the patient's functional and cognitive status, how well they recognize hypoglycemic or hyperglycemic symptoms, and how to respond to them and their other disease states.

Chemical similarities are present among sulfonamides, sulfonylureas, carbonic anhydrase inhibitors, thiazides, and loop diuretics (except ethacrynic acid). Use in patients with sulfonylurea allergy is specifically contraindicated in product labeling, however a risk of cross-reaction exists in patients with allergy to any of these compounds; avoid use when previous reaction has been severe.

Product labeling states oral hypoglycemic drugs may be associated with an increased cardiovascular mortality as compared to treatment with diet alone or diet plus insulin. Data to support this association are limited, and several studies, including a large prospective trial (UKPDS) have not supported an association.

Drug Interactions

Increased Effect/Toxicity: Salicylates, anticoagulants, H_2 antagonists, TCAs, MAO inhibitors, beta-blockers, and thiazides may increase effect of sulfonylureas.

Decreased Effect: Many drugs, including corticosteroids, beta-blockers, and thiazides may alter response to oral hypoglycemics.

Drug Uptake

Onset of action: Oral: 4-6 hours

Duration: 10-24 hours

Half-life, elimination: 7 hours

Pregnancy Risk Factor D

Generic Available Yes

TOLBUTamide (tole BYOO ta mide)

Related Information

Endocrine Disorders and Pregnancy *on page 1331*

U.S. Brand Names Orinase Diagnostic®; Tol-Tab®

Canadian Brand Names Apo®-Tolbutamide

Mexican Brand Names Artosin; Diaval; Rastinon

Pharmacologic Category Antidiabetic Agent, Sulfonylurea

Synonyms Tolbutamide Sodium

Use Adjunct to diet for the management of mild to moderately severe, stable, noninsulin-dependent (type II) diabetes mellitus

Local Anesthetic/Vasoconstrictor Precautions No information available to require special precautions

Effects on Dental Treatment Use salicylates with caution in patients taking tolazamide due to potential increased hypoglycemia; NSAIDs such as ibuprofen and naproxen may be safely used. Tolbutamide-dependent diabetics (noninsulin dependent, type 2) should be appointed for dental treatment in morning in order to minimize chance of stress-induced hypoglycemia.

Dosage Divided doses may increase GI side effects

Adults:

Oral: Initial: 500-1000 mg 1-3 times/day; usual dose should not be >2 g/day

I.V. bolus: 1 g over 2-3 minutes

Elderly: Oral: Initial: 250 mg 1-3 times/day; usual: 500-2000 mg; maximum: 3 g/day

Mechanism of Action Ability to lower elevated blood glucose levels in patients with functional pancreatic beta cells is similar to the other sulfonylurea agents; stimulates synthesis and release of endogenous insulin from pancreatic islet tissue; hypoglycemic effect is attributed to an increased sensitivity of insulin receptors and improved peripheral utilization of insulin. Suppression of glucagon secretion may also contribute to the hypoglycemic effects of tolbutamide.

Other Adverse Effects Frequency not defined:

Cardiovascular: Venospasm

Central nervous system: Headache, dizziness
Dermatologic: Skin rash, urticaria, photosensitivity
Endocrine & metabolic: Hypoglycemia, SIADH
Gastrointestinal: Constipation, diarrhea, heartburn, anorexia, epigastric fullness, taste alteration
Hematologic: Aplastic anemia, hemolytic anemia, bone marrow suppression, thrombocytopenia, leukopenia, agranulocytosis
Hepatic: Cholestatic jaundice
Local: Thrombophlebitis
Otic: Tinnitus
Miscellaneous: Hypersensitivity reaction, disulfiram-like reactions

Warnings/Precautions False-positive response has been reported in patients with liver disease, idiopathic hypoglycemia of infancy, severe malnutrition, acute pancreatitis. Because of its low potency and short duration, it is a useful agent in the elderly if drug interactions can be avoided. How "tightly" an elderly patient's blood glucose should be controlled is controversial; however, a fasting blood sugar <150 mg/dL is now an acceptable end point. Such a decision should be based on the patient's functional and cognitive status, how well they recognize hypoglycemic or hyperglycemic symptoms, and how to respond to them and their other disease states.

Chemical similarities are present among sulfonamides, sulfonylureas, carbonic anhydrase inhibitors, thiazides, and loop diuretics (except ethacrynic acid). Use in patients with sulfonylurea allergy is specifically contraindicated in product labeling, however a risk of cross-reaction exists in patients with allergy to any of these compounds; avoid use when previous reaction has been severe.

Product labeling states oral hypoglycemic drugs may be associated with an increased cardiovascular mortality as compared to treatment with diet alone or diet plus insulin. Data to support this association are limited, and several studies, including a large prospective trial (UKPDS) have not supported an association.

Drug Interactions CYP2C8, 2C9, 2C18, and 2C19 enzyme substrate; CYP2C19 enzyme inhibitor

Increased Effect/Toxicity: A number of drugs increase the effect of first-generation sulfonylureas (tolbutamide) including salicylates, chloramphenicol, anticoagulants, H_2 antagonists, tricyclic antidepressants, MAO inhibitors, beta-blockers, and thiazide diuretics.

Decreased Effect: Drugs with increase glucose (corticosteroids, thiazides) may decrease the effect of tolbutamide.

Drug Uptake

Onset of action: Peak effect: Hypoglycemic action: Oral: 1-3 hours; I.V.: 30 minutes
Absorption: Oral: Rapid
Duration: Oral: 6-24 hours; I.V.: 3 hours
Half-life, plasma: 4-25 hours; Elimination: 4-9 hours
Time to peak: 3-5 hours

Pregnancy Risk Factor D

Generic Available Yes

Tolcapone (TOLE ka pone)

U.S. Brand Names Tasmar®

Mexican Brand Names Tasmar®

Pharmacologic Category Anti-Parkinson's Agent, COMT Inhibitor

Use Adjunct to levodopa and carbidopa for the treatment of signs and symptoms of idiopathic Parkinson's disease

Local Anesthetic/Vasoconstrictor Precautions No information available to require special precautions

Effects on Dental Treatment Dopaminergic therapy in Parkinson's disease (ie, treatment with levodopa) is associated with orthostatic hypotension. Tolcapone enhances levodopa bioavailability and may increase the occurrence of hypotension/syncope in the dental patient. The patient should be carefully assisted from the chair and observed for signs of orthostatic hypotension.

Dosage Adults: Oral: Initial 100 mg 3 times/day, may increase to 200 mg 3 times/day

Mechanism of Action A selective and reversible inhibitor of catechol-o-methyltransferase (COMT)

Other Adverse Effects

>10%:
Cardiovascular: Orthostatic hypotension
Central nervous system: Sleep disorder, excessive dreaming, somnolence, headache
Gastrointestinal: Nausea, diarrhea, anorexia
Neuromuscular & skeletal: Dyskinesia, dystonia, muscle cramps

1% to 10%:
Central nervous system: Hallucinations, fatigue, loss of balance, hyperkinesia
Gastrointestinal: Vomiting, constipation, xerostomia, abdominal pain, flatulence, dyspepsia
Genitourinary: Urine discoloration

(Continued)

Tolcapone *(Continued)*

Neuromuscular & skeletal: Paresthesia, stiffness
Miscellaneous: Diaphoresis (increased)

Warnings/Precautions Due to reports of fatal liver injury associated with use of this drug, the manufacturer is advising that tolcapone be reserved for use only in patients who do not have severe movement abnormalities and who do not respond to or who are not appropriate candidates for other available treatments. It is not recommended that patients receive tolcapone concomitantly with nonselective MAO inhibitors. Selegiline is a selective MAO-B inhibitor and can be taken with tolcapone.

Drug Interactions CYP2A6 and 3A3/4 enzyme substrate

May increase the effect/levels of methyldopa, dobutamine, apomorphine, and isoproterenol due to inhibition of catechol-O-methyl transferase enzymes (COMT)

Drug Uptake

Absorption: Rapid
Half-life, elimination: 2-3 hours
Time to peak: ~2 hours

Pregnancy Risk Factor C

Generic Available No

Tolectin® *see* Tolmetin *on page 1180*
Tolectin® DS *see* Tolmetin *on page 1180*
Tolinase® *see* TOLAZamide *on page 1177*

Tolmetin (TOLE met in)

Related Information

Rheumatoid Arthritis and Osteoarthritis *on page 1340*
Temporomandibular Dysfunction (TMD) *on page 1397*

U.S. Brand Names Tolectin®; Tolectin® DS

Canadian Brand Names Novo-Tolmetin; Tolectin®

Mexican Brand Names Tolectin®

Pharmacologic Category Nonsteroidal Anti-inflammatory Drug (NSAID)

Synonyms Tolmetin Sodium

Use Treatment of rheumatoid arthritis and osteoarthritis, juvenile rheumatoid arthritis

Local Anesthetic/Vasoconstrictor Precautions No information available to require special precautions

Effects on Dental Treatment NSAID formulations are known to reversibly decrease platelet aggregation via mechanisms different than observed with aspirin. The dentist should be aware of the potential of abnormal coagulation. Caution should also be exercised in the use of NSAIDs in patients already on anticoagulant therapy with drugs such as warfarin (Coumadin®).

Dosage Oral:

Children ≥2 years:
Anti-inflammatory: Initial: 20 mg/kg/day in 3 divided doses, then 15-30 mg/kg/day in 3 divided doses
Analgesic: 5-7 mg/kg/dose every 6-8 hours
Adults: 400 mg 3 times/day; usual dose: 600 mg to 1.8 g/day; maximum: 2 g/day

Mechanism of Action Inhibits prostaglandin synthesis by decreasing the activity of the enzyme, cyclo-oxygenase, which results in decreased formation of prostaglandin precursors

Other Adverse Effects 1% to 10%:

Cardiovascular: Chest pain, hypertension, edema
Central nervous system: Headache, dizziness, drowsiness, depression
Dermatologic: Skin irritation
Endocrine & metabolic: Weight gain/loss
Gastrointestinal: Heartburn, abdominal pain, diarrhea, flatulence, vomiting, constipation, gastritis, peptic ulcer, nausea
Genitourinary: Urinary Tract Infection
Hematologic: Elevated BUN, transient decreases in hemoglobin/hematocrit
Ocular: Visual disturbances
Otic: Tinnitus

Warnings/Precautions Use with caution in patients with upper GI disease, impaired renal function, CHF, dehydration, hypertension, and patients receiving anticoagulants; if GI upset occurs with tolmetin, take with antacids other than sodium bicarbonate. Withhold for at least 4-6 half-lives prior to surgical or dental procedures.

Drug Interactions CYP2C9 enzyme inhibitor

ACE-inhibitors: Antihypertensive effects may be decreased by concurrent therapy with NSAIDs; monitor BP.
Angiotensin II antagonists: Antihypertensive effects may be decreased by concurrent therapy with NSAIDs; monitor BP.
Anticoagulants (warfarin, heparin, LMWHs) in combination with NSAIDs can cause increased risk of bleeding.

Other antiplatelet drugs (ticlopidine, clopidogrel, aspirin, abciximab, dipyridamole, eptifibatide, tirofiban) can cause an increased risk of bleeding.

Corticosteroids may increase the risk of GI ulceration; avoid concurrent use.

Cyclosporine: NSAIDs may increase serum creatinine, potassium, BP, and cyclosporine levels; monitor cyclosporine levels and renal function carefully.

Hydralazine's antihypertensive effect is decreased; avoid concurrent use.

Lithium levels can be increased; avoid concurrent use if possible or monitor lithium levels and adjust dose. Sulindac may have the least effect. When NSAID is stopped, lithium will need adjustment again.

Loop diuretics efficacy (diuretic and antihypertensive effect) may be reduced.

Methotrexate: Severe bone marrow suppression, aplastic anemia, and GI toxicity have been reported with concomitant NSAID therapy. Avoid use during moderate or high-dose methotrexate (increased and prolonged methotrexate levels). NSAID use during low-dose treatment of rheumatoid arthritis has not been fully evaluated; extreme caution is warranted.

Thiazides antihypertensive effects are decreased; avoid concurrent use.

Warfarin's INRs may be increased by piroxicam. Other NSAIDs may have the same effect depending on dose and duration. Monitor INR closely. Use the lowest dose of NSAIDs possible and for the briefest duration.

Drug Uptake

Onset of action: Analgesic: 1-2 hours; Anti-inflammatory: Days to weeks

Absorption: Oral: Well absorbed

Time to peak: 30-60 minutes

Pregnancy Risk Factor C/D (3rd trimester or at term)

Generic Available No

Tolnaftate (tole NAF tate)

U.S. Brand Names Absorbine® Antifungal [OTC]; Absorbine® Jock Itch [OTC]; Absorbine Jr.® Antifungal [OTC]; Aftate® for Athlete's Foot [OTC]; Aftate® for Jock Itch [OTC]; Blis-To-Sol® [OTC]; Dr Scholl's Athlete's Foot [OTC]; Dr Scholl's Maximum Strength Tritin [OTC]; Genaspor® [OTC]; NP-27® [OTC]; Quinsana Plus® [OTC]; Tinactin® [OTC]; Tinactin® for Jock Itch [OTC]; Ting® [OTC]

Canadian Brand Names Pitrex

Mexican Brand Names Tinaderm®

Pharmacologic Category Antifungal Agent, Topical

Use Treatment of tinea pedis, tinea cruris, tinea corporis, tinea manuum, tinea versicolor infections

Local Anesthetic/Vasoconstrictor Precautions No information available to require special precautions

Effects on Dental Treatment No effects or complications reported

Dosage Children and Adults: Topical: Wash and dry affected area; apply 1-3 drops of solution or a small amount of cream or powder and rub into the affected areas 2-3 times/day for 2-4 weeks

Mechanism of Action Distorts the hyphae and stunts mycelial growth in susceptible fungi

Other Adverse Effects 1% to 10%:

Dermatologic: Pruritus, contact dermatitis

Local: Irritation, stinging

Drug Uptake Onset of action: 24-72 hours

Pregnancy Risk Factor C

Generic Available Yes

Tol-Tab® *see* TOLBUTamide *on page 1178*

Tolterodine (tole TER oh dine)

U.S. Brand Names Detrol™; Detrol® LA

Canadian Brand Names Detrol™

Mexican Brand Names Detrusitol®

Pharmacologic Category Anticholinergic Agent

Synonyms Tolterodine Tartrate

Use Treatment of patients with an overactive bladder with symptoms of urinary frequency, urgency, or urge incontinence

Local Anesthetic/Vasoconstrictor Precautions No information available to require special precautions

Effects on Dental Treatment The anticholinergic effects of tolterodine are selective for the urinary bladder rather than salivary glands; xerostomia should not be significant.

Dosage Adults: Oral:

Initial: 2 mg twice daily. The dose may be lowered to 1 mg twice daily based on individual response and tolerability.

Dosing adjustment in patients concurrently taking cytochrome P450 3A4 inhibitors: 1 mg twice daily

(Continued)

Tolterodine *(Continued)*

Mechanism of Action A competitive antagonist of muscarinic receptors; in animal models, demonstrates selectivity for urinary bladder receptors over salivary receptors; urinary bladder contraction is mediated by muscarinic receptors. Tolterodine increases residual urine volume and decreases detrusor muscle pressure.

Other Adverse Effects As reported with immediate release tablet, unless otherwise specified

>10%: Gastrointestinal: Dry mouth (35%; extended release capsules 23%)

1% to 10%:

Cardiovascular: Chest pain (2%)

Central nervous system: Headache (7%; extended release capsules 6%), somnolence (3%; extended release capsules 3%), fatigue (4%; extended release capsules 2%), dizziness (5%; extended release capsules 2%), anxiety (extended release capsules 1%)

Dermatologic: Dry skin (1%)

Gastrointestinal: Abdominal pain (5%; extended release capsules 4%), constipation (7%; extended release capsules 6%), dyspepsia (4%; extended release capsules 3%), diarrhea (4%), weight gain (1%)

Genitourinary: Dysuria (2%; extended release capsules 1%)

Neuromuscular & skeletal: Arthralgia (2%)

Ocular: Abnormal vision (2%; extended release capsules 1%), dry eyes (3%; extended release capsules 3%)

Respiratory: Bronchitis (2%), sinusitis (extended release capsules 2%)

Drug Interactions CYP2D6 and CYP3A3/4 enzyme substrate

Serum levels and/or toxicity of tolterodine may be increased by drugs which inhibit CYP2D6; effect was seen with fluoxetine. Inhibitors include amiodarone, cimetidine, delavirdine, paroxetine, propafenone, quinidine, and ritonavir. No dosage adjustment was needed in patients coadministered tolterodine and fluoxetine.

Serum level and/or toxicity of tolterodine may be increased by drugs which inhibit CYP3A3/4, particularly in patients who are poor metabolizers via CYP2D6; effect was seen with ketoconazole. Other inhibitors include amiodarone, cimetidine, clarithromycin, cyclosporine, erythromycin, delavirdine, diltiazem, dirithromycin, disulfiram, fluoxetine, fluvoxamine, indinavir, itraconazole, nefazodone, nevirapine, propoxyphene, quinupristin-dalfopristin, ritonavir, saquinavir, verapamil, vinblastine, zafirlukast, zileuton.

Drug Uptake

Absorption: Immediate release tablet: Rapid

Half-life, elimination:

Immediate release tablet: Extensive metabolizers: ~2 hours; poor metabolizers: ~10 hours

Extended release capsule: Extensive metabolizers: ~7 hours; poor metabolizers: ~18 hours

Time to peak: Immediate release tablet: 1-2 hours; Extended release tablet: 2-6 hours

Pregnancy Risk Factor C

Generic Available No

Tolu-Sed® DM [OTC] *see* Guaifenesin and Dextromethorphan *on page 569*

Tonocard® *see* Tocainide *on page 1176*

Topamax® *see* Topiramate *on page 1182*

Topicort® *see* Desoximetasone *on page 362*

Topicort®-LP *see* Desoximetasone *on page 362*

Topicycline® *see* Tetracycline *on page 1147*

Topiramate (toe PYE ra mate)

U.S. Brand Names Topamax®

Canadian Brand Names Topamax®

Mexican Brand Names Topamax®

Pharmacologic Category Anticonvulsant, Miscellaneous

Use In adults and pediatric patients (ages 2-16 years), adjunctive therapy for partial onset seizures and adjunctive therapy of primary generalized tonic-clonic seizures; treatment of seizures associated with Lennox-Gastaut syndrome in patients ≥2 years of age

Unlabeled/Investigational: Bipolar disorder, infantile spasms, neuropathic pain

Local Anesthetic/Vasoconstrictor Precautions No information available to require special precautions

Effects on Dental Treatment ≤10%: Gingivitis and xerostomia

Dosage Oral:

Children 2-16 years: Partial seizures (adjunctive therapy), primary generalized tonic-clonic seizures (adjunctive therapy), or seizure associated with Lennox-Gastaut syndrome: Initial dose titration should begin at 25 mg (or less, based on a range of 1-3 mg/kg/day) nightly for the first week; dosage may be increased in increments of 1-3 mg/kg/day (administered in 2 divided doses) at 1- or 2-week intervals to a total daily dose of 5-9 mg/kg/day.

Adults: Partial onset seizures (adjunctive therapy), primary generalized tonic-clonic seizures (adjunctive therapy): Initial: 25-50 mg/day; titrate in increments of 25-50 mg per week until an effective daily dose is reached; the daily dose may be increased by 25 mg at weekly intervals for the first 4 weeks; thereafter, the daily dose may be increased by 25-50 mg weekly to an effective daily dose (usually at least 400 mg); usual maximum dose: 1600 mg/day

Note: A more rapid titration schedule has been previously recommended (ie, 50 mg/week), and may be attempted in some clinical situations; however, this may reduce the patient's ability to tolerate topiramate.

Dosing adjustment in renal impairment: Cl_{cr} <70 mL/minute: Administer 50% dose and titrate more slowly

Hemodialysis: Supplemental dose may be needed during hemodialysis

Dosing adjustment in hepatic impairment: Clearance may be reduced

Mechanism of Action Mechanism is not fully understood, it is thought to decrease seizure frequency by blocking sodium channels in neurons, enhancing GABA activity, and by blocking glutamate activity

Other Adverse Effects

>10%:

Central nervous system: Dizziness, ataxia, somnolence, psychomotor slowing, nervousness, memory difficulties, speech problems, fatigue

Gastrointestinal: Nausea

Neuromuscular & skeletal: Paresthesia, tremor

Ocular: Nystagmus, diplopia, abnormal vision

Respiratory: Upper respiratory infections

1% to 10%:

Cardiovascular: Chest pain, edema

Central nervous system: Language problems, abnormal coordination, confusion, depression, difficulty concentrating, hypoesthesia

Endocrine & metabolic: Hot flashes

Gastrointestinal: Dyspepsia, abdominal pain, anorexia, constipation, xerostomia, gingivitis, weight loss

Neuromuscular & skeletal: Myalgia, weakness, back pain, leg pain, rigors

Otic: Decreased hearing

Renal: Nephrolithiasis

Respiratory: Pharyngitis, sinusitis, epistaxis

Miscellaneous: Flu-like symptoms

Warnings/Precautions Avoid abrupt withdrawal of topiramate therapy, withdraw slowly to minimize the potential of increased seizure frequency; the risk of kidney stones is about 2-4 times that of the untreated population; the risk of this event may be reduced by increasing fluid intake; use cautiously in patients with hepatic or renal impairment, during pregnancy, or in nursing mothers.

Drug Interactions CYP2C19 enzyme substrate; CYP2C19 enzyme inhibitor

Increased Effect/Toxicity: Concomitant administration with other CNS depressants will increase its sedative effects. Coadministration with other carbonic anhydrase inhibitors may increase the chance of nephrolithiasis. Topiramate may increase phenytoin concentration by 25%.

Decreased Effect: Phenytoin can decrease topiramate levels by as much as 48%, carbamazepine reduces it by 40%, and valproic acid reduces topiramate by 14%. Digoxin levels and ethinyl estradiol blood levels are decreased when coadministered with topiramate. Topiramate may decrease valproic acid concentration by 11%.

Drug Uptake

Absorption: Good; unaffected by food

Half-life, elimination: Mean: Adults: 21 hours

Time to peak: ~2-4 hours

Pregnancy Risk Factor C

Generic Available No

Toposar® *see* Etoposide *on page 481*

Topotecan (toe poe TEE kan)

U.S. Brand Names Hycamtin™

Canadian Brand Names Hycamtin™

Pharmacologic Category Antineoplastic Agent, Natural Source (Plant) Derivative

Synonyms Hycamptamine; SK and F 104864; SKF 104864; SKF 104864-A; TOPO; Topotecan Hydrochloride; TPT

Use Treatment of ovarian cancer after failure of first-line chemotherapy; treatment of small cell lung cancer sensitive disease after failure of first-line chemotherapy

Unlabeled/Investigational: Treatment of nonsmall cell lung cancer, sarcoma (pediatrics)

Local Anesthetic/Vasoconstrictor Precautions No information available to require special precautions

Effects on Dental Treatment No effects or complications reported

Mechanism of Action Camptothecin (CPT) analogue and potent inhibitor of topoisomerase I, an enzyme which relaxes torsionally strained-coiled duplex DNA; (Continued)

Topotecan *(Continued)*

topotecan acts in S phase preventing DNA replication and translocation. Structure-activity studies have revealed a direct relationship between the ability of CPT analogues to inhibit topoisomerase I catalytic activity and their potency as cytotoxic agents.

Other Adverse Effects

>10%:

Central nervous system: Headache

Dermatologic: Alopecia (reversible)

Gastrointestinal: Nausea, vomiting, diarrhea

Emetic potential: Moderately low (10% to 30%)

Hematologic: Myelosuppressive: Principle dose-limiting toxicity; white blood cell count nadir is 8-11 days after administration and is more frequent than thrombocytopenia (at lower doses); recover is usually within 21 days and cumulative toxicity has not been noted.

WBC: Mild to severe

Platelets: Mild (at low doses)

Nadir: 8-11 days

Recovery: 14-21 days

1% to 10%:

Neuromuscular & skeletal: Paresthesia

Respiratory: Dyspnea

Drug Interactions Decreased Effect: Concurrent administration of TPT and G-CSF in clinical trials results in severe myelosuppression. Concurrent *in vitro* exposure to TPT and the topoisomerase II inhibitor etoposide results in no altered effect; sequential exposure results in potentiation. Concurrent exposure to TPT and 5-azacytidine results in potentiation both *in vitro* and *in vivo*. Myelosuppression was more severe when given in combination with cisplatin.

Drug Uptake

Absorption: Oral: ~30%

Half-life, elimination: 3 hours

Pregnancy Risk Factor D

Generic Available No

Comments Constituted vial: When constituted with 2 mL of sterile water for injection, USP, each mL contains topotecan 2.5 mg and mannitol 50 mg with a pH of approximately 3.5. Final infusion preparation: Topotecan constituted solution should be further diluted in 5% dextrose injection. Topotecan should NOT be diluted in buffered solutions.

Toprol-XL® *see* Metoprolol *on page 803*

Toradol® *see* Ketorolac Tromethamine *on page 676*

Torecan® *see* Thiethylperazine *on page 1157*

Toremifene (TORE em i feen)

U.S. Brand Names Fareston®

Canadian Brand Names Fareston®

Mexican Brand Names Fareston®

Pharmacologic Category Antineoplastic Agent, Estrogen Receptor Antagonist

Synonyms FC1157a; Toremifene Citrate

Use Treatment of advanced breast cancer; management of desmoid tumors and endometrial carcinoma

Local Anesthetic/Vasoconstrictor Precautions No information available to require special precautions

Effects on Dental Treatment No effects or complications reported

Mechanism of Action Nonsteroidal, triphenylethylene derivative. Competitively binds to estrogen receptors on tumors and other tissue targets, producing a nuclear complex that decreases DNA synthesis and inhibits estrogen effects. Nonsteroidal agent with potent antiestrogenic properties which compete with estrogen for binding sites in breast and other tissues; may involve effects on calcium channels, calmodulin, and/or protein kinase C; cells accumulate in the G_0 and G_1 phases; therefore, tamoxifen is cytostatic rather than cytocidal.

Other Adverse Effects

>10%:

Endocrine & metabolic: Vaginal discharge, hot flashes

Gastrointestinal: Nausea, vomiting

Miscellaneous: Diaphoresis

1% to 10%:

Cardiovascular: Thromboembolism: Tamoxifen has been associated with the occurrence of venous thrombosis and pulmonary embolism; arterial thrombosis has also been described in a few case reports; cardiac failure, myocardial infarction, edema

Central nervous system: Dizziness

Endocrine & metabolic: Hypercalcemia may occur in patients with bone metastases; galactorrhea and vitamin deficiency, menstrual irregularities

Genitourinary: Vaginal bleeding or discharge, endometriosis, priapism, possible endometrial cancer
Ocular: Ophthalmologic effects (visual acuity changes, cataracts, or retinopathy), corneal opacities, dry eyes

Contraindications Hypersensitivity to toremifene or any component of the formulation

Warnings/Precautions Toremifene should be used cautiously in patients with anemia or hepatic failure

Drug Interactions CYP3A3/4 enzyme substrate

Increased Effect/Toxicity: Enzyme inhibitors (such as ketoconazole or erythromycin) may increase blood levels of toremifene. Concurrent therapy with warfarin results in significant enhancement of anticoagulant effects; has been speculated that a ↓ in antitumor effect of tamoxifen may also occur due to alterations in the percentage of active tamoxifen metabolites.

Decreased Effect: Phenobarbital, phenytoin, and carbamazepine increase the rate of toremifene metabolism and lower blood levels.

Drug Uptake

Absorption: Well absorbed
Half-life, elimination: N-desmethyltoremifene: 6 days; 4-hydroxytoremifene: 5 days
Time to peak: ~3 hours

Pregnancy Risk Factor D

Generic Available No

Selected Readings

Gams R, "Phase III Trials of Toremifene vs Tamoxifen," *Oncology*, 1997, 11(5 Suppl 4): 23-8.
Hamm JT, "Phase I and II Studies of Toremifene," *Oncology*, 1997, 11(5 Suppl 4):19-22.
Holli K, "Evolving Role of Toremifene in the Adjuvant Setting," *Oncology*, 1997, 11(5 Suppl 4):48-51.
Kangas L, "Review of the Pharmacological Properties of Toremifene," *J Steroid Biochem*, 1990, 36(3):191-5.
Pyrhönen S, Valavaara R, Modig H, et al, "Comparison of Toremifene and Tamoxifen in Postmenopausal Patients With Advanced Breast Cancer: A Randomized Double-Blind, the "Nordic" Phase III Study," *Br J Cancer*, 1997, 76(2):270-7.
Williams GM and Jeffrey AM, "Safety Assessment of Tamoxifen and Toremifene," *Oncology*, 1997, 11(5 Suppl 4):41-7.

Tornalate® *see* Bitolterol *on page 170*

Torsemide (TOR se mide)

Related Information

Cardiovascular Diseases *on page 1308*

U.S. Brand Names Demadex®

Pharmacologic Category Diuretic, Loop

Use Management of edema associated with CHF and hepatic or renal disease; used alone or in combination with antihypertensives in treatment of hypertension; I.V. form is indicated when rapid onset is desired

Local Anesthetic/Vasoconstrictor Precautions No information available to require special precautions

Effects on Dental Treatment No effects or complications reported

Dosage Adults: Oral, I.V.:

Congestive heart failure: 10-20 mg once daily; may increase gradually for chronic treatment by doubling dose until the diuretic response is apparent (for acute treatment, I.V. dose may be repeated every 2 hours with double the dose as needed)
Chronic renal failure: 20 mg once daily; increase as described above
Hepatic cirrhosis: 5-10 mg once daily with an aldosterone antagonist or a potassium-sparing diuretic; increase as described above
Hypertension: 5 mg once daily; increase to 10 mg after 4-6 weeks if an adequate hypotensive response is not apparent; if still not effective, an additional antihypertensive agent may be added

Mechanism of Action Inhibits reabsorption of sodium and chloride in the ascending loop of Henle and distal renal tubule, interfering with the chloride-binding cotransport system, thus causing increased excretion of water, sodium, chloride, magnesium, and calcium; does not alter GFR, renal plasma flow, or acid-base balance

Other Adverse Effects 1% to 10%:

Cardiovascular: Edema (1.1%), EKG abnormality (2%), chest pain (1.2%)
Central nervous system: Headache (7.3%), dizziness (3.2%), insomnia (1.2%), nervousness (1%)
Endocrine & metabolic: Hyperglycemia, hyperuricemia, hypokalemia
Gastrointestinal: Diarrhea (2%), constipation (1.8%), nausea (1.8%), dyspepsia (1.6%), sore throat (1.6%)
Genitourinary: Excessive urination (6.7%)
Neuromuscular & skeletal: Weakness (2%), arthralgia (1.8%), myalgia (1.6%)
Respiratory: Rhinitis (2.8%), cough increase (2%)

Warnings/Precautions Adjust dose to avoid dehydration. In cirrhosis, avoid electrolyte and acid/base imbalances that might lead to hepatic encephalopathy. Ototoxicity is associated with rapid I.V. administration of other loop diuretics and has been seen with oral torsemide. Do not administer I.V. in <2 minutes; single

(Continued)

Torsemide *(Continued)*

doses should not exceed 200 mg. Hypersensitivity reactions can rarely occur. Monitor fluid status and renal function in an attempt to prevent oliguria, azotemia, and reversible increases in BUN and creatinine. Close medical supervision of aggressive diuresis is required. Monitor closely for electrolyte imbalances particularly hypokalemia and correct when necessary. Coadministration with antihypertensives may increase the risk of hypotension.

Chemical similarities are present among sulfonamides, sulfonylureas, carbonic anhydrase inhibitors, thiazides, and loop diuretics (except ethacrynic acid). Use in patients with sulfonylurea allergy is specifically contraindicated in product labeling, however a risk of cross-reaction exists in patients with allergy to any of these compounds; avoid use when previous reaction has been severe.

Drug Interactions CYP2C9 enzyme substrate

Increased Effect/Toxicity: Torsemide-induced hypokalemia may predispose to digoxin toxicity and may increase the risk of arrhythmia with drugs which may prolong QT interval, including type Ia and type III antiarrhythmic agents, cisapride, terfenadine, and some quinolones (sparfloxacin, gatifloxacin, and moxifloxacin). The risk of toxicity from lithium and salicylates (high dose) may be increased by loop diuretics. Hypotensive effects and/or adverse renal effects of ACE inhibitors and NSAIDs are potentiated by bumetanide-induced hypovolemia. The effects of peripheral adrenergic-blocking drugs or ganglionic blockers may be increased by bumetanide.

Torsemide may increase the risk of ototoxicity with other ototoxic agents (aminoglycosides, cis-platinum), especially in patients with renal dysfunction. Synergistic diuretic effects occur with thiazide-type diuretics. Diuretics tend to be synergistic with other antihypertensive agents, and hypotension may occur.

Decreased Effect: Torsemide efficacy may be decreased with NSAIDs. Torsemide action may be reduced with probenecid. Diuretic action may be impaired in patients with cirrhosis and ascites if used with salicylates. Glucose tolerance may be decreased when used with sulfonylureas.

Drug Uptake

Onset of action: Diuresis: 30-60 minutes; Peak effect: 1-4 hours

Absorption: Oral: Rapid

Duration: ~6 hours

Half-life, elimination: 2-4; Cirrhosis: 7-8 hours

Pregnancy Risk Factor B

Generic Available No

Touro™ Allergy *see* Brompheniramine and Pseudoephedrine *on page 180*

Touro Ex® *see* Guaifenesin *on page 568*

Touro LA® *see* Guaifenesin and Pseudoephedrine *on page 570*

T-Phyl® *see* Theophylline *on page 1152*

Trace-4® *see* Trace Metals *on page 1186*

Trace Metals (trase MET als)

U.S. Brand Names Chroma-Pak®; Iodopen®; Molypen®; M.T.E.-4®; M.T.E.-5®; M.T.E.-6®; MulTE-PAK-4®; MulTE-PAK-5®; Neotrace-4®; PedTE-PAK-4®; Pedtrace-4®; P.T.E.-4®; P.T.E.-5®; Sele-Pak®; Selepen®; Trace-4®; Zinca-Pak®

Pharmacologic Category Trace Element, Parenteral

Recommended Daily Parenteral Dosage

Element	Infants	Children	Adults
Chromium[1]	0.2 mcg/kg	0.2 mcg/kg (maximum 5 mcg)	10-15 mcg
Copper[2]	20 mcg/kg	20 mcg/kg (maximum 300 mcg)	0.5-1.5 mg
Manganese[2, 3]	1 mcg/kg	1 mcg/kg (maximum 50 mcg)	150-800 mcg
Molybdenum[1, 4]	0.25 mcg/kg	0.25 mcg/kg (maximum 5 mcg)	20-120 mcg
Selenium[1, 4]	2 mcg/kg	2 mcg/kg (maximum 30 mcg)	20-40 mcg
Zinc		50 mcg/kg (maximum 5 mg)	2.5-4 mg
preterm	400 mcg/kg		
term <3 months	250 mcg/kg		
term >3 monhs	100 mcg/kg		

[1]Omit in patients with renal dysfunction.

[2]Omit in patients with obstructive jaundice.

[3]Current available commercial products are not in appropriate ratios to maintain this recommendation — doses of up to 10 mcg/kg have been used.

[4]Indicated for use in long-term parenteral nutrition patients.

Synonyms Chromium; Copper; Iodine; Manganese; Molybdenum; Neonatal Trace Metals; Selenium; Zinc

Use Prevention and correction of trace metal deficiencies

Local Anesthetic/Vasoconstrictor Precautions No information available to require special precautions

Effects on Dental Treatment No effects or complications reported

Dosage See table on previous page.

Pregnancy Risk Factor C

Generic Available Yes

Comments Persistent diarrhea or excessive GI fluid losses from ostomy sites may grossly increase zinc losses

Tracleer™ *see* Bosentan *on page 171*

Tramadol (TRA ma dole)

U.S. Brand Names Ultram®

Canadian Brand Names Ultram®

Mexican Brand Names Nobligan®; Prontofort®; Tradol

Pharmacologic Category Analgesic, Non-narcotic

Synonyms Tramadol Hydrochloride

Use Relief of moderate to moderately severe pain

Local Anesthetic/Vasoconstrictor Precautions No information available to require special precautions

Effects on Dental Treatment No effects or complications reported

Dosage Oral:

Adults: Moderate to severe chronic pain: 50-100 mg every 4-6 hours, not to exceed 400 mg/day

For patients not requiring rapid onset of effect, tolerability may be improved by starting dose at 25 mg/day and titrating dose by 25 mg every 3 days, until reaching 25 mg 4 times/day. Dose may then be increased by 50 mg every 3 days as tolerated, to reach dose of 50 mg 4 times/day.

Elderly: >75 years: 50-100 mg every 4-6 hours (not to exceed 300 mg/day); see dosing adjustments for renal and hepatic impairment

Dosing adjustment in renal impairment: Cl_{cr} <30 mL/minute: Administer 50-100 mg dose every 12 hours (maximum: 200 mg/day)

Dosing adjustment in hepatic impairment: Cirrhosis: Recommended dose: 50 mg every 12 hours

Mechanism of Action Binds to μ-opiate receptors in the CNS causing inhibition of ascending pain pathways, altering the perception of and response to pain; also inhibits the reuptake of norepinephrine and serotonin, which also modifies the ascending pain pathway

Other Adverse Effects Incidence of some adverse effects may increase over time.

>10%:

Central nervous system: Dizziness, headache, somnolence, vertigo

Gastrointestinal: Constipation, nausea

1% to 10%:

Cardiovascular: Vasodilation

Central nervous system: Agitation, anxiety, confusion, coordination impaired, emotional lability, euphoria, hallucinations, malaise, nervousness, sleep disorder, tremor

Dermatologic: Pruritus, rash

Endocrine & metabolic: Menopausal symptoms

Gastrointestinal: Abdominal pain, anorexia, diarrhea, dyspepsia, flatulence, vomiting, xerostomia

Genitourinary: Urinary frequency, urinary retention

Neuromuscular & skeletal: Hypertonia, spasticity, weakness

Ocular: Miosis, visual disturbance

Miscellaneous: Diaphoresis

<1%: Abnormal gait, allergic reaction, amnesia, anaphylactoid reactions, anaphylaxis, angioedema, bronchospasm, cognitive dysfunction, concentration difficulty, death, depression, dyspnea, dysuria, hallucinations, menstrual disorder, orthostatic hypotension, paresthesia, seizure, serotonin syndrome, Stevens-Johnson syndrome, suicidal tendency, syncope, taste perversion, tachycardia, toxic epidermal necrolysis, tremor, urticaria, vesicles, weight loss

Postmarketing and/or case reports: Abnormal EKG, cataracts, creatinine increased, deafness, gastrointestinal bleeding, hemoglobin decreased, hepatitis, hypertension, hypotension, liver enzymes elevated, liver failure, migraine, myocardial ischemia, palpitations, proteinuria, pulmonary edema, pulmonary embolism, speech disorders, stomatitis, tinnitus

Contraindications Hypersensitivity to tramadol, opioids, or any component of their formulation; opioid-dependency; acute intoxication with ethanol, hypnotics, centrally-acting analgesics, opioids, or psychotropic drugs

Warnings/Precautions Should be used only with extreme caution in patients receiving MAO inhibitors. May cause CNS depression and/or respiratory depression, particularly when combined with other CNS depressants. Use with caution

(Continued)

Tramadol *(Continued)*

and reduce dosage when administered to patients receiving other CNS depressants. An increased risk of seizures may occur in patients receiving serotonin reuptake inhibitors (SSRIs or anorectics), tricyclic antidepressants, other cyclic compounds (including cyclobenzaprine, promethazine), neuroleptics, MAO inhibitors, or drugs which may lower seizure threshold. Patients with a history of seizures, or with a risk of seizures (head trauma, metabolic disorders, CNS infection, or malignancy, or during ethanol/drug withdrawal) are also at increased risk.

Elderly patients and patients with chronic respiratory disorders may be at greater risk of adverse events. Use with caution in patients with increased intracranial pressure or head injury. Use tramadol with caution and reduce dosage in patients with liver disease or renal dysfunction and in patients with myxedema, hypothyroidism, or hypoadrenalism. Not recommended during pregnancy or in nursing mothers. Tolerance or drug dependence may result from extended use; abrupt discontinuation should be avoided. Safety and efficacy in pediatric patients have not been established.

Drug Interactions CYP2D6 and 3A3/4 (minor) enzyme substrate

Amphetamines: May increase the risk of seizures with tramadol.

Carbamazepine: Decreases half-life of tramadol by 33% to 50%.

CYP2D6 inhibitors: May increase tramadol serum concentration.

Digoxin: Rare reports of digoxin toxicity with concomitant tramadol use.

Linezolid: May be associated with increased risk of seizures (due to MAO inhibition)

MAO inhibitors: May increases the risk of seizures.

Naloxone: May increase the risk of seizures (if administered in tramadol overdose)

Neuroleptic agents: May increase the risk of tramadol-associated seizures and may have additive CNS depressant effects.

Opioids: May increase the risk of seizures, and may have additive CNS depressant effects.

Quinidine: May increase the tramadol serum concentration.

Selegiline: An increased risk of seizures has been associated with MAO inhibitors. It is not clear if drugs with selective MAO type B inhibition are safer than nonselective agents.

SSRIs: May increase the risk of seizures with tramadol. Includes citalopram, fluoxetine, paroxetine, sertraline.

Tricyclic antidepressants: May increase the risk of seizures.

Warfarin: Concomitant use may lead to an elevation of prothrombin times; monitor.

Dietary/Ethanol/Herb Considerations

Ethanol: Avoid use; may increase CNS depression.

Food: May be taken with food; absorption unaffected. Fluids, fruit, and fiber may reduce constipation.

Herb/Nutraceutical: Avoid gotu kola, kava, SAMe, St John's wort, and valerian; may increase CNS depression.

Drug Uptake

Onset of action: ~1 hour

Duration of action: 9 hours

Absorption: Rapid and complete

Half-life, elimination: Tramadol: ~6 hours; Active metabolite: 7 hours; prolonged in elderly, hepatic or renal dysfunction

Time to peak: 2 hours

Pregnancy Risk Factor C

Breast-feeding Considerations Not recommended for postdelivery analgesia in nursing mothers.

Dosage Forms TAB: 50 mg

Generic Available No

Comments Literature reports suggest that the efficacy of tramadol in oral surgery pain is equivalent to the combination of aspirin and codeine. One study (Olson et al 1990) showed acetaminophen and dextropropoxyphene combination to be superior to tramadol and another study showed tramadol to be superior to acetaminophen and dextropropoxyphene combination. Tramadol appears to be at least equal to if not better than codeine alone. Seizures have been reported with the use of tramadol.

Selected Readings

Collins M, Young I, Sweeney P, et al, "The Effect of Tramadol on Dento-Alveolar Surgical Pain," *Br J Oral Maxillofac Surg*, 1997, 35(1):54-8.

Kahn LH, Alderfer RJ, and Graham DJ, "Seizures Reported With Tramadol," *JAMA*, 1997, 278(20):1661.

Lewis KS and Han NH, "Tramadol: A New Centrally Acting Analgesic," *Am J Health Syst Pharm*, 1997, 54(6):643-52.

Sunshine A, "New Clinical Experience With Tramadol," *Drugs*, 1994, 47(Suppl 1):8-18.

Sunshine A, Olson NZ, Zighelboim I, et al, "Analgesic Oral Efficacy of Tramadol Hydrochloride in Postoperative Pain," *Clin Pharmacol Ther*, 1992; 51(6):740-6.

Wynn RL, "Tramadol (Ultram) - A New Kind of Analgesic," *Gen Dent*, 1996, 44(3):216-8,220.

Trandate® *see* Labetalol *on page 680*

Trandolapril (tran DOE la pril)

U.S. Brand Names Mavik®

Canadian Brand Names Mavik™

Mexican Brand Names Gopten®

Pharmacologic Category Angiotensin-Converting Enzyme (ACE) Inhibitor

Use Management of hypertension alone or in combination with other antihypertensive agents

Unlabeled/Investigational: As a class, ACE inhibitors are recommended in the treatment of systolic CHF

Local Anesthetic/Vasoconstrictor Precautions No information available to require special precautions

Effects on Dental Treatment No effects or complications reported

Dosage Adults: Oral:

Hypertension: Initial dose in patients not receiving a diuretic: 1 mg/day (2 mg/day in black patients). Adjust dosage according to the BP response. Make dosage adjustments at intervals of ≥1 week. Most patients have required dosages of 2-4 mg/day. There is a little experience with doses >8 mg/day. Patients inadequately treated with once daily dosing at 4 mg may be treated with twice daily dosing. If BP is not adequately controlled with trandolapril monotherapy, a diuretic may be added.

Heart failure postmyocardial infarction or left ventricular dysfunction postmyocardial infarction: Initial: 1 mg/day; titrate patients (as tolerated) towards the target dose of 4 mg/day. If a 4 mg dose is not tolerated, patients can continue therapy with the greatest tolerated dose.

Dosing adjustment in renal impairment: Cl_{cr} ≤30 mL/minute: Recommended starting dose: 0.5 mg/day.

Dosing adjustment in hepatic impairment: Cirrhosis: Recommended starting dose: 0.5 mg/day.

Mechanism of Action An angiotensin-converting enzyme (ACE) inhibitor which prevents the formation of angiotensin II from angiotensin I; trandolapril must undergo enzymatic hydrolysis, mainly in liver, to its biologically active metabolite, trandolaprilat. A CNS mechanism may also be involved in the hypotensive effect as angiotensin II increases adrenergic outflow from the CNS. Vasoactive kallikrein's may be decreased in conversion to active hormones by ACE inhibitors, thus, reducing BP.

Other Adverse Effects Frequency ranges include data from hypertension and heart failure trials. Higher rates of adverse reactions have generally been noted in patients with CHF. However, the frequency of adverse effects associated with placebo is also increased in this population.

>1%:

Cardiovascular: Hypotension (<1% to 11%), bradycardia (<1% to 4.7%), intermittent claudication (3.8%), stroke (3.3%)

Central nervous system: Dizziness (1.3% to 23%), syncope (5.9%), asthenia (3.3%)

Endocrine & metabolic: Elevated uric acid (15%), hyperkalemia (5.3%), hypocalcemia (4.7%)

Gastrointestinal: Dyspepsia (6.4%), gastritis (4.2%)

Neuromuscular & skeletal: Myalgia (4.7%)

Renal: Elevated BUN (9%), elevated serum creatinine (1.1% to 4.7%) Respiratory: Cough (1.9% to 35%)

Warnings/Precautions Neutropenia, agranulocytosis, angioedema, decreased renal function (hypertension, renal artery stenosis, CHF), hepatic dysfunction (elimination, activation), proteinuria, first-dose hypotension (hypovolemia, CHF, dehydrated patients at risk, eg, diuretic use, elderly), elderly (due to renal function changes); use with caution and modify dosage in patients with renal impairment; use with caution in patients with collagen vascular disease, CHF, hypovolemia, valvular stenosis, hyperkalemia (>5.7 mEq/L), anesthesia

Drug Interactions

Increased Effect/Toxicity: Potassium supplements, co-trimoxazole (high dose), angiotensin II receptor antagonists (candesartan, losartan, irbesartan, etc), or potassium-sparing diuretics (amiloride, spironolactone, triamterene) may result in elevated serum potassium levels when combined with trandolapril. ACE inhibitor effects may be increased by phenothiazines or probenecid (increases levels of captopril). ACE inhibitors may increase serum concentration/effects of digoxin, lithium, and sulfonlyureas.

Diuretics have additive hypotensive effects with ACE inhibitors, and hypovolemia increases the potential for adverse renal effects of ACE inhibitors. In patients with compromised renal function, coadministration with nonsteroidal anti-inflammatory drugs may result in further deterioration of renal function. Allopurinol and ACE inhibitors may cause a higher risk of hypersensitivity reaction when taken concurrently.

Decreased Effect: Aspirin (high dose) may reduce the therapeutic effects of ACE inhibitors; at low dosages this does not appear to be significant. Rifampin may decrease the effect of ACE inhibitors. Antacids may decrease the bioavailability

(Continued)

Trandolapril *(Continued)*

of ACE inhibitors (may be more likely to occur with captopril); separate administration times by 1-2 hours. NSAIDs, specifically indomethacin, may reduce the hypotensive effects of ACE inhibitors. More likely to occur in low renin or volume dependent hypertensive patients.

Drug Uptake

Onset of action: 1-2 hours; Peak effect: Reduction in blood pressure: 6 hours

Absorption: Rapid

Duration: Prolonged; 72 hours after single dose

Half-life, elimination: Trandolapril: 6 hours; Trandolaprilat: Effective: 10 hours, Terminal: 24 hours

Time to peak: Parent: 1 hour; Active metabolite trandolaprilat: 4-10 hours

Pregnancy Risk Factor C/D (2nd and 3rd trimesters)

Generic Available No

Comments Patients taking diuretics are at risk for developing hypotension on initial dosing; to prevent this, discontinue diuretics 2-3 days prior to initiating trandolapril; may restart diuretics if blood pressure is not controlled by trandolapril alone

Selected Readings

Bevan EG, McInnes GT, Aldigier JC, et al, "Effect of Renal Function on the Pharmacokinetics and Pharmacodynamics of Trandolapril," *Br J Clin Pharmacol*, 1993, 35(2):128-35.

Conen H and Brunner HR, "Pharmacologic Profile of Trandolapril, A New Angiotensin-Converting Enzyme Inhibitor," *Am J Heart*, 1993, 125(5 Pt 2):1524-31.

Zannad F, "Trandolapril. How Does It Differ From Other Angiotensin-Converting Enzyme Inhibitors?" *Drugs*, 1993, 46(Suppl 2):172-81.

Trandolapril and Verapamil (tran DOE la pril & ver AP a mil)

U.S. Brand Names Tarka®

Pharmacologic Category Antihypertensive Agent Combination

Synonyms Verapamil and Trandolapril

Use Combination drug for the treatment of hypertension, however, not indicated for initial treatment of hypertension; replacement therapy in patients receiving separate dosage forms (for patient convenience); when monotherapy with one component fails to achieve desired antihypertensive effect, or when dose-limiting adverse effects limit upward titration of monotherapy

Local Anesthetic/Vasoconstrictor Precautions No information available to require special precautions

Effects on Dental Treatment No effects or complications reported

Dosage Dose is individualized

Drug Uptake See Trandolapril *on page 1189* and Verapamil *on page 1236*

Pregnancy Risk Factor C/D (2nd and 3rd trimesters)

Generic Available No

Tranexamic Acid (tran eks AM ik AS id)

U.S. Brand Names Cyklokapron®

Canadian Brand Names Cyklokapron®

Pharmacologic Category Antihemophilic Agent

Use Short-term use (2-8 days) in hemophilia patients during and following tooth extraction to reduce or prevent hemorrhage

Unlabeled/Investigational: Has been used as an alternative to aminocaproic acid for subarachnoid hemorrhage

Local Anesthetic/Vasoconstrictor Precautions No information available to require special precautions

Effects on Dental Treatment No effects or complications reported

Dosage Children and Adults: I.V.: 10 mg/kg immediately before surgery, then 25 mg/kg/dose orally 3-4 times/day for 2-8 days

Alternatively:

Oral: 25 mg/kg 3-4 times/day beginning 1 day prior to surgery

I.V.: 10 mg/kg 3-4 times/day in patients who are unable to take oral

Dosing adjustment/interval in renal impairment:

Cl_{cr} 50-80 mL/minute: Administer 50% of normal dose or 10 mg/kg twice daily I.V. or 15 mg/kg twice daily orally

Cl_{cr} 10-50 mL/minute: Administer 25% of normal dose or 10 mg/kg/day I.V. or 15 mg/kg/day orally

Cl_{cr} <10 mL/minute: Administer 10% of normal dose or 10 mg/kg/dose every 48 hours I.V. or 15 mg/kg/dose every 48 hours orally

Mechanism of Action Forms a reversible complex that displaces plasminogen from fibrin resulting in inhibition of fibrinolysis; it also inhibits the proteolytic activity of plasmin

Other Adverse Effects

>10%: Gastrointestinal: Nausea, diarrhea, vomiting

1% to 10%:

Cardiovascular: Hypotension, thrombosis

Ocular: Blurred vision

Contraindications Acquired defective color vision; active intravascular clotting; subarachnoid hemorrhage; concurrent factor IX complex or anti-inhibitor coagulant concentrates

Drug Interactions Increased Effect/Toxicity: Chlorpromazine may increase cerebral vasospasm and ischemia. Coadministration of Factor IX complex or anti-inhibitor coagulant concentrates may increase risk of thrombosis.

Drug Uptake Half-life, elimination: 2-10 hours

Pregnancy Risk Factor B

Generic Available No

Comments Antifibrinolytic drugs are useful for the control of bleeding after dental extractions in patients with hemophilia because the oral mucosa and saliva are rich in plasminogen activators. In a clinical trial, tranexamic acid reduced recurrent bleeding and the amount of clotting-factor-replacement therapy needed. In adults, the oral dose was 20-25 mg/kg tranexamic acid every 8 hours until the dental sockets were completely healed. Mouthwashes containing tranexamic acid are effective for preventing oral bleeding in patients with hemophilia and in patients requiring dental extraction while receiving long-term oral anticoagulant therapy.

Immediately before dental extraction in hemophilic patients, administer 10 mg/kg tranexamic acid I.V. together with replacement therapy. Following surgery, a dose of 25 mg/kg may be given orally 3-4 times/day for 2-8 days.

Selected Readings

Mannucci PM, "Hemostatic Drugs," *N Eng J Med*, 1998, 339(4):245-53.

Sindet-Pedersen S, "Distribution of Tranexamic Acid to Plasma and Saliva After Oral Administration and Mouth Rinsing: A Pharmacokinetic Study," *J Clin Pharmacol*, 1987, 27(12):1005-8.

Sindet-Pedersen S, Ramstron G, Bernvil S, et al, "Hemostatic Effect of Tranexamic Acid Mouthwash in Anticoagulant-Treated Patients Undergoing Oral Surgery," *N Engl J Med*, 1989, 320(13):840-3.

Transderm-Nitro® Patch *see* Nitroglycerin *on page 871*

Transderm Scōp® *see* Scopolamine *on page 1077*

Trans-Ver-Sal® AdultPatch [OTC] *see* Salicylic Acid *on page 1072*

Trans-Ver-Sal® PediaPatch [OTC] *see* Salicylic Acid *on page 1072*

Trans-Ver-Sal® PlantarPatch [OTC] *see* Salicylic Acid *on page 1072*

Tranxene® *see* Clorazepate *on page 311*

Tranylcypromine (tran il SIP roe meen)

U.S. Brand Names Parnate®

Canadian Brand Names Parnate®

Pharmacologic Category Antidepressant, Monoamine Oxidase Inhibitor

Synonyms Transamine Sulphate; Tranylcypromine Sulfate

Use Treatment of major depressive episode without melancholia

Unlabeled/Investigational: Post-traumatic stress disorder

Local Anesthetic/Vasoconstrictor Precautions Attempts should be made to avoid use of vasoconstrictor due to possibility of hypertensive episodes with monoamine oxidase inhibitors

Effects on Dental Treatment

>10%: Orthostatic hypotension

Avoid use as an analgesic due to toxic reactions with MAO inhibitors.

Dosage Adults: Oral: 10 mg twice daily, increase by 10 mg increments at 1- to 3-week intervals; maximum: 60 mg/day

Mechanism of Action Inhibits the enzymes monoamine oxidase A and B which are responsible for the intraneuronal metabolism of norepinephrine and serotonin and increasing their availability to postsynaptic neurons; decreased firing rate of the locus ceruleus, reducing norepinephrine concentration in the brain; agonist effects of serotonin

Other Adverse Effects Frequency not defined:

Cardiovascular: Orthostatic hypotension, edema

Central nervous system: Dizziness, headache, drowsiness, sleep disturbances, fatigue, hyper-reflexia, twitching, ataxia, mania, akinesia, confusion, disorientation, memory loss

Dermatologic: Rash, pruritus, urticaria, localized scleroderma, cystic acne (flare), alopecia

Endocrine & metabolic: Sexual dysfunction (anorgasmia, ejaculatory disturbances, impotence), hypernatremia, hypermetabolic syndrome, SIADH

Gastrointestinal: Xerostomia, constipation, weight gain

Genitourinary: Urinary retention, incontinence

Hematologic: Leukopenia, agranulocytosis

Hepatic: Hepatitis

Neuromuscular & skeletal: Weakness, tremor, myoclonus

Ocular: Blurred vision, glaucoma

Miscellaneous: Diaphoresis

Contraindications Hypersensitivity to tranylcypromine or any component of the formulation; uncontrolled hypertension; pheochromocytoma; hepatic or renal disease; cerebrovascular defect; cardiovascular disease; concurrent use of sympathomimetics (and related compounds), CNS depressants, ethanol, meperidine, bupropion, buspirone, guanethidine, and serotonergic drugs (including SSRIs)

(Continued)

Tranylcypromine *(Continued)*

- do not use within 5 weeks of fluoxetine discontinuation or 2 weeks of other antidepressant discontinuation; general anesthesia, local vasoconstrictors; spinal anesthesia (hypotension may be exaggerated); foods which are high in tyramine, tryptophan, or dopamine, chocolate, or caffeine.

Drug Interactions CYP2A6 and 2C19 enzyme inhibitor

Increased Effect/Toxicity: In general, the combined use of tranylcypromine with TCAs, venlafaxine, trazodone, dexfenfluramine, sibutramine, lithium, meperidine, fenfluramine, dextromethorphan, and SSRIs should be avoided due to the potential for severe adverse reactions (serotonin syndrome, death). Tranylcypromine in combination with amphetamines, other stimulants (methylphenidate), levodopa, metaraminol, buspirone, bupropion, reserpine, and decongestants (pseudoephedrine) may result in severe hypertensive reactions. MAO inhibitors (including tranylcypromine) may inhibit the metabolism of barbiturates and prolong their effect. Tranylcypromine may increase the pressor response of norepinephrine and may prolong neuromuscular blockade produced by succinylcholine. Tramadol may increase the risk of seizures and serotonin syndrome in patients receiving an MAO inhibitor. Tranylcypromine may produce additive hypoglycemic effect in patients receiving hypoglycemic agents and may produce delirium in patients receiving disulfiram.

Decreased Effect: Tranylcypromine inhibits the antihypertensive response to guanadrel or guanethidine.

Drug Uptake

Onset of action: Therapeutic: 2-3 weeks continued dosing

Duration: May continue to have a therapeutic effect and interactions 2 weeks after discontinuing therapy

Half-life, elimination: 90-190 minutes

Time to peak: ~2 hours

Pregnancy Risk Factor C

Generic Available No

Trastuzumab (tras TU zoo mab)

U.S. Brand Names Herceptin®

Canadian Brand Names Herceptin®

Pharmacologic Category Monoclonal Antibody

Use

Single agent for the treatment of patients with metastatic breast cancer whose tumors overexpress the HER-2/*neu* protein and who have received one or more chemotherapy regimens for their metastatic disease

Combination therapy with paclitaxel for the treatment of patients with metastatic breast cancer whose tumors overexpress the HER-2/*neu* protein and who have not received chemotherapy for their metastatic disease

Note: HER-2/*neu* protein overexpression or amplification has been noted in ovarian, gastric, colorectal, endometrial, lung, bladder, prostate, and salivary gland tumors. It is not yet known whether trastuzumab may be effective in these other carcinomas which overexpress HER-2/*neu* protein.

Local Anesthetic/Vasoconstrictor Precautions No information available to require special precautions

Effects on Dental Treatment <1%: Stomatitis

Mechanism of Action A monoclonal antibody which binds to the extracellular domain of the human epidermal growth factor receptor 2 protein (HER2); mediates antibody-dependent cellular cytotoxicity against cells which overproduce HER2

Other Adverse Effects

>10%:

Central nervous system: Pain (47%), fever (36%), chills (32%), headache (26%)

Dermatologic: Rash (18%)

Gastrointestinal: Nausea (33%), diarrhea (25%), vomiting (23%), abdominal pain (22%), anorexia (14%)

Neuromuscular & skeletal: Weakness (42%), back pain (22%)

Respiratory: Cough (26%), dyspnea (22%), rhinitis (14%), pharyngitis (12%)

Miscellaneous: Infection (20%)

1% to 10%:

Cardiovascular: Peripheral edema (10%), CHF (7%), tachycardia (5%)

Central nervous system: Insomnia (14%), dizziness (13%), paresthesia (9%), depression (6%), peripheral neuritis (2%), neuropathy (1%)

Dermatologic: Herpes simplex (2%), acne (2%)

Gastrointestinal: Nausea and vomiting (8%)

Genitourinary: Urinary tract infection (5%)

Hematologic: Anemia (4%), leukopenia (3%)

Neuromuscular & skeletal: Bone pain (7%), arthralgia (6%)

Respiratory: Sinusitis (9%)

Miscellaneous: Flu syndrome (10%), accidental injury (6%), allergic reaction (3%)

Warnings/Precautions Serious adverse events, including hypersensitivity reaction (anaphylaxis), infusion reactions (including fatalities), and pulmonary events (including adult respiratory distress syndrome) have been associated with trastuzumab. Most of these events occur within 24 hours of infusion, however delayed reactions have occurred. Use with caution in pre-existing pulmonary disease. Discontinuation of trastuzumab should be strongly considered in any patient who develops anaphylaxis, angioedema, or acute respiratory distress syndrome. Retreatment of patients who experienced severe hypersensitivity reactions has been attempted (with premedication). Some patients tolerated retreatment, while others experienced a second severe reaction.

Drug Interactions Paclitaxel may result in a decrease in clearance of trastuzumab, increasing serum concentration.

Drug Uptake Half-life, elimination: Mean: 5.8 days; Range: 1-32 days

Pregnancy Risk Factor B

Generic Available No

Trasylol® *see* Aprotinin *on page 109*

Travatan™ *see* Travoprost *on page 1193*

Travoprost (TRA voe prost)

U.S. Brand Names Travatan™

Mexican Brand Names Travatan®

Pharmacologic Category Prostaglandin, Ophthalmic

Use Reduction of elevated intraocular pressure in patients with open-angle glaucoma or ocular hypertension who are intolerant of the other IOP-lowering medications or insufficiently responsive (failed to achieve target IOP determined after multiple measurements over time) to another IOP-lowering medication

Local Anesthetic/Vasoconstrictor Precautions No information available to require special precautions

Effects on Dental Treatment No effects or complications reported

Dosage Ophthalmic: Adults: Glaucoma (open angle) or ocular hypertension: Instill 1 drop into affected eye(s) once daily in the evening; do not exceed once-daily dosing (may decrease IOP-lowering effect). If used with other topical ophthalmic agents, separate administration by at least 5 minutes.

Mechanism of Action A selective FP prostanoid receptor agonist which lowers intraocular pressure by increasing outflow

Other Adverse Effects

>10%: Ocular: Hyperemia (35% to 50%)

5% to 10%: Ocular: Decreased visual acuity, eye discomfort, foreign body sensation, pain, pruritus

1% to 5%:

- Cardiovascular: Angina pectoris, bradycardia, hypotension, hypertension
- Central nervous system: Depression, pain, anxiety, headache
- Endocrine & metabolic: Hypercholesterolemia
- Gastrointestinal: Dyspepsia
- Genitourinary: Prostate disorder, urinary incontinence
- Neuromuscular & skeletal: Arthritis, back pain, chest pain
- Ocular (1% to 4%): Abnormal vision, blepharitis, blurred vision, conjunctivitis, dry eye, iris discoloration, keratitis, lid margin crusting, photophobia, subconjunctival hemorrhage, cataract, tearing, periorbital skin discoloration (darkening), eyelash darkening, eyelash growth increased
- Respiratory: Bronchitis, sinusitis

Contraindications Hypersensitivity to travoprost or any component of the formulation; pregnancy

Drug Interactions Specific drug interactions have not been reported. When using more than one ophthalmic product, wait at least 5 minutes between application of each medication.

Drug Uptake

Onset of action: ~2 hours; Peak effect: 12 hours

Absorption: Via cornea; plasma concentrations ≤25 pg/mL ≤30 minutes

Duration: Plasma levels decrease to <10 pg/mL ≤1 hour

Pregnancy Risk Factor C

Generic Available No

Trazodone (TRAZ oh done)

U.S. Brand Names Desyrel®

Canadian Brand Names Alti-Trazodone; Apo®-Trazodone; Apo®-Trazodone D; Desyrel®; Gen-Trazodone; Novo-Trazodone; Nu-Trazodone; PMS-Trazodone; Trazorel

Pharmacologic Category Antidepressant, Serotonin Reuptake Inhibitor/Antagonist

Synonyms Trazodone Hydrochloride

Use Treatment of depression

Unlabeled/Investigational: Potential augmenting agent for antidepressants, hypnotic

Local Anesthetic/Vasoconstrictor Precautions No information available to require special precautions

(Continued)

Trazodone *(Continued)*

Effects on Dental Treatment

>10%: Xerostomia; especially in the elderly (may contribute to periodontal diseases and oral discomfort)

Trazodone elicits anticholinergic effects; much less frequent than with tricyclic antidepressants.

Dosage Oral: Therapeutic effects may take up to 6 weeks to occur; therapy is normally maintained for 6-12 months after optimum response is reached to prevent recurrence of depression

Children 6-12 years: Depression: Initial: 1.5-2 mg/kg/day in divided doses; increase gradually every 3-4 days as needed; maximum: 6 mg/kg/day in 3 divided doses

Adolescents: Depression: Initial: 25-50 mg/day; increase to 100-150 mg/day in divided doses

Adults:

Depression: Initial: 150 mg/day in 3 divided doses (may increase by 50 mg/day every 3-7 days); maximum: 600 mg/day

Sedation/hypnotic (unlabeled use): 25-50 mg at bedtime (often in combination with daytime SSRIs); may increase up to 200 mg at bedtime

Elderly: 25-50 mg at bedtime with 25-50 mg/day dose increase every 3 days for inpatients and weekly for outpatients, if tolerated; usual dose: 75-150 mg/day

Mechanism of Action Inhibits reuptake of serotonin and norepinephrine by the presynaptic neuronal membrane and desensitization of adenyl cyclase, down regulation of beta-adrenergic receptors, and down regulation of serotonin receptors. Causes adrenoreceptor subsensitivity, and induces significant changes in 5-HT presynaptic receptor adrenoreceptors. Trazodone also significantly blocks histamine (H_1) and alpha$_1$-adrenergic receptors.

Other Adverse Effects

>10%:

Central nervous system: Dizziness, headache, sedation

Gastrointestinal: Nausea, xerostomia

1% to 10%:

Cardiovascular: Syncope, hypertension, hypotension, edema

Central nervous system: Confusion, decreased concentration, fatigue, incoordination

Gastrointestinal: Diarrhea, constipation, weight gain/loss

Neuromuscular & skeletal: Tremor, myalgia

Ocular: Blurred vision

Respiratory: Nasal congestion

Drug Interactions CYP2D6 and 3A3/4 enzyme substrate

Increased Effect/Toxicity: Trazodone, in combination with other serotonergic agents (buspirone, MAO inhibitors), may produce additive serotonergic effects, including serotonin syndrome. Trazodone, in combination with other psychotropics (low potency antipsychotics), may result in additional hypotension. Fluoxetine may inhibit the metabolism of trazodone resulting in elevated plasma concentrations.

Decreased Effect: Trazodone inhibits the hypotensive response to clonidine.

Drug Uptake

Onset of action: Therapeutic: 1-3 weeks

Half-life, elimination: 4-7.5 hours, 2 compartment kinetics

Time to peak: 30-100 minutes; prolonged in presence of food (≤ 2.5 hours)

Pregnancy Risk Factor C

Generic Available Yes

Trecator®-SC *see* Ethionamide *on page 475*

Trelstar™ Depot *see* Triptorelin *on page 1215*

Trelstar™ LA *see* Triptorelin *on page 1215*

Trental® *see* Pentoxifylline *on page 937*

Treprostinil (tre PROST in il)

U.S. Brand Names Remodulin™

Pharmacologic Category Vasodilator

Synonyms Treprostinil Sodium

Use Treatment of pulmonary arterial hypertension (PAH) in patients with NYHA Class II-IV symptoms to decrease exercise-associated symptoms

Local Anesthetic/Vasoconstrictor Precautions No information available to require special precautions

Effects on Dental Treatment No effects or complications reported

Dosage S.C. infusion:

Adults: PAH: Initial: 1.25 ng/kg/minute continuous; if dose cannot be tolerated, reduce to 0.625 ng/kg/minute. Increase at rate not >1.25 ng/kg/minute per week for first 4 weeks, and not >2.5 ng/kg/minute per week for remainder of therapy. Limited experience with doses >40 ng/kg/minute.

Note: Dose must be carefully and individually titrated (symptom improvement with minimal adverse effects).

Elderly: Limited experience in patients >65 years; refer to adult dosing; use caution

Dosage adjustment in hepatic impairment:
Mild to moderate: Initial: 0.625 ng/kg/minute; increase with caution.
Severe: No data available.

Mechanism of Action Direct dilator of both pulmonary and systemic arterial vascular beds; inhibits platelet aggregation

Other Adverse Effects
>10%:
Cardiovascular: Vasodilation (11%)
Central nervous system: Headache (27%)
Dermatologic: Rash (14%)
Gastrointestinal: Diarrhea (25%), nausea (22%)
Local: Infusion site pain (85%), infusion site reaction (83%)
Miscellaneous: Jaw pain (13%)
1% to 10%:
Cardiovascular: Edema (9%), hypotension (4%)
Central nervous system: Dizziness (9%)
Dermatologic: Pruritus (8%)

Drug Interactions Increased Effect/Toxicity: Anticoagulants, antiplatelet agents, and NSAIDs; may increase risk of bleeding

Drug Uptake
Absorption: S.C.: Rapidly and completely
Half-life, elimination: Terminal: 2-4 hours

Pregnancy Risk Factor B

Generic Available No

Tretinoin, Oral (TRET i noyn, oral)

U.S. Brand Names Vesanoid®

Canadian Brand Names Vesanoid™

Pharmacologic Category Antineoplastic Agent, Miscellaneous

Synonyms All-*trans*-Retinoic Acid

Use Acute promyelocytic leukemia (APL): Induction of remission in patients with APL, French American British (FAB) classification M3 (including the M3 variant), characterized by the presence of the t(15;17) translocation or the presence of the PML/RARα gene who are refractory to or who have relapsed from anthracycline chemotherapy, or for whom anthracycline-based chemotherapy is contraindicated. Tretinoin is for the induction of remission only. All patients should receive an accepted form of remission consolidation or maintenance therapy for APL after completion of induction therapy with tretinoin.

Local Anesthetic/Vasoconstrictor Precautions No information available to require special precautions

Effects on Dental Treatment <1%: Bleeding gums, xerostomia

Mechanism of Action Retinoid that induces maturation of acute promyelocytic leukemia (APL) cells in cultures; induces cytodifferentiation and decreased proliferation of APL cells

Other Adverse Effects Virtually all patients experience some drug-related toxicity, especially headache, fever, weakness and fatigue. These adverse effects are seldom permanent or irreversible nor do they usually require therapy interruption
>10%:
Cardiovascular: Arrhythmias, flushing, hypotension, hypertension, peripheral edema, chest discomfort, edema
Central nervous system: Dizziness, anxiety, insomnia, depression, confusion, malaise, pain
Dermatologic: Burning, redness, cheilitis, inflammation of lips, dry skin, pruritus, photosensitivity
Endocrine & metabolic: Increased serum concentration of triglycerides
Gastrointestinal: GI hemorrhage, abdominal pain, other GI disorders, diarrhea, constipation, dyspepsia, abdominal distention, weight gain/loss, xerostomia
Hematologic: Hemorrhage, disseminated intravascular coagulation
Local: Phlebitis, injection site reactions
Neuromuscular & skeletal: Bone pain, arthralgia, myalgia, paresthesia
Ocular: Itching of eye
Renal: Renal insufficiency
Respiratory: Upper respiratory tract disorders, dyspnea, respiratory insufficiency, pleural effusion, pneumonia, rales, expiratory wheezing, dry nose
Miscellaneous: Infections, shivering
1% to 10%:
Cardiovascular: Cardiac failure, cardiac arrest, myocardial infarction, enlarged heart, heart murmur, ischemia, stroke, myocarditis, pericarditis, pulmonary hypertension, secondary cardiomyopathy, cerebral hemorrhage, pallor
Central nervous system: Intracranial hypertension, agitation, hallucination, agnosia, aphasia, cerebellar edema, cerebellar disorders, convulsions, coma, CNS depression, encephalopathy, hypotaxia, no light reflex, neurologic reaction, spinal cord disorder, unconsciousness, dementia, forgetfulness, somnolence, slow speech, hypothermia
Dermatologic: Skin peeling on hands or soles of feet, rash, cellulitis

(Continued)

Tretinoin, Oral *(Continued)*

Endocrine & metabolic: Fluid imbalance, acidosis
Gastrointestinal: Hepatosplenomegaly, ulcer
Genitourinary: Dysuria, polyuria, enlarged prostate
Hepatic: Ascites, hepatitis
Neuromuscular & skeletal: Tremor, leg weakness, hyporeflexia, dysarthria, facial paralysis, hemiplegia, flank pain, asterixis, abnormal gait
Ocular: Dry eyes, photophobia
Renal: Acute renal failure, renal tubular necrosis
Respiratory: Lower respiratory tract disorders, pulmonary infiltration, bronchial asthma, pulmonary/larynx edema, unspecified pulmonary disease
Miscellaneous: Face edema, lymph disorders

Warnings/Precautions Not to be used in women of childbearing potential unless woman is capable of complying with effective contraceptive measures; therapy is normally begun on the second or third day of next normal menstrual period; two reliable methods of effective contraception must be used during therapy and for 1 month after discontinuation of therapy, unless abstinence is the chosen method. Within 1 week prior to the institution of tretinoin therapy, the patient should have blood or urine collected for a serum or urine pregnancy test with a sensitivity of at least 50 mIU/L. When possible, delay tretinoin therapy until a negative result from this test is obtained. When a delay is not possible, place the patient on two reliable forms of contraception. Repeat pregnancy testing and contraception counseling monthly throughout the period of treatment.

Drug Interactions CYP3A3/4 enzyme substrate

Increased Effect/Toxicity: Ketoconazole increases the mean plasma AUC of tretinoin. Other drugs which inhibit CYP3A4 would be expected to increase tretinoin concentrations, potentially increasing toxicity.

Decreased Effect: Metabolized by the hepatic cytochrome P450 system: All drugs that induce this system would be expected to interact with tretinoin.

Drug Uptake

Half-life, elimination: Terminal: Parent drug: 0.5-2 hours
Time to peak: 1-2 hours

Pregnancy Risk Factor D

Generic Available No

Tretinoin, Topical (TRET i noyn, TOP i kal)

U.S. Brand Names Altinac™; Avita®; Renova®; Retin-A®; Retin-A® Micro

Canadian Brand Names Rejuva-A®; Retin-A®; Retinova®

Mexican Brand Names Stieva-A®

Pharmacologic Category Retinoic Acid Derivative

Synonyms Retinoic Acid; *trans*-Retinoic Acid; Vitamin A Acid

Use Treatment of acne vulgaris; photodamaged skin; palliation of fine wrinkles, mottled hyperpigmentation, and tactile roughness of facial skin as part of a comprehensive skin care and sun avoidance program

Unlabeled/Investigational: Some skin cancers

Local Anesthetic/Vasoconstrictor Precautions No information available to require special precautions

Effects on Dental Treatment No effects or complications reported

Dosage Topical:

Children >12 years and Adults: Apply once daily before retiring; if stinging or irritation develops, decrease frequency of application. Relapses normally occur within 3-6 weeks after stopping medication.

Adults ≥18: Palliation of fine wrinkles, mottled hyperpigmentation, and tactile roughness of facial skin: Pea-sized amount of the 0.02% or 0.05% emollient cream applied to entire face once daily in the evening

Elderly: Use of the 0.02% emollient cream in patients 65-71 years of age showed similar improvement in fine wrinkles as seen in patients <65 years. Safety and efficacy of the 0.02% cream have not been established in patients >71 years of age. Safety and efficacy of the 0.05% cream have not been established in patients >50 years of age.

Mechanism of Action Keratinocytes in the sebaceous follicle become less adherent which allows for easy removal; decreases microcomedone formation

Other Adverse Effects 1% to 10%:

Cardiovascular: Edema
Dermatologic: Excessive dryness, erythema, scaling of the skin, hyperpigmentation or hypopigmentation, photosensitivity, initial acne flare-up
Local: Stinging, blistering

Drug Interactions CYP3A3/4 enzyme substrate

Increased Effect/Toxicity: Topical application of sulfur, benzoyl peroxide, salicylic acid, resorcinol, or any product with strong drying effects potentiates adverse reactions with tretinoin. Photosensitizing medications (thiazides, tetracyclines, fluoroquinolones, phenothiazines, sulfonamides) augment phototoxicity and should not be used when treating palliation of fine wrinkles, mottled hyperpigmentation, and tactile roughness of facial skin.

Drug Uptake Absorption: Topical: Minimal
Pregnancy Risk Factor C
Generic Available No

Trexall™ *see* Methotrexate *on page 788*
Triacet™ *see* Triamcinolone *on page 1197*

Triacetin (trye a SEE tin)

U.S. Brand Names Ony-Clear® Nail [OTC]
Pharmacologic Category Antifungal Agent, Topical
Synonyms Glycerol Triacetate
Use Fungistat for athlete's foot and other superficial fungal infections
Local Anesthetic/Vasoconstrictor Precautions No information available to require special precautions
Effects on Dental Treatment No effects or complications reported
Dosage Apply twice daily, cleanse areas with dilute alcohol or mild soap and water before application; continue treatment for 7 days after symptoms have disappeared
Generic Available No

Triacin® [OTC] *see* Triprolidine and Pseudoephedrine *on page 1213*
Triacin-C® *see* Triprolidine, Pseudoephedrine, and Codeine *on page 1214*
Triafed® [OTC] *see* Triprolidine and Pseudoephedrine *on page 1213*
Triam-A® *see* Triamcinolone *on page 1197*

Triamcinolone (trye am SIN oh lone)

Related Information
Oral Nonviral Soft Tissue Ulcerations or Erosions *on page 1384*
Respiratory Diseases *on page 1328*

U.S. Brand Names Amcort®; Aristocort®; Aristocort® A; Aristocort® Forte; Aristocort® Intralesional; Aristospan® Intra-Articular; Aristospan® Intralesional; Atolone®; Azmacort®; Delta-Tritex®; Flutex®; Kenacort®; Kenaject-40®; Kenalog®; Kenalog-10®; Kenalog-40®; Kenalog® H; Kenalog® in Orabase®; Kenonel®; Nasacort®; Nasacort® AQ; Tac™-3; Tac™-40; Triacet™; Triam-A®; Triam Forte®; Triderm®; Tri-Kort®; Trilog®; Trilone®; Tri-Nasal®; Tristoject®
Canadian Brand Names Aristocort®; Aristospan®; Azmacort®; Kenalog®; Kenalog® in Orabase; Nasacort™; Nasacort® AQ; Oracort; Triaderm; Trinasal®
Mexican Brand Names Kenacort®; Ledercort; Triamsicort®; Zamacort®
Pharmacologic Category Corticosteroid, Adrenal; Corticosteroid, Inhalant (Oral); Corticosteroid, Nasal; Corticosteroid, Systemic; Corticosteroid, Topical
Synonyms Triamcinolone Acetonide, Aerosol; Triamcinolone Acetonide, Parenteral; Triamcinolone Diacetate, Oral; Triamcinolone Diacetate, Parenteral; Triamcinolone Hexacetonide; Triamcinolone, Oral
Use
Inhalation: Control of bronchial asthma and related bronchospastic conditions.
Intranasal: Management of seasonal and perennial allergic rhinitis in patients ≥12 years of age
Systemic: Adrenocortical insufficiency, rheumatic disorders, allergic states, respiratory diseases, systemic lupus erythematosus, and other diseases requiring anti-inflammatory or immunosuppressive effects
Topical: Inflammatory dermatoses responsive to steroids

Local Anesthetic/Vasoconstrictor Precautions No information available to require special precautions
Effects on Dental Treatment No effects or complications reported
Dosage In general, single I.M. dose of 4-7 times oral dose will control patient from 4-7 days up to 3-4 weeks.

Children 6-12 years:
- Oral inhalation: 1-2 inhalations 3-4 times/day, not to exceed 12 inhalations/day
- I.M. (acetonide or hexacetonide): 0.03-0.2 mg/kg at 1- to 7-day intervals
- Intra-articular, intrabursal, or tendon-sheath injection: 2.5-15 mg, repeated as needed

Children >12 years and Adults:
- Intranasal: 2 sprays in each nostril once daily; may increase after 4-7 days up to 4 sprays once daily or 1 spray 4 times/day in each nostril
- Topical: Apply a thin film 2-3 times/day
- Oral: 4-48 mg/day
- I.M.: Acetonide or hexacetonide: 60 mg (of 40 mg/mL), additional 20-100 mg doses (usual: 40-80 mg) may be given when signs and symptoms recur, best at 6-week intervals to minimize HPA suppression
- Oral inhalation: 2 inhalations 3-4 times/day, not to exceed 16 inhalations/day
- Intra-articular (hexacetonide): 2-20 mg every 3-4 weeks as hexacetonide salt
- Intralesional (use 10 mg/mL) (diacetate or acetonide): 1 mg/injection site, may be repeated one or more times/week depending upon patients response; maximum; 30 mg at any one time; may use multiple injections if they are >1 cm apart

(Continued)

Triamcinolone *(Continued)*

Intra-articular, intrasynovial, and soft-tissue injection (use 10 mg/mL or 40 mg/mL) (diacetate or acetonide): 2.5-40 mg depending upon location, size of joints, and degree of inflammation; repeat when signs and symptoms recur

Sublesional (as acetonide): Up to 1 mg per injection site and may be repeated one or more times weekly; multiple sites may be injected if they are 1 cm or more apart, not to exceed 30 mg

See table.

Triamcinolone Dosing

	Acetonide	Diacetate	Hexacetonide
Intrasynovial	2.5-40 mg	5-40 mg	
Intralesional	2.5-40 mg	5-40 mg (not >25 mg per lesion)	Up to 0.5 mg/sq inch affected area
Sublesional	1-30 mg		
Systemic I.M.	60 mg/day; 20-100 mg/day upon recurrence	~40 mg/week	
Intra-articular		2-40 mg	2-20 mg average
large joints	15-40 mg		10-20 mg
small joints	2.5-10 mg		2-6 mg
Tendon sheaths	2.5-10 mg		
Intradermal	1 mg/site		

Therapy should be discontinued when control is achieved; if no improvement is seen, reassessment of diagnosis may be necessary.

Mechanism of Action Decreases inflammation by suppression of migration of polymorphonuclear leukocytes and reversal of increased capillary permeability; suppresses the immune system by reducing activity and volume of the lymphatic system; suppresses adrenal function at high doses

Other Adverse Effects

Systemic:

>10%:

Central nervous system: Insomnia, nervousness

Gastrointestinal: Increased appetite, indigestion

1% to 10%:

Central nervous system: Dizziness, lightheadedness, headache

Dermatologic: Hirsutism, hypopigmentation

Endocrine & metabolic: Diabetes mellitus

Neuromuscular & skeletal: Arthralgia

Ocular: Cataracts, glaucoma

Respiratory: Epistaxis

Miscellaneous: Diaphoresis

<1% (Limited to important or life-threatening): Edema, hypertension, seizures, Cushing's syndrome, pituitary-adrenal axis suppression

Topical:

1% to 10%:

Dermatologic: Itching, allergic contact dermatitis, erythema, dryness papular rashes, folliculitis, furunculosis, pustules, pyoderma, vesiculation, hyperesthesia, skin infection (secondary)

Local: Burning, irritation

<1% (Limited to important or life-threatening): Gastric ulcer, glaucoma, cataracts (posterior subcapsular)

Contraindications Hypersensitivity to triamcinolone or any component of the formulation; systemic fungal infections; serious infections (except septic shock or tuberculous meningitis); primary treatment of status asthmaticus

Warnings/Precautions Fatalities have occurred due to adrenal insufficiency in asthmatic patients during and after transfer from systemic corticosteroids to aerosol steroids; several months may be required for recovery from this syndrome; during this period, aerosol steroids do **not** provide the increased systemic steroid requirement needed to treat patients having trauma, surgery or infections; avoid using higher than recommended dose

Use with caution in patients with hypothyroidism, cirrhosis, nonspecific ulcerative colitis and patients at increased risk for peptic ulcer disease. Corticosteroids should be used with caution in patients with diabetes, hypertension, osteoporosis, glaucoma, cataracts, or tuberculosis. Use caution in hepatic impairment. Do not use occlusive dressings on weeping or exudative lesions and general caution with occlusive dressings should be observed; discontinue if skin irritation or contact dermatitis should occur; do not use in patients with decreased skin circulation; avoid the use of high potency steroids on the face.

Because of the risk of adverse effects, systemic corticosteroids should be used cautiously in the elderly, in the smallest possible dose, and for the shortest possible time. Azmacort® (metered dose inhaler) comes with its own spacer device attached and may be easier to use in older patients. Controlled clinical studies have shown that inhaled and intranasal corticosteroids may cause a reduction in growth velocity in pediatric patients. Growth velocity provides a means of comparing the rate of growth among children of the same age.

In studies involving inhaled corticosteroids, the average reduction in growth velocity was approximately 1 cm (about 1/3 of an inch) per year. It appears that the reduction is related to dose and how long the child takes the drug.

FDA's Pulmonary and Allergy Drugs and Metabolic and Endocrine Drugs advisory committees discussed this issue at a July 1998 meeting. They recommended that the agency develop classwide labeling to inform healthcare providers so they would understand this potential side effect and monitor growth routinely in pediatric patients who are treated with inhaled corticosteroids, intranasal corticosteroids or both.

Long-term effects of this reduction in growth velocity on final adult height are unknown. Likewise, it also has not yet been determined whether patients' growth will "catch up" if treatment in discontinued. Drug manufacturers will continue to monitor these drugs to learn more about long-term effects. Children are prescribed inhaled corticosteroids to treat asthma. Intranasal corticosteroids are generally used to prevent and treat allergy-related nasal symptoms.

Patients are advised not to stop using their inhaled or intranasal corticosteroids without first speaking to their healthcare providers about the benefits of these drugs compared to their risks.

Drug Interactions

Increased Effect: The addition of salmeterol has been demonstrated to improve response to inhaled corticosteroids (as compared to increasing steroid dosage).

Increased Toxicity: Salicylates may increase risk of GI ulceration.

Decreased Effect: Barbiturates, phenytoin, rifampin increase metabolism of triamcinolone; vaccine and toxoid effects may be reduced.

Dietary/Ethanol/Herb Considerations

Ethanol: Avoid use; may enhance gastric mucosal irritation.

Food: Administer with food to reduce GI upset; food interferes with calcium absorption.

Herb/Nutraceutical: Avoid cat's claw and echinacea due to immunostimulant properties.

Drug Uptake

Duration: Oral: 8-12 hours

Absorption: Topical: Systemic

Time to peak: I.M.: 8-10 hours

Half-life, elimination: Biologic: 18-36 hours

Pregnancy Risk Factor C

Dosage Forms AERO, oral inhalation (Azmacort®): 100 mcg/metered spray (20 g). **AERO, topical, as acetonide:** 0.2 mg/2 second spray (23 g, 63 g). **CRM, as acetonide:** 0.025% (15 g, 60 g, 80 g, 240 g, 454 g); 0.1% (15 g, 30 g, 60 g, 80 g, 90 g, 120 g, 240 g); 0.5% (15 g, 20 g, 30 g, 240 g). **INJ, as acetonide:** 10 mg/mL (5 mL); 40 mg/mL (1 mL, 5 mL, 10 mL). **INJ, as diacetate:** 25 mg/mL (5 mL); 40 mg/mL (1 mL, 5 mL, 10 mL). **INJ, as hexacetonide:** 5 mg/mL (5 mL); 20 mg/mL (1 mL, 5 mL). **LOTION, as acetonide:** 0.025% (60 mL); 0.1% (15 mL, 60 mL). **OINT, as acetonide:** 0.025% (15 g, 30 g, 60 g, 80 g, 120 g, 454 g); 0.1% (15 g, 30 g, 60 g, 80 g, 120 g, 240 g, 454 g); 0.5% (15 g, 20 g, 30 g, 240 g). **PASTE, oral topical, as acetonide** (Kenalog® in Orabase®): 0.1% (5 g). **SPRAY, intranasal:** (Nasacort®, Nasacort® AQ™): 55 mcg per actuation (15 mL); (Tri-Nasal®): 50 mcg per actuation (15 mL). **SYR:** 2 mg/5 mL (120 mL); 4 mg/5 mL (120 mL). **TAB:** 1 mg, 2 mg, 4 mg, 8 mg

Generic Available Yes

Comments Triamcinolone 16 mg is equivalent to cortisone 100 mg (no mineralocorticoid activity)

Triamcinolone Acetonide Dental Paste

(trye am SIN oh lone a SEE toe nide DEN tal paste)

U.S. Brand Names Kenalog® in Orabase®

Canadian Brand Names Oracort®

Pharmacologic Category Anti-inflammatory Agent; Corticosteroid, Topical

Use

Dental: For adjunctive treatment and for the temporary relief of symptoms associated with oral inflammatory lesions and ulcerative lesions resulting from trauma

Medical: Localized inflammation responsive to steroids

Local Anesthetic/Vasoconstrictor Precautions No information available to require special precautions

Effects on Dental Treatment No effects or complications reported

(Continued)

Triamcinolone Acetonide Dental Paste *(Continued)*

Dosage Press a small dab (about 1/4 inch) to the lesion until a thin film develops. A larger quantity may be required for coverage of some lesions. For optimal results use only enough to coat the lesion with a thin film.

Mechanism of Action Decreases inflammation by suppression of migration of polymorphonuclear leukocytes and reversal of increased capillary permeability; suppresses the immune system by reducing activity and volume of the lymphatic system; suppresses adrenal function at high doses

Contraindications Hypersensitivity to triamcinolone or any component of the formulation; presence of fungal, viral, or bacterial infections of the mouth or throat

Warnings/Precautions Patients with tuberculosis, peptic ulcer or diabetes mellitus should not be treated with any corticosteroid preparation without the advice of the patient's physician. Normal immune responses of the oral tissues are depressed in patients receiving topical corticosteroid therapy. Virulent strains of oral microorganisms may multiply without producing the usual warning symptoms of oral infections. The small amount of steroid released from the topical preparation makes systemic effects very unlikely. If local irritation or sensitization should develop, the preparation should be discontinued. If significant regeneration or repair of oral tissues has not occurred in seven days, re-evaluation of the etiology of the oral lesion is advised.

Dietary/Ethanol/Herb Considerations Herb/Nutraceutical: Avoid cat's claw and echinacea due to immunostimulant properties.

Drug Uptake
Absorption: Systemic
Half-life, elimination: Biological: 18-36 hours

Pregnancy Risk Factor C

Dosage Forms PASTE, dental: 5 g [each g provides 1 mg (0.1%) triamcinolone in emollient dental paste containing gelatin, pectin, and carboxymethylcellulose sodium in a polyethylene and mineral oil gel base]

Generic Available Yes

Comments When applying to tissues, attempts to spread this preparation may result in a granular, gritty sensation and cause it to crumble. This preparation should be applied at bedtime to permit steroid contact with the lesion throughout the night.

Triam Forte® *see* Triamcinolone *on page 1197*
Triaminic® AM Decongestant Formula [OTC] *see* Pseudoephedrine *on page 1022*
Triaminic® Infant Decongestant [OTC] *see* Pseudoephedrine *on page 1022*
Triaminic® Sore Throat Formula [OTC] *see* Acetaminophen, Dextromethorphan, and Pseudoephedrine *on page 34*

Triamterene (trye AM ter een)

Related Information
Cardiovascular Diseases *on page 1308*

U.S. Brand Names Dyrenium®

Canadian Brand Names Dyrenium®

Pharmacologic Category Diuretic, Potassium Sparing

Use Alone or in combination with other diuretics in treatment of edema and hypertension; decreases potassium excretion caused by kaliuretic diuretics

Local Anesthetic/Vasoconstrictor Precautions No information available to require special precautions

Effects on Dental Treatment No effects or complications reported

Dosage Oral:
Children: 2-4 mg/kg/day in 1-2 divided doses; maximum: 300 mg/day
Adults: 100-300 mg/day in 1-2 divided doses; maximum dose: 300 mg/day

Mechanism of Action Competes with aldosterone for receptor sites in the distal renal tubules, increasing sodium, chloride, and water excretion while conserving potassium and hydrogen ions; decreases calcium excretion; increases magnesium loss; may block the effect of aldosterone on arteriolar smooth muscle as well

Other Adverse Effects 1% to 10%:
Cardiovascular: Hypotension, edema, CHF, bradycardia
Central nervous system: Dizziness, headache, fatigue
Gastrointestinal: Constipation, nausea
Respiratory: Dyspnea

Drug Interactions Increased Effect/Toxicity: Angiotensin-converting enzyme inhibitors or spironolactone can cause hyperkalemia, especially in patients with renal impairment, potassium-rich diets, or on other drugs causing hyperkalemia; avoid concurrent use or monitor closely. Potassium supplements may further increase potassium retention and cause hyperkalemia; avoid concurrent use.

Drug Uptake
Onset of action: Diuresis: 2-4 hours
Absorption: Oral: Unreliable
Duration: 7-9 hours

Pregnancy Risk Factor B (manufacturer); D (expert analysis)

Generic Available No

Triavil® *see* Amitriptyline and Perphenazine *on page 77*
Triaz® *see* Benzoyl Peroxide *on page 153*
Triaz® Cleanser *see* Benzoyl Peroxide *on page 153*

Triazolam (trye AY zoe lam)

Related Information

Dental Drug Interactions: Update on Drug Combinations Requiring Special Considerations *on page 1434*

Patients Requiring Sedation *on page 1400*

U.S. Brand Names Halcion®

Canadian Brand Names Apo®-Triazo; Gen-Triazolam; Halcion®

Mexican Brand Names Halcion®

Pharmacologic Category Benzodiazepine

Use

Dental: Oral premedication before dental procedures

Medical: Short-term treatment of insomnia

Local Anesthetic/Vasoconstrictor Precautions No information available to require special precautions

Effects on Dental Treatment No effects or complications reported

Restrictions C-IV

Dosage Oral:

Children <18 years: Dosage not established

Adults: 0.25 mg taken the evening before oral surgery; or 0.25 mg 1 hour before procedure

Mechanism of Action Binds to stereospecific benzodiazepine receptors on the postsynaptic GABA (gamma-aminobutyric acid) neuron at several sites within the CNS, including the limbic system, reticular formation. Enhancement of the inhibitory effect of GABA on neuronal excitability results by increased neuronal membrane permeability to chloride ions. This shift in chloride ions results in hyperpolarization (a less excitable state) and stabilization.

Other Adverse Effects

>10%: Central nervous system: Drowsiness, anteriograde amnesia

1% to 10%:

- Central nervous system: Headache, dizziness, nervousness, lightheadedness, ataxia
- Gastrointestinal: Nausea, vomiting

<1%: Cramps, confusion, depression, euphoria, fatigue, memory impairment, pain, tachycardia, visual disturbance

Contraindications Hypersensitivity to triazolam or any component of the formulation (cross-sensitivity with other benzodiazepines may exist); concurrent therapy with CYP3A3/4 inhibitors (including ketoconazole, itraconazole, and nefazodone); pregnancy

Warnings/Precautions May cause drug dependency; avoid abrupt discontinuance in patients with prolonged therapy or seizure disorders; not considered a drug of choice in the elderly

Drug Interactions CYP3A3/4 and 3A5-7 enzyme substrate

CNS depressants: Sedative effects and/or respiratory depression may be additive with CNS depressants; includes barbiturates, narcotic analgesics, and other sedative agents; monitor for increased effect

CYP3A3/4 inhibitors: Serum level and/or toxicity of some benzodiazepines may be increased; inhibitors include amiodarone, cimetidine, clarithromycin, erythromycin, delavirdine, diltiazem, dirithromycin, disulfiram, fluoxetine, fluvoxamine, grapefruit juice, indinavir, itraconazole, ketoconazole, nefazodone, nevirapine, propoxyphene, quinupristin-dalfopristin, ritonavir, saquinavir, verapamil, zafirlukast, zileuton; monitor for altered benzodiazepine response

Enzyme inducers: Metabolism of some benzodiazepines may be increased, decreasing their therapeutic effect; consider using an alternative sedative/hypnotic agent; potential inducers include phenobarbital, phenytoin, carbamazepine, rifampin, and rifabutin

Levodopa: Therapeutic effects may be diminished in some patients following the addition of a benzodiazepine; limited/inconsistent data

Oral contraceptives: May decrease the clearance of some benzodiazepines (those which undergo oxidative metabolism); monitor for increased benzodiazepine effect

Theophylline: May partially antagonize some of the effects of benzodiazepines; monitor for decreased response; may require higher doses for sedation

Dietary/Ethanol/Herb Considerations

Ethanol: Avoid use; may increase CNS depression.

Food may decrease the rate of absorption. Avoid grapefruit products; may increase serum concentration.

Herb/Nutraceutical: Avoid gotu kola, kava, SAMe, and valerian; may increase CNS depression. Avoid St John's wort; may decrease serum concentration and

(Continued)

Triazolam *(Continued)*

increase CNS depression. Melatonin may increase benzodiazepine binding at receptor sites causing enhancement of activity of triazolam; use cautiously.

Drug Uptake

Onset of action: Hypnotic: 15-30 minutes
Duration: 6-7 hours
Half-life, elimination: 1.7-5 hours

Pregnancy Risk Factor X

Dosage Forms TAB: 0.125 mg, 0.25 mg

Generic Available Yes

Comments Triazolam (0.25 mg) 1 hour prior to dental procedure has been used as an oral pre-op sedative

Selected Readings

Berthold CW, Dionne RA, and Corey SE, "Comparison of Sublingually and Orally Administered Triazolam for Premedication Before Oral Surgery," *Oral Surg Oral Med Oral Pathol Oral Radiol Endod*, 1997, 84(2):119-24.

Berthold CW, Schneider A, and Dionne RA, "Using Triazolam to Reduce Dental Anxiety," *J Am Dent Assoc*, 1993, 124(11):58-64.

Kaufman E, Hargreaves KM, and Dionne RA, "Comparison of Oral Triazolam and Nitrous Oxide With Placebo and Intravenous Diazepam for Outpatient Premedication," *Oral Surg Oral Med Oral Pathol*, 1993, 75(2):156-64.

Kurzrock M, "Triazolam and Dental Anxiety," *J Am Dent Assoc*, 1994, 125(4):358, 360.

Lieblich SE and Horswell B, "Attenuation of Anxiety in Ambulatory Oral Surgery Patients With Oral Triazolam," *J Oral Maxillofac Surg*, 1991, 49(8):792-7.

Milgrom P, Quarnstrom FC, Longley A, et al, "The Efficacy and Memory Effects of Oral Triazolam Premedication in Highly Anxious Dental Patients," *Anesth Prog*, 1994, 41(3):70-6.

Tri-Chlor® *see* Trichloroacetic Acid *on page 1203*

Trichlormethiazide (trye klor meth EYE a zide)

Related Information

Cardiovascular Diseases *on page 1308*

U.S. Brand Names Metahydrin®; Naqua®

Canadian Brand Names Metahydrin®; Metatensin®; Naqua®; Trichlorex®

Pharmacologic Category Diuretic, Thiazide

Use Management of mild to moderate hypertension; treatment of edema in CHF and nephrotic syndrome

Local Anesthetic/Vasoconstrictor Precautions No information available to require special precautions

Effects on Dental Treatment No effects or complications reported

Dosage Oral:

Children >6 months: 0.07 mg/kg/24 hours or 2 mg/m²/24 hours
Adults: 1-4 mg/day

Mechanism of Action The diuretic mechanism of action of the thiazides is primarily inhibition of sodium, chloride, and water reabsorption in the renal distal tubules, thereby producing diuresis with a resultant reduction in plasma volume. The antihypertensive mechanism of action of the thiazides is unknown. It is known that doses of thiazides produce greater reduction in BP than equivalent diuretic doses of loop diuretics. There has been speculation that the thiazides may have some influence on vascular tone mediated through sodium depletion, but this remains to be proven.

Other Adverse Effects 1% to 10%:

Endocrine & metabolic: Hypokalemia
Respiratory: Dyspnea (<5%)

Warnings/Precautions Avoid in severe renal disease (ineffective). Electrolyte disturbances (hypokalemia, hypochloremic alkalosis, hyponatremia) can occur. Use with caution in severe hepatic dysfunction; hepatic encephalopathy can be caused by electrolyte disturbances. Gout can be precipitate in certain patients with a history of gout, a familial predisposition to gout, or chronic renal failure. Cautious use in diabetics; may see a change in glucose control. Hypersensitivity reactions can occur. Can cause SLE exacerbation or activation. Use with caution in patients with moderate or high cholesterol concentrations. Photosensitization may occur. Correct hypokalemia before initiating therapy.

Chemical similarities are present among sulfonamides, sulfonylureas, carbonic anhydrase inhibitors, thiazides, and loop diuretics (except ethacrynic acid). Use in patients with thiazide or sulfonamide allergy is specifically contraindicated in product labeling, however a risk of cross-reaction exists in patients with allergy to any of these compounds; avoid use when previous reaction has been severe.

Drug Interactions

Increased Effect/Toxicity: Increased effect of thiazides with furosemide and other loop diuretics. Increased hypotension and/or renal adverse effects of ACE inhibitors may result in aggressively diuresed patients. Beta-blockers increase hyperglycemic effects of thiazides in type 2 diabetes mellitus. Cyclosporine and thiazides can increase the risk of gout or renal toxicity. Digoxin toxicity can be exacerbated if a thiazide induces hypokalemia or hypomagnesemia. Lithium toxicity can occur with thiazides due to reduced renal excretion of lithium. Thiazides may prolong the duration of action with neuromuscular blocking agents.

Decreased Effect: Effects of oral hypoglycemics may be decreased. Decreased absorption of thiazides with cholestyramine and colestipol. NSAIDs can decrease the efficacy of thiazides, reducing the diuretic and antihypertensive effects.

Drug Uptake

Onset of action: Diuresis: ~2 hours; Peak effect: 4 hours

Duration: 12-24 hours

Pregnancy Risk Factor D

Generic Available Yes

Trichloroacetic Acid (trye klor oh a SEE tik AS id)

U.S. Brand Names Tri-Chlor®

Pharmacologic Category Keratolytic Agent

Use Debride callous tissue

Local Anesthetic/Vasoconstrictor Precautions No information available to require special precautions

Effects on Dental Treatment No effects or complications reported

Dosage Apply to verruca, cover with bandage for 5-6 days, remove verruca, reapply as needed

Generic Available Yes

Triclosan and Fluoride (trye KLOE san & FLOR ide)

Related Information

Periodontal Diseases *on page 1375*

U.S. Brand Names Colgate Total® Toothpaste

Pharmacologic Category Antibacterial, Dental; Mineral, Oral, Topical

Synonyms Fluoride and Triclosan (Dental)

Use Anticavity, antigingivitis, antiplaque toothpaste

Local Anesthetic/Vasoconstrictor Precautions No information available to require special precautions

Effects on Dental Treatment No effects or complications reported

Dosage Brush teeth thoroughly after each meal or at least twice daily

Mechanism of Action Triclosan an antibacterial agent which helps to prevent gingivitis with regular use. Fluoride promotes remineralization of decalcified enamel, inhibits the cariogenic microbial process in dental plaque, and increases tooth resistance to acid dissolution.

Warnings/Precautions Antigingivitis and antiplaque effects have not been determined in children <6 years of age. If an amount greater than used for brushing is swallowed, seek professional assistance of contact a poison control center immediately.

Comments It has been shown that stannous fluoride and triclosan when formulated into a toothpaste vehicle provide plaque inhibitory effects. To provide a longer retention time of the triclosan in plaque, a polymer has been added to the toothpaste vehicle. The polymer is known as PVM/MA which stands for polyvinylmethyl ether/maleic acid copolymer, and is listed as an inactive ingredient (PVM/MA Copolymer) on the manufacturer's label. Studies have reported that the retention of triclosan in plaque (exceeding the minimal inhibitory concentration) after polymer application was 14 hours after brushing. Ongoing studies are evaluating the effects of triclosan/copolymer on alveolar bone loss. Rosling et al. have reported that the daily use of Colgate Total® reduced (1) the frequency of deep periodontal pockets and (2) the number of sites that exhibited additional probing attachment and bone loss.

Selected Readings

Binney A, Addy M, Owens J, et al, "A Comparison of Triclosan and Stannous Fluoride Toothpastes for Inhibition of Plaque Regrowth. A Crossover Study Designed to Access Carry Over," *J Clin Periodontol*, 1997, 24(3):166-70.

Ellwood RP, Worthington HV, Blinkhorn AS, et al, "Effect of a Triclosan/Copolymer Dentifrice on the Incidence of Periodontal Attachment Loss in Adolescents," *J Clin Periodontol*, 1998, 25(5):363-7.

Mandel ID, "The New Toothpastes," *J Calif Dent Assoc*, 1998, 26(3):186-90.

Rosling B, Wannfors B, Volpe AR, et a, "The Use of a Triclosan/Copolymer Dentifrice May Retard the Progression of Periodontitis," *J Clin Periodontol*, 1997, 24(12):873-80.

TriCor® *see* Fenofibrate *on page 490*

Tricosal® *see* Choline Magnesium Trisalicylate *on page 279*

Triderm® *see* Triamcinolone *on page 1197*

Tridesilon® *see* Desonide *on page 362*

Tridihexethyl (trye dye heks ETH il)

U.S. Brand Names Pathilon®

Pharmacologic Category Anticholinergic Agent; Antispasmodic Agent, Gastrointestinal

Synonyms Tridihexethyl Chloride

Use Adjunctive therapy in peptic ulcer treatment

Local Anesthetic/Vasoconstrictor Precautions No information available to require special precautions

Effects on Dental Treatment >10%: Xerostomia

Dosage Adults: Oral: 1-2 tablets 3-4 times/day before meals and 2 tablets at bedtime

(Continued)

Tridihexethyl *(Continued)*

Other Adverse Effects

>10%:

Dermatologic: Dry skin

Gastrointestinal: Constipation, xerostomia, dry throat

Respiratory: Dry nose

Miscellaneous: Decreased diaphoresis

1% to 10%: Gastrointestinal: Dysphagia

Drug Interactions Potassium chloride wax-matrix preparations

Pregnancy Risk Factor C

Generic Available No

Tridil® *see* Nitroglycerin *on page 871*

Tridione® *see* Trimethadione *on page 1209*

Triethanolamine Polypeptide Oleate-Condensate

(trye eth a NOLE a meen pol i PEP tide OH lee ate-KON den sate)

U.S. Brand Names Cerumenex®

Canadian Brand Names Cerumenex®

Pharmacologic Category Otic Agent, Cerumenolytic

Use Removal of ear wax (cerumen)

Local Anesthetic/Vasoconstrictor Precautions No information available to require special precautions

Effects on Dental Treatment No effects or complications reported

Dosage Children and Adults: Otic: Fill ear canal, insert cotton plug; allow to remain 15-30 minutes; flush ear with lukewarm water as a single treatment; if a second application is needed for unusually hard impactions, repeat the procedure

Mechanism of Action Emulsifies and disperses accumulated cerumen

Drug Uptake Onset of action: Slight disintegration of very hard ear wax by 24 hours

Pregnancy Risk Factor C

Generic Available No

Triethanolamine Salicylate (trye eth a NOLE a meen sa LIS i late)

U.S. Brand Names Myoflex® [OTC]; Sportscreme® [OTC]

Canadian Brand Names Antiphlogistine Rub A-535 No Odour; Myoflex®

Pharmacologic Category Analgesic, Topical; Salicylate; Topical Skin Product

Use Relief of pain of muscular aches, rheumatism, neuralgia, sprains, arthritis on intact skin

Local Anesthetic/Vasoconstrictor Precautions No information available to require special precautions

Effects on Dental Treatment No effects or complications reported

Dosage Apply to area as needed

Other Adverse Effects 1% to 10%:

Central nervous system: Confusion, drowsiness

Gastrointestinal: Nausea, vomiting, diarrhea

Respiratory: Hyperventilation

Generic Available No

Tri-Fed® [OTC] *see* Triprolidine and Pseudoephedrine *on page 1213*

Trifluoperazine (trye floo oh PER a zeen)

U.S. Brand Names Stelazine®

Canadian Brand Names Apo®-Trifluoperazine; Stelazine®

Mexican Brand Names Flupazine®; Stelazine®

Pharmacologic Category Antipsychotic Agent, Phenothiazine, Piperazine

Synonyms Trifluoperazine Hydrochloride

Use Treatment of schizophrenia

Unlabeled/Investigational: Management of psychotic disorders

Local Anesthetic/Vasoconstrictor Precautions Most pharmacology textbooks state that in presence of phenothiazines, systemic doses of epinephrine paradoxically decrease the blood pressure. This is the so called "epinephrine reversal" phenomenon. This has never been observed when epinephrine is given by infiltration as part of the anesthesia procedure.

Effects on Dental Treatment

Significant hypotension may occur, especially when the drug is administered parenterally; orthostatic hypotension is due to alpha-receptor blockade, the elderly are at greater risk for orthostatic hypotension.

Tardive dyskinesia: Prevalence rate may be 40% in elderly; development of the syndrome and the irreversible nature are proportional to duration and total cumulative dose over time. Extrapyramidal reactions are more common in elderly with up to 50% developing these reactions after 60 years of age; drug-induced **Parkinson's syndrome** occurs often; **Akathisia** is the most common extrapyramidal reaction in elderly.

Increased confusion, memory loss, psychotic behavior, and agitation frequently occur as a consequence of anticholinergic effects. Antipsychotic associated sedation in nonpsychotic patients is extremely unpleasant due to feelings of depersonalization, derealization, and dysphoria.

Dosage

Children 6-12 years: Schizophrenia/psychoses:

Oral: Hospitalized or well-supervised patients: Initial: 1 mg 1-2 times/day, gradually increase until symptoms are controlled or adverse effects become troublesome; maximum: 15 mg/day

I.M.: 1 mg twice daily

Adults:

Schizophrenia/psychoses:

Outpatients: Oral: 1-2 mg twice daily

Hospitalized or well-supervised patients: Initial: 2-5 mg twice daily with optimum response in the 15-20 mg/day range; do not exceed 40 mg/day

I.M.: 1-2 mg every 4-6 hours as needed up to 10 mg/24 hours maximum

Nonpsychotic anxiety: Oral: 1-2 mg twice daily; maximum: 6 mg/day; therapy for anxiety should not exceed 12 weeks; do not exceed 6 mg/day for longer than 12 weeks when treating anxiety; agitation, jitteriness, or insomnia may be confused with original neurotic or psychotic symptoms

Elderly:

Schizophrenia/psychoses:

Oral: Refer to adult dosing. Dose selection should start at the low end of the dosage range and titration must be gradual.

I.M.: Initial: 1 mg every 4-6 hours; increase at 1 mg increments; do not exceed 6 mg/day

Behavioral symptoms associated with dementia behavior: Oral: Initial: 0.5-1 mg 1-2 times/day; increase dose at 4- to 7-day intervals by 0.5-1 mg/day; increase dosing intervals (bid, tid, etc) as necessary to control response or side effects. Maximum daily dose: 40 mg. Gradual increases (titration) may prevent some side effects or decrease their severity.

Hemodialysis: Not dialyzable (0% to 5%)

Mechanism of Action Blocks postsynaptic mesolimbic dopaminergic receptors in the brain; exhibits a strong alpha-adrenergic blocking effect and depresses the release of hypothalamic and hypophyseal hormones

Other Adverse Effects Frequency not defined:

Cardiovascular: Hypotension, orthostatic hypotension, cardiac arrest

Central nervous system: Extrapyramidal symptoms (pseudoparkinsonism, akathisia, dystonias, tardive dyskinesia), dizziness, headache, neuroleptic malignant syndrome (NMS), impairment of temperature regulation, lowering of seizures threshold

Dermatologic: Increased sensitivity to sun, rash, discoloration of skin (blue-gray)

Endocrine & metabolic: Changes in menstrual cycle, changes in libido, breast pain, hyperglycemia, hypoglycemia, gynecomastia, lactation, galactorrhea

Gastrointestinal: Constipation, weight gain, nausea, vomiting, stomach pain, xerostomia

Genitourinary: Difficulty in urination, ejaculatory disturbances, urinary retention, priapism

Hematologic: Agranulocytosis, leukopenia, pancytopenia, thrombocytopenic purpura, eosinophilia, hemolytic anemia, aplastic anemia

Hepatic: Cholestatic jaundice, hepatotoxicity

Neuromuscular & skeletal: Tremor

Ocular: Pigmentary retinopathy, cornea and lens changes

Respiratory: Nasal congestion

Drug Interactions CYP1A2 enzyme substrate

Aluminum salts: May decrease the absorption of phenothiazines; monitor

Amphetamines: Efficacy may be diminished by antipsychotics; in addition, amphetamines may increase psychotic symptoms; avoid concurrent use

Anticholinergics: May inhibit the therapeutic response to phenothiazines and excess anticholinergic effects may occur; includes benztropine, trihexyphenidyl, biperiden, and drugs with significant anticholinergic activity (TCAs, antihistamines, disopyramide)

Antihypertensives: Concurrent use of phenothiazines with an antihypertensive may produce additive hypotensive effects (particularly orthostasis)

Bromocriptine: Phenothiazines inhibit the ability of bromocriptine to lower serum prolactin concentrations

CNS depressants: Sedative effects may be additive with phenothiazines; monitor for increased effect; includes barbiturates, benzodiazepines, narcotic analgesics, ethanol, and other sedative agents

CYP1A2 inhibitors: Serum concentrations may be increased due to decreased metabolism; includes cimetidine, ciprofloxacin, fluvoxamine, isoniazid, ritonavir, and zileuton.

Enzyme inducers: May enhance the hepatic metabolism of phenothiazines; larger doses may be required; includes rifampin, rifabutin, barbiturates, phenytoin, and cigarette smoking

(Continued)

Trifluoperazine *(Continued)*

Epinephrine: Chlorpromazine (and possibly other low potency antipsychotics) may diminish the pressor effects of epinephrine

Guanethidine and guanadrel: Antihypertensive effects may be inhibited by phenothiazines

Levodopa: Phenothiazines may inhibit the antiparkinsonian effect of levodopa; avoid this combination

Lithium: Phenothiazines may produce neurotoxicity with lithium; this is a rare effect

Metoclopramide: May increase extrapyramidal symptoms (EPS) or risk.

Phenytoin: May reduce serum levels of phenothiazines; phenothiazines may increase phenytoin serum levels

Polypeptide antibiotics: Rare cases of respiratory paralysis have been reported with concurrent use of phenothiazines

Propranolol: Serum concentrations of phenothiazines may be increased; propranolol also increases phenothiazine concentrations

QT_c-prolonging agents: Effects on QT_c interval may be additive with phenothiazines, increasing the risk of malignant arrhythmias; includes type Ia antiarrhythmics, TCAs, and some quinolone antibiotics (sparfloxacin, moxifloxacin, and gatifloxacin)

Sulfadoxine-pyrimethamine: May increase phenothiazine concentrations

Trazodone: Phenothiazines and trazodone may produce additive hypotensive effects

Tricyclic antidepressants: Concurrent use may produce increased toxicity or altered therapeutic response

Valproic acid: Serum levels may be increased by phenothiazines

Drug Uptake Half-life, elimination: >24 hours with chronic use

Pregnancy Risk Factor C

Generic Available Yes

Triflupromazine (trye floo PROE ma zeen)

U.S. Brand Names Vesprin®

Canadian Brand Names Vesprin®

Pharmacologic Category Antipsychotic Agent, Phenothiazine, Aliphatic

Synonyms Triflupromazine Hydrochloride

Use Treatment of psychoses; severe nausea and vomiting

Unlabeled/Investigational: Pain; hiccups

Local Anesthetic/Vasoconstrictor Precautions Most pharmacology textbooks state that in presence of phenothiazines, systemic doses of epinephrine paradoxically decrease the blood pressure. This is the so called "epinephrine reversal" phenomenon. This has never been observed when epinephrine is given by infiltration as part of the anesthesia procedure.

Effects on Dental Treatment

Significant hypotension may occur, especially when the drug is administered parenterally; orthostatic hypotension is due to alpha-receptor blockade, the elderly are at greater risk for orthostatic hypotension.

Tardive dyskinesia: Prevalence rate may be 40% in elderly; development of the syndrome and the irreversible nature are proportional to duration and total cumulative dose over time. Extrapyramidal reactions are more common in elderly with up to 50% developing these reactions after 60 years of age; drug-induced **Parkinson's syndrome** occurs often; **Akathisia** is the most common extrapyramidal reaction in elderly.

Increased confusion, memory loss, psychotic behavior, and agitation frequently occur as a consequence of anticholinergic effects. Antipsychotic associated sedation in nonpsychotic patients is extremely unpleasant due to feelings of depersonalization, derealization, and dysphoria.

Dosage Safety and efficacy have not been established for children <2.5 years of age.

Psychosis:
- Children ≥2.5 years: I.M.: 0.2-0.25 mg/kg, up to a maximum total daily dose of 10 mg
- Adults:
  - I.M.: 5-15 mg every 4 hours; initial dose: 60 mg, up to a maximum total daily dose of 150 mg
  - I.V.: 1 mg, may be repeated every 4 hours, up to a maximum total daily dose of 3 mg

Nausea and vomiting:
- Children ≥2.5 years:
  - I.M.: 0.2-0.25 mg/kg, up to a maximum total daily dose of 10 mg
  - I.V.: Not recommended for use in children
- Adults:
  - I.M.: 5-15 mg, may be repeated every 4 hours, up to a maximum total daily dose of 60 mg
  - I.V.: 1 mg, may be repeated every 4 hours, up to a maximum total daily dose of 3 mg

Elderly: I.M.: 2.5 mg, up to a maximum total daily dose of 15 mg

Mechanism of Action The sites of action appear to be the reticular activity system of the midbrain, limbic system, hypothalamus, globus pallidus, and corpus striatum. Postsynaptic, adrenergic, dopaminergic, and serotonergic receptors are blocked.

Other Adverse Effects Frequency not defined:

Cardiovascular: Hypotension, tachycardia, syncope, peripheral edema, QT prolongation

Central nervous system: Neuroleptic malignant syndrome, extrapyramidal symptoms (dystonia, akathisia, pseudoparkinsonism, tardive dyskinesia), sedation, dizziness, drowsiness, insomnia, anxiety, depression, headache, seizures, NMS hyperpyrexia

Dermatologic: Photosensitivity, dermatitis, urticaria

Endocrine & metabolic: Syndrome of inappropriate antidiuretic hormone, galactorrhea, gynecomastia, hyperglycemia, hypoglycemia, breast engorgement, lactation, mastalgia

Gastrointestinal: Xerostomia, weight gain

Hematologic: Agranulocytosis, leukopenia, eosinophilia, thrombocytopenia, aplastic anemia, hemolytic anemia

Hepatic: Jaundice

Neuromuscular & skeletal: Weakness

Ocular: Nystagmus, blurred vision, keratopathy, lacrimation, pigment deposition

Drug Interactions

Aluminum salts: May decrease the absorption of phenothiazines; monitor

Amphetamines: Efficacy may be diminished by antipsychotics; in addition, amphetamines may increase psychotic symptoms; avoid concurrent use

Anticholinergics: May inhibit the therapeutic response to phenothiazines and excess anticholinergic effects may occur; includes benztropine, trihexyphenidyl, biperiden, and drugs with significant anticholinergic activity (TCAs, antihistamines, disopyramide)

Antihypertensives: Concurrent use of phenothiazines with an antihypertensive may produce additive hypotensive effects (particularly orthostasis)

Bromocriptine: Phenothiazines inhibit the ability of bromocriptine to lower serum prolactin concentrations

CNS depressants: Sedative effects may be additive with phenothiazines; monitor for increased effect; includes barbiturates, benzodiazepines, narcotic analgesics, ethanol, and other sedative agents

CYP inhibitors: Metabolism of phenothiazines may be decreased, increasing clinical effect or toxicity; monitor for increased effect/toxicity

Enzyme inducers: May enhance the hepatic metabolism of phenothiazines; larger doses may be required; includes rifampin, rifabutin, barbiturates, phenytoin, and cigarette smoking

Epinephrine: Chlorpromazine (and possibly other low potency antipsychotics) may diminish the pressor effects of epinephrine

Guanethidine and guanadrel: Antihypertensive effects may be inhibited by phenothiazines

Levodopa: Phenothiazines may inhibit the antiparkinsonian effect of levodopa; avoid this combination

Lithium: Phenothiazines may produce neurotoxicity with lithium; this is a rare effect

Metoclopramide: May increase extrapyramidal symptoms (EPS) or risk.

Phenytoin: May reduce serum levels of phenothiazines; phenothiazines may increase phenytoin serum levels

Polypeptide antibiotics: Rare cases of respiratory paralysis have been reported with concurrent use of phenothiazines

Propranolol: Serum concentrations of phenothiazines may be increased; propranolol also increases phenothiazine concentrations

QT_c-prolonging agents: Effects on QT_c interval may be additive with phenothiazines, increasing the risk of malignant arrhythmias; includes type Ia antiarrhythmics, TCAs, and some quinolone antibiotics (sparfloxacin, moxifloxacin, and gatifloxacin)

Sulfadoxine-pyrimethamine: May increase phenothiazine concentrations

Trazodone: Phenothiazines and trazodone may produce additive hypotensive effects

Tricyclic antidepressants: Concurrent use may produce increased toxicity or altered therapeutic response

Valproic acid: Serum levels may be increased by phenothiazines

Pregnancy Risk Factor C

Generic Available No

Trifluridine (trye FLURE i deen)

Related Information

Systemic Viral Diseases *on page 1354*

U.S. Brand Names Viroptic®

Canadian Brand Names Viroptic®

Pharmacologic Category Antiviral Agent, Ophthalmic

Synonyms F_3T; Trifluorothymidine

(Continued)

Trifluridine *(Continued)*

Use Treatment of primary keratoconjunctivitis and recurrent epithelial keratitis caused by herpes simplex virus types I and II

Local Anesthetic/Vasoconstrictor Precautions No information available to require special precautions

Effects on Dental Treatment No effects or complications reported

Dosage Adults: Instill 1 drop into affected eye every 2 hours while awake, to a maximum of 9 drops/day, until re-epithelialization of corneal ulcer occurs; then use 1 drop every 4 hours for another 7 days; do **not** exceed 21 days of treatment; if improvement has not taken place in 7-14 days, consider another form of therapy

Mechanism of Action Interferes with viral replication by incorporating into viral DNA in place of thymidine, inhibiting thymidylate synthetase resulting in the formation of defective proteins

Other Adverse Effects >10%: Local: Burning, stinging

Drug Uptake Absorption: Ophthalmic: Systemic absorption negligible, corneal penetration adequate

Pregnancy Risk Factor C

Generic Available No

Trihexyphenidyl (trye heks ee FEN i dil)

U.S. Brand Names Artane®

Canadian Brand Names Apo®-Trihex

Mexican Brand Names Hipokinon

Pharmacologic Category Anticholinergic Agent; Anti-Parkinson's Agent, Anticholinergic

Synonyms Benzhexol Hydrochloride; Trihexyphenidyl Hydrochloride

Use Adjunctive treatment of Parkinson's disease; also used in treatment of drug-induced extrapyramidal effects and acute dystonic reactions

Local Anesthetic/Vasoconstrictor Precautions No information available to require special precautions

Effects on Dental Treatment >10%: Xerostomia; normal salivary flow resumes with discontinuation; prolonged xerostomia may contribute to development of caries, periodontal disease, oral candidiasis and discomfort.

Dosage Adults: Oral: Initial: 1-2 mg/day, increase by 2 mg increments at intervals of 3-5 days; usual dose: 5-15 mg/day in 3-4 divided doses

Mechanism of Action Exerts a direct inhibitory effect on the parasympathetic nervous system. It also has a relaxing effect on smooth musculature; exerted both directly on the muscle itself and indirectly through parasympathetic nervous system (inhibitory effect). Thought to act by blocking excess acetylcholine at cerebral synapses; many of its effects are due to its pharmacologic similarities with atropine

Other Adverse Effects Frequency not defined:

Cardiovascular: Tachycardia

Central nervous system: Confusion, agitation, euphoria, drowsiness, headache, dizziness, nervousness, delusions, hallucinations, paranoia

Dermatologic: Dry skin, increased sensitivity to light, rash

Gastrointestinal: Constipation, xerostomia, dry throat, ileus, nausea, vomiting, parotitis

Genitourinary: Urinary retention

Neuromuscular & skeletal: Weakness

Ocular: Blurred vision, mydriasis, increase in intraocular pressure, glaucoma

Respiratory: Dry nose

Miscellaneous: Diaphoresis (decreased)

Drug Interactions

Increased Effect/Toxicity: Central and/or peripheral anticholinergic syndrome can occur when administered with amantadine, rimantadine, narcotic analgesics, phenothiazines and other antipsychotics (especially with high anticholinergic activity), tricyclic antidepressants, quinidine and some other antiarrhythmics, and antihistamines.

Decreased Effect: May increase gastric degradation of levodopa and decrease the amount of levodopa absorbed by delaying gastric emptying; the opposite may be true for digoxin. Therapeutic effects of cholinergic agents (tacrine, donepezil) and neuroleptics may be antagonized.

Drug Uptake

Onset of action: Peak effect: ~1 hour

Half-life, elimination: 3.3-4.1 hours

Time to peak: 1-1.5 hours

Pregnancy Risk Factor C

Generic Available Yes

Tri-K® *see* Potassium Acetate, Potassium Bicarbonate, and Potassium Citrate *on page 975*

Tri-Kort® *see* Triamcinolone *on page 1197*

Trilafon® *see* Perphenazine *on page 941*

Trileptal® *see* Oxcarbazepine *on page 897*

Tri-Levlen® *see* Combination Hormonal Contraceptives *on page 323*
Trilisate® *see* Choline Magnesium Trisalicylate *on page 279*
Trilog® *see* Triamcinolone *on page 1197*
Trilone® *see* Triamcinolone *on page 1197*
Tri-Luma™ *see* Fluocinolone, Hydroquinone, and Tretinoin ***Not Available in U.S.*** *on page 513*

Trimethadione (trye meth a DYE one)

U.S. Brand Names Tridione®

Pharmacologic Category Anticonvulsant, Oxazolidinedione

Synonyms Troxidone

Use Control absence (petit mal) seizures refractory to other drugs

Local Anesthetic/Vasoconstrictor Precautions No information available to require special precautions

Effects on Dental Treatment No effects or complications reported

Dosage Oral:

Children: Initial: 25-50 mg/kg/24 hours in 3-4 equally divided doses every 6-8 hours

Adults: Initial: 900 mg/day in 3-4 equally divided doses, increase by 300 mg/day at weekly intervals until therapeutic results or toxic symptoms appear

Mechanism of Action An oxazolidinedione with anticonvulsant sedative properties; elevates the cortical and basal seizure thresholds, and reduces the synaptic response to low frequency impulses

Other Adverse Effects Frequency not defined:

Central nervous system: Drowsiness, hiccups
Dermatologic: Alopecia, exfoliative dermatitis, rash
Endocrine & metabolic: Porphyria
Gastrointestinal: Anorexia, vomiting, stomach upset, abdominal pain, weight loss
Hematologic: Aplastic anemia, agranulocytosis, thrombocytopenia,
Hepatic: Hepatitis, jaundice
Neuromuscular & skeletal: Myasthenia gravis-like syndrome
Ocular: Diplopia, photophobia, hemeralopia, nystagmus, scotomata
Renal: Nephrosis, proteinuria
Miscellaneous: Lupus

Drug Interactions

Acetylcholinesterase inhibitors: May reduce the antimyasthenic effects of these agents (limited documentation); monitor

CNS depressants: Sedative effects may be additive with other CNS depressants; monitor for increased effect; includes ethanol, sedatives, antidepressants, narcotic analgesics, other anticonvulsants, and benzodiazepines

Pregnancy Risk Factor D

Generic Available No

Trimethobenzamide (trye meth oh BEN za mide)

U.S. Brand Names Benzacot®; Tigan®

Canadian Brand Names Tigan®

Pharmacologic Category Anticholinergic Agent; Antiemetic

Synonyms Trimethobenzamide Hydrochloride

Use Treatment of postoperative nausea and vomiting; nausea associated with gastroenteritis

Local Anesthetic/Vasoconstrictor Precautions No information available to require special precautions

Effects on Dental Treatment No effects or complications reported

Dosage Rectal use is contraindicated in neonates and premature infants.

Children:
- Rectal: <14 kg: 100 mg 3-4 times/day
- Oral, rectal: 14-40 kg: 100-200 mg 3-4 times/day

Adults:
- Oral: 250 mg 3-4 times/day
- I.M., rectal: 200 mg 3-4 times/day

Mechanism of Action Acts centrally to inhibit the medullary chemoreceptor trigger zone

Other Adverse Effects Frequency not defined:

Cardiovascular: Hypotension
Central nervous system: Coma, depression, disorientation, dizziness, drowsiness, extrapyramidal symptoms (EPS), headache, opisthotonos, Parkinson-like syndrome, seizures
Hematologic: Blood dyscrasias
Hepatic: Jaundice
Neuromuscular & skeletal: Muscle cramps
Ocular: Blurred vision
Miscellaneous: Hypersensitivity reactions

Warnings/Precautions May mask emesis due to Reye's syndrome or mimic CNS effects of Reye's syndrome in patients with emesis of other etiologies; use in patients with acute vomiting should be avoided. May cause drowsiness; patient

(Continued)

Trimethobenzamide *(Continued)*

should avoid tasks requiring alertness (eg, driving, operating machinery). May cause extrapyramidal symptoms (EPS) which may be confused with CNS symptoms of primary disease responsible for emesis.

Drug Interactions Antagonism of oral anticoagulants may occur.

Drug Uptake

Onset of action: Antiemetic: Oral: 10-40 minutes; I.M.: 15-35 minutes
Absorption: Rectal: ~60%
Duration: 3-4 hours
Half-life, elimination: 7-9 hours
Time to peak: Oral: 45 minutes; I.M.: 30 minutes

Pregnancy Risk Factor C

Generic Available Yes

Trimethoprim (trye METH oh prim)

U.S. Brand Names Primsol®; Proloprim®; Trimpex®

Canadian Brand Names Proloprim®

Pharmacologic Category Antibiotic, Miscellaneous

Synonyms TMP

Use Treatment of urinary tract infections; acute otitis media in children; acute exacerbations of chronic bronchitis in adults; in combination with other agents for treatment of toxoplasmosis, *Pneumocystis carinii*

Local Anesthetic/Vasoconstrictor Precautions No information available to require special precautions

Effects on Dental Treatment No effects or complications reported

Dosage Oral:

Children: 4 mg/kg/day in divided doses every 12 hours

Adults: 100 mg every 12 hours or 200 mg every 24 hours; in the treatment of *Pneumocystis carinii* pneumonia; dose may be as high as 15-20 mg/kg/day in 3-4 divided doses

Dosing interval in renal impairment: Cl_{cr} 15-30 mL/minute: Administer 50 mg every 12 hours

Hemodialysis: Moderately dialyzable (20% to 50%)

Mechanism of Action Inhibits folic acid reduction to tetrahydrofolate, and thereby inhibits microbial growth

Other Adverse Effects 1% to 10%:

Central nervous system: Headache
Dermatologic: Rash (3% to 7%), pruritus
Gastrointestinal: Nausea, vomiting, epigastric distress
Hematologic: Megaloblastic anemia (with chronic high doses)

Drug Interactions CYP2C8/9 enzyme inhibitor

Increased Effect/Toxicity: Increased effect/toxicity/levels of phenytoin. Concurrent use with ACE inhibitors increases risk of hyperkalemia. Increased myelosuppression with methotrexate. May increase levels of digoxin. Concurrent use with dapsone may increase levels of dapsone and trimethoprim. Concurrent use with procainamide may increase levels of procainamide and trimethoprim.

Drug Uptake

Absorption: Oral: Readily and extensive
Half-life, elimination: 8-14 hours (increases with renal impairment)
Time to peak: 1-4 hours

Pregnancy Risk Factor C

Generic Available Yes

Trimethoprim and Polymyxin B

(trye METH oh prim & pol i MIKS in bee)

U.S. Brand Names Polytrim®

Canadian Brand Names PMS-Polytrimethoprim; Polytrim™

Pharmacologic Category Antibiotic, Ophthalmic

Synonyms Polymyxin B and Trimethoprim

Use Treatment of surface ocular bacterial conjunctivitis and blepharoconjunctivitis

Local Anesthetic/Vasoconstrictor Precautions No information available to require special precautions

Effects on Dental Treatment No effects or complications reported

Dosage Instill 1-2 drops in eye(s) every 4-6 hours

Other Adverse Effects 1% to 10%: Local: Burning, stinging, itching, increased redness

Drug Uptake See Trimethoprim *on page 1210* and Polymyxin B *on page 971*

Pregnancy Risk Factor C

Generic Available No

Trimetrexate Glucuronate (tri me TREKS ate gloo KYOOR oh nate)

U.S. Brand Names Neutrexin®

Pharmacologic Category Antineoplastic Agent, Miscellaneous

Use Alternative therapy for the treatment of moderate-to-severe *Pneumocystis carinii* pneumonia (PCP) in immunocompromised patients, including patients with acquired immunodeficiency syndrome (AIDS), who are intolerant of, or are refractory to, co-trimoxazole therapy or for whom co-trimoxazole and pentamidine are contraindicated (concurrent folinic acid (leucovorin) must always be administered)

Local Anesthetic/Vasoconstrictor Precautions No information available to require special precautions

Effects on Dental Treatment No effects or complications reported

Dosage Adults: I.V.: 45 mg/m^2 once daily over 60 minutes for 21 days; it is necessary to reduce the dose in patients with liver dysfunction, although no specific recommendations exist; concurrent folinic acid 20 mg/m^2 every 6 hours orally or I.V. for at least 24 hours after the last dose of trimetrexate

Mechanism of Action Exerts an antimicrobial effect through potent inhibition of the enzyme dihydrofolate reductase (DHFR)

Other Adverse Effects 1% to 10%:

Central nervous system: Seizures, fever
Dermatologic: Rash
Gastrointestinal: Stomatitis, nausea, vomiting
Hematologic: Neutropenia, thrombocytopenia, anemia
Hepatic: Elevated LFTs
Neuromuscular & skeletal: Peripheral neuropathy
Renal: Increased serum creatinine
Miscellaneous: Flu-like illness, hypersensitivity reactions

Drug Interactions Metabolized by cytochrome isoenzyme, possibly CYP3A3/4

Increased Effect/Toxicity: Cimetidine, clotrimazole, ketoconazole, and acetaminophen have been shown to decrease clearance of trimetrexate resulting in increased serum concentration.

Decreased Effect: Trimetrexate is metabolized by cytochrome P450 enzymes in the liver. Examples of drugs where this interaction may occur are erythromycin, rifampin, rifabutin, ketoconazole, and fluconazole.

Drug Uptake Half-life, elimination: 15-17 hours

Pregnancy Risk Factor D

Generic Available No

Trimipramine (trye MI pra meen)

U.S. Brand Names Surmontil®

Canadian Brand Names Apo®-Trimip; Novo-Tripramine; Nu-Trimipramine; Rhotrimine®; Surmontil®

Pharmacologic Category Antidepressant, Tricyclic (Tertiary Amine)

Synonyms Trimipramine Maleate

Use Treatment of various forms of depression, often in conjunction with psychotherapy

Local Anesthetic/Vasoconstrictor Precautions Use with caution; epinephrine, norepinephrine and levonordefrin have been shown to have an increased pressor response in combination with TCAs

Effects on Dental Treatment

>10%: Xerostomia

Long-term treatment with TCAs such as trimipramine increases the risk of caries by reducing salivation and salivary buffer capacity.

Dosage Adults: Oral: 50-150 mg/day as a single bedtime dose up to a maximum of 200 mg/day outpatient and 300 mg/day inpatient

Mechanism of Action Increases the synaptic concentration of serotonin and/or norepinephrine in the CNS by inhibition of their reuptake by the presynaptic neuronal membrane

Other Adverse Effects Frequency not defined:

Cardiovascular: Arrhythmias, hypotension, hypertension, tachycardia, palpitations, heart block, stroke, myocardial infarction

Central nervous system: Headache, exacerbation of psychosis, confusion, delirium, hallucinations, nervousness, restlessness, delusions, agitation, insomnia, nightmares, anxiety, seizures, drowsiness

Dermatologic: Photosensitivity, rash, petechiae, itching

Endocrine & metabolic: Sexual dysfunction, breast enlargement, galactorrhea, SIADH

Gastrointestinal: Xerostomia, constipation, increased appetite, nausea, unpleasant taste, weight gain, diarrhea, heartburn, vomiting, anorexia, trouble with gums, decreased lower esophageal sphincter tone may cause GE reflux

Genitourinary: Difficult urination, urinary retention, testicular edema

Hematologic: Agranulocytosis, eosinophilia, purpura, thrombocytopenia

Hepatic: Cholestatic jaundice, increased liver enzymes

Neuromuscular & skeletal: Tremors, numbness, tingling, paresthesia, incoordination, ataxia, peripheral neuropathy, extrapyramidal symptoms

Ocular: Blurred vision, eye pain, disturbances in accommodation, mydriasis, increased intraocular pressure

Otic: Tinnitus

Miscellaneous: Allergic reactions

(Continued)

Trimipramine *(Continued)*

Drug Interactions CYP2D6 enzyme substrate

Increased Effect/Toxicity: Trimipramine increases the effects of amphetamines, anticholinergics, other CNS depressants (sedatives, hypnotics), chlorpropamide, tolazamide, and warfarin. When used with MAO inhibitors, hyperpyrexia, hypertension, tachycardia, confusion, seizures, and **deaths have been reported** (serotonin syndrome). The SSRIs (to varying degrees), cimetidine, indinavir, methylphenidate, ritonavir, quinidine, diltiazem, and verapamil inhibit the metabolism of TCAs and clinical toxicity may result. Use of lithium with a TCA may increase the risk for neurotoxicity. Phenothiazines may increase concentration of some TCAs and TCAs may increase concentration of phenothiazines. Pressor response to I.V. epinephrine, norepinephrine, and phenylephrine may be enhanced in patients receiving TCAs (**Note:** Effect is unlikely with epinephrine or levonordefrin dosages typically administered as infiltration in combination with local anesthetics). Combined use of beta-agonists or drugs which prolong QT_c (including quinidine, procainamide, disopyramide, cisapride, sparfloxacin, gatifloxacin, moxifloxacin) with TCAs may predispose patients to cardiac arrhythmias.

Decreased Effect: Carbamazepine, phenobarbital, and rifampin may increase the metabolism of trimipramine resulting in decreased effect of trimipramine. Trimipramine inhibits the antihypertensive response to bethanidine, clonidine, debrisoquin, guanadrel, guanethidine, guanabenz, and guanfacine. Cholestyramine and colestipol may bind TCAs and reduce their absorption; monitor for altered response.

Drug Uptake

Onset of action: Therapeutic: >2 weeks

Half-life, elimination: 20-26 hours

Time to peak, plasma: Oral: ≤6 hours

Pregnancy Risk Factor C

Generic Available No

Selected Readings

Friedlander AH, Mahler ME, "Major Depressive Disorder. Psychopathology, Medical Management, and Dental Implications," *J Am Dent Assoc*, 201, 132(5):629-38.

Ganzberg S, "Psychoactive Drugs," *ADA Guide to Dental Therapeutics*, 2nd ed, Chicago, IL: ADA Publishing, a Division of ADA Business Enterprises, Inc, 2000, 376-405.

Yagiela JA, "Adverse Drug Interactions in Dental Practice: Interactions Associated With Vasoconstrictors. Part V of a Series," *J Am Dent Assoc*, 1999, 130(5):701-9.

Trimox® *see* Amoxicillin *on page 86*

Trimpex® *see* Trimethoprim *on page 1210*

Trinalin® *see* Azatadine and Pseudoephedrine *on page 135*

Tri-Nasal® *see* Triamcinolone *on page 1197*

Tri-Norinyl® *see* Combination Hormonal Contraceptives *on page 323*

Triostat® *see* Liothyronine *on page 715*

Triotann® *see* Chlorpheniramine, Pyrilamine, and Phenylephrine *on page 273*

Trioxsalen (trye OKS a len)

U.S. Brand Names Trisoralen®

Pharmacologic Category Psoralen

Synonyms Trimethylpsoralen

Use In conjunction with controlled exposure to ultraviolet light or sunlight for repigmentation of idiopathic vitiligo; increasing tolerance to sunlight with albinism; enhance pigmentation

Local Anesthetic/Vasoconstrictor Precautions No information available to require special precautions

Effects on Dental Treatment No effects or complications reported

Dosage Children >12 years and Adults: Oral: 10 mg/day as a single dose, 2-4 hours before controlled exposure to UVA (for 15-35 minutes) or sunlight; do not continue for longer than 14 days

Mechanism of Action Psoralens are thought to form covalent bonds with pyrimidine bases in DNA which inhibit the synthesis of DNA. This reaction involves excitation of the trioxsalen molecule by radiation in the long-wave ultraviolet light (UVA) resulting in transference of energy to the trioxsalen molecule producing an excited state. Binding of trioxsalen to DNA occurs only in the presence of ultraviolet light. The increase in skin pigmentation produced by trioxsalen and UVA radiation involves multiple changes in melanocytes and interaction between melanocytes and keratinocytes. In general, melanogenesis is stimulated but the size and distribution of melanocytes is unchanged.

Other Adverse Effects

>10%:

Dermatologic: Itching

Gastrointestinal: Nausea

1% to 10%:

Central nervous system: Dizziness, headache, mental depression, insomnia, nervousness

Dermatologic: Severe burns from excessive sunlight or ultraviolet exposure
Gastrointestinal: Gastric discomfort

Drug Uptake
Onset of action: Peak effect: Photosensitivity: 2 hours
Absorption: Rapid
Duration: Skin sensitivity to light: 8-12 hours
Half-life, elimination: ~2 hours

Pregnancy Risk Factor C

Generic Available No

Tripelennamine (tri pel EN a meen)

U.S. Brand Names PBZ®; PBZ-SR®

Pharmacologic Category Antihistamine

Synonyms Tripelennamine Citrate; Tripelennamine Hydrochloride

Use Perennial and seasonal allergic rhinitis and other allergic symptoms including urticaria

Local Anesthetic/Vasoconstrictor Precautions No information available to require special precautions

Effects on Dental Treatment Chronic use of antihistamines will inhibit salivary flow, particularly in elderly patients; this may contribute to periodontal disease and oral discomfort.

Dosage Oral:
Children: 5 mg/kg/day in 4-6 divided doses, up to 300 mg/day maximum
Adults: 25-50 mg every 4-6 hours, extended release tablets 100 mg morning and evening up to 100 mg every 8 hours

Mechanism of Action Competes with histamine for H_1-receptor sites on effector cells in the GI tract, blood vessels, and respiratory tract

Other Adverse Effects
>10%:
Central nervous system: Slight to moderate drowsiness
Respiratory: Thickening of bronchial secretions
1% to 10%:
Central nervous system: Headache, fatigue, nervousness, dizziness
Gastrointestinal: Appetite increase, weight gain, nausea, diarrhea, abdominal pain, xerostomia
Neuromuscular & skeletal: Arthralgia
Respiratory: Pharyngitis

Drug Interactions Increased effect/toxicity with CNS depressants and MAO inhibitors

Drug Uptake
Onset of action: Antihistaminic: 15-30 minutes
Duration: 4-6 hours; PBZ-SR®: ≤8 hours

Pregnancy Risk Factor B

Generic Available Yes

Triphasil® *see* Combination Hormonal Contraceptives *on page 323*
Triphed® [OTC] *see* Triprolidine and Pseudoephedrine *on page 1213*
Triple Antibiotic® *see* Bacitracin, Neomycin, and Polymyxin B *on page 141*
Triposed® Tablet [OTC] *see* Triprolidine and Pseudoephedrine *on page 1213*

Triprolidine and Pseudoephedrine

(trye PROE li deen & soo doe e FED rin)

U.S. Brand Names Act-A-Med® [OTC]; Actanol® [OTC]; Actedril® [OTC]; Actifed® [OTC]; Allerfed® [OTC]; Allerfrim® [OTC]; Allerphed® [OTC]; Altafed® [OTC]; Aphedrid™ [OTC]; Aprodine® [OTC]; Biofed-PE® [OTC]; Cenafed® Plus Tablet [OTC]; Genac® Tablet [OTC]; Histafed® [OTC]; Hista-Tabs® [OTC]; Pseudocot-T® [OTC]; Ridifed® [OTC]; Ritifed® [OTC]; Silafed® [OTC]; Triacin® [OTC]; Triafed® [OTC]; Tri-Fed® [OTC]; Triphed® [OTC]; Triposed® Tablet [OTC]; Tri-Pseudafed® [OTC]; Tri-Pseudo® [OTC]; Tri-Sofed® [OTC]; Trisudex® [OTC]; Tri-Sudo® [OTC]; Uni-Fed® [OTC]; Vi-Sudo® [OTC]

Canadian Brand Names Actifed®

Pharmacologic Category Alpha/Beta Agonist; Antihistamine

Synonyms Pseudoephedrine and Triprolidine

Use Temporary relief of nasal congestion, decongest sinus openings, running nose, sneezing, itching of nose or throat and itchy, watery eyes due to common cold, hay fever, or other upper respiratory allergies

Local Anesthetic/Vasoconstrictor Precautions Use with caution since pseudoephedrine is a sympathomimetic amine which could interact with epinephrine to cause a pressor response

Effects on Dental Treatment Chronic use of antihistamines will inhibit salivary flow, particularly in elderly patients; this may contribute to periodontal disease and oral discomfort.

(Continued)

Triprolidine and Pseudoephedrine *(Continued)*

Dosage Oral:
Children:
Syrup:
4 months to 2 years: 1.25 mL 3-4 times/day
2-4 years: 2.5 mL 3-4 times/day
4-6 years: 3.75 mL 3-4 times/day
6-12 years: 5 mL every 4-6 hours; do not exceed 4 doses in 24 hours
Tablet: $^1/_2$ every 4-6 hours; do not exceed 4 doses in 24 hours
Children >12 years and Adults:
Syrup: 10 mL every 4-6 hours; do not exceed 4 doses in 24 hours
Tablet: 1 every 4-6 hours; do not exceed 4 doses in 24 hours

Mechanism of Action Refer to Pseudoephedrine *on page 1022*

Triprolidine is a member of the propylamine (alkylamine) chemical class of H_1-antagonist antihistamines. As such, it is considered to be relatively less sedating than traditional antihistamines of the ethanolamine, phenothiazine, and ethylenediamine classes of antihistamines. Triprolidine has a shorter half-life and duration of action than most of the other alkylamine antihistamines. Like all H_1-antagonist antihistamines, the mechanism of action of triprolidine is believed to involve competitive blockade of H_1-receptor sites resulting in the inability of histamine to combine with its receptor sites and exert its usual effects on target cells. Antihistamines do not interrupt any effects of histamine which have already occurred. Therefore, these agents are used more successfully in the prevention rather than the treatment of histamine-induced reactions.

Other Adverse Effects
>10%:
Cardiovascular: Tachycardia
Central nervous system: Slight to moderate drowsiness, nervousness, insomnia, transient stimulation
Respiratory: Thickening of bronchial secretions
1% to 10%:
Central nervous system: Headache, fatigue, dizziness
Gastrointestinal: Appetite increase, weight gain, nausea, diarrhea, abdominal pain, xerostomia
Genitourinary: Dysuria
Neuromuscular & skeletal: Arthralgia, weakness
Respiratory: Pharyngitis
Miscellaneous: Diaphoresis

Drug Interactions
Increased Effect/Toxicity: Increased toxicity with MAO inhibitors or drugs with MAO inhibiting activity such as linezolid or furazolidone (hypertensive crisis). May increase toxicity of sympathomimetics, CNS depressants, and alcohol.
Decreased effect of guanethidine, reserpine, and methyldopa

Drug Uptake Refer to Pseudoephedrine *on page 1022*

Pregnancy Risk Factor C

Generic Available Yes

Triprolidine, Pseudoephedrine, and Codeine

(trye PROE li deen, soo doe e FED rin, & KOE deen)

U.S. Brand Names Aprodine® w/C; Triacin-C®

Canadian Brand Names CoActifed®

Pharmacologic Category Antihistamine/Decongestant/Antitussive

Synonyms Codeine, Pseudoephedrine, and Triprolidine; Pseudoephedrine, Triprolidine, and Codeine Pseudoephedrine, Codeine, and Triprolidine; Triprolidine, Codeine, and Pseudoephedrine; Triprolidine, Pseudoephedrine, and Codeine, Triprolidine, and Pseudoephedrine

Use Symptomatic relief of cough

Local Anesthetic/Vasoconstrictor Precautions Use with caution since pseudoephedrine is a sympathomimetic amine which could interact with epinephrine to cause a pressor response

Effects on Dental Treatment ≤10%: Tachycardia, palpitations, xerostomia; use vasoconstrictor with caution

Restrictions C-V

Dosage Oral:
Children:
2-6 years: 2.5 mL 4 times/day
7-12 years: 5 mL 4 times/day
Children >12 years and Adults: 10 mL 4 times/day

Drug Uptake See Pseudoephedrine and Codeine monographs.

Pregnancy Risk Factor C

Generic Available Yes

Tri-Pseudafed® [OTC] *see* Triprolidine and Pseudoephedrine *on page 1213*
Tri-Pseudo® [OTC] *see* Triprolidine and Pseudoephedrine *on page 1213*

TripTone® Caplets® [OTC] *see* DimenhyDRINATE *on page 396*

Triptorelin (trip toe REL in)

U.S. Brand Names Trelstar™ Depot; Trelstar™ LA

Canadian Brand Names Trelstar™ Depot

Pharmacologic Category Luteinizing Hormone-Releasing Hormone Analog

Synonyms Triptorelin Pamoate

Use Palliative treatment of advanced prostate cancer as an alternative to orchiectomy or estrogen administration

Local Anesthetic/Vasoconstrictor Precautions No information available to require special precautions

Effects on Dental Treatment No effects or complications reported

Dosage I.M.: Adults: 3.75 mg once monthly

Mechanism of Action Causes suppression of ovarian and testicular steroidogenesis due to decreased levels of LH and FSH with subsequent decrease in testosterone (male) and estrogen (female) levels. After chronic and continuous administration, usually 2-4 weeks after initiation, a sustained decrease in LH and FSH secretion occurs.

Other Adverse Effects As reported with Trelstar™ Depot and Trelstar™ LA; frequency of effect may vary by product:

>10%:

Endocrine & metabolic: Hot flashes (59% to 73%), glucose increased, hemoglobin decreased, RBC count decreased

Hepatic: Alkaline phosphatase increased, ALT increased, AST increased

Neuromuscular & skeletal: Skeletal pain (12% to 13%)

Renal: BUN increased

1% to 10%:

Cardiovascular: Leg edema (6%), hypertension (4%), chest pain (2%), peripheral edema (1%)

Central nervous system: Headache (5% to 7%), dizziness (1% to 3%), pain (2% to 3%), emotional lability (1%), fatigue (2%), insomnia (2%)

Dermatologic: Rash (2%), pruritus (1%)

Endocrine & metabolic: Alkaline phosphatase increased (2%), breast pain (2%), gynocomastia (2%), libido decreased (2%)

Gastrointestinal: Nausea (3%), anorexia (2%), constipation (2%), dyspepsia (2%), vomiting (2%), abdominal pain (1%), diarrhea (1%)

Genitourinary: Dysuria (5%), impotence (2% to 7%), urinary retention (1%), urinary tract infection (1%)

Hematologic: Anemia (1%)

Local: Injection site pain (4%)

Neuromuscular & skeletal: Leg pain (2% to 5%), back pain (3%), arthralgia (2%), leg cramps (2%), myalgia (1%), weakness (1%)

Ocular: Conjunctivitis (1%), eye pain (1%)

Respiratory: Cough (2%), dyspnea (1%), pharyngitis (1%)

Drug Interactions Not studied; hyperprolactinemic drugs (dopamine antagonists such as antipsychotics, and metoclopramide) are contraindicated.

Drug Uptake

Absorption: Oral: Not active

Half-life, elimination: 2.8 ± 1.2 hours; Moderate to severe renal impairment: 6.5 ± 1.2 to 7.7 ± 1.3 hours; Hepatic impairment: 7.6 ± 1.2 hours

Time to peak: 1-3 hours

Pregnancy Risk Factor X

Generic Available No

Tri-Sofed® [OTC] *see* Triprolidine and Pseudoephedrine *on page 1213*

Trisoralen® *see* Trioxsalen *on page 1212*

Tristoject® *see* Triamcinolone *on page 1197*

Trisudex® [OTC] *see* Triprolidine and Pseudoephedrine *on page 1213*

Tri-Sudo® [OTC] *see* Triprolidine and Pseudoephedrine *on page 1213*

Tri-Tannate® *see* Chlorpheniramine, Pyrilamine, and Phenylephrine *on page 273*

Tri-Tannate Plus® [OTC] *see* Chlorpheniramine, Ephedrine, Phenylephrine, and Carbetapentane *on page 270*

Tritec® *see* Ranitidine Bismuth Citrate *on page 1041*

Trivagizole 3™ *see* Clotrimazole *on page 312*

Trivora® *see* Combination Hormonal Contraceptives *on page 323*

Trizivir® *see* Abacavir, Lamivudine, and Zidovudine *on page 22*

Trobicin® *see* Spectinomycin *on page 1105*

Trocaine® [OTC] *see* Benzocaine *on page 151*

Trocal® [OTC] *see* Dextromethorphan *on page 372*

Troleandomycin (troe lee an doe MYE sin)

U.S. Brand Names Tao®

Pharmacologic Category Antibiotic, Macrolide

Synonyms Triacetyloleandomycin

(Continued)

Troleandomycin *(Continued)*

Use Adjunct in the treatment of corticosteroid-dependent asthma due to its steroid-sparing properties; antibiotic with spectrum of activity similar to erythromycin

Local Anesthetic/Vasoconstrictor Precautions No information available to require special precautions

Effects on Dental Treatment No effects or complications reported

Dosage Oral:

Children 7-13 years: 25-40 mg/kg/day divided every 6 hours (125-250 mg every 6 hours)

Adjunct in corticosteroid-dependent asthma: 14 mg/kg/day in divided doses every 6-12 hours not to exceed 250 mg every 6 hours; dose is tapered to once daily then alternate day dosing

Children >13 years and adults: 250-500 mg 4 times/day

Mechanism of Action Decreases methylprednisolone clearance from a linear first order decline to a nonlinear decline in plasma concentration. Tao® also has an undefined action independent of its effects on steroid elimination. Inhibits RNA-dependent protein synthesis at the chain elongation step; binds to the 50S ribosomal subunit resulting in blockage of transpeptidation.

Other Adverse Effects

>10%: Gastrointestinal: Abdominal cramping and discomfort

1% to 10%:

Dermatologic: Urticaria, skin rashes

Gastrointestinal: Nausea, vomiting, diarrhea

Drug Interactions CYP3A3/4 enzyme substrate; CYP3A3/4 enzyme inhibitor

Increased Effect/Toxicity: Avoid concomitant use of the following with troleandomycin due to increased risk of malignant arrhythmias: Astemizole, cisapride, gatifloxacin, moxifloxacin, pimozide, sparfloxacin, terfenadine, thioridazine. Other agents that prolong the QT_c interval, including type Ia (eg, quinidine) and type III antiarrhythmic agents, and selected antipsychotic agents (eg, mesoridazine, thioridazine) should be used with extreme caution.

May increase the serum concentrations (and possibly the toxicity) of the following agents: Alfentanil (and possibly other narcotic analgesics), benzodiazepines (alprazolam, diazepam, midazolam, triazolam), buspirone, calcium channel blockers, dihydropyridine (felodipine), carbamazepine, cilostazol, clozapine, colchicine, cyclosporine, digoxin, disopyramide, ergot alkaloids (eg, bromocriptine), HMG-CoA reductase inhibitors (except fluvastatin, pravastatin), loratadine, methylprednisolone, rifabutin, tacrolimus, theophylline, sildenafil, valproate, vinblastine, vincristine, zopiclone.

The effects of neuromuscular-blocking agents and warfarin have been potentiated by troleandomycin. Troleandomycin serum concentrations may be increased by amprenavir (and possibly other protease inhibitors).

Decreased Effect: May decrease the serum concentrations of zafirlukast; may antagonize the therapeutic effects of clindamycin and lincomycin

Drug Uptake Time to peak: ~2 hours

Pregnancy Risk Factor C

Generic Available No

Tromethamine (troe METH a meen)

U.S. Brand Names THAM®

Pharmacologic Category Alkalinizing Agent

Synonyms Tris Buffer; Tris(hydroxymethyl)aminomethane

Use Correction of metabolic acidosis associated with cardiac bypass surgery or cardiac arrest; to correct excess acidity of stored blood that is preserved with acid citrate dextrose (ACD); to prime the pump-oxygenator during cardiac bypass surgery; indicated in severe metabolic acidosis in patients in whom sodium or carbon dioxide elimination is restricted [eg, infants needing alkalinization after receiving maximum sodium bicarbonate (8-10 mEq/kg/24 hours)]

Local Anesthetic/Vasoconstrictor Precautions No information available to require special precautions

Effects on Dental Treatment No effects or complications reported

Dosage

Neonates and Infants: Metabolic acidosis associated with RDS: Initial: Approximately 1 mL/kg for each pH unit below 7.4; additional doses determined by changes in PaO_2, pH, and pCO_2; **Note:** Although THAM® solution does not raise pCO_2 when treating metabolic acidosis with concurrent respiratory acidosis, bicarbonate may be preferred because the osmotic effects of THAM® are greater.

Adults: Dose depends on buffer base deficit; when deficit is known: tromethamine (mL of 0.3 M solution) = body weight (kg) x base deficit (mEq/L); when base deficit is not known: 3-6 mL/kg/dose I.V. (1-2 mEq/kg/dose)

Metabolic acidosis with cardiac arrest:

I.V.: 3.5-6 mL/kg (1-2 mEq/kg/dose) into large peripheral vein; 500-1000 mL if needed in adults

I.V. continuous drip: Infuse slowly by syringe pump over 3-6 hours

Acidosis associated with cardiac bypass surgery: Average dose: 9 mL/kg (2.7 mEq/kg); 500 mL is adequate for most adults; maximum dose: 500 mg/kg in ≤1 hour

Excess acidity of acid citrate dextrose priming blood: 14-70 mL of 0.3 molar solution added to each 500 mL of blood

Dosing comments in renal impairment: Use with caution and monitor for hyperkalemia and EKG

Mechanism of Action Acts as a proton acceptor, which combines with hydrogen ions to form bicarbonate buffer, to correct acidosis

Other Adverse Effects 1% to 10%:

Cardiovascular: Venospasm

Local: Tissue irritation, necrosis with extravasation

Drug Uptake Absorption: 30% of dose is not ionized

Pregnancy Risk Factor C

Generic Available No

Comments 1 mM = 120 mg = 3.3 mL = 1 mEq of THAM®

Tronolane® [OTC] *see* Pramoxine *on page 984*

Tronothane® [OTC] *see* Pramoxine *on page 984*

Tropicacyl® *see* Tropicamide *on page 1217*

Tropicamide (troe PIK a mide)

U.S. Brand Names Mydriacyl®; Opticyl®; Tropicacyl®

Canadian Brand Names Diotrope®; Mydriacyl®

Pharmacologic Category Ophthalmic Agent, Mydriatic

Synonyms Bistropamide

Use Short-acting mydriatic used in diagnostic procedures; as well as preoperatively and postoperatively; treatment of some cases of acute iritis, iridocyclitis, and keratitis

Local Anesthetic/Vasoconstrictor Precautions No information available to require special precautions

Effects on Dental Treatment No effects or complications reported

Dosage Children and Adults (individuals with heavily pigmented eyes may require larger doses):

Cycloplegia: Instill 1-2 drops (1%); may repeat in 5 minutes

Exam must be performed within 30 minutes after the repeat dose; if the patient is not examined within 20-30 minutes, instill an additional drop

Mydriasis: Instill 1-2 drops (0.5%) 15-20 minutes before exam; may repeat every 30 minutes as needed

Mechanism of Action Prevents the sphincter muscle of the iris and the muscle of the ciliary body from responding to cholinergic stimulation

Other Adverse Effects 1% to 10%:

Cardiovascular: Tachycardia, vascular congestion, edema

Central nervous system: Parasympathetic stimulations, drowsiness, headache

Dermatologic: Eczematoid dermatitis

Gastrointestinal: Xerostomia

Local: Transient stinging

Ocular: Blurred vision, photophobia with or without corneal staining, increased intraocular pressure, follicular conjunctivitis

Drug Uptake

Onset of action: Mydriasis: ~20-40 minutes; Cycloplegia: ~30 minutes

Duration: Mydriasis: ~6-7 hours; Cycloplegia: <6 hours

Pregnancy Risk Factor C

Generic Available Yes

Trovafloxacin/Alatrofloxacin (TROE va flox a sin)

U.S. Brand Names Trovan®

Canadian Brand Names Trovan™

Mexican Brand Names Trovan®

Pharmacologic Category Antibiotic, Quinolone

Synonyms Alatrofloxacin Mesylate; CP-99,219-27

Use Treatment of nosocomial pneumonia, community-acquired pneumonia, complicated intra-abdominal infections, gynecologic/pelvic infections, complicated skin and skin structure infections

Note: Should be used only in life- or limb-threatening infections

Local Anesthetic/Vasoconstrictor Precautions No information available to require special precautions

Effects on Dental Treatment No effects or complications reported

Dosage Adults:

Nosocomial pneumonia: I.V.: 300 mg single dose followed by 200 mg/day orally for a total duration of 10-14 days

Community-acquired pneumonia: Oral, I.V.: 200 mg/day for 7-14 days

(Continued)

Trovafloxacin/Alatrofloxacin *(Continued)*

Complicated intra-abdominal infections, including postsurgical infections/gynecologic and pelvic infections: I.V.: 300 mg as a single dose followed by 200 mg/day orally for a total duration of 7-14 days

Skin and skin structure infections, complicated, including diabetic foot infections: Oral, I.V.: 200 mg/day for 10-14 days

Mechanism of Action Unique fluoroquinolone antibiotic with *in vitro* activity against atypical, Gram-negative, Gram-positive including penicillin-resistant pneumococci, intracellular and anaerobic pathogens; it is a fluoroquinolone with a 2-4-difluorophenyl substituent at the N-1 position and a fused pyrolidine substituent at the 7 position. Inhibits DNA-gyrase in susceptible organisms; inhibits relaxation of supercoiled DNA and promotes breakage of double-stranded DNA

Other Adverse Effects Fatalities have occurred in patients developing hepatic necrosis.

1% to 10% (range reported in clinical trials):

- Central nervous system: Dizziness (2% to 11%), lightheadedness (<1% to 4%), headache (1% to 5%)
- Dermatologic: Rash (<1% to 2%), pruritus (<1% to 2%)
- Gastrointestinal: Nausea (4% to 8%), abdominal pain (<1% to 1%), vomiting, diarrhea
- Genitourinary: Vaginitis (<1% to 1%)
- Hepatic: Increased LFTs
- Local: Injection site reaction, pain, or inflammation

Drug Interactions

Increased Effect/Toxicity:

Decreased Effect: Coadministration with antacids containing aluminum or magnesium, citric acid/sodium citrate, sucralfate, and iron markedly reduces absorption of trovafloxacin. Separate oral administration by at least 2 hours. Coadministration of I.V. morphine also reduces absorption. Separate I.V. morphine by 2 hours (when trovafloxacin is taken in fasting state) or 4 hours (when taken with food). Do not administer multivalent cations (eg, calcium, magnesium) through the same I.V. line.

Drug Uptake

Half-life, elimination: ~10 hours

Time to peak, plasma: 1-3 hours

Pregnancy Risk Factor C

Generic Available No

Comments *In vitro* trovafloxacin was more active than sparfloxacin, ofloxacin, ciprofloxacin, ceftriaxone, erythromycin and vancomycin against *S. pneumoniae*. It was also more active against penicillin-resistant strains than ceftriaxone, erythromycin or vancomycin. Trovafloxacin is very effective in bronchitis and pneumonia. It has good activity against resistant organisms, and penetration of the cerebral spinal fluid giving potential in the treatment of CNS infections.

Trovan® *see* Trovafloxacin/Alatrofloxacin *on page 1217*

Truphylline® *see* Aminophylline *on page 71*

Trusopt® *see* Dorzolamide *on page 412*

Truxazole® *see* SulfiSOXAZOLE *on page 1123*

Truxcillin® *see* Penicillin V Potassium *on page 931*

Trypsin, Balsam Peru, and Castor Oil

(TRIP sin, BAL sam pe RUE, & KAS tor oyl)

U.S. Brand Names Granulex

Pharmacologic Category Protectant, Topical

Use Treatment of decubitus ulcers, varicose ulcers, debridement of eschar, dehiscent wounds and sunburn

Local Anesthetic/Vasoconstrictor Precautions No information available to require special precautions

Effects on Dental Treatment No effects or complications reported

Dosage Apply a minimum of twice daily or as often as necessary

Generic Available Yes

T-Stat® *see* Erythromycin, Topical *on page 454*

Tuberculin Purified Protein Derivative (too BER kyoo lin tests)

U.S. Brand Names Aplisol®; Tine Test PPD; Tubersol®

Pharmacologic Category Diagnostic Agent

Synonyms Mantoux; PPD; Tine Test; TST; Tuberculin Skin Test

Use Skin test in diagnosis of tuberculosis, to aid in assessment of cell-mediated immunity; routine tuberculin testing is recommended at 12 months of age and at every 1-2 years thereafter, before the measles vaccination

Local Anesthetic/Vasoconstrictor Precautions No information available to require special precautions

Effects on Dental Treatment No effects or complications reported

Dosage Children and Adults: Intradermal: 0.1 mL about 4" below elbow; use 1/4" to 1/2" or 26- or 27-gauge needle; significant reactions are ≥5 mm in diameter

Interpretation of induration of tuberculin skin test injections: Positive: ≥10 mm; inconclusive: 5-9 mm; negative: <5 mm

Interpretation of induration of Tine test injections: Positive: >2 mm and vesiculation present; inconclusive: <2 mm (give patient Mantoux test of 5 TU/0.1 mL - base decisions on results of Mantoux test); negative: <2 mm or erythema of any size (no need for retesting unless person is a contact of a patient with tuberculosis or there is clinical evidence suggestive of the disease)

Mechanism of Action Tuberculosis results in individuals becoming sensitized to certain antigenic components of the *M. tuberculosis* organism. Culture extracts called tuberculins are contained in tuberculin skin test preparations. Upon intracutaneous injection of these culture extracts, a classic delayed (cellular) hypersensitivity reaction occurs. This reaction is characteristic of a delayed course (peak occurs >24 hours after injection, induration of the skin secondary to cell infiltration, and occasional vesiculation and necrosis). Delayed hypersensitivity reactions to tuberculin may indicate infection with a variety of nontuberculosis mycobacteria, or vaccination with the live attenuated mycobacterial strain of *M. bovis* vaccine, BCG, in addition to previous natural infection with *M. tuberculosis.*

Other Adverse Effects

1% to 10%:

- Central nervous system: Pain
- Gastrointestinal: Ulceration
- Miscellaneous: Necrosis

Frequency not defined:

- Dermatologic: Ulceration, necrosis, vesiculation
- Local: Pain at injection site

Drug Interactions Decreased Effect: Reaction may be suppressed in patients receiving systemic corticosteroids, aminocaproic acid, or within 4-6 weeks following immunization with live or inactivated viral vaccines

Drug Uptake

Onset of action: Delayed hypersensitivity reactions: 5-6 hours; Peak effect: 48-72 hours

Duration: A few days

Pregnancy Risk Factor C

Generic Available No

Comments Test dose: 0.1 mL intracutaneously; examine site at 48-72 hours after administration; whenever tuberculin is administered, a record should be made of the administration technique (Mantoux method, disposable multiple-puncture device), tuberculin used (OT or PPD), manufacturer and lot number of tuberculin used, date of administration, date of test reading, and the size of the reaction in millimeters (mm).

Tubersol® *see* Tuberculin Purified Protein Derivative *on page 1218*

Tuinal® *see* Amobarbital and Secobarbital *on page 84*

Tums® [OTC] *see* Calcium Carbonate *on page 201*

Tums® E-X Extra Strength Tablet [OTC] *see* Calcium Carbonate *on page 201*

Tums® Ultra [OTC] *see* Calcium Carbonate *on page 201*

Tusibron® [OTC] *see* Guaifenesin *on page 568*

Tusibron-DM® [OTC] *see* Guaifenesin and Dextromethorphan *on page 569*

Tussar® SF Syrup *see* Guaifenesin, Pseudoephedrine, and Codeine *on page 570*

Tuss-DM® [OTC] *see* Guaifenesin and Dextromethorphan *on page 569*

Tussend® *see* Hydrocodone, Pseudoephedrine, and Guaifenesin *on page 608*

Tussigon® *see* Hydrocodone and Homatropine *on page 604*

Tussionex® *see* Hydrocodone and Chlorpheniramine *on page 602*

Tussi-Organidin® DM NR *see* Guaifenesin and Dextromethorphan *on page 569*

Tussi-Organidin® NR *see* Guaifenesin and Codeine *on page 568*

Tusstat® *see* DiphenhydrAMINE *on page 398*

Twice-A-Day® Nasal [OTC] *see* Oxymetazoline *on page 907*

Twilite® [OTC] *see* DiphenhydrAMINE *on page 398*

Twin-K® *see* Potassium Citrate and Potassium Gluconate *on page 979*

Twinrix® *see* Hepatitis A Inactivated and Hepatitis B (Recombinant) Vaccine *on page 582*

Tylenol® [OTC] *see* Acetaminophen *on page 26*

Tylenol® Allergy Sinus [OTC] *see* Acetaminophen, Chlorpheniramine, and Pseudoephedrine *on page 33*

Tylenol® Arthritis Pain [OTC] *see* Acetaminophen *on page 26*

Tylenol® Children's [OTC] *see* Acetaminophen *on page 26*

Tylenol® Cold Non-Drowsy [OTC] *see* Acetaminophen, Dextromethorphan, and Pseudoephedrine *on page 34*

Tylenol® Extra Strength [OTC] *see* Acetaminophen *on page 26*

Tylenol® Flu Non-Drowsy Maximum Strength [OTC] *see* Acetaminophen, Dextromethorphan, and Pseudoephedrine *on page 34*

Tylenol® Infants [OTC] *see* Acetaminophen *on page 26*
Tylenol® Junior Strength [OTC] *see* Acetaminophen *on page 26*
Tylenol® PM Extra Strength [OTC] *see* Acetaminophen and Diphenhydramine *on page 30*
Tylenol® Severe Allergy [OTC] *see* Acetaminophen and Diphenhydramine *on page 30*
Tylenol® Sinus Non-Drowsy [OTC] *see* Acetaminophen and Pseudoephedrine *on page 30*
Tylenol® Sore Throat [OTC] *see* Acetaminophen *on page 26*
Tylenol® With Codeine *see* Acetaminophen and Codeine *on page 28*
Tylox® *see* Oxycodone and Acetaminophen *on page 903*
Typhim Vi® *see* Typhoid Vaccine *on page 1220*

Typhoid Vaccine (TYE foid vak SEEN)

U.S. Brand Names Typhim Vi®; Vivotif Berna™

Canadian Brand Names Vivotif Berna®

Pharmacologic Category Vaccine

Synonyms Typhoid Vaccine Live Oral Ty21a

Use Typhoid vaccine: Live, attenuated Ty21a typhoid vaccine should not be administered to immunocompromised persons, including those known to be infected with HIV. Parenteral inactivated vaccine is a theoretically safer alternative for this group.

Oral: For immunization of children >6 years of age and adults who expect intimate exposure of or household contact with typhoid fever, travelers to areas of world with risk of exposure to typhoid fever, and workers in microbiology laboratories with expected frequent contact with *S. typhi*

Parenteral: Promotes active immunity to typhoid fever for patients intimately exposed to a typhoid carrier or foreign travel to a typhoid fever endemic area

Local Anesthetic/Vasoconstrictor Precautions No information available to require special precautions

Effects on Dental Treatment No effects or complications reported

Dosage

S.C. (AKD and H-P):

- Children 6 months to 10 years: 0.25 mL; repeat in ≥4 weeks (total immunization is 2 doses)
- Children >10 years and Adults: 0.5 mL; repeat dose in ≥4 weeks (total immunization is 2 doses)
- Booster: 0.25 mL every 3 years for children 6 months to 10 years and 0.5 mL every 3 years for children >10 years and adults

Oral: Adults:

- Primary immunization: 1 capsule on alternate days (day 1, 3, 5, and 7)
- Booster immunization: Repeat full course of primary immunization every 5 years

Mechanism of Action Virulent strains of *Salmonella typhi* cause disease by penetrating the intestinal mucosa and entering the systemic circulation via the lymphatic vasculature. One possible mechanism of conferring immunity may be the provocation of a local immune response in the intestinal tract induced by oral ingesting of a live strain with subsequent aborted infection. The ability of *Salmonella typhi* to produce clinical disease (and to elicit an immune response) is dependent on the bacteria having a complete lipopolysaccharide. The live attenuate Ty21a strain lacks the enzyme UDP-4-galactose epimerase so that lipopolysaccharide is only synthesized under conditions that induce bacterial autolysis. Thus, the strain remains avirulent despite the production of sufficient lipopolysaccharide to evoke a protective immune response. Despite low levels of lipopolysaccharide synthesis, cells lyse before gaining a virulent phenotype due to the intracellular accumulation of metabolic intermediates.

Other Adverse Effects All serious adverse reactions must be reported to the U.S. Department of Health and Human Services (DHHS) Vaccine Adverse Event Reporting System (VAERS) 1-800-822-7967.

Oral:

1% to 10%:

- Dermatologic: Rash
- Gastrointestinal: Abdominal discomfort, stomach cramps, diarrhea, nausea, vomiting

Injection:

>10%:

- Central nervous system: Headache (9% to 30%), fever
- Dermatologic: Local tenderness, erythema, induration (6% to 40%)
- Neuromuscular & skeletal: Myalgia (14% to 29%)

Drug Interactions

Increased Effect/Toxicity: Simultaneous administration with other vaccines which cause local or systemic adverse effects should be avoided.

Decreased effect with concurrent use of sulfonamides or other antibiotics

Drug Uptake

Onset of action: Immunity to *Salmonella typhi*: Oral: ~1 week

Duration: Immunity: Oral: ~5 years; Parenteral: ~3 years

Pregnancy Risk Factor C

Generic Available No

Comments Inactivated bacteria vaccine; federal law requires that the date of administration, the vaccine manufacturer, lot number of vaccine, and the administering person's name, title and address be entered into the patient's permanent medical record

Tyzine® *see* Tetrahydrozoline *on page 1150*
UAD Otic® *see* Neomycin, Polymyxin B, and Hydrocortisone *on page 857*
Ulcerease® [OTC] *see* Phenol *on page 946*
Ultiva™ *see* Remifentanil *on page 1044*
Ultracet™ *see* Acetaminophen and Tramadol *on page 31*
Ultram® *see* Tramadol *on page 1187*
Ultra Mide® *see* Urea *on page 1221*
Ultrase® *see* Pancrelipase *on page 914*
Ultrase® MT *see* Pancrelipase *on page 914*
Ultra Tears® [OTC] *see* Artificial Tears *on page 117*
Ultravate™ *see* Halobetasol *on page 577*
Unasyn® *see* Ampicillin and Sulbactam *on page 96*

Undecylenic Acid and Derivatives

(un de sil EN ik AS id & dah RIV ah tivs)

U.S. Brand Names Caldesene® [OTC]; Pedi-Pro [OTC]

Pharmacologic Category Antifungal Agent, Topical

Synonyms Zinc Undecylenate

Use Treatment of athlete's foot (tinea pedis), ringworm (except nails and scalp), prickly heat, jock itch (tinea cruris), diaper rash and other minor skin irritations due to superficial dermatophytes

Local Anesthetic/Vasoconstrictor Precautions No information available to require special precautions

Effects on Dental Treatment No effects or complications reported

Dosage Children and Adults: Topical: Apply as needed twice daily after cleansing the affected area for 2-4 weeks

Other Adverse Effects 1% to 10%: Dermatologic: Skin irritation, sensitization

Generic Available Yes

Comments Ointment should be applied at night, powder may be applied during the day or used alone when a drying effect is needed

Uni-Bent® Cough Syrup *see* DiphenhydrAMINE *on page 398*
Unicap® [OTC] *see* Vitamins, Multiple *on page 1246*
Uni-Dur® *see* Theophylline *on page 1152*
Uni-Fed® [OTC] *see* Triprolidine and Pseudoephedrine *on page 1213*
Uniphyl® *see* Theophylline *on page 1152*
Uniretic™ *see* Moexipril and Hydrochlorothiazide *on page 824*
Unithroid™ *see* Levothyroxine *on page 705*
Uni-tussin® [OTC] *see* Guaifenesin *on page 568*
Uni-tussin® DM [OTC] *see* Guaifenesin and Dextromethorphan *on page 569*
Univasc® *see* Moexipril *on page 824*

Urea (yoor EE a)

U.S. Brand Names Amino-Cerv™ Vaginal Cream; Aquacare® [OTC]; Carmol® [OTC]; Gormel® Creme [OTC]; Lanaphilic® [OTC]; Nutraplus® [OTC]; Rea-Lo® [OTC]; Ultra Mide®; Ureacin®-20 [OTC]; Ureaphil®

Canadian Brand Names UltraMide 25™; Uremol®; Urisec®

Mexican Brand Names Derma Keri®; Dermoplast®

Pharmacologic Category Diuretic, Osmotic; Keratolytic Agent; Topical Skin Product

Synonyms Carbamide

Use Reduces intracranial pressure and intraocular pressure; topically promotes hydration and removal of excess keratin in hyperkeratotic conditions and dry skin; mild cervicitis

Local Anesthetic/Vasoconstrictor Precautions No information available to require special precautions

Effects on Dental Treatment No effects or complications reported

Dosage

Children: I.V. slow infusion:
- <2 years: 0.1-0.5 g/kg
- >2 years: 0.5-1.5 g/kg

Adults:
- I.V. infusion: 1-1.5 g/kg by slow infusion (1-2½ hours); maximum: 120 g/24 hours
- Topical: Apply 1-3 times/day
- Vaginal: Insert 1 applicatorful in vagina at bedtime for 2-4 weeks

(Continued)

Urea *(Continued)*

Mechanism of Action Elevates plasma osmolality by inhibiting tubular reabsorption of water, thus enhancing the flow of water into extracellular fluid

Other Adverse Effects 1% to 10%:

Central nervous system: Headache

Endocrine & metabolic: Electrolyte imbalance

Gastrointestinal: Nausea, vomiting

Local: Transient stinging, local irritation, tissue necrosis from extravasation of I.V. preparation

Drug Interactions Decreases effect/toxicity/levels of lithium

Drug Uptake

Onset of action: Therapeutic: I.V.: Maximum: 1-2 hours

Duration: 3-6 hours; diuresis can continue ≤10 hours

Half-life, elimination: 1 hour

Pregnancy Risk Factor C

Generic Available Yes

Urea and Hydrocortisone (yoor EE a & hye droe KOR ti sone)

U.S. Brand Names Carmol-HC®

Canadian Brand Names Ti-U-Lac® H; Uremol® HC

Pharmacologic Category Corticosteroid, Topical

Synonyms Hydrocortisone and Urea

Use Inflammation of corticosteroid-responsive dermatoses

Local Anesthetic/Vasoconstrictor Precautions No information available to require special precautions

Effects on Dental Treatment No effects or complications reported

Dosage Apply thin film and rub in well 1-4 times/day

Therapy should be discontinued when control is achieved; if no improvement is seen, reassessment of diagnosis may be necessary.

Drug Uptake See Urea *on page 1221* and Hydrocortisone *on page 608*

Pregnancy Risk Factor C

Generic Available No

Ureacin®-20 [OTC] *see* Urea *on page 1221*

Ureaphil® *see* Urea *on page 1221*

Urecholine® *see* Bethanechol *on page 162*

Urex® *see* Methenamine *on page 781*

Urimax™ *see* Methenamine, Sodium Biphosphate, Phenyl Salicylate, Methylene Blue, and Hyoscyamine *on page 782*

Urispas® *see* Flavoxate *on page 504*

Uristat® [OTC] *see* Phenazopyridine *on page 943*

Urocit®-K *see* Potassium Citrate *on page 978*

Urodol® [OTC] *see* Phenazopyridine *on page 943*

Urofemme® [OTC] *see* Phenazopyridine *on page 943*

Urofollitropin (yoor oh fol li TROE pin)

U.S. Brand Names Fertinex®; Metrodin®

Canadian Brand Names Fertinorm® H.P.

Mexican Brand Names Fertinorm® H.P.; Follitrin®

Pharmacologic Category Ovulation Stimulator

Use Induction of ovulation in patients with polycystic ovarian disease and to stimulate the development of multiple oocytes

Local Anesthetic/Vasoconstrictor Precautions No information available to require special precautions

Effects on Dental Treatment No effects or complications reported

Dosage Adults: Female: S.C.: 75 units/day for 7-12 days, used with hCG may repeat course of treatment 2 more times

Mechanism of Action Preparation of follicle-stimulating hormone 75 IU with <1 IU of luteinizing hormone (LH) which is isolated from the urine of postmenopausal women. Follicle-stimulating hormone plays a role in the development of follicles. Elevated FSH levels early in the normal menstrual cycle are thought to play a significant role in recruiting a cohort of follicles for maturation. A single follicle is enriched with FSH receptors and becomes dominant over the rest of the recruited follicles. The increased number of FSH receptors allows it to grow despite declining FSH levels. This dominant follicle secretes low levels of estrogen and inhibin which further reduces pituitary FSH output. The ovarian stroma, under the influence of luteinizing hormone, produces androgens which the dominant follicle uses as precursors for estrogens.

Other Adverse Effects

>10%:

Endocrine & metabolic: Ovarian enlargement or ovarian cysts

Local: Edema at injection site, pain at injection site

1% to 10%:
- Cardiovascular: Arterial thromboembolism
- Central nervous system: Fever, chills
- Dermatologic: Rash, urticaria
- Endocrine & metabolic: Breast tenderness
- Gastrointestinal: Nausea, vomiting, abdominal pain, diarrhea
- Miscellaneous: Hyperstimulation syndrome

Drug Uptake Half-life, elimination: 3.9 hours and 70.4 hours (FSH has two half-lives)

Pregnancy Risk Factor X

Generic Available No

Urogesic® *see* Phenazopyridine *on page 943*

Uro-KP-Neutral® *see* Potassium Phosphate and Sodium Phosphate *on page 982*

Uro-Mag® [OTC] *see* Magnesium Oxide *on page 742*

Urso® *see* Ursodiol *on page 1223*

Ursodiol (ER soe dye ole)

U.S. Brand Names Actigall™; Urso®

Canadian Brand Names Urso®

Mexican Brand Names Ursofalk

Pharmacologic Category Gallstone Dissolution Agent

Synonyms Ursodeoxycholic Acid

Use Actigall™: Gallbladder stone dissolution; prevention of gallstones in obese patients experiencing rapid weight loss; Urso®: Primary biliary cirrhosis

Unlabeled/Investigational: Liver transplantation

Local Anesthetic/Vasoconstrictor Precautions No information available to require special precautions

Effects on Dental Treatment No effects or complications reported

Dosage Adults: Oral:
- Gallstone dissolution: 8-10 mg/kg/day in 2-3 divided doses; use beyond 24 months is not established; obtain ultrasound images at 6-month intervals for the first year of therapy; 30% of patients have stone recurrence after dissolution
- Gallstone prevention: 300 mg twice daily
- Primary biliary cirrhosis: 13-15 mg/kg/day in 4 divided doses (with food)

Mechanism of Action Decreases the cholesterol content of bile and bile stones by reducing the secretion of cholesterol from the liver and the fractional reabsorption of cholesterol by the intestines. Mechanism of action in primary biliary cirrhosis is not clearly defined.

Other Adverse Effects

>10%:
- Central nervous system: Headache (up to 25%), dizziness (up to 17%)
- Gastrointestinal: In treatment of primary biliary cirrhosis: Constipation (up to 26%)

1% to 10%:
- Dermatologic: Rash (<1% to 3%), alopecia (<1% to 5%)
- Gastrointestinal:
  - In gallstone dissolution: Most GI events (diarrhea, nausea, vomiting) are similar to placebo and attributable to gallstone disease.
- Hematologic: Leukopenia (3%)
- Miscellaneous: Allergy (5%)

In treatment of primary biliary cirrhosis: Constipation, diarrhea (1%), dyspepsia, headache

Drug Interactions Decreased effect with aluminum-containing antacids, cholestyramine, colestipol, clofibrate, and oral contraceptives (estrogens)

Drug Uptake Half-life, elimination: 100 hours

Pregnancy Risk Factor B

Generic Available Yes

Comments Use beyond 24 months is not established; obtain ultrasound images at 6-month intervals for the first year of therapy; 30% of patients have stone recurrence after dissolution

Uvadex® *see* Methoxsalen *on page 790*

Vagifem® *see* Estradiol *on page 457*

Vagistat®-1 [OTC] *see* Tioconazole *on page 1172*

Valacyclovir (val ay SYE kloe veer)

Related Information

Systemic Viral Diseases *on page 1354*

U.S. Brand Names Valtrex®

Canadian Brand Names Valtrex®

Pharmacologic Category Antiviral Agent, Oral

Synonyms Valacyclovir Hydrochloride

(Continued)

Valacyclovir *(Continued)*

Use Treatment of herpes zoster (shingles) in immunocompetent patients; episodic treatment of recurrent genital herpes in immunocompetent patients; for first episode genital herpes

Local Anesthetic/Vasoconstrictor Precautions No information available to require special precautions

Effects on Dental Treatment No effects or complications reported

Dosage Oral: Adults:

Herpes zoster (shingles): 1 g 3 times/day for 7 days

Genital herpes:

- Initial episode: 1 g 2 times/day for 10 days
- Episodic treatment: 500 mg twice daily for 3 days
- Prophylaxis: 500-1000 mg once daily

Dosing interval in renal impairment:

- Herpes zoster:
  - Cl_{cr} 30-49 mL/minute: 1 g every 12 hours
  - Cl_{cr} 10-29 mL/minute: 1 g every 24 hours
  - Cl_{cr} <10 mL/minute: 500 mg every 24 hours
- Genital herpes:
  - Initial episode:
    - Cl_{cr} 10-29 mL/minute: 1 g every 24 hours
    - Cl_{cr} <10 mL/minute: 500 mg every 24 hours
  - Episodic treatment: Cl_{cr} <10-29 mL/minute: 500 mg every 24 hours
  - Prophylaxis: Cl_{cr} <10-29 mL/minute:
    - For usual dose of 1 g every 24 hours, decrease dose to 500 mg every 24 hours
    - For usual dose of 500 mg every 24 hours, decrease dose to 500 mg every 48 hours

Hemodialysis: Dialyzable (~33% removed during 4-hour session); administer dose postdialysis

Chronic ambulatory peritoneal dialysis/continuous arteriovenous hemofiltration dialysis: Pharmacokinetic parameters are similar to those in patients with ESRD; supplemental dose not needed following dialysis

Mechanism of Action Valacyclovir, the L-valyl ester of acyclovir, is rapidly converted to acyclovir before it exerts its antiviral activity against HSV-1, HSV-2, or VZV. It is most active against HSV-1 and least against VZV due to its varied affinity for thymidine kinase. Thymidine kinase converts it into acyclovir monophosphate; this is then converted into the diphosphate and triphosphate forms. Acyclovir triphosphate inhibits replication of herpes viral DNA via competitive inhibition of herpes viral DNA polymerase, incorporation and termination of the growing viral DNA chain, and inactivation of the viral DNA polymerase.

Other Adverse Effects

>10%:

- Central nervous system: Headache (14% to 38%)
- Gastrointestinal: Nausea (11% to 15%)

1% to 10%:

- Central nervous system: Dizziness (2% to 4%), depression (0% to 7%)
- Endocrine: Dysmenorrhea (≤1% to 8%)
- Gastrointestinal: Abdominal pain (2% to 11%), vomiting (<1% to 6%)
- Hematologic: Leukopenia (≤1%), thrombocytopenia (≤1%)
- Hepatic: AST increased (1% to 4%)
- Neuromuscular & skeletal: Arthralgia (≤1 to 6%)

Warnings/Precautions Thrombotic thrombocytopenic purpura/hemolytic uremic syndrome has occurred in immunocompromised patients (at doses of 8 g/day); use caution and adjust the dose in elderly patients or those with renal insufficiency and in patients receiving concurrent nephrotoxic agents; treatment should begin as soon as possible after the first signs and symptoms (within 72 hours of onset of first diagnosis or within 24 hours of onset of recurrent episodes); safety and efficacy in children have not been established

Drug Interactions

Increased Effect/Toxicity: Valacyclovir and acyclovir have increased CNS side effects with zidovudine and probenecid.

Decreased Effect: Cimetidine and/or probenecid has decreased the rate but not the extent of valacyclovir conversion to acyclovir leading to decreased effectiveness of valacyclovir.

Drug Uptake

Absorption: Rapid

Half-life, elimination (normal renal function): Adults: Acyclovir: 2.5-3.3 hours; End-stage renal disease: 14-20 hours; Valacyclovir: ~30 minutes

Pregnancy Risk Factor B

Generic Available No

Valcyte™ *see* Valganciclovir *on page 1226*

Valdecoxib (val de KOKS ib)

U.S. Brand Names Bextra®

Pharmacologic Category Nonsteroidal Anti-inflammatory Drug (NSAID), COX-2 Selective

Use Relief of signs and symptoms of osteoarthritis and adult rheumatoid arthritis; treatment of primary dysmenorrhea

Local Anesthetic/Vasoconstrictor Precautions No information available to require special precautions

Effects on Dental Treatment No effects or complications reported

Dosage Oral: Adults:

Osteoarthritis and rheumatoid arthritis: 10 mg once daily; **Note:** No additional benefits seen with 20 mg/day

Primary dysmenorrhea: 20 mg twice daily as needed

Dosage adjustment in renal impairment: Not recommended for use in advanced disease

Dosage adjustment in hepatic impairment: Not recommended for use in advanced liver dysfunction (Child-Pugh Class C)

Mechanism of Action Inhibits prostaglandin synthesis by decreasing the activity of the enzyme, cyclooxygenase-2 (COX-2), which results in decreased formation of prostaglandin precursors. Does not affect platelet function.

Other Adverse Effects

2% to 10%:

Cardiovascular: Peripheral edema (2% to 3%), hypertension (2%)

Central nervous system: Headache (5% to 9%), dizziness (3%)

Dermatologic: Rash (1% to 2%)

Gastrointestinal: Dyspepsia (8% to 9%), abdominal pain (7% to 8%), nausea (6% to 7%), diarrhea (5% to 6%), flatulence (3% to 4%), abdominal fullness (2%)

Neuromuscular & skeletal: Back pain (2% to 3%), myalgia (2%)

Otic: Earache, tinnitus

Respiratory: Upper respiratory tract infection (6% to 7%), sinusitis (2% to 3%)

Miscellaneous: Influenza-like symptoms (2%)

<2%: Acne, albuminuria, alkaline phosphatase increased, allergy, ALT increased, alopecia, amenorrhea, anemia, aneurysm, angina, anorexia, anxiety, aortic stenosis, appetite increased, arrhythmia, arthralgia, AST increased, atrial fibrillation, blurred vision, bradycardia, breast neoplasm, bronchitis, bronchospasm, BUN increased, cardiomyopathy, carotid stenosis, cataract, cellulitis, cervical dysplasia, chest pain, chills, colitis, confusion, CHF, conjunctivitis, constipation, convulsion, coronary thrombosis, cough, CPK increased, creatinine increased, cystitis, depression exacerbation, dermatitis (contact), dermatitis (fungal), diabetes mellitus, diverticulosis, dry skin, duodenal ulcer, duodenitis, dysmenorrhea, dysphagia, dyspnea, dysuria, ecchymosis, EKG abnormality, eczema, edema, emphysema, eosinophilia, epistaxis, eructation, esophageal perforation, esophagitis, eye pain, facial edema, fatigue, fecal incontinence, fever, gastric ulcer, gastritis, gastroenteritis, gastroesophageal reflux, gastrointestinal bleeding, glycosuria, goiter, gout, halitosis, heart block, heart murmur, hemangioma, hematemesis, hematuria, hematochezia, hematoma, hemorrhoids, hepatitis, hiatal hernia, hot flushes, hypercholesterolemia, hyperglycemia, hyperkalemia, hyperlipemia, hyperparathyroidism, hypertension exacerbation, hypertensive encephalopathy, hypertonia, hyperuricemia, hypocalcemia, hypoesthesia, hypokalemia, hypotension, intermittent claudication, impotence, insomnia, keratitis, laryngitis, LDH increased, leukopenia, leukocytosis, leukorrhea, lipoma, LFTs increased, lymphadenopathy, lymphangitis, lymphopenia, malaise, mastitis, melena, menorrhagia, menstrual bloating, migraine, micturition frequency increased, mitral insufficiency, morbid dreaming, myocardial infarction, myocardial ischemia, neck stiffness, nervousness, neuralgia, neuropathy, osteoporosis, ovarian cyst (malignant), pain, palpitations, paresthesia, pericarditis, periorbital swelling, pharyngitis, photosensitivity, pleurisy, pneumonia, pruritus, pyuria, rash erythematous, rash maculopapular, rash psoriaform, rhinitis, skin hypertrophy, skin ulceration, somnolence, stomatitis, stool frequency increased, sweating increased, syncope, synovitis, tachycardia, taste perversion, tendonitis, tenesmus, thirst increased, thrombocytopenia, thrombophlebitis, tremor, twitching, unstable angina, urinary incontinence, urinary tract infection, urticaria, vaginal hemorrhage, varicose vein, vasospasm, ventricular fibrillation, vertigo, vomiting, weakness, weight gain/loss, xerostomia, xerophthalmia

Contraindications Hypersensitivity to valdecoxib or any component of the formulation; patients who have experienced asthma, urticaria, or allergic-type reactions to aspirin or NSAIDs; pregnancy (3rd trimester)

Warnings/Precautions Gastrointestinal irritation, ulceration, bleeding, and perforation may occur with NSAIDs (it is unclear whether valdecoxib is associated with rates of these events which are similar to nonselective NSAIDs). Use with caution in patients with a history of GI disease (bleeding or ulcers) or risk factor for GI bleeding, use lowest dose for shortest time possible. Use with caution in patients with decreased renal function, hepatic disease, CHF, hypertension, dehydration, or asthma. Anaphylactoid reactions may occur, even with no prior exposure to

(Continued)

Valdecoxib *(Continued)*

valdecoxib. Use caution in patients with known or suspected deficiency of cytochrome P450 isoenzyme 2C9. Use in patients with severe hepatic impairment (Child-Pugh Class C) is not recommended. Safety and efficacy have not been established for patients <18 years of age.

Drug Interactions CYP3A3/4 and 2C9 enzyme substrate; CYP2C9 enzyme inhibitor (weak *in vitro*), 3A3/4 enzyme inhibitor (weak *in vitro*), 2C19 enzyme inhibitor (moderate *in vitro*), 2D6 enzyme inhibitor (weak at supratherapeutic doses)

ACE inhibitors: Antihypertensive effects may be decreased by concurrent therapy with NSAIDs; monitor BP.

Angiotensin II antagonists: Antihypertensive effects may be decreased by concurrent therapy with NSAIDs; monitor BP.

Anticoagulants (warfarin, heparin, LMWHs): In combination with NSAIDs, can cause increased risk of bleeding.

Antiplatelet drugs (ticlopidine, clopidogrel, aspirin, abciximab, dipyridamole, eptifibatide, tirofiban): Can cause an increased risk of bleeding.

Corticosteroids: May increase the risk of GI ulceration; avoid concurrent use

Cyclosporine: NSAIDs may increase serum creatinine, potassium, BP, and cyclosporine levels; monitor cyclosporine levels and renal function carefully.

CYP2C9 inhibitors: May increase valdecoxib levels. Use caution with concurrent use; inhibitors include amiodarone, cimetidine, fluconazole, fluoxetine, isoniazid, metronidazole, omeprazole, valproic acid.

CYP2D6 substrates: Valdecoxib (40 mg twice daily for 7 days) increased levels of dextromethorphan.

CYP3A3/4 inhibitors: May increase valdecoxib levels. Use caution with concurrent use; inhibitors include amiodarone, cimetidine, clarithromycin, erythromycin, delavirdine, diltiazem, disulfiram, fluoxetine, fluvoxamine, grapefruit juice, nefazodone, nevirapine, propoxyphene, quinupristin-dalfopristin, verapamil, zafirlukast, zileuton

Hydralazine: Antihypertensive effect is decreased; avoid concurrent use

Lithium levels can be increased; avoid concurrent use if possible or monitor lithium levels and adjust dose. Sulindac may have the least effect. When NSAID is stopped, lithium will need adjustment again.

Loop diuretics: Diuretic and antihypertensive efficacy is reduced. May be anticipated with any NSAID.

Methotrexate: Severe bone marrow suppression, aplastic anemia, and GI toxicity have been reported with concomitant NSAID therapy. Selective COX-2 inhibitors appear to have a lower risk of this toxicity, however, caution is warranted.

Thiazides: Diuretic efficacy is reduced.

Warfarin: Valdecoxib (40 mg twice daily) caused a significant increase in plasma warfarin exposure (12% R-warfarin, 15% S-warfarin). May increase the anticoagulant effects of warfarin. Monitor INR closely.

Dietary/Ethanol/Herb Considerations

Ethanol: Avoid use; may enhance gastric mucosal irritation.

Food: May be taken with food; high-fat meal delays time to peak by 1-2 hours. Avoid garlic, ginger, and green tea.

Herb/Nutraceutical: Avoid cat's claw, dong quai, evening primrose, feverfew, garlic, ginger, ginkgo biloba, ginseng, green tea, horse chestnut, and red clover due to additional antiplatelet activity.

Drug Uptake

Onset of action: Dysmenorrhea: 60 minutes

Half-life, elimination: 8-11 hours

Time to peak: 2.25-3 hours

Pregnancy Risk Factor C/D (3rd trimester)

Dosage Forms TAB: 10 mg, 20 mg

Generic Available No

Valertest No.1® *see* Estradiol and Testosterone *on page 461*

Valganciclovir (val gan SYE kloh veer)

U.S. Brand Names Valcyte™

Pharmacologic Category Antiviral Agent

Synonyms Valganciclovir Hydrochloride

Use Treatment of cytomegalovirus (CMV) retinitis in patients with acquired immunodeficiency syndrome (AIDS)

Local Anesthetic/Vasoconstrictor Precautions No information available to require special precautions

Effects on Dental Treatment No effects or complications reported

Dosage Oral: Adults: CMV retinitis:

Induction: 900 mg twice daily for 21 days (with food)

Maintenance: Following induction treatment, or for patients with inactive CMV retinitis who require maintenance therapy: Recommended dose: 900 mg once daily (with food)

Dosage adjustment in renal impairment:

Induction dose (for 21 days):

Cl_{cr} 40-59 mL/minute: 450 mg twice daily

Cl_{cr} 25-39 mL/minute: 450 mg once daily

Cl_{cr} 10-24 mL/minute: 450 mg every 2 days

Maintenance dose:

Cl_{cr} 40-59 mL/minute: 450 mg once daily

Cl_{cr} 25-39 mL/minute: 450 mg every 2 days

Cl_{cr} 10-24 mL/minute: 450 mg twice weekly

Valganciclovir is not recommended in patients receiving hemodialysis. For patients on hemodialysis (Cl_{cr} <10 mL/minute), it is recommended that ganciclovir be used (dose adjusted as specified for ganciclovir).

Mechanism of Action Valganciclovir is rapidly converted to ganciclovir in the body. The bioavailability of ganciclovir from valganciclovir is increased 10-fold compared to the oral ganciclovir. A dose of 900 mg achieved systemic exposure of ganciclovir comparable to that achieved with the recommended doses of I.V. ganciclovir of 5 mg/kg. Ganciclovir is phosphorylated to a substrate which competitively inhibits the binding of deoxyguanosine triphosphate to DNA polymerase resulting in inhibition of viral DNA synthesis.

Other Adverse Effects

>10%:

Central nervous system: Fever (31%), headache (9% to 22%), insomnia (16%)

Gastrointestinal: Diarrhea (16% to 41%), nausea (8% to 30%), vomiting (21%), abdominal pain (15%)

Hematologic: Granulocytopenia (11% to 27%), anemia (8% to 26%)

Ocular: Retinal detachment (15%)

1% to 10%:

Central nervous system: Peripheral neuropathy (9%), paresthesia (8%), seizures (<5%), psychosis, hallucinations (<5%), confusion (<5%), agitation (<5%)

Hematologic: Thrombocytopenia (8%), pancytopenia (<5%), bone marrow depression (<5%), aplastic anemia (<5%), bleeding (potentially life-threatening due to thrombocytopenia <5%)

Renal: Decreased renal function (<5%)

Miscellaneous: Local and systemic infections, including sepsis (<5%); allergic reaction (<5%)

Contraindications Hypersensitivity to valganciclovir, ganciclovir, acyclovir, or any component of their formulation; absolute neutrophil count <500/mm^3; platelet count <25,000/mm^3; hemoglobin <8 g/dL

Drug Interactions

Increased Effect/Toxicity: Reported for ganciclovir: Immunosuppressive agents may increase hematologic toxicity of ganciclovir. Imipenem/cilastatin may increase seizure potential. Oral ganciclovir increases blood levels of zidovudine, although zidovudine decreases steady-state levels of ganciclovir. Since both drugs have the potential to cause neutropenia and anemia, some patients may not tolerate concomitant therapy with these drugs at full dosage. Didanosine levels are increased with concurrent ganciclovir. Other nephrotoxic drugs (eg, amphotericin and cyclosporine) may have additive nephrotoxicity with ganciclovir.

Decreased Effect: Reported for ganciclovir: A decrease in blood levels of ganciclovir AUC may occur when used with didanosine.

Drug Uptake

Absorption: Well absorbed, high-fat meal increases AUC by 30%

Half-life, elimination (increases with renal impairment): Ganciclovir: 4.08 hours; Severe renal impairment: ≤68 hours

Pregnancy Risk Factor C

Generic Available No

Valisone® [DSC] *see* Betamethasone *on page 159*

Valium® *see* Diazepam *on page 373*

Valorin [OTC] *see* Acetaminophen *on page 26*

Valorin Extra [OTC] *see* Acetaminophen *on page 26*

Valproic Acid and Derivatives

(val PROE ik AS id & dah RIV ah tives)

U.S. Brand Names Depacon®; Depakene®; Depakote® Delayed Release; Depakote® ER; Depakote® Sprinkle®

Canadian Brand Names Alti-Divalproex; Apo®-Divalproex; Depakene®; Epival® I.V.; Gen-Divalproex; Novo-Divalproex; Nu-Divalproex; PMS-Valproic Acid; PMS-Valproic Acid E.C.; Rhoxal-valproic

Mexican Brand Names Atemperator-S®; Cryoval®; Depakene®; Epival®; Leptilan®; Valprosid®

Pharmacologic Category Anticonvulsant, Miscellaneous

Synonyms Dipropylacetic Acid; Divalproex Sodium; DPA; 2-Propylpentanoic Acid; 2-Propylvaleric Acid; Valproate Semisodium; Valproate Sodium; Valproic Acid

Use

Mania associated with bipolar disorder (Depakote®)

(Continued)

Valproic Acid and Derivatives *(Continued)*

Migraine prophylaxis (Depakote®, Depakote® ER)
Monotherapy and adjunctive therapy in the treatment of patients with complex partial seizures that occur either in isolation or in association with other types of seizures (Depacon™, Depakote®)
Sole and adjunctive therapy of simple and complex absence seizures (Depacon™, Depakene®, Depakote®)
Adjunctively in patients with multiple seizure types that include absence seizures (Depacon™, Depakene®)

Unlabeled/Investigational: Behavior disorders in Alzheimer's disease

Local Anesthetic/Vasoconstrictor Precautions No information available to require special precautions

Effects on Dental Treatment No effects or complications reported

Dosage

Seizures:

Children >10 years and Adults:

Oral: Initial: 10-15 mg/kg/day in 1-3 divided doses; increase by 5-10 mg/kg/day at weekly intervals until therapeutic levels are achieved; maintenance: 30-60 mg/kg/day in 2-3 divided doses. Adult usual dose: 1000-2500 mg/day

Children receiving more than one anticonvulsant (ie, polytherapy) may require doses up to 100 mg/kg/day in 3-4 divided doses

I.V.: Administer as a 60-minute infusion (≤20 mg/minute) with the same frequency as oral products; switch patient to oral products as soon as possible. Rapid infusions have been given: ≤15 mg/kg over 5-10 minutes. (1.5-3 mg/kg/minute).

Rectal: Dilute syrup 1:1 with water for use as a retention enema; loading dose: 17-20 mg/kg one time; maintenance: 10-15 mg/kg/dose every 8 hours

Mania: Adults: Oral: 750 mg/day in divided doses; dose should be adjusted as rapidly as possible to desired clinical effect; a loading dose of 20 mg/kg may be used; maximum recommended dosage: 60 mg/kg/day

Migraine prophylaxis: Adults: Oral:

Extended release tablets: 500 mg once daily for 7 days, then increase to 1000 mg once daily; adjust dose based on patient response; usual dosage range 500-1000 mg/day

Delayed release tablets: 250 mg twice daily; adjust dose based on patient response, up to 1000 mg/day

Elderly: Elimination is decreased in the elderly. Studies of elderly patients with dementia show a high incidence of somnolence. In some patients, this was associated with weight loss. Starting doses should be lower and increases should be slow, with careful monitoring of nutritional intake and dehydration. Safety and efficacy for use in patients >65 years have not been studied for migraine prophylaxis.

Dosing adjustment in renal impairment: A 27% reduction in clearance of unbound valproate is seen in patients with Cl_{cr} <10 mL/minute. Hemodialysis reduces valproate concentrations by 20%, therefore no dose adjustment is needed in patients with renal failure. Protein binding is reduced, monitoring only total valproate concentrations may be misleading.

Dosing adjustment/comments in hepatic impairment: Reduce dose. Clearance is decreased with liver impairment. Hepatic disease is also associated with increased albumin concentrations and 2- to 2.6-fold increase in the unbound fraction. Free concentrations of valproate may be elevated while total concentrations appear normal.

Mechanism of Action Causes increased availability of gamma-aminobutyric acid (GABA), an inhibitory neurotransmitter, to brain neurons or may enhance the action of GABA or mimic its action at postsynaptic receptor sites

Other Adverse Effects

Adverse reactions reported when used as monotherapy for complex partial seizures:

>10%:

Central nervous system: Somnolence (18% to 30%), dizziness (13% to 18%), insomnia (9% to 15%), nervousness (7% to 11%)

Dermatologic: Alopecia (13% to 24%)

Gastrointestinal: Nausea (26% to 34%), diarrhea (19% to 23%), vomiting (15% to 23%), abdominal pain (9% to 12%), dyspepsia (10% to 11%), anorexia (4% to 11%)

Hematologic: Thrombocytopenia (1% to 24%)

Neuromuscular & skeletal: Tremor (19% to 57%), weakness (10% to 21%)

Respiratory: Respiratory tract infection (13% to 20%), pharyngitis (2% to 8%), dyspnea (1% to 5%)

1% to 10%

Cardiovascular: Hypertension, palpitation, peripheral edema (3% to 8%), tachycardia, chest pain

Central nervous system: Amnesia (4% to 7%), abnormal dreams, anxiety, confusion, depression (4% to 5%), malaise, personality disorder

Dermatologic: Bruising (4% to 5%), dry skin, petechia, pruritus, rash

Endocrine & metabolic: Amenorrhea, dysmenorrhea
Gastrointestinal: Eructation, flatulence, hematemesis, increased appetite, pancreatitis, periodontal abscess, taste perversion, weight gain (4% to 9%)
Genitourinary: Urinary frequency, urinary incontinence, vaginitis
Hepatic: Increased AST and ALT
Neuromuscular & skeletal: Abnormal gait, arthralgia, back pain, hypertonia, incoordination, leg cramps, myalgia, myasthenia, paresthesia, twitching
Ocular: Amblyopia/blurred vision (4% to 8%), abnormal vision, nystagmus (1% to 7%)
Otic: Deafness, otitis media, tinnitus (1% to 7%)
Respiratory: Epistaxis, increased cough, pneumonia, sinusitis

Additional adverse effects: Frequency not defined:
Cardiovascular: Bradycardia
Central nervous system: Aggression, ataxia, behavioral deterioration, cerebral atrophy (reversible), dementia, emotional upset, encephalopathy (rare), fever, hallucinations, headache, hostility, hyperactivity, hypesthesia, incoordination, Parkinsonism, psychosis, vertigo
Dermatologic: Cutaneous vasculitis, erythema multiforme, photosensitivity, Stevens-Johnson syndrome, toxic epidermal necrolysis (rare)
Endocrine & metabolic: Breast enlargement, galactorrhea, hyperammonemia, hyponatremia, inappropriate ADH secretion, irregular menses, parotid gland swelling, polycystic ovary disease (rare), abnormal thyroid function tests
Genitourinary: Enuresis, urinary tract infection
Hematologic: Anemia, aplastic anemia, bone marrow suppression, eosinophilia, hematoma formation, hemorrhage, hypofibrinogenemia, intermittent porphyria, leukopenia, lymphocytosis, macrocytosis, pancytopenia
Hepatic: Bilirubin increased, hyperammonemic encephalopathy (in patients with UCD)
Neuromuscular & skeletal: Asterixis, bone pain, dysarthria
Ocular: Diplopia, "spots before the eyes"
Renal: Fanconi-like syndrome (rare, in children)
Miscellaneous: Anaphylaxis, decreased carnitine, hyperglycinemia, lupus

Drug Interactions CYP2C19 enzyme substrate; CYP2C9 and 2D6 enzyme inhibitor, CYP3A3/4 enzyme inhibitor (weak)

Increased Effect/Toxicity: Absence seizures have been reported in patients receiving VPA and clonazepam. Valproic acid may increase, decrease, or have no effect on carbamazepine and phenytoin levels. Valproic acid may increase serum concentration of carbamazepine - epoxide (active metabolite). Valproic acid may increase serum concentration of diazepam, lamotrigine, nimodipine, and phenobarbital, and tricyclic antidepressants. Chlorpromazine (and possibly other phenothiazines), macrolide antibiotics (clarithromycin, erythromycin, troleandomycin), felbamate, and isoniazid may inhibit the metabolism of valproic acid. Aspirin or other salicylates may displace valproic acid from protein-binding sites, leading to acute toxicity. CYP2C18/19 inhibitors: May increase serum concentration of valproic acid; inhibitors include cimetidine, felbamate, fluoxetine, and fluvoxamine

Decreased Effect: Valproic acid may displace clozapine from protein binding site resulting in decreased clozapine serum concentration. Carbamazepine, lamotrigine, and phenytoin may induce the metabolism of valproic acid. Cholestyramine (and possibly colestipol) may bind valproic acid in GI tract, decreasing absorption. Acyclovir may reduce valproic acid levels.

Drug Uptake
Half-life, elimination: Children: 4-14 hours; Adults: 8-17 hours; increases in neonates and liver dysfunction
Time to peak: 1-4 hours; 3-5 hours after divalproex (enteric coated)

Pregnancy Risk Factor D

Generic Available Yes

Selected Readings Redington K, Wells C, and Petito F, "Erythromycin and Valproic Acid Interaction," *Ann Intern Med*, 1992, 116(10):877-8.

Valrubicin (val ru BYE cin)

U.S. Brand Names Valstar™

Canadian Brand Names Valstar™

Pharmacologic Category Antineoplastic Agent, Anthracycline

Use Intravesical therapy of BCG-refractory carcinoma *in situ* of the urinary bladder

Local Anesthetic/Vasoconstrictor Precautions No information available to require special precautions

Effects on Dental Treatment No effects or complications reported

Mechanism of Action Blocks function of DNA topoisomerase II; inhibits DNA synthesis, causes extensive chromosomal damage, and arrests cell development

Other Adverse Effects
>10%: Genitourinary: Frequency (61%), dysuria (56%), urgency (57%), bladder spasm (31%), hematuria (29%), bladder pain (28%), urinary incontinence (22%), cystitis (15%), urinary tract infection (15%)

(Continued)

Valrubicin *(Continued)*

1% to 10%:

Cardiovascular: Chest pain (2%), vasodilation (2%), peripheral edema (1%)

Central nervous system: Headache (4%), malaise (4%), dizziness (3%), fever (2%)

Dermatologic: Rash (3%)

Endocrine & metabolic: Hyperglycemia (1%)

Gastrointestinal: Abdominal pain (5%), nausea (5%), diarrhea (3%), vomiting (2%), flatulence (1%)

Genitourinary: Nocturia (7%), burning symptoms (5%), urinary retention (4%), urethral pain (3%), pelvic pain (1%), hematuria (microscopic) (3%)

Hematologic: Anemia (2%)

Neuromuscular & skeletal: Weakness (4%), back pain (3%), myalgia (1%)

Respiratory: Pneumonia (1%)

Drug Interactions

Increased Effect/Toxicity: No specific drug interactions studies have been performed. Systemic exposure to valrubicin is negligible, and interactions are unlikely.

Decreased Effect: No specific drug interactions studies have been performed. Systemic exposure to valrubicin is negligible, and interactions are unlikely.

Drug Uptake Absorption: Well absorbed into bladder tissue, negligible systemic absorption. Trauma to mucosa may increase absorption, and perforation greatly increases absorption with significant systemic myelotoxicity.

Pregnancy Risk Factor C

Generic Available No

Valsartan (val SAR tan)

U.S. Brand Names Diovan®

Canadian Brand Names Diovan®

Mexican Brand Names Diovan®

Pharmacologic Category Mineral

Use Treatment of hypertension alone or in combination with other antihypertensives

Local Anesthetic/Vasoconstrictor Precautions No information available to require special precautions

Effects on Dental Treatment No effects or complications reported

Dosage Adults: Initial: 80 mg or 160 mg once daily (in patients who are not volume depleted); majority of effect within 2 weeks, maximal effects in 4-6 weeks; dose may be increased to achieve desired effect; maximum recommended dose: 320 mg/day

Dosing adjustment in renal impairment: No dosage adjustment necessary if Cl_{cr} >10 mL/minute.

Dosing adjustment in hepatic impairment (mild - moderate): ≤80 mg/day

Dialysis: Not significantly removed

Mechanism of Action As a prodrug, valsartan produces direct antagonism of the angiotensin II (AT2) receptors, unlike the angiotensin-converting enzyme inhibitors. It displaces angiotensin II from the AT1 receptor and produces its BP lowering effects by antagonizing AT1-induced vasoconstriction, aldosterone release, catecholamine release, arginine vasopressin release, water intake, and hypertrophic responses. This action results in more efficient blockade of the cardiovascular effects of angiotensin II and fewer side effects than the ACE inhibitors.

Other Adverse Effects Similar incidence to placebo; independent of race, age, and gender.

>1%:

Cardiovascular: Hypotension (6.9%)

Central nervous system: Dizziness (2% to 9%), drowsiness(2.1%), ataxia (1.4%), fatigue (2%)

Endocrine & metabolic: Increased serum potassium (4.4%)

Gastrointestinal: Abdominal pain (2%), dysgeusia (1.4%)

Hematologic: Neutropenia (1.9%)

Hepatic: Increased LFTs

Respiratory: Cough (2.9% versus 1.5% in placebo)

Miscellaneous: Viral infection (3%)

>1% but frequency ≤ placebo: Headache, upper respiratory infection, cough, diarrhea, rhinitis, sinusitis, nausea, pharyngitis, edema, arthralgia

Warnings/Precautions Use extreme caution with concurrent administration of potassium-sparing diuretics or potassium supplements, in patients with mild-moderate hepatic dysfunction (adjust dose), in those who may be sodium/water depleted (eg, on high-dose diuretics), and in the elderly; avoid use in patients with CHF, unilateral renal artery stenosis, aortic/mitral valve stenosis, coronary artery disease, or hypertrophic cardiomyopathy, if possible

Drug Interactions

Increased Effect/Toxicity: Valsartan blood levels may be increased by cimetidine and monoxidine; clinical effect is unknown. Concurrent use of potassium salts/supplements, co-trimoxazole (high dose), ACE inhibitors, and potassium-sparing diuretics (amiloride, spironolactone, triamterene) may increase the risk of hyperkalemia.

Decreased Effect: Phenobarbital, ketoconazole, troleandomycin, sulfaphenazole

Drug Uptake

Onset of action: Peak effect: 4-6 hours

Half-life, elimination: 9 hours

Time to peak: 2 hours

Pregnancy Risk Factor C/D (2nd and 3rd trimesters)

Generic Available No

Valsartan and Hydrochlorothiazide

(val SAR tan & hye droe klor oh THYE a zide)

U.S. Brand Names Diovan HCT®

Canadian Brand Names Diovan HCT®

Pharmacologic Category Antihypertensive Agent Combination

Synonyms Hydrochlorothiazide and Valsartan

Use Treatment of hypertension

Local Anesthetic/Vasoconstrictor Precautions No information available to require special precautions

Effects on Dental Treatment No effects or complications reported

Dosage Adults: Oral: Dose is individualized

Drug Uptake See Valsartan *on page 1230* and Hydrochlorothiazide *on page 595*

Pregnancy Risk Factor C (1st trimester); D (2nd and 3rd trimester)

Generic Available No

Valstar™ *see* Valrubicin *on page 1229*

Valtrex® *see* Valacyclovir *on page 1223*

Vanatrip® *see* Amitriptyline *on page 75*

Vancenase® AQ 84 mcg *see* Beclomethasone *on page 146*

Vancenase® Pockethaler® *see* Beclomethasone *on page 146*

Vanceril® *see* Beclomethasone *on page 146*

Vancocin® *see* Vancomycin *on page 1231*

Vancoled® *see* Vancomycin *on page 1231*

Vancomycin (van koe MYE sin)

Related Information

Cardiovascular Diseases *on page 1308*

U.S. Brand Names Lyphocin®; Vancocin®; Vancoled®

Canadian Brand Names Vancocin®

Mexican Brand Names Balcoran; Vancocin®; Vanmicina®

Pharmacologic Category Antibiotic, Miscellaneous

Synonyms Vancomycin Hydrochloride

Use Treatment of patients with the following infections or conditions:

- Infections due to documented or suspected methicillin-resistant *S. aureus* or beta-lactam resistant coagulase negative *Staphylococcus*
- Serious or life-threatening infections (ie, endocarditis, meningitis) due to documented or suspected staphylococcal or streptococcal infections in patients who are allergic to penicillins and/or cephalosporins
- Empiric therapy of infections associated with gram-positive organisms; used orally for staphylococcal enterocolitis or for antibiotic-associated pseudomembranous colitis produced by *C. difficile*

Local Anesthetic/Vasoconstrictor Precautions No information available to require special precautions

Effects on Dental Treatment No effects or complications reported

Dosage Initial dosage recommendation: I.V.:

Neonates:

- Postnatal age ≤7 days:
  - <1200 g: 15 mg/kg/dose every 24 hours
  - 1200-2000 g: 10 mg/kg/dose every 12 hours
  - >2000 g: 15 mg/kg/dose every 12 hours
- Postnatal age >7 days:
  - <1200 g: 15 mg/kg/dose every 24 hours
  - ≥1200 g: 10 mg/kg/dose divided every 8 hours

Infants >1 month and Children:

- 40 mg/kg/day in divided doses every 6 hours
- Prophylaxis for bacterial endocarditis:
  - Dental, oral, or upper respiratory tract surgery: 20 mg/kg 1 hour prior to the procedure
  - GI/GU procedure: 20 mg/kg plus gentamicin 2 mg/kg 1 hour prior to surgery

Infants >1 month and Children with staphylococcal CNS infection: 60 mg/kg/day in divided doses every 6 hours

Adults:

With normal renal function: 1 g **or** 10-15 mg/kg/dose every 12 hours

(Continued)

Vancomycin *(Continued)*

Prophylaxis for bacterial endocarditis:
Dental, oral, or upper respiratory tract surgery: 1 g 1 hour before surgery
GI/GU procedure: 1 g plus 1.5 mg/kg gentamicin 1 hour prior to surgery

Dosing interval in renal impairment (vancomycin levels should be monitored in patients with any renal impairment):
Cl_{cr} >60 mL/minute: Start with 1 g or 10-15 mg/kg/dose every 12 hours
Cl_{cr} 40-60 mL/minute: Start with 1 g or 10-15 mg/kg/dose every 24 hours
Cl_{cr} <40 mL/minute: Will need longer intervals; determine by serum concentration monitoring

Hemodialysis: Not dialyzable (0% to 5%); generally not removed; exception minimal-moderate removal by some of the newer high-flux filters; dose may need to be administered more frequently; monitor serum concentrations
Continuous ambulatory peritoneal dialysis (CAPD): Not significantly removed; administration via CAPD fluid: 15-30 mg/L (15-30 mcg/mL) of CAPD fluid
Continuous arteriovenous hemofiltration: Dose as for Cl_{cr} 10-40 mL/minute

Antibiotic lock technique (for catheter infections): 2 mg/mL in SWI/NS or D_5W; instill 3-5 mL into catheter port as a flush solution instead of heparin lock (**Note:** Do not mix with any other solutions)

Intrathecal: Vancomycin is available as a powder for injection and may be diluted to 1-5 mg/mL concentration in preservative-free 0.9% sodium chloride for administration into the CSF
Neonates: 5-10 mg/day
Children: 5-20 mg/day
Adults: Up to 20 mg/day

Oral: Pseudomembranous colitis produced by *C. difficile*:
Neonates: 10 mg/kg/day in divided doses
Children: 40 mg/kg/day in divided doses, added to fluids
Adults: 125 mg 4 times/day for 10 days

Mechanism of Action Inhibits bacterial cell wall synthesis by blocking glycopeptide polymerization through binding tightly to D-alanyl-D-alanine portion of cell wall precursor

Other Adverse Effects

Oral:
>10%: Gastrointestinal: Bitter taste, nausea, vomiting
1% to 10%:
Central nervous system: Chills, drug fever
Hematologic: Eosinophilia
<1%: Vasculitis, thrombocytopenia, ototoxicity, renal failure, interstitial nephritis

Parenteral:
>10%:
Cardiovascular: Hypotension accompanied by flushing
Dermatologic: Erythematous rash on face and upper body (red neck or red man syndrome - infusion rate related)
1% to 10%:
Central nervous system: Chills, drug fever
Dermatologic: Rash
Hematologic: Eosinophilia, reversible neutropenia
<1%: Vasculitis, Stevens-Johnson syndrome, ototoxicity (especially with large doses), thrombocytopenia, renal failure (especially with renal dysfunction or pre-existing hearing loss)

Contraindications Hypersensitivity to vancomycin or any component of the formulation; previous severe hearing loss

Warnings/Precautions Use with caution in patients with renal impairment or those receiving other nephrotoxic or ototoxic drugs; dosage modification required in patients with impaired renal function (especially elderly)

Drug Interactions Increased Toxicity: Anesthetic agents and other ototoxic or nephrotoxic agents

Dietary/Ethanol/Herb Considerations Food: Administer with food to reduce GI upset.

Drug Uptake
Absorption: Oral: Poor; I.M.: Erratic; Intraperitoneal: ~38%
Half-life, elimination: Biphasic: Terminal:
Newborns: 6-10 hours
Infants and Children 3 months to 4 years: 4 hours
Children >3 years: 2.2-3 hours
Adults: 5-11 hours; prolonged significantly with reduced renal function
End-stage renal disease: 200-250 hours
Time to peak: I.V.: 45-65 minutes

Pregnancy Risk Factor C

Breast-feeding Considerations Vancomycin is excreted in breast milk but is poorly absorbed from the gastrointestinal tract. Therefore, systemic absorption would not be expected. Theoretically, vancomycin in the GI tract may affect the normal bowel flora in the infant, resulting in diarrhea.

Dosage Forms CAP: 125 mg, 250 mg. **INJ, powder for reconstitution:** 500 mg, 1 g, 2 g, 5 g, 10 g. **POWDER, oral solution:** 1 g, 10 g

Generic Available Yes

Vaniqa™ *see* Eflornithine *on page 431*

Vanoxide-HC® *see* Benzoyl Peroxide and Hydrocortisone *on page 154*

Vanquish® Extra Strength Pain Reliever [OTC] *see* Acetaminophen, Aspirin, and Caffeine *on page 33*

Van R Gingibraid® *see* Epinephrine, Racemic and Aluminum Potassium Sulfate *on page 440*

Vansil™ *see* Oxamniquine *on page 894*

Vantin® *see* Cefpodoxime *on page 241*

Vaponefrin® *see* Epinephrine, Racemic *on page 440*

VAQTA® *see* Hepatitis A Vaccine *on page 583*

Varicella-Zoster Immune Globulin (Human)

(var i SEL a- ZOS ter i MYUN GLOB yoo lin HYU man)

Pharmacologic Category Immune Globulin

Synonyms VZIG

Use Passive immunization of susceptible immunodeficient patients after exposure to varicella; most effective if begun within 96 hours of exposure

VZIG supplies are limited, restrict administration to those meeting the following criteria:

One of the following underlying illnesses or conditions:

- Neoplastic disease (eg, leukemia or lymphoma)
- Congenital or acquired immunodeficiency
- Immunosuppressive therapy with steroids, antimetabolites or other immunosuppressive treatment regimens
- Newborn of mother who had onset of chickenpox within 5 days before delivery or within 48 hours after delivery
- Premature (≥28 weeks gestation) whose mother has no history of chickenpox
- Premature (<28 weeks gestation or ≤1000 g VZIG) regardless of maternal history

One of the following types of exposure to chickenpox or zoster patient(s):

- Continuous household contact
- Playmate contact (>1 hour play indoors)
- Hospital contact (in same 2-4 bedroom or adjacent beds in a large ward or prolonged face-to-face contact with an infectious staff member or patient)
- Susceptible to varicella-zoster

Age of <15 years; administer to immunocompromised adolescents and adults and to other older patients on an individual basis

An acceptable alternative to VZIG prophylaxis is to treat varicella, if it occurs, with high-dose I.V. acyclovir

Local Anesthetic/Vasoconstrictor Precautions No information available to require special precautions

Effects on Dental Treatment No effects or complications reported

Dosage High risk susceptible patients who are exposed again >3 weeks after a prior dose of VZIG should receive another full dose; there is no evidence VZIG modifies established varicella-zoster infections.

I.M.: Administer by deep injection in the gluteal muscle or in another large muscle mass. Inject 125 units/10 kg (22 lb); maximum dose: 625 units (5 vials); minimum dose: 125 units; do not give fractional doses. Do not inject I.V. See table.

VZIG Dose Based on Weight

Weight of Patient		Dose	
(kg)	(lb)	Units	# of Vials
0-10	0-22	125	1
10.1-20	22.1-44	250	2
20.1-30	44.1-66	375	3
30.1-40	66.1-88	500	4
>40	>88	625	5

Mechanism of Action The exact mechanism has not been clarified but the antibodies in varicella-zoster immune globulin most likely neutralize the varicella-zoster virus and prevent its pathological actions

Other Adverse Effects 1% to 10%: Local: Discomfort at the site of injection (pain, redness, edema)

Drug Interactions Decreased Effect: Live virus vaccines (do not administer within 3 months of immune globulin administration)

Pregnancy Risk Factor C

Generic Available No

Comments Should be administered within 96 hours of exposure

Vascor® *see* Bepridil *on page 156*
Vaseretic® 5-12.5 *see* Enalapril and Hydrochlorothiazide *on page 434*
Vaseretic® 10-25 *see* Enalapril and Hydrochlorothiazide *on page 434*
Vasocidin® *see* Sulfacetamide Sodium and Prednisolone *on page 1116*
VasoClear® [OTC] *see* Naphazoline *on page 847*
Vasocon-A® [OTC] *see* Naphazoline and Antazoline *on page 847*
Vasocon Regular® *see* Naphazoline *on page 847*
Vasodilan® *see* Isoxsuprine *on page 664*

Vasopressin (vay soe PRES in)

U.S. Brand Names Pitressin®

Canadian Brand Names Pressyn®

Pharmacologic Category Antidiuretic Hormone Analog; Hormone, Posterior Pituitary

Synonyms ADH; Antidiuretic Hormone; 8-Arginine Vasopressin; Vasopressin Tannate

Use Treatment of diabetes insipidus; prevention and treatment of postoperative abdominal distention; differential diagnosis of diabetes insipidus

Unlabeled/Investigational: Adjunct in the treatment of GI hemorrhage and esophageal varices; pulseless ventricular tachycardia (VT)/ventricular fibrillation (VF)

Local Anesthetic/Vasoconstrictor Precautions No information available to require special precautions

Effects on Dental Treatment No effects or complications reported

Dosage

Diabetes insipidus (highly variable dosage; titrated based on serum and urine sodium and osmolality in addition to fluid balance and urine output):

Children: I.M., S.C.: 2.5-10 units 2-4 times/day as needed

Adults:

I.M., S.C.: 5-10 units 2-4 times/day as needed (dosage range 5-60 units/day)

Intranasal: Administer on cotton pledget or nasal spray

Abdominal distention: Adults: I.M.: 5 mg stat, 10 mg every 3-4 hours

GI hemorrhage: Children and Adults: Continuous I.V. infusion: 0.5 milliunit/kg/hour (0.0005 unit/kg/hour); double dosage as needed every 30 minutes to a maximum of 10 milliunits/kg/hour

Children: 0.01 units/kg/minute; continue at same dosage (if bleeding stops) for 12 hours, then taper off over 24-48 hours

Adults: I.V.: Initial: 0.2-0.4 unit/minute, then titrate dose as needed; if bleeding stops, continue at same dose for 12 hours, taper off over 24-48 hours

Mechanism of Action Increases cyclic adenosine monophosphate (cAMP) which increases water permeability at the renal tubule resulting in decreased urine volume and increased osmolality; causes peristalsis by directly stimulating the smooth muscle in the GI tract

Other Adverse Effects Frequency not defined:

Cardiovascular: Increased BP, arrhythmias, venous thrombosis, vasoconstriction (with higher doses), angina, myocardial infarction

Central nervous system: Pounding in the head, fever, vertigo

Dermatologic: Urticaria, circumoral pallor

Gastrointestinal: Flatulence, abdominal cramps, nausea, vomiting

Genitourinary: Uterine contraction

Neuromuscular & skeletal: Tremor

Respiratory: Bronchial constriction

Miscellaneous: Diaphoresis

Drug Interactions

Increased Effect/Toxicity: Chlorpropamide, urea, clofibrate, carbamazepine, and fludrocortisone potentiate antidiuretic response.

Decreased Effect: Lithium, epinephrine, demeclocycline, and heparin block antidiuretic activity to varying degrees.

Drug Uptake

Onset of action: Nasal: 1 hour

Absorption: Destroyed by trypsin in GI tract, must be administered parenterally or intranasally

Duration: Nasal: 3-8 hours; Parenteral: I.M., S.C.: 2-8 hours

Half-life, elimination: Nasal: 15 minutes; Parenteral: 10-20 minutes

Pregnancy Risk Factor B

Generic Available No

Vasosulf® *see* Sulfacetamide Sodium and Phenylephrine *on page 1116*
Vasotec® *see* Enalapril *on page 432*
Vasotec® I.V. *see* Enalapril *on page 432*
V-Dec-m® *see* Guaifenesin and Pseudoephedrine *on page 570*
Vectrin® [DSC] *see* Minocycline *on page 816*
Veetids® *see* Penicillin V Potassium *on page 931*
Veg-Pancreatin 4X [OTC] *see* Pancreatin *on page 913*
Velban® *see* VinBLAStine *on page 1240*

Velosef® *see* Cephradine *on page 253*
Velosulin® BR (Buffered) *see* Insulin Preparations *on page 639*

Venlafaxine (VEN la faks een)

U.S. Brand Names Effexor®; Effexor® XR
Canadian Brand Names Effexor®; Effexor® XR
Mexican Brand Names Efexor®
Pharmacologic Category Antidepressant, Serotonin/Norepinephrine Reuptake Inhibitor
Use Treatment of depression, generalized anxiety disorder (GAD)
Unlabeled/Investigational: Obsessive-compulsive disorder (OCD), chronic fatigue syndrome; attention-deficit/hyperactivity disorder (ADHD) and autism in children
Local Anesthetic/Vasoconstrictor Precautions No information available to require special precautions
Effects on Dental Treatment >10%: Significant xerostomia; may contribute to oral discomfort, especially in older patients
Dosage Oral:
Children and Adolescents:
ADHD (unlabeled use): 60 mg or 1.4 mg/kg administered in 2-3 divided doses
Autism (unlabeled use): Initial: 12.5 mg/day; adjust to 6.25-50 mg/day
Adults:
Immediate-release tablets: 75 mg/day, administered in 2 or 3 divided doses, taken with food; dose may be increased in 75 mg/day increments at intervals of at least 4 days, up to 225-375 mg/day
Extended-release capsules: 75 mg once daily taken with food; for some new patients, it may be desirable to start at 37.5 mg/day for 4-7 days before increasing to 75 mg once daily; dose may be increased by up to 75 mg/day increments every 4 days as tolerated, up to a maximum of 225 mg/day
Note: When discontinuing this medication, it is imperative to taper the dose. If venlafaxine is used >6 weeks, the dose should be tapered over 2 weeks when discontinuing its use.
Dosing adjustment in renal impairment: Cl_{cr} 10-70 mL/minute: Decrease dose by 25%; decrease total daily dose by 50% if dialysis patients; dialysis patients should receive dosing after completion of dialysis
Dosing adjustment in moderate hepatic impairment: Reduce total daily dosage by 50%
Mechanism of Action Venlafaxine and its active metabolite o-desmethylvenlafaxine (ODV) are potent inhibitors of neuronal serotonin and norepinephrine reuptake and weak inhibitors of dopamine reuptake; causes beta-receptor down regulation and reduces adenylcyclase coupled beta-adrenergic systems in the brain
Other Adverse Effects
≥10%:
Central nervous system: Headache (25%), somnolence (23%), dizziness (19%), insomnia (18%), nervousness (13%)
Gastrointestinal: Nausea (37%), xerostomia (22%), constipation (15%), anorexia (11%)
Genitourinary: Abnormal ejaculation/orgasm (12%)
Neuromuscular & skeletal: Weakness (12%)
Miscellaneous: Diaphoresis (12%)
1% to 10%:
Cardiovascular: Vasodilation (4%), hypertension (dose-related; 3% in patients receiving <100 mg/day, up to 13% in patients receiving >300 mg/day), tachycardia (2%), chest pain (2%), postural hypotension (1%)
Central nervous system: Anxiety (6%), abnormal dreams (4%), yawning (3%), agitation (2%), confusion (2%), abnormal thinking (2%), depersonalization (1%), depression (1%)
Dermatologic: Rash (3%), pruritus (1%)
Endocrine & metabolic: Decreased libido
Gastrointestinal: Diarrhea (8%), vomiting (6%), dyspepsia (5%), flatulence (3%), taste perversion (2%), weight loss (1%)
Genitourinary: Impotence (6%), urinary frequency (3%), impaired urination (2%), orgasm disturbance (2%), urinary retention (1%)
Neuromuscular & skeletal: Tremor (5%), hypertonia (3%), paresthesia (3%), twitching (1%)
Ocular: Blurred vision (6%), mydriasis (2%)
Otic: Tinnitus (2%)
Miscellaneous: Infection (6%), chills (3%), trauma (2%)
Drug Interactions CYP2D6, 2E1, and 3A3/4 enzyme substrate; CYP2D6 enzyme inhibitor (weak)
Increased Effect/Toxicity: Concurrent use of MAO inhibitors (phenelzine, isocarboxazid), or drugs with MAO inhibitor activity (linezolid) may result in serotonin syndrome; should not be used within 2 weeks of each other. Selegiline may have a lower risk of this effect, particularly at low dosages, due to selectivity for MAO type B. In addition, concurrent use of buspirone, lithium, meperidine, nefazodone,
(Continued)

Venlafaxine *(Continued)*

selegiline, serotonin agonists (sumatriptan, naratriptan), sibutramine, SSRIs, trazodone, or tricyclic antidepressants may increase the risk of serotonin syndrome. Neuroleptic malignant syndrome has been described in a patient receiving methylphenidate and venlafaxine. Serum levels of haloperidol may be increased by venlafaxine. Inhibitors of CYP2D6, CYP2E1, or CYP3A3/4 may increase the serum concentration and/or toxicity of venlafaxine.

Decreased Effect: Serum levels of indinavir may be reduced be venlafaxine (AUC reduced by 28%) - clinical significance not determined. Enzyme inducers (carbamazepine, phenytoin, phenobarbital) may reduce the serum concentration of venlafaxine.

Drug Uptake

Absorption: Oral: 92% to 100%; food has no significant effect on the absorption of venlafaxine or formation of the active metabolite O-desmethyl-venlafaxine (ODV); absolute bioavailability is ~45%

Half-life, elimination: Venlafaxine 3-7 hours; ODV 9-13 hours; steady state concentrations of both venlafaxine and ODV in plasma were attained within 3 days of multiple dose therapy. Half-life is prolonged with cirrhosis (Adults: Venlafaxine ~30%, ODV ~60%) and with dialysis (Adults: Venlafaxine ~180%, ODV ~142%)

Time to peak: Venlafaxine: Immediate release: 2 hours, ODV: 3 hours; Extended release: 5.5 hours, ODV: 9 hours

Pregnancy Risk Factor C

Generic Available No

Venofer® *see* Iron Sucrose *on page 656*

Venoglobulin®-S *see* Immune Globulin, Intravenous *on page 630*

Ventolin® *see* Albuterol *on page 45*

Ventolin® HFA *see* Albuterol *on page 45*

Ventolin Rotacaps® [DSC] *see* Albuterol *on page 45*

VePesid® *see* Etoposide *on page 481*

Verapamil (ver AP a mil)

Related Information

Calcium Channel Blockers and Gingival Hyperplasia *on page 1432*

Cardiovascular Diseases *on page 1308*

U.S. Brand Names Calan®; Calan® SR; Covera-HS®; Isoptin®; Isoptin® SR; Verelan®; Verelan® PM

Canadian Brand Names Alti-Verapamil; Apo®-Verap; Calan®; Chronovera®; Covera®; Gen-Verapamil; Gen-Verapamil SR; Isoptin®; Isoptin® I.V.; Isoptin® SR; Novo-Veramil; Novo-Veramil SR; Nu-Verap; Tarka®; Veralan®

Mexican Brand Names Cronovera®; Dilacoran; Veraken; Verdilac

Pharmacologic Category Antiarrhythmic Agent, Class IV; Calcium Channel Blocker

Synonyms Iproveratril Hydrochloride; Verapamil Hydrochloride

Use Orally used for treatment of angina pectoris (vasospastic, chronic stable, unstable) and hypertension; I.V. for supraventricular tachyarrhythmias (PSVT, atrial fibrillation, atrial flutter)

Unlabeled/Investigational: Migraine; hypertrophic cardiomyopathy; bipolar disorder (manic manifestations)

Local Anesthetic/Vasoconstrictor Precautions No information available to require special precautions

Effects on Dental Treatment Calcium channel blockers (CCB) have been reported to cause gingival hyperplasia (GH). Verapamil induced GH has appeared 11 months or more after subjects took daily doses of 240-360 mg. The severity of hyperplastic syndrome does not seem to be dose-dependent. Gingivectomy is only successful if CCB therapy is discontinued. GH regresses markedly 1 week after CCB discontinuance with all symptoms resolving in 2 months. If a patient must continue CCB therapy, begin a program of professional cleaning and patient plaque control to minimize severity and growth rate of gingival tissue.

Dosage

Children: SVT:

I.V.:

<1 year: 0.1-0.2 mg/kg over 2 minutes; repeat every 30 minutes as needed

1-15 years: 0.1-0.3 mg/kg over 2 minutes; maximum: 5 mg/dose, may repeat dose in 15 minutes if adequate response not achieved; maximum for second dose: 10 mg/dose

Oral (dose not well established):

1-5 years: 4-8 mg/kg/day in 3 divided doses **or** 40-80 mg every 8 hours

>5 years: 80 mg every 6-8 hours

Adults:

SVT: I.V.: 2.5-5 mg (over 2 minutes); second dose of 5-10 mg (~0.15 mg/kg) may be given 15-30 minutes after the initial dose if patient tolerates, but does not respond to initial dose; maximum total dose: 20 mg

Angina: Oral: Initial dose: 80-120 mg 3 times/day (elderly or small stature: 40 mg 3 times/day); range: 240-480 mg/day in 3-4 divided doses

Hypertension: Oral: 80 mg 3 times/day or 240 mg/day (sustained release); range: 240-480 mg/day; 120 mg/day in the elderly or small patients (no evidence of additional benefit in doses >360 mg/day).

Note: One time per day dosing is recommended at bedtime with Covera-HS®.

Dosing adjustment in renal impairment: Cl_{cr} <10 mL/minute: Administer at 50% to 75% of normal dose.

Dialysis: Not dialyzable (0% to 5 %) via hemo- or peritoneal dialysis; supplemental dose is not necessary.

Dosing adjustment/comments in hepatic disease: Reduce dose in cirrhosis, reduce dose to 20% to 50% of normal and monitor EKG.

Mechanism of Action Inhibits calcium ion from entering the "slow channels" or select voltage-sensitive areas of vascular smooth muscle and myocardium during depolarization; produces a relaxation of coronary vascular smooth muscle and coronary vasodilation; increases myocardial oxygen delivery in patients with vasospastic angina; slows automaticity and conduction of A-V node.

Other Adverse Effects

>10%: Gastrointestinal: Gingival hyperplasia (19%)

1% to 10%:

Cardiovascular: Bradycardia (1.4% oral, 1.2% I.V.); first-, second-, or third-degree AV block (1.2% oral, unknown I.V.); CHF (1.8% oral); hypotension (2.5% oral, 3% I.V.); peripheral edema (1.9% oral), symptomatic hypotension (1.5% I.V.); severe tachycardia (1% I.V.)

Central nervous system: Dizziness (3.3% oral, 1.2% I.V.), fatigue (1.7% oral), headache (2.2% oral, 1.2% I.V.)

Dermatologic: Rash (1.2% oral)

Gastrointestinal: Constipation (12% up to 42% in clinical trials), nausea (2.7% oral, 0.9% I.V.)

Respiratory: Dyspnea (1.4% oral)

Drug Interactions CYP2C8/9 (minor), 2C18 (minor), 2C19 (minor), 3A3/4, and 1A2 enzyme substrate; CYP3A3/4 inhibitor

Alfentanil's plasma concentration is increased. Fentanyl and sufentanil may be affected similarly.

Amiodarone use may lead to bradycardia and decreased cardiac output. Monitor closely if using together.

Aspirin and concurrent verapamil use may increase bleeding times; monitor closely, especially if on other antiplatelet agents or anticoagulants.

Azole antifungals may inhibit the calcium channel blocker's metabolism; avoid this combination. Try an antifungal like terbinafine (if appropriate) or monitor closely for altered effect of the calcium channel blocker.

Barbiturates reduce the plasma concentration of verapamil. May require much higher dose of verapamil.

Beta-blockers may have increased pharmacodynamic interactions with verapamil.

Buspirone's serum concentration may increase. May require dosage adjustment.

Calcium may reduce the calcium channel blocker's effects, particularly hypotension.

Carbamazepine's serum concentration is increased and toxicity may result; avoid this combination.

Cimetidine reduced verapamil's metabolism; consider an alternative H_2 antagonist.

Cyclosporine's serum concentrations are increased by verapamil; avoid this combination. Use another calcium channel blocker or monitor cyclosporine trough levels and renal function closely.

Digoxin's serum concentration is increased; reduce digoxin's dose when adding verapamil.

Doxorubicin's clearance was reduced; monitor for altered doxorubicin's effect.

Erythromycin may increase verapamil's effects; monitor altered verapamil effect.

Ethanol's effects may be increased by verapamil; reduce ethanol consumption.

Flecainide may have additive negative effects on conduction and inotropy.

Grapefruit juice: Verapamil serum concentrations may be increased by grapefruit juice. Avoid concurrent use.

HMG-CoA reductase inhibitors (atorvastatin, cerivastatin, lovastatin, simvastatin): Serum concentration will likely be increased; consider pravastatin/fluvastatin or a dihydropyridine calcium channel blocker.

Lithium neurotoxicity may result when verapamil is added; monitor lithium levels.

Midazolam's plasma concentration is increased by verapamil; monitor for prolonged CNS depression.

Nafcillin decreases plasma concentration of verapamil; avoid this combination.

Nondepolarizing muscle relaxant: Neuromuscular blockade may be prolonged. Monitor closely.

Prazosin's serum concentration increases; monitor BP.

Quinidine's serum concentration is increased; adjust quinidine's dose as necessary.

Rifampin increases the metabolism of calcium channel blockers; adjust the dose of the calcium channel blocker to maintain efficacy.

(Continued)

Verapamil *(Continued)*

Tacrolimus's serum concentrations are increased by verapamil; avoid the combination. Use another calcium channel blocker or monitor tacrolimus trough levels and renal function closely.

Theophylline's serum concentration may be increased by verapamil. Those at increased risk include children and cigarette smokers.

Drug Uptake

Onset of action: Peak effect: Oral: Immediate release: 2 hours; I.V.: 1-5 minutes

Duration: Oral: Immediate release tablets: 6-8 hours; I.V.: 10-20 minutes

Half-life, elimination (increases with hepatic cirrhosis): Infants: 4.4-6.9 hours; Adults: Single dose: 2-8 hours; Multiple dose: increases ≤12 hours

Pregnancy Risk Factor C

Generic Available Yes

Selected Readings Wynn RL, "Update on Calcium Channel Blocker Induced Gingival Hyperplasia," *Gen Dent*, 1995, 43(3):218-22.

Verelan® *see* Verapamil *on page 1236*

Verelan® PM *see* Verapamil *on page 1236*

Vergon® [OTC] *see* Meclizine *on page 750*

Vermox® *see* Mebendazole *on page 749*

Verr-Canth™ *see* Cantharidin *on page 210*

Versacaps® *see* Guaifenesin and Pseudoephedrine *on page 570*

Versed® *see* Midazolam *on page 809*

Vesanoid® *see* Tretinoin, Oral *on page 1195*

Vesprin® *see* Triflupromazine *on page 1206*

Vexol® *see* Rimexolone *on page 1055*

VFEND® *see* Voriconazole *on page 1248*

Viadur™ *see* Leuprolide Acetate *on page 692*

Viagra® *see* Sildenafil *on page 1086*

Vibramycin® *see* Doxycycline *on page 418*

Vibra-Tabs® *see* Doxycycline *on page 418*

Vicks® 44D Cough & Head Congestion [OTC] *see* Pseudoephedrine and Dextromethorphan *on page 1023*

Vicks® 44E [OTC] *see* Guaifenesin and Dextromethorphan *on page 569*

Vicks® DayQuil® Cold and Flu Non-Drowsy [OTC] *see* Acetaminophen, Dextromethorphan, and Pseudoephedrine *on page 34*

Vicks Formula 44® [OTC] *see* Dextromethorphan *on page 372*

Vicks Formula 44® Pediatric Formula [OTC] *see* Dextromethorphan *on page 372*

Vicks® Pediatric Formula 44E [OTC] *see* Guaifenesin and Dextromethorphan *on page 569*

Vicks Sinex® Nasal [OTC] *see* Phenylephrine *on page 950*

Vicodin® *see* Hydrocodone and Acetaminophen *on page 598*

Vicodin® ES *see* Hydrocodone and Acetaminophen *on page 598*

Vicodin® HP *see* Hydrocodone and Acetaminophen *on page 598*

Vicodin Tuss™ *see* Hydrocodone and Guaifenesin *on page 603*

Vicon-C® [OTC] *see* Vitamin B Complex With Vitamin C *on page 1244*

Vicon Forte® *see* Vitamins, Multiple *on page 1246*

Vicon® Plus [OTC] *see* Vitamins, Multiple *on page 1246*

Vicoprofen® *see* Hydrocodone and Ibuprofen *on page 605*

Vidarabine (vye DARE a been)

Related Information

Oral Viral Infections *on page 1380*

Systemic Viral Diseases *on page 1354*

U.S. Brand Names Vira-A®

Mexican Brand Names Adena a Ungena

Pharmacologic Category Antiviral Agent, Ophthalmic

Synonyms Adenine Arabinoside; Ara-A; Arabinofuranosyladenine; Vidarabine Monohydrate

Use Treatment of acute keratoconjunctivitis and epithelial keratitis due to herpes simplex virus; herpes simplex conjunctivitis

Local Anesthetic/Vasoconstrictor Precautions No information available to require special precautions

Effects on Dental Treatment No effects or complications reported

Dosage Children and Adults: Ophthalmic: Keratoconjunctivitis: Place ½" of ointment in lower conjunctival sac 5 times/day every 3 hours while awake until complete re-epithelialization has occurred, then twice daily for an additional 7 days

Mechanism of Action Inhibits viral DNA synthesis by blocking DNA polymerase

Other Adverse Effects Frequency not defined: Ocular: Burning eyes, lacrimation, keratitis, photophobia, foreign body sensation, uveitis

Drug Interactions Allopurinol may increase vidarabine levels.

Pregnancy Risk Factor C

Generic Available No

ViDaylin® *see* Vitamins, Multiple *on page 1246*

Videx® *see* Didanosine *on page 382*

Videx® EC *see* Didanosine *on page 382*

Vigabatrin *Not Available in U.S.* (vye GA ba trin)

Canadian Brand Names Sabril®

Pharmacologic Category Anticonvulsant, Miscellaneous

Use Active management of partial or secondary generalized seizures not controlled by usual treatments; treatment of infantile spasms

Unlabeled/Investigational: Spasticity, tardive dyskinesia

Local Anesthetic/Vasoconstrictor Precautions No information available to require special precautions

Effects on Dental Treatment No effects or complications reported

Dosage Oral:

Children: **Note:** Administer daily dose in 2 divided doses, especially in the higher dosage ranges:

Adjunctive treatment of seizures: Initial: 40 mg/kg/day; maintenance dosages based on patient weight:

10-15 kg: 0.5-1 g/day

16-30 kg: 1-1.5 g/day

31-50 kg: 1.5-3 g/day

>50 kg: 2-3 g/day

Infantile spasms: 50-100 mg/kg/day, depending on severity of symptoms; higher doses (up to 150 mg/kg/day) have been used in some cases.

Adults: Adjunctive treatment of seizures: Initial: 1 g/day (severe manifestations may require 2 g/day); dose may be given as a single daily dose or divided into 2 equal doses. Increase daily dose by 0.5 g based on response and tolerability. Optimal dose range: 2-3 g/day (maximum dose: 3 g/day)

Elderly: Initiate at low end of dosage range (refer to adult dosing); monitor closely for sedation and confusion

Dosage adjustment in renal impairment: Cl_{cr} <60 mL/minute: Initiate at lower dosage; monitor closely for sedation and confusion

Mechanism of Action Irreversibly inhibits gamma-aminobutyric acid transaminase (GABA-T), increasing the levels of the inhibitory compound gamma amino butyric acid (GABA) within the brain; duration of effect is dependent upon rate of GABA-T resynthesis

Other Adverse Effects

>10%

Central nervous system: Fatigue (27%), headache (26%), drowsiness (22%), dizziness (19%), depression (13%), tremor (11%), agitation (11%). **Note:** In pediatric use, hyperactivity (hyperkinesia, agitation, excitation, or restlessness) was reported in 11% of patients.

Endocrine & metabolic: Weight gain (12%)

Ophthalmic: Visual field defects (33%), abnormal vision (11%)

1% to 10%

Cardiovascular: Edema (dependent), chest pain

Central nervous system: Amnesia, confusion, paresthesia, impaired concentration, insomnia, anxiety, emotional lability, abnormal thinking, speech disorder, vertigo, aggression, nervousness, personality disorder

Dermatologic: Rash (5%, similar to placebo), skin disorder

Endocrine & metabolic: Increased appetite, dysmenorrhea, menstrual disorder

Gastrointestinal: Nausea, diarrhea, abdominal pain, constipation, vomiting

Genitourinary: Urinary tract infection

Hematologic: Purpura

Neuromuscular & skeletal: Ataxia, arthralgia, back pain, abnormal coordination, abnormal gait, weakness, hyporeflexia, arthrosis

Ophthalmologic: Nystagmus, diplopia, eye pain

Otic: Ear pain

Respiratory: Throat irritation, nasal congestion, upper respiratory tract infection, sinusitis

Drug Interactions Increased Effect/Toxicity: May decrease serum concentrations of phenobarbital by 9% to 21% and of phenytoin by 16% to 33%

Drug Uptake

Absorption: Rapid

Duration: Variable (not strictly correlated to serum concentrations); dependent on rate of GABA-T resynthesis

Half-life, elimination: 5-8 hours (≤13 hours in elderly)

Time to peak: 2 hours

Pregnancy Risk Factor Not assigned; contraindicated per manufacturer

Generic Available No

VinBLAStine (vin BLAS teen)

U.S. Brand Names Alkaban-AQ®; Velban®

Canadian Brand Names Velban®

Mexican Brand Names Lemblastine

Pharmacologic Category Antineoplastic Agent, Natural Source (Plant) Derivative

Synonyms Vinblastine Sulfate; Vincaleukoblastine; VLB

Use Palliative treatment of Hodgkin's disease; advanced testicular germinal-cell cancers; non-Hodgkin's lymphoma, histiocytosis, and choriocarcinoma

Local Anesthetic/Vasoconstrictor Precautions No information available to require special precautions

Effects on Dental Treatment No effects or complications reported

Mechanism of Action VLB binds to tubulin and inhibits microtubule formation, therefore, arresting the cell at metaphase by disrupting the formation of the mitotic spindle; it is specific for the M and S phases; binds to microtubular protein of the mitotic spindle causing metaphase arrest

Other Adverse Effects

>10%:

Dermatologic: Alopecia

Gastrointestinal: Nausea and vomiting are most common and are easily controlled with standard antiemetics; constipation, diarrhea (less common), stomatitis, abdominal cramps, anorexia, metallic taste

Emetic potential: Moderate (30% to 60%)

Hematologic: May cause severe bone marrow suppression and is the dose-limiting toxicity of VLB (unlike vincristine); severe granulocytopenia and thrombocytopenia may occur following the administration of VLB and nadir 5-10 days after treatment

Myelosuppressive:

WBC: Moderate - severe

Platelets: Moderate - severe

Onset: 4-7 days

Nadir: 5-10 days

Recovery: 17 days

1% to 10%:

Cardiovascular: Hypertension, Raynaud's phenomenon

Central nervous system: Depression, malaise, headache, seizures

Dermatologic: Rash, photosensitivity, dermatitis

Endocrine & metabolic: Hyperuricemia

Extravasation: VLB is a vesicant and can cause tissue irritation and necrosis if infiltrated; if extravasation occurs, follow institutional policy, which may include hyaluronidase and hot compresses

Vesicant chemotherapy

Gastrointestinal: Paralytic ileus, stomatitis

Genitourinary: Urinary retention

Neuromuscular & skeletal: Jaw pain, myalgia, paresthesia

Respiratory: Bronchospasm

Drug Interactions CYP3A3/4 and 3A5-7 enzyme substrate; CYP2D6 enzyme inhibitor

Increased Effect/Toxicity: Vinblastine levels may be increased when given with drugs that inhibit cytochrome P450 3A enzyme substrate. Previous or simultaneous use with mitomycin-C has resulted in acute shortness of breath and severe bronchospasm within minutes or several hours after *Vinca* alkaloid injection and may occur up to 2 weeks after the dose of mitomycin. Mitomycin-C in combination with administration of VLB may cause acute shortness of breath and severe bronchospasm, onset may be within minutes or several hours after VLB injection.

Decreased Effect: Phenytoin plasma concentrations may be reduced with concomitant combination chemotherapy with vinblastine. Alpha-interferon enhances interferon toxicity; phenytoin may ↓ plasma concentrations.

Drug Uptake

Absorption: Unreliable, from the GI tract; must be given I.V.

Half-life, elimination: Biphasic: Initial 0.164 hours; Terminal: 25 hours

Pregnancy Risk Factor D

Generic Available Yes

Vincasar® PFS™ *see* VinCRIStine *on page 1240*

VinCRIStine (vin KRIS teen)

U.S. Brand Names Oncovin®; Vincasar® PFS™

Canadian Brand Names Oncovin®; Vincasar® PFS™

Mexican Brand Names Citomid®; Vintec®

Pharmacologic Category Antineoplastic Agent, Natural Source (Plant) Derivative

Synonyms LCR; Leurocristine; VCR; Vincristine Sulfate

Use Treatment of leukemias, Hodgkin's disease, neuroblastoma, malignant lymphomas, Wilms' tumor, and rhabdomyosarcoma

Local Anesthetic/Vasoconstrictor Precautions No information available to require special precautions

Effects on Dental Treatment No effects or complications reported

Mechanism of Action Binds to microtubular protein of the mitotic spindle causing metaphase arrest; cell-cycle phase specific in the M and S phases

Other Adverse Effects

>10%:

Dermatologic: Alopecia occurs in 20% to 70% of patients

Extravasation: VCR is a vesicant and can cause tissue irritation and necrosis if infiltrated; if extravasation occurs, follow institutional policy, which may include hyaluronidase and hot compresses

Vesicant chemotherapy

1% to 10%:

Cardiovascular: Orthostatic hypotension or hypertension, hypertension, hypotension

Central nervous system: Motor difficulties, seizures, headache, CNS depression, cranial nerve paralysis, fever

Dermatologic: Rash

Endocrine & metabolic: Hyperuricemia

SIADH: Rarely occurs, but may be related to the neurologic toxicity; may cause symptomatic hyponatremia with seizures; the increase in serum ADH concentration usually subsides within 2-3 days after onset

Gastrointestinal: Constipation and possible paralytic ileus secondary to neurologic toxicity; oral ulceration, abdominal cramps, anorexia, metallic taste, bloating, nausea, vomiting, weight loss, diarrhea

Emetic potential: Low (<10%)

Local: Phlebitis

Neurologic: Alterations in mental status such as depression, confusion, or insomnia; constipation, paralytic ileus, and urinary tract disturbances may occur. All patients should be on a prophylactic bowel management regimen. Cranial nerve palsies, headaches, jaw pain, optic atrophy with blindness have been reported. Intrathecal administration of VCR has uniformly caused death; VCR should **never** be administered by this route. Neurologic effects of VCR may be additive with those of other neurotoxic agents and spinal cord irradiation.

Neuromuscular & skeletal: Jaw pain, leg pain, myalgia, cramping, numbness, weakness

Peripheral neuropathy: Frequently the dose-limiting toxicity of VCR. Most frequent in patients >40 years of age; occurs usually after an average of 3 weekly doses, but may occur after just one dose. Manifested as loss of the deep tendon reflexes in the lower extremities, numbness, tingling, pain, paresthesias of the fingers and toes (stocking glove sensation), and "foot drop" or "wrist drop"

Ocular: Photophobia

Drug Interactions CYP3A3/4 and 3A5-7 enzyme substrate; CYP2D6 enzyme inhibitor

Increased Effect/Toxicity: Vincristine levels may be increased when given with drugs that inhibit cytochrome P450 3A enzyme (itraconazole has been shown to increase onset and severity of neuromuscular adverse effects of vincristine). Digoxin plasma concentrations and renal excretion may decrease with combination chemotherapy including vincristine. Vincristine should be given 12-24 hours before asparaginase to minimize toxicity (may decrease the hepatic clearance of vincristine). Acute pulmonary reactions may occur with mitomycin-C. Previous or simultaneous use with mitomycin-C has resulted in acute shortness of breath and severe bronchospasm within minutes or several hours after *Vinca* alkaloid injection and may occur up to 2 weeks after the dose of mitomycin.

Decreased Effect: Digoxin and phenytoin levels may decrease with combination chemotherapy.

Drug Uptake

Absorption: Oral: Poor

Half-life, elimination: Terminal: 24 hours

Pregnancy Risk Factor D

Generic Available Yes

Vinorelbine (vi NOR el been)

U.S. Brand Names Navelbine®

Canadian Brand Names Navelbine®

Mexican Brand Names Navelbine®

Pharmacologic Category Antineoplastic Agent, Natural Source (Plant) Derivative

Synonyms Vinorelbine Tartrate

Use Treatment of nonsmall cell lung cancer (as a single agent or in combination with cisplatin)

Unlabeled/Investigational: Breast cancer, ovarian carcinoma (cisplatin resistant), Hodgkin's disease

Local Anesthetic/Vasoconstrictor Precautions No information available to require special precautions

Effects on Dental Treatment No effects or complications reported

(Continued)

Vinorelbine *(Continued)*

Mechanism of Action Semisynthetic *Vinca* alkaloid which binds to tubulin and inhibits microtubule formation, therefore, arresting the cell at metaphase by disrupting the formation of the mitotic spindle; it is specific for the M and S phases; binds to microtubular protein of the mitotic spindle causing metaphase arrest

Other Adverse Effects

>10%:

Central nervous system: Fatigue (27%)

Dermatologic: Alopecia (12%)

Gastrointestinal: Nausea (44%, severe <2%) and vomiting (20%) are most common and are easily controlled with standard antiemetics; constipation (35%), diarrhea (17%)

Emetic potential: Moderate (30% to 60%)

Hematologic: May cause severe bone marrow suppression and is the dose-limiting toxicity of vinorelbine; severe granulocytopenia (90%) may occur following the administration of vinorelbine; leukopenia (92%), anemia (83%)

Myelosuppressive:

WBC: Moderate - severe

Onset: 4-7 days

Nadir: 7-10 days

Recovery: 14-21 days

Hepatic: Elevated SGOT (67%), elevated total bilirubin (13%)

Local: Injection site reaction (28%), injection site pain (16%)

Neuromuscular & skeletal: Weakness (36%), peripheral neuropathy (20% to 25%)

1% to 10%:

Cardiovascular: Chest pain (5%)

Gastrointestinal: Paralytic ileus (1%)

Hematologic: Thrombocytopenia (5%)

Local: Extravasation: Vesicant and can cause tissue irritation and necrosis if infiltrated; if extravasation occurs, follow institutional policy, which may include hyaluronidase and hot compresses; phlebitis (7%)

Vesicant chemotherapy

Neuromuscular & skeletal: Mild to moderate peripheral neuropathy manifested by paresthesia and hyperesthesia, loss of deep tendon reflexes (<5%); myalgia (<5%), arthralgia (<5%), jaw pain (<5%)

Respiratory: Dyspnea (3% to 7%)

Drug Interactions CYP2D6 and 3A3/4 enzyme inhibitor

Increased Effect/Toxicity: Previous or simultaneous use with mitomycin-C has resulted in acute shortness of breath and severe bronchospasm within minutes or several hours after *Vinca* alkaloid injection and may occur up to 2 weeks after the dose of mitomycin. Cisplatin: Incidence of granulocytopenia is significantly higher than with single-agent vinorelbine.

Drug Uptake

Absorption: Unreliable; must be given I.V.

Half-life, elimination: Triphasic: Terminal: 27.7-43.6 hours

Pregnancy Risk Factor D

Generic Available No

Vioform® [OTC] *see* Clioquinol *on page 302*

Viokase® *see* Pancrelipase *on page 914*

Vioxx® *see* Rofecoxib *on page 1064*

Vira-A® *see* Vidarabine *on page 1238*

Viracept® *see* Nelfinavir *on page 853*

Viramune® *see* Nevirapine *on page 859*

Virazole® Aerosol *see* Ribavirin *on page 1048*

Viread™ *see* Tenofovir *on page 1139*

Virilon® *see* MethylTESTOSTERone *on page 799*

Viroptic® *see* Trifluridine *on page 1207*

Viscoat® *see* Chondroitin Sulfate-Sodium Hyaluronate *on page 281*

Visicol™ *see* Sodium Phosphates *on page 1098*

Visine® Extra [OTC] *see* Tetrahydrozoline *on page 1150*

Visine® L.R. [OTC] *see* Oxymetazoline *on page 907*

Visken® *see* Pindolol *on page 960*

Vistacot® *see* HydrOXYzine *on page 616*

Vistaril® *see* HydrOXYzine *on page 616*

Vistide® *see* Cidofovir *on page 283*

Vi-Sudo® [OTC] *see* Triprolidine and Pseudoephedrine *on page 1213*

Vita-C® [OTC] *see* Ascorbic Acid *on page 117*

Vitacarn® *see* Levocarnitine *on page 698*

Vitamin A (VYE ta min aye)

U.S. Brand Names Aquasol A®; Palmitate-A® [OTC]

Mexican Brand Names Arovit; A-Vicon; A-Vitex

Pharmacologic Category Vitamin

Synonyms Oleovitamin A

Use Treatment and prevention of vitamin A deficiency; parenteral (I.M.) route is indicated when oral administration is not feasible or when absorption is insufficient (malabsorption syndrome)

Local Anesthetic/Vasoconstrictor Precautions No information available to require special precautions

Effects on Dental Treatment No effects or complications reported

Dosage

RDA:
- <1 year: 375 mcg
- 1-3 years: 400 mcg
- 4-6 years: 500 mcg*
- 7-10 years: 700 mcg*
- >10 years: 800-1000 mcg*
- Male: 1000 mcg
- Female: 800 mcg
- * mcg retinol equivalent (0.3 mcg retinol = 1 unit vitamin A)

Vitamin A supplementation in measles (recommendation of the World Health Organization): Children: Oral: Administer as a single dose; repeat the next day and at 4 weeks for children with ophthalmologic evidence of vitamin A deficiency:
- 6 months to 1 year: 100,000 units
- >1 year: 200,000 units

Note: Use of vitamin A in measles is recommended only for patients 6 months to 2 years of age hospitalized with measles and its complications **or** patients >6 months of age who have any of the following risk factors and who are not already receiving vitamin A: immunodeficiency, ophthalmologic evidence of vitamin A deficiency including night blindness, Bitot's spots or evidence of xerophthalmia, impaired intestinal absorption, moderate to severe malnutrition including that associated with eating disorders, or recent immigration from areas where high mortality rates from measles have been observed

Note: Monitor patients closely; dosages >25,000 units/kg have been associated with toxicity

Severe deficiency with xerophthalmia: Oral:
- Children 1-8 years: 5000-10,000 units/kg/day for 5 days or until recovery occurs
- Children >8 years and Adults: 500,000 units/day for 3 days, then 50,000 units/day for 14 days, then 10,000-20,000 units/day for 2 months

Deficiency (without corneal changes): Oral:
- Infants <1 year: 100,000 units every 4-6 months
- Children 1-8 years: 200,000 units every 4-6 months
- Children >8 years and Adults: 100,000 units/day for 3 days then 50,000 units/day for 14 days

Deficiency: I.M.: **Note:** I.M. route is indicated when oral administration is not feasible or when absorption is insufficient (malabsorption syndrome):
- Infants: 7500-15,000 units/day for 10 days
- Children 1-8 years: 17,500-35,000 units/day for 10 days
- Children >8 years and Adults: 100,000 units/day for 3 days, followed by 50,000 units/day for 2 weeks
- **Note:** Follow-up therapy with an oral therapeutic multivitamin (containing additional vitamin A) is recommended:
  - Low Birth Weight Infants: Additional vitamin A is recommended, however no dosage amount has been established
  - Children ≤8 years: 5000-10,000 units/day
  - Children >8 years and Adults: 10,000-20,000 units/day

Malabsorption syndrome (prophylaxis): Children >8 years and Adults: Oral: 10,000-50,000 units/day of water miscible product

Dietary supplement: Oral:
- Infants up to 6 months: 1500 units/day
- Children:
  - 6 months to 3 years: 1500-2000 units/day
  - 4-6 years: 2500 units/day
  - 7-10 years: 3300-3500 units/day
- Children >10 years and Adults: 4000-5000 units/day

Mechanism of Action Needed for bone development, growth, visual adaptation to darkness, testicular and ovarian function, and as a cofactor in many biochemical processes

Other Adverse Effects 1% to 10%:

Central nervous system: Irritability, vertigo, lethargy, malaise, fever, headache

Dermatologic: Drying or cracking of skin

Endocrine & metabolic: Hypercalcemia

Gastrointestinal: Weight loss

Ocular: Visual changes

(Continued)

Vitamin A *(Continued)*

Miscellaneous: Hypervitaminosis A

Contraindications Hypersensitivity to vitamin A or any component of the formulation; hypervitaminosis A

Warnings/Precautions Evaluate other sources of vitamin A while receiving this product; patients receiving >25,000 units/day should be closely monitored for toxicity

Drug Interactions

Increased Effect/Toxicity: Retinoids may have additive adverse effects.

Decreased Effect: Cholestyramine resin decreases absorption of vitamin A. Neomycin and mineral oil may also interfere with vitamin A absorption.

Drug Uptake Absorption: Vitamin A in dosages **not** exceeding physiologic replacement is well absorbed after oral administration. Water miscible preparations are absorbed more rapidly than oil preparations. Large oral doses, conditions of fat malabsorption, low protein intake, hepatic or pancreatic disease reduce oral absorption.

Pregnancy Risk Factor A/X (dose exceeding RDA recommendation)

Generic Available Yes

Vitamin A and Vitamin D (VYE ta min aye & VYE ta min dee)

U.S. Brand Names A and D™ Ointment [OTC]

Pharmacologic Category Topical Skin Product

Synonyms Cod Liver Oil

Use Temporary relief of discomfort due to chapped skin, diaper rash, minor burns or abrasions, and irritations associated with ostomy skin care

Local Anesthetic/Vasoconstrictor Precautions No information available to require special precautions

Effects on Dental Treatment No effects or complications reported

Dosage Topical: Apply locally with gentle massage as needed

Other Adverse Effects Frequency not defined: Local: Irritation

Pregnancy Risk Factor B

Generic Available Yes

Vitamin B Complex (VYE ta min bee KOM pleks)

U.S. Brand Names Apatate® [OTC]; Gevrabon® [OTC]; Lederplex® [OTC]; Lipovite® [OTC]; Mega B® [OTC]; Megaton™ [OTC]; Mucoplex® [OTC]; NeoVadrin® B Complex [OTC]; Orexin® [OTC]; Surbex® [OTC]

Canadian Brand Names Penta/3B®; Vita 3B

Pharmacologic Category Vitamin, Water Soluble

Use Supportive nutritional supplementation in conditions in which water-soluble vitamins are required like GI disorders, chronic alcoholism, pregnancy, severe burns, and recovery from surgery

Local Anesthetic/Vasoconstrictor Precautions No information available to require special precautions

Effects on Dental Treatment No effects or complications reported

Dosage Dosage is usually 1 tablet or capsule/day; please refer to package insert

Generic Available Yes

Vitamin B Complex With Vitamin C

(VYE ta min bee KOM pleks with VYE ta min see)

U.S. Brand Names Allbee® With C [OTC]; Surbex-T® Filmtabs® [OTC]; Surbex® With C Filmtabs® [OTC]; Thera-Combex® H-P Kapseals® [OTC]; Vicon-C® [OTC]

Canadian Brand Names Penta/3B®+C; Vita 3B+C

Pharmacologic Category Vitamin, Water Soluble

Use Supportive nutritional supplementation in conditions in which water-soluble vitamins are required like GI disorders, chronic alcoholism, pregnancy, severe burns, and recovery from surgery

Local Anesthetic/Vasoconstrictor Precautions No information available to require special precautions

Effects on Dental Treatment No effects or complications reported

Dosage Adults: Oral: 1 every day

Generic Available Yes

Vitamin B Complex With Vitamin C and Folic Acid

(VYE ta min bee KOM pleks with VYE ta min see & FOE lik AS id)

U.S. Brand Names Berocca®; Nephrocaps®

Pharmacologic Category Vitamin, Water Soluble

Use Supportive nutritional supplementation in conditions in which water-soluble vitamins are required like GI disorders, chronic alcoholism, pregnancy, severe burns, and recovery from surgery

Local Anesthetic/Vasoconstrictor Precautions No information available to require special precautions

Effects on Dental Treatment No effects or complications reported

Dosage Adults: Oral: 1 every day

Generic Available Yes

Vitamin E (VYE ta min ee)

U.S. Brand Names Amino-Opti-E® [OTC]; Aquasol E® [OTC]; E-Complex-600® [OTC]; E-Vitamin® [OTC]; Vita-Plus® E Softgels® [OTC]; Vitec® [OTC]; Vite E® Creme [OTC]

Pharmacologic Category Vitamin

Synonyms *d*-Alpha Tocopherol; *dl*-Alpha Tocopherol

Use Prevention and treatment of hemolytic anemia secondary to vitamin E deficiency, dietary supplement

To reduce the risk of bronchopulmonary dysplasia or retrolental fibroplasia in infants exposed to high concentrations of oxygen; prevention and treatment of tardive dyskinesia and Alzheimer's disease

Local Anesthetic/Vasoconstrictor Precautions No information available to require special precautions

Effects on Dental Treatment No effects or complications reported

Dosage One unit of vitamin E = 1 mg *dl*-alpha-tocopherol acetate. Oral:

Recommended daily allowance (RDA):
- Premature infants ≤3 months: 17 mg (25 units)
- Infants:
  - ≤6 months: 3 mg (4.5 units)
  - 7-12 months: 4 mg (6 units)
- Children:
  - 1-3 years: 6 mg (9 units); upper limit of intake should not exceed 200 mg/day
  - 4-8 years: 7 mg (10.5 units); upper limit of intake should not exceed 300 mg/day
  - 9-13 years: 11 mg (16.5 units); upper limit of intake should not exceed 600 mg/day
  - 14-18 years: 15 mg (22.5 units); upper limit of intake should not exceed 800 mg/day
- Adults: 15 mg (22.5 units); upper limit of intake should not exceed 1000 mg/day
- Pregnant female:
  - ≤18 years: 15 mg (22.5 units); upper level of intake should not exceed 800 mg/day
  - 19-50 years: 15 mg (22.5 units); upper level of intake should not exceed 1000 mg/day
- Lactating female:
  - ≤18 years: 19 mg (28.5 units); upper level of intake should not exceed 800 mg/day
  - 19-50 years: 19 mg (28.5 units); upper level of intake should not exceed 1000 mg/day

Vitamin E deficiency:
- Children (with malabsorption syndrome): 1 unit/kg/day of water miscible vitamin E (to raise plasma tocopherol concentrations to the normal range within 2 months and to maintain normal plasma concentrations)
- Adults: 60-75 units/day

Prevention of vitamin E deficiency: Adults: 30 units/day

Prevention of retinopathy of prematurity or BPD secondary to O_2 therapy (AAP considers this use investigational and routine use is not recommended):
- Retinopathy prophylaxis: 15-30 units/kg/day to maintain plasma levels between 1.5-2 µg/mL (may need as high as 100 units/kg/day)

Cystic fibrosis, beta-thalassemia, sickle cell anemia may require higher daily maintenance doses:
- Children:
  - Cystic fibrosis: 100-400 units/day
  - Beta-thalassemia: 750 units/day
- Adults:
  - Sickle cell: 450 units/day
  - Alzheimer's disease: 1000 units twice daily
  - Tardive dyskinesia: 1600 units/day

Mechanism of Action Prevents oxidation of vitamin A and C; protects polyunsaturated fatty acids in membranes from attack by free radicals and protects red blood cells against hemolysis

Other Adverse Effects <1%: Blurred vision, contact dermatitis with topical preparation, diarrhea, fatigue, gonadal dysfunction, headache, intestinal cramps, nausea, weakness

Contraindications Hypersensitivity to vitamin E or any component of the formulation; I.V. route

Warnings/Precautions May induce vitamin K deficiency; necrotizing enterocolitis has been associated with oral administration of large dosages (eg, >200 units/day) of a hyperosmolar vitamin E preparation in low birth weight infants

Drug Interactions

Cholestyramine (and colestipol): May reduce absorption of vitamin E

(Continued)

Vitamin E *(Continued)*

Iron: Vitamin E may impair the hematologic response to iron in children with iron-deficiency anemia; monitor

Orlistat: May reduce absorption of vitamin E

Warfarin: Vitamin E may alter the effect of vitamin K actions on clotting factors resulting in an increase hypoprothrombinemic response to warfarin; monitor

Drug Uptake Absorption: Oral: Depends on presence of bile; reduced in conditions of malabsorption, in low birth weight premature infants, and as dosage increases; water miscible preparations are better absorbed than oil preparations

Pregnancy Risk Factor A/C (dose exceeding RDA recommendation)

Dosage Forms CAP: 100 units, 200 units, 400 units, 500 units, 600 units, 1000 units. **CAP, water miscible:** 73.5 mg, 147 mg, 165 mg, 330 mg, 400 units. **CRM:** 50 mg/g (15 g, 30 g, 60 g, 75 g, 120 g, 454 g). **DROPS, oral:** 50 mg/mL (12 mL, 30 mL). **LIQ, topical:** 10 mL, 15 mL, 30 mL, 60 mL. **LOTION:** 120 mL. **OIL:** 15 mL, 30 mL, 60 mL. **OINT:** 30 mg/g (45 g, 60 g). **TAB:** 200 units, 400 units

Generic Available Yes

Vitamins, Multiple (VYE ta mins, MUL ti pul)

U.S. Brand Names Becotin® Pulvules®; Cefol® Filmtab®; Eldercaps® [OTC]; NeoVadrin® [OTC]; Niferex®-PN; Secran®; Stresstabs® 600 Advanced Formula [OTC]; Therabid® [OTC]; Theragran® [OTC]; Theragran® Hematinic®; Theragran® Liquid [OTC]; Theragran-M® [OTC]; Unicap® [OTC]; Vicon Forte®; Vicon® Plus [OTC]; ViDaylin®

Mexican Brand Names Clanda®; Complan; Suplena; Vi-Syneral

Pharmacologic Category Vitamin

Synonyms B Complex; B Complex With C; Children's Vitamins; Hexavitamin; Multiple Vitamins; Multivitamins, Fluoride; Parenteral Multiple Vitamins; Prenatal Vitamins; Therapeutic Multivitamins; Vitamins, Multiple (Injectable); Vitamins, Multiple (Oral); Vitamins, Multiple (Pediatric); Vitamins, Multiple (Prenatal); Vitamins, Multiple (Therapeutic); Vitamins, Multiple With Iron

Use Dietary supplement

Local Anesthetic/Vasoconstrictor Precautions No information available to require special precautions

Effects on Dental Treatment No effects or complications reported

Dosage

Infants 1.5-3 kg: I.V.: 3.25 mL/24 hours (M.V.I.® Pediatric)

Children:

Oral:

≤2 years: Drops: 1 mL/day (premature infants may get 0.5-1 mL/day)

>2 years: Chew 1 tablet/day

≥4 years: 5 mL/day liquid

I.V.: >3 kg and <11 years: 5 mL/24 hours (M.V.I.® Pediatric)

Adults:

Oral: 1 tablet/day or 5 mL/day liquid

I.V.: >11 years: 5 mL of vials 1 and 2 (M.V.I.®-12)/one TPN bag/day

I.V. solutions: 10 mL/24 hours (M.V.I.®-12)

Other Adverse Effects

1% to 10%: Hypervitaminosis; refer to individual vitamin entries for individual reactions

<1%: Anaphylaxis following parenteral administration (rare), allergic reactions

Rare reports following I.V. administration include: Rash, erythema, pruritus, headache, dizziness, agitation, anxiety, diplopia, urticaria, edema (peripheral)

Contraindications Hypersensitivity to any component of the formulation; pre-existing hypervitaminosis

Warnings/Precautions RDA values are not requirements, but are recommended daily intakes of certain essential nutrients; periodic dental exams should be performed to check for dental fluorosis; use with caution in patients with severe renal or liver failure. Pediatric infusion contains vitamin K (caution in patients receiving coumarin anticoagulants). Additional vitamin A may be required in pediatric patients.

Drug Interactions

Hydralazine: May decrease the effect of pyridoxine

Isoniazid: May decrease the effect of pyridoxine

Levodopa: Pyridoxine may decrease the effect of levodopa.

Methotrexate: Folic acid may decrease response to methotrexate.

Phenytoin: Folic acid may lower serum phenytoin concentrations; phenytoin may lower serum folate concentrations.

Warfarin: Vitamin K (contained in pediatric infusion) may antagonize the effect of warfarin.

Pregnancy Risk Factor A/C (dose exceeding RDA recommendation)

Dosage Forms See table on following page.

Generic Available Yes

Multivitamin Products Comparison

Product	Content Given Per	A IU	D IU	E IU	C mg	FA mg	B_1 mg	B_2 mg	B_3 mg	B_6 mg	B_{12} mcg	Other
Theragran®	5 mL liquid	10,000	400		200		10	10	100	4.1	5	B_5 21.4 mg
Vi-Daylin®	1 mL drops	1500	400	4.1	35		0.5	0.6	8	0.4	1.5	Alcohol <0.5%
Vi-Daylin® Iron	1 mL	1500	400	4.1	35		0.5	0.6	8	0.4		Fe 10 mg
Albee® with C	tablet				300		15	10.2		5		Niacinamide 50 mg, pantothenic acid 10 mg
Vitamin B complex	tablet					400 mcg	1.5	1.7		2	6	Niacinamide 20 mg
Hexavitamin	cap/tab	5000	400		75		2	3	20			
Iberet-Folic-500®	tablet				500	0.8	6	6	30	5	25	B_5 10 mg, Fe 105 mg
Stuartnatal® 1+1	tablet	4000	400	11	120	1	1.5	3	20	10	12	Cu, Zn 25 mg, Fe 65 mg, Ca 200 mg
Theragran-M®	tablet	5000	400	30	90	0.4	3	3.4	30	3	9	Cl, Cr, I, K, B_5 10 mg, Mg, Mn, Mo, P, Se, Zn 15 mg, Fe 27 mg, biotin 30 mcg, beta-carotene 1250 IU
Vi-Daylin®	tablet	2500	400	15	60	0.3	1.05	1.2	13.5	1.05	4.5	
M.V.I.®-12 injection	5 mL	3300	200	10	100	0.4	3	3.6	40	4	5	B_5 15 mg, biotin 60 mcg
M.V.I.®-12 unit vial	20 mL											
M.V.I.® pediatric powder	5 mL	2300	400	7	80	0.14	1.2	1.4	17	1	1	B_5 5 mg, biotin 20 mcg, vitamin K 200 mcg

Vita-Plus® E Softgels® [OTC] *see* Vitamin E *on page 1245*
Vitec® [OTC] *see* Vitamin E *on page 1245*
Vite E® Creme [OTC] *see* Vitamin E *on page 1245*
Vitrasert® *see* Ganciclovir *on page 547*
Vitravene™ *see* Fomivirsen *on page 534*
Vivactil® *see* Protriptyline *on page 1021*
Viva-Drops® [OTC] *see* Artificial Tears *on page 117*
Vivelle® *see* Estradiol *on page 457*
Vivelle-Dot® *see* Estradiol *on page 457*
Vivotif Berna™ *see* Typhoid Vaccine *on page 1220*
Volmax® *see* Albuterol *on page 45*
Voltaren® *see* Diclofenac *on page 378*
Voltaren®-XR *see* Diclofenac *on page 378*

Voriconazole (vor i KOE na zole)

U.S. Brand Names VFEND®

Pharmacologic Category Antifungal Agent, Oral; Antifungal Agent, Parenteral

Synonyms UK109496

Use Treatment of invasive aspergillosis and serious fungal infections caused by *Scedosporium apiospermum* and *Fusarium* spp (including *Fusarium solanae*) in patients intolerant of, or refractory to, other therapy

Local Anesthetic/Vasoconstrictor Precautions No information available to require special precautions

Effects on Dental Treatment No effects or complications reported

Dosage Children >12 years and Adults: I.V.: Initial: Loading dose: 6 mg/kg every 12 hours for 2 doses; followed by maintenance dose of 4 mg/kg every 12 hours

Conversion to oral dosing:

Patients >40 kg: 200 mg every 12 hours

Patients ≤40 kg: 100 mg every 12 hours

Note: Dosage may be increased by 100 mg/dose in patients who fail to respond adequately (50 mg/dose in patients ≤40 kg)

Dosage adjustment in patients unable to tolerate treatment:

I.V.: Dose may be reduced to 3 mg/kg every 12 hours

Oral: Dose may be reduced in 50 mg increments to a minimum dosage of 200 mg every 12 hours in patients weighing >40 kg (100 mg every 12 hours in patients ≤40 kg)

Dosage adjustment in patients receiving concomitant phenytoin:

I.V.: Increase maintenance dosage to 5 mg/kg every 12 hours

Oral: Increase dose from 200 mg to 400 mg every 12 hours in patients >40 kg (100 mg to 200 mg every 12 hours in patients ≤40 kg)

Dosage adjustment in renal impairment: In patients with Cl_{cr} <50 mL/minute, accumulation of the I.V. vehicle (SBECD) occurs. After initial loading dose, oral voriconazole should be administered to these patients, unless an assessment of the benefit:risk to the patient justifies the use of I.V. voriconazole. Monitor serum creatinine and change to oral voriconazole therapy when possible.

Dosage adjustment in hepatic impairment:

Mild to moderate hepatic dysfunction (Child-Pugh class A and B): Following standard loading dose, reduce maintenance dosage by 50%

Severe hepatic impairment: Should only be used if benefit outweighs risk; monitor closely for toxicity

Mechanism of Action Interferes with fungal cytochrome P450 activity, decreasing ergosterol synthesis (principal sterol in fungal cell membrane) and inhibiting fungal cell membrane formation

Other Adverse Effects Includes adverse reactions reported from all trials, including trials conducted in immunocompromised patients; cause:effect relationship not established for many reactions.

>10%: Ocular: Visual changes (photophobia, color changes, increased or decreased visual acuity, or blurred vision occur in ~30%)

1% to 10%:

Cardiovascular: Tachycardia (3%), hypertension (2%), hypotension (2%), vasodilation (2%), peripheral edema (1%)

Central nervous system: Fever (6%), chills (4%), headache (3%), hallucinations (3%), dizziness (1%)

Dermatologic: Rash (6%), pruritus (1%)

Endocrine & metabolic: Hypokalemia (2%), hypomagnesemia (1%)

Gastrointestinal: Nausea (6%), vomiting (5%), abdominal pain (2%), diarrhea (1%), xerostomia (1%)

Hematologic: Thrombocytopenia (1%)

Hepatic: Alkaline phosphatase increased (4%), serum transaminases increased (2%), AST increased (2%), ALT increased (2%), cholestatic jaundice (1%)

Renal: Acute renal failure (1%)

<1% (Limited to important or life-threatening): Acute tubular necrosis, adrenal cortical insufficiency, agranulocytosis, allergic reaction, anaphylactoid reaction,

anemia (aplastic), anemia (macrocytic, megaloblastic, or microcytic), angioedema, aplastic anemia, ataxia, atrial arrhythmia, atrial fibrillation, AV block, bigeminy, bone marrow depression, bone necrosis, bradycardia, brain edema, bundle branch block, cardiac arrest, cerebral hemorrhage, cholecystitis, cholelithiasis, color blindness, coma, CHF, convulsion, delirium, dementia, depersonalization, depression, DIC, discoid lupus erythematosus, duodenal ulcer perforation, dyspnea, encephalopathy, enlarged liver, enlarged spleen, eosinophilia, erythema multiforme, exfoliative dermatitis, extrapyramidal symptoms, fixed drug eruption, gastrointestinal hemorrhage, grand mal seizure, Guillain-Barré syndrome, hematemesis, hemolytic anemia, hepatic coma, hepatic failure, hepatitis, intestinal perforation, intracranial hypertension, leukopenia, lung edema, myasthenia, myocardial infarction, neuropathy, night blindness, optic atrophy, optic neuritis, pancreatitis, pancytopenia, papilledema, paresthesia, photosensitivity, psychosis, pulmonary embolus, QT interval prolongation, respiratory distress syndrome, sepsis, Stevens-Johnson syndrome, suicidal ideation, supraventricular tachycardia, syncope, thrombotic thrombocytopenic purpura, toxic epidermal necrolysis, ventricular arrhythmia, ventricular fibrillation, ventricular tachycardia (including possible torsade de pointes), vertigo, visual field defect

Contraindications Hypersensitivity to voriconazole or any component of the formulation (cross-reaction with other azole antifungal agents may occur but has not been established, use caution); coadministration of CYP3A4 substrates which may lead to QT_c prolongation (terfenadine, astemizole, cisapride, pimozide, or quinidine); coadministration with barbiturates (long acting), carbamazepine, ergot alkaloids, rifampin, rifabutin, and sirolimus; pregnancy (unless risk:benefit ratio justifies use)

Warnings/Precautions Visual changes are commonly associated with treatment, including blurred vision, changes in visual acuity, color changes, and photophobia. Patients should be warned to avoid tasks which depend on vision, including operating machinery or driving. Changes are reversible on discontinuation following brief exposure/treatment regimens (≤28 days); reversibility following long-term administration has not been evaluated.

Serious hepatic reactions (including hepatitis, cholestasis, and fulminant hepatic failure) have occurred during treatment, primarily in patients with serious concomitant medical conditions, including hematological malignancy. However, hepatotoxicity has occurred in patients with no identifiable risk factors. Use caution in patients with pre-existing hepatic impairment (dose adjustment required).

Tablets contain lactose; avoid administration in hereditary galactose intolerance, Lapp lactase deficiency, or glucose-galactose malabsorption. Avoid/limit use of I.V. formulation in patients with renal impairment (I.V. formulation contains excipient SBECD, which may accumulate in renal insufficiency). Infusion-related reactions may occur with I.V. dosing. Consider discontinuation of infusion if reaction is severe.

Avoid use in pregnancy, unless an evaluation of the potential benefit justifies possible risk to the fetus. Safety and efficacy have not been established in children <12 years of age.

Drug Interactions CYP2C19, CYP2C9, and CYP3A3/4 (minor) enzyme substrate; CYP2C19, CYP2C9, and CYP3A3/4 (minor) enzyme inhibitor

Benzodiazepines (metabolized by oxidation): Alprazolam, diazepam, temazepam, triazolam, and midazolam serum concentrations/toxicity may be increased.

Buspirone: Serum concentrations may be increased; monitor for sedation.

Busulfan: Serum concentrations may be increased; avoid concurrent use.

Calcium channel blockers: Serum concentrations may be increased (applies to those agents metabolized by CYP3A3/4, including felodipine, nifedipine, and verapamil).

Cisapride: Serum concentrations may be increased which may lead to malignant arrhythmias; concurrent use is contraindicated.

Docetaxel: Serum concentrations may be increased; avoid concurrent use.

Dofetilide: Serum levels/toxicity may be increased; avoid concurrent use.

Enzyme inducers: Rifampin decreases voriconazole's serum concentration to levels which are no longer effective; concurrent use is contraindicated. Other inducers (barbiturates, carbamazepine, rifabutin) may share this effect. Rifabutin serum levels are increased by voriconazole; concurrent use is contraindicated.

Ergot alkaloids: Serum levels may be increased by voriconazole, leading to ergot toxicity; concurrent use is contraindicated.

Erythromycin (and clarithromycin): Although voriconazole is a substrate for CYP3A3/4, no significant increase in serum levels was noted during concurrent erythromycin, likely reflecting a limited role in voriconazole metabolism.

H_2 antagonists: Changes in gastric acidity do not appear to significantly affect voriconizole absorption.

HMG-CoA reductase inhibitors (except pravastatin and fluvastatin): Serum concentrations may be increased. The risk of myopathy/rhabdomyolysis may be increased. Switch to pravastatin/fluvastatin or monitor for development of myopathy.

(Continued)

Voriconazole *(Continued)*

Immunosuppressants (cyclosporine, sirolimus, and tacrolimus): Serum concentrations may be increased; monitor serum concentrations and renal function. Concurrent use of sirolimus is contraindicated. Decrease cyclosporine dosage by 50% when initiating voriconazole, decrease tacrolimus dosage by 66% when initiating voriconazole.

Methylprednisolone: Serum concentrations may be increased; monitor.

NNRTIs: Effects on serum concentrations may be difficult to predict. Serum levels of voriconazole may be increased by efavirenz or delavirdine. Serum levels may be decreased by efavirenz or nevirapine. Monitor closely for efficacy/toxicity.

Phenytoin: Serum concentrations of voriconazole may be decreased; adjust dose of voriconazole; monitor phenytoin levels and adjust dose as needed.

Pimozide: Serum levels/toxicity may be increased; concurrent use is contraindicated.

Protease inhibitors: Indinavir did not appear to alter voriconizole serum concentrations during concurrent treatment. Other protease inhibitors may result in increased voriconazole concentrations.

Proton pump inhibitors: Changes in gastric acidity do not appear to significantly affect voriconizole absorption. However, voriconazole may significantly increase serum levels of omeprazole. For omeprazole dosages >40 mg/day, reduce omeprazole dosage by 50%. Serum levels of other proton pump inhibitors may also be increased.

Quinidine: Serum levels may be increased; concurrent use is contraindicated.

Sulfonylureas: Serum levels may be increased by voriconazole, potentially leading to hypoglycemia; monitor.

Trimetrexate: Serum concentrations may be increased; monitor.

Warfarin: Anticoagulant effects may be increased; monitor INR.

Vinca alkaloids: Serum concentrations may be increased; consider reduced dosage of vinca alkaloid.

Zolpidem: Serum levels may be increased; monitor.

Dietary/Ethanol/Herb Considerations

Food may decrease absorption; should be taken 1 hour before or 1 hour after a meal. Avoid grapefruit products; may increase voriconazole serum levels.

Herb/Nutraceutical: Avoid St John's wort; may decrease serum concentration.

Drug Uptake

Absorption: Oral: Well absorbed

Half-life, elimination: Variable, dose dependent

Time to peak: 1-2 hours

Pregnancy Risk Factor D

Breast-feeding Considerations Excretion in breast milk has not been investigated; avoid breast-feeding until additional data are available.

Dosage Forms TAB: 50 mg, 200 mg. **INJ, powder for reconstitution:** 200 mg

Generic Available No

VōSol® HC *see* Acetic Acid, Propylene Glycol Diacetate, and Hydrocortisone *on page 37*

Vumon *see* Teniposide *on page 1139*

V.V.S.® *see* Sulfabenzamide, Sulfacetamide, and Sulfathiazole *on page 1114*

Vytone® *see* Iodoquinol and Hydrocortisone *on page 650*

Warfarin (WAR far in)

Related Information

Cardiovascular Diseases *on page 1308*

Dental Drug Interactions: Update on Drug Combinations Requiring Special Considerations *on page 1434*

Dicumarol *on page 381*

U.S. Brand Names Coumadin®

Canadian Brand Names Coumadin®; Taro-Warfarin

Mexican Brand Names Dimantil

Pharmacologic Category Anticoagulant, Coumarin Derivative

Synonyms Warfarin Sodium

Use Prophylaxis and treatment of venous thrombosis, pulmonary embolism and thromboembolic disorders; atrial fibrillation with risk of embolism and as an adjunct in the prophylaxis of systemic embolism after myocardial infarction

Unlabeled/Investigational: Prevention of recurrent transient ischemic attacks and to reduce risk of recurrent myocardial infarction

Local Anesthetic/Vasoconstrictor Precautions No information available to require special precautions

Effects on Dental Treatment Signs of warfarin overdose may first appear as bleeding from gingival tissue; consultation with prescribing physician is advisable prior to surgery to determine temporary dose reduction or withdrawal of medication.

Dosage

Oral:

Infants and Children: 0.05-0.34 mg/kg/day; infants <12 months of age may require doses at or near the high end of this range; consistent anticoagulation may be difficult to maintain in children <5 years of age

Adults: Initial dosing must be individualized based upon patient's end organ function, concurrent therapy, and risk of bleeding; ACCP recommendation: 5 mg/day for 2-5 days, then adjust dose according to results of prothrombin time; usual maintenance dose ranges from 2-10 mg/day (selected sensitive patients may require less; resistant patients may require higher dosages).

Note: Lower starting doses may be required for patients with hepatic impairment, poor nutrition, CHF, elderly, or a high risk of bleeding. Higher initial doses may be reasonable in selected patients (ie, receiving enzyme-inducing agents and with low risk of bleeding).

I.V. (administer as a slow bolus injection): 2-5 mg/day

Dosing adjustment/comments in hepatic disease: Monitor effect at usual doses; the response to oral anticoagulants may be markedly enhanced in obstructive jaundice (due to reduced vitamin K absorption) and also in hepatitis and cirrhosis (due to decreased production of vitamin K-dependent clotting factors); prothrombin index should be closely monitored

Mechanism of Action Interferes with hepatic synthesis of vitamin K-dependent coagulation factors (II, VII, IX, X)

Other Adverse Effects As with all anticoagulants, bleeding is the major adverse effect of warfarin. Hemorrhage may occur at virtually any site. Risk is dependent on multiple variables, including the intensity of anticoagulation and patient susceptibility. Additional adverse effects are often related to idiosyncratic reactions, and the frequency cannot be accurately estimated.

Cardiovascular: Vasculitis, edema, hemorrhagic shock

Central nervous system: Fever, lethargy, malaise, asthenia, pain, headache, dizziness, stroke

Dermatologic: Rash, dermatitis, bullous eruptions, urticaria, pruritus, alopecia

Gastrointestinal: Anorexia, nausea, vomiting, stomach cramps, abdominal pain, diarrhea, flatulence, gastrointestinal bleeding, taste disturbance, mouth ulcers

Genitourinary: Priapism, hematuria

Hematologic: Hemorrhage, leukopenia, unrecognized bleeding sites (eg, colon cancer) may be uncovered by anticoagulation, retroperitoneal hematoma, agranulocytosis

Hepatic: Increased transaminases, hepatic injury, jaundice

Neuromuscular & skeletal: Paresthesia, osteoporosis

Respiratory: Hemoptysis, epistaxis, pulmonary hemorrhage, tracheobronchial calcification

Miscellaneous: Hypersensitivity/allergic reactions

Skin necrosis/gangrene, due to paradoxical local thrombosis, is a known but rare risk of warfarin therapy. Its onset is usually within the first few days of therapy and is frequently localized to the limbs, breast or penis. The risk of this effect is increased in patients with protein C or S deficiency.

"Purple toes syndrome," caused by cholesterol microembolization, also occurs rarely. Typically, this occurs after several weeks of therapy, and may present as a dark, purplish, mottled discoloration of the plantar and lateral surfaces. Other manifestations of cholesterol microembolization may include livedo reticularis, rash, gangrene, abrupt and intense pain in lower extremities, abdominal, flank, or back pain, hematuria, renal insufficiency, hypertension, cerebral ischemia, spinal cord infarction, or other symptom of vascular compromise.

Drug Interactions CYP1A2 enzyme substrate (minor), CYP2C8, 2C9, 2C18, 2C19, and 3A3/4 enzyme substrate; CYP2C9, 2C19 enzyme inhibitor

Increased bleeding tendency: Administration with the following drugs increase the chances of hemorrhage:

Inhibit platelet aggregation: Cephalosporins, dipyridamole, indomethacin, oxyphenbutazone, penicillin (parenteral), phenylbutazone, salicylates, sulfinpyrazone

Inhibit procoagulant factors: Antimetabolites, quinidine, quinine, salicylates

Ulcerogenic drugs: Adrenal corticosteroids, indomethacin, oxyphenbutazone, phenylbutazone, potassium products, salicylates

Enhanced anticoagulant effects:

Decrease vitamin K: Oral antibiotics can increase or decrease INR. Check INR 3 days after patient begins antibiotics to see the INR value and adjust the warfarin dose accordingly.

Displace anticoagulant: Chloral hydrate, clofibrate, diazoxide, ethacrynic acid, miconazole (including intravaginal use), nalidixic acid, phenylbutazone, salicylates, sulfonamides, sulfonylureas

Inhibit metabolism: Allopurinol, amiodarone, azole antibiotics, capecitabine, chloramphenicol, chlorpropamide, cimetidine, ciprofloxacin, disulfiram, flutamide, isoniazid, metronidazole, norfloxacin, ofloxacin, omeprazole, phenylbutazone,

(Continued)

Warfarin *(Continued)*

phenytoin, propafenone, propoxyphene, protease inhibitors, quinidine, sulfamethoxazole and trimethoprim, sulfinpyrazone, sulfonamides, tamoxifen, tolbutamide, zafirlukast, zileuton

Other: Acetaminophen, anabolic steroids, clarithromycin, clofibrate, danazol, erythromycin, gemfibrozil, glucagon, influenza vaccine, propranolol, propylthiouracil, ranitidine, SSRIs, sulindac, tetracycline, thyroid drugs, vitamin E (≥400 int. units)

Decreased anticoagulant effects: May occur when administered with the following drugs:

Induction of enzymes: Barbiturates, carbamazepine, glutethimide, griseofulvin, nafcillin, phenytoin, rifampin

Increased procoagulant factors: Estrogens, oral contraceptives, vitamin K (including nutritional supplements)

Decreased drug absorption: Aluminum hydroxide, cholestyramine*, colestipol*

Other: Ethchlorvynol, griseofulvin, spironolactone**, sucralfate

*Cholestyramine and colestipol may increase the anticoagulant effect by binding vitamin K in the gut; yet, the decreased drug absorption appears to be of more concern.

**Diuretic-induced hemoconcentration with subsequent concentration of clotting factors has been reported to decrease the effects of oral anticoagulants.

Drug Uptake

Onset of action: Anticoagulation: Oral: 36-72 hours

Peak effect: Full therapeutic effect: 5-7 days; INR may increase in 36-72 hours

Absorption: Oral: Rapid

Duration: 2-5 days

Half-life, elimination: 20-60 hours; Mean: 40 hours (highly variable)

Time to peak: Full therapeutic effect: 5-7 days; INR may increase in 36-72 hours

Pregnancy Risk Factor D

Generic Available Yes: Tablet

Wart-Off® [OTC] *see* Salicylic Acid *on page 1072*

4-Way® Long Acting Nasal [OTC] *see* Oxymetazoline *on page 907*

WelChol™ *see* Colesevelam *on page 320*

Wellbutrin® *see* BuPROPion *on page 188*

Wellbutrin SR® *see* BuPROPion *on page 188*

Wellcovorin® *see* Leucovorin *on page 691*

Wesmycin® *see* Tetracycline *on page 1147*

Westcort® *see* Hydrocortisone *on page 608*

Westhroid® *see* Thyroid *on page 1164*

Wigraine® *see* Ergotamine *on page 448*

40 Winks® [OTC] *see* DiphenhydrAMINE *on page 398*

Winstrol® *see* Stanozolol *on page 1107*

Wound Wash Saline™ [OTC] *see* Sodium Chloride *on page 1094*

Wycillin® *see* Penicillin G Procaine *on page 930*

Wydase® *see* Hyaluronidase *on page 592*

Wygesic® *see* Propoxyphene and Acetaminophen *on page 1013*

Wymox® *see* Amoxicillin *on page 86*

Wytensin® *see* Guanabenz *on page 571*

Xalatan® *see* Latanoprost *on page 687*

Xanax® *see* Alprazolam *on page 56*

Xeloda® *see* Capecitabine *on page 210*

Xenical® *see* Orlistat *on page 890*

Xigris™ *see* Drotrecogin Alfa *on page 424*

Xopenex® *see* Levalbuterol *on page 693*

X-Prep® [OTC] *see* Senna *on page 1081*

X-Seb™ T [OTC] *see* Coal Tar and Salicylic Acid *on page 315*

Xylocaine® *see* Lidocaine *on page 706*

Xylocaine® With Epinephrine *see* Lidocaine and Epinephrine *on page 709*

Xylometazoline (zye loe met AZ oh leen)

U.S. Brand Names Otrivin® [OTC]; Otrivin® Pediatric [OTC]

Canadian Brand Names Decongest

Pharmacologic Category Vasoconstrictor, Nasal

Synonyms Xylometazoline Hydrochloride

Use Symptomatic relief of nasal and nasopharyngeal mucosal congestion

Local Anesthetic/Vasoconstrictor Precautions No information available to require special precautions

Effects on Dental Treatment No effects or complications reported

Dosage

Children 2-12 years: Instill 2-3 drops (0.05%) in each nostril every 8-10 hours

Children >12 years and Adults: Instill 2-3 drops or sprays (0.1%) in each nostril every 8-10 hours

Mechanism of Action Stimulates alpha-adrenergic receptors in the arterioles of the conjunctiva and the nasal mucosa to produce vasoconstriction

Other Adverse Effects Frequency not defined:

Cardiovascular: Palpitations

Central nervous system: Drowsiness, dizziness, seizures, headache

Ocular: Blurred vision, ocular irritation, photophobia

Miscellaneous: Diaphoresis

Drug Uptake

Onset of action: Intranasal: Local vasoconstriction: 5-10 minutes

Duration: 5-6 hours

Pregnancy Risk Factor C

Generic Available Yes

Yasmin® *see* Combination Hormonal Contraceptives *on page 323*

Yeast-Gard® Medicated Douche [OTC] *see* Povidone-Iodine *on page 982*

Yocon® *see* Yohimbine *on page 1253*

Yodoxin® *see* Iodoquinol *on page 650*

Yohimbine (yo HIM bine)

U.S. Brand Names Aphrodyne®; Yocon®

Canadian Brand Names PMS-Yohimbine; Yocon®

Pharmacologic Category Miscellaneous Product

Synonyms Yohimbine Hydrochloride

Use No FDA sanctioned indications

Unlabeled/Investigational: Treatment of SSRI-induced sexual dysfunction; weight loss; impotence; sympathicolytic and mydriatic; may have activity as an aphrodisiac

Local Anesthetic/Vasoconstrictor Precautions No information available to require special precautions

Effects on Dental Treatment No effects or complications reported

Dosage Adults: Oral: Impotence: 5.4 mg 3 times/day

Mechanism of Action Derived from the bark of the yohimbe tree (*Corynanthe yohimbe*, Pausinystalia yohimbe), this indole alkaloid produces a presynaptic $alpha_2$-adrenergic blockade; a weak MAO inhibitor; parasympathetic tone is also decreased. Peripheral autonomic effect is to increase cholinergic and decrease adrenergic activity; yohimbine exerts a stimulating effect on the mood and a mild antidiuretic effect.

Other Adverse Effects Frequency not defined:

Cardiovascular: Tachycardia, bradycardia, hypertension, hypotension (orthostatic), flushing, shock, sinus tachycardia, vasodilation, sinus bradycardia

Central nervous system: Anxiety, mania, hallucinations, irritability, dizziness, psychosis, insomnia, headache, panic attacks

Gastrointestinal: Nausea, vomiting, anorexia, salivation

Hematologic: Neutropenia, agranulocytosis

Neuromuscular & skeletal: Tremors, paresthesia

Ocular: Lacrimation, mydriasis

Respiratory: Bronchospasm, sinusitis

Miscellaneous: Antidiuretic action, salivation, diaphoresis

Drug Interactions CYP2D6 and 3A3/4 enzyme substrate; CYP2D6 inhibitor

Increased Effect/Toxicity: Caution with other CNS acting drugs. When used in combination with CYP3A3/4 inhibitors, serum concentration and/or toxicity of yohimbine may be increased; inhibitors include amiodarone, cimetidine, clarithromycin, erythromycin, delavirdine, diltiazem, dirithromycin, disulfiram, fluoxetine, fluvoxamine, indinavir, itraconazole, ketoconazole, metronidazole, nefazodone, nevirapine, propoxyphene, quinupristin-dalfopristin, ritonavir, saquinavir, verapamil, zafirlukast, zileuton; monitor for altered response. MAO inhibitors or drugs with MAO inhibition (linezolid, furazolidone) theoretically may increase toxicity or adverse effects.

Drug Uptake

Absorption: Oral: 33%

Half-life, elimination: 0.6 hour

Generic Available Yes

Yutopar® *see* Ritodrine ***No longer manufactured*** *on page 1058*

Zaditor™ *see* Ketotifen *on page 679*

Zafirlukast (za FIR loo kast)

Related Information

Respiratory Diseases *on page 1328*

U.S. Brand Names Accolate®

Canadian Brand Names Accolate®

Mexican Brand Names Accolate®

Pharmacologic Category Leukotriene Receptor Antagonist

(Continued)

Zafirlukast *(Continued)*

Synonyms ICI 204, 219

Use Prophylaxis and chronic treatment of asthma in adults and children ≥5 years of age

Local Anesthetic/Vasoconstrictor Precautions No information available to require special precautions

Effects on Dental Treatment No effects or complications reported

Dosage Oral:

Children <7 years: Safety and effectiveness has not been established

Children 7-11 years: 10 mg twice daily

Adults: 20 mg twice daily

Elderly: The mean dose (mg/kg) normalized AUC and C_{max} increase and plasma clearance decreases with increasing age. In patients >65 years of age, there is a 2- to 3-fold greater C_{max} and AUC compared to younger adults.

Mechanism of Action A selective and competitive leukotriene-receptor antagonist (LTRA) of leukotriene D4 and E4 (LTD4 and LTE4) which are components of slow-reacting substance of anaphylaxis (SRSA); cysteinyl leukotriene production and receptor occupation have been correlated with the pathophysiology of asthma, including airway edema, smooth muscle constriction and altered cellular activity associated with the inflammatory process, which contribute to the signs and symptoms of asthma.

Other Adverse Effects

>10%: Central nervous system: Headache (12.9%)

1% to 10%:

Central nervous system: Dizziness, pain, fever

Gastrointestinal: Nausea, diarrhea, abdominal pain, vomiting, dyspepsia

Hepatic: SGPT elevation

Neuromuscular & skeletal: Back pain, myalgia, weakness

Drug Interactions CYP2C9 enzyme substrate; CYP2C9 and 3A3/4 enzyme inhibitor

Increased Effect/Toxicity: Zafirlukast concentrations are increased by aspirin. Warfarin effect may be increased with zafirlukast. Zafirlukast may increase theophylline levels.

Decreased Effect: Zafirlukast concentrations may be reduced by erythromycin and terfenadine.

Drug Uptake

Absorption: Food reduces bioavailability by 40%

Half-life, elimination: 10 hours

Time to peak: 3 hours

Pregnancy Risk Factor B

Generic Available No

Zagam® *see* Sparfloxacin *on page 1104*

Zalcitabine (zal SITE a been)

Related Information

HIV Infection and AIDS *on page 1334*

U.S. Brand Names Hivid®

Canadian Brand Names Hivid®

Mexican Brand Names Hivid®

Pharmacologic Category Antiretroviral Agent, Reverse Transcriptase Inhibitor (Nucleoside)

Synonyms ddC; Dideoxycytidine

Use In combination with at least two other antiretrovirals in the treatment of patients with HIV infection; it is not recommended that zalcitabine be given in combination with didanosine, stavudine, or lamivudine due to overlapping toxicities, virologic interactions, or lack of clinical data

Local Anesthetic/Vasoconstrictor Precautions No information available to require special precautions

Effects on Dental Treatment >10%: Oral ulceration

Dosage Oral:

Neonates: Dose unknown

Infants and Children <13 years: Safety and efficacy have not been established; suggested usual dose: 0.01 mg/kg every 8 hours; range: 0.005-0.01 mg/kg every 8 hours

Adolescents and Adults: 0.75 mg 3 times/day

Dosing adjustment in renal impairment: Adults:

Cl_{cr} 10-40 mL/minute: 0.75 mg every 12 hours

Cl_{cr} <10 mL/minute: 0.75 mg every 24 hours

Moderately dialyzable (20% to 50%)

Mechanism of Action Purine nucleoside analogue, zalcitabine or 2′,3′-dideoxycitidine (ddC) has been found to have *in vitro* activity and is reported to be successful against HIV in short-term clinical trials. Intracellularly, ddC is converted to active metabolite ddCTP; lack the presence of the 3′-hydroxyl group necessary for phosphodiester linkages during DNA replication. As a result viral replication is prematurely terminated. ddCTP acts as a competitor for binding sites on the HIV-RNA dependent DNA polymerase (reverse transcriptase) to further contribute to inhibition of viral replication.

Other Adverse Effects

>10%:

- Central nervous system: Fever (5% to 17%), malaise (2% to 13%)
- Neuromuscular & skeletal: Peripheral neuropathy (28%)

1% to 10%:

- Central nervous system: Headache (2%), dizziness (1%), fatigue (4%), seizures (1.3%)
- Dermatologic: Rash (2% to 11%), pruritus (3% to 5%)
- Endocrine & metabolic: Hypoglycemia (2% to 6%), hyponatremia (4%), hyperglycemia (1% to 6%)
- Gastrointestinal: Nausea (3%), dysphagia (1% to 4%), anorexia (4%), abdominal pain (3% to 8%), vomiting (1% to 3%), diarrhea (<1% to 10%), weight loss, oral ulcers (3% to 7%), increased amylase (3% to 8%)
- Hematologic: Anemia (occurs as early as 2-4 weeks), granulocytopenia (usually after 6-8 weeks)
- Hepatic: Abnormal hepatic function (9%), hyperbilirubinemia (2% to 5%)
- Neuromuscular & skeletal: Myalgia (1% to 6%), foot pain
- Respiratory: Pharyngitis (2%), cough (6%), nasal discharge (4%)

Drug Interactions Increased Effect/Toxicity: Amphotericin, foscarnet, and aminoglycosides may potentiate the risk of developing peripheral neuropathy or other toxicities associated with zalcitabine by interfering with the renal elimination of zalcitabine. Other drugs associated with peripheral neuropathy include chloramphenicol, cisplatin, dapsone, disulfiram, ethionamide, glutethimide, gold, hydralazine, iodoquinol, isoniazid, metronidazole, nitrofurantoin, phenytoin, ribavirin, and vincristine. Concomitant use with zalcitabine may increase risk of peripheral neuropathy. Concomitant use of zalcitabine with didanosine is not recommended.

Drug Uptake

Absorption: Well, but variable; decreased 39% with food

Half-life, elimination: 2.9 hours; Renal impairment: ≤8.5 hours

Pregnancy Risk Factor C

Generic Available No

Zaleplon (ZAL e plon)

U.S. Brand Names Sonata®

Canadian Brand Names Sonata®; Starnoc®

Pharmacologic Category Hypnotic, Nonbenzodiazepine

Use Short-term treatment of insomnia

Local Anesthetic/Vasoconstrictor Precautions No information available to require special precautions

Effects on Dental Treatment No effects or complications reported

Restrictions C-IV

Dosage Oral:

Adults: 10 mg at bedtime (range: 5-20 mg); has been used for up to 5 weeks of treatment in controlled trial setting

Elderly: 5 mg at bedtime

Dosage adjustment in hepatic impairment: Mild to moderate impairment: 5 mg; not recommended for use in patients with severe hepatic impairment

Mechanism of Action Zaleplon is unrelated to benzodiazepines, barbiturates, or other hypnotics. However, it interacts with the benzodiazepine GABA receptor complex. Nonclinical studies have shown that it binds selectively to the brain omega-1 receptor situated on the alpha subunit of the GABA-A receptor complex.

Other Adverse Effects 1% to 10%:

- Cardiovascular: Peripheral edema, chest pain
- Central nervous system: Amnesia, anxiety, depersonalization, dizziness, hallucinations, hypesthesia, somnolence, vertigo, malaise, depression, lightheadedness, impaired coordination, fever, migraine
- Dermatologic: Photosensitivity reaction, rash, pruritus
- Gastrointestinal: Abdominal pain, anorexia, colitis, dyspepsia, nausea, constipation, xerostomia
- Genitourinary: Dysmenorrhea
- Neuromuscular & skeletal: Paresthesia, tremor, myalgia, weakness, back pain, arthralgia
- Ocular: Abnormal vision, eye pain
- Otic: Hyperacusis
- Miscellaneous: Parosmia

Contraindications Hypersensitivity to zaleplon or any component of the formulation

Warnings/Precautions Symptomatic treatment of insomnia should be initiated only after careful evaluation of potential causes of sleep disturbance. Failure of sleep disturbance to resolve after 7-10 days may indicate psychiatric and/or medical illness.

(Continued)

Zaleplon *(Continued)*

Use with caution in patients with depression, particularly if suicidal risk may be present. Use with caution in patients with a history of drug dependence. Abrupt discontinuance may lead to withdrawal symptoms. May impair physical and mental capabilities. Patients must be cautioned about performing tasks which require mental alertness (operating machinery or driving). Use with caution in patients receiving other CNS depressants or psychoactive medications. Effects with other sedative drugs or ethanol may be potentiated.

Use with caution in the elderly, those with compromised respiratory function, or renal and hepatic impairment. Because of the rapid onset of action, zaleplon should be administered immediately prior to bedtime or after the patient has gone to bed and is having difficulty falling asleep.

Drug Interactions CYP3A3/4 substrate (minor metabolic pathway)

Increased Effect/Toxicity: Zaleplon potentiates the CNS effects of CNS depressants, including alcohol, imipramine, and thioridazine. Cimetidine increases concentrations of zaleplon. Avoid concurrent use or use 5 mg zaleplon as starting dose in patient receiving cimetidine.

Decreased Effect: CYP3A4 inducers (eg, phenytoin, carbamazepine, phenobarbital) could lead to ineffectiveness of zaleplon.

Drug Uptake

Onset of action: Rapid
Absorption: Rapid and almost complete
Duration: 6-8 hours
Half-life, elimination: 1 hour
Time to peak: 1 hour

Pregnancy Risk Factor C

Generic Available No

Zanaflex® *see* Tizanidine *on page 1174*

Zanamivir (za NA mi veer)

Related Information

Systemic Viral Diseases *on page 1354*

U.S. Brand Names Relenza®

Canadian Brand Names Relenza®

Pharmacologic Category Antiviral Agent; Neuraminidase Inhibitor

Use Treatment of uncomplicated acute illness due to influenza virus in adults and adolescents ≥12 years of age; treatment should only be initiated in patients who have been symptomatic for ≤2 days

Unlabeled/Investigational: Prophylaxis against influenza A/B infections

Local Anesthetic/Vasoconstrictor Precautions No information available to require special precautions

Effects on Dental Treatment No effects or complications reported

Dosage Adolescents ≥12 years and Adults: 2 Inhalations: (10 mg total) twice daily for 5 days. Two doses should be taken on the first day of dosing, regardless of interval, while doses should be spaced by ~ 12 hours on subsequent days.

Mechanism of Action Inhibits influenza virus neuraminidase enzymes, potentially altering virus particle aggregation and release

Other Adverse Effects Most adverse reactions occurred at a frequency which was equal to the control (lactose vehicle).

>1.5%:

- Central nervous system: Headache (2%), dizziness (2%)
- Gastrointestinal: Nausea (3%), diarrhea (3% adults, 2% children), vomiting (1% adults, 2% children)
- Respiratory: Sinusitis (3%), bronchitis (2%), cough (2%), other nasal signs and symptoms (2%), infection (ear, nose, and throat; 2% adults, 5% children)

<1.5%: Malaise, fatigue, fever, abdominal pain, myalgia, arthralgia, and urticaria

Contraindications Hypersensitivity to zanamivir or any component of the formulation

Warnings/Precautions Patients must be instructed in the use of the delivery system. No data are available to support the use of this drug in patients who begin treatment after 48 hours of symptoms, as a prophylactic treatment for influenza, or in patients with significant underlying medical conditions. Use with caution in patients with underlying respiratory disease - bronchospasm may be provoked.

Drug Uptake

Absorption: Inhalation: 4% to 17%
Half-life, elimination: 2.5-5.1 hours

Pregnancy Risk Factor C

Generic Available No

Zanosar® *see* Streptozocin *on page 1112*
Zantac® *see* Ranitidine Hydrochloride *on page 1042*
Zantac® 75 [OTC] *see* Ranitidine Hydrochloride *on page 1042*
Zapzyt® [OTC] *see* Benzoyl Peroxide *on page 153*

Zarontin® *see* Ethosuximide *on page 476*
Zaroxolyn® *see* Metolazone *on page 801*
Zeasorb®-AF [OTC] *see* Miconazole *on page 807*
Zebeta® *see* Bisoprolol *on page 168*
Zemplar™ *see* Paricalcitol *on page 917*
Zenapax® *see* Daclizumab *on page 344*
Zephiran® [OTC] *see* Benzalkonium Chloride *on page 151*
Zephrex® *see* Guaifenesin and Pseudoephedrine *on page 570*
Zephrex LA® *see* Guaifenesin and Pseudoephedrine *on page 570*
Zerit® *see* Stavudine *on page 1108*
Zestoretic® *see* Lisinopril and Hydrochlorothiazide *on page 721*
Zestril® *see* Lisinopril *on page 719*
Zetar® [OTC] *see* Coal Tar *on page 315*
Zevalin™ *see* Ibritumomab *on page 620*
Ziac® *see* Bisoprolol and Hydrochlorothiazide *on page 169*
Ziagen® *see* Abacavir *on page 22*

Zidovudine (zye DOE vyoo deen)

Related Information

HIV Infection and AIDS *on page 1334*
Systemic Viral Diseases *on page 1354*
Zidovudine and Lamivudine *on page 1258*

U.S. Brand Names Retrovir®

Canadian Brand Names Apo®-Zidovudine; AZT™; Novo-AZT; Retrovir®

Mexican Brand Names Dipedyne; Isadol®; Kenamil; Retrovir AZT®

Pharmacologic Category Antiretroviral Agent, Reverse Transcriptase Inhibitor (Nucleoside)

Synonyms Azidothymidine; AZT; Compound S; ZDV

Use Management of patients with HIV infections in combination with at least two other antiretroviral agents; for prevention of maternal/fetal HIV transmission as monotherapy

Local Anesthetic/Vasoconstrictor Precautions No information available to require special precautions

Effects on Dental Treatment No effects or complications reported

Dosage

Prevention of maternal-fetal HIV transmission:

Neonatal: Oral: 2 mg/kg/dose every 6 hours for 6 weeks beginning 6-12 hours after birth; infants unable to receive oral dosing may receive 1.5 mg/kg I.V. infused over 30 minutes every 6 hours

Maternal (may delay treatment until after 10-12 weeks gestation): Oral (per HIV/ATIS 2001 guidelines): 200 mg 3 times/day or 300 mg twice daily until start of labor

During labor and delivery, administer zidovudine I.V. at 2 mg/kg over 1 hour followed by a continuous I.V. infusion of 1 mg/kg/hour until the umbilical cord is clamped

Children 3 months to 12 years for HIV infection:

Oral: 160 mg/m^2/dose every 8 hours; dosage range: 90 mg/m^2/dose to 180 mg/m^2/dose every 6-8 hours; some Working Group members use a dose of 180 mg/m^2 every 12 hours when using in drug combinations with other antiretroviral compounds, but data on this dosing in children is limited

I.V. continuous infusion: 20 mg/m^2/hour

I.V. intermittent infusion: 120 mg/m^2/dose every 6 hours

Adults:

Oral: 300 mg twice daily or 200 mg 3 times/day

I.V.: 1-2 mg/kg/dose (infused over 1 hour) administered every 4 hours around-the-clock (6 doses/day)

Prevention of HIV following needlesticks: 200 mg 3 times/day plus lamivudine 150 mg twice daily; a protease inhibitor (eg, indinavir) may be added for high risk exposures; begin therapy within 2 hours of exposure if possible

Patients should receive I.V. therapy only until oral therapy can be administered

Dosing interval in renal impairment: Cl_{cr} <10 mL/minute: May require minor dose adjustment

Hemodialysis: At least partially removed by hemo- and peritoneal dialysis; administer dose after hemodialysis or administer 100 mg supplemental dose; during CAPD, dose as for Cl_{cr} <10 mL/minute

Continuous arteriovenous or venovenous hemodiafiltration effects: Administer 100 mg every 8 hours

Dosing adjustment in hepatic impairment: Reduce dose by 50% or double dosing interval in patients with cirrhosis

Dosing adjustment in hematologic toxicity: Significant anemia (hemoglobin <7.5 g/dL or >25% decrease from baseline) and/or significant neutropenia (<750 cells/mm^3 or >50% decrease from baseline) may require interruption of therapy until

(Continued)

Zidovudine *(Continued)*

bone marrow recovery is evident. Adjunctive measures (epoetin alfa) may be required when therapy is resumed. If pronounced anemia is experienced during concurrent treatment with drugs known to increase serum concentration of zidovudine (ie, fluconazole, valproate), reduction in zidovudine dose may be considered.

Mechanism of Action A thymidine analog which interferes with the HIV viral RNA dependent DNA polymerase resulting in inhibition of viral replication; nucleoside reverse transcriptase inhibitor

Other Adverse Effects

>10%:

Central nervous system: Severe headache (42%), fever (16%)

Dermatologic: Rash (17%)

Gastrointestinal: Nausea (46% to 61%), anorexia (11%), diarrhea (17%), pain (20%), vomiting (6% to 25%)

Hematologic: Anemia (23% in children), leukopenia, granulocytopenia (39% in children)

Neuromuscular & skeletal: Weakness (19%)

1% to 10%:

Central nervous system: Malaise (8%), dizziness (6%), insomnia (5%), somnolence (8%)

Dermatologic: Hyperpigmentation of nails (bluish-brown)

Gastrointestinal: Dyspepsia (5%)

Hematologic: Changes in platelet count

Neuromuscular & skeletal: Paresthesia (6%)

Drug Interactions CYP3A3/4 enzyme substrate

Increased Effect/Toxicity: Coadministration of zidovudine with drugs that are nephrotoxic (amphotericin B), cytotoxic (flucytosine, vincristine, vinblastine, doxorubicin, interferon), inhibit glucuronidation or excretion (acetaminophen, cimetidine, indomethacin, lorazepam, probenecid, aspirin), or interfere with RBC/WBC number or function (acyclovir, ganciclovir, pentamidine, dapsone). Clarithromycin may increase blood levels of zidovudine (although total body exposure was unaffected, peak plasma concentrations were increased). Valproic acid significantly increases zidovudine's blood levels (believed due to inhibition first pass metabolism).

Drug Uptake

Absorption: Oral: Well absorbed (66% to 70%)

Half-life, elimination: Terminal: 60 minutes

Time to peak: 30-90 minutes

Pregnancy Risk Factor C

Generic Available No

Zidovudine and Lamivudine (zye DOE vyoo deen & la MI vyoo deen)

Related Information

HIV Infection and AIDS *on page 1334*

U.S. Brand Names Combivir®

Canadian Brand Names Combivir®

Pharmacologic Category Antiretroviral Agent, Reverse Transcriptase Inhibitor (Nucleoside)

Synonyms AZT + 3TC; Lamivudine and Zidovudine

Use Management of patients with HIV infections in combination with at least one other antiretroviral agent

Local Anesthetic/Vasoconstrictor Precautions No information available to require special precautions

Effects on Dental Treatment No effects or complications reported

Dosage Children >12 years and Adults: Oral: 1 tablet twice daily

Mechanism of Action The combination of zidovudine and lamivudine are believed to act synergistically to inhibit reverse transcriptase via DNA chain termination after incorporation of the nucleoside analogue as well as to delay the emergence of mutations conferring resistance

Other Adverse Effects See Zidovudine *on page 1257* and Lamivudine *on page 683*

Drug Interactions Drug interactions are listed according to the individual components:

Lamivudine:

Ribavirin: Concomitant use of ribavirin and nucleoside analogues may increase the risk of developing lactic acidosis (includes adefovir, didanosine, lamivudine, stavudine, zalcitabine, zidovudine).

Sulfamethoxazole/trimethoprim: Increased AUC and decreased clearance of lamivudine with concomitant use

Zalcitabine: Intracellular phosphorylation of lamivudine and zalcitabine may be inhibited if used together; concomitant use should be avoided.

Zidovudine: Plasma levels of zidovudine are increased by ~39% with concomitant use.

Zidovudine: CYP3A3/4 enzyme substrate

Atovaquone: Atovaquone may decrease zidovudine clearance, increasing zidovudine AUC ~35%

Bone marrow suppressants/cytotoxic agents: Concomitant use may increase risk of hematologic toxicity. (May be seen with adriamycin, dapsone, flucytosine, vincristine, vinblastine.)

Doxorubicin: May decrease the antiviral activity of zidovudine (based on *in vitro* data). Avoid concurrent use.

Fluconazole: Fluconazole may decrease clearance and metabolism of zidovudine

Ganciclovir: Concomitant use may increase risk of hematologic toxicities; monitor hemoglobin, hematocrit, and white blood cell count with differential frequently; dose reduction or interruption of either agent may be needed

Interferon-alpha: Concomitant use may increase risk of hematologic toxicities; monitor hemoglobin, hematocrit, and white blood cell count with differential frequently; dose reduction or interruption of either agent may be needed

Phenytoin: Decreased plasma levels of phenytoin may be seen. Phenytoin may decrease clearance of zidovudine.

Probenecid: Probenecid may increase zidovudine levels. Myalgia, malaise, and/or fever and maculopapular rash have been reported with concomitant use.

Ribavirin: Concomitant use of ribavirin and nucleoside analogues may increase the risk of developing lactic acidosis (includes adefovir, didanosine, lamivudine, stavudine, zalcitabine, zidovudine). May decrease the antiviral activity of zidovudine (based on *in vitro* data); avoid concurrent use.

Stavudine: May decrease the antiviral activity of zidovudine (based on *in vitro* data). Avoid concurrent use.

Valproic acid: Valproic acid may increase plasma levels of zidovudine; monitor for possible increase in side effects (AUC increased by 80%).

Drug Uptake

Half-life, elimination: Zidovudine: 0.5-3 hours; Lamivudine: 5-7 hours

See Zidovudine *on page 1257* and Lamivudine *on page 683*

Pregnancy Risk Factor C

Generic Available No

Zilactin®-B [OTC] *see* Benzocaine *on page 151*

Zilactin® Baby [OTC] *see* Benzocaine *on page 151*

Zilactin-L® [OTC] *see* Lidocaine *on page 706*

Zileuton (zye LOO ton)

Related Information

Respiratory Diseases *on page 1328*

U.S. Brand Names Zyflo™

Pharmacologic Category 5-Lipoxygenase Inhibitor

Use Prophylaxis and chronic treatment of asthma in adults and children ≥12 years of age

Local Anesthetic/Vasoconstrictor Precautions No information available to require special precautions

Effects on Dental Treatment No effects or complications reported

Dosage Oral:

Children ≥12 years of age and Adults: 600 mg 4 times/day with meals and at bedtime

Elderly: Zileuton pharmacokinetics were similar in healthy elderly subjects (>65 years) compared with healthy younger adults (18-40 years)

Dosing adjustment in hepatic impairment: Contraindicated with active liver disease

Mechanism of Action Specific inhibitor of 5-lipoxygenase and thus inhibits leukotriene (LTB1, LTC1, LTD1 and LTE1) formation. Leukotrienes are substances that induce numerous biological effects including augmentation of neutrophil and eosinophil migration, neutrophil and monocyte aggregation, leukocyte adhesion, increased capillary permeability and smooth muscle contraction.

Other Adverse Effects

>10%:

Central nervous system: Headache (24.6%)

Hepatic: ALT elevation (12%)

1% to 10%:

Cardiovascular: Chest pain

Central nervous system: Pain, dizziness, fever, insomnia, malaise, nervousness, somnolence

Gastrointestinal: Dyspepsia, nausea, abdominal pain, constipation, flatulence

Hematologic: Low white blood cell count

Neuromuscular & skeletal: Myalgia, arthralgia, weakness

Ocular: Conjunctivitis

Warnings/Precautions Elevations of one or more LFTs may occur during therapy. These laboratory abnormalities may progress, remain unchanged or resolve with continued therapy. Use with caution in patients who consume substantial quantities of ethanol or have a past history of liver disease. Zileuton is not indicated for use in

(Continued)

Zileuton *(Continued)*

the reversal of bronchospasm in acute asthma attacks, including status asthmaticus. Zileuton can be continued during acute exacerbations of asthma.

Drug Interactions CYP1A2, 2C9, and 3A3/4 enzyme substrate; CYP1A2 and 3A3/4 enzyme inhibitor

Increased Effect/Toxicity: Zileuton increases concentrations/effects of of beta-blockers (propranolol), terfenadine, theophylline, and warfarin. Potentially, it may increase levels of many drugs, including cisapride, due to inhibition of CYP3A4.

Drug Uptake

Absorption: Oral: Rapid

Half-life, elimination: 2.5 hours

Time to peak: 1.7 hours

Pregnancy Risk Factor C

Generic Available No

Zinacef® *see* Cefuroxime *on page 246*

Zinca-Pak® *see* Trace Metals *on page 1186*

Zincate® Oral *see* Zinc Supplements *on page 1261*

Zinc Chloride (zingk KLOR ide)

Pharmacologic Category Trace Element

Use Cofactor for replacement therapy to different enzymes helps maintain normal growth rates, normal skin hydration and senses of taste and smell

Local Anesthetic/Vasoconstrictor Precautions No information available to require special precautions

Effects on Dental Treatment No effects or complications reported

Dosage Clinical response may not occur for up to 6-8 weeks

Supplemental to I.V. solutions:

- Premature Infants <1500 g, up to 3 kg: 300 mcg/kg/day
- Full-term Infants and Children ≤5 years: 100 mcg/kg/day
- Adults:
  - Stable with fluid loss from small bowel: 12.2 mg zinc/liter TPN or 17.1 mg zinc/kg (added to 1000 mL I.V. fluids) of stool or ileostomy output
  - Metabolically stable: 2.5-4 mg/day, add 2 mg/day for acute catabolic states

Pregnancy Risk Factor C

Generic Available Yes

Comments Clinical response may not occur for up to 6-8 weeks

Zincfrin® [OTC] *see* Phenylephrine and Zinc Sulfate *on page 951*

Zinc Gelatin (zingk JEL ah tin)

U.S. Brand Names Gelucast®

Pharmacologic Category Topical Skin Product

Synonyms Dome Paste Bandage; Unna's Boot; Unna's Paste; Zinc Gelatin Boot

Use Protectant and to support varicosities and similar lesions of the lower limbs

Local Anesthetic/Vasoconstrictor Precautions No information available to require special precautions

Effects on Dental Treatment No effects or complications reported

Dosage Apply externally as an occlusive boot

Other Adverse Effects 1% to 10%: Local: Irritation

Generic Available Yes

Zincon® [OTC] *see* Pyrithione Zinc *on page 1029*

Zinc Oxide (zingk OKS ide)

U.S. Brand Names Ammens® Medicated Deodorant [OTC]; Balmex® [OTC]; Boudreaux's® Butt Paste [OTC]; Critic-Aid Skin Care® [OTC]; Desitin® [OTC]; Desitin® Creamy [OTC]

Canadian Brand Names Zincofax®

Pharmacologic Category Topical Skin Product

Synonyms Base Ointment; Lassar's Zinc Paste

Use Protective coating for mild skin irritations and abrasions; soothing and protective ointment to promote healing of chapped skin, diaper rash

Local Anesthetic/Vasoconstrictor Precautions No information available to require special precautions

Effects on Dental Treatment No effects or complications reported

Dosage Children and Adults: Topical: Apply as required for affected areas several times daily

Mechanism of Action Mild astringent with weak antiseptic properties

Other Adverse Effects 1% to 10%:

Dermatologic: Skin sensitivity

Local: Irritation

Generic Available Yes

Zinc Oxide, Cod Liver Oil, and Talc

(zingk OKS ide, kod LIV er oyl, & talk)

U.S. Brand Names Desitin® [OTC]

Pharmacologic Category Topical Skin Product

Use Relief of diaper rash, superficial wounds and burns, and other minor skin irritations

Local Anesthetic/Vasoconstrictor Precautions No information available to require special precautions

Effects on Dental Treatment No effects or complications reported

Dosage Topical: Apply thin layer as needed

Other Adverse Effects 1% to 10%: Local: Skin sensitivity, irritation

Generic Available Yes

Zinc Supplements (zink)

U.S. Brand Names Orazinc® Oral [OTC]; Zincate® Oral

Pharmacologic Category Electrolyte Supplement; Mineral, Oral; Mineral, Parenteral; Trace Element

Synonyms Zinc Acetate; Zinc Sulfate

Use Cofactor for replacement therapy to different enzymes helps maintain normal growth rates, normal skin hydration and senses of taste and smell; zinc supplement (oral and parenteral); may improve wound healing in those who are deficient. May be useful to promote wound healing in patients with pressure sores.

Local Anesthetic/Vasoconstrictor Precautions No information available to require special precautions

Effects on Dental Treatment No effects or complications reported

Dosage Clinical response may not occur for up to 6-8 weeks

RDA: Oral:
- Birth to 6 months: 3 mg elemental zinc/day
- 6-12 months: 5 mg elemental zinc/day
- 1-10 years: 10 mg elemental zinc/day (44 mg zinc sulfate)
- ≥11 years: 15 mg elemental zinc/day (65 mg zinc sulfate)

Zinc deficiency: Zinc sulfate: Oral:
- Infants and Children: 0.5-1 mg elemental zinc/kg/day divided 1-3 times/day; somewhat larger quantities may be needed if there is impaired intestinal absorption or an excessive loss of zinc
- Adults: 110-220 mg zinc sulfate (25-50 mg elemental zinc)/dose 3 times/day

Zinc supplements:
- Parenteral: TPN: I.V. infusion (chloride or sulfate): Supplemental to I.V. solutions (clinical response may not occur for up to 6-8 weeks):
  - Premature Infants <1500 g, up to 3 kg: 300 mcg/kg/day
  - Full-term Infants and Children ≤5 years: 100 mcg/kg/day

  or
  - Premature Infants: 400 mcg/kg/day
  - Term <3 months: 250 mcg/kg/day
  - Term >3 months: 100 mcg/kg/day
  - Children: 50 mcg/kg/day
  - Adults:
    - Stable with fluid loss from small bowel: 12.2 mg zinc/liter TPN or 17.1 mg zinc/kg (added to 1000 mL I.V. fluids) of stool or ileostomy output
    - Metabolically stable: 2.5-4 mg/day, add 2 mg/day for acute catabolic states

Mechanism of Action Provides for normal growth and tissue repair, is a cofactor for >70 enzymes; ophthalmic astringent and weak antiseptic due to precipitation of protein and clearing mucus from outer surface of the eye

Zinecard® *see* Dexrazoxane *on page 368*
Zithromax® *see* Azithromycin *on page 137*
Zithromax® Z-PAK® *see* Azithromycin *on page 137*
ZNP® Bar [OTC] *see* Pyrithione Zinc *on page 1029*
Zocor® *see* Simvastatin *on page 1088*
Zofran® *see* Ondansetron *on page 887*
Zofran® ODT *see* Ondansetron *on page 887*
Zoladex® Implant *see* Goserelin *on page 565*

Zoledronic Acid (ZOE le dron ik AS id)

U.S. Brand Names Zometa®

Canadian Brand Names Zometa®

Mexican Brand Names Zometa®

Pharmacologic Category Bisphosphonate Derivative

Synonyms CGP-42446; Zoledronate

Use Treatment of hypercalcemia of malignancy, multiple myeloma, and bone metastases of solid tumors in conjunction with standard antineoplastic therapy

Local Anesthetic/Vasoconstrictor Precautions No information to require special precautions

Effects on Dental Treatment No effects or complications reported

(Continued)

Zoledronic Acid *(Continued)*

Dosage I.V.: Adults:

Hypercalcemia of malignancy (albumin-corrected serum calcium ≥12 mg/dL): 4 mg (maximum) given as a single dose infused over **no less than 15 minutes**; patients should be adequately hydrated prior to treatment (restoring urine output to ~2 L/day). Monitor serum calcium and wait at least 7 days before considering retreatment. Dosage adjustment may be needed in patients with decreased renal function following treatment.

Multiple myeloma or metastatic bone lesions from solid tumors: 4 mg given over 15 minutes every 3-4 weeks; duration of treatment ranges from 9-15 months

Note: Patients should receive a daily calcium supplement and multivitamin containing vitamin D

Dosage adjustment for toxicity:

Hypercalcemia of malignancy: Evidence of renal deterioration: Evaluate risk versus benefit.

Bone metastases: Evidence of renal deterioration: Discontinue further dosing until renal function returns to baseline: renal deterioration defined as follows:

Normal baseline creatinine: Increase of 0.5 mg/dL

Abnormal baseline creatinine: Increase of 1 mg/dL

Mechanism of Action A bisphosphonate which inhibits bone resorption via actions on osteoclasts or on osteoclast precursors; inhibits osteoclastic activity and skeletal calcium release induced by tumors.

Other Adverse Effects

>10%:

Cardiovascular: Leg edema (up to 19%)

Central nervous system: Fever (30% to 44%), headache (18%), insomnia (15%), anxiety (9% to 14%), dizziness (14%), agitation (13%)

Dermatologic: Alopecia (11%)

Endocrine & metabolic: Hypophosphatemia (13%), hypokalemia (12%), dehydration (up to 12%)

Gastrointestinal: Diarrhea (17% to 22%), abdominal pain (12% to 16%)

Genitourinary: Urinary tract infection (11% to 14%)

Hematologic: Anemia (22% to 29%), neutropenia (11%)

Neuromuscular & skeletal: Myalgia (21%), paresthesias (18%), arthralgia (18%) skeletal pain (12%)

Respiratory: Dyspnea (22%), coughing (12% to 19%)

1% to 10%:

Cardiovascular: Hypotension (10%), chest pain

Central nervous system: Hypoesthesia (10%)

Dermatologic: Dermatitis (10%)

Endocrine & metabolic: Hypomagnesemia (up to 10%), hypocalcemia, hypophosphatemia (9%), hypermagnesemia (Grade 3: 2%)

Gastrointestinal: Anorexia (9%), mucositis, dysphagia

Genitourinary: Urinary tract infection (14%)

Hematologic: Thrombocytopenia, pancytopenia

Neuromuscular & skeletal: Arthralgia, rigors (10%)

Renal: Serum creatinine increased

Respiratory: Pleural effusion , upper respiratory tract infection (8%)

Symptoms of hypercalcemia include polyuria, nephrolithiasis, anorexia, nausea, vomiting, constipation, weakness, fatigue, confusion, stupor, and coma. These may not be drug-related adverse events, but related to the underlying metabolic condition.

Drug Interactions Increased Effect/Toxicity: Aminoglycosides may also lower serum calcium levels; loop diuretics increase risk of hypocalcemia

Drug Uptake

Onset of action: Maximum effect may not been seen for 7 days

Half-life, elimination (triphasic): Terminal: 167 hours

Pregnancy Risk Factor D

Generic Available No

Zolmitriptan (zohl mi TRIP tan)

U.S. Brand Names Zomig®; Zomig-ZMT™

Canadian Brand Names Zomig®

Mexican Brand Names Zomig®

Pharmacologic Category Serotonin 5-HT_{1D} Receptor Agonist

Synonyms 311C90

Use Acute treatment of adult migraine, with or without auras

Local Anesthetic/Vasoconstrictor Precautions No information available to require special precautions

Effects on Dental Treatment No effects or complications reported

Dosage Oral:

Children: Safety and efficacy have not been established

Adults: Migraine:

Tablet: Initial: ≤2.5 mg at the onset of migraine headache; may break 2.5 mg tablet in half

Orally-disintegrating tablet: Initial: 2.5 mg at the onset of migraine headache

Use the lowest possible dose to minimize adverse events. If the headache returns, the dose may be repeated after 2 hours; do not exceed 10 mg within a 24-hour period. Controlled trials have not established the effectiveness of a second dose if the initial one was ineffective

Elderly: No dosage adjustment needed but elderly patients are more likely to have underlying cardiovascular disease and should have careful evaluation of cardiovascular system before prescribing.

Dosage adjustment in hepatic impairment: Administer with caution in patients with liver disease, generally using doses <2.5 mg. Patients with moderate-to-severe hepatic impairment may have decreased clearance of zolmitriptan, and significant elevation in BP was observed in some patients.

Mechanism of Action A selective 5-hydroxytryptamine (5-HT 1B/1D) receptor agonist. The drug binds tightly and specifically to this receptor. The current theory of migraine headaches suggests that symptoms are due to local cranial vasodilation or to the release of sensory neuropeptides through nerve endings in the trigeminal system. The activity of zolmitriptan can most likely be attributed to its agonist effects at the 5-HT 1B/1D receptors in intracranial blood vessels and sensory nerves, which results in cranial vessel constriction and the inhibition of proinflammatory neuropeptide release.

Other Adverse Effects

1% to 10%:

Cardiovascular: Chest pain (2% to 4%), palpitations (up to 2%)

Central nervous system: Dizziness (6% to 10%), somnolence (5% to 8%), pain (2% to 3%), vertigo (≤2%)

Gastrointestinal: Nausea (4% to 9%), xerostomia (3% to 5%), dyspepsia (1% to 3%), dysphagia (≤2%)

Neuromuscular & skeletal: Paresthesia (5% to 9%), weakness (3% to 9%), warm/cold sensation (5% to 7%), hypesthesia (1% to 2%), myalgia (1% to 2%), myasthenia (up to 2%)

Miscellaneous: Neck/throat/jaw pain (4% to 10%), diaphoresis (up to 3%), allergic reaction (up to 1%)

Events related to other serotonin 5-HT_{1D} receptor agonists: Cerebral hemorrhage, stroke, subarachnoid hemorrhage, peripheral vascular ischemia, colonic ischemia, ventricular fibrillation

Drug Interactions Increased Effect/Toxicity: Ergot-containing drugs may lead to vasospasm; cimetidine, MAO inhibitors, oral contraceptives, propranolol increase levels of zolmitriptan; concurrent use with SSRIs and sibutramine may lead to serotonin syndrome.

Drug Uptake

Onset of action: 0.5-1 hour

Absorption: Well absorbed

Half-life, elimination: 2.8-3.7 hours

Time to peak: Tablet: 1.5 hours; orally-disintegrating tablet: 3 hours

Pregnancy Risk Factor C

Generic Available No

Comments Not intended for the prophylactic therapy of migraine or for use in the management of hemiplegic or basilar migraine. The safety and effectiveness of zolmitriptan for the treatment of cluster headache, have not been confirmed.

Zoloft® *see* Sertraline *on page 1083*

Zolpidem (zole PI dem)

U.S. Brand Names Ambien®

Canadian Brand Names Ambien®

Pharmacologic Category Hypnotic, Nonbenzodiazepine

Synonyms Zolpidem Tartrate

Use Short-term treatment of insomnia

Local Anesthetic/Vasoconstrictor Precautions No information available to require special precautions

Effects on Dental Treatment No effects or complications reported

Restrictions C-IV

Dosage Duration of therapy should be limited to 7-10 days

Adults: Oral: 10 mg immediately before bedtime; maximum dose: 10 mg

Elderly: 5 mg immediately before bedtime

Mechanism of Action Structurally dissimilar to benzodiazepine, however, has much or all of its actions explained by its effects on benzodiazepine (BZD) receptors, especially the omega-1 receptor; retains hypnotic and much of the anxiolytic properties of the BZD, but has reduced effects on skeletal muscle and seizure threshold.

(Continued)

Zolpidem *(Continued)*

Other Adverse Effects

1% to 10%:

Cardiovascular: Palpitations

Central nervous system: Headache, drowsiness, dizziness, lethargy, lightheadedness, depression, abnormal dreams, amnesia

Dermatologic: Rash

Gastrointestinal: Nausea, diarrhea, xerostomia, constipation

Respiratory: Sinusitis, pharyngitis

Drug Interactions CYP3A3/4 enzyme substrate

Antipsychotics: Sedative effects may be additive with antipsychotics, including phenothiazines; monitor for increased effect

CNS depressants: Sedative effects may be additive with other CNS depressants; monitor for increased effect; includes barbiturates, benzodiazepines, narcotic analgesics, ethanol, and other sedative agents

CYP3A3/4 inhibitors: Serum level and/or toxicity of zolpidem may be increased; inhibitors include amiodarone, cimetidine, clarithromycin, erythromycin, delavirdine, diltiazem, dirithromycin, disulfiram, fluoxetine, fluvoxamine, grapefruit juice, indinavir, itraconazole, ketoconazole, metronidazole, nefazodone, nevirapine, propoxyphene, quinupristin-dalfopristin, ritonavir, saquinavir, verapamil, zafirlukast, zileuton; monitor for increased response

Enzyme inducers: May increase the metabolism of zolpidem, reducing its effectiveness; inducers include phenytoin, carbamazepine, phenobarbital, and rifampin

SSRIs: Sertraline and fluoxetine (to a lesser extent) have been demonstrated to increase zaleplon levels; pharmacodynamic effects were not significantly changed; monitor

Drug Uptake

Onset of action: 30 minutes

Absorption: Rapid

Duration: 6-8 hours

Half-life, elimination: 2-2.6 hours; Cirrhosis: ≤9.9 hours

Pregnancy Risk Factor B

Generic Available No

Zometa® *see* Zoledronic Acid *on page 1261*

Zomig® *see* Zolmitriptan *on page 1262*

Zomig-ZMT™ *see* Zolmitriptan *on page 1262*

Zonalon® Cream *see* Doxepin *on page 414*

Zone-A Forte® *see* Pramoxine and Hydrocortisone *on page 984*

Zonegran® *see* Zonisamide *on page 1264*

Zonisamide (zoe NIS a mide)

U.S. Brand Names Zonegran®

Canadian Brand Names Zonegran™

Pharmacologic Category Anticonvulsant, Miscellaneous

Use Adjunct treatment of partial seizures in adults with epilepsy

Local Anesthetic/Vasoconstrictor Precautions No information available to require special precautions

Effects on Dental Treatment Xerostomia and taste perversion have been reported in approximately 2 out of every 100 patients.

Dosage

Children >16 years and Adults: Oral: Adjunctive treatment of partial seizures: Initial dose: 100 mg/day; dose may be increased to 200 mg/day after two weeks. Further dosage increases to 300 mg and 400 mg/day can then be made with a minimum of 2 weeks between adjustments, in order to reach steady-state at each dosage level. Doses of up to 600 mg/day have been studied, however, there is no evidence of increased response with doses >400 mg/day.

Elderly: Data from clinical trials insufficient for patients >65 years of age; begin dosing at the low end of the dosing range

Mechanism of Action The exact mechanism of action is not known. May stabilize neuronal membranes and suppress neuronal hypersynchronization through action at sodium and calcium channels; does not affect GABA activity.

Other Adverse Effects Adjunctive Therapy: Frequencies noted in patients receiving other anticonvulsants:

>10%:

Central nervous system: Somnolence (17%), dizziness (13%)

Gastrointestinal: Anorexia (13%)

1% to 10%:

Central nervous system: Headache (10%), agitation/irritability (9%), fatigue (8%), tiredness (7%), ataxia (6%), confusion (6%), decreased concentration (6%), memory impairment (6%), depression (6%), insomnia (6%), speech disorders (5%), mental slowing (4%), anxiety (3%), nervousness (2%), schizophrenic/schizophreniform behavior (2%), difficulty in verbal expression (2%), status epilepticus (1%), tremor (1%), convulsion (1%), hyperesthesia (1%), incoordination (1%)

Dermatologic: Rash (3%), bruising (2%), pruritus (1%)

Gastrointestinal: Nausea (9%), abdominal pain (6%), diarrhea (5%), dyspepsia (3%), weight loss (3%), constipation (2%), xerostomia (2%), taste perversion (2%), vomiting (1%)

Neuromuscular & skeletal: Paresthesia (4%), weakness (1%), abnormal gait (1%)

Ocular: Diplopia (6%), nystagmus (4%), amblyopia (1%)

Otic: Tinnitus (1%)

Respiratory: Rhinitis (2%), pharyngitis (1%), increased cough (1%)

Miscellaneous: Flu-like syndrome (4%) accidental injury (1%)

Contraindications Hypersensitivity to sulfonamides, zonisamide, or any component of their formulation

Warnings/Precautions Rare, but potentially fatal sulfonamide reactions have occurred following the use of zonisamide. These reactions include Stevens-Johnson syndrome and toxic epidermal necrolysis, usually appearing within 2-16 weeks of drug initiation. Discontinue zonisamide if rash develops. Chemical similarities are present among sulfonamides, sulfonylureas, carbonic anhydrase inhibitors, thiazides, and loop diuretics (except ethacrynic acid). Use in patients with sulfonamide allergy is specifically contraindicated in product labeling, however a risk of cross-reaction exists in patients with allergy to any of these compounds; avoid use when previous reaction has been severe. Decreased sweating and hyperthermia requiring hospitalization have been reported in children. The safety and efficacy in children <16 years of age has not been established.

Discontinue zonisamide in patients who develop acute renal failure or a significant sustained increase in creatinine/BUN concentration. Kidney stones have been reported. Use cautiously in patients with renal or hepatic dysfunction. Do not use if estimated Cl_{cr} <50 mL/minute. Significant CNS effects include psychiatric symptoms, psychomotor slowing, and fatigue or somnolence. Fatigue and somnolence occur within the first month of treatment, most commonly at doses of 300-500 mg/day. Abrupt withdrawal may precipitate seizures; discontinue or reduce doses gradually.

Drug Interactions CYP3A3/4 enzyme substrate

Increased Effect/Toxicity: Sedative effects may be additive with other CNS depressants; monitor for increased effect; includes barbiturates, benzodiazepines, narcotic analgesics, and other sedative agents. Serum level and/or toxicity of zonisamide may be increased by CYP3A3/4 inhibitors; inhibitors include amiodarone, cimetidine, clarithromycin, erythromycin, delavirdine, diltiazem, dirithromycin, disulfiram, fluoxetine, fluvoxamine, indinavir, itraconazole, ketoconazole, metronidazole, nefazodone, nevirapine, propoxyphene, quinupristin-dalfopristin, ritonavir, saquinavir, verapamil, zafirlukast, zileuton; monitor for increased response. **Note:** Zonisamide did NOT affect steady state levels of carbamazepine, phenytoin, or valproate; zonisamide half-life is decreased by carbamazepine, phenytoin, phenobarbital, and valproate

Decreased Effect: Enzyme inducers may increase the metabolism of zonisamide, reducing its effectiveness (phenytoin, carbamazepine, phenobarbital, and rifampin).

Drug Uptake

Half-life, elimination: 63 hours

Time to peak: 2-6 hours

Pregnancy Risk Factor C

Generic Available No

Comments FDA-approved March, 2000; consult product labeling for full prescribing information.

Zopiclone *Not Available in U.S.* (ZOE pi clone)

Canadian Brand Names Alti-Zopiclone; Apo®-Zopiclone; Gen-Zopiclone; Imovane®; Nu-Zopiclone; Rhovane®

Pharmacologic Category Hypnotic, Nonbenzodiazepine

Use Symptomatic relief of transient and short-term insomnia

Local Anesthetic/Vasoconstrictor Precautions No information available to require special precautions

Effects on Dental Treatment No effects or complications reported

Dosage Oral (just before bedtime):

Adults: 5-7.5 mg

Patients with chronic respiratory insufficiency: 3.75 mg; may increase up to 7.5 mg with caution in appropriate cases

Elderly: Initial: 3.75 mg; may increase to 5-7.5 mg

Dosage adjustment in hepatic impairment: 3.75 mg; may increase up to 7.5 mg with caution in appropriate cases

Mechanism of Action A cyclopyrrolone derivative and has a pharmacological profile similar to benzodiazepines; reduces sleep latency, increases duration of sleep, and decreases the number of nocturnal awakenings

(Continued)

Zopiclone *Not Available in U.S.* *(Continued)*

Other Adverse Effects Frequency not defined:

Cardiovascular: Palpitations

Central nervous system: Drowsiness, somnolence, dizziness, confusion, anterograde amnesia, chills, memory impairment, euphoria, nightmares, agitation, anxiety, nervousness, hostility, depression, asthenia, speech abnormalities, headache

Dermatological: Rash, spots on skin

Endocrine & metabolic: Anorexia; libido decreased; alkaline phosphatase, ALT, and AST increased; appetite increased

Gastrointestinal: Constipation, coated tongue, diarrhea, xerostomia, dyspepsia, halitosis, nausea, taste alteration (bitter taste, common), vomiting

Neuromuscular & skeletal: Hypotonia, impaired coordination, limb heaviness, muscle spasms, paresthesia, tremors

Ocular: Amblyopia

Respiratory: Dyspnea

Miscellaneous: Diaphoresis

Drug Interactions Metabolism may involve CYP isoenzymes; profile not defined

Increased Effect/Toxicity: May produce additive CNS depressant effects with sedatives, antihistamines, anticonvulsants, or psychotropic medications. Zopiclone activity may be enhanced by compounds that inhibit cytochrome P450 (specific isoenzymes not defined).

Drug Uptake

Absorption: Elderly: 75% to 94%

Half-life, elimination: 5 hours; Elderly: 7 hours; Hepatic insufficiency: 11.9 hours

Time to peak: <2 hours; Hepatic insufficiency: 3.5 hours

Pregnancy Risk Factor Not assigned; similar agents rated D

Generic Available Yes

ZORprin® *see* Aspirin *on page 119*

Zostrix® [OTC] *see* Capsaicin *on page 212*

Zostrix®-HP [OTC] *see* Capsaicin *on page 212*

Zosyn® *see* Piperacillin and Tazobactam Sodium *on page 963*

Zovia™ *see* Combination Hormonal Contraceptives *on page 323*

Zovirax® *see* Acyclovir *on page 40*

Zyban® *see* BuPROPion *on page 188*

Zydone® *see* Hydrocodone and Acetaminophen *on page 598*

Zyflo™ *see* Zileuton *on page 1259*

Zyloprim® *see* Allopurinol *on page 53*

Zymase® [DSC] *see* Pancrelipase *on page 914*

Zyprexa® *see* Olanzapine *on page 884*

Zyprexa® Zydis® *see* Olanzapine *on page 884*

Zyrtec® *see* Cetirizine *on page 254*

Zyrtec-D 12 Hour™ *see* Cetirizine and Pseudoephedrine *on page 255*

Zyvox™ *see* Linezolid *on page 714*

NATURAL PRODUCTS: HERBAL AND DIETARY SUPPLEMENTS

Medical problem: " I have a toothache."
2000 BC response: "Here, eat this root."
1000 AD: "That root is heathen; here, say this prayer."
1850 AD: "That prayer is superstitious; here, drink this potion."
1940 AD: "That potion is snake oil; here, swallow this pill."
1985 AD: "That pill is ineffective; here, take this new antibiotic."
2000 AD: "That antibiotic is artificial; here, eat this root."

Adapted from an anonymous Internet communication.

INTRODUCTION

For centuries, Eastern and Western civilizations have attributed a large number of medical uses to plants and herbs. Over time, modern scientific methodologies have emerged from some of these remedies. Conversely, some of these agents have fallen into less popularity as more medical knowledge has evolved. In spite of this dichotomy, herbal and natural therapies for treatment of common medical ailments have become exceedingly popular. In America, people consistently seek out natural products that may be able to offset some perceived ailment or assist in the prevention of an ailment. One area of particular interest to those individuals using herbal or natural remedies has commonly been weight loss. There are numerous systemic considerations when some of the natural products that have been attributed weight loss powers are utilized. Many of these products are sold under the blanket of dietary supplements and, therefore, have avoided some of the more stringent Food and Drug Administration legislation. However, in 1994, that legislation was modified to include herbs, vitamins, minerals, and amino acids that may be taken as dietary supplements and the federal guidelines were further modified in 1999. This information must be made available to patients taking these types of products.

The real concern lies in the fact that health claims need not be approved by the FDA, but advertisements must include a disclaimer saying that the product has not yet been fully evaluated. Claims of medicinal use/value are often drawn from popular use, not necessarily from scientific studies. Safety is a concern when these agents are taken in combination with other prescription drugs due to the medical risk which might result. Many of these natural products may have real medicinal value but caution on the part of the dental clinician is prudent. It is impossible to cover all of the natural products, therefore, this chapter has been limited to some of the most popular dietary and herbal supplements and natural remedies used by patients you might treat and what we know about the effects of some of these agents on the body's various systems. An extensive reading list is provided for further research.

POPULAR NATURAL PRODUCTS

This section contains general information on commonly encountered herbal or nutritional products. For each of the natural products described in this section, potential/suspected drug interactions have been compiled from:

- anecdotal reports,
- scientific studies (when available), and
- any known similarities of pharmacologic effects with prescription and OTC drugs.

Most drug interactions between prescription and OTC medications and natural products have not been subject to exhaustive investigation. Readers are encouraged to consult current and comprehensive references, as well as the evolving medical literature on these interactions, for additional data.

(Continued)

ALPHABETICAL LISTING OF NATURAL PRODUCTS

Aloe

Synonyms Aloe vera; Cape

Use Analgesic, anti-inflammatory, emollient/moisturizer, laxative, wound-healing agent; treatment of minor burns, cuts, and skin irritations, including irritant and roentgen dermatitis; promotes healthy GI system and normal muscle/joint function; oral rinse good for gums and soft tissue; historically used orally in India as a laxative and to treat intestinal infections and amenorrhea; root used for colic; gel is used in many cosmetic and pharmaceutical formulations

Effects on Bleeding None reported

Local Anesthetic/Vasoconstrictor Precautions No information available to require special precautions

Dosage

Oral: Drink 4-8 oz/day 100% aloe vera juice plain or mixed with juice; may be used as a rinse to gargle with and swallow

Topical: Apply gel 3-4 times/day to affected area

Mechanism of Action/Effect Has therapeutic value in a wide variety of soft tissue injuries; penetrates injured tissues and dilates capillaries, thereby increasing blood flow to the injury; prevents progressive dermal ischemia following burns, frostbite, and electrical injuries; has antithromboxane activity, yet maintains prostaglandin ratio without causing injured blood vessels to collapse; contains barbaloin (a glycoside of anthraquinone origin), bradykinase (a protease inhibitor), emodin, tannins, and volatile oils

Adverse Reactions Frequency not defined:

Central nervous system: Catharsis

Dermatologic: Contact dermatitis (allergic)

Endocrine & metabolic: Hypokalemia

Gastrointestinal: Abdominal cramps, diarrhea

Renal: Albuminuria, hematuria (may cause red discoloration of urine), proteinuria

Warnings Use with caution in diabetics and those taking hypoglycemic agents or insulin; may lower blood sugar. Some juice products may have high sodium content. Some wound healing may be delayed when administered topically. May alter GI absorption of other herbs or drugs. Avoid other herbs with hypoglycemic or laxative properties (see below).

Potential/Suspected Interactions Increased Effect/Toxicity:

Herbs with hypoglycemic properties: Alfalfa, bilberry, bitter melon, burdock, celery, damiana, fenugreek, garcinia, garlic, ginger, ginseng (American), gymnema, marshmallow, stinging nettle

Herbs with laxative properties: Cascara, eyebright, plantain, psyllium, rhubarb, senna, yellow dock

Alpha-Lipoic Acid

Synonyms Alpha-lipoate; Lipoic Acid; Thioctic acid

Use Antioxidant; treatment of diabetes, diabetic neuropathy, glaucoma; prevention of cataracts and neurologic disorders including stroke

Effects on Bleeding None reported

Local Anesthetic/Vasoconstrictor Precautions No information available to require special precautions

Dosage Oral: Range: 20-600 mg/day; Common dosage: 25-50 mg twice daily

Stage II open angle glaucoma: 150 mg/day (studies showed significant improvement after 2 months)

Mechanism of Action/Effect Sulfur-containing cofactor for pyruvate dehydrogenase (PDH) and alpha-ketoglutarate dehydrogenase; one of the most potent antioxidants and is metabolized to dihydrolipoic acid (DHLA), which also has antioxidant properties. It is fat- and water-soluble and may improve recycling of other antioxidants (eg, coenzyme Q10, glutathione, vitamins C and E). This antioxidant activity may limit development of diabetic complications by increasing muscle cell glucose uptake and insulin sensitivity in (type 2 diabetics), increasing neuronal blood flow and distal nerve conduction, improving glucose utilization and regeneration of glutathione, and reducing oxidative stress. In HIV-infected individuals, it is useful in blocking activation of NF-kappa B (required for HIV virus transcription) and improving T-helper lymphocytes and T-helper/suppressor cell ratio.

Adverse Reactions Frequency not defined: Dermatologic: Rash

Warnings Use with caution in individuals predisposed to hypoglycemia including those receiving antidiabetic agents.

Potential/Suspected Interactions Increased Effect/Toxicity:

Insulin and oral hypoglycemics

Herbs with hypoglycemic properties: Alfalfa, aloe, bilberry, bitter melon, burdock, celery, damiana, fenugreek, garcinia, garlic, ginger, ginseng (American), gymnema, marshmallow, stinging nettle

Herbs with estrogenic activity: Black cohosh, dong quai, evening primrose

Androstenedione

Synonyms Andro

Use Androgenic, anabolic; Athletic performance and libido enhancement; believed to facilitate faster recovery from exercise, increase strength, and promote muscle development in response to training (studies inconclusive)

Effects on Bleeding None reported

Local Anesthetic/Vasoconstrictor Precautions No information available to require special precautions

Dosage Adults: Oral: 50-100 mg/day (usually about 1 hour before exercising)

Mechanism of Action/Effect A weak androgenic steroid hormone produced through natural gonadal and adrenal synthesis; precursor to testosterone and estrone (elevates serum testosterone from 15% to 300%) with androgenic and anabolic properties

Adverse Reactions Frequency not defined:

Cardiovascular: Hypertension

Central nervous system: Aggressive behavior, cerebrovascular accident, depression, euphoria, psychosis

Dermatologic: Acne, edema, exacerbation of psoriasis, hirsutism (increase in pubic hair growth), hypertrichosis, pruritus

Endocrine & metabolic: Amenorrhea, breast enlargement, breast soreness, clitoral enlargement, gynecomastia, hirsutism, hypercalcemia, hypoprolactinemia, increased libido, infertility (males), virilism

Gastrointestinal: GI irritation, nausea, vomiting

Genitourinary: Azoospermia, benign prostatic hyperplasia (BPA), bladder irritability, clitoral enlargement, epididymitis, impotence, testicular atrophy, oligospermia, priapism, prostatic carcinoma

Hematologic: Leukopenia or neutropenia (agranulocytosis, granulocytopenia), polycythemia

Hepatic: Aminotransferase level elevation (asymptomatic), cholestatic hepatitis, cholestatic jaundice, hepatic dysfunction, hepatic necrosis (especially with water-based oral preparations), hepatocellular carcinoma, jaundice

Neuromuscular & skeletal: Piloerection

Miscellaneous: Hypersensitivity reactions

Contraindications Hypertension

Warnings Use with caution in individuals with CHF, prostate conditions, or hormone-sensitive tumors. The FDA requires specific labeling noting that it "contains steroid hormones that may cause breast enlargement, testicular shrinkage, and infertility in males, and increased facial/body hair, voice-deepening, and clitoral enlargement in females." Avoid herbs with hypertensive properties (see below).

Potential/Suspected Interactions

Increased Effect/Toxicity:

Androgenic drugs and estrogens

Herbs with hypertensive properties: Bayberry, blue cohosh, cayenne, ephedra, ginger, ginseng , kola nut (caffeine), licorice

Decreased Effect: Requires cobalt, calcium, and zinc for conversion to testosterone; maintain selenium required for excretion of excess

Astragalus

Synonyms *Astragalus membranaceus*; Milk Vetch

Use Adaptogen, antibacterial, diuretic, immunostimulant/immunosupportive, radioprotective, vasodilator; treatment of cancer (adjunct to chemotherapy/radiation), hepatitis, peripheral vascular diseases, respiratory infections; disease resistance, stamina, tissue oxygenation; promotes adrenal cortical function

Unlabeled/Investigational: Treatment of HIV/AIDS; antiaging

Effects on Bleeding None reported

Local Anesthetic/Vasoconstrictor Precautions No information available to require special precautions

Dosage Oral:

Children: 1/3 of adult dose

Adults: 20-500 mg 4 times/day (standardized to 0.5% glycosides and 70% polysaccharides per dose); Typical dose: 400 mg twice daily; Acute symptoms: 500 mg every 3 hours

Tea: 9-30 g dried root steeped in boiling water for 15 minutes; drink 3 cups/day

Tincture: 30 drops 3 times/day

Mechanism of Action/Effect Contains bioflavonoids, choline, isoflavones, polysaccharides (including astragalan B) saponins, and triterpenoids (including astragalosides I-VIII); astragalan B binds to cholesterol on outer membranes of viruses, allowing the immune system to attack by destabilizing and weakening the invader. Animal studies have shown that astragalan B controls bacterial infections and protects against many toxins. Saponins and triterpenoids have structural similarity to steroid hormone precursors and appear to increase adrenal activity. Polysaccharides stimulate natural killer (NK) cells, augment T-cell function, and increase interferon production; administration has been shown to increase phagocytosis by (Continued)

Astragalus *(Continued)*

reticuloendothelial cells, decrease T-suppressor cell function, and improve T-killer cell function; may decrease cyclophosphamide-induced immune suppression; stabilizes heart rhythms

Warnings Use with caution in individuals with acute infection, especially when fever is present.

Potential/Suspected Interactions

Increased Effect/Toxicity: May enhance effects of immune stimulants

Decreased Effect: May limit effects of immunosuppressants

Bifidobacterium bifidum / Lactobacillus acidophilus

Use Antidiarrheal, digestive aid; treatment of GI complaints. See also Lactobacillus acidophilus and Lactobacillus bulgaricus *on page 682*

B. bifidum: Maintenance of anaerobic microflora in the colon; treatment of Crohn's disease, diarrhea, ulcerative colitis

L. acidophilus: Recolonization of the GI tract with beneficial bacteria during and after antibiotic use; treatment of constipation, infant diarrhea, lactose intolerance

Effects on Bleeding None reported

Local Anesthetic/Vasoconstrictor Precautions No information available to require special precautions

Dosage Oral: 5-10 billion colony forming units (CFU)/day [dairy free] (refrigerate to maintain optimum potency)

Mechanism of Action/Effect Natural components of colonic flora used to facilitate recolonization with benign symbiotic organisms; promotes vitamin K synthesis and absorption

Adverse Reactions No known toxicity or serious side effect

Potential/Suspected Interactions Antibiotics eliminate *B. bifidum* and *L. acidophilus*

Bilberry

Synonyms *Vaccinium myrtillus*

Use Anticoagulant, antioxidant; treatment of ophthalmic disorders (cataracts, diabetic retinopathy, day/night blindness, diminished visual acuity, macular degeneration, myopia) and vascular disorders (phlebitis, varicose veins); helps maintain capillary integrity and reduce hyperpermeability

Effects on Bleeding May see increased bleeding due to inhibition of platelet aggregation

Local Anesthetic/Vasoconstrictor Precautions No information available to require special precautions

Dosage Oral: 80 mg 2-3 times/day

Mechanism of Action/Effect Inhibits a variety of inflammatory mediators, including histamine, proteases, leukotrienes, and prostaglandins; may decrease capillary permeability and inhibit platelet aggregation

Contraindications Active bleeding (eg, intracranial bleeding, peptic ulcer)

Warnings Use with caution in diabetics (may lower blood sugar), individuals with a history of bleeding, hemostatic or drug-related hemostatic disorders, those taking anticoagulants (eg, aspirin or aspirin-containing products, NSAIDs, and warfarin) or antiplatelet agents (eg, ticlopidine, clopidogrel, and dipyridamole), hypoglycemic agents or insulin. Avoid other herbs with anticoagulant/antiplatelet and/or hypoglycemic properties (see below). May alter absorption of calcium, copper, magnesium, and zinc due to tannins. Discontinue at least 14 days prior to dental or surgical procedures.

Potential/Suspected Interactions Increased Effect/Toxicity:

Anticoagulant or antiplatelet agents and insulin or oral hypoglycemics

Herbs with anticoagulant/antiplatelet properties: Alfalfa, anise, bladderwrack, bromelain, cat's claw, celery, coleus, cordyceps, dong quai, evening primrose, fenugreek, feverfew, garliç, ginger, ginkgo biloba, ginseng (American/Panax/Siberian), grape seed, green tea, guggul, horse chestnut seed, horseradish, licorice, prickly ash, red clover, reishi, sweet clover, turmeric, white willow

Herbs with hypoglycemic properties: Alfalfa, aloe, bitter melon, burdock, celery, damiana, fenugreek, garcinia, garlic, ginger, ginseng (American), gymnema, marshmallow, stinging nettle

Black Cohosh

Synonyms *Cimicifuga racemosa*

Use Analgesic, anti-inflammatory, phytoestrogenic; treatment of rheumatoid arthritis, mild depression, vasomotor symptoms of menopause and premenstrual syndrome (PMS)

Effects on Bleeding None reported

Local Anesthetic/Vasoconstrictor Precautions No information available to require special precautions

Dosage Oral: 20-40 mg twice daily (standardized to contain 1 mg triterpenes per dose)

Mechanism of Action/Effect Active components are cimicifugosides (reported to affect hypothalamus/pituitary function) and isoflavones (eg, formononetin); also contains triterpene glycosides (eg, acetin and 27-deoxyactein), aromatic and fatty acids, starches, sugars, resins, small amounts of salicylic acid, and tannins; phytoestrogenic compounds mimic the body's natural estrogen but have not been associated with the adverse effects of synthetic estrogen. Further clinical trials are needed to determine whether black cohosh has significant estrogenic actions in the body.

Adverse Reactions Frequency not defined (high doses):

Cardiovascular: Hypotension

Central nervous system: Headache

Gastrointestinal: Nausea, vomiting

Contraindications History of endometrial cancer or estrogen-dependent tumors, lactation, pregnancy (may stimulate uterine contractions)

Warnings Use with caution in individuals taking hormonal contraceptives or receiving hormone replacement therapy (HRT), those with endometrial cancer, history of estrogen-dependent tumors, hypotension, thromboembolic disease, stroke, or salicylate allergy (unknown whether amount of salicylic acid may affect platelet aggregation or have other effects associated with salicylates). Monitor serum hormone levels after 6 months of therapy. Avoid other hypotensive or phytoestrogenic herbs (see below).

Potential/Suspected Interactions Increased Effect:

Antihypertensive agents, hormonal contraceptives, hormone replacement therapy (HRT), sedatives

Herbs with hypotensive properties: Aconite, arnica, baneberry, bryony, California poppy, choke cherry, coleus, golden seal, green (false) hellebore, hawthorn, immortal, Indian tobacco, jaborandi, mistletoe, night blooming cereus, pasque flower, pleurisy root, quinine, shepherd's purse

Phytoestrogenic herbs: Alfalfa, blood root, hops, kudzu, licorice, pomegranate, red clover, soybean, thyme, yucca

Bromelain

Synonyms *Anas comosus*

Use Anticoagulant, anti-inflammatory, digestive aid; treatment of arthritis, dyspepsia, sinusitis

Effects on Bleeding May cause increased bleeding due to inhibition of platelet aggregation

Local Anesthetic/Vasoconstrictor Precautions No information available to require special precautions

Dosage Oral:

Digestive enzyme: 500 mg 3 times/day with meals

Inflammation: 1000 mg twice daily either 1 hour before or 2 hours after meals

Mechanism of Action/Effect Inhibits the enzyme, thromboxane synthetase, which converts prostaglandin H_2 into proinflammatory prostaglandins and thromboxanes; early reports found ingesting bromelain to be beneficial in inflammatory conditions (arthritis) but research using enteric-coated bromelain at low dosages reported no benefit (studies inconclusive)

Contraindications Active bleeding (eg, peptic ulcer, intracranial bleeding)

Warnings Use with caution in individuals with cardiovascular disease (eg, CHF, hypertension), GI ulceration, history of bleeding, hemostatic or drug-related hemostatic disorders, those taking anticoagulants (eg, aspirin or aspirin-containing products, NSAIDs, warfarin), or antiplatelet agents (eg, ticlopidine, clopidogrel, dipyridamole). Avoid other herbs with anticoagulant/antiplatelet properties (see below). Discontinue at least 14 days prior to dental or surgical procedures.

Potential/Suspected Interactions Increased Effect/Toxicity:

Anticoagulant or antiplatelet agents

Herbs with anticoagulant/antiplatelet properties: Alfalfa, anise, bilberry, bladderwrack, cat's claw, celery, coleus, cordyceps, dong quai, evening primrose, fenugreek, feverfew, garlic, ginger, ginkgo biloba, ginseng (American/Panax/Siberian), grape seed, green tea, guggul, horse chestnut seed, horseradish, licorice, prickly ash, red clover, reishi, sweet clover, turmeric, white willow

Calendula

Synonyms *Calendula officinalis*

Use Analgesic, anti-inflammatory, antimicrobial (antibacterial, antifungal, antiviral), antiprotozoal, antiseptic, antispasmodic, immunostimulant, wound-healing agent; treatment of minor burns, cuts, and other skin irritation

Effects on Bleeding None reported

Local Anesthetic/Vasoconstrictor Precautions No information available to require special precautions

Dosage Topical: Apply to affected area as needed

Mechanism of Action/Effect Stimulates phagocytosis and increases granulation

Warnings Use with caution in individuals with plant allergies.

Carnitine

Synonyms L-Carnitine

Use Treatment of CHF, hyperlipidemia, male infertility; athletic performance enhancement, weight loss

Effects on Bleeding None reported

Local Anesthetic/Vasoconstrictor Precautions No information available to require special precautions

Dosage Oral: ODA: 500-2000 mg/day in divided doses

Mechanism of Action/Effect Normally synthesized in humans from two amino acids, methionine and lysine, physiologically, participates in the transport of long-chain fatty acids across mitochondrial membranes to allow energy production; assists in the oxidation of branched-chain amino acids (a substrate for muscle during stress) and ketones when necessary; may lower serum cholesterol and triglycerides; claimed to improve efficiency of energy production in muscle tissue, including the myocardium. Improved energy generation has been proposed to improve cardiac performance and increase energy and endurance.

Potential/Suspected Interactions Decreased Effect: Depleted by valproic acid and zidovudine

Cat's Claw

Synonyms *Uncaria tomentosa*

Use Anticoagulant, anti-inflammatory, antimicrobial (antibacterial, antifungal, antiviral), antiplatelet, antioxidant, immunosupportive; treatment of allergies and minor infections or inflammatory conditions

Effects on Bleeding May cause increased bleeding due to inhibition of platelet aggregation

Local Anesthetic/Vasoconstrictor Precautions No information available to require special precautions

Dosage 250-1000 mg 3 times/day (standardized to contain ≥3% pentacyclic oxindole alkaloids and ≤0.06% tetracyclic oxindole alkaloids per dose)

Mechanism of Action/Effect Unclear due to the number of potentially active components; immunomodulatory and anti-inflammatory activity may be derived from multiple components. Several glycosides are reported to stimulate phagocytosis. Isopteridine is claimed to have immunostimulatory properties. Triterpenoid alkaloids and quinovic acid glycosides may inhibit replication of some DNA viruses. In animal studies, sterols have demonstrated anti-inflammatory activity, while glycosidic components may reduce inflammation and edema. Rhynchophylline may inhibit platelet aggregation and thrombus formation. Proanthocyanidins (PCOs) appear to be potent antioxidants, improve capillary fragility, and inhibit platelet-activating factor (PAF).

Contraindications Active bleeding (eg, intracranial bleeding, peptic ulcer), pregnancy

Warnings Use with caution in individuals taking anticoagulants (eg, aspirin or aspirin-containing products, NSAIDs, warfarin) or antiplatelet agents (eg, clopidogrel, dipyridamole, ticlopidine), therapeutic immunosuppression or I.V. immunoglobulin therapy (eg, transplant recipients), those with a history of bleeding, and hemostatic or drug-related hemostatic disorders. Avoid other herbs with anticoagulant/antiplatelet properties (see below). Discontinue at least 14 days prior to dental or surgical procedures.

Potential/Suspected Interactions Increased Effect:

Anticoagulant or antiplatelet agents, immunosuppressant therapy, and IV immunoglobulin therapy

Herbs with anticoagulant/antiplatelet properties: Alfalfa, anise, bilberry, bladderwrack, bromelain, celery, coleus, cordyceps, dong quai, evening primrose, fenugreek, feverfew, garlic, ginger, ginkgo biloba, ginseng (American/Panax/Siberian), grape seed, green tea, guggul, horse chestnut seed, horseradish, licorice, prickly ash, red clover, reishi, sweet clover, turmeric, white willow

Cayenne

Synonyms *Capsicum annuum*; *Capsicum frutescens*

Use Analgesic, anti-inflammatory, digestive stimulant, sympathomimetic; treatment of arthritis (osteo and rheumatoid), diabetic neuropathy, postmastectomy pain syndrome, postherpetic neuralgia, pruritus, psoriasis; appetite suppressant, bronchial relaxation, cardiovascular circulatory support, decongestant

Effects on Bleeding None reported

Local Anesthetic/Vasoconstrictor Precautions No information available to require special precautions

Dosage

Oral: 400 mg 3 times/day (standardized to contain ≥0.25% capsaicin per dose)

Topical: Apply as directed by manufacturer's labeling

Mechanism of Action/Effect Contains a resinous and pungent substance known as capsaicin which increases mucosal blood flow and/or vascular permeability and may inhibit gastric motility and activate duodenal motility. Capsaicin selectively activates certain populations of unmyelinated primary afferent sensory neurons (type "C"); many positive cardiovascular effects are due to its excitation of a distinct population of these neurons in the vagus nerve. Gastric and duodenal mucosa are believed to contain capsaicin-sensitive areas that, when stimulated by capsaicin, protect against acid and drug-induced ulcers.

Adverse Reactions Frequency not defined:

Cardiovascular: Hypertension, increased heart rate, vasoconstriction

Central nervous system: Insomnia

High doses:

Central nervous system: Dizziness, headache, hyperactivity, irritability, tremor

Gastrointestinal: Anorexia, xerostomia

Contraindications Anticoagulant or antiplatelet agents, cardiovascular disease (eg, arrhythmias, hypertension), diabetes, hyperthyroidism, pregnancy, psychiatric disorders

Warnings Use with caution in individuals with GI ulceration, hypertension, and those taking MAO inhibitors. May alter GI absorption of other herbs or drugs; avoid other herbs with hypertensive or sympathomimetic properties (see below).

Potential/Suspected Interactions Increased Effect/Toxicity:

Anticoagulant or antiplatelet agents, and MAO inhibitors (due to increased catecholamine secretion), stimulants (eg, OTC decongestants);

Herbs with anticoagulant/antiplatelet properties: Alfalfa, anise, bilberry, bladderwrack, bromelain, cat's claw, celery, coleus, cordyceps, dong quai, evening primrose, fenugreek, feverfew, garlic, ginger, ginkgo biloba, ginseng (American/Panax/Siberian), grape seed, green tea, guggul, horse chestnut seed, horseradish, licorice, prickly ash, red clover, reishi, sweet clover, turmeric, white willow

Herbs with hypertensive properties: Bayberry, blue cohosh, ephedra, ginger, ginseng (American), kola nut (caffeine), licorice

Herbs with sympathomimetic properties: Calamus, ephedra, Fu-tse (Fo-tzu), kola nut (caffeine), guarana, night blooming cereus, peyote (mescal buttons), scotch broom tops, Syrian rue, yellow jasmine, yohimbe

Decreased Effect: Antihypertensives and salicylates

Chamomile

Synonyms *Matricaria chamomilla*; *Matricaria recutita*

Use Antibacterial, anti-inflammatory, antispasmodic, antiulcer agent, anxiolytic, appetite stimulant, carminative, digestive aid, sedative (mild); treatment of eczema and psoriasis, hemorrhoids, inflammatory skin conditions, indigestion and irritable bowel syndrome (IBS), insomnia, leg ulcers, mastitis, premenstrual syndrome (PMS)

Effects on Bleeding None reported

Local Anesthetic/Vasoconstrictor Precautions No information available to require special precautions

Dosage Oral: 400-1600 mg/day in divided doses (standardized to contain 1% apigenin and 0.5% essential oil per dose)

Liquid extract: 1-4 mL 3 times/day

Rinse: Gargle with liquid extract 2-3 times/day as needed

Tea: ±3 g dried flowers steeped in ±150 mL boiling water for 5-10 minutes; drink 3-4 times/day

Topical: Apply to affected area as needed

Mechanism of Action/Effect Contains many active compounds; principle components are the volatile oil, alpha bisabolol which is responsible for the antispasmotic and anti-inflammatory effect, and the flavonoid, apifenin, which provides the anti-anxiety effect; topical ointments containing alpha bisabolol have been reported to be more effective than hydrocortisone in the treatment of inflammatory skin conditions

Adverse Reactions Frequency not defined:

Dermatologic: Contact dermatitis (rare)

Gastrointestinal: Emesis (dried flower buds), GI upset (high doses)

Respiratory: Nasal congestion, sneezing

Miscellaneous: Anaphylaxis, hypersensitivity (atopic individuals)

Contraindications Hypersensitivity to pollen from asters, chrysanthemums, daisies, feverfew, ragweed, or sunflowers; lactation and pregnancy

Warnings Use with caution in individuals with allergies and asthma (cross sensitivity may occur in those with allergies to asters, chrysanthemums, daisies, feverfew, sunflowers, or ragweed), and those taking anticoagulants, antiplatelets, and sedatives. Avoid other herbs with allergenic, anticoagulant, or antiplatelet properties (see below).

Potential/Suspected Interactions Increased Effect:

Anticoagulant/antiplatelet agents (coumarin-type anticoagulants with high doses), anxiolytics, barbiturates, benzodiazepines, CNS depressants, sedatives

Allergenic herbs: Bittersweet, devil's dung, echinacea, feverfew, flaxseed, garlic, ginseng, gotu kola, male fern, propolis, yucca

Herbs with anticoagulant/antiplatelet properties: Alfalfa, anise, bilberry, bladderwrack, bromelain, cat's claw, celery, coleus, cordyceps, dong quai, evening primrose, fenugreek, feverfew, garlic, ginger, ginkgo biloba, ginseng (American/

(Continued)

Chamomile *(Continued)*

Panax/Siberian), grape seed, green tea, guggul, horse chestnut seed, horseradish, licorice, prickly ash, red clover, reishi, sweet clover, turmeric, white willow

Chasteberry

Synonyms Chastetree; *Vitex agnus-castus*

Use Treatment of acne vulgaris, amenorrhea, corpus luteum insufficiency, endometriosis, hyperprolactinemia, lactation insufficiency, menopausal symptoms, premenstrual syndrome [PMS]

Effects on Bleeding None reported

Local Anesthetic/Vasoconstrictor Precautions No information available to require special precautions

Dosage Oral: 400 mg/day in the morning on an empty stomach (standardized to contain 0.5% agnuside and 0.6% aucubin per dose)

Mechanism of Action/Effect Reported to have a significant effect on pituitary function; demonstrates progesterone-like action; may stimulate luteinizing hormone (LH) and inhibit follicle-stimulating hormone (FSH)

Contraindications Lactation and pregnancy (based on case reports of uterine stimulation and emmenagogue effects)

Warnings Use with caution in individuals taking hormonal contraceptives or receiving hormone replacement therapy (HRT). Avoid other phytoprogestogenic herbs (see below).

Potential/Suspected Interactions Increased Effect/Toxicity:

Dopamine antagonists (eg, antipsychotics, levodopa, metoclopramide), hormonal contraceptives, and hormone replacement therapy (HRT)

Phytoprogestogenic herbs: Blood root, oregano, yucca

Chondroitin Sulfate

Use Treatment of osteoarthritis

Effects on Bleeding None reported

Local Anesthetic/Vasoconstrictor Precautions No information available to require special precautions

Dosage Oral: 300-1500 mg/day

Mechanism of Action/Effect Reported to act synergistically with glucosamine to support maintenance of strong, healthy cartilage and joint function (studies inconclusive); inhibits synovial enzymes, elastase and hyaluronidase, which may contribute to cartilage destruction and loss of joint function

Warnings No known toxicity or serious side effects

Chromium

Use Treatment of hyper- and hypoglycemia, hyperlipidemia, hypercholesterolemia, obesity

Effects on Bleeding None reported

Local Anesthetic/Vasoconstrictor Precautions No information available to require special precautions

Dosage Oral: 50-600 mcg/day

Mechanism of Action/Effect In its trivalent form, chromium picolinate (the only active form of chromium), appears to increase insulin sensitivity, improve glucose transport into cells, and improve lipid profile by decreasing total cholesterol and triglycerides, increasing the "good" high-density lipoprotein (HDL). The mechanism of action could include one or more of the following: Enhancing beta cell activity in the pancreas and insulin binding to target tissues, increasing the number of insulin receptors, promoting activation of insulin-receptor tyrosine dinase activity. Picolinic acid causes notable changes in brain chemicals (dopamine, norepinephrine, and serotonin).

Adverse Reactions Frequency not defined:

Central nervous system: Cognitive impairment

Gastrointestinal: Changes in appetite, flatulence, loose stools

Hematologic: Anemia (isolated reports)

Renal: Renal failure

Contraindications Behavioral disorders

Potential/Suspected Interactions Drugs that may affect blood sugar levels (eg, beta blockers, insulin, oral hypoglycemics, thiazides)

Coenzyme Q_{10}

Synonyms CoQ_{10}; Ubiquinone

Use Antioxidant; treatment of angina, breast cancer, cardiovascular diseases (eg, CHF), chronic fatigue syndrome, diabetes, hypertension, muscular dystrophy, obesity, periodontal disease

Effects on Bleeding None reported

Local Anesthetic/Vasoconstrictor Precautions No information available to require special precautions

Dosage Oral: 30-200 mg/day

Breast cancer, cardiovascular disease, and diabetes: >300 mg/day (per case reports)

Mechanism of Action/Effect Involved in ATP generation, the primary source of energy in human physiology; functions as a lipid-soluble antioxidant, providing protection against free radical damage within mitochondria

Warnings Avoid other agents with hypoglycemic properties (see below).

Potential/Suspected Interactions

Increased Effect: Antidiabetic agents

Herbs with hypoglycemic properties: Alfalfa, aloe, bilberry, bitter melon, burdock, celery, damiana, fenugreek, garcinia, garlic, ginger, ginseng (American), gymnema, marshmallow, stinging nettle

Decreased Effect: May decrease response to warfarin; potential of decreased effect with beta blockers, biguanides, chlorpromazine, clonidine, diazoxide, haloperidol, HMG-C_0A reductase inhibitors, hydralazine, methyldopa, sulfonylureas, thiazide diuretics, and tricyclic antidepressants

Cranberry

Synonyms *Vaccinium macrocarpon*

Use Treatment of urinary tract infection and prevention of nephrolithiasis

Effects on Bleeding None reported

Local Anesthetic/Vasoconstrictor Precautions No information available to require special precautions

Dosage Oral: 100% cranberry juice 300-400 mg twice daily or 8-16 oz/day

Mechanism of Action/Effect Current research indicates that a cranberry-derived glycoprotein inhibits *E. coli* adherence to the epithelial cells of the urinary tract.

Creatine

Use Athletic performance enhancement, energy production, and protein synthesis for muscle building

Effects on Bleeding None reported

Local Anesthetic/Vasoconstrictor Precautions No information available to require special precautions

Dosage Oral: Loading dose: 10-20 g/day in divided doses for 1 week; Maintenance: 5 g/day

Mechanism of Action/Effect A naturally occurring crystalline molecule that includes atoms of carbon, hydrogen, nitrogen, and oxygen; enhances formation of polyamines, a powerful growth promoting substance; promotes protein synthesis for quick energy; combines with phosphate to form phosphocreatine released in muscle contraction

Potential/Suspected Interactions Decreased Effect: Caffeine may block effects

Dehydroepiandrosterone

Synonyms DHEA

Use Antiaging; treatment of depression, diabetes, fatigue, lupus

Effects on Bleeding None reported

Local Anesthetic/Vasoconstrictor Precautions No information available to require special precautions

Dosage Oral: 5-50 mg/day; 100 mg/day sometimes used in elderly

Mechanism of Action/Effect Precursor for synthesis of >50 additional hormones (eg, estrogen, testosterone); secreted by adrenal glands; may increase circulating testosterone levels; stimulates production of insulin growth factor-1 (IGF-1), a hormone which enhances insulin sensitivity, energy production, anabolic metabolism, and muscle growth

Adverse Reactions No known toxicity or serious side effects; no long-term studies conducted

Contraindications History of breast or prostate cancer

Warnings Use with caution in individuals with diabetes, hepatic dysfunction, or those predisposed to hypoglycemia (monitor blood glucose and dosage of antidiabetic agents). Avoid other agents with hypoglycemic properties (see below).

Potential/Suspected Interactions Increased Effect/Toxicity:

Androgens, corticosteroids, hormonal contraceptives, hormone replacement therapy (HRT), insulin, oral hypoglycemic agents, and testosterone

Herbs with hypoglycemic properties: Alfalfa, aloe, bilberry, bitter melon, burdock, celery, damiana, fenugreek, garcinia, garlic, ginger, ginseng (American), gymnema, marshmallow, stinging nettle

Devil's Claw

Synonyms *Harpagophytum procumbens*

Use Anti-inflammatory, cardiotonic; treatment of back pain, gout, osteoarthritis, and other inflammatory conditions

Effects on Bleeding May see increased bleeding due to inhibition of platelet aggregation

Local Anesthetic/Vasoconstrictor Precautions No information available to require special precautions

(Continued)

Devil's Claw *(Continued)*

Dosage Oral: 100-200 m 1-2 times/day (standardized to contain 5% harpagosides per dose)

Mechanism of Action/Effect Reportedly improves joint mobility and reduces pain and swelling in arthritis (may be more effective for osteoarthritis and chronic symptoms compared to rheumatoid and acute symptoms). Anti-inflammatory activity has reported for constituents, harpagoside and beta sitosterol; therapeutic effect comparable to phenylbutazone (studies inconclusive); may have chronotropic and inotropic effects

Adverse Reactions Frequency not defined:

Cardiovascular: Cardiomegaly, cardiomyopathy, hypertension, palpitations, tachycardia, vasculitis, vasoconstriction

Central nervous system: Agitation, anxiety, auditory and visual hallucination, CNS-stimulating effects, excitation, fear, headache, insomnia, irritability, nervousness, psychosis, restlessness, sympathetic storm, tension

Endocrine & metabolic: Hypokalemia

Gastrointestinal: Anorexia, nausea

Hepatic: Aminotransferase level elevation (asymptomatic)

Neuromuscular & skeletal: Tremors, weakness

Contraindications Active bleeding (eg, intracranial bleeding, peptic ulcer), GI disorders, lactation, pregnancy (may stimulate uterine contractions)

Warnings Use with caution in individuals with history of bleeding, hemostatic or drug-related hemostatic disorders, and those taking anticoagulants (eg, aspirin or aspirin-containing products, NSAIDs, warfarin) or antiplatelet agents (eg, clopidogrel, dipyridamole, ticlopidine), antiarrhythmic agents, or cardiac glycosides (eg, digoxin). Avoid herbs with anticoagulant/antiplatelet properties (see below). Discontinue at least 14 days prior to dental or surgical procedures.

Potential/Suspected Interactions Increased Effect:

Antiarrhythmics or cardiac glycosides and anticoagulant or antiplatelet agents

Herbs with anticoagulant/antiplatelet properties: Alfalfa, anise, bilberry, bladderwrack, bromelain, cat's claw, celery, coleus, cordyceps, dong quai, evening primrose, fenugreek, feverfew, garlic, ginger, ginkgo biloba, ginseng (American/Panax/Siberian), grape seed, green tea, guggul, horse chestnut seed, horseradish, licorice, prickly ash, red clover, reishi, sweet clover, turmeric, white willow

Docosahexaenoic Acid

Synonyms DHA

Use Treatment of Alzheimer's disease, attention deficit disorder (ADD) and attention deficit hyperactivity disorder (ADHD), Crohn's disease, diabetes, eczema and psoriasis, hypertension, hypertriglyceridemia, and rheumatoid arthritis; coronary heart disease risk reduction

Effects on Bleeding None reported

Local Anesthetic/Vasoconstrictor Precautions No information available to require special precautions

Dosage Oral: 125-250 mg 1-2 times/day

Mechanism of Action/Effect A long-chain, unsaturated, omega-3 fatty acid critical in the development of infants' brains and retinas; highly concentrated in synaptosomes in the brain (the region where nerve cells communicate with each other), photoreceptors (the portion of the retina that receives light stimulation), the cerebral cortex, and the mitochondria. Alpha-linolenic acid (ALA) is the precursor for the other omega-3 fatty acids, however, it is estimated that only a small percentage gets converted to DHA; the primary dietary source of DHA is from cold water or oily fish (herring, mackerel, salmon, sardines, and tuna).

Warnings Use caution with individuals taking anticoagulants (eg, aspirin or aspirin-containing products, NSAIDs, warfarin) or antiplatelet agents (eg, clopidogrel, dipyridamole, ticlopidine), insulin or oral hypoglycemics. Avoid herbs with anticoagulant/antiplatelet properties (see below); may intensify the blood-thinning effect

Potential/Suspected Interactions Increased Effect:

Anticoagulant or antiplatelet agents

Herbs with anticoagulant/antiplatelet properties: Alfalfa, anise, bilberry, bladderwrack, bromelain, cat's claw, celery, coleus, cordyceps, dong quai, evening primrose, fenugreek, feverfew, garlic, ginger, ginkgo biloba, ginseng (American/Panax/Siberian), grape seed, green tea, guggul, horse chestnut seed, horseradish, licorice, prickly ash, red clover, reishi, sweet clover, turmeric, white willow

Dong Quai

Synonyms *Angelica sinensis*; Chinese angelica

Use Anabolic, anticoagulant; treatment of amenorrhea, anemia, dysmenorrhea, hypertension, menopausal symptoms, premenstrual syndrome (PMS); female vitality

Effects on Bleeding Has potential for decreasing platelet aggregation and may increase bleeding

Local Anesthetic/Vasoconstrictor Precautions No information available to require special precautions

Dosage Adults: Oral: 200 mg twice daily (standardized to contain 0.8% to 1.1% ligustilide per dose)

Mechanism of Action/Effect Reported to cause vasodilation; may have hematopoietic properties; rich in phytoestrogens, which may demonstrate similar pharmacological effects, but are less potent than pure estrogenic compounds

Contraindications Active bleeding (eg, peptic ulcer, intracranial bleeding), prolonged exposure to sunlight or other sources of ultraviolet radiation (eg, tanning booths)

Warnings May alter hemostasis, potentiate effects of warfarin, and/or cause photosensitization; use with caution in lactation, pregnancy, cardiovascular or cerebrovascular disease, endometrial cancer, estrogen-dependent tumors, hemostatic or drug-related hemostatic disorders, history of bleeding, hypotension, stroke, thromboembolic disease, and individuals taking anticoagulants (eg, aspirin or aspirin-containing products, NSAIDs, warfarin), antiplatelet agents (eg, clopidogrel, dipyridamole, ticlopidine), antihypertensive medications, hormonal contraceptives or hormone replacement therapy (HRT), or steroids. Avoid other herbs with anabolic, anticoagulant, or antiplatelet properties (see below). Discontinue at least 14 days prior to dental or surgical procedures.

Potential/Suspected Interactions Increased Effect/Toxicity:

Anticoagulant or antiplatelet agents, antihypertensives, hormonal contraceptives, hormone replacement therapy (HRT), photosensitizing agents

Anabolic herbs: Devil's club, ginseng (American/Asian/Siberian), muira puama, sarsparilla, suma, tribulus, wild yam

Herbs with anticoagulant/antiplatelet properties: Alfalfa, anise, bilberry, bladderwrack, bromelain, cat's claw, celery, coleus, cordyceps, evening primrose, fenugreek, feverfew, garlic, ginger, ginkgo biloba, ginseng (American/Panax/Siberian), grape seed, green tea, guggul, horse chestnut seed, horseradish, licorice, prickly ash, red clover, reishi, sweet clover, turmeric, white willow

Echinacea

Synonyms American Coneflower; Black Susans; Comb Flower; *Echinacea angustifolia*; *Echinacea purpurea*; Indian Head; Purple Coneflower; Scury Root; Snakeroot

Use Antibacterial, antihyaluronidase, anti-infective, anti-inflammatory, antiviral, immunostimulant, wound-healing agent; treatment of arthritis, chronic skin complaints, cold, flu, sore throat, tonsillitis, minor upper respiratory tract infections, urinary tract infections

Effects on Bleeding None reported

Local Anesthetic/Vasoconstrictor Precautions No information available to require special precautions

Dosage In addition to forms listed below, there are some products designed to be applied topically; refer to product labeling to ensure formulation is used correctly. Continuous use should not exceed 8 weeks; not to exceed 10 days in immunosuppressed individuals or acute infection therapy. If used for prophylaxis, cycle 3 weeks on and 1 week off.

Oral (with food):

- Capsule, tablet, or tea: 500 mg to 2 g, 3 times/day for 1 day, then 250 mg 4 times/day (standardized to contain 4% sesquiterpene esters per dose)
- Expressed juice of fresh herb: 6-9 mL/day (per Commission E)
- Liquid extract: 0.25-1 mL 3 times/day
- Tincture: 1-2 mL 3 times/day

Topical: Apply to affected areas as needed

Mechanism of Action/Effect Stimulates cytokines, TNF-alfa, and interferons; caffeic acid glycosides and isolutylamides associated with the plant can also cause immune stimulation (leukocyte phagocytosis and T-cell activation)

Adverse Reactions Frequency not defined:

Dermatologic: Allergic reactions (rare; none known for oral and external formulations per Commission E)

Gastrointestinal: Tingling sensation of tongue

Miscellaneous: Immunosuppression (use >6-8 weeks)

Contraindications Hypersensitivity to asters, chamomile, chrysanthemums, daisies, feverfew, ragweed, sunflowers; autoimmune diseases such as collagen vascular disease (lupus, RA), HIV or AIDS, multiple sclerosis, tuberculosis; immunosuppressants; pregnancy (only parenteral administration per Commission E)

Warnings Use as a preventative treatment should be discouraged; may alter immunosuppression; long-term use may cause immunosuppression. Individuals allergic to asters, chamomile, chrysanthemums, daisies, feverfew, sunflowers, or ragweed may display cross-allergy potential (rare but severe); avoid other allergenic herbs (see below). Use with caution in individuals with renal impairment.

Potential/Suspected Interactions

Increased Effect/Toxicity:

Allergenic herbs: Bittersweet, chamomile, devil's dung, echinacea, feverfew, flaxseed, garlic, ginseng, gotu kola, male fern, propolis, yucca

(Continued)

Echinacea (Continued)

Herbs with anticoagulant/antiplatelet properties: Alfalfa, anise, bilberry, bladderwrack, bromelain, cat's claw, celery, coleus, cordyceps, dong quai, evening primrose, fenugreek, feverfew, garlic, ginkgo biloba, ginseng (American/Panax/Siberian), grape seed, green tea, guggul, horse chestnut seed, horseradish, licorice, prickly ash, red clover, reishi, sweet clover, turmeric, white willow

Decreased Effect: Corticosteroids and immunosuppressants; depletes potassium

Ephedra

Synonyms *Ephedra sinica*

Use Appetite-suppressant, stimulant, sympathomimetic (potent), thermogenic, thyroid-stimulant; treatment of allergies, arthritis, asthma, bronchitis, edema, fever, hay fever, headache, obesity, urticaria; euphoria

Effects on Bleeding None reported

Local Anesthetic/Vasoconstrictor Precautions Has potential to interact with epinephrine and levonordefrin to result in increased BP; use vasoconstrictor with caution

Dosage not to exceed 8 mg of total ephedrine alkaloids per dose or <24 mg in 24 hours; per Commission E, herb preparation corresponds to 15-30 mg total alkaloid (calculated as ephedrine)

Adults: Oral:

E. sinica extracts (with 10% alkaloid content): 125-250 mg 3 times/day

Tea: Steep 1 heaping teaspoon in 240 mL of boiling water for 10 minutes (equivalent to 15-30 mg of ephedrine)

Mechanism of Action/Effect Active constituent is ephedrine; stimulates alpha-, beta$_1$-, and beta$_2$-adrenergic receptors and the release of norepinephrine; its activity on the sympathetic nervous system causes vasoconstriction and cardiac stimulation resulting in a temporary rise in both systolic and diastolic BP; causes mydriasis and produces bronchial muscle relaxation; contains the alkaloids, ephedrine and pseudoephedrine, which are routinely isolated and used in OTC products as decongestants

Adverse Reactions Frequency not defined:

Cardiovascular: Hypertension, increased heart rate, vasoconstriction

Central nervous system: Insomnia

High doses:

Central nervous system: Dizziness, headache, hyperactivity, insomnia, irritability, tremor

Gastrointestinal: Anorexia, increased peristalsis, xerostomia

Contraindications Anticoagulant or antiplatelet agents, cardiovascular disease (eg, arrhythmias, hypertension), children, diabetes, hyperthyroidism, MAO inhibitors, pregnancy, psychiatric disorders

Per Commission E: Anxiety, glaucoma, hypertension, impaired cerebral circulation, pheochromocytoma, prostate adenoma (with residual urine accumulation), thyrotoxicosis

Warnings Product labeling contains the following AHPA warning as of March 1994: "Seek advice from two health care professionals prior to use if you are pregnant or nursing, or if you have high BP, heart or thyroid disease, diabetes, difficulty in urination due to prostate enlargement, or if taking two MAO inhibitors or any other prescription drug. Reduce or discontinue use if nervousness, tremor, sleeplessness, loss of appetite, or nausea occur. Not intended for use by person <18 years of age. Keep out of reach of children."

Also use caution in individuals with diabetes (elevates blood glucose), osteoporosis, renal impairment (including nephrolithiasis) and those taking OTC stimulants (eg, caffeine, decongestants). May alter GI absorption of other herbs or drugs; avoid other herbs with hypertensive, thyroid-stimulating, or sympathomimetic properties (see below).

Potential/Suspected Interactions Increased Effect:

Antiarrhythmics, beta-blockers, cardiac glycosides, calcium channel blockers, OTC stimulants, sympathomimetic or thyroid medications

Secale alkaloid derivatives or oxytocin: Development of hypertension

Per Commission E: Guanethidine and MAO inhibitors potentiate ephedra's sympathomimetic effect

Herbs with hypertensive properties: Bayberry, blue cohosh, cayenne, ginger, ginseng (American), kola nut (caffeine), licorice

Thyroid-stimulating herbs: Fu-tse (Fo-tzu), gotu kola, mustard, yohimbe

Evening Primrose

Synonyms Evening Primrose Oil; *Oenothera biennis*

Use Anticoagulant, anti-inflammatory, hormone stimulant; treatment of atopic eczema and psoriasis, attention deficit disorder (ADD) and attention deficit hyperactivity disorder (ADHD), dermatitis, diabetic neuropathy, endometriosis, hyperglycemia, irritable bowel syndrome (IBS), multiple sclerosis (MS), omega-6 fatty acid supplementation, premenstrual syndrome (PMS), menopausal symptoms, rheumatoid arthritis

Effects on Bleeding May see increased bleeding due to inhibition of platelet aggregation

Local Anesthetic/Vasoconstrictor Precautions No information available to require special precautions

Dosage Oral: 500 mg to 8 g/day (standardized to contain 8% to 9% gamma-linolenic acid (GLA) and ≤72% linoleic acid (LA) per dose)

Mechanism of Action/Effect Contains high amounts of gamma-linolenic acid (GLA), and essential omega-6 fatty acid which reportedly stimulates hormone synthesis and reduces generation of arachidonic acid metabolites in short-term use, improving symptoms of various inflammatory and immune conditions

Contraindications Active bleeding (may inhibit platelet aggregation), anticonvulsant or antipsychotic agents, seizure disorders (may lower seizure threshold), schizophrenia

Warnings Use with caution in individuals with a history of bleeding, hemostatic or drug-related hemostatic disorders, those taking anticoagulants (eg, aspirin or aspirin-containing products, NSAIDs, warfarin) or antiplatelet agents (eg, clopidogrel, dipyridamole, ticlopidine). Avoid other herbs with anticoagulant/antiplatelet properties (see below). Discontinue at least 14 days prior to dental or surgical procedures.

Potential/Suspected Interactions Increased Effect/Toxicity:

Anticoagulant or antiplatelet agents, anticonvulsants, phenothiazines, and other drugs which lower seizure threshold

Herbs with anticoagulant/antiplatelet properties: Alfalfa, anise, bilberry, bladderwrack, bromelain, cat's claw, celery, coleus, cordyceps, dong quai, fenugreek, feverfew, garlic, ginger, ginkgo biloba, ginseng (American/Panax/Siberian), grape seed, green tea, guggul, horse chestnut seed, horseradish, licorice, prickly ash, red clover, reishi, sweet clover, turmeric, white willow

Feverfew

Synonyms Altamisa; Bachelor's Button; Featherfew; Featherfoil; Nosebleed; *Tanacetum parthenium*; Wild Quinine

Use Anticoagulant/anti-inflammatory, antiprostaglandin, antispasmodic, digestive aid, emmenagogue, sedative; prophylaxis and treatment of migraine headaches and rheumatoid arthritis; treatment of fever, hypertension, premenstrual syndrome (PMS), tinnitus

Effects on Bleeding May see increased bleeding due to inhibition of platelet aggregation

Local Anesthetic/Vasoconstrictor Precautions No information available to require special precautions

Dosage Oral (standardized to contain 0.2% parthenolide per dose): 125 mg once or twice daily

Inflammation and rheumatoid arthritis: 100-250 mg/day

Mechanism of Action/Effect Active ingredient is parthenolide (~0.2% concentration), a serotonin antagonist; reported to inhibit leukotrinenes, prostaglandins, thromboxanes and platelet aggregation; may have spasmolytic activity

Adverse Reactions

10%:

Gastrointestinal: Bleeding gums (within 3 days)

Frequency not defined:

Central nervous system (upon discontinuation): Headache, insomnia, nervousness

Dermatologic: Contact dermatitis

Gastrointestinal: Abdominal pain, loss of taste, mouth ulcerations, nausea, vomiting

Neuromuscular & skeletal (upon discontinuation): Still joints

Contraindications Active bleeding (eg, intracranial bleeding, peptic ulcer), children <2 years of age; hypersensitivity to asters, chrysanthemums, daisies, sunflowers, chamomile, feverfew, or ragweed pollens; lactation and pregnancy

Warnings Use with caution in individuals with a history of bleeding, hemostatic disorders or drug-related hemostatic problems, and those taking anticoagulants (eg, aspirin or aspirin-containing products, NSAIDs, warfarin), antiplatelet agents (eg, clopidogrel, dipyridamole, ticlopidine), or medications with serotonergic properties. Abrupt discontinuation may increase migraine frequency. May alter absorption of calcium, copper, magnesium, and zinc due to tannins. Avoid other herbs with allergenic, anticoagulant, or antiplatelet properties (see below). Discontinue at least 14 days prior to dental or surgical procedures.

Potential/Suspected Interactions Increased Effect/Toxicity:

Anticoagulant or antiplatelet agents

Allergenic herbs: Bittersweet, chamomile, devil's dung, echinacea, flaxseed, garlic, ginseng, gotu kola, male fern, propolis, yucca

Herbs with anticoagulant/antiplatelet properties: Alfalfa, anise, bilberry, bladderwrack, bromelain, cat's claw, celery, coleus, cordyceps, dong quai, evening primrose, fenugreek, garlic, ginkgo biloba, ginseng (American/Panax/Siberian), grape

(Continued)

Feverfew *(Continued)*

seed, green tea, guggul, horse chestnut seed, horseradish, licorice, prickly ash, red clover, reishi, sweet clover, turmeric, white willow

Fish Oils

Use Antiatherogenic, anticoagulant/antiplatelet, anti-inflammatory; prevention and treatment of cardiovascular diseases; treatment of arteriosclerosis, arthritis, Crohn's disease, diabetes, dyslipidemia, dysmenorrhea, eczema and psoriasis, glaucoma, hypercholesterolemia, hypertension, hypertriglyceridemia; memory enhancement

Effects on Bleeding None reported

Local Anesthetic/Vasoconstrictor Precautions No information available to require special precautions

Dosage Oral: 750 mg 2-3 times/day

Mechanism of Action/Effect Source of eicosapentaenoic acid (EPA) and docosahexaenoic acid (DHA), omega-3 fatty acids which are necessary for the production of cellular membranes, hormones, and nerve tissue; EPA is converted into the series 3 prostaglandins, which have anti-inflammatory activity; although the body synthesizes these fats from alpha-linolenic acid (ALA), conversion in many people is inefficient (most people are deficient in omega-3 fatty acids); prevents atherosclerotic plaque formation

Warnings Use caution with individuals taking anticoagulants (eg, aspirin or aspirin-containing products, NSAIDs, warfarin) or antiplatelet agents (eg, clopidogrel, dipyridamole, ticlopidine), insulin or oral hypoglycemics. Avoid herbs with anticoagulant/antiplatelet properties (see below); may intensify the blood-thinning effect.

Potential/Suspected Interactions Increased Effect/Toxicity:

Anticoagulant or antiplatelet agents and insulin or oral hypoglycemics

Herbs with anticoagulant/antiplatelet properties: Alfalfa, anise, bilberry, bladderwrack, bromelain, cat's claw, celery, coleus, cordyceps, dong quai, evening primrose, fenugreek, feverfew, garlic, ginger, ginkgo biloba, ginseng (American/Panax/Siberian), grape seed, green tea, guggul, horse chestnut seed, horseradish, licorice, prickly ash, red clover, reishi, sweet clover, turmeric, white willow

Flaxseed Oil

Synonyms ALA; Alpha-linolenic Acid

Use Antioxidant, antiatherogenic; treatment of eczema and psoriasis, hypertension, hypercholesterolemia, hypertriglyceridemia; contains 3 times more omega-3 than omega-6 and may be used to help reverse the imbalance between omega-3 and omega-6 (estimated optimal ratio between omega-3 and omega-6 fatty acids is about 1:4 and ratio for many in U.S. is 1:20 to 1:30)

Effects on Bleeding None reported

Local Anesthetic/Vasoconstrictor Precautions No information available to require special precautions

Dosage Oral: 1 Tbsp/day (contains ~58% to 60% omega-3 fatty acid) [available in capsules; must be refrigerated]

Mechanism of Action/Effect The richest source of alpha-linolenic acid (ALA), which contains approximately 58% to 60% omega-3 fatty acids and 18% to 20% omega-6 fatty acids; prevents atherosclerotic plaque formation and plays a critical role in the transport and oxidation of cholesterol; precursor for the omega-3 fatty acids, eicosapentaenoic acid (EPA) and docosahexaenoic acid (DHA), which are an integral part of the production of cellular membranes, hormones, and nerve tissue; EPA is converted into the series 3 prostaglandins, which have anti-inflammatory activity

Contraindications Hypersensitivity to flaxseed, flaxseed oil or any member of the flax plant (*Linaceae*) family

Warnings Use with caution in individuals with plant allergies, those taking anticoagulants (eg, aspirin or aspirin-containing products, NSAIDs, warfarin) or antiplatelet agents (eg, clopidogrel, dipyridamole, ticlopidine), insulin or oral hypoglycemics. Avoid herbs with allergenic, anticoagulant, or antiplatelet properties (see below); may intensify the blood-thinning effect

Potential/Suspected Interactions Increased Effect/Toxicity:

Allergenic herbs: Bittersweet, chamomile, devil's dung, echinacea, feverfew, garlic, ginseng, gotu kola, male fern, propolis, yucca

Anticoagulant or antiplatelet agents and insulin or oral hypoglycemics

Herbs with anticoagulant/antiplatelet properties: Alfalfa, anise, bilberry, bladderwrack, bromelain, cat's claw, celery, coleus, cordyceps, dong quai, evening primrose, fenugreek, feverfew, garlic, ginger, ginkgo biloba, ginseng (American/Panax/Siberian), grape seed, green tea, guggul, horse chestnut seed, horseradish, licorice, prickly ash, red clover, reishi, sweet clover, turmeric, white willow

Folic Acid (FOE lik AS id)

Synonyms Folate

Use Treatment of alcoholism, anemia, atherosclerosis, cervical dysplasia, Crohn's disease, depression, gingivitis, neural tube birth defects, osteoporosis; prevention of breast and colon cancer

Effects on Bleeding None reported

Local Anesthetic/Vasoconstrictor Precautions No information available to require special precautions

Dosage Oral: RDI: 400 mcg/day; ODA: 400-1000 mcg/day

Mechanism of Action/Effect Cofactor in many enzymatic reactions in growth and development; B-vitamin which converts (in humans) to its biologically active form, tetrahydrofolic acid (THFA) which is required for proper neuron cell functioning, closure of the neural tube during pregnancy, and synthesis of amino acids, DNA, and RNA; essential for cell growth and division (especially red blood cells, hair, and skin); participates in methylation reactions, such as the conversion of homocysteine to methionine (elevated homocysteine is a risk factor for accelerated atherosclerosis in some individuals)

Potential/Suspected Interactions Decreased Effect:

Drugs which can deplete folic acid: Antacids, antibiotics, anticoagulants (eg, aspirin or aspirin-containing products, NSAIDs, warfarin), anticonvulsants (eg, barbiturates, carbamazepine, phenytoin, primidone, valproate), biguanides, bile acid sequestrants, corticosteroids (eg, prednisone), cycloserine, ethanol, H_2-receptor antagonists, hormonal contraceptives, potassium-sparing diuretics (triamterene), methotrexate, pyrimethamine, sulfasalazine, trimethoprim-containing antibiotics (co-trimoxazole)

High doses may alter the metabolism of phenobarbital, phenytoin, or primidone; may decrease the efficacy of methotrexate (in cancer therapy) and pyrimethamine; cholestyramine and colestipol may decrease absorption

Garlic

Synonyms *Allium savitum*; Comphor of the Poor; Nectar of the Gods; Poor Mans Treacle; Rustic Treacle; Stinking Rose

Use Antibiotic, anticoagulant/antiplatelet (potent), anti-inflammatory, antioxidant (aged extract improves benefits), antitumor agent, immunosupportive; treatment of hypercholesterolemia, hypertension, hypertriglyceridemia, hypoglycemia; may decrease thrombosis

Effects on Bleeding May see increased bleeding due to potent platelet inhibition

Local Anesthetic/Vasoconstrictor Precautions No information available to require special precautions

Dosage Onset of cholesterol-lowering and hypotensive effects may require months.

Adults: Oral: 400 mg 2-3 times/day (equivalent to 1200 mg of fresh garlic or 10 mg of allicin standardized to contain 4 mg of total allicin potential (TAP) per dose) **or** 600 mg of aged extract 1-3 times/day (standardized to contain 1 mg/g S-allyl cysteine (SAC) per dose)

Cardiovascular benefits: -0.25-1 g/kg or 1-4 cloves/day (in divided doses) in an 80 kg individual

Mechanism of Action/Effect May decrease LDL cholesterol and increase HDL cholesterol, decrease blood glucose levels and triglycerides, increase fibrinolytic activity, and decrease thrombosis; crushed bulb converts to allicin, which may have antioxidant activity. Ajoene, a byproduct of allicin, is potent platelet inhibitor. Per Commission E, antibiotic property is ~1% as active as penicillin.

Adverse Reactions Frequency not defined:

Dermatologic: Eczema, immunologic contact urticaria, skin blistering, systemic contact dermatitis

Gastrointestinal: Changes in intestinal flora (rare per Commission E), GI upset (>5 cloves)

Ocular: Lacrimation

Respiratory: Asthma (due to inhalation of garlic dust)

Miscellaneous: Allergic reactions (rare); change in odor of skin and breath (per Commission E)

Contraindications Active bleeding (eg, intracranial bleeding, peptic ulcer) and pregnancy

Warnings Use with caution in diabetics (may lower blood sugar), individuals taking anticoagulants (eg, aspirin or aspirin-containing products, NSAIDs, warfarin), antihypertensives, antiplatelet agents (eg, clopidogrel, dipyridamole, ticlopidine), hypoglycemic agents or insulin, hypolipidemic agents, and those with a history of bleeding, hemostatic or drug-related hemostatic disorders; may cause GI distress in sensitive individuals. Avoid other herbs with allergenic, anticoagulant/antiplatelet, hypoglycemic, or hypolipidemic properties (see below). Discontinue at least 14 days prior to dental or surgical procedures.

Potential/Suspected Interactions

Increased Effect:

Anticoagulant/antiplatelet agents, antihypertensives, hypoglycemic agents and insulin, amphotericin B (against *Cryptococcus neoformans*)

(Continued)

Garlic *(Continued)*

Allergenic herbs: Bittersweet, chamomile, devil's dung, echinacea, feverfew, flaxseed, ginseng, gotu kola, male fern, propolis, yucca

Herbs with anticoagulant/antiplatelet properties: Alfalfa, anise, bilberry, bladderwrack, bromelain, cat's claw, celery, coleus, cordyceps, dong quai, evening primrose, fenugreek, feverfew, ginger, ginkgo biloba, ginseng (American/Panax/Siberian), grape seed, green tea, guggul, horse chestnut seed, horseradish, licorice, prickly ash, red clover, reishi, sweet clover, turmeric, white willow

Herbs with hypoglycemic properties: Alfalfa, aloe, bilberry, bitter melon, burdock, celery, damiana, fenugreek, garcinia, ginger, ginseng (American), gymnema, marshmallow, stinging nettle

Herbs with hypolipidemic properties: Alfalfa, artichoke, blue cohosh, fenugreek, ginger, guggul, gymnema, plantain, skullcap, myrrh, tansy, red yeast rice

Decreased Effect: May reduce iodine uptake

Ginger

Synonyms *Zingiber officinale*

Use Analgesic, anticoagulant, antiemetic (lack of sedative effects is advantageous over other antiemetics), anti-inflammatory (musculoskeletal), digestive aid; treatment of amenorrhea (Chinese remedy), arthritis, colds, culinary herb, dyspepsia, flu, headaches, motion sickness, nausea/vomiting (eg, from chemotherapy/radiation)

Effects on Bleeding Very high doses may inhibit platelet aggregation.

Local Anesthetic/Vasoconstrictor Precautions No information available to require special precautions

Dosage Oral:

Digestive aid or prevention of motion sickness: 250 mg of ginger root powder 3-4 times/day with food (standardized to contain 4% volatile oils or 5% 6-gingerol and 6-shogaol per dose)

Per Commission E: 2-4 g/day or equivalent preparations

Ale/tea: 8 oz of ginger ale contains ~1 g; 1 cup tea contains ~250 mg

Mechanism of Action/Effect Unknown; antiemetic activity believed to be due to shogaol documented to be comparable to several antiemetic medications, having local effects in the GI tract and/or activity in CNS;. gingerol shown to stimulate gastric secretions and peristalsis; ginger may decrease nausea associated with radiation and chemotherapy and is claimed to be superior to antihistamines for motion sickness due to lack of sedative effects. It may increase GI motility and and thus block nausea feedback from the GI tract; decreases gastric-emptying delays associated with cisplatin; may delay coagulation due to effect on platelet-activating factor and inhibit platelet aggregation (very high doses); may have cardiotonic activity; appears to decrease prostaglandin synthesis

Adverse Reactions Frequency not defined:

Central nervous system: Depression (high doses)

Gastrointestinal: Increased salivation

Contraindications Active bleeding (eg, intracranial bleeding, peptic ulcer) and gallstones (per Commission E)

Warnings Use with caution in diabetics, individuals with a history of bleeding, hemostatic or drug-related hemostatic disorders, those taking anticoagulants (eg, aspirin or aspirin-containing products, NSAIDs, warfarin), antiplatelet agents (eg, clopidogrel, dipyridamole, ticlopidine), cardiac glycosides (eg, digoxin), hypolipidemic agents, hypoglycemic agents, or insulin. Has cardioactive constituents; avoid large and/or prolonged doses. Avoid other herbs with anticoagulant/antiplatelet, hypertensive, hyperlipidemic, or hypoglycemic properties (see below). Discontinue at least 14 days prior to dental or surgical procedures.

Potential/Suspected Interactions Increased Effect/Toxicity:

Anticoagulant or antiplatelet agents, antihypertensives, chemotherapy agents, cisplatin (decreases gastric emptying delays), insulin, oral hypoglycemics

Herbs with anticoagulant/antiplatelet properties: Alfalfa, anise, bilberry, bladderwrack, bromelain, cat's claw, celery, coleus, cordyceps, dong quai, evening primrose, fenugreek, feverfew, garlic, ginkgo biloba, ginseng (American/Panax/Siberian), grape seed, green tea, guggul, horse chestnut seed, horseradish, licorice, prickly ash, red clover, reishi, sweet clover, turmeric, white willow

Herbs with hypertensive properties: Bayberry, blue cohosh, cayenne, ephedra, ginseng (American), kola nut (caffeine), licorice

Herbs with hypoglycemic properties: Alfalfa, aloe, bilberry, bitter melon, burdock, celery, damiana, fenugreek, garcinia, garlic, ginseng (American), gymnema, marshmallow, stinging nettle

Herbs with hypolipidemic properties: Alfalfa, artichoke, blue cohosh, fenugreek, garlic, guggul, gymnema, plantain, skullcap, myrrh, tansy, red yeast rice

Ginkgo Biloba

Synonyms BN-52063; EGb; GBE; ginkgold; Ginkgopowder; Ginkogink; Kaveri; Kew Tree; Maidenhair Tree; Oriental Plum Tree; Rökan; Silver Apricot; Superginkgo; Tanakan; Tanakene; Tebonin; Tramisal; Valverde; Vasan; Vital

Use Anticoagulant/antiplatelet, antioxidant

Per Commission E: Treatment of primary degenerative dementia, vascular dementia, and demential syndromes (eg, memory deficit), depressive emotional conditions, headache, and tinnitus

Treatment of Alzheimer's disease, arterial insufficiency and intermittent claudication (European remedy), cerebral vascular disease (dementia), macular degeneration, resistant depression, traumatic brain injury, tinnitus, visual disorders, vertigo of vascular origin

Effects on Bleeding May see increased bleeding due to inhibition of platelet aggregation; antagonizes platelet activating factor (PAF)

Local Anesthetic/Vasoconstrictor Precautions No information available to require special precautions

Dosage May require 1-2 months of use for therapeutic effect (elderly: 1 month)

Oral (administer with food):

- 40-80 mg twice daily to 3 times/day (standardized to contain 24% to 27% ginkgo flavone glycosides and 6% to 7% triterpenes per dose); Maximum dose: 360 mg/day
- Cerebral ischemia: 120 mg/day extract in 2-3 divided doses (standardized to contain 24% flavonoid-glycoside extract and 6% terpene glycosides)

Mechanism of Action/Effect Extract contains terpenoids and flavonoids reported to inactivate oxygen-free radicals; causes vasodilation and inhibits platelet aggregation; CNS effects may be due to 4-O-methylpyridoxine (an antipyridoxine compound). Reported to increase peripheral blood flow; can increase alpha waves and decrease slow potentials in EEG.

Adverse Reactions Frequency not defined:

Cardiovascular: Bilateral subdural hematomas, palpitations

Central nervous system: Dizziness, headache (rare, per Commission E), restlessness, seizures (in children)

Dermatologic: Allergic skin reactions (rare, per Commission E), cheilitis, urticaria

Gastrointestinal: Diarrhea, GI upset (rare, per Commission E), nausea, proctitis, stomatitis, vomiting

Hematologic: Hyphema

Contraindications Active bleeding (eg, intracranial bleeding, peptic ulcer) or clotting disorders, anticoagulants or antiplatelet agents, hypersensitivity to ginkgo biloba preparations (per Commission E), MAO inhibitors, pregnancy, vasodilators

Warnings Use with caution in individuals with a history of bleeding, hemostatic drug-related hemostatic disorders, those taking anticoagulants (eg, aspirin or aspirin-containing products, NSAIDs, warfarin) or antiplatelet agents (eg, clopidogrel, dipyridamole, ticlopidine), and MAO inhibitors. Cross reactivity for contact dermatitis (due to fruit pulp) exists with poison ivy and poison oak; may last for 10 days (washing skin within 10 minutes may prevent reaction or topical corticosteroids may be helpful). Fruit pulp contains ginkolic acids which are allergens (seeds are not sensitizing). Admit individuals with neurologic abnormalities after ingestion or ingestions >2 pieces of fruit; pyridoxine may be useful after ingestion of ginkgo seeds or kernels. Avoid other herbs with anticoagulant/antiplatelet properties (see below). Discontinue at least 2-3 weeks prior to surgery; use with caution following recent surgery or trauma.

Potential/Suspected Interactions

Increased Effect/Toxicity:

- Anticoagulant/antiplatelet agents and MAO inhibitors
- Herbs with anticoagulant/antiplatelet properties: Alfalfa, anise, bilberry, bladderwrack, bromelain, cat's claw, celery, coleus, cordyceps, dong quai, evening primrose, fenugreek, feverfew, garlic, ginger, ginseng (American/Panax/Siberian), grape seed, green tea, guggul, horse chestnut seed, horseradish, licorice, prickly ash, red clover, reishi, sweet clover, turmeric, white willow

Decreased Effect: Anticonvulsants, fluoxetine (may reverse genital anesthesia and diminished sexual desire induced by drug)

Ginseng, Panax

Synonyms Asian Ginseng; *Panax ginseng*

Use Adaptogen, adrenal tonic, anticoagulant, cardiotonic, hormone stimulant, immunostimulant; support in chemotherapy and radiation (decreases weight loss), postsurgical recovery (stabilize white blood cell counts), endurance

Effects on Bleeding May have antiplatelet effects

Local Anesthetic/Vasoconstrictor Precautions Has potential to interact with epinephrine and levonordefrin to result in increased BP; use vasoconstrictor with caution.

Dosage Oral:

Per Commission E: 1-2 g of dried root or equivalent preparations; for maximum benefit, cycle 4 weeks on, 2 weeks off.

(Continued)

Ginseng, Panax *(Continued)*

100-600 mg/day in divided doses (standardized to contain a minimum of 5% ginsenosides per dose)

Herbal tea: ~1.75 g; 0.5-2 g/day

Mechanism of Action/Effect Ginsenosides, the active agent, stimulate secretion of adrenocorticotropic hormone (ACTH), leading to production of increased release of adrenal hormones (eg, cortisol) and are believed to act via hormone receptors in the hypothalamus, pituitary glands, and other tissues. Panax ginseng may have CNS stimulant and estrogen-like effect; reported to have immunostimulating effects on the reticuloendothelial system. Diols, specific triterpenoid saponins, contribute to sedative and antihypertensive properties; triols reportedly increase BP and function as CNS stimulants. Low doses increase BP while high doses exhibit a hypotensive effect.

Adverse Reactions Frequency not defined:

- Endocrine & metabolic: Mastalgia (prolonged or high dose)
- Genitourinary: Vaginal breakthrough bleeding

Signs/symptoms of Ginseng Abuse Syndrome:

- Cardiovascular: Hypertension, palpitations and tachycardia (in sensitive individuals, after prolonged use, or at high doses)
- Central nervous system: Insomnia, nervousness
- Dermatologic: Eruptions
- Gastrointestinal: Diarrhea

Contraindications Active bleeding (may alter hemostasis), acute infection, lactation, pregnancy, renal failure

Warnings Use with caution in elderly or individuals with cardiovascular disease (eg, hypertension), history of bleeding, hemostatic or drug-related hemostatic disorders, and those receiving anticoagulants (eg, aspirin or aspirin-containing products, NSAIDs, warfarin) or antiplatelet agents (eg, clopidogrel, dipyridamole, ticlopidine), hormonal contraceptives, MAO inhibitors, stimulants (eg, OTC decongestants, caffeine), and those receiving hormonal replacement therapy (HRT). May cause "Ginseng Abuse Syndrome"; monitor for signs/symptoms (see Adverse Reactions). Avoid other herbs with allergenic, anticoagulant/antiplatelet or hypertensive properties (see below). Discontinue at least 14 days prior to dental or surgical procedures.

Potential/Suspected Interactions

Increased Effect/Toxicity:

- Anticoagulant or antiplatelet agents, CNS stimulants, chemotherapy agents, diuretics (eg, furosemide), MAO inhibitors, stimulants (eg, caffeine, decongestants), sympathomimetics
- Allergenic herbs: Bittersweet, chamomile, devil's dung, echinacea, feverfew, flaxseed, garlic, gotu kola, male fern, propolis, yucca
- Herbs with anticoagulant/antiplatelet properties: Alfalfa, anise, bilberry, bladderwrack, bromelain, cat's claw, celery, coleus, cordyceps, dong quai, evening primrose, fenugreek, feverfew, garlic, ginger, ginkgo biloba, grape seed, green tea, guggul, horse chestnut seed, horseradish, licorice, prickly ash, red clover, reishi, sweet clover, turmeric, white willow
- Herbs with hypertensive properties: Bayberry, blue cohosh, cayenne, ephedra, ginger, kola nut (caffeine), licorice

Decreased Effect: Antihypertensive agents, cardiac glycosides (eg, digoxin), hormonal contraceptives, and hormone replacement therapy (HRT)

Ginseng, Siberian

Synonyms *Eleutherococcus senticosus*; Siberian Ginseng

Use Adaptogen, anticoagulant, antiviral, immunosupportive; treatment of arteriosclerosis, chronic inflammatory disease, diabetes, hypertension; adaptation to stress, athletic performance enhancement, energy production

Effects on Bleeding May have antiplatelet effects

Local Anesthetic/Vasoconstrictor Precautions Has potential to interact with epinephrine and levonordefrin to result in increased BP; use vasoconstrictors with caution

Dosage For maximum benefit, cycle 4 weeks on, 2 weeks off.

Oral: 100-200 mg twice daily (standardized to contain 0.8% eleutherosides B and E per dose)

Mechanism of Action/Effect Full mechanism unknown; different from Asian and Panax varieties; similar to Panax in adaptogenic and protective action but without stimulant properties; increases messenger and ribosomal RNA synthesis, lipolysis, and muscle efficiency while protecting glycogen and creatinine phosphate; reported to increase efficiency of natural killer cells and enhance the body's ability to decrease toxicity of certain drugs and pollutants

Adverse Reactions

Frequency not defined:

- Endocrine & metabolic: Mastalgia (prolonged or high dose)
- Genitourinary: Vaginal breakthrough bleeding

Signs/symptoms of Ginseng Abuse Syndrome:
Cardiovascular: Hypertension, palpitations and tachycardia (in sensitive individuals, after prolonged use, or at high doses)
Central nervous system: Insomnia, irritability, nervousness
Dermatologic: Eruptions
Gastrointestinal: Diarrhea

Contraindications Active bleeding (may alter hemostasis); high doses during acute phases of infection (especially when high fever is present)

Warnings Use with caution in the elderly or individuals with cardiovascular disease (eg, CHF, hypertension), history of bleeding, hemostatic or drug-related hemostatic disorders, those taking anticoagulants (eg, aspirin or aspirin-containing products, NSAIDs, warfarin) or antiplatelet agents (eg, clopidogrel, dipyridamole, ticlopidine), antihypertensive agents, digoxin, hexobarbital, hypoglycemic agents or insulin, and steroids. Extensive or prolonged use may heighten estrogenic activity. Avoid other herbs with allergenic, anabolic, anticoagulant/antiplatelet, or hypertensive properties (see below). Discontinue at least 14 days prior to dental or surgical procedures.

Potential/Suspected Interactions
Increased Effect/Toxicity:
Anticoagulant or antiplatelet agents, antihypertensives, barbiturates, digoxin, insulin, oral hypoglycemics, stimulants (eg, OTC decongestants, caffeine)
Allergenic herbs: Bittersweet, chamomile, devil's dung, echinacea, feverfew, flaxseed, garlic, gotu kola, male fern, propolis, yucca
Anabolic herbs: Devil's club, dong quai, ginseng (American/Asian), muira puama, sarsparilla, suma, tribulus, wild yam
Herbs with anticoagulant/antiplatelet properties: Alfalfa, anise, bilberry, bladderwrack, bromelain, cat's claw, celery, coleus, cordyceps, dong quai, evening primrose, fenugreek, feverfew, garlic, ginger, ginkgo biloba, grape seed, green tea, guggul, horse chestnut seed, horseradish, licorice, prickly ash, red clover, reishi, sweet clover, turmeric, white willow
Herbs with hypertensive properties: Bayberry, blue cohosh, cayenne, ephedra, ginger, kola nut (caffeine), licorice
Decreased Effect: May shorten duration of certain sedatives

Glucosamine

Synonyms Glucosamine Hydrochloride; Glucosamine Sulfate

Use Treatment of bursitis, gout, osteoarthritis, rheumatoid arthritis, tendonitis

Effects on Bleeding None reported

Local Anesthetic/Vasoconstrictor Precautions No information available to require special precautions

Dosage Oral: 500 mg sulfate 3 times/day

Mechanism of Action/Effect An amino sugar which is a key component in the synthesis of proteoglycans, a group of proteins found in cartilage; these are negatively charged and attract water so they can produce synovial fluid in the joints. The theory is that supplying the body with these precursors replenishes important synovial fluid and lead to production of new cartilage. Glucosamine also appears to inhibit cartilage-destroying enzymes (eg, collagenase and phospholipase A2), thus stopping the degenerative processes of osteoarthritis. A third mechanism may be glucosamine's ability to prevent production of damaging superoxide radicals, which may lead to cartilage destruction.

Adverse Reactions Frequency not defined: Gastrointestinal: Flatulence, nausea

Warnings Use with caution in diabetics (may cause insulin resistance) and those taking oral anticoagulants (may increase effect). Avoid other herbs with hyperglycemic properties (see Drug Interactions).

Potential/Suspected Interactions
Increased Effect: Oral anticoagulants, insulin or oral hypoglycemics
Herbs with anticoagulant/antiplatelet properties: Alfalfa, anise, bilberry, bladderwrack, bromelain, cat's claw, celery, coleus, cordyceps, dong quai, evening primrose, fenugreek, feverfew, garlic, ginger, ginkgo biloba, ginseng (American/Panax/Siberian), grape seed, green tea, guggul, horse chestnut seed, horseradish, licorice, prickly ash, red clover, reishi, sweet clover, turmeric, white willow
Herbs with hyperglycemic properties: Elecampane, ginseng (American), gotu kola

Golden Seal

Synonyms Eye Balm; Eye Root; *Hydrastis canadensis*; Indian Eye; Jaundice Root; Orange Root; Turmeric Root; Yellow Indian Paint; Yellow Root

Use Antibacterial, antifungal, anti-inflammatory, coagulant; treatment of bronchitis, cystitis, gastritis, infectious diarrhea, inflammation of mucosal membranes, hemorrhoids, postpartum hemorrhage

Effects on Bleeding None reported

Local Anesthetic/Vasoconstrictor Precautions No information available to require special precautions

Dosage Oral: 250 mg 2-4 times/day (standardized to contain 10% alkaloids or 2.5% berberine and 1.5% to 5% hydrastine per dose)
Root: 0.5-1 g 3 times/day
Solid form: 5-10 grains
(Continued)

Golden Seal *(Continued)*

Mechanism of Action/Effect Contains the alkaloids, hydrastine (4%) and berberine (6%), which at higher doses can cause vasoconstriction, hypertension, and mucosal irritation; berberine can produce hypotension

Adverse Reactions Frequency not defined (high doses):

Cardiovascular: Hyper- or hypotension, myocardial damage

Central nervous system: CNS depression, delirium, hallucinations, hyper-reflexia, stimulation/agitation, seizures

Gastrointestinal: Diarrhea, mouth and throat irritation, nausea, vomiting

Neuromuscular & skeletal: Extremity numbness

Respiratory: Respiratory failure

Contraindications Lactation and pregnancy, hypertension, glaucoma, diabetes, history of stroke, heart disease

Warnings Efficacy not established in clinical studies. High doses (2-3 g) may cause hypotension or GI distress; toxic doses (18 g) reported to induce CNS depression. Overdose associated with myocardial damage and respiratory failure; extended use of high doses associated with delirium, GI disorders, hallucinations, and neuroexcitation. May alter liver enzymes. Use with caution in individuals with history of bleeding, hemostatic or drug-related hemostatic disorders, hypotension, those taking anticoagulants (aspirin or aspirin-containing products, NSAIDs, and warfarin) or antiplatelet agents (ticlopidine, clopidogrel, and dipyridamole). Avoid other herbs with coagulant or hypotensive properties (see below).

Potential/Suspected Interactions Increased Effect/Toxicity:

Antihypertensive agents, vasoconstrictors

Coagulant herbs: Agrimony, mistletoe, yarrow

Herbs with hypotensive properties: Aconite, arnica, baneberry, black cohosh, bryony, California poppy, choke cherry, coleus, green (false) hellebore, hawthorn, immortal, Indian tobacco, jaborandi, mistletoe, night blooming cereus, pasque flower, pleurisy root, quinine, shepherd's purse

Decreased Effect: Vitamin B

Gotu Kola

Synonyms *Centella asiatica*

Use Diuretic (mild), sedative (high doses), thermogenic, thyroid-stimulant, wound-healing agent; treatment of hemorrhoids, hypertension, poor circulation, psoriasis, tumors, varicose veins, venous insufficiency, and wounds from infection, inflammation, trauma, or surgery (scar reduction); memory enhancement; modulation/support of connective tissue synthesis; Ayurvedic medicine uses for revitalizing nerves and brain cells; Eastern healers use for emotional disorders (eg, depression) thought to be rooted in physical problems; alcoholic extract was used to treat leprosy in Western medicine

Effects on Bleeding None reported

Local Anesthetic/Vasoconstrictor Precautions No information available to require special precautions

Dosage

Infusion: 600 mg

Oral: 50-250 mg 2-3 times/day (standardized to contain 10% to 30% asiaticosides and 2% to 4% triterpenes per dose)

Topical: Apply a 0.2% to 0.4% preparation to wound areas 2-3 times/day

Mechanism of Action/Effect Extract contains asiaticoside, an active component of *C. asiatica*, in which a trisaccharide moiety is linked to the aglycone asiatic acid; madecassol, the other triterpenoid derivative is used as an ingredient in scar-reducing products. The wound-healing and vascular effects are mostly due to these triterpene saponins and their sapogenins. Many studies found *C. asiatica* acts on certain cells of the epidermis to promote keratinization in areas of infection and stimulates the reticuloendothelial system; reported to increase superoxide dismutase (SOD) and glutathione peroxidase while decreasing lipid peroxide levels. Topical administration improves tissue healing (skin, connective tissue, lymph, and mucous membranes) and may also stabilize connective tissue growth in scleroderma; reportedly stimulates synthesis of hyaluronidase and chondroitin sulfate in connective tissue

Adverse Reactions Frequency not defined:

Cardiovascular: Increased heart rate

Central nervous system: Insomnia

Gastrointestinal: Increased peristalsis

Dermatologic: Dermatitis (topical application)

Contraindications Pregnancy

Warnings Advise caution when driving or operating machinery; large doses may be sedating. Use with caution in individuals taking sedatives (eg, anxiolytics, benzodiazepines); effects may be additive with other CNS depressants. Topical administration may cause contact dermatitis in sensitive individuals. High or prolonged doses may elevate cholesterol levels. Avoid other allergenic, hyperglycemic, or thyroid-stimulating herbs (see below).

Potential/Suspected Interactions Increased Effect/Toxicity:

Anxiolytics, other CNS depressants, and sedatives (eg, benzodiazepines)

Allergenic herbs: Bittersweet, chamomile, devil's dung, echinacea, feverfew, flaxseed, garlic, ginseng, male fern, propolis, yucca

Herbs with hyperglycemic properties: Elecampane and ginseng (American)

Thyroid-stimulating herbs: Fu-tse (Fo-tzu), ephedra, mustard, yohimbe

Grapefruit Seed

Synonyms *Citrus paradisi*; GSE

Use Antibiotic, antimycotic, antiparasitic, antiprotozoan, antimicrobial (antibacterial, antifungal, antiviral), disinfectant, immunostimulant; treatment of GI complaints, herpes, various bacterial and fungal infections (eg, *Candida albicans*, *Salmonella*), inflammatory conditions of the gums, parasites; facial cleanser, water disinfectant

Effects on Bleeding None reported

Local Anesthetic/Vasoconstrictor Precautions No information available to require special precautions

Dosage Oral:

100 mg 1-3 times/day with food

Drops: 5-10 drops 2-3 times/day

Rinse: 5-10 drops 2-3 times/say; dilute in water, swish, and expectorate

Mechanism of Action/Effect Extract is in a highly acidic liquid rich in polyphenolic compounds (eg, apigenin, campherol glycoside, hesperidin, naringin, neohesperidin, poncirin, rutinoside, quercitin) and seems to exert its antimicrobial activity in the cytoplasmic membrane of bacteria by altering cell membrane with a dose-dependent inhibition of cellular respiration; effective against 800 various viruses and species of bacteria and about 100 types of fungi without damaging friendly intestinal bacteria; disinfectant effect and lack of bacterial resistance is believed to be due to the flavonoids

Contraindications Allergy to grapefruit; astemizole, cisapride, and terfenadine

Warnings GSE is not the equivalent of grapefruit juice but since grapefruit juice/pulp has been associated with the inhibition of drug metabolism via cytochrome P450 isoenzyme 3A4 (CYP3A4), resulting in a number of drug interactions, it is reasonable to avoid the concurrent use of grapefruit seed extract in individuals receiving astemizole, cisapride, terfenadine and other medications metabolized by this pathway.

Potential/Suspected Interactions Nonsedating antihistamines, concurrent use of medications metabolized by CYP3A4 (interaction reported with grapefruit juice)

Grape Seed

Synonyms *Vitis vinifera*

Use Anticoagulant/antiplatelet, anti-inflammatory, antioxidant (potent); treatment of allergies and asthma, arterial/venous insufficiency (capillary fragility, intermittent claudication, poor circulation, varicose veins); improves peripheral circulation

Effects on Bleeding May see increase in bleeding due to inhibition of platelet aggregation

Local Anesthetic/Vasoconstrictor Precautions No information available to require special precautions

Dosage Oral: 25-100 mg 1-3 times/day (standardized to contain 40% to 80% proanthocyanidins or 95% polyphenols or a procyanidolic value >95% per dose)

Mechanism of Action/Effect Contains proanthocyanidins reported to neutralize many free radicals, including hydroxyl, lipid peroxides, and iron-induced lipid peroxidation; antioxidant properties are believed to block lipid peroxidation, which stabilizes cell membranes. Proanthocyanidins inhibit destruction of collagen (possibly by stabilizing 1-antitrypsin), which inhibits destructive enzymes such as elastin and hyaluronic acid. Stabilization of collagen allows red blood cells to traverse the capillaries and prevent fluid exudation. Anti-inflammatory activity is due to inhibition of mediators, such as histamine and prostaglandins.

Contraindications Active bleeding; may inhibit platelet aggregation. use with caution in individuals with drug-related hemostatic problems, hemostatic disorders, or history of bleeding, and individuals taking anticoagulants including aspirin, aspirin-containing products, NSAIDs, warfarin, or antiplatelet agents (eg, clopidogrel, dipyridamole, ticlopidine). Discontinue use at least 14 days before dental or surgical procedures.

Warnings Use with caution in individuals with history of bleeding, hemostatic or drug-related hemostatic problems, those taking anticoagulants (eg, aspirin or aspirin-containing products, NSAIDs, warfarin) or antiplatelet agents (eg, clopidogrel, dipyridamole, ticlopidine). Avoid other herbs with anticoagulant/antiplatelet properties (see below). May alter absorption of calcium, copper, magnesium, and zinc due to tannins. Discontinue use at least 14 days before dental or surgical procedures.

Potential/Suspected Interactions Increased Effect/Toxicity:

Anticoagulant or antiplatelet agents, xanthine oxidase inhibitors (*In vitro* studies indicate may increase toxicity of methotrexate)

(Continued)

Grape Seed *(Continued)*

Herbs with anticoagulant/antiplatelet properties: Alfalfa, anise, bilberry, bladderwrack, bromelain, cat's claw, celery, coleus, cordyceps, dong quai, evening primrose, fenugreek, feverfew, garlic, ginger, ginkgo biloba, ginseng (American/Panax/Siberian), green tea, guggul, horse chestnut seed, horseradish, licorice, prickly ash, red clover, reishi, sweet clover, turmeric, white willow

Green Tea

Synonyms *Camellia sinensis*

Use Antibacterial, anticarcinogen, antioxidant, astringent, anticoagulant/antiplatelet, antifungal, antiviral, diuretic, immunosupportive; prophylaxis and treatment of cancer, cardiovascular disease, hypercholesterolemia

Effects on Bleeding May see increased bleeding due to inhibition of platelet aggregation

Local Anesthetic/Vasoconstrictor Precautions No information available to require special precautions

Dosage Recommend decaffeinated products; there are more drug interactions with high doses of caffeine-containing products.

Oral: 250-500 mg/day (standardize to contain 50% to 97% polyphenols per dose, providing ≥50% epigallocatechin-3-gallate)

Mechanism of Action/Effect Reportedly protects against oxidative damage to cells and tissues; demonstrated to increase HDL cholesterol, decrease LDL cholesterol and triglycerides, block peroxidation of LDL, inhibit formation of thromboxane formation, and block platelet aggregation; human studies have noted improvement in prognosis of some forms of breast cancer

Adverse Reactions Frequency not defined: (Nondecaffeinated products):

Cardiovascular: Palpitations, tachycardia

Central nervous system: Insomnia, nervousness

Gastrointestinal: Decreased appetite, gastric irritation

Contraindications Active bleeding (eg, peptic ulcer, intracerebral bleeding)

Warnings Use caffeinated products with caution in individuals with cardiovascular disease, peptic ulcer, and those taking other stimulants (eg, decongestants). Use with caution in individuals with a history of bleeding, hemostatic or drug-related hemostatic disorders, those taking anticoagulants (aspirin or aspirin-containing products, NSAIDS, warfarin) or antiplatelet agents (eg, ticlopidine, clopidogrel, dipyridamole). Addition of milk to any tea may significantly lower antioxidant potential. May alter absorption of calcium, copper, magnesium, and zinc due to tannins. Avoid other herbs with anticoagulant/antiplatelet properties (see below). Discontinue at least 14 days prior to dental or surgical procedures.

Potential/Suspected Interactions Increased Effect/Toxicity:

Anticoagulant or antiplatelet agents, theophylline; reported to enhance doxorubicin's inhibitory effects on tumor growth

Drugs which interact with high doses of caffeine-containing green tea products: Acid and MAO inhibitors, anticoagulant or antiplatelet agents, barbiturates, beta blockers, CNS stimulants, fluconazole, hormonal contraceptives or hormone replacement therapy, phenobarbital, phenytoin, quinidine, quinolones, sympathomimetics, theophylline, sedatives, verapamil

Herbs with anticoagulant/antiplatelet properties: Alfalfa, anise, bilberry, bladderwrack, bromelain, cat's claw, celery, coleus, cordyceps, dong quai, evening primrose, fenugreek, feverfew, garlic, ginger, ginkgo biloba, ginseng (American/Panax/Siberian), grape seed, guggul, horse chestnut seed, horseradish, licorice, prickly ash, red clover, reishi, sweet clover, turmeric, white willow

Hawthorn

Synonyms *Crataegus laevigata*; *Crataegus monogyna*; *Crataegus oxyacantha*; *Crataegus pinnatifida*; English Hawthorn; Haw; Maybush; Whitehorn

Use Cardiotonic, sedative, vasodilator; treatment of cardiovascular abnormalities (eg, arrhythmia, angina, CHF, hyper- or hypotension, peripheral vascular diseases, tachycardia); used synergistically with digoxin (Europe)

Effects on Bleeding None reported

Local Anesthetic/Vasoconstrictor Precautions No information available to require special precautions

Dosage Oral: 250 mg 1-3 times/day (standardized to contain ≥2% vitexin-2-O-rhamnoside or minimum of 10% to 20% procyanidins per dose)

Per Commission E: 160-900 mg native water-ethanol extract (ethanol 45% v/v or methanol 70% v/v, drug-extract ratio: 4-7:1, with defined flavonoid or procyanidin content), corresponding to 30-168.7 mg procyanidins, calculated as epicatechin, or 3.5-19.8 mg flavonoids, calculated as hyperoside in accordance with DAB 10 [German pharmacopoeia #10] in 2 or 3 individual doses; duration of administration: 6 weeks minimum

Mechanism of Action/Effect Contains catechin, epicatechin, and flavonoids, which may be cardioprotective and have vasodilatory properties; dilates coronary vessels

Adverse Reactions Frequency not defined:

Cardiovascular: Bradycardia, hyper- or hypotension,
Central nervous system: Depression, fatigue
Dermatologic: Rash
Gastrointestinal: Nausea

Contraindications Lactation and pregnancy

Warnings Use with caution in individuals taking ACE inhibitors and antihypertensive agents (may lower BP further). Avoid other herbs with hypotensive properties (see below).

Potential/Suspected Interactions Increased Effect:

ACE inhibitors, antiarrhythmics, antihypertensives, cardiac glycosides (eg, digoxin)

Herbs with hypotensive properties: Aconite, arnica, baneberry, black cohosh, bryony, California poppy, choke cherry, coleus, golden seal, green (false) hellebore, immortal, Indian tobacco, jaborandi, mistletoe, night blooming cereus, pasque flower, pleurisy root, quinine, shepherd's purse

Horse Chestnut

Synonyms *Aesculus hippocastanum*

Use Analgesic, anticoagulant/antiplatelet, anti-inflammatory, cardiotonic, sedative, wound-healing agent; treatment of varicose veins, hemorrhoids, other venous insufficiencies, deep vein thrombosis, lower extremity edema

Effects on Bleeding Inhibits platelet aggregation; may see increased bleeding

Local Anesthetic/Vasoconstrictor Precautions No information available to require special precautions

Dosage

Oral: 300 mg 1-2 times/day (standardized to contain 50 mg escin per dose)
Topical: Apply 2% escin gel 1-2 times/day to affected area

Mechanism of Action/Effect Contains flavonoids, sterols, tannins, saponin, and escin (seed) which promotes circulation in the veins; reported to support collagen structures; anti-inflammatory activity may be related to quercetin's reported ability to inhibit cyclo-oxygenase and lipoxygenase, enzymes which form inflammatory prostaglandins and leukotrienes. Quercetin is also an inhibitor of phosphodiesterase; correlated with cardiotonic, hypotensive, spasmolytic, and sedative actions.

Adverse Reactions Frequency not defined:

Cardiovascular: Vasodilation, decreased heart rate
Gastrointestinal: Increased peristalsis, dyspepsia
Respiratory: Bronchial constriction

High dose:

Cardiovascular: Flushing, hypotension
Central nervous system: Headache
Ocular: Decreased visual acuity
Respiratory: Asthmatic attack
Miscellaneous: Sweating

Contraindications Active bleeding (eg, intracranial bleeding, peptic ulcer), asthma, bethanechol, carbachol, coronary insufficiency, hyperthyroidism, lactation, metoclopramide, pilocarpine, pregnancy

Warnings Use with caution in individuals with a history of bleeding, hemostatic or drug-related hemostatic disorders, hepatic or renal impairment, and those taking anticoagulants (eg, aspirin or aspirin-containing products, NSAIDs, warfarin) or antiplatelets (eg, clopidogrel, dipyridamole, ticlopidine). Avoid other herbs with anticoagulant/antiplatelet or parasympathomimetic properties (see below). May alter GI absorption of other herbs, minerals, or drugs (especially calcium, copper, magnesium, and zinc) due to tannins. Discontinue at least 14 days prior to dental or surgical procedures.

Potential/Suspected Interactions Increased Effect/Toxicity:

Anticoagulant or antiplatelet agents

Herbs with anticoagulant/antiplatelet properties: Alfalfa, anise, bilberry, bladderwrack, bromelain, cat's claw, celery, coleus, cordyceps, dong quai, evening primrose, fenugreek, feverfew, garlic, ginger, ginkgo biloba, ginseng (American/Panax/Siberian), grape seed, green tea, guggul, horseradish, licorice, prickly ash, red clover, reishi, sweet clover, turmeric, white willow

Herbs with parasympathomimetic properties: Bittersweet, blood root, blue flag, bryony, dogbane, dogwood, false/green hellebore, huperzineA, immortal, jaborandi, leptandra, pasque flower, pink root, pleurisy root, pokeweed, senega snakeroot, wahoo, yohimbe

HuperzineA

Synonyms *Huperzia serrata*

Use Acetylcholinesterase inhibitor; treatment of senile dementia and Alzheimer's disease

Effects on Bleeding None reported

Local Anesthetic/Vasoconstrictor Precautions No information available to require special precautions

Dosage Oral: 50 mcg 1-3 times/day

(Continued)

HuperzineA *(Continued)*

Mechanism of Action/Effect Purified huperzineA keeps AChE from breaking down into acetylcholine.

Adverse Reactions Frequency not defined:

Cardiovascular: Vasodilation, decreased heart rate
Gastrointestinal: Increased peristalsis, dyspepsia
Respiratory: Bronchial constriction

High dose:

Cardiovascular: Flushing, hypotension
Central nervous system: Headache
Ocular: Decreased visual acuity
Respiratory: Asthmatic attack
Miscellaneous: Sweating

Contraindications Active bleeding (eg, intracranial bleeding, peptic ulcer), asthma, bethanechol, carbachol, coronary insufficiency, hyperthyroidism, metoclopramide, pilocarpine

Warnings Use with caution in individuals taking AChE inhibitors (eg, donepezil or tacrine). Avoid cholinergic drugs and other herbs with parasympathomimetic properties (see below).

Potential/Suspected Interactions Increased Effect/Toxicity:

Acetylcholinesterase inhibitors (donepezil, tacrine)

Herbs with parasympathomimetic properties: Bittersweet, blood root, blue flag, bryony, dogbane, dogwood, false/green hellebore, horse chestnut, immortal, jaborandi, leptandra, pasque flower, pink root, pleurisy root, pokeweed, senega snakeroot, wahoo, yohimbe

Kava

Synonyms Awa; Kava Kava; Kew; *Piper methysticum*; Tonga

Use Anxiolytic, diuretic, sedative; treatment of insomnia, nervous anxiety, postischemic episodes, stress; skeletal muscle relaxation

Effects on Bleeding None reported

Local Anesthetic/Vasoconstrictor Precautions No information available to require special precautions

Dosage

Oral: 100-250 mg 1-3 times/day (standardized to contain 60-120 kavalactones per dose)

Per Commission E: Herb and preparations equivalent to 60-120 mg kavalactones

Mechanism of Action/Effect Extract contains alpha-pyrones and may possess central dopaminergic antagonistic properties.

Adverse Reactions Frequency not defined:

Central nervous system: Depression (prolonged use), euphoria, somnolence
Neuromuscular & skeletal: Muscle weakness
Dermatologic: Allergic skin reactions (rare); temporary discoloration of hair, nails, and skin
Ocular: Visual disturbances (pupil enlargement and oculomotor equilibrium disturbance reported)

Contraindications Parkinson's disease (reported to cause dopamine antagonism)

Per Commission E: Endogenous depression and pregnancy

Warnings The FDA Center for Food Safety and Applied Nutrition (CFSAN) notified healthcare professionals and consumers of the potential risk of severe liver associated with the use of kava-containing dietary supplements. Recently, more than 20 cases of hepatitis, cirrhosis, and liver failure have been reported in Europe, with at least one individual requiring a liver transplant. Given these reports, individuals with hepatic impairment or those taking drugs which can affect the liver, should consult a physician before using supplements containing kava. Physicians are urged to closely evaluate these individuals for potential liver complications. Discontinue if yellow discoloration of skin, hair, or nails occurs (temporary; caused by extended continuous use). Accommodative disturbances (eg, enlargement of the pupils and disturbances of the oculomotor equilibrium) have been described.

Use with caution in individuals taking antianxiety or antidepressant agents, diuretics, hypnotic or sedative agents, alprazolam, or alcohol. May cause sedation; advise caution when driving or operating heavy machinery. Long-term use has resulted in rash. Avoid other herbs with diuretic properties (see below). Discontinue if depression occurs (per Commission E, should not be used >3 months without medical supervision).

Potential/Suspected Interactions Increased Effect/Toxicity:

Alprazolam (coma), barbiturates, CNS depressants, diuretics, psychopharmacological agents

Herbs with diuretic properties: Artichoke, celery seed, corn silk, couchgrass, dandelion, elder flower, horsetail, juniper berry, shepherd's purse, uva ursi, yarrow

Licorice

Synonyms Glycocome; Glycyrrhiza glabra; Lakriment Neu; Liquorice; Sweet Root; Ulgastrin Neo

Use Adaptogen, adrenocorticotropic, antidote, anti-inflammatory, antimicrobial (antibacterial, antifungal, antiviral), antioxidant, antispasmodic, antitussive, detoxification agent, emollient, emmenagogue (high doses), expectorant, immunostimulant, laxative (mild), phytoestrogenic; treatment of abdominal pain, Addison's disease, adrenal insufficiency, age spots, arthritis, asthma, atherosclerosis, benign prostatic hyperplasia (BPH), bronchitis, burns, cancer, candidiasis, carbuncle, chronic gastritis, circulatory disorders, colic, colitis, cold/flu, constipation, contact dermatitis, cough, debility, diabetes, diphtheria, diverticulosis, dizziness, dropsy, duodenal ulcer, dyspepsia, excessive thirst, fever, gastric ulcer, gastritis, hay fever, heart palpitation, heartburn, hemorrhoids, hypercholesterolemia, hyperglycemia, hypotension, inflammation, irritable bowel syndrome (IBS), laryngitis, liver disorders, malaria, menopausal symptoms, menstrual cramps, nausea, peptic ulcer, poisoning (eg, ethanol, atropine, chloral hydrate, cocaine, snakebite), pharyngitis, polyuria, rheumatism, rash, sore throat, stress, tetanus, vertigo; adjunct in long-term cortisone treatment

Per Commission E: GI ulceration, upper/lower respiratory tract infections; foodstuff in candy, chewing gum, chewing tobacco, and cough preparations

Effects on Bleeding None reported

Local Anesthetic/Vasoconstrictor Precautions No information available to require special precautions

Dosage Oral: <250-500 mg 3 times/day (standardized to contain 20% glycyrrhizinic acid per dose)

Liquid extract (dried root): 15-30 drops 3 times/day in juice

Deglycyrrhizinated licorice: Chew 250 mg 3 times/day (standardized to contain ≤2% glycyrrhizin per dose) 1 hour before or 2 hours after meals and at bedtime

Candy twists (2-4) contain 100 g licorice (equivalent to 700 mg of glycyrrhizinic acid); Toxic: 2-3 twists/day for 2-4 weeks

Catarrhs of upper respiratory tract (per Commission E): 5-15 g root/day (equivalent to 200-600 mg glycyrrhizin) or 0.5-1 g juice

Gastric/duodenal ulcers: 1.5-3 g juice

Mechanism of Action/Effect Reportedly inhibits adrenal and thymic atrophy in addition to leukotriene and prostaglandin synthesis; reported to have demulcent and weak phytoestrogenic activity; stimulates the adrenocortical axis and production of mucus, which may cause symptomatic improvements

Adverse Reactions Frequency not defined:

Cardiovascular: Edema, hypertension

Central nervous system: Headache, seizures, tetany

Endocrine & metabolic: Amenorrhea, distal sodium reabsorption, hypokalemia, hypomagnesemia, hyponatremia, potassium loss

Gastrointestinal: Intestinal dilatation (ileus)

Neuromuscular & skeletal: Carpopedal spasms, myopathy, rhabdomyolysis

Ocular: Bilateral pytosis

Renal: Myoglobinuria

Contraindications Cardiovascular disease (eg, arrhythmias, hypertension), diuretics, edema, hepatic or renal disorders, hypernatremia, hypokalemia, lactation, laxatives, nausea or vomiting, obesity (due to possible mineralocorticoid effects from glycyrrhizin content), penicillin, renal impairment; Per Commission E: Hypertonia and pregnancy

Warnings Use caution in diabetics, individuals with plant allergies, hypertension, and those taking antihypertensive agents, cardiac glycosides, corticosteroids, diuretics, hormonal contraceptives, laxatives, nitrofurantoin, or receiving hormone replacement therapy (HRT). Avoid other herbs that may be aldosterone synergistic (eg, horehound), hypertensive, or phytoestrogenic (see below).

Potential/Suspected Interactions

Increased Effect/Toxicity:

Cortisol half-life and progesterone; concomitant use of furosemide can exacerbate hypokalemia; licorice can antagonize the effects of spironolactone

Per Commission E: At daily dosages of glycyrrhizin >100 mg: Potassium loss due to other drugs (eg, thiazide diuretics) can be increased causing increased sensitivity to digitalis glycosides.

On prolonged use and with higher doses, mineral corticoid effects may occur in the form of sodium and water retention; in potassium loss, accompanied by edema, hypertension, and hypokalemia; in rare cases, myoglobinuria

Herbs with anticoagulant/antiplatelet properties: Alfalfa, anise, bilberry, bladderwrack, bromelain, cat's claw, celery, coleus, cordyceps, dong quai, evening primrose, fenugreek, feverfew, garlic, ginger, ginkgo biloba, ginseng (American/Panax/Siberian), grape seed, green tea, guggul, horse chestnut seed, horseradish, prickly ash, red clover, reishi, sweet clover, turmeric, white willow

Herbs with hypertensive properties: Bayberry, blue cohosh, cayenne, ephedra, ginger, ginseng (American), kola nut (caffeine)

(Continued)

Licorice *(Continued)*

Phytoestrogenic herbs: Alfalfa, black cohosh, blood root, hops, kudzu, pomegranate, red clover, soybean, thyme, yucca

Decreased Effect: Barbiturates, cocaine, ephedrine, epinephrine, nicotine, pilocarpine, strychnine, tetrodoxine, and urethane through glucuronic-like conjugation action

Lutein

Use Antioxidant; treatment of cataracts and macular degeneration

Effects on Bleeding None reported

Local Anesthetic/Vasoconstrictor Precautions No information available to require special precautions

Dosage Oral: 2-6 mg/day

Mechanism of Action/Effect A carotenoid present in high concentrations in the central portion of the macula, a highly sensitive area of the retina; within the eye, this pigment filters out blue light and has been claimed to prevent macular degeneration. It protects the visual structures from oxygen free radicals and singlet oxygen, strengthens capillaries, and protects the vessels responsible for nutrient supply to this region

Lycopene

Use Treatment of atherosclerosis, macular degeneration; prevention of cancer (especially prostate)

Effects on Bleeding None reported

Local Anesthetic/Vasoconstrictor Precautions No information available to require special precautions

Dosage Oral: 5 mg 1-3 times/day

Mechanism of Action/Effect A carotenoid which function as natural pigment and antioxidant; supplementation reported to protect against macular degeneration, atherosclerosis, and several types of cancer (eg, prostate cancer); functions as a free radical scavenger which may prevent oxidative damage to subcellular components, protecting from degenerative changes and carcinogenesis

Mastic

Synonyms *Pistacia lentiscus*

Use Antibacterial; treatment of dyspepsia, gastric and duodenal ulcers, halitosis

Effects on Bleeding None reported

Local Anesthetic/Vasoconstrictor Precautions No information available to require special precautions

Dosage Oral: 1000-3000 mg/day in divided doses

Mechanism of Action/Effect Exact mechanism unknown; extract reduces stomach secretions and damage to stomach lining; reported to kill *H. pylori* bacteria, possibly by altering its structure and making it more susceptible to the immune system

Melaleuca Oil

Synonyms *Melaleuca alternifolia*; Tea Tree Oil

Use Analgesic, anti-inflammatory, antibacterial, antifungal, antiseptic, antiviral, disinfectant, immunosupportive, wound-healing agent; treatment of acne, allergy and cold symptoms, minor bruises/burns/cuts, dental plaque, gum inflammation, insect bites, eczema and psoriasis, fungal infections (eg, athlete's foot, oral thrush), hair lice, herpes, muscle pain, respiratory tract infections (eg, bronchitis), toothache, warts; aromatherapy, facial skin toner, household disinfectant (to remove dust mites and lice from laundry), insect repellent, massage oil

Effects on Bleeding None reported

Local Anesthetic/Vasoconstrictor Precautions No information available to require special precautions

Dosage Essential oil should be standardized to contain at least 30% terpinen 4-0l and 15% cineole.

Household disinfectant: 1% solution in laundry water

Inhalant (decongestant, facial toner): Up to 8 drops to be inhaled on handkerchief or pillow case or 5 drops in steaming water

Topical:

- Children: Toxic ≤5 mL
- Adults: <10 mL
  - Eczema and psoriasis: 10 drops in hot bath water
  - Oral rinse: Up to 10 drops in warm water
  - Massage oil: Diluted in carrier oil 1:40 (about 8 drops per tablespoon or 50 drops per 100 mL)
  - Minor skin irritations: 1 drop undiluted oil applied directly to problem area

Mechanism of Action/Effect Unclear; a complex chemical substance consisting of approximately 50 compounds; it is the strongest natural antiseptic, 4-5 times more potent than household disinfectants but can be used daily without damage to surrounding skin; consists of plant terpenes, pinenes, and cineole

Adverse Reactions Frequency not defined:
Central nervous system: CNS depression
Dermatologic: Rash (rare)

Contraindications Oral ingestion; undiluted oil on infants <1 year of age or during pregnancy

Warnings Contains cineole; may cause rash in sensitive individuals if applied directly to skin undiluted. Store in dark glass bottle; may react badly with some polymer plastics.

Melatonin

Use Antioxidant; treatment of sleep disorders (eg, jet lag, insomnia, neurologic problems, shift work), aging, cancer; supports immune system

Effects on Bleeding None reported

Local Anesthetic/Vasoconstrictor Precautions No information available to require special precautions

Dosage Sleep disturbances: Oral: 0.3-5 mg/day; to be taken in the evening

Mechanism of Action/Effect Hormone responsible for regulating the body's circadian rhythm and sleep patterns; receptors are found in blood cells, brain, gut, and ovaries. Release is prompted by darkness and inhibited by light. Secretion appears to peak during childhood, and declines gradually through adolescence and adulthood. Antioxidant properties may also assist in regulating cardiovascular and reproductive function.

Adverse Reactions Frequency not defined: Central nervous system: Drowsiness, fatigue, headache, irritability, sedation

Contraindications Immune disorders, lactation, pregnancy

Warnings Avoid agents that may cause additional CNS depression (see below).

Potential/Suspected Interactions Increased Effect/Toxicity:
Hypnotics, sedatives, or other drugs that induce drowsiness (eg, benzodiazepines, narcotics); CNS depressants (prescription, supplements such as 5-HTP)
Herbs with sedative properties: Gotu kola, kava, SAMe, St John's wort, and valerian

Methyl Sulfonyl Methane

Synonyms Dimethyl Sulfone; $DMSO_2$; MSM

Use Analgesic, anti-inflammatory; treatment of interstitial cystitis, lupus, and osteoarthritis

Effects on Bleeding None reported

Local Anesthetic/Vasoconstrictor Precautions No information available to require special precautions

Dosage Oral: 2000-6000 mg/day

Mechanism of Action/Effect Source of biological sulfur, derived from dimethyl sulfoxide (DMSO); roughly 15% of DMSO is converted metabolically to dimethyl sulfone ($DMSO_2$), another name for MSM. It is an important component of connective tissues, enzymes, hormones, proteins and is required for hepatic detoxification. Pain relief may be due to inhibition of pain impulses along type C nerve fibers, increased blood flow, and reduced muscular spasm.

Milk Thistle

Synonyms *Silybum marianum*

Use Antidote (Death Cap mushroom), antioxidant (hepatoprotective, including drug toxicities); treatment of acute/chronic hepatitis, jaundice, and stimulation of bile secretion/cholagogue

Effects on Bleeding None reported

Local Anesthetic/Vasoconstrictor Precautions No information available to require special precautions

Dosage Oral: 80-120 mg 1-3 times/day (standardized to contain 80% silymarin per dose)

Mechanism of Action/Effect Reported to inhibit inflammatory effects of leukotrienes which could contribute to hepatic damage and be hepatoprotective against acetaminophen, ethanol, psychotropics (eg, butyrophenones, phenothiazines), and other drugs that modify hepatic function. Activity is derived from silymarin, which is composed of three primary flavonoids (silybin, silydianin, and silychristin); silymarin reportedly alters the composition of hepatocytes, limiting entry of hepatotoxins. Silymarin stimulates hepatic regeneration, protein synthesis and increases hepatic glutathione by over 35%. Glutathione is an important antioxidant in detoxification reactions, acting as an important sulfhydryl donor in detoxification reactions.

Nicotinamide Adenine Dinucleotide

Synonyms Coenzyme 1; NADH

Use Treatment of chronic fatigue, Parkinson's disease; increases stamina and energy

Effects on Bleeding None reported

Local Anesthetic/Vasoconstrictor Precautions No information available to require special precautions

(Continued)

Nicotinamide Adenine Dinucleotide *(Continued)*

Dosage Oral: 2.5-5 mg 1-4 times/day

Mechanism of Action/Effect An essential coenzyme in the production of energy in the mitochondria; facilitates DNA-repair mechanisms and stimulates the production of adrenaline and dopamine

Passion Flower

Synonyms *Passiflora* spp

Use Sedative

Effects on Bleeding None reported

Local Anesthetic/Vasoconstrictor Precautions No information available to require special precautions

Dosage Oral (standardized to contain 3.5% isovitexin per dose):

Anxiety: 100 mg 2-3 times/day

Insomnia: 200 mg at bedtime

Mechanism of Action/Effect The constituents, maltol and ethylmaltol, have been shown to produce CNS sedation and reduce spontaneous motor activity (low doses) in laboratory animals. In humans, it may be effective combined with other sedative and antianxiety herbs, such as valerian. These effects may be due to synergism or the potential binding of passion flower constituents to benzodiazepine receptors *in vivo.*

Warnings Advise caution when driving or operating heavy machinery. Use with caution in individuals taking antianxiety agents or antidepressants and other sedatives; reported in animal studies to increase sleeping time induced by hexobarbital.

Potential/Suspected Interactions Increased Effect/Toxicity:

Antidepressants, anxiolytics, barbiturates, sedatives

Herbs with sedative properties: Gotu kola, kava, SAMe, St John's wort, and valerian

Red Yeast Rice

Synonyms *Monascus purpureus*

Use Antibiotic, anti-inflammatory, antioxidant, HMG-CoA reductase inhibitor; treatment of hypercholesterolemia, hypertension, hypertriglyceridemia

Effects on Bleeding None reported

Local Anesthetic/Vasoconstrictor Precautions No information available to require special precautions

Dosage Oral: 1200 mg twice daily (standardized to 0.4% total HMG-Coa reductase inhibitors per dose)

Mechanism of Action/Effect Special form of vitamin E; contains eight compounds with HMG-CoA reductase inhibitory activity; some forms contain large amounts of monacolin K, a natural substance closely related to lovastatin but not identical. Red yeast rice contains additional food-derived accessory factors and seems to be more effective than isolated, purified lovastatin.

Adverse Reactions Frequency not defined: Gastrointestinal: GI upset

Contraindications Active bleeding (eg, intracranial bleeding, peptic ulcer), alcoholics (>1-2 drinks/day), children and individuals <20 years of age, history or risk of hepatic disease, hypersensitivity to rice or yeast, lactation and pregnancy (or if trying to become pregnant), organ transplant recipients, recent major surgery, serious disease or infection

Warnings Use with caution in individuals with a history of bleeding, hemostatic or drug-related hemostatic disorders, and those taking anticoagulants (eg, aspirin or aspirin-containing products, NSAIDs, warfarin) or antiplatelet agents (eg, clopidogrel, dipyridamole, ticlopidine), cyclosporine, erythromycin, itraconazole, niacin, HMG-CoA reductase inhibitors (associated with rare but serious adverse effects, including hepatic and skeletal muscle disorders), and other hyperlipidemic agents. Avoid other herbs with hyperlipidemic properties (see below). Discontinue at the first sign of hepatic dysfunction; discontinue at least 14 days prior to dental or surgical procedures.

Potential/Suspected Interactions Increased Effect/Toxicity:

Anticoagulant and antiplatelet agents, HMG-CoA reductase inhibitors and other cholesterol-lowering agents, clofibrate, cyclosporine, erythromycin, fenofibrate, gemfibrozil, itraconazole, ketoconazole, niacin

Herbs with anticoagulant/antiplatelet properties: Alfalfa, anise, bilberry, bladderwrack, bromelain, cat's claw, celery, coleus, cordyceps, dong quai, evening primrose, fenugreek, feverfew, garlic, ginger, ginkgo biloba, ginseng (American/Panax/Siberian), grape seed, green tea, guggul, horse chestnut seed, horseradish, licorice, prickly ash, red clover, reishi, sweet clover, turmeric, white willow

SAMe

Synonyms S-adenosylmethionine

Use Treatment of depression

Effects on Bleeding None reported

Local Anesthetic/Vasoconstrictor Precautions No information available to require special precautions

Dosage Oral: 400-1600 mg/day

Mechanism of Action/Effect Not defined; functions as a cofactor in many synthetic pathways

Adverse Reactions Frequency not defined:

Central nervous system: Restlessness

Gastrointestinal: Nausea, xerostomia

Contraindications Active bleeding (eg, intracranial bleeding, peptic ulcer)

Warnings Use caution when combining with other antidepressants, tryptophan, or 5-HTP; ineffective in the treatment of depressive symptoms associated with bipolar disorder

Potential/Suspected Interactions Increased Effect/Toxicity: MAO inhibitors, tricyclic antidepressants, or SSRIs; may potentiate the antidepressant effects of 5-HTP, tryptophan, and St John's wort

Sassafras Oil

Synonyms *Laurus Sassafras*; *Sassafras albidum*; *Sassafras radix*; *Sassafras varifolium*; *Sassafrax*

Use Demulcent; treatment of inflammation of the eyes, insect bites, rheumatic pain; used in the past as a flavoring for beer, sauces, and tea

Effects on Bleeding None reported

Local Anesthetic/Vasoconstrictor Precautions No information available to require special precautions

Dosage Adults: Topical: 1-5 drops in distilled water

Mechanism of Action/Effect Contains safrole (up to 80%), one of the heaviest of the volatile oils chemically found to be the methylene ether of allyl-dioxibenene; safrole is slowly absorbed from the alimentary canal, escapes the lungs unaltered, and through the kidneys oxidized into piperonalic acid; inhibits liver microsomal enzymes and its metabolite may cause hepatic tumors

Adverse Reactions Frequency not defined: Dermatologic: Contact dermatitis, diaphoresis

Contraindications Ingestion considered unsafe by the FDA; banned in food by FDA since 1960

Warnings Ingestion can result in poisoning or death (dose-dependent). Sassafras tea can contain as much as 200 mg (3 mg/kg) of safrole; emesis (within 30 minutes) can be considered for ingestion >5 mL (considered lethal).

Saw Palmetto

Synonyms Palmetto Scrub; *Sabal serrulata*; *Sabasilis serrulatae*; *Serenoa repens*

Use Antiandrogen, anti-inflammatory; treatment of benign prostatic hyperplasia (BPH)

Effects on Bleeding None reported

Local Anesthetic/Vasoconstrictor Precautions No information available to require special precautions

Dosage Adults: Oral: 0.5-1 g dried fruit 3 times/day **or** 160 mg twice daily (standardized to contain at least 80% to 90% fatty acids and sterols per dose)

Mechanism of Action/Effect Liposterolic extract of berries may inhibit the enzymes 5α-reductase, along with cyclo-oxygenase and 5-lipoxygenase; does not reduce prostatic enlargement but may help increase urinary flow.

Adverse Reactions Frequency not defined:

Central nervous system: Headache

Endocrine & metabolic: Gynecomastia

Gastrointestinal: Stomach problems (rare, per Commission E)

Contraindications Hormone replacement therapy (HRT), lactation, pregnancy, prostate medications

Warnings Not FDA approved; use with caution in individuals on alpha-adrenergic blocking agents and finasteride.

Potential/Suspected Interactions Increased Effect/Toxicity: Alpha-adrenergic blocking agents, finasteride, hormone replacement therapy (HRT), prostate medications

Schisandra

Synonyms *Schizandra chinensis*

Use Adaptogen, anti-inflammatory, antioxidant, antitussive, hepatoprotective, immunostimulant; treatment of cancer, chronic diarrhea, cough, diabetes, diaphoresis, fatigue, hepatitis; adjunct support for chemotherapy and radiation, detoxification, energy production, health tonic

Effects on Bleeding None reported

Local Anesthetic/Vasoconstrictor Precautions No information available to require special precautions

Dosage Oral: 100 mg twice daily (standardized to contain at least 9% schisandrins per dose)

Mechanism of Action/Effect Reported to lower serum glutamic-pyruvic transaminase (SGPT) concentration, a liver enzyme found in blood when liver damage is

(Continued)

Schisandra *(Continued)*

present; stimulates hepatic glycogen synthesis and protein synthesis and increases microsomal enzyme activity

Contraindications Pregnancy (due to uterine stimulation)

Warnings May alter metabolism of many drugs; use with caution in individuals taking calcium channel blockers.

Potential/Suspected Interactions Cytochrome P450 enzyme induction may alter metabolism of many drugs (calcium channel blockers noted to be decreased). Cardioprotective action reported during administration of doxorubicin.

Shark Cartilage

Use Treatment of cancer, osteoarthritis, and rheumatoid arthritis

Effects on Bleeding None reported

Local Anesthetic/Vasoconstrictor Precautions No information available to require special precautions

Dosage

Oral: Dosage range: 3000 mg 3 times/day, taken 20 minutes before meals

Rectal: Retention enemas; 15-20 g/day

Mechanism of Action/Effect A mixture of glycosaminoglycans (GAGs), including chondroitin sulfate; contains antiangiogenesis factors which inhibit the growth of new blood vessels and may prevent tumors from developing the network of blood vessels they need to supply them with nutrients

Soy Isoflavones

Synonyms Isoflavones

Use Estrogenic (weak); treatment of bone loss, hypercholesterolemia, menopausal symptoms

Effects on Bleeding None reported

Local Anesthetic/Vasoconstrictor Precautions No information available to require special precautions

Dosage Oral: 500-1000 mg soy extract daily

Mechanism of Action/Effect Contains plant-derived estrogenic compounds (potency estimated to be only 1/1000 to 1/100,000 that of estradiol); claimed to inhibit bone reabsorption in postmenopausal women; reported to lower serum lipids, including LDL cholesterol and triglycerides, along with increases in HDL cholesterol

Contraindications History of estrogenic tumors (eg, endometrial or breast cancer)

Warnings May alter response to hormone replacement therapy; use with caution in individuals with history of thromboembolism or stroke

Potential/Suspected Interactions Increased Effect/Toxicity: Estrogen-containing medications, hormonal contraceptives, hormone replacement therapy (HRT)

St John's Wort

Synonyms Amber Touch-and-Feel; Goatweed; *Hypercium perforatum*; Klamath Weed; Rosin Rose

Use Antibacterial, anti-inflammatory, antiviral (high doses), anxiolytic, wound-healing agent; treatment of AIDS (popular due to possible antiretroviral activity), anxiety and stress, insomnia; mild to moderate depression; bruises, muscle soreness, and sprains; vitiligo

Per Commission E: Psychovegetative disorders, depressive moods, anxiety and/or nervous unrest; oily preparations for dyspeptic complaints; oily preparations externally for treatment of post-therapy of acute and contused injuries, myalgia, first degree burns

Effects on Bleeding None reported

Local Anesthetic/Vasoconstrictor Precautions No information available to require special precautions

Dosage

Oral: 300 mg 3 times/day (standardized to contain 0.3% to 0.5% hypericin and/or 3% to 5% hyperforin per dose); minimum of 4-6 weeks therapy recommended

Topical: Apply oil extract to bruises and use for muscle soreness and sprains

Mechanism of Action/Effect Active ingredients are xanthones, flavonoids (hypericin) which can act as MAO inhibitors (although *in vitro* activity is minimal); majority of activity appears to be related to GABA modulation; may also be related to dopamine, serotonin, norepinephrine modulation

Adverse Reactions Frequency not defined:

Cardiovascular: Tachycardia

Dermatologic: Photosensitization (especially in fair-skinned persons per Commission E)

Gastrointestinal: GI upset

Contraindications Children <2 years of age, indinavir, therapeutic immunosuppressants, stimulants, SSRIs, antidepressants, digoxin, endogenous depression, pregnancy

Warnings May be photosensitizing; use caution with drugs metabolized by CYP3A3/4 and tyramine-containing foods (eg, cheese, wine). Use with caution in individuals taking antidepressants, cardiac glycosides, MAO inhibitors, narcotics, reserpine, stimulants, and SSRIs. High does may elevate LFTs (reversible). May alter absorption of calcium, copper, magnesium, and zinc due to tannins. Interacts with many drugs, see below.

Potential/Suspected Interactions

Increased Effect/Toxicity: SSRIs or other antidepressants, tetracycline (photosensitivity)

Decreased Effect: Appears to induce CYP3A3/4 enzymes, potentially reducing effect of many medications (eg, ritonavir, MAO inhibitors, levodopa, 5-hydroxytryptophan, diltiazem, nicardipine, verapamil, etoposide, paclitaxel, vinblastine, vincristine, glucocorticoids, dextromethorphan, ephedrine, lithium, meperidine, pseudoephedrine, selegiline, yohimbine, and ACE inhibitors)

Turmeric

Synonyms *Curcuma longa*

Use Anti-inflammatory, antioxidant, antiplatelet, antirheumatic; treatment of rheumatoid arthritis and other inflammatory conditions, hypercholesterolemia, and hyperlipidemia

Effects on Bleeding May see increased bleeding due to inhibition of platelet aggregation

Local Anesthetic/Vasoconstrictor Precautions No information available to require special precautions

Dosage Oral: 300 mg 3 times/day with meals (standardized to contain 95% curcuminoids per dose)

Mechanism of Action/Effect Anti-inflammatory activity claimed to be comparable to NSAIDs in treatment of rheumatoid arthritis. Antioxidant activity is associated with phenolic fraction, curcuminoids, which also inhibit leukotrienes and prostaglandin synthesis. Curcuminoids reportedly lowered the levels of blood lipid peroxides; may decrease LDL cholesterol and total cholesterol, while increasing HDL cholesterol.

Contraindications Active bleeding (eg, intracranial bleeding, peptic ulcer), biliary obstruction

Warnings Use with caution in individuals with history of bleeding, hemostatic or drug-related hemostatic disorders, and those taking anticoagulants (eg, aspirin or aspirin-containing products, NSAIDs, warfarin) or antiplatelet agents (eg, clopidogrel, dipyridamole, ticlopidine). Discontinue at least 14 days prior to dental or surgical procedures.

Potential/Suspected Interactions Increased Effect/Toxicity:

Anticoagulant/antiplatelet agents and antihyperlipidemics

Herbs with anticoagulant/antiplatelet properties: Alfalfa, anise, bilberry, bladderwrack, bromelain, cat's claw, celery, coleus, cordyceps, dong quai, evening primrose, fenugreek, feverfew, garlic, ginger, ginkgo biloba, ginseng (American/Panax/Siberian), grape seed, green tea, guggul, horse chestnut seed, horseradish, licorice, prickly ash, red clover, reishi, sweet clover, white willow

Uva Ursi

Synonyms *Arctostaphylos uva-ursi*; Bearberry

Use Analgesic, antiseptic, astringent, diuretic; treatment and prevention of urinary tract infections; prevention of kidney stones; treatment of bladder infections, urethritis, and a variety of renal disorders (eg, cystitis, nephritis, nephrolithiasis)

Effects on Bleeding None reported

Local Anesthetic/Vasoconstrictor Precautions No information available to require special precautions

Dosage Oral: 100-200 mg/day (standardized to contain 10% to 25% arbutin per dose)

Mechanism of Action/Effect A potent urinary antiseptic with an astringent effect on the lower digestive tract, reducing general intestinal irritation; contains arbutin, a phenolic glycoside that demonstrates analgesic and antiseptic properties in the urinary tract similar to phenazopyridine; disinfectant properties are most prominent in alkaline urine. Constituents of whole plant preparations are believed to enhance efficacy by contributing to urinary alkalinization. Arbutin is destroyed in the GI tract but additional plant components block its degradation and enhance absorption when whole plant preparations are ingested.

Adverse Reactions Frequency not defined (high doses):

Central nervous system: Convulsions

Gastrointestinal: Vomiting

Contraindications Lactation and pregnancy, renal failure; use >7-10 days

Warnings May cause green-brown discoloration of urine; may alter GI absorption of other herbs, minerals, or drugs (especially calcium, copper, magnesium, and zinc) due to tannins. Use caution with individuals taking diuretics; avoid other herbs with diuretic properties (see below).

Potential/Suspected Interactions May alter absorption of other herbs, minerals, or drugs.

(Continued)

Uva Ursi *(Continued)*

Increased Effect/Toxicity: Herbs with diuretic properties: Artichoke, celery seed, corn silk, couchgrass, dandelion, elder flower, horsetail, juniper berry, kava, shepherd's purse, yarrow

Decreased Effect: Has decreased effect in acidic urine; drinking water with 1 tsp baking soda prior to use may promote conversion of hydroquinones to their active form.

Valerian

Synonyms Radix; Red Valerian; *Valeriana edulis*; *Valeriana wallichi*

Use Antispasmotic, anxiolytic, sedative (mild); treatment of anxiety and panic attacks, headache, intestinal cramps, nervous tension during PMS and menopause, restless motor syndrome and muscle spasms, sleep disorders (eg, insomnia, jet lag)

Per Commission E: Treatment of sleep disorders based on nervous conditions, restlessness

Effects on Bleeding None reported

Local Anesthetic/Vasoconstrictor Precautions No information available to require special precautions

Dosage Oral: 200 mg 1-4 times/day (standardized to contain 0.8% to 1% valerenic acids per dose)

Dried root: 0.3-1 g

Sedative: 1-3 g (1-3 mL of tincture)

Mechanism of Action/Effect May affect neurotransmitter levels (serotonin, GABA, and norepinephrine)

Adverse Reactions Frequency not defined:

Cardiovascular: Cardiac disturbances (unspecified)

Central nervous system: Fatigue, lightheadedness, restlessness

Gastrointestinal: Nausea

Neuromuscular & skeletal: Tremor

Ocular: Blurred vision

Contraindications Children <3 years of age

Warnings Advise caution when driving or operating heavy machinery. Use only valepotriate and baldrinal-free supplements in children <12 years of age due to potential mutagenic properties. Use with caution in individuals taking antianxiety or antidepressant agents, antipsychotics, histamines, and hypnotics/sedatives. Avoid herbs with sedative properties (see below).

Potential/Suspected Interactions Increased Effect/Toxicity:

Antianxiety or antidepressant agents, antipsychotics, antihistamines, barbiturates, other CNS depressants (not synergistic with alcohol), hypnotics/sedatives

Herbs with sedative properties: Gotu kola, kava, SAMe, St John's wort, and valerian

Vanadium

Use Treatment of type 1 and type 2 diabetes

Effects on Bleeding None reported

Local Anesthetic/Vasoconstrictor Precautions No information available to require special precautions

Dosage Oral: RDI: 250 mcg 1-3 times/day

Mechanism of Action/Effect Reported to be a cofactor in nicotinamide adenine dinucleotide phosphate (NADPH) oxidation reactions, lipoprotein lipase activity, amino acid transport, and hematopoiesis; may augment glucose regulation

Adverse Reactions No dietary toxicity or serious side effects have been reported, however, industrial exposure has resulted in toxicity.

Warnings May alter glucose regulation; use with caution in diabetics, those predisposed to hypoglycemia, or taking hypoglycemic agents (eg, insulin). Monitor blood sugar and dosage of these agents; may require adjustment (should be carefully coordinated among the individual's healthcare providers).

Potential/Suspected Interactions Increased Effect:

Oral hypoglycemics, insulin

Herbs with hypoglycemic properties: Alfalfa, aloe, bilberry, bitter melon, burdock, celery, damiana, fenugreek, garcinia, garlic, ginger, ginseng (American), gymnema, marshmallow, stinging nettle

Wild Yam

Synonyms *Dioscorea villosa*

Use Anti-inflammatory, antispasmodic, cholagogue, diuretic (high doses), expectorant (high doses); treatment of diverticulitis, dysmenorrhea, intestinal colic, menopausal symptoms, nausea, premenstrual syndrome (PMS), rheumatic and other inflammatory conditions; female vitality

Effects on Bleeding None reported

Local Anesthetic/Vasoconstrictor Precautions No information available to require special precautions

Dosage Adults:

Oral: 250 mg 1-3 times/day (standardized to contain 10% diosgenin per dose)

Liquid extract: 2-4 mL/day

Tea: 1-2 teaspoons root steeped in 1 cup boiling water for 15 minutes; drink 3 times/day

Topical: Apply as directed

Mechanism of Action/Effect Primarily used for its spasmolytic properties; appears to decrease spasm in the large intestine and uterus; contains the steroidal saponin, diosgenin, but the plant itself is devoid of estrogen and progesterone. Anti-inflammatory action is believed to be due to an affinity for steroid receptors shown by the steroidal saponins present in the plant.

Adverse Reactions Frequency not defined: Gastrointestinal: Emesis (high doses), GI upset (sensitive individuals)

Contraindications Estrogen, progesterone, hormonal contraceptives, hormone replacement therapy (HRT), history of endometrial cancer or estrogen-dependent tumors

Warnings Use with caution in individuals with a history of stroke or thromboembolic disease and those taking steroids, hormonal contraceptives, or receiving hormone replacement therapy (HRT). Use in children, or women during lactation or pregnancy is not recommended. Overdose may result in poisoning. Avoid other anabolic herbs (see below).

Potential/Suspected Interactions Increased Effect:

Androgens, estrogens, hormonal contraceptives, hormone replacement therapy (HRT), steroids

Anabolic herbs: Devil's club, dong quai, ginseng (American/Asian/Siberian), muira puama, sarsparilla, suma, tribulus

Herbs with estrogenic properties: Black cohosh, dong quai, and evening primrose

Yohimbe

Synonyms Johimbe; *Pausinystalia yohimbe*; Yohimbehe cortex

Use Anesthetic (local), antiatherogenic, antiviral, aphrodesiac, stimulant, sympathomimetic, thermogenic, vasodilator, vasopressomimetic; treatment of angina pectoris, arteriosclerosis, exhaustion, male erectile dysfunction

Effects on Bleeding None reported

Local Anesthetic/Vasoconstrictor Precautions Has potential to interact with epinephrine and levonordefrin to result in increased BP; use vasoconstrictor with caution

Dosage Adults: Oral: 500-750 mg twice daily

Mechanism of Action/Effect Alkaloid which contains several other psychoactive alkaloids believed to have an effect similar to yohimbine; has CNS, respiratory, and thyroid stimulatory activity; blocks peripheral 5-HT receptors and prevents accumulation of lipid-containing plaques on innermost layers of arteries; has selective alpha$_2$ adrenergic blocking properties; aphrodisiac activity may be due to enlargement of the vasculature in the genitals, increase of nerve impulses to genital tissue, and an increased transmission of reflex excitability in the sacral region of the spinal cord; may have MAO inhibitor activity

Adverse Reactions Frequency not defined:

Cardiovascular: Cardiac failure, hypertension, tachycardia, vasoconstriction

Central nervous system: Insomnia

Gastrointestinal: Increased peristalsis, dyspepsia

High doses:

Cardiovascular: Hypotension

Central nervous system: Dizziness, headache, hyperactivity, irritability, psychosis, tremor

Gastrointestinal: Anorexia, xerostomia

Ocular: Decreased visual acuity

Respiratory: Asthmatic attack

Miscellaneous: Sweating

Contraindications Alpha$_2$-blockers, anticoagulant or antiplatelet agents, antidepressants, asthma, bethanechol, carbachol, cardiovascular disease (eg, arrhythmias, hypertension), chronic inflammation of genitalia, chronic prostatitis, diabetes, hyperthyroidism, MAO inhibitors, metoclopramide, pilocarpine, pregnancy, psychiatric disorders

Warnings Toxic doses may trigger cardiac failure, hypotension, and psychosis. Use with caution in individuals with diabetes, GI ulceration, or osteoporosis. Avoid other herbs with hypertensive, parasympathomimetic, sympathomimetic, thyroid-stimulating, or vasopressomimetic properties (see below).

Potential/Suspected Interactions Antihypertensives; may cause both hyper- and hypotension (dose-dependent)

Increased Effect/Toxicity:

Alpha$_2$ blockers, MAO inhibitors, naloxone, other sympathomimetics, tricyclic antidepressants

Herbs with hypertensive properties: Bayberry, blue cohosh, cayenne, ephedra, ginger, ginseng, kola nut (caffeine), licorice

(Continued)

Yohimbe *(Continued)*

Herbs with parasympathomimetic properties: Bittersweet, blood root, blue flag, bryony, dogbane, dogwood, false/green hellebore, horse chestnut, huperzineA, immortal, jaborandi, leptandra, pasque flower, pink root, pleurisy root, pokeweed, senega snakeroot, wahoo

Herbs with sympathomimetic properties: Calamus, cayenne, ephedra, Fu-tse (Fo-tzu), guarana, kola nut (caffeine), night blooming cereus, peyote (mescal buttons), scotch broom tops, Syrian rue, yellow jasmine

Thyroid-stimulating herbs: Fu-tse (Fo-tzu), gotu kola, ephedra, mustard

Herbs with vasopressomimetic properties: Goat's head, peyote (mescal buttons)

EFFECTS ON VARIOUS SYSTEMS

CARDIOVASCULAR SYSTEM

CONGESTIVE HEART FAILURE

(Diuretics, Xanthine derivatives, Licorice, Ginseng, Aconite)

Alisma plantago, bearberry (*Arctostaphylos uva-ursi*), buchu (*Barosma betulina*), couch grass, dandelion, horsetail rush, juniper, licorice, and xanthine derivatives exert varying degrees of diuretic action. Many patients with congestive heart failure (CHF) are already taking a diuretic medication. By taking products containing one or more of these components, patients already on diuretic medications may increase their risk for dehydration.

Ginseng and licorice can potentially worsen congestive heart failure and edema by causing fluid retention. Aconite has varying effects on the heart that itself could lead to heart failure. Patients with CHF should be advised to consult with their healthcare provider before using products containing any of these components.

HYPERTENSION/HYPOTENSION

(Diuretics, Ginkgo biloba, Ginseng, Hawthorn, Ma-huang, Xanthine derivatives)

The stimulant properties of ginseng and ma-huang could worsen pre-existing hypertension. Elevated blood pressure has been reported as a side effect of ginseng. Although ma-huang contains ephedrine, a known vasoconstrictor, ma-huang's effect on blood pressure varies between individuals. Ma-huang can cause hypotension or hypertension. Due to its unpredictable effects, patients with pre-existing hypertension should use caution when using natural products containing ma-huang. Providers should caution patients with labile hypertension against the use of ginseng.

The diuretic effect of xanthine derivatives and other diuretic components could increase the effects of antihypertensive medications, increasing the risk for hypotension. Hawthorn and ginkgo biloba can cause vasodilation increasing the hypotensive effects of antihypertensive medication. Patients susceptible to hypotension or patients taking antihypertensive medication should use caution when taking products containing xanthine derivatives or diuretics. Patients with pre-existing hypertension or hypotension who wish to use products containing these components should be closely monitored by a healthcare professional for changes in blood pressure control.

ARRHYTHMIAS

(Ginseng)

It has been reported that ginseng may increase the risk of arrhythmias, although it is unclear whether this effect is due to the actual ingredient (ginseng) or other possible impurities. Patients at risk for arrhythmias should be cautioned against the use of products containing ginseng without first consulting with their healthcare provider.

CENTRAL NERVOUS SYSTEM

(Aconite, Ginseng, Xanthine derivatives)

Aconite and hawthorn have potentially sedating effects, and aconite also contains various alkaloids and traces of ephedrine. Some documented central nervous system (CNS) effects of aconite include sedation, vertigo, and incoordination. Hawthorn has been reported to exert a depressive effect on the CNS leading to sedation.

Ginseng, ma-huang, and xanthine derivatives can exert a stimulant effect on the central nervous system. Some of the CNS effects of ginseng include nervousness, insomnia, and euphoria. The action of ma-huang is due to the presence of ephedrine and pseudoephedrine. Ma-huang exerts a stimulant action on the CNS similar to decongestant/weight loss products (Dexatrim®, etc) thus causing nervousness, insomnia, and anxiety. Kola nut, green tea, guarana, and yerba mate contain varying amounts of caffeine, a xanthine derivative. Stimulant properties exerted by these herbs are expected to be comparable to those of caffeine, including insomnia, nervousness, and anxiety.

Products containing aconite and hawthorn should be used with caution in patients with known history of depression, vertigo, or syncope. Ginseng or xanthine derivatives should be avoided in patients with history of insomnia or anxiety. Use of natural products with these components may contribute to a worsening of a patient's pre-existing medical condition. Patients taking CNS-active medications should avoid or use extreme caution when using preparations containing any of the above components. These components may interact directly or indirectly with CNS-active medications causing an increase or decrease in overall effect.

(Continued)

ENDOCRINE SYSTEM

DIABETES MELLITUS

(Chromium, Glucomannan, Ginseng, Hawthorn, Ma-huang, Periploca, Spirulina)

Ma-huang and spirulina both may increase glucose levels. This could cause a decrease in glucose control, thereby, increasing a patient's risk for hyperglycemia. Patients with diabetes or glucose intolerance should avoid using ma-huang and spirulina containing products.

Chromium, ginseng, glucomannan, periploca (*gymneme sylvestre*), and hawthorn should be used with caution in patients being treated for diabetes. These ingredients may reduce glucose levels increasing the risk for hypoglycemia in patients who are already taking a hypoglycemic agent. Patients with diabetes who wish to use products containing these ingredients should be closely monitored for fluctuations in blood glucose levels.

GASTROINTESTINAL SYSTEM

PEPTIC ULCER DISEASE

(Betaine Hydrochloride, White Willow)

Betaine hydrochloride is a source of hydrochloric acid. The acid released from betaine hydrochloride could aggravate an existing ulcer. White willow, like aspirin, contains salicylates.

Aspirin has been known to induce gastric damage by direct irritation on the gastric mucosa and by an indirect systemic effect. As a result, patients with a history of peptic ulcer disease or gastritis are informed to avoid use of aspirin and other salicylate derivatives. These precautions should also apply to white willow. Patients with a history of peptic ulcer disease or gastritis should not use products containing white willow or betaine hydrochloride as either could exacerbate ulcers.

INFLAMMATORY BOWEL DISEASE

(Cascara Sagrada, Senna, Dandelion)

Cascara sagrada and senna are stimulant laxatives. Their laxative effect is exerted by stimulation of peristalsis in the colon and by inhibition of water and electrolyte secretion. The laxative effect produced by these herbs could induce an exacerbation of inflammatory bowel disease. Patients with a history of inflammatory bowel disease should avoid using products containing cascara sagrada or senna, and use caution when taking products containing dandelion which may also have a laxative effect.

OBSTRUCTION/ILEUS

(Glucomannan, Kelp, Psyllium)

Glucomannan, kelp, and psyllium act as bulk laxatives. In the presence of water, bulk laxatives swell or form a viscous solution adding extra bulk in the gastrointestinal tract. The resulting mass is thought to stimulate peristalsis. In the presence of an ileus, these laxatives could cause an obstruction.

If sufficient water is not consumed when taking a bulk laxative, a semisolid mass can form resulting in an obstruction. Any patient who wishes to take a natural product containing kelp, psyllium, or glucomannan should drink sufficient water to decrease the risk of obstruction. This may be of concern in particular disease states such as CHF or other cases where excess fluid intake may influence the existing disease presentation. Patients with a suspected obstruction or ileus should avoid using products containing kelp, psyllium, or glucomannan without consent of their primary healthcare provider.

HEMATOLOGIC SYSTEM

ANTICOAGULATION THERAPY & COAGULATION DISORDERS

(Horsetail Rush, Ginseng, Ginkgo Biloba, Guarana, White Willow)

Horsetail rush, ginseng, ginkgo biloba, guarana, and white willow can potentially affect platelet aggregation and bleeding time. Ginkgo biloba, ginseng, guarana, and white willow inhibit platelet aggregation resulting in an increase in bleeding time. Horsetail rush, on the other hand, may decrease bleeding time. Patients with coagulation disorders or patients on anticoagulation therapy may be sensitive to the effects on coagulation by these components and should, therefore, avoid use of products containing any of these components.

OTHER

PHENYLKETONURIA

(Aspartame, Spirulina)

Patients with phenylketonuria should not use products containing aspartame or spirulina. Aspartame, a common artificial sweetener, is metabolized to phenylalanine, while spirulina contains phenylalanine.

GOUT

(Diuretics, White Willow)

Patients with a history of gout should avoid using natural products containing components with diuretic action or white willow. By increasing urine output, ingredients with diuretic action may concentrate uric acid in the blood increasing the risk of gout in these patients. White willow, like aspirin, may inhibit excretion of urate resulting in an increase in uric acid concentration. The increase in urate levels could cause precipitation of uric acid resulting in an exacerbation of gout.

ORAL MEDICINE TOPICS

PART I:

DENTAL MANAGEMENT AND THERAPEUTIC CONSIDERATIONS IN MEDICALLY-COMPROMISED PATIENTS

This first part of the chapter focuses on common medical conditions and their associated drug therapies with which the dentist must be familiar. Patient profiles with commonly associated drug regimens are described.

TABLE OF CONTENTS

CARDIOVASCULAR DISEASES

Cardiovascular disease is the most prevalent human disease affecting over 60 million Americans and this group of diseases accounts >50% of all deaths in the United States. Surgical and pharmacological therapy have resulted in many cardiovascular patients living healthy and profitable lives. Consequently, patients presenting to the dental office may require treatment planning modifications related to the medical management of their cardiovascular disease. For the purposes of this text, we will cover coronary artery disease (CAD) including angina pectoris and myocardial infarction, cardiac arrhythmias, heart failure, and hypertension.

CARDIOVASCULAR DRUGS AND DENTAL CONSIDERATIONS

Some of the drug listings are redundant because the drugs are used to treat more than one cardiovascular disorder. As a convenience to the reader, each table has been constructed as a stand alone listing of drugs for the given disorder. The dental implications of these cardiovascular drugs are listed in Tables 8 and 9. Each of these 2 tables is a consolidation of the drugs from Tables 1-7. The more frequent cardiovascular, respiratory, and central nervous system adverse reactions which you may see in the dental patient are described in Table 8 *on page 1321*. Table 9 *on page 1324* describes the effects on dental treatment reported for these drugs. It is suggested that the reader use Tables 8 and 9 to check for potential effects which could occur in the medicated cardiovascular dental patients.

CORONARY ARTERY DISEASE

Any long-term decrease in the delivery of oxygen to the heart muscle can lead to the condition ischemic heart disease. Often arteriosclerosis and atherosclerosis result in a narrowing of the coronary vessels' lumina and are the most common causes of vascular ischemic heart disease. Other causes such as previous infarct, mitral valve regurgitation, and ruptured septa may also lead to ischemia in the heart muscle. The two most common major conditions that result from ischemic heart disease are angina pectoris and myocardial infarction. Sudden death, a third category, can likewise result from ischemia.

To the physician, the most common presenting sign or symptom of ischemic heart disease is chest pain. This chest pain can be of a transient nature as in angina pectoris or the result of a myocardial infarction. It is now believed that sudden death represents a separate occurrence that essentially involves the development of a lethal cardiac arrhythmia or coronary artery spasm leading to an acute shutdown of the heart muscle blood supply. Risk factors in patients for coronary atherosclerosis include cigarette smoking, elevated blood lipids, hypertension, as well as diabetes mellitus, age, and gender (male).

Coronary artery disease (CAD) is the cause of about half of all deaths in the United States. CAD has been shown to be correlated with the levels of plasma cholesterol and/or triacylglycerol-containing lipoprotein particles. Primary prevention focuses on averting the development of CAD. In contrast, secondary prevention of (CAD) focuses on therapies to reduce morbidity and mortality in patients with clinically documented CAD.

Lipid-lowering and cardioprotective drugs provide significant risk-reducing benefits in the secondary prevention of CAD. By reducing the levels of total and low density cholesterol through the inhibition of hydroxymethylglutaryl coenzyme A (HMG-CoA) reductase, statin drugs significantly improve survival. Cardioprotective drug therapy includes antiplatelet/anticoagulant agents to inhibit platelet adhesion, aggregation and blood coagulation; beta-blockers to lower heart rate, contractility and blood pressure; and the angiotensin-converting enzyme (ACE) inhibitors to lower peripheral resistance and workload. For a listing of these drugs, see Table 1 on following page.

Table 1.
DRUGS USED IN THE TREATMENT OF CAD

Reduction of Total and Low-Density Cholesterol Levels	
Bile Acid Sequestrant	
Colesevelam (Welchol™)	*on page 320*
HMG-CoA Reductase Inhibitors	
Fluvastatin (Lescol®)	*on page 527*
Lovastatin (Mevacor®)	*on page 734*
Pravastatin (Pravachol®)	*on page 984*
Simvastatin (Zocor™)	*on page 1088*
Atorvastatin (Lipitor®)	*on page 126*
Fibrate Group	
Clofibrate (Atromid-S®)	*on page 305*
Fenofibrate (TriCor™)	*on page 490*
Gemfibrozil (Lopid®)	*on page 552*
Bile Acid Resins	
Cholestyramine (Prevalite®, Questran®)	*on page 279*
Colestipol (Colestid®)	*on page 320*
Nicotinic Acid	
Cardioprotective Therapy	
Antiplatelet/Anticoagulant Agents	
Aspirin	*on page 119*
Clopidogrel (Plavix®)	*on page 310*
Ticlopidine (Ticlid®)	*on page 1168*
Warfarin (Coumadin®)	*on page 1250*
Beta-Adrenergic Receptor Blockers	
Atenolol (Tenormin®)	*on page 125*
Metoprolol (Lopressor®, Toprol XL®)	*on page 803*
Propranolol (Betachron E-R®, Inderal®)	*on page 1016*
Angiotensin-Converting Enzyme (ACE) Inhibitors	
Captopril (Capoten®)	*on page 213*
Enalapril (Vasotec®)	*on page 432*
Fosinopril (Monopril®)	*on page 539*
Lisinopril (Prinivil®, Zestril®)	*on page 719*
Ramipril (Altace™)	*on page 1040*

ANGINA PECTORIS

(EMPHASIS ON UNSTABLE ANGINA)

Numerous physiologic triggers can initiate the rupture of plaque in coronary blood vessels. Rupture leads to the activation, adhesion and aggregation of platelets, and the activation of the clotting cascade, resulting in the formation of occlusive thrombus. If this process leads to the complete occlusion of the artery, acute myocardial infarction with ST-segment elevation occurs. Alternatively, if the process leads to severe stenosis and the artery remains patent, unstable angina occurs. Triggers which induce unstable angina include physical exertion, mechanical stress due to an increase in cardiac contractility, pulse rate, blood pressure, and vasoconstriction.

Unstable angina accounts for more than 1 million hospital admissions annually. In 1989, Braunwald devised a classification system according to the severity of the clinical manifestations of angina. These manifestations are defined as acute angina while at rest (within the 48 hours before presentation), subacute angina while at rest (within the previous month but not within the 48 hours before presentation), or new onset of accelerated (progressively more severe) angina. The system also classifies angina according to the clinical circumstances in which unstable angina develops, defined as either angina in the presence or absence of other conditions (ie, fever, hypoxia, tachycardia, thyrotoxicosis) and whether or not ECG abnormalities are present. Recently, the term "acute coronary syndrome" has been used to describe the range of conditions that includes unstable angina, non-Q-wave myocardial infarction, and Q-wave myocardial infarction.

Pharmacologic therapy to treat unstable angina includes antiplatelet drugs, antithrombin therapy, and conventional antianginal therapy with beta-blockers, nitrates, and calcium channel blockers. These drug groups and selected agents are listed in Table 2 on following page.

CARDIOVASCULAR DISEASES *(Continued)*

Table 2. DRUGS USED TO MANAGE UNSTABLE ANGINA

Antiplatelet Drugs
- Aspirin *on page 119*
- Clopidogrel (Plavix®) *on page 310*
- Ticlopidine (Ticlid®) *on page 1168*
- **Glycoprotein IIb/IIIa Receptor Antagonists**
  - Abciximab (ReoPro®) *on page 23*
  - Eptifibatide (Integrilin®) *on page 445*
  - Tirofiban (Aggrastat®) *on page 1173*

Antithrombin Drugs
- **Indirect Thrombin Inhibitors**
  - Unfractionated heparin (Heparin) *on page 580*
  - Low molecular weight heparins
    - Dalteparin (Fragmin®) *on page 345*
    - Enoxaparin (Lovenox®) *on page 434*
    - Tinzaparin (Innohep®) *on page 1171*
- **Direct Thrombin Inhibitors**
  - Lepirudin (Hirudin®) *on page 689*
  - Argatroban *on page 110*
  - Argatroban (*Marketed Without Brand Name*) *on page 110*
- **Dicumarols**
  - Warfarin (Coumadin®) *on page 1250*

Conventional Antianginal Drugs
- **Beta-Blockers**
  - Atenolol (Tenormin®) *on page 125*
  - Bisoprolol (Zebeta®) *on page 168*
  - Carteolol (Cartrol®) *on page 226*
  - Nadolol (Corgard®) *on page 839*
  - Propranolol (Inderal®) *on page 1016*
- **Nitrates**
  - Isosorbide Dinitrate (Dilatrate®-SR, Isordil®) *on page 661*
  - Isosorbide Mononitrate (Imdur®) *on page 662*
  - Nitroglycerin (sublingual spray or tablets, oral tablets, transdermal patch) *on page 871*
- **Calcium Channel Blockers**
  - Diltiazem (Cardizem®) *on page 394*
  - Nifedipine (Procardia®, Adalat®) *on page 865*
  - Verapamil (Calan®) *on page 1236*

Antiplatelet Drugs

Aspirin reduces platelet aggregation by blocking platelet cyclo-oxygenase through irreversible acetylation. This action prevents the formation of thromboxane A_2. A number of studies have confirmed that aspirin reduces the risk of death from cardiac causes and fatal and nonfatal myocardial infarction by approximately 50% to 70% in patients presenting with unstable angina. Ticlopidine is a second-line alternative to aspirin in the treatment of unstable angina and is also used as adjunctive therapy with aspirin to prevent thrombosis after placement of intracoronary stents. Ticlopidine blocks ADP-mediated platelet aggregation. Clopidogrel inhibits platelet aggregation by affecting the ADP-dependent activation of the glycoprotein IIb/IIIa complex. Clopidogrel is chemically related to ticlopidine, but has fewer side effects.

Platelet Glycoprotein IIb/IIIa Receptor Antagonists

Antagonists of glycoprotein IIb/IIIa, a receptor on the platelet for adhesive proteins, inhibit the final common pathway involved in adhesion, activation and aggregation. Presently, there exist three classes of inhibitors. One class is murine-human chimeric antibodies of which abciximab is the prototype. The other two classes are the synthetic peptide forms (eg, eptifibatide) and the synthetic nonpeptide forms (eg, tirofiban). These agents, in combination with heparin and aspirin, have been used to treat unstable angina, significantly reducing the incidence of death or myocardial infarction.

Antithrombin Drugs

Unfractionated heparin, in combination with aspirin, is used to treat unstable angina. Unfractionated heparin consists of polysaccharide chains which bind to antithrombin III, causing a conformational change that accelerates the inhibition of thrombin and factor Xa. Unfractionated heparin is therefore an indirect thrombin inhibitor. Unfractionated heparin can only be administered intravenously. Low-molecular-weight heparins (LMWH) have a more predictable pharmacokinetic profile than the unfractionated heparin and can be administered subcutaneously. These heparins have a mechanism of action and use similar to unfractionated heparin.

The direct antithrombins decrease thrombin activity in a manner independent of any actions on antithrombin III. Two such direct antithrombins are lepirudin (also known as recombinant hirudin) and argatroban. These agents are highly specific, direct thrombin inhibitor with each molecule capable of binding to one molecule of thrombin and inhibiting its thrombogenic activity. Direct antithrombins are used for the prevention or reduction of ischemic complications associated with unstable angina.

Warfarin (Coumadin®) elicits its anticoagulant effect by interfering with the hepatic synthesis of vitamin K-dependent coagulation factors II, VII, IX, and X. Although warfarin appears to be somewhat effective after myocardial infarction in preventing death or recurrent myocardial infarction, its effectiveness in the treatment of acute coronary syndrome is questionable. Combination therapy with aspirin and heparin followed by warfarin has resulted in reduced incidence of recurrent angina, myocardial infarction, death, or all three at 14 days as compared with aspirin alone. In contrast, another study however failed to show any additional benefit in the treatment of acute coronary syndrome using a combination of aspirin and warfarin compared to aspirin alone.

Conventional Antianginal Therapy: Beta-Blockers, Nitrates, Calcium Channel Blockers

Current thinking is that there is a definite link between unstable angina and acute myocardial infarction. In this regard, beta-blockers are currently recommended as first-line agents in all acute coronary syndromes. A meta-analysis of studies involving 4700 patients with unstable angina demonstrated a 13% reduction in the risk of myocardial infarction among patients treated with beta-blockers. The various preparations of beta-blockers appear to have equal efficacy. The effects of beta-blockers are thought to be due to their ability to decrease myocardial oxygen demand.

Nitrates, such as nitroglycerin, are widely used in the management of unstable angina. Nitrates elicit a number of effects including a reduction in oxygen demand, arteriolar vasodilation, augmentation of collateral coronary blood flow and frequency of coronary vasospasm. Intravenous nitroglycerin is one of the first line therapies for unstable angina because of the ease of dose titration and the rapid resolution of effects. Continuous nitrate therapy with oral and transdermal patch preparations has resulted in tolerance to the beneficial effects of nitrates. A 6- to 8-hour daily nitrate-free interval will minimize the tolerance phenomenon. Also, supplemental use of vitamin C appears to prevent nitrate tolerance.

Calcium channel blockers such as nifedipine, verapamil, and diltiazem cause coronary vasodilation and reduced blood pressure. Because of these actions, the calcium channel blockers were thought to be a drug group which could be effective in the treatment of unstable angina. However, a meta analysis of studies in which patients with unstable angina were treated with calcium channel blockers found no effect of the drugs on the incidence of death or myocardial infarction. More recently, it has been shown that treatment with diltiazem and verapamil may result in increased survival and reduced rates of reinfarction in patients with acute coronary syndrome. Current thinking suggests that calcium channel blockers should be used in patients in whom beta-blockers are contraindicated or in those with refractory symptoms after treatments with aspirin, nitrates, or beta-blockers.

Dental Management

The dental management of the patient with angina pectoris may include sedation techniques for complicated procedures (see "Patients Requiring Sedation" *on page 1400*), to limit the extent of procedures, and to limit the use of local anesthesia containing 1:100,000 epinephrine to two carpules. Anesthesia without a vasoconstrictor might also be selected. The appropriate use of a vasoconstrictor in anesthesia, however, should be weighed against the necessity to maximize anesthesia. Complete history and appropriate referral and consultation with the patient's physician for those patients who are known to be at risk for angina pectoris is recommended.

MYOCARDIAL INFARCTION

Myocardial infarction is the leading cause of death in the United States. It is an acute irreversible ischemic event that produces an area of myocardial necrosis in the heart tissue. If a patient has a previous history of myocardial infarction, he/she may be taking a variety of drugs (ie, antihypertensives, lipid lowering drugs, ACE inhibitors, and antianginal medications) to not only prevent a second infarct, but to treat the long-term associated ischemic heart disease. Postmyocardial infarction patients are often taking anticoagulants such as warfarin and antiplatelet agents such as aspirin. Consultation with the prescribing physician by the dentist is necessary prior to invasive procedures. Temporary dose reduction may allow the dentist to proceed with very invasive procedures. Most procedures, however, can be accomplished without changing the anticoagulant therapy at all, using local hemostasis techniques.

Aspirin (various products) *on page 119*
Warfarin (Coumadin®) *on page 1250*

CARDIOVASCULAR DISEASES *(Continued)*

Thrombolytic drugs, that might dissolve hemostatic plugs, may also be given on a short-term basis immediately following an infarct and include:

Alteplase (Activase®) *on page 59*
Reteplase (Retavase™) *on page 1047*
Streptokinase (Kabikinase®; Streptase®) *on page 1109*
Tenecteplase (TNKase™) *on page 1138*

Alteplase [tissue plasminogen activator (TPA)] is also currently in use for acute myocardial infarction. Following myocardial infarction and rehabilitation, outpatients may be placed on anticoagulants (such as coumadin), diuretics, beta-adrenergic blockers, ACE inhibitors to reduce blood pressure, and calcium channel blockers. Depending on the presence or absence of continued angina pectoris, patients may also be taking nitrates, beta-blockers, or calcium channel blockers as indicated for treatment of angina.

BETA-ADRENERGIC BLOCKING AGENTS CATEGORIZED ACCORDING TO SPECIFIC PROPERTIES

Alpha-Adrenergic Blocking Activity

Labetalol (Normodyne®, Trandate®) *on page 680*

Intrinsic Sympathomimetic Activity

Acebutolol (Sectral®) *on page 25*
Pindolol (Visken®) *on page 960*

Long Duration of Action and Fewer CNS Effects

Acebutolol (Sectral®) *on page 25*
Atenolol (Tenormin®) *on page 125*
Betaxolol (Kerlone®) *on page 161*
Nadolol (Corgard®) *on page 839*

Beta$_1$-Receptor Selectivity

Acebutolol (Sectral®) *on page 25*
Atenolol (Tenormin®) *on page 125*
Metoprolol (Lopressor®, Toprol XL®) *on page 803*

Non-Selective (blocks both beta$_1$- and beta$_2$-receptors)

Betaxolol (Kerlone®) *on page 161*
Labetalol (Normodyne®, Trandate®) *on page 680*
Nadolol (Corgard®) *on page 839*
Pindolol (Visken®) *on page 960*
Propranolol (Inderal®) *on page 1016*
Timolol (Blocadren®) *on page 1170*

ARRHYTHMIAS

Abnormal cardiac rhythm can develop spontaneously and survivors of a myocardial infarction are often left with an arrhythmia. An arrhythmia is any alteration or disturbance in the normal rate, rhythm, or conduction through the cardiac tissue. This is known as a cardiac arrhythmia. Abnormalities in rhythm can occur in either the atria or the ventricles. Various valvular deformities, drug effects, and chemical derangements can initiate arrhythmias. These arrhythmias can be a slowing of the heart rate (<60 beats/minute) as defined in bradycardia or tachycardia resulting in a rapid heart beat (usually >150 beats/minute). The dentist will encounter a variety of treatments for management of arrhythmias. Usually, underlying causes such as reduced cardiac output, hypertension, and irregular ventricular beats will require treatment. Pacemaker therapy is also sometimes used. Indwelling pacemakers may require supplementation with antibiotics, and consultation with the physician is certainly appropriate. Sinus tachycardia is often treated with drugs such as:

Propranolol (Betachron ER®; Inderal®) *on page 1016*
Quinidine (Cardioquin®; Quinaglute®) *on page 1034*

Beta-blockers are often used to slow cardiac rate and diazepam may be helpful when anxiety is a contributing factor in arrhythmia. When atrial flutter and atrial fibrillation are diagnosed, drug therapy is usually required.

Digitoxin (Crystodigin®) *on page 388*
Digoxin (Lanoxin®) *on page 389*

Atrial fibrillation (AF) is an arrhythmia characterized by multiple electrical activations in the atria resulting in scattered and disorganized depolarization and repolarization of the myocardium. Atrial contraction can lead to an irregular and rapid rate of ventricular contraction. The prevalence of atrial fibrillation within the US population ranges between 1% and 4%, with the incidence increasing with age. It is often associated with rheumatic valvular disease and nonvalvular conditions including coronary artery disease and hypertension. Coronary artery disease is present in about one-half of the patients with atrial fibrillation. Atrial fibrillation is a major risk factor for systemic and cerebral embolism. It is thought that thrombi develop as a result of stasis in the dilated left atrium and is dislodged by sudden changes in cardiac rhythm. About 10% of all strokes in patients >60 years of age are caused by atrial fibrillation.

The cornerstones of drug therapy for atrial fibrillation are the restoration and maintenance of a normal sinus rhythm through the use of antiarrhythmic drugs, ventricular rate control through the use of beta-blockers, digitalis drugs or calcium channel blockers, and stroke prevention through the use of anticoagulants.

Antiarrhythmic Drugs

Cardiac rhythm is conducted through the sinoatrial (SA) and atrioventricular (AV) nodes, bundle branches, and Purkinje fibers. Electrical impulses are transmitted within this system by the opening and closing of sodium and potassium channels. Antiarrhythmic drugs are classified by which channel they act upon, a classification known as Vaughan Williams after the author of the published paper. The Class I agents act primarily on sodium channels, and the Class III agents act on potassium channels. In addition, there are subclassifications within the Class I agents according to effects of the drug on conduction and refractoriness within the Purkinje and ventricular tissues. Class IA agents show moderate depression of conduction and prolongation of repolarization. Class IB agents show modest depression of conduction and shortening of repolarization. Class IC agents show marked depression of conduction and mild or no effect on repolarization. Class IA and IC agents are effective in the treatment of atrial fibrillation. Class IB agents (ie, lidocaine, phenytoin) are not used to treat atrial fibrillation, but are effective in treating ventricular arrhythmias. Class II drugs are the beta-adrenergic blocking drugs and Class IV are the calcium channel blockers. Table 3 lists the drugs and the categories used to treat atrial fibrillation.

Table 3.
DRUGS USED IN THE TREATMENT OF ATRIAL FIBRILLATION

Class I Antiarrhythmic Agents
Disopyramide (Norpace®) *on page 403*
Flecainide (Tambocor®) *on page 505*
Moricizine (Ethmozine®) *on page 828*
Procainamide (Pronestyl®) *on page 997*
Propafenone (Rythmol®) *on page 1009*
Quinidine (Cardioquin®; Quinaglute®; Quinalan®; Quinidex®; Quinora®) *on page 1034*
Class II Antiarrhythmic Agents (Beta-Adrenergic Blockers)
Cardioselective (Beta$_1$-Receptor Block only)
Acebutolol (Sectral®) *on page 25*
Atenolol (Tenormin®) *on page 125*
Betaxolol (Kerlone®) *on page 161*
Metoprolol (Lopressor®) *on page 803*
Noncardioselective (Beta$_1$- and Beta$_2$-Receptor Block)
Nadolol (Corgard®) *on page 839*
Penbutolol (Levatol®) *on page 925*
Pindolol (Visken®) *on page 960*
Propranolol (Inderal®) *on page 1016*
Timolol (Blocadren®) *on page 1170*
Class III Antiarrhythmic Agents
Amiodarone (Cordarone®) *on page 72*
Dofetilide (Tikosyn™) *on page 408*
Ibutilide (Corvert®) *on page 623*
Sotalol (Betapace®) *on page 1102*
Class IV Antiarrhythmic Agents (Calcium Channel Blockers)
Diltiazem (Cardizem®) *on page 394*
Verapamil (Calan®) *on page 1236*
Miscellaneous Agents
Digitalis
Anticoagulants
Aspirin *on page 119*
Warfarin (Coumadin®) *on page 1250*

*Source: USP DI, Volumes I and II, Update, April, 1998.

Restoring and Maintaining Normal Sinus Rhythm

Cardioversion induced by drugs can usually restore sinus rhythm in patients with atrial fibrillation. Class I drugs (moricizine), Class IA drugs (disopyramide, procainamide, quinidine), Class IC drugs (flecainide, propafenone), and Class III antiarrhythmics (amiodarone, sotalol) are all effective in restoring normal sinus rhythm. Success rates may vary greatly and are complicated by the high rate of spontaneous conversion. The drugs used for pharmacologic conversion are also used to maintain sinus rhythm.

CARDIOVASCULAR DISEASES *(Continued)*

Ventricular Rate Control

It is accepted practice to treat patients with medication when the resting ventricular rate is >110 beats/minute. Digoxin, calcium channel blockers, and beta-adrenergic blockers are used in the regulation of ventricular rate. Digoxin increases the vagal tone to the AV node, calcium channel blockers slow the AV nodal conduction, and the beta-adrenergic blocking drugs decrease the sympathetic activation of the AV nodal conduction.

Stroke Prevention

Reports from stroke prevention trials indicate that patients with atrial fibrillation incurred a 4% annual risk of stroke if not treated. Also, patients with heart failure or coronary heart diseases were three times more likely to have a stroke than those without risk factors. Anticoagulation therapy with warfarin reduced the stroke risk by 64%. Warfarin was found to be more effective than aspirin in all age groups in the Stroke Prevention in Atrial Fibrillation II Trial. To achieve optimal levels of anticoagulation with the lowest incidence of bleeding, the INR (international normalized ratio) is usually maintained between 2 and 3. For patients <60 years of age with atrial fibrillation and having no other risk factors, no anticoagulant therapy is needed. Aspirin (325 mg daily) is recommended for those patients >60 years of age.

ANTICOAGULANT THERAPY

Many patients with ischemic heart disease, atherosclerosis, and those with atrial fibrillation are also frequently placed on anticoagulants such as Coumadin®. (See Myocardial Infarction *on page 1311.*)

Large numbers of patients are receiving oral anticoagulation therapy. The dental clinician is often faced with the decision as to how to manage these patients prior to invasive dental procedures. Key factors regarding the patient receiving anticoagulant therapy include: What is the bleeding risk of the procedure planned?, what are the clotting risks (ie, can the medication management be safely altered)?, and what is the patient's current anticoagulant therapy level in terms of bleeding measurements (ie, laboratory evaluations) and their prognosis? The International Normalized Ratio, or INR, is one of the most common coagulation values sought. The INR should be determined the day of the procedure if there is a high risk of bleeding.

Most patients receiving anticoagulant therapy are on one of two regimens. Warfarin, under the name Coumadin®, is the most common long-term outpatient anticoagulant given. Many patients, however, are also on aspirin products to achieve some level of anticoagulation. The mechanisms of the action of these two drugs are different and it is important that the clinician be aware of the appropriate tests and the appropriate time relative to treatment selection.

Partial thromboplastin time and bleeding time (IVY) are appropriate measures for platelet dysfunction. Aspirin, ticlopidine (Ticlid®), and other new drugs, such as Clopidogrel (Plavix®), are actually considered antiplatelet drugs, whereas oral Coumadin® is considered an oral anticoagulant. Aspirin works by inhibiting cyclo-oxygenase which is an enzyme involved in the platelet system associated with clot formation. As little as one aspirin (300 mg dose) can result in an alteration in this enzyme pathway. Although aspirin is cleared from the circulation very quickly (within 15-30 minutes), the effect on the life of the platelet may last up to 7-10 days. Therefore, the clinician planning an extensive invasive procedure on patients with antiplatelet therapy may wish to consider a change prior to one week before the invasive treatment. However, most routine dental procedures can be accomplished with no change in these medications using aggressive local hemostasis efforts and prudent treatment planning.

The effects of Coumadin® on the coagulation within patients, occur by way of the vitamin K-dependent clotting mechanism and are generally monitored by measuring the prothrombin time known as the PT. Often to prevent venous thrombosis, a patient will be maintained at approximately 1.5 times their normal prothrombin time. Other anticoagulant goals such as prevention of arterial thromboembolism, as in patients with artificial heart valves, may require 2-2.5 times the normal prothrombin time. It is important for the clinician to obtain not only the accurate PT but also the International Normalized Ratio (INR) for the patient. This ratio is calculated by dividing the patient's PT by the mean normal PT for the laboratory, which is determined by using the International Sensitivity Index (ISI) to adjust for the lab's reagents.

The response to oral anticoagulants varies greatly in patients and should be monitored regularly. The dental clinician planning an invasive procedure should consider not only what the patient can tell them from a historical point-of-view, but also when the last monitoring test was performed. In general, most dental procedures can be performed in patients that are 1.5 times normal or less. Most researchers suggest that 2.5 times normal poses little risk in most dental patients and procedures, but these values may be misleading unless the INR is also determined. When in doubt, the prudent dental clinician would consult with the patient's physician and obtain current prothrombin time and INR in order to evaluate fully and plan for his patients. The clinician is referred to the excellent review: Herman WW, Konzelman JL, and Sutley SH, "Current Perspectives on

Dental Patients Receiving Coumadin Anticoagulant Therapy," *J Am Dent Assoc*, 1997, 128:327-35.

Coumadin®-like Anticoagulants

Dicumarol *on page 381*
Warfarin (Coumadin®) *on page 1250*

Platelet Aggregation Inhibitors

Aspirin (various products) *on page 119*
Clopidogrel (Plavix®) *on page 310*
Eptifibatide (Integrillin®) *on page 445*
Ticlopidine (Ticlid®) *on page 1168*
Tirofiban (Aggrastat®) *on page 1173*

Anticoagulant, Other

Lepirudin (Refludan®) *on page 689*

Antiplatelet Agent

Aspirin and Extended-Release Dipyridamole *on page 123*

Although not used specifically for this purpose, numerous herbal medicines and natural dietary supplements have been associated with inhibition of platelet aggregation or other anticoagulation effects, and therefore may lead to increased bleeding during invasive dental procedures. Current reports include bilberry, bromelain, cat's claw, devil's claw, dong quai, evening primrose, feverfew, garlic (irreversible inhibition), ginger (only at very high doses), ginkgo biloba, ginseng, grape seed, green tea, horse chestnut, and turmeric.

The basis for anticoagulation therapy is that mitral stenosis may be the result of the long-term arrhythmia and there is concern over the possibility of stroke. Ventricular dysrhythmias are often treated with drugs such as quinidine, procainamide, lidocaine, and beta-adrenergic agents. Quinidine is used for selected arrhythmias. Lidocaine is often used when there are ventricular dysrhythmias. Procainamide (Pronestyl®) is an alternative agent.

Over the past three decades, there has been an increasing use of drugs that relate to the clotting mechanism in patients. These drugs have included the widespread use of aspirin as well as an increasing use of the anticoagulant found in warfarin or Coumadin®. Also, there has been increasing evidence that more patients have a gastrointestinal sensitivity to aspirin. Therefore, alternative analgesics such as acetaminophen and the NSAID products have expanded in utilization tremendously. These factors resulted in numerous potential drug interactions that, until now, have been thought to be quite innocuous. The use of acetaminophen, which is primarily for analgesic and antipyretic properties, has increased dramatically. The drug is available as an over-the-counter medication for a wide range of nonspecific conditions and, in fact, in the United States, acetaminophen is the most frequently ingested medication.

Regarding dental management patients that are already taking warfarin, the use of analgesics is implicated as a potential source of drug interaction. In a recent article by Hayek in *JAMA*, it was found that patients taking warfarin for anticoagulation identified the use of dangerously elevated INRs and the fact was discovered that they concomitantly had been taking acetaminophen (not necessarily with their physician's recommendation). The study of the international normalized ratio (INR) in these patients has indicated that additional factors independently influence the INR, as well as the potential interaction with acetaminophen. Potential effects on the INR are greatest in patients taking acetaminophen at high doses over a protracted time period. Short term pain management with acetaminophen poses little risk. These factors included advanced malignancy, patients who did not take their warfarin properly (therefore, took more than was necessary), changes in oral intake of liquids or solids, acute diarrhea leading to dehydration, alcohol consumption, and vitamin K intake. The mechanisms of these augmenting factors for enhancement of the INR are that the cytochrome P450 system, present in the liver, is also affected by changes in metabolism associated with these factors. For instance, the metabolism of alcohol in the liver alters its ability to manage the CYP450 enzyme system necessary for warfarin, therefore, enhancing its presence and potentially increasing the half-life of warfarin. As oral intake of nutrients declines in patients with either diarrhea or reduced intake of liquids and/or solids, absorption of vitamin K is reduced and the vitamin K dependent system of metabolism of warfarin changes, therefore increasing warfarin blood levels. These factors, along with the liver metabolism of acetaminophen, have resulted in the increased concern that patients, who may be taking acetaminophen as an analgesic or for other reasons, may be at risk for enhancing or elevating, inadvertently, their anticoagulation effect of warfarin. The dentist should be aware of this potential interaction in prescribing any drug containing acetaminophen or in recommending that a patient use an analgesic for relief of even mild pain on a prolonged basis. Therefore, the dentist must be concerned with these factors and is referred to the discussion in the Pain Management section *on page 1360* for more consideration (adapted from *JAMA*, March 4, 1998, Vol 279, No 9).

Acetaminophen *on page 26*

CARDIOVASCULAR DISEASES *(Continued)*

HEART FAILURE

Heart failure is a condition in which the heart is unable to pump sufficient blood to meet the needs of the body. It is caused by impaired ability of the cardiac muscle to contract or by an increased workload imposed on the heart. Most frequently, the underlying cause of heart failure is coronary artery disease. Other contributory causes include hypertension, diabetes, idiopathic dilated cardiomyopathy, and valvular heart disease. It is estimated that heart failure affects approximately 5 million Americans. The New York Heart Association functional classification is regarded as the standard measure to describe the severity of a patient's symptom. Class I is characterized by having no limitation of physical activity. There is no dyspnea, fatigue, palpitations, or angina with ordinary physical activity. There is no objective evidence of cardiovascular dysfunction. Class II includes those patients having slight limitation of physical activity. These patients experience fatigue, palpitations, dyspnea, or angina with ordinary physical activity, but are comfortable at rest. There is evidence of minimal cardiovascular dysfunction. Class III is characterized by marked limitation of activity. Less than ordinary physical activity causes fatigue, palpitations, dyspnea, or angina, but patients are comfortable at rest. There is objective evidence of moderately severe cardiovascular dysfunction. Class IV is characterized by the inability to carry out any physical activity without discomfort. Symptoms of heart failure or anginal syndrome may be present even at rest, and any physical activity undertaken increases discomfort. There is objective evidence of severe cardiovascular dysfunction. Drug classes and the specific agents used to treat heart failure are listed in Table 4.

Table 4.
DRUGS USED IN THE TREATMENT OF HEART FAILURE

Angiotensin-Converting Enzyme Inhibitors (ACE)*
- Benazepril (Lotensin®) *on page 149*
- Captopril (Capoten®) *on page 213*
- Enalapril (Vasotec®) *on page 432*
- Fosinopril (Monopril®) *on page 539*
- Lisinopril (Prinivil®) *on page 719*
- Perindopril Ethumine (Aceon®) *on page 939*
- Quinapril (Accupril®) *on page 1031*
- Ramipril (Altace™) *on page 1040*
- Trandolapril (Mavik®) *on page 1189*

Diuretics
- **Thiazides**
  - Hydrochlorothiazide (HydroDIURIL®) *on page 595*
- **Loop Diuretics**
  - Furosemide (Lasix®) *on page 544*
- **Potassium-Sparing Agents**
  - Spironolactone (Aldactone®) *on page 1106*

Digitalis Glycosides
- Digoxin (Lanoxin®) *on page 389*
- Digitoxin (Crystodigin®) *on page 388*

Beta-Adrenergic Receptor Blockers
- Bisoprolol (Zebeta®) *on page 168*
- Carvedilol (Coreg®) *on page 227*
- Metoprolol (Lopressor®, Toprol XL®) *on page 803*

Catecholamines
- Dobutamine (Dobutrex®) *on page 405*
- Dopamine

Supplemental Agents
- **Direct-Acting Vasodilators**
  - Hydralazine (Apresoline®) *on page 593*
  - Nitroglycerin *on page 871*
  - Nitroprusside (Nitropress®) *on page 872*
- **Phosphodiesterase Inhibitors**
  - Inamrinone (Inocor®) *on page 631*
  - Milrinone (Primacor®) *on page 815*

*Regarded as the cornerstone of treatment of heart failure and should be used routinely and early in all patients.

From USP DI, Volumes I and II, Update, December 1998.

Drug Classes and Specific Agents Used to Treat Heart Failure

Angiotensin-converting enzyme (ACE) inhibitors reduce left ventricular volume and filling pressure while decreasing total peripheral resistance. They induce cardiac output (modestly) and natriuresis. ACE inhibitors are usually used in all patients with heart failure if no contraindication or intolerance exists. This group of drugs is considered the cornerstone of treatment and are used routinely and early if pharmacologic treatment is indicated.

Diuretics increase sodium chloride and water excretion resulting in reduction of preload, thus relieving the symptoms of pulmonary congestion associated with heart failure. They may also reduce myocardial oxygen demand. The thiazides, loop diuretics, and potassium-sparing agents are all useful in reducing preload by way of their diuretic actions.

Digitalis glycosides have been used in the treatment of heart failure for more than 200 years. Digitalis drugs increase cardiac output by a direct positive inotropic action on the myocardium. This increased cardiac output results in decreased venous pressure, reduced heart size, and diminished compensatory tachycardia.

Beta-adrenergic receptor blocking drugs (beta-blockers) are used in the treatment of heart failure because of their beneficial effect in reducing mortality. A meta-analysis of randomized clinical trials showed that the beta-blockers significantly reduced all causes of cardiac-related deaths, with carvedilol (Coreg®) showing the greatest efficacy. The overall risk of death was reduced by over 30%.

Other drugs used in the treatment of heart failure are referred to as supplemental agents. The direct-acting vasodilators reduce excessive vasoconstriction and reduce workload of the failing heart. The catecholamines and phosphodiesterase inhibitors are alternative agents with positive inotropic effects, are effective for short-term therapy, and have not been demonstrated to prolong life during long-term therapy.

Treatment of arrhythmias often can result in oral manifestations including oral ulcerations with drugs such as procainamide, lupus-like lesions, as well as xerostomia.

HYPERTENSION

In the United States, almost 50 million adults, 25-74 years of age, have hypertension. Hypertension is defined as systolic blood pressure ≥140 mm Hg, and/or diastolic pressure >90 mm Hg. People with blood pressure above normal are considered at increased risk of developing damage to the heart, kidney, brain, and eyes, resulting in premature morbidity and mortality. Individuals with high normal blood pressure (systolic blood pressure of 130-139 mm Hg and diastolic blood pressure of 85-89 mm Hg) should be monitored and encouraged to reduce blood pressure by nondrug measures which include weight control, restriction of sodium and alcohol, and participation in an exercise program. Stage 1 hypertension is blood pressure of 140-159/90-99 mm Hg. If the desired blood pressure is not achieved with nondrug measures within 6 months in patients with stage 1 hypertension (without target organ disease and/or clinical cardiovascular disease), pharmacologic therapy is suggested.

The suggested initial goals of drug therapy are the maintenance of an arterial pressure of ≤140/90 mm Hg with concurrent control of other modifiable cardiovascular risk factors. Further reduction to 130/85 mm Hg should be pursued if cardiovascular and cerebrovascular function is not compromised. The Hypertension Optimal Treatment (HOT) randomized trial using patients 50-80 years of age found that the lowest incidence of major cardiovascular events and the lowest risk of cardiovascular mortality occurred at a mean diastolic blood pressure of 82.6 and 86.5 mm Hg respectively.

Table 5.
CLASSIFICATION OF BLOOD PRESSURE FOR ADULTS ≥18 YEARS OF AGE*

Category	Systolic (mm Hg)		Diastolic (mm Hg)
Optimal†	<120	and	<80
Normal	<130	and	<85
High-Normal	130-139	or	85-89
Hypertension‡			
Stage 1	140-159	or	90-99
Stage 2	160-179	or	100-109
Stage 3	≥180	or	≥110

*Not taking antihypertensive drugs and not acutely ill. When systolic and diastolic blood pressures fall into different categories, the higher category should be selected to classify the individual's blood pressure status. For example, 160/92 mm Hg should be classified as stage 2 hypertension, and 174/120 mm Hg should be classified as stage 3 hypertension. Isolated systolic hypertension is defined as SBP of 140 mm Hg or greater and DBP below 90 mm Hg and staged appropriately (ie, 170/82 mm Hg is defined as stage 2 isolated systolic hypertension). In addition to classifying stages of hypertension on the basis of average blood pressure levels, clinicians should specify presence or absence of target organ disease and additional risk factors. The specificity is important for risk classification and treatment.

†Optimal blood pressure with respect to cardiovascular risk is below 120/80 mm Hg. However, unusually low readings should be evaluated for clinical significance.

‡Based on the average of two or more readings taken at each of two or more visits after an initial screening.

CARDIOVASCULAR DISEASES *(Continued)*

Table 6.
RECOMMENDATIONS FOR FOLLOW-UP BASED ON INITIAL BLOOD PRESSURE MEASUREMENTS FOR ADULTS

Initial Blood Pressure (mm Hg)*		Follow-Up Recommended†
Systolic	**Diastolic**	
<130	<85	Recheck in 2 years
130-139	85-89	Recheck in 1 year‡
140-159	90-99	Confirm within 2 months‡
160-179	100-109	Evaluate or refer to source of care within 1 month
≥180	≥110	Evaluate or refer to source of care immediately or within 1 week depending on clinical situation

*If systolic and diastolic categories are different, follow recommendations for shorter time follow-up (eg, 160/86 mm Hg should be evaluated or referred to source of care within 1 month).

†Modify the scheduling of follow-up according to reliable information about past blood pressure measurements, other cardiovascular risk factors, or target organ disease.

‡Provide advice about lifestyle modifications.

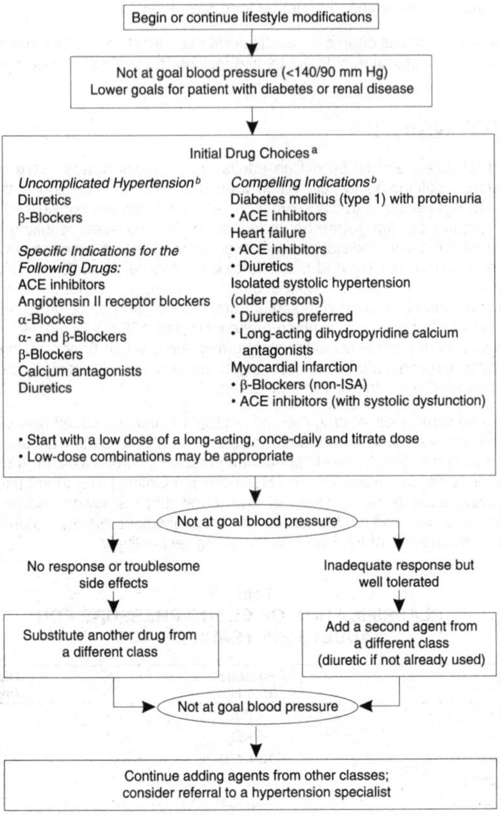

[a] Unless contraindicated. ACE indicates angiotensin-converting enzyme; ISA, intrinsic sympathomimetic activity.
[b] Based on randomized controlled trials.

Adapted from "The Sixth Report of the Joint National Committee on Prevention, Detection, Evaluation, and Treatment of High Blood Pressure," Arch Intern Med, 1997, 157(21):2413-46.

CLASSES OF DRUGS USED IN THE TREATMENT OF HYPERTENSION

- Diuretics
- Beta-adrenergic receptor blocking agents (beta-blockers)
- $Alpha_1$-adrenergic receptor blocking agents ($alpha_1$-blockers)
- Agents which have both alpha- and beta-adrenergic blocking properties (alpha-/beta-blockers)
- Angiotensin-converting enzyme (ACE) inhibitors
- Angiotensin II receptor blockers
- Calcium channel blocking agents
- Supplemental agents such as central-acting $alpha_2$-adrenergic receptor agonists and direct-acting peripheral vasodilators.

Table 7 lists the drug categories and representative agents used to treat hypertension. Combination drugs are now available to supply several classes of these drugs.

Table 7. DRUG CATEGORIES AND REPRESENTATIVE AGENTS USED IN THE TREATMENT OF HYPERTENSION*

Diuretics

Thiazide Types

- Bendroflumethiazide (Naturetin®) *on page 150*
- Chlorothiazide (Diurigen®, Diuril®) *on page 267*
- Chlorthalidone (Hygroton®) *on page 277*
- Hydrochlorothiazide (Esidrix®) *on page 595*
- Indapamide (Lozol®) *on page 632*
- Methyclothiazide (Aquatensen®, Enduron®) *on page 792*
- Metolazone (Mykrox®, Zaroxolyn®) *on page 801*
- Polythiazide (Renese®) *on page 972*
- Quinethazone (Hydromox®) *on page 1033*
- Trichlormethiazide (Metahydrin®; Naqua®) *on page 1202*

Loops

- Bumetanide (Bumex®) *on page 183*
- Ethacrynic Acid (Edecrin®) *on page 471*
- Furosemide (Lasix®) *on page 544*
- Torsemide (Demadex®) *on page 1185*

Potassium-Sparing

- Amiloride (Midamor®) *on page 67*
- Spironolactone (Aldactone®) *on page 1106*
- Triamterene (Dyrenium®) *on page 1200*

Potassium-Sparing Combinations

- Hydrochlorothiazide and Spironolactone (Aldactazide®) *on page 596*
- Hydrochlorothiazide and Triamterene (Dyazide®) *on page 597*

Beta-Blockers

Cardioselective

- Acebutolol (Sectral®) *on page 25*
- Atenolol (Tenormin®) *on page 125*
- Betaxolol (Kerlone®) *on page 161*
- Bisoprolol (Zebeta™) *on page 168*
- Metoprolol (Lopressor®) *on page 803*
- Sotalol (Betapace®) *on page 1102*

Noncardioselective

- Carteolol (Cartrol®) *on page 226*
- Carvedilol (Coreg®) *on page 227*
- Nadolol (Corgard®) *on page 839*
- Penbutolol (Levatol®) *on page 925*
- Pindolol (Visken®) *on page 960*
- Propranolol (Inderal®) *on page 1016*
- Timolol (Blocadren®) *on page 1170*

$Alpha_1$-Blocker

- Doxazosin (Cardura®) *on page 413*
- Guanadrel (Hylorel®) *on page 572*
- Guanethidine (Ismelin®) *on page 573*
- Prazosin (Minipress®) *on page 986*
- Reserpine (Serpalan®, Serpasil®) *on page 1046*
- Terazosin (Hytrin®) *on page 1140*

Alpha-/Beta-Blocker

- Carvedilol (Coreg®) *on page 227*
- Labetalol (Normodyne®, Trandate®) *on page 680*

CARDIOVASCULAR DISEASES *(Continued)*

Angiotensin-Converting Enzyme (ACE) Inhibitors
- Benazepril (Lotensin®) *on page 149*
- Captopril (Capoten®) *on page 213*
- Enalapril (Vasotec®) *on page 432*
- Fosinopril (Monopril®) *on page 539*
- Lisinopril (Prinivil®) *on page 719*
- Moexipril (Univasc®) *on page 824*
- Quinapril (Accupril®) *on page 1031*
- Ramipril (Altace™) *on page 1040*
- Trandolapril (Mavik®) *on page 1189*

Angiotensin-Converting Enzyme (ACE) Inhibitor/Diuretic Combination
- Captopril and Hydrochlorothiazide (Capozide®) *on page 214*
- Enalapril and Hydrochlorothiazide (Vasoretic®) *on page 434*
- Lisinopril and Hydrochlorothiazide (Zestoretic®) *on page 721*

Angiotensin II Receptor Blockers
- Candesartan (Atacand™) *on page 208*
- Eprosartan (Teveten®) *on page 445*
- Irbesartan (Avapro®) *on page 653*
- Losartan (Cozaar®) *on page 732*
- Telmisartan (Micardis®) *on page 1134*
- Valsartan (Diovan®) *on page 1230*

Angiotensin II Receptor Blocker/Diuretic Combination
- Candesartan (Atacand™) + HCTZ *on page 208*
- Irbesartan (Avalide®) + HCTZ *on page 208*
- Valsartan/HCTZ (Diovan®) + HCTZ *on page 1230*

Calcium Channel Blockers
- Amlodipine (Norvasc®) *on page 81*
- Bepridil (Vascor®) *on page 156*
- Diltiazem (Cardizem®, Dilacor™ XR) *on page 394*
- Felodipine (Plendil®) *on page 489*
- Isradipine (DynaCirc®) *on page 665*
- Nicardipine (Cardene®) *on page 862*
- Nifedipine (Adalat®, Procardia®) *on page 865*
- Nisoldipine (Sular™) *on page 868*
- Verapamil (Calan®) *on page 1236*

Supplemental Agents

Central-Acting Alpha$_2$-Agonist
- Clonidine (Catapres®) *on page 308*
- Guanabenz (Wytensin®) *on page 571*
- Guanfacine (Tenex®) *on page 574*
- Methyldopa (Aldomet®) *on page 793*

Direct-Acting Peripheral Vasodilator
- Hydralazine (Apresoline®) *on page 593*
- Minoxidil (Loniten®) *on page 818*

*Source: USP DI, Volumes I and II, Update, November 1998.

Current Thinking Regarding Antihypertensive Drug Selection

Medications in the first eight categories in Table 7 were held to be equally effective in two large-scale studies reported in the *New England Journal of Medicine* and the *Journal of the American Medical Association*, and that any of the medications could be used initially for monotherapy. According to the Sixth Report of the Joint National Committee on Prevention, Detection, Evaluation, and Treatment of High Blood Pressure (JNC VI), diuretics or beta-blockers are recommended as initial therapy for uncomplicated hypertension. If a diuretic is selected as initial therapy, a thiazide diuretic is preferred in patients with normal renal function. If necessary, potassium replacement or concurrent treatment with a potassium-sparing agent may prevent hypokalemia. Loop diuretics are used in patients with impaired renal function or who cannot tolerate thiazides. Diuretics are well tolerated and inexpensive. They are considered the drugs of choice for treating isolated systolic hypertension in the elderly.

Beta-blockers are the agents of choice in patients with coronary artery disease or supraventricular arrhythmia, and in young patients with hyperdynamic circulation. Beta-blockers are alternatives for initial therapy and are more effective in Caucasian patients than in African-American patients. Beta-blockers are not considered first choice drugs in elderly patients with uncomplicated hypertension. The beta-blocking drug carvedilol also selectively blocks alpha$_1$ receptors and has been shown to reduce mortality in hypertensive patients.

Alpha$_1$-adrenergic blocking agents can be used as initial therapy. The alpha$_1$-blocking agent prazosin and related drugs have an added advantage in treating hypertensive patients with coexisting hyperlipidemia since these medications seem to have beneficial effects on lipid levels. Selective blockade of the post-synaptic alpha$_1$-receptors by prazosin and related agents reduces peripheral vascular resistance and systemic blood pressure. In addition, all alpha$_1$-adrenergic blocking agents relieve symptoms of benign prostatic hyperplasia.

ACE inhibitors are the preferred drugs for patients with coexisting heart failure. They are useful as initial therapy in hypertensive patients with kidney damage or diabetes mellitus with proteinuria, and in Caucasian patients. No clinically relevant differences have been found among the available ACE inhibitors. The ACE inhibitors are well tolerated by young, physically active patients, and the elderly. The most common adverse effect of the ACE inhibitors is dry cough. Angiotensin II receptor blockers produce hemodynamic effects similar to ACE inhibitors while avoiding dry cough. These agents are similar to the ACE inhibitors in potency and are useful for initial therapy.

Calcium channel blocking agents are effective as initial therapy in both African-American and Caucasian patients, and are well tolerated by the elderly. These agents inhibit entry of calcium ion into cardiac cells and smooth muscle cells of the coronary and systemic vasculature. Nifedipine (Procardia®) and amlodipine (Norvasc®) are more potent as peripheral vasodilators than diltiazem (Cardizem®). Long-acting formulations of the calcium channel blockers have been shown to be very safe despite some earlier reports that short-acting calcium channel blockers were associated with a 60% increase in heart attacks among hypertensive patients given a short-acting calcium antagonist.

Supplemental antihypertensive agents include the central-acting alpha$_2$ agonists and direct-acting vasodilators. These agents are less commonly prescribed for initial therapy because of the impressive effectiveness of the other drug groups. Clonidine (Catapres®) lowers blood pressure by activating inhibitory alpha$_2$ receptors in the CNS, thus reducing sympathetic outflow. It lowers both supine and standing blood pressure by reducing total peripheral resistance. Hydralazine (Apresoline®) reduces blood pressure by directly relaxing arteriolar smooth muscle. Hydralazine is given orally for the management of chronic hypertension, usually with a diuretic and a beta-blocker.

The most common oral side effects of the management of the hypertensive patient are related to the antihypertensive drug therapy. A dry sore mouth can be caused by diuretics and central-acting adrenergic inhibitors. Occasionally, lichenoid reactions can occur in patients taking quinidine and methyldopa. The thiazides are occasionally also implicated. Lupus-like face rashes can be seen in patients taking calcium channel blockers as well as documented in Calcium Channel Blockers & Gingival Hyperplasia *on page 1432* of the Appendix.

Table 8.
CARDIOVASCULAR / RESPIRATORY / NERVOUS SYSTEM EFFECTS CAUSED BY DRUGS USED FOR CARDIOVASCULAR DISORDERS*

Agent	Incidence	Adverse Effect
Alpha$_1$-Blocker		
Prazosin (Minipress®)	More frequent	Orthostatic hypotension, dizziness
	Less frequent	Heart Palpitations
	Rare	Angina
Alpha-/Beta-Blocker		
Carvedilol (Coreg®)	More frequent	Bradycardia, postural hypotension, dizziness
	Rare	A-V block, hypertension, hypotension, palpitations, vertigo, nervousness, asthma
Angiotensin-Converting Enzyme (ACE) Inhibitors		
Benazepril (Lotensin®)	Less frequent	Dizziness, insomnia, headache
	Rare	Hypotension, bronchitis
Captopril (Capoten®)	Less frequent	Tachycardia, insomnia, transient cough, dizziness, headache
	Rare	Hypotension
Enalapril (Vasotec®)	Less frequent	Chest pain, palpitations, tachycardia, syncope, dizziness, dyspnea
	Rare	Angina pectoris, asthma
Fosinopril (Monopril®)	Less frequent	Orthostatic hypotension, dizziness, cough, headache
	Rare	Syncope, insomnia
Lisinopril (Prinivil®)	Less frequent	Hypotension, dizziness
	Rare	Angina pectoris, orthostatic hypotension, rhythm disturbances, tachycardia
Moexipril (Univasc®)	Less frequent	Hypotension, peripheral edema, headache, dizziness, fatigue, cough, pharyngitis, upper respiratory infection, sinusitis
	Rare	Chest pain, myocardial infarction, palpitations, arrhythmias, syncope, CVA, orthostatic hypotension, dyspnea, bronchospasm
Perindopril (Aceon®)	Less frequent	Headache, dizziness, cough†
	Rare	Hypotension
Quinapril (Accupril®)	Less frequent	Hypotension, dizziness, headache, cough
	Rare	Orthostatic hypotension, angina, insomnia
Ramipril (Altace®)	Less frequent	Tachycardia, dizziness, headache, cough
	Rare	Hypotension

CARDIOVASCULAR DISEASES *(Continued)*

Agent	Incidence	Adverse Effect
Trandolapril (Mavril®)	*Less frequent* *Rare*	Tachycardia, headache, dizziness, cough‡ Hypotension
Angiotensin-Converting Enzyme Inhibitor/Diuretic Combination		
Captopril/HCTZ (Capozide®)	*Less frequent* *Rare*	Tachycardia, palpitations, chest pain, dizziness Hypotension
Angiotensin II Receptor Blockers		
Candesartan (Atacand®)	*Less frequent* *Rare*	Chest pain, flushing Myocardial infarction, tachycardia, angina, palpitations, dyspnea
Losartan (Cozaar®)	*Less frequent* *Rare*	Hypotension without reflex tachycardia, dizziness Orthostatic hypotension, angina, A-V block (second degree), CVA, palpitations, tachycardia, sinus bradycardia, flushing, dyspnea
Angiotensin II Receptor Blocker/Diuretic Combination		
Candesartan (Atacand™ HCT) + HCTZ	*Less frequent* *Rare*	Chest pain, flushing Myocardial infarction, tachycardia, angina, palpitations, dyspnea
Irbesartan/HCTZ (Avalide®)		Effects unavailable
Valsartan/HCTZ (Diovan™ HCT)		Effects unavailable
Antiplatelet/Anticoagulant Agents		
Abciximab (ReoPro®)	*More frequent* *Less frequent*	Hypotension, pain Bradycardia
Aspirin	*Less frequent or Rare*	Anaphylactoid reaction, bronchospastic allergic reaction
Clopidogrel (Plavix®)	*Less frequent*	Chest pain, edema, hypertension, headache, dizziness, depression, fatigue, dyspnea, rhinitis, bronchitis, coughing, upper respiratory infection, syncope, palpitations, cardiac failure, paresthesia, vertigo, atrial fibrillation, neuralgia
Eptifibatide (Integrilin®)	*More frequent*	Hypotension, bleeding
Ticlopidine (Ticlid®)	*Less frequent* *Rare*	Dizziness Peripheral neuropathy, angioedema, vasculitis, allergic pneumonitis
Tirofiban (Aggrastat®)	*More frequent* *Less frequent*	Bleeding Bradycardia, dizziness, headache
Warfarin (Coumadin®)	*Less frequent* *Rare*	Hemoptysis Fever, purple toes syndrome
Beta-Blockers		
Acebutolol (Sectral®)	*Less frequent* *Rare*	Chest pain, bradycardia, hypotension, dizziness, dyspepsia, dyspnea Ventricular arrhythmias
Atenolol (Tenormin®)	*Less frequent* *Rare*	Bradycardia, hypotension, chest pain, dizziness, dyspepsia, dyspnea Ventricular arrhythmias
Betaxolol (Kerlone®)	*Less frequent* *Rare*	Bradycardia, palpitations, dizziness Chest pain
Bisoprolol (Zebeta®)	*More frequent* *Less frequent*	Lethargy Hypotension, chest pain, bradycardia, headache, dizziness, insomnia, cough
Labetalol (Normodyne®, Trandate®)	*Less frequent* *Rare*	Orthostatic hypotension, dizziness, nasal congestion Bradycardia, chest pain
Metoprolol (Lopressor®)	*More frequent* *Less frequent* *Rare*	Dizziness Bradycardia, heartburn, wheezing Chest pain, confusion
Nadolol (Corgard®)	*More frequent* *Less frequent* *Rare*	Bradycardia Dizziness, dyspepsia, wheezing Congestive heart failure, orthostatic hypotension, confusion, paresthesia
Penbutolol (Levatol®)	*Less frequent* *Rare*	Congestive heart failure, dizziness Bradycardia, chest pain, hypotension, confusion
Pindolol (Visken®)	*More frequent* *Less frequent*	Dizziness Congestive heart failure, dyspnea
Propranolol (Inderal®)	*More frequent* *Less frequent* *Rare*	Bradycardia Congestive heart failure, dizziness, wheezing Chest pain, hypotension, bronchospasm
Timolol (Blocadren®)	*Less frequent* *Rare*	Bradycardia, dizziness, dyspnea Chest pain, congestive heart failure

Agent	Incidence	Adverse Effect
Calcium Channel Blockers		
Amlodipine (Norvasc®)	Less frequent	Palpitations, dizziness, dyspnea
	Rare	Hypotension, bradycardia, arrhythmias
Diltiazem (Cardizem®)	Less frequent	Bradycardia, dizziness
	Rare	Dyspepsia, paresthesia, tremor
Nifedipine (Procardia®)	More frequent	Flushing, dizziness
	Less frequent	Palpitations, hypotension, dyspnea
	Rare	Tachycardia, syncope
Verapamil (Calan®)	Less frequent	Bradycardia, congestive heart failure, hypotension
	Rare	Chest pain, hypotension (excessive)
Class I Antiarrhythmics		
Disopyramide (Norpace®)	More frequent	Exacerbation of angina pectoris, dizziness
	Less frequent	Hypotension, hypertension, tachycardia, dyspnea
	Rare	Syncope, flushing, hyperventilation
Flecainide (Tambocor®)	More frequent	Dizziness, dyspnea
	Less frequent	Palpitations, chest pain, tachycardia, tremor
	Rare	Bradycardia, nervousness, paresthesia
Procainimide (Pronestyl®)	Less frequent	Tachycardia, dizziness, lightheadedness
	Rare	Hypotension, confusion, disorientation
Propafenone (Rythmol®)	More frequent	Dizziness
	Less frequent	Palpitations, angina, bradycardia, loss of balance, dyspepsia, dyspnea
	Rare	Paresthesia
Quinidine (Quinaglute®)	Less frequent	Hypotension, syncope, lightheadedness, wheezing
	Rare	Confusion, vertigo, angina, edema
Class III Antiarrhythmics		
Amiodarone (Cordarone®)	More frequent	Dizziness, tremor, paresthesia, dyspnea
	Less frequent	Congestive heart failure, bradycardia, tachycardia
	Rare	Hypotension
Sotalol (Betapace®)	More frequent	Bradycardia, chest pain, palpitations, fatigue, dizziness, lightheadedness, dyspnea
	Less frequent	CHF, hypotension, proarrhythmia, syncope, reduced peripheral circulation, edema, asthma, upper respiratory problems
	Rare	Diaphoresis, clouded sensorium, fever, lack of coordination
Digitalis Glycosides		
Digoxin (Lanoxicaps®, Lanoxin®) Digitoxin (Digitaline®-Canada)	Rare	Atrial tachycardia, sinus bradycardia, ventricular fibrillation, vertigo
Diuretics		
Thiazide type	Rare	Hypotension
Loops	More frequent	Orthostatic hypotension, dizziness
Potassium-sparing	Less frequent	Hypotension, bradycardia, dizziness
	Rare	Flushing
Potassium-sparing combination	Rare	Dizziness
HMG-CoA Reductase Inhibitors		
Atorvastatin Cerivastatin Fluvastatin Lovastatin Pravastatin Simvastatin	Less frequent	Headache, dizziness
Nitrates		
Nitroglycerins	More frequent	Postural hypotension, flushing, headache, dizziness
	Rare	Reflex tachycardia, bradycardia, arrhythmia
Supplemental Drugs for Heart Failure		
Amrinone (Inocor®)	Less frequent	Arrhythmia, chest pain
Dobutamine (Dobutrex®)	Less frequent	Tachycardia, chest pain
	Rare	Headache, dyspnea
Hydralazine (Apresoline®)	More frequent	Tachycardia, headache
	Less frequent	Hypotension, nasal congestion
	Rare	Edema, dizziness
Milrinone (Primacor®)	More frequent	Arrhythmias
	Less frequent	Chest pain
Nitroprusside sodium (Nitropress®)	Less frequent	Palpitations, headache

CARDIOVASCULAR DISEASES *(Continued)*

Agent	Incidence	Adverse Effect
Supplemental Drugs for Hypertension		
Central-Acting Alpha$_2$-Agonists		
Clonidine (Catapres®)	*More frequent*	Dizziness
	Less frequent	Orthostatic hypotension, nervousness/agitation
	Rare	Palpitations, tachycardia, bradycardia, congestive heart failure
Direct-Acting		
Hydralazine (Apresoline®)	*More frequent*	Tachycardia, headache
	Less frequent	Hypotension, nasal congestion
	Rare	Edema, dizziness

Legend: % of Incidence: More frequent = >10%, Less frequent = 1% to 10%, Rare = <1%

*Source: Professional package insert for individual agents or United States Pharmacopeial Dispensing Information. *Drug Information for the Health Care Professional*, Vol I, 19th ed, Rockville, MD: The United States Pharmacopeial Convention, Inc, 1999.

†Incidence greater in women 3:1.

‡More frequent in women.

Table 9.
CARDIOVASCULAR DRUGS DENTAL DRUG INTERACTIONS AND EFFECTS ON DENTAL TREATMENT

Alpha$_1$-Blocker	
Prazosin (Minipress®)	Significant orthostatic hypotension a possibility; monitor patient when getting out of dental chair; significant dry mouth in up to 10% of patients.
Alpha-/Beta-Blocker	
Carvedilol (Coreg®)	See Nonselective Beta-Blockers
ACE Inhibitors	The NSAID indomethacin reduces the hypotensive effects of ACE inhibitors. Effects of other NSAIDs such as ibuprofen not considered significant.
Angiotensin-Converting Enzyme Inhibitor/Diuretic Combination	
Captopril/HCTZ (Capozide®)	No effect or complications on dental treatment reported.
Angiotensin II Receptor Blockers	
Candesartan (Atacand®)	No effect or complications on dental treatment reported.
Losartan (Cozaar®)	
Antiplatelet/Anticoagulant Agents	
Aspirin	May cause a reduction in the serum levels of NSAIDs if they are used to manage post-operative pain.
Clopidogrel (Plavix®)	If a patient is to undergo elective surgery and an antiplatelet effect is not desired, clopidogrel should be discontinued 7 days prior to surgery.
Eptifibatide (Integrilin®)	Bleeding may occur while patient is medicated with eptifibatide; platelet function is restored in about 4 hours following discontinuation.
Warfarin (Coumadin®)	Signs of warfarin overdose may first appear as bleeding from gingival tissue; consultation with prescribing physician is advisable prior to surgery to determine temporary dose reduction or withdrawal of medication.
Beta-Blockers	
Cardioselective	Cardioselective beta-blockers (ie, atenolol) have no effect or complications on dental treatment reported.
Noncardioselective	Any of the noncardioselective beta-blockers (ie, nadolol, penbutolol, pindolol, propranolol, timolol) may enhance the pressor response to vasoconstrictor epinephrine resulting in hypertension and reflex bradycardia. Although not reported, it is assumed that similar effects could be caused with levonordefrin (Neo-Cobefrin®). Use either vasoconstrictor with caution in hypertensive patients medicated with noncardioselective beta-adrenergic blockers.
Calcium Channel Blockers	Cause gingival hyperplasia in approximately 1% of the general population taking these drugs. There have been fewer reports with diltiazem and amlodipine than with other CBs such as nifedipine. The hyperplasia will usually disappear with cessation of drug therapy. Consultation with the physician is suggested
Class I Antiarrhythmics	
Disopyramide (Norpace®)	Increased serum levels and toxicity with erythromycin. High incidence of anticholinergic effect manifested as dry mouth and throat.
Flecainide (Tambocor®)	No effects or complications on dental treatment reported.

Procainimide (Pronestyl®)	Systemic lupus-like syndrome has been reported resulting in joint pain and swelling, pains with breathing, skin rash.
Propafenone (Rythmol®)	Greater than 10 % experience significantly reduced salivary flow; taste disturbance, bitter or metallic taste
Quinidine (Quinaglute®)	Secondary anticholinergic effects may decrease salivary flow, especially in middle-aged and elderly patients; known to contribute to caries, periodontal disease, and oral candidiasis.
Class III Antiarrhythmics	
Amiodarone	Bitter or metallic taste has been reported.
Digitalis Glycosides	Use vasoconstrictor with caution due to risk of cardiac arrhythmias. Sensitive gag reflex induced by digitalis drugs may cause difficulty in taking dental impressions.
Diuretics	
Thiazide type	No effects or complications on dental treatment reported.
Loops	NSAIDs may increase chloride and tubular water reuptake to counter-act loop type diuretics.
Potassium-sparing	No effects or complications on dental treatment reported.
Potassium-sparing combination	No effects or complications on dental treatment reported.
HMG-CoA Reductase Inhibitors	Concurrent use of erythromycin, clarithromycin, and some of the statin drugs may result in rhabdomyolysis.
Nitrates	No effects or complications on dental treatment reported.
Supplemental Drugs for Heart Failure	
Amrinone (Inocor®) Milrinone (Primacor®)	No effects or complications on dental treatment reported
Supplemental Drugs for Hypertension	
Central-Acting $Alpha_2$-Agonists	
Clonidine (Catapres®)	Greater than 10% of patients experience significant dry mouth.
Direct-Acting	
Hydralazine (Apresoline®)	No effect or complications on dental treatment reported.

GASTROINTESTINAL DISORDERS

The oral cavity and related structures comprise the first part of the gastrointestinal tract. Diseases affecting the oral cavity are often reflected in GI disturbances. In addition, the oral cavity may indeed reflect diseases of the GI tract, including ulcers, polyps, and liver and gallbladder diseases. The first oral condition that may reflect or be reflected in GI disturbances is that of taste. Typically, complaints of taste abnormalities are presented to the dentist. The sweet, saline, sour, and bitter taste sensations all vary in quality and intensity and are affected by the olfactory system. Often, anemic conditions are reflected in changes in the tongue, resulting in taste aberrations.

Gastric and duodenal ulcers represent the primary diseases that can reflect themselves in the oral cavity. Gastric reflux and problems with food metabolism often present as acid erosions to the teeth and occasionally, changes in the mucosal surface as well. Patients may be encountered that may be identified, upon diagnosis, as harboring the organism *Helicobacter pylori.* Treatment with antibiotics can oftentimes aid in correcting the ulcerative disease.

Gastric Acid Secretion Inhibitor

Lansoprazole (Prevacid®) *on page 686*
Omeprazole (Prilosec®) *on page 886*
Pantaprazole (Protonix®) *on page 915*

Histamine H_2 Antagonist

Cimetidine (Tagamet®) *on page 286*
Famotidine (Pepcid®) *on page 486*
Nizatidine (Axid®) *on page 874*
Ranitidine Bismuth Citrate (Tritec®) *on page 1041*
Ranitidine Hydrochloride (Zantac®) *on page 1042*

Proton Pump Inhibitors

Lansoprazole (Prevacid®) *on page 686*
Omeprazole (Prilosec®) *on page 886*
Pantaprazole (Protonix®) *on page 915*

The oral aspects of gastrointestinal disease are often nonspecific and are related to the patient's gastric reflux problems. Intestinal polyps occasionally present as part of the "Peutz-Jeghers Syndrome", resulting in pigmented areas of the peri-oral region that resemble freckles. The astute dentist will need to differentiate these from melanin pigmentation, while at the same time encouraging the patient to perhaps seek evaluation for an intestinal disorder.

Diseases of the liver and gallbladder system are complex. Most of the disorders that the dentist is interested in are covered in the section on hepatitis and liver disease *on page 1354.* All of the new drugs, including interferons, are mentioned in this section.

Multiple Drug Regimens for the Treatment of *H. pylori* Infection

Drug	Dosages*	Duration of Therapy
H_2-receptor antagonist	Any one given at appropriate dose	4 weeks
plus		
Bismuth *on page 167*	525 mg 4 times/day	2 weeks
plus		
Metronidazole *on page 804*	250 mg 4 times/day	2 weeks
plus		
Tetracycline *on page 1147*	500 mg 4 times/day	2 weeks
Also see Bismuth Subsalicylate, Metronidazole, and Tetracycline combination product *on page 167*		
Ranitidine bismuth citrate *on page 1041*	400 mg twice daily	2 weeks
plus		
Clarithromycin *on page 296*	500 mg twice daily	2 weeks
plus		
Amoxicillin *on page 86*	1000 mg twice daily	2 weeks
Ranitidine bismuth citrate *on page 1041*	400 mg twice daily	2 weeks
plus		
Clarithromycin *on page 296*	500 mg twice daily	2 weeks
plus		
Metronidazole *on page 804*	500 mg twice daily	2 weeks
Ranitidine bismuth citrate *on page 1041*	400 mg twice daily	2 weeks
plus		
Clarithromycin *on page 296*	500 mg twice daily	2 weeks
plus		
Tetracycline *on page 1147*	500 mg twice daily	2 weeks
Proton pump inhibitor		
Lansoprazole *on page 686*	30 mg twice daily	2 weeks
or		
Omeprazole *on page 886plus*	20 mg twice daily	
Clarithromycin *on page 296*	500 mg twice daily	2 weeks
plus		
Amoxicillin *on page 86*	1000 mg twice daily	2 weeks
Proton pump inhibitor		
Lansoprazole *on page 686*	30 mg twice daily	2 weeks
or		
Omeprazole *on page 886*	20 mg twice daily	
plus		
Clarithromycin *on page 296*	500 mg twice daily	2 weeks
plus		
Metronidazole *on page 804*	500 mg twice daily	2 weeks
Proton pump inhibitor		
Lansoprazole *on page 686*	30 mg twice daily	2 weeks
or		
Omeprazole *on page 886*	20 mg twice daily	
plus		
Bismuth *on page 167*	525 mg 4 times/day	2 weeks
plus		
Metronidazole *on page 804*	500 mg 3 times/day	2 weeks
plus		
Tetracycline *on page 1147*	500 mg 4 times/day	2 weeks
Also see Bismuth Subsalicylate, Metronidazole, and Tetracycline combination product *on page 167*		

From Howden CS and Hunt RH, "Guidelines for the Management of *Helicobacter pylori* Infection," *AJG*, 1998, 93:2336.

RESPIRATORY DISEASES

Diseases of the respiratory system put dental patients at increased risk in the dental office because of their decreased pulmonary reserve, the medications they may be taking, drug interactions between these medications, medications the dentist may prescribe, and in some patients with infectious respiratory diseases, a risk of disease transmission.

The respiratory system consists of the nasal cavity, the nasopharynx, the trachea, and the components of the lung including, of course, the bronchi, the bronchioles, and the alveoli. The diseases that affect the lungs and the respiratory system can be separated by location of affected tissue. Diseases that affect the lower respiratory tract are often chronic, although infections can also occur. Three major diseases that affect the lower respiratory tract are often encountered in the medical history for dental patients. These include chronic bronchitis, emphysema, and asthma. Diseases that affect the upper respiratory tract are usually of the infectious nature and include sinusitis and the common cold. The upper respiratory tract infections may also include a wide variety of nonspecific infections, most of which are also caused by viruses. Influenza produces upper respiratory type symptoms and is often caused by orthomyxoviruses. Herpangina is caused by the Coxsackie type viruses and results in upper respiratory infections in addition to pharyngitis or sore throat. One serious condition, known as croup, has been associated with *Haemophilus influenzae* infections. Other more serious infections might include respiratory syncytial virus, adenoviruses, and parainfluenza viruses.

The respiratory symptoms that are often encountered in both upper respiratory and lower respiratory disorders include cough, dyspnea (difficulty in breathing), the production of sputum, hemoptysis (coughing up blood), a wheeze, and occasionally chest pain. One additional symptom, orthopnea (difficulty in breathing when lying down) is often used by the dentist to assist in evaluating the patient with the condition, pulmonary edema. This condition results from either respiratory disease or congestive heart failure.

No effective drug treatments are available for the management of many of the upper respiratory tract viral infections. However, amantadine (sold under the brand name Symmetrel®) is a synthetic drug given orally (200 mg/day) and has been found to be effective against some strains of influenza. Treatment other than for influenza includes supportive care products available over the counter. These might include antihistamines for symptomatic relief of the upper respiratory congestion, antibiotics to combat secondary bacterial infections, and in severe cases, fluids when patients have become dehydrated during the illness (see Therapeutic Category Index for selection). The treatment of herpangina may include management of the painful ulcerations of the oropharynx. The dentist may become involved in managing these lesions in a similar way to those seen in other acute viral infections (see Viral Infection section).

SINUSITIS

Sinusitis also represents an upper respiratory infection that often comes under the purview of the practicing dentist. Acute sinusitis characterized by nasal obstruction, fever, chills, and midface head pain may be encountered by the dentist and discovered as part of a differential work-up for other facial or dental pain. Chronic sinusitis may likewise produce similar dental symptoms. Dental drugs of choice may include ephedrine or nasal drops, antihistamines, and analgesics. These drugs sometimes require supplementation with antibiotics. Most commonly, broad spectrum antibiotics, such as ampicillin, are prescribed. These are often combined with antral lavage to re-establish drainage from the sinus area. Surgical intervention such as a Caldwell-Luc procedure opening into the sinus is rarely necessary and many of the second generation antibiotics such as cephalosporins are used successfully in treating the acute and chronic sinusitis patient (see "Antibiotic Prophylaxis" *on page 1344*).

Gatifloxacin (Tequin™) *on page 549*
Moxifloxacin (Avelox™) *on page 832*

LOWER RESPIRATORY DISEASES

Lower respiratory tract diseases, including asthma, chronic bronchitis, and emphysema are often identified in dental patients. Asthma is an intermittent respiratory disorder that produces recurrent bronchial smooth muscle spasm, inflammation, swelling of the bronchial mucosa, and hypersecretion of mucus. The incidence of childhood asthma appears to be increasing and may be related to the presence of pollutants such as sulfur dioxide and indoor cigarette smoke. The end result is widespread narrowing of the airways and decreased ventilation with increased airway resistance, especially to expiration. Asthmatic patients often suffer from asthmatic attacks when stimulated by respiratory tract infections, exercise, and cold air. Medications such as aspirin and some nonsteroidal anti-inflammatory agents as well as cholinergic and beta-adrenergic blocking drugs, can also trigger asthmatic attacks in addition to chemicals, smoke, and emotional anxiety.

The classical chronic obstructive pulmonary diseases (COPD) of chronic bronchitis and emphysema are both characterized by chronic airflow obstructions during normal ventilatory efforts. They often occur in combination in the same patient and their treatment is similar. One common finding is that the patient is often a smoker. The dentist can play a role in reinforcement of smoking cessation in patients with chronic respiratory diseases.

Treatments include a variety of drugs depending on the severity of the symptoms and the respiratory compromise upon full respiratory evaluation. Patients who are having acute and chronic obstructive pulmonary attacks may be susceptible to infection and antibiotics such as penicillin, ampicillin, tetracycline, or trimethoprim-sulfamethoxazole are often used to eradicate susceptible infective organisms. Corticosteroids, as well as a wide variety of respiratory stimulants, are available in inhalant and/or oral forms. In patients using inhalant medication, oral candidiasis is occasionally encountered.

Amantadine (Symmetrel®) *on page 64*
Analgesics *on page 1466*
Antibiotics *on page 1467*
Antihistamines *on page 1470*
Decongestants *on page 1475*
Epinephrine (Dental) (Sus-Phrine®) *on page 438*
Gatifloxacin (Tequin™) *on page 549*
Moxifloxacin (Avelox™) *on page 832*

SPECIFIC DRUGS USED IN THE TREATMENT OF CHRONIC RESPIRATORY CONDITIONS

Beta$_2$-Selective Agonists

Albuterol (Proventil®,Ventolin®) *on page 45*
Bitolterol (Tornalate®) *on page 170*
Isoetharine (Bronkosol®, Bronkometer®) *on page 658*
Metaproterenol (Alupent®) *on page 776*
Pirbuterol (Maxair™) *on page 965*
Salmeterol (Serevent®) *on page 1073*
Terbutaline (Brethine®, Brethaire®) *on page 1141*

Methylxanthines

Aminophylline (Somophylline®) *on page 71*
Theophylline (Theo-Dur®, Slo-Bid®) *on page 1152*

Mast Cell Stabilizer

Cromolyn Sodium (Intal®) *on page 330*
Nedocromil Sodium (Tilade®) *on page 851*

Corticosteroids

Beclomethasone (Beclovent®, Vanceril®) *on page 146*
Dexamethasone (Decadron® phosphate Respihaler®) *on page 363*
Flunisolide (AeroBid®; Nasarel®) *on page 511*
Fluticasone (Flovent®, Flonase®) *on page 525*
Mometasone Furoate (Nasonex®) *on page 827*
Prednisone (Deltasone®; Liquid Pred®; Meticorten®; Prednicen-M®; Sterapred®) *on page 990*
Triamcinolone (Azmacort™) *on page 1197*

Anticholinergics

Ipratropium (Atrovent®) *on page 651*

Leukotriene Receptor Antagonists

Montelukast (Singulair®) *on page 827*
Zafirlukast (Accolate®) *on page 1253*

5-Lipoxygenase Inhibitors

Zileuton (Zyflo®) *on page 1259*

Other respiratory diseases include tuberculosis and sarcoidosis which are considered to be restrictive granulomatous respiratory diseases. Tuberculosis is covered in "Nonviral Infectious Diseases" *on page 1342*. Sarcoidosis is a condition that at one time was thought to be similar to tuberculosis, however, it is a multisystem disorder of unknown origin which has as a characteristic lymphocytic and mononuclear phagocytic accumulation in epithelioid granulomas within the lung. It occurs worldwide but shows a slight increased prevalence in temperate climates. The treatment of sarcoidosis is usually one that corresponds to its usually benign course, however, many patients are placed on corticosteroids at the level of 40-60 mg of prednisone daily. This treatment is continued for a protracted period of time. As in any disease requiring steroid therapy, consideration of adrenal suppression is necessary. Alteration of steroid dosage prior to stressful dental procedures may be necessary, usually increasing the steroid dosage prior to and during the stressful procedures and then gradually returning the patient to the original dosage over several days. Many dentists prefer to use the Medrol® Dosepak®, however, consultation with the patient's physician regarding dose selection is always advised. Even in the

RESPIRATORY DISEASES *(Continued)*

absence of evidence of adrenal suppression, consultation with the prescribing physician for appropriate dosing and timing of procedures is advisable.

Prednisone *on page 990*

RELATIVE POTENCY OF ENDOGENOUS AND SYNTHETIC CORTICOSTEROIDS

Agent	Equivalent Dose (mg)
Short-Acting (8-12 h)	
Cortisol	20
Cortisone	25
Intermediate-Acting (18-36 h)	
Prednisolone	5
Prednisone	5
Methylprednisolone (Medrol®[)	4
Triamcinolone	4
Long-Acting (36-54 h)	
Betamethasone	0.75
Dexamethasone	0.75

Potential drug interactions for the respiratory disease patient exist. An acute sensitivity to aspirin-containing drugs and some of the nonsteroidal anti-inflammatory drugs is a threat for the asthmatic patient. Barbiturates and narcotics may occasionally precipitate asthmatic attacks as well. Erythromycin, clarithromycin, and ketoconazole are contraindicated in patients who are taking theophylline due to potential enhancement of theophylline toxicity. Patients that are taking steroid preparations as part of their respiratory therapy may require alteration in dosing prior to stressful dental procedures. The physician should be consulted.

Barbiturates *on page 1473*
Clarithromycin *on page 296*
Erythromycin *on page 450*
Ketoconazole *on page 672*

ENDOCRINE DISORDERS AND PREGNANCY

The human endocrine system manages metabolism and homeostasis. Numerous glandular tissues produce hormones that act in broad reactions with tissues throughout the body. Cells in various organ systems may be sensitive to the hormone, or they release, in reaction to the hormone, a second hormone that acts directly on another organ. Diseases of the endocrine system may have importance in dentistry. For the purposes of this section, we will limit our discussion to diseases of the thyroid tissues, diabetes mellitus, and conditions requiring the administration of synthetic hormones, and pregnancy.

THYROID

Thyroid diseases can be classified into conditions that cause the thyroid to be overactive (hyperthyroidism) and those that cause the thyroid to be underactive (hypothyroidism). Clinical signs and symptoms associated with hyperthyroidism may include goiter, heat intolerance, tremor, weight loss, diarrhea, and hyperactivity. Thyroid hormone production can be tested by TSH levels and additional screens may include radioactive iodine uptake or a pre-T_4 (tetraiodothyronine, thyroxine) assay or iodine index or total serum T_3 (triiodothyronine). The results of thyroid function tests may be altered by ingestion of antithyroid drugs such as propylthiouracil, estrogen-containing drugs, and organic and inorganic iodides. When a diagnosis of hyperthyroidism has been made, treatment usually begins with antithyroid drugs which may include propranolol coupled with radioactive iodides as well as surgical procedures to reduce thyroid tissue. Generally, the beta-blockers are used to control cardiovascular effects of excessive T_4. Propylthiouracil or methimazole are the most common antithyroid drugs used. The dentist should be aware that epinephrine is definitely contraindicated in patients with uncontrolled hyperthyroidism.

Diseases and conditions associated with hypothyroidism may include bradycardia, drowsiness, cold intolerance, thick dry skin, and constipation. Generally, hypothyroidism is treated with replacement thyroid hormone until a euthyroid state is achieved. Various preparations are available, the most common is levothyroxine, commonly known as Synthroid® or Levothroid®, and is generally the drug of choice for thyroid replacement therapy.

Drugs to Treat Hypothyroidism

Levothyroxine (Levothroid®, Levoxyl®, Synthroid®) *on page 705*
Liothyronine (Cytomel®, Triostat™) *on page 715*
Liotrix (Thyrolar®) *on page 718*
Thyroid (Armour® Thyroid, S-P-T, Thyrar®, Thyroid Strong®) *on page 1164*

Drugs to Treat Hyperthyroidism

Methimazole (Tapazole®) *on page 782*
Potassium Iodide (Pima®, SSKI®, Thyro-Block®) *on page 980*
Propranolol (Betachron E-R®, Inderal®) *on page 1016*
Propylthiouracil *on page 1019*

DIABETES

Diabetes mellitus refers to a condition of prolonged hyperglycemia associated with either abnormal production or lack of production of insulin. Commonly known as Type 1 diabetes, insulin-dependent diabetes (IDDM) is a condition where there are absent or deficient levels of circulating insulin therefore triggering tissue reactions associated with prolonged hyperglycemia. The kidney's attempt to excrete the excess glucose and the organs that do not receive adequate glucose essentially are damaged. Small vessels and arterial vessels in the eye, kidney, and brain are usually at the greatest risk. Generally, blood sugar levels between 70-120 mg/dL are considered to be normal. Inadequate insulin levels allow glucose to rise to greater than the renal threshold which is 180 mg/dL, and such elevations prolonged lead to organ damage.

The goals of treatment of the diabetic are to maintain metabolic control of the blood glucose levels and to reduce the morbid effects of periodic hyperglycemia. Insulin therapy is the primary mechanism to attain management of consistent insulin levels. Insulin preparations are categorized according to their duration of action. Generally, NPH or intermediate-acting insulin and long-acting insulin can be used in combination with short-acting or regular insulin to maintain levels consistent throughout the day.

In Type 2 or noninsulin-dependent diabetes (NIDDM), the receptor for insulin in the tissues is generally down regulated and the glucose, therefore, is not utilized at an appropriate rate. There is perhaps a stronger genetic basis for noninsulin-dependent diabetes than for Type 1. Treatment of the diabetes Type 2 patient is generally directed toward early nonpharmacologic intervention, mainly weight reduction, moderate exercise, and lower plasma-glucose concentrations. Oral hypoglycemic agents as seen in the

ENDOCRINE DISORDERS AND PREGNANCY *(Continued)*

list below are often used to maintain blood sugar levels. Thirty percent of Type 2 diabetics require insulin, as well as, oral hypoglycemics in order to manage their diabetes. Generally, the two classes of oral hypoglycemics are the sulfonylureas and the biguanides. The sulfonylureas are prescribed more frequently and they stimulate beta cell production of insulin, increase glucose utilization, and tend to normalize glucose metabolism in the liver. The uncontrolled diabetic may represent a challenge to the dental practitioner.

Glycosylated hemoglobin or glycol-hemoglobin assays have emerged as a "gold standard" by which glycemic control is measured in diabetic patients. The test does not rely on the patient's ability to monitor their daily blood glucose levels and is not influenced by acute changes in blood glucose or by the interval since the last meal. Glyco-hemoglobin is formed when glucose reacts with hemoglobin A in the blood and is composed of several fractions. Numerous assay methods have been developed, however, they vary in their precision. Dental clinicians are advised to be aware of the laboratory's particular standardization procedures when requesting glycosylated hemoglobin values. One major advantage of the glycosylated hemoglobin assay is that it provides an overview of the level of glucose in the life span of the red blood cell population in the patient, and therefore is a measure of overall glycemic control for the previous six to twelve weeks. Thus, clinicians use glycosylated hemoglobin values to determine whether their patient is under good control, on average. These assays have less value in medication dosing decisions. Blood glucose monitoring methods are actually better in that respect. The values of glycosylated hemoglobin are expressed as a percentage of the total hemoglobin in the red blood cell population and a normal value is considered to be <6%. The goal is generally for diabetic patients to remain at <7% and values >8% would constitute a worrisome signal. Medical conditions such as anemias or any red blood cell disease, numerous levels of myelosuppression, or pregnancy can artificially lower glycosylated hemoglobin values.

See Insulin Preparations (various products) *on page 639*

Oral Hypoglycemic Agents

Acarbose (Precose®) *on page 24*
Acetohexamide (Dymelor®) *on page 37*
Chlorpropamide (Diabinese®) *on page 275*
Glimepiride (Amaryl®) *on page 557*
Glipizide (Glucotrol®) *on page 558*
Glyburide (Diaβeta, Glynase™, PresTab™, Micronase®) *on page 560*
Glyburide and Metformin (Glucovance™) *on page 561*
Metformin (Glucophage®) *on page 777*
Miglitol (Glyset®) *on page 814*
Repaglinide (Prandin®) *on page 1045*
Tolazamide (Tolinase®) *on page 1177*
Tolbutamide (Orinase®) *on page 1178*

Adjunct Therapy

Metoclopramide (Clopra®, Maxolon®, Octamide®, Reglan®) *on page 800*

Oral manifestations of uncontrolled diabetes might include abnormal neutrophil function resulting in a poor response to periodontal pathogens. Increased risk of gingivitis and periodontitis in these patients is common. Candidiasis is a frequent occurrence. Denture sore mouth may be more prominent and poor wound healing following extractions may be one of the complications encountered.

HORMONAL THERAPY

Two uses of hormonal supplementation include oral contraceptives and estrogen replacement therapy. Drugs used for contraception interfere with fertility by inhibiting release of follicle stimulating hormone, luteinizing hormone, and by preventing ovulation. There are few oral side effects; however, moderate gingivitis, similar to that seen during pregnancy, has been reported. The dentist should be aware that decreased effect of oral contraceptives has been reported with most antibiotics. See individual monographs for specific details.

The combination estradiol cypionate and medroxyprogesterone acetate has recently been approved. It is a single monthly injection and has similar warnings and guidelines. However, it's use with antibiotics have not been firmly established. Therefore, discussion/consultation with the patient's OB/GYN physician is indicated.

Drugs commonly encountered include:

Combination Hormonal Contraceptives (various products) *on page 323*
Estradiol (various products) *on page 457*

Estradiol Cypionate and Medroxyprogesterone Acetate (Lunelle™) *on page 461*
Levonorgestrel (Norplant®) *on page 703*
Medroxyprogesterone Acetate (Amen®, Curretab®, Cycrin®, Depo-Provera®, Provera®) *on page 753*
Mestranol and Norethindrone (Ortho-Novum™ 1/50) *on page 774*
Norethindrone (Aygestin®, Micronor®, Nor-Q.D.®) *on page 876*
Norgestrel (Ovrette®) *on page 877*

Estrogens or derivatives are usually prescribed as replacement therapy following menopause or cyclic irregularities and to inhibit osteoporosis. The following list of drugs may interact with antidepressants and barbiturates. New tissue-specific estrogens like Evista® may help with the problem of osteoporosis.

Estrogens, Conjugated (Premarin®) *on page 463*
Estrogens, Conjugated (Synthetic) (Cenestin™) *on page 466*
Estrogens, Esterified (Estratab®, Menest®) *on page 467*
Estrogens and Medroxyprogesterone (Prempro®) *on page 465*
Estrogens and Methyltestosterone (Estratest®, Premarin®) *on page 463*
Estrone (Aquest®, Kestrone®) *on page 468*
Estropipate (Ogen®, Ortho-Est®) *on page 469*
Ethinyl Estradiol (Estinyl®) *on page 474*
Quinestrol (Estrovis®) *on page 1033*
Raloxifene (Evista®) *on page 1039*

PREGNANCY

Normal endocrine and physiologic functions are altered during pregnancy. Endogenous estrogens and progesterone increase and placental hormones are secreted. Thyroid stimulating hormone and growth hormone also increase. Cardiovascular changes can result and increased blood volume can lead to blood pressure elevations and transient heart murmurs. Generally, in a normal pregnancy, oral gingival changes will be limited to gingivitis. Alteration of treatment plans might include limiting administration of all drugs to emergency procedures only during the first and third trimesters and medical consultation regarding the patients' status for all elective procedures. Limiting dental care throughout pregnancy to preventive procedures is not unreasonable. The effects on dental treatment of the "morning after pill" (Plan B™ and Preven™) and the abortifacient, mifepristone *on page 813*, have not been documented at this time.

HIV INFECTION AND AIDS

Human immunodeficiency virus (HIV) represents agents HIV-1 and HIV-2 that produce a devastating systemic disease. The virus causes disease by leading to elevated risk of infections in patients and, from our experience over the last 18 years, there clearly are oral manifestations associated with these patients. Also, there has been a revolution in infection control in our dental offices over the last two decades due to our expanding knowledge of this infectious agent. Infection control practices (see "Infectious Disease Information" *on page 1442*) have been elevated to include all of the infectious agents with which dentists often come into contact. These might include in addition to HIV, hepatitis viruses (of which the serotypes include A, B, C, D, E, F, and G), the herpes viruses; sexually transmitted diseases such as syphilis, gonorrhea, papillomavirus, all of which are covered elsewhere in this book.

Acquired immunodeficiency syndrome (AIDS) has been recognized since early 1981 as a unique clinical syndrome manifest by opportunistic infections or by neoplasms complicating the underlying defect in the cellular immune system. These defects are now known to be brought on by infection and pathogenesis with human immunodeficiency virus 1 or 2 (HIV-1 is the predominant serotype identified). The major cellular defect brought on by infection with HIV is a depletion of T-cells, primarily the sub-type, T-helper cells, known as CD4+ cells. Over these years, our knowledge regarding HIV infection and the oral manifestations often associated with patients with HIV or AIDS, has increased dramatically. Populations of individuals known to be at high risk of HIV transmission include homosexuals, intravenous drug abuse patients, transfusion recipients, patients with other sexually transmitted diseases, and patients practicing promiscuous sex.

The definitions of AIDS have also evolved over this period of time. The natural history of HIV infection along with some of the oral manifestations can be reviewed in Table 1. The risk of developing these opportunistic infections increases as the patient progresses to AIDS.

Table 1.
NATURAL HISTORY OF HIV INFECTION/ORAL MANIFESTATIONS

Time From Transmission (Average)	Observation	CD4 Cell Count
0	Viral transmissions	Normal: 1000 (±500/mm³)
2-4 weeks	Self-limited infectious mononucleosis-like illness with fever, rash, leukopenia, mucocutaneous ulcerations (mouth, genitals, etc), thrush	Transient decrease
6-12 weeks	Seroconversion (rarely requires ≥3 months for seroconversion)	Normal
0-8 years	Healthy/asymptomatic HIV infection; peripheral/ persistent generalized lymphadenopathy; HPV, thrush, OHL; RAU, periodontal diseases, salivary gland diseases; dermatitis	≥500/mm³ gradual reduction with average decrease of 50-80/mm³/ year
4-8 years	Early symptomatic HIV infection previously called (AIDS-related complex): Thrush, vaginal candidiasis (persistent, frequent and/or severe), cervical dysplasia/CA Hodgkin's lymphoma, B-cell lymphoma, oral hairy leukoplakia, salivary gland diseases, ITP, xerostomia, dermatitis, shingles; RAU, herpes simplex, HPV, bacterial infections, periodontal diseases, molluscum contagiosum, other physical symptoms: fever, weight loss, fatigue	≥300-500/mm³
6-10 years	AIDS: Wasting syndrome, *Candida* esophagitis, Kaposi's sarcoma, HIV-associated dementia, disseminated *M. avium*, Hodgkin's or B-cell lymphoma, herpes simplex >30 days; PCP; cryptococcal meningitis, other systemic fungal infections; CMV	<200/mm³

Natural history indicates course of HIV infection in absence of antiretroviral treatment. Adapted from Bartlett JG, "A Guide to HIV Care from the AIDS Care Program of the Johns Hopkins Medical Institutions," 2nd ed.

PCP -*Pneumocystis carinii* pneumonia; ITP -idiopathic thrombocytopenia purpura; HPV - human papilloma virus; OHL - oral hairy leukoplakia; RAU - recurrent aphthous ulcer

Patients with HIV infection and/or AIDS are seen in dental offices throughout the country. In general, it is the dentist's obligation to treat HIV individuals including patients of record and other patients who may seek treatment when the office is accepting new patients. These patients are protected under the Americans with Disabilities Act and the dentist has an obligation as described. Two excellent publications, one by the American Dental Association and the other by the American Academy of Oral Medicine, outline the dentist's responsibility as well as a very detailed explanation of dental management protocols for HIV patients. These protocols, however, are evolving just as our knowledge of HIV has evolved. New drugs and their interactions (see Dental Drug Interactions *on page 1434* in Appendix) present the dentist with continuous need for updates regarding the appropriate management of HIV patients. Diagnostic tests, including determining viral load in combination with the CD4 status, now are used to modify a patient's treatment in ways that allow them to remain relatively illness-free for longer periods of time. This places more of a responsibility on the dental practice team to be aware of drug changes, of new drugs, and of the appropriate oral management in such patients.

Our knowledge of AIDS allows us to properly treat these patients while protecting ourselves, our staff, and other patients in the office. All types of infectious disease require consistent practices in our dental offices known as Universal Precautions (see Infectious Disease Information *on page 1442*). The office team that utilizes these precautions appropriately is well protected against passage of infectious agents. These agents include sexually transmitted disease agents, the highly virulent hepatitis viruses, and the less virulent but always worrisome HIV. In general, an office that is practicing universal precautions is one that is considered safe for patients and staff. Throughout this spectrum, HIV is placed somewhere in the middle in terms of infection risk in the dental office. Other sexually transmitted diseases and infectious diseases such as tuberculosis represent a greater threat to the dentist than HIV itself. However, due to the grave danger of HIV infection, many of our precautions have been instituted to assist the dentist in protecting himself, his staff, and other patients in situations where the office may be involved in treating a patient that is HIV positive.

As in the management of all medically compromised patients, the appropriate care of HIV patients begins with a complete and thorough history. This history must allow the dentist to identify risk factors in the development of HIV as well as identify those patients known to be HIV positive. Knowledge of all medications prescribed to patients at risk is also important.

The current antiretroviral therapy used to treat patients with HIV infection and/or AIDS includes three primary classifications of drugs. These are the nucleoside analogs, protease inhibitors, and the non-nucleoside/nucleotide analogs (analogs refers to chemicals that can substitute competitively for naturally produced cell components such as found in DNA, RNA, or proteins). The newest drugs include several nucleoside analogs, abacavir (Ziagen®), subprotease inhibitors, amprenavir, and several non-nucleoside analogs, efavirenz (Sustiva®) and adefovir (Preveon®). Finding the perfect "cocktail" of anti-HIV medications still eludes clinicians. This is partly due to the fact that therapies are still too novel and the patient's years too few to study. Numerous recently published studies have indicated that combinations of drugs are far better than individual drug therapy. Several of these studies have looked at two drug combinations particularly between nucleoside analogs in combination with protease inhibitors. The newer drugs (non-nucleoside analogs) have added the possibility of a triple cocktail. Recently several studies indicated that this three-drug combination may be the best in managing HIV infection.

When HIV was first discovered, the efforts for monitoring HIV infection focused on the CD4 blood levels and the ratios between the helper cells, suppressor cells within the patient's immune system. These markers were used to indicate success or failure of drug therapies as patients moved through HIV pathogenesis toward AIDS. More recently, however, the advent of protease inhibitors has allowed clinicians to monitor the actual presence of viral RNA within the patient and the term viral load has become the focus of therapy monitoring. The availability of better therapies and our rapidly expanding knowledge of molecular biology of the HIV virus have created new opportunities to control the AIDS epidemic. Cases can be monitored quite closely looking at the number of copy units or virions within the patient's bloodstream as an indication in combination with other infections and/or declining or increasing CD4 numbers to establish prognostic values for the patient's success. Long-term survival of patients infected with HIV has been accomplished by monitoring and adjusting therapy to these numbers.

Comprehensive coordinated approaches, that have been advocated by researchers, have sought to establish national standards for HIV reporting, greater access to effective newly approved medications, improved access to individual physicians treating HIV patients, and continued protection of patient's privacy. These goals allow the reporting of studies that suggest that combination therapies, some of which have been tried in less controlled individual patient treatments, may prove useful in larger populations of HIV-infected individuals. As these studies are reported, the dental clinician should be aware that patients' drug therapies change rapidly, various combinations may be tried, and the side effects and interactions as described in the chapter on drug interactions and the CYP system will also emerge. The dentist must be aware of these potential interactions with seemingly innocuous drugs such as clarithromycin, erythromycin, and some of the sedative drugs that a dentist may utilize in their practice as well as some of the analgesics. These drug interactions may be the most important part of monitoring that the dentist provides in helping to manage a situation. Some of the antiviral drugs more commonly used for HIV, AIDS, Asymptomatic, CD4 <500, and the newer drugs (ie, protease inhibitors, nucleoside analogs, and non-nucleoside nucleotide analogs) are listed in Table 2 on following page.

HIV INFECTION AND AIDS *(Continued)*

Table 2. CATEGORIES OF ANTIRETROVIRAL DRUGS

Nucleoside Analogs	Protease Inhibitors	Non-Nucleoside/Nucleotide Analogs
Zidovudine (Retrovir®, AZT, SDV)	Saquinavir (Invirase®)	Nevirapine (Viramune®)
Didanosine (Videx®, ddi)	Ritonavir (Norvir®)	Delavirdine (Rescriptor®)
Zalcitabine (HIVID®, ddc)	Indinavir (Crixivan®)	Efavirenz (Sustiva®)
Stavudine (Zerit®, d4T)	Nelfinavir (Viracept®)	Adefovir (Preveon®)
Lamivudine (Epivir®)	Amprenavir (Agenerase™)	
Abacavir (Ziagen™)		

The presence of other infections is an important part of the health history. Appropriate medical consultation may be mandated after a health history in order to accomplish a complete evaluation of the patients at risk. Uniformity in the taking of a history from a patient is the dentist's best plan for all patients so that no selectivity or discrimination can be implicated.

An appropriate review of symptoms may also identify oral and systemic conditions that may be present in aggressive HIV disease. Medical physical examination may reveal pre-existing or developing intra- or extra-oral signs/symptoms of progressive disease. Aggressive herpes simplex, herpes zoster, papillomavirus, Kaposi's sarcoma or lymphoma are among the disorders that might be identified. In addition to these, intra-oral examination may raise suspicion regarding fungal infections, angular cheilitis, squamous cell carcinoma, and recurrent aphthous ulcers. The dentist should be vigilant in all patients regardless of HIV risk.

It will always be up to the dental practitioner to determine whether testing for HIV should be recommended following the history and physical examination of a new patient. Because of the severe psychological implications of learning of HIV positivity for a patient, the dentist should be aware that there are appropriate referral sites where psychological counseling and appropriate discrete testing for the patient is available. The dentist's office should have these sites available for referral should the patient be interested. Candid discussions, however, with the patient regarding risk factors and/or other signs or symptoms in their history and physical condition that may indicate a higher HIV risk than the normal population, should be an area the dentist feels comfortable in broaching with any new patient. Oftentimes, it is appropriate to recommend testing for other infectious diseases should risk factors be present. For example, testing for hepatitis B may be appropriate for the patient and along with this the dentist could recommend that the patient consider HIV testing. Because of the legal issues involved, anonymity for HIV testing may be appropriate and it is always up to the patient to follow the doctor's recommendations.

When a patient has either given a positive history of knowing that they are HIV positive or it has been determined after referral for consultation, the dentist should be aware of the AIDS-defining illnesses. Of course, current medical status and drug therapy that the patient may be undergoing is of equal importance. The dentist, through medical consultation and regular follow-up with the patient's physician, should be made aware of the CD4 count (Table 3), the viral load, and the drugs that the patient is taking. The presence of other AIDS-defining illnesses as well as complications, such as higher risk of endocarditis and the risk of other systemic infections such as tuberculosis, are extremely important for the dentist. These may make an impact on the dental treatment plan in terms of the selection of preprocedural antibiotics or the use of oral medications to treat opportunistic infections in or around the oral cavity.

Table 3. CD4+ LYMPHOCYTE COUNT AND PERCENTAGE AS RELATED TO THE RISK OF OPPORTUNISTIC INFECTION

CD4+ Cells/mm³	CD4+ Percentage*	Risk of Opportunistic Infection
>600	32-60	No increased risk
400-500	<29	Initial immune suppression
200-400	14-28	Appearance of opportunistic infections, some may be major
<200	<14	Severe immune suppression. AIDS diagnosis. Major opportunistic infections. Although variable, prognosis for surviving greater than 3 years is poor

Table 3. CD4+ LYMPHOCYTE COUNT AND PERCENTAGE AS RELATED TO THE RISK OF OPPORTUNISTIC INFECTION *(continued)*

CD4+ Cells/mm^3	CD4+ Percentage*	Risk of Opportunistic Infection
<50	—	Although variable, prognosis for surviving greater than 1 year is poor

*Several studies have suggested that the CD4+ percentage demonstrates less variability between measurements, as compared to the absolute CD4+ cell count. CD4+ percentages may therefore give a clearer impression of the course of disease.

Adapted from Glick M and Silverman S, "Dental Management of HIV-Infected Patients," *J Am Dent Assoc* (Supplement to Reviewers), 1995.

AIDS-defining illnesses such as candidiasis, recurrent pneumonia, or lymphoma are clearly important to the dentist. Chemotherapy that might be being given to the patient for treatment for any or all of these disorders can have implications in terms of the patient's response to simple dental procedures.

Drug therapies have become complex in the treatment of HIV/AIDS. Because of the moderate successes with protease inhibitors and the drug combination therapies, more patients are living longer and receiving more dental care throughout their lives. Drug therapies are often tailored to the current CD4 count in combination with the viral load. In general, patients with high CD4 counts are usually at lower risk for complications in the dental office than patients with low CD4 counts. However, the presence of a high viral load with or without a stable CD4 count may be indicative or a more rapid progression of the HIV/AIDS disease process than had previously been thought. Patients with a high viral load and a declining CD4 count are considered to have the greatest risk and the poorest prognosis of all the groups.

Other organ damage, such as liver compromise potentially leading to bleeding disorders, can be found as the disease progresses to AIDS. Liver dysfunction may be related to pre-existing hepatic diseases due to previous infection with a hepatitis virus such as hepatitis B or other drug toxicities associated with the treatment of AIDS. The dentist must have available current prothrombin and partial thromboplastin times (PT and PTT) in order to accurately evaluate any risk of bleeding abnormality. Platelet count and liver function studies are also important. Potential drug interactions include some antibiotics, as well as any anticoagulating drugs, which may be contraindicated in such patients. It may be necessary to avoid nonsteroidal anti-inflammatory drugs as well as aspirin. (See the introductory text "Pharmacology of Drug Metabolism and Interactions" *on page 17*).

The use of preprocedural antibiotics is another issue in the HIV patient. As the absolute neutrophil count declines during the progression of AIDS, the use of antibiotics as a preprocedural step prior to dental care may be necessary. If protracted treatment plans are necessary, the dentist should receive updated information as the patient receives such from their physician. It is always important that the dentist have current CD4 counts, viral load assay, as well as liver function studies, AST and ALT, and bleeding indicators including platelet count, PT, and PTT. If any other existing conditions such as cardiac involvement or joint prostheses are involved, antibiotic coverage may also be necessary. However, these determinations are no different than in the non-HIV population and this subject is covered in "Preprocedural Antibiotic Prophylaxis Guidelines for Dental Patients" *on page 1344*. Use the table of Normal Blood Values *on page 1446* as general guidelines for provision of dental care.

The consideration of current blood values is important in long-term care of any medically compromised patient and in particular the HIV-positive patient. Preventive dental care is likewise valuable in these patients, however, the dentist's approach should be no different than as with all patients. See Table 4 for oral lesions commonly associated with HIV disease and a brief description of their usual treatment. The clinician is referred to other sections of the text for more detailed descriptions of these common oral lesions. Other important parts of the text that may be useful for the dentist include the office protocol for universal precautions *on page 1442* and the Frequently Asked Questions at the end of this chapter. The clinician should also be aware that several of the protease inhibitors have now been associated with drug interactions. Some of these drug interactions include therapies that the dentist may be utilizing. The basis for these drug interactions with protease inhibitors is the inhibition of cytochrome P450 isoforms, which are important in normal liver function and metabolism of drugs. A detailed description of the mechanisms of inhibition can be found in "Pharmacology of Drug Metabolism and Interactions" *on page 17*, as well as a table illustrating some known drug interactions with antiviral therapy and drugs commonly prescribed in the dental office. The metabolism of these drugs could be affected by the patient's antiviral therapy. Please see the section on selected references for more information on management of HIV patients.

HIV INFECTION AND AIDS *(Continued)*

Table 4. ORAL LESIONS COMMONLY SEEN IN HIV/AIDS

Condition	Management
Oral candidiasis	See "Oral Fungal Infections" *on page 1377*
Angular cheilitis	See "Oral Fungal Infections" *on page 1377*
Oral hairy leukoplakia	See "Systemic Viral Diseases" *on page 1354*
Periodontal diseases	See "Oral Bacterial Infections" *on page 1367*
Linear gingivitis	
Ulcerative periodontitis	
Herpes simplex	Acyclovir - see "Systemic Viral Diseases" *on page 1354*
Herpes zoster	Acyclovir - see "Systemic Viral Diseases" *on page 1354*
Chronic aphthous ulceration	Palliation / Thalidomide (Thalomid®)
Salivary gland disease	Referral
Human papillomavirus	Laser / Surgical excision
Kaposi's sarcoma	See "Antibiotic Prophylaxis" *on page 1344*; Biopsy / Laser
Non-Hodgkin's lymphoma	Biopsy / Referral
Tuberculosis	Referral

Dapsone (Avlosulfon®) *on page 350*
Delavirdine (Rescriptor™) *on page 355*
Didanosine (Videx®) *on page 382*
Indinavir (Crixivan®) *on page 633*
Lamivudine (Epivir®) *on page 683*
Lopinavir and Ritonavir (Kaletra™) *on page 725*
Nelfinavir (Viracept®) *on page 853*
Ritonavir (Norvir®) *on page 1059*
Stavudine (Zerit®) *on page 1108*
Thalidomide (Thalomid®) *on page 1150*
Tenofovir (Viread™) *on page 1139*
Zalcitabine (Hivid®) *on page 1254*
Zidovudine (Retrovir®) *on page 1257*
Zidovudine and Lamivudine (Combivir®) *on page 1258*

FREQUENTLY ASKED QUESTIONS

How does one get AIDS, aside from having unprotected sex?

Our current knowledge about the immunodeficiency virus is that it is carried via semen, contaminated needles, blood products, transfusion products not tested, and potentially in other fluids of the body. Patients at highest risk include I.V. drug abusers, those receiving multiple transfusions with blood that has not been screened for HIV, or patients practicing unprotected sex with multiple partners, where the history of the partner may not be as clear as the patient would like.

Are patients safe from AIDS or HIV infection when they present to the dentist office?

Our current knowledge indicates that the answer is an unequivocal yes. The patient is protected because dental offices are practicing universal precautions using antimicrobial handwashing agents, gloves, face masks, eye protection, special clothing, aerosol control, and instrument soaking and autoclaving. All of these procedures stop potential transmission to a new patient, as well as, allow for easy disposal of contaminated office supplies for elimination of microbes by an antimicrobial technique, should they be contaminated through treatment of another patient. These precautions are mandated by OSHA requirements and covered in Universal Precautions in the Appendix.

What is the most common opportunistic infection that HIV-positive patients suffer that may be important in dentistry?

The most common opportunistic infection important to dentistry is oral candidiasis. This disease can present as white plaques, red areas, or angular cheilitis occurring at the corners of the mouth. Management of such lesions is appropriate by the dentist and is described in this handbook (see Oral Fungal Infections *on page 1377*). Other oral complications include HIV-associated periodontal disease, as well as the other conditions outlined in Table 4. Of great concern to the dentist is the risk of tuberculosis. In many HIV-positive patients, tuberculosis has become a serious, life-threatening opportunistic infection. The dentist should be aware that appropriate referral for anyone showing such respiratory signs and symptoms would be prudent.

Can one patient infect another through unprotected sex if the other patient has tested negative for HIV?

Yes, there is always the possibility that a sexual partner may be in the early window of time when plasma viremia is not at a detectable level. The antibody response to plasma viremia may be slightly delayed and diagnostic testing may not indicate HIV positivity. This window of time represents a period when the patient may be infectious but not show up yet on normal diagnostic testing.

Can HIV be passed by oral fluids?

As our knowledge about HIV has evolved, we have thought that HIV is inactivated in saliva by an agent possibly associated with secretory leukocyte protease inhibitors known as SLPI. There is, however, a current resurgence in our interest in oral transmission because some research indicates that in moderate to advanced periodontal lesions or other oral lesions where there is tissue damage, the presence of a serous exudate may increase the risk of transmission. The dentist should be aware of this ongoing research and attempt to renew knowledge regularly so that any future breakthroughs will be noted.

RHEUMATOID ARTHRITIS AND OSTEOARTHRITIS

Arthritis and its variations represent the most common chronic musculoskeletal disorders of man. The conditions can essentially be divided into rheumatoid, osteoarthritic, and polyarthritic presentations. Differences in age of onset and joint involvement exist and it is now currently believed that the diagnosis of each may be less clear than previously thought. These autoinflammatory diseases have now been shown to affect young and old alike. Criteria for a diagnosis of rheumatoid arthritis include a positive serologic test for rheumatoid factor, subcutaneous nodules, affected joints on opposite sides of the body, and clear radiographic changes. The hematologic picture includes moderate normocytic hypochromic anemia, mild leukocytosis, and mild thrombocytopenia. During acute inflammatory periods, C-reactive protein is elevated and IgG and IgM (rheumatoid factors) can be detected. Osteoarthritis lacks these diagnostic features.

Other systemic conditions, such as systemic lupus erythematosus and Sjögren's syndrome, are often found simultaneously with some of the arthritic conditions. The treatment of arthritis includes the use of slow-acting and rapid-acting anti-inflammatory agents ranging from the gold salts to aspirin (see following listings). Long-term usage of these drugs can lead to numerous adverse effects including bone marrow suppression, platelet suppression, and oral ulcerations. The dentist should be aware that steroids (usually prednisone) are often prescribed along with the listed drugs and are often used in dosages sufficient to induce adrenal suppression. Adjustment of dosing prior to invasive dental procedures may be indicated along with consultation with the managing physician. Alteration of steroid dosage prior to stressful dental procedures may be necessary, usually increasing the steroid dosage prior to and during the stressful procedures and then gradually returning the patient to the original dosage over several days. Even in the absence of evidence of adrenal suppression, consultation with the prescribing physician for appropriate dosing and timing of procedures is advisable.

Gold Salts

Auranofin (Ridaura®) *on page 132*
Aurothioglucose (Solganol®) *on page 133*

Metabolic Inhibitor

Leflunomide (Arava®) *on page 687*
Methotrexate *on page 788*

Immunomodulator

Etanercept (Enbrel®) *on page 470*

Nonsteroidal Anti-inflammatory Agents

Aminosalicylate Sodium (Sodium P.A.S.) *on page 72*
Choline Magnesium Trisalicylate (Trilisate®) *on page 279*
Choline Salicylate (Arthropan®) *on page 280*
Diclofenac (Cataflam®, Voltaren®) *on page 378*
Diflunisal (Dolobid®) *on page 386*
Etodolac (Lodine®) *on page 479*
Fenoprofen (Nalfon®) *on page 492*
Flurbiprofen (Ansaid®) *on page 522*
Ibuprofen (various products) *on page 621*
Indomethacin (Indocin®) *on page 634*
Ketoprofen (Orudis®) *on page 674*
Ketorolac (Toradol®) *on page 676*
Magnesium Salicylate (Doan's®, Magan®, Mobidin®) *on page 742*
Meclofenamate (Meclomen®) *on page 751*
Mefenamic Acid (Ponstel®) *on page 754*
Nabumetone (Relafen®) *on page 838*
Naproxen (Naprosyn®) *on page 848*
Oxaprozin (Daypro™) *on page 895*
Piroxicam (Feldene®) *on page 965*
Salsalate (various products) *on page 1074*
Sulindac (Clinoril®) *on page 1125*
Tolmetin (Tolectin®) *on page 1180*

COX-2 Inhibitor NSAID

Celecoxib (Celebrex®) *on page 247*
Rofecoxib (Vioxx®) *on page 1064*
Valdecoxib (Bextra®) *on page 1225*

Combination NSAID Product to Prevent GI Distress

Diclofenac and Misoprostol (Arthrotec®) *on page 380*

Salicylates

Aspirin (various products) *on page 119*
Choline Magnesium Trisalicylate (Trilisate®) *on page 279*
Salsalate (Argesic®-SA, Artha-G®, Disalcid®, Marthritic® Mono-Gesic®, Salflex®, Salgesic®, Salsitab®) *on page 1074*

Other

Hydroxychloroquine (Plaquenil®) *on page 613*
Prednisone (various products) *on page 990*

ANTI-INFLAMMATORY AGENTS USED IN THE TREATMENT OF RHEUMATOID ARTHRITIS AND OSTEOARTHRITIS

Drug	Adverse Effects
SLOW-ACTING	
GOLD SALTS	
Aurothioglucose I.M. parenteral injection (Myochrysine®); Auranofin (Ridaura®)	GI intolerance, diarrhea; leukopenia, thrombocytopenia, and/or anemia; skin and oral eruptions; possible nephrotoxicity and hepatotoxicity
METABOLIC INHIBITOR	
Leflunomide (Arava®)	Diarrhea, respiratory tract infection
Methotrexate	Oral ulcerations, leukopenia
IMMUNOMODULATOR	
Etanercept (Enbrel®)	Headache, respiratory tract infection, positive ANA
OTHER	
Hydroxychloroquine (Plaquenil®)	Usually mild and reversible; ophthalmic complications
Prednisone	Insomnia, nervousness, indigestion, increased appetite
RAPID-ACTING	
SALICYLATES	
Aspirin	Inhibition of platelet aggregation; gastrointestinal (GI) irritation, ulceration, and bleeding; tinnitus; teratogenicity
Choline magnesium salicylate (Trilisate®)	GI irritation and ulceration, weakness, skin rash, hemolytic anemia, troubled breathing
Salsalate	
OTHER NONSTEROIDAL ANTI-INFLAMMATORY DRUGS	
Diclofenac (Cataflam®, Voltaren®); Diflunisal (Dolobid®); Etodolac (Lodine®); Fenoprofen calcium (Nalfon®); Flurbiprofen sodium (Ansaid®); Ibuprofen (Motrin®); Indomethacin (Indocin®); Ketoprofen (Orudis®); Ketorolac tromethamine (Toradol®); Meclofenamate (Meclomen®); Nabumetone (Relafen®); Naproxen (Naprosyn®); Oxaprozin (Daypro™); Phenylbutazone; Piroxicam (Feldene®); Salsalate (Argesic®-SA, Artha-G®, Disalcid®, Mono-Gesic®, Salflex®, Salgesic®, Salsitab®); Sulindac (Clinoril®); Tolmetin (Tolectin®)	GI irritation, ulceration, and bleeding; inhibition of platelet aggregation; displacement of protein-bound drugs (eg, oral anticoagulants, sulfonamides, and sulfonylureas); headache; vertigo; mucocutaneous rash or ulceration; parotid enlargement
COX-2 INHIBITOR NSAID	
Celecoxib (Celebrex®) Rofecoxib (Vioxx®) Valdecoxib (Bextra®)	Headache, dyspepsia, upper respiratory tract infection, sinusitis
COMBINATION NSAID PRODUCT TO PREVENT GI DISTRESS	
Diclofenac and Misoprostol (Arthrotec®)	Inhibition of platelet aggregation; displacement of protein-bound drugs (eg, oral anticoagulants, sulfonamides, and sulfonylureas); headache; vertigo; mucocutaneous rash or ulceration; parotid enlargement; diarrhea

NONVIRAL INFECTIOUS DISEASES

Nonviral infectious diseases are numerous. For the purposes of this text, discussion will be limited to tuberculosis, gonorrhea, and syphilis.

TUBERCULOSIS

Tuberculosis is caused by the organism *Mycobacterium tuberculosis* as well as a variety of other mycobacteria including *M. bovis*, *M. avium-intracellulare*, and *M. kansasii*. Diagnosis of tuberculosis can be made from a skin test and a positive chest x-ray as well as acid-fast smears of cultures from respiratory secretions. Nucleic acid probes and polymerase chain reaction (PCR) to identify nucleic acid of *M. tuberculosis* have recently become useful.

The treatment of tuberculosis is based on the general principle that multiple drugs should reduce infectivity within 2 weeks and that failures in therapy may be due to noncompliance with the long-term regimens necessary. General treatment regimens last 6-12 months.

Isoniazid-resistant and multidrug-resistant mycobacterial infections have become an increasingly significant problem in recent years. TB as an opportunistic disease in HIV-positive patients has also risen. Combination drug therapy has always been popular in TB management and the advent of new antibiotics has not diminished this need.

ANTITUBERCULOSIS DRUGS

Bactericidal Agents

Capreomycin (Capastat®) *on page 212*
*Isoniazid (INH™, Laniazid®, Nydrazid®) *on page 659*
Kanamycin (Kantrex®) *on page 669*
*Pyrazinamide *on page 1026*
Rifabutin (Mycobutin®) *on page 1050*
*Rifampin (Rifadin®, Rimactane®) *on page 1051*
*Streptomycin *on page 1111*

Bacteriostatic Agents

Cycloserine (Seromycin® Pulvules®) *on page 336*
*Ethambutol (Myambutol®) *on page 472*
Ethionamide (Trecator®-SC) *on page 475*
Para-Aminosalicylate Sodium *on page 917*

*Drugs of Choice

SEXUALLY TRANSMITTED DISEASES

Sexually transmitted diseases (STDs) represent a group of infectious diseases that include bacterial, fungal, and viral etiologies. Several related infections are covered elsewhere. Gonorrhea and syphilis will be covered here.

The management of a patient with a STD begins with identification. Paramount to the correct management of patients with a history of gonorrhea or syphilis is when the condition was diagnosed, how and with what agent it was treated, did the condition recur, and are there any residual signs and symptoms potentially indicating active or recurrent disease. With universal precautions, the patient with *Neisseria gonorrhoea* or *Treponema pallidum* infection poses little threat to the dentist; however, diagnosis of oral lesions may be problematic. Gonococcal pharyngitis, primary syphilitic lesions (chancre), secondary syphilitic lesions (mucous patch), and tertiary lesions (gumma) may be identified by the dentist.

Drugs used in treatment of gonorrhea/syphilis include:

Cefixime (Suprax®) *on page 237*
Ceftriaxone (Rocephin®) *on page 245*
Ciprofloxacin (Cipro™) *on page 288*
Doxycycline (alternate) (Doryx®, Doxy®, Doxychel®, Vibramycin®, Vibra-Tabs®) *on page 418*
Ofloxacin (Floxin®, Ocuflox™) *on page 883*
Penicillin G Benzathine (Bicillin® L-A; Permapen®) *on page 928*
Penicillin G, Parenteral, Aqueous (Pfizerpen®) *on page 929*
Spectinomycin (alternate) (Trobicin®) *on page 1105*

The drugs listed above are often used alone or in stepped regimens, particularly when there is concomitant *Chlamydia* infection or when there is evidence of disseminated disease. The proper treatment for syphilis depends on the state of the disease.

Current treatment regimens for syphilis include:

1°, 2°, early latent (<1 y)	Benzathine penicillin G I.M.: 2-4 million units x 1 (alternate doxycycline)
Latent (>1 y), gumma, or cardiovascular	As above but once weekly for 3 weeks
Neurosyphilis	Aqueous penicillin G I.V.: 12-24 million units/day for 14 days

ANTIBIOTIC PROPHYLAXIS
PREPROCEDURAL GUIDELINES FOR DENTAL PATIENTS

INTRODUCTION

In dental practice the clinician is often confronted with a decision to prescribe antibiotics. The focus of this chapter is on the use of antibiotics as a preprocedural treatment in the prevention of adverse infectious sequelae in the two most commonly encountered situations: prevention of endocarditis and prosthetic implants.

The criteria for preprocedural decisions begins with patient evaluation. An accurate and complete medical history is always the initial basis for any prescriptive treatments on the part of the dentist. These prescriptive treatments can include ordering appropriate laboratory tests, referral to the patient's physician for consultation, or immediate decision to prescribe preprocedural antibiotics. The dentist should also be aware that antibiotic coverage of the patient might be appropriate due to diseases that are covered elsewhere in this text, such as human immunodeficiency virus, cavernous thrombosis, undiagnosed or uncontrolled diabetes, lupus, renal failure, and periods of neutropenia as are often associated with cancer chemotherapy. In these instances, medical consultation is almost always necessary in making antibiotic decisions in order to tailor the treatment and dosing to the individual patient's needs.

All tables or figures in this chapter were adapted from the ADA Advisory Statement: "Antibiotic Prophylaxis for Dental Patients With Total Joint Replacement," *J Am Dent Assoc*, 1997, 128:1004-8 or from Dajani AS, Taubert KA, Wilson W, et al, "Prevention of Bacterial Endocarditis. Recommendations by the American Heart Association," *JAMA*, 1997, 7(22):1794-801.

PREVENTION OF BACTERIAL ENDOCARDITIS

Guidelines for the prevention of bacterial endocarditis have been updated by the American Heart Association with approval by the Council of Scientific Affairs of the American Dental Association. These guidelines supercede those issued and published in 1990. They were developed to more clearly define the situations of antibiotic use, to reduce costs to the patient, to reduce gastrointestinal adverse effects, and to improve patient compliance. Highlights of the current recommendations are shown in Table 1 and the specific antibiotic regimens are listed in Table 2 and further illustrated in Figure 1 found at the end of this chapter. Amoxicillin is an amino-type penicillin with an extended spectrum of antibacterial action compared to penicillin VK. The pharmacology of amoxicillin as a dental antibiotic has been reviewed previously in *General Dentistry*. The suggested regimen for standard general prophylaxis is a dose of 2 g 1 hour before the procedure. A follow-up dose is no longer necessary. This dose of amoxicillin is lower than the previous dosing regimen of 3 g 1 hour before the procedure and then 1.5 g 6 hours after the initial dose. Dajani, et al, stated that the 2 g dose of amoxicillin resulted in adequate serum levels for several hours making the second dose unnecessary, both because of a prolonged serum level of amoxicillin above the minimal inhibitory concentration for oral streptococci, and an inhibitory activity of 6-14 hours by amoxicillin against streptococci. The new pediatric dose is 50 mg/kg orally 1 hour before the procedure and not to exceed the adult dose. Amoxicillin is available in capsules (250 mg and 500 mg), chewable tablets (125 mg, 250 mg, 400 mg), and liquid suspension (400 mg/5 mL). The retail cost of generic capsules and tablets ranges from 20-30 cents each and suspension is approximately $12 per 100 mL.

Table 1.
HIGHLIGHTS OF THE NEWEST GUIDELINES FOR ENDOCARDITIS PREVENTION

No.	Change From Old Guidelines
1.	Oral initial dosing for amoxicillin reduced to 2 g
2.	Follow-up antibiotic dose is no longer recommended
3.	Erythromycin is no longer recommended for penicillin-allergic patients
4.	Clindamycin and other alternatives have been recommended to replace the erythromycin regimens
5.	Clearer guidelines for prophylaxis decisions for patients with mitral valve prolapse have been developed

For individuals unable to take oral medications, intramuscular or intravenous ampicillin is recommended for both adults and children (Table 2). It is to be given 30 minutes before the procedure at the same doses used for the oral amoxicillin medication. Ampicillin is also an amino-type penicillin having an antibacterial spectrum similar to amoxicillin. Ampicillin is not absorbed from the gastrointestinal tract as effectively as amoxicillin and, therefore, is not recommended for oral use.

Table 2. PROPHYLACTIC REGIMENS FOR BACTERIAL ENDOCARDITIS FOR DENTAL PROCEDURES

Situation	Agent	Regimen*
Standard general prophylaxis	Amoxicillin *on page 86*	Adults: 2 g orally 1 hour before procedure Children: 50 mg/kg orally 1 hour before procedure
Unable to take oral medications	Ampicillin *on page 94*	Adults: 2 g I.M. or I.V. within 30 minutes before procedure Children: 50 mg/kg I.M. or I.V. within 30 minutes before procedure
Allergic to penicillin	Clindamycin *on page 300* or	Adults: 600 mg orally 1 hour before procedure Children: 20 mg/kg orally 1 hour before procedure
	Cephalexin *on page 251* or Cefadroxil *on page 232*	Adults: 2 g orally 1 hour before procedure Children: 50 mg/kg orally 1 hour before procedure
	Azithromycin *on page 137* or Clarithromycin *on page 296*	Adults: 500 mg orally 1 hour before procedure Children: 15 mg/kg orally 1 hour before procedure
Allergic to penicillin and unable to take oral medications	Clindamycin *on page 300* or	Adults: 600 mg I.V. within 30 minutes before procedure Children: 20 mg/kg I.V. within 30 minutes before procedure
	Cefazolin *on page 234*	Adults: 1 g I.M. or I.V. within 30 minutes before procedure Children: 25 mg/kg I.M. or I.V. within 30 minutes before procedure

*Total children's dose should not exceed adult dose.

Note: Cephalosporins should not be used in individuals with immediate-type hypersensitivity reaction (urticaria, angioedema, or anaphylaxis) to penicillins

Individuals who are allergic to the penicillins such as amoxicillin or ampicillin should be treated with an alternate antibiotic. The new guidelines have suggested a number of alternate agents including clindamycin, cephalosporins, azithromycin, and clarithromycin. Clindamycin (Cleocin®) occupies an important niche in dentistry as a useful and effective antibiotic and it was a recommended alternative agent for the prevention of bacterial endocarditis in the previous guidelines. In the new guidelines, the oral adult dose is 600 mg 1 hour before the procedure. A follow-up dose is not necessary. Clindamycin is available as 300 mg capsules; thus 2 capsules will provide the recommended dose. The children's oral dose for clindamycin is 20 mg/kg 1 hour before the procedure. Clindamycin is available as pediatric-flavored granules for oral solution. When reconstituted with water, each bottle yields a solution containing 75 mg/5 mL. Intravenous clindamycin is recommended in adults and children who are allergic to penicillin and unable to take oral medications. Refer to Table 2 for the intravenous doses of clindamycin.

Clindamycin was developed in the 1960s as a semisynthetic derivative of lincomycin which was found in the soil organism, *Streptomyces lincolnensis*, near Lincoln, Nebraska. It is commercially available as the hydrochloride salt to improve solubility in the gastrointestinal tract. Clindamycin is antibacterial against most aerobic Gram-positive cocci including staphylococci and streptococci, and against many types of anaerobic Gram-negative and Gram-positive organisms. It has been used over the years in dentistry as an alternative to penicillin and erythromycins for the treatment of oral-facial infections. For a review, see Wynn and Bergman.

The mechanism of antibacterial action of clindamycin is the same as erythromycin. It inhibits protein synthesis in susceptible bacteria resulting in the inhibition of bacterial growth and replication. Following oral administration of a single dose of clindamycin (150 mg, 300 mg, or 600 mg) on an empty stomach, 90% of the dose is rapidly absorbed into the bloodstream and peak serum concentrations are attained within 45-80 minutes. Administration with food does not markedly impair absorption into the bloodstream. Clindamycin serum levels exceed the minimum inhibitory concentration (MIC) for bacterial growth for at least 6 hours after the recommended dose of 600 mg. The serum half-life is 2-3 hours.

Adverse effects of clindamycin after a single dose are virtually nonexistent. Although it is estimated that 1% of patients taking clindamycin will develop symptoms of pseudomembranous colitis, these symptoms usually develop after 9-14 days of clindamycin therapy. These symptoms have never been reported in patients taking an acute dose for the prevention of endocarditis.

In lieu of clindamycin, penicillin-allergic individuals may receive cephalexin (Keflex®) or cefadroxil (Duricef®) provided that they have not had an immediate-type sensitivity reaction such as anaphylaxis, urticaria, or angioedema to penicillins. These antibiotics are first-generation cephalosporins having an antibacterial spectrum of action similar to

ANTIBIOTIC PROPHYLAXIS *(Continued)*

amoxicillin and ampicillin. They elicit a bactericidal action by inhibiting cell wall synthesis in susceptible bacteria. The recommended adult prophylaxis dose for either of these drugs is 2 g 1 hour before the procedure. Again, no follow-up dose is needed. The children's oral dose for cephalexin and cefadroxil is 50 mg/kg 1 hour before the procedure. Cephalexin is supplied as capsules (250 mg and 500 mg) and tablets (250 mg, 500 mg, 1 g). Cefadroxil is supplied as 500 mg capsules and 1 g tablets. Both antibiotics are available in the form of powder for oral suspension at concentrations of 125 mg and 250 mg (cefadroxil also available as 500 mg/5 mL).

For those individuals (adults and children) allergic to penicillin and unable to take oral medicines, parenteral cefazolin (Ancef®) may be used provided that they do not have the sensitivities described previously and footnoted in Table 2. Cefazolin is also a first-generation cephalosporin. Please note that the parenteral cefazolin can be given I.M. or I.V. Refer to Table 2 for the adult and children's doses of parenteral cefazolin.

Azithromycin (Zithromax®) and clarithromycin (Biaxin®) are members of the erythromycin-class of antibiotics known as the macrolides. The pharmacology of these drugs has been reviewed previously in *General Dentistry*. The erythromycins have been available for use in dentistry and medicine since the mid 1950s. Azithromycin and clarithromycin represent the first additions to this class in >40 years. The adult prophylactic dose for either drug is 500 mg 1 hour before the procedure with no follow-up dose. The pediatric prophylactic dose of azithromycin and clarithromycin is 15 mg/kg orally 1 hour before the procedure. Although the erythromycin family of drugs are known to inhibit the hepatic metabolism of theophylline and carbamazepine to enhance their effects, azithromycin has not been shown to affect the liver metabolism of these drugs.

Azithromycin is well absorbed from the gastrointestinal tract and is extensively taken up from the circulation into tissues with a slow release from those tissues. It reaches peak serum levels in 2-4 hours and serum half-life is 68 hours. Zithromax® is supplied as 250 mg (retail cost ranges from $7-$8 each) and 600 mg tablets (approximately $15 each). It is also available for oral suspension, supplied as single-dose packets containing 1 g each (approximately $60 for 3 packets). Azithromycin is not yet available as a generic drug.

Clarithromycin (Biaxin®) achieves peak plasma concentrations in 3 hours and maintains effective serum concentrations over a 12-hour period. Reports indicate that it probably interacts with theophylline and carbamazepine by elevating the plasma concentrations of the two drugs. Biaxin® is supplied as 250 mg and 500 mg tablets (retail cost approximately $4 each) and 500 mg extended release tablets (approximately $5 each). It is also available as suspension, supplied as 125 mg/100 mL and 125 mg/50 mL (approximately $20 per 50 mL). Clarithromycin is not yet available as a generic drug.

Amoxicillin (Amoxil®, Biomox®, Larotid®, Polymox®, Trimox®, Utimox®, Wymox®) *on page 86*

Ampicillin (Amcill®, Marcillin®, Omnipen®, Polycillin®, Principen®, Totacillin®) *on page 94*

Azithromycin (Zithromax®) *on page 137*

Cefadroxil (Duricef®, Ultracef®) *on page 232*

Cefazolin (Ancef®) *on page 234*

Cephalexin (Keflex®) *on page 251*

Clarithromycin (Biaxin®) *on page 296*

Clindamycin (Cleocin®) *on page 300*

Clinical Considerations for Dentistry

See Figure 1 algorithm at the end of this chapter.

The clinician should review carefully those detailed dental procedures in Table 3 to determine those treatment conditions where prophylaxis is, or is not, recommended. In general, in patients with cardiac conditions where prophylaxis is recommended (Table 4), invasive dental procedures where bleeding is likely to be induced from hard or soft tissues (Table 3) should be preceded by antibiotic coverage (Table 2). Clearly, the production of significant bacteremia during a dental procedure is the major risk factor. Patients with a suspicious history of a cardiac condition who are in need of an immediate dental procedure should be prophylaxed with an appropriate antibiotic prior to the procedure(s) until medical evaluation has been completed and the risk level determined. If unanticipated bleeding develops during a procedure in an at-risk patient, appropriate antibiotics should be given immediately. The efficacy of this action is based on animal studies and is possibly effective ≤ 2 hours after the bacteremia.

Table 3. DENTAL PROCEDURES AND PREPROCEDURAL ANTIBIOTICS

Endocarditis or Prosthesis Prophylaxis Recommended Due to Likely Significant Bacteremia*
Dental extractions
Periodontal procedures including surgery, subgingival placement of antibiotic fibers/strips, scaling and root planing, probing, recall maintenance
Dental implant placement and reimplantation of avulsed teeth
Endodontic (root canal) instrumentation or surgery only beyond the apex
Initial placement of orthodontic bands but not brackets
Intraligamentary local anesthetic injections
Prophylactic cleaning of teeth or implants where bleeding is anticipated
Endocarditis Prophylaxis Not Recommended Due to Usually Insignificant Bacteremia
Restorative dentistry† (operative and prosthodontic) with or without retraction cord‡
Local anesthetic injections (nonintraligamentary)
Intracanal endodontic treatment; postplacement and build-up‡
Placement of rubber dam‡
Postoperative suture removal
Placement of removable prosthodontic/orthodontic appliances
Oral impressions‡
Fluoride treatments
Taking of oral radiographs
Orthodontic appliance adjustment
Shedding of primary teeth
‡In general, the presence of moderate to severe gingival inflammation may elevate these procedures to a higher risk of bacteremia.

*Prophylaxis is recommended for patients with high- and moderate-risk cardiac as well as high-risk prosthesis conditions

†This includes restoration of decayed teeth and replacement of missing teeth

‡Clinical judgment may indicate antibiotic use in any circumstances that may create significant bleeding.

Patients with moderate to advanced gingival inflammatory disease and/or periodontitis should be considered at greater risk of bacteremia. However, the ongoing daily risk of self-induced bacteremia in these patients is currently thought to be minimal as compared to the bacteremia during dental procedures. The clinician may wish to consider the use of a preprocedural antimicrobial rinse in addition to antibiotic prophylaxis and, of course, efforts should always focus on improving periodontal health during dental care. If a series of dental procedures is planned, the clinician must judge whether an interval between procedures, requiring prophylaxis, should be scheduled. The literature supports 9- to 14-day intervals as ideal to minimize the risk of emergence of resistant organisms. Since serum levels of the standard amoxicillin dose may be adequate for 6-14 hours depending on the specific organism challenge, the clinician may have to consider the efficacy of a second dose if multiple procedures are planned over the course of a single day.

Table 4. CARDIAC CONDITIONS PREDISPOSING TO ENDOCARDITIS

Endocarditis Prophylaxis Recommended
High-Risk Category
Prosthetic cardiac valves, including bioprosthetic and homograft valves
Previous bacterial endocarditis
Complex cyanotic congenital heart disease (eg, single ventricle states, transposition of the great arteries, tetralogy of Fallot)
Surgically constructed systemic pulmonary shunts or conduits
Moderate-Risk Category
Most other congenital cardiac malformations (other than above and below)
Acquired valvar dysfunction (eg, rheumatic heart disease)
Hypertrophic cardiomyopathy
Mitral valve prolapse with valvar regurgitation and/or thickened leaflets*
Endocarditis Prophylaxis Not Recommended
Negligible-Risk Category (no greater risk than the general population)
Isolated secundum atrial septal defect
Surgical repair of atrial septal defect, ventricular septal defect, or patent ductus arteriosus (without residual defects beyond 6 mo)
Previous coronary artery bypass graft surgery
Mitral valve prolapse without valvar regurgitation
Physiologic, functional, or innocent heart murmurs
Previous Kawasaki disease without valvar dysfunction
Previous rheumatic fever without valvar dysfunction
Cardiac pacemakers (intravascular and epicardial) and implanted defibrillators
****Specific risk for patients with a history of fenfluramine or dexfenfluramine (fen-phen or Redux®) use, has not been determined. Such patients should have medical evaluation for potential cardiac damage, as currently recommended by the FDA.**

ANTIBIOTIC PROPHYLAXIS *(Continued)*

For patients with suspected or confirmed mitral valve prolapse (MVP), the risk of infection as well as other complications such as tachycardia, syncope, congestive heart failure, or progressive regurgitation are variable. The risk depends on age and severity of MVP. The decision to recommend prophylaxis in such patients is oftentimes controversial but it is generally agreed that the determination of regurgitation is the most predictive (see Algorithm Figure 2 at the end of this chapter). Therefore, patients with MVP with mitral regurgitation require prophylaxis. If the regurgitation is undetermined and the patient is in need of an immediate procedure, then prophylaxis should be given in any case and the patient referred for further evaluation. If echocardiographic or Doppler studies demonstrate regurgitation, then prophylaxis would be recommended routinely. If no regurgitation can be demonstrated by these studies, then MVP alone does not require prophylaxis.

PREPROCEDURAL ANTIBIOTICS FOR PROSTHETIC IMPLANTS

A significant number of dental patients have had total joint replacements or other implanted prosthetic devices. Prior to performing dental procedures that might induce bacteremia, the dentist must consider the use of antibiotic prophylaxis in these patients. Until recently, only the American Heart Association had taken a formal stance on implanted devices by suggesting guidelines for the use of antibiotic prophylaxis in patients with prosthetic heart valves. These guidelines and the recent guidelines for prevention of bacterial endocarditis have been published in *General Dentistry.*

The use of antibiotics in patients with other prosthetic devices, including total joint replacements has remained controversial because of several issues. Late infections of implanted prosthetic devices have rarely been associated with microbial organisms of oral origin. Secondly, since late infections in such patients are often not reported, data is lacking to substantiate or refute this potential. Also, there is general acceptance that patients with acute infections at distant sites such as the oral cavity may be at greater risk of infection of an implanted prosthetic device. Periodontal disease has been implicated as a distant site infection. Since antibiotics are associated with allergies and other adverse reactions, and because the frequent use of antibiotics may lead to emergence of resistant organisms, any perceived benefit of antibiotic prophylaxis must always be weighed against known risks of toxicity, allergy, or potential microbial resistance.

Recently, an advisory group made up of representatives from the American Dental Association and the American Academy of Orthopaedic Surgeons published a statement in the *Journal of the American Dental Association* on the use of antibiotics prior to dental procedures in patients with total joint replacements. The statement concluded that antibiotic prophylaxis should not be prescribed routinely for most dental patients with total joint replacements or for any patients with pins, plates, and screws. However, in an attempt to base the guidelines on available scientific evidence, the advisory group stated that certain patients may be potential risks for joint infection thus justifying the use of prophylactic antibiotics. Those conditions considered by the advisory group to be associated with potential elevated risk of joint infections are listed in Table 5. The dentist should carefully review the patient's history to ensure identification of those medical problems leading to potential elevated risks of joint infections as listed in Table 5. Where appropriate, medical consultation with the patient's internist or orthopedist may be prudent to assist in this determination. The orthopedist should be queried specifically, as to the status of the joint prosthesis itself.

Table 5. PATIENTS WITH POTENTIAL ELEVATED RISK OF JOINT INFECTION

Inflammatory arthropathies: Rheumatoid arthritis, systemic lupus erythematosus
Disease-, drug-, or radiation-induced immunosuppression
Insulin-dependent diabetes
First 2 years following joint replacement
Previous prosthetic joint infections
Patients with acute infections at a distant site
Hemophilia

Patients who present with elevated risks of joint infections, in which the dentist is going to perform any procedures associated with a high risk of bacteremia, need to receive preprocedural antibiotics. Those dental procedures associated with high risk of bacteremia are listed in Table 3. Patients undergoing dental procedures involving low risk of bacteremia, probably do not require premedication even though the patient may be in the category of elevated risk of joint infections. Patients with an acute oral infection or moderate to severe gingival inflammation and/or periodontitis must be considered at higher risk for bacteremia during dental procedures than those without active dental disease. In these patients, as in all patients, the dental clinician should aggressively treat these oral conditions striving for optimum oral health. The listing of low bacteremia risks in Table 3 may need to be reconsidered, depending on the patient's oral health.

ANTIBIOTIC REGIMENS

The antibiotic prophylaxis regimens as suggested by the advisory panel are listed in Table 6. These regimens are not exactly the same as those listed in Table 2 (for prevention of endocarditis) and must be reviewed carefully to avoid confusion. Cephalexin, cephradine, or amoxicillin may be used in patients not allergic to penicillin. The selected antibiotic is given as a single 2 g dose 1 hour before the procedure. A follow-up dose is not recommended. Cephalexin (Keflex®) and amoxicillin have been described earlier in this chapter. Cephradine (Velosef®) is a first-generation cephalosporin-type antibiotic effective against anaerobic bacteria and aerobic Gram-positive bacteria. It is used in medicine predominantly to treat infections of the bones and joints, infections of the lower respiratory tract, urinary tract, and skin and soft tissues.

Parenteral cefazolin (Ancef®) or ampicillin are the recommended antibiotics for those patients unable to take oral medications; see Table 6 for doses. Cefazolin is a first-generation cephalosporin effective against anaerobes and aerobic Gram-positive bacteria. Ampicillin is an aminopenicillin described earlier. For patients allergic to penicillin, clindamycin is the recommended antibiotic of choice. Clindamycin is active against aerobic and anaerobic streptococci, most staphylococci, the *Bacteroides*, and the *Actinomyces* families of bacteria. The recommended oral and parenteral doses of clindamycin in the joint prosthetic patient are listed in Table 6.

Table 6. ANTIBIOTIC REGIMENS FOR PATIENTS WITH PROSTHETIC IMPLANTS

Patients not allergic to penicillin:	Cephalexin, cephradine, or amoxicillin:	2 g orally 1 hour prior to the procedure
Patients not allergic to penicillin and unable to take oral medications:	Cefazolin: or Ampicillin:	1 g I.M. or I.V. 1 hour prior to the procedure 2 g I.M. or I.V. 1 hour prior to the procedure
Patients allergic to penicillin:	Clindamycin:	600 mg orally 1 hour prior to dental procedure
Patients allergic to penicillin and unable to take oral medications:	Clindamycin:	600 mg I.V. 1 hour prior to the procedure

Amoxicillin (Amoxil®, Biomox®, Larotid®, Polymox®, Trimox®, Utimox®, Wymox®) *on page 86*

Ampicillin (Amcill®, Marcillin®, Omnipen®, Polycillin®, Principen®, Totacillin®) *on page 94*

Cefazolin (Ancef®) *on page 234*

Cephalexin (Keflex®) *on page 251*

Cephradine (Velosef®) *on page 253*

Clindamycin (Cleocin®) *on page 300*

Clinical Considerations for Dentistry

See Algorithm Figure 3 at the end of this chapter.

The frequency of postinsertion infections in patients who have undergone total joint replacement or prosthetic device placement is variable. The most common cause of infection with all devices is found to be from contamination at the time of surgical insertions. The presence of an acute distant infection at a site other than the joint, however, appears to be a risk factor for late infection of these devices. The rationale by the American Dental Association and the American Academy of Orthopedic Surgeons in their advisory statement has been to provide guidelines to minimize the use of antibiotics to the first 2 years following total joint replacement. As more data are collected, these recommendations may be revised. However, it is thought to be prudent for the dental clinician to fully evaluate all patients with respect to history and or physical findings prior to determining the risk.

If a procedure considered to be low risk for bacteremia is performed in a patient at risk for joint complications, and inadvertent bleeding occurs, then an appropriate antibiotic should be given immediately. Although this is not ideal, animal studies suggest that it may be useful. Likewise, in patients where concern exists over joint complications and a medical consultation cannot be immediately obtained, the patient should be treated as though antibiotic coverage is necessary until such time that an appropriate consultation can be completed. The presence of an acute oral infection, in addition to any pre-existing dental conditions, may increase the risk of late infection at the prosthetic joint. Even though most late joint infections are caused by *Staphylococcus* sp, the risk of bacteremia involving another organism, predominant in an acute infection, may increase the risk of joint infection.

ANTIBIOTIC PROPHYLAXIS *(Continued)*

The dentist may also need to consider the question of multiple procedures over a period of time. Procedures planned over a period of several days would best be rescheduled at intervals of 9-14 days. The risk of emergence of resistant organisms in patients receiving multiple short-term doses of antibiotics has been shown to be greater than those receiving antibiotics over longer intervals of time.

FREQUENTLY ASKED QUESTIONS

Can erythromycin still be used to prevent bacterial endocarditis in dental patients?

If the clinician has successfully used erythromycin in the past, this form of prophylaxis can be continued using the regimen included in the recommendation of 1990. Erythromycin has, however, been excluded for the vast majority of patients due to gastric upset.

If the patient is presently taking antibiotics for some other ailment, is prophylaxis still necessary?

If a patient is already taking antibiotics for another condition, prophylaxis should be accomplished with a drug from another class. For example, in the patient who is not allergic to penicillin who is taking erythromycin for a medical condition such as mycoplasma infection, amoxicillin would be the drug of choice for prophylaxis. Also, in the penicillin-allergic patient taking clindamycin, prophylaxis would best be accomplished with azithromycin or clarithromycin. The new guidelines restated the position that doses of antibiotics for prevention of recurrence of rheumatic fever are thought to be inadequate to prevent bacterial endocarditis and prophylaxis should be accomplished with the full dose of a drug from another class.

Can clindamycin be used safely in patients with gastrointestinal disorders?

If a patient has a history of inflammatory bowel disease and is allergic to penicillin, azithromycin or clarithromycin should be selected over clindamycin. In patients with a negative history of inflammatory bowel disease, clindamycin has not been shown to induce colitis following a single-dose administration.

Why do the suggested drug regimens for patients with joint prostheses resemble so closely the regimens for the prevention of bacterial endocarditis?

Bacteremia is the predisposing risk factor for the development of endocarditis in those patients at risk due to a cardiac condition. Likewise, the potential of bacteremia during dental procedures is considered to be the risk factor in some late joint prostheses infections, even though this risk is presumed to be much lower.

How do we determine those patients who have had joint replacement complications?

Patients who have had complications during the initial placement of a total joint would be those who had infection following placement, those with recurrent pain, or those who have had previous joint replacement failures. If the patient reports even minor complications, a medical consultation with the orthopedist would be the most appropriate action for the dentist.

Is prophylaxis required in patients with pins, screws, or plates often used in orthopedic repairs?

There is currently no evidence supporting use of antibiotics following the placement of pins, plates, or screws. Breast implants, dental implants, and implanted lenses in the eye following cataract surgery are also all thought to be at minimal risk for infection following dental procedures. Therefore, no antibiotic prophylaxis is recommended in these situations. There is, however, some evidence indicating elevated risk of infection following some types of penile implants and some vascular access devices, used during chemotherapy. It is recommended that the dentist discuss such patients with the physician prior to determining the need for antibiotics.

What should I do if medical consultation results in a recommendation that differs from the published guidelines endorsed by the American Dental Association?

The dentist is ultimately responsible for treatment recommendations. Ideally, by communicating with the physician, a consensus can be achieved that is either in agreement with the guidelines or is based on other established medical reasoning.

What is the best antibiotic modality for treating dental infections?

Penicillin is still the drug of choice for treatment of infections in and around the oral cavity. Phenoxy-methyl penicillin (Pen VK®) has long been the most commonly selected antibiotic. In penicillin-allergic individuals, erythromycin may be an appropriate consideration. If another drug is sought, clindamycin prescribed 300 mg as a loading dose followed by 150 mg 4 times/day would be an appropriate regimen for a dental infection. In general, if there is no response to Pen VK®, then Augmentin® may be a good alternative in the nonpenicillin-allergic patient because of its slightly altered spectrum. Recommendations would include that the patient should take the drug with food.

Is there cross-allergenicity between the cephalosporins and penicillin?

The incidence of cross-allergenicity is 5% to 8% in the overall population. If a patient has demonstrated a Type I hypersensitivity reaction to penicillin, namely urticaria or anaphylaxis, then this incidence would increase to 20%.

Is there definitely an interaction between contraception agents and antibiotics?

There are well founded interactions between contraceptives and antibiotics. The best instructions that a patient could be given by their dentist are that should an antibiotic be necessary and the dentist is aware that the patient is on contraceptives, and if the patient is using chemical contraceptives, the patient should seriously consider additional means of contraception during the antibiotic management.

Are antibiotics necessary in diabetic patients?

In the management of diabetes, control of the diabetic status is the key factor relative to all morbidity issues. If a patient is well controlled, then antibiotics will likely not be necessary. However, in patients where the control is questionable or where they have recently been given a different drug regimen for their diabetes or if they are being titrated to an appropriate level of either insulin or oral hypoglycemic agents during these periods of time, the dentist might consider preprocedural antibiotics to be efficacious.

Do nonsteroidal anti-inflammatory drugs interfere with blood pressure medication?

At the current time there is no clear evidence that NSAIDs interfere with any of the blood pressure medications that are currently in use.

Is a patient who has taken phentermine at risk for cardiac problems just like a patient who took "fen-phen"?

No, there is often confusion with these drug names. "Fen-phen" referred to a combined use of fenfluramine and phentermine and it is this combination that has led to the FDA statement (see Table 4). The single drug phentermine has not been implicated in this current concern over cardiac complications.

ANTIBIOTIC PROPHYLAXIS *(Continued)*

Figure 1
Preprocedural Dental Action Plan for Patients With a History Indicative of Elevated Endocarditis Risk

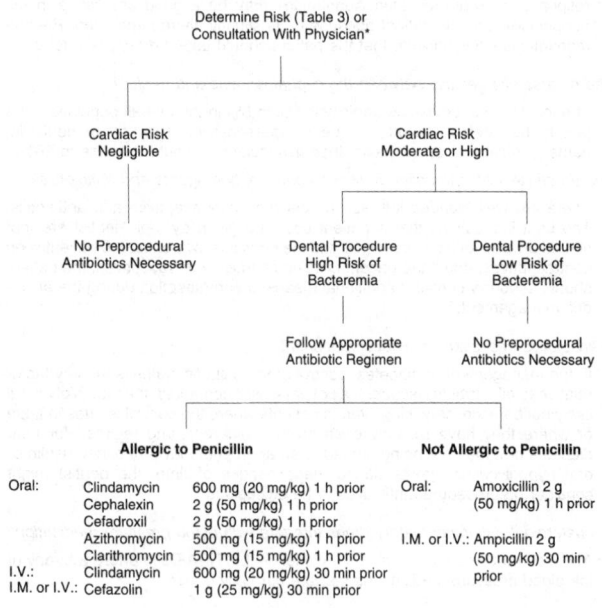

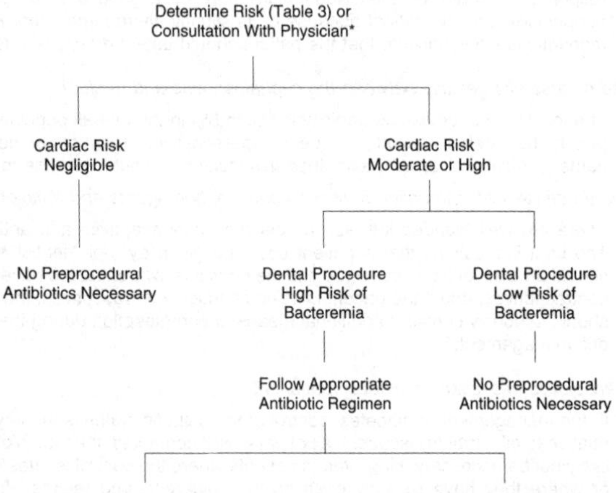

Allergic to Penicillin

Oral:	Clindamycin	600 mg (20 mg/kg) 1 h prior
	Cephalexin	2 g (50 mg/kg) 1 h prior
	Cefadroxil	2 g (50 mg/kg) 1 h prior
	Azithromycin	500 mg (15 mg/kg) 1 h prior
	Clarithromycin	500 mg (15 mg/kg) 1 h prior
I.V.:	Clindamycin	600 mg (20 mg/kg) 30 min prior
I.M. or I.V.:	Cefazolin	1 g (25 mg/kg) 30 min prior

Not Allergic to Penicillin

Oral:	Amoxicillin 2 g (50 mg/kg) 1 h prior
I.M. or I.V.:	Ampicillin 2 g (50 mg/kg) 30 min prior

Dosages for children are in parentheses and should never exceed adult dose. Cephalosporins should be avoided in patients with previous Type I hypersensitivity reactions to penicillin due to some evidence of cross allergenicity.

* For Emergency Dental Care, the clinician should attempt phone consultation. If unable to contact patient's physician or determine risk, the patient should be treated as though there is moderate or high risk of cardiac complication and follow the algorithm.

Figure 2
Patient With Suspected Mitral Valve Prolapse

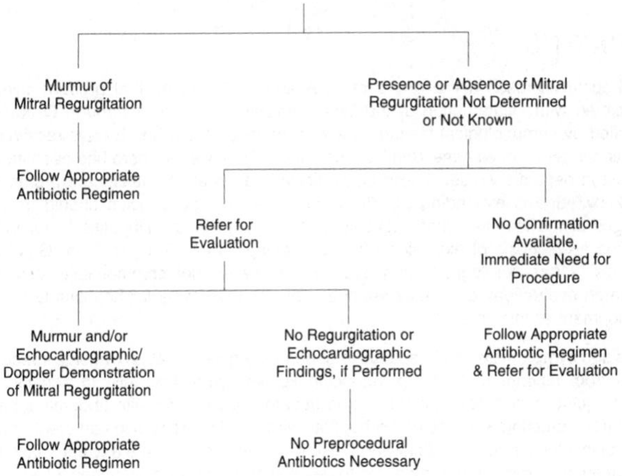

Figure 3
Preprocedural Dental Action Plan for Patients With Prosthetic Implants

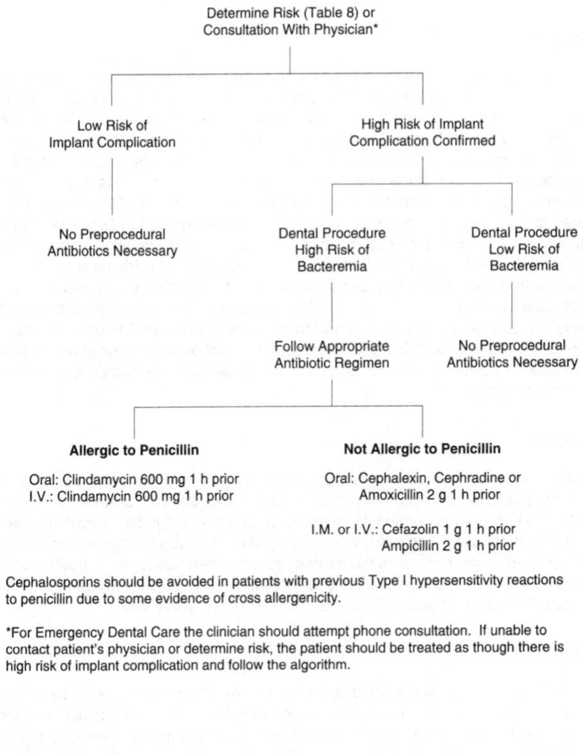

Cephalosporins should be avoided in patients with previous Type I hypersensitivity reactions to penicillin due to some evidence of cross allergenicity.

*For Emergency Dental Care the clinician should attempt phone consultation. If unable to contact patient's physician or determine risk, the patient should be treated as though there is high risk of implant complication and follow the algorithm.

SYSTEMIC VIRAL DISEASES

HEPATITIS

The hepatitis viruses are a group of DNA and RNA viruses that produce symptoms associated with inflammation of the liver. Currently, hepatitis A through G have been identified by immunological testing; however, hepatitis A through E have received most attention in terms of disease identification. Recently, however, there has been increased interest in hepatitis viruses F and G, particularly as relate to healthcare professionals. Our knowledge is expanding rapidly in this area and the clinician should be alert to changes in the literature that might update their knowledge. Hepatitis F, for instance, remains a diagnosis of exclusion effectively being non-A, B, C, D, E, or G. Whereas, hepatitis G has serologic testing available, however, not commercially at this time. Research evaluations of various antibody and RT-PCR tests for hepatitis G are under development at this time.

Signs and symptoms of viral hepatitis in general are quite variable. Patients infected may range from asymptomatic to experiencing flu-like symptoms only. In addition, fever, nausea, joint muscle pain, jaundice, and hepatomegaly along with abdominal pain can result from infection with one of the hepatitis viruses. The virus also can create an acute or chronic infection. Usually following these early symptoms or the asymptomatic period, the patient may recover or may go on to develop chronic liver dysfunction. Liver dysfunction may be represented primarily by changes in liver function tests known as LFTs and these primarily include aspartate aminotransferase known as AST and alanine aminotransferase known as ALT. In addition, for A, B, C, D, and E there are serologic tests for either antigen, antibody, or both. Of hepatitis A through G, five forms have both acute and chronic forms whereas A and E appear to only create acute disease. There are differences in the way clinicians may approach a known postexposure to one of the hepatitis viruses. In many instances, gamma globulin may be used, however, the indications for gamma globulin as a drug limit their use to several of the viruses only. The dental clinician should be aware that the gastroenterologist may choose to give gamma globulin off-label.

Hepatitis A

Hepatitis A virus is an enteric virus that is a member of the Picornavirus family along with Coxsackie viruses and poliovirus. Previously known as infectious hepatitis, hepatitis A has been detected in humans for centuries. It causes acute hepatitis, often transmitted by oral-fecal contamination and having an incubation period of approximately 30 days. Typically, constitutional symptoms are present and jaundice may occur. Drug therapy that the dentist may encounter in a patient being treated for hepatitis A would primarily include immunoglobulin. Hepatitis A vaccine (inactivated) is an FDA-approved vaccine indicated in the prevention of contracting hepatitis A in exposed or high-risk individuals. Candidates at high risk for HAV infection include persons traveling internationally to highly endemic areas, individuals with chronic liver disease, individuals engaging in high-risk sexual behavior, illicit drug users, persons with high-risk occupational exposure, hemophiliacs or other persons receiving blood products, pediatric populations, and food handlers in high-risk environments. Two formulations of hepatitis A vaccine are available, Havrix® and VAQTA®. Each is administered as an injection in the deltoid region and both are available in pediatric and adult dosages. For additional information, refer to Hepatitis A Vaccine *on page 583.*

Hepatitis B

Hepatitis B virus is previously known as serum hepatitis and has particular trophism for liver cells. Hepatitis B virus causes both acute and chronic disease in susceptible patients. The incubation period is often long and the diagnosis might be made by serologic markers even in the absence of symptoms. No drug therapy for acute hepatitis B is known; however, chronic hepatitis has recently been successfully treated with alfa-interferon. There are vaccines available for hepatitis A and B. See Hepatitis A Inactivated and Hepatitis B (Recombinant) Vaccine (Twinrex®) *on page 582.*

Hepatitis C

Hepatitis C virus was described in 1988 and has been formerly classified as non-A/non-B. It is clear that hepatitis C represents a high percentage of the transfusion-associated hepatitis that is seen. Treatment of acute hepatitis C infection is generally supportive. Interferon Alfa-2a therapy has been used with some success recently and interferon-alfa may be beneficial with hepatitis C related chronic hepatitis.

Hepatitis D

Hepatitis D, previously known as the delta agent, is a virus that is incomplete in that it requires previous infection with hepatitis B in order to be manifested. Currently, no antiviral therapy is effective against hepatitis D.

Hepatitis E

Hepatitis E virus is an RNA virus that represents a proportion of the previously classified non-A/non-B diagnoses. There is currently no antiviral therapy against hepatitis E.

Hepatitis F

Hepatitis F, as was mentioned, remains a diagnosis of exclusion. There are no known immunological tests available for identification of hepatitis F at present and currently the Centers for Disease Control have not come out with specific guidelines or recommendations. It is thought, however, that hepatitis F is a bloodborne virus and it has been used as a diagnosis in several cases of post-transfusion hepatitis.

Hepatitis G

Hepatitis G virus (HGV) is the newest hepatitis and is also assumed to be a bloodborne virus. Similar in family to hepatitis C, it is thought to occur concomitantly with hepatitis C and appears to be even more prevalent in some blood donors than hepatitis C. Occupational transmission of HGV is currently under study (see the references for updated information) and currently there are no specific CDC recommendations for postexposure to an HGV individual as the testing for identification remains experimental.

Hepatitis A Vaccine (Havrix®) *on page 583*
Hepatitis A Inactivated and Hepatitis B (Recombinant) Vaccine (Twinrex®) *on page 582*
Hepatitis B Immune Globulin (H-BIG®, HyperHep®) *on page 584*
Hepatitis B Vaccine (Engerix-B®, Recombivax HB®) *on page 584*
Immune Globulin, Intramuscular (Gamastan®, Gammar®) *on page 629*
Immune Globulin, Intravenous (Gamimune® N, Gammagard®, Gammagard® S/D, Gammar®-P, Polygam®, Polygam® S/D, Sandoglobulin®, Venoglobulin®-I, Venoglobulin®-S) *on page 630*
Interferon Alfa-2a (Roferon-A®) *on page 641*
Interferon Alfa-2a (Roferon-A®) *on page 641*
Peginterferon Alfa-2b (PEG-Intron™) *on page 922*

TYPES OF HEPATITIS VIRUS

Features	A	B	C	D	E	F	G
Incubation Period	2-6 wks	8-24 wks	2-52 wks	3-13 wks	3-6 wks	Unknown	Unknown
Onset	Abrupt	Insidious	Insidious	Abrupt	Abrupt	Insidious	Insidious
Symptoms							
Jaundice	Adults: 70% to 80%; Children: 10%	25%	25%	Varies	Unknown	Unknown	Unknown
Asymptomatic patients	Adults: 50%; Children: Most	~75%	~75%	Rare	Rare	Common	Common
Routes of Transmission							
Fecal/Oral	Yes	No	No	No	Yes	Unknown	Unknown
Parenteral	Rare	Yes	Yes	Yes	No		
Sexual	No	Yes	Possible	Yes	No		
Perinatal	No	Yes	Possible	Possible	No		
Water/Food	Yes	No	No	No	Yes		
Sequelae (% of patients)							
Chronic state	No	Adults: 6% to 10%; Children: 25% to 50%; Infants: 70% to 90%	>75%	10% to 15%	No	Unknown	Likely
Case-Fatality Rate	0.6%	1.4%	1% to 2%	30%	1% to 2% Pregnant women: 20%	Unknown	Unknown

SYSTEMIC VIRAL DISEASES *(Continued)*

PRE-EXPOSURE RISK FACTORS FOR HEPATITIS B

Healthcare factors:

Healthcare workers*

Special patient groups (eg, adolescents, infants born to HB_sAg–positive mothers, military personnel, etc)

Hemodialysis patients†

Recipients of certain blood products‡

Lifestyle factors:

Homosexual and bisexual men

Intravenous drug abusers

Heterosexually active persons with multiple sexual partners or recently acquired sexually transmitted diseases

Environmental factors:

Household and sexual contacts of HBV carriers

Prison inmates

Clients and staff of institutions for the mentally handicapped

Residents, immigrants and refugees from areas with endemic HBV infection

International travelers at increased risk of acquiring HBV infection

*The risk of hepatitis B virus (HBV) infection for healthcare workers varies both between hospitals and within hospitals. Hepatitis B vaccination is recommended for all healthcare workers with blood exposure.

†Hemodialysis patients often respond poorly to hepatitis B vaccination; higher vaccine doses or increased number of doses are required. A special formulation of one vaccine is now available for such persons (Recombivax HB®, 40 mcg/mL). The anti-HB_s (antibody to hepatitis B surface antigen) response of such persons should be tested after they are vaccinated, and those who have not responded should be revaccinated with 1-3 additional doses.

Patients with chronic renal disease should be vaccinated as early as possible, ideally before they require hemodialysis. In addition, their anti- HB_s levels should be monitored at 6- to 12-month intervals to assess the need for revaccination.

‡Patients with hemophilia should be immunized subcutaneously, not intramuscularly.

POSTEXPOSURE PROPHYLAXIS FOR HEPATITIS B*

Exposure	Hepatitis B Immune Globulin	Hepatitis B Vaccine
Perinatal	0.5 mL I.M. within 12 hours of birth	0.5 mL† I.M. within 12 hours of birth (no later than 7 days), and at 1 and 6 months‡; test for HB_sAg and anti-HB_s at 12-15 months
Sexual	0.06 mL/kg I.M. within 14 days of sexual contact; a second dose should be given if the index patient remains HB_sAg-positive after 3 months and hepatitis B vaccine was not given initially	1 mL I.M. at 0, 1, and 6 months for homosexual and bisexual men and regular sexual contacts of persons with acute and chronic hepatitis B
Percutaneous; exposed person unvaccinated		
Source known HB_sAg-positive	0.06 mL/kg I.M. within 24 hours	1 mL I.M. within 7 days, and at 1 and 6 months§
Source known, HB_sAg status not known	Test source for HB_sAg; if source is positive, give exposed person 0.06 mL/kg I.M. once within 7 days	1 mL I.M. within 7 days, and at 1 and 6 months§
Source not tested or unknown	Nothing required	1 mL I.M. within 7 days, and at 1 and 6 months
Percutaneous; exposed person vaccinated		
Source known HB_sAg-positive	Test exposed person for anti-HB_s¶. If titer is protective, nothing is required; if titer is not protective, give 0.06 mL/kg within 24 hours	Review vaccination status#
Source known, HB_sAg status not known	Test source for HB_sAg and exposed person for anti-HB_s. If source is HB_sAg-negative, or if source is HB_sAg-positive but anti-HB_s titer is protective, nothing is required. If source is HB_sAg-positive and anti-HB_s titer is not protective or if exposed person is a known nonresponder, give 0.06 mL/kg I.M. within 24 hours. A second dose of hepatitis B immune globulin can be given 1 month later if a booster dose of hepatitis B vaccine is not given.	Review vaccination status#

POSTEXPOSURE PROPHYLAXIS FOR HEPATITIS B* *(continued)*

Exposure	Hepatitis B Immune Globulin	Hepatitis B Vaccine
Source not tested or unknown	Test exposed person for anti-HB_s. If anti-HB_s titer is protective, nothing is required. If anti-HB_s titer is not protective, 0.06 mL/kg may be given along with a booster dose of hepatitis B vaccine.	Review vaccination status#

*HB_sAg = hepatitis B surface antigen; anti-HB_s = antibody to hepatitis B surface antigen; I.M. = intramuscularly; SRU = standard ratio units.

†Each 0.5 mL dose of plasma-derived hepatitis B vaccine contains 10 mcg of HB_sAg; each 0.5 mL dose of recombinant hepatitis B vaccine contains 5 mcg or 10 mcg of HB_sAg.

‡If hepatitis B immune globulin and hepatitis B vaccine are given simultaneously, they should be given at separate sites.

§If hepatitis B vaccine is not given, a second dose of hepatitis B immune globulin should be given 1 month later.

¶Anti-HB_s titers <10 SRU by radioimmunoassay or negative by enzyme immunoassay indicate lack of protection. Testing the exposed person for anti-HB_s is not necessary if a protective level of antibody has been shown within the previous 24 months.

#If the exposed person has not completed a three-dose series of hepatitis B vaccine, the series should be completed. Test the exposed person for anti-HB_s. If the antibody level is protective, nothing is required. If an adequate antibody response in the past is shown on retesting to have declined to an inadequate level, a booster dose (1 mL) of hepatitis B vaccine should be given. If the exposed person has inadequate antibody or is a known nonresponder to vaccination, a booster dose can be given along with one dose of hepatitis B immune globulin.

HERPES

The herpes viruses not only represent a topic of specific interest to the dentist due to oral manifestations, but are widespread as systemic infections. Herpes simplex virus is also of interest because of its central nervous system infections and its relationship as one of the viral infections commonly found in AIDS patients. Oral herpes infections will be covered elsewhere. Treatment of herpes simplex primary infection includes acyclovir. Ganciclovir is an alternative drug and foscarnet is also occasionally used. Epstein-Barr virus is a member of the herpesvirus family and produces syndromes important in dentistry, including infectious mononucleosis with the commonly found oral pharyngitis and petechial hemorrhages, as well as being the causative agent of Burkitt's lymphoma. The relationship between Epstein-Barr virus to oral hairy leukoplakia in AIDS patients has not been shown to be one of cause and effect; however, the presence of Epstein-Barr in these lesions is consistent. Currently, there is no accepted treatment for Epstein-Barr virus, although acyclovir has been shown in *in vitro* studies to have some efficacy. Varicella-zoster virus is another member of the herpesvirus family and is the causative agent of two clinical entities, chickenpox and shingles or herpes zoster. Oral manifestations of both chickenpox and herpes zoster include vesicular eruptions often leading to confluent mucosal ulcerations. Acyclovir is the drug of choice for treatment of herpes zoster infections.

There are other herpes viruses that produce disease in man and animals. These viruses have no specific treatment, therefore, incidence is thought to be less common than those mentioned and the specific treatment is not determined at present. The role of some of these viruses in concomitant infection with the HIV and other coinfection viruses is still under study.

SYSTEMIC VIRAL DISEASES *(Continued)*

ANTIVIRALS

AGENTS OF ESTABLISHED EFFECTIVENESS

Viral Infection	Drug
Cytomegalovirus	
Retinitis	Ganciclovir Foscarnet
Pneumonia	Ganciclovir
Hepatitis viruses	
Chronic hepatitis A & B	Hepatitis A Inactivated & Hepatitis B (Recombinant) vaccine
Chronic hepatitis C	Interferon Alfa-2a
Chronic hepatitis B	Interferon Alfa-2b Peginterferon Alfa-2b
Herpes simplex virus	
Orofacial herpes	
First episode	Acyclovir*
Recurrence	Acyclovir* Penciclovir*
Genital herpes	
First episode	Acyclovir
Recurrence	Acyclovir
Suppression	Acyclovir
Encephalitis	Acyclovir
Mucocutaneous disease in immunocompromised	Acyclovir
Neonatal	Acyclovir
Keratoconjunctivitis	Trifluridine Vidarabine
Influenza A virus	Amantadine Oseltamivir Rimantadine Zanamivir
Papillomavirus	
Condyloma acuminatum	Interferon Alfa-2b Imiquimod (Aldara®): (use for oral lesions is under study)
Respiratory syncytial virus	Ribavirin
Varicella-zoster virus	
Varicella in normal children	Acyclovir
Varicella in immunocompromised	Acyclovir
Herpes zoster in immunocompromised	Acyclovir
Herpes zoster in normal hosts	Acyclovir Famciclovir Valacyclovir

*Although acyclovir is often used for these infections, penciclovir is specifically approved for herpes labialis. The clinician is referred to the monographs for more discussion.

Acyclovir (Zovirax®) *on page 40*
Amantadine (Symmetrel®) *on page 64*
Atovaquone (Mepron™) *on page 128*
Cidofovir (Vistide®) *on page 283*
Famciclovir (Famvir™) *on page 485*
Fomivirsen (Virtravene®) *on page 534*
Foscarnet (Foscavir®) *on page 537*
Ganciclovir (Cytovene®, Vitrasert®) *on page 547*
Hepatitis B Immune Globulin (H-BIG®, HyperHep®) *on page 584*
Imiquimod (Aldara®) *on page 628*
Immune Globulin, Intramuscular (Gamastan®, Gammar®) *on page 629*
Interferon Alfa-2a (Roferon-A®) *on page 641*
Interferon Alfa-2b (Intron® A) *on page 642*
Interferon Alfa-n3 (Alferon® N) *on page 646*
Oseltamivir (Tamiflu™) *on page 892*
Penciclovir (Denavir®) *on page 926*
Rifabutin (Mycobutin®) *on page 1050*
Rimantadine (Flumadine®) *on page 1055*
Trifluridine (Viroptic®) *on page 1207*
Valacyclovir (Valtrex®) *on page 1223*
Vidarabine (Vira-A®) *on page 1238*
Zanamivir (Relenza®) *on page 1256*

ORAL MEDICINE TOPICS

PART II:

DENTAL MANAGEMENT AND THERAPEUTIC CONSIDERATIONS IN PATIENTS WITH SPECIFIC ORAL CONDITIONS AND OTHER MEDICINE TOPICS

This second part of the chapter focuses on therapies the dentist may choose to prescribe for patients suffering from oral disease or who are in need of special care. Some overlap between these sections has resulted from systemic conditions that have oral manifestations and vice-versa. Cross-references to the descriptions and the monographs for individual drugs described elsewhere in this handbook allow for easy retrieval of information. Example prescriptions of selected drug therapies for each condition are presented so that the clinician can evaluate alternate approaches to treatment, since there is seldom a single drug of choice.

Drug prescriptions shown represent prototype drugs and popular prescriptions and are examples only. The pharmacologic category index is available for cross-referencing if alternatives and additional drugs are sought.

TABLE OF CONTENTS

ORAL PAIN

PAIN PREVENTION

For the dental patient, the prevention of pain aids in relieving anxiety and reduces the probability of stress during dental care. For the practitioner, dental procedures can be accomplished more efficiently in a "painless" situation. Appropriate selection and use of local anesthetics is one of the foundations for success in this arena. Local anesthetics listed below include drugs for the most commonly confronted dental procedures. Ester anesthetics are no longer available in dose form for dental injections, and historically had a higher incidence of allergic manifestations due to the formation of the metabolic byproduct, para-aminobenzoic acid. Articaine, which has an ester side chain, is rapidly metabolized to a non-PABA acid and, hence, functions as an amide and has a low allergic potential. The amides, in general, have an almost negligible allergic rate, and only one well-documented case of amide allergy has been reported by Seng, et al. Although injectable diphenhydramine (Benadryl®) has been used in an attempt to provide anesthesia in patients allergic to all the local anesthetics, it is no longer recommended in this context. The vehicle for injectable diphenhydramine can cause tissue necrosis.

The potential interaction between acetaminophen and warfarin has been recently raised in the literature. The cytochrome P450 system of drug metabolism for these vitamin K dependent metabolic pathways has raised the possibility that prolonged use of acetaminophen may inadvertently enhance, to dangerous levels, the anticoagulation effect of warfarin. As monitored by the INR, the effects of these drugs may be one and one-half to two times greater than as expected from the warfarin dosage alone. This potential interaction could be of importance in selecting an analgesic/antipyretic drug for the dental patient.

LOCAL ANESTHETICS

Articaine and Epinephrine [U.S.] (Septocaine™) *on page 114*

Articaine and Epinephrine [Canada] (Septanest®, Ultracaine DS®) *on page 113*

Bupivacaine (Marcaine®, Sensorcaine® MPF) *on page 184*

Bupivacaine and Epinephrine (Marcaine® with Epinephrine; Sensorcaine®) *on page 186*

Chloroprocaine (Nesacaine®) *on page 265*

Etidocaine With Epinephrine (Duranest® with Epinephrine) *on page 477*

Levobupivacaine (Chirocaine®) *on page 696*

Lidocaine and Epinephrine (Lignospan® Standard; Lignospan® Forte; Octocaine® 50; Octocaine® 100; Xylocaine® with Epinephrine) *on page 709*

Lidocaine (Dilocaine®, Duo-Trach®, Nervocaine®, Octocaine®, Xylocaine®) *on page 706*

Lidocaine Transoral (Dentipatch®) *on page 713*

Mepivacaine Dental Anesthetic (Carbocaine® 3%; Isocaine® 3%; Polocaine® 3%; Scandonest® 3% Plain) *on page 767*

Mepivacaine and Levonordefrin (Carbocaine® 2% with Neo-Cobefrin®, Isocaine® 2%; Polocaine® 2%; Scandonest® *on page 765*

Prilocaine (Citanest® Plain 4%) *on page 992*

Prilocaine With Epinephrine (Citanest Forte® with Epinephrine) *on page 993*

Ropivacaine (Naropin®) *on page 1068*

Tetracaine (Pontocaine®, Viractin®) *on page 1146*

Tetracaine and Dextrose (Pontocaine® with Dextrose Injection) *on page 1147*

The selection of a vasoconstrictor with the local anesthetic must be based on the length of the procedure to be performed, the patient's medical status (epinephrine is contraindicated in patients with uncontrolled hyperthyroidism), and the need for hemorrhage control. The following table lists some of the common drugs with their duration of action. Transoral patches with lidocaine are now available (Dentipatch®) and the new long-acting amide injectable, Ropivacaine (Naropin®) may be useful for postoperative pain management.

DENTAL ANESTHETICS
(Average Duration by Route)

Product	Infiltration	Inferior Alveolar Block
Articaine HCl 4% and epinephrine 1:100,000	60 minutes	60 minutes
Carbocaine® HCl 3% (mepivacaine)	20 minutes	40 minutes
Carbocaine® HCl 2% with Neo-Cobefrin® 1:20,000 (mepivacaine HCl and levonordefrin)	50 minutes	60-75 minutes
Duranest® Injection (etidocaine)	5-10 hours	5-10 hours
Citanest® Plain 4% (prilocaine)	20 minutes	2.5 hours
Citanest Forte® with Epinephrine (prilocaine with epinephrine)	2.25 hours	3 hours
Lidocaine HCl 2% and epinephrine 1:100,000	60 minutes	90 minutes
Marcaine® HCl 0.5% with epinephrine 1:200,000 (bupivacaine and epinephrine)	60 minutes	5-7 hours

The use of preinjection topical anesthetics can assist in pain prevention (see also "Oral Viral Infections" *on page 1380* and "Oral Nonviral Soft Tissue Ulcerations or Erosions" *on page 1384*). Some clinicians are also using EMLA® (eutectic mixture of local anesthetic with lidocaine and prilocaine) as a topical. Skin patch available by Astra not currently approved for oral use.

Benzocaine (Hurricaine®, Numzident®, various other products) *on page 151*

Lidocaine (Dilocaine®, Duo-Trach®, Nervocaine®, Octocaine®, Xylocaine®) *on page 706*

Lidocaine Transoral (Dentipatch®) *on page 713*

Tetracaine (Pontocaine®, Viractin®) *on page 1146*

PAIN MANAGEMENT

The patient with existing acute or chronic oral pain requires appropriate treatment and sensitivity on the part of the dentist, all for the purpose of achieving relief from the oral source of pain. Pain can be divided into mild, moderate, and severe levels and requires a subjective assessment by the dentist based on knowledge of the dental procedures to be performed, the presenting signs and symptoms of the patient, and the realization that most dental procedures are invasive often leading to pain once the patient has left the dental office. The practitioner must be aware that the treatment of the source of the pain is usually the best management. If infection is present, treatment of the infection will directly alleviate the patient's discomfort. However, a patient who is not in pain tends to heal better and it is wise to adequately cover the patient for any residual or recurrent discomfort suffered. Likewise, many of the procedures that the dentist performs have pain associated with them. Much of this pain occurs after leaving the dentist office due to an inflammatory process or a healing process that has been initiated. It is difficult to assign specific pain levels (mild, moderate, or severe) for specific procedures; however, the dentist should use his or her prescribing capacity judiciously so that overmedication is avoided.

The following categories of drugs and appropriate example prescriptions for each follow. These include management of mild pain with aspirin products, acetaminophen, and some of the nonsteroidal noninflammatory agents. Management of moderate pain includes codeine, Vicodin®, Vicodin ES®, Lorcet® 10/650; and Motrin® in the 800 mg dosage. Severe pain may require treatment with Percodan®, Percocet®, or Demerol®. All prescription pain preparations should be closely monitored for efficacy and discontinued if the pain persists or requires a higher level formulation.

The chronic pain patient represents a particular challenge for the practitioner. Some additional drugs that may be useful in managing the patient with chronic pain of neuropathic origin are covered in the temporomandibular dysfunction section *on page 1397.* It is always incumbent on the practitioner to reevaluate the diagnosis, source of pain, and treatment, whenever prolonged use of analgesics (narcotic or non-narcotic) is contemplated. Drugs such as Dilaudid® are not recommended for management of dental pain in most states.

Narcotic analgesics can be used on a short-term basis or intermittently in combination with non-narcotic therapy in the chronic pain patient. Judicious prescribing, monitoring, and maintenance by the practitioner is imperative, particularly whenever considering the use of a narcotic analgesic due to the abuse and addiction liabilities.

ORAL PAIN *(Continued)*

MILD PAIN

Acetaminophen (various products) *on page 26*

Aspirin (various products) *on page 119*

Diflunisal (Dolobid®) *on page 386*

Ibuprofen (various products) *on page 621*

Ketoprofen (Actron®, Orudis®, Orudis KT®, Oruvail®) *on page 674*

Naproxen (Naprosyn®), Naproxen sodium (Aleve®, Anaprox®) *on page 848*

OVER-THE-COUNTER PRESCRIPTION EXAMPLES

Rx

Aspirin 325 mg

Disp: To be determined by practitioner

Sig: Take 2-3 tablets every 4 hours

Rx

Ibuprofen 200 mg

Disp: To be determined by practitioner

Sig: Take 2-3 tablets every 4 hours, not to exceed 16 tablets in 24 hours

Note: Ibuprofen is available over-the-counter as Motrin IB®, Advil®, Nuprin®, and many other brands in 200 mg tablets.

Note: NSAIDs should **never** be taken together, nor should they be combined with aspirin. NSAIDs have anti-inflammatory effects as well as analgesics. An allergy to aspirin constitutes a contradiction to all the new NSAIDs. Aspirin and the NSAIDs may increase post-treatment bleeding.

Note: Use with caution in patients with CHF, hypertension, decreased renal or hepatic function, history of GI disease, or those receiving anticoagulants; withhold for at least 4-6 half-lives prior to surgical or dental procedures

Rx

Acetaminophen 325 mg

Disp: To be determined by practitioner

Sig: Take 2-3 tablets every 4 hours

Note: Products include: Tylenol®, Datril®, Anacin® 3, and many others.

Note: Acetaminophen can be given if patient has allergy, bleeding problems, or stomach upset secondary to aspirin or NSAIDs.

Rx

Aleve® 220 mg

Disp: To be determined by practitioner

Sig: 1-2 tablets every 8 hours

Ingredient: Naproxen sodium

Rx

Orudis KT® 12.5 mg

Disp: To be determined by practitioner

Sig: 1-2 tablets every 8 hours

Ingredient: Ketoprofen

PRESCRIPTION ONLY EXAMPLES

Rx

Ketoprofen 25 mg

Disp: To be determined by practitioner

Sig: 1-2 tablets every 8 hours

Rx

Dolobid® 500 mg

Disp: 16 tablets

Sig: Take 2 tablets initially, then 1 tablet every 8-12 hours as needed for pain

Ingredient: Diflunisal

MODERATE/MODERATELY SEVERE PAIN

Aspirin and Codeine (Empirin® with Codeine) *on page 122*

Dihydrocodeine Compound (Synalgos® DC) *on page 392*

Hydrocodone and Acetaminophen (Lortab®, Vicodin®, various products) *on page 598*

Hydrocodone and Ibuprofen (Vicoprofen®) *on page 605*

Acetaminophen and Tramadol (Ultracet™) *on page 31*

Ibuprofen (various products) *on page 621*

A new class of NSAIDs has been approved and indicated in the treatment of arthritis, COX-2 inhibitors (celecoxib, Celebrex®; rofecoxib, Vioxx®). Rofecoxib (Vioxx®) is indicated for use in short-term oral pain management. Celecoxib (Celebrex®) has recently been approved for use in oral pain management. Valdecoxib (Bextra®) is a COX-2 inhibitor also recently indicated for acute pain but its use in dental management is still under evaluation.

The following is a guideline to use when prescribing codeine with either aspirin or acetaminophen (Tylenol®):

Codeine No. 2 = codeine 15 mg

Codeine No. 3 = codeine 30 mg

Codeine No. 4 = codeine 60 mg

Example: ASA No. 3 = aspirin 325 mg + codeine 30 mg

PRESCRIPTION EXAMPLES

Not Controlled:

Rx

Motrin® 800 mg*
Disp: 16 tablets
Sig: Take 1 tablet 3 times/day as needed for pain

Ingredient: Ibuprofen

Note: May be taken up to 4 times/day for more severe pain.

***Note:** Also available as 600 mg

Rx

Ultracet™
Disp: 36 tablets
Sig: Take 2 tablets every 4-6 hours as needed for pain, not to exceed 8 tablets in 24 hours

Ingredients: Acetaminophen 325 mg and tramadol 37.5 mg

ORAL PAIN *(Continued)*

Controlled:

Rx

Tylenol® No. 3*
Disp: 16 tablets
Sig: Take 1 tablet every 4 hours as needed for pain

Ingredients: Acetaminophen and codeine

***Note:** Also available as #2 and #4

Rx

Synalgos® DC
Disp: 16 capsules
Sig: Take 1 capsule every 4 hours as needed for pain

Ingredients: Dihydrocodeine 16 mg, aspirin 356.4 mg, and caffeine 30 mg

Rx

Vicodin®
Disp: 16 tablets
Sig: Take 1 tablet every 4 hours as needed for pain

Ingredients: Hydrocodone 5 mg and acetaminophen 500 mg

Note: Available as Vicodin ES®; take 1 tablet every 8-12 hours

Rx

Lortab® 5 mg*
Disp: 16 tablets
Sig: Take 1 or 2 tablets every 4 hours as needed for pain, not to exceed 8 tablets in 24 hours

Ingredients: Hydrocodone 5 mg and acetaminophen 500 mg

Rx

Darvocet–N 100®
Disp: 36 tablets
Sig: Take 1 tablet every 4 hours as needed for pain, not to exceed 6 tablets in 24 hours

Ingredients: Propoxyphene 100 mg and acetaminophen 650 mg

Rx

Vicoprofen®
Disp: 16 tablets
Sig: Take 1-2 tablets every 4-6 hours as needed for pain   No Refills

Ingredients: Hydrocodone 7.5 mg and ibuprofen 200 mg

HYDROCODONE PRODUCTS

Available hydrocodone oral products are listed in the following table and are scheduled as C-III controlled substances, indicating that prescriptions may either be oral or written. Thus, the prescriber may call–in a prescription to the pharmacy for any of these hydrocodone products. All the formulations are combined with acetaminophen except for Vicoprofen®, which contains ibuprofen, and Lortab® ASA, Alor® 5/500, and Damason–P®, which all contain aspirin. Most of these brand name drugs are available generically and the pharmacist will dispense the generic equivalent if available, unless the prescriber indicates otherwise.

HYDROCODONE ANALGESIC COMBINATION ORAL PRODUCTS (All Products DEA Schedule C-III)

Hydrocodone is available under numerous brand names with varying dosages and in combination with aspirin or ibuprofen.					
Hydrocodone Bitartrate	**Acetaminophen (APAP*)**	**Other**	**Brand Name**	**Generic Available**	**Form**
2.5 mg	500 mg	–	Lortab® 2.5/500	Yes	Tablet
5 mg	400 mg	–	Zydone®	No	Tablet
5 mg	500 mg	–	Vicodin®; Dolagesic®; Hy-Phen®; Hydrocet®; Anexsia® 5/500; Lortab®5/500	Yes	Tablet
5 mg	500 mg	–	Polygesic®; Lorcet-HD®	Yes	Capsule
7.5 mg	400 mg	–	Zydone®	No	Tablet
7.5 mg	500 mg	–	Lortab® 7.5/500	Yes	Tablet
7.5 mg	650 mg	–	Anexsia® 7.5/650; Lorcet Plus®	Yes	Tablet
7.5 mg	750 mg	–	Vicodin ES®	Yes	Tablet
10 mg	400 mg	–	Zydone®	No	Tablet
10 mg	325 mg	–	Norco®	No	Tablet
10 mg	500 mg	–	Lortab® 10/500	Yes	Tablet
10 mg	650 mg	–	Lorcet®	Yes	Tablet
10 mg	660 mg	–	Vicodin HP®; Anexsia® 10/660	Yes	Tablet
10 mg	750 mg		Maxidone™	No	Tablet
7.5 mg/15 mL	500 mg/15 mL	–	Lortab® Elixir	Yes	Elixir
5 mg	–	Aspirin 500 mg	Lortab® ASA; Alor® 5/500; Damason–P®	Yes	Tablet
7.5 mg	–	Ibuprofen 200 mg	Vicoprofen®	No	Tablet

*APAP is the common acronym for acetaminophen and is the abbreviation of the chemical name N-acetylparaminophenol.

The following are the usual adult doses of the hydrocodone oral products as listed by the most recent edition of the Drug Information for the Health Care Professional (USPDI).

1 or 2 tablets containing 2.5 mg of hydrocodone and 500 mg of acetaminophen every 4-6 hours; or

1 tablet containing 5 mg of hydrocodone and 500 mg acetaminophen every 4-6 hours as needed, with dosage being increased to 2 tablets every 6 hours, if necessary; or

1 capsule containing 5 mg of hydrocodone and 500 mg of acetaminophen every 4-6 hours as needed, with dosage being increased to 2 capsules every 6 hours if necessary; or

1 tablet containing 7.5 mg hydrocodone and 650 mg of acetaminophen every 4-6 hours as needed, with dosage being increased to 2 tablets every 6 hours if necessary; or

1 tablet containing 7.5 mg hydrocodone and 750 mg of acetaminophen every 4-6 hours as needed; or

1 tablet containing 10 mg of hydrocodone and 650 mg acetaminophen every 4-6 hours as needed.

For the elixir (Lortab®), the recommended dose is 1 tablespoonful every 4-6 hours when necessary for pain.

For the aspirin products (Lortab® ASA, Alor® 5/500, and Damason-P®), the recommended dose is 1 or 2 tablets every 4-6 hours as needed.

For the ibuprofen product (Vicoprofen®), the recommended dose is 1 or 2 tablets every 4-6 hours as needed. The manufacturer recommends that the maximum dose of Vicoprofen® should not exceed 5 tablets in 24 hours.

The usual adult prescribing limits for the combination hydrocodone-acetaminophen products is up to 40 mg of hydrocodone and up to 4000 mg (4 g) of acetaminophen in a 24-hour period.

ORAL PAIN *(Continued)*

SEVERE PAIN

Meperidine (Demerol®) *on page 760*

Oxycodone (OxyContin®, OxyIR®, Roxicodone™) *on page 901*

Oxycodone and Acetaminophen (Percocet®, Roxicet®, Roxilox®, Tylox®) *on page 903*

Oxycodone and Aspirin (Codoxy®, Percodan®, Roxiprin®) *on page 905*

Oxycodone is available in a variety of dosages and combinations under numerous brand names. A new combination of Oxycodone hydrochloride with ibuprofen has been used in Phase III clinical trials at Forest Laboratories and is currently awaiting approval.

PRESCRIPTION EXAMPLES

Rx

Demerol® 50 mg*

Disp: 16 tablets

Sig: Take 1 tablet every 4 hours as needed for pain — No Refills

Ingredient: Meperidine

***Note:** Triplicate prescription required in some states.

Rx

Roxicodone™ 5 mg

Disp: 24 tablets

Sig: Take 1 tablet every 6 hours as needed for pain — No Refills

Ingredient: Oxycodone

Note: Some formulations available as controlled release.

Rx

Percodan®*

Disp: 16 tablets

Sig: Take 1 tablet every 4 hours as needed for pain — No Refills

Ingredients: Oxycodone 4.88 mg and aspirin 325 mg

***Note:** Triplicate prescription required in some states.

Note: See monograph *on page 905* for contraindications and precautions for aspirin or narcotic medications.

Rx

Percocet® tablets or Tylox® capsules*

Disp: 16 tablets or capsules

Sig: Take 1 tablet every 4 hours as needed for pain — No Refills

Ingredients: Oxycodone 5 mg and acetaminophen 325 mg (Tylox® contains acetaminophen 500 mg)

***Note:** Triplicate prescription required in some states.

ORAL BACTERIAL INFECTIONS

Dental infection can occur for any number of reasons, primarily involving pulpal and periodontal infections. Secondary infections of the soft tissues as well as sinus infections pose special treatment challenges. The drugs of choice in treating most oral infections have been selected because of their efficacy in providing adequate blood levels for delivery to the oral tissues and their proven usefulness in managing dental infections. Penicillin remains the primary drug for treatment of dental infections of pulpal origin. The management of soft tissue infections may require the use of additional drugs.

OROFACIAL INFECTIONS

The basis of all infections is the successful multiplication of a microbial pathogen on or within a host. The pathogen is usually defined as any microorganism that has the capacity to cause disease. If the pathogen is bacterial in nature, antibiotic therapy is often indicated.

DIFFERENTIAL DIAGNOSIS OF ODONTOGENIC INFECTIONS

In choosing the appropriate antibiotic for therapy of a given infection, a number of important factors must be considered. First, the identity of the organism must be known. In odontogenic infections involving dental or periodontal structures, this is seldom the case. Secondly, accurate information regarding antibiotic susceptibility is required. Again, unless the organism has been identified, this is not possible. And thirdly, host factors must be taken into account, in terms of ability to absorb an antibiotic, to achieve appropriate host response. When clinical evidence of cellulitis or odontogenic infection has been found and the cardinal signs of swelling, inflammation, pain, and perhaps fever are present, the selection by the clinician of the appropriate antibiotic agent may lead to eradication.

CAUSES OF ODONTOGENIC INFECTIONS

Most acute orofacial infections are of odontogenic origin. Dental caries, resulting in infection of dental pulp, is the leading cause of odontogenic infection.

The major causative organisms involved in dental caries have been identified as members of the viridans (alpha-hemolytic) streptococci and include *Streptococcus mutans, Streptococcus sobrinus,* and *Streptococcus milleri.* Once the bacteria have breached the enamel they invade the dentin and eventually the dental pulp. An inflammatory reaction occurs in the pulp tissue resulting in necrosis and a lower tissue oxidation-reduction potential. At this point, the bacterial flora changes from predominantly aerobic to a more obligate anaerobic flora. The anaerobic gram-positive cocci *(Peptostreptococcus* species), and the anaerobic gram-negative rods, including *Bacteroides, Prevotella, Porphyromonas,* and *Fusobacterium* are most frequently present. An abscess usually forms at the apex of the involved tooth resulting in destruction of bone. Depending on the effectiveness of the host resistance and the virulence of the bacteria, the infection may spread through the marrow spaces, perforate the cortical plate, and enter the surrounding soft tissues.

The other major source of odontogenic infection arises from the anaerobic bacterial flora that inhabits the periodontal and supporting structures of the teeth. The most important potential pathogenic anaerobes within these structures are *Actinobacillus actinomycetemcomitans, Prevotella intermedius, Porphyromonas gingivalis, Fusobacterium nucleatum,* and *Eikenella corrodens.*

Most odontogenic infections (70%) have mixed aerobic and anaerobic flora. Pure aerobic infections are much less common and comprise ~5% incidence. Pure anaerobic infections make up the remaining 25% of odontogenic infections. Clinical correlates suggest that early odontogenic infections are characterized by rapid spreading and cellulitis with the absence of abscess formation. The bacteria are predominantly aerobic with gram-positive, alpha-hemolytic streptococci *(S. viridans)* the predominant pathogen. As the infection matures and becomes more severe, the microbial flora becomes a mix of aerobes and anaerobes. The anaerobes present are determined by the characteristic flora associated with the site of origin, whether it be pulpal or periodontal. Finally, as the infectious process becomes controlled by host defenses, the flora becomes primarily anaerobic. For example, Lewis and MacFarlane found a predominance of facultative oral streptococci in the early infections (<3 days of symptoms) with the later predominance of obligate anaerobes.

In a review of severe odontogenic infections, it was reported that Brook, et al, observed that 50% of odontogenic deep facial space infections yielded anaerobic bacteria only. Also, 44% of these infections yielded a mix of aerobic and anaerobic flora. The results of a study published in 1998 by Sakamoto, et al, were also described in the review. The study confirmed that odontogenic infections usually result from a synergistic interaction among several bacterial species and usually consist of an oral streptococcus and an oral anaerobic gram-negative rod. Sakamoto and his group reported a high level of the *Streptococcus milleri* group of aerobic gram-positive cocci, and high levels of oral

ORAL BACTERIAL INFECTIONS *(Continued)*

anaerobes, including the *Peptostreptococcus* species and the *Prevotella, Porphyromonas,* and *Fusobacterium* species.

Oral streptococci, especially of the *Streptococcus milleri* group, can invade soft tissues initially, thus preparing an environment conducive to growth of anaerobic bacteria. Obligate oral anaerobes are dependent on nutrients synthesized by the aerobes. Thus the anaerobes appear approximately 3 days after onset of symptoms. Early infections are thus caused primarily by the aerobic streptococci (exquisitely sensitive to penicillin) and late infections are caused by the anaerobes (frequently resistant to penicillin).

It appears logical, as Flynn has noted, to separate infections presenting early in their course from those presenting later when selecting empiric antibiotics of choice for odontogenic infections.

If the patient is not allergic to penicillin, penicillin VK still remains the empiric antibiotic of first choice to treat mild or early odontogenic infections (see Table 1). In penicillin allergy, clindamycin clearly remains the alternative antibiotic for treatment of mild or early infections. Secondary alternative antibiotics still recognized as useful in these conditions are cephalexin (Keflex®), or other first generation cephalosporins available in oral dose forms. The first generation cephalosporins can be used in both penicillin-allergic and nonallergic patients, providing that the penicillin allergy is not the anaphylactoid type.

PENICILLIN VK

The spectrum of antibacterial action of penicillin VK is consistent with most of the organisms identified in odontogenic infections (see Table 2). Penicillin VK is a beta-lactam antibiotic, as are all the penicillins and cephalosporins, and is bactericidal against gram-positive cocci and the major pathogens of mixed anaerobic infections. It elicits virtually no adverse effects in the absence of allergy and is relatively low in cost. Adverse drug reactions occurring in >10% of patients include mild diarrhea, nausea, and oral candidiasis. To treat odontogenic infections and other orofacial infections, the usual dose for adults and children >12 years of age is 500 mg every 6 hours for at least 7 days (see Table 4). The daily dose for children ≤12 years of age is 25-50 mg/kg of body weight in divided doses every 6-8 hours (see Table 4). The patient must be instructed to take the penicillin continuously for the duration of therapy.

After oral dosing, penicillin VK achieves peak serum levels within 1 hour. Penicillin VK may be given with meals, however, blood concentrations may be slightly higher when penicillin is given on an empty stomach. The preferred dosing is 1 hour before meals or 2 hours after meals to ensure maximum serum levels. Penicillin VK diffuses into most body tissues, including oral tissues, soon after dosing. Hepatic metabolism accounts for <30% of the elimination of penicillins. Elimination is primarily renal. The nonmetabolized penicillin is excreted largely unchanged in the urine by glomerular filtration and active tubular secretion. Penicillins cross the placenta and are distributed in breast milk. Penicillin VK, like all beta-lactam antibiotics, causes death of bacteria by inhibiting synthesis of the bacterial cell wall during cell division. This action is dependent on the ability of penicillins to reach and bind to penicillin-binding proteins (PBPs) located on the inner membrane of the bacterial cell wall. PBPs (which include transpeptidases, carboxypeptidases, and endopeptidases) are enzymes that are involved in the terminal stages of assembling and reshaping the bacterial cell wall during growth. Penicillins and beta-lactams bind to and inactivate PBPs resulting in lysis of the cell due to weakening of the cell wall.

Penicillin VK is considered a "narrow spectrum" antibiotic. This class of antibiotics produces less alteration of normal microflora thereby reducing the incidence of superinfection. Also, its bactericidal action will reduce the numbers of microorganisms resulting in less reliance on host-phagocyte mechanisms for eradication of the pathogen.

Among patients, 0.7% to 10% are allergic to penicillins. There is no evidence that any single penicillin derivative differs from others in terms of incidence or severity when administered orally. About 85% of allergic reactions associated with penicillin VK are delayed and take >2 days to develop. This allergic response manifests as skin rashes characterized as erythema and bullous eruptions. This type of allergic reaction is mild, reversible, and usually responds to concurrent antihistamine therapy, such as diphenhydramine (Benadryl®). Severe reactions of angioedema have occurred, characterized by marked swelling of the lips, tongue, face, and periorbital tissues. Patients with a history of penicillin allergy must never be given penicillin VK for treatment of infections. The alternative antibiotic is clindamycin. If the allergy is the delayed type and not the anaphylactoid type, a first generation cephalosporin may be used as an alternate antibiotic.

CLINDAMYCIN

In the event of penicillin allergy, clindamycin is clearly an alternative of choice in treating mild or early odontogenic infections (see Table 1). It is highly effective against almost all oral pathogens. Clindamycin is active against most aerobic gram-positive cocci, including staphylococci, *S. pneumoniae,* other streptococci, and anaerobic gram-negative and gram-positive organisms, including bacteroides (see Table 3). Clindamycin is not effective against mycoplasma or gram-negative aerobes. It inhibits protein synthesis in bacteria through binding to the 50 S subunit of bacterial ribosomes. Clindamycin has bacteriostatic actions at low concentrations, but is known to elicit bactericidal effects against susceptible bacteria at higher concentrations of drug at the site of infection.

The usual adult oral dose of clindamycin to treat orofacial infections of odontogenic origin is 150-450 mg every 6 hours for 7-10 days. The usual daily oral dose for children is 8-25 mg/kg in 3-4 equally divided doses (see Table 4).

Following oral administration of a 150 mg or a 300 mg dose on an empty stomach, 90% of the dose is rapidly absorbed into the bloodstream and peak serum concentrations are attained in 45-60 minutes. Administration with food does not markedly impair absorption into the bloodstream. Clindamycin serum levels exceed the minimum inhibitory concentration for bacterial growth for at least 6 hours after the recommended doses. The serum half-life is 2-3 hours. Clindamycin is distributed effectively to most body tissues, including saliva and bone. Its small molecular weight enables it to more readily enter bacterial cytoplasm and to penetrate bone. It is partially metabolized in the liver to active and inactive metabolites and is excreted in the urine, bile, and feces.

Adverse effects caused by clindamycin can include abdominal pain, nausea, vomiting, and diarrhea. Hypersensitivity reactions are rare, but have resulted in skin rash. Approximately 1% of clindamycin users develop pseudomembranous colitis characterized by severe diarrhea, abdominal cramps, and excretion of blood or mucus in the stools. The mechanism is disruption of normal bacterial flora of the colon, which leads to colonization of the bacterium *Clostridium difficile*. This bacterium releases endotoxins that cause mucosal damage and inflammation. Symptoms usually develop 2-9 days after initiation of therapy, but may not occur until several weeks after taking the drug. If significant diarrhea develops, clindamycin therapy should be discontinued immediately. Theoretically, any antibiotic can cause antibiotic-associated colitis and clindamycin probably has an undeserved reputation associated with this condition.

Sandor, et al, also notes that odontogenic infections are typically polymicrobial and that anaerobes outnumber aerobes by at least four-fold. The penicillins have historically been used as the first-line therapy in these cases, but increasing rates of resistance have lowered their usefulness. Bacterial resistance to penicillins is predominantly achieved through production of beta-lactamases. Clindamycin, because of its relatively broad spectrum of activity and resistance to beta-lactamase degradation, is an attractive first-line therapy in treatment of odontogenic infections.

FIRST GENERATION CEPHALOSPORINS

Antibiotics of this class, which are available in oral dosage forms, include cefadroxil (Duricef®), cephalexin (Keflex®), and cephradine (Velosef®). The first generation cephalosporins are alternates to penicillin VK in the treatment of odontogenic infections based on bactericidal effectiveness against the oral streptococci. These drugs are most active against gram-positive cocci, but are not very active against many anaerobes. First generation cephalosporins are indicated as alternatives in early infections because they are effective in killing the aerobes. First generation cephalosporins are active against gram-positive staphylococci and streptococci, but not enterococci. They are active against many gram-negative aerobic bacilli, including *E. coli, Klebsiella,* and *Proteus mirabilis.* They are inactive against methicillin-resistant *S. aureus* and penicillin-resistant *S. pneumoniae.* The gram-negative aerobic cocci, *Moraxella catarrhalis,* portrays variable sensitivity to first generation cephalosporins.

Cephalexin (Keflex®) is the first generation cephalosporin often used to treat odontogenic infections. The usual adult dose is 250-1000 mg every 6 hours with a maximum of 4 g/day. Children's dose is 25-50 mg/kg/day in divided doses every 6 hours; for severe infections: 50-100 mg/kg/day in divided doses every 6 hours with a maximum dose of 3 g/day (see Table 4).

Cephalexin (Keflex®) causes diarrhea in about 1% to 10% of patients. About 90% of the cephalexin is excreted unchanged in urine.

SECOND GENERATION CEPHALOSPORINS

The second generation cephalosporins such as cefaclor (Ceclor®) have better activity against some of the anaerobes including some *Bacteroides, Peptococcus,* and *Peptostreptococcus* species. Cefaclor (Ceclor®) and cefuroxime (Ceftin®) have been used to treat early stage infections. These antibiotics have the advantage of twice-a-day dosing. The usual oral adult dose of cefaclor is 250-500 mg every 8 hours (or daily dose can be given in 2 divided doses) for at least 7 days. Children's dose is 20-40 mg/kg/day divided every 8-12 hours with a maximum dose of 2 g/day. The usual adult oral dose of cefuroxime is 250-500 mg twice daily. Children's dose is 20 mg/kg/day (maximum 500 mg/day) in 2 divided doses.

The cephalosporins inhibit bacterial cell wall synthesis by binding to one or more of the penicillin-binding proteins (PBPs), which in turn inhibits the final transpeptidation step of peptidoglycan synthesis in bacterial cell walls, thus inhibiting cell wall biosynthesis. Bacteria eventually lyse due to ongoing activity of cell wall autolytic enzymes while cell wall assembly is arrested.

ORAL BACTERIAL INFECTIONS *(Continued)*

BACTERIAL RESISTANCE TO ANTIBIOTICS

If a patient with an early stage odontogenic infection does not respond to penicillin VK within 24-36 hours, it is evidence of the presence of resistant bacteria. Bacterial resistance to the penicillins is predominantly achieved through the production of beta-lactamase. A switch to beta-lactamase-stable antibiotics should be made. For example, Kuriyama, et al, reported that past beta-lactam administration increases the emergence of beta-lactamase-producing bacteria and that beta-lactamase-stable antibiotics should be prescribed to patients with unresolved infections who have received beta-lactams. These include either clindamycin or amoxicillin/clavulanic acid (Augmentin®). Doses are listed in Table 4.

In the past, all *S. viridans* species were uniformly susceptible to beta-lactam antibiotics. However, over the years, there has been a significant increase in resistant strains. Resistance may also be due to alteration of penicillin-binding proteins. Consequently, drugs which combine a beta-lactam antibiotic with a beta-lactamase inhibitor, such as amoxicillin/clavulanic acid (Augmentin®), may no longer be more effective than the penicillin VK alone. In these situations, clindamycin is the recommended alternate antibiotic.

Evidence suggests that empirical use of penicillin VK as the first-line drug in treating early odontogenic infections is still the best way to ensure the minimal production of resistant bacteria to other classes of antibiotics, since any overuse of clindamycin or amoxicillin/clavulanic acid (Augmentin®) is minimized in these situations. There is concern that overuse of clindamycin could contribute to development of clindamycin-resistant pathogens.

In late odontogenic infections, it is suggested that clindamycin be considered the first-line antibiotic to treat these infections. The dose of clindamycin would be the same as that used to treat early infections (see Table 4). In these infections, anaerobic bacteria usually predominate. Since penicillin spectrum includes anaerobes, penicillin VK is also useful as an empiric drug of first choice in these infections. It has been reported, however, that the penicillin resistance rate among patients with serious and late infections is in the 35% to 50% range. Therefore, if penicillin is the drug of first choice and the patient does not respond within 24-36 hours, a resistant pathogen should be suspected and a switch to clindamycin be made. Clindamycin, because of its relatively broad spectrum of activity and resistance to beta-lactamase degradation, is an attractive first-line therapy in the treatment of these infections. Another alternative is to add a second drug to the penicillin (eg, metronidazole [Flagyl®]). Consequently, for those infections not responding to treatment with penicillin, the addition of a second drug (eg, metronidazole), not a beta-lactam or macrolide, is likely to be more effective. Bacterial resistance to metronidazole is very rare. The metronidazole dose is listed in Table 4.

Nonionized metronidazole is readily taken up by anaerobic organisms. Its selectivity for anaerobic bacteria is a result of the ability of these organisms to reduce metronidazole to its active form within the bacterial cell. The electron transport proteins necessary for this reaction are found only in anaerobic bacteria. Reduced metronidazole then disrupts DNA's helical structure, thereby inhibiting bacterial nucleic acid synthesis leading to death of the organism. Consequently, metronidazole is not effective against gram-positive aerobic cocci and most *Actinomyces, Lactobacillus,* and *Proprionibacterium* species. Since most odontogenic infections are mixed aerobic and anaerobic, metronidazole should rarely be used as a single agent. Alternatively, one can switch to a beta-lactamase resistant drug (eg, amoxicillin/clavulanic acid [Augmentin®]). The beta-lactamase resistant penicillins including methicillin, oxacillin, cloxacillin, dicloxacillin, and nafcillin, are only effective against gram-positive cocci and have no activity against anaerobes, hence, should not be used to treat the late stage odontogenic infections.

RESISTANCE IN ODONTOGENIC INFECTIONS

Recently, there has been an alarming increase in the incidence of resistant bacterial isolates in odontogenic infections. Many anaerobic bacteria have developed resistance to beta-lactam antibiotics via production of beta-lactamase enzymes. These include several species of *Prevotella, Porphyromonas, Fusobacterium nucleatum,* and *Campylobacter gracilus. Fusobacterium,* especially in combination with *S. viridans* species, has been associated with severe odontogenic infections. Often, they are resistant to macrolides. Clindamycin is the empiric drug of first choice in these patients.

SEVERE INFECTIONS

In patients hospitalized for severe odontogenic infections, I.V. antibiotics are indicated and clindamycin is the clear empiric antibiotic of choice. Alternative antibiotics include an I.V. combination of penicillin and metronidazole or I.V. ampicillin-sulbactam (Unasyn®). Clindamycin, I.V. cephalosporins (if penicillin allergy is not the anaphylactoid type), and ciprofloxacin have been used in patients allergic to penicillins. Flynn notes that *Eikenella corrodens*, an occasional oral pathogen, is resistant to clindamycin. Ciprofloxacin is an excellent antibiotic for this organism.

ERYTHROMYCIN, CLARITHROMYCIN, AND AZITHROMYCIN

In the past, erythromycins were considered highly effective antibiotics for treating odontogenic infections, especially in penicillin allergy. At the present time, however, the current high resistance rates of both oral streptococci and oral anaerobes have rendered the entire macrolide family of antibiotics obsolete for odontogenic infections. Montgomery has noted that resistance develops rapidly to macrolides and there may be cross-resistance between erythromycin and newer macrolides, particularly among streptococci and staphylococci. Hardee has stated that erythromycin is no longer very useful because of resistant pathogens. The antibacterial spectrum of the erythromycin family is similar to penicillin VK. Erythromycins are effective against streptococcus, staphylococcus, and gram-negative aerobes, such as *H. influenzae, M. catarrhalis, N. gonorrhoeae, Bordetella pertussis,* and *Legionella pneumophilia.* Erythromycins are considered narrow spectrum antibiotics.

Both azithromycin and clarithromycin have been used to treat acute odontogenic infections. This is because of the following spectrum of actions: Clarithromycin shows good activity against many gram-positive and gram-negative aerobic and anaerobic organisms. It is active against methicillin-sensitive *S. aureus* and most streptococcus species. *S. aureus* strains resistant to erythromycin are resistant to clarithromycin. Clarithromycin is active against *H. influenzae.* It is similar to erythromycin in effectiveness against anaerobic gram-positive cocci and *Bacteroides sp.* Clarithromycin has been suggested as an alternative antibiotic if the prescriber wants to give an antibiotic from the macrolide family (see Table 3). The recommended oral adult dose is 500 mg twice daily for 7 days.

Azithromycin is active against staphylococci, including *S. aureus* and *S. epidermidis*, as well as streptococci, such as *S. pyogenes* and *S. pneumoniae.* Erythromycin-resistant strains of staphylococcus, enterococcus, and streptococcus, including methicillin-resistant *S. aureus*, are also resistant to azithromycin. It has excellent activity against *H. influenzae.* Inhibition of anaerobes, such as *Clostridium perfringens*, is better with azithromycin than with erythromycin. Inhibition of *Bacteroides fragilis* and other bacteroides species by azithromycin is comparable to erythromycin. Both azithromycin and clarithromycin are presently recommended as alternatives in the prophylactic regimen for prevention of bacterial endocarditis.

AMOXICILLIN

Some clinicians select amoxicillin over penicillin VK as the penicillin of choice to empirically treat odontogenic infections. Except for coverage of *Haemophilus influenzae* in acute sinus and otitis media infections, amoxicillin does not offer any advantage over penicillin VK for treatment of odontogenic infections. It is less effective than penicillin VK for aerobic gram-positive cocci, and similar to penicillin for coverage of anaerobes. Although it does provide coverage against gram-negative enteric bacteria, this is not needed to treat odontogenic infections, except in immunosuppressed patients where these organisms may be present. If one adheres to the principle of using the most effective narrow spectrum antibiotic, amoxicillin should not be favored over penicillin VK.

The following tables have been adapted from Wynn RL, Bergman SA, Meiller TF, et al. "Antibiotics in Treating Orofacial Infections of Odontogenic Origin," *Gen Dent*, 2001, 47(3): 238-52.

Amoxicillin and Clavulanate Potassium (Augmentin®) *on page 88*
Amoxicillin Trihydrate (various products) *on page 86*
Cephalexin (Biocef®, Cefanex®, Keflet®, Keflex®, Keftab®) *on page 251*
Ceftibuten (Cedax®) *on page 243*
Cefditoren (Spectracef™) *on page 235*
Chlorpheniramine (Chlor-Trimeton®, various products) *on page 268*
Chlorhexidine (Peridex®, PerioGard®) *on page 263*
Clarithromycin (Biaxin®) *on page 296*
Clindamycin (Cleocin®) *on page 300*
Dicloxacillin (Dycill®, Dynapen®, Pathocil®) *on page 380*
Erythromycin (various products) *on page 450*
Gatifloxacin (Tequin™) *on page 549*
Loratadine and Pseudoephedrine (Claritin-D®) *on page 729*
Metronidazole (Flagyl®, MetroGel®, Protostat®) *on page 804*
Mouthwash, Antiseptic (Listerine®) *on page 831*
Moxifloxacin (Avelox®) *on page 832*
Oxymetazoline (Afrin®, various products) *on page 907*
Penicillin V Potassium (various products) *on page 931*
Pseudoephedrine (Sudafed®, various products) *on page 1022*
Tetracycline (Achromycin®, Sumycin®, Tetracyn®) *on page 1147*

ORAL BACTERIAL INFECTIONS *(Continued)*

Table 1. EMPIRIC ANTIBIOTICS OF CHOICE FOR ODONTOGENIC INFECTIONS

Type of Infection	Antibiotic of Choice
Early (first 3 days of symptoms)	Penicillin VK
	Clindamycin
	Cephalexin (or other first generation cephalosporin)*
No improvement in 24-36 hours	Beta-lactamase-stable antibiotic:
	Clindamycin or amoxicillin / clavulanic acid
Penicillin allergy	Clindamycin
	Cephalexin (if penicillin allergy is not anaphylactoid type)
	Clarithromycin (Biaxin®)†
Late (>3 days)	Clindamycin
	Penicillin VK-metronidazole
Penicillin allergy	Clindamycin

*For better patient compliance, second generation cephalosporins (cefaclor; cefuroxime) at twice daily dosing have been used; see text.

†A macrolide useful in patients allergic to penicillin, given as twice daily dosing for better patient compliance; see text.

Table 2. PENICILLIN VK: ANTIBACTERIAL SPECTRUM

Gram-positive cocci	Oral anaerobes
Streptococci	*Bacteriodes*
Nonresistant staphylococci*	*Porphyromonas*
Pneumococci	*Prevotella*
	Peptococci
Gram-negative cocci	Peptostreptococci
Neisseria meningitides	*Actinomyces*
Neiserria gonorrhoeae	*Veillonella*
	Eubacterium
Gram-positive rods	*Eikenella*
Bacillus	*Capnocytophaga*
Corynebacterium	*Campylobacter*
Clostridium	*Fusobacterium*
	Others

*Nonresistant staphylococcus represents a small portion of community-acquired strains of *S. aureus* (5% to 15%). Most strains of *S. aureus* and *S. epidermidis* produce beta-lactamases, which destroy penicillins.

Table 3. CLINDAMYCIN: ANTIBACTERIAL SPECTRUM*

Gram-Positive Cocci	Anaerobes†
Streptococci‡	Gram-negative bacilli
S. aureus¶	*Bacteriodes* species including *B. fragilis*
Penicillinase and nonpenicillinase-producing staphylococcus	*B. melaninogenicus* *Fusobacterium species*
S. epidermidis	Gram-positive nonsporeforming bacilli
Pneumococci	*Propionibacterium*
	Eubacterium
	Actinomyces species
	Gram-positive cocci
	Peptococcus
	Peptostreptococcus
	Microaerophilic streptococci

**In vitro* activity against isolates; information from manufacturer's package insert

†*Clostridia* are more resistant than most anaerobes to clindamycin. Most *Clostridium perfringens* are susceptible but *C. sporogens* and *C. tertium* are frequently resistant.

‡Except *S. faecalis*

¶Some staph strains originally resistant to erythromycin rapidly develop resistance to clindamycin.

Table 4.
ORAL DOSE RANGES OF ANTIBIOTICS USEFUL IN TREATING ODONTOGENIC INFECTIONS*

Clinicians must select specific dose and regimen from ranges available to be prescribed based on clinical judgment		
Antibiotic	Dosage	
	Children	Adults
Penicillin VK	≤12 years: 25-50 mg/kg body weight in equally divided doses q6-8h for at least 7 days; maximum dose: 3 g/day	>12 years: 500 mg q6h for at least 7 days
Clindamycin	8-25 mg/kg in 3-4 equally divided doses	150-450 mg q6h for at least 7 days; maximum dose: 1.8 g/day
Cephalexin (Keflex®)	25-50 mg/kg/d in divided doses q6h severe infection: 50-100 mg/kg/d in divided doses q6h; maximum dose: 3 g/24 h	250-1000 mg q6h; maximum dose: 4 g/day
Amoxicillin/ clavulanic acid (Augmentin®)	<40 kg: 20-40 mg (amoxicillin)/kg/d in divided doses q8h >40 kg: 250-500 mg q8h or 875 mg q12h for at least 7 days; maximum dose 2 g/day	>40 kg: 250-500 mg q8h or 875 mg q12h for at least 7 days; maximum dose: 2 g/day
Metronidazole (Flagyl®)		500 mg q6-8h for 7-10 days; maximum dose: 4 g/day

*For doses of other antibiotics, see monographs

SINUS INFECTION TREATMENT

Sinus infections represent a common condition which may present with confounding dental complaints. Treatment is sometimes instituted by the dentist, but due to the often chronic and recurrent nature of sinus infections, early involvement of an otolaryngologist is advised. These infections may require antibiotics of varying spectrum as well as requiring the management of sinus congestion. Although amoxicillin is usually adequate, many otolaryngologists go directly to Augmentin®. Second-generation cephalosporins and clarithromycin are sometimes used depending on the chronicity of the problem.

PRESCRIPTION EXAMPLES FOR SINUS INFECTIONS

The selected antibiotic should be used with a nasal decongestant and possibly an antihistamine.

Antibiotics:

Rx

Amoxicillin 500 mg

Disp: 21 capsules

Sig: Take 1 capsule 3 times/day

OR

Rx

Augmentin® 250, 500, or 875 mg

Disp: Appropriate quantity for 7-10 days

Sig: Take 1 tablet 3 times/day for 250 or 500 mg; twice daily for 875 mg

Ingredients: Amoxicillin 500 mg and clavulanate potassium 125 mg

AND

Decongestants/Antihistamine:

Rx

Afrin® Nasal Spray (OTC)

Disp: 15 mL

Sig: Spray once in each nostril every 6-8 hours for no more than 3 days

Ingredient: Oxymetazoline

ORAL BACTERIAL INFECTIONS *(Continued)*

OR

Rx	
	Sudafed® 60 mg tablets (OTC)
	Disp: 30 tablets
	Sig: Take 1 tablet every 4-6 hours as needed for congestion

Ingredient: Pseudoephedrine

AND

Rx	
	Chlor-Trimeton® 4 mg (OTC)
	Disp: 14 tablets
	Sig: Take 1 tablet twice daily

Ingredient: Chlorpheniramine

FREQUENTLY ASKED QUESTIONS

What is the best antibiotic modality for treating dental infections?

Penicillin is still the drug of choice for treatment of infections in and around the oral cavity. Phenoxy-methyl penicillin (Pen VK) long has been the most commonly selected antibiotic. In penicillin-allergic individuals, erythromycin may be an appropriate consideration. If another drug is sought, clindamycin prescribed 300 mg as a loading dose followed by 150 mg 4 times/day would be an appropriate regimen for a dental infection. In general, if there is no response to Pen VK, then Augmentin® may be a good alternative in the nonpenicillin-allergic patient because of its slightly altered spectrum. Recommendations would include that the patient should take the drug with food.

Is there cross-allergenicity between the cephalosporins and penicillin?

The incidence of cross-allergenicity is 5% to 8% in the overall population. If a patient has demonstrated a Type I hypersensitivity reaction to penicillin, namely urticaria or anaphylaxis, then this incidence would increase to 20%.

Is there definitely an interaction between contraception agents and antibiotics?

There are well founded interactions between contraceptives and antibiotics. The best instructions that a patient could be given by their dentist are that should an antibiotic be necessary and the dentist is aware that the patient is on contraceptives, and if the patient is using chemical contraceptives, the patient should seriously consider additional means of contraception during the antibiotic management.

Are antibiotics necessary in diabetic patients?

In the management of diabetes, control of the diabetic status is the key factor relative to all morbidity issues. If a patient is well controlled, then antibiotics will likely not be necessary. However, in patients where the control is questionable or where they have recently been given a different drug regimen for their diabetes or if they are being titrated to an appropriate level of either insulin or oral hypoglycemic agents during these periods of time, the dentist might consider preprocedural antibiotics to be efficacious.

Do nonsteroidal anti-inflammatory drugs interfere with blood pressure medication?

At the current time there is no clear evidence that NSAIDs interfere with any of the blood pressure medications that are currently in usage.

PERIODONTAL DISEASES

Periodontal diseases are common to mankind affecting, according to some epidemiologic studies, greater than 80% of the worldwide population. The conditions refer primarily to diseases that are caused by accumulations of dental plaque and the subsequent immune response of the host to the bacteria and toxins present in this plaque. Although most of the organisms that have been implicated in advanced periodontal diseases are anaerobic in nature, some aerobes contribute by either coaggregation with the anaerobic species or direct involvement with specific disease types.

Periodontal condition, as a group of diseases, affects the soft tissues supporting the teeth (ie, gingiva) leading to the term gingivitis or inflammation of gingival structures and those conditions that affect the bone and ligament supporting the teeth (ie, periodontitis) resulting from the infection and/or inflammation of these structures. Diseases of the periodontia can be further subdivided into various types including adult periodontitis, early onset periodontitis, prepubertal periodontitis, and rapidly progressing periodontitis. In addition, specific conditions associated with predisposing immunodeficiency disease, such as those found in HIV-infected patients, create further subclassifications of the periodontal diseases, some of which are covered in those chapters associated with those conditions.

It is well accepted that control of most periodontal diseases requires, at the very minimum, appropriate mechanical cleansing of the dentition and the supporting structures by the patient. These efforts include brushing, some type of interdental cleaning, preferably with either floss or other aids, as well as appropriate sulcular cleaning usually with a brush.

Following appropriate dental treatment by the general dental practitioner and/or the periodontist, aids to these efforts by the patient might include the use of chemical agents to assist in the control of the periodontal diseases, or to prevent periodontal diseases. There are many available chemical agents on the market, only some of which are approved by the American Dental Association. Several have been tested utilizing guidelines published in 1986 by the American Dental Association for assessment of agents that claim efficacy in the management of periodontal diseases. These chemical agents include chlorhexidine (Peridex®, PerioGard®), which are bisbiguanides and benzalkonium chloride, which is a quarternary compound. Chlorhexidine, in various concentrations, has shown efficacy in reducing plaque and gingivitis in patients with short-term utilization. Some side effects include staining of the dentition which is reversible by dental prophylaxis. Chlorhexidine demonstrates the concept of substantivity, indicating that after its use, it has a continued effect in reducing the ability of plaque to form. It has been shown to be useful in a variety of periodontal conditions including acute necrotizing ulcerative gingivitis and healing studies. Some disturbances in taste and accumulation of calculus have been reported, however, chlorhexidine is the most applicable chemical agent of the bisbiguanides that has been studied to date.

Other chemical agents available as mouthwashes include the phenol compound Listerine Antiseptic®. These compounds are primarily restricted to prototype agents; the first to be approved by the ADA being Listerine Antiseptic®. Listerine Antiseptic® has been shown to be effective against plaque and gingivitis in long-term studies and comparable to chlorhexidine in these long-term investigations. However, chlorhexidine performs better than Listerine Antiseptic® in short-term investigations. Triclosan, the chemical agent found in the toothpaste Total®, has been recently approved by the FDA and is an aid in the prevention of gingivitis. Antiplaque activity of triclosan is enhanced with the addition of zinc citrate and there are no serious side effects to the use of triclosan. Sanguinarine is a principle herbal extract used for antiplaque activity. It is an alkyloid from the plant *Sanguinaria canadensis* and has some antimicrobial properties perhaps due to its enzyme activity. Zinc citrate and zinc chloride have often been added to toothpastes as well as enzymes such as mucinase, mutanase, and dextrinase which have demonstrated varying results in studies. Some commercial anionic surfactants are available on the market which include aminoalcohols and the agent Plax® which essentially is comprised of sodium thiosulfate as a surfactant. Recent studies have shown Plax® to have some efficacy when it is added to triclosan.

Long-term use of prescription medications, including antibiotics, is seldom recommended and is not in any way a substitute for general dental/periodontal therapies. As adjunctive therapy, however, benefit has been shown and the new formulations of doxycycline (Periostat® and Atridox®), are recommended for long-term or repetitive treatments. It should be noted that the manufacturer's claims indicate that Periostat® functions as a collagenase inhibitor not as an antibiotic at recommended low doses for long-term therapy. Atridox®, however, functions as an antibiotic and is not recommended for constant long-term therapy, but rather in repetitive applications as necessary. Prescription medications used in efforts to treat periodontal diseases have historically included the use of antibiotics such as tetracycline although complications with use with young patients have often precluded their prescription. Doxycycline is often preferred to tetracycline in low doses. This broad-spectrum bacteriostatic agent has shown efficacy against a wide variety of bacterial organisms found in periodontal disease. Minocycline slow-release (Arestin™) has recently been approved.

PERIODONTAL DISEASES *(Continued)*

The drug metronidazole is a nitromidazole. It is an agent that was originally used in treatment of protozoan infections and some anaerobic bacteria. It is bactericidal and has a good absorption and distribution throughout the body. The studies using metronidazole have suggested that it has a variety of uses in periodontal treatment and can be used as adjunct in both acute necrotizing ulcerative gingivitis and has specific efficacy against spirochetes, bacteria, and some *Porphyromonas* species. Clindamycin is a derivative of vancomycin and has been useful in treatment of suppurative periodontal lesions. However, long-term use is precluded by its complicating toxicities associated with colitis and gastrointestinal problems.

Research has also shown that various combination therapies of metronidazole and tetracycline for juvenile periodontitis and metronidazole with amoxicillin for rapidly progressive disease can be useful. The use of other prescription drugs including nonsteroidal anti-inflammatory, as well as other antibacterial agents, have been under study. Effects on prostaglandins of NSAIDs may indirectly slow periodontal disease progression. New research is currently underway in this regard. Perhaps, in combination therapy with some of the antibiotics, these drugs may assist in reducing the patient's immune response or inflammatory response to the presence of disease-causing bacteria.

Of greatest interest has been the improvement in technology for delivery of chemical agents to the periodontally-diseased site. These systems include biodegradable gelatins and biodegradable chips that can be placed under the gingiva and deliver antibacterial agents directly to the site as an adjunct to periodontal treatment. The initial therapy of mechanical debridement by the periodontal therapist is essential prior to using any chemical agent, and the dentist should be aware that the development of newer agents does not substitute for appropriate periodontal therapy and maintenance. The trade names of the gelatin chips and subgingival delivery systems include Periochip®, Atridox®, and Periostat®.

In addition to the periodontal therapy, consideration of the patient's pre-existing or developing medical conditions are important in the management of the periodontal patient. Several diseases illustrate these points most acutely. The reader is referred to the chapters on Diabetes, Cardiovascular Disease, Pregnancy, Respiratory Disease, HIV, and Cancer Chemotherapy. It has long been accepted that uncontrolled diabetes may predispose to periodontal lesions. Now, under current investigation is the hypothesis that pre-existing periodontal diseases may make it more difficult for a diabetic patient to come under control. In addition, the inflammatory response and immune challenge that is ongoing in periodontal disease appears to be implicated in the development of coronary artery disease as well as an increased risk of myocardial infarction and/or stroke. The accumulation of intra-arterial plaques appears enhanced by the presence of the inflammatory response often seen systemically in patients suffering with periodontal disease. The American Heart Association is currently considering recommendations regarding antibiotic prophylaxis in patients with cardiovascular disease. In addition, the clinician is referred to the section on preprocedural antibiotics in the text for a consideration of antibiotic usage in patients that may be at risk for infective endocarditis. Other conditions including pregnancy and respiratory diseases such as COPD, HIV, and cancer therapy must be considered in the overall view of periodontal diseases. The reader is referred to the sections within the text.

Amoxicillin *on page 86*
Minocycline (Arestin™) *on page 817*
Benzalkonium chloride *on page 151*
Chlorhexidine (Peridex®, PerioGard®, Periochip®) *on page 263*
Clindamycin *on page 300*
Doxycycline (Periostat®, Atridox®) *on page 421*
Listerine Antiseptic® *on page 831*
Metronidazole *on page 804*
NSAIDs see Oral Pain section *on page 1360*
Tetracycline *on page 1147*
Triclosan and Fluorides (Total®) *on page 1203*

ORAL FUNGAL INFECTIONS

Oral fungal infections can result from alteration in oral flora, immunosuppression, and underlying systemic diseases that may allow the overgrowth of these opportunistic organisms. These systemic conditions might include diabetes, long-term xerostomia, adrenal suppression, anemia, and chemotherapy-induced myelosuppression for the management of cancer. Drugs of choice in treating fungal infections are amphotericin B, ciclopirox olamine, clotrimazole, itraconazole, ketoconazole, fluconazole, naftifine hydrochloride, nystatin, and oxiconazole. Patients being treated for fungal skin infections may also be using topical antifungal preparations coupled with a steroid such as triamcinolone. Clinical presentation might include pseudomembranous, atrophic, and hyperkeratotic forms. Fungus has also been implicated in denture stomatitis and symptomatic geographic tongue.

Nystatin (Mycostatin®) is effective topically in the treatment of candidal infections of the skin and mucous membrane. The drug is extremely well tolerated and appears to be nonsensitizing. In persons with denture stomatitis in which monilial organisms play at least a contributory role, it is important to soak the prosthesis overnight in a nystatin suspension. Nystatin ointment can be placed in the denture during the daytime much like a denture adhesive. Medication should be continued for at least 48 hours after disappearance of clinical signs in order to prevent relapse. Patients must be re-evaluated after 14 days of therapy. Predisposing systemic factors must be reconsidered if the oral fungal infection persists. Topical applications rely on contact of the drug with the lesions. Therefore, 4-5 times daily with a dissolving troche or pastille is appropriate. Concern over the presence of sugar in the troches and pastilles has led practitioners to sometimes prescribe the vaginal suppository formulation for off-labeled oral use.

Voriconazole (VFEND®) is indicated for treatment of serious fungal infections in patients intolerant of, or refractory to, other therapy.

Amphotericin B (Fungizone®) *on page 91*
Clotrimazole (Mycelex®) troches *on page 312*
Fluconazole (Diflucan®) *on page 506*
Ketoconazole (Nizoral®) *on page 672*
Nystatin (Mycostatin®) ointment or cream *on page 880*
Nystatin (Mycostatin®) oral suspension *on page 880*
Nystatin (Mycostatin®) pastilles *on page 880*
Nystatin (Mycostatin®) powder *on page 880*
Nystatin and Triamcinolone (Mycolog®–II) cream *on page 881*
Voriconazole (VFEND®)*on page 1248* tablet or injection

Note: Consider Peridex® oral rinse, or Listerine® antiseptic oral rinse for long-term control in immunosuppressed patients.

PRESCRIPTION EXAMPLES

Rx

Mycostatin® pastilles

Disp: 70 pastilles

Sig: Dissolve 1 tablet in mouth until gone, 4-5 times/day for 14 days

Ingredient: 200,000 units of nystatin per tablet

Note: Pastille is more effective than oral suspension due to prolonged contact.

Rx

Mycostatin® oral suspension

Disp: 60 mL (2 oz)

Sig: Use 1 teaspoonful 4-5 times/day; rinse and hold in mouth as long as possible before swallowing or spitting out (2 minutes); do not eat or drink for 30 minutes following application

Ingredients: Nystatin 100,000 units/mL; vehicle contains 50% sucrose and not more than 1% alcohol

ORAL FUNGAL INFECTIONS *(Continued)*

Rx

Mycostatin® ointment or cream

Disp: 15 g or 30 g tube

Sig: Apply liberally to affected areas 4-5 times/day; do not eat or drink for 30 minutes after application

Ingredients:

Cream: 100,000 units nystatin per g, aqueous vanishing cream base

Ointment: 100,000 units nystatin per g, polyethylene, and mineral oil gel base

Note: Denture wearers should apply to dentures prior to each insertion; for edentulous patients, Mycostatin® powder (15 g) can also be prescribed to be sprinkled on dentures.

OR

Rx

Mycelex® troche 10 mg

Disp: 70 tablets

Sig: Dissolve 1 tablet in mouth 5 times/day

Ingredient: Clotrimazole

Note: Tablets contain sucrose, risk of caries with prolonged use (>3 months); care must be exercised in diabetic patients.

Rx

Fungizone® oral suspension 100mg/mL

Disp: 50 mL

Sig: 1 mL; swish and swallow 4 times/day between meals

Ingredient: Amphotericin B (Conventional)

MANAGEMENT OF FUNGAL INFECTIONS REQUIRING SYSTEMIC MEDICATION

If the patient is refractory to topical treatment, consideration of a systemic route might include Diflucan® or Nizoral®. Also, when the patient cannot tolerate topical therapy, ketoconazole (Nizoral®) is an effective, well tolerated, systematic drug for mucocutaneous candidiasis. Concern over liver function and possible drug interactions must be considered.

PRESCRIPTION EXAMPLES

Rx

Nizoral® 200 mg

Disp: 10 or 28 tablets

Sig: Take 1 tablet/day for 10-14 days

Ingredient: Ketoconazole

Note: To be used if *Candida* infection does not respond to mycostatin; potential for liver toxicity; liver function should be monitored with long-term use (>3 weeks)

Rx

Diflucan® 100 mg

Disp: 15 tablets

Sig: Take 2 tablets the first day and 1 tablet/day for 10-14 days

Ingredient: Fluconazole

MANAGEMENT OF ANGULAR CHEILITIS

Angular cheilitis may represent the clinical manifestation of a multitude of etiologic factors. Cheilitis-like lesions may result from local habits, from a decrease in the intermaxillary space, or from nutritional deficiency. More commonly, angular cheilitis represents a mixed infection coupled with an inflammatory response involving *Candida albicans* and other organisms. The drug of choice is now formulated to contain nystatin and triamcinolone and the effect is excellent.

PRESCRIPTION EXAMPLE

Rx

Mycolog®–II cream

Disp: 15 g tube

Sig: Apply to affected area after each meal and before bedtime

Ingredients: Nystatin 100,000 units and triamcinolone acetonide 0.1%

ORAL VIRAL INFECTIONS

Oral viral infections are most commonly caused by herpes simplex viruses and Coxsackie viruses. Oral pharyngeal infections and upper respiratory infections are commonly caused by the Coxsackie group A viruses. Soft tissue viral infections, on the other hand, are most often caused by the herpes simplex viruses. Herpes zoster or varicella-zoster virus, which is one of the herpes family of viruses, can likewise cause similar viral eruptions involving the mucosa.

The diagnosis of an acute viral infection is one that begins by ruling out bacterial etiology and having an awareness of the presenting signs and symptoms associated with viral infection. Acute onset and vesicular eruption on the soft tissues generally favors a diagnosis of viral infection. Unfortunately, vesicles do not remain for a great length of time in the oral cavity; therefore, the short-lived vesicles rupture leaving ulcerated bases as the only indication of their presence. These ulcers, however, are generally small in size and only when left unmanaged, coalesce to form larger, irregular ulcerations. Distinction should be made between the commonly occurring intraoral ulcers (aphthous ulcerations) which do not have a viral etiology and the lesions associated with intraoral herpes. The management of an oral viral infection may be palliative for the most part; however, with the advent of acyclovir we now have a family of drugs that can assist in managing primary and secondary infection. Human *Papillomavirus* is implicated in a number of oral lesions, the most common of which is *Condyloma acuminatum.* Recently, Aldara® has been approved for genital warts; oral use is under study.

It should be noted that herpes can present as a primary infection (gingivostomatitis), recurrent lip lesions (herpes labialis), and intraoral ulcers (recurrent intraoral herpes), involving the oral and perioral tissues. Primary infection is a systemic infection that leads to acute gingivostomatitis involving multiple tissues of the buccal mucosa, lips, tongue, floor of the mouth, and the gingiva. Treatment of primary infections utilizes acyclovir in combination with supportive care. Topical anesthetic used in combination with Benadryl® 0.5% in a saline vehicle was found to be an effective oral rinse in the symptomatic treatment of primary herpetic gingivostomatitis; however, Dyclone® is no longer available. Other agents for symptomatic and supportive treatment include commercially available elixir of Benadryl®, Xylocaine® viscous, Orajel® (OTC), Camphophenique® (OTC), and antibiotics to prevent secondary infections. Systemic supportive therapy should include forced fluids, high concentration protein, vitamin and mineral food supplements, and rest.

Antivirals

Abreva ™(OTC) *on page 406*
Acyclovir (Zovirax®) *on page 40*
Imiquimod (Aldara®) *on page 628*
Lysine® (OTC) *on page 738*
Nelfinavir (Viracept®) *on page 853*
Penciclovir (Denavir®) *on page 926*
Vidarabine (Vira-A®) *on page 1238*
Valacyclovir (Valtrex®) *on page 1223*

Supportive Therapy

Diphenhydramine (Benadryl®, various products) *on page 398*
Lidocaine (Xylocaine®) *on page 706*

Prevention of Secondary Bacterial Infection

Penicillin V Potassium (various products) *on page 931*

PRIMARY INFECTION

PRESCRIPTION EXAMPLE

Rx

Zovirax® 200 mg

Disp: 70 capsules

Sig: Take 1 capsule every 4 hours for 2 weeks, not to exceed 5 in 24 hours

Ingredient: Acyclovir

SUPPORTIVE CARE FOR PAIN AND PREVENTION OF SECONDARY INFECTION

Primary infections often become secondarily infected with bacteria, requiring antibiotics. Dietary supplement may be necessary. Options are presented due to variability in patient compliance and response.

PRESCRIPTION EXAMPLES

Rx

Benadryl® elixir 12.5 mg/5 mL

Disp: 4 oz bottle

Sig: Rinse with 1 teaspoonful for 2 minutes before each meal

Ingredient: Diphenhydramine

Rx

Benadryl® elixir 12.5 mg/5 mL with Kaopectate®, 50% mixture by volume

Disp: 8 oz

Sig: Rinse with 1 teaspoonful every 2 hours

Ingredients: Diphenhydramine and attapulgite

Rx

Xylocaine® viscous 2%

Disp: 450 mL bottle

Sig: Swish with 1 tablespoon 4 times/day and spit out

Ingredient: Lidocaine

Rx

Meritene®

Disp: 1 lb can (plain, chocolate, eggnog flavors)

Sig: Take 3 servings/day; prepare as indicated on can

Ingredient: Protein/vitamin/mineral food supplement

ORAL VIRAL INFECTIONS *(Continued)*

RECURRENT HERPETIC INFECTIONS

Following this primary infection, the herpesvirus remains latent until such time as it has the opportunity to recur. The etiology of this latent period and the degree of viral shedding present during latency is currently under study; however, it is thought that some trigger in the mucosa or the skin causes the virus to begin to replicate. This process may involve Langerhans cells which are immunocompetent antigen-presenting cells resident in all epidermal surfaces. The virus replication then leads to eruptions in tissues surrounding the mouth. The most common form of recurrence is the lip lesion or herpes labialis, however, intraoral recurrent herpes also occurs with some frequency. Prevention of recurrences has been attempted with lysine (OTC) 500-1000 mg/day but response has been variable. Herpes zoster outbreaks, although uncommon, can involve the oral and facial tissues. Valacyclovir is the drug of choice.

Water-soluble bioflavonoid-ascorbic acid complex, now available as Peridin-C®, may be helpful in reducing the signs and symptoms associated with recurrent herpes simplex virus infections. As with all agents used, the therapy is more effective when instituted in the early prodromal stage of the disease process.

PREVENTION PRESCRIPTION EXAMPLES

Rx

Lysine (OTC) 500 mg

Sig: Take 2 tablets/day as preventive; increase to 4 tablets/day if prodrome or recurrence begins

Rx

Citrus bioflavonoids and ascorbic acid tablets 400 mg (Peridin-C®)

Disp: 10 tablets

Sig: Take 2 tablets at once, then 1 tablet 3 times/day for 3 days

Where a recurrence is usually precipitated by exposure to sunlight, the lesion may be prevented by the application to the area of a sunscreen, with a high skin protection factor (SPF) in the range of 10-15.

PRESCRIPTION EXAMPLE

Rx

PreSun® (OTC) 15 sunscreen lotion

Disp: 4 fluid oz

Sig: Apply to susceptible area 1 hour before sun exposure

TREATMENT

Acyclovir (Zovirax®) and vidarabine (Vira-A®) possess antiviral activity against herpes simplex types 1 and 2. Historically, ophthalmic ointments were used topically to treat recurrent mucosal and skin lesions. These do not penetrate well on the skin lesions, thereby providing questionable relief of symptoms. If recommended, use should be closely monitored. Penciclovir, an active metabolite of famciclovir, has been specifically approved in a cream for treatment of recurrent herpes lesions (see acyclovir *on page 40* and penciclovir *on page 926*).

PRESCRIPTION EXAMPLES

Rx

Zovirax® ointment 5% (3%)

Disp: 15 g tube

Sig: Apply thin layer to lesions 6 times/day for 7 days

Ingredient: Acyclovir

Rx

Zovirax® 200 mg

Disp: 70 capsules

Sig: Take 1 capsule every 4 hours for 2 weeks, up to 5 capsules within 24 hours

Ingredient: Acyclovir

Rx

Denavir™

Disp: 2 g tube

Sig: Apply locally every 2 hours, during waking hours, for 4 days

Ingredient: Penciclovir 1%

Note: Denavir™ is approved for use in treating recurrent herpes labialis.

Rx

Abreva™ (OTC) cream

Sig: Apply locally as directed 5 times/day

Ingredient: Docosanol 10%

PRESCRIPTION EXAMPLE FOR HERPES ZOSTER

Rx

Valtrex®

Sig: Take 2 caplets 3 times/day for 7 days

Ingredient: Valacyclovir 500 mg

Note: Reevaluate after 7 days; may require dose reduction in patients with altered renal function, consult with patient's physician(s).

ORAL NONVIRAL SOFT TISSUE ULCERATIONS OR EROSIONS

RECURRENT APHTHOUS STOMATITIS

Kenalog® in Orabase is indicated for the temporary relief of symptoms associated with infrequent recurrences of minor aphthous lesions and ulcerative lesions resulting from trauma. More severe forms of recurrent aphthous stomatitis may be treated with an oral suspension of tetracycline. The agent appears to reduce the duration of symptoms and decrease the rate of recurrence by reducing secondary bacterial infection. Its use is contraindicated during the last half of pregnancy, infancy, and childhood to the age of 8 years. *Lactobacillus acidophilus* preparations (Bacid®, Lactinex®) are occasionally effective for reducing the frequency and severity of the lesions. Debacterol® has recently been approved. Patients with long-standing history of recurrent aphthous stomatitis should be evaluated for iron, folic acid, and vitamin B_{12} deficiencies. Regular use of Listerine® antiseptic has been shown in clinical trials to reduce the severity, duration, and frequency of aphthous stomatitis. Debacterol® has recently been approved. Chlorhexidine oral rinses 20 mL for 30 seconds 2-3 times/day have also demonstrated efficacy in reducing the duration of aphthae. With both of these products, however, patient intolerance of the burning from the alcohol content is of concern. Viractin® has been approved for symptomatic relief. Immunocompromised patients such as those with AIDS may have severe ulcer recurrences and the drug thalidomide has been approved for these patients.

Amlexanox (Aphthasol®) *on page 80*
Attapulgite (Diasorb®, Kaopectate®, Rheaban®) *on page 132*
Chlorhexidine (Peridex®, PerioGard®) *on page 263*
Clobetasol (Temovate®) *on page 303*
Dexamethasone (Decadron®) *on page 363*
Diphenhydramine (Benadryl®, various products) *on page 398*
Fluocinonide (Lidex®) ointment with Orabase *on page 513*
Debacterol® *on page 1124*
Lactobacillus acidophilus and *Lactobacillus bulgaricus* (Bacid®, Lactinex®) *on page 682*
Metronidazole (Flagyl®) *on page 804*
Mouthwash, Antiseptic (Listerine®) *on page 831*
Prednisone (various products) *on page 990*
Tetracaine (Pontocaine®, Viractin®) *on page 1146*
Tetracycline liquid *on page 1147*
Thalidomide (Thalomid®) *on page 1150*
Triamcinolone (Kenalog®) Acetonide Dental Paste *on page 1199*

PRESCRIPTION EXAMPLES FOR MINOR APHTHAE, BURNING TONGUE SYNDROME, GEOGRAPHIC TONGUE, MILD FORMS OF ORAL LICHEN PLANUS

Rx

Listerine® antiseptic (OTC)

Sig: 20 mL for 30 seconds twice daily

Ingredients: Thymol 0.064%, eucalyptus 0.092%, methyl salicylate 0.060%, menthol 0.042%, and alcohol 26.9%

Rx

Peridex® oral rinse

Disp: 1 bottle

Sig: 20 mL for 30 seconds 3 times/day

Ingredients: Chlorhexidine gluconate 0.12% and alcohol 11.6%

Rx

PerioGard® oral rinse

Disp: 1 bottle

Sig: 20 mL for 30 seconds 3 times/day

Ingredients: Chlorhexidine gluconate 0.12% and alcohol 11.6%

Rx

Tetracycline capsules 250 mg

Disp: 40 capsules

Sig: Suspend contents of 1 capsule in a teaspoonful of water; rinse for 2 minutes 4 times/day and swallow

Note: Also available as liquid (125 mg/5 mL), which is convenient to use; swish 5 mL for 2 minutes 4 times/day

Rx

Kenalog® in Orabase 0.1%

Disp: 5 g tube

Sig: Coat the lesion with a film after each meal and at bedtime

Ingredient: Triamcinolone

Rx

Benadryl® elixir 12.5 mg/5 mL

Disp: 4 oz bottle

Sig: Rinse with 1 teaspoonful for 2 minutes before each meal and swallow

Ingredient: Diphenhydramine

Note: Elixir of Benadryl®, a potent antihistamine, is used in the oral cavity primarily as a mild topical anesthetic agent for the symptomatic relief of certain allergic deficiencies which should be ruled out as possible etiologies for the oral condition under treatment. It is often used alone and in solutions with agents such as Kaopectate® or Maalox® to assist in coating the oral mucosa. Benadryl® is also available in capsules.

Rx

Benadryl® syrup (mix 50/50) with Kaopectate®*

Disp: 8 oz total

Sig: Rinse with 2 teaspoons as needed to relieve pain or burning (use after meals)

Ingredient: Diphenhydramine and attapulgite

***Note:** May be mixed with Maalox® if constipation is a problem.

Rx

Lidex® ointment mixed 50/50 with Orabase®

Disp: 30 g total

Sig: Apply thin layer to oral lesions 4-6 times/day

Ingredient: Fluocinonide 0.05%

Note: To be used for oral inflammatory lesions that do not respond to Kenalog® in Orabase®.

ORAL NONVIRAL SOFT TISSUE ULCERATIONS OR EROSIONS *(Continued)*

EROSIVE LICHEN PLANUS AND MAJOR APHTHAE

Elixir of dexamethasone (Decadron®), a potent anti-inflammatory agent, is used topically in the management of acute episodes of erosive lichen planus and major aphthae. Continued supervision of the patient during treatment is essential.

PRESCRIPTION EXAMPLE

Rx

Decadron® elixir 0.5 mg/5 mL

Disp: 100 mL bottle

Sig: Rinse with 1 teaspoonful for 2 minutes 4 times/day; do not swallow

Ingredient: Dexamethasone

Note: Other regimens altering topical and systemic uptake including swish-and-swallow can be designed by the dentist depending upon the severity and usual duration of the lesions.

For severe cases and when the oropharynx is involved, some practitioners have the patient swallow after a 2-minute rinse.

Allergy	Benadryl®
Aphthous	Benadryl®/Maalox® (compounded prescription) Benadryl®/Kaopectate® (compounded prescription) Lidex® in Orabase (compounded prescription) Kenalog® in Orabase Tetracycline mouth rinse
Oral inflammatory disease	Lidex® in Orabase (compounded prescription) Kenalog® in Orabase Prednisone Temovate® cream

The use of long-term steroids is always a concern due to possible adrenal suppression. If systemic steroids are contemplated for a protracted time, medical consultation is advisable.

PRESCRIPTION EXAMPLE FOR SYSTEMIC STEROID

Rx

Prednisone 5 mg

Disp: 60 tablets

Sig: Take 4 tablets in morning with food and 4 tablets at noon with food for 4 day, then decrease the total number of tablets by 1 each day until down to zero

Note: Medrol® (methylprednisolone) dose packs (2-60 mg/day) are an alternative choice; see Methylprednisolone *on page 797*

PRESCRIPTION EXAMPLE FOR HIGH POTENCY TOPICAL CORTICOSTEROID

Rx

Temovate® cream 0.05%

Disp: 15 g tube

Sig: Apply locally 4-6 times/day

Ingredient: Clobetasol

NECROTIZING ULCERATING PERIODONTITIS (HIV Periodontal Disease)

Initial Treatment *(In-Office)*

Gentle debridement

Note: Ensure patient has no iodine allergies

Betadine® rinse *on page 982*

At-Home Treatment

Listerine® antiseptic rinse (20 mL for 30 seconds twice daily)

Peridex® rinse *on page 263*

Metronidazole (Flagyl®) 7-10 days *on page 804*

Follow-Up Therapy

Proper dental cleaning, including scaling and root planing (repeat as needed)

Continue Peridex® and Listerine® rinse (indefinitely)

DENTIN HYPERSENSITIVITY, HIGH CARIES INDEX, AND XEROSTOMIA

DENTIN HYPERSENSITIVITY

Suggested steps in resolving dentin hypersensitivity when a thorough exam has ruled-out any other source for the problem:

Treatment Steps

- Home treatment with a desensitizing toothpaste containing potassium nitrate (used to brush teeth as well as a thin layer applied, each night for 2 weeks)
- If needed, in office potassium oxalate (Protect® by Butler) and/or in office fluoride iontophoresis
- If sensitivity is still not tolerable to the patient, consider pumice then dentin adhesive and unfilled resin or composite restoration overlaying a glass ionomer base

Home Products (all contain nitrate as active ingredient):

Promise®
Denquel®
Sensodyne®

Dentifrice Products *on page 1447*

ANTICARIES AGENTS

Fluoride (Gel 0.4%, Rinse 0.05%) *on page 514*

New toothpastes with triclosan such as Colgate Total® show promise for combined treatment/prevention of caries, plaque, and gingivitis.

FLUORIDE GELS

Oral Rinse Products *on page 1462*

Used for the prevention of demineralization of the tooth structure secondary to xerostomia. For patients with long-term or permanent xerostomia, daily application is accomplished using custom gel applicator trays. Patients with porcelain crowns should use a neutral pH fluoride.

OVER-THE-COUNTER (OTC) PRODUCTS

Form	Brand Name	Strength / Size
Gel, topical (stannous fluoride)	Gel-Kam® (cinnamon, fruit, mint flavors)	0.4% [0.1%] (65 g, 105 g, 122 g)
	Gel-Tin® (lime, grape, cinnamon, raspberry, mint, orange flavors)	0.4% [0.1%] (60 g, 120 g)
	Stop® (grape, cinnamon, bubblegum, piña colada, mint flavors)	0.4% [0.1%] (60 g, 120 g)
Rinse, topical (as sodium)	ACT®, Fluorigard®	0.05% [0.02%] (90 mL, 180 mL, 300 mL, 360 mL, 480 mL)
	Listermint® with Fluoride	0.02% [0.01%] (180 mL, 300 mL, 360 mL, 480 mL, 540 mL, 720 mL, 960 mL, 1740 mL)

PRESCRIPTION ONLY (Rx) PRODUCTS

Form	Brand Name	Strength / Size
Drops, oral (as sodium)		0.275 mg/drop [0.125 mg/drop]
	Fluoritab®, Flura-Drops®	0.55 mg/drop [0.25 mg/drop] (22.8 mL, 24 mL)
	Karidium®, Luride®	0.275 mg/drop [0.125 mg/drop] (30 mL, 60 mL)
	Pediaflor®	1.1 mg/mL [0.5 mg/mL] (50 mL)
Gel-Drops	Thera-Flur® (lime flavor), Thera-Flur-N®	1.1% [0.55%] (24 mL)
Gel, topical Acidulated phosphate fluoride	Minute-Gel® (spearmint, strawberry, grape, apple-cinnamon, cherry cola, bubblegum flavors)	1.23% (480 mL)

PRESCRIPTION ONLY (Rx) PRODUCTS *(continued)*

Form	Brand Name	Strength / Size
Sodium fluoride	Karigel® (orange flavor)	1.1% [0.5%]
	Karigel®-N	1.1% [0.5%]
	PreviDent® (mint, berry, cherry, fruit sherbet flavors)	1.1% [0.5%] (24 g, 30 g, 60 g, 120 g, 130 g, 250 g)
Lozenge (as sodium)	Flura-Loz® (raspberry flavor)	2.2 mg [1 mg]
Rinse, topical (as sodium)	Fluorinse®, Point-Two®	0.2% [0.09%] (240 mL, 480 mL, 3780 mL)
Solution, oral (as sodium)	Phos-Flur® (cherry, cinnamon, grape, wintergreen flavors)	0.44 mg/mL [0.2 mg/mL] (250 mL, 500 mL, 3780 mL)
Tablet (as sodium)		1.1 mg [0.5 mg]; 2.2 mg [1 mg]
Chewable	Fluor-A-Day®	0.55 mg [0.25 mg]
	Fluor-A-Day®, Fluoritab®, Luride® Lozi-Tab®, Pharmaflur®	1.1 mg [0.5 mg]
	Fluor-A-Day®, Fluoritab®, Karidium®, Luride® Lozi-Tab®, Luride®-SF Lozi-Tab®, Pharmaflur®	2.2 mg [1 mg]
Oral	Flura®, Karidium®	2.2 mg [1 mg]
Varnish	Duraflor®	5% [50 mg/mL] (10 mL)

Tables copied from Newland, JR, Meiller, TF, Wynn, RL, et al, *Oral Soft Tissue Diseases,* 2nd ed, Hudson (Cleveland), OH: Lexi-Comp, Inc, 2002.

REMINERALIZING GEL

In addition to fluoride gel to remineralize enamel breakdown in severely xerostomic patients, applicator trays may be used.

Revive®

Note: Many preparations are available over-the-counter, so prescriptions are not always required. If caries is severe, use fluoride gel in custom tray once daily as long as needed (years).

ANTIPLAQUE AGENTS

PRESCRIPTION EXAMPLES

Rx

Listerine® antiseptic mouthwash (OTC)

Sig: 20 mL, swish for 30 seconds twice daily

Ingredients: Thymol 0.064%, eucalyptus 0.092%, methyl salicylate 0.060%, menthol 0.042%, and alcohol 26.9%

Rx

Peridex® oral rinse

Disp: 3 times 16 oz

Sig: 1/2 oz, swish for 30 seconds 2-3 times/day

Ingredients: Chlorhexidine gluconate 0.12% and alcohol 11.6%

Rx

PerioGard® oral rinse

Disp 3 times 16 oz

Sig: 1/2 oz, swish for 30 seconds 2-3 times/day

Ingredients: Chlorhexidine gluconate 0.12% and alcohol 11.6%

Note: Peridex® may stain teeth yellow to brown (removable with dental cleaning), temporarily alter taste, and increase the deposition of calculus (reversible).

Chlorhexidine (Peridex®) *on page 263*

DENTIN HYPERSENSITIVITY, HIGH CARIES INDEX, AND XEROSTOMIA *(Continued)*

MANAGEMENT OF SIALORRHEA

In patients suffering with medical conditions that result in hypersalivation, the dentist may determine that it is appropriate to use an atropine sulfate medication to achieve a dry field for dental procedures or to reduce excessive drooling. Currently there is one ADA approved medication sold under the name of Sal-Tropine™. See Atropine Sulfate Dental Tablets *on page 131*

XEROSTOMIA

Xerostomia refers to the subjective sensation of a dry mouth. Numerous factors can play a role in the patient's perception of dry mouth. Changes in salivary function caused by drugs, surgical intervention, or treatment of cancer are among the leading causes of xerostomia. Other factors including aging, smoking, mouth breathing, and the immune complex of disorders, Sjögren's syndrome, can also be implicated in a patient's perception of xerostomia. Human immunodeficiency virus (HIV) may produce xerostomia when viral changes in salivary glands are present. Xerostomia affects women more frequently than men and is also more common in older individuals. Some alteration in salivary function naturally occurs with age, but it is extremely difficult to quantify the effects. Xerostomia and salivary gland hypofunction in the elderly population are contributory to deterioration in the quality of life.

Once a diagnosis of xerostomia or salivary gland hypofunction is made and possible causes confirmed, treatment for the condition usually involves management of the underlying disease and avoidance of unnecessary medications. In addition, good hydration is essential and water is the drink of choice. Also, the use of artificial saliva substitutes, selected chewing gums, and/or toothpastes formulated to treat xerostomia, is often warranted. In more difficult cases, such as patients receiving radiotherapy for cancer of the head and neck regions or patients with Sjögren's syndrome, systemic cholinergic stimulants may be administered if no contraindications exist.

CLINICAL PRODUCT USE

Because of the complex nature of xerostomia, management by the dental clinician is difficult. Treatment success is also difficult to assess and is often unsatisfactory. The salivary stimulants, pilocarpine and cevimeline, may aid in some conditions but are only approved for use as sialogogues in patients receiving radiotherapy and in Sjögren's patients, specifically as described above. Artificial salivas are available as over-the-counter products and represent the potential for continuous application by the patient to achieve comfort for their xerostomic condition.

The role of the clinician in attempting treatment of dry mouth is to first achieve a differential diagnosis and to ensure that other conditions are not simultaneously present. For example, many patients suffer burning mouth syndrome or painful oral tissues with no obvious etiology accompanying dry mouth. Also, higher caries incidence may be associated with changes in salivary flow. As previously mentioned, Sjögren's syndrome represents an immune complex of disorders that can affect the eyes, oral tissues, and other organ systems. The reader is referred to current oral pathology or oral medicine text for review of signs and symptoms of Sjögren's syndrome.

Treatment of cancer often leads to dry mouth. Surgical intervention removing salivary tissue due to the presence of a salivary gland tumor results in loss of salivary function. Also, many of the chemotherapeutic agents produce transitory changes in salivary flow, such that the patient may perceive a dry mouth during chemotherapy. Most notably related to salivary dysfunction is the use of radiation regimens to head and neck tissues. Tumors in or about salivary gland tissue, the oral cavity, and oropharynx are most notably sensitive to radiation therapy and subsequent dry mouth. In the head and neck, therapeutic radiation is commonly used in treatment of squamous cell carcinomas and lymphomas. The radiation level necessary to destroy malignant cells ranges from 40-70 Gy. Salivary tissue is extremely sensitive to radiation changes. Radiation dosages >30 Gy are sufficient to permanently change salivary function. In addition to the mucositis and subsequent secondary infection by fungal colonization or viral exacerbation, oral tissues can become exceptionally dry due to the effects of radiation on salivary glands. In fact, permanent damage to salivary gland tissue within the beam path produces significant levels of xerostomia in most patients. Some recovery may be noted by the patient. Most often, the effects are permanent and even progressive as the radiation dosage increases.

Artificial salivas do not produce any protectant or stimulation of the salivary gland. The use of pilocarpine and cevimeline as salivary stimulants in pre-emptive treatment, as well as postradiation treatment, have been shown to have some efficacy in management of dry mouth. The success rate, however, still is often unsatisfactory and post-treatment management by the dentist usually requires fluoride supplements to prevent radiation-induced caries due to dry mouth. Also, management of dry mouth through patient use of the artificial salivary gel, solutions and sprays, or other over-the-counter products for dry mouth (eg, chewing gum, toothpaste, mouthwash, swab-sticks) is highly recommended. The use of pilocarpine or cevimeline should only be considered by the dentist in consultation with the managing physician. The oftentimes severe and widespread cholinergic side effects of pilocarpine and cevimeline mandate close monitoring of the patient.

The use of artificial salivary substitutes is less problematic for the dentist. The dentist should, in considering selection of a drug, base his or her decision on patient compliance and comfort. Salivary substitutes presently on the market may have some benefit in terms of electrolyte balance and salivary consistency. However, the ultimate decision needs to be based on patients' taste, their willingness to use the medication ad libitum, and improvement in their comfort related to dry mouth. Many of the drugs are pH balanced to reduce additional risk of dental demineralization or caries. Oftentimes, the dentist must try numerous medications, one at a time, prior to finding one which gives the patient some comfort. Another gauge of acceptability is to investigate whether the artificial saliva substitute has the American Dental Association's seal of approval. Most of the currently accepted saliva substitute products have been evaluated by the ADA.

In general, considerations that the clinician might use in a prescribed regimen would be that saliva substitutes are meant to be used regularly throughout the day by the patient to achieve comfort during meals, reduce tissue abrasion, and prevent salivary stagnation on teeth. Other than these, there are no specific recommendations for patients. Recommendations by the dentist need to be tailored to the patient's acceptance. Salivary substitutes may provide an allergic potential in patients who are sensitive to some of the preservatives present in artificial saliva products. In addition to this allergic potential, there is a risk of microbial contamination by placement of the salivary substitute container in close contact with the oral cavity.

Patient education regarding the use of saliva substitutes is also part of the clinical approach. The patient with chronic xerostomia should be educated about regular professional care, high performance in dental hygiene, the need to re-evaluate oral soft tissue pathology, and any changes that might occur long term. In patients with severe xerostomia, artificial salivary medications should be given in combination with topical fluoride treatment programs designed by the dentist to reduce caries.

DENTIN HYPERSENSITIVITY, HIGH CARIES INDEX, AND XEROSTOMIA *(Continued)*

PRODUCTS AND DRUGS TO TREAT DRY MOUTH

Medication	Manufacturer and Phone Number	Product Type	Manufacturer's Description	Indication	Ingredients	Directions for Use	Form and Availability
ARTIFICIAL SALIVAS (OTC)							
Moi-Stir® Moistening Solution	Kingswood Laboratories, Inc (800) 968-7772	Pump spray	Saliva supplement for moistening of mouth and mucosal area	Nontherapeutic treatment of dry mouth; intended for comfort only	Water, sorbitol, sodium carboxymethylcellulose, methylparaben, propylparaben, potassium chloride, sodium chloride, flavoring	Spray directly into mouth as necessary to treat drying conditions	4 oz spray bottle; order directly from manufacturer or various distributors
MouthKote® Oral Moisturizer	Parnell Pharmaceuticals, Inc (800) 457-4276	Aqueous solution	Pleasant lemon-lime-flavored oral moisturizer to lubricate and protect oral tissue	Treats the discomfort of oral dryness caused by medications, disease, surgery, irradiation, aging	Water, xylitol, sorbitol, yerba santa, citric acid, ascorbic acid, flavor, sodium benzoate, sodium saccharin	Swirl 1 or 2 teaspoonfuls in mouth for 8-10 seconds; swallow or spit out; shake well before using	2 oz and 8 oz bottles; available at drugstores or order directly from manufacturer
BreathTech™ Plaque Fighter Mouth Spray	Omnii Oral Pharmaceuticals (800) 445-3386	Pump dispenser	Plaque inhibitor in vanilla-mint flavor for breath malodor or reduced salivary flow	Treats the discomfort of oral dryness	Microdent® patented plaque-inhibitor formula	Spray directly into mouth; spread over teeth and tissue with tongue	18 mL pump dispenser; order directly from manufacturer
Optimoist™ Oral Moisturizer	Colgate Oral Pharmaceuticals (800) 225-3756	Oral moisturizer, aqueous solution	Pleasant tasting saliva substitute for instant relief of dry mouth and throat without demineralizing tooth enamel	Treats the discomfort of oral dryness	Deionized water, xylitol, calcium phosphate monobasic, citric acid, sodium hydroxide, sodium benzoate, flavoring, acesulfame potassium, hydroxyethylcellulose, polysorbate 20 and sodium monofluorophosphate (fluoride concentration is 2 parts per million)	Spray directly into mouth to relieve dry mouth discomfort; may be swallowed or expectorated; use as needed	2 oz and 12 oz bottles; available at mass merchandise stores, food stores, and drugstores

PRODUCTS AND DRUGS TO TREAT DRY MOUTH *(continued)*

Medication	Manufacturer and Phone Number	Product Type	Manufacturer's Description	Indication	Ingredients	Directions for Use	Form and Availability
Biotene® OralBalance® Mouth Moisturizing Gel	Laclede Professional Products, Inc (800) 922-5856	Gel	Sugar-free oral lubricant; relieves dry mouth symptoms up to 8 hours; soothes and protects oral tissue to promote healing; helps to inhibit harmful bacteria; improves retention under dentures	Relieves symptoms of dry mouth: burning, itching, cotton palate, sore tissue swallowing difficulties	Contains the "Biotene®" protective salivary enzyme system Active: Glucose oxidase (2000 units), lactoperoxidase (3000 units), lysozyme (5 mg), lactoferrin (5 mg) Other: Hydrogenated starch, xylitol, hydroxyethyl cellulose, glycerate polyhydrate, aloe vera	Using a clean fingertip, apply a 1" ribbon of gel on tongue; add additional amount of gel on other dry; use as needed	1.4 oz tube; available at mass merchandise stores, food stores, and drugstores
Salivart® Synthetic Saliva, Aqueous Solution	Gebauer Co (800) 321-9348	Aerosol aqueous spray	Oral moisturizer for patients with reduced salivary flow	Replacement therapy for patients complaining of xerostomia	Sodium carboxymethylcellulose, sorbitol, sodium chloride, potassium chloride, calcium chloride dihydrate, magnesium chloride hexahydrate, potassium phosphate dibasic, purified water, nitrogen (propellant)	Spray directly into mouth or throat for 1-2 seconds; use as needed	2.48 fl oz (75 g); available at most drugstores or directly from manufacturer
OTHER DRY MOUTH PRODUCTS (OTC)							
Biotene® Dry Mouth Gum	Laclede Professional Products, Inc (800) 922-9348	Chewing gum	Sugar-free; helps stimulate saliva flow; fights cause/effect of bad breath; reduces plaque	Treats oral dryness	Active: Lactoperoxidase (0.11 Units), glucose oxidase (0.15 Units) Other: Sorbitol, gum base, xylitol, hydrogenated glucose, potassium thiocyanate	Chew 1 or 2 pieces; use as needed	Each package contains 17 pieces; available at drugstores or directly from manufacturer
Biotene® Dry Mouth Toothpaste	Laclede Professional Products, Inc (800) 922-9348	Toothpaste	Reduces harmful bacteria which cause cavities, periodontal disease, and oral infections	Use in place of regular toothpaste for dry mouth	Active: Lactoperoxidase (15,000 Units), glucose oxidase (10,000 Units), lysozyme (16 mg), sodium monofluorophosphate Other: Sorbitol, glycerin, calcium pyrophosphate, hydrated silica, xylitol, isoceteth-20, cellulose gum, flavoring, sodium benzoate, beta-d-glucose, potassium thiocyanate	Use in place of regular toothpaste; rinse toothbrush before applying; brush for 2 minutes; rinse lightly	4.5 oz tube; available at drugstores or directly from manufacturer

DENTIN HYPERSENSITIVITY, HIGH CARIES INDEX, AND XEROSTOMIA *(Continued)*

PRODUCTS AND DRUGS TO TREAT DRY MOUTH *(continued)*

Medication	Manufacturer and Phone Number	Product Type	Manufacturer's Description	Indication	Ingredients	Directions for Use	Form and Availability
Biotene® Gentle Mouthwash	Laclede Professional Products, Inc (800) 922-9348	Mouthwash	Alcohol-free; strong antibacterial formula neutralizes mouth odors; soothes as it cleans to protect teeth and oral tissue	Treats dry mouth or oral irritations	Lysozyme, lactoferrin, glucose oxidase, lactoperoxidase	Use 15 mL (1 tablespoonful); swish thoroughly for 30 seconds and spit out; for dry throat, sip 1 tablespoonful of mouthwash 2-3 times/day	Available at drugstores or directly from manufacturer
Moi-Stir® Oral Swabsticks	Kingswood Laboratories, Inc (800) 968-7772	Swabsticks	Lubricates and moistens mouth and mucosal area	Lubricates and moistens mouth and mucosal area	Water, sorbitol, sodium carboxymethylcellulose, methylparaben, propylparaben, potassium chloride, sodium chloride, flavoring	Gently swab all intraoral surfaces of mouth, gums, tongue, palate, buccal mucosa, gingival, teeth, and lips where uncomfortable dryness exists	3 swabsticks/packet, 100 packets/case; order directly from manufacturer or from various distributors.
CHOLINERGIC SALIVARY STIMULANTS (Rx)							
Cevimeline (Evoxac®)	Snow Brand Pharmaceuticals (800) 475-6473			Treats symptoms of dry mouth in patients with Sjögren's syndrome	Active: Cevimeline 30 mg Other: Lactose monohydrate, hydroxypropyl cellulose, magnesium stearate	1 capsule (30 mg) 3 times/day	30 mg capsules
Pilocarpine (Salagen®)	MGI Pharmaceuticals, Inc (800) 562-5580			Treats xerostomia caused by radiation therapy in patients with head/neck cancer, Sjögren's syndrome	Active: Pilocarpine 5 mg Other: Carnauba wax, hydroxypropyl methylcellulose, iron oxide, microcrystalline cellulose, stearic acid, titanium dioxide	1-2 tablets (5 mg) 3-4 times/day, not to exceed 30 mg/day	5 mg tablets

CHOLINERGIC SALIVARY STIMULANTS (PRESCRIPTION ONLY)

Pilocarpine (Salagen® *on page 955*), approved in 1994, and cevimeline (Evoxac® *on page 256*), approved in 2000, are cholinergic drugs which stimulate salivary flow. They stimulate muscarinic-type acetylcholine receptors in salivary glands within the parasympathetic division of the autonomic nervous system, causing an increase in serous-type saliva. Thus, they are considered cholinergic, muscarinic-type (parasympathomimetic) drugs. Due to significant side effects caused by these drugs, they are available by prescription only.

Pilocarpine (Salagen®) is indicated for the treatment of xerostomia caused by radiation therapy in patients with head and neck cancer and xerostomia in patients suffering from Sjögren's syndrome. The usual adult dosage is 1-2 tablets (5 mg) 3-4 times/day, not to exceed 30 mg/day. Patients should be treated for a minimum of 90 days for optimum effect. The most frequent adverse side effect is perspiration, which occurs in about 30% of patients who use 5 mg 3 times/day. Other adverse effects (in about 10% of patients) are nausea, rhinitis, chills, frequent urination, dizziness, headache, lacrimation, and pharyngitis. Salagen® is contraindicated for patients with uncontrolled asthma and narrow-angle glaucoma.

The salivary-stimulative effects of oral pilocarpine have been documented since the late 1960s and 1970s. Pilocarpine has been documented to overcome xerostomia from different causes. More recent studies confirm its effectiveness in improving salivary flow in patients undergoing irradiation therapy for head and neck cancer. A capstone study by Johnson, et al, reported the effects of pilocarpine in 208 irradiation patients at 39 different treatment sites. Salagen®, at a dose of 5 mg 3 times/day, improved salivation in 44% of patients, compared with 25% in the placebo group. They concluded that treatment with pilocarpine (Salagen®) produced the best overall outcome with respect to saliva production and relief of symptoms of xerostomia in patients undergoing irradiation therapy.

Additional studies have been published showing the effectiveness of pilocarpine (Salagen®) in stimulating salivary flow in patients suffering from Sjögren's syndrome and the FDA has recently approved the use of Salagen® for this indication.

Recent reports suggest that pre-emptive use of pilocarpine may be effective in protecting salivary glands during therapeutic irradiation; further studies are needed to confirm this. As of this publication date, the use of pilocarpine has not been approved to treat xerostomia induced by chronic medication. Pilocarpine could be used as a sialagogue for individuals with xerostomia induced by antidepressants and other medications. However, the potential for serious drug interactions is a concern and more studies are needed to clarify the safety and effectiveness of pilocarpine when given in the presence of other medications.

Cevimeline (Evoxac®) is indicated for treatment of symptoms of dry mouth in patients with Sjögren's syndrome. The usual dosage in adults is 1 capsule (30 mg) 3 times/day. Cevimeline (Evoxac®) is supplied in 30 mg capsules. Some adverse effects reported for Evoxac® include increased sweating (19%), rhinitis (11%), sinusitis (12%), and upper respiratory infection (11%). Evoxac® is contraindicated for patients with uncontrolled asthma, narrow-angle glaucoma, acute iritis, and other conditions where miosis is undesirable.

DENTIN HYPERSENSITIVITY, HIGH CARIES INDEX, AND XEROSTOMIA *(Continued)*

OTHER DRUGS IMPLICATED IN XEROSTOMIA

>10%	1% to 10%
Alprazolam	Acrivastine and Pseudoephedrine
Amitriptyline hydrochloride	Albuterol
Amoxapine	Amantadine hydrochloride
Anisotropine methylbromide	Amphetamine sulfate
Atropine sulfate	Astemizole (withdrawn from market)
Belladonna and Opium	Azatadine maleate
Benztropine mesylate	Beclomethasone dipropionate
Bupropion	Bepridil hydrochloride
Chlordiazepoxide	Bitolterol mesylate
Clomipramine hydrochloride	Brompheniramine maleate
Clonazepam	Carbinoxamine and Pseudoephedrine
Clonidine	Chlorpheniramine maleate
Clorazepate dipotassium	Clemastine fumarate
Cyclobenzaprine	Clozapine
Desipramine hydrochloride	Cromolyn sodium
Diazepam	Cyproheptadine hydrochloride
Dicyclomine hydrochloride	Dexchlorpheniramine maleate
Diphenoxylate and Atropine	Dextroamphetamine sulfate
Doxepin hydrochloride	Dimenhydrinate
Ergotamine	Diphenhydramine hydrochloride
Estazolam	Disopyramide phosphate
Flavoxate	Doxazosin
Flurazepam hydrochloride	Dronabinol
Glycopyrrolate	Ephedrine sulfate
Guanabenz acetate	Flumazenil
Guanfacine hydrochloride	Fluvoxamine
Hyoscyamine sulfate	Gabapentin
Interferon Alfa-2a	Guaifenesin and Codeine
Interferon Alfa-2b	Guanadrel sulfate
Interferon Alfa-N3	Guanethidine sulfate
Ipratropium bromide	Hydroxyzine
Isoproterenol	Hyoscyamine, Atropine, Scopolamine, and Phenobarbital
Isotretinoin	Imipramine
Loratadine	Isoetharine
Lorazepam	Levocabastine hydrochloride
Loxapine	Levodopa
Maprotiline hydrochloride	Levodopa and Carbidopa
Methscopolamine bromide	Levorphanol tartrate
Molindone hydrochloride	Meclizine hydrochloride
Nabilone	Meperidine hydrochloride
Nefazodone	Methadone hydrochloride
Oxybutynin chloride	Methamphetamine hydrochloride
Oxazepam	Methyldopa
Paroxetine	Metoclopramide
Phenelzine sulfate	Morphine sulfate
Prochlorperazine	Nortriptyline hydrochloride
Propafenone hydrochloride	Ondansetron
Protriptyline hydrochloride	Oxycodone and Acetaminophen
Quazepam	Oxycodone and Aspirin
Reserpine	Pentazocine
Selegiline hydrochloride	Phenylpropanolamine hydrochloride
Temazepam	Prazosin hydrochloride
Thiethylperazine maleate	Promethazine hydrochloride
Trihexyphenidyl hydrochloride	Propoxyphene
Trimipramine maleate	Pseudoephedrine
Venlafaxine	Risperidone
	Sertraline hydrochloride
	Terazosin
	Terbutaline sulfate

TEMPOROMANDIBULAR DYSFUNCTION (TMD)

Temporomandibular dysfunction comprises a broad spectrum of signs and symptoms. Although TMD presents in patterns, diagnosis is often difficult. Evaluation and treatment is time-intensive and no single therapy or drug regimen has been shown to be universally beneficial.

The thorough diagnostician should perform a screening examination for the temporomandibular joint on all patients. Ideally, a baseline maximum mandibular opening along with lateral and protrusive movement evaluation should be performed. Secondly, the joint area should be palpated and an adequate exam of the muscles of mastication and the muscles of the neck and shoulders should be made. These muscle would include the elevators of the mandible (masseter, internal pterygoid, and temporalis); the depressors of the mandible (including the external pterygoid and digastric); etrusive muscles (including the temporalis and digastric), and protrusive muscles (including the external and internal pterygoids). These muscles also account for lateral movement of the mandible. The clinician should also be alert to indicators of dysfunction, primarily a history of pain with jaw function, chronic history of joint noise (although this can often be misinterpreted), pain in the muscles of the neck, limited jaw movement, pain in the actual muscles of mastication, and headache or even earache. The signs and symptoms are extremely variable and the clinician should be alert for any or all of these areas of interest. Because of the complexity of both evaluation and diagnosis, the general dentist often finds it too time consuming to spend the countless hours evaluating and treating the temporomandibular dysfunction patient. Therefore, oral medicine specialists trained in temporomandibular evaluation and treatment often accept referrals for the management of these complicated patients.

The Oral Medicine specialist in TMD management, the physical therapist interested in head and neck pain, and the Oral and Maxillofacial surgeon will all work together with the referring general dentist to accomplish successful patient treatment. Table 1 lists the wide variety of treatment alternatives available to the team. Depending on the diagnosis, one or more of the therapies might be selected. For organic diseases of the joint not responding to nonsurgical approaches, a wide variety of surgical techniques are available (Table 2).

ACUTE TMD

Acute TMD oftentimes presents alone or as an episode during a chronic pattern of signs and symptoms. Trauma, such as a blow to the chin or the side of the face, can result in acute TMD. Occasionally, similar symptoms will follow a lengthy wide open mouth dental procedure.

The condition usually presents as continuous deep pain in the TMJ. If edema is present in the joint, the condyle sometimes can be displaced which will cause abnormal occlusion of the posterior teeth on the affected side. The diagnosis is usually based on the history and clinical presentation. Management of the patient includes:

1. Restriction of all mandibular movement to function in a pain-free range of motion
2. Soft diet
3. NSAIDs (eg, Anaprox® DS 1 tablet every 12 hours for 7-10 days)
4. Moist heat applications to the affected area for 15-20 minutes, 4-6 times/day
5. Consideration of a muscle relaxant, such as methocarbamol (Robaxin®) *on page 783*, adult patient of average height/weight, two (500 mg) tablets at bedtime; daytime dose can be tailored to patient

Additional therapies could include referral to a physical therapist for ultrasound therapy 2-4 times/week and a single injection of steroid in the joint space. A team approach with an oral maxillofacial surgeon for this procedure may be helpful. Spray and stretch with Fluori-methane® is often helpful for rapid relief of trismus.

Dichlorodifluoromethane and Trichloromonofluoromethane (Fluori-methane®) *on page 377*

TEMPOROMANDIBULAR DYSFUNCTION (TMD) *(Continued)*

CHRONIC TMD

Following diagnosis which is often problematic, the most common therapeutic modalities include:

- Explaining the problem to the patient
- Recommending a soft diet:
  - diet should consist of soft foods (eg, eggs, yogurt, casseroles, soup, ground meat)
  - avoid chewing gum, salads, large sandwiches, and hard fruit
- Reducing stress; moist heat application 4-6 times/day for 15-20 minutes coupled with a monitored exercise program will be beneficial. Usually, working with a physical therapist is ideal.
- Medications include analgesics, anti-inflammatories, tranquilizers, and muscle relaxants

MEDICATION OPTIONS

Most commonly used medication (NSAIDs)

Aminosalicylate Sodium (Sodium P.A.S.) *on page 72*
Choline Magnesium Trisalicylate (Trilisate®) *on page 279*
Choline Salicylate (Arthropan®) *on page 280*
Diclofenac (Cataflam®, Voltaren®) *on page 378*
Diflunisal (Dolobid®) *on page 386*
Etodolac (Lodine®) *on page 479*
Fenoprofen (Nalfon®) *on page 492*
Flurbiprofen (Ansaid®) *on page 522*
Ibuprofen (various products) *on page 621*
Indomethacin (Indocin®) *on page 634*
Ketoprofen (Orudis®) *on page 674*
Ketorolac (Toradol®) *on page 676*
Magnesium Salicylate (Doan's®, Magan®, Mobidin®) *on page 742*
Meclofenamate (Meclomen®) *on page 751*
Mefenamic Acid (Ponstel®) *on page 754*
Nabumetone (Relafen®) *on page 838*
Naproxen (Naprosyn®) *on page 848*
Oxaprozin (Daypro™) *on page 895*
Piroxicam (Feldene®) *on page 965*
Salsalate (various products) *on page 1074*
Sulindac (Clinoril®) *on page 1125*
Tolmetin (Tolectin®) *on page 1180*

Tranquilizers and muscle relaxants, when used appropriately, can provide excellent adjunctive therapy. These drugs should be primarily used for a short period of time to manage acute pain. In low dosages, amitriptyline is often used to treat chronic pain and occasionally migraine headache. Two new drugs similar to the prototype drug, amitriptyline, have recently been approved for use in adults only, for treatment of acute migraine with or without aura: Almotriptan malate (Axert™ ; Pharmacia Corp) and Frovatriptan succinate (Frova™ ; Elan). Selective serotonin reuptake inhibitors (SSRIs) are sometimes used in the management of chronic neuropathic pain, particularly in patients not responding to amitriptyline. Recently, gabapentin (Neurontin®) has been approved for chronic pain. Problems of inducing bruxism with SSRIs, however, have been reported and may preclude their use. Clinicians attempting to evaluate any patient with bruxism or involuntary muscle movement, who is simultaneously being treated with an SSRI, should be aware of this potential association.

See individual monographs for dosing instructions.

Common minor tranquilizers include:

Alprazolam (Xanax®) *on page 56*

Diazepam (Valium®) *on page 373*

Lorazepam (Ativan®) *on page 729*

Chronic neuropathic pain management:

Amitriptyline (Elavil®) *on page 75*

Carbamazepine (Tegretol®) *on page 216*

Gabapentin (Neurontin®) *on page 546*

Acute migraine management:

Almotriptan (Axert™) *on page 54*

Frovatriptan (Frova™) *on page 542*

Rizatriptan (Maxalt®) *on page 1063*

Common muscle relaxants include:

Chlorzoxazone (Parafon® Forte DSC) *on page 277*

Cyclobenzaprine (Flexeril®) *on page 333*

Methocarbamol (Robaxin®) *on page 783*

Orphenadrine (Norgesic® Forte) *on page 891*

Note: Muscle relaxants and tranquilizers should generally be prescribed with an analgesic or NSAID to relieve pain as well.

Narcotic analgesics can be used on a short-term basis or intermittently in combination with non-narcotic therapy in the chronic pain patient. Judicious prescribing, monitoring, and maintenance by the practitioner is imperative whenever considering the use of narcotic analgesics due to the abuse and addiction liabilities.

Table 1.
TMD - NONSURGICAL THERAPIES

1. Moist heat and cold spray
2. Injections in muscle trigger areas (procaine)
3. Exercises (passive, active)
4. Medications
   a. Muscle relaxants
   b. Minerals
   c. Multiple vitamins (Ca, B_6, B_{12})
5. Orthopedic craniomandibular repositioning appliance (splints)
6. Biofeedback, acupuncture
7. Physiotherapy: TMJ muscle therapy
8. Myofunctional therapy
9. TENS (transcutaneous electrical neural stimulation), Myo-Monitor
10. Dental therapy
    a. Equilibration (coronoplasty)
    b. Restoring occlusion to proper vertical dimension of maxilla to mandible by orthodontics, dental restorative procedures, orthognathic surgery, permanent splint, or any combination of these

Table 2.
TMD - SURGICAL THERAPIES

1. Cortisone injection into joint (with local anesthetic)
2. Bony and/or fibrous ankylosis: requires surgery (osteoarthrotomy with prosthetic appliance)
3. Chronic subluxation: requires surgery, depending on problem (possibly eminectomy and/or prosthetic implant)
4. Osteoarthritis: requires surgery, depending on problem
   a. Arthroplasty with implant
   b. Meniscectomy with implant
   c. Arthroplasty with repair of disc and/or implant
   d. Implant with Silastic insert
5. Rheumatoid arthritis
   a. Arthroplasty with implant with Silastic insert
   b. "Total" TMJ replacement
6. Tumors: require osteoarthrotomy — removal of tumor and restoring of joint when possible
7. Chronic disc displacement: requires repair of disc and possible removal of bone from condyle

PATIENTS REQUIRING SEDATION

Anxiety constitutes the most frequently found psychiatric problem in the general population. Anxiety can range from simple phobias to severe debilitating anxiety disorders. Functional results of this anxiety can, therefore, range from simple avoidance of dental procedures to panic attacks when confronting stressful situations such as seen in some patients regarding dental visits. Many patients claim to be anxious over dental care when in reality they simply have not been managed with modern techniques of local anesthesia, the availability of sedation, or the caring dental practitioner.

The dentist may detect anxiety in patients during the treatment planning evaluation phase of the care. The anxious person may appear overly alert, may lean forward in the dental chair during conversation or may appear concerned over time, possibly using this as a guise to require that they cut short their dental visit. Anxious persons may also show signs of being nervous by demonstrating sweating, tension in their muscles including their temporomandibular musculature, or they may complain of being tired due to an inability to obtain an adequate night's sleep.

The management of such patients requires a methodical approach to relaxing the patient, discussing their dental needs, and then planning, along with the patient the best way to accomplish dental treatment in the presence of their fears, both real or imagined. Consideration may be given to sedation to assist with managing the patient. This sedation can be oral or parenteral, or inhalation in the case of nitrous oxide. The dentist must be adequately trained in administering the sedative of choice, as well as in monitoring the patient during the sedated procedures. Numerous medications are available to achieve the level of sedation usually necessary in the dental office: Valium®, Ativan®, Xanax®, Vistaril®, Serax®, and BuSpar® represent a few. BuSpar® is soon to be available as a transdermal patch. These oral sedatives can be given prior to dental visits as outlined in the following prescriptions. They have the advantage of allowing the patient a good night's sleep prior to the day of the procedures and providing on-the-spot sedation during the procedures. Nitrous oxide represents an in the office administered sedative that is relatively safe, but requires additional training and carefully planned monitoring protocols of any auxiliary personnel during the inhalation procedures. Both the oral and the inhalation techniques can, however, be applied in a very useful manner to manage the anxious patient in the dental office.

Alprazolam (Xanax®) *on page 56*
Buspirone (BuSpar®) *on page 189*
Diazepam (Valium®) *on page 373*
Hydroxyzine (Vistaril®, various products) *on page 616*
Lorazepam (Ativan®) *on page 729*
Nitrous Oxide *on page 873*
Oxazepam (Serax®) *on page 896*
Triazolam (Halcion®) *on page 1201*

Note: Although various sedatives have been used for preprocedure sedation, no specific regimens or protocols have been established. Guidelines for use are still under study.

Fluoxetine (Prozac®) *on page 517*
Fluvoxamine (Luvox®) *on page 528*
Paroxetine (Paxil™) *on page 918*
Sertraline (Zoloft®) *on page 1083*

PRESCRIPTION EXAMPLES

Rx

Valium® 5 mg*

Disp: 6 tablets

Sig: Take 1 tablet in evening before going to bed and 1 tablet 1 hour before appointment

Ingredient: Diazepam

***Note:** Also available as 2 mg and 10 mg

Rx

Ativan® 1 mg*

Disp: 4 tablets

Sig: Take 2 tablets in evening before going to bed and 2 tablets 1 hour before appointment

Ingredient: Lorazepam

***Note:** Also available as 0.5 mg and 2 mg

Rx

Xanax® 0.5 mg

Disp: 4 tablets

Sig: Take 1 tablet in evening before going to bed and 1 tablet 1 hour before appointment

Ingredient: Alprazolam

Rx

Vistaril® 25 mg

Disp: 16 capsules

Sig: Take 2 capsules in evening before going to bed and 2 capsules 1 hour before appointment

Ingredient: Hydroxyzine

Rx

Halcion® 0.25 mg

Disp: 4 tablets

Sig: Take 1 tablet in evening before going to bed and 1 tablet 1 hour before appointment

Ingredient: Triazolam

Rx

Serax® 10 mg

Disp: 2 capsules

Sig: Take 1 capsule before bed and 1 capsule 30 minutes before appointment.

Ingredient: Oxazepam

MANAGEMENT OF PATIENTS UNDERGOING CANCER THERAPY

CANCER PATIENT DENTAL PROTOCOL

The objective in treatment of a patient with cancer is eradication of the disease. Oral complications, such as mucosal ulceration, xerostomia, bleeding, and infections can cause significant morbidity and may compromise systemic treatment of the patient. With proper oral evaluation before systemic treatment, many of the complications can be minimized or prevented.

MUCOSITIS

Normal oral mucosa acts as a barrier against chemical and food irritants and oral microorganisms. Disruption of the mucosal barrier can therefore lead to secondary infection, increased pain, delayed healing, and decreased nutritional intake.

Mucositis is inflammation of the mucous membranes. It is a common reaction to chemotherapy and radiation therapy. It is first seen as an erythematous patch. The mucosal epithelium becomes thin as a result of the killing of the rapidly dividing basal layer mucosal cells. Seven to ten days after cytoreduction chemotherapy and between 1000 cGy and 3000 cGy of radiation to the head and neck, mucosal tissues begin to desquamate and eventually develop into frank ulcerations. The mucosal integrity is broken and is secondarily infected by normal oral flora. The resultant ulcerations can also act as a portal of entry for pathogenic organisms into the patient's bloodstream and may lead to systemic infections. These ulcerations often force interruption of therapy.

Certain chemotherapeutic agents, such as 5-fluorouracil, methotrexate, and doxorubicin, are more commonly associated with the development of oral mucositis. Treatment of oral mucositis is mainly palliative, but steps should be taken to minimize secondary pathogenic infections. Culture and sensitivity data should be obtained to select appropriate therapy for the bacterial, viral, or fungal organisms found.

Prevention of radiation mucositis is difficult. Stents can be constructed to prevent irradiation of uninvolved tissues. The use of multiple ports and fractionation of therapy into smaller doses over a longer period of time can reduce the severity. Fractured restorations, sharp teeth, and ill-fitted prostheses can damage soft tissues and lead to additional interruption of mucosal barriers. Correction of these problems before radiation therapy can diminish these complications.

CHEMOTHERAPY

Chemotherapy for neoplasia also frequently results in oral complications. Infections and mucositis are the most common complications seen in patients receiving chemotherapy. Also occurring frequently are pain, altered nutrition, and xerostomia, which can significantly affect the quality of life.

RADIATION CARIES

Dental caries that sometimes follows radiation therapy is called radiation caries. It usually develops in the cervical region of the teeth adjacent to the gingiva, often affecting many teeth. It is secondary to the damage done to the salivary glands and is initiated by dental plaque, but its rapid progress is due to changes in saliva. In addition to the diminution in the amount of saliva, both the salivary pH and buffering capacity are diminished, which decreases anticaries activity of saliva. Oral bacteria also change with xerostomia leading to the increase in caries activity.

SALIVARY CHANGES

Chemotherapy is not thought to directly alter salivary flow, but alterations in taste and subjective sensations of dry mouth are relatively common complaints. Patients with mucositis and graft-vs-host disease following bone marrow or stem cell transplantation often demonstrate signs and symptoms of xerostomia. Radiation does directly affect salivary production. Radiation to the salivary glands produces fibrosis and alters the production of saliva. If all the major salivary glands are in the field, the decrease in saliva can be dramatic and the serous portion of the glands seems to be most severely affected. The saliva produced is increased in viscosity, which contributes to food retention and increased plaque formation. These xerostomic patients have difficulty in managing a normal diet. Normal saliva also has bacteriostatic properties that are diminished in these patients.

The dental management recommendations for patients undergoing chemotherapy, bone marrow transplantation, and/or radiation therapy for the treatment of cancer are based primarily on clinical observations. The following protocols will provide a conservative, consistent approach to the dental management of patients undergoing chemotherapy or bone marrow transplantation. Many of the cancer chemotherapy drugs produce oral side effects including mucositis, oral ulceration, dry mouth, acute infections, and taste aberrations. Cancer drugs include antibiotics, alkylating agents, antimetabolites, DNA inhibitors, hormones, and cytokines.

All patients undergoing chemotherapy or bone marrow transplantation for malignant disease should have the following baseline:

A. Panoramic radiograph

B. Dental consultation and examination

C. Dental prophylaxis and cleaning (if the neutrophil count is >1500/mm³ and the platelet count is >50,000/mm³)

   – Prophylaxis and cleaning will be deferred if the patient's neutrophil count is <1500 and the platelet count is <50,000. Oral hygiene recommendations will be made. These levels are arbitrary guidelines and the dentist should consider the patient's oral condition and planned procedure relative to hemorrhage and level of bacteremia.

D. Oral Hygiene: Patients should be encouraged to follow normal hygiene procedures. Addition of a chlorhexidine mouth rinse such as Peridex® or PerioGard® *on page 263* is usually helpful. If the patient develops oral mucositis, tolerance of such alcohol-based products may be limited.

E. If the patient develops mucositis, bacterial, viral, and fungal cultures should be obtained. Sucralfate suspension in either a pharmacy-prepared form or Carafate® suspension, as well as Benadryl® *on page 398* or Xylocaine® viscous, *on page 706*can assist in helping the patient to tolerate food. Patients may also require systemic analgesics for pain relief depending on the presence of mucositis. Positive fungal cultures may require a nystatin swish-and-swallow prescription.

F. The determination of performing dental procedures must be based on the goal of preventing infection during periods of neutropenia. Timing of procedures must be coordinated with the patient's hematologic status.

G. If oral surgery is required, at least 7-10 days of healing should be allowed before the anticipated date of bone marrow suppression (eg, ANC <1000/mm³ and/or platelet count of 50,000/mm³).

H. Daily use of topical fluorides is recommended for those who have received radiation therapy to the head and neck region involving salivary glands. Any patients with prolonged xerostomia subsequent to graft-vs-host disease and/or chemotherapy can also be considered for fluoride supplement. Use the fluoride-containing mouthwashes (Act®, Fluorigard®, etc) each night before going to sleep; swish, hold 1-2 minutes, spit out or use prescription fluorides (gels or rinses); apply daily for 3-4 minutes as directed; if mouth is sore (mucositis), use flavorless/colorless gels (Thera-Flur®, Gel-Kam®). Improvement in salivary flow following radiation therapy to the head and neck has been noted with Salagen® *on page 955* or Evoxac™ *on page 256.*

Benzonatate (Tessalon® Perles) *on page 153*
Cevimeline (Evoxac®) *on page 256*
Chlorhexidine (Peridex®, PerioGard®) *on page 263*
Diphenhydramine (Benadryl® elixir) *on page 398*
Lidocaine (Xylocaine®) *on page 706*
Pilocarpine (Dental) (Salagen®) *on page 956*
Povidone-Iodine (Betadine®) *on page 982*
Sucralfate (Carafate®) *on page 1113*

PRESCRIPTION EXAMPLES

Rx

Peridex® or PerioGard® oral rinse

Disp: 3 bottles

Sig: 20 mL for 30 seconds 3 times/day; swish and expectorate

Ingredient: Chlorhexidine gluconate 0.12% and alcohol 11.6%

Rx

Xylocaine® viscous 2%

Disp: 450 mL bottles

Sig: 1 tablespoonful; swish 4 times/day

Ingredient: Lidocaine

MANAGEMENT OF PATIENTS UNDERGOING CANCER THERAPY *(Continued)*

Rx

Betadine® mouthwash

Disp: 6 oz bottle

Sig: 1 tablespoonful, rinse 4 times/day; do not swallow

Ingredient: Povidone iodine 0.8%

Rx

Mycostatin® oral suspension

Disp: 60 mL bottle

Sig: 2 mL 4 times/day; hold in mouth for 2 minutes and swallow

Ingredient: Nystatin 100,000 units/mL

Note: When the oral mucous membranes are especially sensitive, nystatin "popsicles" can be made by adding 2 mL of nystatin oral suspension to the water in ice cube trays.

Rx

Tessalon Perles®

Disp: 50

Sig: Squeeze contents of capsule and apply to lesion

Ingredient: Benzonatate

Note: Tessalon Perles® have been used ad lib to provide relief in painful mucositis.

ORAL CARE PRODUCTS

BACTERIAL PLAQUE CONTROL

Patients should use an extra soft bristle toothbrush and dental floss for removal of plaque. Sponge/foam sticks and lemon-glycerine swabs do not adequately remove bacterial plaque.

PRESCRIPTION EXAMPLE

Rx

Ultra Suave® toothbrush

Biotene Supersoft® toothbrush

Note: Chlorhexidine 0.12% (Peridex® or other preparations available in Canada and Europe) may be used to assist with bacterial plaque control.

CHOLINERGIC AGENTS

See Products for Xerostomia *on page 1388*

Used for the treatment of xerostomia caused by radiation therapy in patients with head and neck cancer and from Sjögren's syndrome

Cevimeline (Evoxac®) *on page 256*
Pilocarpine (Dental) (Salagen®) *on page 956*

FLUORIDE GELS

See Oral Rinse Products *on page 1388*

Used for the prevention of demineralization of the tooth structure secondary to xerostomia. For patients with long-term or permanent xerostomia, daily application is accomplished using custom gel applicator trays. Patients with porcelain crowns should use a neutral pH fluoride.

REMINERALIZING GEL

In addition to fluoride gel to remineralize enamel breakdown in severely xerostomic patients, applicator trays may be used.

Revive®

SALIVA SUBSTITUTES

See Products for Xerostomia *on page 1388*

ORAL AND LIP MOISTURIZERS/LUBRICANTS

See Mouth Pain, Cold Sore, and Canker Sore Products *on page 1458*

Note: Water-based gels should first be used to provide moisture to dry oral tissues.

Surgi-Lube®
K-Y Jelly®
Oral Balance®
Mouth Moisturizer®

PALLIATION OF PAIN

See Mouth Pain, Cold Sore, and Canker Sore Products *on page 1458*

Note: Palliative pain preparations should be monitored for efficacy.

- For relief of pain associated with isolated ulcerations, topical anesthetic and protective preparations may be used.
  - Orabase-B® with 20% benzocaine *on page 151*
- For generalized oral pain:
  - Chloraseptic Spray® (OTC) anesthetic spray without alcohol *on page 946*
  - Ulcer-Ease® anesthetic/analgesic mouthrinse
  - Xylocaine® 2% viscous *on page 706*
    - **Note:** May anesthetize swallowing mechanism and cause aspiration of food; caution patient against using too close to eating; lack of sensation may also allow patient to damage intact mucosa
  - Tantum Mouthrinse® (benzydamine hydrochloride); may be diluted as required
    - **Note:** Available only in Canada and Europe

PATIENT PREPARED PALLIATIVE MIXTURES

Coating agents:

Maalox® *on page 62*
Mylanta® *on page 63*
Kaopectate® *on page 132*

These products can be mixed with Benadryl® elixir (50:50):

Diphenhydramine (Benadryl®) *on page 398*

Mouth Pain, Cold Sore, and Canker Sore Products *on page 1458*

Topical anesthetics (diphenhydramine chloride):

Benadryl® elixir or Benylin® cough syrup *on page 398*

Note: Choose product with lowest alcohol and sucrose content; ask pharmacist for assistance

PHARMACY PREPARATIONS

A pharmacist may also prepare the following solutions for relief of generalized oral pain:

Benadryl-Lidocaine Solution

Diphenhydramine injectable 1.5 mL (50 mg/mL) *on page 398*
Xylocaine viscous 2% (45 mL) *on page 706*
Magnesium aluminum hydroxide solution (45 mL)

Swish and hold 1 teaspoonful in mouth for 30 seconds; do not use too close to eating

Rx

Carafate suspension 1 g/10 mL

Disp: 420 mL

Sig: 1 teaspoonful; swish and hold in mouth for 30 seconds

Ingredient: Sucralfate

ORAL MEDICINE TOPICS

PART III:
OTHER ORAL MEDICINE TOPICS

TABLE OF CONTENTS

DENTIST'S ROLE IN RECOGNIZING DOMESTIC VIOLENCE

Recognition of the signs and symptoms of domestic violence is becoming an important topic for dental and medical professionals throughout the world. Unfortunately, statistics related to domestic abuse of women and children appear to be on the rise, perhaps, in part, due to this increased recognition.

Some statistics are indeed staggering. In the United States, a woman or child is physically abused every five to fifteen seconds. In fact, violence is cited as one of the common causes of emergency room admissions for women 15-44 years of age. Furthermore, 50,000 deaths occur annually, which are attributable to violence in the form of homicide or suicide.

The dentist is in a unique position to recognize many of the signs and symptoms of domestic violence, including child abuse and neglect. The dentist's responsibilities and professional role in this arena are not clear in all states. However, each professional has the responsibility to understand the current state laws regarding the reporting of domestic violence, child abuse, and/or neglect within his/her state. Many states have existing codes defining the role of the professional in these regards. The overall problem of domestic violence, including child abuse, neglect, and other forms of abuse are indeed public health issues. The costs of domestic violence, such as medical, dental, psychiatric, hospital, and emergency care fees are borne to a great extent by the community in addition to the individual.

Domestic abuse is defined as "controlling behavior." Although this often includes physical injury, the primary focus of domestic abuse is one person being in control of another person, making that person do something against his/her will. Women are often abused both physically and mentally in relationships that have existed for many years. Children are often the focus of domestic violence; however, the pattern for an entire family's abuse may be present. Abuse comes in many forms and many victims do not even realize that abuse is occurring. Some victims simply "chalk it up" to things that happen within families. Abuse can include the following: battery and physical assault, such as throwing objects, pushing, hitting, slapping, kicking, or attacking with a weapon; sexual assault including the abuser forcing sexual activities upon another; and, psychological abuse, such as forcing a victim to perform degrading or humiliating acts, threatening harm to a female or male partner or child, or destroying valued possessions of another. Verbal abuse can also be included; however, the psychological forms of abuse are very difficult to ascertain and the signs and symptoms may be difficult to separate from other psychological traits. Abuse tends to have a cyclic pattern, often where a partner, or the controlling individual within the domestic situation, is extremely friendly, intimate, and a good household member. However, due to unknown reasons, as tension develops, family violence often erupts. Once battering has begun, it often increases in frequency and in severity with time. Early recognition by those around the domestic situation can often prevent serious effects. However, until physical violence becomes part of the domestic abuse situation, recognition is usually difficult.

Since nearly 65% of abuse cases (where physical injury is involved) involve injury to the head, neck, or mouth, dental professionals are in a unique position to detect and perhaps, if appropriate in their state, report suspected abuse. In children, these percentages are even higher. Much of our information and beliefs about domestic abuse stem from our knowledge regarding the dental professional in the arena of child abuse and neglect. Being wards of adults, children are vulnerable. Child abuse includes any act that is nonaccidental, endangering or impairing a child's safety or emotional health. Types of child abuse would include physical abuse, emotional abuse and neglect, including health care neglect. Any child suffering from an emotional injury, including sexual abuse or neglect, should be brought to the attention of the social welfare system. Occasionally, "Munchausen syndrome," which is defined as the guardians fabricating or inducing illness in the child, can be observed. Intentional poisoning and safety neglect are also included.

From a medical point-of-view, neglect is much more difficult to determine than abuse. The role of the dentist may be in defining the state of normal and customary pediatric health within a locality. However, due to parents and families moving about the country, sometimes one standard may not be appropriate for all locations.

To detect abuse, or to detect domestic patterns of abuse in the family, the medical or dental professional must be aware of several key behavioral indicators: when the child or adult in question avoids eye contact, is wary of their guardian or spouse, demonstrates fear of touch, or dramatic mood changes. Reports of any history of suicide attempts or running away would also be indicators. Any unexplained injury or injuries that are inconsistent with explanation, including delays in seeking care for such an injury, could represent an abusive situation. The guardian or spouse may also give specific indicators. When it is determined that they cannot explain the injury or that the explanation offered is inconsistent or changes, abuse may be suspected. Nonspecific indicators might include hostile or aggressive behavior or if the queried individual wants to go to a different practitioner when the questioning becomes too intense.

The principles of head-neck examination for the dentist are important and include gathering an overall visual impression of general cleanliness, dress, and stature and examining for any specific physical indicators such as bruises, welts, bite marks, abrasions, lacerations, or other injuries to the head or neck. Contusions or bruises represent the highest percentage of abuse injuries to the young child. The extremely young child or infant often suffers fractures, which fall to second place in terms of incidence as the child matures. In the adult, fractures are much less common. The dentist needs to document the location since often this represents the characteristic that may be difficult for the person to explain. Common areas for injuries include the bony eminences over the knees, shins, and elbows, but could also be on the face, including the zygomatic arch and the chin. Burns are more rare but represent one of the most serious types of injuries. Intraoral injuries including trauma to the oral mucosa, tooth fractures, palatal lesions, ecchymoses, and fractures represent serious evidence of domestic or child abuse. Physical indicators of sexual abuse may not be obvious to the dentist, however, bruising of the hard palate or other evidence of sexual dysfunction may sometimes be found.

The dentist has the responsibility to document from a forensic point-of-view the characteristics that are observed. If necessary, evidence including impressions for bite marks or photographs to document unexplained injuries to the head, neck, and face may be necessary. The legal liability for the dentist is determined by the state laws governing the dental practice. The dental practitioner's failure to diagnose child abuse and neglect is another consideration which goes along with ethical and legal considerations. In the area of child abuse, the states are generally much more clear than they are regarding spousal abuse or overall domestic violence. The dentist has a responsibility to refer a patient for a second opinion if there are concerns that abuse is taking place. Unfortunately, there is no uniformity in the state laws regarding either the responsibility for reporting adult domestic violence or abuse, nor is there uniformity in protecting the health professional by reporting, in good faith, abuse situations. When spousal abuse or other domestic violence is suspected, the definitions become even less clear. They are very similar in ambiguity to those that are faced by the professional regarding neglect as opposed to direct physical or mental abuse. The American Dental Association code is clear on principles and ethics regarding professional conduct regarding the responsibility for recognition of child abuse. They are much less clear on spousal or other abuse and it is likely that in the future as some consistency is noted between and among the various state laws, the ADA Council will undoubtedly take a position.

It is clearly up to the individual states to take the lead in establishing strict guidelines for recognition and reporting of domestic abuse, including protection under the "good faith" statutes for the practitioner. Rules and regulations regarding malicious reporting should also be better defined by the states. The national position is difficult to define because of the extreme variation among states. Dentists are encouraged to use their best judgement in proceeding in any situation of domestic abuse. They should primarily know their state laws and join in the discussion of the topic so that appropriate state actions and formation of legal codes can be undertaken.

CHEMICAL DEPENDENCY AND SMOKING CESSATION

INTRODUCTION

As long as history has been recorded, every society has used drugs that alter mood, thought, and feeling. In addition, pharmacological advances sometimes have been paralleled by physical as well as unfortunate behavioral dependence on agents initially consumed for therapeutic purposes.

In 1986, the American Dental Association passed a policy statement recognizing chemical dependency as a disease. In recognizing this disease, the Association mandated that dentists have a responsibility to include questions relating to a history of chemical dependency, or more broadly, substance abused in their health history questionnaire. A positive response may require the dentist to alter the treatment plan for the patient's dental care. This includes patients who are actively abusing alcohol, drugs, or patients who are in recovery. The use and abuse of drugs is not a topic that is usually found in the dental curriculum. Information about substance abuse is usually gleaned from newspapers, magazines, or just hearsay.

This chapter reviews street drugs, where they come from, signs and symptoms of the drug abuser, and some of the dental implications of treating patients actively using or in recovery from these substances. There are many books devoted to this topic that provide greater detail. The intent is to provide an overview of some of the most prevalent drugs, how patients abusing these drugs may influence dental treatment, and how to recognize some signs and symptoms of use and withdrawal.

Street drugs, like other drugs, can come from various sources. They may be derived from natural sources (ie, morphine and codeine). They may be semisynthetic, that is a natural product is chemically modified to produce another molecule (ie, morphine conversion to heroin). Street drugs may also be synthetic with no natural origin.

BENZODIAZEPINES AND OTHER NONALCOHOL SEDATIVES

Benzodiazepines are the most commonly prescribed drugs worldwide. These drugs are used mainly for treatment of anxiety disorders and, in some instances, insomnia. Even though they are used in high quantities throughout the world, intentional abuse is not that common. These drugs, however, have the ability to induce a strong physical dependency on the use of the medication. As tolerance builds up to the drug, the physical dependency increases dramatically. Unlike street drugs, where addiction is a primary consideration, the overuse of benzodiazepine lies in their ability to induce physical dependency. When these drugs are taken for several weeks, there is relatively little tolerance induced. However, after several months, the proportion of patients who become tolerant increases and reducing the dose or stopping the medication produces severe withdrawal symptoms.

Benzodiazepine Withdrawal Symptoms	
Craving for benzodiazepines	Irritability
Anxiety	Sleep disturbances

It is extremely difficult for the physician to distinguish between the withdrawal symptoms and the reappearance of the myriad anxiety symptoms that cause the drug to be prescribed initially. Many patients increase their dose over time because tolerance develops to at least the sedative effects of the drug. The antianxiety benefits of the benzodiazepines continue to occur long after tolerance to the sedating effects. Patients often take these drugs for many years with relatively few ill effects other than the risk of withdrawal. The dentist should be keenly aware of the signs and symptoms and the historical pattern in patients taking benzodiazepines.

BARBITURATES AND NONBENZODIAZEPINE SEDATIVES

The use of barbiturates as sedative medications has declined over the years due to the increased safety and efficacy of benzodiazepines. Abuse problems with barbiturates resemble those with benzodiazepines in many ways. Drugs in this category are frequently prescribed as hypnotics for patients complaining of insomnia. The physician should, therefore, be aware of the problems that can develop when the hypnotic agent is withdrawn. The underlying problem that has lead to the insomnia is not treated directly by the use of barbiturates and the patient seeking a sleep medication may have altered ability to sleep normally because of the medication. The withdrawal symptoms for the barbiturates are similar to the benzodiazepine sedatives.

ALCOHOL

The chronic use of alcohol, as well as that of other sedatives, is associated with the development of depression. The risk of suicide among alcoholics is one of the highest of any diagnostic category. Cognitive deficits have been reported in alcoholics tested while sober. These deficits usually improve after weeks to months of abstinence. More severe recent memory impairment is associated with specific brain damage caused by nutritional deficiencies common in alcoholics.

Alcohol is toxic to many organ systems. As a result, the medical complications of alcohol abuse and dependence include liver disease, cardiovascular disease, endocrine and gastrointestinal effects, and malnutrition, in addition to CNS dysfunctions. Ethanol readily crosses the placental barrier, producing the *fetal alcohol syndrome*, a major cause of mental retardation.

Alcohol Withdrawal Syndrome Signs and Symptoms	
Alcohol craving	Hypertension
Tremor, irritability	Sweating
Nausea	Perceptual distortion
Sleep disturbance	Seizures (12-48 hours after last drink)
Tachycardia	
Delirium tremens (rare in uncomplicated withdrawal):	
Severe agitation	Tachycardia
Confusion	Nausea, diarrhea
Visual hallucinations	Dilated pupils
Fever, profuse sweating	

NICOTINE

Cigarette (nicotine) addiction is influenced by multiple variables. Nicotine itself produces reinforcement; users compare nicotine to stimulants such as cocaine or amphetamine, although its effects are of lower magnitude.

Nicotine is absorbed readily through the skin, mucous membranes, and of course, through the lungs. The pulmonary route produces discernible central nervous system effects in as little as 7 seconds. Thus, each puff produces some discrete reinforcement. With 10 puffs per cigarette, the 1 pack per day smoker reinforces the habit 200 times daily. The timing, setting, situation, and preparation all become associated repetitively with the effects of nicotine.

Nicotine has both stimulant and depressant actions. The smoker feels alert, yet there is some muscle relaxation. Nicotine activates the nucleus accumbens reward system in the brain. Increased extracellular dopamine has been found in this region after nicotine injections in rats. Nicotine affects other systems as well, including the release of endogenous opioids and glucocorticoids.

Nicotine Withdrawal Syndrome Signs and Symptoms	
Irritability, impatience, hostility	Restlessness
Anxiety	Decreased heart rate
Dysphoric or depressed mood	Increased appetite or weight gain
Difficulty concentrating	

Medications to assist users in breaking a nicotine habit:

Bupropion (Zyban®) *on page 188*

Nicotine (Habitrol®, Nicoderm®, Nicorette® (polacrilex gum - OTC), Nicotrol® (OTC), ProStep®) *on page 863*

SMOKING CESSATION PRODUCTS

Several years ago, the journal, *Science*, stated that approximately 80% of smokers say they want to quit, but each year <1 in 10 actually succeed. Nicotine transdermal delivery preparations (or nicotine patches) were approved by the U.S. Food and Drug Administration in 1992 as aids to smoking cessation for the relief of nicotine withdrawal symptoms. Four preparations were approved simultaneously: Habitrol®, Nicoderm®, Nicotrol®, and ProStep®. These products differ in how much nicotine is released and whether they provide a 24- or 16-hour release time.

Studies are still being reported on the effectiveness of nicotine patches on smoking cessation. Most previous studies had good entry criteria including definition of the Fagerstrom score. Dr Fred Cowan of Oregon Health Sciences University described these Fagerstrom criteria in a previous report on nicotine substitutes in AGD *Impact*. Abstinence of smoking cessation has usually been assessed by self-report, measurement of carbon monoxide in breath, and plasma or urine nicotine products.

In numerous protocols, percentages of study subjects who abstained from smoking after 3-10 weeks of patch treatment with nicotine compared to placebo, have never exceeded 40%. After the initial assessment, six studies continued to follow the study subjects

CHEMICAL DEPENDENCY AND SMOKING CESSATION *(Continued)*

through 24-52 weeks of patch treatment. The results were even poorer with <25% sustained success. A review of these and additional studies, reveals some general conclusions regarding the effectiveness of nicotine patches in smoking cessation. In every study, many smokers abstained after treatment with placebo patches; nicotine treatment was initially more effective than placebo; and improved abstinence rates were more marked in the short term (10 weeks) than in the long term (52 weeks). Subjects undergoing smoking cessation trials tended to gain weight irrespective of whether placebo or nicotine patches were worn. Patients often favor the nicotine polacrilex gum (Nicorette®) which releases nicotine into the blood stream via the oral mucosa.

Data are now available from smoking cessation studies carried out in general medical practices. The effectiveness of nicotine patch substitution under these conditions is similar to the results described above. Most patch systems and gum are now available as over-the-counter products; only Habitrol® remains prescription. Practitioners and patients should remain skeptical since these aids appear to work best only when supplemented with psychological counseling and a single-minded effort on the part of the patient. New products (eg, Zyban®) are now also being marketed as smoking cessation aids. These drugs are norepinephrine serotonin reuptake inhibitors and their action directly affects the craving for tobacco.

OPIATES

The opiates are most often called narcotics. The most common opiate found on the street is heroin. Heroin is the diacetyl derivative of morphine which is extracted from opium. Although commercial production of morphine involves extraction from the dried opium plant which grows in many parts of the world, some areas still harvest opium by making slits in the unripened seed pod. The pod secretes a white, viscous material which upon contact with the air turns a blackish-brown color. It is this off-white material that is called opium. The opium is then dried and smoked or processed to yield morphine and codeine. Actually, the raw opium contains several chemicals that are used medicinally or commercially. Much (approximately 50%) of morphine is converted chemically into heroin which finds its way into the United States and then on the street. Heroin is a Schedule I drug and as such has no acceptable use in the United States today. In fact, possession is a violation of the Controlled Substances Act of 1970. The majority of the heroin found on the streets is from Southeast Asia and can be as concentrated as 100%.

The heroin user goes through many phases once the drug has been administered. When administered intravenously, the user initially feels a "rush" often described as an "orgasmic rush". This initial feeling is most likely due to the release of histamine resulting in cutaneous vasodilation, itching, and a flushed appearance. Shortly after this "rush" the user becomes euphoric. This euphoric stage often called "stoned" or being "high" lasts approximately 3-4 hours. During this stage, the user is lethargic, slow to react to stimuli, speech is slurred, pain reaction threshold is elevated, he/she exhibits xerostomia, slowed heart rate, and the pupils may be constricted. Following the "high", the abuser is "straight" for about 2 hours, with no tell-tale signs of abuse. Approximately 6-8 hours following the last injection of heroin, the user begins to experience a runny nose, lacrimation, and abdominal muscle cramps as he/she begins the withdrawal from the drug. During this stage and the one that follows, the person may become agitated as he/she develops anxiety about where the next "hit" will come from. The withdrawal signs and symptoms become more intense. For the next 3 days, the abuser begins to sweat profusely in combination with cutaneous vasoconstriction. The skin becomes cold and clammy, hence the term "cold turkey". Tachycardia, pupillary dilation, diarrhea, and salivation occur for 3 days following the last injection. Withdrawal signs and symptoms may last longer than the average of 3 days or they may be more abrupt.

Opioid Withdrawal Signs and Symptoms

Symptoms	Signs
Regular Withdrawal	
Craving for opioids Restlessness, irritability Increased sensitivity to pain Nausea, cramps Muscle aches Dysphoric mood Insomnia, anxiety	Pupillary dilation Sweating Piloerection ("gooseflesh") Tachycardia Vomiting, diarrhea Increased blood pressure Yawning Fever
Protracted Withdrawal	
Anxiety Insomnia Drug craving	Cyclic changes in weight, pupil size, respiratory center sensitivity

Many patients who have been abusing opiates for any length of time will exhibit multiple carious lesions, particularly class V lesions. This increased caries rate is probably a result of the heroin-induced xerostomia, high intake of sweets, and lack of daily oral hygiene. Patients who are recovering from heroin or any opiate addiction should not be given any kind of opiate analgesic, whether it be for sedation or as a postoperative analgesic because of the increased chance of relapse. The nonsteroidal anti-inflammatory drugs (NSAIDs) should be used to control any postoperative discomfort. Patients who admit to a past history of intravenous heroin use, or any intravenous drug for that matter, are at higher risk for subacute bacterial endocarditis (SBE), HIV disease, and hepatitis but with the exception of postoperative analgesia should present no special problem for dental care.

OxyContin®, a synthetic opiate, has gained popularity as a street drug in recent years. The drug manufacturer has tried to salvage its name, however, OxyContin® is one of the most widely abused pain medications in use today. It is an excellent analgesic, widely used and is, therefore, available for abuse potential. As with the other opiates, clinical signs and symptoms that the dentist should recognize are consistent with opiate addiction and usage.

MARIJUANA

The number one most abused illegal drug by high school students today is marijuana. Marijuana is a plant that grows throughout the world, but is particularly suited for a warm, humid environment. There are three species of plant but the two most frequently cited are *Cannabis sativa* and *Cannabis indica*. All species possess a female and male plant. Although approximately 450 chemicals have been isolated from the plant, the major psychoactive ingredient is delta-9-tetrahydrocannabinol (THC). Of these 450 chemicals, there are approximately 23 psychoactive chemicals, THC being the most abundant. The highest concentration of THC is found in the bud of the female plant. The concentration of THC varies according to growing conditions and location on the plant but has increased from approximately 2% to 3% in marijuana sold in the 1950s to approximately 30% sold on the streets today. Marijuana can be smoked in cigarettes (joints), pipes, water pipes (bongs), or baked in brownies, cakes, etc, and then ingested. However, smoking marijuana is more efficient and the "high" has a quicker onset. Marijuana is a Schedule I drug but has been promoted as a medicinal for the treatment of glaucoma, for increasing appetite in patients who have HIV disease, and to prevent the nausea associated with cancer chemotherapy. In response to this request, the FDA approved dronabinol (Marinol®), a synthetic THC and placed this drug in Schedule II to be prescribed by physicians for the indicated medical conditions.

Dronabinol (Marinol®) *on page 423*

An individual under the influence of marijuana may exhibit no signs or symptoms of intoxication. The pharmacologic effects are dose-dependent and depend to a large extent on the set and setting of the intoxicated individual. As the dose of THC increases, the person experiences euphoria or a state of well-being, often referred to as "mellowing out". Everything becomes comical, problems disappear, and their appetite for snack foods increases. This is called the "munchies". The marijuana produces time and spatial distortion, which contribute, as the dose increases, to a dysphoria characterized by paranoia and fear. Although there has never been a death reported from marijuana overdose, certainly the higher doses may produce such bizarre circumstances as to increase the chances of accidental death. THC is fat soluble. Daily consumption of marijuana will result in THC being stored in body fat which will result in detectable amounts of THC being found in the urine for as long as 60 days in some cases.

Marijuana Withdrawal Syndrome Signs and Symptoms	
Restlessness	Restlessness
Irritability	Sleep EEG disturbance
Mild agitation	Nausea, cramping
Insomnia	

Because of anxiety associated with dental visits, marijuana would be the most likely drug, after alcohol, to be used when coming to the dental office. But, unlike alcohol, marijuana may not produce any detectable odor on the breath nor signs of intoxication. Fortunately, local anesthetics, analgesics, and antibiotics used by the general dentist do not interact with marijuana. The major concern with the marijuana-intoxicated patient is a failure to follow directions while in the chair, and the inability to follow postoperative instructions.

COCAINE

Cocaine, referred to on the street as "snow", "nose candy", "girl", and many other euphemisms, has created an epidemic. This drug is like no other local anesthetic. Known for about the last 2000 years, cocaine has been used and abused by politicians, scientists, farmers, warriors, and of course, on the street. Cocaine is derived from the leaves

CHEMICAL DEPENDENCY AND SMOKING CESSATION *(Continued)*

of a plant called *Erythroxylon coca* which grows in South America. Ninety percent of the world's supply of cocaine originates in Peru, Bolivia, and Colombia. At last estimate, the United States consumes 75% of the world's supply. The plant grows to a height of approximately 4 feet and produces a red berry. Farmers go through the fields stripping the leaves from the plant three times a year. During the working day, the farmers chew the coca leaves to suppress appetite and fight the fatigue of working the fields. The leaves are transported to a laboratory site where the cocaine is extracted by a process called maceration. It takes approximately 7-8 pounds of leaves to produce 1 ounce of cocaine.

On the streets of the United States, cocaine can be found in two forms – one is the hydrochloride salt which can be "snorted" or dissolved in water and injected intravenously, the other is the free base form which can be smoked and is sometimes referred to as "crack", "rock", or "free base". It is called crack because it cracks or pops when large pieces are smoked. It is called rock because it is hard and difficult to break into smaller pieces. The most popular method of administration of cocaine is "snorting" in which small amounts of cocaine hydrochloride are divided into segments or "lines" and any straw-like device can be used to inhale one or more lines of the cocaine into the nose. Although cocaine does not reach the lungs, enough cocaine is absorbed through nasal mucosa to provide a "high" within 3-5 minutes. Rock or crack, on the other hand, is heated and inhaled from any device available. This form of cocaine does reach the lungs and provides a much faster onset of action as well as a more intense stimulation. There are dangers to the user with any form of cocaine. Undoubtedly, the most dangerous form is the intravenous route.

Cocaine Withdrawal Signs and Symptoms	
Dysphoria, depression	Cocaine craving
Sleepiness, fatigue	Bradycardia

The cocaine user, regardless of how the cocaine was administered, presents a potential life-threatening situation in the dental operatory. The patient under the influence of cocaine could be compared to a car going 100 miles per hour. Blood pressure is elevated and heart rate is likely increased. Use of a local anesthetic with epinephrine in such a patient may result in a medical emergency. Such patients can be identified by jitteriness, irritability, talkativeness, tremors, and short abrupt speech patterns. These same signs and symptoms may also be seen in a normal dental patient with preoperative dental anxiety; therefore, the dentist must be particularly alert to identify the potential cocaine abuser. If a patient is suspected, they should never be given a local anesthetic with vasoconstrictor for fear of exacerbating cocaine-induced sympathetic response. Life-threatening episodes of cardiac arrhythmias and hypertensive crises have been reported when local anesthetic with vasoconstrictor was administered to a patient under the influence of cocaine. No local anesthetic used by any dentist can interfere with, nor test positive for cocaine in any urine testing screen. Therefore, the dentist need not be concerned with any false drug use accusations associated with dental anesthesia.

PSYCHEDELIC AGENTS

Perceptual distortions that include hallucinations, illusions, and disorders of thinking such as paranoia can be produced by toxic doses of many drugs. These phenomena also may be seen during toxic withdrawal from sedatives such as alcohol. There are, however, certain drugs that have as their primary effect the production of perception, thought, or mood disturbances at low doses with minimal effects on memory and orientation. These are commonly called *hallucinogenic drugs*, but their use does not always result in frank hallucinations.

Ecstasy (MDMA) and Phenylethylamines (MDA): MDA and MDMA have stimulant, as well as, psychedelic effects and produce degeneration of serotonergic nerve cells and axons. While nerve degeneration has not been well-demonstrated in human beings, the potential remains. Thus, there is possible neurotoxicity with overuse of these drugs. Ecstasy became popular during the 1980s on college campuses and it is still recommended by some psychotherapists as an aid to the process of therapy, although very little controlled data is available. Acute effects are dose-dependent and include dry mouth, jaw clinching, muscle aches, and tachycardia. At higher doses, effects include agitation, hyperthermia, panic attacks, and visual hallucinations. Frequent, repeated use of psychedelic drugs is unusual and, therefore, tolerance is not commonly seen. However, tolerance does develop to the behavioral effects of various psychedelic drugs, and after numerous doses, the tendency towards behavioral tolerance can be observed.

LSD: LSD is the most potent hallucinogenic drug and produces significant psychedelic effects with a total dose of as little as 25-50 mcg. This drug is over 3000 times more potent than mescaline. LSD is sold on the illicit market in a variety of forms. A popular contemporary system involves postage stamp-sized papers impregnated with varying doses of LSD (≥50-300 mcg). A majority of street samples sold as LSD actually contain LSD. In contrast, the samples of mushrooms and other botanicals sold as sources of psilocybin and other psychedelics have a low probability of containing the advertised hallucinogenics.

Phencyclidine (PCP): PCP deserves special mention because of its widespread availability and because its pharmacological effects are different from LSD. PCP was originally developed as an anesthetic in the 1950s and later abandoned because of a high frequency of postoperative delirium with hallucinations. It was classed as a dissociative anesthetic because, in the anesthetized state, the patient remains conscious with staring gaze, flat facies, and rigid muscles. It was discovered as a drug of abuse in the 1970s, first in an oral form and then in a smoked version enabling a better control over the dose.

INHALANTS

Anesthetic gases such as nitrous oxide or halothane are sometimes used as intoxicants by medical personnel. Nitrous oxide also is abused by food service employees because it is supplied for use as a propellant in disposable aluminum minitanks for whipping cream canisters. Nitrous oxide produces euphoria and analgesia and then loss of consciousness. Compulsive use and chronic toxicity rarely are reported, but there are obvious risks of overdose associated with the abuse of this anesthetic. Chronic use has been reported to cause peripheral neuropathy.

The dental team should be alert to the signs and symptoms of drug abuse and withdrawal. Further reading is recommended.

ANIMAL AND HUMAN BITES GUIDELINES

The dentist is often confronted with early management of animal and human bites. The following protocols may assist in appropriate care and referral.

WOUND MANAGEMENT

Irrigation: Critically important; irrigate all penetration wounds using 20 mL syringe, 19-gauge needle and >250 mL 1% povidone-iodine solution. This method will reduce wound infection by a factor of 20. When there is high risk of rabies, use viricidal 1% benzalkonium chloride in addition to the 1% povidone-iodine. Irrigate wound with normal saline after antiseptic irrigation.

Debridement: Remove all crushed or devitalized tissue remaining after irrigation; minimize removal on face and over thin skin areas or anywhere you would create a worse situation than the bite itself already has; do not extend puncture wounds surgically — rather, manage them with irrigation and antibiotics.

Suturing: Close most dog bites if <8 hours (<12 hours on face); do not routinely close puncture wounds, or deep or severe bites on the hands or feet, as these are at highest risk for infection. Cat and human bites should not be sutured unless cosmetically important. Wound edge freshening, where feasible, reduces infection; minimize sutures in the wound and use monofilament on the surface.

Immobilization: Critical in all hand wounds; important for infected extremities.

Hospitalization/I.V. Antibiotics: Admit for I.V. antibiotics all significant human bites to the hand, especially closed fist injuries, and bites involving penetration of the bone or joint (a high index of suspicion is needed). Consider I.V. antibiotics for significant established wound infections with cellulitis or lymphangitis, any infected bite on the hand, any infected cat bite, and any infection in an immunocompromised or asplenic patient. Outpatient treatment with I.V. antibiotics may be possible in selected cases by consulting with infectious disease.

LABORATORY ASSESSMENT

Gram's Stain: Not useful prior to onset of clinically apparent infection; examination of purulent material may show a predominant organism in established infection, aiding antibiotic selection; not warranted unless results will change your treatment.

Culture: Not useful or cost-effective prior to onset of clinically apparent infection.

X-ray: Whenever you suspect bony involvement, especially in craniofacial dog bites in very small children or severe bite/crush in an extremity; cat bites with their long needle-like teeth may cause osteomyelitis or a septic joint, especially in the hand or wrist.

IMMUNIZATIONS

Tetanus: All bite wounds are contaminated. If not immunized in last 5 years, or if not current in a child, give DPT, DT, Td, or TT as indicated. For absent or incomplete primary immunization, give 250 units tetanus immune globulin (TIG) in addition.

Rabies: In the U.S. 30,000 persons are treated each year in an attempt to prevent 1-5 cases. Domestic animals should be quarantined for 10 days to prove need for prophylaxis. High-risk animal bites (85% of cases = bat, skunk, raccoon) usually receive treatment consisting of:

- human rabies immune globulin (HRIG): 20 units/kg I.M. (unless previously immunized with HDCV)
- human diploid cell vaccine (HDCV): 1 mL I.M. on days 0, 3, 7, 14, and 28 (unless previously immunized with HDCV - then give only first 2 doses)

Rabies Immune Globulin, Human *on page 1038*
Rabies Virus Vaccine *on page 1038*
Tetanus Immune Globulin, Human *on page 1145*

BITE WOUNDS AND PROPHYLACTIC ANTIBIOTICS

Parenteral vs Oral: If warranted, consider an initial I.V. dose to rapidly establish effective serum levels, especially if high risk, delayed treatment, or if patient reliability is poor.

Dog Bite:

1. Rarely get infected (~5%)
2. Infecting organisms: Staph coag negative, staph coag positive, alpha strep, diphtheroids, beta strep, *Pseudomonas aeruginosa*, gamma strep, *Pasteurella multocida*
3. Prophylactic antibiotics are seldom indicated. Consider for high risk wounds such as distal extremity puncture wounds, severe crush injury, bites occurring in cosmetically sensitive areas (eg, face), or in immunocompromised or asplenic patients.

Cat Bite:

1. Often get infected (~25% to 50%)
2. Infecting organisms: *Pasteurella multocida* (first 24 hours), coag positive staph, anaerobic cocci (after first 24 hours)
3. Prophylactic antibiotics are indicated in all cases.

Human Bite:

1. Intermediate infection rate (~15% to 20%)
2. Infecting organisms: Coag positive staph α, β, γ strep, *Haemophilus*, *Eikenella corrodens*, anaerobic streptococci, *Fusobacterium*, *Veillonella*, bacteroides.
3. Prophylactic antibiotics are indicated in almost all cases except superficial injuries.

Amoxicillin (various products) *on page 86*
Amoxicillin and Clavulanate Potassium (Augmentin®) *on page 88*
Cefazolin (Ancef®; Kefzol®; Zolicef®) *on page 234*
Cefotetan (Cefotan®) *on page 240*
Ceftriaxone (Rocephin®) *on page 245*
Clindamycin (Cleocin®) *on page 300*
Doxycycline (various products) *on page 418*
Imipenem/Cilastatin (Primaxin®) *on page 626*
Trimethoprim and Sulfamethoxazole (various products) *on page 1120*

BITE WOUND ANTIBIOTIC REGIMENS

	Dog Bite	Cat Bite	Human Bite
Prophylactic Antibiotics			
Prophylaxis	No routine prophylaxis, consider if involves face or hand, or immunosuppressed or asplenic patients	Routine prophylaxis	Routine prophylaxis
Prophylactic antibiotic	Amoxicillin	Amoxicillin	Amoxicillin
Penicillin allergy	Doxycycline if >10 y or co-trimoxazole	Doxycycline if >10 y or co-trimoxazole	Doxycycline if >10 y or erythromycin and cephalexin*
Outpatient Oral Antibiotic Treatment (mild to moderate infection)			
Established infection	Amoxicillin and clavulanic acid	Amoxicillin and clavulanic acid	Amoxicillin and clavulanic acid
Penicillin allergy (mild infection only)	Doxycycline if >10 y	Doxycycline if >10 y	Cephalexin* or clindamycin
Outpatient Parenteral Antibiotic Treatment (moderate infections – single-drug regimens)			
	Ceftriaxone	Ceftriaxone	Cefotetan
Inpatient Parenteral Antibiotic Treatment			
Established infection	Ampicillin + cefazolin	Ampicillin + cefazolin	Ampicillin + clindamycin
Penicillin allergy	Cefazolin*	Ceftriaxone*	Cefotetan* or imipenem
Duration of Prophylactic and Treatment Regimens			
Prophylaxis: 5 days			
Treatment: 10-14 days			

*Contraindicated if history of immediate hypersensitivity reaction (anaphylaxis) to penicillin.

DENTAL OFFICE EMERGENCIES

All dentists would like to avoid the problems associated with managing dental office medical emergencies. As practitioners, we cannot be certain that these situations will not occur. It is hoped that with preparation, most if not all dental office emergencies can be avoided.

The American Dental Association's publication on dental therapeutics describes the incidence of medical emergencies in the dental office. Most of the problems that the dentist encounters are not life-threatening, but any emergency can become serious if not properly managed. If the dentist and dental office personnel can identify the signs and symptoms of a developing potential office emergency, many emergencies can be aborted and treated within the dental office.

Occasionally, life-threatening office emergencies occur and it is incumbent upon the dentist to be well prepared, to not only evaluate, but to act to stabilize, activate EMS, and manage/refer these patients to an appropriate medical facility for more definitive emergency care.

THIS CHAPTER PRESENTS ONLY THE MOST BASIC GUIDELINES FOR ANY OFFICE EMERGENCY. SPECIFIC PROTOCOLS CAN BE FOUND IN OUR COMPANION MANUAL: *Dental Office Medical Emergencies, A Manual of Office Response Protocols,* 1st ed (revised), Hudson, OH: Lexi-Comp, Inc, 2000.

In addition, a recent statement update from the American Dental Association on Scientific Affairs has been published in the March 2002 Journal of the American Dental Association (Vol 133, pp. 364-5). Briefly, it states: Though rare, life-threatening medical emergencies occasionally occur in the dental office. Recently, the American Dental Association on Scientific Affairs published a preparedness statement to update its pre-existing statements on the subject.

Preparedness to recognize and appropriately manage medical emergencies in the dental environment includes the following:

- Current basic life support certification for all office staff
- Didactic and clinical courses in emergency medicine
- Periodic office emergency drills
- Telephone numbers of EMS or other appropriately trained health care providers
- Emergency drug kit and equipment and knowledge to properly use all items

HISTORY AND PHYSICAL EXAMINATION

The best tool to reduce the risk of a medical emergency occurring in the dental office is the patient's history and record. The dentist should collect adequate information to establish a complete baseline history on all new patients and an adequate updated history on all recall or patients returning to the office.

History and physical examination on all new patients should include:

- Baseline history
- Medications
- Past/current medical conditions
- Allergies
- Need for and results of medical consultation
- Baseline vital signs – pulse, blood pressure, respirations, temperature

Having this information available in the patient record in a format that is easily accessible by trained dental office personnel, allows quick reference of baseline values should a medical emergency occur during the delivery of dental care.

In today's dental practice, some clinicians believe that patient care has become more complicated due to increased use of over-the-counter and prescription medications, as well as the increased complexity of medical diagnoses and management. Other clinicians believe that technological and medical care advances have actually simplified patient care. For the most part, patients seeking elective dental care are adequately managed medically. Patients often appear to have complications based on history, but may be quite stable. New patients and patients with dental emergencies require special attention on the part of the practitioner. It is incumbent upon the dentist to be able to adequately evaluate complete histories and the current medical status of patients, so patients can be assessed for any potential risk while undergoing dental procedures. Each dental office should design a history format that works best for them.

Obtaining the history is usually the first and often the most important interaction with any new patient and with any patient of record that is being re-evaluated after a period of time. Many techniques can be used when addressing sensitive or complicated medical information. Most commonly, the medical history addresses major medical problems in the form of a questionnaire; it follows a review-of-systems format in addressing other symptomatology, which might be present, but remains undiagnosed to-date. This style is often supplemented with a narrative description by the interviewer. Regardless of the technique used, all dental office personnel should be familiar with how to access the information and should have adequate medical knowledge to alert the dentist to any known pre-existing conditions.

A review of current medications must also be included. The review must include home remedies, nonprescription drugs, vitamins or dietary supplements, and medications not prescribed to the patient (but available from friends or relatives) that may have been used by the patient. Doses and frequency of use are important. Drugs that have known associations with some medical emergencies are described with each protocol.

Certain drug classes are associated with potential dental office medical emergencies. Syncope can be caused by alpha$_1$-adrenergic receptor blockers (used to treat hypertension), nitroglycerin, some tricyclic antidepressants, and those antipsychotics which inhibit dopamine type 2 receptors and block alpha$_1$-adrenergic receptors (ie, clozapine). Orthostatic or postural hypotension can also be caused by medication in these drug classes. In addition, this condition has occurred in patients taking angiotensin-converting enzyme (ACE) inhibitors, calcium channel blockers, or beta-adrenergic receptor blockers for hypertension. Hypoglycemia is associated with the oral antidiabetic drugs. These associations are not always obvious, but the dentist should be attentive to the increased risk when patients are taking drugs in these therapeutic categories.

Allergies must be covered in some detail so the dentist is made aware of any known pre-existing allergies, either to environmental agents or medications. Medical reactions or toxicities in the dental office can result in serious life-threatening symptoms. Recognizing any predisposing history may allow the dentist to avoid these interactions or recognize them should they occur. Previous substance abuse might predispose the patient to drug reactions, and untoward medical response, during the delivery of dental care.

If the past history and general state of health, as well as the current physical evaluation, determines that a patient requires medical consultation, this should be noted in the patient's record. The reason for the consultation and the outcome should be clearly indicated in the record so the dentist is aware of the result of such consultation at each subsequent visit. This readiness may reduce risk.

As part of the normal physical examination that the dentist provides for each new patient and each recall patient, vital signs should be recorded. In most instances, these procedures are limited to measurements of pulse and blood pressure; however, in instances where any predisposing conditions might warrant or suggest more detailed evaluation, baseline respiratory rate and temperature might also be recorded. These data should be available and readily accessible in each patient's record so that, should an office emergency occur, the dental office personnel can compare the status during the emergency with the baseline data.

Elaborate schemes are available in oral medicine texts that assign risk by a variety of classifications. One method is to use the American Society of Anesthesiologists classification scheme to evaluate whether a patient's pre-existing medical condition places them at high risk during the delivery of anesthesia. Another mechanism is to assign the risk of dental procedures based on an analysis of pre-existing medical conditions matched with the complexity of the planned dental procedure. This protocol takes into account the potential invasiveness of the dental procedure. Simple procedures in complicated patients may have low total risk, whereas complex procedures in simple patients may place the patient at significant risk for an office emergency. Each dental practitioner should design or adapt a patient analysis plan for their own office.

EQUIPMENT

The dental office should be adequately equipped to not only deliver routine care to each new patient and each returning patient, but also should be set up for appropriate management and stabilization of any potential office emergency. This requires that each patient and treatment area should be equipped with a minimum of a blood pressure cuff and a stethoscope. The office should also have available:

- Appropriately-sized blood pressure cuffs
- Tourniquets
- Stethoscopes
- First-aid kits
- Emergency number call list
- Emergency cabinet
- Oxygen tank (size E portable with low flow regulator)
- Nasal cannula
- Masks (non-rebreather and a bag-valve mask [Ambu®])
- Syringes (intramuscular: I.M. 3 cc disposable, subcutaneous: S.C. tuberculin)

The emergency call list should be properly posted so office personnel need not search other operatories or the reception area for such information. Centrally located emergency cabinets, which include tourniquets, emergency medical care drugs, instruments, and supplies, are essential.

DENTAL OFFICE EMERGENCIES *(Continued)*

DENTAL OFFICE EMERGENCY DRUGS

Protocols should be established for most office emergencies. Recognition and rapid diagnosis lead to appropriate management. Major drugs usually available in the emergency drug cabinet are listed below.

Albuterol *on page 45*
Ammonia Spirit, Aromatic *on page 82*
Dexamethasone *on page 363*
(Alternative is Solu-Cortef® Mix-O-Vials for I.M.; has a longer shelf life)
Diazepam (Valium®) *on page 373*
Diphenhydramine (Benadryl®) *on page 398*
Epinephrine *on page 438*
(AnaKit® includes preloaded Tubex® syringes, which have measured dosing in increments)
Flumazenil *on page 511*
Glucose *on page 559*
(Emergency kit should also have oral carbohydrate source, such as Glutose 15™ oral gel and injectable glucagon)
Hydrocortisone *on page 608*
Morphine *on page 829*
Naloxone (Narcan®) *on page 844*
Nitroglycerin *on page 871*
Oxygen *on page 906*

Drug cabinet supplies should be in dose forms which the dentist is comfortable administering. Typical routes of administration could include oral (eg, diphenhydramine), inhalation (eg, albuterol), intramuscular/I.M. (eg, hydrocortisone), subcutaneous/S.C. (eg, epinephrine), or intravenous/I.V. (eg, epinephrine). Sublingual/S.L. injection can be substituted for some I.V. administrations in situations (ie, anaphylaxis) where a drug such as epinephrine may be life-saving. Oral mucosal absorption (eg, nitroglycerin) is also useful.

STAFF TRAINING

Office personnel, including the dentist, dental hygienists, and dental assistants, should all be trained in measurement of vital signs. Primarily, this includes measurement of pulse and evaluation of blood pressure. Proper technique for evaluating vital signs is necessary so information is accurate, and in the event of an emergency situation, ongoing measurements could be made by assisting personnel. The dentist should be able to provide this training to new employees, however, continuing education courses in proper techniques are available.

Dental office personnel should all be trained in basic life support first-aid, although the dentist is ultimately in charge of delivering care to either patient or personnel. Each office member should be aware of basic principles for management of nonlife-threatening injuries. All office personnel should be trained in cardiopulmonary resuscitation (CPR) or basic life support (BLS). Training courses are readily available through the American Heart Association and/or hospital facilities in most areas. Training should include not only basic initial training, but also renewal of skills should be a requirement for continued employment. One to two years is a reasonable time for updating such skills in cardiopulmonary resuscitation. Applicable state requirements or recommendations should be reviewed.

GENERAL PRINCIPLES OF RECOGNITION

As a practicing dentist, you should be familiar with:

- Altered states or loss of consciousness
- Cardiovascular emergencies (often associated with chest pain), including heart attack and stroke
- Respiratory emergencies, including asthmatic bronchospasm and obstruction
- Allergic reactions, including signs of anaphylaxis
- Other potential emergencies:
  - Diabetes, including acute hypo- and hyperglycemic states/reactions
  - Acute neurologic disturbances, including convulsive disorders such as epilepsy, stress-induced panic attacks, and acute headaches
  - Abdominal distress, including the abdominal disorders and diseases classified as acute (sudden onset) abdominal distress
  - Communicable diseases, including the major bacteria- and virus-induced illnesses of our society

Although symptoms can be very specific, detecting medical emergencies usually means recognizing some general changes in the state of the patient:

- Acute changes in affect or consciousness
- Sudden onset of pain, anywhere in the body
- Feelings of fever and chills
- Tight feeling in the chest
- Difficulty in expiration or inspiration
- Choking
- Dizziness or feelings of faintness
- Numbness or tingling sensations

The dental practitioner must be familiar with several basic diagnostic signs that should be compared to baseline measurements in the patient's record:

- Pulse rate and character — remember that a pulse rate >120 or <50 beats per minute can indicate a true emergency for the adult patient
- Blood pressure — a systolic pressure <70 may indicate shock and pressures >200/100 may present a hypertensive crisis (pre-CVA)
- Breathing rate and character — a true emergency may exist when the adult patient's respirations are >30 per minute
- Skin temperature, condition, and color
- Diaphoresis — often associated with anxiety, but can indicate ischemia
- Pupil size, equality, and response
- Color of the lips, tongue, earlobes, and nailbeds
- Breath odors
- Muscular activity — spasms and paralysis or weakness such as seen in ischemic attacks or CVA
- Bleeding or discharges from the body

ALL PRACTITIONERS MUST BE PREPARED TO CARRY OUT A BASIC PLAN FOR STABILIZATION

These steps are the basic action plan for stabilization in every office emergency. They should be activated within the first seconds following recognition of any developing problem. Sometimes, based on the initial recognition signs, activation of the emergency medical system (EMS) will occur immediately, usually by calling 911 (if available in your area). If the dentist is unsure of the underlying reason for the medical emergency or does not feel adequately trained, then basic life support (BLS) procedures should be the extent of the treatment until the emergency medical team arrives.

BASIC ACTION PLAN FOR STABILIZATION

PATIENT PLACEMENT	→ **UPRIGHT / SEMI-RECLINING?**
	→ **SUPINE?**
	→ **TRENDELENBURG (FEET UP, HEAD DOWN)*?**
AIRWAY AND BREATHING	→ **IS THE AIRWAY OPEN?**
	→ **CLEAR OF OBSTRUCTIONS?**
	→ **IS THE PATIENT BREATHING ON THEIR OWN?**
	→ **DOES THE SITUATION REQUIRE OXYGEN TO INCREASE PERFUSION?**
	→ **ACTIVATE CPR IF NECESSARY**
CIRCULATION	→ **MONITOR PULSE**
	→ **PROCEED WITH CPR, IF APPROPRIATE**

DENTAL OFFICE EMERGENCIES *(Continued)*

ADDITIONAL MANAGEMENT†

→ **ALWAYS CONSIDER ACTIVATING EMS IMMEDIATELY**

→ **CONTINUALLY OBSERVE, MONITOR VITAL SIGNS, AND EVALUATE FOR ANY SIGNS OF RECOVERY OR DETERIORATION**

→ **ASSIGN SOMEONE IN THE OFFICE TO QUICKLY RE-EVALUATE PATIENT'S HISTORY AND RECORD FOR CLUES TO THE CAUSE OF THE INCIDENT OR DRUGS THE PATIENT MAY BE TAKING**

→ **DETERMINE, IF POSSIBLE, THE TENTATIVE MEDICAL CONDITION CAUSING THE SYMPTOMS**

→ **DELIVER SPECIFIC CARE IF APPROPRIATE**

→ **BE PREPARED TO ACTIVATE EMS CALL FOR ASSISTANCE IF PATIENT'S CONDITION DETERIORATES**

→ **ALWAYS CONSIDER THE NEED FOR FOLLOW-UP MEDICAL EVALUATION AS PATIENT RECOVERS**

*Trendelenburg's position is a supine position which is inclined at an angle so that the pelvis and legs are slightly higher than the head.

†Although these management suggestions are essentially the same for each of the protocols, the order and specific care will vary.

SUGGESTED READINGS

ANTIBIOTICS IN TREATMENT OF ODONTOGENIC INFECTIONS

Doern GV, Ferraro MJ, Breuggemann AB, et al, "Emergence of High Rates of Antimicrobial Resistance Among Viridans Group Streptococci in the United States," *Antimicrob Agents Chemother,* 1996, 40(4):891-84.

Flynn TR, "The Swollen Face. Severe Odontogenic Infections," *Emerg Med Clin North Am,* 2000, 18(3):481-519.

Hardee WM, "Tried-and-True Medication," *Practical Endodontics,* 1997, 7(5):38.

Johnson BS, "Principles and Practice of Antibiotic Therapy," *Infect Dis Clin North Am,* 1999, 13(4):851-70.

Kuriyama T, Nakagawa K, Karasawa T, et al, "Past Administration of Beta-lactam Antibiotics and Increase in the Emergence of Beta-lactamase-producing Bacteria in Patients With Orofacial Odontogenic Infections," *Oral Surg Oral Med Oral Path Oral Radiol Endod,* 2000, 89(2):186-92.

Lee CY, "Management of Odontogenic Infections With Microbial, Anatomic and Antibiotic Considerations," *Hawaii Dent J,* 1993, 24(8):8-11.

Mandell GM, Bennett JE, Douglas GR, et al, eds, *Mandell, Douglas, and Bennett's Principles and Practice of Infectious Disease,* 5th ed, Philadelphia, PA: Churchill Livingstone, Inc, 2000, 2567-8.

Montgomery EH, "Antimicrobial Agents in the Prevention and Treatment of Infection," *Pharmacology and Therapeutics for Dentistry,* 4th ed, Yagiela JA, Neidle EA, Dowd FJ, eds, St. Louis, MO: Mosby-Year Book, Inc, 1998, 637.

Palacios E and Valvassori G, "Deep Facial Infection of Odontogenic Origin," *Ear Nose Throat J,* 2001, 80(1):15.

Storoe W, Haug RH, and Lillich TT, "The Changing Face of Odontogenic Infections," *J Oral Maxillofac Surg,* 2001, 59(7):739-48

Wynn RL and Bergman SA, "Antibiotics and Their Use in the Treatment of Orofacial Infections, Part I," *Gen Dent,* 1994, 42(5):398, 400-2.

Wynn RL and Bergman SA, "Antibiotics and Their Use in the Treatment of Orofacial Infections, Part II," *Gen Dent,* 1994, 42(6):498-502.

Wynn RL and Bergman SA, Meiller TF, et al, "Antibiotics in Treating Oral-Facial Infections of Odontogenic Origin," *Gen Dent,* 2001, 47(3):238-52.

CANCER

Al-Balawi SA and Nwoku AL, "Management of Oral Cancer in a Tertiary Care Hospital," *Saudi Med J,* 2002, 23(2):156-9.

Carl W, "Oral Complications of Local and Systemic Cancer Treatment," *Curr Opin Oncol,* 1995, 7(4):320-4.

Chambers MS, Toth BB, Martin JW, et al, "Oral and Dental Management of the Cancer Patient: Prevention and Treatment of Complications," *Support Care Cancer,* 1995, 3(3):168-75.

Dutton JM, Graham SM, and Hoffman HT, "Metastatic Cancer to the Floor of Mouth: The Lingual Lymph Nodes, "*Head Neck,* 2002 24(4):401-5.

Flaitz CM, "Persistent White Lesion of the Lateral Tongue," *Am J Dent,* 2001, 14(6):402-3.

Gellrich NC, Schramm A, Bockmann R, et al, "Follow-Up in Patients With Oral Cancer," *J Oral Maxillofac Surg,* 2002, 60(4):380-6.

Hobson RS and Clark JD, "Management of the Orthodontic Patient at Risk From Infective Endocarditis," *Br Dent J,* 1995, 179(2):48.

Jullien JA, Downer MC, Zakrzewska JM, et al, "Evaluation of a Screening Test for the Early Detection of Oral Cancer and Precancer," *Community Dent Health,* 1995, 12(1):3-7.

Messer NC, Yant WR, and Archer RD, "Developing Provider Partnerships in the Detection of Oral Cancer and the Prevention of Smokeless Tobacco Use," *Md Med J,* 1995, 44(10):788-91.

Takinami S, Yahata H, Kanoshima A, et al, "Hepatocellular Carcinoma Metastatic to the Mandible," *Oral Surg Oral Med Oral Pathol Oral Radiol Endod,* 1995, 79(5):649-54.

Vigneswaran N, Tilashalski K, Rodu B, et al, "Tobacco Use and Cancer. A Reappraisal," *Oral Surg Oral Med Oral Pathol Oral Radiol Endod,* 1995, 80(2):178-82.

Weaver RG, Whittaker L, Valachovic RW, et al, "Tobacco Control and Prevention Effort in Dental Education," *J Dent Educ,* 2002, 66(3):426-9.

CARDIOVASCULAR

"Adjusted-Dose Warfarin Versus Low-Intensity, Fixed-Dose Warfarin Plus Aspirin for High-Risk Patients With Atrial Fibrillation: Stroke Prevention in Atrial Fibrillation III Randomized Clinical Trial," *Lancet,* 1996, 348(9028):633-8.

American Heart Association, "Heart and Stroke Facts: 1996 Statistical Supplement," Dallas, Texas: National Center of the American Heart Association, 1996, 15.

Ayala C, Croft JB, Greenlund KJ, et al, "Sex Differences in US Mortality Rates for Stroke and Stroke Subtypes by Race/Ethnicity and Age, 1995-1998," *Stroke,* 2002, 33(5):1197-201.

Frazier OH, "Mechanical Circulatory Support: New Advances, New Pumps, New Ideas," *Semin Thorac Cardiovasc Surg,* 2002, 14(2):178-86.

Garcia R, "Floss or Die: The Link Between Oral Health and Cardiac Disease," *Harv Dent Bull,* 1998, 7(2):16-7.

SUGGESTED READINGS *(Continued)*

Gilligan DM, Ellenbogen KA, and Epstein AE, "The Management of Atrial Fibrillation," *Am J Med*, 1996, 101:413-21.

Giuliani ER, Gersh BJ, McGoon MD, et al, *Mayo Clinic Practice of Cardiology*, 3rd ed, St Louis, MO: Mosby-Year Book, Inc, 1996, 1698-814.

Glick M, "Screening for Traditional Risk Factors for Cardiovascular Disease: A Review for Oral Health Care Providers," *J Am Dent Assoc*, 2002, 133(3):291-300.

Hansson L, Zanchetti A, Carruthers SG, et al, "Effects of Intensive Blood Pressure Lowering and Low-Dose Aspirin in Patients With Hypertension: Principal Results of the Hypertension Optimal Treatment (HOT) Randomized Trial. HOT Study Group," *Lancet*, 1998, 351:1755-62.

Heidenreich PA, Lee TT, and Massie BM, "Effect of Beta-Blockade on Mortality in Patients With Heart Failure: A Meta-analysis of Randomized Clinical Trials," *J Am Coll Cardiol*, 1997, 30(1):27-34.

Hylek EM, Skates SJ, Sheehan MA, et al, "An Analysis of the Lowest Effective Intensity of Prophylactic Coagulation for Patients With Nonrheumatic Atrial Fibrillation," *N Engl J Med*, 1996, 335:540-6.

Kannel WB, "Blood Pressure as a Cardiovascular Risk Factor. Prevention and Treatment," *JAMA*, 1996, 275:1571-6.

Kaplan NM, "Hypertension and Diabetes," *J Hum Hypertens*, 2002, 16(Suppl 1):S56-60.

Kaplan NM, "Perspectives on the New JNC VI Guidelines for the Treatment of Hypertension," *Formulary*, 1997, 32:1224-31.

Kerpen SJ, Kerpen HO, and Sachs SA, "Mitral Valve Prolapse: A Significant Cardiac Defect in the Development of Infective Endocarditis," *Spec Care Dentist*, 1984, 4(4):158-9.

Lopaschuk GD, "Metabolic Abnormalities in the Diabetic Heart," *Heart Fail Rev*, 2002, 7(2):149-59.

Morley J, Marinchak R, Rials SJ, et al, "Atrial Fibrillation, Anticoagulation, and Stroke," *Am J Cardiol*, 1996, 77:38A-44A.

Reyes AJ, "Diuretics in the Treatment of Patients who Present Congestive Heart Failure and Hypertension," *J Hum Hypertens*, 2002, 16(Suppl 1):S104-13.

"The Sixth Report of the Joint National Committee on Prevention, Detection, Evaluation, and Treatment of High Blood Pressure (JNC VI)," *Arch Intern Med*, 1997, 157:2413-46.

CHEMICAL DEPENDENCY AND SMOKING CESSATION

Abelin T, Buehler A, Muller P, et al, "Controlled Trial of Transdermal Nicotine Patch in Tobacco Withdrawal," *Lancet*, 1989, 1(8628):7-10.

Alterman AI, Droba M, Antelo RE, et al, "Amantadine May Facilitate Detoxification of Cocaine Addicts," *Drug Alcohol Depend*, 1992, 31(1):19-29.

Ciancio SG, ed, *ADA Guide to Dental Therapeutics*, 1st ed, Chicago, IL: ADA Publishing Co, 1998.

Fiester S, Goldstein M, Resnick M, et al, "Practice Guideline for the Treatment of Patients With Nicotine Dependence," *Am J Psych*, 1996, 15(Suppl 10):31.

Gelskey SC, "Tobacco-Use Cessation Programs and Policies at the University of Manitoba's Faculty of Dentistry," *J Can Dent Assoc*, 2001, 67(3):145-8.

Herkenham MA, "Localization of Cannabinoid Receptors in Brain: Relationship to Motor and Reward Systems," *Biological Basis of Substance Abuse*, Korenman SG and Barchas JD, eds, New York, NY: Oxford University Press, 1993, 187-200.

Kausch O and McCormick RA, "Suicide Prevalence in Chemical Dependency Programs: Preliminary Data from a National Sample, and an Examination of Risk Factors," *J Subst Abuse Treat*, 2002, 22(2):97-102.

Kreek MJ, "Rationale for Maintenance Pharmacotherapy of Opiate Dependence," O'Brien CP and Barchas JD, eds, *Addictive States*, New York, NY: Raven Press, 1992, 205-30.

Leshner AI, "Molecular Mechanisms of Cocaine Addiction," *N Engl J Med*, 1996, 335(2):128-9.

Mendelson JH and Mello NK, "Management of Cocaine Abuse and Dependence," *N Engl J Med*, 1996, 334(15):965-72.

O'Brien CP, "Drug Addiction and Drug Abuse," *The Pharmacological Basis of Therapeutics*, 9th ed, Molinoff PB and Ruddon R, eds, New York, NY: McGraw-Hill, 1996, 557-77.

O'Brien CP, "Treatment of Alcoholism as a Chronic Disorder," *Toward a Molecular Basis of Alcohol Use and Abuse*, Jansson B, Jornvall H, Rydberg U, et al, eds, Basel, Switzerland: Birkhauser Verlag, 1994, Vol 71, EXS, 349-59.

Ostroff JS, Hay JL, Primavera LH, et al, "Motivating Smoking Cessation Among Dental Patients: Smokers' Interest in Biomarker Testing for Susceptibility to Tobacco-Related Cancers," *Nicotine Tob Res*, 1999, 1(4):347-55.

Ostrowski DJ and DeNelsky GY, "Pharmacologic Management of Patients Using Smoking Cessation Aids," *Dental Clin North Am*, 1996, 40(3):779-801.

Schydlower M, "Adolescent Substance Use and Abuse: Current Issues," *Tex Med*, 2002, 98(2):31-5.

Self DW, Barnhart WJ, Lehman DA, et al, "Opposite Modulation of Cocaine-Seeking Behavior by D1- and D2-Like Dopamine Receptor Agonists," *Science*, 1996 271(5255):1586-9.

The Smoking Cessation Clinical Practice Guideline Panel and Staff, The Agency for Health Care Policy and Research Smoking Cessation Clinical Practice Guideline *JAMA*, 1996, 275(1):1270-80.

Tomar SL, "Dentistry's Role in Tobacco Control," *J Am Dent Assoc*, 200, 132 (Suppl):S30-35.
Weisner C, Mertens J, Tam T, et al, "Factors Affecting the Initiation of Substance Abuse Treatment in Managed Care," *Addiction*, 2001, 96(5):705-16.

DENTIST'S ROLE IN RECOGNIZING DOMESTIC ABUSE

World Wide Web Sites

American Academy of Pediatrics — http://www.aap.org
American College of Emergency Physicians — http://www.acep.org
American Dental Association — http://www.ada.org
National Clearinghouse on Child Abuse and Neglect Information — http://www.calib.com/nccanch
National Data Archive on Child Abuse and Neglect — http://www.ndacan.cornell.edu
Prevent Child Abuse America (formerly National Committee to Prevent Child Abuse) — http://www.childabuse.org
University of Medicine and Dentistry - New Jersey — http://www.umdnj.edu/~baum/famvio.htm
USDHHS Agency of Children and Families — http://www.acf.dhhs.gov

Toll-Free Hotlines

Bureau of Indian Affairs Federal Hotline — 800-633-5155
Child Abuse Hotlines (24-Hour) — 800-4-ACHILD
Covenant House Nineline — 800-999-9999
National Family Violence Helpline — 800-222-2000

Books and Journal Articles (available at a local library or through interlibrary loan)

Besharov DJ, *Recognizing Child Abuse*, New York, NY, Free Press, 1990.
Chiodo GT, Tolle SW, and Tilden VP, "The Dentist and Family Violence," *Gen Dent*, 1998, 46(1):20-5.
Davidhizar R, Dowd S, and Giger JN, "Recognizing Abuse in Culturally Diverse Clients," *Health Care Superv*, 1998, 17(2):10-20.
Domestic Violence: A Directory of Protocols for Health Care Providers, Children's Safety Network, Newton, MA: Education Development Center, Inc, 1992.
Erickson MJ, Hill TD, and Siegel RM, "Barriers to Domestic Violence Screening in the Pediatric Setting," *Pediatrics*, 2001, 108(1):98-102.
"Health and Human Rights: A Call to Action on the 50th Anniversary of the Universal Declaration of Human Rights. The Writing Group for the Consortium for Health and Human Rights," *JAMA*, 1998, 280(5).
LaCerva V, *Pathways to Peace: Forty Steps to a Less Violent America*, Tesuque, NM: Heartsongs Publications, 1996.
McDowell JD, Kassebaum DK, and Stromboe SE, "Recognizing and Reporting Victims of Domestic Violence," *J Am Dent Assoc*, 1992, 123(9):44-50.
Mouden LD and Bross DC, "Legal Issues Affecting Dentistry's Role in Preventing Child Abuse and Neglect," *J Am Dent Assoc*, 1995, 126(8):1173-80.
"Protecting Children From Abuse and Neglect," Center for the Future of Children, The David and Lucille Packard Foundation, *The Future of Children*, 1998, 8(1):1-142. (Electronic version: http://www.futureofchildren.org)
Reece RM, *Child Abuse: Medical Diagnosis and Management*, Philadelphia, PA: Lea and Febiger, 1994.
Rupp RP, "Conditions to Be Considered in the Differential Diagnosis of Child Abuse and Neglect," *Gen Dent*, 1998, 46(1):96-9.
Salber PR and Talliaferro EH, *The Physicians' Guide to Domestic Violence: How to Ask the Right Questions and Recognize Abuse...Another Way to Save a Life*, Volcano, CA: Volcano Press, 1995.
Silva C, McFarlane J, Socken K, et al, "Symptoms of Post-Traumatic Stress Disorder in Abused Women in a Primary Care Setting," *J Women's Health*, 1997, 6:543-52.
Sweet D, "Recognizing and Intervening in Domestic Violence: Proactive Role for Dentistry," *Medscape Womens Health*, 1996, 1(6):3.
Watts C and Zimmerman C, "Violence Against Women: Global Scope and Magnitude," *Lancet*, 2002, 359(9313):1232-7.

DIAGNOSIS AND MANAGEMENT OF PAIN

Brown RS, Hinderstein B, Reynolds DC, et al, "Using Anesthetic Localization to Diagnose Oral and Dental Pain," *J Am Dent Assoc*, 1995, 126(5):633-4, 637-41.
Denson DD and Katz JA, "Nonsteroidal Anti-inflammatory Agents," *Practical Management of Pain*, 2nd ed, PP Raj, ed, St Louis, MO: Mosby Year Book, 1992.
Henry G, "Postoperative Pain Experience With Flurbiprofen and Acetaminophen With Codeine," *J Dent Res*, 1992, 71:952.
Jaffe JH and Martin WR, "Opioid Analgesic and Antagonists," *The Pharmacological Basis of Therapeutics*, 8th ed, Gilman AG, Rall TW, Nies AD, et al, eds, New York, NY: Maxwell Pergamon MacMillan Publishing, 1990.
Kalso E and Vainio A, "Morphine and Oxycodone Hydrochloride in the Management of Cancer Pain," *Clin Pharmacol Ther*, 1990, 47(5):639-46.
McQuay H, Carroll D, Jadad AR, et al, "Anticonvulsant Drugs for Management of Pain: A Systemic Review," *BMJ*, 1995, 311(7012):1047-52.
Robertson S, Goodell H, and Wolff HG, "The Teeth as a Source of Headache and Other Pain," *Arch Neurol Psychiatry*, 1947, 57:277.

SUGGESTED READINGS *(Continued)*

Sandler NA, Ziccardi V, and Ochs M, "Differential Diagnosis of Jaw Pain in the Elderly," *J Am Dent Assoc* 1995, 126(9):1263-72.

Seng GF, Kraus K, Cartwright G, et al, "Confirmed Allergic Reactions to Amide Local Anesthetics," *Gen Dent*, 1996, 44(1):52-4.

Stoller EP, Gilbert GH, Pyle MA, et al, "Coping With Tooth Pain: A Qualitative Study of Lay Management Strategies and Professional Consultation," *Spec Care Dentist*, 2001, 21(6):208-15.

Wright EF and Schiffman EL, "Treatment Alternatives for Patients With Masticatory Myofascial Pain," *J Am Dent Assoc*, 1995, 126(7):1030-9.

HIV INFECTION AND AIDS

Alsakka H, "Dental Management of HIV/AIDS Patients," *Northwest Dent*, 2001, 80(3):33-4.

Center for Disease Control (CDC), CfDC, "Update: AIDS Cases in Males Who Have Sex With Males," *MMWR Morb Mortal Wkly Rep*, 1995, 44(29):401-2.

Center for Disease Control (CDC), CfDC, "First 500,000 AIDS Cases," *MMWR Morb Mortal Wkly Rep*, 1995, 44(46):849-53.

Center for Disease Control (CDC), CfDC, "Update: HIV Exposures in HCWs," *MMWR Morb Mortal Wkly Rep*, 1995, 44(50):929.

Center for Disease Control (CDC), CfDCaP, "Recommended Infection-Control Practices for Dentistry," *MMWR Morb Mortal Wkly Rep*, 1993, 42(RR-8).

Glick M, *Clinicians Guide to Treatment of HIV-Infected Patients*, Academy of Oral Medicine, 1996.

Greenspan D, Greenspan JS, Schiodt M, et al, *AIDS and the Mouth*, Munksgaard, Copenhagen, 1990.

Greenspan JS and Greenspan D, "Oral Manifestations of HIV Infection," *The Proceedings of the Second International Workshop*, Chicago, IL: Quintessence Publishing Co, 1995.

Lyles AM, "What the Dentist Should Know About a Patient With HIV/AIDS," *J Calif Dent Assoc*, 2001, 29(2):158-69.

"Oral Health Care for Adults With HIV Infection," New York, NY: AIDS Institute, New York State Department of Health, 1993.

Ryder MI, "Periodontal Management of HIV-infected Patients."*Periodontol 2000*, 2000, 23:85-93.

Silverman S, *Color Atlas of Oral Manifestations of AIDS*, 2nd ed, St Louis, MO: Mosby, 1996.

Squassi A, Khaszki C, Blanco B, et al, "Relation Between Demographic and Epidemiological Characteristics and Permanency Under a Dental Health Care Program for HIV Infected Patients," *Acta Odontol Latinoam*, 1998, 11(1):3-13.

NATURAL PRODUCTS: HERBALS AND DIETARY SUPPLEMENTS

1995 Martindale - The Extra Pharmacopoeia, Vol 86, Roy Pharm Soc, GB, 1996.

Blumenthal M, Goldberg A, Gruenwald J, et al, *German Commission E Monographs: Therapeutic Monographs on Medicinal Plants for Human Use*, Austin, TX: American Botanical Council, 1997.

Cohan RP and Jacobsen PL, "Herbal Supplements: Considerations in Dental Practice," *J Calif Dent Assoc*, 2000, 28(8):600-10.

D'Arcy PF, "Adverse Reactions and Interactions With Herbal Medicines: Part 1. Adverse Reactions," *Adverse Drug Reaction Toxicol Rev*, 1991, 10(4):189-208.

D'Arcy PF, McEmay JC, and Welling PG, *Mechanisms of Drug Interactions*, New York, NY: Springer-Verlag, 1996.

DeSmet PA, "Health Risks of Herbal Remedies," *Drug Saf*, 1995, 13(2):81-93.

Ernst E and DeSmet PA, "Risks Associated With Complementary Therapies," *Meyler's Side Effects of Drugs*, 13th ed, Dukes MN ed, New York, NY: Elsevier Science, 1996.

Heber D, Yip I, Ashley JM, et al, "Cholesterol-lowering Effects of a Proprietary Chinese Red Yeast Rice Dietary Supplement," *Am J Clin Nutr*, 1999, 69:231-6.

Keller K, "Therapeutic Use of Herbal Drugs and Their Potential Toxicity, Problems and Results of the Revision of Herbal Medicines in the EEC," *Proceedings of the 3rd International Conference on Pharmacopoeias and Quality Control of Drugs*, Rome, November, 1992, published in Bologna, Fondazione Rhone-Poulenc Rorer per le Scienze Mediche, 1993.

McGuffin M, Hobbs C, Upton R, et al, *American Herbal Product Association's Botanical Safety Handbook: Guidelines for the Safe Use and Labeling for Herbs of Commerce*, Boca Raton, FL: CRC Press, 1997.

Mistry MG and Mays DA, "Precautions Against Global Use of Natural Products for Weight Loss: A Review of Active Ingredients and Issues Concerning Concomitant Disease States," *Therapeutic Perspectives*, 1996, 10(1):2.

Moynihan P, "The British Nutrition Foundation Oral Task Force Report - Issues Relevant to Dental Health Professionals," *Br Dent J*, 2000, 188(6):308-12.

ORAL INFECTIONS

Caufield PW and Griffen AL, "Dental Caries. An Infectious and Transmissible Disease," *Pediatr Clin North Am*, 2000, 47(5):1001-19.

Chow AW, "Infections of the Oral Cavity, Neck, and Head," *Principles and Practice of Infectious Diseases*, 4th ed, Mandell GL, Bennett JE, Dolin R, eds, New York, NY: Churchill Livingstone, 1995, 593-605.

Dajani A, Taubert K, Ferrieri P, et al, "Treatment of Acute Streptococcal Pharyngitis and Prevention of Rheumatic Fever: A Statement for Health Professionals," *Pediatrics*, 1995, 96(4):758-64.

Diz Dios P, Ocampo Hermida A, Miralles Alvarez C, et al, "Fluconazole-Resistant Oral Candidiasis in HIV-Infected Patients," *AIDS*, 1995, 9(7):809-10.

Dobson RL, "Antimicrobial Therapy for Cutaneous Infections," *J Am Acad Dermatol*, 1990, 22(5):871-3.

Goldberg MH and Topazian R, "Odontogenic Infections and Deep Facial Space Infections of Dental Origin," *Oral and Maxillofacial Infections*, 3rd ed, Philadelphia, PA: WB Saunders, 1994, 232-6.

Lewis MA, Parkhurst CL, Douglas CW, et al, "Prevalence of Penicillin Resistant Bacteria in Acute Suppurative Oral Infection," *J Antimicrob Chemother*, 1995, 35(6):785-91.

Muzyka BC and Glick M, "A Review of Oral Fungal Infections and Appropriate Therapy," *J Am Dent Assoc*, 1995, 126(1):63-72.

Shay K, "Infectious Complications of Dental and Periodontal Diseases in the Elderly Population," *Clin Infect Dis*, 2002, 34(9):1215-23.

Sykes LM and Sukha A, " Potential Risk of Serious Oral Infections in the Diabetic Patient: a Clinical Report," *J Prosthet Dent*, 2001, 86(6):569-73.

ORAL LEUKOPLAKIA

Barker JN, Mitra RS, Griffiths CE, et al, "Keratinocytes as Initiators of Inflammation," *Lancet*, 1991, 337(8735):211-4.

Boehncke WH, Kellner I, Konter U, et al, "Differential Expression of Adhesion Molecules on Infiltrating Cells in Inflammatory Dermatoses," *J Am Acad Dermatol*, 1992, 26(6):907-13.

Corso B, Eversole LR, and Hutt-Fletcher L, "Hairy Leukoplakia: Epstein-Barr Virus Receptors on Oral Keratinocyte Plasma Membranes," *Oral Surg Oral Med Oral Pathol*, 1989, 67(4):416-21.

Flaitz CM, "Persistent White Lesion of the Lateral Tongue," *Am J Dent*, 2001, 14(6):402-3.

Greenspan D, Greenspan JS, Overby G, et al, "Risk Factors for Rapid Progression From Hairy Leukoplakia to AIDS: A Nested Case-Control Study, *J Acquir Immune Defic Syndr*, 1991, 4(7):652-8.

McGuff HS, Otto RA, and Aufdemorte TB, "Clinical Warning Signs and Symptoms of Head and Neck Cancer," *Tex Dent J*, 2000, 117(6):14-9.

Regezi JA, Stewart JC, Lloyd RV, et al, "Immunohistochemical Staining of Langerhans Cells and Macrophages in Oral Lichen Planus," *Oral Surg Oral Med Oral Pathol*, 1985, 60(4):396-402.

Sciubba JJ, "Oral Leukoplakia," *Crit Rev Oral Biol Med*, 1995, 6(2):147-60.

Sciubba JJ, "Oral Precancer and Cancer: Etiology, Clinical Presentation, Diagnosis, and Management," *Compend Contin Educ Dent* 2000, 21(10A):892-8, 900-2.

ORAL SOFT TISSUE DISEASES

Antenucci EL, "Integration of Lasers Into a Soft Tissue Management Program," *Dent Clin North Am*, 2000, 44(4):811-9.

Delaney JE and Keels MA, "Pediatric Oral Pathology. Soft Tissue and Periodontal Conditions," *Pediatr Clin North Am*, 2000, 47(5):1125-47.

Goupil MT, "Occupational Health and Safety Emergencies," *Dent Clin North Am*, 1995, 39(3):637-47.

Haddad AJ, Avon SL, Clokie CM, et al, "Nodular Fasciitis in the Oral Cavity," *J Can Dent Assoc*, 2001, 67(11):664-7.

MacPhail LA, Greenspan D, Greenspan JS, et al, "Recurrent Aphthous Ulcers in Association With HIV Infection. Diagnosis and Treatment," *Oral Surg Oral Med Oral Pathol*, 1992, 73(3):283-8.

Meiller TF, Kutcher MJ, Overholser CD, et al, "Effect of an Antimicrobial Mouthrinse on Recurrent Aphthous Ulcerations," *Oral Surg Oral Med Oral Pathol*, 1991, 72(4):425-9.

Moncarz V, Ulmansky M, and Lustmann J, "Lichen Planus: Exploring Its Malignant Potential," *J Am Dent Assoc*, 1993, 124(3):102-8.

Rodu B and Mattingly G, "Oral Mucosal Ulcers: Diagnosis and Management," *J Am Dent Assoc*, 1992, 123(10):83-6.

Van Dis ML and Vincent SD, "Diagnosis and Management of Autoimmune and Idiopathic Mucosal Diseases," *Dent Clin North Am*, 1992, 36(4):897-917.

Vincent SD and Lilly GE, "Clinical, Historic, and Therapeutic Features of Aphthous Stomatitis. Literature Review and Open Clinical Trial Employing Steroids," *Oral Surg, Oral Med, Oral Pathol*, 1992, 74(1):79-86.

Wactawski-Wende J, " Periodontal Diseases and Osteoporosis: Association and Mechanisms, "*Ann Periodontol*, 2001, (1):197-208.

ORAL VIRAL DISEASES

Balfour HH, Rotbart HA, Feldman S, et al, "Acyclovir Treatment of Varicella in Otherwise Healthy Adolescents. The Collaborative Acyclovir Varicella Study Group," *J Pediatr*, 1992, 120(4):627-33.

Chang Y, Cesarman E, Pessin MS, et al, "Identification of Herpesvirus-Like DNA Sequences in AIDS-Associated Kaposi's Sarcoma," *Science*, 1994, 266(5192):1865-9.

Farquharson A, Ajagbe O, and Brown RS, "Differential Diagnosis of Severe Recurrent Oral Ulceration," *Dent Today*, 2002, 21(3):74-9.

SUGGESTED READINGS *(Continued)*

Ficarra G and Shillitoe EJ, "HIV-Related Infections of the Oral Cavity," *Oral Biol Med*, 1992, 3(3):207-31.

Moore TO, Moore AY, Carrasco D, et al, "Human Papillomavirus, Smoking, and Cancer," *J Cutan Med Surg*, 2001, 5(4):323-8.

Skegg DC, "Oral Contraceptives, Parity, and Cervical Cancer," *Lancet*, 2002, 359(9312):1080-1.

Spruance SL, Stewart JC, Rowe NH, et al, "Treatment of Recurrent Herpes Simplex Labialis With Oral Acyclovir," *J Infect Dis*, 1990, 161(2):185-90.

Woldeamanuel Y and Abate D, "Characterization of *Candida albicans* Isolates from the Oral Cavity of HIV-Positive Patients," *Ethiop Med J*, 1998, 36(4):235-43.

PERIODONTAL DISEASE

Bollen CM and Quirynen M, "Microbiological Response to Mechanical Treatment in Combination With Adjunctive Therapy. A Review of the Literature," *J Periodontol*, 1996, 67(11):1143-58.

Brecx M, Netuschil L, Reichart B, et al, "Efficacy of Listerine®, Meridol®, and Chlorhexidine Mouthrinses on Plaque, Gingivitis, and Plaque Bacteria Vitality," *J Clin Periodontol*, 1990, 17(1):292-7.

Ciancio SG, "Medications as Risk Factors for Periodontal Disease," *J Periodontol*, 1996, 67(Suppl 10):S1055-9.

Crout RJ, Lee HM, Schroeder K, et al, "The Cyclic Regimen of Low-Dose Doxycycline for Adult Periodontitis. A Preliminary Study," *J Periodontol*, 1996, 67(5):506-14.

DePaola LG, Overholser CD, Meiller TF, et al, "Chemotherapeutic Inhibition of Supragingival Dental Plaque and Gingivitis Development," *J Clin Periodontol*, 1989, 16(1):311-5.

Desvarieux M, "Periodontal Disease, Race, and Vascular Disease," *Compend Contin Educ Dent*, 2001, 22(3):34-41.

Elter JR, White BA, Gaynes BN, et al, "Relationship of Clinical Depression to Periodontal Treatment Outcome," *J Periodontol*, 2002, 73(4):441-9.

Genco RJ, "Current View of Risk Factors for Periodontal Diseases," *J Periodontol*, 1996, 67(Suppl 10):S1041-9.

Graves DT, Jiang Y, and Genco C, "Periodontal Disease: Bacterial Virulence Factors, Host Response and Impact on Systemic Health," *Curr Opin Infect Dis*, 2000, 13(3):227-232.

Greenstein G and Hart TC, "Clinical Utility of a Genetic Susceptibility Test for Severe Chronic Periodontitis: A Critical Evaluation," *J Am Dent Assoc*, 2002, 133(4):452-9.

Hitzig C, Charbit Y, Bitton C, et al, "Topical Metronidazole as an Adjunct to Subgingival Debridement in the Treatment of Chronic Periodontitis," *J Clin Periodontol*, 1994, 21(2):146-51.

Kjaerheim V, Skaare A, Barkvoll P, et al, "Antiplaque, Antibacterial, and Anti-inflammatory Properties of Triclosan Mouthrinses in Combination With Zinc Citrate or Polyvinylmethylether Maleic Acid (PVM-MA) Copolymer," *Eur J Oral Sci*, 1996, 104(5-6):529-34.

Loesche WJ, Giordano J, Soehren S, et al, "Nonsurgical Treatment of Patients With Periodontal Disease," *Oral Surg, Oral Med Oral Pathol*, 1996, 81(5):533-43.

Michalowicz BS, Pihlstrom BL, Drisko CL, et al, "Evaluation of Periodontal Treatments Using Controlled-Release Tetracycline Fibers: Maintenance Response," *J Periodontol*, 1995, 66(8):708-15.

Landry RG and Jean M, "Periodontal Screening and Recording (PSR) Index: Precursors, Utility and Limitations in a Clinical Setting," *Int Dent J*, 2002, 52(1):35-40.

Mealey BL, "Diabetes and Periodontal Disease: Two Sides of a Coin," *Compend Contin Educ Dent*, 2000, 21(11):943-6, 948, 950, passim.

Moseley R, Waddington RJ, and Embery G, "Hyaluronan and Its Potential Role in Periodontal Healing," *Dent Update*, 2002, 29(3):144-8.

Palomo F, Wantland L, Sanchez A, et al, "The Effect of Three Commercially Available Dentifrices Containing Triclosan on Supragingival Plaque Formation and Gingivitis: A Six Month Clinical Study," *Int Dent J*, 1994, 44(I Suppl 1):75-81.

Pavici MJ, van Winkelhoff AJ, Steures NH, et al, "Microbiological and Clinical Effects of Metronidazole and Amoxicillin in *Actinobacillus actinomycetemcomitans*-Associated Periodontitis. A 2-Year Evaluation," *J Clin Periodontol*, 1994, 21(2):107-12.

Ross NM, Mankodi SM, Mostler KL, et al, "Effects of Rinsing Time on Antiplaque Antigingivitis Efficacy of Listerine®, *J Clin Periodontol*, 1993, 20(1):279-81.

Seymour RA and Heasman PA, "Tetracyclines in the Management of Periodontal Diseases. A Review," *J Clin Periodontol*, 1995, 22(1):22-35.

Seymour RA and Heasman PA, "Pharmacological Control of Periodontal Disease. II Antimicrobial Agents," *J Dent*, 1995, 23(1):5-14.

Slots J and Ting M, "Systemic Antibiotics in the Treatment of Periodontal Disease," *Periodontol 2000*, 2002, 28:106-76.

PERIODONTOLOGY

Listgarten MA, "Pathogenesis of Periodontitis," *J Clin Periodontol*, 1986, 13(5):418-30.

Loesche WJ, Syed SA, Laughon BE, et al, "The Bacteriology of Acute Necrotizing Ulcerative Gingivitis," *J Periodontol*, 1982, 53(4):223-30.

PHARMACOLOGY OF DRUG METABOLISM AND INTERACTIONS

DeVane CL, "Pharmacogenetics and Drug Metabolism of Newer Antidepressant Agents," *J Clin Psychiatry*, 1994, 55(Suppl 12):38-45.

Hupp WS, " Seizure Disorders," *Oral Surg Oral Med Oral Pathol Oral Radiol Endod*, 2001, 92(6):593-6.

Ketter TA, Flockhart DA, Post RM, et al, "The Emerging Role of Cytochrome P450 3A in Psychopharmacology,"*J Clin Psychopharmacol*, 1995, 15(6):387-98.

Michalets EL, "Update: Clinically Significant Cytochrome P450 Drug Interactions," *Pharmacotherapy*, 1998, 18(1):84-112.

Moore PA, "Dental Therapeutic Indications for the Newer Long-Acting Macrolide Antibiotics," *J Am Dent Assoc*, 1999, 130(9):1341-3.

Nemeroff CB, DeVane CL, and Pollock BG, "Newer Antidepressants and the Cytochrome P450 System," *Am J Psychiatry*, 1996, 153(3):311-20.

Schmider J, Greenblatt DJ, von Moltke LL, et al, "Relationship of *In Vitro* Data on Drug Metabolism to *In Vivo* Pharmacokinetics and Drug Interactions: Implications for Diazepam Disposition in Humans," *J Clin Psychopharmacol*, 1996, 16(4):267-72.

Watkins PB, "Role of Cytochrome P450 in Drug Metabolism and Hepatotoxicity," *Semin Liver Dis*, 1990, 10(4):235-50.

Weinberg MA and Fine JB, "The Importance of Drug Interactions in Dental Practice," *Dent Today*, 2001, 20(9):88-93.

PREPROCEDURAL ANTIBIOTICS

"Advisory Statement. Antibiotic Prophylaxis for Dental Patients With Total Joint Replacement. American Dental Association; American Academy of Orthopaedic Surgeons," *J Am Dent Assoc*, 1997, 128(7):1004-8.

Bartzokas CA, Johnson R, Jane M, et al, "Relation Between Mouth and Haematogenous Infection in Total Joint Replacements," *BMJ*, 1994, 309(6953):506-8.

Berney P and Francioli P, "Successful Prophylaxis of Experimental Streptococcal Endocarditis With Single-Dose Amoxicillin Administered After Bacterial Challenge," *J Infect Dis*, 1990, 161(2):281-5.

Brause BD, "Infections Associated With Prosthetic Joints," *Clin Rheum Dis*, 1986, 12(2):523-36.

Chenoweth CE and Burket JS, "Antimicrobial Prophylaxis: Principles and Practice," *Formulary*, 1997, 32:692-708.

Ching DW, Gould IM, Rennie JA, et al, "Prevention of Late Haematogenous Infection in Major Prosthetic Joints," *J Antimicrob Chemother*, 1989, 23(5):676-80.

Clauzel AM, Visier S, and Michel FB, "Efficacy and Safety of Azithromycin in Lower Respiratory Tract Infections," *Eur Respir J*, 1990, 3(Suppl 10):S89.

Clemens JD and Ransohoff DF, "A Quantitative Assessment of Predental Antibiotic Prophylaxis for Patients With Mitral-Valve Prolapse," *J Chron Dis*, 1984, 37(7):531-44.

Dajani AS, Taubert KA, Wilson W, et al, "Prevention of Bacterial Endocarditis. Recommendations by the American Heart Association," *JAMA*, 1997, 277(22):1794-801.

Doern GV, Ferraro MJ, Brueggemann AB, et al, "Emergence of High Rates of Antimicrobial Resistance Among Viridans Group Streptococci in the United States," *Antimicrob Agents Chemother*, 1996, 40(4):891-4.

Durack DT, "Antibiotics for Prevention of Endocarditis During Dentistry: Time to Scale Back?" *Ann Intern Med*, 1998, 129(10):829-31.

Durack DT, "Prevention of Infective Endocarditis," *N Engl J Med*, 1995, 332(1):38-44.

Fluckiger U, Francioli P, Blaser J, et al, "Role of Amoxicillin Serum Levels for Successful Prophylaxis of Experimental Endocarditis Due to Tolerant Streptococci," *J Infect Dis*, 1994, 169(6):1397-400.

Hanssen AD, Osmon DR, and Nelson CL, "Prevention of Deep Prosthetic Joint Infection," *J Bone Joint Surg*, 1996, 78:458-71.

Little J, "The American Heart Association's Guidelines for the Prevention of Bacterial Endocarditis: A Critical Review," *Gen Dent*, 1998, 46:508-15.

"Risks for and Prevention of Infective Endocarditis," *Cardiology Clinics - Diagnosis and Management of Infective Endocarditis*, Child JS, ed, Philadelphia, PA: WB Saunders Co, 1996, 14:327-43.

Sale L, "Some Tragic Results Following Extraction of Teeth. II." *J Am Dent Assoc*, 1939, 26:1647-51.

Strom BL, Abrutyn E, Berlin JA, et al, "Dental and Cardiac Risk Factors for Infective Endocarditis. A Population-Based, Case-Control Study," *Ann Intern Med*, 1998, 129(10):761-9.

Strom BL, Abrutyn E, Berlin JA, et al, "Prophylactic Antibiotics to Prevent Infective Endocarditis? Relative Risks Reassessed," *J Investig Med*, 1996, 44:229.

Wahl M, "Myths of Dental-Induced Prosthetic Joint Infections," *Clin Infect Dis*, 1995, 20(5):1420-5.

Wynn RL, "Amoxicillin Update," *Gen Dent*, 1991, 39(5):322, 324, 326.

Wynn RL and Bergman SA, "Antibiotics and Their Use in the Treatment of Orofacial Infections, Part I," *Gen Dent*, 1994, 42(5): 398, 400, 402.

Wynn RL, "New Erythromycins," *Gen Dent*, 1996, 44(4):304-7.

Wynn RL, Meiller TF, and Crossley HL, "New Guidelines for the Prevention of Bacterial Endocarditis. American Heart Association," *Gen Dent*, 1997, 45(5):426-8, 430-4.

TEMPOROMANDIBULAR DYSFUNCTION

Amir I, Hermesh H, and Gavish A, "Bruxism Secondary to Antipsychotic Drug Exposure: A Positive Response to Propranolol," *Clin Neuropharmacol*, 1997, 20(1):86-9.

SUGGESTED READINGS *(Continued)*

Becker IM, "Occlusion as a Causative Factor in TMD. Scientific Basis to Occlusal Therapy," *NY State Dent J*, 1995, 61(9):54-7.

Bell WE, *Temporomandibular Disorders: Classification Diagnosis, Management*, 3rd ed, Chicago IL: Year Book Medical Publishers, 1990.

Bostwick JM and Jaffee MS, "Buspirone as an Antidote to SSRI-Induced Bruxism in 4 Cases," *J Clin Psychiatry*, 1999, 60(12):857-60.

Brown ES and Hong SC, "Antidepressant-Induced Bruxism Successfully Treated With Gabapentin," *J Am Dent Assoc*, 1999, 130(10):1467-9.

Carlson CR, Bertrand PM, Ehrlich AD, et al, "Physical Self-Regulation Training for the Management of Temporomandibular Disorders," *J Orofac Pain*, 2001, 15(1):47-55.

Canavan D and Gratt BM, "Electronic Thermography for the Assessment of Mild and Moderate Temporomandibular Joint Dysfunction," *Oral Surg Oral Med Oral Pathol Oral Radiol Endod*, 1995, 79(6):778-86.

Clark GT and Takeuchi H, "Temporomandibular Dysfunction, Chromic Orofacial Pain and Oral Motor Disorders in the 21st Century," *J Calif Dent Assoc*, 1995, 23(4):44-6, 48-50.

Dos Santos J Jr, "Supportive Conservative Therapies for Temporomandibular Disorders," *Dent Clin North Am*, 1995, 39(2):459-77.

Felicio CM, Mazzetto MO, and Perri Angote Dos Santos C, "Masticatory Behavior in Individuals With Temporomandibular Disorders," *Minerva Stomatol*, 2002, 51(4):111-20.

Gerber PE and Lynd LD, "Selective Serotonin Reuptake Inhibitor-Induced Movement Disorders," *Ann Pharmacother*, 1998, 32(6):692-8.

Maini S, Osborne JE, Fadl HM, et al, "Temporomandibular Joint Dysfunction Following Tonsillectomy," *Clin Otolaryngol*, 2002, 27(1):57-60.

Nicolakis P, Erdogmus B, Kopf A, et al, "Effectiveness of Exercise Therapy in Patients With Myofascial Pain Dysfunction Syndrome," *J Oral Rehabil*, 2002, 29(4):362-8.

Okeson JP, "Occlusion and Functional Disorders of the Masticatory System," *Dent Clin North Am*, 1995, 39(2):285-300.

Quinn JH, "Mandibular Exercises to Control Bruxism and Deviation Problems," *Cranio*, 1995, 13(1):30-4.

Schiffman E, Haley D, Baker C, et al, "Diagnostic Criteria for Screening Headache Patients for Temporomandibular Disorders," *Headache*, 1995, 35(3):121-4.

Thayer T, "Acupuncture TMD and Facial Pain," *SAAD Dig*, 2001, 18(3):3-7.

XEROSTOMIA

American Dental Association. ADA Guide to Dental Therapeutics, 2nd ed, Chicago, IL: ADA Publishing Co, Inc, 2001.

"Cevimeline (Evoxac) for Dry Mouth," *Med Lett Drugs Ther,* 2000, 42(1084):70.

Fox PC, Atkinson JC, Macynski AA, et al, "Pilocarpine Treatment of Salivary Gland Hypofunction and Dry Mouth (Xerostomia)," *Arch Intern Med,* 1991, 151(6):1149-52.

Johnson JT, Ferretti GA, Nethery WJ, et al, "Oral Pilocarpine for Post-Irradiation Xerostomia in Patients With Head and Neck Cancer," *N Eng J Med,* 1993, 329(6):390-5.

Johnstone PA, Niemtzow RC, and Riffenburgh RH, "Acupuncture for Xerostomia: Clinical Update," *Cancer*, 2002, 94(4):1151-6.

Nusair S and Rubinow A, "The Use of Oral Pilocarpine in Xerostomia and Sjögren's Sundrome," *Semin Arthritis Rheum,* 1999, 28(6):360-7.

Rhodus NL and Schuh MJ, "Effects of Pilocarpine on Salivary Flow in Patients With Sjögren's Syndrome," *Oral Surg Oral Med Oral Pathol,* 1991, 72(5):545-9.

Sanchez-Guerrero J, Aguirre-Garcia E, Perez-Dosal MR, et al, "The Wafer Test: A Semi-Quantitative Test to Screen for Xerostomia," *Rheumatology (Oxford)*, 2002, 41(4):381-9.

Ship JA, Pillemer SR, and Baum BJ, "Xerostomia and the Geriatric Patient," *J Am Geriatr Soc*, 2002, 50(3):535-43.

Sugerman PB and Barber MT, "Patient Selection for Endosseous Dental Implants: Oral and Systemic Considerations," *Int J Oral Maxillofac Implants*, 2002, 17(2):191-201.

Taylor SE and Miller EG, "Pre-emptive Pharmacologic Intervention in Radiation-Induced Salivary Dysfunction," *Proc Soc Exp Biol Med,* 1999, 221(1):14-26.

Tenovuo J, "Clinical Applications of Antimicrobial Host Proteins Lactoperoxidase, Lysozyme and Lactoferrin in Xerostomia: Efficacy and Safety," *Oral Dis*, 2002, 8(1):23-9.

Wray D, Lowe GD, Dagg JH, et al, *Textbook of General and Oral Medicine,* London, England: Churchill Livingstone, 1999.

Wynn RL, Meiller TF, and Crossley HL, *Drug Information Handbook for Dentistry,* 6th ed, Hudson (Cleveland), OH: Lexi-Comp, Inc, 2000.

Valdez IH, Wolff A, Atkinson JC, et al, "Use of Pilocarpine During Head and Neck Radiation Therapy to Reduce Xerostomia and Salivary Dysfunction," *Cancer,* 1993, 71(5):1848-51.

APPENDIX

TABLE OF CONTENTS

CALCIUM CHANNEL BLOCKERS AND GINGIVAL HYPERPLASIA

Drug	FDA Approval	Cases Cited in Literature
Amlodipine (Norvasc®)	1992	3
Bepridil (Vascor®)	1993	0
Diltiazem (Cardizem®, Dilacor®)	1982	>20
Felodipine (Plendil®)	1992	1
Isradipine (DynaCirc®)	1991	1
Nicardipine (Cardene®)	1989	0
Nifedipine (Adalat®, Procardia®)	1982	>120
Nimodipine (Nimotop®)	1989	0
Nisoldipine (Sular®)	1995	0
Nitrendipine[1] (Baypress®)		1
Verapamil (Calan®, Isoptin®, Verelan®)	1982	7

[1]Not yet approved for use in the United States.

SOME GENERAL OBSERVATIONS OF CCB-INDUCED GH

Calcium channel blockers (CCBs) are well known to cause gingival enlargement. In the early 1990s, it was thought that this class of drugs caused a true hyperplasia of the gingiva. Current thinking is that the term "hyperplasia" is inappropriate since the drug-induced effect results in an increase in extracellular tissue volume rather than an increase in the number of cells. Most of the reported cases of CCB-induced gingival enlargement have involved patients >50 years of age taking CCBs for postmyocardial infarction syndrome, angina pain, essential hypertension, and Raynaud's syndrome. Nifedipine (Procardia®) is associated with the highest number of reported cases in the literature, followed by diltiazem (Cardizem®). Depending on the CCB in question, gingival enlargement has appeared any time between 1-24 months after daily dosing. Discontinuance of the CCB usually results in complete disappearance or marked regression of symptoms, with symptoms reappearing upon remedication. The time required after drug discontinuance for marked regression of enlargement has been 1 week. Complete disappearance of all symptoms usually takes 2 months. If gingivectomy is performed and the drug retained or resumed, the gingival enlargement can recur. Only when the CCB is discontinued or a switch to a non-CCB occurs, will the gingivectomy usually be successful. One study of Nishikawa et al, showed that if nifedipine could not be discontinued, gingival enlargement did not recur after gingivectomy when extensive plaque control was carried out. If the CCB is changed to another class of cardiovascular drug, the enlargement will probably regress and disappear. A switch to another CCB, however, will probably result in continued gingival enlargement. For example, Giustiniani et al, reported disappearance of symptoms within 15 days after discontinuance of verapamil, with recurrence of symptoms after resumption with diltiazem. One case report described a nonsurgical management of a patient presenting with nifedipine-induced gingival overgrowth. Establishment and maintenance of a considerably improved standard of plaque control led to complete resolution of the overgrowth without recurrence, even though the medication dose was increased. The reader is referred to the review of 1991 for descriptive clinical and histological findings of CCB-induced gingival enlargement. A more recent review has been authorized by Silverstein et al, and published in 1997.

Two reports described the prevalence of amlodipine (Norvasc®)-induced gingival overgrowth. The study by Ellis et al, examined a sample of patients taking 1 of 3 CCBs who were drawn from a community-based population in northeastern England. Out of 911 patients, 442 were taking nifedipine, 181 amlodipine, and 186 diltiazem. In addition, 102 control subjects were included. It was found that 6.3% of subjects taking nifedipine were seen to have significant overgrowth, which was significantly greater than the overgrowth seen with the other two drug groups or the control group. The prevalence of gingival overgrowth induced by amlodipine or diltiazem was not significantly different compared to the control group. This study concluded that the prevalence of significant gingival overgrowth related to CCBs was low. Also, males were 3 times as likely as females to develop significant overgrowth.

In a second study by Jorgensen, a large group of patients taking amlodipine was studied in order to determine the prevalence of, what he called, "gingival hyperplasia". Out of 150 dentate patients who volunteered to undergo a screening examination, mild hyperplasia was found in 5 patients (3.3%). This was significantly less than rates reported for patients taking nifedipine and not significantly different from rates reported in control groups of cardiac patients not taking CCBs. Jorgensen concluded that amlodipine, at a dose of 5 mg daily, did not induce gingival hyperplasia.

There have been reports of verapamil-induced gingival enlargement in the literature with at least 7 cases listed in the review by this author. The prevalence of verapamil-induced enlargement, however, has not been investigated.

References

Bullon P, Machuca G, Armas JR, et al, "The Gingival Inflammatory Infiltrate in Cardiac Patients Treated With Calcium Antagonists," *J Clin Periodontol*, 2001, 28(10):897-903.

Ciantar M, "Nifedipine-Induced Gingival Overgrowth: Remission Following Nonsurgical Therapy," *Dent Update*, 1997, 45(4):371-6.

Desai P and Silver JG, "Drug-Induced Gingival Enlargements," *J Can Dent Assoc*, 1998, 64(4):263-8.

Ellis JS, Seymour RA, Steele JG, et al, "Prevalence of Gingival Overgrowth Induced by Calcium Channel Blockers: A Community-Based Study," *J Periodontol*, 1999, 70(1):63-7.

Giustiniani S, Robestelli della Cuna F, and Marieni M, "Hyperplastic Gingivitis During Diltiazem Therapy," *Int J Cardiol*, 1987, 15(2):247-9.

Hood KA, "Drug-Induced Gingival Hyperplasia in Transplant Recipients," *Prog Transplant*, 2002, 12(1):17-21.

Jorgensen MG, "Prevalence of Amlodipine-Related Gingival Hyperplasia, *J Periodontol*, 1997, 68(7):676-8.

Missouris GG, Kalaitzidis RG, Cappuccio FP, et al, "Gingival Hyperplasia Caused by Calcium Channel Blockers," *J Hum Hypertens.* , 2000, 14(2):155-6.

Nishikawa S, Tada H, Hamasaki A, et al, "Nifedipine-Induced Gingival Hyperplasia: A Clinical and *In Vitro* Study," *J Periodontol*, 1991, 62(1):30-5.

Silverstein LH, Garnick JJ, Szikman M, et al, "Medication-Induced Gingival Enlargement: A Clinical Review," *Gen Dent*, 1997, 45(4):371-6.

Wynn RL, "Calcium Channel Blockers and Gingival Hyperplasia," *Gen Dent*, 1991, 39(4):240-3.

Wynn RL, "Update on Calcium Channel Blocker-Induced Gingival Hyperplasia," *Gen Dent*, 1995, 43(3):218-20, 222.

DENTAL DRUG INTERACTIONS: UPDATE ON DRUG COMBINATIONS REQUIRING SPECIAL CONSIDERATIONS

This update discussion includes 16 drug interaction monographs describing clinically important drug combinations requiring special considerations in dental practice. The actions which have resulted from these combinations range from life-threatening adverse effects to attenuation of the therapeutic effects of the interacting drug. The monographs are organized according to the four major groups of drugs used in dentistry: antibiotics, nonsteroidal anti-inflammatory drugs (including aspirin), epinephrine (vasoconstrictors), and narcotic analgesics. An additional monograph on Valium® and alcohol is included.

ANTIBIOTICS - ORAL CONTRACEPTIVES

Description of the Interaction

Case reports suggest that antibiotics used in dentistry can reduce the effectiveness of oral contraceptives resulting in breakthrough ovulation and unplanned pregnancies.

Mechanism

Estrogens, which are components of oral contraceptives, are activated in the intestine by bacteria and reabsorbed into the blood stream as active compounds to inhibit ovulation. Antibiotics reduce the bacteria population in the intestine, which may result in less activated estrogen available to inhibit ovulation.

Background Reports

Tetracyclines: One report described a woman on an estrogen-type oral contraceptive who became pregnant after a 5-day course of tetracycline.[1] Also, several cases of unintended pregnancy and menstrual irregularities have been reported following concurrent use of tetracyclines and oral contraceptives.[2,3]

Penicillins: Ampicillin has been shown to reduce estrogen levels in women not taking oral contraceptives and there are reports of unplanned pregnancies in women taking ampicillin with oral contraceptives.[4,5] Concomitant use of penicillin with estrogen-containing oral contraceptives decreased the efficacy of the contraceptive and increased the incidence of breakthrough bleeding.[6,7] Since amoxicillin is closely related to other penicillins, it may also interact with oral contraceptives.

Cephalosporins: Cephalexin (Keflex®) has been reported to interact with oral contraceptives resulting in an unplanned pregnancy.[8]

Erythromycins: Unlike ampicillin and tetracyclines, erythromycins have been implicated in only a few cases of oral contraceptive failure over the last 15 years and it is questionable whether erythromycin was the cause of those reported failures.

Management

If antibiotics are prescribed to oral contraceptive users, it is suggested that the patients be advised to use additional methods of birth control during both 7- to 10-day dosing, and the two-dose prophylaxis regimens. Any additional method of birth control should be continued through the remaining oral contraceptive cycle.

1. Bacon JF and Shenfield GM, "Pregnancy Attributable to Interaction Between Tetracycline and Oral Contraceptives," *Br Med J*, 1980, 280(6210):293.
2. Orme ML, "The Clinical Pharmacology of Oral Contraceptive Steroids," *Br J Clin Pharmacol*, 1982, 14:31.
3. Back DJ, Grimmer SF, Orme ML, et al, "Evaluation of Committee on Safety of Medicines Yellow Card Reports on Oral Contraceptive-Drug Interactions With Anticonvulsants and Antibiotics," *Br J Clin Pharmacol*, 1988, 25(5):527-32.
4. Trybuchowski H, "Effect of Ampicillin on the Urinary Output of Steroidal Hormones in Pregnant and Nonpregnant Women," *Clin Chim Acta*, 1973, 45:9-18.
5. Aldercreutz H, Martin F, Lehtinen T, et al, "Effect of Ampicillin Administration on Plasma Conjugated and Unconjugated Estrogen and Progesterone Levels in Pregnancy," *Am J Obstet Gynecol*, 1977, 128(3):266-71.
6. Proudfit CW, "Concurrent Oral Contraceptive and Antibiotic Therapy," *JAMA*, 1981, 246:2076.
7. True RJ, "Interactions Between Antibiotics and Oral Contraceptives," *JAMA*, 1982, 247(10):1408.
8. Bainton R, "Interaction Between Antibiotic Therapy and Contraceptive Medication," *Oral Surg Oral Med Oral Pathol*, 1986, 61(5):453-5.

TETRACYCLINES - ANTACIDS (Containing Divalent or Trivalent Ions)

Description of the Interaction

Concomitant therapy with a tetracycline and an antacid containing aluminum, calcium, or magnesium can reduce serum concentration and the efficacy of the tetracycline.

Mechanism

Aluminum, calcium, and magnesium ions can combine with the tetracycline molecule in the gastrointestinal tract to form a larger ionized molecule unable to be absorbed into the blood stream.

Background

The interaction between tetracyclines and antacids containing aluminum, calcium, and magnesium is well documented. Foods and dairy products containing calcium will also impair the absorption of tetracyclines. Some reports suggest that doxycycline and minocycline are minimally affected by antacids and dairy products.[1,2]

Management

Tetracyclines should be given as far apart as possible from antacids and dairy products.

1. Welling PG, Koch PA, Lau CC, et al, "Bioavailability of Tetracycline and Doxycycline in Fasted and Nonfasted Subjects," *Antimicrob Agents Chemother*, 1977, 11(3):462-9.
2. "Anti-Infective Drug Interactions," *Drug Interactions and Updates*, Hansten PD and Horn JR, eds, Malvern, PA: Lea and Febiger.

TETRACYCLINE - PENICILLIN

Description of the Interaction

Simultaneous tetracycline-penicillin therapy may impair the efficacy of penicillin.

Mechanism

Penicillin kills bacteria by inhibiting cell wall synthesis. Tetracycline inhibits protein synthesis in bacteria and this action has been shown to antagonize the cell wall inhibiting effect of penicillin.

Background

Most of the manufacturers product information contains warnings against using tetracyclines and penicillins together.

Management

Tetracycline-penicillin combination should never be used to treat oral infections. For penicillin two-dose prophylaxis, it would be prudent not to give to patients taking tetracycline. Reappoint if possible.

ERYTHROMYCIN - PENICILLIN

Description of the Interaction

Simultaneous erythromycin-penicillin therapy may impair the efficacy of penicillin.

Mechanism

Penicillin kills bacteria by inhibiting cell wall synthesis. Erythromycin inhibits protein synthesis in bacteria and this action may antagonize the cell wall inhibiting effect of penicillin.

Background

This interaction has not been sufficiently documented in clinical studies.

Management

Erythromycin-penicillin combination should not be used to treat oral infections. For penicillin two-dose prophylaxis, it would be prudent not to give to patients taking erythromycin. Reappoint if possible.

ERYTHROMYCIN - THEOPHYLLINE

Description of the Interaction

Erythromycins interact with theophylline, a bronchodilator, to result in symptoms suggestive of a relative overdose of theophylline. Resulting symptoms were nausea, vomiting, and seizures.

DENTAL DRUG INTERACTIONS: UPDATE ON DRUG COMBINATIONS REQUIRING SPECIAL CONSIDERATIONS
(Continued)

Mechanism

A recent study showed that erythromycin forms complexes with a specific enzyme that metabolizes theophylline and that this complex may explain the impairment of theophylline metabolic inactivation resulting in symptoms of theophylline overdose.[1]

Background

An erythromycin regimen of 5- to 20-day daily dosing in theophylline patients caused increased blood levels, a longer half-life, and decreased urinary clearance of the theophylline.[2] A more recent review indicated that many patients did not experience any interactions between the two drugs with 8 out of 22 studies reporting no change in theophylline kinetics after erythromycin dosing.[3] The interactions which have occurred have included all formulations of erythromycin. There have been no reported interactions between erythromycin and theophylline when using the prophylaxis dosing schedule.

Management

Patients taking theophylline and who may be at increased risk for theophylline toxicity should be given erythromycin with caution and only if there is absolutely no alternative to erythromycin. These patients should be monitored closely.

1. Delaforge M and Sartori E, "In Vivo Effects of Erythromycin, Oleandomycin, and Erythralosamine Derivatives on Hepatic Cytochrome P-50," *Biochem Pharmacol*, 1990, 40(2):223-8.
2. Cummins LH, et al, "Erythromycin's Effect on Theophylline Blood Levels. Correspondence," *Pediatrics*, 1977, 59:144-5.
3. Ludden TM, "Pharmacokinetic Interactions of the Macrolide Antibiotics," *Clin Pharmacokinet*, 1985, 10(1):63-79.

ERYTHROMYCIN - CARBAMAZEPINE (Tegretol®)

Description of the Interaction

Erythromycin has interacted with carbamazepine (Tegretol®), an antiepileptic, to cause increased blood levels resulting in carbamazepine toxicity.[1] Symptoms were drowsiness, dizziness, nausea, headache, and blurred vision.

Mechanism

This interaction is suggestive of an inhibition of the hepatic metabolizing enzymes by erythromycin which normally convert carbamazepine to inactive products.

Background

The increased blood levels of carbamazepine have occurred within 1 day of concomitant erythromycin therapy.[1] This effect has not been reported with the two-dose erythromycin, prophylaxis regimen.

Management

Patients taking carbamazepine and who may be at increased risk for carbamazepine toxicity should be given erythromycin with caution and only if there is absolutely no alternative to erythromycin. These patients should be monitored closely.

1. Ludden TM, "Pharmacokinetic Interactions of the Macrolide Antibiotics," *Clin Pharmacokinet*, 1985, 10(1):63.

ERYTHROMYCIN - TRIAZOLAM (Halcion®)

Description of the Interaction

Erythromycin has interacted with triazolam (Halcion®), a hypnotic type antianxiety agent, to cause increased blood levels resulting in triazolam toxicity. Resulting effects were psychomotor impairment and memory dysfunction.

Mechanism

This interaction is suggestive of an inhibition of the hepatic metabolizing enzymes by erythromycin which normally convert triazolam to inactive products.

Background

Erythromycin has caused significant increases in triazolam blood concentrations within 3 days after 333 mg erythromycin base 3 times/day and triazolam 0.5 mg daily.[1]

Management

Patients taking triazolam should be given erythromycin with caution and only if there is absolutely no alternative to erythromycin. These patients should be closely monitored.

1. Phillips JP, "A Pharmacokinetic Drug Interaction Between Erythromycin and Triazolam," *J Clin Psychopharmacol*, 1986, 6(5):297-9.

IBUPROFEN (Motrin®, Advil®, Nuprin®) - ORAL ANTICOAGULANTS (Coumarins)

Description of the Interaction

Bleeding may occur when ibuprofen is administered to patients taking coumarin-type anticoagulants.

Mechanism

Inhibition of prostaglandins by ibuprofen results in decreased platelet aggregation and interference with blood clotting, resulting in an enhancement of the anticoagulant effect of coumarins.

Background

Product information on ibuprofen states that Motrin® inhibits platelet aggregation, but the effect is quantitatively less and of shorter duration than aspirin. It goes on to state that bleeding has been reported when Motrin® had been administered to patients on coumarin-type anticoagulants and the clinician should use caution in these circumstances. Caution is advised when using naproxen with coumarins since interactions have been seen with other NSAIDs of this class; diflunisal, when given with warfarin, has resulted in prolongation of prothrombin time and serious clinical bleeding has been reported in patients taking flurbiprofen together with coumarins. Product information states that ibuprofen, naproxen, and diflunisal may be responsible for increased prothrombin time response of warfarin (flurbiprofen was not mentioned).

Management

It is suggested that ibuprofen (Motrin®, Advil®, Nuprin®) and other dental NSAIDs such as naproxen (Naprosyn®), naproxen sodium (Anaprox®, Aleve®), diflunisal (Dolobid®), flurbiprofen (ANSAID®), and ketorolac (Toradol® Oral), be used with caution (if at all) in patients taking coumarin-type anticoagulants. Use of other analgesics is preferred.

IBUPROFEN (Motrin®, Advil®, Nuprin®) - LITHIUM

Description of the Interaction

Concurrent administration of ibuprofen with lithium produces symptoms of lithium toxicity including nausea, vomiting, slurred speech, and mental confusion.

Mechanism

Prostaglandins stimulate renal lithium tubular secretion. NSAIDs inhibit prostaglandin-induced renal secretion of lithium, which increases lithium plasma levels and produces symptoms of lithium toxicity.

Background

Lithium is used for the treatment of acute mania and to prevent recurrent episodes of bipolar (manic-depressive) illness. The therapeutic lithium plasma concentration is extremely narrow (0.8-1.2 mEq/L) and drugs that cause lithium plasma levels to go outside this narrow therapeutic range will result in lithium toxicity. Of the four NSAIDs used in dentistry (ibuprofen, naproxen, diflunisal, and flurbiprofen) the former two have been well documented to interact with lithium. In 1980, Ragheb et al, reported that a patient taking 2400 mg ibuprofen daily experienced nausea and drowsiness while stabilized on lithium.[1] The lithium plasma level increased from 0.8-1.0 mEq/L. Subsequently, in a study of 11 healthy volunteers, Kristoff et al, observed that 400 mg of ibuprofen 4 times/day combined with 450 mg of lithium carbonate every 12 hours, increased lithium plasma levels within several days.[2] Decreased ability to concentrate, lightheadedness, and fatigue resulted from this interaction.

Ragheb reported that concomitant administration of lithium and ibuprofen (1.8 g/day) in nine patients with bipolar- or schizoid-type disorders resulted in significant increases (average 34%) in lithium plasma concentrations as well as decreases in lithium clearance.[3] Individual variations were observed, with increases in lithium levels ranging from 12% to 66% within 6 days of concomitant administration of ibuprofen. In this study, tremors occurred in three patients as a result of this interaction. Ragheb reported that patients older than 50 years were more susceptible to

DENTAL DRUG INTERACTIONS: UPDATE ON DRUG COMBINATIONS REQUIRING SPECIAL CONSIDERATIONS *(Continued)*

lithium toxicity. Concomitant use of ibuprofen and lithium citrate or carbonate may elevate lithium plasma concentration and reduce renal lithium clearance.

In a 1986 study by Ragheb and Powell, concomitant administration of naproxen and lithium resulted in individual variations in plasma lithium concentration (from increases of 0% to 42%.[4] In that study, lithium renal clearance decreased in patients who were taking daily doses of lithium (900 mg) and naproxen (750 mg) for 6 days. Concomitant use of naproxen and lithium may increase lithium plasma concentration.

Interactions between diflunisal (Dolobid®) and lithium, flurbiprofen (Ansaid®) and lithium, and between these two NSAIDs and lithium have not been reported. However, lack of documentation about diflunisal and flurbiprofen does not mean these agents are safe to use with lithium. Interestingly, aspirin has been shown to affect plasma lithium concentration in healthy subjects.[5] NSAIDs should be used with caution by dental patients who are taking lithium. Substitution of NSAIDs with acetaminophen preparations may be warranted.

Management

Extreme caution is necessary in administering NSAIDs to lithium patients; use of analgesics other than NSAIDs is preferred.

1. Ragheb M, Ban TA, Buchanan D, et al, "Interaction of Indomethacin and Ibuprofen With Lithium in Manic Patients Under a Steady-State Lithium Level," *J Clin Psychiatry*, 1980, 41(11):397-8.
2. Kristoff CA, Hayes PE, Barr WH, et al, "Effect of Ibuprofen on Lithium Plasma and Red Blood Cell Concentrations," *Clin Pharm*, 1986, 5(1):51-5.
3. Ragheb M, "Ibuprofen Can Increase Serum Lithium Level in Lithium-Treated Patients," *J Clin Psychiatry*, 1987, 48(4):161-3.
4. Ragheb M and Powell AL, "Lithium Interaction With Sulindac and Naproxen," *J Clin Psychopharmacol*, 1986, 6(3):150-4.
5. Reimann IW, Diener U, and Frolich JC, "Indomethacin But Not Aspirin Increases Plasma Lithium Ion Levels," *Arch Gen Psychiatry*, 1983, 40(3):283-6.

ASPIRIN - ORAL ANTICOAGULANTS (Coumarins)

Description of the Interaction

Aspirin increases the risk of bleeding in patients taking oral anticoagulants.

Mechanism

Small doses of aspirin inhibit platelet function. Larger doses (>3 g/day) elicit a hypoprothrombinemic effect. Aspirin may also displace oral anticoagulants from plasma protein-binding sites. These actions of aspirin all contribute to increase the risk of bleeding in patients taking oral anticoagulants.

Background

There is much documentation in the literature confirming this interaction. One study using over 500 patients showed that excessive bleeding was about 3 times more common with warfarin (Coumadin®) plus aspirin (500 mg/day) than with warfarin alone.[1] Another study showed enhanced hypoprothrombinemia in warfarin patients during the first few days of aspirin therapy (1 g/day).[2] There are other reports describing bleeding episodes due to concurrent therapy with aspirin and oral anticoagulants.[3,4]

Management

Patients receiving oral anticoagulants should avoid aspirin and aspirin-containing products.

1. Chesebro JH, Fuster V, Elveback LR, et al, "Trial of Combined Warfarin Therapy Plus Dipyridamole or Aspirin Therapy in Prosthetic Heart Valve Replacement: Danger of Aspirin Compared With Dipyridamole," *Am J Cardiol*, 1983, 51(9):1537-41.
2. Donaldson DR, Sreeharan N, Crow MJ, et al, "Assessment of the Interaction of Warfarin With Aspirin and Dipyridamole," *Thromb Haemost*, 1982, 47(1):77.
3. Starr KJ and Petrie JC, "Drug Interactions in Patients on Long-Term Oral Anticoagulant and Antihypertensive Adrenergic Neuron-Blocking Drugs," *Br Med J*, 1972, 4(833):133-5.
4. Udall JA, "Drug Interference With Warfarin Therapy," *Clin Med*, 1970, 77:20.

ASPIRIN - PROBENECID (Benemid®)

Description of the Interaction

Aspirin inhibits the uricosuric action of probenecid.

Mechanism

Unknown

Background

The inhibition of probenecid-induced uricosuria by aspirin is dose-dependent. Doses of aspirin of 1 g or less do not appear to affect probenecid uricosuria. Larger doses, however, appear to considerably inhibit uricosuria. Conversely, probenecid appears to inhibit uricosuria following large doses of aspirin. Aspirin does not interfere with the actions of probenecid to inhibit the renal elimination of penicillins.

Management

It appears prudent to use a nonsalicylate-type analgesic (ie, acetaminophen or NSAID) in patients receiving probenecid as a uricosuric agent (treatment of gouty arthritis).

EPINEPHRINE (Vasoconstrictor) - TRICYCLIC ANTIDEPRESSANTS

Description of the Interaction

Use of epinephrine as vasoconstrictor in local anesthetic injections may cause a hypertensive interaction in patients taking tricyclic antidepressants.

Mechanism

Tricyclic antidepressants cause increases of norepinephrine in synaptic areas in the central nervous system and periphery. Epinephrine may add to the effects of norepinephrine resulting in vasoconstriction and transient hypertension.

Background

There is adequate information in the literature to confirm a hypertensive interaction between epinephrine, norepinephrine, and levonordefrin with TCAs. An I.V. infusion of epinephrine to healthy subjects receiving imipramine resulted in two- to fourfold increases in the pressor response to epinephrine.[1,2] Also cardiac dysrhythmias were reported. Although these effects were seen with I.V. infusions, these reports suggested that caution should certainly be exercised if epinephrine is administered by other routes. I.V. infusions of norepinephrine to healthy subjects receiving imipramine resulted in a four- to eightfold increase in the pressor response to norepinephrine,[1,2] and a later study showed a twofold increase in pressor response to norepinephrine.[3] Other tricyclics were associated with a threefold increase in pressor response to norepinephrine.[4] This increased pressor response was probably due to tricyclic antidepressant-induced inhibition of norepinephrine reuptake. Similar effects have been reported with levonordefrin.[5]

Management

The use of epinephrine in patients taking tricyclic type antidepressants is potentially dangerous. Use minimum amounts of vasoconstrictor with caution in patients on tricyclic antidepressants.

1. Boakes AJ, Laurence DR, Teoh PC, et al, "Interactions Between Sympathomimetic Amines and Antidepressant Agents in Man," *Br Med J*, 1973, 1(849):311-5.
2. Svedmyr N, "The Influence of a Tricyclic Antidepressive Agent (Protriptyline) on Some of the Circulatory Effects of Noradrenaline and Adrenaline in Man," *Life Sci*, 1968, 7(1):77-84.
3. Larochelle P, Hamet P, and Enjalbert M, "Response to Tyramine and Norepinephrine After Imipramine and Trazodone," *Clin Pharmacol Ther*, 1979, 26(1):24-30.
4. Mitchell JR, Cavanaugh JH, Arias L, et al, "Guanethidine and Related Agents. III. Antagonism by Drugs Which Inhibit the Norepinephrine Pump in Man," *J Clin Invest*, 1970, 49(8):1596-604.
5. Jastak JT and Yagiela JA, "Vasoconstrictors and Local Anesthesia: A Review and Rationale for Use," *J Am Dent Assoc*, 1983, 107(4):623-30.

DENTAL DRUG INTERACTIONS: UPDATE ON DRUG COMBINATIONS REQUIRING SPECIAL CONSIDERATIONS *(Continued)*

EPINEPHRINE (Vasoconstrictor) - MONOAMINE OXIDASE INHIBITORS

Description of the Interaction

Use of epinephrine as vasoconstrictor in local anesthetic injections may cause a hypertensive interaction in patients taking monoamine oxidase inhibitors.

Mechanism

Drugs which inhibit monoamine oxidase cause increases in the concentration of endogenous norepinephrine, serotonin, and dopamine in storage sites throughout the central nervous system. Epinephrine may add to the effects of norepinephrine resulting in vasoconstriction and transient hypertension.

Background

One study reported on four healthy subjects taking MAOIs and given I.V. epinephrine. There was no significant effect on heart rate or blood pressure.[1] This same study also showed a lack of interaction with norepinephrine and MAOIs. Nevertheless, it is advisable that vasoconstrictors be used with caution in these patients. Hansten and Horn[2] report that MAOIs may slightly increase the pressor response to norepinephrine and epinephrine, an action which appeared to be due to receptor sensitivity by the MAOI.

Management

There is a potential for unexpected increases in blood pressure when using epinephrine vasoconstrictor in patients taking monoamine oxidase inhibitors. Use vasoconstrictor with caution in these patients.

1. Boakes AJ, Laurence DR, Teoh PC, et al, "Interactions Between Sympathomimetic Amines and Antidepressant Agents in Man," *Br Med J*, 1973, 1(849):311-5.
2. Hansten PD and Horn JR, eds, "Monoamine Oxidase Inhibitor Interactions," *Drug Interactions and Updates*, Malvern, PA: Lea and Febiger, 1990, 387-8.

NARCOTIC ANALGESICS - CIMETIDINE (Tagamet®)

Description of the Interaction

Cimetidine may increase the adverse effects of narcotic analgesics.

Mechanism

The hepatic metabolism of narcotic analgesics to inactive products may be inhibited by cimetidine. The central nervous system effects of narcotic analgesics and cimetidine may be additive.

Background

One study reported that cimetidine, when given to patients taking meperidine (Demerol®), reduced the rate of renal excretion of the narcotic, resulting in increased sedation and an increase in respiratory depression.[1] Additional studies showed that cimetidine may inhibit the liver metabolism of meperidine and fentanyl, another narcotic analgesic thus exacerbating the sedative effects of both of these narcotics.[2,3]

Management

Although the side effects of cimetidine on codeine, hydrocodone, and oxycodone are unknown, it is advised to use caution in prescribing these narcotic analgesics in dental patients taking cimetidine. Ranitidine (Zantac®) is probably less likely to interact with narcotic analgesics.

1. Guay DR, Meatherall RC, Chalmers JL, et al, "Cimetidine Alters Pethidine Disposition in Man," *Br J Clin Pharmacol*, 1984, 18(6):907-14.
2. Knodell RG, Holtzman JL, Crankshaw DL, et al, "Drug Metabolism by Rat and Human Hepatic Microsomes in Response to Interaction With H_2-Receptor Antagonists," *Gastroenterology*, 1982, 82(1):84-8.
3. Lee HR, et al, "Effect of Histamine H_2-Receptors on Fentanyl Metabolism," *Pharmacologist*, 1982, 24:145.

BENZODIAZEPINES - Diazepam (Valium®) - ALCOHOL

Description of the Interaction

Alcohol may enhance the adverse psychomotor effects of benzodiazepines such as Valium®. Combined use may result in dangerous inebriation, ataxia, and respiratory depression.

Mechanism

Alcohol and benzodiazepines have additive central nervous system depressant activity. Also, alcohol may increase the gastrointestinal absorption of diazepam[1,2] leading to symptoms of diazepam overdose.

Background

There is much documentation in the literature to confirm the serious interaction between alcohol and benzodiazepines. Many controlled studies have shown that benzodiazepines, such as diazepam, enhance the detrimental effects of alcohol on simulated driving, reaction times, and other psychomotor skills.[3-6].

Management

Patients receiving benzodiazepines such as diazepam (Valium®) should be warned against consuming any alcohol until the benzodiazepine is cleared from the body. This is usually 48-72 hours after the last dose. This interaction has been unpredictable and significant CNS depression and ataxia have occurred with only a single dose of diazepam (5 mg) along with a moderate amount of alcohol.

1. Hayes SL, Pablo G, Radomski T, et al, "Ethanol and Oral Diazepam Absorption," *N Engl J Med*, 1977, 296(4)-186-9.
2. MacLeod SM, Giles HG, Parzalek G, et al, "Diazepam Actions and Plasma Concentrations Following Ethanol Ingestion," *Eur J Clin Pharmacol*, 1977, 11(5):345-9.
3. Linnoila M and Hakkinen S, "Effects of Diazepam and Codeine, Alone and in Combination With Alcohol, on Simulated Driving," *Clin Pharmacol Ther*, 1974, 15(4):368-73.
4. Linnoila M, "Effects of Diazepam, Chlordiazepoxide, Thioridazine, Haloperidol, Flupenthixole, and Alcohol on Psychomotor Skills Related to Driving," *Ann Med Exp Biol Fenn*, 1973, 51(3):125-32.
5. Linnoila M, "Drug Interaction on Psychomotor Skills Related to Driving: Diazepam and Alcohol," *Eur J Clin Pharmacol*, 1973, 5:186.
6. Morland J, Setekleiv J, Haffner JF, et al, "Combined Effects of Diazepam and Ethanol on Psychomotor Functions," *Acta Pharmacol Toxicol*, 1975, 34(1):5-15.

OCCUPATIONAL EXPOSURE TO BLOODBORNE PATHOGENS (UNIVERSAL PRECAUTIONS)

OVERVIEW AND REGULATORY CONSIDERATIONS

Every healthcare employee, from nurse to housekeeper, has some (albeit small) risk of exposure to HIV and other viral agents such as hepatitis B and Jakob-Creutzfeldt agent. The incidence of HIV-1 transmission associated with a percutaneous exposure to blood from an HIV-1 infected patient is approximately 0.3% per exposure.[1] In 1989, it was estimated that 12,000 United States healthcare workers acquired hepatitis B annually.[2] An understanding of the appropriate procedures, responsibilities, and risks inherent in the collection and handling of patient specimens is necessary for safe practice and is required by Occupational Safety and Health Administration (OSHA) regulations.

The Occupational Safety and Health Administration published its "Final Rule on Occupational Exposure to Bloodborne Pathogens" in the Federal Register on December 6, 1991. OSHA has chosen to follow the Center for Disease Control (CDC) definition of universal precautions. The Final Rule provides full legal force to universal precautions and requires employers and employees to treat blood and certain body fluids as if they were infectious. The Final Rule mandates that healthcare workers must avoid parenteral contact and must avoid splattering blood or other potentially infectious material on their skin, hair, eyes, mouth, mucous membranes, or on their personal clothing. Hazard abatement strategies must be used to protect the workers. Such plans typically include, but are not limited to, the following:

- safe handling of sharp items ("sharps") and disposal of such into puncture resistant containers
- gloves required for employees handling items soiled with blood or equipment contaminated by blood or other body fluids
- provisions of protective clothing when more extensive contact with blood or body fluids may be anticipated (eg, surgery, autopsy, or deliveries)
- resuscitation equipment to reduce necessity for mouth to mouth resuscitation
- restriction of HIV- or hepatitis B-exposed employees to noninvasive procedures

OSHA has specifically defined the following terms: **Occupational exposure** means reasonably anticipated skin, eye mucous membrane, or parenteral contact with blood or other potentially infectious materials that may result from the performance of an employee's duties. **Other potentially infectious materials** are human body fluids including semen, vaginal secretions, cerebrospinal fluid, synovial fluid, pleural fluid, pericardial fluid, peritoneal fluid, amniotic fluid, saliva in dental procedures, and body fluids that are visibly contaminated with blood, and all body fluids in situations where it is difficult or impossible to differentiate between body fluids; any unfixed tissue or organ (other than intact skin) from a human (living or dead); and HIV-containing cell or tissue cultures, organ cultures, and HIV- or HBV-containing culture medium or other solutions, and blood, organs, or other tissues from experimental animals infected with HIV or HBV. An **exposure incident** involves specific eye, mouth, other mucous membrane, nonintact skin, or parenteral contact with blood or other potentially infectious materials that results from the performance of an employee's duties.[3] It is important to understand that some exposures may go unrecognized despite the strictest precautions.

A written Exposure Control Plan is required. Employers must provide copies of the plan to employees and to OSHA upon request. Compliance with OSHA rules may be accomplished by the following methods.

- **Universal precautions (UPs)** means that all human blood and certain body fluids are treated as if known to be infectious for HIV, HBV, and other bloodborne pathogens. UPs do not apply to feces, nasal secretions, saliva, sputum, sweat, tears, urine, or vomitus unless they contain visible blood.
- **Engineering controls (ECs)** are physical devices which reduce or remove hazards from the workplace by eliminating or minimizing hazards or by isolating the worker from exposure. Engineering control devices include sharps disposal containers, self-resheathing syringes, etc.
- **Work practice controls (WPCs)** are practices and procedures that reduce the likelihood of exposure to hazards by altering the way in which a task is performed. Specific examples are the prohibition of two-handed recapping of needles, prohibition of storing food alongside potentially contaminated material, discouragement of pipetting fluids by mouth, encouraging handwashing after removal of gloves, safe handling of contaminated sharps, and appropriate use of sharps containers.
- **Personal protective equipment (PPE)** is specialized clothing or equipment worn to provide protection from occupational exposure. PPE includes gloves, gowns, laboratory coats (the type and characteristics will depend upon the task and degree of exposure anticipated), face shields or masks, and eye protection. Surgical caps or hoods and/or shoe covers or boots are required in instances in

which gross contamination can reasonably be anticipated (eg, autopsies, orthopedic surgery). If PPE is penetrated by blood or any contaminated material, the item must be removed immediately or as soon as feasible. **The employer must provide and launder or dispose of all PPE at no cost to the employee**. Gloves must be worn when there is a reasonable anticipation of hand contact with potentially infectious material, including a patient's mucous membranes or nonintact skin. Disposable gloves must be changed as soon as possible after they become torn or punctured. Hands must be washed after gloves are removed. OSHA has revised the PPE standards, effective July 5, 1994, to include the requirement that the employer certify in writing that it has conducted a hazard assessment of the workplace to determine whether hazards are present that will necessitate the use of PPE. Also, verification that the employee has received and understood the PPE training is required.[4]

Housekeeping protocols: OSHA requires that all bins, cans, and similar receptacles, intended for reuse which have a reasonable likelihood for becoming contaminated, be inspected and decontaminated immediately or as soon as feasible upon visible contamination and on a regularly scheduled basis. Broken glass that may be contaminated must not be picked up directly with the hands. Mechanical means (eg, brush, dust pan, tongs, or forceps) must be used. Broken glass must be placed in a proper sharps container.

Employers are responsible for teaching appropriate clean-up procedures for the work area and personal protective equipment. A 1:10 dilution of household bleach is a popular and effective disinfectant. It is prudent for employers to maintain signatures or initials of employees who have been properly educated. If one does not have written proof of education of universal precautions teaching, then by OSHA standards, such education never happened.

Pre-exposure and postexposure protocols: OSHA's Final Rule includes the provision that employees, who are exposed to contamination, be offered the hepatitis B vaccine at no cost to the employee. Employees may decline; however, a declination form must be signed. The employee must be offered free vaccine if he/she changes his/her mind. Vaccination to prevent the transmission of hepatitis B in the healthcare setting is widely regarded as sound practice.[5] In the event of exposure, a confidential medical evaluation and follow-up must be offered at no cost to the employee. Follow-up must include collection and testing of blood from the source individual for HBV and HIV if permitted by state law if a blood sample is available. If a postexposure specimen must be specially drawn, the individual's consent is usually required. Some states may not require consent for testing of patient blood after accidental exposure. One must refer to state and/or local guidelines for proper guidance.

The employee follow-up must also include appropriate postexposure prophylaxis, counseling, and evaluation of reported illnesses. The employee has the right to decline baseline blood collection and/or testing. If the employee gives consent for the collection but not the testing, the sample must be preserved for 90 days in the event that the employee changes his/her mind within that time. Confidentiality related to blood testing must be ensured. **The employer does not have the right to know the results** of the testing of either the source individual or the exposed employee.

MANAGEMENT OF OCCUPATIONAL EXPOSURE TO HIV IN THE WORKPLACE[6]

1. Likelihood of transmission of HIV-1 from occupational exposure is 0.2% per parenteral exposure (eg, needlestick) to blood from HIV infected patients.
2. Factors that increase risk for occupational transmission include advanced stages of HIV in source patient, hollow bore needle puncture, a poor state of health or inexperience of healthcare worker (HCW).
3. Immediate actions an exposed healthcare worker should take include aggressive first aid at the puncture site (eg, scrubbing site with povidone-iodine solution for 10 minutes) or at mucus membrane site (eg, saline irrigation of eye for 15 minutes). Then immediate reporting to the hospital's occupational medical service. The authors indicate that there is no direct evidence for the efficacy of their recommendations. Other institutions suggest rigorous scrubbing with soap.
4. After first aid is initiated, the healthcare worker should report exposure to a supervisor and to the institution's occupational medical service for evaluation.
5. Occupational medicine should perform a thorough investigation including identifying the HIV and hepatitis B status of the source, type of exposure, volume of inoculum, timing of exposure, extent of injury, appropriateness of first aid, as well as psychological status of the healthcare worker. HIV serologies should be performed on the healthcare worker. HIV risk counselling should begin at this point.
6. All parenteral exposures should be treated equally until they can be evaluated by the occupational medicine service, who will then determine the actual risk of exposure. Follow-up counselling sessions may be necessary.
7. Although the data are not clear, antiviral prophylaxis may be offered to healthcare workers who are parenterally or mucous membrane exposed. If used, antiretroviral prophylaxis should be initiated within 1-2 hours after exposure.

OCCUPATIONAL EXPOSURE TO BLOODBORNE PATHOGENS (UNIVERSAL PRECAUTIONS) *(Continued)*

8. Counselling regarding risk of exposure, antiviral prophylaxis, plans for follow up, exposure prevention, sexual activity, and providing emotional support and response to concerns are necessary to support the exposed healthcare worker. Follow-up should consist of periodic serologic evaluation and blood chemistries and counts if antiretroviral prophylaxis is initiated. Additional information should be provided to healthcare workers who are pregnant or planning to become pregnant.

HAZARDOUS COMMUNICATION

Communication regarding the dangers of bloodborne infections through the use of labels, signs, information, and education is required. Storage locations (eg, refrigerators and freezers, waste containers) that are used to store, dispose of, transport, or ship blood or other potentially infectious materials require labels. The label background must be red or bright orange with the biohazard design and the word biohazard in a contrasting color. The label must be part of the container or affixed to the container by permanent means.

Education provided by a qualified and knowledgeable instructor is mandated. The sessions for employees must include:

- accessible copies of the regulation
- general epidemiology of bloodborne diseases
- modes of bloodborne pathogen transmission
- an explanation of the exposure control plan and a means to obtain copies of the written plan
- an explanation of the tasks and activities that may involve exposure
- the use of exposure prevention methods and their limitations (eg, engineering controls, work practices, personal protective equipment)
- information on the types, proper use, location, removal, handling, decontamination, and disposal of personal protective equipment)
- an explanation of the basis for selection of personal protective equipment
- information on the HBV vaccine, including information on its efficacy, safety, and method of administration and the benefits of being vaccinated (ie, the employee must understand that the vaccine and vaccination will be offered free of charge)
- information on the appropriate actions to take and persons to contact in an emergency involving exposure to blood or other potentially infectious materials
- an explanation of the procedure to follow if an exposure incident occurs, including the method of reporting the incident
- information on the postexposure evaluation and follow-up that the employer is required to provide for the employee following an exposure incident
- an explanation of the signs, labels, and color coding
- an interactive question-and-answer period

RECORD KEEPING

The OSHA Final Rule requires that the employer maintain both education and medical records. The medical records must be kept confidential and be maintained for the duration of employment plus 30 years. They must contain a copy of the employee's HBV vaccination status and postexposure incident information. Education records must be maintained for 3 years from the date the program was given.

OSHA has the authority to conduct inspections without notice. Penalties for cited violation may be assessed as follows:

Serious violations. In this situation, there is a substantial probability of death or serious physical harm, and the employer knew, or should have known, of the hazard. A violation of this type carries a mandatory penalty of up to $7000 for each violation.

Other-than-serious violations. The violation is unlikely to result in death or serious physical harm. This type of violation carries a discretionary penalty of up to $7000 for each violation.

Willful violations. These are violations committed knowingly or intentionally by the employer and have penalties of up to $70,000 per violation with a minimum of $5000 per violation. If an employee dies as a result of a willful violation, the responsible party, if convicted, may receive a personal fine of up to $250,000 and/or a 6-month jail term. A corporation may be fined $500,000.

Large fines frequently follow visits to laboratories, physicians' offices, and healthcare facilities by OSHA Compliance Safety and Health Offices (CSHOS). Regulations are vigorously enforced. A working knowledge of the final rule and implementation of appropriate policies and practices is imperative for all those involved in the collection and analysis of medical specimens.

Effectiveness of universal precautions in averting exposure to potentially infectious materials has been documented.[7] Compliance with appropriate rules, procedures, and policies, including reporting exposure incidents, is a matter of personal professionalism and prudent self-preservation.

Footnotes

1. Henderson DK, Fahey BJ, Willy M, et al, "Risk for Occupational Transmission of Human Immunodeficiency Virus Type 1 (HIV-1) Associated With Clinical Exposures. A Prospective Evaluation," *Ann Intern Med*, 1990, 113(10):740-6.
2. Niu MT and Margolis HS, "Moving Into a New Era of Government Regulation: Provisions for Hepatitis B Vaccine in the Workplace, *Clin Lab Manage Rev*, 1989, 3:336-40.
3. Bruning LM, "The Bloodborne Pathogens Final Rule — Understanding the Regulation," *AORN Journal*, 1993, 57(2):439-40.
4. "Rules and Regulations," *Federal Register*, 1994, 59(66):16360-3.
5. Schaffner W, Gardner P, and Gross PA, "Hepatitis B Immunization Strategies: Expanding the Target," *Ann Intern Med*, 1993, 118(4):308-9.
6. Fahey BJ, Beekmann SE, Schmitt JM, et al, "Managing Occupational Exposures to HIV-1 in the Healthcare Workplace," *Infect Control Hosp Epidemiol*, 1993, 14(7):405-12.
7. Wong ES, Stotka JL, Chinchilli VM, et al, "Are Universal Precautions Effective in Reducing the Number of Occupational Exposures Among Healthcare Workers?" *JAMA*, 1991, 265(9):1123-8.

References

Buehler JW and Ward JW, "A New Definition for AIDS Surveillance," *Ann Intern Med*, 1993, 118(5):390-2.

Brown JW and Blackwell H, "Complying With the New OSHA Regs, Part 1: Teaching Your Staff About Biosafety," *MLO*, 1992, 24(4)24-8. Part 2: "Safety Protocols No Lab Can Ignore," 1992, 24(5):27-9. Part 3: "Compiling Employee Safety Records That Will Satisfy OSHA," 1992, 24(6):45-8.

Department of Labor, Occupational Safety and Health Administration, "Occupational Exposure to Bloodborne Pathogens; Final Rule (29 CFR Part 1910.1030), "*Federal Register*, December 6, 1991, 64004-182.

Gold JW, "HIV-1 Infection: Diagnosis and Management," *Med Clin North Am*, 1992, 76(1):1-18.

"Hepatitis B Virus: A Comprehensive Strategy for Eliminating Transmission in the United States Through Universal Childhood Vaccination," Recommendations of the Immunization Practices Advisory Committee (ACIP), *MMWR Morb Mortal Wkly Rep*, 1991, 40(RR-13):1-25.

"Mortality Attributable to HIV Infection/AIDS — United States", *MMWR Morb Mortal Wkly Rep*, 1991, 40(3):41-4.

National Committee for Clinical Laboratory Standards, "Protection of Laboratory Workers From Infectious Disease Transmitted by Blood, Body Fluids, and Tissue," NCCLS Document M29-T, Villanova, PA: NCCLS, 1989, 9(1).

"Nosocomial Transmission of Hepatitis B Virus Associated With a Spring-Loaded Fingerstick Device — California," *MMWR Morb Mortal Wkly Rep*, 1990, 39(35):610-3.

Polish LB, Shapiro CN, Bauer F, et al, "Nosocomial Transmission of Hepatitis B Virus Associated With the Use of a Spring-Loaded Fingerstick Device," *N Engl J Med*, 1992, 326(11):721-5.

"Recommendations for Preventing Transmission of Human Immunodeficiency Virus and Hepatitis B Virus to Patients During Exposure-Prone Invasive Procedures," *MMWR Morb Mortal Wkly Rep*, 1991, 40(RR-8):1-9.

"Update: Acquired Immunodeficiency Syndrome — United States," *MMWR Morb Mortal Wkly Rep*, 1992, 41(26):463-8.

"Update: Transmission of HIV Infection During an Invasive Dental Procedure — Florida," *MMWR Morb Mortal Wkly Rep*, 1991, 40(2):21-7, 33.

"Update: Universal Precautions for Prevention of Transmission of Human Immunodeficiency Virus, Hepatitis B Virus, and Other Bloodborne Pathogens in Healthcare Settings," *MMWR Morb Mortal Wkly Rep*, 1988, 37(24):377-82, 387-8.

NORMAL BLOOD VALUES

Test	Range of Normal Values
Complete blood count (CBC)	
White blood cells	4,500-11,000
Red blood cells (male)	4.6-6.2 x 10^6 μL
Red blood cells (female)	4.2-5.4 x 10^6 μL
Platelets	150,000-450,000
Hematocrit (male)	40% to 54%
Hematocrit (female)	38% to 47%
Hemoglobin (male)	13.5-18 g/dL
Hemoglobin (female)	12-16 g/dL
Mean corpuscular volume (MCV)	80-96 μm^3
Mean corpuscular hemoglobin (MCH)	27-31 pg
Mean corpuscular hemoglobin concentration (MCHC)	32% to 36%
Differential white blood cell count (%)	
Segmented neutrophils	56
Bands	3.0
Eosinophils	2.7
Basophils	0.3
Lymphocytes	34.0
Monocytes	4.0
Hemostasis	
Bleeding time (BT)	2-8 minutes
Prothrombin time (PT)	10-13 seconds
Activated partial thromboplastin time (aPTT)	25-35 seconds
Serum chemistry	
Glucose (fasting)	70-110 mg/dL
Blood urea nitrogen (BUN)	8-23 mg/dL
Creatinine (male)	0.1-0.4 mg/dL
Creatinine (female)	0.2-0.7 mg/dL
Bilirubin, indirect (unconjugated)	0.3 mg/dL
Bilirubin, direct (conjugated)	0.1-1 mg/dL
Calcium	9.2-11 mg/dL
Magnesium	1.8-3 mg/dL
Phosphorus	2.3-4.7 mg/dL
Serum electrolytes	
Sodium (Na^+)	136-142 mEq/L
Potassium (K^+)	3.8-5 mEq/L
Chloride (Cl^-)	95-103 mEq/L
Bicarbonate (HCO_3^-)	21-28 mmol/L
Serum enzymes	
Alkaline phosphatase	20-130 IU/L
Alanine aminotransferase (ALT) (formerly called SGPT)	4-36 units/L
Aspartate aminotransferase (AST) (formerly called SGOT)	8-33 units/L
Amylase	16-120 Somogyi units/dL
Creatine kinase (CK) (male)	55-170 units/L
Creatine kinase (CK) (female)	30-135 units/L

DENTIFRICE PRODUCTS

Brand Name	Abrasive Ingredient	Therapeutic Ingredient	Foaming Agent
Aim® Baking Soda Gel	Hydrated silica, sodium bicarbonate	Sodium monofluorophosphate 0.7% (fluoride 0.14%)	Sodium lauryl sulfate
	Other Ingredients: Sorbitol and related polyols, water, glycerin, SD alcohol 38B, flavor, cellulose gum, sodium saccharin, blue #1, yellow #10		
Aim® Extra Strength Gel	Hydrated silica	Sodium monofluorophosphate 1.2%	Sodium lauryl sulfate
	Other Ingredients: Sorbitol, water, PEG-32, SD alcohol 38B, flavor, cellulose gum, sodium saccharin, sodium benzoate, blue #1, yellow #10		
Aim® Regular Strength	Hydrated silica	Sodium monofluorophosphate 0.8% (fluoride 0.14%)	Sodium lauryl sulfate
	Other Ingredients: Sorbitol and other related polyols, water, glycerin, SD alcohol 38B, flavor, cellulose gum, sodium saccharin, blue #1, yellow #10		
Aim® Tartar Control Gel	Hydrated silica	Sodium monofluorophosphate 0.8% (fluoride 0.14%)	Sodium lauryl sulfate
	Other Ingredients: Sorbitol and related polyols, water, glycerin, zinc citrate trihydrate, SD alcohol 38B, flavor, cellulose gum, sodium saccharin, blue #1, yellow #10		
Aquafresh® Baking Soda Toothpaste	Calcium carbonate, hydrated silica, sodium bicarbonate	Sodium monofluorophosphate	Sodium lauryl sulfate
	Other Ingredients: Calcium carrageenan, cellulose gum, colors, flavor, glycerin, PEG-8, sodium benzoate, sodium saccharin, sorbitol, titanium dioxide, water		
Aquafresh® Extra Fresh Toothpaste*	Hydrated silica, calcium carbonate	Sodium monofluorophosphate	Sodium lauryl sulfate
	Other Ingredients: Sorbitol, water, glycerin, PEG-8, titanium dioxide, cellulose gum, flavor, sodium saccharin, sodium benzoate, calcium carrageenan, colors		
Aquafresh® for Kids Toothpaste*	Hydrated silica, calcium carbonate	Sodium monofluorophosphate	Sodium lauryl sulfate
	Other Ingredients: Sorbitol, water, glycerin, PEG-8, titanium dioxide, cellulose gum, flavor, sodium saccharin, calcium carrageenan, sodium benzoate, colors		
Aquafresh® Gum Care Toothpaste	Hydrated silica, calcium carbonate	Sodium monofluorophosphate	Sodium lauryl sulfate
	Other Ingredients: Calcium carrageenan, cellulose gum, colors, flavor, PEG-8, sodium benzoate, sodium saccharin, sorbitol, titanium dioxide, water		
Aquafresh® Sensitive Toothpaste	Hydrated silica	Potassium nitrate, sodium fluoride	Sodium lauryl sulfate
	Other Ingredients: Colors, flavor, glycerin, sodium benzoate, sodium saccharin, sorbitol, titanium dioxide, water, xanthan gum		
Aquafresh® Tartar Control Toothpaste*	Hydrated silica	Sodium fluoride	Sodium lauryl sulfate
	Other Ingredients: Tetrapotassium pyrophosphate, tetrasodium pyrophosphate, sorbitol, glycerin, PEG-8, flavor, xanthan gum, sodium saccharin, sodium benzoate, colors, titanium dioxide, water		
Aquafresh® Triple Protection Toothpaste*	Hydrated silica, calcium carbonate	Sodium monofluorophosphate	Sodium lauryl sulfate
	Other Ingredients: PEG-8, sorbitol, cellulose gum, sodium benzoate, titanium dioxide, calcium carrageenan, flavor, sodium saccharin, colors, water		
Aquafresh® Whitening Gel or Toothpaste	Hydrated silica	Sodium fluoride	Sodium lauryl sulfate
	Other Ingredients: Colors, flavor, glycerin, PEG-8, sodium benzoate, sodium hydroxide, sodium saccharin, sodium tripolyphosphate, sorbitol, titanium dioxide, water, xanthan gum		
Biotene® Antibacterial Dry Mouth Toothpaste	Hydrated silica, calcium pyrophosphate	Lactoperoxidase, glucose oxidase, lysozyme, sodium monofluorophosphate (0.76%)	
	Other Ingredients: Sorbitol, glycerin, xylitol, isoceteth-20, cellulose gum, flavor, sodium benzoate, beta-d-glucose, potassium thiocyanate		
Close-Up® Baking Soda Toothpaste (mint)	Hydrated silica, sodium bicarbonate	Sodium monofluorophosphate 0.79% (fluoride 0.15%)	Sodium lauryl sulfate

DENTIFRICE PRODUCTS *(Continued)*

Brand Name	Abrasive Ingredient	Therapeutic Ingredient	Foaming Agent
	Other Ingredients: Sorbitol and related polyols, water, glycerin, SD alcohol 38B, flavor, cellulose gum, sodium saccharin, sodium benzoate, red #33, red #40, titanium dioxide		
Close-Up® Classic Red Gel	Hydrated silica	Sodium monofluorophosphate 0.8% (fluoride 0.14%)	Sodium lauryl sulfate
	Other Ingredients: Sorbitol and related polyols, water, glycerin, SD alcohol 38B, flavor, cellulose gum, sodium saccharin, sodium chloride, red #33, red #40		
Close-Up® Cool Mint Gel	Hydrated silica	Sodium monofluorophosphate 0.79% (fluoride 0.15%)	Sodium lauryl sulfate
	Other Ingredients: Sorbitol, water, glycerin, SD alcohol 38B, flavor, cellulose gum, sodium saccharin, polysorbate 20, blue #1, mica, red #33, titanium dioxide		
Close-Up® Original Red Whitening Toothpaste	Hydrated silica	Sodium monofluorophosphate 0.8% (fluoride 0.14%)	Sodium lauryl sulfate
	Other Ingredients: Sorbitol and related polyols, water, glycerin, SD alcohol 38B, flavor, cellulose gum, sodium saccharin, sodium chloride, red #30 lake, titanium dioxide, blue #1		
Close-Up® Tartar Control Gel (mint)	Hydrated silica	Sodium monofluorophosphate 0.79% (fluoride 0.15%)	Sodium lauryl sulfate
	Other Ingredients: Sorbitol and related polyols, water, glycerin, zinc citrate trihydrate, SD alcohol 38B, flavor, cellulose gum, sodium saccharin, red #33, red #40, **caffeine free**		
Close-Up® Tartar Control Whitening Toothpaste	Hydrated silica	Sodium monofluorophosphate 0.8% (fluoride 0.14%)	Sodium lauryl sulfate
	Other Ingredients: Sorbitol and related polypols, water, glycerin, SD alcohol 38B, flavor, zinc citrate trihydrate, cellulose gum, sodium saccharin, titanium dioxide, blue #1, yellow #10		
Colgate® Baking Soda & Peroxide Tartar Control Toothpaste*	Hydrated silica, sodium bicarbonate	Sodium monofluorophosphate 0.76%	Sodium lauryl sulfate
	Other Ingredients: Glycerin, propylene glycol, water, pentasodium triphosphate, tetrasodium pyrophosphate, titanium dioxide, flavor, sodium hydroxide, calcium peroxide, sodium saccharin, carrageenan, cellulose gum, FD&C blue #1, D&C yellow #10		
Colgate® Baking Soda & Peroxide Whitening Toothpaste*	Hydrated silica, sodium bicarbonate, aluminum oxide	Sodium monofluorophosphate 0.76%	Sodium lauryl sulfate
	Other Ingredients: Glycerin, polypylene glycol, water, pentasodium triphosphate, tetrasodium pyrophosphate, titanium dioxide, flavor, sodium hydroxide, calcium peroxide, sodium saccharin, carrageenan, cellulose gum, **dietetically sucrose free**		
Colgate® Baking Soda Tartar Control Gel or Toothpaste	Hydrated silica, sodium bicarbonate	Sodium fluoride 0.243%	Sodium lauryl sulfate
	Other Ingredients: Glycerin, tetrasodium pyrophosphate, PVM/MA copolymer, cellulose gum, flavor, sodium saccharin, sodium hydroxide, titanium dioxide (paste), FD&C blue #1, D&C yellow #10 (gel), **dietetically sucrose free**		
Colgate® Junior Gel*	Hydrated silica	Sodium fluoride 0.243%	Sodium lauryl sulfate
	Other Ingredients: Sorbitol, water, PEG-12, flavor, tetrasodium pyrophosphate, cellulose gum, sodium saccharin, mica, titanium dioxide, colorants, **dietetically sucrose free**		
Colgate® Platinum™ Whitening Toothpaste*	Silica, aluminum oxide	Sodium monofluorophosphate	Sodium lauryl sulfate
	Other Ingredients: Water, hydrated silica, sorbitol, glycerin, PEG-12, tetrapotassium pyrophosphate, PVM/MA copolymer, flavor, sodium hydroxide, sodium saccharin, titanium dioxide		
Colgate® Platinum™ Whitening with Baking Soda Toothpaste*	Sodium bicarbonate, aluminum oxide	Sodium monofluorophosphate 0.76%	Sodium lauryl sulfate
	Other Ingredients: Water, glycerin, PEG-12, tetrapotassium pyrophosphate, PVM/MA copolymer, flavor, sodium hydroxide, sodium saccharin, titanium dioxide, cellulose gum		
Colgate® Sensitive Maximum Strength Toothpaste	Hydrated silica, sodium bicarbonate	Potassium nitrate 5%, stannous fluoride 0.45%	Sodium lauryl sulfate

Brand Name	Abrasive Ingredient	Therapeutic Ingredient	Foaming Agent
	Other Ingredients: Glycerin and/or sorbitol, water, PEG-40 castor oil, PEG-12, poloxamer 407, sodium citrate, flavor, titanium dioxide, sodium hydroxide, cellulose gum, xanthan gum, sodium saccharin, stannous chloride, citric acid, tetrasodium pyrophosphate, FD&C Blue No. 1		
Colgate® Sensitive Plus Whitening	Hydrated silica, Sodium bicarbonate	Potassium nitrate 5% antisensitivity (FDA required amount), Stannous Fluoride 0.45% (0.15% w/v fluoride ion)	Sodium lauryl sulfate
	Other Ingredients: Glycerin and/or sorbitol, water, PEG-40 castor oil, PEG-12, poloxamer 405, sodium citrate, flavor, titanium dioxide, sodium hydroxide, cellulose gum, xanthan gum, sodium saccharin, stannous chloride, citric acid, tetrasodium pyrophosphate, mica, FD&C blue No.1, D&C yellow No. 10		
Colgate® Tartar Control Micro Cleansing Gel or Toothpaste*	Hydrated silica	Sodium fluoride 0.243%	Sodium lauryl sulfate
	Other Ingredients: Water, sorbitol, glycerin, PEG-12, tetrasodium pyrophosphate, PVM/MA copolymer, cellulose gum, flavor, sodium hydroxide, titanium dioxide, sodium saccharin, carrageenan, **dietetically sucrose free**		
Colgate® Tartar Control Plus Whitening	Hydrated silica, aluminum oxide	Sodium monofluorophosphate 0.76%	Sodium lauryl sulfate
	Other Ingredients: Water, sorbitol, glycerin, pentasodium triphosphate, tetrasodium pyrophosphate, PVM/MA copolymer, cellulose gum, flavor, sodium hydroxide, titanium dioxide, sodium saccharin, carrageenan		
Colgate® Toothpaste*	Dicalcium phosphate dihydrate	Sodium monofluorophosphate 0.76%	Sodium lauryl sulfate
	Other Ingredients: Glycerin, cellulose gum, tetrasodium pyrophosphate, sodium saccharin, flavor, **dietetically sucrose free**		
Colgate Total® Toothpaste	Hydrated silica	Sodium fluoride 0.243%, triclosan 0.3%	Sodium lauryl sulfate
	Other Ingredients: Water, glycerin, sorbitol, PVM/MA copolymer, cellulose gum, flavor, sodium hydroxide, propylene glycol, carrageenan, sodium saccharin, titanium dioxide		
Colgate Total® Fresh Stripe Toothpaste	Hydrated silica	Sodium fluoride 0.243%, triclosan 0.3%	Sodium lauryl sulfate
	Other Ingredients: Water, glycerin, sorbitol, PVM/MA copolymer, cellulose gum, flavor, sodium hydroxide, propylene glycol, carrageenan, sodium saccharin, mica, titanium dioxide, FD&C blue #1, D&C yellow #10		
Colgate® Winterfresh Gel*	Hydrated silica	Sodium fluoride 0.243%	Sodium lauryl sulfate
	Other Ingredients: Sorbitol, water, PEG-12, flavor, tetrasodium pyrophosphate, cellulose gum, sodium saccharin, FD&C blue #1, **dietetically sucrose free**		
Crest® Baking Soda Tartar Protection Gel or Toothpaste (mint)*	Hydrated silica, sodium bicarbonate	Sodium fluoride 0.243%	Sodium lauryl sulfate
	Other Ingredients: Water, glycerin, sorbitol, tetrasodium pyrophosphate, PEG-6, flavor, cellulose gum, sodium saccharin, titanium dioxide (paste), FD&C blue #1 (gel), disodium pyrophosphate, tetrapotassium pyrophosphate, carbomer 956, xanthan gum, FD&C yellow #5 (gel)		
Crest® Cavity Protection with Baking Soda Gel or Toothpaste (mint)*	Hydrated silica, sodium bicarbonate	Sodium fluoride 0.243%	Sodium lauryl sulfate
	Other Ingredients: Sorbitol, water, glycerin, sodium carbonate, flavor, cellulose gum, sodium saccharin, titanium dioxide (paste), FD&C blue #1 (gel)		
Crest® Cavity Protection Gel (cool mint)*	Hydrated silica	Sodium fluoride 0.243%	Sodium lauryl sulfate
	Other Ingredients: Sorbitol, water, trisodium phosphate, flavor, sodium phosphate, xanthan gum, sodium saccharin, carbomer 956, FD&C blue #1, carbomer 940A		
Crest® Cavity Protection Toothpaste* (icy mint or regular)	Hydrated silica	Sodium fluoride 0.243%	Sodium lauryl sulfate

DENTIFRICE PRODUCTS *(Continued)*

Brand Name	Abrasive Ingredient	Therapeutic Ingredient	Foaming Agent
	Other Ingredients: Sorbitol, water, glycerin (mint), trisodium phosphate, flavor, sodium phosphate, cellulose gum (mint), xanthan gum (regular), sodium saccharin, carbomer 956, titanium dioxide, FD&C blue #1. carbomer 940A		
Crest® Extra Whitening Gel or Toothpaste	Hydrated silica	Sodium fluoride 0.15%	Sodium lauryl sulfate, poloxamer 407
	Other Ingredients: Sorbitol, water, glycerin, tetrasodium pyrophosphate, sodium carbonate, carboxymethylcellulose sodium, titanium dioxide, carnauba wax, sodium saccharin, flavor, FD&C blue #1, FD&C yellow #5, PEG-6, sodium bicarbonate†		
Crest® for Kids Cavity Protection Gel	Hydrated silica	Sodium fluoride 0.243%	Sodium lauryl sulfate
	Other Ingredients: Sorbitol, water, trisodium phosphate, sodium phosphate, xanthan gum, flavor, sodium saccharin, carbomer 956, mica, titanium dioxide, FD&C blue #1		
Crest® Gum Care Gel or Toothpaste	Hydrated silica	Stannous fluoride 0.454%	Sodium lauryl sulfate
	Other Ingredients: Sorbitol, water, stannous chloride, titanium dioxide (paste), flavor, sodium hydroxide, sodium saccharin, sodium carrageenan, FD&C blue #1 (gel), sodium gluconate, hydroxyethylcellulose		
Crest® Multicare Gel or Toothpaste (cool mint, fresh mint)	Hydrated silica, sodium bicarbonate	Sodium fluoride 0.243%	Sodium lauryl sulfate
	Other Ingredients: Tetrasodium pyrophosphate, xylitol, water, glycerin, PEG-6, poloxamer 407, sodium carbonate, flavor, cellulose gum, xanthan gum, sodium saccharin, titanium dioxide, FD&C blue #1, FD&C yellow #5 (cool mint)		
Crest® Sensitivity Protection Toothpaste* (mild mint)	Hydrated silica	Potassium nitrate 5%, sodium fluoride 0.15%	Sodium lauryl sulfate
	Other Ingredients: Water, glycerin, sorbitol, trisodium phosphate, cellulose gum, flavor, xanthan gum, sodium saccharin, titanium dioxide, **dye free**		
Crest® Tartar Protection Gel* (fresh mint, smooth mint)		Sodium fluoride 0.243%	Sodium lauryl sulfate
	Other Ingredients: Water, sorbitol, glycerin, tetrapotassium pyrophosphate, PEG-6, disodium pyrophosphate, tetrasodium pyrophosphate, flavor, xanthan gum, sodium saccharin, carbomer 956, FD&C blue #1, FD&C yellow #5 (smooth mint)		
Crest® Tartar Protection Toothpaste* (original flavor)	Silica	Sodium fluoride 0.243%	Sodium lauryl sulfate
	Other Ingredients: Water, sorbitol, glycerin, tetrapotassium pyrophosphate, PEG-6, disodium pyrophosphate, tetrasodium pyrophosphate, flavor, xanthan gum, sodium saccharin, carbomer 956, titanium dioxide, FD&C blue #1		
Crest® Whitening Plus Scope®	Hydrated silica	Sodium fluoride 0.243% (0.15% w/v fluoride ion)	Sodium lauryl sulfate
	Other ingredients: Water, sorbitol, glycerin, tetrapotassium pyrophosphate, PEG-6, disodium pyrophosphate, tetrasodium pyrophosphate, flavor, alcohol (1.14%), xanthan gum, sodium saccharin, carbomer 956, polysorbate 80, sodium benzoate, cetylpyridinium chloride, benzoic acid, domiphen bromide (.0002 w/v%)		
Dr. Tichenor's Toothpaste	Hydrated silica	Sodium fluoride	Sodium lauryl sulfate
	Other Ingredients: Water, glycerin, sorbitol, insoluble sodium metaphosphate, peppermint oil, cellulose gum, sodium saccharin, sodium phosphate, titanium dioxide, magnesium aluminum silicate, **dye free**		
Enamelon® All-Family Toothpaste	Hydrated silica	Sodium fluoride (fluoride 0.14%)	Sodium lauryl sulfate
	Other Ingredients: Water, glycerin, sorbitol, monoammonium phosphate, calcium sulfate, xanthan gum, flavor, PEG-60 hydrogenated castor oil, sodium saccharin, ammonium chloride, cellulose gum, titanium dioxide, magnesium chloride, methylparaben, propylparaben, FD&C blue #1		
First Teeth™ Baby Gel		Lactoperoxidase 0.7 units/g, lactoferrin, glucose oxidase	Sodium lauryl sulfate
	Other Ingredients: Water, glycerin, sorbitol, pectin, xylitol, flavor, aloe vera, propylene glycol		

Brand Name	Abrasive Ingredient	Therapeutic Ingredient	Foaming Agent
Fluoride Foam™*‡	**Ingredients:** Fluoride 1.23% (from sodium fluoride and hydrogen fluoride), water, phosphoric acid, poloxamer, sodium saccharin, flavor		
Fluorigard® Anti-Cavity Liquid*‡	**Ingredients:** Sodium fluoride 0.05%, ethyl alcohol, pluronic F108 and F127, sweetener, flavor, glycerin, sorbitol, preservatives, **dye free, gluten free**		
Gleem® Toothpaste	Hydrated silica	Sodium fluoride 0.243%	Sodium lauryl sulfate
	Other Ingredients: Sorbitol, water, trisodium phosphate, flavors, sodium phosphate, xanthan gum, sodium saccharin, carbomer 956, titanium dioxide, **dye free**		
Listerine® Essential Care Gel	Hydrated silica	Anticavity: Sodium monofluorophosphate 0.76% (0.13% W/V fluoride ion Antiplaque/ Antigingivitis: Eucalyptol 0.738%, menthol 0.340%, methyl salicylate 0.480%, thymol 0.511%	Sodium lauryl sulfate
	Other Ingredients: Water, sorbitol, glycerin, flavors, cellulose gum, sodium saccharin, phosphoric acid, FD&C blue #1, D&C yellow #10, sodium phosphate, benzoic acid, PEG-32, and xanthan gum		
Listerine® Gel or Toothpaste (cool mint)	Hydrated silica	Sodium monofluorophosphate	Sodium lauryl sulfate
	Other Ingredients: Water, sorbitol, glycerin, flavors, cellulose gum, sodium saccharin, phosphoric acid, FD&C blue #1, D&C yellow #10, sodium phosphate, benzoic acid, titanium dioxide (paste), xanthan gum		
Listerine® Tartar Control Gel or Toothpaste (cool mint)	Hydrated silica	Sodium fluoride	Sodium lauryl sulfate
	Other Ingredients: Water, sorbitol, glycerin, PEG-32, flavor, cellulose gum, sodium saccharin, tetrapotassium pyrophosphate, FD&C blue #1, D&C yellow #10, titanium dioxide (paste)		
Mentadent® Advanced Whitening Gel or Toothpaste	Hydrated silica, sodium bicarbonate	Sodium fluoride 0.15%	Sodium lauryl sulfate, hydrogen peroxide
	Other Ingredients: Zinc citrate trihydrate, water, sorbitol, glycerin, poloxamer 407, PEG-32, SD alcohol 38B, flavor, cellulose gum, sodium saccharin, phosphoric acid, blue #1, titanium dioxide		
Mentadent® Gum Care Gel or Toothpaste	Hydrated silica, sodium bicarbonate	Sodium fluoride 0.24% (fluoride 0.15%)	Sodium lauryl sulfate, hydrogen peroxide
	Other Ingredients: Zinc citrate trihydrate (1.8%), water, sorbitol, glycerin, poloxamer 407, PEG-32, SD alcohol 38B, flavor, cellulose gum, sodium saccharin, menthol, methyl salicylate, phosphoric acid, green #3, titanium dioxide		
Mentadent® Tartar Control Gel or Toothpaste	Hydrated silica, sodium bicarbonate	Sodium fluoride 0.24%	Sodium lauryl sulfate, hydrogen peroxide
	Other Ingredients: Water, sorbitol, glycerin, poloxamer 407, PEG-32, zinc citrate, SD alcohol 38B, flavor, cellulose gum, sodium saccharin, phosphoric acid, blue #1, titanium dioxide, menthol		
Mentadent® with Baking Soda & Peroxide Gel or Toothpaste*	Hydrated silica, sodium bicarbonate	Sodium fluoride 0.24% (fluoride 0.15%)	Sodium lauryl sulfate, hydrogen peroxide
	Other Ingredients: Water, sorbitol, glycerin, poloxamer 407, PEG-32, SD alcohol 38B, flavor, cellulose gum, sodium saccharin, phosphoric acid, blue #1, titanium dioxide		
My First Colgate® Gel*	Hydrated silica	Sodium fluoride 0.243%	Sodium lauryl sulfate
	Other Ingredients: Water, sorbitol, PEG-12, flavor, tetrasodium pyrophosphate, cellulose gum, sodium saccharin, FD&C red #40, D&C red #33, **dietetically sucrose free**		
Natural White® Toothpaste	Hydrated silica	Sodium fluoride	Sodium lauryl sulfate
	Other Ingredients: Sorbitol, water, glycerin, sodium benzoate, titanium dioxide, flavor, cellulose gum, **dietetically sucrose free**		
Natural White® Baking Soda Toothpaste	Calcium carbonate	Sodium monofluorophosphate	Sodium lauryl sulfate
	Other Ingredients: Sorbitol, water, glycerin, sodium bicarbonate†, carrageenan, natural flavor, **dietetically sucrose free**		
Natural White® Fights Plaque Toothpaste	Hydrated silica	Sodium fluoride	Sodium lauryl sulfate

DENTIFRICE PRODUCTS *(Continued)*

Brand Name	Abrasive Ingredient	Therapeutic Ingredient	Foaming Agent
	Other Ingredients: Sorbitol, water, glycerin, sodium benzoate, titanium dioxide, flavor, cellulose gum, **dietetically sucrose free**		
Natural White® Sensitive Toothpaste	Hydrated silica	Sodium monofluorophosphate, potassium nitrate	Sodium lauryl sulfate
	Other Ingredients: Sorbitol, water, glycerin, flavor, FD&C red #40, sodium benzoate, titanium dioxide, sodium saccharin, **dietetically sucrose free**		
Natural White® Tartar Control Toothpaste	Hydrated silica	Sodium fluoride	Sodium lauryl sulfate
	Other Ingredients: Sorbitol, water, glycerin, xanthan gum, tetrapotassium pyrophosphate, titanium dioxide, cellulose gum, flavor, sodium benzoate, FD&C blue #1, D&C yellow #10, **dietetically sucrose free**		
Natural White® with Peroxide Gel		Hydrogen peroxide	
	Other Ingredients: Water, glycerin, flavor, dipotassium phosphate, sodium saccharin, phosphoric acid, poloxamer, **dietetically sucrose free**		
Orajel® Baby Tooth & Gum Cleanser Gel			
	Other Ingredients: Poloxamer 407 (2%), simethicone (0.12%), Microdent, carboxymethylcellulose, sodium, citric acid, flavor, glycerin, methylparaben, potassium sorbate, propylene glycol, propylparaben, water, sodium saccharin, sorbitol, **fluoride free**		
Orajel® Gold Sensitive Teeth Gel for Adults	Hydrated silica	Potassium nitrate 5%, sodium monofluorophosphate 0.2%	Sodium lauryl sulfate
	Other Ingredients: FD&C blue #1, flavor, glycerin, sodium lauroyl sarcosinate, sodium saccharin, sorbitol, xanthan gum		
Pearl Drops® Toothpolish Paste	Hydrated silica, calcium pyrophosphate, dicalcium phosphate, aluminum hydroxide	Sodium monofluorophosphate	Sodium lauryl sulfate
	Other Ingredients: Water, sorbitol, glycerin, PEG-12, flavor, cellulose gum, trisodium phosphate, sodium phosphate, sodium saccharin, **dietetically sucrose free**, **dye free**		
Pearl Drops® Toothpolish Gel	Hydrated silica	Sodium monofluorophosphate	Sodium lauryl sulfate
	Other Ingredients: Sorbitol, water, glycerin, PEG-12, flavor, cellulose gum, sodium saccharin, FD&C blue #1, FD&C yellow #10, **dietetically sucrose free**		
Pearl Drops® Whitening Extra Strength Paste	Hydrated silica, calcium pyrophosphate, dicalcium phosphate	Sodium monofluorophosphate	Sodium lauryl sulfate
	Other Ingredients: Water, sorbitol, glycerin, PEG-12, flavor, cellulose gum, trisodium phosphate, sodium phosphate, sodium saccharin, titanium dioxide, **dietetically sucrose free**, **dye free**		
Pearl Drops® Whitening Gel (icy cool mint)	Hydrated silica	Sodium monofluorophosphate	Sodium lauryl sulfate
	Other Ingredients: Sorbitol, water, glycerin, PEG-12, flavor, cellulose gum, sodium saccharin, FD&C blue #1, FD&C yellow #10, **dietetically sucrose free**		
Pepsodent® Baking Soda Toothpaste	Hydrated silica	Sodium monofluorophosphate 0.8% (fluoride (0.14%)	Sodium lauryl sulfate
	Other Ingredients: Sorbitol, water, sodium bicarbonate†, PEG-32, SD alcohol 38B, flavor, cellulose gum, sodium saccharin, titanium dioxide		
Pepsodent® Original Toothpaste	Hydrated silica	Sodium monofluorophosphate 0.8% (fluoride 0.14%)	Sodium lauryl sulfate
	Other Ingredients: Sorbitol and related polyols, water, glycerin, SD alcohol 38B, flavor, cellulose gum, sodium saccharin, titanium dioxide		
Pepsodent® Tartar Control Toothpaste	Hydrated silica	Sodium monofluorophosphate 0.8% (fluoride 0.14%)	Sodium lauryl sulfate
	Other Ingredients: Sorbitol and related polyols, water, glycerin, SD alcohol 38B, zinc citrate trihydrate, flavor, cellulose gum, sodium saccharin, titanium dioxide, blue #1, yellow #1		
Pete & Pam™ Gel (premeasured strips)	Hydrated silica	Sodium monofluorophosphate 0.76%	Sodium lauryl sarcosinate

Brand Name	Abrasive Ingredient	Therapeutic Ingredient	Foaming Agent
	Other Ingredients: Sorbitol, water, glycerin, xanthan gum, polysorbate 20, sodium benzoate, pluronic P84, FD&C blue #1, FD&C red #33, FD&C yellow #5, flavor, xylitol		
Promise® Toothpaste	Dicalcium phosphate	Potassium nitrate, sodium monofluorophosphate	Sodium lauryl sulfate
	Other Ingredients: Water, hydroxyethylcellulose, flavor, sodium saccharin, methylparaben, propylparaben, D&C yellow #10, FD&C blue #1, glycerin, sorbitol, silicon dioxide, **dietetically sucrose free**		
Reach Act Adult Anti-Cavity Treatment Liquid (cinnamon, mint)‡	**Ingredients:** Sodium fluoride 0.05%, cetylpyridinium chloride, D&C red #33 (cinnamon), EDTA calcium disodium, FD&C yellow #5, flavor, glycerin, monobasic sodium phosphate, dibasic sodium phosphate, poloxamer 407, polysorbate 80 (cinnamon), polysorbate 20 (mint), propylene glycol, sodium benzoate, sodium saccharin, water, FD&C green #3 (mint), menthol (mint), methyl salicylate (mint), potassium sorbate (mint), **alcohol free**		
Reach Act for Kids*‡	**Ingredients:** Sodium fluoride 0.05%, cetylpyridinium chloride, D&C red #33, EDTA calcium disodium, flavor, glycerin, monobasic sodium phosphate, dibasic sodium phosphate, poloxamer 407, polysorbate 80, propylene glycol, sodium benzoate, sodium saccharin, water, **alcohol free**		
Rembrandt® Age-Defying Adult Toothpaste (original or mint)	Dicalcium orthophosphate, soft silica	Sodium monofluorophosphate (fluoride 0.15%)	
	Other Ingredients: Trihydroxy propane, perhydrol urea, aluminum oxide, acetylated pectins, sodium citrate, iridium, papain, carboxyl polymethylene, saccharin, propylene glycol, flavor		
Rembrandt® Age-Defying Adult Formula Mouthwash‡	**Ingredients:** Sodium fluoride 0.05%, water, glycerin, hydrogen peroxide solution, sodium citrate, polyoxyl 40 hydrogenated castor oil, flavor, cocamidopropyl betaine, citric acid, sodium benzoate, sodium saccharin, sodium hydroxide, **alcohol free**		
Rembrandt® Daily Whitening Gel	Silica	Sodium monofluorophosphate (fluoride 0.15%)	Carbamide peroxide, sodium lauryl sulfate
	Other Ingredients: Glycerin, sodium citrate, carbopol, triethanolamine, flavor		
Rembrandt® Naturals Toothpaste	Silica	0.15% fluoride ion from sodium monofluorophosphate wt/vol%	None
	Other ingredients: Water (artesian springs), dicalcium phosphate (from monetite, a mineral), glycerine (by-product of vegetable soap), xylitol (from birch trees), cocamidopropyl betaine (from coconut), flavor (spearmint, peppermint, other natural sources), sodium citrate (from citrus fruit), stevia (from stevia plant), papain (from papaya plant), sodium carrageenan (from seaweed), citric acid and vitamin C (from citrus fruit), ginkgo extract, raspberry leaf extract. Also available containing aloe vera and echinacea or papaya and ginseng.		
Rembrandt® Whitening Baking Soda Toothpaste	Sodium bicarbonate, silica	Sodium monofluorophosphate (fluoride 0.15%)	Sodium lauryl sulfate
	Other Ingredients: Glycerin, sorbitol, alumina, water, sodium citrate, sodium carrageenan, papain, flavor, sodium hydroxide, FD&C blue #1, sodium saccharin		
Rembrandt® Whitening Canker Sore Prevention Toothpaste	Dicalcium phosphate, silica	Sodium monofluorophosphate (fluoride 0.15%)	
	Other Ingredients: Water, glycerin, xylitol, sodium citrate, natural flavors, sodium carrageenan, papain, citric acid, **dye free**		
Rembrandt® Whitening Natural Toothpaste	Dicalcium phosphate, silica	Sodium monofluorophosphate	
	Other Ingredients: Water, glycerin, xylitol, sodium citrate, natural flavors, sodium carrageenan, papain, citric acid, **dye free**		
Rembrandt® Whitening Sensitive Toothpaste	Dicalcium phosphate dihydrate	Potassium nitrate 5%, sodium monofluorophosphate 0.76%	Sodium lauryl sulfate
	Other Ingredients: Glycerin, sorbitol, water, alumina, papain, sodium citrate, flavor, carboxymethylcellulose sodium, sodium saccharin, methylparaben, FD&C red #40, citric acid		
Rembrandt® Whitening Toothpaste (mint or original)	Dicalcium phosphate dihydrate	Sodium monofluorophosphate 0.76%	Sodium lauryl sulfate
	Other Ingredients: Glycerin, sorbitol, water, alumina, sodium citrate, flavor, sodium carrageenan, papain, sodium saccharin, methylparaben, citric acid, FD&C blue #1, FD&C yellow #5		

DENTIFRICE PRODUCTS *(Continued)*

Brand Name	Abrasive Ingredient	Therapeutic Ingredient	Foaming Agent
Revelation® Toothpowder	Calcium carbonate		Vegetable soap powder
	Other Ingredients: Methyl salicylate, menthol, **dye free**		
Sensodyne® Baking Soda Toothpaste	Sodium bicarbonate, silica	Potassium nitrate, sodium fluoride	Sodium lauryl sulfate
	Other Ingredients: Water, glycerin, flavor, hydroxyethylcellulose, titanium dioxide, sodium saccharin, **dietetically sucrose free, dye free**		
Sensodyne® Cool Gel	Silica	Potassium nitrate, sodium fluoride	Sodium methyl cocoyl taurate
	Other Ingredients: Water, sorbitol, glycerin, sodium carboxymethylcellulose, flavor, sodium saccharin, FD&C blue #1, trisodium phosphate, **dietetically sucrose free**		
Sensodyne® Extra Whitening Toothpaste	Silica	Potassium nitrate, sodium monofluorophosphate	Sodium lauryl sulfate
	Other Ingredients: Water, flavor, glycerin, PEG-12, PEG-75, sodium carbonate, sodium saccharin, titanium dioxide, calcium peroxide, **dietetically sucrose free**		
Sensodyne® Tartar Control Toothpaste	Hydrated silica, silica, sodium bicarbonate	Potassium nitrate, sodium fluoride	Cocamidopropyl betaine
	Other Ingredients: Cellulose gum, flavor, glycerin, sodium saccharin, tetrasodium pyrophosphate, titanium dioxide, water		
Sensodyne® Toothpaste* (fresh mint)	Dicalcium phosphate	Potassium nitrate, sodium monofluorophosphate	Sodium lauryl sulfate
	Other Ingredients: Water, glycerin, sorbitol, hydroxmethylcellulose, flavor, sodium saccharin, methylparaben, propylparaben, D&C yellow #10, FD&C blue #1, silicon dioxide, **dietetically sucrose free**		
Sensodyne® Toothpaste (original)	Silica	Potassium nitrate, sodium fluoride	Sodium methyl cocoyl taurate
	Other Ingredients: Water, glycerin, sorbitol, cellulose gum, titanium dioxide, sodium saccharin, flavor, D&C red #28, trisodium phosphate		
Slimer® Gel*	Hydrated silica	Sodium fluoride 0.15%	
	Other Ingredients: Sorbitol, water, glycerin, PEG-32, flavor, ethyl alcohol, propylene glycol, glyceryl triacetate, cellulose gum, sodium saccharin, sodium benzoate, FD&C blue #1, FD&C red #33, **dietetically sucrose free**		
Thermodent Toothpaste	Diatomaceous earth, silica	Strontium chloride hexahydrate	Sodium methyl cocoyl taurate
	Other Ingredients: Sorbitol, glycerin, titanium dioxide, guar gum, PEG-40 stearate, hydroxyethylcellulose, flavor, preservative, water		
Tom's® Natural Baking Soda with Propolis & Myrrh Toothpaste	Calcium carbonate, sodium bicarbonate		Sodium lauryl sulfate
	Other Ingredients: Glycerin, water, carrageenan, peppermint oil, myrrh, propolis, **fluoride free**		
Tom's® Natural Baking Soda, Calcium, and Fluoride Toothpaste	Calcium carbonate, sodium bicarbonate	Sodium monofluorophosphate	Sodium lauryl sulfate
	Other Ingredients: Glycerin, water, carrageenan, peppermint oil, xylitol		
Tom's® Natural Calcium and Fluoride Toothpaste*	Calcium carbonate	Sodium monofluorophosphate	Sodium lauryl sulfate
	Other Ingredients: Glycerin; water; carrageenan; xylitol (spearmint); cinnamon, fennel oil, or spearmint; peppermint oil (cinnamon, spearmint)		
Tom's® Natural Calcium and Fluoride Toothpaste	Calcium carbonate, hydrated silica	Sodium monofluorophosphate	Sodium lauryl sulfate
	Other Ingredients: Glycerin, water, carrageenan, xylitol, natural wintergreen oil		
Tom's® Natural for Children with Calcium and Fluoride Toothpaste	Calcium carbonate, hydrated silica	Sodium monofluorophosphate	Sodium lauryl sulfate
	Other Ingredients: Glycerin, fruit extracts, carrageenan, water		
Tom's® Natural with Propolis and Myrrh Toothpaste	Calcium carbonate		Sodium lauryl sulfate
	Other Ingredients: Glycerin; water; carrageenan; spearmint, peppermint, cassia, or fennel oil; propolis; myrrh, **fluoride free**		
Ultra Brite® Baking Soda & Peroxide Toothpaste	Hydrated silica, sodium bicarbonate	Sodium monofluorophosphate 0.76%	Sodium lauryl sulfate

Brand Name	Abrasive Ingredient	Therapeutic Ingredient	Foaming Agent
	Other Ingredients: Glycerin, water, propylene glycol, cellulose gum, flavor, sodium saccharin, titanium dioxide, sodium hydroxide, calcium peroxide, carrageenan, **dietetically sucrose free**		
Ultra Brite® Gel	Hydrated silica	Sodium monofluorophosphate 0.76%	Sodium lauryl sulfate
	Other Ingredients: Sorbitol, water, PEG-12, flavor, cellulose gum, sodium saccharin, FD&C blue #1, D&C red #33		
Ultra Brite® Toothpaste	Hydrated silica, alumina	Sodium monofluorophosphate 0.76%	Sodium lauryl sulfate
	Other Ingredients: Glycerin, cellulose gum, sorbitol, carrageenan gum, titanium dioxide, sodium saccharin, flavor, tetrasodium pyrophosphate, **dietetically sucrose free**		
Viadent® Fluoride Gel	Hydrated silica	Sodium monofluorophosphate 0.8%	Sodium lauryl sulfate
	Other Ingredients: Sodium saccharin, zinc chloride, teaberry flavor, sodium carboxymethylcellulose, sorbitol, sanguinaria extract		
Viadent® Fluoride Toothpaste	Hydrated silica	Sodium monofluorophosphate 0.8%	Sodium lauryl sulfate
	Other Ingredients: Sorbitol, titanium dioxide, carboxymethylcellulose, flavor, sodium saccharin, citric acid, zinc chloride, anhydrous sanguinaria extract, citric acid		
Viadent® Original Toothpaste	Dicalcium phosphate		Sodium lauryl sulfate
	Other Ingredients: Glycerin, sorbitol, titanium dioxide, zinc chloride, carrageenan, flavor, sodium saccharin, citric acid, sanguinaria extract, **fluoride free**		
Vince Tooth Powder	Calcium carbonate, sodium carbonate, tricalcium phosphate		
	Other Ingredients: Sodium alum, sodium perborate monohydrate, magnesium trisilicate, sodium saccharin, flavor, D&C red		

*Carries American Dental Association (ADA) seal indicating safety and efficacy.

†Sodium bicarbonate can also be considered an abrasive.

‡Topical fluoride product

Adapted with permission from *Nonprescription Products: Formulations & Features, Companion to the Handbook of Nonprescription Drugs*, 11th ed,, Washington, DC, American Pharmaceutical Association, 1998, 344-58.

DENTURE ADHESIVE PRODUCTS

Brand Name	Product Form / Ingredients
Confident®	**Cream** / Carboxymethylcellulose gum 32%, ethylene oxide polymer 13%, petrolatum, liquid petrolatum, propylparaben
Cushion Grip®	**Gel** / Alcohol 26.2%, triacetin, polyvinyl acetate
Dentlock®	**Powder** / Karaya gum
Dentrol®	**Liquid** / Carboxymethylcellulose sodium, ethylene oxide polymer, mineral oil, polyethylene, flavor, propylparaben
Denturite®	**Liquid** / Butyl phthalyl butyl glycolate, vinyl acetate, SDA alcohol **Powder** / Polyethyl methacrylate polymer
Effergrip®*	**Cream** / Carboxymethylcellulose sodium, polyvinyl methyl ether maleic acid calcium sodium double salt, color, flavor, preservatives, vehicle
Ezo® Cushions	**Pad** / Paraffin wax, cotton
Fixodent®	**Cream** / Carboxymethylcellulose sodium, calcium zinc gantrez (PVA/MA copolymer), mineral oil, petrolatum, color **Powder** / Carboxymethylcellulose sodium, calcium zinc gantrez (PVM/MA copolymer), peppermint oil
Fixodent® Extra Hold	**Powder** / Carboxymethylcellulose sodium, calcium zinc gantrez (PVA/MA copolymer), peppermint oil
Fixodent® Free	**Cream** / Carboxymethylcellulose sodium, calcium zinc gantrez (PVM/MA copolymer), mineral oil, petrolatum
Fixodent® Fresh	**Cream** / Carboxymethylcellulose sodium, calcium zinc gantrez (PVM/MA copolymer), mineral oil, petrolatum, color, peppermint flavor
Orafix® Special	**Cream** / Carboxymethylcellulose sodium, calcium/sodium polyvinyl methyl ether anhydride copolymer, polyvinyl pyrolidone
Orafix® Ultra	**Cream** / Polyvinyl methyl ether copolymer, carboxymethylcellulose
Plasti-Liner®	**Strip** / Polyethyl methacrylate polymer, butyl phthalyl butyl glycolate, triacetin
Poli-Grip®	**Cream** / Carboxymethylcellulose sodium gum 32%, ethylene oxide polymer 13%, petrolatum 36.7%, liquid petrolatum, propylparaben, flavor, dye
Poli-Grip® Free	**Cream** / Carboxymethylcellulose sodium, methyl vinyl ether maleic acid salt, petrolatum, mineral oil
Poli-Grip® Super	**Cream** / Carboxymethylcellulose sodium, methyl vinyl ether maleic acid salt copolymer, petrolatum, mineral oil, flavor, dye **Powder** / Carboxymethylcellulose sodium, methyl vinyl ether maleic salt copolymer, flavor
Poli-Grip® Ultra Fresh	**Cream** / Carboxymethylcellulose sodium, methyl vinyl ether maleic acid salt copolymer, petrolatum, mineral oil, flavor, dye
Polident® Dentu-Grip	**Powder** / Carboxymethylcellulose gum 49%, methyl vinyl ether maleic acid salt copolymer, flavor
Quik-Fix®	**Liquid** / Methyl methacrylate monomer, hydroxyethyl methacrylate monomer, color stable concentrate, triacetin **Powder** / Polyethyl methacrylate polymer
Sea-Bond®	**Pad** / Ethylene oxide polymer, sodium alginate
Snug® Cushion	**Sponge** / Acrylate resin, propylene glycol monolaurate
Wernet's®	**Powder** / Karaya gum 94.6%, water-soluble ethylene oxide polymer 5%, flavor

*Carries American Dental Association (ADA) seal indicating safety and efficacy.

Adapted with permission from *Nonprescription Products: Formulations & Features, Companion to the Handbook of Nonprescription Drugs*, 11th ed,, Washington, DC, American Pharmaceutical Association, 1998, 358-9.

DENTURE CLEANSER PRODUCTS

Brand Name	Product Form / Ingredients
Ban-A-Stain®	**Liquid** / Phosphoric acid 25%, deionized water, methylparaben, xanthan gum, alkyl phenoxy polyethoxy ethanol, oil of cassis, FD&C red #40, imidurea
Dentu-Creme®	**Paste** / Dicalcium phosphate dihydrate, propylene glycol, calcium carbonate, sodium lauryl sulfate, glycerin, aluminum silicate, hydroxyethylcellulose, flavor, magnesium aluminum silicate, sodium saccharin, methylparaben, propylparaben, water. FD&C blue #1
Efferdent® Antibacterial*	**Tablet** / Potassium monopersulfate, sodium carbonate, sodium perborate, sodium bicarbonate, fragrance, colors
Efferdent® Plus	**Tablet** / Potassium monopersulfate, sodium perborate, sodium bicarbonate, fragrance, colors, (including FD&C yellow #5), sodium saccharin, chelating agents, detergents
Efferdent®, 2 Layer	**Tablet** / Potassium monopersulfate, sodium bicarbonate, sodium carbonate, detergents, fragrance, colors, sodium saccharin, chelating agents
Stain Away® Plus	**Powder** / Effervescent, high-oxygenating powder (at the time of publication, the manufacturer had not responded to a request for ingredients of this product)

* Carries American Dental Association (ADA) seal indicating safety and efficacy.

Adapted with permission from *Nonprescription Products: Formulations & Features, Companion to the Handbook of Nonprescription Drugs*, 11th ed,, Washington, DC, American Pharmaceutical Association, 1998, 357.

MOUTH PAIN, COLD SORE, AND CANKER SORE PRODUCTS

Brand Name	Anesthetic/ Analgesic	Other Ingredients
Abreva™ [OTC]		**Cream**: Docosanol 10%, benzyl alcohol, light mineral oil, propylene glycol, purified water, sucrose distearate, sucrose stearate
Anbesol® Baby Gel (grape, original)	Benzocaine 7.5%	Benzoic acid (grape), carbomer 934P, D&C red #33, EDTA disodium, FD&C blue #1 (grape), flavor (grape), glycerin, methylparaben (grape), PEG, propylparaben (grape), saccharin, purified water, clove oil (original)
Anbesol® Gel or Liquid	Benzocaine 6.3% (gel), 6.4% (liquid); phenol 0.5%	**Gel**: Alcohol 70%, glycerin, carbomer 934P, D&C red #33, D&C yellow #10, FD&C blue #1, FD&C yellow #6, flavor, camphor **Liquid:** Alcohol 70%, potassium iodide, povidone iodine, camphor, menthol, glycerin
Anbesol® Maximum Strength Gel or Liquid	Benzocaine 20%	Alcohol 60%, carbomer 934P (gel), D&C yellow #10, FD&C blue #1, FD&C red #40, flavor, PEG, saccharin
Baby® Gumz	Benzocaine 10%	PEG 8 and 32, **alcohol free, dietetically sucrose free**
Benzodent® Denture Analgesic Ointment*	Benzocaine 20%	8-hydroxyquinoline sulfate, petrolatum, sodium carboxymethycellulose, color, eugenol
Blistex® Lip Medex Ointment	Camphor 1%, menthol 1%, phenol 0.5%	Petrolatum, cocoa butter, flavor, lanolin, mixed waxes, oil of cloves
Blistex® Medicated Ointment	Menthol 0.6%, camphor 0.5%, phenol 0.5%	Water, mixed waxes, mineral oil, petrolatum, lanolin
Campho-Phenique® Cold Sore Gel†	Camphor 10.8%, phenol 4.7%	Eucalyptus oil, colloidal silicon dioxide, glycerin, light mineral oil, **alcohol free**
Cankaid® Liquid		Carbamide peroxide 10%‡, citric acid monohydrate, sodium citrate, dihydrate, EDTA disodium
Carmex Lip Balm Ointment	Menthol, camphor, salicylic acid, phenol	Alum, fragrance, petrolatum, lanolin, cocoa butter, wax, **alcohol free**, **dye free**, **gluten free**, **dietetically sucrose free**
Chap Stick® Medicated Lip Balm (stick, ointment)	Camphor 1%, menthol 0.6%, phenol 0.5%	**Stick:** Petrolatum 41%, paraffin wax, mineral oil, cocoa butter, 2-octyl dodecanol, arachidyl propionate, polyphenylmethylsiloxane 556, white wax, isopropyl lanolate, carnauba wax, isopropyl myristate, lanolin, fragrance, methylparaben, propylparaben, oleyl alcohol, cetyl alcohol **Ointment**: Petrolatum (jar 60%, tube 67%), microcrystalline wax, mineral oil, cocoa butter, lanolin, paraffin war (jar), fragrance, methylparaben, propylparaben
Dent's® Double-Action Kit (tablets, drops)	Benzocaine 20% (drops), acetaminophen 325 mg (tablet)	**Drops:** Denatured alcohol 74%, chlorobutanol anhydrous 0.09%, propylene glycol, FD&C red #40, eugenol

Brand Name	Anesthetic/ Analgesic	Other Ingredients
Dent's® Extra Strength Toothache Gum	Benzocaine 20%	Petrolatum, cotton and wax base, beeswax, FD&C red #40 aluminum lake, eugenol
Dent's® Maxi-Strength Toothache Treatment Drops	Benzocaine 20%	Denatured alcohol 74%, chlorobutanol anhydrous 0.09%, propylene glycol, FD&C red #40, eugenol
Dent-Zel-Ite® Oral Mucosal Analgesic Liquid	Benzocaine 5%, camphor	Alcohol 81%, wintergreen, glycerin, **dye free**
Dent-Zel-Ite® Temporary Dental Filling Liquid	Camphor	Alcohol 56.18%, sandarac gum, methyl salicylate
Dent-Zel-Ite® Toothache Relief Drops	Eugenol 85%, camphor	Alcohol 13.5%, wintergreen
Dentapaine® Gel	Benzocaine 20%	Glycerin, oil of cloves, sodium saccharin, methylparaben, PEG 400 and 4000, water, **alcohol free**, **dye free**, **gluten free, dietetically sucrose free**
Dr. Hand's® Teething Gel or Lotion	Menthol	SD alcohol 38B (gel 10%, lotion 11%), sterilized water, carbomer 940, witch hazel, polysorbate 80, sodium hydroxide, simethicone, D&C red #33, FD&C red #3
Gly-Oxide® Liquid		Carbamide peroxide 10%‡, citric acid, flavor, glycerin, propylene glycol, sodium stannate, water
Herpecin-L® Cold Sore Lip Balm Stick†		Padimate O 7%, allantoin 0.5%, titanium dioxide, beeswax, cetyl esters, flavor, octyldodecanol, paraffin, petrolatum, sesame oil, vitamins B_6, C, and E
Hurricaine® Aerosol* (wild cherry)	Benzocaine 20%	PEG, saccharin, flavor, alcohol, **dye free**, **gluten free, sulfite free**
Hurricaine® Gel* (wild cherry, pina colada, watermelon)	Benzocaine 20%	PEG, saccharin, flavor, **alcohol free**, **dye free**, **gluten free, sulfite free**
Hurricaine® Liquid* (wild cherry, pina colada)	Benzocaine 20%	PEG, saccharin, flavor, **alcohol free**, **dye free**, **gluten free, dietetically sucrose free**
Kank-A® Professional Strength Liquid*	Benzocaine 20%	Benzoin tincture compound, cetylpyridinium chloride, ethylcellulose, SD alcohol 24%, dimethyl isosorbide, castor oil, flavor, tannic acid, propylene glycol, saccharin, benzyl alcohol
Lip-Ex® Ointment	Phenol, camphor, salicylic acid, menthol	Petrolatum, cherry flavor
Lipmagik® Liquid	Benzocaine 6.3%, phenol 0.5%	Alcohol 70%, **dye free**, **sulfite free**, **gluten free**
Little Teethers® Oral Pain Relief Gel	Benzocaine 7.5%	Carbomer, glycerin, flavor, potassium sorbate, acesulfame K, PEGs, **alcohol free**, **dye free**, **dietetically sodium free, dietetically sucrose free**
Medadyne® Liquid	Benzocaine 10%, menthol, camphor, benzyl alcohol	Benzalkonium chloride, tannic acid, flavor, SD alcohol, thymol
Numzident® Adult Strength Gel	Benzocaine 10%	PEG-8, glycerin, PEG-75, sodium saccharin, purified water, flavor
Numzit® Teething Gel	Benzocaine 7.5%	PEG-8, PEG-75, sodium saccharin, clove oil, peppermint oil, purified water

MOUTH PAIN, COLD SORE, AND CANKER SORE PRODUCTS *(Continued)*

Brand Name	Anesthetic/ Analgesic	Other Ingredients
Orabase® Baby Gel*	Benzocaine 7.5%	Glycerin, PEG, carbopol, preservative, sweetener, flavor, **alcohol free**
Orabase® Gel	Benzocaine 15%	Ethanol, propylene glycol, ethylcellulose, tannic acid, salicylic acid, flavor, sodium saccharin
Orabase® Lip Cream	Benzocaine 5%, menthol 0.5%, camphor, phenol	Allantoin 1%, carboxymethylcellulose sodium, veegum, Tween 80, phenonip, PEG, biopure, talc, kaolin, lanolin, petrolatum, oil of clove, hydrated silica, **alcohol free**
Orabase® Plain Paste*		Pectin, gelatin, carboxymethylcellulose sodium, polyethylene, mineral oil, flavor, preservative, guar, tragacanth, **alcohol free**
Orabase-B® with Benzocaine Paste*	Benzocaine 20%	Plasticized hydrocarbon gel, guar, carboxymethylcellulose, tragacanth, pectin, preservatives, flavor, **alcohol free**
Oragesic Solution	Benzyl alcohol 2%, menthol	Water, sorbitol, polysorbate 20, sodium chloride, yerba santa, saccharin, flavor, **sulfite free**
Orajel® Baby Gel or Liquid	Benzocaine 7.5%	**Gel:** FD&C red #40, flavor, glycerin, PEGs, sodium saccharin, sorbic acid, sorbitol, **alcohol free** **Liquid:** Not applicable
Orajel® Baby Nighttime Gel	Benzocaine 10%	FD&C red #40, flavor, glycerin, PEGs, sodium saccharin, sorbic acid, sorbitol, **alcohol free**
Orajel® CoverMed Cream (tinted light, medium)	Dyclonine HCl 1%	Allantoin 0.5%
Orajel® Denture Gel	Benzocaine 20%	Cellulose gum, gelatin, menthol, methyl salicylate, pectin, plasticized hydrocarbon gel, PEG, sodium saccharin
Orajel® Maximum Strength Gel	Benzocaine 20%	Clove oil, flavor, PEGs, sodium saccharin, sorbic acid
Orajel® Mouth-Aid Gel or Liquid	Benzocaine 20%	**Gel**: Zinc chloride 0.1%, benzalkonium chloride 0.02%. allantoin, carbomer, EDTA disodium, peppermint oil, PEG, polysorbate 60, propyl gallate, propylene glycol, purified water, povidone, sodium saccharin, sorbic acid, stearyl alcohol **Liquid:** Ethyl alcohol 44.2%
Orajel® PM Cream	Benzocaine 20%	
Orajel® Periostatic Spot Treatment Oral Cleanser		Carbamide peroxide 15%‡, citric acid, EDTA disodium, flavor, methylparaben, PEG, purified water, sodium chloride, sodium saccharin
Orajel® Periostatic Super Cleaning Oral Rinse		Hydrogen peroxide 1.5%‡, ethyl alcohol 4%
Orajel® Regular Strength Gel	Benzocaine 10%	Clove oil, flavor, PEGs, sodium saccharin, sorbic acid
Peroxyl® Hygienic Dental Rinse		Hydrogen peroxide 1.5%‡, alcohol 5%, pluronic F108, sorbitol, sodium saccharin, dye, polysorbate 20, mint flavor, **gluten free**, **sulfite free**

Brand Name	Anesthetic/ Analgesic	Other Ingredients
Peroxyl® Oral Spot Treatment Gel		Hydrogen peroxide 1.5%‡, ethyl alcohol 5%, pluronic F108, sorbitol, sodium saccharin, dye, polysorbate 20, mint flavor, dye, pluronic F127, **gluten free**, **dietetically sucrose free**
Proxigel® Gel†	Menthol	Carbamide peroxide 10%‡, glycerin, carbomer, phosphoric acid, triethanolamine, flavor, **dye free**, **gluten free**, **dietetically sucrose free**
Red Cross® Canker Sore Medication Ointment†	Benzocaine 20%, phenol	Carbomer 974P, mineral oil, petrolatum, propylparaben
Red Cross® Toothache Medication Drops	Eugenol 85%	Sesame oil
Retre-Gel®†	Benzocaine 5%, menthol 1%	Glycerin 20%
Tanac® Medicated Gel	Dyclonine HCl 1%	Allantoin 0.5%
Tanac® No Sting Liquid	Benzocaine 10%	Benzalkonium chloride 0.125%, saccharin
Zilactin® Gel	Benzyl alcohol 10%	**Gluten free**
Zilactin® Baby Gel	Benzocaine 10%	**Alcohol free, dye free, gluten free**
Zilactin®-B Gel	Benzocaine 10%	**Gluten free**
Zilactin®-L Liquid	Lidocaine 2.5%	**Gluten free**

*Carries American Dental Association (ADA) seal indicating safety and efficacy

†Agent for cold sore treatment only

‡Agent for debridement or wound cleansing

Adapted with permission from *Nonprescription Products: Formulations & Features, Companion to the Handbook of Nonprescription Drugs*, 11th ed,, Washington, DC, American Pharmaceutical Association, 1998, 338-40.

ORAL RINSE PRODUCTS

Brand Name	Antiseptic	Other Ingredients
Astring-O-Sol® Liquid	SD alcohol 38B 75.6%, methyl salicylate	Water, myrrh extract, zinc chloride, citric acid
Betadine® Mouthwash/Gargle	Alcohol 8.8%	Povidone-iodine 0.5%, glycerin, sodium saccharin, flavor
Biotene® Mouthwash	Lysozyme (6 mg), lactoferrin (6 mg) glucose oxidase (4000 units)	Water, xylitol, hydrogenated starch, propylene glycol, hydroxyethylcellulose, aloe vera, natural peppermint, poloxamer 407, calcium lactate, zinc gluconate, sodium benzoate, benzoic acid
Cepacol® Mouthwash/Gargle	Alcohol 14%, cetylpyridinium chloride 0.05%	EDTA disodium, color, flavor, glycerin, polysorbate 80, saccharin, sodium biphosphate, sodium phosphate, water, **gluten free, dietetically sucrose free**
Cepacol® Mouthwash/Gargle (mint)	Alcohol 14.5%, cetylpyridinium chloride 0.5%	Color, flavor, glucono delta-lactone, glycerin, poloxamer 407, sodium saccharin, sodium gluconate, water, **gluten free, dietetically sucrose free**
Dr. Tichenor's® Antiseptic Liquid	SDA alcohol 38B 70%	Oil of peppermint, extract of arnica, water, **dye free, gluten free**
Listerine®* Liquid	Alcohol 26.9%, eucalyptol 0.092%, thymol 0.064%, methyl salicylate 0.06%, menthol 0.042%	Benzoic acid, poloxamer 407, caramel, water, sodium benzoate
Listerine®* Liquid (freshburst, cool mint)	Alcohol 21.6%, eucalyptol 0.092%, thymol 0.064%, methyl salicylate 0.06%, menthol 0.042%	Water, sorbitol solution, poloxamer 407, benzoic acid, flavor, sodium saccharin, sodium citrate, citric acid, FD&C green #3, D&C yellow #10 (freshburst)
Mentadent® Mouthwash (cool mint, fresh mint)	Alcohol 10%	Water, sorbitol, sodium bicarbonate, hydrogen peroxide, poloxamer 407, sodium lauryl sulfate, flavor, polysorbate 20, methyl salicylate (cool mint), sodium saccharin, phosphoric acid, blue #1, yellow #5 (cool mint)
Plax® Advanced Formula (mint sensation)	Alcohol 8.7%	Water, sorbitol solution, tetrasodium pyrophosphate, benzoic acid, flavor, poloxamer 407, sodium benzoate, sodium lauryl sulfate, sodium saccharin, xanthan gum, FD&C blue #1
Plax® Advanced Formula (original, SoftMINT)	Alcohol 8.7%	Sodium lauryl sulfate, water, sorbitol solution, sodium benzoate, tetrasodium pyrophosphate, benzoic acid, poloxamer 407, sodium saccharin, flavor (SoftMINT), xanthan gum (SoftMINT), flavor enhancer (SoftMINT), FD&C blue #1 (SoftMINT), FD&C yellow #5 (SoftMINT)

Brand Name	Antiseptic	Other Ingredients
Rembrandt® Naturals Mouthwash		Spring water, glycerin, xylitol, sodium citrate, vitamin C, stevia, citric acid, dicalcium phosphate, cocamidopropyl betain, flavor, ginkgo extract, raspberry leaf extract, alcohol free. Also available with papaya and ginseng or aloe and echinacea
S.T. 37® Solution	Hexylresorcinol 0.1%	Glycerin, propylene glycol, citric acid, EDTA disodium, sodium bisulfite, sodium citrate
Scope® Baking Soda	SD alcohol 38F 9.9%, cetylpyridinium chloride, domiphen bromide	Sorbitol, sodium bicarbonate, sodium saccharin, flavor
Scope® (cool peppermint)	SD alcohol 38F 14%, cetylpyridinium chloride, domiphen bromide	Purified water, glycerin, poloxamer 407, sodium saccharin, sodium benzoate, N-ethylmethylcarboxamide, benzoic acid, FD&C blue #1, flavor
Targon® Smokers' Mouthwash (clean taste)	SDA alcohol 38B 15.6%	Water, glycerin, polyoxyl 40 hydrogenated caster oil, sodium lauryl sulfate, dibasic sodium phosphate, benzoic acid, sodium saccharin, caramel powder, **dietetically sucrose free**
Targon® Smokers' Mouthwash (original)	SDA alcohol 38B 16%	Water, sodium saccharin, sodium benzoate, glycerin, sodium lauryl sulfate, FD&C green #3, FD&C yellow #5, polyoxyl 40 hydrogenated castor oil, **dietetically sucrose free**
Tom's of Maine® Natural Mouthwash (cinnamon, original)	Menthol	Water, glycerin, aloe vera juice, witch hazel, poloxamer 335, spearmint oil, ascorbic acid, **alcohol free**

*Carries American Dental Association (ADA) seal indicating safety and efficacy

Note: SD alcohol refers to "specially denatured" alcohol

Adapted with permission from *Nonprescription Products: Formulations & Features, Companion to the Handbook of Nonprescription Drugs*, 11th ed,, Washington, DC, American Pharmaceutical Association, 1998, 341-2.

TOP 50 MOST PRESCRIBED DRUGS IN 2001*

1. Hydrocodone/acetaminophen
2. Lipitor®
3. Premarin®
4. Atenolol
5. Synthroid ®
6. Zithromax®
7. Furosemide
8. Amoxicillin
9. Norvasc®
10. Alprazolam
11. Albuterol (aerosol)
12. Claritin®
13. Hydrochlorothiazide
14. Prilosec®
15. Zoloft®
16. Paxil®
17. Triamterene/hydrochlorothiazide
18. Prevacid®
19. Ibuprofen
20. Celebrex®
21. Zocor®
22. Cephalexin
23. Glucophage®
24. Vioxx®
25. Zestril®
26. Augmentin®
27. Propoxyphene N/acetaminophen
28. Prempro™
29. Prednisone
30. Ortho Tri-Cyclen®
31. Acetaminophen/codeine
32. Zyrtec®
33. Allegra®
34. Levoxyl®
35. Trimox®
36. Metoprolol tartrate
37. Lorazepam
38. Toprol-XL®
39. Prozac®
40. Ranitidine hydrochloride
41. Ambien®
42. Celexa™
43. Amitriptyline
44. Fosamax®
45. Accupril®
46. Viagra®
47. Pravachol®
48. Naproxen
49. Neurontin®
50. Coumadin®

*Based on more than 3.1 billion prescriptions dispensed in U.S.
Source: NDC Health

PHARMACOLOGIC CATEGORY INDEX

ALPHABETICAL INDEX

NOTES

NOTES

NOTES

NOTES

NOTES

NOTES

Other titles offered by

LEXI-COMP, INC

DRUG INFORMATION HANDBOOK (International edition available)

by Charles Lacy, RPh, PharmD, FCSHP; Lora L. Armstrong, RPh, PharmD, BCPS; Morton P. Goldman, PharmD, BCPS; and Leonard L. Lance, RPh, BSPharm

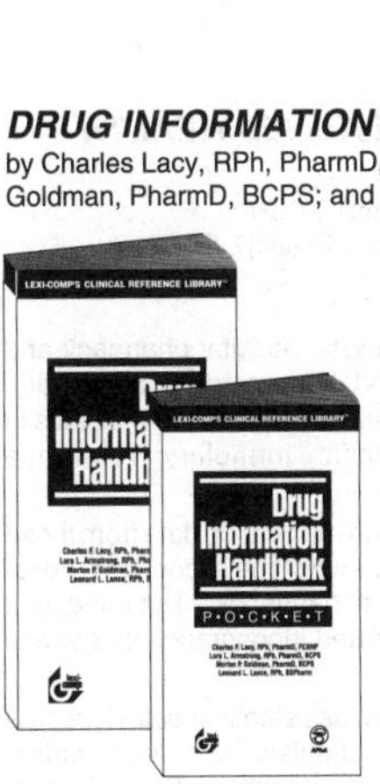

Specifically compiled and designed for the healthcare professional requiring quick access to concisely-stated comprehensive data concerning clinical use of medications. *The Drug Information Handbook* is an ideal portable drug information resource, providing the reader with up to 34 key points of data concerning clinical use and dosing of the medication. Material provided in the Appendix section is recognized by many users to be, by itself, well worth the purchase of the handbook.

All medications found in the *Drug Information Handbook,* are included in the abridged *Pocket* edition (select fields were extracted to maintain portability).

PEDIATRIC DOSAGE HANDBOOK (International edition available)

by Carol K. Taketomo, PharmD; Jane Hurlburt Hodding, PharmD; and Donna M. Kraus, PharmD

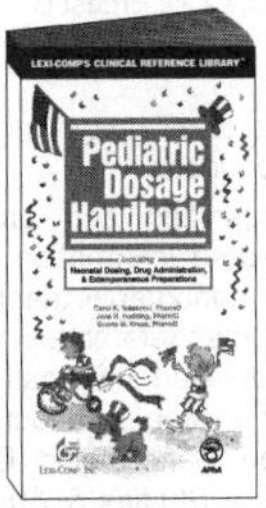

Special considerations must frequently be taken into account when dosing medications for the pediatric patient. This highly regarded quick reference handbook is a compilation of recommended pediatric doses based on current literature, as well as the practical experience of the authors and their many colleagues who work every day in the pediatric clinical setting.

Includes neonatal dosing, drug administration, and (in select monographs) extemporaneous preparations for medications used in pediatric medicine.

GERIATRIC DOSAGE HANDBOOK

by Todd P. Semla, PharmD, BCPS, FCCP; Judith L. Beizer, PharmD, FASCP; and Martin D. Higbee, PharmD, CGP

2000 "Book of the Year" — *American Journal of Nursing*

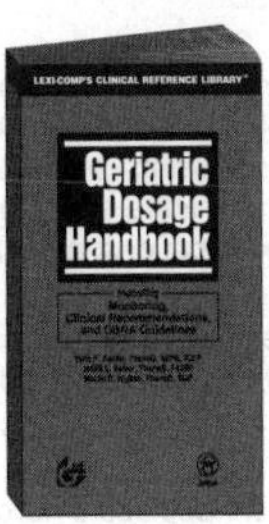

Many physiologic changes occur with aging, some of which affect the pharmacokinetics or pharmacodynamics of medications. Strong consideration should also be given to the effect of decreased renal or hepatic functions in the elderly, as well as the probability of the geriatric patient being on multiple drug regimens.

Healthcare professionals working with nursing homes and assisted living facilities will find the drug information contained in this handbook to be an invaluable source of helpful information.

An International Brand Name Index with names from 22 different countries is also included.

To order call toll free anywhere in the U.S.: 1-800-837-LEXI (5394)

Outside of the U.S. call: 330-650-6506 or online at www.lexi.com

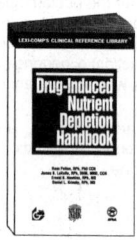

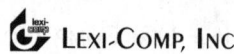

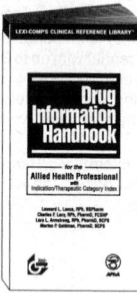

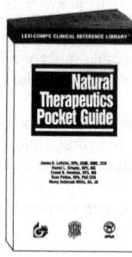

Other titles offered by

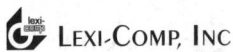

LEXI-COMP, INC

DRUG INFORMATION HANDBOOK FOR ADVANCED PRACTICE NURSING

by Beatrice B. Turkoski, RN, PhD; Brenda R. Lance, RN, MSN; and Mark F. Bonfiglio, PharmD
Foreword by: Margaret A. Fitzgerald, MS, RN, CS-FNP

1999 "Book of the Year" — *American Journal of Nursing*
Advanced Practice Nursing Category

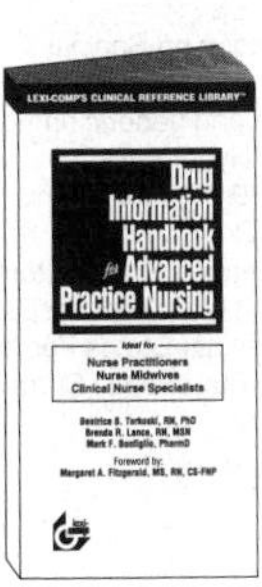

Designed specifically to meet the needs of nurse practitioners, clinical nurse specialists, nurse midwives, and graduate nursing students. The handbook is a unique resource for detailed, accurate information, which is vital to support the advanced practice nurse's role in patient drug therapy management. Over 4750 U.S., Canadian, and Mexican medications are covered in the 1000 monographs. Drug data is presented in an easy-to-use, alphabetically organized format covering up to 46 key points of information (including dosing for pediatrics, adults, and geriatrics). Cross-referenced to Appendix of over 230 pages of valuable comparison tables and additional information. Also included are two indexes, Pharmacologic Category and Controlled Substance, which facilitate comparison between agents.

DRUG INFORMATION HANDBOOK FOR NURSING

by Beatrice B. Turkoski, RN, PhD; Brenda R. Lance, RN, MSN; and Mark F. Bonfiglio, PharmD

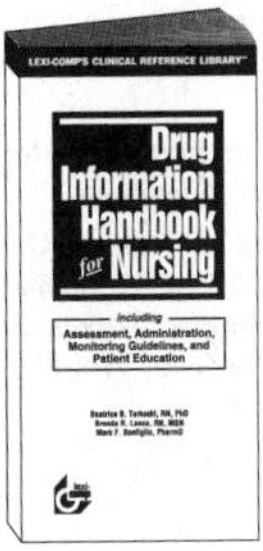

Registered Professional Nurses and upper-division nursing students involved with drug therapy will find this handbook provides quick access to drug data in a concise easy-to-use format.

Over 4000 U.S., Canadian, and Mexican medications are covered with up to 43 key points of information in each monograph. The handbook contains basic pharmacology concepts and nursing issues such as patient factors that influence drug therapy (ie, pregnancy, age, weight, etc) and general nursing issues (ie, assessment, administration, monitoring, and patient education). The Appendix contains over 230 pages of valuable information.

DRUG INFORMATION HANDBOOK FOR PHYSICIAN ASSISTANTS

by Michael J. Rudzinski, RPA-C, RPh and J. Fred Bennes, RPA, RPh

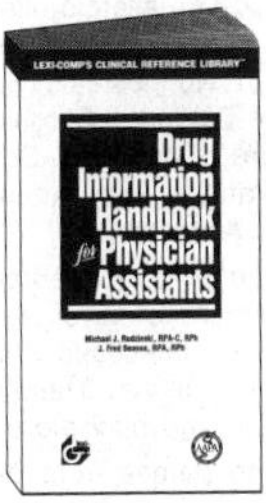

This comprehensive and easy-to-use handbook covers over 4100 drugs and also includes monographs on commonly used herbal products. There are up to 26 key fields of information per monograph, such as Pediatric and Adult Dosing With Adjustments for Renal/Hepatic Impairment, Labeled and Unlabeled Uses, Drug & Alcohol interactions, and Education & Monitoring Issues. Brand (U.S. and Canadian) and generic names are listed alphabetically for rapid access. It is fully cross-referenced by page number and includes alphabetical and pharmacologic indexes.

To order call toll free anywhere in the U.S.: 1-800-837-LEXI (5394)
Outside of the U.S. call: 330-650-6506 or online at www.lexi.com

Other titles offered by

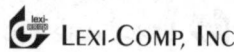

LEXI-COMP, INC

DRUG INFORMATION HANDBOOK FOR CARDIOLOGY

by Bradley G. Phillips, PharmD and Virend K. Somers, MD, Dphil

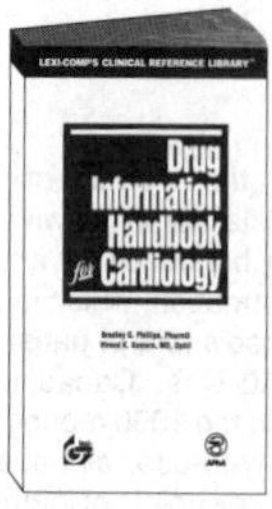

An ideal resource for physicians, pharmacists, nurses, residents, and students. This handbook was designed to provide the most current information on cardiovascular agents and other ancillary medications.

- Each monograph includes information on Special Cardiovascular Considerations and I.V. to Oral Equivalency
- Alphabetically organized by brand and generic name
- Appendix contains information on Hypertension, Anticoagulation, Cytochrome P-450, Hyperlipidemia, Antiarrhythmia, and Comparative Drug Charts
- Special Topics/Issues include Emerging Risk Factors for Cardiovascular Disease, Treatment of Cardiovascular Disease in the Diabetic, Cardiovascular Stress Testing, and Experimental Cardiovascular Therapeutic Strategies in the New Millenium, *and much more . . .*

DRUG INFORMATION HANDBOOK FOR ONCOLOGY

by Dominic A. Solimando, Jr, MA; Linda R. Bressler, PharmD, BCOP; Polly E. Kintzel, PharmD, BCPS, BCOP; and Mark C. Geraci, PharmD, BCOP

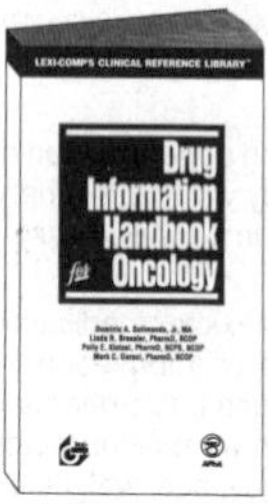

Presented in a concise and uniform format, this book contains the most comprehensive collection of oncology-related drug information available. Organized like a dictionary for ease of use, drugs can be found by looking up the *brand or generic name*!

This book contains individual monographs for both Antineoplastic Agents and Ancillary Medications.

The fields of information per monograph include: Use, U.S. Investigational, Bone Marrow/Blood Cell Transplantation, Vesicant, Emetic Potential. A Special Topics Section, Appendix, and Therapeutic Category & Key Word Index are valuable features to this book, as well.

ANESTHESIOLOGY & CRITICAL CARE DRUG HANDBOOK

by Andrew J. Donnelly, PharmD; Francesca E. Cunningham, PharmD; and Verna L. Baughman, MD

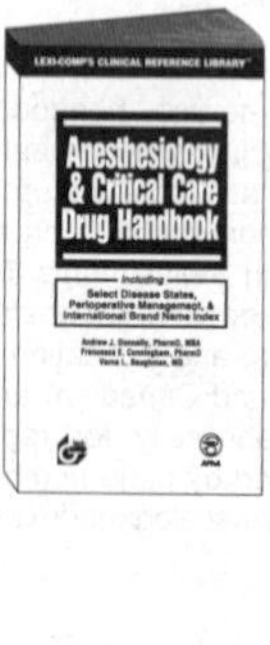

Contains the most commonly used drugs in the perioperative and critical care setting. This handbook also contains the following Special Issues and Topics: Allergic Reaction, Anesthesia for Cardiac Patients in Noncardiac Surgery, Anesthesia for Obstetric Patients in Nonobstetric Surgery, Anesthesia for Patients With Liver Disease, Chronic Pain Management, Chronic Renal Failure, Conscious Sedation, Perioperative Management of Patients on Antiseizure Medication, and Substance Abuse and Anesthesia.

The Appendix includes Abbreviations & Measurements, Anesthesiology Information, Assessment of Liver & Renal Function, Comparative Drug Charts, Infectious Disease-Prophylaxis & Treatment, Laboratory Values, Therapy Recommendations, Toxicology information, *and much more.*

International Brand Name Index with names from over 22 different countries is also included.

To order call toll free anywhere in the U.S.: 1-800-837-LEXI (5394)

Outside of the U.S. call: 330-650-6506 or online at www.lexi.com

Other titles offered by

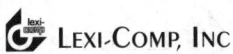

LEXI-COMP, INC

DRUG INFORMATION HANDBOOK FOR PSYCHIATRY

by Matthew A. Fuller, PharmD and Martha Sajatovic, MD

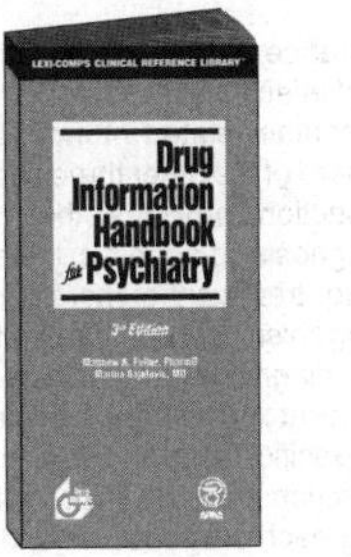

The source for comprehensive and clinically relevant drug information for the mental health professional. Alphabetically arranged by generic and brand name for ease-of-use. There are up to 35 key fields of information including these unique fields: "Effect on Mental Status" and "Effect on Psychiatric Treatment".

A special topics/issues section includes psychiatric assessment, major psychiatric disorders, major classes of psychotropic medications, psychiatric emergencies, special populations, enhanced patient education information section, and DSM-IV classification. Also contains a valuable appendix section, Pharmacologic Index, and Alphabetical Index.

RATING SCALES IN MENTAL HEALTH

by Martha Sajatovic, MD and Luis F. Ramirez, MD

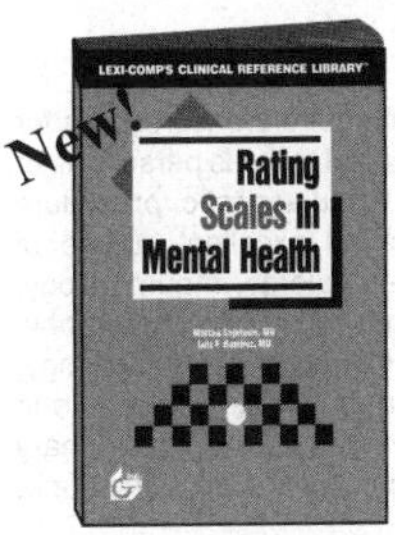

A basic guide to the rating scales in mental health, this is an ideal reference for psychiatrists, nurses, residents, psychologists, social workers, healthcare administrators, behavioral healthcare organizations, and outcome committees. It is designed to assist clinicians in determining the appropriate rating scale when assessing their client. A general concepts section provides text discussion on the use and history of rating scales, statistical evaluation, rating scale domains, and two clinical vignettes. Information on over 80 rating scales used in mental health organized in 6 categories. Appendix contains tables and charts in a quick reference format allowing clinicians to rapidly identify categories and characteristics of rating scales.

PSYCHOTROPIC DRUG INFORMATION HANDBOOK

by Matthew A. Fuller, PharmD and Martha Sajatovic, MD

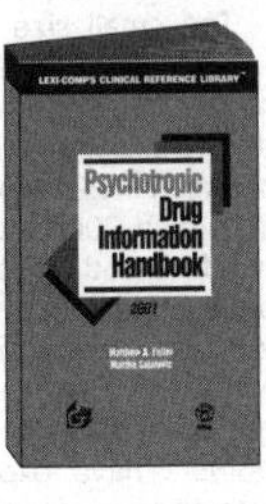

This portable, yet comprehensive guide to psychotropic drugs provides healthcare professionals with detailed information on use, drug interactions, pregnancy risk factors, warnings/precautions, adverse reactions, mechanism of action, and contraindications. Alphabetically organized by brand and generic name this concise handbook provides quick access to the information you need and includes patient education sheets on the psychotropic medications. It is the perfect pocket companion to the *Drug Information for Mental Health*.

To order call toll free anywhere in the U.S.: 1-800-837-LEXI (5394)

Outside of the U.S. call: 330-650-6506 or online at www.lexi.com

Other titles offered by

LEXI-COMP, INC

INFECTIOUS DISEASES HANDBOOK

by Carlos M. Isada, MD; Bernard L. Kasten Jr., MD; Morton P. Goldman, PharmD; Larry D. Gray, PhD; and Judith A. Aberg, MD

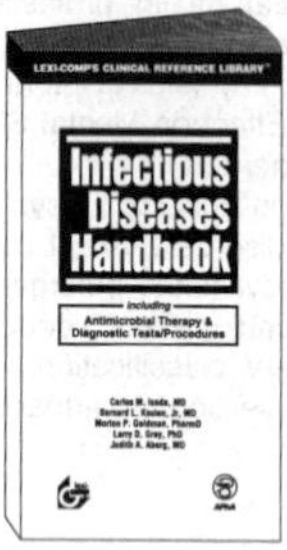

A four-in-one quick reference concerned with the identification and treatment of infectious diseases. Each of the four sections of the book contain related information and cross-referencing to one or more of the other three sections. The Disease Syndrome section provides the clinical presentation, differential diagnosis, diagnostic tests, and drug therapy recommended for treatment of more common infectious diseases. The Organism section presents the microbiology, epidemiology, diagnosis, and treatment of each organism. The Laboratory Diagnosis section describes performance of specific tests and procedures. The Antimicrobial Therapy section presents important facts and considerations regarding each drug recommended for specific diseases of organisms. Also contains an International Brand Name Index with names from 22 different countries.

DIAGNOSTIC PROCEDURE HANDBOOK by Frank Michota, MD

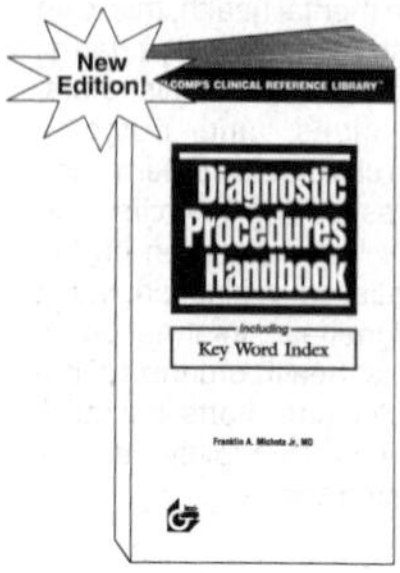

A comprehensive, yet concise, quick reference source for physicians, nurses, students, medical records personnel, or anyone needing quick access to diagnostic procedure information. This handbook is an excellent source of information in the following areas: allergy, rheumatology, and infectious disease; cardiology; computed tomography; diagnostic radiology; gastroenterology; invasive radiology; magnetic resonance imaging; nephrology, urology, and hematology; neurology; nuclear medicine; pulmonary function; pulmonary medicine and critical care; ultrasound; and women's health.

POISONING & TOXICOLOGY HANDBOOK

by Jerrold B. Leikin, MD and Frank P. Paloucek, PharmD

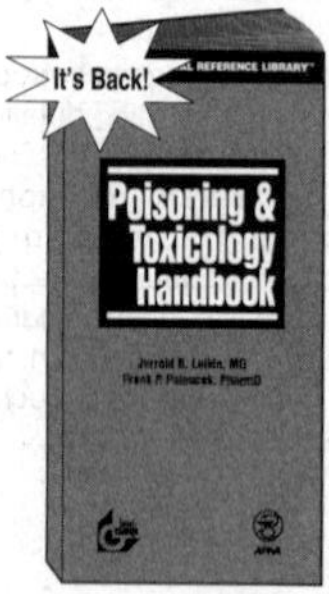

It's back by popular demand! The small size of our Poisoning & Toxicology Handbook is once again available. Better than ever, this comprehensive, portable reference contains 80 antidotes and drugs used in toxicology with 694 medicinal agents, 287 nonmedicinal agents, 291 biological agents, 57 herbal agents, and more than 200 laboratory tests. Monographs are extensively referenced and contain valuable information on overdose symptomatology and treatment considerations, as well as, admission criteria and impairment potential of select agents. Designed for quick reference with monographs arranged alphabetically, plus a cross-referencing index. The authors have expanded current information on drugs of abuse and use of antidotes, while providing concise tables, graphics, and other pertinent toxicology text.

To order call toll free anywhere in the U.S.: 1-800-837-LEXI (5394)
Outside of the U.S. call: 330-650-6506 or online at www.lexi.com

Other titles offered by

LEXI-COMP, INC

CLINICIAN'S GUIDE TO DIAGNOSIS—A Practical Approach
by Samir Desai, MD

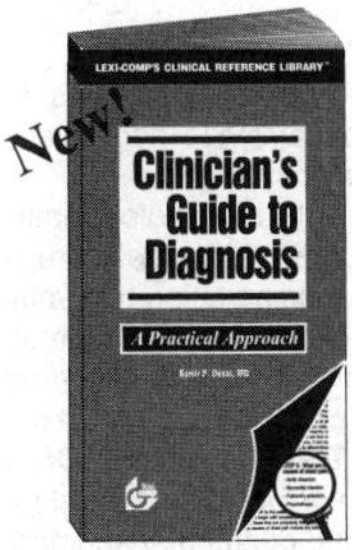

Symptoms are what prompt patients to seek medical care. In the evaluation of a patient's symptom, it is not unusual for healthcare professionals to ask "What do I do next?" This is precisely the question for which the *Clinician's Guide to Diagnosis: A Practical Approach* provides the answer. It will lead you from symptom to diagnosis through a series of steps designed to mimic the logical thought processes of seasoned clinicians. For the young clinician, this is an ideal book to help bridge the gap between the classroom and actual patient care. For the experienced clinician, this concise handbook offers rapid answers to the questions that are commonly encountered on a day-to-day basis. Let this guide become your companion, providing you with the tools necessary to tackle even the most challenging symptoms.

CLINICIAN'S GUIDE TO LABORATORY MEDICINE—A Practical Approach by Samir P. Desai, MD and Sana Isa-Pratt, MD

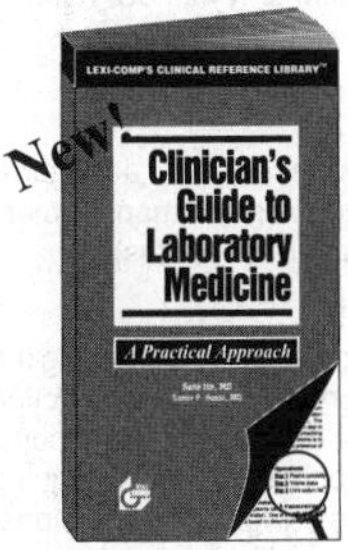

When faced with the patient presenting with abnormal laboratory tests, the clinician can now turn to the *Clinician's Guide to Laboratory Medicine: A Practical Approach.* This source is unique in its ability to lead the clinician from laboratory test abnormality to clinical diagnosis. Written for the busy clinician, this concise handbook will provide rapid answers to the questions that busy clinicians face in the care of their patients. No longer does the clinician have to struggle in an effort to find this information - *it's all here.*

LABORATORY TEST HANDBOOK & CONCISE version
by David S. Jacobs MD, FACP; Wayne R. DeMott, MD, FACP; and Dwight K. Oxley, MD, FACP

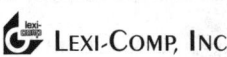

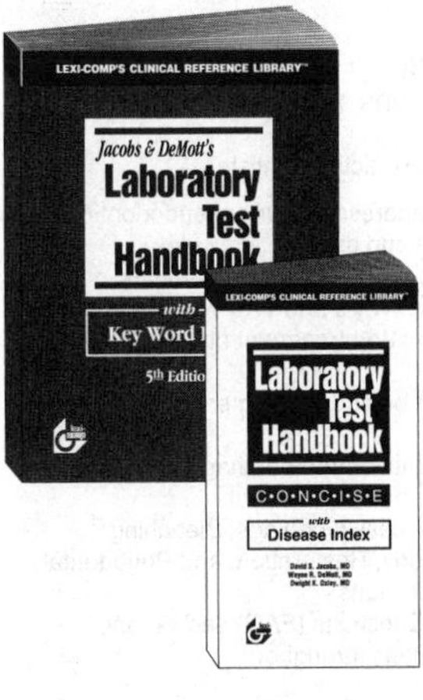

Contains over 900 clinical laboratory tests and is an excellent source of laboratory information for physicians of all specialties, nurses, laboratory professionals, students, medical personnel, or anyone who needs quick access to most routine and many of the more specialized testing procedures available in today's clinical laboratory.

Each monograph contains test name, synonyms, patient care, specimen requirements, reference ranges, and interpretive information with footnotes, references, and selected websites.

The *Laboratory Test Handbook Concise* is a portable, abridged (800 tests) version and is an ideal, quick reference for anyone requiring information concerning patient preparation, specimen collection and handling, and test result interpretation.

To order call toll free anywhere in the U.S.: 1-800-837-LEXI (5394)
Outside of the U.S. call: 330-650-6506 or online at www.lexi.com

Other titles offered by

LEXI-COMP, INC

DRUG INFORMATION HANDBOOK FOR DENTISTRY

by Richard L. Wynn, BSPharm, PhD; Timothy F. Meiller, DDS, PhD; and Harold L. Crossley, DDS, PhD

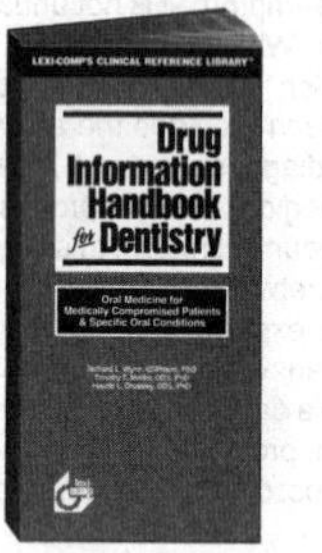

For all dental professionals requiring quick access to concisely-stated drug information pertaining to medications commonly prescribed by dentists and physicians.

Designed and written by dentists for all dental professionals as a portable, chair-side resource. Includes drugs commonly prescribed by dentists or being taken by dental patients and written in an easy-to-understand format. There are 24 key points of information for each drug including **Local Anesthetic/Vasoconstrictor, Precautions, Effects on Dental Treatment, and Drug Interactions**. Includes information on dental treatment for medically compromised patients and dental management of specific oral conditions.

Also contains Canadian & Mexican brand names.

ORAL SOFT TISSUE DISEASES

by J. Robert Newland, DDS, MS; Timothy F. Meiller, DDS, PhD; Richard L. Wynn, BSPharm, PhD; and Harold L.Crossley, DDS, PhD

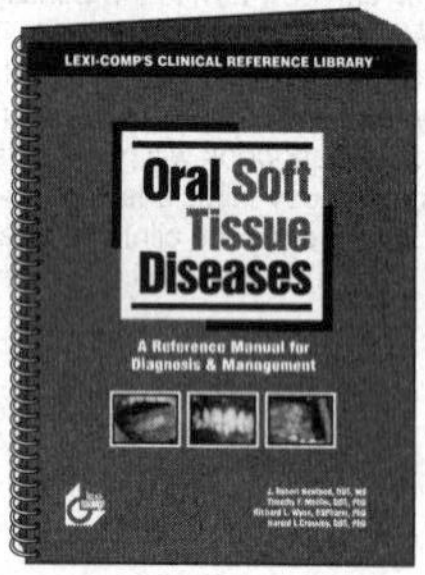

Designed for all dental professionals, a pictorial reference to assist in the diagnosis and management of oral soft tissue diseases, (over 160 photos).

Easy-to-use, sections include:

Diagnosis process: obtaining a history, examining the patient, establishing a differential diagnosis, selecting appropriate diagnostic tests, interpreting the results, etc.; White lesions; Red lesions; Blistering-sloughing lesions; Ulcerated lesions; Pigmented lesions; Papillary lesions; Soft tissue swelling (each lesion is illustrated with a color representative photograph); Specific medications to treat oral soft tissue diseases; Sample prescriptions; and Special topics.

CLINICIAN'S ENDODONTIC HANDBOOK

by Thom C. Dumsha, MS, DDS and James L. Gutmann, DDS, FACD, FICD

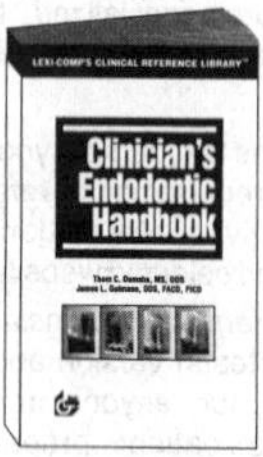

Designed for all general practice dentists.

- A quick reference addressing current endodontics
- Easy-to-use format and alphabetical index
- Latest techniques, procedures, and materials
- Root canal therapy: Why's and Why Nots
- A guide to diagnosis and treatment of endodontic emergencies
- Facts and rationale behind treating endodontically-involved teeth
- Straight-forward dental trauma management information
- Pulpal Histology, Access Openings, Bleaching, Resorption, Radiology, Restoration, and Periodontal / Endodontic Complications
- Frequently Asked Questions (FAQ) section and "Clinical Note" sections throughout.

To order call toll free anywhere in the U.S.: 1-800-837-LEXI (5394)

Outside of the U.S. call: 330-650-6506 or online at www.lexi.com

Other titles offered by

LEXI-COMP, INC

DENTAL OFFICE MEDICAL EMERGENCIES

by Timothy F. Meiller, DDS, PhD; Richard L. Wynn, BSPharm, PhD; Ann Marie McMullin, MD; Cynthia Biron, RDH, EMT, MA; and Harold L. Crossley, DDS, PhD

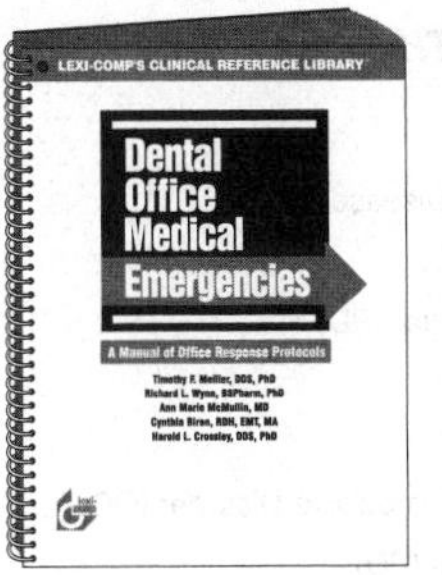

Designed specifically for general dentists during times of emergency. A tabbed paging system allows for quick access to specific crisis events. Created with urgency in mind, it is spiral bound and drilled with a hole for hanging purposes.

- Basic Action Plan for Stabilization
- Allergic / Drug Reactions
- Loss of Consciousness / Respiratory Distress / Chest Pain
- Altered Sensation / Changes in Affect
- Management of Acute Bleeding
- Office Preparedness / Procedures and Protocols
- Automated External Defibrillator (AED)
- Oxygen Delivery

POISONING & TOXICOLOGY COMPENDIUM

by Jerrold B. Leikin, MD and Frank P. Paloucek, PharmD

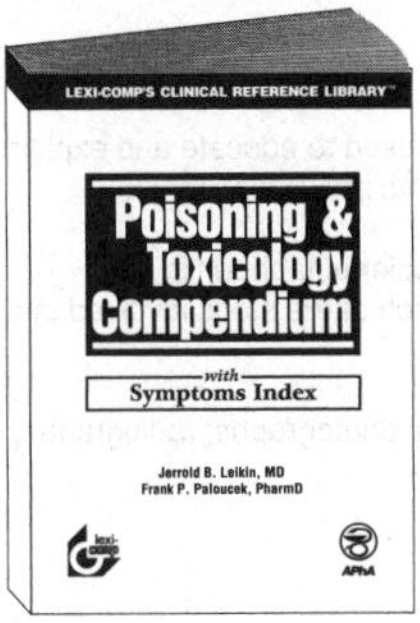

A six-in-one reference wherein each major entry contains information relative to one or more of the other sections. This compendium offers comprehensive, concisely-stated monographs covering 645 medicinal agents, 256 nonmedicinal agents, 273 biological agents, 49 herbal agents, 254 laboratory tests, 79 antidotes, and 222 pages of exceptionally useful appendix material.

A truly unique reference that presents signs and symptoms of acute overdose along with considerations for overdose treatment. Ideal reference for emergency situations.

DRUG INFORMATION HANDBOOK FOR THE CRIMINAL JUSTICE PROFESSIONAL

by Marcelline Burns, PhD; Thomas E. Page, MA; and Jerrold B. Leikin, MD

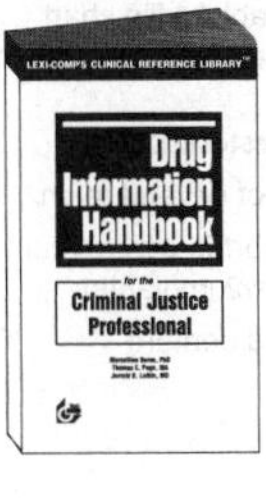

Compiled and designed for police officers, law enforcement officials, and legal professionals who are in need of a reference which relates to information on drugs, chemical substances, and other agents that have abuse and/or impairment potential. Contains over 450 medications, agents, and substances. Contains up to 33 fields of information including Scientific Name, Commonly Found In, Abuse Potential, Impairment Potential, Use, When to Admit to Hospital, Mechanism of Toxic Action, Signs & Symptoms of Acute Overdose, Drug Interactions, Reference Range, and Warnings/Precautions. There is a glossary of medical terms for the layman along with a slang street drug listing and an Appendix includes Chemical, Bacteriologic, and Radiologic Agents - Effects and Treatment; Controlled Substances - Uses and Effects; Medical Examiner Data; Federal Trafficking Penalties, *and much more.*

To order call toll free anywhere in the U.S.: 1-800-837-LEXI (5394)

Outside of the U.S. call: 330-650-6506 or online at www.lexi.com

Other titles offered by

LEXI-COMP, INC

New!

Patient Education Desk Charts

A PATIENT GUIDE TO MENTAL HEALTH ISSUES

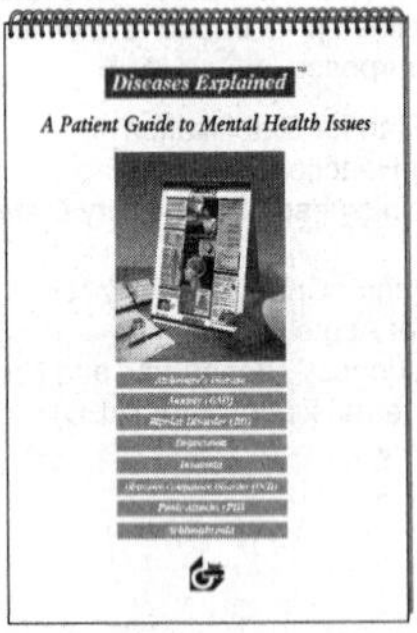

- ▶ Alzheimer's Disease
- ▶ Anxiety (GAD)
- ▶ Bipolar Disorder (BD)
- ▶ Depression
- ▶ Insomnia
- ▶ Obsessive-Compulsive Disorder (OCD)
- ▶ Panic Attacks (PD)
- ▶ Schizophrenia

A PATIENT GUIDE TO ROOT THERAPY

Contributor Thom C. Dumsha, M.S., D.D.S., M.S.

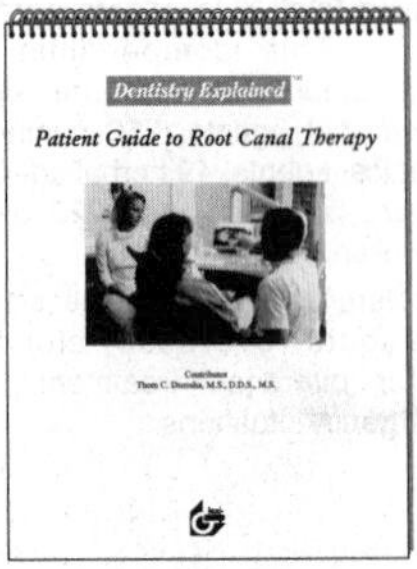

- An ideal tool used to educate and explain to your patients about root canals
- 8 1/2" x 11" colorful tabbed flip chart explaining each of the steps involved in a root canal
- Actual clinical photographs, radiographs, and diagrams

PATIENT GUIDE TO DENTAL IMPLANTS

Contributor Marvin L. Baer, D.D.S., M.Sc.

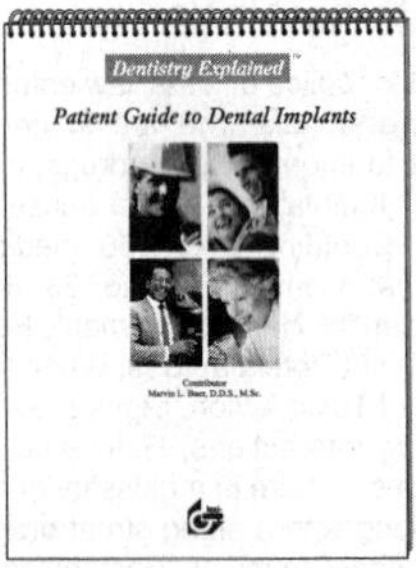

- An ideal tool used to educate and explain to your patients about dental implants
- 8 1/2" x 11" colorful tabbed flip chart explaining each of the steps involved in:
  1.) Single tooth restoration
  2.) Replacement of several teeth
  3.) Implants supported overdenture (4 implants/2 implants)
  4.) Screw-retained denture

To order call toll free anywhere in the U.S.: 1-800-837-LEXI (5394)

Outside of the U.S. call: 330-650-6506 or online at www.lexi.com

Other titles offered by

LEXI-COMP, INC

PATIENT EDUCATION Wall Posters

Ideal for Waiting Rooms and Examination Rooms.

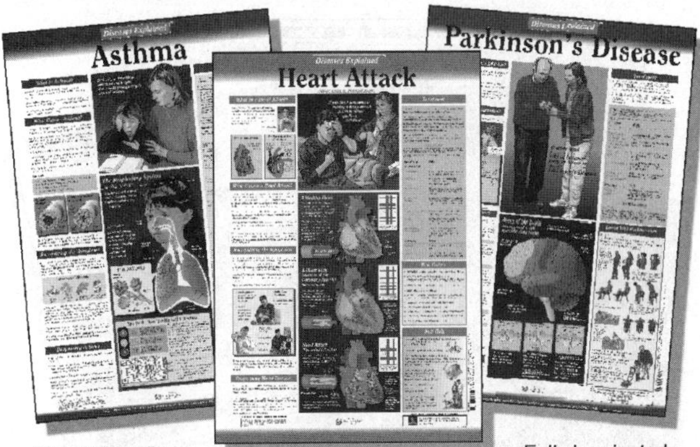

Size 20"x 28"

Fully Laminated

Written in a layman's language and presented in an easy-to-follow, graphic style. Each condition is carefully described, along with the treatments available, and complex medical terms are explained.

Titles available

Acne
Alzheimer's Disease
Anemia
Angina
Anxiety
Asthma
Bipolar Disorder
Breast Cancer
Congestive Heart Failure
Cholesterol
COPD
Depression
Diabetes
Deep Vein Thrombosis
Enlarged Prostate (BPH)
Epilepsy
Essential Tremor
Glaucoma
Heart Attack
HIV and AIDS
Hypertension
Irritable Bowel Syndrome
Incontinence
Insomnia
Menopause
Migraine
Multiple Sclerosis
OCD
Osteoporosis
Otitis Media
Panic Attacks
Parkinson's Disease
Schizophrenia
Spasticity
Stroke
Thyroid Disease

To order a catalog, call Toll Free at: 1-877-837-5394
or visit us online at - **www.diseases-explained.com**

LEXI-COMP, INC

Diseases Explained ™

Outside of the U.S. call: 330-650-6506